Meyler's Side Effects of Drugs Used in Cancer and Immunology

Meyler's Side Effects of Drugs Used in Cancer and Immunology

Editor

J K Aronson, MA, DPhil, MBChB, FRCP, FBPharmacolS, FFPM (Hon)
Oxford, United Kingdom

ELSEVIER

AMSTERDAM • BOSTON • HEIDELBERG • LONDON • NEW YORK • OXFORD
PARIS • SAN DIEGO • SAN FRANCISCO • SINGAPORE • SYDNEY • TOKYO

Elsevier
Radarweg 29, PO Box 211, 1000 AE Amsterdam, The Netherlands
The Boulevard, Langford Lane, Kidlington, Oxford OX5 1GB, UK
525 B Street, Suite 1900, San Diego, CA 92101-4495, USA

Notice
No responsibility is assumed by the publisher for any injury and/or damage to persons
or property as a matter of products liability, negligence or otherwise, or from any use or operation
of any methods, products, instructions or ideas contained in the material herein. Because of rapid
advances in the medical sciences, in particular, independent verification of diagnoses and drug
dosages should be made

Medicine is an ever-changing field. Standard safety precautions must be followed, but as new
research and clinical experience broaden our knowledge, changes in treatment and drug therapy
may become necessary or appropriate. Readers are advised to check the most current product
information provided by the manufacturer of each drug to be administered to verify the
recommended dose, the method and duration of administrations, and contraindications. It is the
responsibility of the treating physician, relying on experience and knowledge of the patient, to
determine dosages and the best treatment for each individual patient. Neither the publisher nor the
authors assume any liability for any injury and/or damage to persons or property arising from this
publication.

British Library Cataloguing in Publication Data
A catalogue record for this book is available from the British Library

Library of Congress Cataloging in Publication Data
A catalog record for this book is available from the Library of Congress

ISBN: 978-044-453267-1

For information on all Elsevier publications
visit our web site at http://www.elsevierdirect.com

Typeset by Integra Software Services Pvt. Ltd, Pondicherry, India www.integra-india.com
Printed and bound in the UK

08 09 10 10 9 8 7 6 5 4 3 2 1

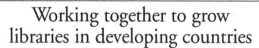

Contents

Preface

This volume covers the adverse effects of drugs used in cancer chemotherapy and in immunology. The material has been collected from *Meyler's Side Effects of Drugs: The International Encyclopedia of Adverse Drug Reactions and Interactions* (15th edition, 2006, in six volumes), which was itself based on previous editions of *Meyler's Side Effects of Drugs* and *Side Effects of Drugs Annuals,* and from later *Side Effects of Drugs Annuals* (SEDA) 28, 29, 30, and 31. The main contributors of this material were JK Aronson, M Behrend, F Braun, DC Broering, G Chevrel, J Costa, J Descotes, MNG Dukes, M Farré, PI Folb, FA Goumas, JT Hartmann, HP Lipp, A Stanley, and T Vial. For contributors to earlier editions of *Meyler's Side Effects of Drugs and the Side Effects of Drugs Annuals,* see http://www.elsevier.com/wps/find/bookseriesdescription.cws_home/BS_SED/description.

A brief history of the Meyler series

Leopold Meyler was a physician who was treated for tuberculosis after the end of the Nazi occupation of The Netherlands. According to Professor Wim Lammers, writing a tribute in Volume VIII (1975), Meyler got a fever from para-aminosalicylic acid, but elsewhere Graham Dukes has written, based on information from Meyler's widow, that it was deafness from dihydrostreptomycin; perhaps it was both. Meyler discovered that there was no single text to which medical practitioners could look for information about unwanted effects of drug therapy; Louis Lewin's text "Die Nebenwirkungen der Arzneimittel" ("The Untoward Effects of Drugs") of 1881 had long been out of print (SEDA-27, xxv-xxix). Meyler therefore determined to make such information available and persuaded the Netherlands publishing firm of Van Gorcum to publish a book, in Dutch, entirely devoted to descriptions of the adverse effects that drugs could cause. He went on to agree with the Elsevier Publishing Company, as it was then called, to prepare and issue an English translation. The first edition of 192 pages (*Schadelijke Nevenwerkingen van Geneesmiddelen*) appeared in 1951 and the English version (*Side Effects of Drugs*) a year later.

The book was a great success, and a few years later Meyler started to publish what he called surveys of unwanted effects of drugs. Each survey covered a period of two to four years. They were labelled as volumes rather than editions, and after Volume IV had been published Meyler could no longer handle the task alone. For subsequent volumes he recruited collaborators, such as Andrew Herxheimer. In September 1973 Meyler died unexpectedly, and Elsevier invited Graham Dukes to take over the editing of Volume VIII.

Dukes persuaded Elsevier that the published literature was too large to be comfortably encompassed in a four-yearly cycle, and he suggested that the volumes should be produced annually instead. The four-yearly volume could then concentrate on providing a complementary critical encyclopaedic survey of the entire field. The first *Side Effects of Drugs Annual* was published in 1977. The first encyclopaedic edition of *Meyler's Side Effects of Drugs,* which appeared in 1980, was labelled the ninth edition, and after that new encyclopaedic edition appeared every four years until 2000. The 15th edition was published in 2006, in both hard and electronic versions.

Monograph structure

The monographs in this volume are arranged in the following sections:

Drugs used in cancer chemotherapy
- Alkylating agents
- Antimetabolites
- Cytostatic antibiotics
- Hormone agonists and antagonists
- Photodynamic therapy
- Platinum-containing compounds
- Retinoids
- Taxanes
- Topoisomerase inhibitors
- Tyrosine kinase inhibitors
- Vinca alkaloids
- Other anticancer drugs

Corticosteroids and prostaglandins
Cytokines and cytokine modulators
- Interferons
- Interleukins
- Myeloid colony-stimulating factors
- Tumor necrosis factor alfa and its antagonists

Monoclonal antibodies
Immune modulators
- Immunosuppressants
- Immunostimulants and other immune modulators

The volume ends with three sections containing information about the mutagenic, tumorigenic, and adverse immunological effects of drugs that are not covered in the first sections of the book.

In each monograph in the Meyler series the information is organized into sections as shown below (although not all the sections are covered in each monograph).

Drug names

Drugs have usually been designated by their recommended or proposed International Non-proprietary Names (rINN or pINN); when these are not available, chemical names have been used. In some cases brand names have been used.

Spelling

For indexing purposes, American spelling has generally been used, e.g. anemia, estrogen, rather than anaemia, oestrogen.

Cross-references

The various editions of *Meyler's Side Effects of Drugs* are cited in the text as SED-l3, SED-14, etc; the *Side Effects of Drugs Annuals* are cited as SEDA-1, SEDA-2, etc.

J K Aronson
Oxford, October 2009

Organization of material in monographs in the Meyler series (not all sections are included in each monograph)

General information
Drug studies
  Observational studies
  Comparative studies
  Drug-combination studies
  Placebo-controlled studies
  Systematic reviews
Organs and systems
  Cardiovascular
  Respiratory
  Ear, nose, throat
  Nervous system
  Neuromuscular function
  Sensory systems
  Psychological
  Psychiatric
  Endocrine
  Metabolism
  Nutrition
  Electrolyte balance
  Mineral balance
  Metal metabolism
  Acid-base balance
  Fluid balance
  Hematologic
  Mouth
  Teeth
  Salivary glands
  Gastrointestinal
  Liver
  Biliary tract
  Pancreas
  Urinary tract
  Skin
  Hair
  Nails
  Connective tissues
  Sweat glands
  Serosae
  Musculoskeletal
  Sexual function
  Reproductive system
  Breasts
  Immunologic
  Autacoids
  Infection risk
  Body temperature

  Multiorgan failure
  Trauma
  Death
Long-term effects
  Drug abuse
  Drug misuse
  Drug tolerance
  Drug resistance
  Drug dependence
  Drug withdrawal
  Genotoxicity
  Cytotoxicity
  Mutagenicity
  Tumorigenicity
Second-generation effects
  Fertility
  Pregnancy
  Teratogenicity
  Fetotoxicity
  Lactation
  Breast feeding
Susceptibility factors
  Genetic factors
  Age
  Sex
  Physiological factors
  Diseases
  Other features of the patient
Drug administration
  Drug formulations
  Drug additives
  Drug contamination and adulteration
  Drug dosage regimens
  Drug administration route
  Drug overdose
Interactions
  Drug-drug interactions
  Food-drug interactions
  Drug-device interactions
  Drug-smoking interactions
  Other environmental interactions
Interference with diagnostic tests
Diagnosis of adverse drug reactions
Management of adverse drug reactions
Monitoring therapy
References

DRUGS USED IN CANCER CHEMOTHERAPY

General Information

Drugs that are used to treat cancers generally have both anticancer and immunosuppressive properties, while immunosuppressant drugs have more specific immunosuppressive effects, although this is a somewhat arbitrary distinction. The following list of drugs is based on the classification used in the *British National Formulary*. Monoclonal antibodies are not included in this list, although they are covered in this volume.

1. **Alkylating drugs**

   - Nitrosoureas—carmustine (BCNU), lomustine (CCNU), nimustine (ACNU), streptozocin
   - N-lost derivatives—bendamustine, chlorambucil, chlormethine (mechlorethamine, mustine, nitrogen mustard), melphalan, oxazaphosphorines (cyclophosphamide, ifosfamide, trofosfamide), estramustine
   - Others—busulfan, dacarbazine and temozolomide, mitobronitol, mitomycin, procarbazine, thiotepa, treosulfan

2. **Antimetabolites**

   - Folic acid antagonists—lometrexol, methotrexate, pemetrexed, piritrexim, raltitrexed, trimetrexate
   - Purine derivatives—cladribine (2-chlorodeoxyadenosine), clofarabine, fludarabine, mercaptopurine, pentostatin (deoxycoformycin), tioguanine
   - Pyrimidine derivatives—azacytidine, capecitabine, cytarabine, decitabine, doxifluridine, floxuridine, fluorouracil, gemcitabine, tegafur, troxacitabine
   - Phosphatidylcholine antagonists—miltefosine

3. **Cytostatic antibiotics**

   - Anthracyclines—aclarubicin, daunorubicin, doxorubicin, epirubicin, idarubicin
   - Others—acivicin, amsacrine, bleomycin, dactinomycin (actinomycin D), mitoxantrone

4. **Hormones agonists and antagonists used in cancer treatment**

   - Antiandrogens—bicalutamide, cyproterone, flutamide
   - Aromatase inhibitors—anastrozole, exemestane, letrozole
   - Selective estrogen receptor modulators (SERMs)

5. **Photodynamic therapy**

   - Aminolevulinic acid, hematoporphyrin derivatives, porfimer, temoporfin

6. **Platinum compounds**

   Carboplatin, cisplatin, oxaliplatin

7. **Retinoids and retinoid receptor agonists (bexarotene)**

8. **Taxanes**

   Docetaxel, paclitaxel

9. **Topoisomerase inhibitors**

   - Inhibitors of topoisomerase type 1—irinotecan, topotecan
   - Inhibitors of topoisomerase type 2—etoposide, teniposide

10. **Tyrosine kinase inhibitors**

    Dasatinib, erlotinib, gefitinib, imatinib, lapatinib, nilotinib, pazopanib, sorafenib, sunitinib

11. **Vinca alkaloids**

    Vinblastine, vincristine, vindesine, vinorelbine

12. **Other anticancer drugs**

    Asparaginase (colaspase and crisantaspase), bortezomib, hydroxycarbamide (hydroxyurea), miltefosine

General adverse effects

There are several types of adverse effects that many anticancer drugs have in common. These include hyperuricemia (as a result of tumor lysis syndrome), bone marrow suppression, oral mucositis, gastrointestinal discomfort, and alopecia. These are dealt with under the relevant headings below.

Individual drugs also have specific adverse effects. However, one of the difficulties in attributing adverse effects to individual cytostatic and immunosuppressant drugs is the common use of multidrug or multi-intervention studies. A good example of this is the Phase I Study of Foscan-Mediated Photodynamic Therapy and Surgery in Patients with Mesothelioma, in which the authors could not separate the adverse effects, which included local effects, cardiotoxicity, and hepatotoxicity, according to causative drug or procedure (1).

Extravasation of cytostatic drugs
Extravasation is leakage of intravenous drugs from a vein into the surrounding tissues. This can cause local pain accompanied by burning or stinging, erythema, swelling, and tenderness. Not all cytostatic drugs are harmful to the tissues after extravasation. The different types of drugs are classified in Table 1.

The management of extravasation of cytostatic drugs has been reviewed (2–5) and guidelines have been suggested (http://www.ucht.n-i.nhs.uk/pubinfo/Extravasation_of_intravenous_drugs).

Local extravasation
- Stop administering the drug and explain to the patient that extravasation may have occurred.
- Put on gloves and goggles.
- Leave the cannula in place.
- Attach a 20 ml syringe and try to withdraw residual drug.
- Give specific antidotes for specific cytostatic drugs Table 2.
- Remove the cannula.
- Do not apply pressure, which increases the area of extravasation.
- Apply a thermal pack (for vesicant, exfoliant, and irritant drugs only) Table 2.
- Raise the limb for 48 hours for vesicant drugs.
- Review vesicant extravasation in 24 hours.
- Consult a plastic surgeon if necessary.

Table 1   Classification of cytostatic drugs according to their ability to cause tissue damage after extravasation (from http://www.ucht.n-i.nhs.uk/pubinfo/Extravasation_of_intravenous_drugs)

Vesicants[a]	Exfoliants[b]	Irritants[c]	Inflammatory agents[d]	Neutral agents[e]
Amsacrine	Aclarubicin	Carboplatin	Etoposide phosphate	Asparaginase
Chlormethine	Carmustine	Daunorubicin liposomal	Fluorouracil	Bleomycin
Dactinomycin	Cisplatin	Doxorubicin liposomal	Methotrexate	Cladribine
Daunorubicin	Dacarbazine	Etoposide	Raltitrexed	Cyclophosphamide
Doxorubicin	Docetaxel	Irinotecan		Cytarabine
Epirubicin	Floxuridine	Teniposide		Fludarabine
Idarubicin	Mitoxantrone			Gemcitabine
Mitomycin	Oxaliplatin			Ifosfamide
Streptozocin	Paclitaxel			Interleukin-2
Vinca alkaloids	Topotecan			Melphalan
	Treosulfan			Pentostatin
				Thiotepa
				Interferon alfa

[a]Vesicants cause pain, inflammation, and blistering of the skin and underlying tissues, leading to tissue death and necrosis
[b]Exfoliants cause inflammation and shedding of the skin, but are less likely to cause tissue death
[c]Irritants cause inflammation and irritation, but rarely cause tissue damage
[d]Inflammatory agents cause mild to moderate inflammation and flare in local tissues
[e]Neutral agents do not cause inflammation or tissue damage

Table 2   Specific antidotes for cytostatic drugs after extravasation

Drug	Antidote	Instructions	Comments
Anthracyclines	Dimethylsulfoxide + dexrazoxane	Apply dimethylsulfoxide 99% topically Give intravenous dexrazoxane 1000 mg/m^2 on days 1 and 2 and 500 mg/m^2 on day 3; most effective if the first dose is given within 6 hours	Apply a cold pack for 15 minutes, four times a day. Inspect after 24 hours and 7 days. If there are signs of erythema or ulceration after 7 days, discuss with a plastic surgeon
Chlormethine	Sodium thiosulfate	Dilute 0.6 ml of sodium thiosulfate 50% with 9.4 ml of water for injection. Inject 4 ml through the cannula, then remove the cannula. Infiltrate with 0.2 ml subcutaneously over and around the affected area	Apply a cold pack for 15 minutes, four times a day. Inspect after 24 hours and 7 days. If there are signs of erythema or ulceration after 7 days, discuss with a plastic surgeon
Cisplatin[a,b]	Sodium thiosulfate	Dilute 0.6 ml of sodium thiosulfate 50% with 9.4 ml of water for injection. Inject 4 ml through the cannula, then remove the cannula. Infiltrate with 0.2 ml subcutaneously over and around the affected area	Apply a warm pack for 15 minutes, four times a day. Inspect after 24 hours and 7 days. If there are signs of erythema or ulceration after 7 days, discuss with a plastic surgeon
Vinca alkaloids	Hyaluronidase	Mix 1500 units of hyaluronidase with 1 ml of sodium chloride 0.9% for injection. Inject 0.5 ml through the cannula. Remove the cannula. Infiltrate with 0.2 ml subcutaneously over and around the affected area	Apply a warm pack for 15 minutes, four times a day. Inspect after 24 hours and 7 days. If there are signs of erythema or ulceration after 7 days, discuss with a plastic surgeon

[a]High concentration only
[b]Sodium thiosulfate should only be used if a large volume (greater than 20 ml) of concentrated cisplatin (that is a concentration over 0.5 mg/ml) has extravasated

Extravasation from a central venous catheter

If the patient complains of altered sensation, pain, burning, or swelling at the central venous catheter site or in the ipsilateral chest, or if there is a change in intravenous flow rate, extravasation may have occurred.

- Stop administering the drug and explain to the patient that extravasation may have occurred.
- Put on gloves and goggles.
- Attach a 20 ml syringe and try to withdraw residual drug from the line.

- If the reason for extravasation is needle dislodgement, and if aspiration through the needle was unsuccessful, remove the needle and try to aspirate subcutaneously in the pocket and surrounding tissues.
- Give specific antidotes for specific cytostatic drugs Table 2.
- If a needle is still in situ it should be removed after instillation of the antidote; the antidote can also be injected into the surrounding tissues if needed.
- Do not apply pressure, which increases the area of extravasation.
- Apply a thermal pack (for vesicant, exfoliant, and irritant drugs only) Table 2.

Table 3 Some review articles in cytostatic drug therapy

	Topic	Reference
Adverse effects	The relation between a drug's adverse effects spectrum and its pharmacological action	(6)
	Adverse effects profiles of individual drugs	(7)
	Prognostic factors	(8)
	Anemia	(9)
	Nausea and vomiting	(10)
	The relation between toxicity and efficacy	(11,12)
Treatment of specific cancers	Colorectal cancers	(13)
	Lymphomas	(14)
	Melanoma	(15)
	Metastatic breast cancer	(16)
	Prostate cancer	(17)
	Soft tissue sarcomas	(18)
	Testicular carcinoma, non-seminomatous	(19)
Administration	The relation between a drug's adverse effects spectrum and its dosage regimen	(20–22)
	Effects of dosage regimens in combined therapy	(23,24,25)
	Effects of the route of administration	(26,27)
	Dose-finding techniques	(28)
	Preventing dose-limiting adverse effects in patients with nasopharyngeal carcinoma	(96)
	Oral versus intravenous therapy in small cell lung cancer	(29)
Susceptibility factors	Effects of sex	(30)
	The expression and prognostic significance of P glycoprotein in adult solid tumors	(31)

Table 4 Neurotoxic effects of cytostatic drugs

Drug	Neurotoxicity
Asparaginase	Acute encephalopathy
Bortezomib	Peripheral neuropathy
Busulfan	Seizures
Carmustine	Brain damage in conventional doses when combined with radiation
Chlorambucil	Disorientation, cognitive dysfunction
Chlormethine	Rare encephalopathy following high doses
Cisplatin	Peripheral neuropathy, deafness, cerebral cortical blindness, seizures
Cytarabine	Cerebellar ataxia in high doses
Fluorouracil	Cerebellar ataxia in high doses
Ifosfamide	Mild memory disturbances
Methotrexate	Acute meningitis; acute fatal cerebral dysfunction; chronic leukoencephalopathy
Oxaliplatin	Acute and chronic sensory neuropathy
Taxanes	Peripheral neuropathy
Vinblastine	Jaw pain, myopathy, inappropriate ADH secretion
Vincristine	Peripheral neuropathy, abdominal pain, constipation
Vindesine	Overdose or accidental intrathecal injection is usually fatal
Vinorelbine	Sensorimotor distal symmetrical axonal neuropathy

- Review vesicant extravasation in 24 hours.
- Extravasation in the deep part of a central venous catheter will require referral to a plastic surgeon.

Review articles

Some review articles on the adverse effects of cytostatic drugs and related topics are listed in Table 3.

Organs and Systems

Nervous system

Neurological symptoms occur in more than 20% of patients with cancer and can be increased by cytostatic drugs. Acute and late neurotoxic syndromes involve a number of cytostatic agents Table 4.

The late nervous system effects in survivors 7 years after treatment for childhood acute lymphoblastic leukemia include impaired concentration, attention, and memory (32).

The late effect of chemotherapy and radiotherapy for nervous system lymphoma has been studied in 15 patients; 10 had severe symptomatic diffuse changes in the white matter within 8 months of completing treatment (33).

Endocrine

Combined cytostatic drug therapy for Hodgkin's disease in childhood often results in abnormal endocrine function, particularly increases in follicle-stimulating hormone, prolactin, and thyroid-stimulating hormone (34).

Metabolism

Hyperglycemia was reported in 21 of 56 patients who received weekly paclitaxel with oral estramustine and carboplatin (4-weekly); under 10% required pharmacological intervention (35). There was mild hyperphosphatemia in 24.

There was fasting hypoglycemia in 19 of 35 children with acute lymphoblastic leukemia receiving maintenance therapy of daily oral mercaptopurine and weekly oral methotrexate; all the children improved on withdrawal of chemotherapy and 10 of 15 normalized (36).

There have been cases of acute tumor lysis syndrome in patients with melanoma (37) and light-chain amyloidosis (38). The authors reviewed the incidence of acute tumor lysis syndrome in these diseases, which are less typically associated with it.

Hematologic

The authors of a study in 101 patients concluded that in addition to the dose of chemotherapy and the administration of hemopoietic growth factors, poor performance status and a high concentration of soluble p75-R-TNF can predict the occurrence of chemotherapy-induced myelosuppression in lymphoma (39).

In 43 patients, raised plasma concentrations of FLT3-L (an fms-like tyrosine kinase) in patients who had previously received chemotherapy predicted the stage of recovery of the bone-marrow compartment (40). FLT3-L seems to identify the likelihood that the patient will have severe thrombocytopenia if additional cytostatic therapy is given. Knowledge of bone-marrow activity should permit more aggressive therapy, by establishing the earliest possible time for dosing with any cytostatic agent for which myelosuppression is the dose-limiting toxic effect.

Mouth

Cytostatic drugs can cause oral mucositis, which characteristically affects the whole buccal mucosa (41). It is caused by damage to the oropharyngeal epithelium which has a rapid turnover. The oral mucosa can also be affected by infection. Susceptibility factors include age, nutritional status, tumor type, oral hygiene, and neutrophil count.

Oral mucositis causes pain, interferes with nutrition, and can lead to systemic infection and other complications that increase morbidity and mortality (42). Interventions that have been used to prevent oral mucositis or reduce its severity and sequelae include meticulous pretransplantation and continuing mouth care, calcium phosphate solution, treatment with near-infrared light and lower-energy laser light, interleukin-11, sucralfate, oral glutamine, rinsing with granulocyte-macrophage colony-stimulating factor, tretinoin, keratinocyte growth factor, and amifostine. However, very few interventions have been shown to be effective compared with placebo.

In a retrospective analysis over 13 years of cytostatic therapy for various conditions, six doses of etoposide each of 250 mg/m² caused grade 4 mucositis and 50% of patients who received epirubicin 120 mg/m² developed grade 2 or 3 mucositis (43). Severe stomatitis complicated epirubicin 1250 mg/m² (44).

A scoring system for mucositis has been proposed and validated (45) and multivariate analysis has been used to identify contributory factors (46). A diagnosis of leukemia, the use of total body irradiation or allogenic transplantation in treatment, or delayed neutrophil recovery were associated with an increased incidence of oral mucositis.

It has been proposed that a change in serum diamine oxidase activity is a very sensitive surrogate for early signs of upper gastrointestinal tract mucositis (47).

Gastrointestinal

Nausea and vomiting are common adverse effects of cytostatic drugs (48). They can be acute (occurring within 24 hours of therapy), delayed (persisting for 6–7 days after therapy), or anticipatory (occurring before chemotherapy) (49). Their treatment has been reviewed (50,51).

Diarrhea can also occur (52) and is particularly problematic with some drugs, such as irinotecan (53). Its management has been reviewed (54).

In a retrospective analysis over 13 years of cytostatic therapy for various conditions there were 12 cases in which chemotherapy had caused gastrointestinal perforation (43). Six doses of etoposide each of 250 mg/m² induced an advanced stage (grade 4) of mucositis. Fifty percent of patients receiving epirubicin 120 mg/m² developed grade 2 or 3 mucositis. Severe stomatitis complicated epirubicin 1250 mg/m² (44).

Increased intestinal permeability has been shown in children receiving low-dose methotrexate therapy (44).

Liver

Of 54 patients with non-small-cell lung cancers treated with a combination of gemcitabine 1000 mg/m² on days 1 and 8 and paclitaxel 200 mg/m² on day 1, six had abnormal but significantly raised transaminases (55). The authors believed that this was drug-induced, but could not rule out underlying liver disease.

Urinary tract

Hemolytic-uremic syndrome in association with thrombotic thrombocytopenic purpura has been reported in a patient receiving pentostatin (deoxycoformycin) after exposure to only 15 mg/m² given over 3 days (56).

Skin

There has been a report of six cases of a variant of the palmar-plantar erythrodysesthesia syndrome (hand-foot syndrome), in which patients who had previously reported the syndrome developed it again when they were treated with completely different chemotherapeutic drugs (57). The recall syndrome was of mild to moderate intensity, less severe than the primary syndrome, and self-limiting in all cases.

Four cases of hyperkeratotic seborrheic warts appearing over a 2-year period, 25 years after the patients had been started on azathioprine 2.5 mg/kg, have been reported (58).

Calciphylaxis is a rare, often fatal disease, characterized clinically by progressive cutaneous necrosis and ulceration and histologically by vascular calcification and thrombosis. It has been described in association with end-stage renal disease and hyperparathyroidism.

- A 64-year-old woman who 3 months before had finished a course of cyclophosphamide, doxorubicin, and fluorouracil chemotherapy for breast carcinoma developed calciphylaxis (59). She had no renal disease and had normal renal function and parathyroid hormone concentrations.

The authors speculated that the cause may have been chemotherapy-induced functional deficiency of protein C and protein S.

Musculoskeletal

Bone mineral density has been used to help predict which children who have had chemotherapy may subsequently develop osteoporosis (60).

Reproductive system

Gynecomastia is frequent in men with testicular tumors that produce large amounts of human chorionic gonadotrophin (HCG), and its appearance after completion of chemotherapy may indicate residual or recurrent disease. However, not uncommonly, gynecomastia is a harmless, although troubling, late adverse effect of chemotherapy. In 16 patients who developed gynecomastia 2–9 months after treatment, and who were in complete remission, estradiol concentrations were raised; follicle-stimulating hormone (FSH) produced a higher estradiol/testosterone ratio than similarly treated patients without gynecomastia (61). It is likely that this was due to increased secretion of testicular estrogen in response to a compensatory increase in pituitary gonadotrophins after cytostatic damage to Leydig cells and spermatogenesis.

The gonadal effects of MOPP (mechlorethamine + Oncovin (vincristine) + procarbazine + prednisone/prednisolone) and MVPP (mustine + vinblastine + procarbazine + prednisone/prednisolone) in patients with Hodgkin's disease have been described (SEDA-11, 397; SEDA-11, 403). Similar studies have been conducted in patients treated with ABVD (adriamycin +bleomycin Adjust-vinblastine + dacarbazine) and COPP (cyclophosphamide + vincristine + procarbazine + prednisone) (62). The results suggested that all men have irreversible sterility with preservation of normal Leydig cell function after COPP, which is more spermatotoxic than MOPP and much more so than ABVD. Ovarian failure was age-related after COPP, occurring in 86% of those over 24 years of age at the time of therapy, compared with 28% in women patients less than 24 years old. In contrast to men, sterility in women was always associated with ovarian endocrine failure requiring estrogen replacement. Pregnancies and normal births did occur: 14 women became pregnant and five healthy children were born. It has been proposed that analogues of gonadotropin-releasing hormone preserve gonadal function during the administration of anticancer drugs to premenopausal women.

Infection risk

Infections are major causes of morbidity and mortality in the period after transplantation, whichever immunosuppressive regimen is used, in particular bacterial infections and viral infections (cytomegalovirus, *Herpes simplex* virus, Epstein–Barr virus), but also protozoal and fungal infections (63–65). Based on an analysis of medical and autopsy records, infections were the cause of death in 70% of transplant patients, with bacteria (50%) or fungi (29%) as the most common pathogens (66).

Long-Term Effects

Mutagenicity

An increased incidence of gene aberration is to be expected in the offspring of men being treated at the time of conception with chemotherapy for testicular tumors (67). Various drug regimens for Hodgkin's disease and high-grade non-Hodgkin's lymphoma produce different patterns of changes in sister chromatid exchange frequency, and the changes may reflect the potential of the drugs concerned to induce second malignancies (68).

Tumorigenicity

Malignant tumors have been documented with increasing frequency over the last 35 years as a long-term complication of cytostatic and immunosuppressant therapy.

Alkylating agents have been implicated in the causation of secondary tumors, including acute myeloid leukemia, myelodysplastic syndromes (69), solid tumors (70,71), Hodgkin's disease (72,73), ovarian cancer (74,75), and gastric cancer (69). Survival from the time of diagnosis of secondary malignancies is usually very short (69).

Risks in patients with Hodgkin's disease
The actuarial risks of developing secondary malignancies and/or myelodysplastic syndrome at 5, 10, and 15 years after treatment for Hodgkin's disease have been calculated (76).

In a multicenter, case-control study, the incidence of acute myeloid leukemia in treated Hodgkin's disease was 64 times higher than in the general population, the risk being greater in men. There was also a significant association between the development of acute myeloid leukemia in those patients and the use of extensive radiotherapy, vincristine + procarbazine, splenectomy, and the dose of chlormethine (73). The problem is thought to be the result of chromosomal aberrations developing in patients treated with alkylating agents (77), although there is no general agreement about this (75).

Among 679 patients receiving chemotherapy for advanced Hodgkin's disease, there were four deaths due to secondary malignancies (78). There were 75 deaths in all during 3 years, of which the vast majority were related to disseminated Hodgkin's disease.

The increased incidence of breast cancer after treatment of Hodgkin's disease may be related to supradiaphragmatic irradiation, but the risk was higher in patients with ovarian cancer, which is consistent with a common predisposition to breast and ovarian cancer. However, cytostatic drugs may have contributed to the risk.

Risks in patients with leukemias

The nucleoside analogues fludarabine, pentostatin, and cladribine have not traditionally been associated with secondary malignancies. Long-term follow-up for 5–7.5 years of 2014 patients who had received these agents for chronic lymphoid leukemia and hairy cell leukemia has been reviewed (79). Of 111 malignancies that were detected, the three most common were lymphoma ($n = 25$), prostate cancer ($n = 19$), and lung cancer ($n = 15$). While these incidences suggested significant additional risks beyond those in the normal population, the authors could not conclude beyond a reasonable doubt that the increased risks were greater than expected.

Chemotherapy-related myelodysplastic syndrome has been reported in association with adult T cell leukemia (80).

Risks in patients with Wilms' tumor

The National Wilms' Tumor Study Group has reported the incidence of second malignant neoplasms in 5278 patients treated over 22 years (81). There were 43 second malignant neoplasms, whereas only five were expected. Fifteen years after the diagnosis of Wilms' tumor, the cumulative incidence of a second malignant neoplasm was 1.6% and increasing steadily. Abdominal irradiation, given as part of the initial therapy, increased the risk, and doxorubicin potentiated the radiation effect. Among 234 patients who received doxorubicin and over 35 Gy of abdominal radiation, eight second malignant neoplasms were observed, whereas only 0.22 were expected. Treatment for relapse further increased the risk by a factor of 4–5.

Risks in patients with other tumors

Lymphoblastic leukemia has been described after treatment of a malignant germ cell tumor; it was suggested that this was related to the etoposide component of the treatment, and that development of secondary leukemia after etoposide may not be confined to the myeloid cell lineage (82).

A large international collaborative study by cancer registries has published the incidence of second malignancies following testicular cancer, ovarian cancer, and Hodgkin's disease (83): 3157 second cancers were observed among 133 411 patients diagnosed between 1945 and 1984. Patients with Hodgkin's disease were at particular risk, having an 80% excess of cancers. It confirms the high incidence of this complication noted in other reports involving smaller numbers of patients (84,85).

Other conclusions deriving from the international collaborative study (83) include the following:

- patients with testicular cancer had a 30% greater probability of developing cancers than the general population, and those with ovarian cancer 20%;
- leukemia, previously linked to alkylating agents, occurred in excess after testicular cancer, ovarian cancer, and Hodgkin's disease (relative risk 6.1), as did non-Hodgkin's lymphoma (relative risk 1.8) (the latter particularly after Hodgkin's disease);

- other cancers with significant excesses were lung cancer following Hodgkin's disease (relative risk 1.9), breast cancer following Hodgkin's disease (relative risk 1.4), and bladder cancer following ovarian cancer and Hodgkin's disease (relative risks 1.7 and 2.2 in women, respectively);
- a marked excess in incidence of secondary malignancies was found in the salivary gland, thyroid, bone, and connective tissue (there was a smaller excess for colorectal cancers following ovarian cancer).

It is likely that there is a casual relation between treatment of a first malignancy and development of a second. Alkylating agents are strongly implicated in the pathogenesis of the leukemias. Non-Hodgkin's lymphoma occurred after a 10-year latency in patients with ovarian cancer, suggesting a possible radiation effect, but early in patients with testicular tumors or Hodgkin's disease, possibly related to the immunosuppressive effect of cytostatic drugs. The excess of bladder cancers in patients with Hodgkin's disease and ovarian cancer may be related to radiotherapy (subdiaphragmatic in the former), and/or cyclophosphamide, which is widely used in the treatment of both and is a human bladder carcinogen.

Risks in transplant recipients

Although the risk of secondary malignancy clearly outweighs that of under-treatment in transplant patients, increasing periods of survival extend the importance of this problem and the need for close monitoring. Considerable amounts of data are accumulating based on multicenter or single-center experience, but they reflect the use of various immunosuppressive regimens and prophylactic antiviral treatments, and use different approaches to the calculation of risk incidence. Estimates of risk therefore vary widely between studies and no direct comparison is as a rule possible. However, updated data from the Cincinnati Transplant Tumor Registry, published in 1993, have helped to define comprehensively the characteristics of neoplasms observed in organ transplant recipients (86). Skin and lip cancers were the most common, and non-Hodgkin's lymphomas represent the majority of lymphoproliferative disorders with an incidence some 30- to 50-fold higher than in controls. An excess of Kaposi's sarcomas, carcinomas of the vulva and perineum, hepatobiliary tumors, and various sarcomas is also reported. By contrast, the incidence of common neoplasms encountered in the general population is not increased. In renal transplant patients, the actuarial cumulative risk of cancer is 14–18% at 10 years and 40–50% at 20 years (87,88). Skin cancers accounted for about half of the cases.

There is controversy about which factors (duration of treatment, total dosage, the degree of immunosuppression, or the type of immunosuppressive regimen) are the most relevant to determining risk. Partial or complete regression of lymphoproliferative disorders and Kaposi's sarcomas after reduction of immunosuppressive therapy argues strongly for the role of the degree of immunosuppression (86). The incidence of cancer was also significantly higher in renal transplant patients receiving triple therapy regimens compared with double therapy (89). Similarly, aggressive immunosuppressive therapy may account for the higher incidence of lymphomas in cardiac versus renal allograft patients. In a large, multicenter study involving more than 52 000 kidney or heart transplant patients between 1983 and 1991, the rate of non-Hodgkin's lymphomas in the first year after transplantation was 0.2% in kidney recipients and 1.2% in heart recipients, and fell substantially thereafter (90). Initial immunosuppression with azathioprine and ciclosporin, and prophylactic treatment with antilymphocyte antibodies or muromonab was associated with a significantly increased incidence of non-Hodgkin's lymphomas compared with other immunosuppressive regimens, which confirmed the major role of the degree of immunosuppression. Other studies have confirmed that immunosuppression per se rather than a single agent is responsible for the increased risk of cancer (SEDA-20, 340). Finally, the most striking difference between conventional and modern immunosuppressive regimens, including ciclosporin, was the average time to the appearance of tumors, in particular skin cancers and lymphomas, which was shorter in ciclosporin-treated patients (91,92).

The risk of malignant disease in renal transplant recipients increases with time after the transplant. The commonest cancers in this setting are squamous carcinoma of the skin and lip, in situ carcinoma of the cervix, and non-Hodgkin's lymphoma. An increased incidence of hepatocellular carcinoma has been reported (93). In Australia and New Zealand tumors of the urogenital tract, especially of the kidney and bladder, are the commonest non-cutaneous tumors encountered in renal transplant recipients (94). Severe metaplastic and dysplastic changes, suggestive of premalignancy, have been found in the lining epithelium of collecting ducts and tubules of cadaveric renal transplants in two patients receiving azathioprine and prednisolone (95).

Second-Generation Effects

Fertility

A reduced chance of paternity has been reported in 67% of patients who had been treated with MOPP/ABVD for Hodgkin's disease. This included oligospermia, asthenozoospermia, and/or teratozoospermia. The recovery of spermatogenesis was documented in only 40% (97).

Teratogenicity

The outcomes of pregnancies after the use of immunosuppressive drugs, in particular in renal transplant patients, have been reported, and hundreds of pregnancies have been analysed (98). The largest experience is that derived from the National Transplantation Pregnancy Registry, which has been built up in the USA since 1991 (99). This registry has accumulated data on more than 900 pregnancies, of which 83% followed kidney transplantation. Overall, the immunosuppressive regimens commonly used in transplant patients (that is azathioprine-based or ciclosporin-based programmes) do not appear to increase the overall risk of congenital malformations or to produce a specific pattern of malformation. There was no difference in the rate of malformations

when comparing ciclosporin to other immunosuppressive regimens or to the baseline risk of malformations (100,101). Ectopic pregnancies and miscarriages seemed to occur at a similar rate as in the general population. The most common complications were frequent prematurity and more frequent intrauterine growth retardation with low birth weight. Susceptibility factors associated with adverse pregnancy outcomes included a short interval between transplantation and pregnancy (less than 1–2 years), graft dysfunction before or during pregnancy, and hypertension (102). Possible long-term effects of in utero exposure to immunosuppressive drugs are still seldom investigated. There is no evidence that physical and mental development or renal function are altered in children. In one study, there were changes in T lymphocyte development in seven children born to mothers who had taken azathioprine or ciclosporin, but immune function assays were normal, suggesting that fetal immune system development is not affected (103).

References

1. Friedberg JS, Mick R, Stevenson J, Metz J, Zhu T, Buyske J, Sterman DH, Pass HI, Glatstein E, Hahn SM. A phase I study of Foscan-mediated photodynamic therapy and surgery in patients with mesothelioma. Ann Thorac Surg 2003;75(3):952–9.
2. Dorr RT. Antidotes to vesicant chemotherapy extravasations. Blood Rev 1990;4(1):41–60.
3. Nogler-Semenitz E, Mader I, Furst-Weger P, Terkola R, Wassertheurer S, Giovanoli P, Mader RM. Paravasation von Zytostatika. [Extravasation of cytotoxic agents.] Wien Klin Wochenschr 2004;116(9–10):289–95.
4. Rauh J, Pluntke S, Muller Ch. Paravenose Zytostatikainjektion: Prophylaxe und Sofortmassnahmen im Notfall. [Treatment of perivascular extravasation of cytostatic agents.] MMW Fortschr Med 2004;146(31–32):23–426–7.
5. Jordan K, Grothe W, Schmoll HJ. Paravasation von Zytostatika: Prävention und Therapie. [Extravasation of chemotherapeutic agents: prevention and therapy.] Dtsch Med Wochenschr 2005;130(1–2):33–7.
6. Booser DJ, Hortobagyi GN. Anthracycline antibiotics in cancer therapy. Focus on drug resistance. Drugs 1994;47(2):223–58.
7. Safra T, Groshen S, Jeffers S, Tsao-Wei DD, Zhou L, Mudersbach L, Roman L, Morrow CP, Burnett A, Muggia FM. Treatment of patients with ovarian carcinoma with pegylated liposomal doxorubicin: analysis of toxicities and predictors of outcome. Cancer 2001;91(1):90–100.
8. Freyer G, Rougier P, Bugat R, Droz JP, Marty M, Bleiberg H, Mignard D, Awad L, Herait P, Culine S, Trillet-Lenoir V. Prognostic factors for tumour response, progression-free survival and toxicity in metastatic colorectal cancer patients given irinotecan (CPT-11) as second-line chemotherapy after 5FU failure. CPT-11 F205, F220, F221 and V222 study groups. Br J Cancer 2000;83(4):431–7.
9. Barrett-Lee PJ, Bailey NP, O'Brien ME, Wager E. Large-scale UK audit of blood transfusion requirements and anaemia in patients receiving cytotoxic chemotherapy. Br J Cancer 2000;82(1):93–7.
10. Tsavaris N, Kosmas C, Mylonakis N, Bacoyiannis C, Kalergis G, Vadiaka M, Boulamatsis D, Iakovidis V, Kosmidis P. Parameters that influence the outcome of

nausea and emesis in cisplatin based chemotherapy. Anticancer Res 2000;20(6C):4777–83.

11. Jodrell DI, Stewart M, Aird R, Knowles G, Bowman A, Wall L, Cummings J, McLean C. 5-fluorouracil steady state pharmacokinetics and outcome in patients receiving protracted venous infusion for advanced colorectal cancer. Br J Cancer 2001;84(5):600–3.

12. Mayers C, Panzarella T, Tannock IF. Analysis of the prognostic effects of inclusion in a clinical trial and of myelosuppression on survival after adjuvant chemotherapy for breast carcinoma. Cancer 2001;91(12):2246–57.

13. Lavery IC, Lopez-Kostner F, Pelley RJ, Fine RM. Treatment of colon and rectal cancer. Surg Clin North Am 2000;80(2):535–69.

14. Carrion JR, Garcia Arroyo FR, Salinas P. Infusional chemotherapy (EPOCH) in patients with refractory or relapsed lymphoma. Am J Clin Oncol 1995;18(1):44–6.

15. Reeves ME, Coit DG. Melanoma. A multidisciplinary approach for the general surgeon. Surg Clin North Am 2000;80(2):581–601.

16. Hayes DF, Henderson IC, Shapiro CL. Treatment of metastatic breast cancer: present and future prospects. Semin Oncol 1995;22(2 Suppl 5):5–21.

17. Klein EA. Hormone therapy for prostate cancer: a topical perspective. Urology 1996;47(Suppl 1A):3–12.

18. Demetri GD, Elias AD. Results of single-agent and combination chemotherapy for advanced soft tissue sarcomas. Implications for decision making in the clinic. Hematol Oncol Clin North Am 1995;9(4):765–85.

19. Kennedy BJ, Torkelson J, Fraley EE. Optimal number of chemotherapy courses in advanced nonseminomatous testicular carcinoma. Am J Clin Oncol 1995;18(6):463–8.

20. Cure H, Chevalier V, Pezet D, Bousquet J, Focan C, Levi F, Garufi C, Chipponi J, Chollet P. Phase II trial of chronomodulated infusion of 5-fluorouracil and folinic acid in metastatic colorectal cancer. Anticancer Res 2000;20(6C):4649–53.

21. Hartmann JT, Kanz L, Bokemeyer C. Phase II study of continuous 120-hour-infusion of mitomycin C as salvage chemotherapy in patients with progressive or rapidly recurrent gastrointestinal adenocarcinoma. Anticancer Res 2000;20(2B):1177–82.

22. Bogliolo G, Pannacciulli I, Desalvo L, Barsotti B, Lerza R, Mencoboni M, Arboscello E. Advanced colorectal cancer: quality of life and toxicity in patients after weekly 24-hour continuous infusions of biomodulated 5-fluorouracil. Anticancer Res 2000;20(1B):501–4.

23. Cardoso F, Ferreira Filho AF, Crown J, Dolci S, Paesmans M, Riva A, Di Leo A, Piccart MJ. Doxorubicin followed by docetaxel versus docetaxel followed by doxorubicin in the adjuvant treatment of node positive breast cancer: results of a feasibility study. Anticancer Res 2001;21(1B):789–95.

24. Spielmann M, Tubiana-Hulin M, Namer M, Mansouri H, Bougnoux P, Tubiana-Mathieu N, Lotz V, Eymard JC. Sequential or alternating administration of docetaxel (Taxotere) combined with FEC in metastatic breast cancer: a randomised phase II trial. Br J Cancer 2002;86(5):692–7.

25. Gelderblom H, Mross K, ten Tije AJ, Behringer D, Mielke S, van Zomeren DM, Verweij J, Sparreboom A. Comparative pharmacokinetics of unbound paclitaxel during 1- and 3-hour infusions. J Clin Oncol 2002;20(2):574–81.

26. Vogl TJ, Engelmann K, Mack MG, Straub R, Zangos S, Eichler K, Hochmuth K, Orenberg E. CT-guided intratumoural administration of cisplatin/epinephrine gel for treatment of malignant liver tumours. Br J Cancer 2002;86(4):524–9.

27. Kovacs AF, Obitz P, Wagner M. Monocomponent chemoembolization in oral and oropharyngeal cancer using an aqueous crystal suspension of cisplatin. Br J Cancer 2002;86(2):196–202.

28. Miller VA, Rigas JR, Francis PA, Grant SC, Pisters KM, Venkatraman ES, Woolley K, Heelan RT, Kris MG. Phase II trial of a 75-mg/m2 dose of docetaxel with prednisone premedication for patients with advanced non-small cell lung cancer. Cancer 1995;75(4):968–72.

29. Miller AA, Herndon JE 2nd, Hollis DR, Ellerton J, Langleben A, Richards F 2nd, Green MR. Schedule dependency of 21-day oral versus 3-day intravenous etoposide in combination with intravenous cisplatin in extensive-stage small-cell lung cancer: a randomized phase III study of the Cancer and Leukemia Group B. J Clin Oncol 1995;13(8):1871–9.

30. Sloan JA, Goldberg RM, Sargent DJ, Vargas-Chanes D, Nair S, Cha SS, Novotny PJ, Poon MA, O'Connell MJ, Loprinzi CL. Women experience greater toxicity with fluorouracil-based chemotherapy for colorectal cancer. J Clin Oncol 2002;20(6):1491–8.

31. Leighton JC Jr, Goldstein LJ. P-glycoprotein in adult solid tumors. Expression and prognostic significance. Hematol Oncol Clin North Am 1995;9(2):251–73.

32. Langer T, Martus P, Ottensmeier H, Hertzberg H, Beck JD, Meier W. CNS late-effects after ALL therapy in childhood. Part III. Neuropsychological performance in long-term survivors of childhood ALL: impairments of concentration, attention, and memory. Med Pediatr Oncol 2002;38(5):320–8.

33. Herrlinger U, Schabet M, Brugger W, Kortmann RD, Kanz L, Bamberg M, Dichgans J, Weller M. Primary central nervous system lymphoma 1991–1997: outcome and late adverse effects after combined modality treatment. Cancer 2001;91(1):130–5.

34. Perrone L, Sinisi AA, Tullio M, et al. Endocrine function in subjects treated for childhood Hodgkin's disease. J Pediatr Endocrinol 1989;3:175.

35. Kelly WK, Curley T, Slovin S, Heller G, McCaffrey J, Bajorin D, Ciolino A, Regan K, Schwartz M, Kantoff P, George D, Oh W, Smith M, Kaufman D, Small EJ, Schwartz L, Larson S, Tong W, Scher H. Paclitaxel, estramustine phosphate, and carboplatin in patients with advanced prostate cancer. J Clin Oncol 2001;19(1):44–53.

36. Halonen P, Salo MK, Makipernaa A. Fasting hypoglycemia is common during maintenance therapy for childhood acute lymphoblastic leukemia. J Pediatr 2001;138(3):428–31.

37. Castro MP, VanAuken J, Spencer-Cisek P, Legha S, Sponzo RW. Acute tumor lysis syndrome associated with concurrent biochemotherapy of metastatic melanoma: a case report and review of the literature. Cancer 1999;85(5):1055–9.

38. Akasheh MS, Chang CP, Vesole DH. Acute tumour lysis syndrome: a case in AL amyloidosis. Br J Haematol 1999;107(2):387.

39. Voog E, Bienvenu J, Warzocha K, Moullet I, Dumontet C, Thieblemont C, Monneret G, Gutowski MC, Coiffier B, Salles G. Factors that predict chemotherapy-induced myelosuppression in lymphoma patients: role of the tumor necrosis factor ligand-receptor system. J Clin Oncol 2000;18(2):325–31.

40. Blumenthal RD, Lew W, Juweid M, Alisauskas R, Ying Z, Goldenberg DM. Plasma FLT3-L levels predict bone

marrow recovery from myelosuppressive therapy. Cancer 2000;88(2):333–43.

41. Amadio P, Ferrau F, Priolo D, Toscano G, Colina P, Mare M, Zavettieri M, La Torre F, Mesiti M, Maisano R. Prevenzione e trattamento della mucosite da chemioterapici antiblastici. [Prevention and treatment of mucositis from cytotoxic chemotherapy.] Clin Ter 2002;153(2):127–34.

42. Gabriel DA, Shea T, Olajida O, Serody JS, Comeau T. The effect of oral mucositis on morbidity and mortality in bone marrow transplant. Semin Oncol 2003;30(6 Suppl 18):76–83.

43. Ricci JL, Turnbull AD. Spontaneous gastroduodenal perforation in cancer patients receiving cytotoxic therapy. J Surg Oncol 1989;41(4):219–21.

44. Vorobiof DA, Falkson G. Phase II study of high-dose 4'-epidoxorubicin in the treatment of advanced gastrointestinal cancer. Eur J Cancer Clin Oncol 1989;25(3):563–4.

45. Sonis ST, Eilers JP, Epstein JB, LeVeque FG, Liggett WH Jr, Mulagha MT, Peterson DE, Rose AH, Schubert MM, Spijkervet FK, Wittes JPMucositis Study Group. Validation of a new scoring system for the assessment of clinical trial research of oral mucositis induced by radiation or chemotherapy. Cancer 1999;85(10):2103–13.

46. Rapoport AP, Miller Watelet LF, Linder T, Eberly S, Raubertas RF, Lipp J, Duerst R, Abboud CN, Constine L, Andrews J, Etter MA, Spear L, Powley E, Packman CH, Rowe JM, Schwertschlag U, Bedrosian C, Liesveld JL. Analysis of factors that correlate with mucositis in recipients of autologous and allogeneic stem-cell transplants. J Clin Oncol 1999;17(8):2446–53.

47. Tsujikawa T, Uda K, Ihara T, Inoue T, Andoh A, Fujiyama Y, Bamba T. Changes in serum diamine oxidase activity during chemotherapy in patients with hematological malignancies. Cancer Lett 1999;147(1–2):195–8.

48. Freeman AJ, Cullen MH. Advances in the management of cytotoxic drug-induced nausea and vomiting. J Clin Pharm Ther 1991;16(6):411–21.

49. Schnell FM. Chemotherapy-induced nausea and vomiting: the importance of acute antiemetic control. Oncologist 2003;8(2):187–98.

50. de Wit R, van Alphen MM. Nieuwe ontwikkelingen in de behandeling van misselijkheid en braken door chemotherapie. [New developments in the treatment of nausea and vomiting caused by chemotherapy.] Ned Tijdschr Geneeskd 2003;147(15):690–4.

51. Tonato M, Clark-Snow RA, Osoba D, Del Favero A, Ballatori E, Borjeson S. Emesis induced by low or minimal emetic risk chemotherapy. Support Care Cancer 2005;13(2):109–11.

52. Arnold RJ, Gabrail N, Raut M, Kim R, Sung JC, Zhou Y. Clinical implications of chemotherapy-induced diarrhea in patients with cancer. J Support Oncol 2005;3(3):227–32.

53. Kobayashi K. [Chemotherapy-induced diarrhea.]Gan To Kagaku Ryoho 2003;30(6):765–71.

54. O'Brien BE, Kaklamani VG, Benson AB 3rd. The assessment and management of cancer treatment-related diarrhea. Clin Colorectal Cancer 2005;4(6):375–81.

55. Douillard JY, Lerouge D, Monnier A, Bennouna J, Haller AM, Sun XS, Assouline D, Grau B, Riviere A. Combined paclitaxel and gemcitabine as first-line treatment in metastatic non-small cell lung cancer: a multicentre phase II study. Br J Cancer 2001;84(9):1179–84.

56. Leach JW, Pham T, Diamandidis D, George JN. Thrombotic thrombocytopenic purpura–hemolytic uremic syndrome (TTP–HUS) following treatment with deoxycoformycin in a patient with cutaneous T cell lymphoma (Sézary syndrome): A case report. Am J Hematol 1999;61(4):268–70.

57. Hui YF, Giles FJ, Cortes JE. Chemotherapy-induced palmar–plantar erythrodysesthesia syndrome—recall following different chemotherapy agents. Invest New Drugs 2002;20(1):49–53.

58. Moens C, Moens P, Philippart G. Azathioprine and warts. Ann Rheum Dis 1990;49(4):269.

59. Goyal S, Huhn KM, Provost TT. Calciphylaxis in a patient without renal failure or elevated parathyroid hormone: possible aetiological role of chemotherapy. Br J Dermatol 2000;143(5):1087–90.

60. Arikoski P, Komulainen J, Riikonen P, Jurvelin JS, Voutilainen R, Kroger H. Reduced bone density at completion of chemotherapy for a malignancy. Arch Dis Child 1999;80(2):143–8.

61. Saeter G, Fossa SD, Norman N. Gynaecomastia following cytotoxic therapy for testicular cancer. Br J Urol 1987;59(4):348–52.

62. Kreuser ED, Xiros N, Hetzel WD, Heimpel H. Reproductive and endocrine gonadal capacity in patients treated with COPP chemotherapy for Hodgkin's disease. J Cancer Res Clin Oncol 1987;113(3):260–6.

63. Garcia VD, Keitel E, Almeida P, Santos AF, Becker M, Goldani JC. Morbidity after renal transplantation: role of bacterial infection. Transplant Proc 1995;27(2):1825–6.

64. Wade JJ, Rolando N, Hayllar K, Philpott-Howard J, Casewell MW, Williams R. Bacterial and fungal infections after liver transplantation: an analysis of 284 patients. Hepatology 1995;21(5):1328–36.

65. Singh N, Yu VL. Infections in organ transplant recipients. Curr Opin Infect Dis 1996;9:223–9.

66. Reis MA, Costa RS, Ferraz AS. Causes of death in renal transplant recipients: a study of 102 autopsies from 1968 to 1991. J R Soc Med 1995;88(1):24–7.

67. Schubert J, Tolkendorf E, Held HJ, et al. Can the genetic risk be evaluated for offspring of testicular cancer patients exposed to chemotherapy treatment? Aktuel Urol 1989;20:199.

68. Brown T, Dawson AA, Bennett B, Moore NR. The effects of four drug regimens on sister chromatid exchange frequency in patients with lymphomas. Cancer Genet Cytogenet 1988;36(1):89–102.

69. Bennett JM, Moloney WC, Greene MH, Boice JD Jr. Acute myeloid leukemia and other myelopathic disorders following treatment with alkylating agents. Hematol Pathol 1987;1(2):99–104.

70. Pedersen-Bjergaard J, Ersbal J, Hansen V, et al. Blasenkarzinom nach Cyclophosphamid-Langzeittherapie. Aktuel Urol 1988;19:275.

71. O'Keane JC. Carcinoma of the urinary bladder after treatment with cyclophosphamide. N Engl J Med 1988;319(13):871.

72. Mahe M, Raffi F, Rojouan J, et al. Cancers secondaires après maladie de Hodgkin. Semin Hop Paris 1988;64:3013.

73. van der Velden JW, van Putten WL, Guinee VF, Pfeiffer R, van Leeuwen FE, van der Linden EA, Vardomskaya I, Lane W, Durand M, Lagarde C, et al. Subsequent development of acute non-lymphocytic leukemia in patients treated for Hodgkin's disease. Int J Cancer 1988;42(2):252–5.

74. Guyotat D, Coiffier B, Campos L, Archimbaud E, Treille D, Ehrsam A, Fiere D. Acute leukaemia following high-dose chemoradiotherapy with bone marrow rescue for ovarian teratoma. Acta Haematol 1988;80(1):52–3.

75. Einhorn N, Eklund G, Lambert B. Solid tumours and chromosome aberrations as late side effects of melphalan therapy in ovarian carcinoma. Acta Oncol 1988;27(3):215–9.

76. Hoppe RT. Secondary leukemia and myelodysplastic syndrome after treatment for Hodgkin's disease. Leukemia 1992;6(Suppl 4):155–7.

77. Genuardi M, Zollino M, Serra A, Leone G, Mancini R, Mango G, Neri G. Long-term cytogenetic effects of antineoplastic treatment in relation to secondary leukemia. Cancer Genet Cytogenet 1988;33(2):201–11.

78. Hancock BW, Gregory WM, Cullen MH, Hudson GV, Burton A, Selby P, Maclennan KA, Jack A, Bessell EM, Smith P, Linch DC. British National Lymphoma Investigation; Central Lymphoma Group. ChlVPP alternating with PABlOE is superior to PABlOE alone in the initial treatment of advanced Hodgkin's disease: results of a British National Lymphoma Investigation/Central Lymphoma Group randomized controlled trial. Br J Cancer 2001;84(10):1293–300.

79. Cheson BD, Vena DA, Barrett J, Freidlin B. Second malignancies as a consequence of nucleoside analogue therapy for chronic lymphoid leukemias. J Clin Oncol 1999;17(8):2454–60.

80. Kawabata H, Utsunomiya A, Hanada S, Makino T, Takatsuka Y, Takeuchi S, Suzuki S, Suzumiya J, Ohshima K, Horiike S. Myelodysplastic syndrome in a patient with adult T cell leukaemia. Br J Haematol 1999;106(3):702–5.

81. Breslow NE, Takashima JR, Whitton JA, Moksness J, D'Angio GJ, Green DM. Second malignant neoplasms following treatment for Wilms' tumor: a report from the National Wilms' Tumor Study Group. J Clin Oncol 1995;13(8):1851–9.

82. Bokemeyer C, Freund M, Schmoll HJ, Rieder H, Fonatsch C. Secondary lymphoblastic leukemia following treatment of a malignant germ cell tumour. Ann Oncol 1992;3(9):772.

83. Kaldor JM, Day NE, Band P, Choi NW, Clarke EA, Coleman MP, Hakama M, Koch M, Langmark F, Neal FE, et al. Second malignancies following testicular cancer, ovarian cancer and Hodgkin's disease: an international collaborative study among cancer registries. Int J Cancer 1987;39(5):571–85.

84. Pedersen-Bjergaard J, Specht L, Larsen SO, Ersboll J, Struck J, Hansen MM, Hansen HH, Nissen NI. Risk of therapy-related leukaemia and preleukaemia after Hodgkin's disease. Relation to age, cumulative dose of alkylating agents, and time from chemotherapy. Lancet 1987;2(8550):83–8.

85. Blayney DW, Longo DL, Young RC, Greene MH, Hubbard SM, Postal MG, Duffey PL, DeVita VT Jr. Decreasing risk of leukemia with prolonged follow-up after chemotherapy and radiotherapy for Hodgkin's disease. N Engl J Med 1987;316(12):710–4.

86. Penn I. Tumors after renal and cardiac transplantation. Hematol Oncol Clin North Am 1993;7(2):431–45.

87. Gaya SB, Rees AJ, Lechler RI, Williams G, Mason PD. Malignant disease in patients with long-term renal transplants. Transplantation 1995;59(12):1705–9.

88. London NJ, Farmery SM, Will EJ, Davison AM, Lodge JP. Risk of neoplasia in renal transplant patients. Lancet 1995;346(8972):403–16.

89. Kehinde EO, Petermann A, Morgan JD, Butt ZA, Donnelly PK, Veitch PS, Bell PR. Triple therapy and incidence of de novo cancer in renal transplant recipients. Br J Surg 1994;81(7):985–6.

90. Opelz G, Henderson R. Incidence of non-Hodgkin lymphoma in kidney and heart transplant recipients. Lancet 1993;342(8886–8887):1514–6.

91. Gruber SA, Gillingham K, Sothern RB, Stephanian E, Matas AJ, Dunn DL. De novo cancer in cyclosporine-treated and non-cyclosporine-treated adult primary renal allograft recipients. Clin Transplant 1994;8(4):388–95.

92. Hiesse C, Kriaa F, Rieu P, Larue JR, Benoit G, Bellamy J, Blanchet P, Charpentier B. Incidence and type of malignancies occurring after renal transplantation in conventionally and cyclosporine-treated recipients: analysis of a 20-year period in 1600 patients. Transplant Proc 1995;27(1):972–4.

93. Gruber S, Dehner LP, Simmons RL. De novo hepatocellular carcinoma without chronic liver disease but with 17 years of azathioprine immunosuppression. Transplantation 1987;43(4):597–600.

94. Mittal BV, Cotton RE. Severely atypical changes in renal epithelium in biopsy and graft nephrectomy specimens in two cases of cadaver renal transplantation. Histopathology 1987;11(8):833–41.

95. Kelly G, Scheibner A, Murray E, Sheil R, Tiller D, Horvath J. T6+ and HLA-DR+ cell numbers in epidermis of immunosuppressed renal transplant recipients. J Cutan Pathol 1987;14(4):202–6.

96. Schwarz LR. Elimination of dose limiting toxicities of cisplatin, 5-fluorouracil, and leucovorin using a weekly 24-hour infusion schedule for the treatment of patients with nasopharyngeal carcinoma. Cancer 1996;78(3):566–7.

97. Viviani S, Ragni G, Santoro A, Perotti L, Caccamo E, Negretti E, Valagussa P, Bonadonna G. Testicular dysfunction in Hodgkin's disease before and after treatment. Eur J Cancer 1991;27(11):1389–92.

98. Ramsey-Goldman R, Schilling E. Immunosuppressive drug use during pregnancy. Rheum Dis Clin North Am 1997;23(1):149–67.

99. Armenti VT, Moritz MJ, Davison JM. Drug safety issues in pregnancy following transplantation and immunosuppression: effects and outcomes. Drug Saf 1998;19(3):219–32.

100. Armenti VT, Ahlswede KM, Ahlswede BA, Jarrell BE, Moritz MJ, Burke JF. National Transplantation Pregnancy Registry—outcomes of 154 pregnancies in cyclosporine-treated female kidney transplant recipients. Transplantation 1994;57(4):502–6.

101. Cararach V, Carmona F, Monleon FJ, Andreu J. Pregnancy after renal transplantation: 25 years experience in Spain. Br J Obstet Gynaecol 1993;100(2):122–5.

102. Armenti VT, Ahlswede BA, Moritz MJ, Jarrell BE. National Transplantation Pregnancy Registry: analysis of pregnancy outcomes of female kidney recipients with relation to time interval from transplant to conception. Transplant Proc 1993;25(1 Pt 2):1036–7.

103. Pilarski LM, Yacyshyn BR, Lazarovits AI. Analysis of peripheral blood lymphocyte populations and immune function from children exposed to cyclosporine or to azathioprine in utero. Transplantation 1994;57(1):133–44.

ALKYLATING AGENTS

Alkylating agents—Nitrosoureas

General Information

The nitrosourea cytostatic drugs are alkylating agents that include carmustine, lomustine, nimustine, and streptozocin.

Carmustine (BCNU) is used to treat myeloma, lymphomas, breast cancer, and brain tumors, Topical carmustine has been used to treat mycosis fungoides (1).

Lomustine (CCNU) is used to treat lymphomas and some solid tumors, particularly brain tumors, often in combination with procarbazine and vincristine (2). In contrast to other nitrosoureas, lomustine can be given orally.

Nimustine (ACNU) is used to treat malignant glioma (3).

Streptozocin (streptozotocin) is produced by *Streptomyces achromogenes*. It is used to treat metastatic islet cell carcinoma of the pancreas, but because of its high nephrotoxic and emetogenic potential it should be reserved for patients with symptomatic or progressive disease.

Organs and Systems

Respiratory

Carmustine pulmonary toxicity is well documented. Eight patients developed interstitial pulmonary fibrosis 12–17 years after exposure to carmustine in a total dose of carmustine of 770–1410 mg/m^2 (4).

Lung fibrosis has been described in a long-term follow up 13–17 years after treatment of 31 children given carmustine for brain tumors; six died, and of eight still available for study, six had upper zone fibrotic changes of their lungs on X-ray (5).

Lomustine can cause pulmonary infiltrates and fibrosis (6–8), and fatal pulmonary toxicity has occasionally occurred (9).

Sensory systems

A 2.7% ocular complication rate in 112 patients treated with a cumulative dose of carmustine 370 mg/m^2 for intracranial tumors has been recorded (10).

Eye pain and blindness due to retinal and optic nerve damage are recognized hazards of intracarotid carmustine therapy reference. They are thought to be due, at least in part, to the ethanol content of the diluent. Nimustine (ACNU) is water-soluble and ethanol-free. In a study of 30 patients with malignant gliomas, 123 infusions of nimustine and 53 of carmustine were administered (11). Eye pain was experienced during all carmustine infusions but not with nimustine, and one patient developed unilateral blindness after carmustine. In another study, carmustine was administered in solution with 5% dextrose in water (12). All the patients experienced ipsilateral orbital pain and scleral erythema, suggesting that carmustine itself contributes to the toxicity. Seven additional patients were treated wearing an ocular compression device to decrease blood flow and had not experienced any ocular complications.

Hematologic

Delayed myelosuppression is an important adverse effect of the nitrosoureas (13). It usually occurs 4–6 weeks after administration and can last for about 1–2 weeks. Thrombocytopenia occurs after about 4 weeks and leukopenia after 5–6 weeks.

Of 91 patients treated with topical carmustine, three developed reversible bone marrow suppression (14).

Urinary tract

Nephrotoxicity can rarely occur with lomustine, and all cases have been associated with cumulative doses greater than 1500 mg/m^2 (15).

Streptozocin is highly nephrotoxic, and renal function must be monitored carefully in all patients who are receiving it. Its effects include uremia, proteinuria, anuria, and proximal renal tubular acidosis (16). Uric acid nephropathy has also been reported (17). Adequate hydration has been recommended to reduce the risk of nephrotoxicity (18).

Skin

Local adverse effects of topical carmustine include tender erythema, superficial denudation or bullae, contact allergy, pigment alterations, and patchy telangiectasia (1).

Immunologic

Topical carmustine can cause hypersensitivity reactions, and three previous cases have been supplemented by a fourth (19).

- A 67-year-old woman used topical carmustine for a stage I cutaneous T cell lymphoma. A second course was started after 6 months and resulted in severe erosive inflammation at the site of treatment. Patch tests with carmustine 0.1, 0.5, and 1% in water all gave positive results; 22 controls were tested with 0.1% carmustine and lomustine and were all negative.

The most common adverse effect of chlormethine is an allergic contact dermatitis (20). Neither reducing the concentration of drug applied nor shortening the time of contact appreciably reduces the frequency of this adverse effect, which occurs in 30–80% of patients, although in one study of 203 patients with mycosis fungoides, the use of chlormethine ointment was associated with contact hypersensitivity in under 10% of cases. In an open, prospective study in 39 patients with cutaneous T cell lymphomas or parapsoriasis, chlormethine was applied topically and then washed off after 1 hour (21). There was cutaneous intolerance in 19 patients, six of whom had an allergic contact dermatitis after a mean period of 9.3 weeks, while the other 13 developed irritant contact dermatitis after a longer period. Cutaneous intolerance did not differ significantly according to the number of applications per week or the extent of body area treated. Comparison with published studies showed no significant difference in the number of cases of cutaneous intolerance after short-term application, although their occurrence was delayed. Therapeutic response was decreased appreciably by short-term application as compared with results in the literature.

Second-Generation Effects

Fertility

In 21 boys treated with carmustine or lomustine alone or in combination with procarbazine and vincristine for brain tumors, there were 20 cases of persistent testicular damage (22). From assessment of testicular size it was thought that most of those affected would remain infertile. This supports the idea that germinal epithelium is more susceptible than Leydig cells to cytostatic-induced damage.

Drug–Drug Interactions

Cimetidine

Bone marrow suppression by carmustine may be enhanced by cimetidine (23,24).

References

1. Zackheim HS. Topical carmustine (BCNU) in the treatment of mycosis fungoides. Dermatol Ther 2003;16(4):299–302.
2. Prados MD, Seiferheld W, Sandler HM, Buckner JC, Phillips T, Schultz C, Urtasun R, Davis R, Gutin P, Cascino TL, Greenberg HS, Curran WJ Jr. Phase III randomized study of radiotherapy plus procarbazine, lomustine, and vincristine with or without BUdR for treatment of anaplastic astrocytoma: final report of RTOG 9404. Int J Radiat Oncol Biol Phys 2004;58(4):1147–52.
3. Weller M, Muller B, Koch R, Bamberg M, Krauseneck PNeuro-Oncology Working Group of the German Cancer Society. Neuro-Oncology Working Group 01 trial of nimustine plus teniposide versus nimustine plus cytarabine chemotherapy in addition to involved-field radiotherapy in the first-line treatment of malignant glioma. J Clin Oncol 2003;21(17):3276–84.
4. Hasleton PS, O'Driscoll BR, Lynch P, Webster A, Kalra SJ, Gattamaneini HR, Woodcock AA, Poulter LW. Late BCNU lung: a light and ultrastructural study on the delayed effect of BCNU on the lung parenchyma. J Pathol 1991;164(1):31–6.
5. O'Driscoll BR, Hasleton PS, Taylor PM, Poulter LW, Gattameneni HR, Woodcock AA. Active lung fibrosis up to 17 years after chemotherapy with carmustine (BCNU) in childhood. N Engl J Med 1990;323(6):378–82.
6. Tucci E, Verdiani P, Di Carlo S, Sforza V. Lomustine (CCNU)-induced pulmonary fibrosis. Tumori 1986;72(1):95–8.
7. Vats TS, Trueworthy RC, Langston CM. Pulmonary fibrosis associated with lomustine (CCNU): a case report. Cancer Treat Rep 1982;66(10):1881–2.
8. Stone MD, Richardson MG. Pulmonary toxicity of lomustine. Cancer Treat Rep 1987;71(7–8):786–7.
9. Dent RG. Fatal pulmonary toxic effects of lomustine. Thorax 1982;37(8):627–9.
10. Elsas T, Watne K, Fostad K, Hager B. Ocular complications after intracarotid BCNU for intracranial tumors. Acta Ophthalmol (Copenh) 1989;67(1):83–6.
11. Papavero L, Loew F, Jaksche H. Intracarotid infusion of ACNU and BCNU as adjuvant therapy of malignant gliomas. Clinical aspects and critical considerations. Acta Neurochir (Wien) 1987;85(3–4):128–37.
12. Johnson DW, Parkinson D, Wolpert SM, Kasdon DL, Kwan ES, Laucella M, Anderson ML. Intracarotid chemotherapy with 1,3-bis-(2-chloroethyl)-1-nitrosourea (BCNU) in 5% dextrose in water in the treatment of malignant glioma. Neurosurgery 1987;20(4):577–83.
13. Wakui A. [Cancer chemotherapy with special reference to pharmacokinetics of nitrosoureas.]Gan To Kagaku Ryoho 1982;9(8):1327–38.
14. Zackheim HS, Epstein EH Jr, McNutt NS, Grekin DA, Crain WR. Topical carmustine (BCNU) for mycosis fungoides and related disorders: a 10-year experience. J Am Acad Dermatol 1983;9(3):363–74.
15. Ellis ME, Weiss RB, Kuperminc M. Nephrotoxicity of lomustine. A case report and literature review. Cancer Chemother Pharmacol 1985;15(2):174–5.
16. Hall-Craggs M, Brenner DE, Vigorito RD, Sutherland JC. Acute renal failure and renal tubular squamous metaplasia following treatment with streptozotocin. Hum Pathol 1982;13(6):597–601.
17. Hricik DE, Goldsmith GH. Uric acid nephrolithiasis and acute renal failure secondary to streptozotocin nephrotoxicity. Am J Med 1988;84(1):153–6.
18. Tobin MV, Warenius HM, Morris AI. Forced diuresis to reduce nephrotoxicity of streptozotocin in the treatment of advanced metastatic insulinoma. BMJ (Clin Res Ed) 1987;294(6580):1128.
19. Thomson KF, Sheehan-Dare RA, Wilkinson SM. Allergic contact dermatitis from topical carmustine. Contact Dermatitis 2000;42(2):112.
20. Goday JJ, Aguirre A, Raton JA, Diaz-Perez JL. Local bullous reaction to topical mechlorethamine (mustine). Contact Dermatitis 1990;22(5):306–7.
21. Foulc P, Evrard V, Dalac S, Guillot B, Delaunay M, Verret JL, Dreno B. Evaluation of a 1-h exposure time to mechlorethamine in patients undergoing topical treatment. Br J Dermatol 2002;147(5):926–30.
22. Clayton PE, Shalet SM, Price DA, Campbell RH. Testicular damage after chemotherapy for childhood brain tumors. J Pediatr 1988;112(6):922–6.
23. Selker RG, Moore P, Lodolce D. Bone-marrow depression with cimetidine plus carmustine. N Engl J Med 1978;299(15):834.
24. Volkin RL, Shadduck RK, Winkelstein A, Zeigler ZR, Selker RG. Potentiation of carmustine—cranial irradiation-induced myelosuppression by cimetidine. Arch Intern Med 1982;142(2):243–5.

Alkylating agents — *N*-lost derivatives

General Information

The *N*-lost cytostatic drugs are alkylating agents that include chlormethine (mechlorethamine, mustine, nitrogen mustard), cyclophosphamide, and estramustine (all rINNs). Chlormethine is mainly used topically in the early stages of mycosis fungoides (1). Estramustine is a conjugated derivative of estradiol and chlormethine, mainly used to treat prostate cancer (2).

Organs and Systems

Mineral balance

A patient with androgen-independent prostate cancer developed hypocalcemia during treatment with estramustine (3). The total serum calcium concentrations before and after the initiation of estramustine were 2.1 and 1.1 mmol/l respectively. This prompted a retrospective survey of hypocalcemia in 135 consecutive patients taking estramustine; 20% were affected. The authors speculated that estramustine may cause hypocalcemia by inhibiting mobilization of calcium and the action of parathyroid hormone on the skeleton.

Reproductive system

Gynecomastia severe enough to necessitate withdrawal of therapy was the main adverse effect of estramustine 560 mg/day for more than 1 year in prostatic carcinoma (4).

Breast pain with vaginal bleeding and diarrhea were dose-limiting when estramustine 840 mg/day was given for breast cancer (5).

Immunologic

The most common adverse effect of chlormethine is an allergic contact dermatitis (6). Neither reducing the concentration of drug applied nor shortening the time of contact appreciably reduces the frequency of this adverse effect, which occurs in 30–80% of patients, although in one study of 203 patients with mycosis fungoides, the use of chlormethine ointment was associated with contact hypersensitivity in under 10% of cases (1). In an open, prospective study in 39 patients with cutaneous T cell lymphomas or parapsoriasis, chlormethine was applied topically and then washed off after 1 hour (7). There was cutaneous intolerance in 19 patients, six of whom had an allergic contact dermatitis after a mean period of 9.3 weeks, while the other 13 developed irritant contact dermatitis after a longer period. Cutaneous intolerance did not differ significantly according to the number of applications per week or the extent of body area treated.

Comparison with published studies showed no significant difference in the number of cases of cutaneous intolerance after short-term application, although their occurrence was delayed. Therapeutic response was decreased appreciably by short-term application as compared with results in the literature.

Long-Term Effects

Tumorigenicity

Chlormethine can act as a tumor promotor. In most cases squamous cell carcinomas and basal cell carcinomas have been reported. Two cases of small malignant melanoma, 3 mm in diameter, have been reported in patients with mycosis fungoides stage 1a, with latency intervals of 18 and 10 months after withdrawal of local application, which had been conducted for 18 months and almost 3 years respectively (8).

References

1. Kim YH, Martinez G, Varghese A, Hoppe RT. Topical nitrogen mustard in the management of mycosis fungoides: update of the Stanford experience. Arch Dermatol 2003;139(2):165–73.
2. Eastham JA, Kelly WK, Grossfeld GD, Small EJCancer and Leukemia Group B. Cancer and Leukemia Group B (CALGB) 90203: a randomized phase 3 study of radical prostatectomy alone versus estramustine and docetaxel before radical prostatectomy for patients with high-risk localized disease. Urology 2003;62(Suppl 1):55–62.
3. Park DS, Vassilopoulou Sellin R, Tu S. Estramustine-related hypocalcemia in patients with prostate carcinoma and osteoblastic metastases. Urology 2001;58(1):105.
4. Asakawa M, Wada S, Hayahara N, Yayumoto R, Kishimoto T, Maekawa M, Morikawa Y, Kawakita J, Umeda M, Horii A, et al. [Clinical study of estramustine phosphate disodium (Estracyt) on prostatic cancer—results of long-term therapy for 38 patients with prostatic cancer.]Hinyokika Kiyo 1990;36(11):1361–9.
5. Wada T, Morikawa E, Houjou T, Kadota K, Mori N, Matsunami N, Watatani M, Yasutomi M. [Clinical evaluation of estramustine phosphate in the treatment of patients with advanced breast cancers.]Gan To Kagaku Ryoho 1990;17(9):1901–4.
6. Goday JJ, Aguirre A, Raton JA, Diaz-Perez JL. Local bullous reaction to topical mechlorethamine (mustine). Contact Dermatitis 1990;22(5):306–7.
7. Foulc P, Evrard V, Dalac S, Guillot B, Delaunay M, Verret JL, Dreno B. Evaluation of a 1-h exposure time to mechlorethamine in patients undergoing topical treatment. Br J Dermatol 2002;147(5):926–30.
8. Amichai B, Grunwald MH, Goldstein J, Finkelstein E, Halevy S. Small malignant melanoma in patients with mycosis fungoides. J Eur Acad Dermatol Venereol 1998;11(2):155–7.

Busulfan

General Information

Busulfan is an alkylating agent that is used to treat myeloproliferative disorders and to produce myeloablation before bone marrow or stem cell transplantation. Busulfan is metabolized by hepatic glutathione S-transferase, the activity of which correlates negatively with busulfan maximum and minimum concentrations and positively with busulfan clearance (1).

General adverse effects

Leukemic patients receiving marrow from HLA-identical sibling donors were randomized to either oral busulfan 16 mg/kg ($n = 88$) or total body irradiation ($n = 79$), plus cyclophosphamide 120 mg/kg (2). Over 5–9 years the following adverse effects occurred in the two groups:

- obstructive bronchiolitis (26 versus 5%).
- cataracts (6 versus 2%).
- veno-occlusive disease of the liver (12 versus 1%).
- complete or partial alopecia (28 versus 6%).
- hemorrhagic cystitis (32 versus 10%).
- acute graft-versus-host disease (cumulative incidence at 7 years, 59 versus 47%); death from graft-versus-host disease was more common with busulfan (22 versus 3%).

Organs and Systems

Cardiovascular

Pericardial fibrosis has been reported after busulfan treatment in a man with chronic myeloid leukemia (3). Endocardial fibrosis has also been reported (4).

Respiratory

Busulfan can cause interstitial fibrosing lung disease ("busulfan lung") with an estimated incidence of 6% (5). It begins gradually, causes dyspnea and cough, and is often accompanied by skin pigmentation. It usually occurs after prolonged treatment (on average 41 months, cumulative dose 2900 mg). The respiratory function pattern is characterized by reduced lung volumes with hypoxemia and hypocapnic respiratory failure. Radiology shows interstitial and predominantly basal shadows.

Various authors have discussed the differences in busulfan-induced idiopathic pneumonia syndrome, as a result of either chronic low-dose or short-course high-dose therapy. One group found that chronic low-dose therapy (even at cumulative doses of busulfan of up to 3 g) caused different lung damage from the clinical characteristics, radiological, and pathological features of the idiopathic pneumonia syndrome (6).

Three patients with busulfan-induced interstitial pneumonitis each had circulating immune complexes and alveolitis, and histology demonstrated consistent abnormalities of type I pneumocytes and depletion of type II pneumocytes (7).

Nervous system

Busulfan can cause generalized seizures (8).

High concentrations of busulfan in the cerebrospinal fluid have been correlated with development of myoclonic epilepsy and/or other electroencephalographic changes after high-dose busulfan conditioning regimens for acute leukemia (9).

- A 21-year-old woman with acute lymphoblastic leukemia underwent bone marrow transplantation after a conditioning regimen consisting of busulfan and cyclophosphamide (10). The day after starting busulfan, she had a generalized tonic-clonic seizure and electroencephalography showed diffuse polyspikes and spike-and-wave discharges, with persistent abnormalities (slowing of background activity intermixed with diffuse slow waves and isolated delta and theta bursts) for about 20 days and complete normalization 1 month after the seizure.

Phenytoin and benzodiazepines have been successfully used to prevent seizures during busulfan therapy; benzodiazepines may be preferable, because phenytoin can induce the metabolism of busulfan, reducing its efficacy. In 29 children undergoing hemopoietic stem cell transplantation who received high-dose busulfan, intravenous or oral lorazepam (median dose 0.022 mg/kg) before each dose of busulfan and for 24 hours after the last dose was used as seizure prophylaxis; drowsiness was the only significant adverse effect and there were no seizures (11). There were no tonic-clonic or myoclonic seizures in a prospective study in 16 patients with leukemia receiving busulfan before autologous bone marrow transplantation who were given phenobarbital and clonazepam, despite electroencephalographic changes in two patients after busulfan (12).

Sensory systems

Cataract due to busulfan has been reported after long-term administration (SEDA-1, 341; 13).

- A 42-year-old Japanese woman received busulfan 212 mg/day for only 4 days and developed reduced visual acuity and blurred vision in both eyes; she had a posterior polar subcapsular opacity in the lenses in both eyes (14).
- A 49-year-old man with chronic myelogenous leukemia developed dense posterior subcapsular cataracts and punctate cortical opacities after taking busulfan for 5 years (15). Ultrastructural examination showed cortical liquefaction, with Morgagnian droplets involving primarily the region from the equator to the posterior subcapsular space, crystalloid rays, and abundant degenerate lens fiber membranes.

Hematologic

Aplastic anemia developed in 84 patients with chronic myeloid leukemia receiving busulfan; three patients died (16). The time interval until pancytopenia was detected varied considerably, ranging between 6 and 126 months. The effect did not correlate with the initial doses of busulfan.

Colony-stimulating factors have been used to treat and prevent the adverse hematological effects of busulfan (17,18).

- In a 91-year-old woman with essential thrombocythemia and marked bone marrow suppression induced by long-term busulfan, G-CSF and M-CSF increased the neutrophil and platelet counts but only transiently; there was transient eosinophilia after withdrawal of M-CSF (19).
- A 63-year-old woman with thrombocythemia was given busulfan 2 mg/day and later developed pancytopenia (20). She was given metenolone acetate 15 mg/day and G-CSF 300 µg/day, and frequent blood transfusions without effect. She was then given metenolone acetate, G-CSF 600 µg/day, and erythropoietin 24 000 units twice a week, and her pancytopenia gradually improved over several months.

One patient with busulfan-induced pancytopenia and recurrent thrombocytopenic bleeding was successfully treated prophylactically with random-donor platelet transfusions and later with HLA-matched platelets from a sibling (21).

- A patient with polycythemia vera who had undergone splenectomy received six courses of busulfan for recurrent thrombocytosis over 19 years (22). Severe pancytopenia followed and persisted for 4 months. There was marked erythroid hyperplasia in the bone marrow, with striking dyserythropoiesis, PAS-positive erythrocyte precursors, moderate numbers of circulating normoblasts, and evidence of chronic and acute hemolysis.

Of 39 patients taking busulfan 16 mg/kg/day and cyclophosphamide 120 mg/kg/day for leukemias, who received non-T cell depleted, HLA-matched sibling or unrelated donor marrow transplants 2 days after the end of chemotherapy followed by ciclosporin and methylprednisolone given to prevent graft-versus-host disease, 11 developed eosinophilia, of whom only 2 were still taking methylprednisolone (23). At the onset of eosinophilia, five of these 11 patients had graft-versus-host disease that worsened within 2 months. In the other six patients, graft-versus-host disease was not present initially but developed in all cases at a median of 4 months after the onset of eosinophilia.

Liver

In 66 patients who received busulfan in combination with cyclophosphamide, etoposide, and/or cytarabine in preparation for bone marrow transplantation, there was a higher incidence of veno-occlusive disease of the liver (sinusoidal obstruction syndrome) in those who received busulfan + cyclophosphamide (four of 10) than in those who received busulfan + cyclophosphamide + cytarabine (one of 18) or busulfan + cyclophosphamide + etoposide (seven of 38) (24). The risk of veno-occlusive disease was higher in those whose busulfan AUC was over 1500 minute.µmol/l (relative risk = 11). Other pharmacokinetic parameters, age, sex, type of bone marrow transplantation,

previous therapy, or pretransplant liver function tests were not predictive of veno-occlusive disease.

In 30 patients who received oral busulfan 1 mg/kg, all six of those who developed hepatic veno-occlusive disease had a busulfan AUC greater than the mean, and five had an AUC that was greater than 1 standard deviation above the mean; veno-occlusive disease correlated with an increased AUC (25).

- Intrahepatic cholestasis has been attributed to busulfan in a 57-year-old man with chronic megakaryocytic granulocytic myelosis (26).
- Cholestatic hepatitis occurred in a 61-year-old man with chronic myelocytic leukemia who had taken busulfan for 8 years (27). He presented with fever, abdominal pain, and raised liver enzymes. A liver biopsy showed cellular cholestasis with focal liver cell necrosis accompanied by a mild inflammatory infiltrate. When busulfan was withdrawn, his liver enzymes normalized and his fever resolved.

Urinary tract

Busulfan can rarely cause hemorrhagic cystitis (28,29).

Skin

Busulfan can cause hyperpigmentation (30,31), often in combination with interstitial lung disease (5).

Hair

Of 65 patients who survived for at least 6 months after bone marrow transplantation, 31 had some degree of alopecia and 19 had extensive alopecia (32). The mean minimum busulfan concentration was 656 ng/ml in patients who developed alopecia, compared with 507 ng/ml in those who did not. Patients with more extensive alopecia had higher busulfan concentrations. In multivariate analysis, alopecia was associated with busulfan concentrations higher than the median (OR = 3.43; 95% CI = 3.04, 3.88), allogeneic transplantation (OR = 2.56; CI = 2.28, 2.88), and female sex (OR = 1.96; CI = 1.73, 2.88). There was no association between alopecia and chronic graft-versus-host disease.

Reproductive system

Busulfan can cause ovarian failure.

- A 26-year-old woman with chronic myeloid leukemia developed busulfan-induced ovarian failure, with amenorrhea, climacteric symptoms, raised plasma concentrations of luteinizing and follicle-stimulating hormones, and low 17 beta-estradiol concentrations (33). However, 1 year later she became pregnant, the busulfan was stopped, and amniocentesis showed a normal karyotype. The remainder of the pregnancy was unremarkable and ended with the normal delivery of a healthy child.

Of 21 girls aged 11–21 years who had received high-dose chemotherapy and autologous bone marrow transplantation without total body irradiation for malignant tumors

1.2–13 years before (median 7 years), 10 were given busulfan 600 mg/m^2 and melphalan (140 mg/m^2) with or without cyclophosphamide (3.6 g/m^2) (34). Eleven others did not receive busulfan. Twelve girls (57%) had clinical and hormonal evidence of ovarian failure. Among nine others who had had normal puberty, six had normal gonadotropin concentrations, one had raised gonadotropin concentrations, and two had gonadotropin concentrations at the upper limit of the reference range. All 10 girls who received busulfan developed severe persistent ovarian failure.

Second-Generation Effects

Teratogenicity

Retinal degeneration and microphthalmia have been described in the infants of women who have taken busulfan during pregnancy (35).

- Myeloschisis occurred in a 6-week-old human embryo whose 39-year-old mother had taken busulfan before and during the early stages of gestation for chronic lymphatic leukemia (36). Histology showed reduced mesenchymal elements together with somite disorganization in the affected area of the embryo.

Drug Administration

Drug overdose

A 4.6 kg infant with Wiskott–Aldrich syndrome received an accidental overdose of busulfan during preparation for allogeneic stem cell transplantation (37). Hemodialysis was immediately performed and resulted in accelerated clearance of busulfan. There were no acute neurological or hepatic adverse effects, and after cough and by rales for 2 months pulmonary symptoms resolved. There was stable partial donor chimerism after transplantation, but the patient was well 12 months later.

Drug–Drug Interactions

Cyclophosphamide

In bone marrow transplant recipients, prior administration of busulfan, which itself causes hemorrhagic cystitis, can increase the risk of cyclophosphamide-induced damage (38).

Busulfan reduces the clearance of cyclophosphamide to its active metabolite 4-hydroperoxycyclophosphamide (39). The first dose of high-dose cyclophosphamide should therefore be delayed for at least 24 hours after the last dose of busulfan.

Hydroxycarbamide

During long-term follow-up of patients treated with busulfan and hydroxycarbamide for essential thrombocythemia, seven patients (13%) taking hydroxycarbamide developed secondary acute leukemia, myelodysplasia, or solid tumors, compared with only one of the control group; none of the 20 patients who had never been treated with chemotherapy developed secondary malignancies compared with three of the 77 given hydroxycarbamide only and five of the 15 given busulfan plus hydroxycarbamide. This suggests that the combination of busulfan plus hydroxycarbamide causes a significantly increased risk of secondary malignancies (44).

Itraconazole

In 13 patients given bone marrow transplantation, the clearance of busulfan was reduced by an average of 20% in patients taking itraconazole compared with control patients and patients taking fluconazole (40).

Reduced elimination and increased toxicity of busulfan co-administered with itraconazole has been postulated (43).

Melphalan

The possibility that melphalan and busulfan may cause additive lung damage has been discussed in the light of a 59-year-old patient with chronic myeloid leukemia who developed severe interstitial lung fibrosis after short-term sequential treatment with the two drugs (45).

Metronidazole

In 24 patients with graft-versus-host disease, metronidazole significantly increased busulfan plasma concentrations from 452 to 807 ng/ml (41). The authors concluded that metronidazole should not be administered simultaneously with busulfan, because of the risk of severe toxicity and/or mortality.

Phenytoin

In 17 patients given busulfan during conditioning before bone marrow transplantation, phenytoin increased the clearance of busulfan and shortened its half-life; diazepam did not have the same effect (42). There were reductions in the steady-state concentrations of busulfan in four of seven patients who took phenytoin and in only one of eight patients who took diazepam. This effect of phenytoin is probably due to induction of glutathione transferase.

References

1. Poonkuzhali B, Chandy M, Srivastava A, Dennison D, Krishnamoorthy R. Glutathione S-transferase activity influences busulfan pharmacokinetics in patients with beta thalassemia major undergoing bone marrow transplantation. Drug Metab Dispos 2001;29(3):264–7.
2. Ringden O, Remberger M, Ruutu T, Nikoskelainen J, Volin L, Vindelov L, Parkkali T, Lenhoff S, Sallerfors B, Mellander L, Ljungman P, Jacobsen N. Increased risk of chronic graft-versus-host disease, obstructive bronchiolitis, and alopecia with busulfan versus total body irradiation: long-term results of a randomized trial in allogeneic marrow recipients with leukemia. Nordic Bone Marrow Transplantation Group. Blood 1999;93(7):2196–201.
3. Terpstra W, de Maat CE. Pericardial fibrosis following busulfan treatment. Neth J Med 1989;35(5–6):249–52.

4. Weinberger A, Pinkhas J, Sandbank U, Shaklai M, de Vries A. Endocardial fibrosis following busulfan treatment. JAMA 1975;231(5):495.

5. Massin F, Fur A, Reybet-Degat O, Camus P, Jeannin L. La pneumopathie du busulfan. [Busulfan-induced pneumopathy.] Rev Mal Respir 1987;4(1):3–10.

6. Bilgrami SF, Metersky ML, McNally D, Naqvi BH, Kapur D, Raible D, Bona RD, Edwards RL, Feingold JM, Clive JM, Tutschka PJ. Idiopathic pneumonia syndrome following myeloablative chemotherapy and autologous transplantation. Ann Pharmacother 2001;35(2):196–201.

7. Vergnon JM, Boucheron S, Riffat J, Guy C, Blanc P, Emonot A. Pneumopathies interstitielles au busulfan: analyse histologique, évolutive et par lavage broncho-alvéolaire de trois observations. [Interstitial pneumopathies caused by busulfan. Histologic, developmental and bronchoalveolar lavage analysis of 3 cases.] Rev Med Interne 1988;9(4):377–83.

8. Murphy CP, Harden EA, Thompson JM. Generalized seizures secondary to high-dose busulfan therapy. Ann Pharmacother 1992;26(1):30–1.

9. Meloni G, Raucci U, Pinto RM, Spalice A, Vignetti M, Iannetti P. Pretransplant conditioning with busulfan and cyclophosphamide in acute leukemia patients: neurological and electroencephalographic prospective study. Ann Oncol 1992;3(2):145–8.

10. La Morgia C, Mondini S, Guarino M, Bonifazi F, Cirignotta F. Busulfan neurotoxicity and EEG abnormalities: a case report. Neurol Sci 2004;25(2):95–7.

11. Chan KW, Mullen CA, Worth LL, Choroszy M, Koontz S, Tran H, Slopis J. Lorazepam for seizure prophylaxis during high-dose busulfan administration. Bone Marrow Transplant 2002;29(12):963–5.

12. Meloni G, Nasta L, Pinto RM, Spalice A, Raucci U, Iannetti P. Clonazepam prophylaxis and busulfan-related myoclonic epilepsy in autografted acute leukemia patients. Haematologica 1995;80(6):532–4.

13. Honda A, Dake Y, Amemiya T. [Cataracts in a patient treated with busulfan (Mablin powder) for eight years.] Nippon Ganka Gakkai Zasshi 1993;97(10):1242–5.

14. Kaida T, Ogawa T, Amemiya T. Cataract induced by short-term administration of large doses of busulfan: a case report. Ophthalmologica 1999;213(6):397–9.

15. Hamming NA, Apple DJ, Goldberg MF. Histopathology and ultrastructure of busulfan-induced cataract. Albrecht Von Graefes Arch Klin Exp Ophthalmol 1976;200(2):139–147.

16. Krug K, Stenzel L. Verlaufsvarianten von Panzytopenien nach Busulfanbehandlung der chronischen myeloischen Leukämie (CML). [Varying course of pancytopenia after busulfan treatment of chronic myelocytic leukemia (CML).] Folia Haematol Int Mag Klin Morphol Blutforsch 1978;105(2):181–7.

17. Fiedler W, Goetz G, Weh HJ, Hossfeld DK. GM-CSF in busulfan overdosage. Eur J Haematol 1990;45(3):183–4.

18. Openshaw H, Lund BT, Kashyap A, Atkinson R, Sniecinski I, Weiner LP, Forman S. Peripheral blood stem cell transplantation in multiple sclerosis with busulfan and cyclophosphamide conditioning: report of toxicity and immunological monitoring. Biol Blood Marrow Transplant 2000;6(5A):563–75.

19. Take H, Tamura K, Kurabayashi H, Kubota K, Shirakura T. [Effect of G-CSF and M-CSF on busulfan-induced marrow failure in a 91-year old patient with essential thrombocythemia.] Nippon Ronen Igakkai Zasshi 1993;30(10):901–5.

20. Yamamoto K, Nagata K, Hamaguchi H. [Complete remission of essential thrombocythemia after recovery from severe bone marrow aplasia induced by busulfan treatment.]Gan To Kagaku Ryoho 1997;24(3):365–9.

21. Stuart JJ, Crocker DL, Roberts HR. Treatment of busulfan-induced pancytopenia. Arch Intern Med 1976;136(10):1181–3.

22. Pezzimenti JF, Kim HC, Lindenbaum J. Erythroleukemia-like syndrome due to busulfan toxicity in polycythemia vera. Cancer 1976;38(6):2242–6.

23. Kalaycioglu ME, Bolwell BJ. Eosinophilia after allogeneic bone marrow transplantation using the busulfan and cyclophosphamide preparative regimen. Bone Marrow Transplant 1994;14(1):113–5.

24. Dix SP, Wingard JR, Mullins RE, Jerkunica I, Davidson TG, Gilmore CE, York RC, Lin LS, Devine SM, Geller RB, Heffner LT, Hillyer CD, Holland HK, Winton EF, Saral R. Association of busulfan area under the curve with veno-occlusive disease following BMT. Bone Marrow Transplant 1996;17(2):225–30.

25. Grochow LB, Jones RJ, Brundrett RB, Braine HG, Chen TL, Saral R, Santos GW, Colvin OM. Pharmacokinetics of busulfan: correlation with veno-occlusive disease in patients undergoing bone marrow transplantation Cancer Chemother Pharmacol 1989;25(1):55–61.

26. Adang RP, Breed WP. Leverbeschadiging tijdens gebruik van busulfan. [Liver damage during use of busulfan.] Ned Tijdschr Geneeskd 1989;133(30):1515–8. Erratum in: Ned Tijdschr Geneeskd 1989;133(37):1864.

27. Morris LE, Guthrie TH Jr. Busulfan-induced hepatitis. Am J Gastroenterol 1988;83(6):682–3.

28. Millard RJ. Busulfan-induced hemorrhagic cystitis. Urology 1981;18(2):143–4.

29. Pode D, Perlberg S, Steiner D. Busulfan-induced hemorrhagic cystitis. J Urol 1983;130(2):347–8.

30. Adam BA, Ismail R, Sivanesan S. Busulfan hyperpigmentation: light and electron microscopic studies. J Dermatol 1980;7(6):405–11.

31. Simonart T, Decaux G, Gourdin JM, Peny MO, Noel JC, Leclercq-Smekens M, De Dobbeleer G. Hyperpigmentation induite par le busulfan: une observation avec õtude ultrastructurale. [Hyperpigmentation induced by busulfan: a case with ultrastructure examination.] Ann Dermatol Venereol 1999;126(5):439–40.

32. Ljungman P, Hassan M, Bekassy AN, Ringden O, Oberg G. Busulfan concentration in relation to permanent alopecia in recipients of bone marrow transplants. Bone Marrow Transplant 1995;15(6):869–71.

33. Shalev O, Rahav G, Milwidsky A. Reversible busulfan-induced ovarian failure. Eur J Obstet Gynecol Reprod Biol 1987;26(3):239–42.

34. Teinturier C, Hartmann O, Valteau-Couanet D, Benhamou E, Bougneres PF. Ovarian function after autologous bone marrow transplantation in childhood: high-dose busulfan is a major cause of ovarian failure. Bone Marrow Transplant 1998;22(10):989–94.

35. Saraux H, Lefrancois A. Degenerative Netzhauter krankungen nach Behandlung der Mutter mit Busulfan während der Schwangerschaft. [Degenerative retinal conditions after treatment with Busulfan during pregnancy.] Klin Monatsbl Augenheilkd 1977;170(6):818–20.

36. Abramovici A, Shaklai M, Pinkhas J. Myeloschisis in a six weeks embryo of a leukemic woman treated by busulfan. Teratology 1978;18(2):241–6.

37. Stein J, Davidovitz M, Yaniv I, Ben-Ari J, Gamzu Z, Hoffer E, Bentur Y, Tabak A, Krivoy N. Accidental busulfan overdose: enhanced drug clearance with hemodialysis in a child with Wiskott–Aldrich syndrome. Bone Marrow Transplant 2001;27(5):551–3.

38. Thomas AE, Patterson J, Prentice HG, Brenner MK, Ganczakowski M, Hancock JF, Pattinson JK, Blacklock HA, Hopewell JP. Haemorrhagic cystitis in bone marrow transplantation patients: possible increased risk associated with prior busulphan therapy. Bone Marrow Transplant 1987;1(4):347–55.
39. Hassan M, Ljungman P, Ringden O, Hassan Z, Oberg G, Nilsson C, Bekassy A, Bielenstein M, Abdel-Rehim M, Georen S, Astner L. The effect of busulphan on the pharmacokinetics of cyclophosphamide and its 4-hydroxy metabolite: time interval influence on therapeutic efficacy and therapy-related toxicity. Bone Marrow Transplant 2000;25(9):915–24.
40. Buggia I, Zecca M, Alessandrino EP, Locatelli F, Rosti G, Bosi A, Pession A, Rotoli B, Majolino I, Dallorso A, Regazzi MB. Itraconazole can increase systemic exposure to busulfan in patients given bone marrow transplantation. GITMO (Gruppo Italiano Trapianto di Midollo Osseo). Anticancer Res 1996;16(4A):2083–8.
41. Nilsson C, Aschan J, Hentschke P, Ringden O, Ljungman P, Hassan M. The effect of metronidazole on busulfan pharmacokinetics in patients undergoing hematopoietic stem cell transplantation. Bone Marrow Transplant 2003;31(6):429–435.
42. Hassan M, Oberg G, Bjorkholm M, Wallin I, Lindgren M. Influence of prophylactic anticonvulsant therapy on high-dose busulphan kinetics. Cancer Chemother Pharmacol 1993;33(3):181–6.
43. Buggia I, Zecca M, Alessandrino EP, Locatelli F, Rosti G, Bosi A, Pession A, Rotoli B, Majolino I, Dallorso A, Regazzi MB. Itraconazole can increase systemic exposure to busulfan in patients given bone marrow transplantation. GITMO (Gruppo Italiano Trapianto di Midollo Osseo). Anticancer Res 1996;16(4A):2083–8.
44. Finazzi G, Ruggeri M, Rodeghiero F, Barbui T. Second malignancies in patients with essential thrombocythaemia treated with busulphan and hydroxyurea: long-term follow-up of a randomized clinical trial. Br J Haematol 2000;110(3):577–83.
45. Schallier D, Impens N, Warson F, Van Belle S, De Wasch G. Additive pulmonary toxicity with melphalan and busulfan therapy. Chest 1983;84(4):492–3.

Cyclophosphamide

See also Ifosfamide

General Information

Cyclophosphamide is an alkylating nitrogen mustard derivative mainly used in oncology patients (1) or in conditioning regimens for bone marrow transplantation. Its immunosuppressant properties have been used in organ transplantation and more often in chronic inflammatory disorders or autoimmune diseases.

Observational studies

Cyclophosphamide has been investigated in a wide range of diseases, but results in aplastic anemia and idiopathic pulmonary fibrosis have been disappointing. In a low dose (2 mg/kg/day), it produced minimal efficacy in 19 patients with idiopathic pulmonary fibrosis who had failed to respond to a glucocorticoid or who had had adverse effects (2). Moreover, 13 patients had cyclophosphamide-induced adverse effects, which required drug withdrawal in 9. The most frequent were severe gastrointestinal effects, leukopenia, and skin rashes. In another study, high-dose cyclophosphamide plus ciclosporin (50 mg/kg/day for 4 days) was compared with antithymocyte globulin plus ciclosporin in patients with severe aplastic anemia, but the trial was prematurely stopped after only 31 patients had been enrolled because of three early deaths in patients taking cyclophosphamide (3). Subsequent analysis showed excess morbidity and mortality in patients taking cyclophosphamide, with six proven or suspected cases of systemic fungal infection (including the three deaths) compared with no cases in the other group, but no significant difference in the hematological response rates between the groups. In addition, the durations of hospital stay, neutropenia, and antibacterial treatment were longer with cyclophosphamide. Based on these results, the authors concluded that cyclophosphamide should not be used in aplastic anemia.

General adverse effects

Common adverse effects observed at low doses of cyclophosphamide are similar to, but less frequent than, those observed in oncology patients. They include gastrointestinal disturbances (mostly nausea), hematological toxicity (mostly leukopenia), alopecia, and infectious complications (4,5).

Organs and Systems

Cardiovascular

Cardiac toxicity can be observed at high doses of cyclophosphamide (usually over 1.5 $g/m^2/day$), and acute myocardial necrosis or severe cardiac failure have been anecdotally reported after smaller dosages (SEDA-21, 386).

High-dose cyclophosphamide (120–200 mg/kg) can cause lethal cardiotoxicity, and severe congestive heart failure can develop 1–10 days after the first dose. Severe congestive heart failure is accompanied by electrocardiographic findings of diffuse voltage loss, cardiomegaly, pulmonary vascular congestion, and pleural and pericardial effusions. Pathological findings include hemorrhagic myocardial necrosis, thickening of the left ventricular wall, and fibrinous pericarditis.

Of 80 patients who received cyclophosphamide 50 mg/kg/day for 4 days in preparation for bone marrow grafting 17% had symptoms consistent with cyclophosphamide cardiotoxicity (6). Six died from congestive heart failure. Older patients were at greatest risk of developing cardiotoxicity.

In six patients who developed heart failure after high-dose conditioning therapy before stem cell transplantation, cyclophosphamide was suspected, despite the possible involvement of four drugs (7). The authors suggested monitoring high-risk patients.

Corrected QT dispersion was a predictor of acute heart failure after high-dose cyclophosphamide chemotherapy (5.6 g/m^2 over 4 days) in 19 patients (8).

Respiratory

Cyclophosphamide-induced pneumonitis has been described in 29 cases (9). Considering the widespread use of this drug over many years, this is a rare adverse effect. It does not clearly correlate with dosage (SED-8, 1112; SED-13, 1122). From a review of 12 case reports and a retrospective analysis of six other patients (including four with Wegener's granulomatosis), in whom cyclophosphamide was thought to be the only causative factor, two distinct clinical patterns of pneumonitis with different prognoses were identified (10). Early-onset pneumonitis ($n = 8$) occurred acutely within 1–8 months of treatment, and complete recovery was noted after cyclophosphamide withdrawal and prednisone treatment. In contrast, late-onset pneumonitis ($n = 10$) developed insidiously over several months (eventually after cyclophosphamide withdrawal) in patients maintained taking low daily doses for months to years. These patients had progressive pulmonary fibrosis unresponsive to glucocorticoid therapy, and six died of respiratory failure. Radiological pleural thickening may be an early sign of late-onset lung toxicity.

Nervous system

Progressive multifocal leukoencephalopathy is sometimes associated with Wegener's granulomatosis, but one case occurred in a patient who was taking low-dose cyclophosphamide, with subsequent significant improvement on withdrawal of the drug (SEDA-19, 347).

Sensory systems

Blurred vision is sometimes reported after high intravenous doses of cyclophosphamide, and there has been one report of transient myopia that recurred after each monthly intravenous pulse (11).

Endocrine

Even low-dose intravenous cyclophosphamide can cause a syndrome that resembles inappropriate secretion of antidiuretic hormone, with severe hyponatremia and symptoms of water intoxication (SEDA-19, 347) (SEDA-21, 386). A direct effect on the renal tubules is likely, but no other nephrotoxic effects have been documented.

Hematologic

Leukopenia, and less commonly thrombocytopenia or anemia, due to cyclophosphamide are typically dose-related in the therapeutic range. Cyclophosphamide-induced anemia has led to retinopathy presenting as striated hemorrhage of the retina (12).

Relative eosinophilia and increased interleukin-4 secretion were found in one study, suggesting that an immune deviation toward a type-2 T helper cell (Th2) response can occur (13). The clinical relevance of these findings as regards hypersensitivity reactions is unknown.

The idea that the degree of leukocyte suppression can be used to predict the success of adjuvant chemotherapy has been applied to combined treatment with

cyclophosphamide, methotrexate, and 5-fluorouracil for breast cancer; the lower the nadir leukocyte count, the greater the incidence of metastatic disease-free survival (14).

Mouth and teeth

Unilateral necrosis of the tongue has been attributed to cyclophosphamide (15).

- A 62-year-old woman with invasive ductal carcinoma of the breast was treated with epirubicin and cyclophosphamide. She rapidly developed swelling and necrosis of the tongue and consequent airway obstruction necessitating tracheostomy. After excision of the necrosis, the swelling of the tongue and the airway obstruction resolved.

Because of the temporal connection between the necrosis and the chemotherapy, the authors suspected an adverse effect, although they could not exclude a paraneoplastic pathogenesis.

Gastrointestinal

Nausea and vomiting are infrequent with daily low-dose cyclophosphamide (4).

Two-thirds of patients treated with cyclophosphamide orally for 4 months plus intravenous 5-fluorouracil and methotrexate for breast cancer developed Barrett's epithelium (16), perhaps as a result of esophagitis, rather than through mucosal re-epithelialization by undifferentiated stem cells (17).

Toxic megacolon occurred after five cycles of epirubicin 70 mg/m^2, 5-fluorouracil 500 mg/m^2, and oral cyclophosphamide 75 mg/m^2 for 14 days (18). The clinical presentation included a raised erythrocyte sedimentation rate and a colonic diameter of greater than 9 cm; the outcome can be fatal.

Liver

Cyclophosphamide-induced, dose-related liver damage is probably caused as a result of impaired clearance of its metabolite acrolein (19). This causes raised serum transaminases (20) and can be aggravated by prior exposure to azathioprine.

Acute reversible cytolytic or cholestatic jaundice can also occur after low-dose cyclophosphamide in adults and children (SED-13, 1122; SEDA-19, 347; SEDA-20, 342; SEDA-21, 386). Acute liver failure required liver transplantation in one patient (21). Although glucocorticoids were given concomitantly in most of these patients, no data are available to indicate a possibly increased hepatotoxic potential of this drug combination.

Hepatic veno-occlusive disease was attributed to low-dose cyclophosphamide in a 2-year-old child, and in repeated episodes of serum transaminase fluctuations in a patient with hepatitis C virus infection (SEDA-19, 347).

Late hepatotoxicity has also been reported with low-dose cyclophosphamide (22).

- A 67-year-old man with Sjögren's syndrome took cyclophosphamide for 2 years, a cumulative dose of 40.5 g. He then developed severe progressive jaundice due to acute hepatocellular injury. Gallstones and acute viral hepatitis were excluded, and only anti-smooth muscle antibodies were weakly positive. Liver histology showed marked ballooning of the hepatocytes and cell loss, cytoplasmic and canalicular cholestasis, and infiltration of the portal tract with inflammatory cells. Complete resolution occurred 6 weeks after cyclophosphamide withdrawal.

The authors emphasized this was the first case suggesting a cumulative hepatotoxic effect of low-dose cyclophosphamide. Previous rare cases of low-dose cyclophosphamide-induced acute hepatitis have usually occurred within the first 2 months.

Urinary tract

Hemorrhagic cystitis and bladder cancer are well-known complications of cyclophosphamide. The damage to the urinary bladder epithelium is caused by acrolein, a metabolite of cyclophosphamide that is excreted in the urine. In bone marrow transplant recipients, prior administration of busulfan, which itself causes hemorrhagic cystitis, can increase this risk (23). Mesna (2-mercaptoethane sodium sulfonate) is used to prevent this adverse effect. It is excreted by the kidney, and it binds and detoxifies acrolein in the urine; mesna also prevents the breakdown of acrolein precursors. Intravesical prostaglandin E_2 has been suggested as an alternative treatment (23).

The incidence of cystitis and/or dysuria was only 8% in 531 women with breast cancer who were given oral cyclophosphamide 60 mg/m^2/day for 1 year; the majority of cases were only grade 1 (24).

Upper renal tract disorders with ureteric reflux and bilateral hydronephrosis has been briefly reported in a patient with a history of cyclophosphamide-induced cystitis (SEDA-22, 410–411).

In 155 patients with Wegener's granulomatosis, of whom 142 took daily oral cyclophosphamide, the most frequent long-term cyclophosphamide-related adverse effects were cystitis despite mesna therapy (12%) and myelodysplasia (8%) (25). Patients who took a cumulative dose of over 100 g had a two-fold greater risk of cystitis and/or myelodysplasia than patients who took under 100 g. The authors emphasized that cyclophosphamide therapy should be as short as possible, with mesna and close surveillance in order to reduce treatment-associated morbidity.

Cyclophosphamide was thought to have favored the development of emphysematous cystitis in a 73-year-old man (26).

Skin

High doses of cyclophosphamide can cause the erythrodysesthesia syndrome, that is erythema of the hands and feet (27).

Stevens–Johnson syndrome developed in two patients, including one with positive rechallenge (SEDA-20, 342).

Five of thirty-two patients treated with the alternating drug regimen CAMBO-VIP (cyclophosphamide, doxorubicin, methotrexate, bleomycin, vincristine, etoposide, ifosfamide, and prednisolone) for non-Hodgkin's lymphoma developed blisters under the thickened skin of the palms and/or soles, followed by desquamation (28).

Discrete cutaneous hyperpigmentation occurred in two patients after high-dose chemotherapy with cyclophosphamide, etoposide, and carboplatin (29).

Hair

Alopecia occurs in patients taking cyclophosphamide, but it is less common and less severe in patients taking low doses. Mild to moderate alopecia was observed in 17% of patients with Wegener's granulomatosis (4).

Nails

Beau's lines (transverse ridging of the nails) developed after multiple drug therapy for Hodgkin's disease, including cyclophosphamide (30).

Reproductive system

In autoimmune diseases cyclophosphamide can cause menstrual disorders (oligomenorrhea or sustained amenorrhea) and ultimately sterility or premature menopause. This has been particularly exemplified in lupus erythematosus, and several studies have shown a high prevalence of menstrual disorders or premature ovarian failure in cyclophosphamide-treated patients, or a significantly higher incidence of both complications compared with other immunosuppressive regimens or healthy controls (31–33).

Of 17 adult men who had been treated before puberty for sarcoma with high-dose pulse cyclophosphamide (median dose 20.5 m/m^2) as part of regimens containing vincristine, dactinomycin, and cyclophosphamide, with or without doxorubicin, 10 had azoospermia, five had oligospermia, and only two had normal sperm counts (34). The authors concluded that a previous suggestion that puberty acts as a protection to infertility was not borne out and that the risk of infertility was proportional to the cumulative dose of cyclophosphamide.

Susceptibility factors have been investigated in a large retrospective study of 274 patients aged under 45 years, of whom 70 had received cyclophosphamide, 84 azathioprine but not cyclophosphamide, and 88 either no drug or hydroxychloroquine alone (35). The overall incidence of ovarian failure, defined as sustained amenorrhea for at least 12 months and documented by reduced estradiol concentrations, was 26, 1, and 0% respectively. The mean delay to onset of the first missed menses was 4.4 months. A higher age at the start of treatment and cumulative dose were independent risk factors for cyclophosphamide-induced ovarian failure. The incidences were 14, 28, and 50% in patients aged under 30 years, 30–39 years, and over 40 years respectively, and 4, 26, 31, 70%

for cumulative doses of under 10, 10–20, 20–30, and over 40 g, respectively.

Immunologic

Type I hypersensitivity

Anaphylactic reactions have very rarely occurred after intravenous cyclophosphamide (SED-8, 1126) (SEDA-17, 522) (36), and positive skin tests to the parent drug and/or 4-hydroxycyclophosphamide were found in several well-documented case reports (SEDA-19, 347). Although other mechanisms could be considered, a possible IgE antibody-mediated reaction was substantiated by the positivity of immediate skin tests to cyclophosphamide metabolites in five patients, and the recurrence of symptoms following intravenous or oral rechallenge in several of them (37).

Cyclophosphamide reportedly caused a type I hypersensitivity reaction in a patient with systemic lupus erythematosus (38).

- A 17-year-old Chinese girl with systemic lupus erythematosus developed acute angioedema over the neck, chest, and larynx, and required mechanical ventilation. She had received two previous courses of cyclophosphamide without incident. She developed urticaria 30 minutes after an infusion of cyclophosphamide, without angioedema, stridor, wheezing, or hypotension. Skin prick testing with cyclophosphamide was negative. Four weeks later, 15 minutes after the start of an infusion of cyclophosphamide, she developed generalized urticaria. Further infusions were given with diphenhydramine premedication.

In the absence of drug-induced angioedema or anaphylaxis, monthly therapy with cyclophosphamide can be continued with antihistamine premedication in patients who have allergic reactions.

Infection risk

Owing to its effects on cellular and humoral immune responses, and independently of leukopenia, cyclophosphamide can induce more frequent and more severe infectious complications (SED-13, 1123) (SEDA-20, 343). Older age and total cumulative dose are possible susceptibility factors for severe infectious episodes. More specifically, an increased risk of severe, life-threatening *Pneumocystis jiroveci* pneumonia has been identified, particularly in patients with lymphopenia (39,40). There was also a 10- to 20-fold increase in *Herpes zoster* infections (41,42). Fatal aspergillosis and disseminated cryptococcosis have been sometimes reported (SEDA-20, 343) (43). Infections were mostly reported in patients who were also taking glucocorticoids, and a synergistic effect with glucocorticoids is likely to be relevant in causation (41,44); all the same, there is direct evidence that cyclophosphamide itself is involved. Its role was investigated in a retrospective study of 100 patients with systemic lupus erythematosus: 45% developed serious bacterial infections (58%), opportunistic infections (24%), or *H. zoster* infections (18%), compared with 12% in 43 patients taking high-dose glucocorticoids alone (45). Infections were

more frequent with sequential intravenous and oral cyclophosphamide (68%) than with intravenous cyclophosphamide (39%) or oral cyclophosphamide (40%), and leukopenia was an additional risk factor. Other investigators have similarly adduced evidence of more frequent infections, particularly *P. jiroveci* pneumonia, in patients receiving cyclophosphamide plus glucocorticoids daily rather than alternate-day glucocorticoids (41).

- A 72-year-old man with autoimmune thrombocytopenia had taken prednisone (30 mg/day) for 1 year, when he was found to have systemic lupus erythematosus (46). Prednisone was continued and he started to take chloroquine (250 mg/day) and monthly cyclophosphamide (0.75 g/m^2). Three weeks after the first bolus of cyclophosphamide, he complained of fever and dyspnea, and chest X-rays showed bilateral pulmonary infiltrates. Despite prompt medical management, he died 5 days after admission with cytomegalovirus-induced interstitial pneumonia.

In addition to cyclophosphamide, this patient had several susceptibility factors for fatal infection, namely age (older than 50 years) and a low leukocyte nadir (2900 × 10^6/l) after treatment with cyclophosphamide and prednisone.

Long-Term Effects

Tumorigenicity

Although tumor induction has mostly been documented in patients treated for cancer, long-term cyclophosphamide treatment for non-neoplastic conditions can also increase the incidence of certain neoplasms. Whether this oncogenic effect is a consequence of drug-induced chromosomal aberrations rather than immunosuppression is unclear. An increased incidence of bladder cancers, skin cancers, and myeloproliferative disorders was found in a 20-year follow-up study of 119 patients with rheumatoid arthritis, and a high dose of cyclophosphamide (mean total dose of 80 g) was the main susceptibility factor (47).

In another study in patients with Wegener's granulomatosis there was an 11-fold increase in the incidence of lymphomas compared with the general population (41). In contrast, previous exposure to cyclophosphamide did not appear to be associated with a significantly higher risk of cancer in patients with systemic lupus erythematosus, but the number of cases was very low (48).

Myelodysplastic syndromes

Cyclophosphamide can cause myelodysplastic syndromes, particularly after prolonged treatment. The type of myelodysplastic syndromes and cytogenetic abnormalities that developed after treatment with alkylating agents for rheumatic diseases have been described in eight patients (mean age 57 years), of whom seven had taken oral cyclophosphamide and one chlorambucil (49). The mean cumulative dose of cyclophosphamide was 118 g for a mean cumulative duration of 4.4 years, and the myelodysplastic syndrome was diagnosed 0–4 years (mean 2.4 years) after the end of treatment. Concomitant immunosuppressive drugs were given in four of seven cyclophosphamide-treated patients. Cytogenetic abnormalities of chromosome 5 and/or 7, which are characteristic of treatment-related myelodysplastic syndromes, were found in all patients. Only two patients were still alive at the time of the report, and the outcome was remarkably poor in patients with chromosome 5 deletion. This study suggested that a high cumulative dose of cyclophosphamide is a risk factor for hematological malignancies, and that patients require long-term surveillance.

Urinary tract tumors

Squamous cell carcinoma of the bladder has been reported 4 years after pulsed cyclophosphamide therapy (50). However, the authors noted that other susceptibility factors, such as bladder diverticula and human papilloma virus infection, occurred in the intervening period and they speculated on the cumulative risk.

- A 72-year old woman who received 1400 mg cyclophosphamide over 2 weeks for Wegener's granulomatosis had gross hematuria and dysuria (51). Cystoscopy was normal, but there was marked irregularity of the mucosa of the upper ureteric mucosa, the renal pelvis, and the renal calyces on retrograde ureteropyelography. Nephroscopy showed a gray necrotic uroepithelium with dystrophic calcification.

The risk of bladder cancer persists for as long as 20 years after cyclophosphamide withdrawal. In a retrospective analysis, half of the 145 patients on long-term treatment for Wegener's granulomatosis had microscopic or gross hematuria, among whom 70% had cystoscopic features compatible with cyclophosphamide-induced bladder injury (52). Seven patients (5%) developed bladder cancer, a 31-fold higher incidence than in the general population. As previous episodes of hematuria were found in all seven patients and the drug was the only significant risk factor for bladder cancer, prompt cystoscopy should be done in any patient who develops gross hematuria, even after treatment withdrawal. Another study showed an excess in the incidence of bladder cancer in patients with multiple sclerosis who received cyclophosphamide and who also had an indwelling catheter (53).

Renal adenocarcinoma has been reported in a 50-year-old man after 3 years of cyclophosphamide treatment for hepatic sarcoidosis (54).

Other tumors

It has been suggested that cyclophosphamide can contribute to the risk of cervical dysplasia. In a retrospective study of 110 patients with systemic lupus erythematosus, cervical dysplasia was significantly more frequent in patients who had received intravenous cyclophosphamide (10 of 61) than in a control group who did not receive cyclophosphamide (two of 49) (55). In addition, cervical pathology worsened during cyclophosphamide therapy in all four patients with pre-existing cervical dysplasia, and one patient developed in situ cervical carcinoma.

- A 54-year-old man with polyarteritis nodosa developed hepatic angiosarcoma after taking cyclophosphamide for 13 years (56). Although this may have been coincidental, the authors found two other published reports of this very rare tumor in patients taking long-term cyclophosphamide.

To determine the frequency and types of malignancies that occur in children with end-stage renal insufficiency who required renal replacement therapy, data from 249 patients were analysed retrospectively (57). There were 22 malignancies in 21 patients; skin cancers accounted for 59% and non-Hodgkin's lymphomas for 23%. At 25 years after first renal replacement therapy, the probability of developing a malignancy was 17%. The incidence of cancers overall was 10-fold higher than in the general population. For cancers other than melanoma and non-Hodgkin's lymphoma, the standardized risks were 222 and 46 respectively. The use of more than 20 mg/kg cyclophosphamide was associated with an increased risk of malignancy. Six patients died as a result of their malignancy, accounting for 9.5% of overall mortality. The long-term risk of certain malignancies is significantly increased in children who have undergone renal replacement therapy, especially after treatment with cyclophosphamide.

Second-Generation Effects

Fertility

Cyclophosphamide, or testicular and cranial irradiation, in the treatment of childhood malignancies can lead to small testicular size and decreased sperm production in adulthood (58). Of 17 adult male survivors of childhood sarcomas treated before puberty with high-dose cyclophosphamide, only two had normal sperm counts, 10 had azoospermia, and five had oligospermia (34). The two patients with normal sperm counts had taken the lowest doses of cyclophosphamide.

Gonadal toxicity has been documented in both men and women receiving cyclophosphamide (4). In men, the incidence of transient or permanent oligospermia/azoospermia is 50–90%, and in prepubertal patients spermatogenesis will more readily return to normal than adults. In one study, testosterone prophylaxis given at the same time as cyclophosphamide reduced the incidence of disorders of spermatogenesis and accelerated spermatogenesis recovery after cyclophosphamide discontinuation, but few patients were evaluable (59).

Of 23 men treated with either cyclophosphamide or non-alkylating agent combinations, there was a dose-related disturbance of gonadotrophin secretion in the cyclophosphamide group (60). The chances of maintaining normal gonadal function after combined treatment of Hodgkin's disease are significantly greater among girls than boys at 9-year follow-up (61). Pre- and post-pubescent boys were affected by six cycles of MOPP, whether or not pelvic radiation was administered; on the other hand, in girls similarly treated, ovarian function was directly affected by the number of courses of chemotherapy and the ovarian radiation dose (62). In a study of male gonadal function at 9 years follow-up after regimens containing cyclophosphamide, mechlorethamine, vincristine, or procarbazine, there was azoospermia, whereas regimens containing dactinomycin and vinblastine did not have a toxic effect on spermatogenesis (63). Testicular volume and sperm count in 18 patients, 1–3 years after chemotherapy, showed that all those who had received chemotherapy that did not include cisplatin had normal testicular size and sperm counts, whereas of seven who had received cisplatin, six had small testes and azoospermia and one was oligozoospermic with normal-sized testes (64).

The risk of ovarian failure and infertility has been studied in 84 women with an underlying inflammatory disease receiving intravenous cyclophosphamide (65). The incidence of sustained amenorrhea was 22% and was independent of the underlying inflammatory disease. After treatment with cyclophosphamide following bone marrow transplantation, ovarian function can occasionally recover, resulting in a successful pregnancy up to 7 years after treatment (66). No specific factors correlated with recovery of normal ovarian function. However, recovery was rare if the patient had undergone concurrent total body irradiation (67).

Pregnancy

Cyclophosphamide crosses the placenta and reaches an amniotic fluid concentration of 25%. Six pregnancies occurred in women taking cyclophosphamide; three had induced abortions, one had a spontaneous abortion, and two had normal pregnancies. After withdrawal of cyclophosphamide, 16 women became pregnant; three had induced abortions for severe morphological anomalies, three had spontaneous miscarriages, and 10 delivered healthy infants. Contraception during intravenous cyclophosphamide therapy is recommended, and after withdrawal, pregnancy is possible, with a favourable outcome in two-thirds of cases.

Teratogenicity

The FDA has classified cyclophosphamide as a pregnancy risk factor D drug: it is teratogenic in animals, but population studies have not conclusively shown teratogenicity in humans. However, in a study of in utero first-trimester exposure to four doses of cyclophosphamide 20 mg/kg it was concluded that cyclophosphamide is a human teratogen, that there is a distinct embryopathic phenotype, and that there are serious doubts about the safety of cyclophosphamide in pregnancy (68). The congenital malformation rate has been estimated at 10–44% (69).

Reported congenital abnormalities are many and include facial and palate defects, skin and skeletal anomalies, and visceral malformations. Based on one case and a review of six previous reports of malformations after in utero exposure to cyclophosphamide in the first trimester, a distinct embryopathy due to cyclophosphamide has been suggested (68). The proposed phenotype included growth deficiency, developmental delay, craniosynostosis,

blepharophimosis, flat nasal bridge, abnormal ears, and distal limb defects; chromosomes were normal.

In one case of first-trimester exposure to cyclophosphamide in a woman pregnant with twins, the male twin was born with multiple congenital abnormalities and developed papillary thyroid cancer at 11 years of age and stage III neuroblastoma at 14 years of age; the female twin was unaffected (70).

Most cases have been reported in patients with cancer who were also exposed to other antineoplastic drugs or to irradiation. The potential for congenital abnormalities in the offspring of men treated with cyclophosphamide is yet unknown.

Fetotoxicity

The effects of second- or third-trimester exposure to cyclophosphamide are poorly documented, although normal children have been described (71). However, in other cases growth retardation and neutropenia have been reported (72).

Drug Administration

Drug dosage regimens

In inflammatory or autoimmune diseases, both daily oral and cyclic pulse intravenous cyclophosphamide regimens are used, but it is unclear whether one route of administration should be preferred to another. The cumulative dose obtained in those given an intravenous pulse regimen is consistently lower than in those given daily oral administration, and the incidence of bladder cancer or infection is expected to be lower in the former. However, the choice of the maintenance regimen remains a dilemma as regards efficacy and toxicity (73). For example, in one study in 50 patients with Wegener's granulomatosis there was a similar overall incidence of adverse effects in patients treated with prednisone plus oral cyclophosphamide compared with those who received prednisone plus intravenous pulse cyclophosphamide (74). Patients in the oral group had a higher incidence of severe or fatal infectious complications, but a lower incidence of cumulative relapse rates at 4.5 years.

In 47 patients intravenous pulsed cyclophosphamide was as effective as daily oral cyclophosphamide, but caused fewer adverse effects (75). The patients were randomized to receive monthly intravenous pulses of cyclophosphamide (0.75 g/m^2, $n = 22$) or daily oral cyclophosphamide (2 mg/kg/day, $n = 25$) for at least 1 year. Both groups received glucocorticoids. Whereas efficacy end-points did not show significant differences between the two groups, leukopenia (18 versus 60%) and severe infections (14% with no deaths versus 40% with three deaths) were significantly less frequent with intravenous pulsed cyclophosphamide. As a result, the probability of freedom from adverse effects (no deaths, severe infections, leukopenia, or thrombocytopenia) over a 12-month period was only about 25% in the oral group, compared with 70% in the intravenous group. In addition, and based on the findings of a significantly lower serum follicle-stimulating hormone concentration at 3 and 6 months and a 57% reduction in the total dose in the intravenous pulse group, the intravenous pulse regimen was expected to produce fewer adverse gonadal effects and a reduced risk of malignancies.

Drug–Drug Interactions

Amiodarone

Both amiodarone and cyclophosphamide can cause lung damage.

- Interstitial pneumonitis has been reported in a 59-year-old man, who had taken amiodarone for 18 months, 18 days after a single dose of cyclophosphamide; 1 year before he had also received six cycles of chemotherapy containing cyclophosphamide, vincristine, and prednisone, followed by four cycles of cisplatin, cytarabine, and dexamethasone (253).

The authors suggested that the lung damage had been due to the cyclophosphamide, enhanced by the presence of amiodarone, but in view of the fact that previous similar exposure on six occasions had not resulted in the same effect, it is perhaps more likely that this was a long-term adverse effect of amiodarone alone. The presence of foamy histiocytes in the lung biopsy was consistent with this interpretation (SEDA-15, 168). It is true, however, that lung damage due to amiodarone is usually of a more insidious onset than was reported in this case, although a more rapid onset can occur in patients who are given high concentrations of inspired oxygen. On the other hand, lung damage has occasionally been reported to occur rapidly (71).

Busulfan

In bone marrow transplant recipients, prior administration of busulfan, which itself causes hemorrhagic cystitis, can increase the risk of cyclophosphamide-induced damage (79).

Busulfan reduces the clearance of cyclophosphamide to its active metabolite 4-hydroperoxycyclophosphamide (80). The first dose of high-dose cyclophosphamide should therefore be delayed for at least 24 hours after the last dose of busulfan.

Chloramphenicol

Chloramphenicol inhibits the biotransformation of cyclophosphamide(81).

Cisplatin

A 4-year follow-up of comparison of a combination of cyclophosphamide with either 50 mg/m^2 or 100 mg/m^2 of cisplatin in ovarian cancer has been reported (76). Peripheral neuropathy was dose-limiting and persistent. Ten of thirty-one patients had significant toxicity in the high-dose group compared with one of 24 in the low-dose group.

Corticosteroids—glucocorticoids

The effect of prednisone 1 mg/kg on the pharmacokinetics of cyclophosphamide and its initial metabolites 4-hydroxycyclophosphamide and aldophosphamide (the acyclic tautomer of 4-hydroxycyclophosphamide) has been studied between the first and sixth cycles in seven patients (two men) with systemic vasculitis receiving intravenous cyclophosphamide 0.6 g/m2 as a 1-hour intravenous infusion every 3 weeks for six cycles (82). Prednisone reduced the clearance of cyclophosphamide from 5.8 to 4.0 l/hour, reducing the amount of initial metabolites formed. Although the clinical significance of this interaction is unclear, 4-hydroxycyclophosphamide and aldophosphamide are probably responsible for the cytotoxic activity of cyclophosphamide, and increased cyclophosphamide dosages should be considered in patients taking prednisone.

Fluconazole

Cyclophosphamide is a prodrug that requires cytochrome P_{450}-dependent hepatic activation to produce alkylating species and several inactive by-products. However, very few metabolic interactions involving cyclophosphamide have been reported. In a retrospective study of 22 children treated with cyclophosphamide for cancer or bone marrow transplantation, cyclophosphamide clearance was significantly lower in nine patients taking fluconazole compared with 13 patients not taking it (77). In vitro studies in human liver microsomes confirmed that the rate of 4-hydroxylation of cyclophosphamide was inhibited by fluconazole.

Cyclophosphamide is a prodrug that is metabolized by CYP450 enzymes to produce alkylating species, which are cytotoxic, and the extent of cyclophosphamide metabolism correlates with both treatment efficacy and toxicity. In vitro studies in six human liver microsomes showed that the IC50 of fluconazole for reduction of 4-hydroxy-cyclophosphamide production was 980 mmol/l (83).

A retrospective study in 22 children with cancers addressed the potential interaction between fluconazole and cyclophosphamide. Children with an established profile of cyclophosphamide metabolism who were not receiving other drugs known to affect drug metabolism were selected; 9 were taking fluconazole and 13 were controls. The plasma clearance was significantly lower in patients taking concomitant fluconazole (2.4 versus 4.2 l/hour/m2). It is unclear whether this interaction is associated with a reduction in the therapeutic efficacy of cyclophosphamide.

Indometacin

Synergy between indometacin and cyclophosphamide has been advanced as the cause of a life-threatening acute water intoxication and severe hyponatremia observed in a patient with multiple myeloma and normal renal function (SEDA-15, 99).

Interferon alfa

Depending on the timing of exposure, interferon alfa may adversely affect the pharmacokinetic and hematological effects of cyclophosphamide. In 10 patients with multiple myeloma, interferon alfa given 2 hours before cyclophosphamide infusion significantly reduced cyclophosphamide clearance and produced less exposure to its metabolite 4-hydroxycyclophosphamide compared with interferon administration 24 hours after cyclophosphamide (84). This resulted in a significantly greater fall in white blood cell count in patients who received interferon alfa after cyclophosphamide.

Phenytoin and fosphenytoin

In three patients treated with cyclophosphamide, phenytoin co-medication increased the formation of the S-enantiomer (but not the R-enantiomer) of the dechloroethylated cyclophosphamide metabolite (85). The findings also suggested that phenytoin increased the clearance of both R- and S-cyclophosphamide to 4-hydroxycyclophosphamide (the activation pathway). The clinical relevance of these findings is unclear.

Prednisolone

Daily prednisolone significantly reduced the total clearance of cyclophosphamide and the peak concentration and AUC of 4-hydroxycyclophosphamide (78). It is not known whether this interaction has clinical consequences.

Management of adverse drug reactions

Mesna is used to prevent or ameliorate hemorrhagic cystitis produced by the anticancer drugs cyclophosphamide and ifosfamide. It is excreted by the kidney and binds and detoxifies acrolein in the urine; mesna also prevents the breakdown of acrolein precursors. It is also used as a mucolytic.

Endotracheal instillation of mesna was compared with instillation of saline in mechanically ventilated patients. Following instillation of mesna, there was a significant increase in maximal airway resistance and impairment of oxygenation with a slight increase in $PaCO_2$ (SEDA-20, 183). A single episode of bronchorrhea occurred 10 minutes after the instillation of mesna.

In a randomized, crossover study, 25 volunteers received single doses of intravenous mesna and four different formulations of oral mesna (86). One subject withdrew from the study because of ocular inflammation followed by loss of appetite, nausea, and vomiting. Another developed a rash during the period in which three of his four oral doses were given. Two further subjects developed loose stools after one of the oral doses. Another reported dizziness after an oral dose. One reported pain at the site of the intravenous infusion. The adverse effects were all considered to be mild or moderate and resolved spontaneously without treatment.

Bronchorrhea due to inhaled mesna may be the result of mucolysis, but could also be caused by stimulation of bronchial secretions. Application by aerosol or nebulizer is occasionally followed by bronchospasm, but mesna is usually well tolerated by people with asthma (SEDA-20, 183).

Platinum agents are now combined with ifosfamide in the treatment of cancer. The possibility that mesna may interfere with the anticancer effects of platinum has been investigated using cultured malignant glioma cells (87). Mesna protected tumor cell lines from the cytotoxic effect of the platinum agents. This in vitro study emphasizes the importance of specifying in detail the infusion schedules of mesna and platinum agents.

References

1. Fraiser LH, Kanekal S, Kehrer JP. Cyclophosphamide toxicity. Characterising and avoiding the problem. Drugs 1991;42(5):781–95.
2. Zisman DA, Lynch JP 3rd, Toews GB, Kazerooni EA, Flint A, Martinez FJ. Cyclophosphamide in the treatment of idiopathic pulmonary fibrosis: a prospective study in patients who failed to respond to corticosteroids. Chest 2000;117(6):1619–26.
3. Tisdale JF, Dunn DE, Geller N, Plante M, Nunez O, Dunbar CE, Barrett AJ, Walsh TJ, Rosenfeld SJ, Young NS. High-dose cyclophosphamide in severe aplastic anaemia: a randomised trial. Lancet 2000;356(9241):1554–9.
4. Langford CA. Complications of cyclophosphamide therapy. Eur Arch Otorhinolaryngol 1997;254(2):65–72.
5. Omdal R, Husby G, Koldingsnes W. Intravenous and oral cyclophosphamide pulse therapy in rheumatic diseases: side effects and complications. Clin Exp Rheumatol 1993;11(3):283–8.
6. Goldberg MA, Antin JH, Guinan EC, Rappeport JM. Cyclophosphamide cardiotoxicity: an analysis of dosing as a risk factor. Blood 1986;68(5):1114–8.
7. Mugitani A, Yamane T, Park K, Im T, Tatsumi N, Tatsumi Y. Cardiac complications after high-dose chemotherapy with peripheral blood stem cell transplantation. J Jpn Soc Cancer Ther 1996;31:255–62.
8. Nakamae H, Tsumura K, Hino M, Hayashi T, Tatsumi N. QT dispersion as a predictor of acute heart failure after high-dose cyclophosphamide. Lancet 2000;355(9206):805–6.
9. Glatt E, Henke M, Sigmund G, Costabel U. Cyclophosphamid-induzierte Pneumonitis. [Cyclophosphamide-induced pneumonitis.] Rofo 1988;148(5):545–9.
10. Malik SW, Myers JL, DeRemee RA, Specks U. Lung toxicity associated with cyclophosphamide use. Two distinct patterns. Am J Respir Crit Care Med 1996;154(6 Pt 1):1851–6.
11. Arranz JA, Jimenez R, Alvarez-Mon M. Cyclophosphamide-induced myopia. Ann Intern Med 1992;116(1):92–3.
12. Kadoya K, Suda Y, Tonaki M, et al. Two cases of anemic retinopathy. Folia Ophthalmol Jpn 1989;40:148.
13. Smith DR, Balashov KE, Hafler DA, Khoury SJ, Weiner HL. Immune deviation following pulse cyclophosphamide/methylprednisolone treatment of multiple sclerosis: increased interleukin-4 production and associated eosinophilia. Ann Neurol 1997;42(3):313–8.
14. Poikonen P, Saarto T, Lundin J, Joensuu H, Blomqvist C. Leucocyte nadir as a marker for chemotherapy efficacy in node-positive breast cancer treated with adjuvant CMF. Br J Cancer 1999;80(11):1763–6.
15. Buch RS, Schmidt M, Reichert TE. Akute Nekrose der Zunge unter Epirubicin-Cyclophosphamid-Therapie bei einem invasiv duktalen Mammakarzinom. [Acute tongue necrosis provoked by epirubicin–cyclophosphamide

treatment for invasive ductal breast cancer.] Mund Kiefer Gesichtschir 2003;7(3):175–9.

16. Spechler S. Columnar-lined (Barrett's) esophagus. Curr Opin Gastroenterol 1991;7:557–61.

17. Mullai N, Sivarajan KM, Shiomoto G. Barrett esophagus. Ann Intern Med 1991;114(10):913.

18. de Gara CJ, Gagic N, Arnold A, Seaton T. Toxic megacolon associated with anticancer chemotherapy. Can J Surg 1991;34(4):339–41.

19. Honjo I, Suou T, Hirayama C. Hepatotoxicity of cyclophosphamide in man: pharmacokinetic analysis. Res Commun Chem Pathol Pharmacol 1988;61(2):149–65.

20. Shaunak S, Munro JM, Weinbren K, Walport MJ, Cox TM. Cyclophosphamide-induced liver necrosis: a possible interaction with azathioprine. Q J Med 1988;67(252):309–17.

21. Gustafsson LL, Eriksson LS, Dahl ML, Eleborg L, Ericzon BG, Nyberg A. Cyclophosphamide-induced acute liver failure requiring transplantation in a patient with genetically deficient debrisoquine metabolism: a causal relationship? J Intern Med 1996;240(5):311–4.

22. Mok CC, Wong WM, Shek TW, Ho CT, Lau CS, Lai CL. Cumulative hepatotoxicity induced by continuous low-dose cyclophosphamide therapy. Am J Gastroenterol 2000;95(3):845–6.

23. Thomas AE, Patterson J, Prentice HG, Brenner MK, Ganczakowski M, Hancock JF, Pattinson JK, Blacklock HA, Hopewell JP. Haemorrhagic cystitis in bone marrow transplantation patients: possible increased risk associated with prior busulphan therapy. Bone Marrow Transplant 1987;1(4):347–55.

24. Budd GT, Green S, O'Bryan RM, Martino S, Abeloff MD, Rinehart JJ, Hahn R, Harris J, Tormey D, O'Sullivan J, et al. Short-course FAC-M versus 1 year of CMFVP in node-positive, hormone receptor-negative breast cancer: an intergroup study. J Clin Oncol 1995;13(4):831–9.

25. Reinhold-Keller E, Beuge N, Latza U, de Groot K, Rudert H, Nolle B, Heller M, Gross WL. An interdisciplinary approach to the care of patients with Wegener's granulomatosis: long-term outcome in 155 patients. Arthritis Rheum 2000;43(5):1021–32.

26. Abuzarad H, Gadallah MF, Rabb H, Vermess M, Ramirez G. Emphysematous cystitis: possible side-effect of cyclophosphamide therapy. Clin Nephrol 1998;50(6):394–6.

27. Matsuyama JR, Kwok KK. A variant of the chemotherapy-associated erythrodysesthesia syndrome related to high-dose cyclophosphamide. DICP 1989;23(10):776778–9.

28. Hirano M, Okamoto M, Maruyama F, Ezaki K, Shimizu K, Ino T, Matsui T, Sobue R, Shinkai K, Miyazaki H, et al. Alternating non-cross-resistant chemotherapy for non-Hodgkin's lymphoma of intermediate-grade and high-grade malignancy. A pilot study. Cancer 1992;69(3):772–7.

29. Singal R, Tunnessen WW Jr, Wiley JM, Hood AF. Discrete pigmentation after chemotherapy. Pediatr Dermatol 1991;8(3):231–5.

30. Requena L. Chemotherapy-induced transverse ridging of the nails. Cutis 1991;48(2):129–30.

31. Wang CL, Wang F, Bosco JJ. Ovarian failure in oral cyclophosphamide treatment for systemic lupus erythematosus. Lupus 1995;4(1):11–4.

32. Gonzalez-Crespo MR, Gomez-Reino JJ, Merino R, Ciruelo E, Gomez-Reino FJ, Muley R, Garcia-Consuegra J, Pinillos V, Rodriguez-Valverde V. Menstrual disorders in girls with systemic lupus erythematosus treated with cyclophosphamide. Br J Rheumatol 1995;34(8):737–41.

33. McDermott EM, Powell RJ. Incidence of ovarian failure in systemic lupus erythematosus after treatment with pulse cyclophosphamide. Ann Rheum Dis 1996;55(4):224–9.

34. Kenney LB, Laufer MR, Grant FD, Grier H, Diller L. High risk of infertility and long term gonadal damage in males treated with high dose cyclophosphamide for sarcoma during childhood. Cancer 2001;91(3):613–21.

35. Mok CC, Lau CS, Wong RW. Risk factors for ovarian failure in patients with systemic lupus erythematosus receiving cyclophosphamide therapy. Arthritis Rheum 1998;41(5):831–7.

36. Salles G, Vial T, Archimbaud E. Anaphylactoid reaction with bronchospasm following intravenous cyclophosphamide administration. Ann Hematol 1991;62(2–3):74–5.

37. Popescu N, Sheehan M, Kouides P, Loughner JE, Condemi JJ, Looney RJ, Leddy JP. Allergic reactions to cyclophosphamide: delayed clinical expression associated with positive immediate skin tests to drug metabolites in five patients. J Allerg Clin Immunol 1995;95:288.

38. Thong BY, Leong KP, Thumboo J, Koh ET, Tang CY. Cyclophosphamide type I hypersensitivity in systemic lupus erythematosus. Lupus 2002;11(2):127–9.

39. Jarrousse B, Guillevin L, Bindi P, Hachulla E, Leclerc P, Gilson B, Remy P, Rossert J, Jacquot C, Gilson B. Increased risk of *Pneumocystis carinii* pneumonia in patients with Wegener's granulomatosis. Clin Exp Rheumatol 1993;11(6):615–21.

40. Porges AJ, Beattie SL, Ritchlin C, Kimberly RP, Christian CL. Patients with systemic lupus erythematosus at risk for *Pneumocystis carinii* pneumonia. J Rheumatol 1992;19(8):1191–4.

41. Hoffman GS, Kerr GS, Leavitt RY, Hallahan CW, Lebovics RS, Travis WD, Rottem M, Fauci AS. Wegener granulomatosis: an analysis of 158 patients. Ann Intern Med 1992;116(6):488–98.

42. Kahl LE. *Herpes zoster* infections in systemic lupus erythematosus: risk factors and outcome. J Rheumatol 1994;21(1):84–6.

43. Kattwinkel N, Cook L, Agnello V. Overwhelming fatal infection in a young woman after intravenous cyclophosphamide therapy for lupus nephritis. J Rheumatol 1991;18(1):79–81.

44. Bradley JD, Brandt KD, Katz BP. Infectious complications of cyclophosphamide treatment for vasculitis. Arthritis Rheum 1989;32(1):45–53.

45. Pryor BD, Bologna SG, Kahl LE. Risk factors for serious infection during treatment with cyclophosphamide and high-dose corticosteroids for systemic lupus erythematosus. Arthritis Rheum 1996;39(9):1475–82.

46. Garcia-Porrua C, Gonzalez-Gay MA, Perez de Llano LA, Alvarez-Ferreira J. Fatal interstitial pneumonia due to cytomegalovirus following cyclophosphamide treatment in a patient with systemic lupus erythematosus. Scand J Rheumatol 1998;27(6):465–6.

47. Radis C, Kwoh C, Morgan M, et al. Risk of malignancy in cyclophosphamide treated patients with rheumatoid arthritis: a 20-year follow-up study. Arthr Rheum 1993;36(Suppl):R19.

48. Pettersson T, Pukkala E, Teppo L, Friman C. Increased risk of cancer in patients with systemic lupus erythematosus. Ann Rheum Dis 1992;51(4):437–9.

49. McCarthy CJ, Sheldon S, Ross CW, McCune WJ. Cytogenetic abnormalities and therapy-related myelodysplastic syndromes in rheumatic disease. Arthritis Rheum 1998;41(8):1493–6.

50. Wang JS, Hsieh SP, Jiaan BP, Tseng HH. Human papillomavirus in cyclophosphamide and diverticulum-associated squamous cell carcinoma of urinary bladder: a case report. Zhonghua Yi Xue Za Zhi (Taipei) 1996;57(4):305–9.

51. Aviles RJ, Vlahakis SA, Elkin PL. Cyclophosphamide-associated uroepithelial toxicity. Ann Intern Med 1999;131(7):549.

52. Talar-Williams C, Hijazi YM, Walther MM, Linehan WM, Hallahan CW, Lubensky I, Kerr GS, Hoffman GS, Fauci AS, Sneller MC. Cyclophosphamide-induced cystitis and bladder cancer in patients with Wegener granulomatosis. Ann Intern Med 1996;124(5):477–84.

53. De Ridder D, van Poppel H, Demonty L, D'Hooghe B, Gonsette R, Carton H, Baert L. Bladder cancer in patients with multiple sclerosis treated with cyclophosphamide. J Urol 1998;159(6):1881–4.

54. Das D, Smith A, Warnes TW. Hepatic sarcoidosis and renal carcinoma. J Clin Gastroenterol 1999;28(1):61–3.

55. Bateman H, Yazici Y, Leff L, Peterson M, Paget SA. Increased cervical dysplasia in intravenous cyclophosphamide-treated patients with SLE: a preliminary study. Lupus 2000;9(7):542–4.

56. Rosenthal AK, Klausmeier M, Cronin ME, McLaughlin JK. Hepatic angiosarcoma occurring after cyclophosphamide therapy: case report and review of the literature. Am J Clin Oncol 2000;23(6):581–3.

57. Coutinho HM, Groothoff JW, Offringa M, Gruppen MP, Heymans HS. De novo malignancy after paediatric renal replacement therapy. Arch Dis Child 2001;85(6):478–83.

58. Siimes MA, Rautonen J. Small testicles with impaired production of sperm in adult male survivors of childhood malignancies. Cancer 1990;65(6):1303–6.

59. Masala A, Faedda R, Alagna S, Satta A, Chiarelli G, Rovasio PP, Ivaldi R, Taras MS, Lai E, Bartoli E. Use of testosterone to prevent cyclophosphamide-induced azoospermia. Ann Intern Med 1997;126(4):292–5.

60. Hoorweg-Nijman JJ, Delemarre-van de Waal HA, de Waal FC, Behrendt H. Cyclophosphamide-induced disturbance of gonadotropin secretion manifesting testicular damage. Acta Endocrinol (Copenh) 1992;126(2):143–8.

61. Jackson DV Jr, Craig JB, Spurr CL, White DR, Muss HB, Cruz JM, Richards F, Powell BL. Vincristine infusion in CHOP-CCNU in diffuse large-cell lymphoma. Cancer Invest 1990;8(1):7–12.

62. Ortin TT, Shostak CA, Donaldson SS. Gonadal status and reproductive function following treatment for Hodgkin's disease in childhood: the Stanford experience. Int J Radiat Oncol Biol Phys 1990;19(4):873–80.

63. Aubier F, Flamant F, Brauner R, Caillaud JM, Chaussain JM, Lemerle J. Male gonadal function after chemotherapy for solid tumors in childhood. J Clin Oncol 1989;7(3):304–9.

64. Siimes MA, Elomaa I, Koskimies A. Testicular function after chemotherapy for osteosarcoma. Eur J Cancer 1990;26(9):973–5.

65. Huong du L, Amoura Z, Duhaut P, Sbai A, Costedoat N, Wechsler B, Piette JC. Risk of ovarian failure and fertility after intravenous cyclophosphamide. A study in 84 patients. J Rheumatol 2002;29(12):2571–6.

66. Sanders JE, Buckner CD, Amos D, Levy W, Appelbaum FR, Doney K, Storb R, Sullivan KM, Witherspoon RP, Thomas ED. Ovarian function following marrow transplantation for aplastic anemia or leukemia. J Clin Oncol 1988;6(5):813–8.

67. Gradishar WJ, Schilsky RL. Effects of cancer treatment on the reproductive system. Crit Rev Oncol Hematol 1988;8(2):153–71.

68. Enns GM, Roeder E, Chan RT, Ali-Khan Catts Z, Cox VA, Golabi M. Apparent cyclophosphamide (Cytoxan) embryopathy: a distinct phenotype? Am J Med Genet 1999;86(3):237–41.

69. Roubenoff R, Hoyt J, Petri M, Hochberg MC, Hellmann DB. Effects of antiinflammatory and immunosuppressive drugs on pregnancy and fertility. Semin Arthritis Rheum 1988;18(2):88–110.

70. Zemlickis D, Lishner M, Erlich R, Koren G. Teratogenicity and carcinogenicity in a twin exposed in utero to cyclophosphamide. Teratog Carcinog Mutagen 1993;13(3):139–43.

71. Peretz B, Peretz T. The effect of chemotherapy in pregnant women on the teeth of offspring. Pediatr Dent 2003;25(6):601–4.

72. Kerr JR. Neonatal effects of breast cancer chemotherapy administered during pregnancy. Pharmacotherapy 2005;25(3):438–41.

73. Werth VP. Pulse intravenous cyclophosphamide for treatment of autoimmune blistering disease. Is there an advantage over oral routes? Arch Dermatol 1997;133(2):229–30.

74. Guillevin L, Cordier JF, Lhote F, Cohen P, Jarrousse B, Royer I, Lesavre P, Jacquot C, Bindi P, Bielefeld P, Desson JF, Detree F, Dubois A, Hachulla E, Hoen B, Jacomy D, Seigneuric C, Lauque D, Stern M, Longy-Boursier M. A prospective, multicenter, randomized trial comparing steroids and pulse cyclophosphamide versus steroids and oral cyclophosphamide in the treatment of generalized Wegener's granulomatosis. Arthritis Rheum 1997;40(12):2187–98.

75. Haubitz M, Schellong S, Gobel U, Schurek HJ, Schaumann D, Koch KM, Brunkhorst R. Intravenous pulse administration of cyclophosphamide versus daily oral treatment in patients with antineutrophil cytoplasmic antibody-associated vasculitis and renal involvement: a prospective, randomized study. Arthritis Rheum 1998;41(10):1835–44.

76. Kaye SB, Paul J, Cassidy J, Lewis CR, Duncan ID, Gordon HK, Kitchener HC, Cruickshank DJ, Atkinson RJ, Soukop M, Rankin EM, Davis JA, Reed NS, Crawford SM, MacLean A, Parkin D, Sarkar TK, Kennedy J, Symonds RP. Mature results of a randomized trial of two doses of cisplatin for the treatment of ovarian cancer. Scottish Gynecology Cancer Trials Group. J Clin Oncol 1996;14(7):2113–9.

77. Yule SM, Walker D, Cole M, McSorley L, Cholerton S, Daly AK, Pearson AD, Boddy AV. The effect of fluconazole on cyclophosphamide metabolism in children. Drug Metab Dispos 1999;27(3):417–21.

78. Belfayol-Pisante L, Guillevin L, Tod M, Fauvelle F. Possible influence of prednisone on the pharmacokinetics of cyclophosphamide in systemic vasculitis. Clin Drug Invest 1999;18:225–31.

78. Bhagat R, Sporn TA, Long GD, Folz RJ. Amiodarone and cyclophosphamide: potential for enhanced lung toxicity. Bone Marrow Transplant 2001;27(10):1109–11.

79. Thomas AE, Patterson J, Prentice HG, Brenner MK, Ganczakowski M, Hancock JF, Pattinson JK, Blacklock HA, Hopewell JP. Haemorrhagic cystitis in bone marrow transplantation patients: possible increased risk associated with prior busulphan therapy. Bone Marrow Transplant 1987;1(4):347–55.

80. Hassan M, Ljungman P, Ringden O, Hassan Z, Oberg G, Nilsson C, Bekassy A, Bielenstein M, Abdel-Rehim M, Georen S, Astner L. The effect of busulphan on the pharmacokinetics of cyclophosphamide and its 4-hydroxy metabolite: time interval influence on therapeutic efficacy and therapy-related toxicity. Bone Marrow Transplant 2000;25(9):915–24.

81. Williams ML, Wainer IW, Embree L, Barnett M, Granvil CL, Ducharme MP. Enantioselective induction of cyclophosphamide metabolism by phenytoin. Chirality 1999;11(7):569–74.

82. Belfayol-Pisante L, Guillevin L, Tod M, Fauvelle F. Possible influence of prednisone on the pharmacokinetics of cyclophosphamide in systemic vasculitis. Clin Drug Invest 1999;18:225–31.

83. Yule SM, Walker D, Cole M, McSorley L, Cholerton S, Daly AK, Pearson AD, Boddy AV. The effect of fluconazole on cyclophosphamide metabolism in children. Drug Metab Dispos 1999;27(3):417–21.

84. Hassan M, Nilsson C, Olsson H, Lundin J, Osterborg A. The influence of interferon-alpha on the pharmacokinetics of cyclophosphamide and its 4-hydroxy metabolite in patients with multiple myeloma. Eur J Haematol 1999;63(3):163–70.

85. Halpert J, Naslund B, Betner I. Suicide inactivation of rat liver cytochrome P-450 by chloramphenicol in vivo and in vitro. Mol Pharmacol 1983;23(2):445–52.

86. Cudmore MA, Silva J Jr, Fekety R, Liepman MK, Kim KH. Clostridium difficile colitis associated with cancer chemotherapy. Arch Intern Med 1982;142(2):333–5.

87. Abe H, Tsunaga N, Yamashita S, Ishiguro K, Mitani I. [Anticancer drug-induced colitis—case report and review of the literature.] Gan To Kagaku Ryoho 1997;24(5):619–24.

Dacarbazine and temozolomide

General Information

Dacarbazine is converted to an active metabolite that is thought to be an alkylating agent. It has been used to treat metastatic melanoma and, in combination regimens, soft-tissue sarcomas and Hodgkin's disease.

Temozolomide is structurally related to dacarbazine and is thought to act via the same active metabolite. It has been used to treat malignant gliomas and malignant melanoma.

Organs and Systems

Hematologic

- Temozolomide-related myelodysplastic syndrome has been reported in a 44-year-old woman with recurrent anaplastic astrocytoma in association with a cytogenetic deletion in chromosome 3 (1).

Liver

Hepatotoxicity has been reported with single-dose dacarbazine (2,3), presenting as acute liver necrosis with hepatic venous thrombosis, which can be fatal.

- Severe hepatic insufficiency in a 69-year-old man after two courses of dacarbazine, 250 mg/m^2/day for 5 days, was successfully treated with intravenous hydrocortisone 300 mg/m^2/day (4).

Fatal hepatotoxicity has also been associated with dacarbazine 500 mg/day for 5 days (5). The cause of this effect is unclear; an allergic hepatic vasculitis with thrombosis is possible.

Skin

Phototoxic reactions occurred in 10 patients with malignant melanoma when they were given dacarbazine (6). In five patients who were tested there was increased sensitivity to ultraviolet A; patch-testing in six showed no type IV allergies. In five patients oral temozolomide did not cause phototoxicity.

References

1. Su YW, Chang MC, Chiang MF, Hsieh RK. Treatment-related myelodysplastic syndrome after temozolomide for recurrent high-grade glioma. J Neurooncol 2005;71(3):315–8.

2. Ceci G, Bella M, Melissari M, Gabrielli M, Bocchi P, Cocconi G. Fatal hepatic vascular toxicity of DTIC. Is it really a rare event? Cancer 1988;61(10):1988–91.

3. Lejeune FJ, Macher E, Kleeberg U, Rumke P, Prade M, Thomas D, Sucin S. An assessment of DTIC vs levamisole or placebo in treatment of high risk stage I patients after surgical removal of a primary melanoma of the skin: a phase III adjuvant study. EORTC protocol 18761. Eur J Cancer Clin Oncol 1988;24(Suppl 2):581–90.

4. Herishanu Y, Lishner M, Kitay-Cohen Y. The role of glucocorticoids in the treatment of fulminant hepatitis induced by dacarbazine. Anticancer Drugs 2002;13(2):177–9.

5. McClay E, Lusch CJ, Mastrangelo MJ. Allergy-induced hepatic toxicity associated with dacarbazine. Cancer Treat Rep 1987;71(2):219–20.

6. Treudler R, Georgieva J, Geilen CC, Orfanos CE. Dacarbazine but not temozolomide induces phototoxic dermatitis in patients with malignant melanoma. J Am Acad Dermatol 2004;50(5):783–5.

Ifosfamide

See also Cyclophosphamide

General Information

Ifosfamide is an alkylating agent belonging to the group of oxazaphosphorines. It is used to treat a variety of solid tumors in children, including rhabdomyosarcoma, soft tissue sarcomas, Wilms' tumor, bone sarcomas, and neuroblastoma, and leukemias and lymphomas in adults. It is also sometimes used in combination with other drugs, such as doxorubicin or cisplatin and etoposide.

Organs and Systems

Cardiovascular

Atrial fibrillation has been attributed to ifosfamide after a dose of only 1800 mg/m^2, with mesna, in a regimen for metastatic breast cancer (1).

Nervous system

Convulsions, severe facial spasms, and trismus occurred 7 hours after an infusion of ifosfamide in a dose of 7 g/m^2, having not occurred at a dose of 5 g/m^2, during a phase II study in patients with solid tumors (2).

Severe encephalopathy has been noted in children treated with ifosfamide (1.8 g/m^2) alone. There were no susceptibility factors, such as impaired renal function or lowered albumin. Electroencephalographic abnormalities and seizures were reversible, despite prolonged coma (3).

In an evaluation of ifosfamide in 57 children with malignant solid tumors, all received 1.6 g/m^2/day for 5 days followed by mesna 400 mg/m^2 at 0.25, 4, and 6 hours after ifosfamide (4). Neurological toxicity occurred in 13 patients. The usual symptoms were somnolence and general weakness followed by confusion, tremors, ataxia, aphasia, urinary incontinence, and cranial nerve paralysis. The symptoms of neurotoxicity disappeared spontaneously within 72 hours of completion of the 5-day course. Some patients had recurrent neurotoxicity on rechallenge. In an analysis of the incidence and features of electroencephalographic changes associated with Ifosfamide/mesna therapy there was no significant association between the electroencephalographic record before and during treatment; electroencephalographic changes developed 12–24 hours before clinical toxicity. Discriminant analysis identified low serum albumin, high serum creatinine concentrations, and pelvic involvement by the underlying malignant disease as susceptibility factors for severe encephalopathy (5).

In 12 of 52 patients treated with ifosfamide there was neurocortical toxicity greater than grade 2 (6). They were successfully treated with intravenous methylthioninium chloride (methylene blue) 50 mg 3-hourly, which was also prophylactic in three patients.

Vitamin B$_1$ (thiamine) has also been suggested to be beneficial in treating ifosfamide-associated neurotoxicity (7).

Urinary tract

It has been thought that the metabolism of ifosfamide to chloroacetaldehyde is the mechanism whereby ifosfamide causes renal damage. However, this was not confirmed in a study of repeated doses of 6–9 g/m^2 in 15 children, in whom there was no correlation between the pharmacokinetics of ifosfamide or its metabolites and either acute renal toxicity or chronic renal toxicity at either 1 or 6 months after treatment (8). However, there were changes in the metabolism of ifosfamide with time, particularly a reduction in dechloroethylation, which correlated with the risk of chronic nephrotoxicity.

Children and adolescents given cumulative doses of 32–112 g/m^2 had only transient disturbances in renal function (9). In five children with renal tubular Fanconi syndrome caused by ifosfamide, all went on to develop rickets in the face of declining renal function. None had had pre-existing tubular damage and the syndrome developed at cumulative doses of ifosfamide of 39–99 g/m^2. There were low serum bicarbonate and phosphate concentrations, and

supplementation of these resulted in bone healing but not renal recovery (10).

The susceptibility factors associated with chronic ifosfamide nephrotoxicity up to 28 months after treatment have been studied in 23 children. The authors concluded that cumulative doses of 100 g/m^2 or higher should be avoided in children with cancers (11).

Like cyclophosphamide, ifosfamide causes a hemorrhagic cystitis in a high proportion of patients, with an occasionally fatal outcome. The damage to urinary bladder epithelium is caused by acrolein, a metabolite that is excreted in the urine. In bone marrow transplant recipients, prior administration of busulfan, which itself causes hemorrhagic cystitis, can increase this risk of oxazaphosphorines (12). Mesna (sodium mercaptoethanesulfonate) is used to prevent this adverse effect. It is excreted by the kidney, and it binds and detoxifies acrolein in the urine; mesna also prevents the breakdown of acrolein precursors.

The phosphate disturbance that leads to Fanconi syndrome is well documented with ifosfamide. Of 43 children who received ifosfamide 3.5 g/m^2/day for 5 days for metastatic osteosarcoma, three developed the syndrome (13).

Second-Generation Effects

Fetotoxicity

The effects of second-trimester or third-trimester exposure to ifosfamide are poorly documented, although normal children have been described (14). In a 17-year-old pregnant woman with Ewing's sarcoma doxorubicin and ifosfamide during the 25th to 30th weeks of gestation did not affect the child, which was delivered at 32 weeks (15).

Drug Administration

Drug dosage regimens

There is a higher incidence of ifosfamide encephalopathy associated with the oral form compared with the intravenous form of ifosfamide; this has been attributed to metabolic differences between the two (16).

Drug–Drug Interactions

Cisplatin

Ifosfamide is associated with a peripheral neuropathy when it is given in combination with cisplatin (17). These symptoms improved within a few days after treatment with haloperidol.

Ketoconazole

The effect of ketoconazole on the CYP-mediated metabolism of ifosfamide to 4-hydroxyifosfamide and the ultimate cytotoxic ifosforamide mustard, and its deactivation to 2- and 3-dechloroethylifosfamide has been studied in a randomized, crossover study in 16 patients, who received intravenous ifosfamide 3 g/m^2/day, either alone or in combination with ketoconazole 200 mg bd 1 day before treatment and during 3 days of concomitant administration(18). Ketoconazole did not affect the fraction metabolized or exposure to the dechloroethylated metabolites and thus did not alter the pharmacokinetics of ifosfamide or its metabolism.

Management of adverse drug reactions

See cyclophosphamide (p.27).

References

1. Ingle JN, Krook JE, Mailliard JA, Hartmann LC, Wieand HS. Evaluation of ifosfamide plus mesna as first-line chemotherapy in women with metastatic breast cancer. Am J Clin Oncol 1995;18(6):498–501.
2. Pinkerton CR, Pritchard J. A phase II study of ifosfamide in paediatric solid tumours. Cancer Chemother Pharmacol 1989;24(Suppl 1):S13–5.
3. Gieron MA, Barak LS, Estrada J. Severe encephalopathy associated with ifosfamide administration in two children with metastatic tumors. J Neurooncol 1988;6(1):29–30.
4. Pratt CB, Horowitz ME, Meyer WH, Etcubanas E, Thompson EI, Douglass EC, Wilimas JA, Hayes FA, Green AA. Phase II trial of ifosfamide in children with malignant solid tumors. Cancer Treat Rep 1987;71(2):131–5.
5. Meanwell CA, Blake AE, Kelly KA, Honigsberger L, Blackledge G. Prediction of ifosfamide/mesna associated encephalopathy. Eur J Cancer Clin Oncol 1986;22(7):815–9.
6. Pelgrims J, De Vos F, Van den Brande J, Schrijvers D, Prove A, Vermorken JB. Methylene blue in the treatment and prevention of ifosfamide-induced encephalopathy: report of 12 cases and a review of the literature. Br J Cancer 2000;82(2):291–4.
7. Buesa JM, Garcia-Teijido P, Losa R, Fra J. Treatment of ifosfamide encephalopathy with intravenous thiamin. Clin Cancer Res 2003;9(12):4636–7.
8. Boddy AV, English M, Pearson AD, Idle JR, Skinner R. Ifosfamide nephrotoxicity: limited influence of metabolism and mode of administration during repeated therapy in paediatrics. Eur J Cancer 1996;32A(7):1179–84.
9. Goren MP, Pratt CB, Viar MJ. Tubular nephrotoxicity during long-term ifosfamide and mesna therapy. Cancer Chemother Pharmacol 1989;25(1):70–2.
10. Burk CD, Restaino I, Kaplan BS, Meadows AT. Ifosfamide-induced renal tubular dysfunction and rickets in children with Wilms tumor. J Pediatr 1990;117(2 Pt 1):331–5.
11. Skinner R, Pearson AD, English MW, Price L, Wyllie RA, Coulthard MG, Craft AW. Risk factors for ifosfamide nephrotoxicity in children. Lancet 1996;348(9027):578–80.
12. Thomas AE, Patterson J, Prentice HG, Brenner MK, Ganczakowski M, Hancock JF, Pattinson JK, Blacklock HA, Hopewell JP. Haemorrhagic cystitis in bone marrow transplantation patients: possible increased risk associated with prior busulphan therapy. Bone Marrow Transplant 1987;1(4):347–55.
13. Goorin AM, Harris MB, Bernstein M, Ferguson W, Devidas M, Siegal GP, Gebhardt MC, Schwartz CL, Link M, Grier HE. Phase II/III trial of etoposide and high-dose ifosfamide in newly diagnosed metastatic osteosarcoma: a pediatric oncology group trial. J Clin Oncol 2002;20(2):426–33.
14. Merimsky O, Le Chevalier T, Missenard G, Lepechoux C, Cojean-Zelek I, Mesurolle B, Le Cesne A. Management of cancer in pregnancy: a case of Ewing's sarcoma of the pelvis in the third trimester. Ann Oncol 1999;10(3):345–50.
15. Nakajima W, Ishida A, Takahashi M, Hirayama M, Washino N, Ogawa M, Takahashi S, Okada K. Good outcome for infant of mother treated with chemotherapy for Ewing sarcoma at 25 to 30 weeks' gestation. J Pediatr Hematol Oncol 2004;26(5):308–11.
16. Lind MJ, Margison JM, Cerny T, Thatcher N, Wilkinson PM. Comparative pharmacokinetics and alkylating activity of fractionated intravenous and oral ifosfamide in patients with bronchogenic carcinoma. Cancer Res 1989;49(3):753–7.
17. Drings P, Abel U, Bulzebruck H, Stiefel P, Kleckow M, Manke HG. Experience with ifosfamide combinations (etoposide or DDP) in non-small cell lung cancer. Cancer Chemother Pharmacol 1986;18(Suppl 2):S34–9.
18. Kerbusch T, Jansen RL, Mathot RA, Huitema AD, Jansen M, van Rijswijk RE, Beijnen JH. Modulation of the cytochrome P450-mediated metabolism of ifosfamide by ketoconazole and rifampin. Clin Pharmacol Ther 2001;70(2):132–41.

Melphalan

General Information

Melphalan (L-phenylalanine mustard) is an alkylating agent that has been used to treat a wide variety of solid malignancies, including cancers of the breast and ovary, and multiple myeloma. Intravenous melphalan has been used to treat rhabdomyosarcoma, lymphomas, multiple myeloma, and neuroblastoma (1).

The adverse effects of high-dose intravenous melphalan have been reviewed (2). Two patients who received less than 100 mg/m^2 recovered from marrow aplasia within 3 weeks without major complications. A third patient died 6 days after injection of 290 mg/m^2, probably because of a cardiac dysrhythmia before complete marrow failure had become established. After intravenous administration of more than 125 mg/m^2, gastrointestinal adverse effects, such as hemorrhagic diarrhea, or bowel perforation, can occur. These, together with reduced ADH secretion and electrolyte disturbances are the predominant clinical problems and the reasons for early death before the occurrence of infectious or bleeding complications from prolonged marrow aplasia.

Organs and Systems

Respiratory

Melphalan can cause an acute interstitial pneumonia with hypoxemia (3). This is probably due to a hypersensitivity mechanism and should be distinguished from fibrosing pneumonitis, which melphalan can also cause (4).

Fatal pulmonary fibrosis and atypical epithelial proliferation has been reported in patients with multiple myeloma treated with melphalan (4).

Urinary tract

Acute renal insufficiency has been attributed to melphalan in a patient with third stage ovarian cancer (5).

Reproductive system

Primary ovarian failure has been recognized in adults after intermittent low-dose melphalan, and has also been reported in three adolescents after high-dose melphalan (6).

Drug–Drug Interactions

Busulfan

The possibility that melphalan and busulfan may cause additive lung damage has been discussed in the light of a 59-year-old patient with chronic myeloid leukemia who developed severe interstitial lung fibrosis after short-term sequential treatment with the two drugs (7).

Fludarabine

Cardiotoxicity has rarely been reported with melphalan or fludarabine alone, but severe left ventricular failure developed in three of 21 patients treated with a combination of these two drugs (9).

Interferon alfa

Interferon-induced fever has been thought to increase the cytotoxicity of melphalan (8).

References

1. Sarosy G, Leyland-Jones B, Soochan P, Cheson BD. The systemic administration of intravenous melphalan. J Clin Oncol 1988;6(11):1768–82.
2. JostLM. Uberdosierung von Melphalan (Alkeran): Symptome und Behandlung. [Overdose with melphalan (Alkeran): symptoms and treatment. A review.] Onkologie 1990;13(2):96–101.
3. Liote H, Gauthier JF, Prier A, Gauthier-Rahman S, Kaplan G, Akoun G. Pneumopathie interstitielle, aiguë, reversible, induite par le melphalan. [Acute, reversible, interstitial pneumopathy induced by melphalan.] Rev Mal Respir 1989;6(5):461–4.
4. Taetle R, Dickman PS, Feldman PS. Pulmonary histopathologic changes associated with melphalan therapy. Cancer 1978;42(3):1239–45.
5. Kashimura M, Kondo M, Abe T, Shinohara M, Baba S. [A case report of acute renal failure induced by melphalan in a patient with ovarian cancer.]Gan No Rinsho 1988;34(14):2015–8.
6. Kellie SJ, Kingston JE. Ovarian failure after high-dose melphalan in adolescents. Lancet 1987;1(8547):1425.
7. Schallier D, Impens N, Warson F, Van Belle S, De Wasch G. Additive pulmonary toxicity with melphalan and busulfan therapy. Chest 1983;84(4):492–3.
8. Ehrsson H, Eksborg S, Wallin I, Osterborg A, Mellstedt H. Oral melphalan pharmacokinetics: influence of interferon-induced fever. Clin Pharmacol Ther 1990;47(1):86–90.
9. Ritchie DS, Seymour JF, Roberts AW, Szer J, Grigg AP. Acute left ventricular failure following melphalan and fludarabine conditioning. Bone Marrow Transplant 2001;28(1):101–3.

Mitomycin

General Information

Mitomycin is an alkylating agent that is used intravenously to treat upper gastrointestinal and breast cancers and by direct instillation to treat superficial bladder tumors. Its main adverse effects are thrombocytopenia and leukopenia. Rare but severe adverse effects are hemolytic–uremic syndrome, pneumonitis, and cardiac failure.

Organs and Systems

Respiratory

Biopsy-proven mitomycin pneumonitis occurred in five of 44 patients who were given mitomycin in conjunction with low-dose doxorubicin 20 mg/week (1). The picture was of pulmonary infiltrates clinically and radiologically, progressive dyspnea, and hypoxia, and improvement with glucocorticoids. The mean total dose of mitomycin that had been given in the five patients was 89 mg. Mitomycin-induced interstitial pneumonitis occurs in 2–38% of cases (2,3) and at cumulative doses of 20 mg/m^2 or greater, although doses up to 30 mg/m^2 have been used safely. It is characteristically of slow-onset (3).

A fatal case of mitomycin C-induced pneumonitis has been reported in a radiotherapy/chemotherapy trial in 43 patients (4). The dose was 8 mg/m^2 on days 1 and 29, radiotherapy and vindesine being given on the intervening days.

Urinary tract

Hemolytic–uremic syndrome has often been described in patients treated with mitomycin (5–7). Up to 1990 the United States National Cancer Registry received 85 reports of cancer-associated hemolytic–uremic syndrome and 84 had received a cumulative dose of 60 mg mitomycin or more as part of their treatment (8).

Hemolytic–uremic syndrome presents as a Coombs-negative microangiopathic hemolytic anemia, thrombocytopenia, and renal insufficiency, and the outcome is often fatal. The underlying pathology is thought to be vascular endothelial damage. It occurs 4–7 months after the start of chemotherapy. Blood transfusion can cause clinical deterioration in those affected (9). Histology of the kidney in the hemolytic–uremic syndrome caused by mitomycin shows mesangial proliferative glomerulonephritis with partial thickening and/or splitting of the basement membrane. On electron microscopy there is accumulation of non-homogeneous material in the subendothelial spaces. Neither immunoglobulin nor complement deposition is found (10). Treatment with hemodialysis and immunosuppressive drugs is not always successful. Plasmapheresis is commonly used (11). Prophylactic glucocorticoids can reduce the severity and prevent hemolytic–uremic syndrome in patients receiving mitomycin (12). Erythropoietin is also reportedly beneficial (13).

Mitomycin when administered intravesically causes cystitis of variable severity, which can lead to mucosal ulceration in the worst cases. However, there has also been a report of bladder fibrosis and loss of function in a 74-year-old man who had received 20 mg/week for 8 weeks (14).

Ten cases of bladder wall calcification have been reported after intravesicular administration of mitomycin. These lesions can resemble tumor recurrence in the bladder, and biopsy is advocated to distinguish between the two (15).

Skin

There have been several reports of erythematous blistering skin eruption of the palms and soles affecting patients treated with intravesical mitomycin. This has been attributed to contact dermatitis, but more widespread skin involvement and an association with eosinophilic interstitial cystitis suggest that it may be a more generalized allergic reaction (16–20).

Local extravasation of mitomycin causes inflammation and ulceration, starting within 7–10 days and lasting several weeks. In four cases the onset of tissue necrosis was delayed several weeks or months after exposure (21,22). In one case, ulceration seemed to have been precipitated by drinking ethanol, and in another by exposure to the sun.

Three cases of allergic dermatitis have been described after intravesical mitomycin (23). A type IV hypersensitivity reaction was demonstrated on patch-testing. Six cases of purpuric allergic drug eruption from intravesicular mitomycin have been reported (24).

References

1. Colozza M, Tonato M, Grignani F, Davis S. Low-dose mitomycin and weekly low-dose doxorubicin combination chemotherapy for patients with metastatic breast carcinoma previously treated with cyclophosphamide, methotrexate, and 5-fluorouracil. Cancer 1988;62(2):262–5.
2. Verweij J, van Zanten T, Souren T, Golding R, Pinedo HM. Prospective study on the dose relationship of mitomycin C-induced interstitial pneumonitis. Cancer 1987;60(4):756–61.
3. Linette DC, McGee KH, McFarland JA. Mitomycin-induced pulmonary toxicity: case report and review of the literature. Ann Pharmacother 1992;26(4):481–4.
4. Furuse K, Kubota K, Kawahara M, Kodama N, Ogawara M, Akira M, Nakajima S, Takada M, Kusunoki Y, Negoro S, et alSouthern Osaka Lung Cancer Study Group. Phase II study of concurrent radiotherapy and chemotherapy for unresectable stage III non-small-cell lung cancer. J Clin Oncol 1995;13(4):869–75.
5. Mackintosh J, Tattersal M. Mitomycin-C induced hemolytic–uraemic syndrome. Aust NZ J Med 1988;18:182.
6. Verwey J, de Vries J, Pinedo HM. Mitomycin C-induced renal toxicity, a dose-dependent side effect? Eur J Cancer Clin Oncol 1987;23(2):195–9.
7. Sheldon R, Slaughter D. A syndrome of microangiopathic hemolytic anemia, renal impairment, and pulmonary edema in chemotherapy-treated patients with adenocarcinoma. Cancer 1986;58(7):1428–36.
8. Lesesne JB, Rothschild N, Erickson B, Korec S, Sisk R, Keller J, Arbus M, Woolley PV, Chiazze L, Schein PS, et al. Cancer-associated hemolytic–uremic syndrome: analysis of 85 cases from a national registry. J Clin Oncol 1989;7(6):781–9.
9. Ries F. Nephrotoxicity of chemotherapy. Eur J Cancer Clin Oncol 1988;24(6):951–3.
10. Hayano K, Fukui H, Otsuka Y, Hattori S. [Three cases of renal failure associated with microangiopathic hemolytic anemia after mitomycin C therapy.]Nippon Jinzo Gakkai Shi 1988;30(7):835–42.
11. Poch E, Almirall J, Nicolas JM, Torras A, Revert L. Treatment of mitomycin-C-associated hemolytic uremic syndrome with plasmapheresis. Nephron 1990;55(1):89–90.
12. Hartmann JT, Quietzsch D, Daikeler T, Kollmannsberger C, Mayer F, Kanz L, Bokemeyer C, Mitomycin C. continuous infusion as salvage chemotherapy in pretreated patients with advanced gastric cancer. Anticancer Drugs 1999;10(8):729–33.
13. Catalano C, Gianesini C, Fabbian F. Erythropoietin is beneficial in mitomycin-induced hemolytic–uremic syndrome. Nephron 2002;91(2):324–6.
14. Katz G, Hackett RL, Wajsman Z. Bladder wall fibrosis following intravesical mitomycin treatment for superficial bladder cancer. Urology 1996;47(6):928–9.
15. Garrigos J, Auladell A, Perez P, Garcia J, Matoses M, Marcos M, Linares A. Lesiones vesicales calcificades secundarias a instilacion de mitomicina C. [Calcified bladder lesions secondary to the instillation of mitomycin C.] Arch Esp Urol 1991;44:1057–60.
16. Inglis JA, Tolley DA, Grigor KM. Allergy to mitomycin C complicating topical administration for urothelial cancer. Br J Urol 1987;59(6):547–9.
17. Sala F, Crosti C, Bencini PL, Perotta E, Mansi M. Esantema tossiallergico da instillazione endovesicale di mitomicina C. [Toxicoallergic exanthema caused by intravesical instillation of mitomycin C.] G Ital Dermatol Venereol 1987;122(5):265–7.
18. Mobley WC, Loening SA, Narayana AS, Culp DA. Use of intravesical cisplatin and mitomycin-C for recurrent transitional cell carcinoma of bladder refractory to thiotepa. Urology 1986;27(4):335–9.
19. Ausfeld R, Beer M, Muhlethaler JP, Bartlome F, Widmer R, Tscholl R. Adjuvant intravesical chemotherapy of superficial bladder cancer with monthly doxorubicin or intensive mitomycin. A comparison of two consecutive series. Eur Urol 1987;13(1–2):10–4.
20. Hetherington JW, Newling DW, Robinson MR, Smith PH, Adib RS, Whelan P. Intravesical mitomycin C for the treatment of recurrent superficial bladder tumours. Br J Urol 1987;59(3):239–41.
21. Aizawa H, Tagami H. Delayed tissue necrosis due to mitomycin C. Acta Derm Venereol 1987;67(4):364–6.
22. Bikkers TH, Verweij J, van Geel AN, Stoter G. Ernstige weefselnecrose ten gevolge van extravasatie van mitomycine. [Severe tissue necrosis due to extravasation of mitomycin.] Ned Tijdschr Geneeskd 1987;131(14):588–590.
23. Vidal C, de la Fuente R, Gonzalez Quintela A. Three cases of allergic dermatitis due to intravesical mitomycin C. Dermatology 1992;184(3):208–9.
24. De Groot A, van der Meyden A. Purpuric allergic drug eruption from intravesicle instillation of the antitumor antibiotic mitomycin C. Dermatosen 1991;39:84–6.

Procarbazine

General Information

Procarbazine is an alkylating agent that is used in the treatment of Hodgkin's disease in regimens such as MOPP (chlormethine (mechlorethamine), vincristine (Oncovin), procarbazine, and prednisolone) and BEACOPP (bleomycin, etoposide, doxorubicin (Adriamycin), cyclophosphamide, vincristine, procarbazine, and prednisone) (1). It is also used to treat glioblastoma multiforme.

Organs and Systems

Respiratory

The permanent and acute reversible forms of lung disease attributed to procarbazine have been reviewed (2). Pneumonitis has rarely been reported (3).

Drug–Drug Interactions

Antiepileptic drugs

In a retrospective cohort study in 83 patients with primary brain tumors who were treated with procarbazine, 20 patients had procarbazine hypersensitivity reactions (4). There was a significant association between exposure to antiepileptic drugs and the development of procarbazine hypersensitivity reactions. The authors suggested that this association may have been due to a reactive intermediate generated by induction of CYP3A.

References

1. Massoud M, Armand JP, Ribrag V. Procarbazine in haematology: an old drug with a new life? Eur J Cancer 2004;40(13):1924–7.
2. Millward MJ, Cohney SJ, Byrne MJ, Ryan GF. Pulmonary toxicity following MOPP chemotherapy. Aust NZ J Med 1990;20(3):245–8.
3. Mahmood T, Mudad R. Pulmonary toxicity secondary to procarbazine. Am J Clin Oncol 2002;25(2):187–8.
4. Lehmann DF, Hurteau TE, Newman N, Coyle TE. Anticonvulsant usage is associated with an increased risk of procarbazine hypersensitivity reactions in patients with brain tumors. Clin Pharmacol Ther 1997;62(2):225–9.

ANTIMETABOLITES

Cytarabine

General Information

Cytarabine is a pyrimidine nucleoside that is used to treat acute myelogenous leukemia and lymphocytic leukemias. It is activated intracellularly by deoxycytidine kinase to phosphorylated nucleotides that interfere with DNA synthesis in the S phase of the cell, and is rapidly deaminated intracellularly to the inactive metabolite uracil arabinoside.

Organs and Systems

Respiratory

Two cases of respiratory failure occurred during induction chemotherapy for acute myelomonocytic leukemia with cytarabine and all-*trans*-retinoic acid (1). The authors attributed this to a manifestation of the retinoic acid syndrome. Both patients developed acute respiratory failure with widespread pulmonary infiltrates about 60 hours after starting chemotherapy. Both were managed successfully using high-dose dexamethasone and ventilation.

Nervous system

Central nervous system disturbances, especially impaired cerebellar function, limit doses of cytarabine, and age is an important predictive factor. Of 418 patients who received 36–48 g/m^2 only 35 (8%) had severe cerebellar toxicity, which was irreversible or fatal in 4 (1%) (2). Patients over 50 years of age were significantly more likely to develop cerebellar problems than younger patients (26/137, 19%, compared with 9/281, 3%); a second course did not increase the incidence, implying that it is the individual rather than the cumulative dose that is important.

The cerebellar syndrome is the most common complication of high-dose cytarabine therapy. In a study of the cerebellar syndrome caused by cytarabine (3), in which it was found in seven of 30 patients treated, symptoms of toxicity appeared between the third and seventh days of chemotherapy, manifesting first as lethargy and confusion (3). Within the next 24 hours there were signs of cerebellar dysfunction, including dysarthria, ataxia, tremor, nystagmus, and dysmetria. In most patients in whom neurotoxicity developed, liver function worsened during chemotherapy. Abnormal liver function at the start of therapy and the development of neurotoxicity appear to be linked. The symptoms of neurotoxicity resolved within 4–49 days.

Aseptic meningitis can also occur in patients given cytarabine (4,5), and signs of cerebellar dysfunction after the administration of cytarabine 24 g/m^2 have been reported in association with aseptic meningitis (6).

Sensory systems

Keratoconjunctivitis is a complication of cytarabine therapy, with a reported incidence of 30–100% and commonly associated with high doses (3 g/m^2). Corneal and conjunctival toxicity have been described after therapy for 4 days with 235 mg (100 mg/m^2) daily (7).

Gastrointestinal

The addition of cytarabine 10 mg/m^2/day subcutaneously for 10 days to interferon monotherapy more than doubled the incidence of gastrointestinal toxicity in the treatment of chronic myeloid leukemia in 139 patients (8).

Skin

Acute, painful, swollen, and self-limiting erythema of the hands and soles has been reported after induction therapy for acute myeloid leukemia and attributed to cytarabine (9).

Immunologic

A hypersensitivity reaction has been ascribed to cytarabine (10).

Drug Administration

Drug administration route

The safe intrathecal administration of a long-acting formulation of cytarabine has been reported (11).

Drug–Drug Interactions

Daunorubicin

Hepatotoxicity, with either hyperbilirubinemia or increased alkaline phosphatase activity, occurred in five of 14 patients in a trial of cytarabine 200 mg/m^2/day for 9 days by continuous infusion and daunorubicin 70 mg/m^2/day for 3 days (12).

Flucytosine

The suggested interaction of cytarabine with flucytosine, in which there is competitive inhibition of antifungal activity, has not been confirmed (13).

References

1. Lester WA, Hull DR, Fegan CD, Morris TC. Respiratory failure during induction chemotherapy for acute myelomonocytic leukaemia (FAB M4Eo) with ara-C and all-trans retinoic acid. Br J Haematol 2000;109(4):847–50.
2. Herzig RH, Hines JD, Herzig GP, Wolff SN, Cassileth PA, Lazarus HM, Adelstein DJ, Brown RA, Coccia PF, Strandjord S, et al. Cerebellar toxicity with high-dose cytosine arabinoside. J Clin Oncol 1987;5(6):927–32.

3. Nand S, Messmore HL Jr, Patel R, Fisher SG, Fisher RI. Neurotoxicity associated with systemic high-dose cytosine arabinoside. J Clin Oncol 1986;4(4):571–5.

4. Pease CL, Horton TM, McClain KL, Kaplan SL. Aseptic meningitis in a child after systemic treatment with high dose cytarabine. Pediatr Infect Dis J 2001;20(1):87–9.

5. van den Berg H, van der Flier M, van de Wetering MD. Cytarabine-induced aseptic meningitis. Leukemia 2001;15(4):697–9.

6. Thordarson H, Talstad I. Acute meningitis and cerebellar dysfunction complicating high-dose cytosine arabinoside therapy. Acta Med Scand 1986;220(5):493–5.

7. Thaler J, Hilbe WAustrian CML Study Group. Comparative analysis of two consecutive phase II studies with IFN-alpha and IFN-alpha + ara-C in untreated chronic-phase CML patients Bone Marrow Transplant 1996;17(Suppl 3):S25–8.

8. Shall L, Lucas GS, Whittaker JA, Holt PJ. Painful red hands: a side-effect of leukaemia therapy. Br J Dermatol 1988;119(2):249–53.

9. Barletta JP, Fanous MM, Margo CE. Corneal and conjunctival toxicity with low-dose cytosine arabinoside. Am J Ophthalmol 1992;113(5):587–8.

10. Williams SF, Larson RA. Hypersensitivity reaction to high-dose cytarabine. Br J Haematol 1989;73(2):274–5.

11. Jaeckle KA, Phuphanich S, Bent MJ, Aiken R, Batchelor T, Campbell T, Fulton D, Gilbert M, Heros D, Rogers L, O'Day SJ, Akerley W, Allen J, Baidas S, Gertler SZ, Greenberg HS, LaFollette S, Lesser G, Mason W, Recht L, Wong E, Chamberlain MC, Cohn A, Glantz MJ, Gutheil JC, Maria B, Moots P, New P, Russell C, Shapiro W, Swinnen L, Howell SB. Intrathecal treatment of neoplastic meningitis due to breast cancer with a slow-release formulation of cytarabine. Br J Cancer 2001;84(2):157–63.

12. Kouides PA, Rowe JM. A dose intensive regimen of cytosine arabinoside and daunorubicin for chronic myelogenous leukemia in blast crisis. Leuk Res 1995;19(10):763–70.

13. Wingfield HJ. Absence of fungistatic antagonism between flucytosine and cytarabine in vitro and in vivo. J Antimicrob Chemother 1987;20(4):523–7.

Doxifluridine

General Information

Doxifluridine is a derivative of 5-fluorouracil. It has been used to treat a variety of solid tumors, including cancers of the breast, pancreas, stomach (1), and large bowel.

Organs and Systems

Nervous system

In a neurological evaluation of 17 patients treated with doxifluridine 3 or 5 g/m^2/day for 5 days every 4 weeks for 3 months, 10 developed symptoms of central nervous system toxicity. The neurological symptoms, cerebellar and encephalopathic, developed simultaneously and were commonly first noted during the second week of the first cycle. The neurotoxicity was dose-related and

worsened during subsequent treatment. The symptoms of cerebellar disease ranged from a subjective feeling of unsteady gait to disability, while the encephalopathy resulted in difficulties with concentration and memory. Patients with marked weight loss and with generalized electrocardiographic dysrhythmias are at greatest risk of developing neurotoxicity with doxifluridine (2).

Gastrointestinal

Anorexia has been reported with doxifluridine in the absence of nausea or vomiting (3).

References

1. Nakagawa H, Kobayashi K, Tono T, Fukuda K, Shinn E, Mishima H, Yagyu T, Kobayashi T, Kikkawa N. [Combination of intra-hepatic arterial infusion of low-dose cisplatin and oral administration of high-dose doxyfluridine for patients with liver metastases of gastric cancer.] Gan To Kagaku Ryoho 1996;23(6):783–5.

2. Heier MS, Fossa SD. Wernicke–Korsakoff-like syndrome in patients with colorectal carcinoma treated with high-dose doxifluridine (5′-dFUrd). Acta Neurol Scand 1986;73(5):449–57.

3. Tamaki Y, Tono T, Kobayashi K, Yagyu T, Takatsuka Y, Shin E, Mishima H, Kikkawa N. [Combination with intra-hepatic arterial infusion of low-dose cisplatin and oral administration of high-dose doxyfluridine in patients with liver metastases of gastric cancer.] Gan To Kagaku Ryoho 1994;21(13):2140–2.

Floxuridine

General Information

Floxuridine is a pyrimidine analogue that is used in regional arterial chemotherapy for primary and metastatic malignancies, delivered using an implantable pump.

Organs and Systems

Gastrointestinal

Nine patients who received hepatic arterial infusion chemotherapy developed gastritis heralded by epigastric pain and tenderness, nausea, vomiting, weakness, and anorexia (1). In 7 patients, 18 gastric ulcers were detected endoscopically. Mucosal damage developed despite prophylactic antiulcer therapy and healed only on withdrawal. In 17 biopsy specimens there were variously inflammatory changes, reactive glandular changes, and cell necrosis, even in patients without ulcers. In addition, there was floxuridine-induced glandular atypia in eight biopsy samples from six patients; the crowded glands were distorted and lined by large cells that included bizarre forms with pleomorphic nuclei.

• A patient who received regional intrahepatic chemotherapy from a continuous infusion pump for 31 months developed a gastroduodenal artery–duodenal fistula, and presented with signs and symptoms of upper gastrointestinal bleeding.

Six patients who had received an infusion of floxuridine, either via the hepatic artery or intravenously, developed severe diarrhea (2). In four, the entire ileum or its more distal part was markedly narrowed and in the other two there was thickening or effacement of the mucosal folds in the distal ileum. The symptoms resolved and the radiographic appearances improved after withdrawal.

Biliary tract

The principle of hepatic arterial infusion is based on the fact that hepatic tumors derive much of their blood supply from the hepatic artery, whereas the liver parenchyma receives its supply from the portal venous circulation.

• Acute and chronic cholecystitis has been reported after floxuridine hepatic artery infusion (3). Chemotherapy in this patient was associated with persistent epigastric pain with radiation to the back which was not accompanied by any fever or white blood cell elevation. Cholecystectomy showed a shrunken, thickened fibrotic gallbladder that was filled with thick, pasty, hemorrhagic material. There were no gallstones.

In 27 patients who received intrahepatic floxuridine, total dose 20–41 mg/kg extrahepatic biliary sclerosis was discovered by CT scan and ultrasound, followed by endoscopic retrograde cholangiopancreatography and/or percutaneous cholangiography in three cases (4). Radiological findings included complete obstruction of the common hepatic duct in one case, common hepatic duct stenosis in two cases, common bile duct obstruction in one case, and intrahepatic bile duct dilatation without identifiable obstruction in one case

References

1. Doria MI Jr, Doria LK, Faintuch J, Levin B. Gastric mucosal injury after hepatic arterial infusion chemotherapy with floxuridine. A clinical and pathologic study. Cancer 1994;73(8):2042–7.
2. Kelvin FM, Gramm HF, Gluck WL, Lokich JJ. Radiologic manifestations of small-bowel toxicity due to floxuridine therapy. Am J Roentgenol 1986;146(1):39–43.
3. Pietrafitta JJ, Anderson BG, O'Brien MJ, Deckers PJ. Cholecystitis secondary to infusion chemotherapy. J Surg Oncol 1986;31(4):287–93.
4. Aldrighetti L, Arru M, Ronzoni M, Salvioni M, Villa E, Ferla G. Extrahepatic biliary stenoses after hepatic arterial infusion (HAI) of floxuridine (FUdR) for liver metastases from colorectal cancer. Hepatogastroenterology 2001;48(41):1302–7.

Fludarabine

General Information

Fludarabine phosphate is a purine nucleoside antitumor agent, which inhibits adenosine deaminase. It is mainly used to treat chronic lymphocytic leukemia. Dose-limiting myelotoxicity, nausea and vomiting, and raised liver enzymes were observed during early clinical studies. The most common adverse effect is myelosuppression (WHO grade 3 or 4), and other common adverse effects include infections and gastrointestinal disturbances, although these are usually of mild to moderate intensity (WHO grade 1 or 2) (1).

Organs and Systems

Respiratory

Fludarabine can cause interstitial pneumonitis (2,3).

• A 73-year-old woman developed fever and cough 2 weeks after completing a third cycle of fludarabine for chronic lymphocytic leukemia. A chest X-ray showed multiple pulmonary nodules and a biopsy showed a mononuclear interstitial infiltrate without evidence of malignant, infectious, granulomatous, or vascular causes. Her symptoms and pulmonary nodules resolved after treatment with glucocorticoids (4).

There has also been a report of an acute eosinophilic pneumonia associated with peripheral blood eosinophilia in a patient with follicular lymphoma (5).

Nervous system

Dose-intensified fludarabine causes severe central nervous system toxicity. In 70 patients with acute leukemia who received 95 courses of fludarabine 20–220 mg/m^2 for 5–7 days there was neurotoxicity in 36% of those who received doses over 96 mg/m^2/day, but in only 0.2% of those who received lower doses (6). The onset of neurological symptoms was at 21–60 days after the last course of fludarabine. Visual symptoms were the most common. There was progressive deterioration of mental state or encephalopathy leading to a vegetative state in 11 patients. Progressive demyelination in the central nervous system was the main factor causing the neurotoxic symptoms; this can occur as a result of viral complications during drug-related immunosuppression.

Hematologic

Fludarabine can cause or exacerbate autoimmune thrombocytopenia in chronic lymphocytic leukemia. Two patients with chronic lymphatic leukemia who developed thrombocytopenia while taking fludarabine were treated with high-dose glucocorticoids and initially responded with recovery of platelet counts (7). One developed recurrent thrombocytopenia on two occasions after re-exposure to fludarabine when his disease had become refractory to all other treatments. Of 45 patients with lymphoproliferative disorders treated with fludarabine over the previous 6 years, retrospectively reviewed, 2 had developed autoimmune thrombocytopenia and 3 had developed autoimmune hemolytic anemia.

In three patients with chronic lymphatic leukemia, fludarabine-associated thrombocytopenia responded to rituximab 375 mg/m^2/week for 4 weeks (8). Other similar cases have been reported (9). However, when rituximab was added to a regimen of fludarabine plus cyclophosphamide in patients with relapsed follicular lymphoma, there was unexpected severe hematological toxicity, with significant, prolonged thrombocytopenia WHO grade 3/4 in six of 17 patients (10). Older patients (mean age 65 versus 57 years) were significantly more likely to have this adverse effect, and no other clinical or hematological parameters differed between the patients with thrombocytopenia and those without.

Peripheral blood eosinophilia, in one case up to 7.9 × 10^9/l, has been attributed to fludarabine (11).

- A 58-year-old man who took fludarabine for 5 months developed a peripheral eosinophilia with a peak value of 1.7 × 10^9/l; thorough investigation for other causes of eosinophilia was negative (12).

A patient with a high-grade B cell non-Hodgkin's lymphoma treated with fludarabine developed a high-titer antibody to factor VIII while the lymphoma was in remission; the authors speculated that the occurrence of the inhibitor was an autoimmune adverse effect of fludarabine (13).

Gastrointestinal

Intestinal pseudo-obstruction has been attributed to fludarabine in a 66-year-old man with non-Hodgkin's lymphoma; it was successfully managed with a combination of parasympathomimetic drugs and mechanical decompression (14).

Immunologic

Treatment with fludarabine results in prolonged immunosuppression lasting over 6 months (15). Patients who are immunocompromised are at risk of infection with chemotherapy. Infection with JC virus, a human polyoma virus, occurred in two patients after fludarabine treatment of a low-grade lymphoma, which led to a progressive multifocal leukoencephalopathy (16). In one series of 27 patients who received fludarabine, serious infections developed in 24 (17).

Drug–Drug Interactions

Melphalan

Cardiotoxicity has rarely been reported with melphalan or fludarabine alone, but severe left ventricular failure

developed in three of 21 patients treated with a combination of these two drugs (18).

References

1. Plosker GL, Figgitt DP. Oral fludarabine. Drugs 2003;63(21):2317–23.
2. Hurst PG, Habib MP, Garewal H, Bluestein M, Paquin M, Greenberg BR. Pulmonary toxicity associated with fludarabine monophosphate. Invest New Drugs 1987;5(2):207–10.
3. Levin M, Aziz M, Opitz L. Steroid-responsive interstitial pneumonitis after fludarabine therapy. Chest 1997;111(5):1472–3.
4. Garg S, Garg MS, Basmaji N. Multiple pulmonary nodules: an unusual presentation of fludarabine pulmonary toxicity: case report and review of literature. Am J Hematol 2002;70(3):241–5.
5. Trojan A, Meier R, Licht A, Taverna C. Eosinophilic pneumonia after administration of fludarabine for the treatment of non-Hodgkin's lymphoma. Ann Hematol 2002;81(9):535–537.
6. Chun HG, Leyland-Jones BR, Caryk SM, Hoth DF. Central nervous system toxicity of fludarabine phosphate. Cancer Treat Rep 1986;70(10):1225–8.
7. Leach M, Parsons RM, Reilly JT, Winfield DA. Autoimmune thrombocytopenia: a complication of fludarabine therapy in lymphoproliferative disorders. Clin Lab Haematol 2000;22(3):175–8.
8. Hegde UP, Wilson WH, White T, Cheson BD. Rituximab treatment of refractory fludarabine-associated immune thrombocytopenia in chronic lymphocytic leukemia. Blood 2002;100(6):2260–2.
9. Fernandez MJ, Llopis I, Pastor E, Real E, Grau E. Immune thrombocytopenia induced by fludarabine successfully treated with rituximab. Haematologica 2003;88(2):ELT02.
10. Leo E, Scheuer L, Schmidt-Wolf IG, Kerowgan M, Schmitt C, Leo A, Baumbach T, Kraemer A, Mey U, Benner A, Parwaresch R, Ho AD. Significant thrombocytopenia associated with the addition of rituximab to a combination of fludarabine and cyclophosphamide in the treatment of relapsed follicular lymphoma. Eur J Haematol 2004;73(4):251–7.
11. Sezer O, Schmid P, Hallek M, Schweigert M, Beinert T, Langelotz C, Mergenthaler HG, Possinger K. Eosinophilia during fludarabine treatment of chronic lymphocytic leukemia. Ann Hematol 1999;78(10):475–7.
12. Voutsadakis IA. Fludarabine-induced eosinophilia: case report. Ann Hematol 2002;81(5):292–3.
13. Tiplady CW, Hamilton PJ, Galloway MJ. Acquired haemophilia complicating the remission of a patient with high grade non-Hodgkin's lymphoma treated by fludarabine. Clin Lab Haematol 2000;22(3):163–5.
14. Campbell S, Thomas R, Parker A, Ghosh S. Fludarabine induced intestinal pseudo-obstruction: case report and literature review. Eur J Gastroenterol Hepatol 2000;12(6):711–3.
15. Samonis G, Kontoyiannis DP. Infectious complications of purine analogue therapy. Curr Opin Infect Dis 2001;14(4):409–13.
16. Vidarsson B, Mosher DF, Salamat MS, Isaksson HJ, Onundarson PT. Progressive multifocal leukoencephalopathy after fludarabine therapy for low-grade lymphoproliferative disease. Am J Hematol 2002;70(1):51–4.
17. Perkins JG, Flynn JM, Howard RS, Byrd JC. Frequency and type of serious infections in fludarabine-refractory B-cell chronic lymphocytic leukemia and small lymphocytic lymphoma: implications for clinical trials in this patient population. Cancer 2002;94(7):2033–9.
18. Ritchie DS, Seymour JF, Roberts AW, Szer J, Grigg AP. Acute left ventricular failure following melphalan and

fludarabine conditioning. Bone Marrow Transplant 2001;28(1):101–3.

Fluorouracil

General Information

Fluorouracil is a fluorinated pyrimidine, which is converted intracellularly to the active form, fluorodeoxyuridine monophosphate, which inhibits thymidylate synthetase and hence reduces the production of thymidylic acid, the deoxyribonucleotide of thymine (5-methyluracil), a DNA pyrimidine base, blocking DNA synthesis. In addition, intracellular conversion to 5-fluorouridine monophosphate results in incorporation of the activated antimetabolite into RNA and consequent RNA dysfunction.

Fluorouracil is specific to the S phase of the cell cycle. It is primarily used intravenously to treat carcinoma of the breast and adenocarcinomas of the gastrointestinal tract (1). In addition, topical fluorouracil is used to treat actinic keratoses.

General adverse effects

The dose-limiting toxic effects of fluorouracil vary with the dose and mode of administration.

- With five consecutive daily bolus injections of 450–600 mg/m^2, the dose-limiting effects are myelosuppression, mucositis, and diarrhea.
- With weekly injections of 450–600 mg/m^2, myelosuppression is dose-limiting.
- With continuous five-day infusion of 1000 mg/m^2/day, mucositis and diarrhea are dose-limiting.
- With protracted continuous infusion of 200–400 mg/m^2/day, mucositis and palmar–plantar erythrodysesthesia syndrome are the most common dose-limiting adverse effects (2).

Some very high-dose, short-exposure studies have been reported, including 14 g over 24 hours (3) and 2.6 g/m^2 weekly (4); in the latter study, neurotoxicity was dose-limiting; with 24-hour infusion of 2.6 g/m^2 weekly, palmar–plantar erythrodysesthesia syndrome is a major adverse effect.

Relation of toxicity to pharmacokinetics

The pharmacokinetics of fluorouracil have been determined in 19 patients receiving fluorouracil by protracted intravenous infusion of 190–600 mg/m^2/day (5). The steady-state fluorouracil plasma concentration and AUC were significantly lower in the nine patients who had WHO grade 2 toxicity or less compared with the nine patients who had greater than grade 2 toxicity. In contrast, there was no difference in fluorouracil plasma concentrations between the 10 responders and the nine patients who had no evidence of a clinical response. These investigations confirm previous observations that

correlations can be drawn between fluorouracil pharmacokinetics and clinical toxicity (6). Furthermore, the data suggest that pharmacokinetic monitoring might permit identification of patients at increased risk of toxicity.

Organs and Systems

Cardiovascular

Fluorouracil can cause anginal chest pain, with nonspecific ST–T electrocardiographic changes, during infusion (7). The outcome is favourable if the drug is withdrawn. Re-introduction of the drug has been associated with occasional fatal outcomes and is not recommended (8). The cardiotoxicity of 5-fluorouracil in 135 reported cases has been reviewed (9).

Presentation
More frequent use of fluorouracil by continuous infusion, increased awareness of the problems, and more sophisticated monitoring have increased the reported incidence. By 1990, more than 67 clinical cases had been described (10) and an incidence ranging up to 68% of silent ischemic electrocardiographic changes was identified in patients monitored by continuous 24-hour ambulatory electrocardiography during fluorouracil infusion (11). The clinical features include the following:

- Precordial pain (both non-specific and anginal) (10).
- Electrocardiographic ST–T wave changes (non-specific and ischemic) (10,11).
- Acute myocardial infarction (rare) (12,13).
- Atrial dysrhythmias (including atrial fibrillation) and less often, ventricular extra beats (including refractory ventricular tachycardia and fibrillation) (11–13).
- Ventricular dysfunction (usually global, less frequently segmental).
- Cardiac failure, pulmonary edema, and cardiogenic shock (with and without ischemic symptoms) (13–16).
- Sudden death, presumed to be caused by ventricular fibrillation (13,17,18).

In most patients with chest pain, with or without electrocardiographic changes, the creatinine kinase MB fraction remained normal (10,13,15).

Acute dilated cardiomyopathy with left ventricular dysfunction related temporally to fluorouracil and cisplatin infusion, with subsequent complete recovery, has been tentatively linked to fluorouracil (19). Other similar events have been reported (20,21). The association is more striking in patients who receive a continuous infusion of fluorouracil and in patients who receive concomitant cisplatin (22,23). For example, myocardial ischemia and infarction occur in about 10% of patients who receive fluorouracil by infusion and sudden death has occurred (24).

Five cases of paroxysmal atrial fibrillation and sinus bradycardia attributed to fluorouracil have been reported (25).

Acute pulmonary edema leading to lethal cardiogenic shock has been reported with fluorouracil. This occurred despite the fact that the patient had received eight infusions of leucovorin 100 mg/m^2 at weekly intervals (26).

Most often, cardiotoxicity develops during the second or later course of treatment, but some patients have problems during the first course (10). Those who develop cardiac toxicity and recover usually have symptoms again when re-challenged with another infusion (10,13).

Fluorouracil has also been associated with a number of vascular effects, particularly thromboembolic or circulatory in nature (27). Although Raynaud's phenomenon has been reported after cisplatin-based chemotherapy, the first case of digital ischemia and Raynaud's phenomenon has been reported with fluorouracil given in a De Gramond type schedule (28).

Mechanisms and pathophysiology
The mechanisms of fluorouracil cardiotoxicity are not known. Those that have been suggested include:

- direct uncoupling of electromechanical myocardial function at the level of ATP generation (20);
- an immunoallergic reaction following sensitization by a complex of fluorouracil and cardiac cells;
- vasospasm secondary either to fluorouracil or to released products;
- a direct toxic effect of the drug on the myocardium.

Most reports have attributed chest pain to vasospasm (29). Certainly, the ischemic-like pains and electrocardiographic findings, lack of changes in creatine kinase, and frequent responses to nitrates and at times to calcium antagonists in the setting of anatomically normal coronary angiography, plus reversible contractility defects suggest coronary vasospasm as a mechanism of fluorouracil cardiotoxicity. However, global dysfunction possibly due to stunned myocardium and the lack of universal response to coronary vasodilators leaves some questions about this hypothesis. Some investigators have postulated myocarditis or myocardiopathy (30–32). In 43 patients it did not interfere with the electrical properties of myocardial fibers (33).

Findings on autopsy and endomyocardial biopsy have shown diffuse, interstitial edema, intracytoplasmic vacuolization of myocytes, and no inflammatory infiltrate (34). Acute myocardial infarction has been demonstrated pathologically in some, but not all, patients with clinical infarction (10).

In patients with fluorouracil cardiotoxicity endothelin plasma concentrations were raised (35).

Susceptibility factors
With regard to susceptibility factors for cardiotoxicity with fluorouracil, there was no effect of age or sex on incidence (10). Symptoms have been reported in a 38-year-old man (16) and in several women in their forties (10,14) with no prior cardiac history. Cardiac findings have occurred when fluorouracil was given by infusion or bolus as a single agent or with cisplatin and other drugs (10,21). Although some felt that cardiac irradiation and pre-existing heart disease were susceptibility factors (11,36), others did not (10,37). Several investigators have

documented normal coronary arteries in patients with severe symptoms (13,14).

Frequency
The cardiotoxicity of fluorouracil was first identified in 1975 (38). Of 140 patients treated with intravenous 5-fluorouracil, 4 developed ischemic chest pain within 18 hours of either the second or third dose. In three of these patients the pain recurred after subsequent doses. Predose electrocardiograms in two cases were normal. None of the four patients had a history of ischemic heart disease, although all had received left ventricular irradiation (39).

A 5% incidence of cardiotoxicity-complicating high-dose infusion of fluorouracil 1000 mg/m^2/day for 4 days has been reported and correlated with plasma fluorouracil concentrations in excess of 450 mg/ml (40).

In 910 patients toxicity was life-threatening in 0.55% (41). A combination of cisplatin, fluorouracil, and etoposide given for advanced non-small cell cancer of the lung caused only the expected amount of hematological toxicity, but was associated with a higher than expected incidence of cardiac, pulmonary, and cerebrovascular toxicity, including two myocardial infarctions, two cases of congestive heart failure, one pulmonary embolus, and one cerebrovascular accident in a study of 35 patients (42).

In 1083 patients there was cardiotoxicity in 1.1% of all patients and in 4.6% of patients with prior evidence of heart disease (36).

Management
Some investigators have reported success in preventing cardiotoxicity with calcium antagonists, such as nifedipine and diltiazem (29), while others had less success (15,43). Two patients with proven fluorouracil cardiotoxicity did not have cardiotoxicity when treated with the specific thymidylate synthase inhibitor raltitrexed 3 mg/m^2 every 3 weeks (44). The authors commented that fluorouracil cardiotoxicity is therefore not mediated via thymidylate synthase.

In most cases, fluorouracil-induced dysrhythmias were treatable and the ischemic-like symptoms and electrocardiographic changes disappeared if the infusion was discontinued or responded to nitrates, allowing the infusion to continue. The abnormalities of segmental and global ventricular function reverted to normal within days to weeks of withdrawal. In some patients intravenous inotropic and vasodilator support was needed during the initial period (14–16,19).

However, in one case, both oral nitrates and calcium antagonists failed to prevent chest pain associated with 5-fluorouracil (45).

- About 48 hours after starting her first course of 5-fluorouracil (1000 mg/m^2/day) a woman developed anginal chest pain and electrocardiographic changes that eventually normalized. She was readmitted for her second cycle whilst taking amlodipine 10 mg/day and isosorbide dinitrate 40 mg/day, and after 42 hours into the second cycle had the same chest pain and electrocardiographic changes. These were only controlled by withdrawal of the 5-fluorouracil and the intravenous administration of glyceryl trinitrate.

Respiratory

Pulmonary toxicity in the form of fibrosing alveolitis has been attributed to fluorouracil.

- A 55-year-old man with gastric adenocarcinoma received fluorouracil 1 g intravenously each week for 9 weeks and mitomycin 10 mg intravenously every 3 weeks (46). After 12 treatments he developed severe dyspnea.

Although mitomycin C was most likely the agent responsible for pulmonary toxicity in this patient, combined use with fluorouracil as a contributing factor cannot be ruled out. Necropsy confirmed that the patient had interstitial fibrosis (47).

Nervous system

Fluorouracil can cause neurotoxicity (48), with an incidence of 5–15% and with all schedules of administration in common use (49,50). The toxicity is acute in onset and cumulative dose-dependency has not been observed.

Acute cerebellar dysfunction, with gait ataxia, nystagmus, dysmetria, and dysarthria, is the most common form of neurotoxicity (48,49). A rare problem is optic neuropathy and impaired vision (51).

The acute cerebellar syndrome is considered to be associated with peak concentrations of fluorouracil (48,52). Continuous 5-day infusions appear not to cause neurological toxicity, even when the total dose is higher, although high-dose infusions can cause encephalopathy, with symptoms varying from lethargy to coma (53).

Cerebral demyelination has been reported in a patient receiving fluorouracil and levamisole (54).

Two patients with some of the classic neurological complications of fluorouracil have been reported. One had a cerebellar syndrome in association with global motor weakness and bulbar palsy and the other a bilateral third cranial nerve palsy (55).

Peripheral neuropathy, possibly caused by fluorouracil, has been reported (56).

Five patients developed ischemic stroke within 2–5 days of finishing a 4-day course of fluorouracil plus low-dose cisplatin by continuous infusion (57). Whilst cisplatin has been implicated as having produced central ischemic events, most commonly in combination with vindesine and bleomycin, there has only been one other report involving fluorouracil. Although the causal link was not conclusive, the circumstantial evidence was strong.

The cause of neurotoxicity is not well understood. Acute neurological symptoms, including somnolence, cerebellar ataxia, and upper motor neuron signs, are primarily seen in patients receiving intracarotid infusions for head and neck tumors and also in patients receiving fluorouracil monotherapy in high doses. This syndrome has been reproduced in animals by a neurotoxic metabolite of fluorouracil, fluorocitrate, which has been believed to cause neurotoxicity (52,58). However, several patients have developed severe toxic symptoms due to deficiency

of dihydropyrimidine dehydrogenase, the enzyme that is mainly responsible for metabolizing fluorouracil (59). This toxicity appears to be due to the parent compound and not metabolites. Patients with complete or partial deficiency of the enzyme are particularly subject to fluorouracil neurotoxicity.

The neurotoxicity is usually reversible by withdrawing fluorouracil. Since there is no cumulative effect, therapy can be resumed later if desired, usually with either a lower dose or a less frequent dosing schedule to prevent recurrence.

Sensory systems

Fluorouracil-containing regimens have been linked with several ocular adverse effects, including marked lacrimation, ocular pruritus, and a burning sensation in the eyes (60).

Striate melanokeratosis of the retina has been associated with 5-fluorouracil in reports from a number of centers; there has been no consistent explanation of the pathogenesis of this adverse effect (61–63).

Excessive lacrimation and other ocular disturbances have been reported secondary to intravenous fluorouracil (64–66). In a review of this subject, blurred vision, excessive lacrimation, excessive nasal discharge, and conjunctivitis were the most commonly reported ocular effects of fluorouracil (67). The symptoms, eye irritation and excessive tear production, can be aggravated by cold weather. The onset of symptoms varies from 15 minutes to 14 months after the start of treatment (64). The symptoms usually resolve 2–3 weeks after withdrawal of therapy, with or without the use of topical antibiotic-glucocorticoid combinations (64,67).

More severe toxic effects, including tear duct fibrosis and eversion of the lower eye lid, have been reported (64). Tear duct fibrosis develops in one of six patients with excessive lacrimation from fluorouracil (66). The eversion of the lower eyelid is reversible with conservative management (68) while the tear duct fibrosis may not be (69). Persistent lacrimation has been described in six patients receiving intravenous fluorouracil weekly for 6–10 months (69). Lacrimation persisted in five patients after the withdrawal of fluorouracil, suggesting an irreversible dacryostenosis. Lacrimal duct stenosis has also been reported (70). Bilateral cicatricial ectropion was also reported in a patient after topical administration of fluorouracil for the treatment of multiple facial actinic keratoses (71). If ectropion and tear duct stenosis progress, surgical correction may be required.

Three women developed lacrimal outflow obstruction while receiving fluorouracil, cyclophosphamide, and methotrexate for breast cancer (72). The authors commented on both the high incidence of excessive tearing in patients given fluorouracil, a probable precondition, and the rarity of permanent damage (12 patients reported worldwide), but counselled on the need for vigilance and early referral to an ophthalmologist. Others have suggested that the prevalence of tearing and canalicular fibrosis in patients receiving fluorouracil is related to total dose and duration of treatment, and that the risks become significant at 20–60 weeks of therapy and a total fluorouracil dose of 20–50 g (73).

- Ankyloblepharon (adherence of the eyelids resulting in narrowing of palpebral apertures) was reported in a 59-year-old man during fluorouracil therapy for metastatic adenocarcinoma of the stomach (74). It appeared that bilateral conjunctival ulcers, secondary to fluorouracil and ulcerative blepharitis, resulted in ankyloblepharon. Withdrawal of chemotherapy resulted in improvement and re-initiation of therapy resulted in recurrence of ocular lesions.

Transient, non-infectious, crystalline, intrastromal corneal deposits have been reported after subconjunctival administration of 5-fluorouracil (75). The deposits were treated with glucocorticoids and completely resolved in 4 days.

Psychological, psychiatric

Confusion and cerebral cognitive defects have been attributed to fluorouracil (49,76).

Metabolism

Patients with poorly controlled diabetes are at risk of greater or more severe fluorouracil toxicity, causing hyperglycemia, which has been fatal. This effect seems to be independent of previous diabetic control and or fluorouracil dosage schedules (77).

There have been attempts to unravel the mechanism of fluorouracil-induced hyperammonemia, lactic acidosis, and encephalopathy, a rare adverse effect associated with high-dose therapy. The cause is not known, although Krebs cycle metabolism is almost certainly involved (78,79).

Hematologic

The hematological toxicity of fluorouracil is dose- and schedule-related (80). Leukocytes and platelets are affected, although the latter less so. Myelosuppression begins 4–7 days after the first dose, with recovery usually 14 days after the last dose (2). With continued treatment, anemia can develop in 3–4 months (81). Severe bone marrow depression causing death has been reported (82).

Leukopenia is the most common blood dyscrasia secondary to fluorouracil and usually occurs after every course. The lowest white cell counts are usually seen at 9–14 days after the first course of treatment, but can be delayed for up to 20 days (83,84). Leukopenia usually resolves after drug withdrawal. Leukopenia is often followed by megaloblastic anemia (85). Agranulocytosis has been reported during fluorouracil therapy (84).

Thrombocytopenia has occurred during fluorouracil therapy but is much less frequent than leukopenia (59).

The following summarizes the dose-relatedness of the hematological effects of fluorouracil (86,87):

- With a daily bolus of 12 mg/kg for 5 days, leukopenia (under $4 \times 10^9/l$) occurred in all of 70 patients; 31% had marked leukopenia (under $2 \times 10^9/l$).

- With a continuous infusion of 30 mg/kg/day for 5 days, the leukopenia was mild and occurred in only 12% of patients.
- A protracted continuous infusion of 300 mg/m^2/day caused one case of moderate leukopenia and four cases of mild/moderate thrombocytopenia.
- With a daily bolus of 500 mg/m^2 for 5 days there was a 38% incidence of leukopenia (with 20% below $2 \times 10^9/l$ and an 8% incidence of thrombocytopenia (1% severe).

Gastrointestinal

The gastrointestinal toxicity of 5-fluorouracil is well documented and often dose-limiting. However, in a retrospective 10-year survey of gastrointestinal function in 19 patients who also had inflammatory bowel disease, although it did appear to increase the risk of exacerbation of diarrhea, it was not totally conclusive, as it was difficult to evaluate the contribution of other potentially causative factors, such as radiation (88).

Any site along the gastrointestinal tract can be affected, resulting in symptoms such as nausea and vomiting, stomatitis, dysphagia, retrosternal burning, abdominal pain, diarrhea, and proctitis.

Stomatitis is common and can be severe and life-threatening (84). Stomatitis may be preceded by a dry mouth and erythema of the mucosa followed by a white patchy membrane. In severe cases this is followed by ulceration and necrosis. Breakdown of the mucosa is very painful and can act as a focus for infection (2). Xerostomia at the start of therapy and a baseline neutrophil count of under $4 \times 10^9/l$ are significantly associated with dose-limiting oral mucositis later in chemotherapy, according to the results of a logistic regression analysis of 63 patients (89). Mouth-cooling with oral ice chips for 30 minutes starting immediately before fluorouracil substantially reduced the severity of mucositis.

Nausea and vomiting are common but generally mild (84).

Gastric ulceration has been reported in patients receiving fluorouracil by intrahepatic infusion via percutaneous catheterization in doses of 20–30 mg/kg for 4 days followed by 15 mg/kg over 17 days. Symptoms were observed from 4 to 20 days after starting therapy (90). Gastrointestinal bleeding in three patients and death in one patient were also reported following intra-arterial fluorouracil (91).

Diarrhea is common, particularly in patients who receive a 5-day regimen. The diarrhea can be watery or bloody and life-threatening in severe cases. Repeated episodes of watery diarrhea (more than three movements per day) for several days should alert the oncologist to the potential dangers of dehydration and sepsis, which are potentially fatal adverse effects. Life-threatening diarrhea, with hematemesis, high intestinal obstruction, melena, septicemia, and shock, have been reported after total doses of 4–4.5 g of fluorouracil (92). Similarly, diarrhea followed by neutropenia and life-threatening or fatal sepsis occurred in two of 55 patients with advanced colorectal carcinoma in a pilot study of continuous infusion of fluorouracil (750 mg/m^2/day for 5 days) plus subcutaneous recombinant interferon alfa-2a (6–18 million units/day) (93). Severe diarrhea and mucosal ulceration of the colon with necrosis has also been reported (94).

- A 53-year-old man had a side-to-side ileo-descending colostomy for disseminated carcinoma. Fluorouracil was given in doses of 15 mg/kg for 4 days, then 7.5 mg/kg intravenously on days 6 and 8. He developed severe diarrhea and severe ulceration of the by-passed portion of the colon, resulting in necrosis, and death occurred as the result of bronchopneumonia. Autopsy showed ulcers from the ileocecal valve to the ileocolostomy site. The mucosa of the stomach, small intestine, and colon distal to the colostomy were not involved.

In two cases the diarrhea and colitis associated with fluorouracil therapy were caused by toxigenic *Clostridium difficile*. Both patients responded to oral vancomycin (95).

Colitis has been reported as a rare complication of fluorouracil treatment. Two cases have been reported after intra-arterial chemotherapy (96). A further case has been reported, described by the authors as neutropenic enterocolitis, presenting as abdominal pain, diarrhea, and neutropenia (97). Proven pseudomembranous colitis followed 36 weekly doses of fluorouracil (700 mg) and folinic acid (150 mg); the authors believed that this was only the second reported case (98).

Liver

It has been suggested that handling cytostatic agents can insidiously cause hepatic damage and possibly irreversible fibrosis. Three case reports of hepatic injury in nurses after years of handling cytotoxic drugs (bleomycin, vincristine, cyclophosphamide, doxorubicin, dacarbazine, fluorouracil, and methotrexate) have been described (99). All had neurological symptoms associated with raised serum alanine transaminase and alkaline phosphatase activities. Liver biopsy showed portal hepatitis, with piecemeal necrosis in one and hepatic fibrosis and fat accumulation in the others.

- Diffuse hepatic necrosis has been described in a 29-year-old man receiving 500 mg/day fluorouracil for 4 days (route of administration unspecified) for adenocarcinoma (100). He developed nausea, vomiting, diarrhea, and massive and diffuse hepatic necrosis. The drug was withdrawn and he died 2 days later (6 days after starting medication).

However, the role of fluorouracil in inducing hepatic disease in this patient is unclear.

In a retrospective analysis of a study of *N*-phosphonoacetyl-L-aspartate (250 mg/m^2) followed by weekly boluses of fluorouracil (600–800 mg/m^2) in 44 patients with metastatic colorectal cancer, five of 17 patients with complete or partial responses to therapy developed transient ascites (with or without associated hypoalbuminemia) compared with one of 27 without such a response (101). Other significant findings in some of the responders included raised bilirubin concentrations and

transaminase activities from metastasis. The authors cautioned that the adverse effects observed do not necessarily represent disease progression.

Biliary tract

Intrahepatic infusion of fluorouracil can cause biliary sclerosis (102), believed to result from perfusion of the blood supply to the gall bladder and upper bile duct with high local concentrations of the drug. The median time to onset of biliary sclerosis is three treatment cycles, and although fluorouracil may be restarted at a lower dose after normalization of serum hepatic enzyme activities, most patients become progressively less tolerant.

Of 57 consecutive patients treated with implanted hepatic arterial infusion pumps with a regimen of alternating floxuridine (0.1 mg/kg/day for 7 days) followed by a weekly pump bolus of 5-fluorouracil (15 mg/kg for 3 weeks), two developed biliary sclerosis and 12 had mild transient liver function abnormalities (103). The liver alone or in combination with another area was the site of first progression of disease in 40 patients.

Skin

Two types of skin rashes occur with fluorouracil. The more common form involves erythema of exposed skin areas. With continued fluorouracil therapy the skin becomes hyperpigmented, thin, and atrophic (82). Patients treated with fluorouracil also have an increased susceptibility to sunburn (104). Less commonly (about 1.5%), a severe seborrheic pruritic dermatitis occurs (82). These rashes are usually reversible on withdrawal of fluorouracil. Acute, painful, swollen, and self-limiting erythema of the hands and soles has been reported in association with protracted infusion of fluorouracil (105).

Fluorouracil commonly causes hyperpigmentation and multiple pigmented macules (106). Serpentine supravenous hyperpigmentation is a peculiar dermatological effect seen with continuous infusions of fluorouracil (82,107). Residual macular pigmentation can persist for 3 months after withdrawal. Hyperpigmentation occurs only in the tissues overlying the veins proximal to the infusion site in the limb used. The veins are not sclerosed and usually remain patent (108). This has also been reported in a 56-year-old black man after intravenous fluorouracil 750 mg/m^2/week over 24 weeks for stage-D prostatic carcinoma (109). The patient developed nasal mucosal friability, diffuse pigmentation of the face and hands, and markedly increased pigmentation of the skin immediately overlying the veins that had been used for multiple fluorouracil infusions. Many irregular dark streaks were noted, extending from the hand to the shoulder. These streaks were 1–1.5 cm wide and serpiginous in their course.

Fluorouracil, alone or in combination regimens, via continuous or intermittent infusions or bolus doses, has been associated with hand–foot syndrome or palmar–plantar erythrodysesthesia, a rare syndrome of unknown cause, characterized by varying degrees of painful, erythematous, swollen palms of the hand and soles of the feet (110). Tingling, tenderness, and desquamation can also occur. The pain can be so severe as to inhibit walking and hand grasping (110). The onset of the reaction has ranged from 3 days to 10 months (110,111). Severity appeared to be dose-related in one case (112). The condition gradually subsides over 5–7 days when the drug is withdrawn (112). However, it may recur on rechallenge (111). Pyridoxine 100–150 mg/day has been used to manage this syndrome, allowing continued treatment in a small number of patients (113,114). Topical 5-fluorouracil often causes skin irritation. However, allergic contact dermatitis is only infrequently reported, although it may be underdiagnosed.

- A 64-year-old man was treated with Efudix ointment (containing 5% fluorouracil) for actinic keratosis (115). Patch-testing with the constituents of the cream showed a doubtful reaction to fluorouracil 5% in petroleum jelly; however, intradermal injection of fluorouracil 10 mg/ml gave a positive reaction.

Topical fluorouracil has been associated with allergic contact dermatitis in patients with actinic keratosis and basal cell epitheliomas (116). Topical fluorouracil ointment (5%) was reported to exacerbate dermatitis when it was mistakenly given instead of fluocinonide ointment (117).

Telangiectasia and herpes labialis have been reported in four patients receiving topical 1% fluorouracil in propylene glycol applied three times a day for 7–28 days. Two patients developed herpes labialis 7–10 days after the start of therapy and two developed persistent telangiectasia at the application site (118).

- Bullous pemphigoid has been reported in an 84-year-old man after topical therapy with fluorouracil 1% solution daily over several days for actinic keratosis. All treated lesions became bullous, with the development of a few bullae on untreated areas of normal skin. Bullous lesions were pruritic and sore and some contained hemorrhagic fluid. There was a leukocytosis (11.7×10^9/l). The blister fluid contained predominantly eosinophils, and immunofluorescent studies of the serum and blister fluid showed anti-basement membrane antibody titers of 1:640 and 1:160 respectively. Fluorouracil was discontinued and the patient was treated with steroids and saline compresses, with abatement of symptoms (119).

Fluorouracil not only augments the therapeutic effect of ionizing radiation on tumors, but also increases its mucocutaneous toxicity. The likelihood of severe toxicity within the radiation field is increased significantly and relates to the area irradiated (for example oral stomatitis, esophagitis, enteritis, and skin desquamation). The onset of these effects is within 7 days of the start of radiation.

Hair

Partial reversible alopecia is common after systemic fluorouracil therapy (84).

Nails

Diffuse blue superficial pigmentation, onycholysis, dystrophy, pain and thickening of the nail bed, transverse striations, paronychial inflammation, hyperpigmentation, and nail loss have all been reported with fluorouracil therapy (120–122). It has further been reported that the blue pigment may be scraped off (120).

Sexual function

Vaginitis (shedding of the vaginal epithelium) may be nearly as common as mucositis in women receiving systemic fluorouracil-based chemotherapy regimens (123).

Immunologic

- An anaphylactic reaction with shock after a 10th dose of fluorouracil 900 mg intravenously was reported in a 60-year-old man with colorectal adenocarcinoma (124). Two minutes after his 10th dose of fluorouracil, he became cyanotic and collapsed, with a rapid thready pulse of 120. His blood pressure was 30/0 mmHg. Adrenaline 1:1000, 1 ml, was given, with immediate and prompt signs of recovery. Within 25 minutes, his blood pressure, pulse, and skin color had returned to normal.

Second-Generation Effects

Pregnancy

Fluorouracil is contraindicated throughout pregnancy. The literature on pregnancy and cytotoxic drugs is necessarily limited, but it appears in general that risk of teratogenesis diminishes with the advancement of pregnancy. Therefore, most cytotoxic drugs are absolutely contraindicated in the first trimester, and when fluorouracil has been used in the first trimester it has been reported to cause multiple congenital abnormalities (125).

Administration of fluorouracil to pregnant rats on day 14 of gestation resulted in dose-dependent growth retardation and numerous malformations in near-term fetuses, including hind limb defects and cleft palate (126). After treatment, a number of rapid biochemical and cellular alterations were detectable in embryonic hind limbs and in craniofacial and other tissues, including inhibition of thymidylate synthetase and altered cell cycle progression. In order to assess the importance of these early events in fluorouracil-induced dysmorphogenesis, embryonic midfacial tissues and hind limbs were dissected 3 or 6 hours after administration of fluorouracil to the dam and placed in explant culture. After 5 days in culture, craniofacial explants were evaluated morphologically for palatal closure, and growth was assessed by measuring total protein and DNA contents. Hind-limb explants were stained for cartilage using Alcian blue to evaluate development of digits. Craniofacial explants cultured at either 3 or 6 hours after exposure showed dose-dependent growth retardation and defects of palatal fusion at the end of the culture period. Deficits in protein and DNA content were similar to those in craniofacial tissues that continued to develop in utero after treatment, although morphological defects in cultured explants did not correlate well with the incidence of cleft palate in vivo. Dose-dependent deficits in metatarsal and phalanx development were observed in hind-limb explants dissected either 3 or 6 hours after maternal treatment.

Susceptibility Factors

Genetic factors

Anabolism of fluorouracil to pyrimidine nucleotide analogues is required for its cytotoxic effects and pyrimidine catabolism is important in the regulation of fluorouracil availability and its subsequent anabolism. Dihydropyrimidine dehydrogenase is the initial enzyme of pyrimidine catabolism, accounting for degradation of greater than 80% of a dose of fluorouracil. The importance of catabolism and particularly dihydropyrimidine dehydrogenase in fluorouracil chemotherapy has previously been demonstrated in studies with competitive inhibitors of dihydropyrimidine dehydrogenase and in patients with suspected or proven dihydropyrimidine dehydrogenase deficiency. Before 1991, only two cases of dihydropyrimidine dehydrogenase deficiency associated with fluorouracil toxicity in adults were reported, and in both cases it was the fluorouracil toxicity that focused attention on pyrimidine catabolism. In 1991 a third case of dihydropyrimidine dehydrogenase deficiency was reported (127), suggesting that it may be more frequent than initially thought. There was complete deficiency of dihydropyrimidine dehydrogenase in the affected patient, with evidence of partial deficiency in the patient's parents, daughter, brother, and the brother's children. This pattern of dihydropyrimidine dehydrogenase activity was consistent with the previous two reports, suggesting an autosomal recessive pattern of inheritance.

- A 35-year-old woman with breast carcinoma treated with doses of fluorouracil that were not unusually high. Chemotherapy with cyclophosphamide, fluorouracil, and methotrexate started 3 weeks after surgery. Following day 8 of the protocol, the patient had severe gastrointestinal adverse effects (nausea, prolonged vomiting, diarrhea, stomatitis), hematological toxicity (neutropenia), and fever. She also had mild neurological toxicity causing unsteadiness and difficulty in spelling simple words, which persisted for about 2 weeks.

The neurotoxicity of fluorouracil seems to be more prolonged and severe in patients with dihydropyrimidine dehydrogenase deficiency (128).

Only a few cases of dihydropyrimidine dehydrogenase deficiency have been identified: however, all cases exhibited remarkable toxicity. Enhanced toxicity occurring at normal doses is what usually sets these patients apart. The authors suggested that monitoring dihydropyrimidine dehydrogenase activity may be appropriate in the management of those who have severe toxicity from fluorouracil (127).

Additional studies are needed to characterize this genetic defect, in order to answer the following questions:

- What is the frequency of this gene defect in the general population?
- Does dihydropyrimidine dehydrogenase deficiency correlate with the occurrence of severe fluorouracil toxicity?
- Do individuals with partial dihydropyrimidine dehydrogenase deficiency (that is heterozygotes) have altered metabolism of fluorouracil?
- Is monitoring dihydropyrimidine dehydrogenase activity helpful in the management of patients experiencing severe toxicity to fluorouracil chemotherapy?

Age

Cancer is most common in older people, but little information is available with regard to the impact of age on the toxicity of chemotherapy. A study has been undertaken to determine if age is an independent risk factor for fluorouracil toxicity (129). Toxicity data from a prospective, randomized, multi-institution trial of fluorouracil-based treatment for advanced colorectal carcinoma were analysed. Toxicity for each organ system was graded. The results showed that advanced age was significantly associated with the occurrence of any severe toxicity (58 versus 36%), leukopenia (24 versus 10%), diarrhea (24 versus 14%), vomiting (15 versus 5%), severe toxicity in more than two organ systems (10 versus 3%), and treatment mortality (9 versus 2%). Age and sex were independent predictors of severe toxicity. Advanced age does not contraindicate the use of this type of chemotherapy, but monitoring for multiple organ toxicity and vigorous supportive care of those with toxicity are required.

Dosing decisions in older patients are difficult and must integrate assessments of organ function, co-morbidity, overall physical status, and goals of treatment, in an effort to ensure the best possible outcome for these patients.

Other features of the patient

Circadian variation in toxicity

If the rhythm in fluorouracil toxicity is linked to the asleep–awake circadian cycle across species, the least toxic time in man would correspond to 0400 hours. This hypothesis has been tested using a single-reservoir, programmable-in-time, external ambulatory pump (Chronopump, Autosyringe, Hooksett, USA) in 35 patients with metastatic colorectal cancer (130). Fluorouracil was infused for 5 days via an implanted venous access port, with peak drug delivery at 0400 hours and no infusion from 1800 to 2200 hours. Each course was repeated after a drug-free interval of 16 days. Intrapatient dose escalation was planned from 4 to 9 g/m^2/course (800–1800 mg/m^2/day for 5 days) if toxicity was less than grade 2 according to the World Health Organization (WHO). There was grade 2 or greater toxicity in under 5% of the courses, indicating adequate control of toxicity via dose escalation, and their incidence was dose-dependent. The median maximal tolerated dose was 7.5 mg/m^2/course in 30 patients assessed for this end point.

Cellular glutathione concentrations and fluorouracil toxicity

Little is known about whether components of the diet can modulate the efficacy of fluorouracil in patients with colon carcinoma. Glutathione, an important antioxidant and anticarcinogen, is present in many foods in varying amounts.

The effect of cellular glutathione concentration on the growth of human colon adenocarcinoma cells HT-29 and on the cytotoxic activity of fluorouracil in these cells has been studied (131). Glutathione and buthionine sulfoximine were used respectively to enhance or reduce the glutathione concentration in these cells. A 34% increase in cellular glutathione concentration had no effect on the growth of HT-29 cells, nor on the cytotoxic activity of fluorouracil. A 50% reduction in the cellular glutathione concentration enhanced fluorouracil cytotoxicity by 20–31%, depending on the fluorouracil concentration.

Drug Administration

Drug dosage regimens

Stomatitis and diarrhea are particularly frequent in patients who received a 5-day regimen. An alternative regimen using continuous intravenous infusion of fluorouracil at doses of 30 mg/kg/day for 5 days gives equivalent therapeutic results but a different pattern of toxicity (132). Gastrointestinal symptoms, such as stomatitis and diarrhea, are the principal dose-limiting toxic effects, but myelosuppression is less intense. When fluorouracil is given in combination with leucovorin in patients with metastatic colon cancer, there is enhanced gastrointestinal toxicity, irrespective of the fluorouracil schedule.

Drug administration route

Intravenous administration of fluorouracil 1 g has been compared with hepatic arterial infusion (133). When fluorouracil was administered over 2 hours, systemic drug exposure was 0.7 times lower and clearance 1.5 times higher with hepatic arterial infusion. When the duration of infusion was extended to 24 hours, systemic drug exposure was 0.4 times lower and the clearance was two- to three-fold higher with hepatic arterial infusion. For the 24-hour infusion, co-treatment with angiotensin II (given temporarily to increase tumor blood flow) and albumin microspheres, given to increase drug uptake by the liver via the hepatic artery produced an additional two-fold reduction in systemic fluorouracil exposure. Further evaluation is planned to determine if this will improve the therapeutic index of regionally administered fluorouracil.

Intraperitoneal administration of fluorouracil has been reported to produce a desirable regional advantage (134). The results of a phase I trial of intraperitoneal fluorouracil in escalating concentrations for 4 hours, along with a fixed dose of cisplatin 90 mg/m^2 every 28 days, has been used (135). There was dose-limiting neutropenia at a fluorouracil concentration of 20 mmol/l, although individual patients tolerated concentrations as high as 30 mmol/l. Other toxic effects included mild-to-moderate nausea and vomiting; diarrhea occurred less often. Peak plasma concentrations occurred 1 hour after instillation and there was a significant linear relation between the intraperitoneal fluorouracil dose and the peak plasma fluorouracil

concentration. At every dose, the mean peak intraperitoneal fluorouracil concentration exceeded that in the plasma by two to three log units.

Drug overdose

Cases of deliberate overdosage are unknown, but excessive duration or dosage of therapy will produce life-threatening toxicity because of the hematological effects and other symptoms and signs that are qualitatively similar to the adverse effects. There is no specific antidote to fluorouracil toxicity; treatment consists of supportive care, including G-CSF and antidiarrheal agents.

Drug–Drug Interactions

Allopurinol

Concurrent administration of allopurinol with fluorouracil inhibits the intracellular formation of fluorouridine monophosphate from fluorouracil in normal tissues. In tumor cells that activate fluorouracil by alternative pathways, antitumor responses are still seen (2). Allopurinol increased the half-life of high-dose fluorouracil when it was given by intravenous bolus but not when it was given by 5-day continuous infusion (2).

Allopurinol ameliorates fluorouracil-induced granulocytopenia and possibly lessens the severity of mucositis (136). Allopurinol mouthwash (450 mg total in methylcellulose) given immediately and 1, 2, and 3 hours after fluorouracil reduced the incidence and severity of mucositis in six patients (137) and in another study of 42 patients there was significant reduction of oral toxicity and prolonged pain relief (138). In a randomized, double-blind, placebo-controlled trial, in 44 patients, allopurinol mouthwashes resolved stomatitis in nine of 22 treated patients, and diminished its intensity in 10 (139). However, in another randomized, double-blind, crossover study of allopurinol, mouthwash in 77 patients did not ameliorate fluorouracil-induced mucositis (140), nor did allopurinol reduce the toxicity of intravenously administered fluorouracil (141). Allopurinol is not currently recommended in the prophylaxis of fluorouracil-induced mucositis.

Cimetidine

Pre-treatment for 4 weeks with cimetidine 1 g/day increased the oral systemic availability of fluorouracil by 74%; the AUC was increased by 27% and total body clearance was reduced by 28% (142).

Dipyridamole

The pharmacokinetics of fluorouracil have been studied with escalating doses as a 72-hour intravenous infusion alone or in combination with a fixed dose of dipyridamole, a nucleoside transport inhibitor, and an enhancer of fluorouracil cytotoxicity (143). Stomatitis was dose-limiting at a fluorouracil dose of 2300 mg/m^2/day. For courses given with fluorouracil alone, the pharmacokinetics were linear for doses of 185–2300 mg/m^2/day; however, above this dose total body clearance fell significantly. Dipyridamole increased the total body clearance of fluorouracil, resulting in significantly lower mean steady-state fluorouracil plasma concentrations over the dose range studied. The clinical observation that dipyridamole did not appear to modulate fluorouracil-induced mucositis or leukopenia can be explained by lower exposure to fluorouracil. The basis for this pharmacokinetic interaction is not understood but it serves to underscore the importance of incorporating pharmacokinetic analysis in clinical trials involving new drug combinations.

Folic acid, folinic acid, and calcium folinate

Reduced folates are co-factors for the 5-fluorodeoxyuridine monophosphate-thymidilate synthetase reaction. Leucovorin (calcium folinate) therefore potentiates the toxicity of 5-fluorouracil, and fatal adverse effects have been reported in patients over 65 years of age receiving high-dose treatment with leucovorin simultaneously with fluorouracil. DNA-directed toxicity is increased, whilst RNA-directed toxicity is not affected (146). A qualitative alteration in toxicity is reported with increased gastrointestinal toxicity (2). This has led some groups to recommend that initial dose of fluorouracil should be lowered by 20% and that therapy be stopped temporarily at the first sign of distal gastrointestinal adverse effects (SEDA-15, 414).

Interferons

Initial studies have suggested that interferons may have synergistic activity with fluorouracil (144,145). Interferon alfa-2b has also been associated with an 80% increase in fluorouracil AUC (146).

Interferon alfa

One would expect drugs with myelosuppressive effects to exacerbate the hematological toxicity of interferon alfa. However, even though interferon alfa is increasingly used with other cytotoxic drugs, no specific and unexpected adverse effects have been reported, except for the combination of interferon alfa with 5-fluorouracil, which produced increased serum concentrations of fluorouracil and a significantly higher incidence of severe adverse effects, namely gastrointestinal and myelosuppressive adverse effects (152,153).

Methotrexate

There is sequence-dependent synergy between fluorouracil and methotrexate. Pretreatment with methotrexate enhances the formation of fluorouridine monophosphate and hence fluorouridine triphosphate and RNA-directed toxicity. In studies in which methotrexate has been given 1 hour before fluorouracil, response rates did not differ significantly. However, when it was given 4 hours or more before, there were significantly better response rates (147).

There is sequence-dependent synergy between fluorouracil and methotrexate. Pre-treatment with methotrexate enhances the formation of fluorouridine monophosphate and hence fluorouridine triphosphate; this enhances RNA-directed toxicity. In studies in which methotrexate has been given 1 hour before fluorouracil, response rates did not differ significantly. However, when it was given 4 hours or more before, there were significantly better response rates (154).

Metronidazole

Pretreatment with metronidazole increased the toxicity of fluorouracil given by daily bolus dose (148). The clinical significance of this is yet to be determined.

Pretreatment with metronidazole increased the toxicity of fluorouracil given by a daily bolus dose (151). The clinical significance of this is yet to be determined.

Platinum-containing cytostatic drugs

The combination of cisplatin 100 mg/m^2 with 5-fluorouracil 1000 mg/m^2 for 7 days caused angina and ischemic electrocardiographic changes, suggesting synergistic cardiotoxicity (155). There have also been cases of arterial occlusive events (156) and myocardial infarction (157,158), in some cases with evidence of coronary vascular spasm (159,160).

In 39 patients given low-dose continuous fluorouracil and cisplatin 20 mg/m^2/week for 8 weeks, there was a very low incidence of renal toxicity, although electrolyte abnormalities, particularly hyponatremia and hypomagnesemia, were as expected (161).

Pyridoxine

The dose and duration of protracted infusional fluorouracil is limited by mucositis, diarrhea, and/or palmar–plantar erythrodysesthesia. Typically, palmar–plantar dysesthesia begins several weeks to months after starting treatment. Although the dysesthesia abates within several weeks of discontinuing the infusion, it rapidly recurs when the infusion is resumed. Five patients who developed palmar–plantar dysesthesia during infusion of fluorouracil were treated with oral pyridoxine, 50 or 150 mg/day, once it reached moderate severity (149). The severity of the skin toxicity improved, with resolution of pain in four of the five patients, despite continued administration of fluorouracil. The ability of pyridoxine to modulate fluorouracil-induced cutaneous toxicity is currently undergoing evaluation in the randomized trial (150).

Topoisomerase inhibitors

If irinotecan is combined with 5-fluorouracil and calcium folinate, an infusion regimen of fluorouracil rather than bolus administration is associated with a lower incidence of severe toxicity (leukopenia and life-threatening sepsis) (162).

Other Environmental Interactions

Ionizing radiation

Fluorouracil increases the activity and toxicity of ionizing radiation (2).

References

1. Leichman CG, Fleming TR, Muggia FM, Tangen CM, Ardalan B, Doroshow JH, Meyers FJ, Holcombe RF, Weiss GR, Mangalik A, et al. Phase II study of fluorouracil and its modulation in advanced colorectal cancer: a Southwest Oncology Group study. J Clin Oncol 1995;13(6):1303–11.
2. Chabner BA, Myers CE. Clinical pharmacology of cancer chemotherapy. In: Devita VT, Hellman S, Rosenberg SA, editors. Cancer: Principles and Practice of Oncology. 3rd ed.. Philadelphia: Lippincoft, 1990:349–95.
3. Sullivan RD, Young CW, Miller E, Glatstein N, Clarkson B, Burchenal JH. The clinical effects of the continuous administration of fluorinated pyrimidines (5-fluorouracil and 5-fluoro-2'-deoxyuridine). Cancer Chemother Rep 1960;8:77–83.
4. Ardalan B, Singh G, Silberman H. A randomized phase I and II study of short-term infusion of high-dose fluorouracil with or without N-(phosphonacetyl)-L-aspartic acid in patients with advanced pancreatic and colorectal cancers. J Clin Oncol 1988;6(6):1053–8.
5. Yoshida T, Araki E, Iigo M, Fujii T, Yoshino M, Shimada Y, Saito D, Tajiri H, Yamaguchi H, Yoshida S, Ohkura H, Yoshimori M, Okazaki N. Clinical significance of monitoring serum levels of 5-fluorouracil by continuous infusion in patients with advanced colonic cancer. Cancer Chemother Pharmacol 1990;26(5):352–4.
6. Thyss A, Milano G, Renee N, Vallicioni J, Schneider M, Demard F. Clinical pharmacokinetic study of 5-FU in continuous 5-day infusions for head and neck cancer. Cancer Chemother Pharmacol 1986;16(1):64–6.
7. Farooqi IS, Aronson JK. Iatrogenic chest pain: a case of 5-fluorouracil cardiotoxicity. QJM 1996;89(12):953–5.
8. Clavel M, Simeone P, Grivet B. Toxicité cardiaqué du 5-fluorouracile. Revue de la litterature, cinq nouveaux cas. [Cardiac toxicity of 5-fluorouracil. Review of the literature, 5 new cases.] Presse Méd 1988;17(33):1675–8.
9. Robben NC, Pippas AW, Moore JO. The syndrome of 5-fluorouracil cardiotoxicity. An elusive cardiopathy. Cancer 1993;71(2):493–509.
10. Lomeo AM, Avolio C, Iacobellis G, Manzione L. 5-Fluorouracil cardiotoxicity. Eur J Gynaecol Oncol 1990;11(3):237–41.
11. Rezkalla S, Kloner RA, Ensley J, al-Sarraf M, Revels S, Olivenstein A, Bhasin S, Kerpel-Fronious S, Turi ZG. Continuous ambulatory ECG monitoring during fluorouracil therapy: a prospective study. J Clin Oncol 1989;7(4):509–14.
12. Collins C, Weiden PL. Cardiotoxicity of 5-fluorouracil. Cancer Treat Rep 1987;71(7–8):733–6.
13. Freeman NJ, Costanza ME. 5-Fluorouracil-associated cardiotoxicity. Cancer 1988;61(1):36–45.
14. McKendall GR, Shurman A, Anamur M, Most AS. Toxic cardiogenic shock associated with infusion of 5-fluorouracil. Am Heart J 1989;118(1):184–6.
15. Patel B, Kloner RA, Ensley J, Al-Sarraf M, Kish J, Wynne J. 5-Fluorouracil cardiotoxicity: left ventricular dysfunction and effect of coronary vasodilators. Am J Med Sci 1987;294(4):238–43.
16. Misset B, Escudier B, Leclercq B, Rivara D, Rougier P, Nitenberg G. Acute myocardiotoxicity during 5-fluorouracil therapy. Intensive Care Med 1990;16(3):210–1.
17. Eskilsson J, Albertsson M, Mercke C. Adverse cardiac effects during induction chemotherapy treatment with cisplatin and 5-fluorouracil. Radiother Oncol 1988;13(1):41–6.
18. Mortimer JE, Higano C. Continuous infusion 5-fluorouracil and folinic acid in disseminated colorectal cancer. Cancer Invest 1988;6(2):129–32.
19. Coronel B, Madonna O, Mercatello A, Caillette A, Moskovtchenko JF. Myocardiotoxicity of 5 fluorouracil. Intensive Care Med 1988;14(4):429–30.
20. Chaudary S, Song SY, Jaski BE. Profound, yet reversible, heart failure secondary to 5-fluorouracil. Am J Med 1988;85(3):454–6.
21. Jakubowski AA, Kemeny N. Hypotension as a manifestation of cardiotoxicity in three patients receiving cisplatin and 5-fluorouracil. Cancer 1988;62(2):266–9.
22. de Forni M, Malet-Martino MC, Jaillais P, Shubinski RE, Bachaud JM, Lemaire L, Canal P, Chevreau C, Carrie D, Soulie P, Roche H, Boudjema B, Mihura J, Martino R, Bernadet P, Bugat R. Cardiotoxicity of high-dose continuous infusion fluorouracil: a prospective clinical study. J Clin Oncol 1992;10(11):1795–801.
23. Ensley J, Kish J, Tapazoglou E, et al. 5-FU infusions associated with an ischaemic cardiotoxicity syndrome. Proc Am Soc Clin Oncol 1986;5:142.
24. Gradishar WJ, Vokes EE. 5-Fluorouracil cardiotoxicity: a critical review. Ann Oncol 1990;1(6):409–14.
25. Aziz SA, Tramboo NA, Mohi-ud-Din K, Iqbal K, Jalal S, Ahmad M. Supraventricular arrhythmia: a complication of 5-fluorouracil therapy. Clin Oncol (R Coll Radiol) 1998;10(6):377–8.
26. Wang WS, Hsieh RK, Chiou TJ, Liu JH, Fan FS, Yen CC, Tung SL, Chen PM. Toxic cardiogenic shock in a patient receiving weekly 24-h infusion of high-dose 5-fluorouracil and leucovorin. Jpn J Clin Oncol 1998;28(9):551–4.
27. Doll DC, Yarbro JW. Vascular toxicity associated with chemotherapy and hormonotherapy. Curr Opin Oncol 1994;6(4):345–50.
28. Papamichael D, Amft N, Slevin ML, D'Cruz D. 5-Fluorouracil-induced Raynaud's phenomenon. Eur J Cancer 1998;34(12):1983.
29. Kleiman NS, Lehane DE, Geyer CE Jr, Pratt CM, Young JB. Prinzmetal's angina during 5-fluorouracil chemotherapy. Am J Med 1987;82(3):566–8.
30. Liss RH, Chadwick M. Correlation of 5-fluorouracil (NSC-19893) distribution in rodents with toxicity and chemotherapy in man. Cancer Chemother Rep 1974;58(6):777–86.
31. Suzuki T, Nakanishi H, Hayashi A, et al. Cardiac toxicity of 5-FU in rabbits. Jpn J Pharmacol 1972;27(Suppl):137.
32. Matsubara I, Kamiya J, Imai S. Cardiotoxic effects of 5-fluorouracil in the guinea pig. Jpn J Pharmacol 1980;30(6):871–9.
33. Orditura M, De Vita F, Sarubbi B, Ducceschi V, Auriemma A, Infusino S, Iacono A, Catalano G. Analysis of recovery time indexes in 5-fluorouracil-treated cancer patients. Oncol Rep 1998;5(3):645–7.
34. Martin M, Diaz-Rubio E, Furio V, Blazquez J, Almenarez J, Farina J. Lethal cardiac toxicity after cisplatin and 5-fluorouracil chemotherapy. Report of a case with necropsy study. Am J Clin Oncol 1989;12(3):229–34.
35. Thyss A, Gaspard MH, Marsault R, Milano G, Frelin C, Schneider M. Very high endothelin plasma levels in patients with 5-FU cardiotoxicity. Ann Oncol 1992;3(1):88.
36. Labianca R, Beretta G, Clerici M, Fraschini P, Luporini G. Cardiac toxicity of 5-fluorouracil: a study on 1083 patients. Tumori 1982;68(6):505–10.
37. Jeremic B, Jevremovic S, Djuric L, Mijatovic L. Cardiotoxicity during chemotherapy treatment with 5-fluorouracil and cisplatin. J Chemother 1990;2(4):264–7.

38. Dent RG, McColl I. Letter: 5-Fluorouracil and angina. Lancet 1975;1(7902):347–8.

39. Pottage A, Holt S, Ludgate S, Langlands AO. Fluorouracil cardiotoxicity. BMJ 1978;1(6112):547.

40. Gamelin E, Gamelin L, Larra F, Turcant A, Alain P, Maillart P, Allain YM, Minier JF, Dubin J. Toxicité cardiaque aiguë du 5-fluorouracile: correlation pharmacocinétique. [Acute cardiac toxicity of 5-fluorouracil: pharmacokinetic correlation.] Bull Cancer 1991;78(12):1147–53.

41. Keefe DL, Roistacher N, Pierri MK. Clinical cardiotoxicity of 5-fluorouracil. J Clin Pharmacol 1993;33(11):1060–70.

42. Lynch TJ Jr, Kass F, Kalish LA, Elias AD, Strauss G, Shulman LN, Sugarbaker DJ, Skarin A, Frei E 3rd. Cisplatin, 5-fluorouracil, and etoposide for advanced non-small cell lung cancer. Cancer 1993;71(10):2953–7.

43. Burger AJ, Mannino S. 5-Fluorouracil-induced coronary vasospasm. Am Heart J 1987;114(2):433–6.

44. Kohne CH, Thuss-Patience P, Friedrich M, Daniel PT, Kretzschmar A, Benter T, Bauer B, Dietz R, Dorken B. Raltitrexed (Tomudex): an alternative drug for patients with colorectal cancer and 5-fluorouracil associated cardiotoxicity. Br J Cancer 1998;77(6):973–7.

45. Akpek G, Hartshorn KL. Failure of oral nitrate and calcium channel blocker therapy to prevent 5-fluorouracil-related myocardial ischemia: a case report. Cancer Chemother Pharmacol 1999;43(2):157–61.

46. Fielding JW, Stockley RA, Brookes VS. Interstitial lung disease in a patient treated with 5-fluorouracil and mitomycin C. BMJ 1978;2(6137):602.

47. Fielding JW, Crocker J, Stockley RA, Brookes VS. Interstitial fibrosis in a patient treated with 5-fluorouracil and mitomycin C. BMJ 1979;2(6189):551–2.

48. Moertel CG, Reitemeier RJ, Bolton CF, Shorter RG. Cerebellar ataxia associated with fluorinated pyrimidine therapy. Cancer Chemother Rep 1964;41:15–8.

49. Tuxen MK, Hansen SW. Neurotoxicity secondary to antineoplastic drugs. Cancer Treat Rev 1994;20(2):191–214.

50. Ranuzzi M, Taddei A. Neurotoxicity of antineoplastic agents in chemotherapy. Nuova Riv Neurol 1996;6:55–63.

51. Adams JW, Bofenkamp TM, Kobrin J, Wirtschafter JD, Zeese JA. Recurrent acute toxic optic neuropathy secondary to 5-FU. Cancer Treat Rep 1984;68(3):565–6.

52. Weiss HD, Walker MD, Wiernik PH. Neurotoxicity of commonly used antineoplastic agents. N Engl J Med 1974;291(2):75–811974;291(3):127–33.

53. Shapiro WR, Young DF. Neurological complications of antineoplastic therapy. Acta Neurol Scand Suppl 1984;100:125–32.

54. Fassas AB, Gattani AM, Morgello S. Cerebral demyelination with 5-fluorouracil and levamisole. Cancer Invest 1994;12(4):379–83.

55. Bygrave HA, Geh JI, Jani Y, Glynne-Jones R. Neurological complications of 5-fluorouracil chemotherapy: case report and review of the literature. Clin Oncol (R Coll Radiol) 1998;10(5):334–6.

56. Stein ME, Drumea K, Yarnitsky D, Benny A, Tzuk-Shina T. A rare event of 5-fluorouracil-associated peripheral neuropathy: a report of two patients. Am J Clin Oncol 1998;21(3):248–9.

57. El Amrani M, Heinzlef O, Debroucker T, Roullet E, Bousser MG, Amarenco P. Brain infarction following 5-fluorouracil and cisplatin therapy. Neurology 1998;51(3):899–901.

58. Koenig H, Patel A. Biochemical basis for fluorouracil neurotoxicity. The role of Krebs cycle inhibition by fluoroacetate. Arch Neurol 1970;23(2):155–60.

59. Diasio RB, Beavers TL, Carpenter JT. Familial deficiency of dihydropyrimidine dehydrogenase. Biochemical basis for familial pyrimidinemia and severe 5-fluorouracil-induced toxicity. J Clin Invest 1988;81(1):47–51.

60. Loprinzi CL, Love RR, Garrity JA, Ames MM. Cyclophosphamide, methotrexate, and 5-fluorouracil (CMF)-induced ocular toxicity. Cancer Invest 1990;8(5):459–65.

61. Peterson MR, Skuta GL, Phelan MJ, Stanley SA. Striate melanokeratosis following trabeculectomy with 5-fluorouracil. Arch Ophthalmol 1990;108(9):1216–7.

62. Stank TM, Krupin T, Feitl ME. Subconjunctival 5-fluorouracil-induced transient striate melanokeratosis. Arch Ophthalmol 1990;108(9):1210.

63. Lemp MA. Striate melanokeratosis. Arch Ophthalmol 1991;109(7):917.

64. Christophidis N, Vajda FJ, Lucas I, Louis WJ. Ocular side effects with 5-fluorouracil. Aust NZ J Med 1979;9(2):143–4.

65. Hamersley J, Luce JK, Florentz TR, Burkholder MM, Pepper JJ. Excessive lacrimation from fluorouracil treatment. JAMA 1973;225(7):747–8.

66. Griffin JD, Garnick MB. Eye toxicity of cancer chemotherapy: a review of the literature. Cancer 1981;48(7):1539–49.

67. Imperia PS, Lazarus HM, Lass JH. Ocular complications of systemic cancer chemotherapy. Surv Ophthalmol 1989;34(3):209–30.

68. Straus DJ, Mausolf FA, Ellerby RA, McCracken JD. Cicatricial ectropion secondary to 5-fluorouracil therapy. Med Pediatr Oncol 1977;3(1):15–9.

69. Haidak DJ, Hurwitz BS, Yeung KY. Tear-duct fibrosis (dacryostenosis) due to 5-fluorouracil. Ann Intern Med 1978;88(5):657.

70. Prasad S, Kamath GG, Phillips RP. Lacrimal canalicular stenosis associated with systemic 5-fluorouacil therapy. Acta Ophthalmol Scand 2000;78(1):110–3.

71. Galentine P, Sloas H, Hargett N, Cupples HP. Bilateral cicatricial ectropion following topical administration of 5-fluorouracil. Ann Ophthalmol 1981;13(5):575–7.

72. Lee V, Bentley CR, Olver JM. Sclerosing canaliculitis after 5-fluorouracil breast cancer chemotherapy. Eye 1998;12(Pt 3a):343–9.

73. Hassan A, Hurwitz JJ, Burkes RL. Epiphora in patients receiving systemic 5-fluorouracil therapy. Can J Ophthalmol 1998;33(1):14–9.

74. Insler MS, Helm CJ. Ankyloblepharon associated with systemic 5-fluorouracil treatment. Ann Ophthalmol 1987;19(10):374–5.

75. Rothman RF, Liebmann JM, Ritch R. Noninfectious crystalline keratopathy after postoperative subconjunctival 5-fluorouracil. Am J Ophthalmol 1999;128(2):236–7.

76. Lynch HT, Droszcz CP, Albano WA, Lynch JF. "Organic brain syndrome" secondary to 5-fluorouracil toxicity. Dis Colon Rectum 1981;24(2):130–1.

77. Sadoff L. Overwhelming 5-fluorouracil toxicity in patients whose diabetes is poorly controlled. Am J Clin Oncol 1998;21(6):605–7.

78. Yeh KH, Cheng AL. High-dose 5-fluorouracil infusional therapy is associated with hyperammonaemia, lactic acidosis and encephalopathy. Br J Cancer 1997;75(3):464–5.

79. Valik D, Yeh KH, Cheng AL. Encephalopathy, lactic acidosis, hyperammonaemia and 5-fluorouracil toxicity. Br J Cancer 1998;77(10):1710–2.

80. Grem JL. Fluorinated pyrimidines. In: Chabner BA, Collins JM, editors. Cancer Chemotherapy: Principles and Practice. Philadelphia: Lippincoft, 1990:180–225.

81. Vaitkevicius VK, Brennan MJ, Beckett VL, Kelly JE, Talley RW. Clinical evaluation of cancer chemotherapy with 5-fluorouracil. Cancer 1961;14:131–52.

82. Reitemeier RJ, Moertel CG, Hahn RG. Comparison of 5-fluorouracil (NSC-19893) and 2'-deoxy-5-fluorouridine (NSC-27640) in treatment of patients with advanced adenocarcinoma of colon or rectum. Cancer Chemother Rep 1965;44:39–43.

83. Piro AJ, Wilson RE, Hall TC, Aliapoulios MA, Nevinny HB, Moore FD. Toxicity studies of fluorouracil used with adrenalectomy in breast cancer. Arch Surg 1972;105(1):95–9.

84. Cohn I Jr. Complications and toxic manifestations of surgical adjuvant chemotherapy for breast cancer. Surg Gynecol Obstet 1968;127(6):1201–9.

85. Scott JM, Weir DG. Drug-induced megaloblastic change. Clin Haematol 1980;9(3):587–606.

86. Seifert P, Baker LH, Reed ML, Vaitkevicius VK. Comparison of continuously infused 5-fluorouracil with bolus injection in treatment of patients with colorectal adenocarcinoma. Cancer 1975;36(1):123–8.

87. Lokich JJ, Ahlgren JD, Gullo JJ, Philips JA, Fryer JG. A prospective randomized comparison of continuous infusion fluorouracil with a conventional bolus schedule in metastatic colorectal carcinoma: a Mid-Atlantic Oncology Program Study. J Clin Oncol 1989;7(4):425–32.

88. Tiersten A, Saltz LB. Influence of inflammatory bowel disease on the ability of patients to tolerate systemic fluorouracil-based chemotherapy. J Clin Oncol 1996;14(7):2043–6.

89. McCarthy GM, Awde JD, Ghandi H, Vincent M, Kocha WI. Risk factors associated with mucositis in cancer patients receiving 5-fluorouracil. Oral Oncol 1998;34(6):484–90.

90. Narsete T, Ansfield F, Wirtanen G, Ramirez G, Wolberg W, Jarrett F. Gastric ulceration in patients receiving intrahepatic infusion of 5-fluorouracil. Ann Surg 1977;186(6):734–6.

91. Rousselot LM, Cole DR, Grossi CE. Gastrointestinal bleeding as a sequel to cancer chemotherapy. Am J Gastroenterol 1965;43:311–6.

92. Biran S, krasnokuki D, Brufman G. [Life-threatening gastrointestinal toxicity during 5-fluorouracil therapy.]Harefuah 1977;93(3–4):77.

93. Wadler S, Lyver A, Wiernik PH. Clinical toxicities of the combination of 5-fluorouracil and recombinant interferon alfa-2a: an unusual toxicity profile. Oncol Nurs Forum 1989;16(Suppl 6):12–5.

94. Barrett O Jr, Bourgeois C, Plecha FR. Fluorouracil toxicity following gastrointestinal surgery. Arch Surg 1965;91(6):1002–4.

95. Cudmore MA, Silva J Jr, Fekety R, Liepman MK, Kim KH. Clostridium difficile colitis associated with cancer chemotherapy. Arch Intern Med 1982;142(2):333–5.

96. Abe H, Tsunaga N, Yamashita S, Ishiguro K, Mitani I. [Anticancer drug-induced colitis—case report and review of the literature.]Gan To Kagaku Ryoho 1997;24(5):619–24.

97. Kronawitter U, Kemeny NE, Blumgart L. Neutropenic enterocolitis in a patient with colorectal carcinoma: unusual course after treatment with 5-fluorouracil and leucovorin—a case report. Cancer 1997;80(4):656–60.

98. Trevisani F, Simoncini M, Alampi G, Bernardi M. Colitis associated to chemotherapy with 5-fluorouracil. Hepatogastroenterology 1997;44(15):710–2.

99. Sotaniemi EA, Sutinen S, Arranto AJ, Sutinen S, Sotaniemi KA, Lehtola J, Pelkonen RO. Liver damage in nurses handling cytostatic agents. Acta Med Scand 1983;214(3):181–9.

100. Vestfrid MA, Castelleto L, Gimenez PO. Necrosis hepatica diffusa en el tratamiento con 5-fluorouracilo. [Diffuse liver necrosis in treatment with 5-fluorouracil.] Rev Clin Esp 1972;125(6):549–50.

101. Kemeny N, Seiter K, Martin D, Urmacher C, Niedzwiecki D, Kurtz RC, Costa P, Murray M. A new syndrome: ascites, hyperbilirubinemia, and hypoalbuminemia after biochemical modulation of fluorouracil with N-phosphonacetyl-L-aspartate (PALA). Ann Intern Med 1991;115(12):946–51.

102. Lorenz M, Hottenrott C, Reimann-Kirkowa M, Encke A. Regionale Therapie von isolierten Mamma-karzinom-Lebermetastasen. [Regional therapy of isolated liver metastases from breast cancer.] Geburtshilfe Frauenheilkd 1988;48(6):425–9.

103. Davidson BS, Izzo F, Chase JL, DuBrow RA, Patt Y, Hohn DC, Curley SA. Alternating floxuridine and 5-fluorouracil hepatic arterial chemotherapy for colorectal liver metastases minimizes biliary toxicity. Am J Surg 1996;172(3):244–7.

104. Falkson G, Schulz EJ. Skin changes in patients treated with 5-fluorouracil. Br J Dermatol 1962;74:229–36.

105. Bellmunt J, Navarro M, Hidalgo R, Sole LA. Palmar-plantar erythrodysesthesia syndrome associated with short-term continuous infusion (5 days) of 5-fluorouracil. Tumori 1988;74(3):329–31.

106. Cho KH, Chung JH, Lee AY, Lee YS, Kim NK, Kim CW. Pigmented macules in patients treated with systemic 5-fluorouracil. J Dermatol 1988;15(4):342–6.

107. Pujol RM, Rocamora V, Lopez-Pousa A, Taberner R, Alomar A. Persistent supravenous erythematous eruption: a rare local complication of intravenous 5-fluorouracil therapy. J Am Acad Dermatol 1998;39(5 Pt 2):839–42.

108. Dunagin WO. Dermatologic toxicity. In: Perry MC, Yarbro JW, editors. Toxicity of Chemotherapy. Orlando: Grune and Stratton, 1984:125–54.

109. Hrushesky WJ. Unusual pigmentary changes associated with 5-fluorouracil therapy. Cutis 1980;26(2):181–2.

110. Curran CF, Luce JK. Fluorouracil and palmar-plantar erythrodysesthesia. Ann Intern Med 1989;111(10):858.

111. Jorda E, Galan A, Betlloch I, Ramon D, Revert A, Torres V. Painful, red hands. A side effect of 5-fluorouracil by continuous perfusion. Int J Dermatol 1991;30(9):653.

112. Feldman LD, Ajani JA. Fluorouracil-associated dermatitis of the hands and feet. JAMA 1985;254(24):3479.

113. Vukelja SJ, Lombardo FA, James WD, Weiss RB. Pyridoxine for the palmar-plantar erythrodysesthesia syndrome. Ann Intern Med 1989;111(8):688–9.

114. Molina R, Fabian C, Slavik M, et al. Reversal of palmar-plantar erythrodysesthesia SPPE by B6 without loss of response in colon cancer patients receiving 200 mg/m²/day continuous 5-FU Proc Am Soc Clin Oncol 1987;6:90.

115. Sanchez-Perez J, Bartolome B, del Rio MJ, Garcia-Diez A. Allergic contact dermatitis from 5-fluorouracil with positive intradermal test and doubtful patch test reactions. Contact Dermatitis 1999;41(2):106–7.

116. Sams WM. Untoward response with topical fluorouracil. Arch Dermatol 1968;97(1):14–22.

117. Clemons DE, Aeling JL, Nuss DD. Dermatitis medicamentosa: a pitfall for the unwary. Arch Dermatol 1976;112(8):1179.

118. Burnett JW. Letter: Two unusual complications of topical fluorouracil therapy. Arch Dermatol 1975;111(3):398.

119. Bart BJ, Bean SF. Bullous pemphigoid following the topical use of fluorouracil. Arch Dermatol 1970;102(4):457–60.

120. Nixon DW, Pirozzi D, York RM, Black M, Lawson DH. Dermatologic changes after systemic cancer therapy. Cutis 1981;27(2):181–94.

121. Norton LA. Nail disorders. A review. J Am Acad Dermatol 1980;2(6):451–67.

122. Katz ME, Hansen TW. Nail plate-nail bed separation. An unusual side effect of systemic fluorouracil administration. Arch Dermatol 1979;115(7):860–1.

123. Moroni M, Porta C. Possible efficacy of allopurinol vaginal washings in the treatment of chemotherapy-induced vaginitis. Cancer Chemother Pharmacol 1998;41(2):171–2.

124. DeBeer R, Kabakow B. Anaphylactoid reaction. Associated with intravenous administration of 5-fluorouracil. NY State J Med 1979;79(11):1750–1.

125. Stephens JD, Golbus MS, Miller TR, Wilber RR, Epstein CJ. Multiple congenital anomalies in a fetus exposed to 5-fluorouracil during the first trimester. Am J Obstet Gynecol 1980;137(6):747–9.

126. Shuey DL, Buckalew AR, Wilke TS, Rogers JM, Abbott BD. Early events following maternal exposure to 5-fluorouracil lead to dysmorphology in cultured embryonic tissues. Teratology 1994;50(6):379–86.

127. Harris BE, Carpenter JT, Diasio RB. Severe 5-fluorouracil toxicity secondary to dihydropyrimidine dehydrogenase deficiency. A potentially more common pharmacogenetic syndrome. Cancer 1991;68(3):499–501.

128. Shehata N, Pater A, Tang SC. Prolonged severe 5-fluorouracil-associated neurotoxicity in a patient with dihydropyrimidine dehydrogenase deficiency. Cancer Invest 1999;17(3):201–5.

129. Stein BN, Petrelli NJ, Douglass HO, Driscoll DL, Arcangeli G, Meropol NJ. Age and sex are independent predictors of 5-fluorouracil toxicity. Analysis of a large scale phase III trial. Cancer 1995;75(1):11–7.

130. Levi F, Soussan A, Adam R, Caussanel JP, Metzger G, Jasmin C, Bismuth H, Smolensky M, Misset JL. A phase I–II trial of five-day continuous intravenous infusion of 5-fluorouracil delivered at circadian rhythm modulated rate in patients with metastatic colorectal cancer. J Infus Chemother 1995;5(3 Suppl 1):153–8.

131. Chen MF, Chen LT, Boyce HW Jr. 5-Fluorouracil cytotoxicity in human colon HT-29 cells with moderately increased or decreased cellular glutathione level. Anticancer Res 1995;15(1):163–7.

132. Lokich J, Bothe A, Fine N, Perri J. Phase I study of protracted venous infusion of 5-fluorouracil. Cancer 1981;48(12):2565–8.

133. Goldberg JA, Kerr DJ, Watson DG, Willmott N, Bates CD, McKillop JH, McArdle CS. The pharmacokinetics of 5-fluorouracil administered by arterial infusion in advanced colorectal hepatic metastases. Br J Cancer 1990;61(6):913–5.

134. Speyer JL, Collins JM, Dedrick RL, Brennan MF, Buckpitt AR, Londer H, DeVita VT Jr, Myers CE. Phase I and pharmacological studies of 5-fluorouracil administered intraperitoneally. Cancer Res 1980;40(3):567–72.

135. Schilsky RL, Choi KE, Grayhack J, Grimmer D, Guarnieri C, Fullem L. Phase I clinical and pharmacologic study of intraperitoneal cisplatin and fluorouracil in patients with advanced intraabdominal cancer. J Clin Oncol 1990;8(12):2054–61.

136. Woolley PV, Ayoob MJ, Smith FP, Lokey JL, DeGreen P, Marantz A, Schein PS. A controlled trial of the effect of 4-hydroxypyrazolopyrimidine (allopurinol) on the toxicity of a single bolus dose of 5-fluorouracil. J Clin Oncol 1985;3(1):103–9.

137. Clark PI, Slevin ML. Allopurinol mouthwashes and 5-fluorouracil induced oral toxicity. Eur J Surg Oncol 1985;11(3):267–8.

138. Tsavaris NB, Komitsopoulou P, Tzannou I, Loucatou P, Tsaroucha-Noutsou A, Kilafis G, Kosmidis P. Decreased oral toxicity with the local use of allopurinol in patients who received high dose 5-fluorouracil. Sel Cancer Ther 1991;7(3):113–7.

139. Porta C, Moroni M, Nastasi G. Allopurinol mouthwashes in the treatment of 5-fluorouracil-induced stomatitis. Am J Clin Oncol 1994;17(3):246–7.

140. Loprinzi CL, Cianflone SG, Dose AM, Etzell PS, Burnham NL, Therneau TM, Hagen L, Gainey DK, Cross M, Athmann LM, et al. A controlled evaluation of an allopurinol mouthwash as prophylaxis against 5-fluorouracil-induced stomatitis. Cancer 1990;65(8):1879–82.

141. Howell SB, Pfeifle CE, Wung WE. Effect of allopurinol on the toxicity of high-dose 5-fluorouracil administered by intermittent bolus injection. Cancer 1983;51(2):220–5.

142. Harvey VJ, Slevin ML, Dilloway MR, Clark PI, Johnston A, Lant AF. The influence of cimetidine on the pharmacokinetics of 5-fluorouracil. Br J Clin Pharmacol 1984;18(3):421–30.

143. Remick SC, Grem JL, Fischer PH, Tutsch KD, Alberti DB, Nieting LM, Tombes MB, Bruggink J, Willson JK, Trump DL. Phase I trial of 5-fluorouracil and dipyridamole administered by seventy-two-hour concurrent continuous infusion. Cancer Res 1990;50(9):2667–72.

144. Elias L, Crissman HA. Interferon effects upon the adenocarcinoma 38 and HL-60 cell lines: antiproliferative responses and synergistic interactions with halogenated pyrimidine antimetabolites. Cancer Res 1988;48(17):4868–73.

145. Wadler S, Wiernik PH. Clinical update on the role of fluorouracil and recombinant interferon alfa-2a in the treatment of colorectal carcinoma. Semin Oncol 1990;17(1 Suppl 1):16–21.

146. Schuller J, Czejka M, Miksche M, et al. Influence of interferon alpha-2b leucovorin on pharmacokinetics of 5-fluorouracil. Proc Am Soc Clin Oncol 1991;10:98.

147. Damon LE, Cadman E, Benz C. Enhancement of 5-fluorouracil antitumor effects by the prior administration of methotrexate. Pharmacol Ther 1989;43(2):155–85.

148. Bardakji Z, Jolivet J, Langelier Y, Besner JG, Ayoub J. 5-Fluorouracil–metronidazole combination therapy in metastatic colorectal cancer. Clinical, pharmacokinetic and in vitro cytotoxicity studies. Cancer Chemother Pharmacol 1986;18(2):140–4.

149. Fabian CJ, Molina R, Slavik M, Dahlberg S, Giri S, Stephens R. Pyridoxine therapy for palmar-plantar erythrodysesthesia associated with continuous 5-fluorouracil infusion. Invest New Drugs 1990;8(1):57–63.

150. Beveridge RA, Kales AN, Binder RA, Miller JA, Virts SG. Pyridoxine (B6) and amelioration of hand/foot syndrome. Proc Am Soc Clin Oncol 1990;9:102.

151. Bardakji Z, Jolivet J, Langelier Y, Besner JG, Ayoub J. 5-Fluorouracil–metronidazole combination therapy in metastatic colorectal cancer. Clinical, pharmacokinetic and in vitro cytotoxicity studies. Cancer Chemother Pharmacol 1986;18(2):140–4.

152. Czejka MJ, Schuller J, Jager W, Fogl U, Weiss C. Influence of different doses of interferon-alpha-2b on the blood plasma levels of 5-fluorouracil. Eur J Drug Metab Pharmacokinet 1993;18(3):247–50.

153. Greco FA, Figlin R, York M, Einhorn L, Schilsky R, Marshall EM, Buys SS, Froimtchuk MJ, Schuller J, Schuchter L, Buyse M, Ritter L, Man A, Yap AK. Phase III randomized study to compare interferon alfa-2a in combination with fluorouracil versus fluorouracil alone in patients with advanced colorectal cancer. J Clin Oncol 1996;14(10):2674–81.

154. Damon LE, Cadman E, Benz C. Enhancement of 5-fluorouracil antitumor effects by the prior administration of methotrexate. Pharmacol Ther 1989;43(2):155–85.

155. Coninx P, Nasca S, Lebrun D, Panis X, Lucas P, Garbe E, Legros M. Sequential trial of initial chemotherapy for advanced cancer of the head and neck. DDP versus DDP + 5-fluorouracil Cancer 1988;62(9):1888–92.

156. Stefenelli T, Kuzmits R, Ulrich W, Glogar D. Acute vascular toxicity after combination chemotherapy with cisplatin, vinblastine, and bleomycin for testicular cancer. Eur Heart J 1988;9(5):552–6.

157. Sasaki M, Suzuki A, Ishihara T. [A case of acute myocardial infarction after treatment with cisplatin.]Gan To Kagaku Ryoho 1989;16(6):2289–91.

158. Tsutsumi I, Ozawa Y, Kawakami A, Fujii H, Asamoto H. [Acute myocardial infarction induced by lung cancer chemotherapy with cisplatin and eto poside.]Gan To Kagaku Ryoho 1990;17(3 Pt 1):413–7.

159. Murin J, Kasper J, Danko J, Cerna M, Bulas J, Uhliar R. Vznik infarktu myokardu u choreho lieceneho 5-fluorouracilom. [The development of myocardial infarct in a patient treated with 5-fluorouracil.] Vnitr Lek 1989;35(10):1020–4.

160. Mazoyer G, Assouline D, Fourchard V, Kalb JC. Cardiotoxicité du 5 fluoro-uracile. A propos d'une observation. [Cardiotoxicity of 5 fluoro-uracil. Apropos of a case.] Rev Mal Respir 1989;6(6):551–3.

161. Williamson SK, Tangen CM, Maddox AM, Spiridonidis CH, Macdonald JS. Phase II evaluation of low-dose continuous 5-fluorouracil and weekly cisplatin in advanced adenocarcinoma of the stomach. A Southwest Oncology Group study. Am J Clin Oncol 1995;18(6):484–7.

162. Kohne CH, Van Cutsem E, Wils JA, Bokemeyer C, El-Serafi M, Lutz M, Lorenz M, Anak O, Genicot B, Nordlinger Bthe EORTC GI Group. Irinotecan improves the activity of the AIO regimen in metastatic colorectal cancer: results of EORTC GI-group study 40986. Proc Am Soc Clin Oncol 2003;22:A1018.

Gemcitabine

General Information

Gemcitabine is an S-phase-specific pyrimidine nucleoside analogue of deoxycytidine (2′,2′-difluorodeoxycytidine) that is structurally similar to cytosine arabinoside. It has been used to treat metastatic urothelial carcinoma of the bladder, pancreatic cancer, and some other solid tumors.

General adverse effects

In a retrospective study of the adverse effects of gemcitabine 1000 mg/m^2 on days 1 and 8 in patients with non-small cell lung cancers, the adverse effects of gemcitabine involved the gastrointestinal system (nausea, vomiting, and diarrhea) and the hemopoietic system (leukopenia, neutropenia, thrombocytopenia, and anemia), but only in the last (8th–11th) cycles (1). There was grade 4 vomiting in three patients, grade 4 thrombocytopenia in two, and grade 3 leukopenia in three. Other adverse effects were mild. None of the patients died during chemotherapy.

Organs and Systems

Cardiovascular

In a retrospective chart review of patients with gemcitabine-associated thrombotic microangiopathy diagnosed between January 1997 and February 2002, the cumulative incidence was 0.31% (8 cases among 2586 patients), higher than previously reported (0.015%) (2). The median age was 53 years, the median time to development was 8 (range 3–18) months, and the cumulative dose was 9–56 g/m^2. New or exacerbated hypertension was a prominent feature in seven of nine patients and preceded the diagnosis by 0.5–10 weeks. Treatment included withdrawal of gemcitabine, antihypertensive therapy, plasma exchange, and dialysis. Six patients survived and three died of disease progression; none died as a direct result of thrombotic microangiopathy, but two developed renal insufficiency requiring dialysis, and one developed chronic renal insufficiency.

Gemcitabine can occasionally cause systemic capillary leak syndrome (3,4).

Respiratory

Gemcitabine can cause pulmonary toxicity. The clinical presentation is subacute and often non-specific. Chest X-ray usually shows reticulonodular interstitial infiltrates (5).

- A 75-year-old man with non-small cell lung cancer developed acute respiratory distress syndrome after intravenous gemcitabine monotherapy (6). The total dose of gemcitabine was 1500 mg, and the latent period was 3 days. Chest X-rays and a high resolution CT scan showed bilateral ground-glass opacity. He died on the fourteenth postchemotherapeutic day in respiratory failure. Postmortem examination of the lung showed mixed exudative and fibrotic stages of diffuse alveolar damage.

In one study, the incidence was as high as 15%, even with low-dose gemcitabine 600 mg/m^2 on days 1, 8, and 15 and docetaxel 60 mg/m^2 on day 1; all resolved after withdrawal of treatment and administration of glucocorticoids (7).

In a retrospective review pulmonary toxicity was defined as dyspnea, interstitial pneumonitis, lung disorder, lung edema, lung fibrosis, pneumonia, respiratory disorder, and respiratory distress syndrome (8). Based on 4448 patients, the incidences of dyspnea and other serious pulmonary toxicity were 0.45 and 0.27% respectively. Based on an estimated 217 400 patients treated with commercial gemcitabine worldwide, the crude incidences of dyspnea and other serious pulmonary toxicity were 0.02 and 0.06% respectively.

In a retrospective study of 312 patients treated with gemcitabine over 5 years, 18 developed episodes of acute dyspnea; 6 were attributed to the drug; 4 had a notifiable industrial disease secondary to asbestos exposure (OR = 85, 95% CI = 13, 546); and 5 were active smokers (5).

Liver

- Fatal cholestatic liver failure occurred in a 45-year-old woman with metastatic breast cancer who was given gemcitabine and carboplatin and pre-existing liver damage. After four courses of gemcitabine + carboplatin she developed severe decompensated cholestatic hepatitis (9). Liver biopsy showed marked cholestasis and hepatocellular injury consistent with drug-induced hepatotoxicity.

Urinary tract

Hemolytic–uremic syndrome has occasionally been attributed to gemcitabine (10–12). The manufacturers reviewed their database of 78 800 patient exposures, which confirmed that gemcitabine causes hemolytic–uremic syndrome with a crude overall incidence rate of 0.015% (13).

Skin

Erythema multiforme has been attributed to gemcitabine (14). Toxic epidermal necrolysis has been reported in an elderly man receiving gemcitabine for a transitional cell carcinoma of the bladder (15).

- Scleroderma-like changes of the legs occurred after treatment with gemcitabine in a patient with metastatic carcinoma of the bladder (16). There was initial inflammatory edema and subsequent scleroderma-like changes after 2 cycles of gemcitabine. Cutaneous biopsies showed diffuse sclerosis without involvement of the fascia or muscle. Withdrawal of gemcitabine resulted in resolution of the edema, softening of the skin, and partial reversibility of the fibrotic process.

Patients occasionally develop erysipeloid skin reactions, often, although not always, associated with previous radiotherapy or lymphedema (17).

A cutaneous reaction mimicking acute lipodermato-sclerosis has been attributed to gemcitabine (18).

Immunologic

Two patients developed necrotizing enterocolitis after a first cycle of chemotherapy for epithelial ovarian/peritoneal cancer; both were due to vasculitis (19).

- In a 56-year-old man with a transitional cell carcinoma of the bladder gemcitabine plus cisplatin caused extensive necrotizing vasculitis with muscle damage after the second course of therapy (20). Chemotherapy was withdrawn immediately but the symptoms of severe myalgia and swelling persisted, and he needed additional treatment, consisting of cyclophosphamide and prednisolone.

Other cases of vasculitis have been reported (21).

- A 70-year-old woman with a bladder cancer was given gemcitabine 1700 mg on days 1 and 8 and 3–4 days later developed paresthesia of the fingers, Raynaud's phenomenon, an intermittent fever, digital necrosis, and fingertip gangrene (22). Angiography showed occlusion

of the digital arteries of the second, third, and fourth fingers. Skin biopsy showed hyperkeratosis, acanthosis, and papillomatosis, with endothelioangiitis and non-specific arterial inflammation.

Radiation recall consists of inflammatory reactions triggered by cytotoxic drugs in previously irradiated areas; most are skin reactions. Gemcitabine has been implicated in several cases. The authors of a literature review discovered 12 cases of radiation recall caused by gemcitabine and reported a case of myositis in the rectus abdominis muscle of a patient with pancreatic adenocarcinoma as an effect of radiation recall (23). Most of the cases had inflammation of internal organs or tissues and 30% had dermatitis or mucositis. This is different from the effect of other agents that commonly cause radiation recall (anthracyclines and taxanes), with which 63% are skin reactions. Compared with anthracyclines and taxanes, the interval from the completion of radiation therapy to the start of chemotherapy is less with gemcitabine (median time 56 days, compared with 218 days for the taxanes and 646 days for doxorubicin).

References

1. Gallelli L, Nardi M, Prantera T, Barbera S, Raffaele M, Arminio D, Pirritano D, Colosimo M, Maselli R, Pelaia G, De Gregorio P, De Sarro GB. Retrospective analysis of adverse drug reactions induced by gemcitabine treatment in patients with non-small cell lung cancer. Pharmacol Res 2004;49(3):259–63.
2. Humphreys BD, Sharman JP, Henderson JM, Clark JW, Marks PW, Rennke HG, Zhu AX, Magee CC. Gemcitabine-associated thrombotic microangiopathy. Cancer 2004;100(12):2664–70.
3. De Pas T, Curigliano G, Franceschelli L, Catania C, Spaggiari L, de Braud F. Gemcitabine-induced systemic capillary leak syndrome. Ann Oncol 2001;12(11):1651–2.
4. Pulkkanen K, Kataja V, Johansson R. Systemic capillary leak syndrome resulting from gemcitabine treatment in renal cell carcinoma: a case report. J Chemother 2003;15(3):287–9.
5. Barlesi F, Villani P, Doddoli C, Gimenez C, Kleisbauer JP. Gemcitabine-induced severe pulmonary toxicity. Fundam Clin Pharmacol 2004;18(1):85–91.
6. Maniwa K, Tanaka E, Inoue T, Kato T, Sakuramoto M, Minakuchi M, Maeda Y, Noma S, Kobashi Y, Taguchi Y. An autopsy case of acute pulmonary toxicity associated with gemcitabine. Intern Med 2003;42(10):1022–5.
7. Ryan DP, Kulke MH, Fuchs CS, Grossbard ML, Grossman SR, Morgan JA, Earle CC, Shivdasani R, Kim H, Mayer RJ, Clark JW. A Phase II study of gemcitabine and docetaxel in patients with metastatic pancreatic carcinoma. Cancer 2002;94(1):97–103.
8. Roychowdhury DF, Cassidy CA, Peterson P, Arning M. A report on serious pulmonary toxicity associated with gemcitabine-based therapy. Invest New Drugs 2002;20(3):311–5.
9. Robinson K, Lambiase L, Li J, Monteiro C, Schiff M. Fatal cholestatic liver failure associated with gemcitabine therapy. Dig Dis Sci 2003;48(9):1804–8.
10. Dilhuydy MS, Delclaux C, Pariente A, De Precigout V, Aparicio M. Syndrome hémolytique et urémique compliquant un traitement au long cours par gemcitabine. A propos d'un cas, revue de la litterature. [Hemolytic–uremic syndrome complicating a long-term treatment with

gemcitabine. Report of a case and review of the literature.] Rev Med Interne 2002;23(2):189–92.

11. Citarrella P, Gebbia V, Teresi M, Miceli S, Sciortino G, Vaglica M, Pizzardi N, Palmeri S. Hemolytic uremic syndrome after chemotherapy with gemcitabine and taxotere: a case report. Anticancer Res 2002;22(2B):1183–5.

12. Serke S, Riess H, Oettle H, Huhn D. Elevated reticulocyte count—a clue to the diagnosis of haemolytic–uraemic syndrome (HUS) associated with gemcitabine therapy for metastatic duodenal papillary carcinoma: a case report. Br J Cancer 1999;79(9–10):1519–21.

13. Fung MC, Storniolo AM, Nguyen B, Arning M, Brookfield W, Vigil J. A review of hemolytic uremic syndrome in patients treated with gemcitabine therapy. Cancer 1999;85(9):2023–32.

14. Sommers KR, Kong KM, Bui DT, Fruehauf JP, Holcombe RF. Stevens–Johnson syndrome/toxic epidermal necrolysis in a patient receiving concurrent radiation and gemcitabine. Anticancer Drugs 2003;14(8):659–62.

15. Mermershtain W, Cohen AD, Lazarev I, Grunwald M, Ariad S. Toxic epidermal necrolysis associated with gemcitabine therapy in a patient with metastatic transitional cell carcinoma of the bladder. J Chemother 2003;15(5):510–1.

16. Bessis D, Guillot B, Legouffe E, Guilhou JJ. Gemcitabine-associated scleroderma-like changes of the lower extremities. J Am Acad Dermatol 2004;51(Suppl 2):S73–6.

17. Kuku I, Kaya E, Sevinc A, Aydogdu I. Gemcitabine-induced erysipeloid skin lesions in a patient with malignant mesothelioma. J Eur Acad Dermatol Venereol 2002;16(3):271–2.

18. Chu CY, Yang CH, Chiu HC. Gemcitabine-induced acute lipodermatosclerosis-like reaction. Acta Dermatol Venereol 2001;81(6):426–8.

19. Geisler JP, Schraith DF, Manahan KJ, Sorosky JI. Gemcitabine associated vasculitis leading to necrotizing enterocolitis and death in women undergoing primary treatment for epithelial ovarian/peritoneal cancer. Gynecol Oncol 2004;92(2):705–7.

20. Birlik M, Akar S, Tuzel E, Onen F, Ozer E, Manisali M, Kirkali Z, Akkoc N. Gemcitabine-induced vasculitis in advanced transitional cell carcinoma of the bladder. J Cancer Res Clin Oncol 2004;130(2):122–5.

21. Voorburg AM, van Beek FT, Slee PH, Seldenrijk CA, Schramel FM. Vasculitis due to gemcitabine. Lung Cancer 2002;36(2):203–5.

22. D'Alessandro V, Errico M, Varriale A, Greco A, De Cata A, Carnevale V, Grilli M, De Luca P, Brucoli I, Susi M, Camagna A. Acronecrosi degli arti superiori da gemcitabina: segnalazione di un caso clinico. [Case report: Acro-necrosis of the upper limbs caused by gemcitabine therapy.] Clin Ter 2003;154(3):207–10.

23. Friedlander PA, Bansal R, Schwartz L, Wagman R, Posner J, Kemeny N. Gemcitabine-related radiation recall preferentially involves internal tissue and organs. Cancer 2004;100(9):1793–9.

Meraptopurine

See Azathioprine (p. 493)

Methotrexate

General Information

Methotrexate is a folic acid antagonist that acts by inhibiting dihydrofolate reductase. Owing to its immunosuppressive and anti-inflammatory properties, low-dosage methotrexate (7.5–15 mg/week) has been extensively investigated for other therapeutic purposes characterized by inflammation or cellular proliferation. Since the mid-1980s, methotrexate has become one of the most widely used disease-modifying anti-rheumatic drugs (DMARDs) in rheumatoid arthritis. It also has a significant degree of efficacy in psoriasis, asthma, and inflammatory bowel disease, and may also be effective in systemic lupus erythematosus, giant cell arteritis, and Wegener's granulomatosis. The exact mechanisms by which methotrexate affects these diseases are still uncertain, and its clinical effects probably result from multiple biochemical events at a variety of cellular sites (1).

General adverse effects

Most of the experience regarding the adverse effects of low-dose methotrexate has accumulated in patients with rheumatoid arthritis. Adverse effects are very common during the first year of treatment and reach an incidence of 60–70%. However, they are rarely severe enough to require permanent drug withdrawal, even after very long-term treatment. Based on a cohort study of 152 patients with rheumatoid arthritis, the probability of methotrexate continuation was 30% at 10 years, and adverse effects were the most frequent reason (50%) for drug withdrawal (2). Even though the overall withdrawal rate for methotrexate-induced adverse effects is 7–16%, long-term methotrexate treatment required drug withdrawal because of adverse effects less often than several other second-line DMARDs (SEDA-22, 416). In a retrospective analysis of 437 rheumatoid arthritis patients treated for 3–106 months (mean = 35 months), the most common adverse effects were gastrointestinal disorders (20%), raised liver function tests (13%), respiratory disorders (6.4%), hematological abnormalities (4.4%), weakness (3.4%), central nervous system disorders (2.8%), infections (2.3%), mucocutaneous disorders (2.3%), and arthralgia (1.8%) (3). A Ritchie's index of 10 or less, a low polymorphonuclear leukocyte count, and the absence of rheumatoid factor predicted the occurrence of adverse effects.

In one study, 10 patients (of an original 29) were still taking methotrexate after a mean of 13 years and a mean cumulative dose of 9.7 g (4). The overall drug withdrawal rate was 48%, and the rate of adverse effects, particularly on the gut and central nervous system, fell with time (85% at baseline, 90% at 90 months, 62% at 160 months). It was felt that routine folate supplementation might have contributed to the observed reduction in toxicity, except for mouth ulcers or soreness. Very similar findings were found in another long-term (132 months) prospective study (5).

Raised methotrexate serum concentrations (over 100 nmol/l at 36–42 hours after ingestion) are expected to increase the likelihood of several adverse effects, that is, gastrointestinal and hematological effects, but similar adverse effects can be found even with low methotrexate serum concentrations. Reduced red cell folate concentrations during methotrexate treatment also related to adverse effects and rises in liver enzymes, and red cell folate concentrations above 800 nmol/l protected against common adverse effects and treatment withdrawal (6). Several investigators now advocate the concomitant use of folic acid (5–7 mg/week and up to 27.5 mg/week) to reduce some of methotrexate-associated adverse effects without reducing its efficacy (7).

Prevention of adverse effects

It is possible to reduce the incidence of several adverse effects of methotrexate by using folic or folinic acid. The usual practice is to give weekly folic acid in patients who are taking weekly methotrexate (on a different day) and daily folinic acid in those who are taking daily methotrexate. Folic acid supplementation is now commonly given to reduce the adverse effects of methotrexate, in particular its mucosal and gastrointestinal toxic effects (SED-14, 1297) (SEDA-23, 406), but less is known about how long this should be continued in patients taking long-term treatment.

In a meta-analysis of 307 patients with rheumatoid arthritis from seven randomized clinical trials, of whom 147 took folate supplementation, hematological adverse effects were not significantly reduced in the folate group (8). However, there was a 79% reduction in mucosal and gastrointestinal adverse effects in patients taking folic acid and a non-significant trend toward a reduction (42%) in patients taking folinic acid. Disease activity was not modified by low doses of folate. Finally, the authors noted that folinic acid is more expensive.

In 75 patients with rheumatoid arthritis taking methotrexate (up to 20 mg/week) and folic acid (5 mg/day), folic acid was withdrawn and the patients were randomized to restart folic acid ($n = 38$) or to take placebo ($n = 37$) double-blind, and were regularly assessed for 1 year (9). There were more withdrawals with placebo (46%) than with folic acid (21%) and more nausea. There were no obvious differences in efficacy. This suggests that folic acid supplementation is still helpful in the long term.

Organs and Systems

Cardiovascular

Cardiovascular adverse effects of methotrexate are extremely rare.

- There has been one detailed report of ventricular dysrhythmias and myocardial infarction, with recurrence of

frequent ventricular extra beats on each readministration of methotrexate in a 36-year-old man (10).

It has been suggested that methotrexate increases mortality in patients with rheumatoid arthritis with cardiovascular co-morbidity (11). This assumption was based on a retrospective analysis of 632 patients with rheumatoid arthritis, of whom 73 died. The simultaneous presence of methotrexate and evidence of cardiovascular disease was an independent predictor of mortality. There was no such association with other DMARDs. The authors suggested that this effect may result from a methotrexate-induced increase in serum homocysteine, encouraging atherosclerosis.

Respiratory

Isolated and sustained cough is an unusual adverse effect of methotrexate. Among 13 patients who had a cough, only three met the criteria for methotrexate-induced pneumonitis (12). An irritant effect of methotrexate on the airways was therefore suggested.

Pneumonitis

Acute or subacute interstitial pneumonitis is an important but unpredictable and potentially life-threatening adverse effect of low-dose methotrexate (13–16).

Presentation

In patients with definite or probable methotrexate-induced lung injury, the predominant clinical features include shortness of breath, cough, and fever (13). Pathological examination usually shows an interstitial inflammatory cell infiltrate (sometimes granulomatous or with alveolar damage), and variable degrees of interstitial fibrosis. Unfortunately, confirmatory evidence is sometimes hard to obtain, particularly in patients with rheumatoid arthritis in whom rheumatoid interstitial lung disease can also occur. Infectious pneumonias, particularly viral or *Pneumocystis jiroveci* pneumonia, which resemble methotrexate pneumonitis and can occur as a result of immunosuppression, should also be carefully excluded.

- Pulmonary endoalveolar hemorrhage was a possible complication of pneumonitis in a 57-year-old woman who voluntarily increased her dosage of methotrexate from 7.5 mg once a week to 7.5 mg/day for 15 days (17).

The potential severity of methotrexate pneumonitis was finally exemplified in a careful retrospective multicenter study of 29 patients with definite or probable criteria for methotrexate-induced lung injury (13). Overall, five patients (17%) died, two of them after methotrexate rechallenge.

Frequency

The prevalence of methotrexate pneumonitis has been variably estimated from 0.3 to 18%, with a mean estimated prevalence of 3.3% (14,16). In a review of the respiratory complications of methotrexate, the authors concluded that pneumonitis occurs in 7% of patients, in

25% of whom it is fatal as a result of respiratory failure (18). This can occur with any dose of methotrexate, given via any route; it has occurred after the intrathecal administration of 12 mg given for central nervous system prophylaxis (19). In a review of 194 patients with rheumatoid arthritis and 38 with psoriatic arthritis, the prevalences of pneumonitis were 2.1 and 0.03% respectively (14), which is similar to the 3.2% incidence in a prospective study of 124 patients with rheumatoid arthritis (20). Another analysis performed over 5 years showed that the estimated prevalence of definite or probable pneumonitis was only 0.86% in 1162 patients (10 patients, of whom three died), but this conclusion was based on a limited retrospective identification of cases (21).

Mechanism

Even though methotrexate pneumonitis was first described about 30 years ago, very little is known about the mechanism, and whether it is due to direct cumulative toxicity, hypersensitivity, or an idiosyncratic reaction. In one case, interleukin-8 was speculated to play an important role in the pathogenesis (22).

Susceptibility factors

Susceptibility factors for methotrexate pneumonitis are still poorly understood. In one study, no risk factors were identified and periodic pulmonary function tests were not predictive (20). In contrast, advanced age, diabetes, pre-existing rheumatoid pleuropulmonary involvement or previous lung disease, previous use of DMARDs, and hypoalbuminemia were suggested as the most reliable predictors of methotrexate-induced pneumonitis in a large historical case-control study (15,23). The weekly dose, the cumulative dose, and the duration of treatment were not related to its occurrence. A history of drug-induced pulmonary disorders was also thought to favor methotrexate pneumonitis, but this was based on a single case report in a patient who previously had aminorex-induced primary pulmonary hypertension (SEDA-22, 416).

Management

The management of methotrexate pneumonitis primarily requires methotrexate withdrawal and supportive care. Although glucocorticoids are commonly used, there is as yet no evidence that they positively influence the outcome. Any readministration of methotrexate is dangerous, and four of six patients treated again with methotrexate developed recurrent lung toxicity, of whom two died (13).

Based on a report of 9 cases and a careful reanalysis of 123 previously published cases, the clinical spectrum and histopathology of methotrexate-induced pneumonitis have been reviewed (24). The authors stressed that methotrexate pneumonitis should be promptly recognized to avoid a severe outcome, although no specific features could be identified compared with other drug-induced adverse lung effects and no definite pathological findings compared with rheumatoid lung. Diagnostic criteria therefore mostly included a history of exposure, the exclusion of other pulmonary diseases, especially

infections, and the presence of pulmonary infiltrates on the chest X-ray. Once methotrexate pneumonitis developed, 13% of the patients died from respiratory failure, clearly underlining the fact that methotrexate pneumonitis is potentially life-threatening. Methotrexate reintroduction should also be strongly discouraged in such cases, because about 25% of patients experience recurrence.

Nervous system

Reports of necrotizing leukoencephalopathy in association with methotrexate have been verified by biopsy or autopsy (25,26). Serial electroencephalography can predict this, since slow-wave activity develops during the administration of high-dose methotrexate. Autopsy has shown widespread necrosis and spongiosis in the cerebral and cerebellar white matter in such cases (25).

Chronic brain edema, multifocal white matter necrosis, and deep brain atrophy have been reported in patients who received high-dose methotrexate therapy, with an incidence of 4% (27). All patients received methotrexate $8-9$ g/m^2 intravenously over 4 hours. The encephalopathy began abruptly, an average of 6 days after the second or third weekly treatment, presenting with behavioral abnormalities. These ranged from laughter to lethargy or unresponsiveness. In some patients, there were focal sensorimotor or reflex signs and generalized seizures. The disorder lasted from 15 minutes to 72 hours, and it disappeared as abruptly as it began, without specific treatment.

A rare case of a reversible neurological disturbance associated with focal subcortical white matter pathology has been described after administration of methotrexate 3 g/m^2. In patients who received $8-12.5$ g/m^2, the incidence of neurological abnormalities was 4%. All of these patients were also receiving methotrexate intrathecally as well, but the relevance of this is not known (28).

In one case, low-dose methotrexate was implicated in leukoencephalopathy (29).

Treatment with intrathecal methotrexate of children under 5 years of age with acute lymphoblastic leukemia (irrespective of other drugs) has structural and functional effects on the developing neocerebellar–frontal subsystem (30).

Acute dysarthria has been attributed to methotrexate (31).

- A 71-year-old man was given oral methotrexate (15 mg/week) for a cutaneous T cell lymphoma. Within 3 weeks he developed progressive dysarthria and incoordination, and neurological examination showed mild buccofacial dyskinesia. Complete examination was otherwise normal, and he fully recovered 6–8 weeks after methotrexate withdrawal.

This case is reminiscent of other previously reported neurological abnormalities with low-dose methotrexate.

Psychological, psychiatric

There was a significantly higher risk of late cognitive impairment (concentration and memory) in patients

($n = 39$) taking adjuvant cyclophosphamide, fluorouracil, and methotrexate than in controls matched for age, disease, surgery, and radiation dose (32).

In studies of the neurotoxic effects of low-dose methotrexate treatment, dizziness, headache, visual disturbances or hallucinations, lack of concentration, cognitive dysfunction, and depression-like symptoms were detected in 1–35% of patients (33,34). Advanced age and mild renal insufficiency were possible susceptibility factors (34).

Nutrition

Of patients receiving high-dose methotrexate (5–8 g/m^2), 95% developed a significant increase in serum phenylalanine concentrations, probably due to inhibition of dihydropteridine reductase (35). The clinical significance of this is not obvious, although it is possible that it may contribute to the transient neurological disturbance observed in some patients taking high-dose methotrexate.

Hematologic

Significant hematological abnormalities occur in 10–24% of patients who take methotrexate. Mild to moderate leukopenia is the most frequent, followed by thrombocytopenia. Isolated thrombocytopenia and anemia are uncommon (SEDA-22, 416) (36). In a retrospective study in 315 patients, 13 had thrombocytopenia, two of whom also had pancytopenia (37). Thrombocytopenia correlated with the weekly dosage of methotrexate administered on the same day as NSAIDs, and methotrexate was safely reintroduced in patients who developed thrombocytopenia as a result of concomitant administration of both drugs, provided that NSAIDs were withheld at least on the day of methotrexate administration.

Pancytopenia is a rare but potentially fatal complication, and numerous reports have been published. The characteristics and incidence of pancytopenia have been carefully re-evaluated from case reports and clinical trials published from 1980 to 1995 (38). Of 70 reported cases, 12 patients died (17%). Impaired renal function was the most important contributing factor (54%), particularly in fatal cases (10/12). Other important susceptibility factors included advanced age (over 65 years), hypoalbuminemia, concurrent infection, and/or concomitant multiple medications (particularly co-trimoxazole). The mean cumulative dosage was 675 (10–4800) mg, and the minimal cumulative methotrexate dose leading to fatal pancytopenia was 10 mg. This confirms that pancytopenia can occur at any time during treatment, even in the absence of known susceptibility factors. Bone marrow biopsy showed megaloblastosis and hypocellularity. Eosinophilia and increased mean corpuscular volume were rarely observed. In an overall review of five long-term prospective studies (511 patients), the calculated incidence of methotrexate-induced pancytopenia was 1.4%. Although severe myelosuppression sometimes required folinic acid, there are as yet no data to determine whether prophylactic folate supplementation can reduce the incidence of pancytopenia.

In a double-blind, placebo-controlled study of the safety and efficacy of methotrexate therapy combined with glucocorticoids in patients with giant cell arteritis over 24 months, adverse events were defined as a new diagnosis of any condition during treatment (39). The combination of methotrexate plus prednisolone reduced the number of relapses and improved the course of the disease. Methotrexate was withdrawn in three patients who had adverse events that were clearly drug-related. One had leukopenia, anemia, and mucositis, one developed pancytopenia, and one oral ulcers. These patients were not taking folic acid or folinic acid supplements.

Gastrointestinal

Gastrointestinal adverse effects (stomatitis, anorexia, abdominal pain, dyspepsia, nausea, vomiting, diarrhea, and weight loss) are very common, particularly after oral administration of methotrexate (up to 50%), and often require dosage adjustment (3). Folic acid supplementation reduces the incidence of several gastrointestinal adverse effects.

Stomatitis can sometimes be particularly harmful and has been reported as the cause of transient or permanent treatment withdrawal in 4.5 and 1.1% of 1539 patients respectively (40). However, one study did not show significant differences in the number of oral lesions or the duration or frequency of stomatitis between patients with rheumatoid arthritis taking methotrexate and those not taking methotrexate (19/51 versus 9/46), although the prevalence of ulceration was higher in the methotrexate group (41).

Liver

Cytolytic hepatitis has been reported in a 58-year-old man being treated with intramuscular methotrexate 10 mg/ week (total dose over the previous 4 years 2.3 g); it resolved within 2 weeks of stopping therapy (42).

Hepatic fibrosis and cirrhosis

The main concern over long-term treatment with methotrexate is hepatic fibrosis and cirrhosis. Methotrexate hepatotoxicity was initially reported in children given high daily dose methotrexate for leukemia. After its introduction for the treatment of psoriasis, several papers published in the late 1960s pointed out the possible risk of severe hepatic fibrosis and cirrhosis in patients taking moderate daily doses. Since then many studies have focused on the extent of long-term methotrexate hepatotoxicity in patients taking low-dose methotrexate for psoriasis and rheumatoid arthritis. However, the evidence on the frequency and severity of severe liver disease in these patients is still highly controversial, since there may be liver histological changes before methotrexate treatment, particularly in patients with psoriasis. Furthermore, there are numerous confounding factors (Table 1) which can contribute to histological liver changes, leading several authors to suggest as early as 1990 that methotrexate-induced hepatic fibrosis and cirrhosis is uncommon and only occurs in patients with other susceptibility factors (43).

Frequency

The incidence of liver cirrhosis after a mean dose of 2 g is 7–10%. Once 1.5 g has been administered (44), or 2 years after starting long-term treatment, biopsy should be discussed (45).

Liver failure or cirrhosis were identified among 24 patients in a retrospective survey of more than 16 600 patients with rheumatoid arthritis who had taken methotrexate for at least 5 years, giving an estimated 5-year frequency of one in 1000 (46).

No morphological features of methotrexate hepatotoxicity were demonstrated after 2 years of methotrexate treatment in 48 patients with primary biliary cirrhosis (47).

Collectively, the available data suggest that methotrexate rarely causes significant serious liver damage in patients who have been otherwise carefully selected, who present no risk factors for methotrexate-induced hepatotoxicity, and who have received lower weekly dosages with strict monitoring of liver function (for example transaminases) in order to reduce methotrexate doses when liver enzymes are persistently raised (48).

Diagnosis and monitoring

Routine liver function tests do not reliably indicate liver damage, and they may not become abnormal until there is already considerable liver damage. It is therefore common practice to monitor patients by conducting annual liver biopsies. Measurement of the serum amino-terminal propeptide of type III procollagen (PIII PI) has been used as an alternative to liver biopsy; high concentrations correlate with fibrosis on liver biopsy (49). No patient with a normal serum concentration had an abnormal biopsy. An increase in the plasma phenylalanine/tyrosine ratio in children and adolescents can provide clinical evidence of liver damage before the appearance of symptoms in patients who have taken high doses of methotrexate (50).

Methods of monitoring patients for possible methotrexate hepatotoxicity and guidelines have been reviewed (48,51,52). It should be mentioned that the frequent rise in serum transaminases (involving 30–80% of patients) after the start of treatment is transient and does not predict liver damage; only persistently abnormal transaminases are potential indicators of methotrexate hepatotoxicity.

Mechanism

Folate depletion may be a factor in the pathogenesis of methotrexate-induced liver disease. In 30 patients on long-term methotrexate therapy, aimed at determining whether erythrocyte concentrations of folate and methotrexate might provide an indication for liver biopsy, there was no difference between red cell folate concentrations in patients with cirrhosis or progressive liver fibrosis and patients without fibrosis or with non-progressive hepatic fibrosis. Erythrocyte methotrexate concentrations were higher in patients with progressive hepatic disease, but cumulative dose and length of treatment were stronger predictors. In individual cases, erythrocyte folate and methotrexate concentrations were not a reliable guide (53).

Pathology

In patients with rheumatoid arthritis, baseline histological liver abnormalities were less common, with mild fibrosis only in 0–15% of patients. In retrospective studies with no

Table 1 Susceptibility factors for hepatotoxicity of methotrexate

Strong association	Previous or concurrent heavy alcohol use
	Pre-existing liver disease
	Daily methotrexate administration
	Renal insufficiency
Probable association	Duration of methotrexate treatment (over 2 years)
	Cumulative methotrexate dose (over 1500 mg)
	Prior treatment with arsenicals
	Obesity with diabetes mellitus
Possible or potential association	Maximum weekly dose over 25 mg
	Obesity alone
	Diabetes mellitus alone
	Heterozygous alpha$_1$ -antitrypsin deficiency
	Felty's syndrome
	Prior treatment with vitamin A
	Concurrent NSAID use
	Concurrent treatment with ciclosporin
	Concurrent PUVA treatment
No association	Sex
	HLA phenotype
	Extent of psoriatic skin involvement
	Duration of rheumatoid arthritis
	Glucocorticoid therapy
Negative association	Concurrent folate supplementation
	Concurrent hydroxychloroquine use

pre-methotrexate liver biopsies, mild fibrosis was found in 3–35% of patients taking methotrexate, moderate or severe fibrosis in 0–10%, and cirrhosis in 0–2%. However, no case of cirrhosis was identified in studies which compared pre- and postmethotrexate biopsies or sequential biopsies while on long-term methotrexate, that is, a mean cumulative dose of 1200–5000 mg (52). Again, both worsening and improvement of histological lesions occurred. The application of guidelines to prevent methotrexate hepatotoxicity may account for these reassuring results. Liver biopsy changes were moderate or absent in patients with juvenile rheumatoid arthritis who took a cumulative dose of over 3000 mg (SEDA-21, 388; 52).

In 22 of 29 patients (76%) who were treated with low-pulse doses of methotrexate for rheumatoid arthritis, liver biopsy specimens showed variability in liver cell nuclear size, glycogenated nuclei, and fatty change. Occasionally there was mild portal infiltration with lymphocytes. There were no significant differences in age, duration of treatment, or cumulative dose amongst the cases. Serial increases in serum transaminases and/or alkaline phosphatase activity and development of hypoalbuminemia during treatment were indicators of development of liver disease (54).

In another study, the pathological lesions found in liver biopsies from patients treated with methotrexate were non-specific, consisting usually of macrovesicular steatosis, nuclear pleomorphism, chronic inflammatory infiltrates in the portal tracts, focal liver cell necrosis, fibrosis, and cirrhosis (52).

The pathological features of methotrexate-induced liver damage have been comprehensively reviewed (52). In patients with psoriasis, baseline liver biopsies were often abnormal, with mild fibrosis, moderate or severe fibrosis, and cirrhosis in 0–30, 0–7, and 0–1.5% respectively. These figures increased after methotrexate use, with fibrosis and cirrhosis in 14–34 and 0–21% respectively.

Ultrastructural studies have sometimes identified Ito cell prominence and collagen deposition in the perisinusoidal space of Disse during the first months of treatment and before the appearance of any signs of fibrosis, but these findings have been disputed in rheumatoid arthritis patients. Using immunohistochemical quantification, increased matrix proteins, collagen and transforming growth factor alpha were also found as possible early markers of methotrexate hepatotoxicity (55).

Susceptibility factors

The susceptibility factors for methotrexate-induced hepatotoxicity are listed in Table 1.

In a meta-analysis of 636 patients from 15 studies, who took chronic low-dose methotrexate for rheumatoid arthritis or psoriasis, the risk of liver toxicity increased with cumulative dose and heavy alcohol intake (56).

In one study, the risk of developing cirrhosis progressively increased with the total cumulative dose of methotrexate, from 13% at 2200 mg to 26% at 4000 mg (57). However, studies that compared sequential liver biopsies in patients on treatment and included specific recommendations for patient selection and the monitoring of methotrexate hepatotoxicity, gave contrasting results, with a lower incidence of cirrhosis even after high cumulative methotrexate doses (up to 5100 mg) (52). In addition, although histological lesions can worsen during treatment, improvement or absence of progression of prior fibrosis/cirrhosis has been found in very long-term follow-up of patients still taking methotrexate after 10 years (58).

The incidence and susceptibility factors of rises in serum transaminases have been detailed from a retrospective analysis of 66 patients with rheumatoid arthritis (59). There was an asymptomatic increase in serum transaminases in 42 and 49% of patients respectively, an incidence 4–5 times greater than that found in 21 patients taking other DMARDs. Although most of the rises in transaminases were transient and spontaneously reversible, 14 patients had sustained rises. There was a close relation between the incidence of high transaminases and the weight-adjusted dose of methotrexate. In a multivariate regression analysis, only obesity, methotrexate dose (over 0.15 mg/kg/week), and the concomitant presence of gastrointestinal adverse effects were significantly and independently associated with the likelihood of a rise in alanine transaminase. In the 14 patients who had persistently high transaminases, weekly folic acid 5 mg produced a sustained fall in serum alanine transaminase within 3 months, but three patients had to be withdrawn because of exacerbation of rheumatoid arthritis.

Urinary tract

Low-dose methotrexate is usually not regarded as nephrotoxic, and one report of nephrotic syndrome with minimal change disease on renal biopsy should be regarded with caution, since there was recovery after glucocorticoid treatment and withdrawal of concomitant NSAIDs (SEDA-22, 416).

However, renal toxicity occurs with high-dose methotrexate and more likely to occur with concomitant administration of other nephrotoxic agents, such as aminoglycosides, cephalosporins, NSAIDs, and diuretics (60).

The pathogenesis of methotrexate-induced nephrotoxicity is not understood, but it is thought to result from crystallization of methotrexate in the renal tubules. Adequate hydration and urinary alkalinization are necessary to minimize this effect (61). Urinary beta$_2$ microglobulin may be a useful marker of methotrexate nephrotoxicity (62).

When serum methotrexate concentrations are high, leucovorin (folinic acid) rescue may protect against renal damage. Methotrexate concentrations are only transiently lowered by hemoperfusion, and they are unaffected by peritoneal dialysis once there is acute renal insufficiency. Sustained reductions in drug concentrations and recovery of renal function have been reported after charcoal hemoperfusion followed by hemodialysis (63,64).

Co-administration of methotrexate and procarbazine in the treatment of medulloblastomas increases the risk of methotrexate nephrotoxicity. Delayed administration of methotrexate until 72 hours after procarbazine therapy has been given may reduce this risk (65).

Skin

Since the first descriptions of the rapid development of a large number of nodules, also termed "accelerated nodulosis," in methotrexate-treated patients, a number of such reports have accumulated in patients with rheumatoid arthritis or, more rarely, psoriatic arthritis (66–68). Nodulosis is characterized by the development of small, painful, multiple nodules, sometimes disseminated; pulmonary, meningeal, or pericardial nodulosis has also been reported in a few patients (SEDA-21, 387; 67,69,70). Four cases of nodulosis and four of cutaneous vasculitis were noted during a long-term follow-up of 437 rheumatoid arthritis patients (3), but the estimated incidence of accelerated nodulosis was found to be higher in other studies: that is, 8–12% (5,66,70).

The nodules can appear at any time during treatment, with or without concomitant cutaneous vasculitis, and are usually found in patients with erosive disease and a high titer of rheumatoid factor. This has raised the question as to whether they are a reason to modify treatment, and whether they are rheumatic or represent a true adverse effect of methotrexate; certainly, methotrexate-associated nodulosis is very similar to idiopathic rheumatoid arthritis nodulosis and sometimes disappears despite continuation of methotrexate. However, prompt regression on methotrexate withdrawal and recurrence on rechallenge in several patients strongly argue for a causal drug-related effect.

There was a characteristic clinical and histopathological spectrum of skin lesions, distinct from rheumatoid papules, in four patients who took low-dose methotrexate for acute flares of collagen vascular disease (71). These so-called methotrexate-induced rheumatoid papules developed shortly after methotrexate administration consisted of erythematous indurated papules mostly affecting the proximal limbs, and disappeared after methotrexate was withdrawn or tapered. Histology showed inflammatory infiltrates of interstitially arranged histiocytes and a few neutrophils, but no features of leukocytoclastic vasculitis.

Isolated cutaneous leukocytoclastic vasculitis occurs infrequently in patients taking methotrexate, and an immediate-type hypersensitivity reaction has been thought to be involved, in view of prompt recurrence after drug readministration or a positive mast cell degranulation test as recorded in several patients (SEDA-21, 388; SEDA-22, 417; 72).

Other isolated reports included the occurrence of skin ulceration (SEDA-22, 388) and one fatal case of toxic epidermal necrolysis (SEDA-21, 388).

Persistent hyperpigmentation is an unusual manifestation of weekly administration of methotrexate (73).

- Severely ulcerated psoriatic plaques and acute extensive exfoliative dermatitis occurred in a 37-year-old man who had taken methotrexate for 5 years for psoriasis (74).

In the context of a case of severe reactivation of recent sunburn after a single injection of methotrexate for ectopic pregnancy in a 40-year-old woman, the authors reviewed the literature on methotrexate photosensitivity (75). Photodermatitis reactivation is the only well-documented type of photosensitivity associated with methotrexate. It can occur if methotrexate is given at 2–5 days after excessive exposure to ultraviolet or X-radiation.

A previously unreported skin reaction mimicking Stevens–Johnson syndrome has been reported (76).

- A 61-year-old woman inadvertently took a high dose of methotrexate (10 mg/day) for psoriasis, and developed mucosal ulcers after 3 months. One month later, methotrexate (20 mg/week) was restarted, but she developed painful oral ulceration and burning skin lesions 3 days later. She had an erythema multiform-like rash and several buccal ulcers. There was a moderate pancytopenia. Histological examination of the skin showed features consistent with an acute graft-versus-host reaction. All medications except aspirin were withdrawn, and she recovered fully after treatment with calcium folinate and prednisolone.

The authors speculated that concomitant aspirin may have contributed to this severe reaction.

Hair

Mild alopecia is common in patients taking methotrexate (77,78).

Nails

Yellow nail pigmentation without paronychia has been noted in a patient with psoriasis taking methotrexate (79).

Musculoskeletal

Arthralgia and myalgia sometimes occur within 24 hours of methotrexate injections in patients with rheumatoid arthritis. These transient effects, which can be accompanied by fatigue, malaise, and various neuropsychological disorders, have escaped recognition, but they occurred in 10% of patients over 18 months and sometimes resulted in treatment withdrawal (80).

Leg pain and spontaneous fractures attributed to prolonged high-dose methotrexate therapy in pediatric oncology have been recognized since the 1970s, but there have been some cases in patients taking low-dose methotrexate (81,82). All the same, it is still controversial as to whether methotrexate can actually cause changes in bone metabolism (83). There was a significant reduction in bone mineral density in 11 postmenopausal women taking methotrexate for primary biliary cirrhosis compared with 11 matched controls not taking methotrexate (84). Among 133 patients with rheumatoid arthritis, methotrexate without glucocorticoids was not associated with changes in the bone mineral density after 3 years of treatment, but methotrexate plus prednisone (over 5 mg/day) produced greater bone loss than prednisone alone (85). In contrast, another study failed to show accelerated bone loss in methotrexate users compared with non-users, but the study was limited to 10 patients in each group (86).

The possible effects of methotrexate on bone metabolism and bone loss have been discussed in the context of two adults (87) and in relation to a study in children with juvenile rheumatoid arthritis (88) who had delayed bone healing after surgery. The two adults, aged 52 and 62 years, had been taking methotrexate (7.5 and 15 mg/week) for 14 and 15 months when they underwent metatarsal and tibial osteotomy. Because X-ray examination 5 and 6 months after surgery showed non-union, methotrexate was withdrawn; the bone healed promptly in both patients within 2 months. The authors thought that the outcome in these patients without risk factors for bone fragility suggested that temporary methotrexate withdrawal should be considered in cases of delayed bone healing after surgery.

In contrast, in a longitudinal study of 32 patients with juvenile rheumatoid arthritis, there was no evidence of deleterious effects of long-term, low-dose methotrexate on bone mass density (88). The cumulative dose of glucocorticoids, weight, and height were the main determinants of bone mass changes.

Furthermore, there is evidence that it is disease activity rather than methotrexate that accounts for changes in bone mass (89). This 2-year longitudinal study involved 22 patients taking methotrexate and 18 patients taking other DMARDs; it was strictly controlled for the use of glucocorticoids. There were significant and equal reductions in trabecular bone mineral density in both groups. Bone loss was most marked in patients with active disease.

Sexual function

Impotence has very rarely been attributed to methotrexate (90).

Reproductive system

Although the occurrence of gynecomastia requiring surgical excision in two patients might have been coincidental (91), in another patient it disappeared after methotrexate withdrawal and recurred on rechallenge (92).

Immunologic

Immediate hypersensitivity reactions are rare after low-dose methotrexate.

• A 53-year-old woman had three episodes of angioedema while taking methotrexate, with no recurrence after withdrawal (93).

Vasculitis has been infrequently reported in patients taking low-dose methotrexate (SEDA-21, 388; SEDA-22, 417; 94). Although most cases have been observed in patients with rheumatoid arthritis, suggesting that the underlying disease plays a part, vasculitis has also been described in a patient with ankylosing spondylitis (95). Methotrexate was also reported to have exacerbated pre-existing urticarial vasculitis in a 32-year-old woman; the lesions recurred after rechallenge (96).

Infection risk

Methotrexate-related immunosuppression can be expected to increase the likelihood of infections. The infection rate reported in patients taking low-dose methotrexate has varied from one study to another. In a literature review focusing on patients with rheumatoid arthritis taking methotrexate, the mean infection rate was 1.8% in retrospective studies, 4.6% in open studies, and 11.6% in double-blind studies (97). Infections usually occurred within 1.5 years of starting treatment and mostly comprised common respiratory or cutaneous bacterial infections, *Herpes zoster*, and, more rarely, opportunistic infections. In one comparative study, the overall risk of infections was considered to be low and similar in patients taking methotrexate and azathioprine (97), but others have found a higher prevalence of infections and an increase in antibiotic use in patients with rheumatoid arthritis taking methotrexate as compared to other DMARDs, except cyclophosphamide (98,99).

An accumulating series of case reports has focused on the possible more frequent occurrence of opportunistic infections despite normal leukocyte counts in patients treated for rheumatoid arthritis or, less often, psoriasis (97,100,101). Various bacterial, fungal, and viral opportunistic infections have been described, with *Pneumocystis jiroveci* pneumonia as the most frequently reported (SEDA-21, 389; SEDA-22, 417). Although the most severe, sometimes fatal, infectious diseases were usually observed in patients also taking glucocorticoids (SEDA-22, 417; 102,103), severe infections can also occur in occasional patients not taking concomitant glucocorticoids (SEDA-21, 389; 101,104–107).

Acute reactivation of a presumed quiescent chronic hepatitis B infection in one reported case after methotrexate withdrawal suggests that T cell-mediated immunological rebound might lead to rapid destruction of infected hepatocytes (108).

Long-Term Effects

Tumorigenicity

The evidence that methotrexate is carcinogenic is inconclusive and mostly based on case reports or analyses of cohort studies without control groups (100,109). For example, malignant neoplasms (urothelial carcinoma of the bladder, a malignant teratoma, and a dermal squamous cell carcinoma) have been described in three patients taking prolonged courses of methotrexate 7.5–15 mg/week (110).

From a retrospective study in more than 16 000 rheumatoid arthritis patients, the risk of hematological malignancy in methotrexate-treated patients was thought to be very small and not different from that observed in patients who used other DMARDs (111). In 426 patients with rheumatoid arthritis who took methotrexate for a mean of 37 months (follow-up period 4.6 years), the incidence rate of new cancers (4 cases/1000 person-years) was similar to that found in the general population (2.8 cases/1000 person-years) (112). Another preliminary study did not show an excess in the risk of lymphoproliferative disorders in patients with rheumatoid arthritis receiving long-term methotrexate maintenance (113). Earlier studies in patients with psoriasis did not show a higher incidence of cancers in patients on methotrexate compared with the general population (100,114).

In contrast, there have been several isolated reports of methotrexate-induced lymphomas (SEDA-21, 388; SEDA-22, 417; 115,116). The pathological features in these cases have ranged from benign lymphoid hyperplasia to non-Hodgkin's lymphoma, and more rarely Hodgkin's disease (115), and patients usually had the typical features of lymphoproliferative disorders as found in immunosuppressed patients, that is, transplant patients or patients with congenital or acquired immune deficiency syndromes. Exceptionally, cases of pseudolymphoma have also been reported (SEDA-21, 389).

- Two patients developed lymphomas within 3 years of methotrexate treatment, and the authors suggested that an increase in serum IgE concentrations might anticipate the development of lymphoma in patients with rheumatoid arthritis treated with methotrexate (117).
- A cutaneous B cell lymphoma occurred in a 58-year-old man who had been treated with intramuscular methotrexate 10 mg/week for 4 years (total dose 2.3 g); the lymphoma resolved spontaneously 2 weeks after withdrawal of therapy (118).

A convincing argument implicating methotrexate as the cause of lymphomas is the possible spontaneous remission of lymphoproliferation after methotrexate withdrawal, as reported in several cases (SEDA-22, 389; 115,116). However, the putative pathophysiological mechanisms of methotrexate-induced lymphomas are unclear, and the drug's precise role, as well as that of the underlying disease as a confounding factor, needs to be investigated. The risk of a lymphoma in rheumatoid arthritis probably has more to do with the disease and its activity than with methotrexate treatment (113,119).

Low-dosage methotrexate is also a possible factor in the development of Epstein–Barr virus-associated lymphoproliferative disease, but the role of the Epstein–Barr virus in these cases is unclear. Epstein–Barr virus infection does not appear to be mandatory for the development of lymphoproliferation in patients taking methotrexate, but it was nevertheless found in about one-half of patients who developed lymphomas (SEDA-22, 389; 115,120).

Lymphoproliferative disorders have been observed during treatment of sarcoidosis and connective tissue diseases with low-dose methotrexate.

- A 51-year-old man with systemic sarcoidosis took methotrexate for 36 months and developed a large anal fissure with a diffuse polymorphic infiltrate containing large Epstein–Barr virus-positive lymphoid cells, similar to the classical B cell lymphoproliferative disorders that occur in immunosuppressed transplant recipients of solid organs (121).

This case supports the hypothesis that immunosuppressant therapy may contribute to an increased risk of Epstein–Barr virus-associated lymphoproliferative disorders.

Some of the mechanisms and risk factors of methotrexate-associated non-Hodgkin's lymphoma in patients with rheumatoid arthritis have been reviewed, including an analysis of the characteristic features of 25 detailed published cases (122). Although the epidemiological evidence is limited, several reports of spontaneous remission of lymphomas after methotrexate withdrawal strongly support a cause-and-effect relation.

A second malignancy in a patient taking methotrexate for chronic lymphatic leukemia has been described (123).

- A 55-year-old man with chronic lymphocytic leukemia and rheumatoid arthritis took methotrexate for 4 years and developed a B cell non-Hodgkin's lymphoma in the shoulder and axillary lymph nodes; he had Epstein–Barr viral antigens in the serum. After radiation and chemotherapy had failed, complete remission was achieved with a combination of rituximab and EPOCH (etoposide + prednisone + vincristine + cyclophosphamide + doxorubicin).

The authors thought that T cell deficiency induced by methotrexate, chronic lymphatic leukemia, and rheumatoid arthritis may have contributed to the development of the B cell lymphoma.

Other malignancies, such as malignant melanoma, multiple myeloma, leukemia or solid cancers, have been seldom reported (SEDA-21, 389; SEDA-22, 389; 90,124), and the association with methotrexate therapy is uncertain.

Second-Generation Effects

Teratogenicity

Owing to its known teratogenic effects, methotrexate is usually considered to be contraindicated in pregnancy, and several authors have recommended withdrawing methotrexate at least 3 months before a planned pregnancy. Most of our knowledge on the consequences of in utero exposure to methotrexate is derived from oncology patients. In this setting, the fetal methotrexate syndrome mimics the aminopterin syndrome, with central nervous system abnormalities, skeletal defects, and more rarely cardiac abnormalities. The critical period of exposure is 6–8 weeks after conception and the minimal weekly dose is 10 mg (125), but one report suggested that the critical period may extend to week 11 in patients exposed to high-dose methotrexate (SEDA-22, 417).

- A 3-year-old infant born to a woman who had taken methotrexate 37.5 mg/week throughout the first 8 weeks after conception had significant developmental delay with mental retardation, which might therefore be a feature of the fetal methotrexate syndrome (126).

The developmental effects of in utero exposure to methotrexate have been reviewed, including a brief mention of three original cases (127), and a series of pregnancy outcomes in four patients exposed to low-dose methotrexate during early pregnancy has been reported more extensively (128). Of 24 patients available for evaluation, who took 2.5–35 mg/week and were accidentally exposed from the beginning of pregnancy up to 19 weeks gestation, pregnancy ended in spontaneous abortion in four and elective abortion in three (including one case of major malformation). Of the 17 neonates, three had major malformations. The malformations mostly consisted of central nervous system or craniofacial abnormalities and skeletal defects. Three patients had been exposed up to 8 weeks of gestation and one from 8 to 10 weeks, and the methotrexate doses were 12.5–35 mg/week. This is consistent with the threshold dose of 10 mg/week and the timing of exposure previously suggested for fetal methotrexate syndrome.

Susceptibility Factors

Renal disease

Impaired renal function is a susceptibility factor for methotrexate-induced pancytopenia.

- A 57-year-old man who had been on hemodialysis for the past 5 years developed severe pancytopenia 12 days after a single dose of methotrexate 5 mg (129).
- Severe complications, mostly bone marrow suppression and related complications, occurred in three patients on regular hemodialysis for end-stage renal disease (130).

Drug–Drug Interactions

Acetylsalicylic acid

Aspirin displaces methotrexate from its binding sites and also inhibits its renal tubular elimination (131), so that the dosage of concurrently used methotrexate should be reduced (except once-a-week low-dose treatment in rheumatoid arthritis) (159). However, in are study, aspirin (mean dose 4.5 g) in 12 patients did not cause more toxicity than other NSAIDs taken by 22 other patients (132).

Azathioprine and mercaptopurine

In 43 patients with rheumatoid arthritis, methotrexate was thought to have increased the risk of the azathioprine-induced hypersensitivity syndrome (154).

Ciprofloxacin

Methotrexate elimination can be delayed by ciprofloxacin. Two adolescents with malignant diseases had reduced elimination of methotrexate (12 g/m² 4-hourly) when they took ciprofloxacin 500 mg bd (150).

Deferoxamine

In 21 children the liberation of "catalytic iron" in acute myeloid leukemia appeared to aggravate the adverse effects of high-dose methotrexate chemotherapy (168). This finding suggests that the toxicity of chemotherapy might be reduced by the co-administration of iron chelators.

Doxycycline

Doxycycline can be added to the long list of drugs (SEDA-18, 262; SEDA-23, 253) that can interact with methotrexate (169).

- A 17-year-old girl with a femoral osteosarcoma received her 11th cycle of methotrexate and simultaneously oral doxycycline 100 mg bd for a palpebral abscess. As in previous cycles, pharmacokinetic monitoring of methotrexate was performed. On this occasion the half-life of methotrexate was more than doubled. She developed hematological and gastroenterological toxicity.

The authors recommended that in patients receiving methotrexate an alternative to doxycycline should be used.

Etacrynic acid

Etacrynic acid interacts with human serum albumin and modifies its binding properties (146). Since it binds to two binding sites on albumin, the benzodiazepine binding site and the warfarin binding site, it can displace drugs that bind at those sites (147). It competitively displaced 7-hydroxymethotrexate from its binding proteins in vitro (148). The clinical significance of this effect is not known.

Etretinate

A case of severe hepatitis has been attributed to the combination of methotrexate with etretinate (134), a finding that was not explained by a pharmacokinetic interaction between the two drugs (135).

Fluorouracil

There is sequence-dependent synergy between fluorouracil and methotrexate. Pre-treatment with methotrexate enhances the formation of fluorouridine monophosphate and hence fluorouridine triphosphate; this enhances RNA-directed toxicity. In studies in which methotrexate has been given 1 hour before fluorouracil, response rates did not differ significantly. However, when it was given 4 hours or more before, there were significantly better response rates (136).

There is sequence-dependent synergy between fluorouracil and methotrexate. Pretreatment with methotrexate enhances the formation of fluorouridine monophosphate and hence fluorouridine triphosphate and RNA-directed toxicity. In studies in which methotrexate has been given 1 hour before fluorouracil, response rates did not differ significantly. However, when it was given 4 hours or more before, there were significantly better response rates (157).

Folic acid, folinic acid, and calcium folinate

Methotrexate is an antagonist of folic acid and is used for treating neoplastic diseases and non-neoplastic diseases such as rheumatoid arthritis and psoriasis. As methotrexate reduces the activity of dihydrofolate reductase, supplementation with folic acid and especially with folinic acid could reduce the beneficial effects of methotrexate. This assumption has been supported by the results of an intervention study (155). Patients with rheumatoid arthritis treated with methotrexate (15 g/week) had an increase in symptoms. An open intervention trial of folinic acid 45 mg/week also showed an increase in arthritis symptoms (156). However, other trials showed no effects of this sort, and administration of folic acid or folinic acid is important in preventing methotrexate-induced blood dyscrasias.

Glafenine

An interaction of glafenine with methotrexate has been described in a patient with rheumatoid arthritis (SEDA-14, 95).

Glucocorticoids

Dexamethasone increased the hepatotoxicity of methotrexate in 57 children with brain tumors (137). The hepatotoxicity was not related to differences in serum concentrations and was independent of bone marrow toxicity or mucositis.

There have been conflicting studies on the interaction between low-dose methotrexate and long-term glucocorticoids. In one study, there was a significantly increased AUC and a reduction in methotrexate clearance compared with patients not taking glucocorticoids (138), and in another there was no change (139). Collectively, the data suggest that the interaction, if any, is of little clinical significance.

Ibuprofen

Ibuprofen can potentiate methotrexate-induced renal toxicity (160).

Meloxicam

In 13 patients with rheumatoid arthritis, oral meloxicam for 1 week had no effect on the pharmacokinetics of a single dose of intravenous methotrexate 15 mg (161).

Non-steroidal anti-inflammatory drugs (NSAIDs)

See also Rofecoxib below

Interactions of NSAIDs with methotrexate have been reviewed (SEDA-20, 89). Severe toxicity has been attributed to different dosages of methotrexate in concomitant use with several NSAIDs. Both methotrexate and the NSAIDs are secreted by the organic acid secretory pathway in the kidney and both are highly bound to plasma albumin. Theoretically, NSAIDs can increase methotrexate serum concentrations by competition for renal tubular secretion (140). In a study on the pharmacokinetics of methotrexate in patients with rheumatoid arthritis there was no significant interaction between a single low dose of methotrexate and piroxicam (162). A second study in patients with rheumatoid arthritis showed no significant

differences in the pharmacokinetics of methotrexate 7.5 mg/week with or without NSAIDs. At higher dosages (10–25 mg/week) the renal clearance of methotrexate was reduced by both salicylate and non-salicylate NSAIDs (142).

Since the publication of case histories reporting severe toxic effects in patients taking methotrexate and NSAIDs, there has been much concern among patients taking low-dose methotrexate (SEDA-20, 89) (SEDA-21, 100). However, most of the reports related to patients taking doses of methotrexate higher than those recommended in rheumatoid arthritis. From often mutually contradictory data, it appears that co-administration of most NSAIDs and stable low-dose methotrexate is relatively safe and that the supposed risks have little clinical significance in patients with normal renal function who are regularly monitored for hepatic, hematological, and renal toxicity (141).

Naproxen

Methotrexate alters naproxen kinetics and vice versa (164). Differences between NSAIDs in interactions with methotrexate require other studies (163).

Penicillin

Concomitant penicillin administration has been reported to exacerbate the hematological toxicity of low-dose methotrexate (143). This could have been due to inhibition of the tubular secretion of methotrexate.

Beta-lactams are weak organic acids that compete with the renal tubular secretion of methotrexate and its metabolites and reduce their clearance, leading to methotrexate toxicity (170,171). Consecutive aplastic crises have been described, particularly in patients with impaired renal clearance (172–174). In contrast, co-administration of flucloxacillin in another study produced a significant but not clinically important reduction in methotrexate AUC (175).

The more basic interactions between piperacillin and methotrexate and its major metabolite 7-hydroxymethotrexate have been studied in rabbits (176). The interaction was mainly caused by reduced renal clearance of both methotrexate and its metabolite. The authors concluded that renal function in patients taking this combination should be monitored, with adequate fluid intake, especially in elderly patients, because dehydration may accelerate the occurrence of toxicity.

Platinum-containing anticancer drugs

A patient with no other risk factors developed irreversible nephrotoxicity after four cycles of carboplatin 300 mg/m^2 and methotrexate 50 mg/m^2 (158). This appears to have been an additive effect of drugs that are not individually nephrotoxic until much higher doses.

Probenecid

Probenecid competes with methotrexate for renal tubular secretion, and can cause severe hematological toxicity.

- Severe pancytopenia occurred in an elderly patient taking low-dose methotrexate and probenecid (144).

Probenecid reduces the renal tubular secretion of methotrexate, enhancing its effect (166) and may reduce its plasma protein binding (167).

Rofecoxib

Methotrexate is often prescribed for the management of rheumatoid arthritis, and some NSAIDs have been reported to interact with it, causing increased plasma methotrexate concentrations, associated with impaired renal function. The safety of concurrent rofecoxib and oral methotrexate has been studied for 3 weeks in 25 patients with rheumatoid arthritis (165). Rofecoxib 12.5–50 mg/day had no effect on the plasma concentrations or renal clearance of methotrexate, but supratherapeutic doses of rofecoxib (75 and 250 mg) caused a significant increase in the plasma methotrexate AUC and reduced its renal clearance.

Triamterene

Drugs that inhibit folate metabolism increase the likelihood of serious adverse reactions to methotrexate, particularly hematological toxicity. Bone marrow suppression and reduced plasma folate concentrations resulted from the concomitant administration of triamterene with methotrexate (145).

An interaction between triamterene and methotrexate (also an inhibitor of dihydrofolate reductase), leading to pancytopenia, has been reported (149). Dehydration due to diuretic treatment may have contributed to renal impairment and reduced clearance of methotrexate, further increasing the risk of bone marrow suppression.

Trimethoprim and co-trimoxazole

Methotrexate, a folic acid antagonist, is used in the treatment of several disorders. Its major action is inhibition of dihydrofolate reductase, a critical enzyme in intracellular folate metabolism. Co-trimoxazole competes with methotrexate in inhibiting dihydrofolate reductase and further impairs DNA synthesis (133). This should also be taken into account in patients taking trimethoprim alone (SEDA-22, 418).

- A fatal case of toxic epidermal necrolysis that involved 90% of the total body surface has been described in a 15-year-old boy with T cell acute lymphoblastic leukemia treated concomitantly with co-trimoxazole and methotrexate (151).

The authors suggested that methotrexate toxicity was precipitated by co-trimoxazole.

- Fatal bone marrow suppression has been reported in an 82-year-old woman who took methotrexate 7.5 mg/week for one year for rheumatoid arthritis without hematological problems. She was given trimethoprim 100 mg/day at first and later 200 mg/day. One week later, she developed severe pancytopenia. The bone marrow failed to recover despite treatment

with folinic acid and G-CSF, and she died of bronchopneumonia.

In a literature review, the authors found two other cases of bone marrow suppression after treatment with methotrexate and trimethoprim with full recovery of both. This interaction is also listed in the British National Formulary 1997 (152,153).

References

1. Cronstein BN. Molecular therapeutics. Methotrexate and its mechanism of action. Arthritis Rheum 1996;39(12):1951–60.
2. Alarcon GS, Tracy IC, Strand GM, Singh K, Macaluso M. Survival and drug discontinuation analyses in a large cohort of methotrexate treated rheumatoid arthritis patients. Ann Rheum Dis 1995;54(9):708–12.
3. Bologna C, Viu P, Picot MC, Jorgensen C, Sany J. Long-term follow-up of 453 rheumatoid arthritis patients treated with methotrexate: an open, retrospective, observational study. Br J Rheumatol 1997;36(5):535–40.
4. Kremer JM. Safety, efficacy, and mortality in a long-term cohort of patients with rheumatoid arthritis taking methotrexate: followup after a mean of 13.3 years Arthritis Rheum 1997;40(5):984–5.
5. Weinblatt ME, Maier AL, Fraser PA, Coblyn JS. Longterm prospective study of methotrexate in rheumatoid arthritis: conclusion after 132 months of therapy. J Rheumatol 1998;25(2):238–42.
6. Andersen LS, Hansen EL, Knudsen JB, Wester JU, Hansen GV, Hansen TM. Prospectively measured red cell folate levels in methotrexate treated patients with rheumatoid arthritis: relation to withdrawal and side effects. J Rheumatol 1997;24(5):830–7.
7. Morgan SL, Baggott JE, Vaughn WH, Austin JS, Veitch TA, Lee JY, Koopman WJ, Krumdieck CL, Alarcon GS. Supplementation with folic acid during methotrexate therapy for rheumatoid arthritis. A double-blind, placebo-controlled trial. Ann Intern Med 1994;121(11):833–41.
8. Ortiz Z, Shea B, Suarez-Almazor ME, Moher D, Wells GA, Tugwell P. The efficacy of folic acid and folinic acid in reducing methotrexate gastrointestinal toxicity in rheumatoid arthritis. A metaanalysis of randomized controlled trials. J Rheumatol 1998;25(1):36–43.
9. Griffith SM, Fisher J, Clarke S, Montgomery B, Jones PW, Saklatvala J, Dawes PT, Shadforth MF, Hothersall TE, Hassell AB, Hay EM. Do patients with rheumatoid arthritis established on methotrexate and folic acid 5 mg daily need to continue folic acid supplements long term? Rheumatology (Oxford) 2000;39(10):1102–9.
10. Kettunen R, Huikuri HV, Oikarinen A, Takkunen JT. Methotrexate-linked ventricular arrhythmias. Acta Derm Venereol 1995;75(5):391–2.
11. Landewe RB, van den Borne BE, Breedveld FC, Dijkmans BA. Methotrexate effects in patients with rheumatoid arthritis with cardiovascular comorbidity. Lancet 2000;355(9215):1616–7.
12. Schnabel A, Dalhoff K, Bauerfeind S, Barth J, Gross WL. Sustained cough in methotrexate therapy for rheumatoid arthritis. Clin Rheumatol 1996;15(3):277–82.
13. Kremer JM, Alarcon GS, Weinblatt ME, Kaymakcian MV, Macaluso M, Cannon GW, Palmer WR, Sundy JS, St Clair EW, Alexander RW, Smith GJ, Axiotis CA. Clinical, laboratory, radiographic,

and histopathologic features of methotrexate-associated lung injury in patients with rheumatoid arthritis: a multicenter study with literature review. Arthritis Rheum 1997;40(10):1829–37.

14. Salaffi F, Manganelli P, Carotti M, Subiaco S, Lamanna G, Cervini C. Methotrexate-induced pneumonitis in patients with rheumatoid arthritis and psoriatic arthritis: report of five cases and review of the literature. Clin Rheumatol 1997;16(3):296–304.

15. Golden MR, Katz RS, Balk RA, Golden HE. The relationship of pre-existing lung disease to the development of methotrexate pneumonitis in patients with rheumatoid arthritis. J Rheumatol 1995;22(6):1043–7.

16. Barrera P, Laan RF, van Riel PL, Dekhuijzen PN, Boerbooms AM, van de Putte LB. Methotrexate-related pulmonary complications in rheumatoid arthritis. Ann Rheum Dis 1994;53(7):434–9.

17. Kokelj F, Plozzer C, Muzzi A, Ciani F. Endoalveolar haemorrhage due to methotrexate overdosage in a patient treated for psoriatic arthritis. J Dermatol Treat 1999;10:67–9.

18. Massin F, Coudert B, Marot JP, Foucher P, Camus P, Jeannin L. La pneumopathie du methotrexate. [Pneumopathy caused by methotrexate.] Rev Mal Respir 1990;7(1):5–15.

19. Martins da Cunha AC, Bartsch CH, Gadner H. Acute respiratory failure after intrathecal methotrexate administration. Pediatr Hematol Oncol 1990;7(2):189–92.

20. Cottin V, Tebib J, Massonnet B, Souquet PJ, Bernard JP. Pulmonary function in patients receiving long-term low-dose methotrexate. Chest 1996;109(4):933–8.

21. Bartram SA. Experience with methotrexate-associated pneumonitis in northeastern England: comment on the article by Kremer et al. Arthritis Rheum 1998;41(7):1327–8.

22. Yoshida S, Onuma K, Akahori K, Sakamoto H, Yamawaki Y, Shoji T, Nakagawa H, Hasegawa H, Amayasu H. Elevated levels of IL-8 in interstitial pneumonia induced by low-dose methotrexate. J Allergy Clin Immunol 1999;103(5 Pt 1):952–4.

23. Alarcon GS, Kremer JM, Macaluso M, Weinblatt ME, Cannon GW, Palmer WR, St Clair EW, Sundy JS, Alexander RW, Smith GJ, Axiotis CAMethotrexate-Lung Study Group. Risk factors for methotrexate-induced lung injury in patients with rheumatoid arthritis. A multicenter, case-control study. Ann Intern Med 1997;127(5):356–64.

24. Imokawa S, Colby TV, Leslie KO, Helmers RA. Methotrexate pneumonitis: review of the literature and histopathological findings in nine patients. Eur Respir J 2000;15(2):373–81.

25. Fujii Y, Mizuno Y, Hongo T, Igarashi Y, Arai T, Kino I, Okamoto K. [Serial spectral EEG analysis in a patient with non-Hodgkin's lymphoma complicated by leukoencephalopathy induced by high-dose methotrexate.]Gan To Kagaku Ryoho 1988;15(4 Pt 1):713–7.

26. Poskitt KJ, Steinbok P, Flodmark O. Methotrexate leukoencephalopathy mimicking cerebral abscess on CT brain scan. Childs Nerv Syst 1988;4(2):119–21.

27. Ebner F, Ranner G, Slavc I, Urban C, Kleinert R, Radner H, Einspieler R, Justich E. MR findings in methotrexate-induced CNS abnormalities. Am J Neuroradiol 1989;10(5):959–64.

28. Borgna-Pignatti C, Battisti L, Marradi P, Balter R, Caudana R. Transient neurologic disturbances in a child treated with moderate-dose methotrexate. Br J Haematol 1992;81(3):448.

29. Worthley SG, McNeil JD. Leukoencephalopathy in a patient taking low dose oral methotrexate therapy for rheumatoid arthritis. J Rheumatol 1995;22(2):335–7.

30. Lesnik PG, Ciesielski KT, Hart BL, Benzel EC, Sanders JA. Evidence for cerebellar–frontal subsystem changes in children treated with intrathecal chemotherapy for leukemia: enhanced data analysis using an effect size model. Arch Neurol 1998;55(12):1561–8.

31. Aplin CG, Russell-Jones R. Acute dysarthria induced by low dose methotrexate therapy in a patient with erythrodermic cutaneous T cell lymphoma: an unusual manifestation of neurotoxicity. Clin Exp Dermatol 1999;24(1):23–4.

32. Schagen SB, van Dam FS, Muller MJ, Boogerd W, Lindeboom J, Bruning PF. Cognitive deficits after postoperative adjuvant chemotherapy for breast carcinoma. Cancer 1999;85(3):640–50.

33. Rau R, Schleusser B, Herborn G, Karger T. Longterm combination therapy of refractory and destructive rheumatoid arthritis with methotrexate (MTX) and intramuscular gold or other disease modifying antirheumatic drugs compared to MTX monotherapy. J Rheumatol 1998;25(8):1485–92.

34. Wernick R, Smith DL. Central nervous system toxicity associated with weekly low-dose methotrexate treatment. Arthritis Rheum 1989;32(6):770–5.

35. Dhondt JL, Farriaux JP, Millot F, Taret S, Hayte JM, Mazingue F. Methotrexate a haute close et hyperphenylalaninennie. [High-dose methotrexate and hyperphenylalaninemia.] Arch Fr Pediatr 1991;48(4):249–51.

36. Lapadula G, De Bari C, Acquista CA, Dell'Accio F, Covelli M, Iannone F. Isolated thrombocytopenia associated with low dose methotrexate therapy. Clin Rheumatol 1997;16(4):429–30.

37. Franck H, Rau R, Herborn G. Thrombocytopenia in patients with rheumatoid arthritis on long-term treatment with low dose methotrexate. Clin Rheumatol 1996;15(3):266–70.

38. Gutierrez-Urena S, Molina JF, Garcia CO, Cuellar ML, Espinoza LR. Pancytopenia secondary to methotrexate therapy in rheumatoid arthritis. Arthritis Rheum 1996;39(2):272–6.

39. Jover JA, Hernandez-Garcia C, Morado IC, Vargas E, Banares A, Fernandez-Gutierrez B. Combined treatment of giant-cell arteritis with methotrexate and prednisone. a randomized, double-blind, placebo-controlled trial. Ann Intern Med 2001;134(2):106–14.

40. Carpenter EH, Plant MJ, Hassell AB, Shadforth MF, Fisher J, Clarke S, Hothersall TE, Dawes PT. Management of oral complications of disease-modifying drugs in rheumatoid arthritis. Br J Rheumatol 1997;36(4):473–8.

41. Ince A, Yazici Y, Hamuryudan V, Yazici H. The frequency and clinical characteristics of methotrexate (MTX) oral toxicity in rheumatoid arthritis (RA): a masked and controlled study. Clin Rheumatol 1996;15(5):491–4.

42. Fisher A, Mor E, Hytiroglou P, Emre S, Boccagni P, Chodoff L, Sheiner P, Schwartz M, Thung SN, Miller C. FK506 hepatotoxicity in liver allograft recipients. Transplantation 1995;59(11):1631–2.

43. Kaplan MM. Methotrexate hepatotoxicity and the premature reporting of Mark Twain's death: both greatly exaggerated. Hepatology 1990;12(4 Pt 1):784–6.

44. Lin Y, Huang Y, Lee S, Wu J, Chang C, Chen C, Hwang S. [Clinical study of methotrexate-induced hepatic injury in patients with psoriasis.] Chin J Gastroenterol 1991;8:277–81.

45. Cunliffe RN, Scott BB. Review article: monitoring for drug side-effects in inflammatory bowel disease. Aliment Pharmacol Ther 2002;16(4):647–62.

46. Walker AM, Funch D, Dreyer NA, Tolman KG, Kremer JM, Alarcon GS, Lee RG, Weinblatt ME. Determinants of serious liver disease among patients receiving low-dose methotrexate for rheumatoid arthritis. Arthritis Rheum 1993;36(3):329–35.

47. Bach N, Thung SN, Schaffner F. The histologic effects of low-dose methotrexate therapy for primary biliary cirrhosis. Arch Pathol Lab Med 1998;122(4):342–5.

48. Kremer JM, Alarcon GS, Lightfoot RW Jr, Willkens RF, Furst DE, Williams HJ, Dent PB, Weinblatt ME. Methotrexate for rheumatoid arthritis. Suggested guidelines for monitoring liver toxicity. American College of Rheumatology. Arthritis Rheum 1994;37(3):316–28.

49. Risteli J, Sogaard H, Oikarinen A, Risteli L, Karvonen J, Zachariae H. Aminoterminal propeptide of type III procollagen in methotrexate-induced liver fibrosis and cirrhosis. Br J Dermatol 1988;119(3):321–5.

50. Hilton MA, Bertolone S, Patel CC. Daily profiles of plasma phenylalanine and tyrosine in patients with osteogenic sarcoma during treatment with high-dose methotrexate-citrovorum rescue. Med Pediatr Oncol 1989;17(4):265–70.

51. Roenigk HH Jr, Auerbach R, Maibach HI, Weinstein GD. Methotrexate in psoriasis: revised guidelines. J Am Acad Dermatol 1988;19(1 Pt 1):145–56.

52. West SG. Methotrexate hepatotoxicity. Rheum Dis Clin North Am 1997;23(4):883–915.

53. Zachariae H, Schroder H, Foged E, Sogaard H. Methotrexate hepatotoxicity and concentrations of methotrexate and folate in erythrocytes—relation to liver fibrosis and cirrhosis. Acta Dermatol Venereol 1987;67(4):336–40.

54. Tolman KG, Clegg DO, Lee RG, Ward JR. Methotrexate and the liver. J Rheumatol Suppl 1985;12(Suppl 12):29–34.

55. Jaskiewicz K, Voigt H, Blakolmer K. Increased matrix proteins, collagen and transforming growth factor are early markers of hepatotoxicity in patients on long-term methotrexate therapy. J Toxicol Clin Toxicol 1996;34(3):301–5.

56. Whiting-O'Keefe QE, Fye KH, Sack KD. Methotrexate and histologic hepatic abnormalities: a meta-analysis. Am J Med 1991;90(6):711–6.

57. Zachariae H, Kragballe K, Sogaard H. Methotrexate induced liver cirrhosis. Studies including serial liver biopsies during continued treatment. Br J Dermatol 1980;102(4):407–12.

58. Zachariae H, Sogaard H, Heickendorff L. Methotrexate-induced liver cirrhosis. Clinical, histological and serological studies—a further 10-year follow-up. Dermatology 1996;192(4):343–6.

59. Suzuki Y, Uehara R, Tajima C, Noguchi A, Ide M, Ichikawa Y, Mizushima Y. Elevation of serum hepatic aminotransferases during treatment of rheumatoid arthritis with low-dose methotrexate. Risk factors and response to folic acid. Scand J Rheumatol 1999;28(5):273–81.

60. Maiche AG, Lappalainen K, Teerenhovi L. Renal insufficiency in patients treated with high dose methotrexate. Acta Oncol 1988;27(1):73–4.

61. Christensen ML, Rivera GK, Crom WR, Hancock ML, Evans WE. Effect of hydration on methotrexate plasma concentrations in children with acute lymphocytic leukemia. J Clin Oncol 1988;6(5):797–801.

62. Amino K, Kawaguchi N, Matsumoto S, Manabe J, Ishii Y, Tabata D, Machida M. [Urinary beta 2-microglobulin as an indicator for impaired excretion of methotrexate.]Gan To Kagaku Ryoho 1988;15(11):3103–7.

63. Molina R, Fabian C, Cowley B Jr. Use of charcoal hemoperfusion with sequential hemodialysis to reduce serum methotrexate levels in a patient with acute renal insufficiency. Am J Med 1987;82(2):350–2.

64. Relling MV, Stapleton FB, Ochs J, Jones DP, Meyer W, Wainer IW, Crom WR, McKay CP, Evans WE. Removal of methotrexate, leucovorin, and their metabolites by combined hemodialysis and hemoperfusion. Cancer 1988;62(5):884–8.

65. Price P, Thompson H, Bessell EM, Bloom HJ. Renal impairment following the combined use of high-dose methotrexate and procarbazine. Cancer Chemother Pharmacol 1988;21(3):265–7.

66. Kerstens PJ, Boerbooms AM, Jeurissen ME, Fast JH, Assmann KJ, van de Putte LB. Accelerated nodulosis during low dose methotrexate therapy for rheumatoid arthritis. An analysis of ten cases. J Rheumatol 1992;19(6):867–71.

67. Falcini F, Taccetti G, Ermini M, Trapani S, Calzolari A, Franchi A, Cerinic MM. Methotrexate-associated appearance and rapid progression of rheumatoid nodules in systemic-onset juvenile rheumatoid arthritis. Arthritis Rheum 1997;40(1):175–8.

68. Muzaffer MA, Schneider R, Cameron BJ, Silverman ED, Laxer RM. Accelerated nodulosis during methotrexate therapy for juvenile rheumatoid arthritis. J Pediatr 1996;128(5 Pt 1):698–700.

69. Alarcon GS, Koopman WJ, McCarty MJ. Nonperipheral accelerated nodulosis in a methotrexate-treated rheumatoid arthritis patient. Arthritis Rheum 1993;36(1):132–3.

70. Combe B, Didry C, Gutierrez M, Anaya JM, Sany J. Accelerated nodulosis and systemic manifestations during methotrexate therapy for rheumatoid arthritis. Eur J Med 1993;2(3):153–6.

71. Goerttler E, Kutzner H, Peter HH, Requena L. Methotrexate-induced papular eruption in patients with rheumatic diseases: a distinctive adverse cutaneous reaction produced by methotrexate in patients with collagen vascular diseases. J Am Acad Dermatol 1999;40(5 Pt 1):702–7.

72. Halevy S, Giryes H, Avinoach I, Livni E, Sukenik S. Leukocytoclastic vasculitis induced by low-dose methotrexate: in vitro evidence for an immunologic mechanism. J Eur Acad Dermatol Venereol 1998;10(1):81–5.

73. Toussirot E, Wendling D. Methotrexate-induced hyperpigmentation in a rheumatoid arthritis patient. Clin Exp Rheumatol 1999;17(6):751.

74. Peters T, Theile-Ochel S, Chemnitz J, Sohngen D, Hunzelmann N, Scharffetter-Kochanek K. Exfoliative dermatitis after long-term methotrexate treatment of severe psoriasis. Acta Derm Venereol 1999;79(5):391–2.

75. Khan AJ, Brook S, Marghoob AA, Prestia AE, Spector IJ. Methotrexate and the photodermatitis reactivation reaction: a case report and review of the literature. Cutis 2000;66(5):379–82.

76. Hani N, Casper C, Groth W, Krieg T, Hunzelmann N. Stevens–Johnson syndrome-like exanthema secondary to methotrexate histologically simulating acute graft-versus-host disease. Eur J Dermatol 2000;10(7):548–50.

77. Basu TK, Williams DC, Raven RW. Methotrexate and alopecia. Lancet 1973;2(7824):331.

78. Weinblatt ME. Toxicity of low dose methotrexate in rheumatoid arthritis. J Rheumatol Suppl 1985;12(Suppl 12):35–9.

79. Malka N, Reichert S, Trechot P, Barbaud A, Schmutz JL. Yellow nail pigmentation due to methotrexate. Dermatology 1998;197(3):276.

80. Halla JT, Hardin JG. Underrecognized postdosing reactions to methotrexate in patients with rheumatoid arthritis. J Rheumatol 1994;21(7):1224–6.

81. Singwe M, Le Gars L, Karneff A, Prier A, Kaplan G. Multiple stress fractures in a scleroderma patient on methotrexate therapy. Rev Rhum Engl Ed 1998;65(7–9):508–10.

82. Zonneveld IM, Bakker WK, Dijkstra PF, Bos JD, van Soesbergen RM, Dinant HJ. Methotrexate osteopathy in long-term, low-dose methotrexate treatment for psoriasis and rheumatoid arthritis. Arch Dermatol 1996;132(2):184–7.

83. Mazzantini M, Di Munno O. Methotrexate and bone mass. Clin Exp Rheumatol 2000;18(Suppl 1):S87–92.

84. Blum M, Wallenstein S, Clark J, et al. Effect of methotrexate treatment on bone in postmenopausal women with primary biliary cirrhosis. J Bone Min Res 1996;11:S436.

85. Buckley LM, Leib ES, Cartularo KS, Vacek PM, Cooper SM. Effects of low dose methotrexate on the bone mineral density of patients with rheumatoid arthritis. J Rheumatol 1997;24(8):1489–94.

86. Carbone LD, Kaeley G, McKown KM, Cremer M, Palmieri G, Kaplan S. Effects of long-term administration of methotrexate on bone mineral density in rheumatoid arthritis. Calcif Tissue Int 1999;64(2):100–1.

87. Gerster JC, Bossy R, Dudler J. Bone non-union after osteotomy in patients treated with methotrexate. J Rheumatol 1999;26(12):2695–7.

88. Bianchi ML, Cimaz R, Galbiati E, Corona F, Cherubini R, Bardare M. Bone mass change during methotrexate treatment in patients with juvenile rheumatoid arthritis. Osteoporos Int 1999;10(1):20–5.

89. Mazzantini M, Di Munno O, Incerti-Vecchi L, Pasero G. Vertebral bone mineral density changes in female rheumatoid arthritis patients treated with low-dose methotrexate. Clin Exp Rheumatol 2000;18(3):327–31.

90. Blackburn WD Jr, Alarcon GS. Impotence in three rheumatoid arthritis patients treated with methotrexate. Arthritis Rheum 1989;32(10):1341–2.

91. Thomas E, Leroux JL, Blotman F. Gynecomastia in patients with rheumatoid arthritis treated with methotrexate. J Rheumatol 1994;21(9):1777–8.

92. Del Paine DW, Leek JC, Jakle C, Robbins DL. Gynecomastia associated with low dose methotrexate therapy. Arthritis Rheum 1983;26(5):691–2.

93. Freeman AM, Dasgupta B. Angio-neurotic oedema associated with methotrexate treatment in rheumatoid arthritis. Rheumatology (Oxford) 1999;38(9):908.

94. Fondevila Carlos G, Milone Gustavo A, Santiago P. Cutaneous vasculitis after intermediate dose of methotrexate (IDMTX). Br J Haematol 1989;72(4):591–2.

95. Borman P, Bodur H, Gulec AT, Ucan H, Seckin U, Mocan G. Atypical methotrexate dermatitis and vasculitis in a patient with ankylosing spondylitis. Rheumatol Int 2000;19(5):191–3.

96. Borcea A, Greaves MW. Methotrexate-induced exacerbation of urticarial vasculitis: an unusual adverse reaction. Br J Dermatol 2000;143(1):203–4.

97. Boerbooms AM, Kerstens PJ, van Loenhout JW, Mulder J, van de Putte LB. Infections during low-dose methotrexate treatment in rheumatoid arthritis. Semin Arthritis Rheum 1995;24(6):411–21.

98. Singh G, Fries JF, Williams CA, Zatarain E, Spitz P, Bloch DA. Toxicity profiles of disease modifying antirheumatic drugs in rheumatoid arthritis. J Rheumatol 1991;18(2):188–94.

99. van der Veen MJ, van der Heide A, Kruize AA, Bijlsma JW. Infection rate and use of antibiotics in patients with rheumatoid arthritis treated with methotrexate. Ann Rheum Dis 1994;53(4):224–8.

100. Kanik KS, Cash JM. Does methotrexate increase the risk of infection or malignancy? Rheum Dis Clin North Am 1997;23(4):955–67.

101. LeMense GP, Sahn SA. Opportunistic infection during treatment with low dose methotrexate. Am J Respir Crit Care Med 1994;150(1):258–60.

102. Gatnash AA, Connolly CK. Fatal chickenpox pneumonia in an asthmatic patient on oral steroids and methotrexate. Thorax 1995;50(4):422–3.

103. Wallace JR, Luchi M. Fatal cytomegalovirus pneumonia in a patient receiving corticosteroids and methotrexate for mixed connective tissue disease. South Med J 1996;89(7):726–8.

104. Hayem G, Meyer O, Kahn MF. *Listeria monocytogenes* infection in a patient treated with methotrexate for rheumatoid arthritis. J Rheumatol 1996;23(1):198–9.

105. Krebs S, Gibbons RB. Low-dose methotrexate as a risk factor for *Pneumocystis carinii* pneumonia. Mil Med 1996;161(1):58–60.

106. Lyon CC, Thompson D. *Herpes zoster* encephalomyelitis associated with low dose methotrexate for rheumatoid arthritis. J Rheumatol 1997;24(3):589–91.

107. Roux N, Flipo RM, Cortet B, Lafitte JJ, Tonnel AB, Duquesnoy B, Delcambre B. *Pneumocystis carinii* pneumonia in rheumatoid arthritis patients treated with methotrexate. A report of two cases. Rev Rhum Engl Ed 1996;63(6):453–6.

108. Narvaez J, Rodriguez-Moreno J, Martinez-Aguila MD, Clavaguera MT. Severe hepatitis linked to B virus infection after withdrawal of low dose methotrexate therapy. J Rheumatol 1998;25(10):2037–8.

109. Beauparlant P, Papp K, Haraoui B. The incidence of cancer associated with the treatment of rheumatoid arthritis. Semin Arthritis Rheum 1999;29(3):148–58.

110. Trenkwalder P, Eisenlohr H, Prechtel K, Lydtin H. Three cases of malignant neoplasm, pneumonitis, and pancytopenia during treatment with low-dose methotrexate. Clin Investig 1992;70(10):951–5.

111. Moder KG, Tefferi A, Cohen MD, Menke DM, Luthra HS. Hematologic malignancies and the use of methotrexate in rheumatoid arthritis: a retrospective study. Am J Med 1995;99(3):276–81.

112. Bologna C, Picot MC, Jorgensen C, Viu P, Verdier R, Sany J. Study of eight cases of cancer in 426 rheumatoid arthritis patients treated with methotrexate. Ann Rheum Dis 1997;56(2):97–102.

113. Wolfe F. Inflammatory activity, but not methotrexate or prednisone use predicts non-Hodgkin's lymphoma in rheumatoid arthritis: a 25-year study of 1767 RA patients. Arthritis Rheum 1998;41(Suppl):S188.

114. Bailin PL, Tindall JP, Roenigk HH Jr, Hogan MD. Is methotrexate therapy for psoriasis carcinogenic? A modified retrospective–prospective analysis. JAMA 1975;232(4):359–62.

115. Georgescu L, Quinn GC, Schwartzman S, Paget SA. Lymphoma in patients with rheumatoid arthritis: association with the disease state or methotrexate treatment. Semin Arthritis Rheum 1997;26(6):794–804.

116. Salloum E, Cooper DL, Howe G, Lacy J, Tallini G, Crouch J, Schultz M, Murren J. Spontaneous regression of lymphoproliferative disorders in patients treated with methotrexate for rheumatoid arthritis and other rheumatic diseases. J Clin Oncol 1996;14(6):1943–9.

117. Kono H, Inokuma S, Matsuzaki Y, Nakayama H, Yamazaki J, Hishima T, Maeda Y. Two cases of methotrexate induced lymphomas in rheumatoid arthritis: an association with increased serum IgE. J Rheumatol 1999;26(10):2249–53.

118. Viraben R, Brousse P, Lamant L. Reversible cutaneous lymphoma occurring during methotrexate therapy. Br J Dermatol 1996;135(1):116–8.

119. Baecklund E, Ekbom A, Sparen P, Feltelius N, Klareskog L. Disease activity and risk of lymphoma in patients with rheumatoid arthritis: nested case-control study. BMJ 1998;317(7152):180–1.

120. Kamel OW, van de Rijn M, LeBrun DP, Weiss LM, Warnke RA, Dorfman RF. Lymphoid neoplasms in patients with rheumatoid arthritis and dermatomyositis: frequency of Epstein–Barr virus and other features associated with immunosuppression. Hum Pathol 1994;25(7):638–43.

121. Theate I, Michaux L, Dardenne S, Guiot Y, Briere J, Emile FJ, Fabiani B, Detry R, Gaulard P. Groupe d'Etude des Lymphomes de l'Adulte (GELA). Epstein-Barr virus-associated lymphoproliferative disease occurring in a patient with sarcoidosis treated by methotrexate and methylprednisolone. Eur J Haematol 2002;69(4):248–53.

122. Georgescu L, Paget SA. Lymphoma in patients with rheumatoid arthritis: what is the evidence of a link with methotrexate? Drug Saf 1999;20(6):475–87.

123. Stewart M, Malkovska V, Krishnan J, Lessin L, Barth W. Lymphoma in a patient with rheumatoid arthritis receiving methotrexate treatment: successful treatment with rituximab. Ann Rheum Dis 2001;60(9):892–3.

124. Dubin Kerr L, Troy K, Isola L. Temporal association between the use of methotrexate and development of leukemia in 2 patients with rheumatoid arthritis. J Rheumatol 1995;22(12):2356–8.

125. Ostensen M, Ramsey-Goldman R. Treatment of inflammatory rheumatic disorders in pregnancy: what are the safest treatment options? Drug Saf 1998;19(5):389–410.

126. Del Campo M, Kosaki K, Bennett FC, Jones KL. Developmental delay in fetal aminopterin/methotrexate syndrome. Teratology 1999;60(1):10–2.

127. Lloyd ME, Carr M, McElhatton P, Hall GM, Hughes RA. The effects of methotrexate on pregnancy, fertility and lactation. QJM 1999;92(10):551–63.

128. Ostensen M, Hartmann H, Salvesen K. Low dose weekly methotrexate in early pregnancy. A case series and review of the literature. J Rheumatol 2000;27(8):1872–5.

129. Nakamura M, Sakemi T, Nagasawa K. Severe pancytopenia caused by a single administration of low dose methotrexate in a patient undergoing hemodialysis. J Rheumatol 1999;26(6):1424–5.

130. Chatham WW, Morgan SL, Alarcon GS. Renal failure: a risk factor for methotrexate toxicity. Arthritis Rheum 2000;43(5):1185–6.

131. Stewart CF, Fleming RA, Germain BF, Seleznick MJ, Evans WE. Aspirin alters methotrexate disposition in rheumatoid arthritis patients. Arthritis Rheum 1991;34(12):1514–20.

132. Rooney TW, Furst DE, Koehnke R, Burmeister L. Aspirin is not associated with more toxicity than other nonsteroidal antiinflammatory drugs in patients with rheumatoid arthritis treated with methotrexate. J Rheumatol 1993;20(8):1297–302.

133. Jeurissen ME, Boerbooms AM, van de Putte LB. Pancytopenia and methotrexate with trimethoprim–sulfamethoxazole. Ann Intern Med 1989;111(3):261.

134. Beck HI, Foged EK. Toxic hepatitis due to combination therapy with methotrexate and etretinate in psoriasis. Dermatologica 1983;167(2):94–6.

135. Larsen FG, Nielsen-Kudsk F, Jakobsen P, Schroder H, Kragballe K. Interaction of etretinate with methotrexate pharmacokinetics in psoriatic patients. J Clin Pharmacol 1990;30(9):802–7.

136. Damon LE, Cadman E, Benz C. Enhancement of 5-fluorouracil antitumor effects by the prior administration of methotrexate. Pharmacol Ther 1989;43(2):155–85.

137. Wolff JE, Hauch H, Kuhl J, Egeler RM, Jurgens H. Dexamethasone increases hepatotoxicity of MTX in children with brain tumors. Anticancer Res 1998;18(4B):2895–2899.

138. Lafforgue P, Monjanel-Mouterde S, Durand A, Catalin J, Acquaviva PC. Is there an interaction between low doses of corticosteroids and methotrexate in patients with rheumatoid arthritis? A pharmacokinetic study in 33 patients. J Rheumatol 1993;20(2):263–7.

139. Koerber H, Gross WL, Iven H. Do steroids influence low dose methotrexate pharmacokinetics? J Rheumatol 1994;21(6):1170–2.

140. van Meerten E, Verweij J, Schellens JH. Antineoplastic agents. Drug interactions of clinical significance. Drug Saf 1995;12(3):168–82.

141. Miles SM, Bird HA. Clinical signifiance of drug interactions with antirheumatic agents. Clin Immunother 1996;5:205–13.

142. Kremer JM, Hamilton RA. The effects of nonsteroidal antiinflammatory drugs on methotrexate (MTX) pharmacokinetics: impairment of renal clearance of MTX at weekly maintenance doses but not at 7.5 mg J Rheumatol 1995;22(11):2072–7.

143. Mayall B, Poggi G, Parkin JD. Neutropenia due to low-dose methotrexate therapy for psoriasis and rheumatoid arthritis may be fatal. Med J Aust 1991;155(7):480–4.

144. Basin KS, Escalante A, Beardmore TD. Severe pancytopenia in a patient taking low dose methotrexate and probenecid. J Rheumatol 1991;81(4):609–10.

145. Richmond R, McRorie ER, Ogden DA, Lambert CM. Methotrexate and triamterene—a potentially fatal combination? Ann Rheum Dis 1997;56(3):209–10.

146. Bertucci C, Wainer IW. Improved chromatographic performance of a modified human albumin based stationary phase. Chirality 1997;9(4):335–40.

147. Fehske KJ, Muller WE. High-affinity binding of ethacrynic acid is mediated by the two most important drug binding sites of human serum albumin. Pharmacology 1986;32(4):208–13.

148. Slordal L, Sager G, Jaeger R, Aarbakke J. Interactions with the protein binding of 7–hydroxy-methotrexate in human serum in vitro. Biochem Pharmacol 1988;37(4):607–11.

149. Richmond R, McRorie ER, Ogden DA, Lambert CM. Methotrexate and triamterene—a potentially fatal combination? Ann Rheum Dis 1997;56(3):209–10.

150. Dalle JH, Auvrignon A, Vassal G, Leverger G, Kalifa C. Interaction methotrexate–ciprofloxacine: à propos de deux cas d'intoxication sévère. [Methotrexate–ciprofloxacin interaction: report of two cases of severe intoxication.] Arch Pediatr 2001;8(10):1078–81.

151. Yang CH, Yang LJ, Jaing TH, Chan HL. Toxic epidermal necrolysis following combination of methotrexate and trimethoprim-sulfamethoxazole. Int J Dermatol 2000;39(8):621–3.

152. Steuer A, Gumpel JM. Methotrexate and trimethoprim: a fatal interaction. Br J Rheumatol 1998;37(1):105–6.

153. Richards AJ. Re: Interaction between methotrexate and trimethoprim. Br J Rheumatol 1998;37(7):806.

154. Blanco R, Martinez-Taboada VM, Gonzalez-Gay MA, Armona J, Fernandez-Sueiro JL, Gonzalez-Vela MC, Rodriguez-Valverde V. Acute febrile toxic reaction in patients with refractory rheumatoid arthritis who are receiving combined therapy with methotrexate and azathioprine. Arthritis Rheum 1996;39(6):1016–20.

155. Joyce DA, Will RK, Hoffman DM, Laing B, Blackbourn SJ. Exacerbation of rheumatoid arthritis in patients treated with methotrexate after administration of folinic acid. Ann Rheum Dis 1991;50(12):913–4.

156. Tishler M, Caspi D, Fishel B, Yaron M. The effects of leucovorin (folinic acid) on methotrexate therapy in rheumatoid arthritis patients. Arthritis Rheum 1988;31(7):906–8.

157. Damon LE, Cadman E, Benz C. Enhancement of 5-fluorouracil antitumor effects by the prior administration of methotrexate. Pharmacol Ther 1989;43(2):155–85.

158. Dogliotti L, Bertetto O, Berruti A, Clerico M, Fanchini L, Sicora W, Faggiuolo R. Combination chemotherapy with carboplatin and methotrexate in the treatment of advanced urothelial carcinoma. A phase II study. Am J Clin Oncol 1995;18(1):78–82.

159. Offerhaus L. Drug interactions at excretory mechanisms. Pharmacol Ther 1981;15(1):69–78.

160. Cassano WF. Serious methotrexate toxicity caused by interaction with ibuprofen. Am J Pediatr Hematol Oncol 1989;11(4):481–2.

161. Hubner G, Sander O, Degner FL, Turck D, Rau R. Lack of pharmacokinetic interaction of meloxicam with methotrexate in patients with rheumatoid arthritis. J Rheumatol 1997;24(5):845–51.

162. Combe B, Edno L, Lafforgue P, Bologna C, Bernard JC, Acquaviva P, Sany J, Bressolle F. Total and free methotrexate pharmacokinetics, with and without piroxicam, in rheumatoid arthritis patients. Br J Rheumatol 1995;34(5):421–8.

163. Tracy TS, Worster T, Bradley JD, Greene PK, Brater DC. Methotrexate disposition following concomitant administration of ketoprofen, piroxicam and flurbiprofen in patients with rheumatoid arthritis. Br J Clin Pharmacol 1994;37(5):453–6.

164. Wallace CA, Smith AL, Sherry DD. Pilot investigation of naproxen/methotrexate interaction in patients with juvenile rheumatoid arthritis. J Rheumatol 1993;20(10):1764–8.

165. Schwartz JI, Agrawal NG, Wong PH, Bachmann KA, Porras AG, Miller JL, Ebel DL, Sack MR, Holmes GB, Redfern JS, Gertz BJ. Lack of pharmacokinetic interaction between rofecoxib and methotrexate in rheumatoid arthritis patients. J Clin Pharmacol 2001;41(10):1120–30.

166. Liegler DG, Henderson ES, Hahn MA, Oliverio VT. The effect of organic acids on renal clearance of methotrexate in man. Clin Pharmacol Ther 1969;10(6):849–57.

167. Evans WE, Christensen ML. Drug interactions with methotrexate. J Rheumatol Suppl 1985;12(Suppl 12):15–20.

168. Carmine TC, Evans P, Bruchelt G, Evans R, Handgretinger R, Niethammer D, Halliwell B. Presence of iron catalytic for free radical reactions in patients undergoing chemotherapy: implications for therapeutic management. Cancer Lett 1995;94(2):219–26.

169. Tortajada-Ituren JJ, Ordovas-Baines JP, Llopis-Salvia P, Jimenez-Torres NV. High-dose methotrexate–doxycycline interaction. Ann Pharmacother 1999;33(7–8):804–8.

170. Ronchera CL, Hernandez T, Peris JE, Torres F, Granero L, Jimenez NV, Pla JM. Pharmacokinetic interaction between high-dose methotrexate and amoxycillin. Ther Drug Monit 1993;15(5):375–9.

171. Yamamoto K, Sawada Y, Matsushita Y, Moriwaki K, Bessho F, Iga T. Delayed elimination of methotrexate associated with piperacillin administration. Ann Pharmacother 1997;31(10):1261–2.

172. Mayall B, Poggi G, Parkin JD. Neutropenia due to low-dose methotrexate therapy for psoriasis and rheumatoid arthritis may be fatal. Med J Aust 1991;155(7):480–4.

173. Dawson JK, Abernethy VE, Lynch MP. Methotrexate and penicillin interaction. Br J Rheumatol 1998;37(7):807.

174. Herrick AL, Grennan DM, Griffen K, Aarons L, Gifford LA. Lack of interaction between flucloxacillin and methotrexate in patients with rheumatoid arthritis. Br J Clin Pharmacol 1996;41(3):223–7.

175. Najjar TA, Abou-Auda HS, Ghilzai NM. Influence of piperacillin on the pharmacokinetics of methotrexate and 7-hydroxymethotrexate. Cancer Chemother Pharmacol 1998;42(5):423–8.

176. Najjar TA, Abou-Auda HS, Ghilzai NM. Influence of piperacillin on the pharmacokinetics of methotrexate and 7-hydroxymethotrexate. Cancer Chemother Pharmacol 1998;42(5):423–8.

Miltefosine

General Information

Miltefosine is an alkylphospholipid that affects cell-signaling pathways and membrane synthesis; it was originally developed as an oral antineoplastic agent but is now licensed for use in visceral leishmaniasis in India (1,2).

Observational studies

In an open, multicenter trial in 120 patients, aged 12–50 years, who took 50, 100, or 150 mg/day of miltefosine for 4 or 6 weeks, there was an initial parasitological cure in all cases (3). Six patients had clinical and parasitological relapses by 6 months after initial treatment. There was a 97% cure rate with miltefosine 100 mg/day. Gastrointestinal adverse effects were frequent (in 62%) but mild to moderate in intensity, and no patient discontinued therapy as a result. In one patient, treatment was withdrawn because of raised aspartate transaminase activity, and in 12 others the aspartate transaminase activity increased to 100–150 U/l during treatment. In one patient, treatment was withdrawn because of a raised creatinine concentration.

Comparative studies

Miltefosine has been compared with the most effective standard treatment, amphotericin, in a randomized, open comparison in India, in which 299 patients, aged 12 years or over, received oral miltefosine (50 or 100 mg) and 99 patients received intravenous amphotericin deoxycholate (1 mg/kg every other day to a total of 15 injections) (4). Vomiting and diarrhea were more common with miltefosine. However, the effects were mild in almost all cases, and only 3–4% of patients needed antiemetic drugs in both groups. One patient who took miltefosine withdrew because of gastrointestinal intolerance and one developed Stevens–Johnson syndrome.

Second-Generation Effects

Fertility

Miltefosine caused infertility in male rats, but not in 211 men (4).

References

1. Murray HW. Kala-azar—progress against a neglected disease. N Engl J Med 2002;347(22):1793–4.
2. Guerin PJ, Olliaro P, Sundar S, Boelaert M, Croft SL, Desjeux P, Wasunna MK, Bryceson AD. Visceral leishmaniasis: current status of control, diagnosis, and treatment, and a proposed research and development agenda. Lancet Infect Dis 2002;2(8):494–501.
3. Jha TK, Sundar S, Thakur CP, Bachmann P, Karbwang J, Fischer C, Voss A, Berman J. Miltefosine, an oral agent, for the treatment of Indian visceral leishmaniasis. N Engl J Med 1999;341(24):1795–800.
4. Sundar S, Jha TK, Thakur CP, Engel J, Sindermann H, Fischer C, Junge K, Bryceson A, Berman J. Oral miltefosine for Indian visceral leishmaniasis. N Engl J Med 2002;347(22):1739–46.

Piritrexim

General Information

Piritrexim is a lipid-soluble analogue of methotrexate that has been used to treat methotrexate-resistant tumors (1). It is given with leucovorin (folinic acid) to minimize hematological toxicity. Myelosuppression is the major dose-limiting adverse effect. In 35 patients with urothelial carcinomas there was WHO grade 3/4 thrombocytopenia in four, granulocytopenia in one, and anemia in three; grade 3 non-hematological toxicity consisted of neuropathy in five patients, hepatotoxicity in two, nausea in two, and pulmonary toxicity and rash in one each (2). Piritrexim also causes facial flushing, periorbital edema, and pruritus, and anaphylactic shock has been reported (SEDA-18, 289).

References

1. Liu G, Bailey HH, Arzoomanian RZ, Alberti D, Binger K, Volkman J, Feierabend C, Marnocha R, Wilding G, Thomas JP. Gemcitabine, Paclitaxel, and Piritrexim: a phase I study. Am J Clin Oncol 2003;26(3):280–4.
2. Roth BJ, Manola J, Dreicer R, Graham D, Wilding GEastern Cooperative Oncology Group. Piritrexim in advanced, refractory carcinoma of the urothelium (E3896): a phase II trial of the Eastern Cooperative Oncology Group. Invest New Drugs 2002;20(4):425–9.

Raltitrexed

General Information

Raltitrexed is a specific inhibitor of thymidylate synthase. It is used to treat colorectal cancers.

In about 1000 patients with advanced colorectal cancer, the dose-limiting toxic effects in phase 1 studies were gastrointestinal toxicity, myelosuppression, and weakness; adverse events during phase 2 and 3 studies were similar to those seen during phase 1 (1). In all comparative studies, mucositis and leukopenia were markedly less common and less severe in patients treated with raltitrexed than with bolus fluorouracil + leucovorin. Thrombocytopenia was more common with raltitrexed but it was not associated with an increase in clinically significant hemorrhage. In contrast, raltitrexed-related myelosuppression was more severe than with fluorouracil + leucovorin when the antimetabolite was given by continuous infusion. Raised transaminases were common with raltitrexed but were usually reversible with continued dosing and were not associated with clinical sequelae.

Organs and Systems

Hematologic

In 21 patients with advanced colorectal cancer, intravenous raltitrexed 3 mg/m^2 plus mitomycin 6 mg/m^2 was associated with WHO grade 3/4 anemia in 2, and neutropenia and thrombocytopenia in one each (2).

Liver

Raltitrexed-induced hepatotoxicity is usually characterized by a transient and self-limiting increase in transaminases. However, it can occasionally be fatal.

- A woman aged 76 years and a man aged 56 years were given raltitrexed as adjuvant treatment of colorectal carcinoma and as palliative therapy for advanced biliary carcinoma respectively (3). Both developed fulminant liver failure with rapid deterioration after the second and sixth cycles of chemotherapy respectively, and both died within 24 hours. Autopsy showed signs of acute necrosis involving roughly 50% of the liver without signs of subacute liver damage.

In 130 patients treated with raltitrexed 3 mg/m^2 ($n = 52$) or raltitrexed plus oxaliplatin ($n = 78$), of whom 78 had liver metastases and 25 had raised transaminases, hepatotoxicity caused delays of a week or more in 60 of 584 chemotherapy cycles and was the reason for withdrawal of chemotherapy in eight patients (4). Raised baseline transaminases, the number of chemotherapy cycles, the cumulative dose of raltitrexed, short intervals between courses, and the addition of oxaliplatin predicted hepatotoxicity, while sex, age, creatinine clearance, previous chemotherapy, and the presence of liver metastases did not. Whether glutathione and ademethionine are hepatoprotective is unclear.

Skin

Two patients, aged 75 and 65 years, were given raltitrexed for colorectal cancers. After 5 and 7 days they developed erythematous, edematous, and purpuric skin reactions associated with weakness, diarrhea, and moderate fever (5). The lesions were painful and pseudocellulitic. They were generalized in the first case and localized to the legs in the second. They subsided 15 days after drug withdrawal.

Immunologic

Of 52 patients with colorectal cancer treated with a median of six 3-weekly cycles of raltitrexed 1.5–3.0 mg/m^2 combined with oral carmofur 300–400 mg/m^2 on cycle days 2–14, 39 had a fever on days 2–9 after receiving raltitrexed, 49 had fatigue, and 49 had a raised serum C-reactive protein concentration without a documented infection (6). Median concentrations of C-reactive protein, interleukin-6, interleukin-8, and tumor necrosis factor-alfa were higher 7 days after raltitrexed or raltitrexed + carmofur than at baseline. The authors suggested that patients with colorectal cancer treated with raltitrexed may develop drug-related systemic inflammation, which may be difficult to distinguish from infection.

Susceptibility Factors

Age

Of 90 patients treated with raltitrexed 3 mg/m^2 every 3 weeks, of whom 50 were aged over 70 years, 437 cycles of chemotherapy were administered and grade 3–4 toxicity was reported in under 10% (7). There were no significant differences between younger and older patients, apart from grade 3–4 weakness, which was reported by three of the older patients and none of the younger. This was despite a significantly lower calculated mean creatinine clearance in the older patients.

Renal disease

The pharmacokinetics of raltitrexed, and hence its toxic effects, particularly on the bone marrow and gut, are directly related to creatinine clearance (8). It is recommended that the dose be reduced and dosage interval increased in patients with mild to moderate renal impairment, based on the fact that raltitrexed is mainly excreted unchanged in the urine.

References

1. Zalcberg J. Overview of the tolerability of "Tomudex" (raltitrexed): collective clinical experience in advanced colorectal cancer. Anticancer Drugs 1997;8(Suppl 2):S17–22.
2. Rosati G, Rossi A, Germano D, Reggiardo G, Manzione L. Raltitrexed and mitomycin-C as third-line chemotherapy for colorectal cancer after combination regimens including 5-fluorouracil, irinotecan and oxaliplatin: a phase II study. Anticancer Res 2003;23(3C):2981–5.
3. Raderer M, Fiebiger W, Wrba F, Scheithauer W. Fatal liver failure after the administration of raltitrexed for cancer chemotherapy: a report of two cases. Cancer 2000;89(4):890–2.
4. Massacesi C, Santini D, Rocchi MB, La Cesa A, Marcucci F, Vincenzi B, Delprete S, Tonini G, Bonsignori M. Raltitrexed-induced hepatotoxicity: multivariate analysis of predictive factors. Anticancer Drugs 2003;14(7):533–41.
5. Topard D, Hellier I, Ychou M, Guillot B. Toxidermie au raltitrexed: 2 cas. [Raltitrexed-induced skin reaction.] Ann Dermatol Venereol 2000;127(12):1080–2.
6. Osterlund P, Orpana A, Elomaa I, Repo H, Joensuu H. Raltitrexed treatment promotes systemic inflammatory reaction in patients with colorectal carcinoma. Br J Cancer 2002;87(6):591–9.
7. Romiti A, Tonini G, Santini D, Di Seri M, Masciangelo R, Mezi S, Veri A, Santuari L, Vincenzi B, Brescia A, Marchei P, Frati L, Tomao S. Tolerability of raltitrexed ("Tomudex") in elderly patients with colorectal cancer. Anticancer Res 2002;22(5):3071–6.
8. Judson I, Maughan T, Beale P, Primrose J, Hoskin P, Hanwell J, Berry C, Walker M, Sutcliffe F. Effects of impaired renal function on the pharmacokinetics of raltitrexed (Tomudex ZD1694). Br J Cancer 1998;78(9):1188–93.

Tioguanine

General Information

Tioguanine is an analogue of the physiological purines, guanine and hypoxanthine, and is a purine antimetabolite. It is incorporated into DNA and RNA, resulting in a variety of cytotoxic effects. It has been used to treat hematological malignancies, psoriasis, and more recently, inflammatory bowel disease, such as Crohn's disease. Its main adverse effects are liver damage and hemotoxicity.

Among 111 patients taking tioguanine for inflammatory bowel disease, 29 had laboratory abnormalities, most commonly rises in liver enzymes and reduced platelet counts (1). Of the patients who underwent liver biopsy, there was nodular regenerative hyperplasia in 76% of those with laboratory abnormalities and 33% of those without.

Organs and Systems

Hematologic

Tioguanine can cause blood dyscrasias, in particular thrombocytopenia (2).

In 23 children taking tioguanine and a matched group taking mercaptopurine, there was no difference in the pattern of anemia or neutropenia between the two groups, but dose-limiting thrombocytopenia was more common in those taking tioguanine, four of whom had a fall in platelet count to below 20 × 10^9/l compared with only one taking mercaptopurine (3).

Liver

Nodular regenerative hyperplasia of the liver has been reported in three patients with inflammatory bowel disease who had taken tioguanine for more than a year and who had raised serum liver enzymes; all three had histological foci of nodular regenerative hyperplasia, which was best seen with reticulin silver impregnation (4).

The United Kingdom Medical Research Council Chronic Myeloid Leukemia Group reported 18 cases of tioguanine-induced non-cirrhotic portal hypertension, commonly associated with deterioration in liver function (5).

A patient developed acute sinusoidal obstruction syndrome after taking tioguanine for 14 months for Crohn's disease (6).

- A patient with acute myeloblastic leukemia, who took tioguanine for 2 months, developed severe peliosis hepatis associated with mild lesions of the centrilobular veins; withdrawal was followed by progressive improvement of liver dysfunction (7).

Several cases of hepatic veno-occlusive disease have been reported (8–11).

- A 23-year-old man with acute lymphocytic leukemia took tioguanine for 10 months and developed intense sinusoidal engorgement which resolved on withdrawal with some residual subintimal fibrosis around the terminal hepatic veins (12).

Of 12 patients aged 3–10 years, who had taken tioguanine 25–77 mg/m^2/day for acute lymphoblastic leukemia, one had persistent pancytopenia and intermittent splenomegaly. MRI/MRA scans showed a dilated splenic vein and collaterals, consistent with portal hypertension; esophagoscopy showed esophageal varices (13). A liver biopsy showed periportal fibrosis and marked dilatation of veins and venules. Of the other 12 patients, nine had abnormal MRI/MRA scans with evidence of varices in four. Liver biopsies in two cases showed periportal fibrosis, dilatation of venules and sinusoids, and minimal focal fatty changes.

References

1. Dubinsky MC, Vasiliauskas EA, Singh H, Abreu MT, Papadakis KA, Tran T, Martin P, Vierling JM, Geller SA, Targan SR, Poordad FF. 6-thioguanine can cause serious liver injury in inflammatory bowel disease patients. Gastroenterology 2003;125(2):298–303.
2. Wenzl HH, Hogenauer C, Fickert P, Petritsch W. Thioguanine-induced symptomatic thrombocytopenia. Am J Gastroenterol 2004;99(6):1195.
3. Lancaster DL, Lennard L, Rowland K, Vora AJ, Lilleyman JS. Thioguanine versus mercaptopurine for therapy of childhood lymphoblastic leukaemia: a comparison of haematological toxicity and drug metabolite concentrations. Br J Haematol 1998;102(2):439–43.
4. Shastri S, Dubinsky MC, Fred Poordad F, Vasiliauskas EA, Geller SA. Early nodular hyperplasia of the liver occurring with inflammatory bowel diseases in association with thioguanine therapy. Arch Pathol Lab Med 2004;128(1):49–53.
5. Shepherd PC, Fooks J, Gray R, Allan NC. Thioguanine used in maintenance therapy of chronic myeloid leukaemia causes non-cirrhotic portal hypertension. Results from MRC CML. II. Trial comparing busulphan with busulphan and thioguanine. Br J Haematol 1991;79(2):185–92.
6. Kane S, Cohen SM, Hart J. Acute sinusoidal obstruction syndrome after 6-thioguanine therapy for Crohn's disease. Inflamm Bowel Dis 2004;10(5):652–4.
7. Larrey D, Freneaux E, Berson A, Babany G, Degott C, Valla D, Pessayre D, Benhamou JP. Peliosis hepatis induced by 6-thioguanine administration. Gut 1988;29(9):1265–9.
8. Krivoy N, Raz R, Carter A, Alroy G. Reversible hepatic veno-occlusive disease and 6-thioguanine. Ann Intern Med 1982;96(6 Pt 1):788.
9. Satti MB, Weinbren K, Gordon-Smith EC. 6-thioguanine as a cause of toxic veno-occlusive disease of the liver. J Clin Pathol 1982;35(10):1086–91.
10. Kao NL, Rosenblate HJ. 6-Thioguanine therapy for psoriasis causing toxic hepatic venoocclusive disease. J Am Acad Dermatol 1993;28(6):1017–8.
11. Romagosa R, Kerdel F, Shah N. Treatment of psoriasis with 6-thioguanine and hepatic venoocclusive disease. J Am Acad Dermatol 2002;47(6):970–2.
12. Gill RA, Onstad GR, Cardamone JM, Maneval DC, Sumner HW. Hepatic veno-occlusive disease caused by 6-thioguanine. Ann Intern Med 1982;96(1):58–60.
13. Broxson EH, Dole M, Wong R, Laya BF, Stork L. Portal hypertension develops in a subset of children with standard risk acute lymphoblastic leukemia treated with oral 6-thioguanine during maintenance therapy. Pediatr Blood Cancer 2005;44(3):226–31.

Trimetrexate

General Information

Trimetrexate is a lipid-soluble analogue of methotrexate that has been used in the management of *Pneumocystis jiroveci* in patients with AIDS when other therapy has proved ineffective. It has also been used as an antineoplastic drug in the management of various solid tumors. It is given with leucovorin (folinic acid) to minimize hematological toxicity. Trimetrexate can cause neutropenia and/or thrombocytopenia (SEDA-12, 704) (1,2). Fever and raised liver transaminases, while uncommon, have been noticed. The efficacy of trimetrexate is not as high as that of co-trimoxazole and the recurrence rate is markedly higher (3).

References

1. Hughes WT. *Pneumocystis carinii* pneumonitis. N Engl J Med 1987;317(16):1021–3.
2. Allegra CJ, Chabner BA, Tuazon CU, Ogata-Arakaki D, Baird B, Drake JC, Simmons JT, Lack EE, Shelhamer JH, Balis F, et al. Trimetrexate for the treatment of *Pneumocystis carinii* pneumonia in patients with the acquired immunodeficiency syndrome. N Engl J Med 1987;317(16):978–85.
3. Masur H. Prevention and treatment of *Pneumocystis* pneumonia. N Engl J Med 1992;327(26):1853–60.

CYTOSTATIC ANTIBIOTICS

Acivicin

General Information

Acivicin is a cytostatic antibiotic, a glutamine analogue, which is a potent inhibitor of l-asparagine synthetase and other l-glutamine amidotransferases and has its cytotoxic action by blocking nucleotide biosynthesis.

Besides myelotoxicity, acivicin is neurotoxic, and can cause lethargy and auditory and visual hallucinations. Some patients have nystagmus, incontinence, and severe depression (1,2).

References

1. Willson JK, Knuiman MW, Skeel RT, Wolter JM, Pandya KJ, Falkson G, Chang YC. Phase II clinical trial of acivicin in advanced breast cancer: an Eastern Cooperative Oncology Group Study. Cancer Treat Rep 1986;70(10):1237–8.
2. Booth BW, Korzun AH, Weiss RB, Ellison RR, Budman D, Khojasteh A, Wood W. Phase II trial of acivicin in advanced breast carcinoma: a Cancer and Leukemia Group B Study. Cancer Treat Rep 1986;70(10):1247–8.

Anthracyclines and related compounds

General Information

Anthracyclines form a broad group of antitumor drugs within the group of cytotoxic antibiotics. The lead compounds were doxorubicin and daunorubicin; analogues include epirubicin, idarubicin, and aclarubicin. Mitoxantrone and pixantrone are related compounds of the anthracenedione family. Amsacrine is a related compound of the aminoacridine family.

Liposomal forms of doxorubicin (Caelyx, Myocet) and daunorubicin (DaunoXome) are in use. These drugs are licensed for the treatment of a wide range of tumors (Table 1). Much information regarding the anthracyclines has been previously published in major reviews and textbooks (1,2). With this in mind, their major toxic effects are outlined here, but concentrating in more detail on new findings, such as the interaction with trastuzumab.

Organs and Systems

Cardiovascular

Cardiomyopathy
Anthracyclines can cause the late complication of a cardiomyopathy, which can be irreversible and can proceed to congestive cardiac failure, ventricular dysfunction, conduction disturbances, or dysrhythmias several months or years after the end of treatment (3,4). Doxorubicin can cause abnormalities of right ventricular wall motion (5). A significant number of patients receiving anthracyclines develop cardiac autonomic dysfunction (6).

Dose-relatedness
The development of anthracycline-induced cardiomyopathy is closely related to the cumulative lifetime dose of the anthracycline. The recommended maximum cumulative lifetime dose of doxorubicin is 450–550 mg/m^2 (7) and of daunorubicin 400–550 mg/m^2 intravenously in adults (1,2). About 5% of doxorubicin-treated patients develop congestive cardiac failure at this dose; however, the incidence approaches 50% at cumulative doses of 1000 mg/m^2 (7–9). These figures are derived from experience with doxorubicin administered as a bolus or by infusion of very short duration (under 30 minutes). The incidence of clinical cardiotoxicity falls dramatically with other schedules of administration (that is weekly doses or continuous infusion for more than 24 hours).

In a randomized study of adjuvant chemotherapy comparing bolus against continuous intravenous infusion of doxorubicin 60 mg/m^2, cardiotoxicity, defined as a 10% or greater reduction in left ventricular ejection fraction, occurred in 61% of patients on a bolus median dose equal to 420 mg/m^2 compared with 42% on the continuous infusion schedule with a median dose of 540 mg/m^2; the rate of cardiotoxicity as a function of the cumulative dose of doxorubicin was significantly higher in the bolus treatment arm (10).

In 11 patients with anthracycline cardiotoxicity studied by heart catheterization and endomyocardial biopsy, myocytic damage correlated linearly with cumulative dose (11). There was a non-linear relation between electron microscopic changes and the extent of hemodynamic impairment. There was pronounced fibrous thickening of the endocardium in most patients, especially in the left ventricle. Endocardial fibrosis may be the first morphological sign of cardiotoxicity.

Susceptibility factors
The risk of cardiotoxicity is greater in children and patients with pre-existing cardiac disease or concomitant or prior mediastinal or chest wall irradiation (12,13).

Table 1 Licensed indications for anthracyclines

Drug	Where licensed	Licensed for the treatment of
Doxorubicin	USA and EU	Acute leukemia, lymphomas, soft tissue and osteogenic sarcomas, pediatric malignancies, and adult solid tumors (particularly lung and breast cancers)
Epirubicin	EU	Breast, ovarian, gastric, and lung cancers; malignant lymphomas, leukemias, and multiple myeloma; superficial and in-situ bladder carcinomas
Daunorubicin	USA and EU	Acute leukemias
Idarubicin	USA and EU	Relapsed or first-line treatment refractory advanced breast cancer, acute leukemias
Liposomal doxorubicin (Caelyx, Doxil)	USA and EU	Kaposi's sarcoma in AIDS
Liposomal pegylated daunorubicin (DaunoXome)	USA and EU	Kaposi's sarcoma in AIDS
Liposomal doxorubicin (Myocet)	EU	Breast cancer

Of 682 patients, 144 who were over 65 years of age all had doses up to but not exceeding the usual cumulative dose for doxorubicin (14). The authors concluded that older patients without cardiovascular co-morbidity are at no greater risk of congestive heart failure.

The use of doxorubicin in childhood impairs myocardial growth, resulting in a progressive increase in left ventricular afterload, sometimes associated with impaired myocardial contractility (15). Of 201 children who received doxorubicin and/or daunorubicin 200–1275 mg/m^2, 23% had abnormal cardiac function 4–20 years afterwards. Of those who were followed for more than 10 years, 38% had abnormal cardiac function compared with 18% in those who were followed for less than 10 years (16,17). In another study, more than half of the children studied by serial echocardiography after doxorubicin therapy for acute lymphoblastic leukemia developed increased left ventricular wall stress due to reduced wall thickness. This stress progressed with time (18).

Predisposing factors to mitoxantrone cardiotoxicity include increasing age, prior anthracycline therapy, previous cardiovascular disease, mediastinal radiotherapy, and a cumulative dose of the drug exceeding 120 mg/m^2. In 801 patients treated with mitoxantrone, prior treatment with doxorubicin and mitoxantrone was significantly associated with risk of cardiotoxicity; however, age, sex, and prior mediastinal radiotherapy were not useful predictors (19).

Anesthesia is difficult in patients with cumulative anthracycline-induced cardiotoxicity, and it has proved fatal on occasions (20).

Comparative studies of anthracyclines

All anthracyclines have cardiotoxic potential. However, because only a few cycles of treatment are administered in most regimens, few patients reach the cardiotoxic threshold of cumulative anthracycline dose. There is therefore limited information about the comparative cardiotoxic potential of these agents.

Epirubicin is considered to cause substantially less cardiotoxicity than doxorubicin on a molar basis (4,21). This has been attributed to its more rapid clearance rather than a different action (22). In a randomized, double-blind comparison of epirubicin and doxorubicin, there was a significant reduction in left ventricle ejection fraction with doxorubicin but not with epirubicin (23). However, data from large clinical series and from morphological examination of endomyocardial biopsies in smaller series of patients suggest that the incidence and severity of cumulative cardiac toxicity associated with epirubicin 900 mg/m^2 is similar to that associated with doxorubicin 450–550 mg/m^2 (24). In 29 patients treated with epirubicin in cumulative doses ranging from 147 to 888 mg/m^2 the ultrastructural myocardial lesions were similar to those produced by doxorubicin (partial and total myofibrillar loss in individual myocytes) (25). With both drugs, severe lesions were associated with replacement fibrosis. None of the patients who received epirubicin in the study developed congestive cardiac failure.

Both mitoxantrone and the oral formulation of idarubicin have been thought to be less cardiotoxic than doxorubicin (26,27). The South West Oncology Group reported on 801 patients treated with mitoxantrone; 1.5% developed congestive cardiac failure, an additional 1.5% had a reduced left ventricular ejection fraction (LVEF), and 0.25% developed acute myocardial infarction (19). Idarubicin has been reported to cause short-term cardiac toxicity when used in high doses in leukemia, and there is no doubt that it causes cumulative dose-related toxicity as well (28). Electrocardiographic changes occurred in 7% of adults with acute leukemia receiving aclarubicin (29).

Presentation

The main effects of anthracycline-induced cardiotoxicity are reduced left ventricular function and chronic congestive heart failure. Other cardiotoxic events occur only rarely. Occasionally, acute transient electrocardiographic changes (ST–T wave changes, prolongation of the QT interval) and dysrhythmias can occur. Acute conduction disturbances, acute myopericarditis, and acute cardiac failure are also rare. In a study of the effects of anthracyclines on myocardial function in 50 long-term survivors of childhood cancer, there was cardiac failure in one patient and electrocardiographic abnormalities (non-specific ST segment and T wave changes) in two (13). In one patient with a VVI pacemaker, who received the combination of vincristine, doxorubicin, and dexamethasone, the pacemaker had to be reset after each cycle of treatment, as the pacing threshold had increased, resulting in bradycardia (30).

Hypokinetic heart wall motion abnormalities and early signs of chronic cardiomyopathy have been identified as a significant toxic effect of mitoxantrone in patients who received cumulative doses of 32–174 mg (31). Electrocardiographic T wave inversion and cardiac complications have been described from intensive therapy with mitoxantrone 40 mg/m^2 over 5 days and cyclophosphamide 1550 mg/m^2 for 4 days, given before bone marrow transplantation for metastatic breast cancer. All the patients had had previous exposure to doxorubicin in cumulative doses that did not exceed 442 mg/m^2 (19).

The authors of a study of the use of MRI scans to assess the subclinical effects of the anthracyclines concluded that increased MRI enhancement equal to or greater than 5 on day 3 compared with the baseline predicted significant reduction in ejection fraction at day 28 (32). In 1000 patients given doxorubicin chemotherapy and irradiation there were six cases of congestive heart failure and three cases of myocardial infarction; there was a cumulative cardiac mortality of 0.4% in all anthracycline-exposed patients (33).

Diagnosis

The diagnosis of anthracycline cardiomyopathy is based on the clinical presentation and investigations such as radionuclide cardiac angiography, which can show a reduced ejection fraction (34), and echocardiography, which can show reduced or abnormal ventricular function (35,36). Dysrhythmias can be detected by electrocardiography, and QT$_c$ interval prolongation may offer an easy, non-invasive test to predict patients who are at special risk of late cardiac decompensation after anthracycline treatment for childhood cancer (37). Radioimmunoscintigraphy can be used to highlight damaged myocytes, and changes such as myocardial fibrosis are characteristic on endomyocardial biopsy (13,38,39).

The subtle chronic abnormalities in myocardial function that occur 10–20 years after anthracycline exposure in childhood are best detected by exercise echocardiography, since these patients may have normal resting cardiac function (40).

It has been suggested that monitoring B type natriuretic peptide concentrations after anthracycline administration can reflect cardiac tolerance, and through serial monitoring allow a picture of the degree of left ventricular dysfunction to be established (41).

Mechanisms

Several mechanisms contribute to anthracycline cardiotoxicity. The principal mechanism is thought to be oxidative stresses placed on cardiac myocytes by reactive oxygen species. Amelioration of this toxicity is possible using dexrazoxane, an intracellular metal-chelating agent of the dioxopiperazine class (3). Dexrazoxane acts by depleting intracellular iron, thus reducing the formation of cardiotoxic hydroxyl anions and radicals. In patients without heart failure, in-vivo measurements of myocardial oxidative metabolism and blood flow did not change in patients with cancer receiving doxorubicin (42).

Anthracyclines have the ability inherent in their quinone structure to form free-radical semiquinones which result in very reactive oxygen species, causing peroxidation of the lipid membranes of the heart. However, this reaction has not been demonstrated with mitoxantrone, and the mechanism of its cardiotoxicity is unknown.

Abnormalities of left ventricular ejection fraction have been described in 46% of patients ($n = 14$) treated with mitoxantrone (14 mg/m^2) and with vincristine and prednisolone (43). A history of cardiac disease or of previous anthracycline exposure was excluded. Only one patient developed clinically overt congestive cardiac failure. Other reports have described less cardiotoxicity compared with the parent compound, doxorubicin (4,44).

Management

Anthracycline cardiomyopathy, although reportedly difficult to treat, often responds to current methods used to manage congestive cardiac failure.

Severe anthracycline-induced cardiotoxicity is generally considered irreversible, and it is associated with a poor prognosis and high mortality. However, in four cases the advanced cardiac dysfunction associated with doxorubicin recovered completely after withdrawal (45). Of 19 patients with anthracycline-induced congestive cardiac failure, 12 recovered after withdrawal, although reversal was modest (46).

The prolongation of the QT interval that occurs in patients who have recently finished doxorubicin therapy is slowly reversible over at least 3 years and the degree of prolongation is related to the cumulative dose (47).

Heart transplantation has been successful in patients with late, progressive cardiomyopathy without recurrence of the underlying malignant disease (48).

Cardiac dysrhythmias

Cardiac dysrhythmias have been reported after amsacrine therapy in association with hypokalemia. Pre-existing supraventricular dysrhythmias or ventricular extra beats are not absolute contraindications to its use (49). Of 5430 patients treated with amsacrine, 65 developed cardiotoxicity, including prolongation of the QT interval, non-specific ST–T wave changes, ventricular tachycardia, and ventricular fibrillation (50). There were serious ventricular dysrhythmias resulting in cardiopulmonary arrest in 31 patients; 14 died as a result. The dysrhythmias occurred within minutes to several hours after drug administration. The cardiotoxicity was not related to total cumulative dose, and hypokalemia was possibly a risk factor for dysrhythmias.

Sensory systems

Doxorubicin can cause conjunctivitis, periorbital edema, lacrimation, blepharospasm, keratitis, and reduced visual acuity (51). There have been two reports of persistent photophobia and chronic inflammation of the eye following accidental topical exposure to doxorubicin (52).

Hematologic

Myelosuppression, principally neutropenia, occurs in 60–80% of patients who receive conventional doses of anthracyclines (single-agent standard doses: doxorubicin 60–75 mg/m^2, epirubicin 60–90 mg/m^2 given 3-weekly) (53). On an equimolar basis, in both the single-agent and combination regimens, epirubicin causes less hematological toxicity than doxorubicin (24). The incidence and severity of myelosuppression is related to dose; it has been suggested that severe neutropenia occurs in all patients who are given high-dose anthracyclines (doxorubicin 100 mg/m^2 or more and epirubicin 120 mg/m^2 or more) (54). Neutrophil nadirs occur at 7–10 days after treatment, and full neutrophil recovery usually occurs by day 21 (24). Platelets are less affected; about 35% of patients receiving epirubicin 120 mg/m^2 have grade-3 thrombocytopenia (55). Anemia occurs rarely (24).

Although the extent of leukopenia is not related to cumulative anthracycline dose, patients who have received extensive prior chemotherapy develop more severe leukopenia, possibly because of diminished bone marrow reserve (24). There was a strong correlation between dose and both leukocyte nadirs and platelet nadirs in 287 patients who received single-agent epirubicin 40, 60, 90, or 135 mg/m^2 every 3 weeks (56). Myelosuppression correlates with exposure to epirubicin, as reflected by the plasma AUC (57).

Myelosuppression is not prevented by prolonged doxorubicin infusion (53), although this can mitigate other adverse effects. Hematological toxicity associated with high-dose regimens can be partially ameliorated by giving hemopoietic growth factors, with or without autologous bone marrow or peripheral blood progenitor cell rescue (58–60). However, other adverse effects, mainly mucositis, then become dose-limiting. It has been suggested that mitoxantrone 14 mg/m^2 is more myelosuppressive than doxorubicin 70 mg/m^2, which in turn is more myelosuppressive than epirubicin 70 mg/m^2, each given at 3-week intervals (61).

Secondary acute myeloid leukemia, with or without a preleukemic phase, has been rarely reported in patients being concurrently treated with epirubicin or doxorubicin in association with DNA-damaging antineoplastic agents; such cases have a short latency period (1–3 years) (62,63). In one study, three of 77 patients who received epirubicin plus cisplatin and two who received other epirubicin-containing combinations developed acute myelogenous leukemia 15–33 months after the start of epirubicin treatment for advanced breast cancer (62). However, all had received prior treatment with alkylating agents and/or radiotherapy, which are recognized independent leukemogenic risk factors. Despite high mean lifetime

epirubicin doses in this study (mean 800 mg/m^2), there was no relation between cumulative dose and the risk of acute myelogenous leukemia. In a second study, four of 351 patients with metastatic breast cancer who received fluorouracil + epirubicin + cyclophosphamide, but none of 359 who received cyclophosphamide + methotrexate + 5-fluorouracil, developed leukemia (three acute myelogenous leukemia, one acute lymphoblastic leukemia) (63). No secondary leukemias were documented in other large comparative studies of epirubicin-containing regimens (64,65). Nevertheless, a retrospective analysis of case reports, published in abstract form without references or methods, concluded that when epirubicin was combined with alkylating agents it was associated with an increased risk of secondary acute myelogenous leukemia in women with breast cancer (66).

Prolongation of the prothrombin time after the use of amsacrine 1200 mg/m^2 for acute myeloid leukemia was related to transient deficiency of factor X (67).

Mouth

Mucositis is a well-documented toxic effect of anthracyclines; it has been reported in 8% of combination chemotherapeutic courses including epirubicin in a dose of 180 mg/m^2 (68).

Gastrointestinal

The anthracyclines are classed as moderately to strongly emetogenic. Nausea and vomiting occurs in 21–55% of patients, but is substantially reduced by pretreatment with antiemetic drugs (53,55). In one randomized study, epirubicin 70 mg/m^2, doxorubicin 70 mg/m^2, and mitoxantrone 14 mg/m^2 were compared (61). The first cycles of epirubicin and mitoxantrone were given without antiemetic drugs, unless specifically requested, but thereafter antiemetic drugs were given as required; doxorubicin was given with antiemetic drugs from cycle one. Doxorubicin and epirubicin were significantly more emetogenic than mitoxantrone; there was grade 3 nausea and vomiting in 22% of those who received doxorubicin, 18% of those who received epirubicin, and none of those who received mitoxantrone. Oral idarubicin may cause more emesis, which is quoted as occurring in 25–86% of patients; however, these effects are said to be usually mild to moderate (27).

With the advent of the 5-hydroxytryptamine (5-HT$_3$) receptor antagonists (ondansetron, granisetron, tropisetron), used in conjunction with dexamethasone, nausea and vomiting can be ameliorated in most patients.

Mucositis and stomatitis are potentially severe and dose-limiting adverse effects of the anthracyclines. Both the frequency and the severity are dose-dependent (56,69). Their onset and recovery generally parallel the hematological toxicity, but they can occur earlier (5–10 days after treatment starts). Areas of painful erosions, mainly along the side of the tongue and on the sublingual mucosa, are common. Mucositis occurs in about 9% of patients who receive oral idarubicin in standard doses (27).

Diarrhea has also been reported with the anthracyclines. In a typical study, in which epirubicin 100 mg/m^2

was given for 1–8 cycles, one of 39 patients had grade 1/2 diarrhea and two of 39 had grade 3/4 diarrhea (70). Of patients who take oral idarubicin 10–38% are said to develop diarrhea, again generally mild to moderate (27).

Urinary tract

All anthracyclines can cause discoloration of the urine and other body fluids (that is tears) (1,2).

Skin

Anthracyclines can cause local irritant reactions. These range from erythema and phlebitis at the injection site to potentially severe vesicant reactions requiring skin grafting (24). Care appropriate to the administration of a vesicant must be observed during infusion. Various treatments have been used immediately after extravasation in an attempt to lessen the injury, including ice, steroids, vitamin E, and bicarbonate. The current recommended treatment is by intermittent cooling of the affected area, together with intermittent use of topical dimethylsulfoxide 99% (71). There is also evidence of the efficacy of intravenous dexrazoxane, and the first dose should preferably be given within 6 hours (72). In three patients who had extravasation of epirubicin or doxorubicin, healing occurred without sequelae (73,74); all three received three doses of intravenous dexrazoxane over 3 days (1000 mg/m^2 on the first two days and 500 mg/m^2 on day 3), the first dose being administered at 2–5 hours after extravasation. A fourth patient received dexrazoxane 1500 mg 1 hour after extravasation of doxorubicin and repeated 5 hours later, and 750 mg on day 2; the wound healed slowly and required surgery after 3 months (75). A fifth patient received dexrazoxane more than 6 hours after extravasation of epirubicin; the wound healed slowly and with a crusted center (76).

Reactivation of skin damage can also occur at sites of prior radiation therapy ("radiation recall") (77).

- Widespread allergic contact dermatitis occurred in a 73-year-old man after intravesical administration of epirubicin; a patch test with an aqueous solution of the drug (0.1%) was positive (78).

A syndrome of palmar–plantar erythema (progressing in some patients to blistering and desquamation) has been reported in seven of eight patients with advanced breast or ovarian cancer who received high-dose doxorubicin (125–150 mg/m^2) (79). By contrast, in a similar dose intensification study in which patients received epirubicin 200 mg/m^2 with cyclophosphamide and growth factor support, the palmar–plantar syndrome did not occur (80).

In 60 patients receiving polyethylene glycol-coated liposomal doxorubicin (Doxil) 35–70 mg/m^2 by infusion over 1–2 hours there were four patterns of skin eruption: hand–foot syndrome (40%), a diffuse follicular rash (10%), an intertrigo-like eruption (8%), and new melanotic macules (0.5%) (81).

Hair

Complete or partial alopecia occurs in the majority (60–90%) of patients who receive anthracyclines, and although it is reversible it can be distressing (24). Scalp cooling during chemotherapy to minimize hair loss is now little used, because of limited efficacy, the discomfort of scalp cooling techniques, and concern about the potential creation of a "sanctuary" for circulating tumor cells. Alopecia is less frequent (about 35% of patients) in patients who take oral idarubicin 40–45 mg/m^2 every 3 weeks (27).

Nails

Painful onycholysis, blue discoloration of the nails (82), and reversible loss of fingernails (83) have been attributed to mitoxantrone.

Sweat glands

There has been a single report of hidradenitis associated with mitoxantrone (84).

Long-Term Effects

Mutagenicity

There was an increased number of chromosomally aberrant lymphocytes in nurses who handled cytostatic agents (doxorubicin, cyclophosphamide, vincristine, fluorouracil, and methotrexate) many years ago, before modern facilities for the preparation of chemotherapeutic drugs were in use (85). No long-term fertility problems were identified in 205 men who were treated with doxorubicin during childhood (86).

Tumorigenicity

In 604 women who were given six cycles of epirubicin after 4 years of tamoxifen, there were 12 non-breast second malignancies (87). Although the authors did not analyse these in respect to population expectation, they thought that the frequency was relatively high.

Second-Generation Effects

Teratogenicity

There is no conclusive evidence about whether anthracyclines adversely affect human fertility or are teratogenic. In 26 of 28 pregnancies, three or more chemotherapeutic agents were used to treat acute leukemia (n = 20), non-Hodgkin's lymphoma (n = 3), Ewing's sarcoma (n = 2), breast cancer (n = 2), and myoblastoma (n = 1) (88). The anthracyclines were introduced at various gestational ages, ranging from time of conception to 38 weeks, but in most cases chemotherapy was started in the second trimester. The outcomes were 24 normal infants, including a set of twins. Four of the five cases of infant death occurred in those with hematological malignancies (acute leukemia and non-Hodgkin's lymphoma), one each due to maternal death and therapeutic abortion and two resulting from spontaneous abortion. Neonatal pathological examination showed no congenital anomalies or organ defects, one case of marrow hypoplasia, and one case of neonatal sepsis. These findings suggest that anthracyclines have no detectable effect on the offspring up to the age of 54 months. However, bias inherent in reporting pregnancies with a successful outcome is obvious, so extreme caution must be exercised in the use of anthracyclines in pregnancy, and they should be avoided if at all possible.

Fetotoxicity

Cardiac failure occurred in a 3-day-old neonate whose mother had been given idarubicin 9 mg/m^2 as part of induction therapy for acute lymphoblastic leukemia at 22 weeks; the baby was delivered at 28 weeks (89). In the absence of another known cause, the cardiotoxicity was attributed to idarubicin exposure 6 weeks before.

Susceptibility Factors

Hepatic disease

Since the main route of metabolism and elimination of anthracyclines is via the bile, dosage reduction is recommended if there is hepatic impairment. This was first suggested after a report of increased toxicity in patients with liver metastases who received full-dose anthracycline treatment, followed by a second report that suggested that the clearance of anthracyclines is reduced in patients with hepatic metastases (90,91). These reports led to the current recommendations for anthracycline doses, based on serum bilirubin concentration or sulfobromophthalein clearance. However, the question of whether liver dysfunction significantly affects anthracycline clearance is unclear, and the dosage modifications suggested (see Table 2) have never been validated. Indeed, there is evidence that anthracycline kinetics are altered in patients with raised serum transaminases alone, which may be a better basis for dosage modification (92). In practice, many clinicians make empirical dosage modifications in patients with abnormal liver biochemistry tests (57).

Drug Administration

Drug formulations

The anthracyclines have been formulated in liposomal formulations in order to alter their pharmacokinetics and improve their therapeutic index. Examples include:

- pegylated liposomal doxorubicin (Caelyx/Doxil);
- liposomal doxorubicin (Myocet);
- liposomal daunorubicin (DaunoXome).

These formulations are dealt with in a separate monograph.

Drug administration route

The anthracyclines are most commonly given intravenously, either as bolus doses or, less often, as infusions over varying lengths of time. Alternative routes have been tried, such as the intraperitoneal, intrapleural, and intravesical routes (93,94).

Intraperitoneal
Intraperitoneal instillation of doxorubicin has been used in the early postoperative period in patients with retroperitoneal or visceral sarcoma, in an attempt to eradicate microscopic residual disease after complete macroscopic surgical excision (95). Three of 17 patients had pyrexia, one peritoneal sclerosis, one a pancreatic fistula, and two abdominal pain. There were no anastomotic disruptions or intra-abdominal hemorrhages.

Intrapleural
Adverse effects associated with the intrapleural instillation of doxorubicin in doses of 10–40 mg consist of fever (11–15%), anorexia (24–29%), nausea (20–29%), and chest pain (28–29%) (94,96). Cardiomyopathy and myelosuppression were not reported (96).

Intravesical
Intravesical epirubicin has been used to treat superficial bladder cancers. At a dose of 50 mg, the overall incidence of adverse events was 16–25% (93). The frequency of adverse events tended to increase with dose but not the number of instillations. Most adverse events were mild and transient; the commonest were localized to the bladder and included chemical cystitis (10–38%), urinary tract infection (2–13%), and hematuria (2–33%). Contracted bladder or hemorrhagic cystitis have been reported in 1–6% of patients (93).

Table 2   Effects of liver function on doses of doxorubicin and epirubicin

Drug	Serum bilirubin concentration	BSP retention	Recommended dose
Doxorubicin	20–50 µmol/l	9–15%	50% of normal
	>50 µmol/l	>15%	25% of normal
Epirubicin	20–50 µmol/l		50% of normal
	>50 µmol/l		25% of normal

Adverse events occurred in 31 of 194 patients who received epirubicin 80 mg intravesically compared with 12 of 205 who received placebo after transurethral resection (97). Systemic adverse events (usually cardiac or hematological adverse events or hypersensitivity) generally occurred in under 5% of patients. In two studies of intravesical epirubicin, there were reports of myocardial infarction (9%), stroke (3%), angina pectoris (3%), or atrioventricular block (2%) (98,99). There were no reports of myelosuppression in clinical trials of intravesical epirubicin, apart from thrombocytopenia in one of 37 patients in one cancer trial (98) and hemoglobinemia in two of 40 patients in another (100).

Biochemical abnormalities have been reported in trials of intravesical epirubicin. In one trial, liver function tests were impaired in seven of 40 patients who received epirubicin and in 10 of 35 patients who received epirubicin and verapamil concomitantly (101). In another study, liver function tests were impaired in one of 69 patients who received combination prophylaxis with epirubicin 50 mg and BCG 150 mg after transurethral resection (102).

Hypersensitivity has been reported in 0–8% of patients in trials of intravesical epirubicin; the symptoms included generalized skin rash, vulval irritation, or urinary frequency and dysuria, or were not stated (100,103,104). One of 34 patients developed symptoms characterized as allergic (dizziness, nausea, hypotension) 1 hour after instillation of epirubicin (105). Two patients who received epirubicin developed severe allergic reactions and one died (106,107).

Non-specific systemic adverse events (flu-like symptoms, malaise, fever, nausea, vomiting, anorexia, rash) occurred in under 5% of patients who received intravesical epirubicin (98,103,108). Alopecia was reported in one of 37 patients (98).

Intravesical epirubicin and doxorubicin appear to have similar tolerability profiles (104,109–112).

Valrubicin (a novel N-trifluoroacetyl, 14-valerate derivative of doxorubicin) is currently licensed in the USA for intravesical use in prophylaxis in patients with BCG-refractory carcinoma in situ after transurethral resection. It has a similar toxicity profile to that of epirubicin and doxorubicin (113).

Drug overdose

Very high single doses of anthracyclines can cause acute myocardial degeneration within 24 hours and severe myelosuppression within 10–14 days. Treatment should aim to support the patient during this period and should include such measures as blood transfusion and reverse barrier nursing. Delayed cardiac failure can occur up to 6 months after overdosage.

Drug–Drug Interactions

Etoposide

The combination of idarubicin plus etoposide (total doses 180 mg and 5760 mg respectively) was associated with a case of acute promyelocytic leukemia (114).

Taxanes

The combination of doxorubicin plus paclitaxel is cardiotoxic.

Of 57 patients who had received at least three courses of chemotherapy with a combination of doxorubicin 50 mg/m^2 plus paclitaxel 175–225 mg/m^2, left ventricular ejection fraction did not fall overall but was significantly reduced in eight patients; it fell by more than 14% in three cases and by 33–48% in the other five; none of the patients developed clinical heart failure (115).

Two studies of the combination of epirubicin plus paclitaxel have shown less reduction in left ventricular ejection fraction and no clinical evidence of cardiac failure (116,117).

Clinically significant cardiac insufficiency has been reported in a patient who was given epirubicin (316 mg/m^2) followed by six cycles of docetaxel (100 mg/m^2/cycle) (118).

Trastuzumab

An interaction of doxorubicin with the anti-HER$_2$ receptor humanized monoclonal antibody, trastuzumab (Herceptin), has been reported. Most patients who received trastuzumab in early trials had been pretreated with anthracyclines. Despite this, preliminary information suggested that reduced systolic cardiac function was an adverse effect of trastuzumab (119). More recently, this problem has been further highlighted in a study of women with metastatic breast cancer (120). Patients who had not received prior anthracycline-containing adjuvant chemotherapy were at greater risk of cardiotoxicity when they received trastuzumab in combination with doxorubicin or cyclophosphamide (27 and 75% respectively), compared with only 11% of patients who received trastuzumab in combination with paclitaxel (120,121). The risk of cardiac events in patients treated with doxorubicin, cyclophosphamide, and trastuzumab increased markedly after a cumulative doxorubicin dose of 360 mg/m^2. This suggests synergistic cardiotoxicity with trastuzumab and doxorubicin. Trastuzumab is therefore currently licensed only for use in conjunction with paclitaxel or docetaxel and not with conventional doxorubicin.

The mechanism of trastuzumab-induced cardiotoxicity and its synergy with doxorubicin is as yet unknown. However, the cardiac failure responds to standard medical management (122).

Since trastuzumab is active as a single agent and in combination with chemotherapy in patients whose tumors overexpress HER$_2$, the interaction with doxorubicin is clearly of concern. Although it is possible to avoid this problem by not combining trastuzumab with doxorubicin, there are compelling reasons for further exploring its use with anthracyclines. For example, follow-up results from the CALGB 8541 study have shown that patients who received high and moderate (standard) doses of cyclophosphamide plus doxorubicin plus fluorouracil survived longer than those who received low doses (123). Moreover, examination of patients' HER$_2$ status in this trial showed that those whose tumors expressed large amounts of the HER_2 protein had a significantly worse survival if treated with moderate or low doses of cyclophosphamide plus doxorubicin plus fluorouracil, compared with high doses (124). These results suggest that patients whose tumors express large amounts of the HER_2 receptor protein may require high-dose anthracyclines, presenting the problem of how then to treat them with trastuzumab without causing cardiotoxicity.

In an attempt to avoid cardiotoxicity after the administration of trastuzumab with doxorubicin, alternative adjuvant regimens have been suggested. Trastuzumab could be combined with other anthracyclines (epirubicin or liposomal formulations), which are inherently less cardiotoxic, or given sequentially rather than concomitantly with the anthracycline. Alternatively, non-anthracycline combinations, such as cyclophosphamide plus doxorubicin plus fluorouracil or based around taxanes, cisplatin, and vinorelbine are being investigated (125).

Caution should of course be exercised when giving other cytotoxic drugs, especially myelotoxic agents or agents that cause significant mucositis/stomatitis, in combination with anthracyclines.

References

1. Chabner BA, Longo DL. Cancer Chemotherapy and Biotherapy: Principles and Practice. 2nd ed.. Lippincott Williams and Wilkins;. 2001.
2. Souhami RL, Tannock I, Hohenberger P, Horiot JC. Oxford Textbook of Oncology. 2nd ed.. Oxford: Oxford University Press;. 2002.
3. Wiseman LR, Spencer CM. Dexrazoxane. A review of its use as a cardioprotective agent in patients receiving anthracycline-based chemotherapy. Drugs 1998;56(3):385–403.
4. Okuma K, Ariyoshi Y, Ota K. [Clinical study of acute cardiotoxicity of anti-cancer agents—analysis using Holter ECG monitoring.]Gan To Kagaku Ryoho 1988;15(6):1893–900.
5. Barendswaard EC, Prpic H, Van der Wall EE, Camps JA, Keizer HJ, Pauwels EK. Right ventricle wall motion abnormalities in patients treated with chemotherapy. Clin Nucl Med 1991;16(7):513–6.
6. Viniegra M, Marchetti M, Losso M, Navigante A, Litovska S, Senderowicz A, Borghi L, Lebron J, Pujato D, Marrero H, et al. Cardiovascular autonomic function in anthracycline-treated breast cancer patients. Cancer Chemother Pharmacol 1990;26(3):227–31.
7. Launchbury AP, Habboubi N. Epirubicin and doxorubicin: a comparison of their characteristics, therapeutic activity and toxicity. Cancer Treat Rev 1993;19(3):197–228.
8. Shan K, Lincoff AM, Young JB. Anthracycline-induced cardiotoxicity. Ann Intern Med 1996;125(1):47–58.
9. Von Hoff DD, Layard MW, Basa P, Davis HL Jr, Von Hoff AL, Rozencweig M, Muggia FM. Risk factors for doxorubicin-induced congestive heart failure. Ann Intern Med 1979;91(5):710–7.
10. Casper ES, Gaynor JJ, Hajdu SI, Magill GB, Tan C, Friedrich C, Brennan MF. A prospective randomized trial of adjuvant chemotherapy with bolus versus continuous infusion of doxorubicin in patients with high-grade extremity soft tissue sarcoma and an analysis of prognostic factors. Cancer 1991;68(6):1221–9.
11. Mortensen SA, Olsen HS, Baandrup U. Chronic anthracycline cardiotoxicity: haemodynamic and histopathological manifestations suggesting a restrictive endomyocardial disease. Br Heart J 1986;55(3):274–82.
12. Pihkala J, Saarinen UM, Lundstrom U, Virtanen K, Virkola K, Siimes MA, Pesonen E. Myocardial function in children and adolescents after therapy with anthracyclines and chest irradiation. Eur J Cancer 1996;32A(1):97–103.
13. Hesseling PB, Kalis NN, Wessels G, van der Merwe PL. The effect of anthracyclines on myocardial function in 50 long-term survivors of childhood cancer. Cardiovasc J South Afr 1999;89(Suppl 1):C25–8.
14. Ibrahim NK, Hortobagyi GN, Ewer M, Ali MK, Asmar L, Theriault RL, Fraschini G, Frye DK, Buzdar AU. Doxorubicin-induced congestive heart failure in elderly patients with metastatic breast cancer, with long-term follow-up: the M.D. Anderson experience Cancer Chemother Pharmacol 1999;43(6):471–8.
15. Lipshultz SE, Colan SD, Gelber RD, Perez-Atayde AR, Sallan SE, Sanders SP. Late cardiac effects of doxorubicin therapy for acute lymphoblastic leukemia in childhood. N Engl J Med 1991;324(12):808–15.
16. Steinherz LJ, Steinherz PG, Tan CT, Heller G, Murphy ML. Cardiac toxicity 4 to 20 years after completing anthracycline therapy. JAMA 1991;266(12):1672–7.
17. Drug news. Anthracycline cardiotoxicity uncovered. Drug Ther 1991;57Dec.
18. Fahey J. Cardiovascular function in children with acquired and congenital heart disease. Curr Opin Cardiol 1992;7:111–5.
19. Mather FJ, Simon RM, Clark GM, Von Hoff DD. Cardiotoxicity in patients treated with mitoxantrone: Southwest Oncology Group phase II studies. Cancer Treat Rep 1987;71(6):609–13.
20. McQuillan PJ, Morgan BA, Ramwell J. Adriamycin cardiomyopathy. Fatal outcome of general anaesthesia in a child with adriamycin cardiomyopathy. Anaesthesia 1988;43(4):301–4.
21. Coukell AJ, Faulds D. Epirubicin. An updated review of its pharmacodynamic and pharmacokinetic properties and therapeutic efficacy in the management of breast cancer. Drugs 1997;53(3):453–82.
22. Camaggi CM, Comparsi R, Strocchi E, Testoni F, Angelelli B, Pannuti F. Epirubicin and doxorubicin comparative metabolism and pharmacokinetics. A cross-over study. Cancer Chemother Pharmacol 1988;21(3):221–8.
23. Lahtinen R, Kuikka J, Nousiainen T, Uusitupa M, Lansimies E. Cardiotoxicity of epirubicin and doxorubicin: a double-blind randomized study. Eur J Haematol 1991;46(5):301–5.
24. Plosker GL, Faulds D. Epirubicin. A review of its pharmacodynamic and pharmacokinetic properties, and therapeutic use in cancer chemotherapy. Drugs 1993;45(5):788–856.
25. Torti FM, Bristow MM, Lum BL, Carter SK, Howes AE, Aston DA, Brown BW Jr, Hannigan JF Jr, Meyers FJ, Mitchell EP, et al. Cardiotoxicity of epirubicin and doxorubicin: assessment by endomyocardial biopsy. Cancer Res 1986;46(7):3722–7.
26. Booser DJ, Hortobagyi GN. Anthracycline antibiotics in cancer therapy. Focus on drug resistance. Drugs 1994;47(2):223–58.
27. Buckley MM, Lamb HM. Oral idarubicin. A review of its pharmacological properties and clinical efficacy in the treatment of haematological malignancies and advanced breast cancer. Drugs Aging 1997;11(1):61–86.

28. Petti MC, Mandelli F. Idarubicin in acute leukemias: experience of the Italian Cooperative Group GIMEMA. Semin Oncol 1989;16(1 Suppl 2):10–5.

29. Ota K. Clinical review of aclacinomycin A in Japan. Drugs Exp Clin Res 1985;11(1):17–21.

30. Wilke A, Hesse H, Gorg C, Maisch B. Elevation of the pacing threshold: a side effect in a patient with pacemaker undergoing therapy with doxorubicin and vincristine. Oncology 1999;56(2):110–1.

31. Lai KH, Tsai YT, Lee SD, Ng WW, Teng HC, Tam TN, Lo GH, Lin HC, Lin HJ, Wu JC, et al. Phase II study of mitoxantrone in unresectable primary hepatocellular carcinoma following hepatitis B infection. Cancer Chemother Pharmacol 1989;23(1):54–6.

32. Wassmuth R, Lentzsch S, Erdbruegger U, Schulz-Menger J, Doerken B, Dietz R, Friedrich MG. Subclinical cardiotoxic effects of anthracyclines as assessed by magnetic resonance imaging—a pilot study. Am Heart J 2001;141(6):1007–13.

33. Zambetti M, Moliterni A, Materazzo C, Stefanelli M, Cipriani S, Valagussa P, Bonadonna G, Gianni L. Long-term cardiac sequelae in operable breast cancer patients given adjuvant chemotherapy with or without doxorubicin and breast irradiation. J Clin Oncol 2001;19(1):37–43.

34. Dey HM, Kassamali H. Radionuclide evaluation of doxorubicin cardiotoxicity: the need for cautious interpretation. Clin Nucl Med 1988;13(8):565–8.

35. Solymar L, Marky I, Mellander L, Sabel KG. Echocardiographic findings in children treated for malignancy with chemotherapy including adriamycin. Pediatr Hematol Oncol 1988;5(3):209–16.

36. Nakamura K, Miyake T, Kawamura T, Maekawa I. [Prospective monitoring of adriamycin cardiotoxicity with systolic time intervals.]Nippon Gan Chiryo Gakkai Shi 1988;23(8):1633–7.

37. Schwartz CL, Hobbie WL, Truesdell S, Constine LC, Clark EB. Corrected QT interval prolongation in anthracycline-treated survivors of childhood cancer. J Clin Oncol 1993;11(10):1906–10.

38. Vici P, Ferraironi A, Di Lauro L, Carpano S, Conti F, Belli F, Paoletti G, Maini CL, Lopez M. Dexrazoxane cardioprotection in advanced breast cancer patients undergoing high-dose epirubicin treatment. Clin Ter 1998;149(921):15–20.

39. Rowan RA, Masek MA, Billingham ME. Ultrastructural morphometric analysis of endomyocardial biopsies. Idiopathic dilated cardiomyopathy, anthracycline cardiotoxicity, and normal myocardium. Am J Cardiovasc Pathol 1988;2(2):137–44.

40. Weesner KM, Bledsoe M, Chauvenet A, Wofford M. Exercise echocardiography in the detection of anthracycline cardiotoxicity. Cancer 1991;68(2):435–8.

41. Suzuki T, Hayashi D, Yamazaki T, Mizuno T, Kanda Y, Komuro I, Kurabayashi M, Yamaoki K, Mitani K, Hirai H, Nagai R, Yazaki Y. Elevated B-type natriuretic peptide levels after anthracycline administration. Am Heart J 1998;136(2):362–3.

42. Nony P, Guastalla JP, Rebattu P, Landais P, Lievre M, Bontemps L, Itti R, Beaune J, Andre-Fouet X, Janier M. In vivo measurement of myocardial oxidative metabolism and blood flow does not show changes in cancer patients undergoing doxorubicin therapy. Cancer Chemother Pharmacol 2000;45(5):375–80.

43. Cassidy J, Merrick MV, Smyth JF, Leonard RC. Cardiotoxicity of mitozantrone assessed by stress and resting nuclear ventriculography. Eur J Cancer Clin Oncol 1988;24(5):935–8.

44. Brusamolino E, Bertini M, Guidi S, Vitolo U, Inverardi D, Merante S, Colombo A, Resegotti L, Bernasconi C, Ferrini PR, et al. CHOP versus CNOP (N = mitoxantrone) in non-Hodgkin's lymphoma: an interim report comparing efficacy and toxicity Haematologica 1988;73(3):217–22.

45. Saini J, Rich MW, Lyss AP. Reversibility of severe left ventricular dysfunction due to doxorubicin cardiotoxicity. Report of three cases. Ann Intern Med 1987;106(6):814–6.

46. Moreb JS, Oblon DJ. Outcome of clinical congestive heart failure induced by anthracycline chemotherapy. Cancer 1992;70(11):2637–41.

47. Ferrari S, Figus E, Cagnano R, Iantorno D, Bacci G. The role of corrected QT interval in the cardiologic follow-up of young patients treated with Adriamycin. J Chemother 1996;8(3):232–6.

48. Goenen M, Baele P, Lintermans J, Lecomte C, Col J, Ponlot R, Schoevardts JC, Chalant C. Orthotopic heart transplantation eleven years after left pneumonectomy. J Heart Transplant 1988;7(4):309–11.

49. Puccio CA, Feldman EJ, Arlin ZA. Amsacrine is safe in patients with ventricular ectopy. Am J Hematol 1988;28(3):197–8.

50. Weiss RB, Grillo-Lopez AJ, Marsoni S, Posada JG Jr, Hess F, Ross BJ. Amsacrine-associated cardiotoxicity: an analysis of 82 cases. J Clin Oncol 1986;4(6):918–28.

51. Curran CF, Luce JK. Ocular adverse reactions associated with adriamycin (doxorubicin). Am J Ophthalmol 1989;108(6):709–11.

52. Curran CF, Luce JK. Accidental acute exposure to doxorubicin. Cancer Nurs 1989;12(6):329–31.

53. Abraham R, Basser RL, Green MD. A risk-benefit assessment of anthracycline antibiotics in antineoplastic therapy. Drug Saf 1996;15(6):406–29.

54. Zuckerman KS. Efficacy of intensive, high-dose anthracycline-based therapy in intermediate- and high-grade non-Hodgkin's lymphomas. Semin Oncol 1994;21(1 Suppl 1):59–64.

55. Lissoni A, Cormio G, Colombo N, Gabriele A, Landoni F, Zanetta G, Mangioni C. High-dose epirubicin in patients with advanced or recurrent uterine sarcoma. Int J Gynaecol Cancer 1997;7:241–4.

56. Bastholt L, Dalmark M, Gjedde SB, Pfeiffer P, Pedersen D, Sandberg E, Kjaer M, Mouridsen HT, Rose C, Nielsen OS, Jakobsen P, Bentzen SM. Dose–response relationship of epirubicin in the treatment of postmenopausal patients with metastatic breast cancer: a randomized study of epirubicin at four different dose levels performed by the Danish Breast Cancer Cooperative Group. J Clin Oncol 1996;14(4):1146–55.

57. Dobbs NA, Twelves CJ. Anthracycline doses in patients with liver dysfunction: do UK oncologists follow current recommendations? Br J Cancer 1998;77(7):1145–8.

58. Scinto AF, Ferraresi V, Campioni N, Tonachella R, Piarulli L, Sacchi I, Giannarelli D, Cognetti F. Accelerated chemotherapy with high-dose epirubicin and cyclophosphamide plus r-met-HUG-CSF in locally advanced and metastatic breast cancer. Ann Oncol 1995;6(7):665–71.

59. Hansen F, Stenbygaard L, Skovsgaard T. Effect of granulocyte-macrophage colony-stimulating factor (GM-CSF) on hematologic toxicity induced by high-dose chemotherapy in patients with metastatic breast cancer. Acta Oncol 1995;34(7):919–24.

60. Chevallier B, Chollet P, Merrouche Y, Roche H, Fumoleau P, Kerbrat P, Genot JY, Fargeot P, Olivier JP, Fizames C, et al. Lenograstim prevents morbidity from

intensive induction chemotherapy in the treatment of inflammatory breast cancer. J Clin Oncol 1995;13(7):1564–71.

61. Lawton PA, Spittle MF, Ostrowski MJ, Young T, Madden F, Folkes A, Hill BT, MacRae K. A comparison of doxorubicin, epirubicin and mitozantrone as single agents in advanced breast carcinoma. Clin Oncol (R Coll Radiol) 1993;5(2):80–4.

62. Pedersen-Bjergaard J, Sigsgaard TC, Nielsen D, Gjedde SB, Philip P, Hansen M, Larsen SO, Rorth M, Mouridsen H, Dombernowsky P. Acute monocytic or mye-lomonocytic leukemia with balanced chromosome translo-cations to band 11q23 after therapy with 4-epi-doxorubicin and cisplatin or cyclophosphamide for breast cancer. J Clin Oncol 1992;10(9):1444–51.

63. Shepherd L, Ottaway J, Myles J, Levine M. Therapy-related leukemia associated with high-dose 4-epi-doxoru-bicin and cyclophosphamide used as adjuvant chemother-apy for breast cancer. J Clin Oncol 1994;12(11):2514–5.

64. Coombes RC, Bliss JM, Wils J, Morvan F, Espie M, Amadori D, Gambrosier P, Richards M, Aapro M, Villar-Grimalt A, McArdle C, Perez-Lopez FR, Vassilopoulos P, Ferreira EP, Chilvers CE, Coombes G, Woods EM, Marty M. Adjuvant cyclophosphamide, meth-otrexate, and fluorouracil versus fluorouracil0, epirubicin, and cyclophosphamide chemotherapy in premenopausal women with axillary node-positive operable breast cancer: results of a randomized trial. The International Collaborative Cancer Group. J Clin Oncol 1996;14(1):35–45.

65. Marty M. Epirubicin and the risk of leukemia: not sub-stantiated? International Collaborative Cancer Group Steering Committee. J Clin Oncol 1993;11(7):1431–3.

66. Ragaz J, Yun J, Spinelli J. Analysis of incidence of second-ary acute myelogenous leukemias (2nd AML) in breast cancer patients (BCP) treated with adjuvant therapy (AT)-association with therapeutic regimens. (Abstract no. 147). Proc Am Soc Clin Oncol 1995;14:112.

67. Carter C, Winfield DA. Factor X deficiency during treat-ment of relapsed acute myeloid leukaemia with amsacrine. Clin Lab Haematol 1988;10(2):225–8.

68. Zuckerman KS, Case DC Jr, Gams RA, Prasthofer EF. Chemotherapy of intermediate- and high-grade non-Hodgkin's lymphomas with an intensive epirubicin-con-taining regimen. Blood 1993;82(12):3564–73.

69. Focan C, Andrien JM, Closon MT, Dicato M, Driesschaert P, Focan-Henrard D, Lemaire M, Lobelle JP, Longree L, Ries F. Dose–response relationship of epirubicin-based first-line chemotherapy for advanced breast cancer: a prospective randomized trial. J Clin Oncol 1993;11(7):1253–63.

70. Bissett D, Paul J, Wishart G, Jodrell D, Machan MA, Harnett A, Canney P, George WD, Kaye S. Epirubicin chemotherapy and advanced breast cancer after adjuvant CMF chemotherapy. Clin Oncol (R Coll Radiol) 1995;7(1):12–5.

71. Bertelli G, Gozza A, Forno GB, Vidili MG, Silvestro S, Venturini M, Del Mastro L, Garrone O, Rosso R, Dini D. Topical dimethylsulfoxide for the prevention of soft tissue injury after extravasation of vesicant cytotoxic drugs: a pro-spective clinical study. J Clin Oncol 1995;13(11):2851–5.

72. Langer SW, Sehested M, Jensen PB. Treatment of anthra-cycline extravasation with dexrazoxane. Clin Cancer Res 2000;6(9):3680–6.

73. Jensen JN, Lock-Andersen J, Langer SW, Mejer J. Dexrazoxane—a promising antidote in the treatment of accidental extravasation of anthracyclines. Scand J Plast Reconstr Surg Hand Surg 2003;37(3):174–5.

74. Langer SW, Sehested M, Jensen PB. Protection against anthracycline induced extravasation injuries with dexra-zoxane: Elucidation of the possible mechanism. Proc Am Soc Clin Oncol 2000;38:492.

75. El-Saghir N, Otrock Z, Mufarrij A, Abou-Mourad Y, Salem Z, Shamseddine A, Abbas J. Dexrazoxane for anthracycline extravasation and GM-CSF for skin ulcera-tion and wound healing. Lancet Oncol 2004;5(5):320–1.

76. Bos AM, van der Graaf WT, Willemse PH. A new con-servative approach to extravasation of anthracyclines with dimethylsulfoxide and dexrazoxane. Acta Oncol 2001;40(4):541–2.

77. Perry MC. Complications of chemotherapy. In: Moosa AR, Schimpff SC, Robson MC, editors. Comprehensive Textbook of Oncology. 2nd ed.. Baltimore, Maryland: Williams and Wilkins, 1991:1706–19.

78. Ventura MT, Dagnello M, Di Corato R, Tursi A. Allergic contact dermatitis due to epirubicin. Contact Dermatitis 1999;40(6):339.

79. Bronchud MH, Howell A, Crowther D, Hopwood P, Souza L, Dexter TM. The use of granulocyte colony-sti-mulating factor to increase the intensity of treatment with doxorubicin in patients with advanced breast and ovarian cancer. Br J Cancer 1989;60(1):121–5.

80. Green M. Dose-intensive chemotherapy with cytokine support. Semin Oncol 1994;21(1 Suppl 1):1–6.

81. Lotem M, Hubert A, Lyass O, Goldenhersh MA, Ingber A, Peretz T, Gabizon A. Skin toxic effects of poly-ethylene glycol-coated liposomal doxorubicin. Arch Dermatol 2000;136(12):1475–80.

82. Speechly-Dick ME, Owen ER. Mitozantrone-induced ony-cholysis. Lancet 1988;1(8577):113.

83. Hansen SW, Nissen NI, Hansen MM, Hou-Jensen K, Pedersen-Bjergaard J. High activity of mitoxantrone in previously untreated low-grade lymphomas. Cancer Chemother Pharmacol 1988;22(1):77–9.

84. Burg G, Bieber T, Langecker P. Lokalisierte neutrophile ekkrine Hidradenitis unter Mitroxantron: eine typische Zytostatikanebenwirkung. [Localized neutrophilic eccrine hidradenitis in mitoxantrone therapy: a typical side-effect of cytostatic drugs.] Hautarzt 1988;39(4):233–6.

85. Nikula E, Kiviniitty K, Leisti J, Taskinen PJ. Chromosome aberrations in lymphocytes of nurses handling cytostatic agents. Scand J Work Environ Health 1984;10(2):71–4.

86. Aubier F, Patte C, de Vathaire F, Tournade MF, Oberlin O, Sakiroglu O, Lemerle J. Fertilité masculine après chimiotherapie dans l'enfance. [Male fertility after chemotherapy during childhood.] Ann Endocrinol (Paris) 1995;56(2):141–2.

87. Wils JA, Bliss JM, Marty M, Coombes G, Fontaine C, Morvan F, Olmos T, Perez-Lopez FR, Vassilopoulos P, Woods E, Coombes RC. Epirubicin plus tamoxifen versus tamoxifen alone in node-positive postmenopausal patients with breast cancer: a randomized trial of the International Collaborative Cancer Group. J Clin Oncol 1999;17(7):1988–98.

88. Turchi JJ, Villasis C. Anthracyclines in the treatment of malignancy in pregnancy. Cancer 1988;61(3):435–40.

89. Gessini L, Jandolo B, Pollera C, et al. Neuropatia da cisplatino: un nuovo tipo di polineuropatia assonale ascen-dente progressiva. Riv Neurobiol 1987;33:75.

90. Benjamin RS, Wiernik PH, Bachur NR. Adriamycin che-motherapy—efficacy, safety, and pharmacologic basis of an intermittent single high-dosage schedule. Cancer 1974;33(1):19–27.

91. Camaggi CM, Strocchi E, Tamassia V, Martoni A, Giovannini M, Lafelice G, Canova N, Marraro D, Martini A, Pannuti F. Pharmacokinetic studies of 4'-epi-doxorubicin in cancer patients with normal and impaired renal function and with hepatic metastases. Cancer Treat Rep 1982;66(10):1819–24.

92. Twelves CJ, Dobbs NA, Michael Y, Summers LA, Gregory W, Harper PG, Rubens RD, Richards MA. Clinical pharmacokinetics of epirubicin: the importance of liver biochemistry tests. Br J Cancer 1992;66(4):765–9.

93. Onrust SV, Wiseman LR, Goa KL. Epirubicin: a review of its intravesical use in superficial bladder cancer. Drugs Aging 1999;15(4):307–33.

94. Masuno T, Kishimoto S, Ogura T, Honma T, Niitani H, Fukuoka M, Ogawa N. A comparative trial of LC9018 plus doxorubicin and doxorubicin alone for the treatment of malignant pleural effusion secondary to lung cancer. Cancer 1991;68(7):1495–500.

95. Sugarbaker PH, Sweatman TW, Graves T, Cunliffe W, Israel M. Early postoperative intraperitoneal adriamycin. Pharmacological studies and a preliminary report. Reg Cancer Treat 1991;4:127–31.

96. Walker-Renard PB, Vaughan LM, Sahn SA. Chemical pleurodesis for malignant pleural effusions. Ann Intern Med 1994;120(1):56–64.

97. Oosterlinck W, Kurth KH, Schroder F, Bultinck J, Hammond B, Sylvester R. A prospective European Organization for Research and Treatment of Cancer Genitourinary Group randomized trial comparing transurethral resection followed by a single intravesical instillation of epirubicin or water in single stage Ta, T1 papillary carcinoma of the bladder. J Urol 1993;149(4):749–52.

98. Cumming JA, Kirk D, Newling DW, Hargreave TB, Whelan P. A multi-centre phase two study of intravesical epirubicin in the treatment of superficial bladder tumour. Eur Urol 1990;17(1):20–2.

99. Okamura K, Murase T, Obata K, Ohshima S, Ono Y, Sakata T, Hasegawa Y, Shimoji T, Miyake K. A randomized trial of early intravesical instillation of epirubicin in superficial bladder cancer. The Nagoya University Urological Oncology Group. Cancer Chemother Pharmacol 1994;35(Suppl):S31–5.

100. Bono AV, Hall RR, Denis L, Lovisolo JA, Sylvester R. Chemoresection in Ta-T1 bladder cancer. Members of the EORTC Genito-Urinary Group. Eur Urol 1996;29(4):385–90.

101. Lukkarinen O, Paul C, Hellstrom P, Kontturi M, Nurmi M, Puntala P, Ottelin J, Tammela T, Tidefeldt U. Intravesical epirubicin with and without verapamil for the prophylaxis of superficial bladder tumours. Scand J Urol Nephrol 1991;25(1):25–8.

102. Bono AV, Lovisolo JA, Saredi G. Conservative treatment of primary T1G3 bladder carcinoma: results from a phase II trial. Br J Urol 1997;80(Suppl 2):117.

103. Melekos MD, Dauaher H, Fokaefs E, Barbalias G. Intravesical instillations of 4-epi-doxorubicin (epirubicin) in the prophylactic treatment of superficial bladder cancer: results of a controlled prospective study. J Urol 1992;147(2):371–5.

104. Ali-el-Dein B, el-Baz M, Aly AN, Shamaa S, Ashamallah A. Intravesical epirubicin versus doxorubicin for superficial bladder tumors (stages pTa and pT1): a randomized prospective study. J Urol 1997;158(1):68–74.

105. Kurth K, Vijgh WJ, ten Kate F, Bogdanowicz JF, Carpentier PJ, Van Reyswoud I. Phase 1/2 study of intravesical epirubicin in patients with carcinoma in situ of the bladder. J Urol 1991;146(6):1508–13.

106. Hermenegildo Caudevilla M, Climente Marti M, Polo i Peris A, Poveda Andres JL, Gasso Matoses M. Fatal adverse reaction after intravesical administration of epirubicin. Farm Hosp 1996;20:395–6.

107. Michelena Hernandez L, Iruin Sanz A, Martinez Lopez de Castro N, Sarobe Carricas M, Oderiz Mendioroz N, Vivanco Arana M, Alfaro Basarte J. Systemic reaction due to intravesical epirubicin. Farm Hosp 1996;20:393–4.

108. Melekos MD, Zarakovitis IE, Fokaefs ED, Dandinis K, Chionis H, Bouropoulos C, Dauaher H. Intravesical bacillus Calmette-Guérin versus epirubicin in the prophylaxis of recurrent and/or multiple superficial bladder tumours. Oncology 1996;53(4):281–8.

109. Gohji K, Hara I, Taguchi I, Ueno K, Yamada Y, Eto H, Arakawa S, Kamidono S, Obe S, Ogawa T, et al. Long-term results of a randomised study of intravesical instillation of epirubicin and doxorubicin as a prophylaxis against superficial bladder recurrence. Nishinihon J Urol 1997;59:785–91.

110. Schon G, Merkle W. Epirubicin vs doxorubicin for the treatment of superficial bladder cancer: a randomised study (Abstract no P1.13) Urologe A 1998;(Suppl 1):S18.

111. Shuin T, Kubota Y, Noguchi S, Hosaka M, Miura T, Kondo I, Fukushima S, Ishizuka E, Furuhata A, Moriyama M, et al. A phase II study of prophylactic intravesical chemotherapy with 4'-epirubicin in recurrent superficial bladder cancer: comparison of 4'-epirubicin and adriamycin. Cancer Chemother Pharmacol 1994;35(Suppl):S52–6.

112. Eto H, Oka Y, Ueno K, Nakamura I, Yoshimura K, Arakawa S, Kamidono S, Obe S, Ogawa T, Hamami G, et al. Comparison of the prophylactic usefulness of epirubicin and doxorubicin in the treatment of superficial bladder cancer by intravesical instillation: a multicenter randomized trial. Kobe University Urological Oncology Group. Cancer Chemother Pharmacol 1994;35(Suppl):S46–51.

113. Onrust SV, Lamb HM. Valrubicin. Drugs Aging 1999;15(1):69–75.

114. De Renzo A, Santoro LF, Notaro R, Pane F, Buonaiuto MR, Luciano L, Rotoli B. Acute promyelocytic leukemia after treatment for non-Hodgkin's lymphoma with drugs targeting topoisomerase II. Am J Hematol 1999;60(4):300–4.

115. Martin M, Lluch A, Ojeda B, Barnabas A, Colomer R, Massuti B, Benito D. Paclitaxel plus doxorubicin in metastatic breast cancer: preliminary analysis of cardiotoxicity. Semin Oncol 1997;24(5 Suppl 17):S17–26–17–30.

116. Rischin D, Smith J, Millward M, Lewis C, Boyer M, Richardson G, Toner G, Gurney H, McKendrick J. A phase II trial of paclitaxel and epirubicin in advanced breast cancer. Br J Cancer 2000;83(4):438–42.

117. Lalisang RI, Voest EE, Wils JA, Nortier JW, Erdkamp FL, Hillen HF, Wals J, Schouten HC, Blijham GH. Dose-dense epirubicin and paclitaxel with G-CSF: a study of decreasing intervals in metastatic breast cancer. Br J Cancer 2000;82(12):1914–9.

118. Salminen E, Bergman M, Huhtala S, Jekunen A, Ekholm E. Docetaxel, a promising novel chemotherapeutic agent in advanced breast cancer. Anticancer Res 2000;20(5C):3663–8.

119. Cobleigh MA, Vogel CL, Tripathy D, Robert NJ, Scholl S, Fehrenbacher L, Wolter JM, Paton V, Shak S, Lieberman G, Slamon DJ. Multinational study of the efficacy and safety of humanized anti-HER2 monoclonal

antibody in women who have HER2-overexpressing metastatic breast cancer that has progressed after chemotherapy for metastatic disease. J Clin Oncol 1999;17(9):2639–48.

120. Slamon DJ, Leyland-Jones B, Shak S, Fuchs H, Paton V, Bajamonde A, Fleming T, Eiermann W, Wolter J, Pegram M, Baselga J, Norton L. Use of chemotherapy plus a monoclonal antibody against HER2 for metastatic breast cancer that overexpresses HER2. N Engl J Med 2001;344(11):783–92.

121. Slamon D, Leyland-Jones B, Shak S, Paton V, Bajamonde A, Flemiong T, Eiermann W, Wolter J, Baselga J, Norton L. Addition of Herceptin (humanized anti-HER2 antibody) to first line chemotherapy for HER2 overexpressing metastatic breast cancer (HER2+/MBC) markedly increases anticancer activity: a randomised, multinational, controlled phase III trial (Abstract 377). Proc Am Soc Clin Oncol 1998;17:98a.

122. Gianni L. Tolerability in patients receiving trastuzumab with or without chemotherapy. Ann Oncol 2001;12(Suppl 1):S63–8.

123. Budman DR, Berry DA, Cirrincione CT, Henderson IC, Wood WC, Weiss RB, Ferree CR, Muss HB, Green MR, Norton L, Frei E 3rd. Dose and dose intensity as determinants of outcome in the adjuvant treatment of breast cancer. The Cancer and Leukemia Group B. J Natl Cancer Inst 1998;90(16):1205–11.

124. Thor AD, Berry DA, Budman DR, Muss HB, Kute T, Henderson IC, Barcos M, Cirrincione C, Edgerton S, Allred C, Norton L, Liu ET. erbB-2, p53, and efficacy of adjuvant therapy in lymph node-positive breast cancer. J Natl Cancer Inst 1998;90(18):1346–60.

125. Smith I. Future directions in the adjuvant treatment of breast cancer: the role of trastuzumab. Ann Oncol 2001;12(Suppl 1):S75–9.

Anthracyclines—liposomal formulations

See also Anthracyclines

General Information

Liposomes are microscopic particles composed of a lipid bilayer membrane enclosing active drug in a central aqueous compartment (1). The aim of liposomal encapsulation of a drug is to alter its pharmacokinetics, thus improving efficacy and/or reducing toxicity (2). Current formulations of liposomal formulations of anthracyclines are as follows:

- pegylated liposomal doxorubicin (Caelyx/Doxil)
- liposomal doxorubicin (Myocet)
- liposomal daunorubicin (DaunoXome).

Sterically stabilized liposomal doxorubicin (pegylated liposomal doxorubicin; Caelyx/Doxil) is coated with polyethylene glycol (3), which results in so-called "stealth liposomes." In liposomal daunorubicin the liposome consists of a lipid bilayer of distearoylphosphatidylcholine and cholesterol in a 2:1 molar ratio (4). Both formulations have a hydrophilic outer layer, which attracts a coating of water around the liposomal shell. This increases the

circulation time by making the formulation virtually invisible to the reticuloendothelial system.

The second liposome system (Myocet) was designed to preserve the antitumor effects of doxorubicin but with reduced cardiotoxicity. This type of liposome is readily recognized and phagocytosed by the mononuclear phagocyte system. In animals most of the injected cytotoxic agent is rapidly taken up by phagocytes, minimizing exposure of normal tissues, and thus diminishing some acute and chronic adverse effects (5,6). The doxorubicin is then released by the phagocytes in a controlled fashion, similar to a slow infusion.

Pharmacokinetics

The differences between liposomal doxorubicin and liposomal daunorubicin are due to the differences in their liposomal packaging.

Pegylated liposomal doxorubicin (Caelyx/Doxil) and liposomal daunorubicin (DaunoXome) produce lower peak plasma concentrations and longer circulation times than free drug (7).

Liposomal doxorubicin in Myocet has systemic availability, metabolism, and excretion similar to that of conventional doxorubicin, but at a slower rate (8). In dogs, the plasma concentrations of doxorubicin from Myocet were 1000-fold greater than conventional doxorubicin at 6 hours, but the difference diminished at 24 hours (9). This distinguishes Myocet from Doxil, which persists in the circulation for significantly longer.

Caelyx has linear pharmacokinetics and its disposition occurs in two phases, the first relatively short (5 hours) and the second prolonged (55 hours). Unlike free doxorubicin, most of the pegylated liposomal doxorubicin is confined to the vascular fluid volume, and its blood clearance depends on the liposomal carrier. Liposomal daunorubicin acts similarly to Caelyx, but produces a lower AUC and has a higher clearance and a shorter terminal half-life (10).

Pegylated liposomes (diameter about 70–100 nm) and liposomal daunorubicin (diameter 45 nm) are small enough to pass intact through defective blood vessels that supply tumors. This, rather than any particular affinity for tumor cells, is the reason for their accumulation in tumor tissue (2). Caelyx provides a greater concentration of doxorubicin in Kaposi's sarcoma tumors than in normal skin.

Organs and Systems

Cardiovascular

The incidence of cardiotoxicity in anthracycline-treated patients has been related to the peak plasma drug concentration (11,12). One of the aims in developing pegylated liposomal doxorubicin was to reduce plasma concentrations of free doxorubicin and restrict myocardial penetration, to minimize cardiotoxicity. Preclinical data suggested that the liposomal formulation was indeed less cardiotoxic than the free drug: about 50% more pegylated liposomal doxorubicin than free doxorubicin can be given to rabbits without producing the same frequency of cardiotoxicity (13).

Cardiac adverse events that have been considered probably or possibly related to pegylated liposomal doxorubicin have been reported in 3–9% of patients (14–16). These include hypotension, pericardial effusion, thrombophlebitis, heart failure, and tachycardia (14,15).

Left ventricular failure has been reported in a few patients, particularly those who received high cumulative lifetime doses of pegylated liposomal doxorubicin (over 550 mg/m^2) (14,15). However, cumulative doses of 450 mg/m^2 or more and 550 mg/m^2 have been administered without significant reduction in ejection fraction or the development of cardiac failure (17,18). To date, no or minimal cardiotoxicity has been observed in patients with AIDS-related Kaposi's sarcoma who received pegylated liposomal doxorubicin in high cumulative doses (19).

Both peak and overall concentrations of doxorubicin in myocardial tissue are reduced by 30–40% after Myocet relative to conventional doxorubicin (9). This reduced myocardial exposure resulted in a significant reduction in cardiotoxicity, assessed both functionally and histologically (5,6). Compared with free doxorubicin 75 mg/m^2 given 3-weekly, Myocet 75 mg/m^2 caused significantly less congestive cardiac failure (1 versus 6%) (20). However, a high dose of Myocet (135 mg/m^2, median cumulative dose 405 mg/m^2) caused a significant increase in cardiac toxicity: 38% of patients had a protocol-defined cardiac event, including 13% who developed congestive heart failure (21).

In one study there was a significant (over 20%) reduction in the shortening fraction with liposomal daunorubicin measured by echocardiography (22). In contrast, in another study there was no significant fall in cardiac function, even after cumulative doses of liposomal daunorubicin over 1000 mg/m^2 (23).

Women with metastatic breast cancer were randomized to receive either liposomal doxorubicin (Myocet) 75 mg/m^2 ($n = 108$) or conventional doxorubicin 75 mg/m^2 ($n = 116$) (24). The liposomal formulation was less cardiotoxic than the conventional one, and the cumulative doses before the onset of cardiotoxicity were 780 versus 570 mg/m^2 respectively; the liposomal formulation provided comparable antitumor activity. In another study the authors tried to define the cumulative toxic intravenous dose of daunorubicin (DaunoXome) and concluded that it may be 750–900 mg/m^2 or even higher (exceeding 1000 mg/m^2) (25).

Respiratory

Acute dyspnea, low back pain, and/or pain at the site of tumor have been described, beginning within 1–5 minutes of the start of infusion of pegylated liposomal doxorubicin (26). Three of 35 patients were described as suffering acute dyspnea, two with back pain and two with abdominal pain. In each case the symptoms resolved within 5–15 minutes of stopping the infusion, which was restarted without adverse effects. The mechanism of these symptoms was unclear. However, because the dyspnea was reminiscent of that seen in hemodialysis neutropenia, complete blood counts were obtained from four patients about 2 minutes after the onset of symptoms. All four had relative neutropenia (neutrophil counts of 3–46% of pretreatment), which resolved by the end of the infusion. In vitro, pegylated liposomal doxorubicin, in concentrations predicted to be present in the plasma during the start of treatment, stimulates neutrophil adhesion to human umbilical vein endothelial cells (26). Thus, pegylated liposomal doxorubicin may cause transient sequestration of neutrophils in the pulmonary circulation, resulting in reduced lung compliance and associated dyspnea.

Hematologic

In a phase I dose-finding study of pegylated liposomal doxorubicin, myelosuppression was not a major problem with the doses tested (20–80 mg/m^2, re-dosing every 3–4 weeks). Median nadir white cell and platelet counts were well above 2×10^9/l and 100×10^9/l respectively. In the occasional patient in whom profound granulocytopenia developed there was quick recovery of the cell counts within less than 7 days. Neutropenic fever was documented in only one patient at the top dose of 80 mg/m^2 (17). There was no significant indication of cumulative myelosuppression. Treatment-related anemia was generally mild and blood transfusions were not required. However, two patients with head and neck malignancies and extensive pretreatment were given erythropoietin to maintain hemoglobin concentrations above 9.0 g/dl (17).

Pooled data from 12 phase I or II studies, in 308 patients with solid tumors who received pegylated liposomal doxorubicin in doses of 10–80 mg/m^2, showed that there was neutropenia (neutrophil count below 1×10^9/l) in 50%, anemia in 19%, and thrombocytopenia in 9.2% (27).

Of 71 patients with metastatic breast cancer treated with pegylated liposomal doxorubicin in doses of 45–60 mg/m^2 given 3- or 4-weekly, grade 3/4 neutropenia occurred in 10% and thrombocytopenia in 1% (27).

If pegylated liposomal doxorubicin and liposomal daunorubicin are used to treat AIDS-related Kaposi's sarcoma, one has to consider additional factors that affect the white cell count. In patients with HIV/AIDS, myelosuppression was the most frequent dose-limiting adverse effect of liposomal anthracyclines (22,23). In one study of 30 patients with Kaposi's sarcoma given liposomal daunorubicin 40 mg/m^2, 53% developed granulocytopenia (white cell count below 1×10^9/l); 17% had a hemoglobin concentration below 8.0 g/dl, but none had thrombocytopenia (22).

In another study in 53 patients with AIDS-related Kaposi's sarcoma given pegylated liposomal doxorubicin 20 mg/m^2 every 3 weeks, 21 had leukopenia and three had thrombocytopenia (28).

At doses of 20 mg/m^2 liposomal doxorubicin, combined tolerability data from 705 patients with AIDS-related Kaposi's sarcoma showed that neutropenia (below 1×10^9/l) and anemia were the most common adverse events, affecting 50 and 19% of patients respectively (14).

In summary, myelosuppression after treatment with pegylated liposomal doxorubicin does not appear to be a major problem in patients with solid tumors and relatively intact immunological systems, but is the dose-limiting adverse effect in immunocompromised patients with HIV/AIDS.

High-dose Myocet (135 mg/m^2) caused significant hematological toxicity, namely grade 4 neutropenia in 98% and thrombocytopenia in 46 of 52 patients (21). However, Myocet 75 mg/m^2 3-weekly caused less hematological toxicity than conventional doxorubicin (20).

Gastrointestinal

Stomatitis and pharyngitis have been confirmed, along with hand–foot syndrome, as dose-limiting adverse effects of pegylated liposomal anthracyclines (17). Stomatitis was dose-limiting at high single doses over 70 mg/m^2. Similarly, 12 of 35 patients who received pegylated liposomal doxorubicin 50 mg/m^2 every 3 weeks for advanced ovarian carcinoma required dose reduction (to 40 mg/m^2) or treatment delay (to 4 weeks) because of mucositis (18). Stomatitis and mucositis are dose-dependent (29). In the treatment of Kaposi's sarcoma in patients with HIV/AIDS, mucositis and stomatitis are rarely problematic and are not dose-limiting. Presumably this is because significantly lower doses of pegylated liposomal doxorubicin are used in these patients.

Nausea and vomiting have been reported but appear to be mild and infrequent adverse effects of pegylated liposomal anthracyclines and liposomal daunorubicin (23,30). In most patients pegylated liposomal doxorubicin can be given without prophylactic antiemetics. In one study there was only mild nausea and vomiting in eight of 53 patients who had not received prophylactic antiemetics (28). Further reviews in patients with AIDS-related Kaposi's sarcoma have reported nausea and vomiting in 17 and 8% of patients respectively (29). Pooled data from 12 phase I and II studies in patients with solid tumors showed that 3.6% of patients had had grade 3/4 nausea or vomiting (27). Diarrhea has similarly been recognized as a mild and infrequent adverse effect of pegylated liposomal doxorubicin (three of 53 patients) (28).

Myocet (75 mg/m^2) causes significantly less vomiting (11 versus 23%) than conventional free doxorubicin (75 mg/m^2) (20). It also leads to lower peak-free doxorubicin concentrations in the gastrointestinal mucosa compared with conventional doxorubicin, and less gastrointestinal toxicity (5). However, high-dose Myocet (135 mg/m^2) caused grade 4 mucositis in 10 of 52 patients (21).

Liver

The authors of a case report suggested that pegylated liposomal doxorubicin was the probable cause of hepatic failure in a patient who, 2 weeks after treatment with pegylated liposomal doxorubicin 10 mg/m^2 (cumulative dose 20 mg/m^2) (15), developed jaundice and ascites (31). Despite withdrawal of other potentially hepatotoxic drugs, the patient died of hepatorenal failure 12 weeks later. This may have been an idiosyncratic effect augmented by hepatitis B viral infection (15,32), as there have been no other reports of hepatorenal failure (14,33).

Skin

Skin toxicity, manifesting primarily as palmar–plantar erythrodysesthesia or hand–foot syndrome, is one of the principal dose-limiting adverse effects of pegylated liposomal anthracyclines (for example Caelyx 50 mg/m^2 given every 4 weeks) and may warrant dosage modification, depending on the severity of the symptoms (17,18). In pooled tolerability data, grade 3/4 hand–foot syndrome was reported in 54 (17.5%) of 308 patients (27). The median time to the development of grade 3/4 hand–foot syndrome was 51 days, corresponding to the second or third cycle of treatment (27). Myocet, even when given in a high dose (135 mg/m^2), was not associated with the hand–foot syndrome characteristic of pegylated liposomal doxorubicin (20,21). This was presumed to be due to differences in the liposomal formulation. Pegylated liposomes circulate for prolonged periods and may undergo some eccrine excretion, particularly in cases of hyperhidrosis, whereas with Myocet the liposome is phagocytosed by the reticuloendothelial system and the active drug is then slowly released into the circulation, similar to a slow infusion. Severe forms of hand–foot syndrome may need acute intervention with oral dexamethasone and topical dimethylsulfoxide; oral vitamin B$_6$ has not been proven to be useful.

Conjunctivitis and skin pigmentation have been reported but are mild (23,27,28).

Unlike extravasation of conventional doxorubicin, which can cause severe local inflammation and tissue damage, extravasation of liposomal doxorubicin was associated with only mild transient irritation at the infusion site in the eight documented cases (34,35).

Four cases of extravasation of liposomal daunorubicin have been reported and were associated with only mild irritation and transient erythema and swelling, similar to pegylated liposomal doxorubicin (36).

In 60 patients receiving polyethylene glycol-coated liposomal doxorubicin (Doxil) 35–70 mg/m^2 by infusion over 1–2 hours there were four patterns of skin eruption: hand–foot syndrome (40%), a diffuse follicular rash (10%), an intertrigo-like eruption (8%), and new melanotic macules (0.5%) (37).

Hair

Alopecia can occur during treatment with doxorubicin (38). It is generally mild during treatment with Caelyx and occurs in 6–9% of patients. The incidence of alopecia with single-agent Myocet is higher.

Immunologic

Acute hypersensitivity reactions have been reported with the first infusion of pegylated liposomal doxorubicin (14,15). The symptoms included flushing, shortness of breath, facial swelling, headache, chills, back pain, tightness in the chest and throat, and hypotension. Similar reactions have been reported after the intravenous administration of colloid imaging agents and unloaded liposomes.

Acute reactions to infusion have been observed on first exposure to the drug in six of 56 patients treated with pegylated doxorubicin 20–60 mg/m^2 (17). The reactions developed at 3–25 minutes after the start of the infusion and were characterized by flushing, sensation of choking, back pain, and in one instance hypotension. All the symptoms disappeared shortly after discontinuation of the infusion. Three patients were re-treated successfully using premedication (hydrocortisone, cimetidine, and diphenhydramine) and a slower infusion rate (initial rate 1 mg/minute). Similarly, acute onset symptoms of dyspnea, back pain, and tumor site pain have been reported in other studies (26). Since this reaction generally improves on rechallenge with or without premedication, it has been termed pseudoallergic.

Long-Term Effects

Tumorigenicity

Two patients with acute promyelocytic leukemia developed therapy-related myelodysplasia 2.0–2.5 years after complete remission and then acute myeloid leukemia; both had received anthracyclines (39). In both cases the cytogenetic changes that usually occur after the use of alkylating agents were observed. There has only been one previous similar report after successful therapy with anthracyclines, but these observations suggest that anthracyclines can cause acute myeloid leukemia similar to that caused by alkylating agents.

A flare phenomenon is a well-documented effect of hormonal therapies and/or hormone-responsive tumors. A prostate-specific antigen flare occurred in four of 28 patients who received liposomal doxorubicin (Caelyx) for symptomatic androgen-independent prostate cancer (40).

Second-Generation Effects

Teratogenicity

Pegylated liposomal doxorubicin is embryotoxic in rats and embryotoxic and abortifacient in rabbits. Teratogenicity cannot therefore be ruled out, but there is no reported experience in pregnant women. Equally, it is not known if the drug is excreted into human breast milk, so breastfeeding should be discontinued before the administration of pegylated liposomal doxorubicin.

Susceptibility Factors

Since Caelyx has activity in Kaposi's sarcoma, many studies have been performed in patients with HIV/AIDS. Thus, assessment of the tolerability of Caelyx and Doxil has been complicated by underlying immune suppression, neutropenia, and co-morbidity commonly present in patients with HIV/AIDS. This has led to a difference in

the dose-limiting adverse effects in patients with solid tumors compared to those with Kaposi's sarcoma. Tolerance differs in patients with HIV/AIDS (standard dose 20 mg/m^2 Caelyx every 3 weeks) and those with solid tumors (standard dose 50 mg/m^2 every 4 weeks).

Drug Administration

Drug administration route

Pegylated liposomal doxorubicin has been given to three patients via a catheter located in the hepatic artery (41). No severe adverse effects, such as nausea, vomiting, stomatitis, alopecia, or cardiotoxicity, were observed. There was mild leukopenia (2.8×10^9/l) in one patient; neither anemia nor thrombocytopenia were reported.

Drug overdose

Acute overdose with pegylated liposomal doxorubicin worsens the toxic effects of mucositis, leukopenia, and thrombocytopenia. There have been no reports of overdose of liposomal daunorubicin, but the primary anticipated toxic effect would be myelosuppression.

Drug–Drug Interactions

General

No formal drug interaction studies have been conducted with pegylated liposomal doxorubicin, liposomal daunorubicin, or Myocet. Caution should be exercised when using drugs known to interact with doxorubicin or daunorubicin. Equally, caution should be exercised when giving any other cytotoxic drugs, especially myelotoxic agents, at the same time.

References

1. Kim S. Liposomes as carriers of cancer chemotherapy. Current status and future prospects. Drugs 1993;46(4):618–38.
2. Gabizon AA. Liposomal anthracyclines. Hematol Oncol Clin North Am 1994;8(2):431–50.
3. Verrill M. Anthracyclines in breast cancer: therapy and issues of toxicity. Breast 2001;(Suppl 2):S8–S15.
4. Forssen EA, Ross ME. DaunoXome treatment of solid tumours: preclinical and clinical investigations. J Liposome Res 1994;4:481–512.
5. Kanter PM, Bullard GA, Pilkiewicz FG, Mayer LD, Cullis PR, Pavelic ZP. Preclinical toxicology study of liposome encapsulated doxorubicin (TLC D-99): comparison with doxorubicin and empty liposomes in mice and dogs. In Vivo 1993;7(1):85–95.
6. Kanter PM, Bullard GA, Ginsberg RA, Pilkiewicz FG, Mayer LD, Cullis PR, Pavelic ZP. Comparison of the cardiotoxic effects of liposomal doxorubicin (TLC D-99) versus free doxorubicin in beagle dogs. In Vivo 1993;7(1):17–26.
7. Schuller J, Czejka M, Bandak S, Borow D, Pietrzak C, Marei I, Schernthaner G. Comparison of pharmacokinetics (PK) of free and liposome encapsulated doxorubicin in advanced cancer patients. Onkologie 1995;18(Suppl 2):184.

8. Batist G, Ramakrishnan G, Rao CS, Chandrasekharan A, Gutheil J, Guthrie T, Shah P, Khojasteh A, Nair MK, Hoelzer K, Tkaczuk K, Park YC, Lee LW. Reduced cardiotoxicity and preserved antitumor efficacy of liposome-encapsulated doxorubicin and cyclophosphamide compared with conventional doxorubicin and cyclophosphamide in a randomized, multicenter trial of metastatic breast cancer. J Clin Oncol 2001;19(5):1444–54.

9. Kanter PM, Klaich G, Bullard GA, King JM, Pavelic ZP. Preclinical toxicology study of liposome encapsulated doxorubicin (TLC D-99) given intraperitoneally to dogs. In Vivo 1994;8(6):975–82.

10. Sparano JA, Winer EP. Liposomal anthracyclines for breast cancer. Semin Oncol 2001;28(4 Suppl 12):32–40.

11. Legha SS, Benjamin RS, Mackay B, Ewer M, Wallace S, Valdivieso M, Rasmussen SL, Blumenschein GR, Freireich EJ. Reduction of doxorubicin cardiotoxicity by prolonged continuous intravenous infusion. Ann Intern Med 1982;96(2):133–9.

12. Workman P. Infusional anthracyclines: is slower better? If so, why? Ann Oncol 1992;3(8):591–4.

13. Working PK, Dayan AD. Pharmacological–toxicological expert report. CAELYX. (Stealth liposomal doxorubicin HCl). Hum Exp Toxicol 1996;15(9):751–85.

14. Dezube BJ. Safety assessment: Doxil (doxorubicin HCl liposome injection) in refractory AIDS-related Kaposi's sarcoma. Doxil Clinical Series, Vol. 1, No. 2. Menlo Park, California: SEQUUS Pharmaceuticals Inc, 1996.

15. Goebel FD, Goldstein D, Goos M, Jablonowski H, Stewart JS The International SL-DOX Study Group. Efficacy and safety of Stealth liposomal doxorubicin in AIDS-related Kaposi's sarcoma. Br J Cancer 1996;73(8):989–94.

16. Harrison M, Tomlinson D, Stewart S. Liposomal-entrapped doxorubicin: an active agent in AIDS-related Kaposi's sarcoma. J Clin Oncol 1995;13(4):914–20.

17. Uziely B, Jeffers S, Isacson R, Kutsch K, Wei-Tsao D, Yehoshua Z, Libson E, Muggia FM, Gabizon A. Liposomal doxorubicin: antitumor activity and unique toxicities during two complementary phase I studies. J Clin Oncol 1995;13(7):1777–85.

18. Muggia FM, Hainsworth JD, Jeffers S, Miller P, Groshen S, Tan M, Roman L, Uziely B, Muderspach L, Garcia A, Burnett A, Greco FA, Morrow CP, Paradiso LJ, Liang LJ. Phase II study of liposomal doxorubicin in refractory ovarian cancer: antitumor activity and toxicity modification by liposomal encapsulation. J Clin Oncol 1997;15(3):987–93.

19. Gabizon A, Martin F. Polyethylene glycol-coated (pegylated) liposomal doxorubicin. Rationale for use in solid tumours. Drugs 1997;54(Suppl 4):15–21.

20. Harris L, Winer E, Batist G, Rovira D, Navari R, Lee L the TLC D-99 Study Group. Phase III study of TLC D-99 (liposome encapsulated doxorubicin) vs. free doxorubicin in patients with metastatic breast cancer (Abstract 26). Proc Am Soc Clin Oncol 1998;17:A474.

21. Shapiro CL, Ervin T, Welles L, Azarnia N, Keating J, Hayes DFTLC D-99 Study Group. Phase II trial of high-dose liposome-encapsulated doxorubicin with granulocyte colony-stimulating factor in metastatic breast cancer. J Clin Oncol 1999;17(5):1435–41.

22. Girard PM, Bouchaud O, Goetschel A, Mukwaya G, Eestermans G, Ross M, Rozenbaum W, Saimot AG. Phase II study of liposomal encapsulated daunorubicin in the treatment of AIDS-associated mucocutaneous Kaposi's sarcoma. AIDS 1996;10(7):753–7.

23. Gill PS, Espina BM, Muggia F, Cabriales S, Tulpule A, Esplin JA, Liebman HA, Forssen E, Ross ME, Levine AM. Phase I/II clinical and pharmacokinetic evaluation of liposomal daunorubicin. J Clin Oncol 1995;13(4):996–1003.

24. Harris L, Batist G, Belt R, Rovira D, Navari R, Azarnia N, Welles L, Winer ETLC D-99 Study Group. Liposome-encapsulated doxorubicin compared with conventional doxorubicin in a randomized multicenter trial as first-line therapy of metastatic breast carcinoma. Cancer 2002;94(1):25–36.

25. Fassas A, Buffels R, Anagnostopoulos A, Gacos E, Vadikolia C, Haloudis P, Kaloyannidis P. Safety and early efficacy assessment of liposomal daunorubicin (DaunoXome) in adults with refractory or relapsed acute myeloblastic leukaemia: a phase I–II study. Br J Haematol 2002;116(2):308–15.

26. Skubitz KM, Skubitz AP. Mechanism of transient dyspnea induced by pegylated-liposomal doxorubicin (Doxil). Anticancer Drugs 1998;9(1):45–50.

27. SEQUUS Pharmaceuticals Inc. Doxil safety report (07 Apr 1997). Menlo Park, California, USA.

28. Northfelt DW, Dezube BJ, Thommes JA, Levine R, Von Roenn JH, Dosik GM, Rios A, Krown SE, DuMond C, Mamelok RD. Efficacy of pegylated-liposomal doxorubicin in the treatment of AIDS-related Kaposi's sarcoma after failure of standard chemotherapy. J Clin Oncol 1997;15(2):653–9.

29. Alberts DS, Garcia DJ. A safety review of pegylated liposomal doxorubicin in the treatment of various malignancies. Oncology 1997;11(Suppl 11):54–62.

30. Ranson MR, Carmichael J, O'Byrne K, Stewart S, Smith D, Howell A. Treatment of advanced breast cancer with sterically stabilized liposomal doxorubicin: results of a multi-center phase II trial. J Clin Oncol 1997;15(10):3185–91.

31. Hengge UR, Brockmeyer NH, Rasshofer R, Goos M. Fatal hepatic failure with liposomal doxorubicin. Lancet 1993;341(8841):383–4.

32. Coker RJ, James ND, Stewart JS. Hepatic toxicity of liposomal encapsulated doxorubicin. Lancet 1993;341(8847):756.

33. Stewart S, Jablonowski H, Goebel FD, Arasteh K, Spittle M, Rios A, Aboulafia D, Galleshaw J, Dezube BJInternational Pegylated Liposomal Doxorubicin Study Group. Randomized comparative trial of pegylated liposomal doxorubicin versus bleomycin and vincristine in the treatment of AIDS-related Kaposi's sarcoma. J Clin Oncol 1998;16(2):683–91.

34. Madhavan S, Northfelt DW. Lack of vesicant injury following extravasation of liposomal doxorubicin. J Natl Cancer Inst 1995;87(20):1556–7.

35. Madhavan S, Northfelt DW. Lack of vesicant injury following extravasation of liposomal doxorubicin. Breast Cancer Res Treat 1996;37(Suppl):77.

36. Cabriales S, Bresnahan J, Testa D, Espina BM, Scadden DT, Ross M, Gill PS. Extravasation of liposomal daunorubicin in patients with AIDS-associated Kaposi's sarcoma: a report of four cases. Oncol Nurs Forum 1998;25(1):67–70.

37. Lotem M, Hubert A, Lyass O, Goldenhersh MA, Ingber A, Peretz T, Gabizon A. Skin toxic effects of polyethylene glycol-coated liposomal doxorubicin. Arch Dermatol 2000;136(12):1475–80.

38. Dean JC, Griffith KS, Cetas TC, Mackel CL, Jones SE, Salmon SE. Scalp hypothermia: a comparison of ice packs and the Kold Kap in the prevention of doxorubicin-induced alopecia. J Clin Oncol 1983;1(1):33–7.

39. Zompi S, Legrand O, Bouscary D, Blanc CM, Picard F, Casadevall N, Dreyfus F, Marie JP, Viguie F. Therapy-

related acute myeloid leukaemia after successful therapy for acute promyelocytic leukaemia with t(15;17): a report of two cases and a review of the literature. Br J Haematol 2000;110(3):610–3.

40. Fossa SD, Vaage S, Letocha H, Iversen J, Risberg T, Johannessen DC, Paus E, Smedsrud T. Norwegian Urological Cancer Group. Liposomal doxorubicin (Caelyx) in symptomatic androgen-independent prostate cancer (AIPC)—delayed response and flare phenomenon should be considered. Scand J Urol Nephrol 2002;36(1):34–9.
41. Konno H, Maruo Y, Matsuda I, Nakamura S, Baba S. Intra-arterial liposomal adriamycin for metastatic adenocarcinoma of the liver. Eur Surg Res 1995;27(5):301–6.

Bleomycin

General Information

Bleomycin is a cytostatic drug that causes double-strand breaks in DNA. It has been used to treat Hodgkin's disease and a variety of solid cancers. It is often used in combination with other anticancer drugs, for example in the regimens known as ABVD (doxorubicin + bleomycin + vinblastine + dacarbazine) and BEP (bleomycin + etoposide + cisplatin). It has also been injected intrapleurally in the management of malignant effusions.

Organs and Systems

Respiratory

Bleomycin can cause diffuse interstitial pneumonitis, with significant mortality. Bleomycin is more slowly degraded in the lungs than in other tissues, such as the bone marrow or liver, because of lower bleomycin hydrolase activity. The mechanisms of lung damage include the formation of highly reactive oxygen species; lipid peroxidation of cell membranes has been suggested, but not confirmed (1). Others have suggested a role for angiotensin-converting enzyme in production of the lung damage (2), but the data are unconvincing.

Because this is a severe adverse effect it is generally recommended that a total dose of more than 400 mg of bleomycin should be avoided in patients with normal renal function. In those over 70 years of age reduced creatinine clearance makes dosage reduction necessary.

Estimates of the incidence of bleomycin pulmonary toxicity range from 11 to 23% (3). Of 99 patients previously treated with bleomycin together with other cytostatic drugs for testicular tumors, 16 developed abnormal lung function tests; amongst those who received more than 500 mg of bleomycin cumulatively, 75% had abnormal lung function tests, Raynaud's phenomenon, or both (4). Rapid progression to fatal pulmonary fibrosis has been documented previously and, in all but one instance, there had been previous or concurrent chest radiotherapy. Two cases have been reported of rapidly progressive fatal pulmonary fibrosis in patients receiving bleomycin who had had no previous lung disease, and who had not undergone radiotherapy to the chest (5). Lung toxicity can occur at low cumulative doses of bleomycin during concurrent treatment with cyclophosphamide (which independently causes pulmonary toxicity). In 19 patients (6) there was a high (26%) incidence of fatal pulmonary toxicity in patients receiving the combination of these two drugs, which warrants special caution.

Transient but significant reductions in pulmonary function tests have been reported within 8–12 months in 35 children treated with polychemotherapy who had received a cumulative dose of 120 mg/m^2 up to 12 years after diagnosis (7). However, there were no long-term abnormalities.

In 194 patients there was a fatality rate of 2.8% from pulmonary toxicity. The incidence of fatal pulmonary toxicity increased with each decade of life above 30 and the lower the glomerular filtration rate at the time of administration the greater the death rate; the death rate may exceed 10% in those over 40 years of age (8).

Bleomycin is also associated with a hypersensitivity pneumonitis. This should be considered when interpreting cytological swabs in patients treated with the drug, since the acute cytological changes can be misinterpreted (9).

A syndrome of acute chest pain occurring during bleomycin infusion has been described in 10 patients with features that could not be ascribed to pulmonary fibrosis, hypersensitivity pneumonitis, or cardiovascular toxicity (10). The pain was sudden in onset and occurred during the first or second course, usually on the second or third day. There was retrosternal pressure or pleuritic pain, in some cases severe enough to require narcotic analgesics. Stopping or slowing the infusion produced marked improvement. In two of seven patients who received a subsequent course of treatment, the pain recurred. One patient had dyspnea and two developed an erythematous rash. One had a pleural friction rub and one a pericardial friction rub. There was fever during five episodes. There were no other physical abnormalities. There were electrocardiographic changes suggestive of pericarditis in two patients; one patient developed transient blunting of a costophrenic angle on a chest X-ray, and another a transient and small retrocardiac pulmonary infiltrate. The pain resolved spontaneously with analgesics, and there were no long-term pulmonary or cardiac sequelae. Possible underlying mechanisms include pleuropericarditis due to serosal inflammation or vascular pathology.

Severe morbidity has been reported after the use of regimens containing bleomycin: 10% of patients developed adult respiratory distress syndrome and a further 9% needed prolonged ventilation (11). The authors thought that these rates were higher than expected and attributed this to a combination of the toxic effects of bleomycin on the lung and a large retroperitoneal and/ or pulmonary tumor burden.

Skin

Bleomycin can occasionally cause scleroderma-like changes in the skin (12,13), an effect that may be enhanced by radiotherapy (14).

Body temperature

When bleomycin is used as a sclerosing agent in adults, a dose of up to 1 mg/kg is generally instilled into the chest through a thoracostomy tube. Bleomycin 60 mg intrapleurally caused a fever over 39°C in two of 21 patients with malignant pleural effusions; it settled without treatment and was not associated with local discomfort (15).

Drug Administration

Drug administration route

Several antineoplastic agents have been introduced into the pleural space to achieve pleurodesis, but the largest reported experience is with bleomycin. Intrapleural bleomycin has an efficacy similar to that of tetracycline and doxycycline (16). About 45% of a dose of bleomycin is absorbed systemically, but significant adverse events are uncommon (17). Chest pain is reported in about 28% of patients, fever in 24%, and nausea in about 11% (18). A randomized comparison of bleomycin with tetracycline in 85 patients with malignant pleural effusions showed that toxicity, predominantly in the form of chest pain and fever, was similar with the two drugs (7–17%) (19). Nearly half the patients (34) died within 90 days owing to disease progression. However, one patient died within 2 days of intrapleural bleomycin, and the investigators could not exclude a contribution from the bleomycin. In another comparison of bleomycin with doxycycline there was fever in 13%, chest pain in 11%, and chills in 4% of patients treated with bleomycin (20).

References

1. Jenkinson S, Duncan C, Lawrence R, Collins J. Lack of enhancement of bleomycin lung injury in vitamin E-deficient rats. J Crit Care 1987;2:264.
2. Nussinovitch N, Peleg E, Yaron A, Ratt P, Rosenthal T. Angiotensin converting enzyme in bleomycin-treated patients. Int J Clin Pharmacol Ther Toxicol 1988;26(6):310–3.
3. Potash RJ. Acute dyspnoea in a chemotherapy recipient. Respir Care 1987;32:279.
4. Creutzig A, Polking W, Schmoll HJ, Fabel H, Alexander K. Raynaud-Syndrom und Veranderungen der Lungenfunktion als Folgen einer zytostatischen Therapie von Hodentumoren. [Raynaud syndrome and changes in lung function as sequelae of cytostatic therapy of testicular tumors.] Med Klin (Munich) 1987;82(4):131–4.
5. Dee GJ, Austin JH, Mutter GL. Bleomycin-associated pulmonary fibrosis: rapidly fatal progression without chest radiotherapy. J Surg Oncol 1987;35(2):135–8.
6. Quigley M, Brada M, Heron C, Horwich A. Severe lung toxicity with a weekly low dose chemotherapy regimen in patients with non-Hodgkin's lymphoma. Hematol Oncol 1988;6(4):319–24.
7. Kharasch VS, Lipsitz S, Santis W, Hallowell JA, Goorin A. Long-term pulmonary toxicity of multiagent chemotherapy including bleomycin and cyclophosphamide in osteosarcoma survivors. Med Pediatr Oncol 1996;27(2):85–91.
8. Simpson AB, Paul J, Graham J, Kaye SB. Fatal bleomycin pulmonary toxicity in the west of Scotland 1991–95: a review of patients with germ cell tumours. Br J Cancer 1998;78(8):1061–6.
9. Hartmann CA, Weise I, Voigt D, Reichle G. Gefahr zytologischer Fehlinterpretation bei Zytostatikapneumopathie. [Danger of false cytologic interpretation in cytostatic pneumopathy.] Prax Klin Pneumol 1987;41(6):223–6.
10. White DA, Schwartzberg LS, Kris MG, Bosl GJ. Acute chest pain syndrome during bleomycin infusions. Cancer 1987;59(9):1582–5.
11. Baniel J, Foster RS, Rowland RG, Bihrle R, Donohue JP. Complications of post-chemotherapy retroperitoneal lymph node dissection. J Urol 1995;153(3 Pt 2):976–80.
12. Kerr LD, Spiera H. Scleroderma in association with the use of bleomycin: a report of 3 cases. J Rheumatol 1992;19(2):294–6.
13. Kim KH, Yoon TJ, Oh CW, Ko GH, Kim TH. A case of bleomycin-induced scleroderma. J Korean Med Sci 1996;11(5):454–6.
14. Marck Y, Meunier L, Barneon G, Meynadier J. Sclerose cutanée en pèlerine au decours d'un traitement par l'association bleomycine et radiothérapie. [Scleroderma of the shoulders after treatment with combined bleomycin and radiotherapy.] Ann Dermatol Venereol 1994;121(10):712–4.
15. Hsu NY, Chen C. Intrapleural bleomycin in the management of malignant pleural effusion. J Surg Assoc ROC 1988;21:302.
16. Martinez-Moragon E, Aparicio J, Rogado MC, Sanchis J, Sanchis F, Gil-Suay V. Pleurodesis in malignant pleural effusions: a randomized study of tetracycline versus bleomycin. Eur Respir J 1997;10(10):2380–3.
17. Alberts DS, Chen HS, Mayersohn M, Perrier D, Moon TE, Gross JF. Bleomycin pharmacokinetics in man. II. Intracavitary administration. Cancer Chemother Pharmacol 1979;2(2):127–32.
18. Walker-Renard PB, Vaughan LM, Sahn SA. Chemical pleurodesis for malignant pleural effusions. Ann Intern Med 1994;120(1):56–64.
19. Ruckdeschel JC, Moores D, Lee JY, Einhorn LH, Mandelbaum I, Koeller J, Weiss GR, Losada M, Keller JH. Intrapleural therapy for malignant pleural effusions. A randomized comparison of bleomycin and tetracycline. Chest 1991;100(6):1528–35.
20. Patz EF Jr, McAdams HP, Erasmus JJ, Goodman PC, Culhane DK, Gilkeson RC, Herndon J. Sclerotherapy for malignant pleural effusions: a prospective randomized trial of bleomycin vs doxycycline with small-bore catheter drainage. Chest 1998;113(5):1305–11.

Dactinomycin

General Information

Dactinomycin is used to treat cancers in children, in particular Wilms' tumor. It has similar adverse effects to doxorubicin.

Organs and Systems

Respiratory

Dactinomycin increases the pulmonary toxic effects of radiation by an estimated 30%, and reduces the radiation tolerance of the lung by at least 20% (1).

Liver

Several cases of hepatotoxicity have been reported in children receiving dactinomycin for Wilms' tumor (2–5). The hepatotoxicity of dactinomycin is dose- and schedule-related; mild hepatotoxicity is described in up to 12% of patients (6).

Five of 40 patients, who received a pulsed regimen of 60 µg/kg of dactinomycin every 3 weeks up to and including week 15, developed severe hepatotoxicity, with sharp rises in liver function test values, ascites, and liver enlargement. One child with complicating factors died and the others recovered. All five had possible contributing factors, such as repeated anesthesia (3).

References

1. Cohen IJ, Loven D, Schoenfeld T, Sandbank J, Kaplinsky C, Yaniv Y, Jaber L, Zaizov R. Dactinomycin potentiation of radiation pneumonitis: a forgotten interaction. Pediatr Hematol Oncol 1991;8(2):187–92.
2. Green DM, Finklestein JZ, Norkool P, D'Angio GJ. Severe hepatic toxicity after treatment with single-dose dactinomycin and vincristine. A report of the National Wilms' Tumor Study. Cancer 1988;62(2):270–3.
3. D'Angio GJ. Hepatotoxicity with actinomycin D. Lancet 1987;2(8550):104.
4. Pritchard J, Raine J, Wallendszus K. Hepatotoxicity of actinomycin-D. Lancet 1989;1(8630):168.
5. White L, Tobias V, Hughes DW. Actinomycin D-induced hepatotoxicity. Pediatr Hematol Oncol 1989;6(1):53–7.
6. D'Angio GJ. Hepatotoxicity and actinomycin D. Lancet 1990;335(8700):1290.

HORMONE AGONISTS AND ANTAGONISTS

Antiandrogens

General Information

Antiandrogens include steroids, such as cyproterone acetate, and non-steroidal agents, such as bicalutamide, flutamide, and nilutamide. They have different endocrine effects and therefore different adverse effects (1). Cyproterone acetate tends to result in a loss of sexual interest and erectile dysfunction, whereas most men experience this only moderately or not at all during non-steroidal treatment. The most common adverse effects of the non-steroidal agents are gynecomastia and breast pain. Although the incidence of these events varies considerably between studies, and it is tempting for a reviewer to revise his preferences as new work appears, there is probably no real difference in the incidence of hormonal adverse effects between the three non-steroidal agents. However, there are important differences between them in other respects. Cyproterone acetate has been linked to adverse changes in serum lipids as well as significant, and in some cases fatal, cardiovascular events; it can also induce hepatotoxic effects. Nilutamide is associated with delayed adaptation to darkness, alcohol intolerance, and interstitial pneumonitis. Flutamide is associated with a greater risk of serious hepatotoxicity than bicalutamide or nilutamide. Diarrhea is also more likely to occur during therapy with flutamide than the other antiandrogens. In contrast, no specific non-pharmacological complications have been linked to bicalutamide, while diarrhea and abnormal liver function occur less often than with flutamide. Bicalutamide is a useful alternative to castration in men with prostatic cancer, especially since it appears somewhat less likely to cause impotence or loss of libido (2,3,4).

Antiandrogens are widely used in treating benign prostatic hyperplasia, but there is a tendency for patients to abandon treatment early. A Dutch group has sought to develop optimal treatment strategies for lower urinary tract symptoms suggestive of benign prostatic hyperplasia (5). Within a large general practice database all men aged 45 years and over with new diagnoses of benign prostatic hyperplasia were followed up; 26% discontinued therapy; discontinuation was not in the first place due to adverse reactions. The probability of early discontinuation was higher if the patients were primarily concerned by symptoms related to voiding, post-micturition, or storage rather than if they experienced a range of symptoms. The risk of early discontinuation was higher if patients had a normal prostate-specific antigen concentration. Older age and a higher chronic disease score protected against early treatment.

Finasteride is a selective inhibitor of 5-alpha-reductase. It thereby reduces prostatic concentrations of dihydrotestosterone and so reduces prostatic size (6,7,8). It is therefore used to treat benign prostatic hyperplasia (9,10,11,12) and in the prevention and treatment of prostate cancer (13). It is poorly effective in patients with prostatic obstruction and small prostate glands (14), but in patients with glands larger than 40 ml it produces significant symptomatic improvement.

The ability of finasteride to block the conversion of testosterone to dihydrotestosterone also makes it useful in both male-pattern baldness (15) and hirsutism related to hyperandrogenism (for example, in polycystic ovary syndrome) in women (16).

In the normal daily dose of 1 mg, which is sufficient to treat male pattern hair loss, finasteride is well tolerated over long periods. There is a very slightly higher incidence of impaired sexual function in users compared with placebo (17). In women too, low doses of finasteride (2.5 mg/day) are well tolerated when used to treat hirsutism (18). However, many of the problems seen with finasteride have undoubtedly been due to its use in unnecessarily high doses. Particularly when it is used for cosmetic purposes there has been doubt as to how far dosages can be reduced while maintaining acceptable effects. Long-term information on its safety in women with hirsutism is sparse, and in principle it might adversely affect an unborn child (16). The dose should certainly be kept as low as possible.

Observational studies

Hirsutism

In women with hirsutism low doses of finasteride (2.5 mg/day) are generally well tolerated (19). However, in a randomized study in 38 hirsute women finasteride 2.5 mg every 3 days was as effective as 2.5 mg/day and better tolerated (20).

Prostate cancer

The effect of adding finasteride 5 mg/day to high-dose bicalutamide 150 mg/day has been studied in 41 men with advanced prostate cancer treated over a mean of 3.9 years (21). The serum prostate-specific antigen (PSA) concentration was measured every 2 weeks until disease progression. At the first nadir of PSA, the median fall from baseline was 96.5%; a second nadir occurred in 30 of 41 patients, with a median fall of 98.5% from baseline. The median times to each nadir were 3.7 and 5.8 weeks respectively. The median time to treatment failure was 21 months. Adverse effects were minor, including gynecomastia. Sex drive was normal in 17 of 29 men at baseline and in 12 of 24 men at the second PSA nadir, but one-third of the men had spontaneous erections at both times. The authors concluded that finasteride provided additional intracellular androgen blockade when added to bicalutamide. The duration of control was comparable to that achieved with castration, with preserved sexual function in some patients.

Comparative studies

Androgenetic alopecia

In an open comparative study of androgenetic alopecia in 90 men oral finasteride (1 mg/day for 12 months; n = 65) was compared with 5% topical minoxidil solution twice daily (n = 25) (22). The cure rates were 80% for oral finasteride and 52% for topical minoxidil. The adverse effects were all mild, and did not lead to withdrawal of treatment. Of the 65 men given oral finasteride, six had loss of libido, and one had an increase in body hair at other sites; irritation of the scalp was seen in one of those who used minoxidil. These adverse events disappeared as soon as the treatment was withdrawn. The laboratory data did not show any statistically or clinically significant changes from baseline values to the endpoint, except for the serum total testosterone concentration, which was increased, and free testosterone and serum prostate-specific antigen in the finasteride group which were reduced from baseline values.

Benign prostatic hyperplasia

The benefit of combining an alpha-adrenoceptor antagonist with a 5-alpha-reductase inhibitor has been assessed in men with benign prostatic hyperplasia (23). Modified-release alfuzosin was more effective than finasteride, with no additional benefit in combining the drugs. The adverse effects of alpha-blockade were postural hypotension, hypotension, headache, dizziness, and malaise; the adverse effects of finasteride were ejaculatory disorders and impotence.

The therapeutic and adverse effects of dibenyline, finasteride, and a combination of the two in 190 patients with symptomatic benign prostatic hyperplasia have been evaluated (24). Adverse effects were more common with dibenyline than with finasteride alone or in combination with dibenyline. The drop-out rate was higher with dibenyline (16%) than finasteride alone (7.5%) or the two in combination (4.6%). The reported adverse effects are listed in Table 1.

In short-term studies the herbal preparation saw palmetto (*Serenoa repens*) and finasteride seem to give a similar degree of relief in benign prostatic hyperplasia (25). However, in a prospective 1-year comparative randomized trial in 64 men with category III prostatitis or chronic pelvic pain syndrome, in which finasteride 5 mg/day was compared with saw palmetto 325 mg/day, the mean NIH Chronic Prostatitis Symptom Index score fell from 24 to 18 with finasteride, but scarcely or not at all with saw palmetto (26). Adverse events included headache (n = 3) with saw palmetto and reduced libido (n = 2) with finasteride. Although one might envisage even more prolonged studies, these findings hardly suggest that saw palmetto is a serious replacement for finasteride, even though it is well tolerated.

In a prospective 1-year comparative randomized trial in 64 men with category III prostatitis or chronic pelvic pain syndrome, finasteride was 5 mg/day was compared with

Table 1 Adverse effect of finasteride with or without dibenyline in benign prostatic hyperplasia

Adverse effect	Finasteride	Dibenyline	Combination
Light-headedness	1.9%	25%	19%
Nasal stuffiness	–	9.9%	11%
Impotence	9.3%	17%	17%

saw palmetto 325 mg/day (27). At 1 year the mean NIH Chronic Prostatitis Symptom Index score fell from 24 to 18 in the finasteride group, but scarcely or not at all in the saw palmetto group. Adverse events included headache (n = 3) in the saw palmetto group and reduced libido (n = 2) in the finasteride group. Although one might envisage even more prolonged studies these findings hardly suggest that saw palmetto is a serious replacement for finasteride even though it is well tolerated.

Prostate cancer

Although flutamide is sufficiently well tolerated in prostatic cancer, the much older drug cyproterone acetate continues to show up favorably. In a direct comparison between the two drugs in 310 men the two were equally effective in delaying progression of the cancer and prolonging survival; however, adverse effect profiles were more favorable for cyproterone acetate overall and in particular with respect to gynecomastia, diarrhea, and nausea (28).

Polycystic ovary syndrome

In 44 women with polycystic ovary syndrome treated with finasteride or flutamide for 6 months the adverse effects of flutamide were reduced libido, gastrointestinal disorders, and dry skin (29). Finasteride caused reduced libido, headache, and dry skin. Dry skin was reported in 68% of users of flutamide and in only 27% of users of finasteride.

Placebo-controlled studies

Androgenetic alopecia

In an unusual study, finasteride 1 mg/day was used for 1 year to treat male-pattern baldness in nine subjects; each had an identical twin who received placebo (30). Finasteride significantly improved hair growth. There were no drug-related adverse events, either clinical or biochemical.

Of 1553 men with male-pattern baldness who took finasteride 1 mg/day, all of whom had initially taken part in one of two 1-year placebo-controlled studies, 1215 continued into further controlled studies over another 4 years (31). There was durable improvement in scalp hair over 5 years and no new safety concerns were identified.

Hirsutism

The effects of finasteride for 9 months on hirsutism and serum concentrations of basal gonadotropins, androgens, estrogen, and sex hormone-binding globulin have been studied in 18 women with idiopathic hirsutism (32). Nine took oral finasteride 7.5 mg/day and the other nine took placebo. Hirsutism improved significantly with finasteride after 6 and 9 months; placebo had no significant effect. Adverse effects were headache and modest depression during the first month. Libido did not change. Hirsute patients who took finasteride had a marked fall in dihydrotestosterone from the third month and a significant increase in serum testosterone concentrations from the sixth month of treatment.

Benign prostatic hyperplasia

The effects of finasteride and placebo on quality of life have been evaluated for 12 months in a diverse population of 2342 men with benign prostatic hyperplasia (33). Symptom scores fell significantly at month 3 in those taking finasteride and continued to improve throughout the study. The incidence of drug-related sexual adverse experiences was significantly higher in the finasteride group, but led to withdrawal in only 1.5% of patients.

Prostate cancer

The effects of bicalutamide 150 mg/day, in addition to standard non-medicinal care, have been tested in an internationally co-ordinated series of randomized placebo-controlled studies in more than 8000 patients with localized or locally advanced prostate cancer (34). At this dosage, sufficient to increase the length of progression-free survival, patients with locally advanced disease gained most benefit from bicalutamide. Overall survival was similar with bicalutamide and placebo. Survival appeared to be improved by bicalutamide in those with locally advanced disease, whereas it was reduced by bicalutamide in those with localized disease. The most common adverse events with bicalutamide were gynecomastia and breast pain.

In 9060 men who had participated in the randomized, placebo-controlled Prostate Cancer Prevention Trial in the USA for 7 years, finasteride 5 mg/day either prevented or delayed the appearance of prostate cancer, with an overall reduction in cancer incidence of 25% (35). However, of the 757 tumors that occurred with finasteride, no less than 37% were classified as relatively malignant (Gleason grades 7, 8, 9, or 10), whereas in the placebo group of 1068 tumors only 22% received this grading. The absolute number of high-grade tumors was also rather higher in the finasteride group (n = 280) than in the placebo group (n = 237). Sexual adverse effects (reduced volume of ejaculate, erectile dysfunction, loss of libido, gynecomastia) were also significantly more common in the treated group than in those taking placebo, but in the finasteride group urinary problems, such as prostatic hyperplasia or problems with micturition, were markedly reduced. The authors suggested that "physicians can use these results to counsel men regarding the use of finasteride" but it is hard to see that it provides a simple choice.

Systematic reviews

In a Spanish systematic review of the world literature there were firm conclusions about the value of finasteride in reducing the symptoms of benign prostatic hyperplasia in doses that are well tolerated in all respects (36).

Organs and Systems

Cardiovascular

The long-term effects and adverse effects of finasteride have been studied in a multicenter study of 3270 men (37). There was a background history of cardiovascular disease in 40% of the patients at baseline, and myocardial infarction was reported in 1.5% of those who took finasteride and 0.5% of those who took placebo, a significant difference.

Respiratory

An 88-year-old man developed interstitial pneumonitis while taking flutamide 375 mg/day for prostatic cancer (38). After 3 weeks he developed dyspnea and bilateral pulmonary interstitial infiltrates; glucocorticoid therapy and withdrawal of flutamide resulted in clinical improvement.

Special senses

Cataract has been associated with finasteride therapy (39).

- A 43-year-old man developed impaired vision in both eyes over 3 months. Anterior subcapsular opacities were found in both eyes, necessitating cataract extraction. He had been taking finasteride 1 mg/day for 3 years to treat the early stage of androgenic alopecia. It was suspected that the drug was responsible and the treatment was therefore withdrawn.

Endocrine

In men finasteride had no affect on serum concentrations of luteinizing hormone, follicle-stimulating hormone, cortisol, or estradiol (40). In women finasteride had no effect on basal and gonadorelin-stimulated gonadotropin secretion, the pulsatility of luteinizing hormone secretion, or the concentrations of estradiol, prolactin, free testosterone, androstenedione, dehydroepiandrosterone sulfate, or sex hormone-binding globulin; there were significant reductions in plasma concentrations of cortisol, dihydrotestosterone, and 3-alpha-androstanediol glucuronide (41).

Thyroid function has been studied in 183 patients with prostate cancer who were being treated with continuous androgen deprivation therapy; 64 were being treated with a luteinizing hormone-releasing hormone (LHRH) agonist alone and 119 others with an LHRH agonist + bicalutamide 50 mg/day (42). Treatment lasted an average of 43 months. Mean concentrations of T3 and free T4 were very similar to those in a control group of post-surgical patients without medicinal treatment or recurrence. However, the mean TSH concentration was 16 (4.4–120) mU/l in the controls and 18 (1.5–66) mU/l in the treated group, and the serum concentration of TSH was higher than 5 mU/l in six treated patients (2.1%). There was also a mild reduction in the free T4 serum concentration in treated patients. It therefore seems that androgen deprivation therapy with bicalutamide alters some thyroid function tests.

Metabolism

A marked rise in blood glucose concentration must be a very rare effect of anti-androgen therapy, but a Japanese group has described two patients with prostate cancer with this complication (43).

- A 61-year-old man with a 7-year history of diabetes, well-controlled with diet and acarbose, developed prostate cancer and was given leuprorelin acetate and flutamide. After the second injection of leuprorelin his fasting glucose and hemoglobin A_{1c} concentrations were markedly raised (23 mmol/l and 11% respectively).
- An 81-year-old man with no history of diabetes developed diabetes mellitus after using leuprorelin for prostate carcinoma for 6 months. His fasting glucose was 19 mmol/l and his HbA_{1c} was 9.9%.

In both cases the blood glucose concentration was successfully corrected with a brief course of insulin and was thereafter maintained in the reference range using pioglitazone. This is encouraging, but the toxicity of pioglitazone must surely be borne in mind (see Chapter 42), especially in this type of elderly patient.

In men finasteride did not affect serum lipids, including total cholesterol, low density lipoproteins, high density lipoproteins, or triglycerides (40).

Hematologic

The use of androgen blockade in the treatment of prostatic cancer is, at least for a period, highly effective, but it commonly causes anemia or aggravates the anemia that is often already present in such patients. The onset and degree of the anemia in such cases has been studied in 42 patients with adenocarcinoma of the prostate, stage C, who underwent combined androgen blockage using LH-RH-A and antiandrogen treatment (leukopride acetate 3.75 mg intramuscularly every month plus oral flutamide 250 mg every 8 hours) (44). Patients who developed severe symptomatic anemia were treated with erythropoietin. Observations continued over 6 months. The mean hemoglobin concentration fell significantly from 14.2 g/dl at the start to 12.7 g/dl at 6 months, but there was severe and clinically evident anemia (less than 11 g/dl) in only six patients (14%). The development of severe anemia did not correlate with testosterone baseline values, age, or clinical stage. Its approach was detectable by the third month. The condition was readily correctable with recombinant erythropoietin.

Gastrointestinal

Gastrointestinal effects are common when flutamide is used to treat advanced cases of prostate cancer. At doses of 250 mg every 8 hours or 500 mg/day, 23 of 106 men had gastrointestinal problems, irrespective of the dosage regimen (45). There was no difference in the incidence of these effects in the 56 men who had previously received external beam radiation and 50 others who had undergone radical prostatectomy. This suggests that the gastrointestinal adverse effects of flutamide are not due to a local toxic effect.

Enterocolic lymphocytic phlebitis has been temporally associated with flutamide treatment (46). Although the association could have been coincidental, the facts suggest that the report should be taken seriously.

- A 53-year-old man developed ileocecal intussusception due to an edematous ischemic cecum, due to enterocolic lymphocytic phlebitis, with numerous associated thrombi. The phlebitis involved not only the ischemic area but also other sites, notably the entire right colon, terminal ileum, and appendix. All layers of the bowel wall were involved. The mesenteric veins were also prominently affected, but the arteries were spared. There was a marked lymphocytic infiltrate involving the epithelium of the entire right colon, ileum, and appendix.

This is the first reported case of enterocolic lymphocytic phlebitis, a rare form of vasculitis, in conjunction with lymphocytic colitis, lymphocytic enteritis, and lymphocytic appendicitis. The fact that the patient was taking flutamide at the same time suggests that this peculiar form of lymphocytic inflammation of the veins and mucosa could represent a drug reaction. It should be recalled that diarrhea is a common complication of flutamide use, and perhaps occurs in severe degree in some 15% of men taking full-dose treatment.

Liver

Flutamide causes hepatotoxicity in some 0.36% of patients, and for this reason alone it should not be used in the absence of a serious indication. Whether bulimia nervosa in women justifies its use is open to doubt, since non-pharmacological methods of treatment are available. Furthermore, bulimia nervosa in women can be associated with raised serum testosterone concentrations. In a small double-blind study of the use of flutamide, citalopram, a combination of the two, or placebo in 31 women over 3 months, all the active treatments reduced the tendency to binge eating (47). However, there was a moderate and reversible increase in serum transaminase activities, leading to withdrawal in two of the 19 subjects who were taking flutamide either alone or in combination.

Pancreas

The incidence of acute pancreatitis as a suspected complication of finasteride treatment has been examined in a case-control study in a Danish regional population of 490 000 over 7 years. Of 302 men aged 60 and older with incident acute pancreatitis, three had been exposed to finasteride; of 2994 controls 37 had been exposed to finasteride. After adjustment for alcohol-related diseases, gallstone disease, hyperlipidemia, hypercalcemia, and hyperparathyroidism, the authors found no evidence of an increased risk of acute pancreatitis in users of finasteride (48).

Skin

Cutaneous adverse effects of flutamide, which as a whole are common, include some cases of photosensitivity.

- A 70-year-old man who had taken flutamide for 4 months for prostatic carcinoma photosensitivity was associated with a positive rechallenge test (49). The authors provided evidence that this might have represented an early form of lupus erythematosus. The theory was supported by histology and by the fact that in the literature there is at least one case of flutamide-induced lupus.

Photosensitivity as a complication of flutamide treatment has been described; in one unusually severe case, erythroderma proceeded to extensive vitiligo (50).

Musculoskeletal

Androgen deprivation therapy for prostatic cancer, whether it is carried out surgically or medicinally, carries a substantial risk of osteoporosis and spinal fractures. These risks have been quantified to some extent (51). In 87 elderly men treated in this way over a long period, 38 had radiographic evidence of spinal fractures. They had an initial mean prostate specific antigen of 53 ng/ml and had received androgen deprivation therapy for a mean of 40 months. Mean spinal and femoral neck bone mineral densities were significantly lower than in men without spinal fractures. The duration of androgen deprivation therapy, low serum 25-hydroxycole-calciferol concentrations, and a history of alcohol excess (defined as more than four standard drinks daily) were the main determinants of spinal fractures.

Reversible severe myopathy during treatment with finasteride has been described in a 70-year-old man (52).

Sexual function

Very long-term treatment of prostatic enlargement with finasteride, for example over 10 years, continues to be sufficiently well tolerated, although adverse effects, mostly relating to sexual function, do occur (53,54). The incidence and nature of these adverse effects has been well documented in The Proscar Long-term Efficacy and Safety Study (PLESS), a 4-year, randomized, double-blind, placebo-controlled trial in 3040 men, all of whom took finasteride 5 mg/day (55). At screening, 46% of all the patients reported some history of sexual dysfunction. During the first year of the study, 15% of the finasteride-treated patients and 7% of the placebo-treated patients had sexual adverse events that were considered drug related; during years 2-4, there was no between-group difference in the incidence of new sexual adverse events (7% in each group). Sexual adverse events resolved while continuing therapy in 12% of those taking finasteride and 19% of those taking placebo.

The incidence of erectile dysfunction induced by finasteride is difficult to estimate, since in many users of the drug other causes are present; they include advanced age, heart disease, diabetes, hypertension, smoking, and hypercholesterolemia. Benign prostatic hyperplasia itself can also aggravate or even induce erectile dysfunction. Analysis of a questionnaire study in New Jersey suggested that such pathological factors can have a greater role in inducing erectile dysfunction than drugs such as finasteride and alpha-blockers, although the latter can clearly contribute (56).

At an oral dose of 1 mg/day finasteride has no major adverse effects on measures of semen production or quality (57), although it can cause a slight reduction in the volume of ejaculate (15).

There is a higher incidence of impaired sexual function in men who take finasteride compared with placebo (58,59). The incidence of erectile dysfunction has been estimated at 5% (60), but it is difficult to estimate, since in many users of the drug other causes are present, including advanced age, heart disease, diabetes, hypertension, smoking, and hypercholesterolemia. Benign prostatic hyperplasia itself can also aggravate or even induce erectile dysfunction. A questionnaire study in New Jersey suggested that such pathological factors have a greater role in inducing erectile dysfunction than drugs such as finasteride and alpha-adrenoceptor antagonists, although the latter can clearly contribute (61).

The long-term efficacy and safety of finasteride have been studied in 102 patients with benign prostatic hyperplasia (62). Adverse experiences due to sexual dysfunction continued throughout the study, but the low continuous dropout rate may have reflected a natural process in this aged population, and not necessarily a drug-related effect.

The incidence and nature of adverse effects of finasteride on sexual function have been documented in The Proscar Long-term Efficacy and Safety Study (PLESS), a 4-year, randomized, double-blind, placebo-controlled trial in 3040 men, all of whom took finasteride 5 mg/day (63). At screening, 46% of all the patients reported some history of sexual dysfunction. During the first year of the study, 15% of the finasteride-treated patients and 7% of the placebo-treated patients had sexual adverse events that were considered to be drug-related; during years 2–4 there was no between-group difference in the incidence of new sexual adverse events (7% in each group). Sexual adverse events resolved during continued therapy in 12% of those taking finasteride and 19% of those taking placebo.

In a long-term multicenter study of finasteride in 3270 men the numbers of serious adverse events and withdrawals because of adverse events were significantly higher with placebo (37). Drug-related adverse effects in 1% or more of patients were reduced libido, ejaculation disorders, and impotence. A total of 273 patients, 165 (10%) taking finasteride and 108 (7%) taking placebo, reported a sexual adverse event during the treatment period, including change in libido, ejaculation disorders, impotence, or orgasmic dysfunction.

The effects of finasteride (n = 545), tamsulosin, or the proprietary herbal remedy Permixon on sexual function have been studied in patients with lower urinary tract symptoms due to benign prostatic hyperplasia (64). At 6 months tamsulosin and finasteride caused slight increases in sexual disorders and Permixon caused a slight improvement. Ejaculation disorders were the most frequently reported adverse effects after tamsulosin or finasteride.

However, an Italian investigation of sexual and erectile function, using questionnaires directed to 186 patients treated at various centers with finasteride 1 mg/day for 4–6 months has challenged the accepted wisdom; the authors concluded that (as judged by the five-item International Index of Erectile Function) there was no adverse effect on erection after this period of time (65).

Reproductive system

Of 65 women with idiopathic hirsutism who took either finasteride 5 mg/day or the long-acting gonadorelin agonist leuprorelin (3.75 mg monthly as an intramuscular depot), none had either menstrual abnormalities or other adverse effects (66). However, adequate doses may not have been used, since the hirsutism score improved in only 36% of the patients who took leuprorelin and 14% of those who took finasteride. Serum concentrations of total testosterone, free testosterone, androstenedione, and dehydroepiandrosterone fell in patients treated with leuprorelin, but only serum total testosterone and free testosterone concentrations fell significantly with finasteride.

Breasts

Reversible painful gynecomastia has been reported as an adverse effect of finasteride in a dose as low as 1 mg/day (67); it can be unilateral (68) or bilateral (69). Some reports of gynecomastia in users of finasteride relate to doses as low as 1 mg/day (70).

- A 23-year-old man who was taking finasteride 1 mg/day for 2 months for androgenetic alopecia developed painful enlargement of his right breast (71). Treatment was withdrawn and resolution occurred after 2 months.

However, breast cancer can be misdiagnosed as benign gynecomastia (see below).

In a series of studies from Italy an attempt was made to determine whether giving anastrozole 1 mg/day and/or tamoxifen 20 mg/day could prevent gynecomastia and breast pain due to bicalutamide 150 mg/day (72). In a 48-week double-blind study tamoxifen reduced the symptoms but anastrozole did not.

It is possible to reduce the incidence of gynecomastia in men taking antiandrogens by prophylactic irradiation of the breast. In a major randomized clinical study of antiandrogen use in Scandinavia, breast irradiation, generally using single-fraction electrons (12 to 15 Gy), was given to 174 (69%) of 253 patients (73). After 1 year physician evaluations suggested some form of gynecomastia in 71% and 28% of the non-irradiated and irradiated patients respectively, some form of breast enlargement in 78% and 44%, and some degree of breast tenderness in 75% and 43%.

Long-Term Effects

Tumorigenicity

Striking evidence of the association of finasteride with male breast cancer comes from the Medical Therapy of Prostatic Symptoms (MTOPS) study, a National Institutes of Health (NIH)-sponsored study of about 3047 men that compared finasteride, doxazosin, and the combination for the treatment of benign prostatic hyperplasia. The rate of breast cancer in this trial for men

taking finasteride either alone or with doxazosin was four in 1554, or nearly 200 times that of the general population; one man in the finasteride + doxazosin group and three in the finasteride-alone group developed male breast cancer (74).

- A 53-year-old man developed unilateral gynecomastia following finasteride therapy for alopecia (75). On needle biopsy the mammary mass was diagnosed as adenocarcinoma on the basis of nuclear atypia and particularly because of cytoplasmic vacuolization, but excision biopsy showed only benign gynecomastia with no evidence of malignant change.

In one case a man taking bicalutamide developed gynecomastia, which proceeded to breast cancer (76).

An elderly man with prostate cancer took long-term flutamide and developed adenocarcinoma of the breast (77). There could have been several reasons for this complication. Unlike LH-releaser-based hormonal therapy for prostatic cancer, antiandrogens cause hyperestrogenemia owing to suppressed negative feedback of androgens on LHRH and LH production, stimulation of testicular androgen production, and transformation to estrogens in peripheral target tissues. It is true that, in this particular individual, there were other susceptibility factors, namely BRCA-1 mutation and chromosome 9 inversion, which has been previously shown to impinge upon testicular function and intracrine balance of androgens versus estrogens. However, the authors stressed that men with prostate cancer who take antiandrogens may be at risk of breast cancer and they advised caution in the use of the treatment in men with risk factors for male breast cancer.

Susceptibility factors

Age

In 3040 men with benign prostatic hyperplasia the effects of finasteride 5 mg/day for 4 years were studied in those over and under 65 years (78). In both groups the drug was effective and there were no significant differences in cardiovascular adverse events between placebo and finasteride. There were significant differences between placebo and finasteride in the overall incidence of typical drug-related adverse events, but there were no specific differences associated with age. The principal events were impotence (8.8%), reduced libido (6.8%), reduced volume of ejaculate (3.5%), other disorders of ejaculation (1.5%), rash (0.6%), breast enlargement (0.5%), and breast tenderness (0.2%).

Drug Administration

Drug dosage regimens

The difficulty in weighing benefit against harm when selecting a regimen for patients with hormone-refractory prostate carcinoma is compounded by the fact that patients differ markedly in their needs and responses. This is underlined by the outcome of a panel study undertaken by the Society of Urologic Oncology (79). However, its only firm recommendation, after considering all the medicinal alternatives, was that "management strategies should be targeted toward the individual patient".

In a phase II study of androgen suppression therapy for prostate cancer, 95 patients with recurrent or metastatic prostate cancer received cyclical 8-month periods of treatment with leuprolide acetate and nilutamide, with intermittent rest periods (80). Recovery periods were progressively lengthened until the treatment failed to achieve normal prostate-specific antigen (PSA) concentrations. The 95 subjects received 245 cycles of treatment. The median duration of rest periods was 8 months and the median time to treatment failure was 47 months. There was testosterone recovery during rest periods in 117 cycles (61%). There was mild anemia in 33%, 44%, and 67% of cycles 1, 2, and 3 respectively. Sexual function recovered during the rest periods in 47% of cycles. There was no significant overall change in body mass index at the end of the treatment period. Osteoporosis was documented in at least one site, evaluated in 41 patients (37%). The results of this study suggest that intermittent use of androgen suppression has the potential to reduce adverse effects, allowing recovery of the hemoglobin concentration, permitting return of sexual function, and avoiding weight gain.

Many of the problems seen with finasteride have undoubtedly been due to its use in unnecessarily high doses. Particularly when used for cosmetic ends there has been doubt as to how far dosage can be reduced while maintaining an acceptable effect. Finasteride continues to be used to treat hirsutism in women and is effective, although long-term information on safety is sparse, and in principle it might adverse affect an unborn child (81). The dose should certainly be kept as low as possible.

In a randomized study in 38 hirsute women finasteride 2.5 mg every 3 days was as effective as the higher daily dose formerly used and better tolerated (82).

Drug-drug interactions

Cyproterone acetate

Sequential administration of flutamide and cyproterone acetate has been associated with toxic hepatitis (83).

Sibutramine

An interaction of finasteride with sibutramine has been described (84).

- A 30-year man who was being successfully treated for obesity with sibutramine started to take finasteride to treat alopecia. Soon afterwards he developed paranoid psychotic behavior. The reaction abated and disappeared when finasteride was withdrawn.

The suggested mechanism of this interaction was that finasteride inhibited the hepatic metabolism of sibutramine, which then displaced finasteride from its plasma protein binding sites; inhibition of 5HT (serotonin) and noradrenaline reuptake by sibutramine then triggering the psychotic event.

Interference with diagnostic routines

Finasteride reduces serum prostate-specific antigen concentrations (60). In participants in the Prostate Cancer Prevention Trial who had an end of study biopsy (928 with cancer and 8620 with a negative biopsy) or an interim diagnosis of prostate cancer (n = 671) those who took finasteride had a median fall in PSA of 2% after year 1, while the controls had an increase of 3% (85). By the end of the study PSA had increased annually by 6% (placebo) and 7% (finasteride). In those with interim diagnoses PSA increased by 11% (placebo) and 15% (finasteride) each year before diagnosis. Cases with high grade disease (Gleason 7 and above) had greater increases in PSA than cases with low grade disease. The authors concluded that in men who have taken finasteride for more than 1 year the PSA concentration will need to be adjusted to determine whether it is in the reference range. In the Prostate Cancer Prevention Trial the adjustment factor required to preserve a median PSA concentration increased from 2 at 24 months to 2.5 at 7 years after the start of finasteride treatment.

References

1. Fourcade R-O, McLeod D. Tolerability of antiandrogens in the treatment of prostate cancer. UroOncol 2004;4:5–13.
2. Fradet Y. Bicalutamide (Casodex) in the treatment of prostate cancer. Exp Rev Anticancer Ther 2004;4:37–48.
3. Ciarra A, Cardi A, Di Silverio F. Antiandrogen monotherapy: recommendations for the treatment of prostate cancer. Urol Int 2004;72:91–8.
4. Schellhammer PF, Davis JW. An evaluation of bicalutamide in the treatment of prostate cancer. Clin Prost Cancer 2004;2:213–9.
5. Verhamme KMC, Dieleman JP, Bleumink GS, Bosch JLHR, Stricker BHCh, Sturkenboom MCJM. Treatment strategies, patterns of drug use and treatment discontinuation in men with LUTS suggestive of benign prostatic hyperplasia: the Triumph Project. Eur Urol 2003;44:539–45.
6. Peters DH, Sorkin EM. Finasteride. A review of its potential in the treatment of benign prostatic hyperplasia. Drugs 1993;46(1):177–208.
7. Steiner JF. Finasteride: a 5 alpha-reductase inhibitor. Clin Pharm 1993;12(1):15–23.
8. Steiner JF. Clinical pharmacokinetics and pharmacodynamics of finasteride. Clin Pharmacokinet 1996;30(1):16–27.
9. Nickel JC, Fradet Y, Boake C, Pommerville PJ, Perreault J-P, Afridi SK, Elhilali MM, Barr RE, Beland GA, Bertrand PE, et al. Efficacy and safety of finasteride therapy for benign prostatic hyperplasia: results of a 2-year randomized controlled trial (the PROSPECT study). Can Med Assoc J 1996;155:1251–9.
10. Nickel JC. Long-term implications of medical therapy on benign prostatic hyperplasia end points. Urology 1998;51 Suppl A:50–7.
11. Edwards JE, Moore RA. Finasteride in the treatment of clinical benign prostatic hyperplasia: a systematic review of randomised trials. BMC Urol 2002;2:14.

12. Jimenez Cruz J.F, Quecedo Gutierrez L, Del Llano Senaris J. Finasterida. Diez anos de uso clinico. Revision sistematica de la literatura. Actas Urol Esp 2003;27:202–15.

13. Reddy GK. Finasteride, a selective 5-alpha-reductase inhibitor, in the prevention and treatment of human prostate cancer. Clin Prostate Cancer 2004;2(4):206–8.

14. Ekman P. A risk-benefit assessment of treatment with finasteride in benign prostatic hyperplasia. Drug Saf 1998;18:161–70.

15. Libecco JF, Bergfeld WF. Finasteride in the treatment of alopecia. Expert Opin Pharmacother 2004;5(4):933–40.

16. Townsend KA, Marlowe KF. Relative safety and efficacy of finasteride for treatment of hirsutism. Ann Pharmacother 2004;38(6):1070–3.

17. Whiting DA, Olsen EA, Savin R, Halper L, Rodgers A, Wang L, Hustad C, Palmisano J. Efficacy and tolerability of finasteride 1 mg in men aged 41 to 60 years with male pattern hair loss. Eur J Dermatol 2003;13:150–60.

18. Bayram F, Muderris I, Guven M, Ozcelik B, Kelestimur F. Low-dose 2.5 mg/day) finasteride treatment in hirsutism. Gynecol Endocrinol 2003;17:419–22.

19. Bayram F, Muderris I, Guven M, Ozcelik B, Kelestimur F. Low-dose 2.5 mg/day) finasteride treatment in hirsutism. Gynecol Endocrinol 2003;17:419–22.

20. Tartagni M, Schonauer MM, Cicinelli E, Petruzzelli F, De Pergola G, De Salvia MA, Loverro G. Intermittent low-dose finasteride is as effective as daily administration for the treatment of hirsute women. Fertil Steril 2004;82:752–5.

21. Tay M-H, Kaufman DS, Regan MM, Leibowitz SB, George DJ, Febbo PG, Manola J, Smith MR, Kaplan ID, Kantoff PW, Oh WK. Finasteride and bicalutamide as primary hormonal therapy in patients with advanced adenocarcinoma of the prostate Ann Oncol 2004;15:974–8.

22. Arca E, Acikgoz G, Tastan HB, Kose O, Kurumlu Z. An open, randomized, comparative study of oral finasteride and 5% topical minoxidil in male androgenetic alopecia. Dermatology 2004;209:117–25.

23. De Bruyne FMJ, Jardin A, Colloi D, Resel L, Witjes WPJ, Delauche-Cavallier MC, McCarthy C, Geffriaud-Ricouard C. Sustained release alfuzosin, finasteride and the combination of both in the treatment of benign prostatic hyperplasia. Eur Urol 1998;34:169–75.

24. Kuo HC. Comparative study for therapeutic effect of dibenyline, finasteride and combination drugs for symptomatic benign prostatic hyperplasia. Urol Int 1998;60:85–91.

25. Carraro JC, Raynaud JP, Koch G, Chisholm GD, Di Silverio F, Teillac P, Da Silva FC, Cauquil J, Chopin DK, Hamdy FC, Hanus M, Hauri D, Kalinteris A, Marencak J, Perier A, Perrin P. Comparison of phytotherapy (Permixon) with finasteride in the treatment of benign prostate hyperplasia: a randomized international study of 1,098 patients. Prostate 1996;29(4):231–40.

26. Kaplan SA, Volpe MA, Te AE. A prospective 1-year trial using saw palmetto versus finasteride in the treatment of category III prostatitis/chronic pelvic pain syndrome. J Urol 2004;171:284–8.

27. Kaplan SA, Volpe MA, Te AE. A prospective 1-year trial using saw palmetto versus finasteride in the treatment of category III prostatitis/chronic pelvic pain syndrome. J Urol 2004;171:284–8.

28. Schroder FH, Whelan P, De Reijke TM., Kurth KH, Pavone-Macaluso M, Mattelaer J, Van Velthoven RF, Debois M, Collette L. Metastatic prostate cancer treated by flutamide versus cyproterone acetate: final analysis of the "European Organization for Research and Treatment of Cancer" (EORTC) protocol 30892. Eur Urol 2004;45:457–64.

29. Falsetti L, De Fusco D, Eleftheriou G, Rosina B. Treatment of hirsutism by finasteride and flutamide in women with polycystic ovary syndrome Gynaecol Endosc 1997;6:251–7.

30. Stough DB, Rao NA, Kaufman KD, Mitchell C. Finasteride improves male pattern hair loss in a randomized study in identical twins. Eur J Dermatol 2003;12:32–7.

31. Kaufman KD. Long-term (5-year) multinational experience with finasteride 1 mg in the treatment of men with androgenetic alopecia. Eur J Dermatol 2002;12:38–49.

32. Ciotta L, Cianci A, Calogero AE, Palumbo MA, Marletta E, Sciuto A, Palumbo G. Clinical and endocrine effects of finasteride, a 5α-reductase inhibitor in women with idiopathic hirsutism. Fertil Steril 1995;64:299–306.

33. Byrnes CA, Morton AS, Liss CL, Lippert MC, Gillenwater JY. Efficacy, tolerability, and effect on health-related quality of life of finasteride versus placebo in men with symptomatic benign prostatic hyperplasia: a community based study. CUSP Investigators. Community based study of Proscar. Clin Ther 1995;17:956–69.

34. Wirth MP, See WA, McLeod DG, Iversen P, Morris T, Carroll K; Casodex Early Prostate Cancer Trialists' Group. Bicalutamide 150 mg in addition to standard care in patients with localized or locally advanced prostate cancer: results from the second analysis of the early prostate cancer program at median followup of 5.4 years. J Urol 2004;172:1865–70.

35. Thompson IM, Goodman PJ, Tangen CM, Lucia MS, Miller GJ, Ford LG, Lieber MM, Cespedes RD, Atkins JN, Lippman SM, Carlin SM, Ryan A, Szczepanek CM, Crowley JJ, Coltman CA Jr. The influence of finasteride on the development of prostate cancer. New Engl J Med 2003;349:215–24.

36. Jimenez Cruz J.F, Quecedo Gutierrez L, Del Llano Senaris J. Finasterida: Diez anos de uso clinico. Revision sistematica de la literatura. Actas Urol Esp 2003;27:202–15.

37. Margerger MJ. Long-term effects of finasteride in patients with benign prostatic hyperplasia: a double-blind, placebo-controlled multicenter study. Urology 1998;51:677–86.

38. Nomura M, Sato H, Fujimoto N, Matsumoto T. Interstitial pneumonitis related to flutamide monotherapy for prostate cancer. Int J Urol 2004;11:798–800.

39. Chou S-Y, Kao S-C, Hsu W-M. Propecia-associated bilateral cataract. Clin Exp Ophthalmol 2004;32:106–8.

40. Gormley GJ, Stoner E, Rittmaster RS, Gregg H, Thompson DL, Lasseter KC, Vlasses PH, Stein EA. Effects of finasteride (MK-906), a 5 alpha-reductase inhibitor, on circulating androgens in male volunteers. J Clin Endocrinol Metab 1990;70(4):1136–41.

41. Fruzzetti F, de Lorenzo D, Parrini D, Ricci C. Effects of finasteride, a 5 alpha-reductase inhibitor, on circulating androgens and gonadotropin secretion in hirsute women. J Clin Endocrinol Metab 1994;79(3):831–5.

42. Morote J, Esquena S, Orsola A, Salvador C, Trilla E, Cecchini L, Raventos CX, Planas J, Catalan R, Reventos J. Effect of androgen deprivation therapy in the thyroid function test of patients with prostate cancer Anti-Cancer Drugs 2005;16:863–6.

43. Inaba M, Otani Y, Nishimura K, Takaha N, Okuyama A, Koga M, Azuma J, Kawase I, Kasayama S. Combination therapy with rofecoxib and finasteride in the treatment of men with lower urinary tract symptoms (LUTS) and benign prostatic hyperplasia. Metab Clin Exp 2005;54:55–9.

44. Bogdanos J, Karamanolakis D, Milathianakis C, Repousis P, Tsintavis A, Koutsilieris M. Combined androgen blockade-induced anemia in prostate cancer patients without bone involvement. Anticancer Res 2003;23:1757–62.

45. Langenstroer P, Porter HJ, McLeod DG, Thrasher JB. Direct gastrointestinal toxicity of flutamide: comparison of irradiated and nonirradiated cases. J Urol 2004;171:684–6.

46. Wright CL, Cacala S. Enterocolic lymphocytic phlebitis with lymphocytic colitis, lymphocytic appendicitis, and lymphocytic enteritis. Am J Surg Pathol 2004;28:542–7.

47. Sundblad C, Landen M, Eriksson T, Bergman L, Eriksson E. Effects of the androgen antagonist flutamide and the serotonin reuptake inhibitor citalopram in bulimia nervosa: a placebo-controlled pilot study. J Clin Psychopharmacol 2005;25:85–8.

48. Floyd A, Pedersen L, Nielsen GL, Thorlacius-Ussing O, Sorensen HT. Risk of acute pancreatitis in users of finasteride: a population-based case-control study. J Clin Gastroenterol 2004;38:276–8.

49. Kaur C, Thami GP. Flutamide-induced photosensitivity: is it a forme fruste of lupus? Br J Dermatol 2003;148:603–4.

50. Rafael JP, Manuel GG, Antonio V, Carlos MJ. Widespread vitiligo after erythroderma caused by photosensitivity to flutamide. Contact Dermatitis 2004;50:98–100.

51. Diamond TH, Bucci J, Kersley JH, Aslan P, Lynch WB, Bryant C. Osteoporosis and spinal fractures in men with prostate cancer: risk factors and effects of androgen deprivation therapy. J Urol 2004;172:529–32.

52. Haan J, Hollander JMR, van Duinen SG, Saxena PR, Wintzen AR. Reversible severe myopathy during treatment with finasteride. Muscle Nerve 1997;20:502–4.

53. Lam JS, Romas NA, Lowe FC. Long-term treatment with finasteride in men with symptomatic benign prostatic hyperplasia: 10-year follow-up. Urology 2003;61:354–8.

54. Lowe FC, McConnell JD, Hudson PB, Romas NA, Boake R, Lieber M, Elhilali M, Geller J, Imperto-McGinely J, Andriole GL, Bruskewitz RC, Walsh PC, Bartsch G, Nacey JN, Shah S, Pappas F, Ko A, Cook T, Stoner E, Waldstreicher J. Long-term 6-year experience with finasteride in patients with benign prostatic hyperplasia. Urology 2003;61:791–6.

55. Wessells H, Roy J, Bannow J, Grayhack J, Matsumoto AM, Tenover L, Herlihy R, Fitch W, Labasky R, Auerbach S, Parra R, Rajfer J, Culbertson J, Lee M, Bach MA, Waldstreicher J. Incidence and severity of sexual adverse experiences in finasteride and placebo-treated men with benign prostatic hyperplasia. Urology 2003;61:579–84.

56. Sadeghi-Nejad H, Sherman N, Lue J. Comparison of finasteride and alpha-blockers as independent risk factors for erectile dysfunction. Int J Clin Pract 2003;57:484–7.

57. McClellan KJ, Markham A. Finasteride. A review of its use in male pattern hair loss. Drugs 1999;57:111–26.

58. Lam JS, Romas NA, Lowe FC. Long-term treatment with finasteride in men with symptomatic benign prostatic hyperplasia: 10-year follow-up. Urology 2003;61:354–8.

59. Lowe FC, McConnell JD, Hudson PB, Romas NA, Boake R, Lieber M, Elhilali M, Geller J, Imperto-McGinely J, Andriole GL, Bruskewitz RC, Walsh PC, Bartsch G, Nacey JN, Shah S, Pappas F, Ko A, Cook T, Stoner E, Waldstreicher J. Long-term 6-year experience with finasteride in patients with benign prostatic hyperplasia. Urology 2003;61:791–6.

60. Neal DE. Drugs in focus: finasteride. Presc J 1995;35:89–95.

61. Sadeghi-Nejad H, Sherman N, Lue J. Comparison of finasteride and alpha-blockers as independent risk factors for erectile dysfunction. Int J Clin Pract 2003;57:484–7.

62. Ekman P. Maximum efficacy of finasteride is obtained within 6 months and maintained over 6 years. Eur Urol 1998;33:312–7.

63. Wessells H, Roy J, Bannow J, Grayhack J, Matsumoto AM, Tenover L, Herlihy R, Fitch W, Labasky R, Auerbach S, Parra R, Rajfer J, Culbertson J, Lee M, Bach MA, Waldstreicher J. Incidence and severity of sexual adverse experiences in finasteride and placebo-treated men with benign prostatic hyperplasia. Urology 2003;61:579–84.

64. Zlotta AR, Teillac P, Raynaud JP, Schulman CC. Evaluation of male sexual function in patients with lower urinary tract symptoms (LUTS) associated with benign prostatic hyperplasia (BPH) treated with a phytotherapeutic agent (Permixon®), tamsulosin or finasteride. Eur Urol 2005;48:269–76.

65. Tosti A, Pazzaglia M, Soli M, Rossi A, Rebora A, Atzori L, Barbareschi M, Benci M, Voudouris S, Vena GA. Evaluation of sexual function with an International Index of Erectile Function in subjects taking finasteride for androgenetic alopecia. Arch Dermatol 2004;140:857–8.

66. Bayhan G, Bahceci M, Demirkol T, Ertem M, Yalinkaya A, Erden AC. A comparative study of a gonadotropin-releasing hormone agonist and finasteride on idiopathic hirsutism. Clin Exp Obstet Gynecol 2000;27:203–6.

67. Wade MS, Sinclair RD. Reversible painful gynaecomastia induced by low dose finasteride (1 mg/day). Australas J Dermatol 2000;41:55.

68. Ferrando J, Grimalt R, Alsina M, Bulla F, Manasievska E. Unilateral gynecomastia induced by treatment with 1 mg of oral finasteride. Arch Dermatol 2002;138:543–4.

69. Kim BJ, Kim YJ, Ro BI. Two cases of reversible bilateral painful gynecomastia induced by 1 mg oral finasteride (Propecia). Korean J Dermatol 2003;41:232–4.

70. Kim BJ, Kim YJ, Ro BI. Two cases of reversible bilateral painful gynecomastia induced by 1 mg oral finasteride (Propecia). Korean J Dermatol 2003;41:232–4.

71. Kim H, Kye K, Seo Y, Suhr K, Lee J, Park J. A case of unilateral idiopathic gynecomastia aggravated by low-dose finasteride. Korean J Dermatol 2004;42:643–5.

72. Boccardo F, Rubagotti A, Battaglia M, Di Tonno P, Selvaggi F.P, Conti G, Comeri G, Bertaccini A, Martorana G, Galassi P, Zattoni F, Macchiarella A, Siragusa A, Muscas G, Durand F, Potenzoni D, Manganelli A, Ferraris V, Montefiore F, Trump DL. Evaluation of tamoxifen and anastrozole in the prevention of gynecomastia and breast pain induced by bicalutamide monotherapy of prostate cancer. Urol Oncol 2005;23:377.

73. Widmark A, Fossa SD, Lundmo P, Damber J-E, Vaage S, Damber L, Wiklund F, Klepp O. Does prophylactic breast irradiation prevent antiandrogen-induced gynecomastia? Evaluation of 253 patients in the randomized Scandinavian trial SPCG-7/SFUO-3. Urology 2003;61:145–51.

74. See SC, Ellis RJ. Male breast cancer during finasteride therapy. J Natl Cancer Inst 2004;96:338–9.

75. Zimmerman RL, Fogt F, Cronin D, Lynch R. Cytologic atypia in a 53-year-old man with finasteride-induced gynecomastia. Arch Pathol Lab Med 2000;124:625–7.

76. Chianakwalam C.I, McCahy P, Griffiths N.J. A case of male breast cancer in association with bicalutamide-induced gynaecomastia. Breast 2005;14:163–4.

77. Karamanakos P, Mitsiades CS, Lembessis P, Kontos M, Trafalis D, Koutsilieris M. Male breast adenocarcinoma in a prostate cancer patient following prolonged anti-androgen monotherapy. Anticancer Res 2004;24:1077–81.

78. Kaplan SA, Holtgrewe HL, Bruskewitz R, Saltzman B, Mobley D, Narayan P, Lund RH, Weiner S, Wells G, Cook TJ, Meehan A, Waldstreicher J. Comparison of the

efficacy and safety of finasteride in older versus younger men with benign prostatic hyperplasia. Urology 2001;57:1073–7.

79. Chang SS, Benson MC, Campbell SC, Crook J, Dreicer R, Evans CP, Hall MC, Higano C, Kelly WK, Sartor O, Smith Jr JA. Society of Urologic Oncology position statement. Redefining the management of hormone-refractory prostate carcinoma. Cancer 2005;103:11–21.

80. Malone S, Perry G, Segal R, Dahrouge S, Crook J. Long-term side-effects of intermittent androgen suppression therapy in prostate cancer. Results of a phase II study. BJU Int 2005;96:514–20.

81. Townsend KA, Marlowe KF. Relative safety and efficacy of finasteride for treatment of hirsutism. Ann Pharmacother 2004;38:1070–3.

82. Tartagni M, Schonauer MM, Cicinelli E, Petruzzelli F, De Pergola G, De Salvia MA, Loverro G. Intermittent low-dose finasteride is as effective as daily administration for the treatment of hirsute women. Fertil Steril 2004;82:752–5.

83. Manolakopoulos S, Bethanis S, Armonis A, Economou M, Avgerinos A, Tzourmakliotis D. Toxic hepatitis after sequential administration of flutamide and cyproterone acetate. Dig Dis Sci 2004;49:462–5.

84. Dogol Sucar D, Botelho Sougey E, Brandao Neto J. Psychotic episode induced by potential drug interaction of sibutramine and finasteride. Rev Bras Psiquiatr 2002;24:30–3.

85. Etzioni RD, Howlader N, Shaw PA, Ankerst DP, Penson DF, Goodman PJ, Thompson IM. Long-term effects of finasteride on prostate specific antigen levels: results from the prostate cancer prevention trial. J Urol 2005;174(3):877–81 [erratum 2071].

Flutamide

General Information

Flutamide is a non-steroidal antiandrogen that is used to treat prostatic cancer. Its most common adverse effects are liver damage and photosensitivity.

Organs and Systems

Respiratory

Flutamide has been associated with interstitial pneumonitis.

- An 88-year-old man with prostate cancer took flutamide 375 mg/day for 3 weeks and developed dyspnea and bilateral pulmonary interstitial infiltrates; glucocorticoid therapy and withdrawal of flutamide resulted in clinical improvement (1).

Metabolism

Flutamide has been implicated in cases of pseudoporphyria (2,3).

- A 75-year-old man with prostatic carcinoma took flutamide for 18 months and developed blisters on the back of the hands and fingers after exposure to the sun (4).

The bullae were associated with skin fragility and atrophic scarring. Histopathology and direct immunofluorescence showed ultrastructural features similar to those described in porphyria cutanea tarda. However, porphyrin concentrations in the urine and blood were normal. Flutamide was withdrawn and the lesions healed, without relapse after 11 months.

Hematologic

Although it is the commonest of all antineoplastic adverse effects, there are sometimes peculiarities of hematological toxicity that make it worthy of comment (5).

Flutamide can cause methemoglobinemia (6–8) or sulfhemoglobinemia (5). The latter occurred in a 70-year-old man who had taken flutamide 150 mg tds for 1 month and developed cyanosis and anemia that was not responsive to methylthioninium chloride (methylene blue).

In 45 patients with prostatic cancer taking flutamide 250 mg tds, there was no evidence of methemoglobinemia (9). It is possible that anecdotal reports of this adverse effect are in patients with a particular susceptibility that was not represented in this study.

Gastrointestinal

Among 440 patients taking flutamide, gastrointestinal adverse effects (abdominal pain/distension, diarrhea, constipation, nausea/vomiting, and anorexia) occurred in about 22% (10).

Ischemic colitis has been attributed to flutamide (11).

Liver

Flutamide can cause liver damage, which can occasionally be fatal (12).

- A 74-year-old man developed life-threatening acute liver failure while taking flutamide (13). Other causes of acute liver failure were ruled out and there was no evidence of active prostate cancer or liver metastases.

The authors suggested that mitochondrial dysfunction is implicated in flutamide-associated liver damage.

Three patients with advanced prostate carcinoma who took flutamide 250 mg tds for 20–22 weeks developed signs of liver damage (jaundice, anorexia, nausea, dark urine) and changes in liver function tests (high transaminases and bilirubin), indicative of acute hepatitis; flutamide was withdrawn and there was spontaneous remission over the next 8 weeks (14).

In a retrospective study of 185 patients who had taken flutamide for 151 (range 4–443) days, 9 had liver damage (15). The most common features were weakness, anorexia, weight loss, nausea, vomiting, and jaundice. No patient had evidence of hypersensitivity. In two patients there was fulminant liver failure; one had a liver transplant and the other died. The authors suggested that liver function tests should be monitored during the first months of flutamide therapy and that the drug should be withdrawn if transaminases begin to rise.

Of 123 patients who had taken flutamide, 33 had liver disorders, mostly within 9 months (16). Three variables, body mass index, a past history of liver disorders, and raised transaminases were significantly related to the incidence of liver disorders. Smoking was related to a lower incidence.

Urinary tract

Flutamide rarely causes renal damage.

- A 54-year-old man with metastatic prostate cancer developed non-oliguric acute renal insufficiency while taking flutamide; after withdrawal his renal function returned to normal within 4 weeks (17). After rechallenge his blood urea nitrogen and serum creatinine rose again and recovered completely after withdrawal.

Skin

Flutamide can cause photosensitivity reactions (18–20) and can cause residual vitiligo (21,22). The spectrum of the effect is in the UVA range (23).

- A 68-year-old man had a photosensitive drug eruption while taking flutamide (24). The minimal erythema dose with ultraviolet A light was reduced to 2 J/cm^2 and recovered to over 16 J/cm^2 after withdrawal, without changing reactivity to ultraviolet B. The absorption spectrum of flutamide was not altered after ultraviolet A irradiation.

The authors thought that flutamide has low potency to act as a photohapten, and that a non-photohaptenic mechanism is responsible for this photosensitivity or that its active metabolite may act as a photosensitizer.

Musculoskeletal

In 26 men who took androgen deprivation therapy for prostate cancer for 10 years there was reduced bone mineral density with increasing duration of androgen deprivation therapy across the whole 10-year period (25). The authors also noted that patients taking intermittent therapy had similar loss of bone mineral density at years 2 and 4, but less bone loss from year 6 onwards.

Susceptibility Factors

Renal disease

The pharmacokinetics of flutamide and its pharmacologically active metabolite, hydroxyflutamide, have been studied in 26 men with normal or reduced renal function, some of whom were undergoing hemodialysis; the pharmacokinetics were not altered by renal impairment or hemodialysis (26).

References

1. Nomura M, Sato H, Fujimoto N, Matsumoto T. Interstitial pneumonitis related to flutamide monotherapy for prostate cancer. Int J Urol 2004;11(9):798–800.
2. Schmutz JL, Barbaud A, Trechot P. Flutamide et pseudoporphyrie. [Flutamide and pseudoporphyria.] Ann Dermatol Venereol 1999;126(4):374.
3. Borroni G, Brazzelli V, Baldini F, Borghini F, Gaviglio MR, Beltrami B, Nolli G. Flutamide-induced pseudoporphyria. Br J Dermatol 1998;138(4):711–2.
4. Mantoux F, Bahadoran P, Perrin C, Bermon C, Lacour JP, Ortonne JP. Pseudo-porphyrie cutanée tardive induite par le flutamide. [Flutamide-induced late cutaneous pseudoporphyria.] Ann Dermatol Venereol 1999;126(2):150–2.
5. Kouides PA, Abboud CN, Fairbanks VF. Flutamide-induced cyanosis refractory to methylene blue therapy. Br J Haematol 1996;94(1):73–5.
6. Schott AM, Vial T, Gozzo I, Chareyre S, Delmas PD. Flutamide-induced methemoglobinemia. DICP 1991;25(6):600–1.
7. Jackson SH, Barker SJ. Methemoglobinemia in a patient receiving flutamide. Anesthesiology 1995;82(4):1065–7.
8. Khan AM, Singh NT, Bilgrami S. Flutamide induced methemoglobinemia. J Urol 1997;157(4):1363.
9. Schulz M, Schmoldt A, Donn F, Becker H. Lack of methemoglobinemia with flutamide. Ann Pharmacother 2001;35(1):21–5.
10. Langenstroer P, Porter HJ 2nd, McLeod DG, Thrasher JB. Direct gastrointestinal toxicity of flutamide: comparison of irradiated and nonirradiated cases. J Urol 2004;171(2 Pt 1):684–6.
11. Barouk J, Doubremelle M, Faroux R, Schnee M, Lafargue JP. Colite ischémique après prise de flutamide. [Ischemic colitis after taking flutamide.] Gastroenterol Clin Biol 1998;22(10):841.
12. Lubbert C, Wiese M, Haupt R, Ruf BR. Ikterus und schwere Leberfunktionsstorung bei der hormonablativen Behandlung des Prostatakarzinoms. [Toxic hepatitis and liver failure under therapy with flutamide.] Internist (Berl) 2004;45(3):333–40.
13. Famularo G, De Simone C, Minisola G, Nicotra GC. Flutamide-associated acute liver failure. Ann Ital Med Int 2003;18(4):250–3.
14. Kraus I, Vitezic D, Oguic R. Flutamide-induced acute hepatitis in advanced prostate cancer patients. Int J Clin Pharmacol Ther 2001;39(9):395–9.
15. Garcia Cortes M, Andrade RJ, Lucena MI, Sanchez Martinez H, Fernandez MC, Ferrer T, Martin-Vivaldi R, Pelaez G, Suarez F, Romero-Gomez M, Montero JL, Fraga E, Camargo R, Alcantara R, Pizarro MA, Garcia-Ruiz E, Rosemary-Gomez M. Flutamide-induced hepatotoxicity: report of a case series. Rev Esp Enferm Dig 2001;93(7):423–32.
16. Wada T, Ueda M, Abe K, Kobari T, Yamazaki H, Nakata J, Ikemoto I, Ohishi Y, Aizawa Y. [Risk factor of liver disorders caused by flutamide—statistical analysis using multivariate logistic regression analysis.] Hinyokika Kiyo 1999;45(8):521–6.
17. Altiparmak MR, Bilici A, Kisacik B, Ozguroglu M. Flutamide-induced acute renal failure in a patient with metastatic prostate cancer. Med Oncol 2002;19(2):117–9.
18. Tsien C, Souhami L. Flutamide photosensitivity. J Urol 1999;162(2):494.
19. Kaur C, Thami GP. Flutamide-induced photosensitivity: is it a forme fruste of lupus? Br J Dermatol 2003;148(3):603–4.
20. Martin-Lazaro J, Bujan JG, Arrondo AP, Lozano JR, Galindo EC, Capdevila EF. Is photopatch testing useful in the investigation of photosensitivity due to flutamide? Contact Dermatitis 2004;50(5):325–6.
21. Vilaplana J, Romaguera C, Azon A, Lecha M. Flutamide photosensitivity—residual vitiliginous lesions. Contact Dermatitis 1998;38(2):68–70.

22. Rafael JP, Manuel GG, Antonio V, Carlos MJ. Widespread vitiligo after erythroderma caused by photosensitivity to flutamide. Contact Dermatitis 2004;50(2):98–100.
23. Leroy D, Dompmartin A, Szczurko C. Flutamide photosensitivity. Photodermatol Photoimmunol Photomed 1996;12(5):216–8.
24. Yokote R, Tokura Y, Igarashi N, Ishikawa O, Miyachi Y. Photosensitive drug eruption induced by flutamide. Eur J Dermatol 1998;8(6):427–9.
25. Kiratli BJ, Srinivas S, Perkash I, Terris MK. Progressive decrease in bone density over 10 years of androgen deprivation therapy in patients with prostate cancer. Urology 2001;57(1):127–32.
26. Anjum S, Swan SK, Lambrecht LJ, Radwanski E, Cutler DL, Affrime MB, Halstenson CE. Pharmacokinetics of flutamide in patients with renal insufficiency. Br J Clin Pharmacol 1999;47(1):43–7.

Aromatase inhibitors

General Information

The development of newer antiestrogens continues in the hope of attaining a better benefit to harm balance, particularly in the adjuvant treatment of early breast cancer after the menopause (1,2). The third-generation aromatase inhibitors inhibit the production of estrogen (3). Anastrozole and letrozole are non-steroids, and exemestane (a steroid with some androgenic activity) is a derivative of the androgen androstenedione, the natural substrate of aromatase. Early findings were positive, as demonstrated by a first analysis of the ATAC ("Arimidex, Tamoxifen Alone or in Combination") trial, with a median follow-up of 33 months and a safety analysis after as many as 37 months of treatment (4). The latest safety analysis seemed to confirm that endometrial cancer vaginal bleeding and discharge, cerebrovascular events, venous thromboembolic events, and hot flushes all occurred less often in the anastrozole group, whereas musculoskeletal disorders and fractures continued to occur less often in the tamoxifen group. However, there is still debate about whether the aromatase inhibitors have significant advantages over tamoxifen (5); proponents argue that they are associated with fewer adverse effects (including endometrial cancer as well as those listed above) than tamoxifen (6). However, although they may cause fewer hot flushes, gynaecological, and thromboembolic adverse effects than tamoxifen, they may cause more musculoskeletal complications and sexual dysfunction. There is also variability in the actions of the different aromatase inhibitors, and they are not interchangeable (7).

Organs and Systems

Cardiovascular

Of 8028 postmenopausal women with receptor-positive early breast cancer who were randomly assigned double-

blind to letrozole, tamoxifen, or a sequence of these agents for 5 years, 7963 were included in an analysis of cardiovascular events over a median follow-up time of 30 months (8). There was a similar overall incidence of cardiac adverse events (letrozole 4.8%; tamoxifen 4.7%), but more grade 3–5 events with letrozole (2.4% versus 1.4%), an excess that was only partly attributable to prior hypercholesterolemia. There were more thromboembolic events with tamoxifen (3.9% versus 1.7% overall and 2.3% versus 0.9% for grade 3–5 events). There were no significant differences between tamoxifen and letrozole in the incidence of hypertension or cerebrovascular events.

The risk of venous thromboembolism in women taking anastrozole is lower than that in women taking tamoxifen (1.6% versus 2.4%) (9), but still higher than in the untreated population. Cases of pulmonary embolism have been reported in an 80-year-old woman taking anastrozole (10) and a 72-year-old woman taking letrozole (11).

Sensory systems

Retinal hemorrhages were sought in 35 women taking anastrozole 1 mg/day, 38 taking tamoxifen 20 mg/day, and 53 controls (12). There were retinal hemorrhages within the posterior pole in four of those taking anastrozole and none of the controls or those taking tamoxifen. Two of those taking anastrozole had a flame hemorrhage in the retinal nerve fiber layer and two had a blot hemorrhage deeper in the retina.

Metabolism

In 55 overweight or obese postmenopausal women w ho took tamoxifen (n = 27) or exemestane (n = 28) for 1 year, frat mass fell significantly with exemestane but not tamoxifen. Triglycerides and high-density lipoprotein cholesterol fell significantly and low-density lipoprotein cholesterol rose significantly with exemestane (13).

In 147 postmenopausal women with early breast cancer who took exemestane in a placebo-controlled study, exemestane caused modest reductions in high-density lipoprotein cholesterol and apolipoprotein, but had no major effect on lipid profile, homocysteine concentrations, or coagulation (14).

In 122 postmenopausal patients with metastatic breast cancer who were randomized to exemestane 25 mg/day (n = 62) or tamoxifen 20 mg/day (n = 60), neither exemestane nor tamoxifen had adverse effects at 8, 24 or 48 weeks on concentrations of total cholesterol, HDL cholesterol, apolipoproteins A1 or B, or lipoprotein a (15). Exemestane lowered triglyceride concentrations while tamoxifen increased them.

Hematologic

Reversible thrombocytopenia occurred in a 64-year-old woman with recurrent breast cancer taking letrozole 2.5 mg/day (16).

Liver

Acute hepatitis has been attributed to anastrozole (17).

Urinary tract

Sclerosing glomerulonephritis has been attributed to anastrozole in a 73-year-old postmenopausal woman with breast cancer (18).

Skin

- A 54-year-old Chinese woman developed a rapidly evolving vesicobullous eruption on her face, trunk, and legs, covering 50% of her body surface area, 2 weeks after she had taken letrozole on two separate occasions; histology was consistent with toxic epidermal necrolysis (19).
- Diffuse non-scarring alopecia occurred in a 37-year-old premenopausal woman with relapsed breast cancer 6 months after she had started to take letrozole 2.5 mg/ day and triptorelin 3.75 mg every 28 days; it resolved with topical minoxidil (20).

Musculoskeletal

Myalgia occurred in 12% of patients in a study of letrozole (21). In 12 patients with non-metastatic breast cancer who reported severe musculoskeletal pain while taking letrozole (n = 11) or exemestane (n = 1), the most common reported symptoms were severe early morning stiffness and hand/wrist pain causing impaired ability to completely close/stretch the hand/fingers and to perform daily activities and work-related skills (22). Six had to discontinue treatment owing to severe symptoms. Trigger finger and carpal tunnel syndrome were the most frequently reported clinical signs. Ultrasound examination showed fluid in the tendon sheath surrounding the digital flexor tendons. MRI scans showed enhancement and thickening of the tendon sheath in all 12.

Joint pain, which can be disabling, is common in women taking aromatase inhibitors (5–40%) (23). In 24 women mean age 59 years with joint pain of greater than 5/10 on a visual analogue scale, pain was due to osteoarthritis, shoulder tendinitis, or paraneoplastic aponeurositis in five cases; the other 19 had inflammatory pain of the fingers, wrists, shoulders, forefeet, ankles, or knees, with slight synovial thickening of the proximal interphalangeal joints and metacarpophalangeal joints (24). Nine had antinuclear antibodies and four had rheumatoid factor. Ten had sicca syndrome of the eyes or mouth, seven had probable Sjögren's syndrome according to the San Diego criteria, and one had definite Sjögren's syndrome. One had rheumatoid arthritis, one had Hashimoto thyroiditis, and two had positive hepatitis C serology.

Of 53 postmenopausal women with estrogen receptor-positive breast cancer taking anastrozole, 14 had joint symptoms (13 with digital stiffness and three with arthralgias of wrist and shoulders) (25). Joint symptoms tended to occur in the patients who had previously undergone chemotherapy, but there was no relation between prior hormonal therapy and joint symptoms. Seven patients who stopped taking anastrozole improved. Five who had grade 1 digital stiffness continued taking anastrozole. Two who had with grade 1 stiffness took a Chinese herbal medicine, improved, and continued to take anastrozole.

Aromatase inhibitors increase bone turnover by near complete estrogen depletion, leading to reduced bone mineral density and an increased risk of fractures. Bisphosphonates plus calcium and vitamin D supplementation mitigate this (26). In an open, multicenter, randomized study in 602 women with early-stage breast cancer taking letrozole 2.5 mg/day, zoledronic acid 4 mg every 6 months prevented bone loss (27).

In 70 postmenopausal women with completely resected breast cancers who were disease-free after taking tamoxifen for 2–3 years, a switch to exemestane resulted in increases in serum bone alkaline phosphatase and the carboxy-terminal telopeptide of type I collagen and a fall in parathormone; bone mineral density worsened (28).

In 147 postmenopausal women with early breast cancer who took exemestane in a placebo-controlled study, the mean annual rate of bone mineral density loss was 2.17% versus 1.84% in the lumbar spine and 2.72% versus 1.48% in the femoral neck with exemestane versus placebo. The mean changes in T score after 2 years were −0.21 versus −0.11 in the hip and −0.30 versus −0.21 in the lumbar spine (14).

Carpal tunnel syndrome has been reported in six patients taking aromatase inhibitors (29). Most subsequently experienced relief after withdrawal and/or switching to tamoxifen. In clinical trials of anastrozole and exemestane, carpal tunnel syndrome occurred in about 3% (30,31,32).

Immunologic

Subacute cutaneous lupus erythematosus has been attributed to anastrozole (33).

A 67-year-old woman developed Henoch-Schönlein purpura, with a leukocytoclastic vasculitis and joint pains, after taking anastrozole for 10 months; the symptoms resolved within 2 weeks of withdrawal (34).

Long-Term Effects

Tumorigenicity

In four patients with prostate tumors who were treated with exemestane (two with and two without bicalutamide) there was progression of the tumor after 4 weeks, assessed by measurement of prostate-specific antigen and radiological signs (35). Three of the four had a significant increase in bone pain only a few days after starting treatment and a clear improvement in these symptoms after withdrawal. The study was stopped prematurely and the authors concluded that exemestane has no role to play in the treatment of prostate cancer.

Susceptibility Factors

Renal and hepatic disease

The pharmacokinetics of a single oral dose of exemestane 25 mg have been studied in postmenopausal subjects with normal hepatic function (n = 9), moderately impaired hepatic function (n = 9), severely impaired hepatic function (n = 8), normal renal function (n = 6), moderately impaired renal function (n = 6), and severely impaired renal function (n = 7) (36). Exposure to exemestane was increased two- to three-fold in patients with hepatic impairment; the apparent oral clearance and apparent volume of distribution of exemestane were reduced. Renal impairment was also associated with two- to three-fold increases in exposure due to reduced clearance. However, because exemestane has a relatively large safety margin, the authors considered that these effects were of no clinical significance.

Drug-Drug Interactions

Gefitinib

Liver toxicity attributed to gefitinib in a 63-year-old woman was thought to have been due to inhibition of the metabolism of gefitinib by anastrozole (37).

Tamoxifen

In 34 post-menopausal women with early breast cancer anastrozole 1 mg/day for 28 days had no effect on the pharmacokinetics of tamoxifen 20 mg/day (38).

However, in 12 patients who took letrozole 2.5 mg/day for 6 weeks with and without tamoxifen 20 mg/day plasma concentrations of letrozole were reduced by 38% during combination therapy (39). Tamoxifen did not significantly alter the effect of letrozole in suppressing estradiol, estrone, and estrone sulfate. The authors suggested that sequential therapy might be preferable with these two drugs.

References

1. Powles TJ. Anti-oestrogenic chemoprevention of breast cancer—the need to progress. Eur J Cancer 2003;39:572–9.
2. Miller WR, Jackson J. The therapeutic potential of aromatase inhibitors. Exp Opin Invest Drugs 2003;12:337–51.
3. Smith RE, Good BC. Chemoprevention of breast cancer and the trials of the National Surgical Adjuvant Breast and Bowel Project and others. Endocr Relat Cancer 2003;10:347–57.
4. Baum M, Buzdar A, Cuzick J, Forbes J, Houghton J, Howell A, Sahmoud T; the ATAC (Arimidex, Tamoxifen Alone or in Combination) Trialists' Group. Anastrozole alone or in combination with tamoxifen versus tamoxifen alone for adjuvant treatment of postmenopausal women with early-stage breast cancer: results of the ATAC (Arimidex, Tamoxifen Alone or in Combination) trial efficacy and safety update analyses. Cancer 2003;98:1802–10.
5. Nabholtz JM. Long-term safety of aromatase inhibitors in the treatment of breast cancer. Ther Clin Risk Manag 2008;4(1):189–204.
6. Aapro MS, Forbes JF. Three years' follow-up from the ATAC trial is sufficient to change clinical practice: a debate. Breast Cancer Res Treat 2003;80:S3–11.
7. Miller WR, Bartlett J, Brodie AM, Brueggemeier RW, di Salle E, Lønning PE, Llombart A, Maass N, Maudelonde T, Sasano H, Goss PE. Aromatase inhibitors: are there differences between steroidal and nonsteroidal aromatase inhibitors and do they matter? Oncologist 2008;13(8):829–37.
8. Mouridsen H, Keshaviah A, Coates AS, Rabaglio M, Castiglione-Gertsch M, Sun Z, Thürlimann B, Mauriac L, Forbes JF, Paridaens R, Gelber RD, Colleoni M, Smith I, Price KN, Goldhirsch A. Cardiovascular adverse events during adjuvant endocrine therapy for early breast cancer using letrozole or tamoxifen: safety analysis of BIG 1-98 trial. J Clin Oncol 2007;25(36):5715–22.
9. Howell A, Cuzick J, Baum M, Buzdar A, Dowsett M, Forbes JF, Hoctin-Boes G, Houghton J, Locker GY, Tobias JS. Results of the ATAC (Arimidex, Tamoxifen, Alone or in Combination) trial after completion of 5 years' adjuvant treatment for breast cancer. Lancet 2005;365(9453):60–2.
10. Lycette JL, Luoh SW, Beer TM, Deloughery TG. Acute bilateral pulmonary emboli occurring while on adjuvant aromatase inhibitor therapy with anastrozole: Case report and review of the literature. Breast Cancer Res Treat 2006;99(3):249–55.
11. Oyan B, Altundag K, Ozisik Y. Does letrozole have any place in adjuvant setting in breast cancer patients with documented hypercoagulability? Am J Clin Oncol 2004;27(2):210–1.
12. Eisner A, Falardeau J, Toomey MD, Vetto JT. Retinal hemorrhages in anastrozole users. Optom Vis Sci 2008;85(5):301–8.
13. Francini G, Petrioli R, Montagnani A, Cadirni A, Campagna S, Francini E, Gonnelli S. Exemestane after tamoxifen as adjuvant hormonal therapy in postmenopausal women with breast cancer: effects on body composition and lipids. Br J Cancer 2006;95(2):153–8.
14. Lønning PE, Geisler J, Krag LE, Erikstein B, Bremnes Y, Hagen AI, Schlichting E, Lien EA, Ofjord ES, Paolini J, Polli A, Massimini G. Effects of exemestane administered for 2 years versus placebo on bone mineral density, bone biomarkers, and plasma lipids in patients with surgically resected early breast cancer. J Clin Oncol 2005;23(22):5126–37.
15. Atalay G, Dirix L, Biganzoli L, Beex L, Nooij M, Cameron D, Lohrisch C, Cufer T, Lobelle JP, Mattiaci MR, Piccart M, Paridaens R. The effect of exemestane on serum lipid profile in postmenopausal women with metastatic breast cancer: a companion study to EORTC Trial 10951, 'Randomized phase II study in first line hormonal treatment for metastatic breast cancer with exemestane or tamoxifen in postmenopausal patients'. Ann Oncol 2004;15(2):211–7.
16. Sperone P, Gorzegno G, Berruti A, Familiari U, Dogliotti L. Reversible pancytopenia caused by oral letrozole assumption in a patient with recurrent breast cancer. J Clin Oncol 2002;20(17):3747–8.
17. de la Cruz L, Romero-Vazquez J, Jiménez-Sáenz M, Padron JR, Herrerias-Gutierrez JM. Severe acute hepatitis in a patient treated with anastrozole. Lancet 2007;369(9555):23–4.

18. Kalender ME, Sevinc A, Camci C, Turk HM, Karakok M, Akgul B. Anastrozole-associated sclerosing glomerulonephritis in a patient with breast cancer. Oncology 2007;73(5-6):415–8.

19. Chia WK, Lim YL, Greaves MW, Ang P. Toxic epidermal necrolysis in patient with breast cancer receiving letrozole. Lancet Oncol 2006;7(2):184–5.

20. Carlini P, Di Cosimo S, Ferretti G, Papaldo P, Fabi A, Ruggeri EM, Milella M, Cognetti F. Alopecia in a premenopausal breast cancer woman treated with letrozole and triptorelin. Ann Oncol 2003;14(11):1689–90.

21. Goss PE, Ingle JN, Martino S, Robert NJ, Muss HB, Piccart MJ, Castiglione M, Tu D, Shepherd LE, Pritchard KI, Livingston RB, Davidson NE, Norton L, Perez EA, Abrams JS, Therasse P, Palmer MJ, Pater JL. A randomized trial of letrozole in postmenopausal women after five years of tamoxifen therapy for early-stage breast cancer. N Engl J Med 2003;349(19):1793–802.

22. Morales L, Pans S, Paridaens R, Westhovens R, Timmerman D, Verhaeghe J, Wildiers H, Leunen K, Amant F, Berteloot P, Smeets A, Van Limbergen E, Weltens C, Van den Bogaert W, De Smet L, Vergote I, Christiaens MR, Neven P. Debilitating musculoskeletal pain and stiffness with letrozole and exemestane: associated tenosynovial changes on magnetic resonance imaging. Breast Cancer Res Treat 2007;104(1):87–91.

23. Khanduri S, Dodwell DJ. Aromatase inhibitors and musculoskeletal symptoms. Breast 2008;17(1):76–9.

24. Laroche M, Borg S, Lassoued S, De Lafontan B, Roché H. Joint pain with aromatase inhibitors: abnormal frequency of Sjögren's syndrome. J Rheumatol 2007;34(11):2259–63.

25. Ohsako T, Inoue K, Nagamoto N, Yoshida Y, Nakahara O, Sakamoto N. Joint symptoms: a practical problem of anastrozole. Breast Cancer 2006;13(3):284–8.

26. Coleman RE, Body JJ, Gralow JR, Lipton A. Bone loss in patients with breast cancer receiving aromatase inhibitors and associated treatment strategies. Cancer Treat Rev 2008;34 Suppl 1:S31–42.

27. Brufsky A, Harker WG, Beck JT, Carroll R, Tan-Chiu E, Seidler C, Hohneker J, Lacerna L, Petrone S, Perez EA. Zoledronic acid inhibits adjuvant letrozole-induced bone loss in postmenopausal women with early breast cancer. J Clin Oncol 2007;25(7):829–36.

28. Gonnelli S, Cadirni A, Caffarelli C, Petrioli R, Montagnani A, Franci MB, Lucani B, Francini G, Nuti R. Changes in bone turnover and in bone mass in women with breast cancer switched from tamoxifen to exemestane. Bone 2007;40(1):205–10.

29. Nishihori T, Choi J, DiGiovanna MP, Thomson JG, Kohler PC, McGurn J, Chung GG. Carpal tunnel syndrome associated with the use of aromatase inhibitors in breast cancer. Clin Breast Cancer 2008;8(4):362–5.

30. ATAC Trialists' Group results of the ATAC (Arimidex, Tamoxifen, Alone or in Combination) trial after completion of 5 years' adjuvant treatment for breast cancer. Lancet 2005;365:60–2.

31. The Arimidex, Tamoxifen, Alone or in Combination (ATAC) Trialists Group. Comprehensive side effect profile of anastrozole and tamoxifen as adjuvant treatment for early stage breast cancer: long term safety analysis of the ATAC trial. Lancet Oncol 2006;7:633–43.

32. Coombes RC, Hall E, Gibson LJ, Paridaens R, Jassem J, Delozier T, Jones SE, Alvarez I, Bertelli G, Ortmann O, Coates AS, Bajetta E, Dodwell D, Coleman RE, Fallowfield LJ, Mickiewicz E, Andersen J, Lønning PE, Cocconi G, Stewart A, Stuart N, Snowdon CF, Carpentieri M, Massimini G, Bliss JM, van de Velde C; Intergroup Exemestane Study. A randomized trial of exemestane after two to three years of tamoxifen therapy in postmenopausal women with primary breast cancer. N Engl J Med 2004;350(11):1081–92.

33. Trancart M, Cavailhes A, Balme B, Skowron F. Anastrozole-induced subacute cutaneous lupus erythematosus. Br J Dermatol 2008;158(3):628–9.

34. Conti-Beltraminelli M, Pagani O, Ballerini G, Richetti A, Graffeo R, Ruggeri M, Forni V, Pianca S, Schönholzer C, Mainetti C, Cavalli F, Goldhirsch A. Henoch-Schönlein purpura (HSP) during treatment with anastrozole. Ann Oncol 2007;18(1):205–7.

35. Bonomo M, Mingrone W, Brauchli P, Hering F, Goldhirsch A; Swiss Group for Clinical Cancer Cancer Research, a member of the Swiss Institute of Applied Cancer Research. Exemestane seems to stimulate tumour growth in men with prostate carcinoma. Eur J Cancer 2003;39(14):2111–2.

36. Jannuzzo MG, Poggesi I, Spinelli R, Rocchetti M, Cicioni P, Buchan P. The effects of degree of hepatic or renal impairment on the pharmacokinetics of exemestane in postmenopausal women. Cancer Chemother Pharmacol 2004;53(6):475–81.

37. Carlini P, Papaldo P, Fabi A, Felici A, Ruggeri EM, Milella M, Ciccarese M, Nuzzo C, Cognetti F, Ferretti G. Liver toxicity after treatment with gefitinib and anastrozole: drug-drug interactions through cytochrome P450? J Clin Oncol 2006;24(35):e60–1.

38. Dowsett M, Tobias JS, Howell A, Blackman GM, Welch H, King N, Ponzone R, von Euler M, Baum M. The effect of anastrozole on the pharmacokinetics of tamoxifen in postmenopausal women with early breast cancer. Br J Cancer 1999;79(2):311–5.

39. Dowsett M, Pfister C, Johnston SR, Miles DW, Houston SJ, Verbeek JA, Gundacker H, Sioufi A, Smith IE. Impact of tamoxifen on the pharmacokinetics and endocrine effects of the aromatase inhibitor letrozole in postmenopausal women with breast cancer. Clin Cancer Res 1999;5(9):2338–43.

Diethylstilbestrol

General Information

For a complete account of the adverse effects of estrogens, readers should consult the following monographs in Meyler's Side Effects of Endocrine and Metabolic Drugs:

- Estrogens
- Hormonal contraceptives—emergency contraception
- Hormonal contraceptives—oral
- Hormone replacement therapy—estrogens
- Hormone replacement therapy—estrogens + androgens
- Hormone replacement therapy—estrogens + progestogens.

Diethylstilbestrol and other non-steroidal estrogens came into vogue at a time when the cost of producing steroidal estrogens, whether synthetic or of natural origin, was still prohibitive. They have largely fallen out of favor, in view of the association between the use of diethylstilbestrol in pregnancy and second-generation injury. There seems to be no reason for believing that the short-term acute adverse reactions to these non-steroidal compounds differ from those of estrogenic steroids.

Diethylstilbestrol continues to be recommended in some centers as one of the agents of last resort when prostate cancer proves refractory to steroid hormones or androgen deprivation therapy has done all it can (1). In a Japanese study in which 16 patients were given a daily intravenous injection of diethylstilbestrol diphosphate 250 mg for 28 days, the short-term response was favorable and the drug was well tolerated (2).

Organs and Systems

Cardiovascular

In a randomized study of men treated hormonally for prostatic cancer (3), cardiovascular adverse effects were reported more often in patients treated with diethylstilbestrol than in those treated with cyproterone acetate. The risk was highest during the first 6 months of treatment.

Mineral balance

Profound hypocalcemia occurred in a patient with osteoblastic metastatic carcinoma of the prostate after treatment with diethylstilbestrol 15 mg/day for 7 days (SED-12, 1032) (4).

Immunologic

In 13 women exposed to diethylstilbestrol in utero compared with similar control subjects with respect to the in vitro T cell response to the mitogens phytohemagglutinin, concanavalin A, and interleukin-2, incorporation of tritiated thymidine into T cells from diethylstilbestrol-exposed women was increased three-fold over a range of concentrations in response to concanavalin A, increased by 50% over a range of concentrations in response to phytohemagglutinin, and increased two-fold in response to the endogenous mitogen interleukin-2 (5). This in vitro evidence of a change in T cell-mediated immunity clearly raises questions about the clinical consequences.

Long-Term Effects

Tumorigenicity

Exposure to diethylstilbestrol during pregnancy in 4836 women has been reported to carry a relative risk of 1.27 of breast cancer later in life. However, the authors found no evidence to support the link between diethylstilbestrol exposure and ovarian, endometrial, or other cancers.

In a 25-year follow-up study there were very slightly more breast tumors in women using diethylstilbestrol in pregnancy and significantly more cancer deaths (6).

In one study there was a six-fold risk of endometrial cancer among estrogen users compared with non-users; long-term users (over 5 years) had a 15-fold risk; there were excess risks for both diethylstilbestrol and conjugated estrogens (7).

Diethylstilbestrol can cause hepatic adenomas and carcinomas in experimental animals (8), and hepatocellular carcinoma has been reported in a man who took a total of 668 g over 12 years for suspected carcinoma of the prostate (9).

Second-Generation Effects

Teratogenicity

Diethylstilbestrol was used extensively in pregnancies between 1940 and about 1975, in the belief that it could protect threatened pregnancies and counter the risk of spontaneous abortion. Toward the end of that period, increasingly clear evidence emerged that diethylstilbestrol could have an adverse effect on the second generation that did not become apparent until puberty or adulthood, and perhaps could also appear in the third generation (10). It appears to be the only estrogen with this effect, but it is naturally not excluded that some structurally related non-steroidal estrogens might carry the same risk, although these have never been used in the same way in pregnancy.

History

Diethylstilbestrol provides several illustrations of how societies cope with the risks of harm from a drug. Under different brand names diethylstilbestrol has been given to a wide range of patients over many years, mostly pregnant women and aging men with prostate cancer. The history of iatrogenic disease as a result of the use of diethylstilbestrol in pregnant women shows that patients can play an important role in securing legitimacy for research and the publication of data on the harmful effects of a drug.

Diethylstilbestrol was given to pregnant women in many countries, mainly in the 1940s to 1970s, in the mistaken belief that it would prevent miscarriage and provide strong healthy babies (11,12). The application to market diethylstilbestrol in the USA was the first new drug application submitted to the FDA shortly after the 1938 Food, Drugs, and Cosmetics Act had been passed; permission was granted, although diethylstilbestrol had already been identified as a carcinogen in animals (13). Diethylstilbestrol was especially popular in some maternity clinics in North America, serving middle-class and upper-middle class women, and in the Netherlands, where the Queen's gynecologist promoted it. In other countries it was dispensed through public health maternity centers.

In the USA, evidence showing that it was ineffective for its intended purpose appeared by the 1950s. However, conclusions based on animal experiments, as well as a major double-blind, controlled clinical trial (14), remained unheeded, partly because prescribing physicians trusted their collegial loyalty more than data that implicitly threw doubt on their practice.

In 1971, a rare form of aggressive cancer in the vagina of young girls was attributed to the girls' exposure to diethylstilbestrol in utero in a report that was based on a case-control study of eight young women, two of whom had died, at the Massachusetts General Hospital (15). It was already clear from this small study that monitoring young women exposed to diethylstilbestrol would save lives. However, months and even years were to pass before the discovery led to any public action, at different times in different countries. Only after 5 months, when the risk of cancer in patients exposed to diethylstilbestrol was featured at hearings in the US Congress, did the FDA react. The FDA's Administrator then announced that diethylstilbestrol products were to be labelled with a warning that diethylstilbestrol was contraindicated in pregnancy and should not be given to pregnant women because of risk of the cancer in the offspring (16).

Drug regulatory agencies in other countries in which diethylstilbestrol had also been commonly used in pregnancy delayed taking action. In the Netherlands, the first change of labelling to include a warning to physicians that diethylstilbestrol given to pregnant women might harm the fetus was implemented in 1972. A similar change in labelling was introduced in France in 1977. In many other countries, the news that some daughters of women who had taken diethylstilbestrol while pregnant were at risk of developing a potentially lethal cancer was passed over in silence.

In Britain, the medical community was alerted to the risks by an editorial in the British Medical Journal in 1971, but it was only in 1973 that the Committee on Safety of Medicines advised against the use of diethylstilbestrol during pregnancy (17). In Britain, drugs were commonly not labelled with information about their contents, nor with warnings of risk until well into the 1990s; thus, patients were kept in ignorance. No measures have yet been taken in Britain to alert the public to the need for medical surveillance of women who have been exposed to diethylstilbestrol in utero.

It is estimated that in the USA, the Netherlands, and France, diethylstilbestrol was given to over 5.3 million pregnant women, and it is known that it has been given to pregnant women in most parts of the world. Single cases of clear-cell vaginal carcinoma from many countries are known, but systematic studies have not been conducted everywhere.

One in a thousand young women exposed to diethylstilbestrol before birth have been estimated to be at risk of developing clear-cell vaginal adenocarcinoma (18). Exposure to diethylstilbestrol in utero also has a range of other effects on exposed women, including malformations of the reproductive organs and difficulties in conception and carrying a pregnancy to term. Some of the men exposed to diethylstilbestrol in utero have urogenital malformations and an increased risk of testicular cancer (19).

Most of the women who suspected that they had taken diethylstilbestrol were to learn of the problems from the media, and they had to guess that their daughters might be at risk of developing cancer. When they tried to discover whether they had been given diethylstilbestrol during pregnancy, many of the women found that their obstetricians were not willing to give them access to their own medical records. In a report from a nationwide US survey intended to locate pregnant women who had been given diethylstilbestrol during 1940–72, the investigators complained that at some clinics they had encountered extreme difficulties in getting access to the records (20). Women who have been exposed to diethylstilbestrol sometimes say that never have so many medical files

reportedly been lost through fire and inundation, as when they asked for access to records that might document the use of diethylstilbestrol during pregnancy.

Many doctors did not notice or did not heed warnings in the early 1970s about the risks of giving diethylstilbestrol to pregnant women. As late as 1974, according to one writer, some 11 000 prescriptions for diethylstilbestrol to be used during pregnancy were written in the USA (21). In 1976, it was observed that diethylstilbestrol was given to unsuspecting pregnant women in several Latin-American countries (21). In other countries, prescribing physicians' responses to reports that linked the use of diethylstilbestrol during pregnancy with cancer risks in their daughters were even slower. The latest documented prescription of diethylstilbestrol in Europe was in Spain in 1983 (22).

The first batches of educational material for physicians, with warnings and advice regarding health care for women who had been exposed to diethylstilbestrol, were distributed in the USA in 1971, in the Netherlands in 1974, and in France in 1989. No such material has been distributed in Britain.

Mothers in the USA who had taken diethylstilbestrol formed an organization, DES Action, to inform the public about the risks and to alert exposed mothers that their daughters needed regular medical examinations, so that potential tumor development would be detected early. Through DES Action they also gave each other mutual support during litigation against the manufacturers and acted politically to ensure that health care would be available for their daughters. DES Action groups outside the USA were formed in Australia, Belgium, Canada, France, Great Britain, Italy, Ireland, and the Netherlands. DES Action was still in the 1990s a prime mover in securing resources for research and follow-up of women who had been exposed to diethylstilbestrol, and in promoting educational programs for those women and for medical professionals.

Initiatives by medical researchers, by DES Action, and by the Public Citizen's Health Research Group secured funding in the USA for medical research on the prevalence of cancer and other effects in the young women who had been exposed in utero, and eventually also the men. The US National Institute for Environmental Health Sciences (NIEHS) has been one of the centers for toxicological studies of the effects of diethylstilbestrol. A substantial amount of research on the effects of diethylstilbestrol— animal experiments as well as epidemiological studies— has produced a valuable body of knowledge about how hormones affect the development of the fetus and prime the individual for disease later in life.

As in the case of thalidomide, the emotional engagement evoked by the harm caused by diethylstilbestrol in pregnancy led to committed action. Some physicians have devoted a major part of their careers to finding out why and how diethylstilbestrol produced adverse effects. The anger over the harm caused by diethylstilbestrol inspired patients to a commitment to prevent further harm by engaging in political action and achieving an effective response from legislators and governmental administrators. Despite the abandonment of diethylstilbestrol in pregnancy for habitual or threatened abortion, its late effects continue to be reported. Essentially, the female offspring of these pregnancies tend to develop vaginal changes (adenosis, with cervical ectropion) when reaching adolescence or adulthood and these can subsequently give rise to a clear-cell adenocarcinoma. Whereas carcinomas are a late and infrequent event, even in exposed subjects, cervical vaginal adenosis is common, the incidence probably being some 30% (23). The estimated tumor risk is only 0.14–1.4 per 1000 diethylstilbestrol-exposed subjects, but since up to 6 million fetuses were exposed to diethylstilbestrol between 1940 and 1970 the total number affected in some way may be very high indeed. There is also a high incidence of fertility disturbances among these daughters, and their own pregnancies apparently stand a high chance of not going normally to term (SED-12, 1023) (24). Analogous changes were found in male offspring (25). As in the case of thalidomide, an important element in determining cause and effect was the characteristic nature of the defect: the vaginal pathology does occur spontaneously but is highly unusual. A major problem has been the fact that the defect is as a rule only recognizable so many years after birth, by which time the history of the original treatment may be difficult or impossible to reconstruct. Even today the material is not homogeneous and strict statistical analysis of some of the epidemiological data has been claimed to point to a series of shortcomings. This does not undermine the clear conclusion that the drug is indeed responsible for the effects described (26).

Epidemiological studies on the complications of the use of diethylstilbestrol in pregnancy will certainly produce new data as time goes on: most of the data will probably continue to come from the USA and the Netherlands, where diethylstilbestrol was much more widely used to treat habitual or threatened abortion than elsewhere. In France 150 000–200 000 pregnancies were involved; in the Netherlands, with a much smaller population, 180 000–380 000 pregnant women were treated with diethylstilbestrol up to 1976.

Vaginal adenosis and adenocarcinoma
Second-generation (and possible third-generation) effects of diethylstilbestrol continue to be reported (27,28). Typical is a 1987 update analysing 519 cases of clear-cell carcinoma of the vagina and cervix identified by the Registry for Research on Hormonal Transplacental Carcinogenesis of the University of Chicago (18); in 60% of all cases the patient's mother could be shown to have used diethylstilbestrol during pregnancy. The median age at diagnosis was 19 years. The authors argued that in view of the relative rarity of the tumors, even in exposed women, one could consider that diethylstilbestrol is not a complete carcinogen and that some other factor is also involved in the pathogenesis of this type of carcinoma. The particular question of third-generation injury has actually been the subject of judicial proceedings in the USA (27,28); on the balance of evidence it seems that it can occur, although the mechanism is not clear.

Evidence has also emerged on long-term survival in young women with a clear-cell adenocarcinoma of the vagina, 20% of whom had been exposed to diethylstilbestrol and 80% had not (29). The probabilities of survival at 5 and 10 years for diethylstilbestrol-associated cases were 84 and 78% respectively, compared with 69 and 60% for those not associated with diethylstilbestrol. These differences were not due to differences in clinical prognostic factors, but suggest differences in tumor behavior for as yet undetermined reasons.

Although it is more than 30 years since the full extent of the injury to offspring by the ill-advised use of diethylstilbestrol during pregnancy became clear, details of that injury are still being filled in as the individuals concerned grow older. The picture will continue to develop as long as this generation of individuals lives, and it is even possible that findings in the third generation will throw light on the persisting injury to the family.

Psychological research among "DES daughters" has shown how traumatic it can be for a woman to learn of her prenatal exposure to diethylstilbestrol, and the extent to which this creates persistent uncertainty about her health; the failure of a physician to provide reliable information and continuing support can severely undermine her faith in health care (30).

Long-term studies of the pregnancy experiences of women exposed to diethylstilbestrol in utero, compared with unexposed women, now include one in the US National Collaborative Diethylstilbestrol Adenosis cohort and one in the Chicago cohort and their respective non-exposed comparison groups. A review of questionnaire replies from 3373 exposed daughters and from controls has confirmed that diethylstilbestrol-exposed women were less likely than unexposed women to have had full-term live births and more likely to have had premature births, spontaneous pregnancy losses, or ectopic pregnancies (31). The data are shown in Table 1. Second-trimester spontaneous pregnancy losses were much more common in diethylstilbestrol-exposed women.

Other cancers
Long-term data are also accumulating on the actual incidence of genital cancer in women exposed to diethylstilbestrol in utero (32). In the Netherlands, a country in which diethylstilbestrol was used intensively in pregnancy, there is evidence that the risk of cervical cancer in these women is trebled, rather than doubled as was previously supposed (33).

Table 1 Outcomes in pregnancies exposed and not exposed to diethylstilbestrol

Outcome	Exposed (%)	Non-exposed (%)
Full-term delivery	64	85
Spontaneous abortion	19	10
Preterm delivery	12	4.1
Ectopic pregnancy	4.2	0.8

- A diethylstilbestrol-exposed woman developed concurrent primary cancers of both the vagina and the endometrium at the age of 39 (34).

However, it is important to bear in mind that cases occur in which there is no history of the mother's having taken diethylstilbestrol during pregnancy. In one such case, HIV/AIDS infection was also a predisposing factor for vaginal carcinoma and this could explain a proportion of new cases that are being reported today (35).

A further follow-up and analysis of 3879 women, taken from two earlier US studies, who had been exposed to diethylstilbestrol during pregnancy has been presented (36). The results showed a modest association between diethylstilbestrol exposure and the risk of breast cancer (RR = 1.27; 95% CI = 1.07, 1.52). The increased risk was not further aggravated by a family history of breast cancer, by use of oral contraceptives, or by HRT. There was no evidence that diethylstilbestrol was associated with a raised risk of ovarian, endometrial, or other hormone-associated cancers.

Sensory systems
A study in the USA has produced some evidence that in people with amblyopia, those who were exposed to diethylstilbestrol before birth may be more likely to develop myopia (37).

Menstrual and vaginal disturbances
The effects of in-utero exposure to diethylstilbestrol on the menstrual cycle have been studied prospectively in 198 women and in 162 unexposed controls (38). A major limitation of this study was the exclusion of women with a severe menstrual abnormality. Exposure to diethylstilbestrol was associated with a statistical significantly lower duration of menstrual bleeding but not with dysmenorrhea. For most women exposed to diethylstilbestrol, any effects on reproductive hormonal function are in all probability minor, if present at all.

Even the classic genital manifestations of diethylstilbestrol in women who have been exposed to it in fetal life may be overlooked unless one is alert to them; vaginal discharge with ectropion should cause one to enquire as to possible prenatal diethylstilbestrol exposure (39).

Autoimmune disease
During the last 15 years, various additional aspects of the diethylstilbestrol problem have given rise to concern. One emerged in 1988 from a large multicenter epidemiological cohort study established by the US National Cancer Institute (DESAD Project), in which it was found that women exposed in utero to diethylstilbestrol had a 50% increased incidence of autoimmune disease (40).

Drug Administration

Drug formulations
The parenteral formulation diethylstilbestrol diphosphate is less commonly used than the oral formulation. In Japan, 24 elderly patients with advanced relapsed prostatic cancer were treated with high doses supplemented with ethinylestradiol (doses unclear); there was some slight therapeutic effect, but there were gastrointestinal symptoms and fluid retention (41). Also in Japan, a few patients with advanced disease were treated using intravenous diethylstilbestrol diphosphate 500 mg/day for 20 consecutive days to a total dose of 10 g; the authors' conclusion was more positive but adverse events were not specified (42).

Drug contamination
Contamination of isoniazid tablets with diethylstilbestrol was the cause of several cases of precocious puberty in a children's tuberculosis ward (43).

References

1. Lonning PE, Taylor PD, Anker G, Iddon J, Wie L, Jorgensen LM, Mella O, Howell A. High-dose estrogen treatment in postmenopausal breast cancer patients heavily exposed to endocrine therapy. Breast Cancer Res Treat 2001;67(2):111–16.
2. Takezawa Y, Nakata S, Kobayashi M, Kosaku N, Fukabori Y, Yamanaka H. Moderate dose diethylstilbestrol diphosphate therapy in hormone refractory prostate cancer. Scand J Urol Nephrol 2001;35(4):283–7.
3. Pavone-Macaluso M, de Voogt HJ, Viggiano G, Barasolo E, Lardennois B, de Pauw M, Sylvester R. Comparison of diethylstilbestrol, cyproterone acetate and medroxyprogesterone acetate in the treatment of advanced prostatic cancer: final analysis of a randomized phase III trial of the European Organization for Research on Treatment of Cancer Urological Group. J Urol 1986;136(3):624–31.
4. Harley HA, Mason R, Phillips PJ. Profound hypocalcaemia associated with oestrogen treatment of carcinoma of the prostate. Med J Aust 1983;2(1):41–2.
5. Burke L, Segall-Blank M, Lorenzo C, Dynesius-Trentham R, Trentham D, Mortola JF. Altered immune response in adult women exposed to diethylstilbestrol in utero. Am J Obstet Gynecol 2001;185(1):78–81.
6. Herbst AL, editor. Intrauterine exposure to diethylstilbestrol in the human. Proceedings, "Symposium on DES". Chicago: American College of Obstetricians and Gynecologists, 1977349–95.
7. Antunes CM, Strolley PD, Rosenshein NB, Davies JL, Tonascia JA, Brown C, Burnett L, Rutledge A, Pokempner M, Garcia R. Endometrial cancer and estrogen use. Report of a large case-control study. N Engl J Med 1979;300(1):9–13.
8. Williams GM, Iatropoulos M, Cheung R, Radi L, Wang CX. Diethylstilbestrol liver carcinogenicity and modification of DNA in rats. Cancer Lett 1993;68(2–3):193–8.

9. Rosinus V, Maurer R. [Diättylstilböstrol-induziertes Leberzellkarzinom? Diethylstilbestrol-induced liver cancer?] Schweiz Med Wochenschr 1981;111(30):1139–42.
10. Martino MA, Nevadunsky NS, Magliaro TJ, Goldberg MI. The DES (diethylstilbestrol) years: bridging the past into the future. Prim Care Update Ob Gyns 2002;9:7–12.
11. Smith OW. Diethylstilbestrol in prevention of complications of pregnancy. Am J Obstet Gynecol 1948;56:821–34.
12. Smith OW, Smith GV. The influence of diethylstilbestrol on the progress and outcome of pregnancy as based on a comparison of treated with untreated primigravidas. Am J Obstet Gynecol 1949;58(5):994–1009.
13. Lacassagne A. Apparition d'adénocarcinomes mammaires chez des souris mâles traités par une substance oestrogène synthétique. Comptes Rend Séances Soc Biol 1938;129:641–3.
14. Dieckmann WJ, Davis ME, Rynkiewicz LM, Pottinger RE. Does the administration of diethylstilbestrol during pregnancy have therapeutic value? Am J Obstet Gynecol 1953;66(5):1062–81.
15. Herbst AL, Ulfelder H, Poskanzer DC. Adenocarcinoma of the vagina. Association of maternal stilbestrol therapy with tumor appearance in young women. N Engl J Med 1971;284(15):878–81.
16. US Department of Health, Education and Welfare, Food and Drug Administration. Certain estrogens for oral or parenteral use. Drugs for human use. Drug efficacy study implementation. Federal Register 1971;36(217):21537–8.
17. Mitchell S, producer, Wait J, presenter. Face the Facts. BBC Radio 4, 21 February 2000.
18. Melnick S, Cole P, Anderson D, Herbst A. Rates and risks of diethylstilbestrol-related clear-cell adenocarcinoma of the vagina and cervix. An update. N Engl J Med 1987;316(9):514–16.
19. Palmlund I. Exposure to a xenoestrogen before birth: the diethylstilbestrol experience. J Psychosom Obstet Gynaecol 1996;17(2):71–84.
20. Nash S, Tilley BC, Kurland LT, Gundersen J, Barnes AB, Labarthe D, Donohew PS, Kovacs L. Identifying and tracing a population at risk: the DESAD Project experience. Am J Public Health 1983;73(3):253–9.
21. Norwood C. At highest risk: environmental hazards to young and unborn children. New York: McGraw-Hill, 1980:141.
22. Direcks A, Figueroa S, Mintzes B, Banta D. DES European Study: DES Action the Netherlands for the European Commission Programme "Europe Against Cancer". Utrecht: DES Action the Netherlands, 1991:13, 25.
23. Sopena-Bonnet B. L'adénose cervico-vaginale: l'une des conséquences possibles de l'exposition in utero au DES. Contracept Fertil Sex 1989;17:461.
24. Senekjian EK, Potkul RK, Frey K, Herbst AL. Infertility among daughters either exposed or not exposed to diethylstilbestrol. Am J Obstet Gynecol 1988;158(3 Pt 1):493–8.
25. Hembree WC, Nagler HM, Fang JS, Myles EL, Jagiello GM. Infertility in a patient with abnormal spermatogenesis and in utero DES exposure. Int J Fertil 1988;33(3):173–7.
26. Buitendijk S. Diethylstilbestrol and the next generation—a challenge to the evidence? In: Dukes MNG, editor. Side Effects of Drugs, Annual 12. Amsterdam: Elsevier, 1988:346–8.
27. Lynch HT, Quinn T, Severin MJ. Diethylstilbestrol, teratogenesis and carcinogenesis: medical/legal implications of its long-term sequelae, including third-generation effects. Int J Risk Safety Med 1990;1:171.
28. Curran WJ. The DES product liability story in America: the third generation litigation. Int J Risk Safety Med 1992;3:229.
29. Waggoner SE, Mittendorf R, Biney N, Anderson D, Herbst AL. Influence of in utero diethylstilbestrol exposure on the prognosis and biologic behavior of vaginal clear-cell adenocarcinoma. Gynecol Oncol 1994;55(2):238–44.
30. Duke SS, McGraw SA, Avis NE, Sherman A. A focus group study of DES daughters: implications for health care providers. Psychooncology 2000;9(5):439–44.
31. Kaufman RH, Adam E, Hatch EE, Noller K, Herbst AL, Palmer JR, Hoover RN. Continued follow-up of pregnancy outcomes in diethylstilbestrol-exposed offspring. Obstet Gynecol 2000;96(4):483–9.
32. Herbst AL. Behavior of estrogen-associated female genital tract cancer and its relation to neoplasia following intrauterine exposure to diethylstilbestrol (DES). Gynecol Oncol 2000;76(2):147–56.
33. Verloop J, Rookus MA, van Leeuwen FE. Prevalence of gynecologic cancer in women exposed to diethylstilbestrol in utero. N Engl J Med 2000;342(24):1838–9.
34. Keller C, Nanda R, Shannon RL, Amit A, Kaplan AL. Concurrent primaries of vaginal clear cell adenocarcinoma and endometrial adenocarcinoma in a 39-year old woman with in utero diethylstilbestrol exposure. Int J Gynecol Cancer 2001;11(3):247–50.
35. Izquierdo Mendez N, Herraiz Martinez MA, Furio Bacete V, Cristobal Garcia I, Vidart Aragon JA, Escudero Fernandez M. Adenocarcinoma de celulas claras de cupula vaginal sin relacion con des (dietilestilbestrol): a proposito de un caso y revision de la literatura. Acta Ginecol 2001;58:21–6.
36. Titus-Ernstoff L, Hatch EE, Hoover RN, Palmer J, Greenberg ER, Ricker W, Kaufman R, Noller K, Herbst AL, Colton T, Hartge P. Long-term cancer risk in women given diethylstilbestrol (DES) during pregnancy. Br J Cancer 2001;84(1):126–33.
37. Lempert P. Myopia in diethylstilboestrol exposed amblyopic subjects. Br J Ophthalmol 1999;83(1):126.
38. Hornsby PP, Wilcox AJ, Weinberg CR, Herbst AL. Effects on the menstrual cycle of in utero exposure to diethylstilbestrol. Am J Obstet Gynecol 1994;170(3):709–15.
39. Wingfield M. Not just a cervical ectropion. Three case reports of diethylstilbestrol (DES) exposed women presenting with vaginal discharge and cervical ectropion. J Obstet Gynaecol 1999;19(6):649–51.
40. Noller KL, Blair PB, O'Brien PC, Melton LJ 3rd, Offord JR, Kaufman RH, Colton T. Increased occurrence of autoimmune disease among women exposed in utero to diethylstilbestrol. Fertil Steril 1988;49(6):1080–2.
41. Hisamatsu H, Sakai H, Kanetake H. High-dose intravenous diethylstilbestrol diphosphate (DES-DP) in the treatment of prostatic cancer during relapse. Nioshinihon J Urol 2002;64:199–202.
42. Michinaga S, Ariyoshi A. High-dose intravenous diethylstilbestrol diphosphate therapy for hormone-refractory prostate cancer. Nishinihon J Urol 2002;64:203–5.
43. Weber WW, Grossman M, Thom JV, Sax J, Chan JJ, Duffy M. Drug contamination with diethylstilbestrol. Outbreak of precocious puberty due to contaminated isonicocinic acid hydrazide (INH). N Engl J Med 1963;268:411–15.

Gonadorelin and analogues

General Information

The effects of gonadorelin depend on the duration of use. Gonadotropin release is stimulated in the short term, but is later suppressed owing to down-regulation of hypophyseal receptors. Its therapeutic indications have been summarized (SEDA-13, 1311; 1). Long-acting and depot formulations have the same adverse effects as shorter-acting analogues. The available gonadorelin analogues include buserelin, goserelin, leprorelin, nafarelin, and triptorelin (all rINNs).

Gonadorelin and its analogues cause an initial surge in follicle-stimulating hormone (FSH), luteinizing hormone (LH), and gonadal steroids. Receptor down-regulation and gonadotropin suppression occur after prolonged administration. Thus, both the clinical and adverse effects depend on the duration of administration. Biological activity and adverse effects also vary between gonadorelin agonists.

Comparative studies

In 67 premenopausal Japanese women randomized to 4-weekly, low-dose buserelin 1.8 mg or leuprorelin 1.88 mg, women given leuprorelin had a more rapid clinical response and a higher rate of hot flushes (2).

Adverse effects and quality of life have been compared in 431 men with prostate cancer treated with a gonadorelin agonist or orchidectomy (3). Of the men who reported normal sexual function before treatment, 51% had reduced libido and 69% became impotent. Of those given gonadorelin, 57% had hot flushes. Breast swelling was more common in those given gonadorelin (25% compared with 10% after orchidectomy).

Of 547 men randomized to leuprorelin plus flutamide for 3 or 8 months, those treated for 8 months had a higher overall rate of adverse events, and 87% had hot flushes, compared with 72% of those who were treated for 3 months (4).

Placebo-controlled studies

In a randomized, placebo-controlled study in women who received leuprolide acetate depot 11.25 mg intramuscularly with tibolone 2.5 mg/day (n = 36), leuprolide acetate depot 11.25 mg with placebo (n = 37), or a placebo injection with placebo tablets (n = 39), irritable bowel syndrome related to the menstrual cycle improved in those who received leuprolide (5). There were hot flushes in those who took leuprolide compared with placebo; no data were given about the frequency of hot flushes, but there were no withdrawals because of this symptom. Amenorrhea also occurred. Both flushing and amenorrhea are expected adverse effects of leuprolide.

Organs and Systems

Cardiovascular

Gonadorelin inhibits nitric oxide-mediated arterial relaxation, which disappears within 3 months after stopping treatment. This effect was abolished with "add-back" hormone replacement in a prospective, randomized study of 50 women treated for 6 months (6).

Respiratory

- A 75-year-old man developed a high fever and cough immediately after an injection of leuprorelin acetate 3.75 mg and 8 days after starting flutamide 375 mg/day (7). He died of respiratory failure after a month, and interstitial pneumonitis was confirmed postmortem.

There have been two other reports of pneumonitis associated with gonadorelin agonists.

Ear, nose, throat

Local irritation or rhinitis occurs uncommonly when gonadorelin agonists are taken intranasally.

- A 34-year-old woman had to stop using nafarelin nasal spray after 14 days because of exacerbation of maxillary sinusitis (8).

Nervous system

Pituitary apoplexy (hemorrhagic infarction presenting with sudden severe headache, often followed by pituitary hormone deficiency) has been reported after intravenous gonadorelin testing to investigate a pituitary macroadenoma and in several patients with gonadotropin-secreting pituitary macroadenomas who were given gonadorelin to treat prostate cancer (9). It may be advisable to assess gonadotropin status prior to therapy in such patients.

- A 43-year-old woman with a pituitary macroadenoma, who took quinagolide 37.5 micrograms/day for 33 months, developed a severe headache, nausea and vomiting, and photophobia 30 minutes after diagnostic testing with gonadorelin 50 micrograms intravenously (10). Although a CT scan at the time showed no evidence of hemorrhage, an MRI scan 18 months later showed a partial empty sella.
- A 67-year-old man with prostate cancer and an unsuspected pituitary macroadenoma developed a severe frontal headache, nausea and vomiting, and blindness within 12 hours of insertion of a goserelin implant (11).

Two further cases have been reported, in which gonadorelin was administered either alone (12) or with insulin (13). The mechanism of pituitary apoplexy in these cases is unclear. Gonadorelin may have a direct effect on vascular tone or may increase tumor metabolic activity.

There has been one previous report of seizure exacerbation during leuprorelin treatment, in a girl with pre-existing brain damage (14), and a case of de novo seizures has also been reported (15).

- A 13-year-old girl, who had previously had surgery and radiotherapy for a medulloblastoma, developed atypical absence seizures for the first time after 3 months of therapy with leuprorelin. The seizures stopped 1 month after treatment was withdrawn and did not recur until 30 months later. The seizures were not related to estradiol concentrations or the menstrual cycle.

Neuromuscular function

Prolonged administration of gonadorelin is commonly associated with reduced muscle bulk and voluntary muscle function. In a prospective, uncontrolled study of 62 men with prostate cancer, treatment with cyproterone acetate and goserelin caused an increase in fatigue scores and increased muscle fatiguability on objective testing within 6 weeks, in 66% of subjects (16). Fatigue was unrelated to psychological complaints or to self-reported functional ability.

Sensory systems

Blurred vision, sometimes associated with headache and dizziness, is common soon after the commencement of treatment and usually resolves within 2–3 weeks. It has recurred in some patients after rechallenge (17).

Psychological, psychiatric

Depressed mood and emotional lability occur in up to 75% of gonadorelin recipients, and there are rare reports of more severe mood disturbances (18). Defects of verbal memory have been described and may be reversed by "add-back" estrogen treatment (18) and sertraline (19).

- A 32-year-old woman had psychotic symptoms of persecutory delusions, agitation, and auditory hallucinations a few days after her second injection of triptorelin (20). Her symptoms recurred after a pregnancy, suggesting that they were due to the rapid fall in estrogen in both instances.

During a 6-month, randomized trial, men randomized to gonadorelin agonists had reduced attention and memory test scores, compared with men who were not given gonadorelin agonists but were closely monitored, in whom there was no change (21).

Endocrine

Gonadotropin-releasing hormone analogues initially stimulate the pituitary gland, resulting in increased concentrations of luteinizing hormone and testosterone in men. Subsequently, the pituitary receptors down-regulate and testosterone concentrations fall. On withdrawal of the agonist the effects have been thought to be reversible. However, they can be sustained for substantial periods in men receiving prolonged courses for prostate cancer (22). Patients receiving intermittent androgen therapy for prostate cancer were treated with leuprolide acetate 7.5 mg monthly and nilutamide orally for 8 months. Full testosterone recovery during the off treatment period was documented in 61% of cycles. In cycles during which

recovery occurred, the median time to recovery was 23 (4–61) weeks (23).

Of 247 men with prostate cancer who received goserelin 3.6 mg subcutaneously every 28 days or 10.8 mg every 84 days, 27% and 18% respectively had a rise in serum testosterone concentration to above the castrate range [24]. Only 1.7% had a testosterone concentration within the age-specific reference range. There were no clinical symptoms of tumor flare reaction.

In Japanese children with precocious puberty treated with leuprolide the time between the last injection and the median onset of menarche was 15 (range 3.6–63) months (25). The age at menarche was higher than that of the healthy population (13 versus 12 years).

For in vitro fertilization the use of triptorelin 0.1 mg/day, with early withdrawal, caused suppressed endogenous luteinizing hormone for 10–14 days after withdrawal (26).

Symptoms of hypoestrogenism, including hot flushes, vaginal dryness, reduced libido, and mood changes, occur in almost all women on long-term gonadorelin. Men also experience hypogonadal symptoms with prolonged gonadorelin administration, including hot flushes and reduced libido, although this is a therapeutic effect rather than an adverse effect. Gynecomastia occasionally occurs in men.

"Add-back" estrogen replacement reduces the frequency and severity of these symptoms without apparently compromising the effectiveness of gonadorelin in women with endometriosis (19,27). In a randomized, multicenter, double-blind comparison of intranasal nafarelin twice daily and depot leuprolide acetate monthly for 6 months in 192 young women with endometriosis, nafarelin caused fewer hypoestrogenic symptoms, although the difference between the two groups was statistically significant only after 3 months of therapy (28).

"Draw-back" therapy, in which the dosage of nafarelin was reduced after 4 weeks, had similar efficacy, but a smaller degree of bone loss and fewer vasomotor adverse effects compared with full-dose therapy, in a randomized study in 15 premenopausal women (29).

- A 47-year-old woman developed symptoms of thyrotoxicosis (palpitation, tremor, tachycardia, and goiter) due to Graves' disease, after using goserelin acetate for 13 months (30).
- A 45-year-old woman developed transient thyroiditis associated with antithyroid antibodies in taking leuprorelin (31).

The second patient had other risk factors for autoimmune thyroid disease, and the association was probably coincidental, but the episode may have been precipitated by low estrogen concentrations, as is hypothesized in postpartum thyroiditis.

Further reports of autoimmune thyroid disease in association with gonadorelin analogues have appeared (32).

- A 49-year-old woman developed Graves' disease after receiving buserelin acetate for 4 months.
- A 41-year-old woman developed painless thyroiditis after receiving leuprolide acetate for 4 months.

- A 29-year-old woman developed Graves' disease 4 months after starting to receive buserelin acetate.

Metabolism

In 20 premenopausal women treated with triptorelin for 8 weeks, the mean LDL concentration rose from 2.7 to 3.9 mmol/l and HDL fell from 1.6 to 1.5 mmol/l (33). Although the change in HDL was not clinically relevant in isolation, the increases in LDL and LDL:HDL ratio were significant, suggesting an increased risk of atherogenesis. "Add-back" conjugated equine estrogen did not reverse these changes over 24 weeks.

- A woman with type 2 diabetes had worse glycemic control while receiving buserelin (34). Her blood glucose returned to its previous concentration after withdrawal.

Two men developed hyperglycemia after using leuprolide acetate (35).

- A 61-year-old Japanese man with prostate cancer had had well controlled diabetes for 6 years (Hb_{A1c} less than 6.4%). He received leuprolide acetate subcutaneously 3.75 mg/month and oral flutamide 250 mg/day. Three weeks after the second injection his fasting glucose was 18 mmol/l and Hb_{A1c} 8.0%.
- An 81-year-old Japanese man not known to have diabetes developed prostate cancer. His Hb_{A1c} concentration was 5.1%. He received three injections of leuprolide acetate 3.75 mg/month subcutaneously then 11.25 mg every 3 months. After 7 months he complained of thirst and his blood glucose had increased to 19 mmol/l and Hb_{A1c} to 9.9%.

There is increasing evidence of a link between low testosterone concentrations and type 2 diabetes mellitus.

Hematologic

The relation between androgens and erythropoiesis is well known. In 42 patients with adenocarcinoma of the prostate, leuprolide acetate and flutamide (an antiandrogen) were used in combination (36). Hemoglobin concentrations fell by more than 25% in six patients who developed symptomatic anemia. Checking the hemoglobin at 3 months was thought to be useful in predicting those who would become symptomatic.

Leuprolide acetate has been reported to cause normochromic normocytic anemia in patients with benign prostatic hyperplasia (37). The anemia is usually transient, and the hemoglobin returns to baseline 6 months after stopping androgen suppression. There is a single case report of more serious red cell aplasia in a patient receiving gonadorelin, with resolution after treatment was withdrawn (38).

A coagulopathy has been attributed to leuprolide (39).

- A 65-year-old man, with metastatic carcinoma of the prostate was treated with flutamide 250 mg/day orally followed after 6 days by 7.5mg leuprolide intramuscularly. Two days later he developed bleeding and

hematomas. His hemoglobin fell from 12.4 to 7.8 g/dl and he had a disseminated intravascular coagulopathy.

The timing in this case suggested that testosterone release may have occurred despite androgen blockade by flutamide. As a result, tumor cell growth and coagulopathy may have occurred. In some patients with prostate cancer taking fluoxymesterone (an androgenic hormone) there was activation of clotting (40).

Skin

Injection site reactions are common with gonadorelin receptor agonists. In 119 women randomized to subcutaneous triptorelin a local reaction (redness, pain, or bruising) was present after 1 hour in 24% and persisted for 24 hours in 9.5% (41). In another study in 105 women randomized to leuprorelin acetate, moderate local reactions occurred in 24% and severe reactions in 1% (42).

- A 48-year-old woman developed an itchy skin eruption and spotted dark brown pigmentation 3 weeks after starting nasal buserelin 900 micrograms/day. The lesions resolved when buserelin was withdrawn, and recurred with rechallenge; some persisted for up to 2 years (43).
- A 78-year-old man treated with subcutaneous leuprorelin acetate had repeated local reactions, with erythema, induration, abscesses, and an ulcer on one hip (44).

Altered skin pigmentation has been previously reported in pregnancy and after sex hormone administration, so the initial surge in gonadotropins after gonadorelin treatment was a probable cause for the first patient's presentation. In the second case the lactic acid/glycolic acid vehicle may have caused the reaction rather than leuprorelin.

Epithelioid granulomata have been attributed to leuprorelin (45).

- A 73-year-old man with prostate cancer received leuprorelin acetate injections and developed a subcutaneous nodule at the injection site. Histology showed epithelioid granulomata with multinuclear giant cells.

These lesions were suggested to have been caused by a type IV allergic response to the co-polymer of lactic and glycolic acids used as a vehicle.

Three further cases of granulomatous reactions at leuprorelin injection sites in Japanese men have led to speculation that they occur more often in Japan because of the use of subcutaneous injection rather than intramuscular injection, which is used in Western countries (46). The exact mechanism of this reaction is unknown, and whether it is due to the co-polymer or leuprorelin itself is debated. Local reactions can cause reduced efficacy (47).

Musculoskeletal

Osteoporosis, trabecular bone being most affected, has been regularly observed in both sexes with chronic gonadorelin agonist treatment (48), and the duration of therapy for prostate cancer is inversely related to bone mineral density (49,50). Intravenous pamidronate may prevent bone loss in these patients (51,52).

- A 44-year-old woman with no previous history of widespread pain, depression, or anxiety developed a diffuse pain syndrome consistent with fibromyalgia after leuprorelin treatment. Her symptoms increased in severity with three successive monthly injections, and persisted for several months (53).

In 47 children treated with depot leuprolide acetate for precocious puberty for 2 years, bone mineral density decreased significantly and markers of bone turnover increased significantly during treatment but were normal for age 2 years after treatment was withdrawn (54).

Of 25 girls with idiopathic precocious puberty, 11 had not been treated and 14 had received leuprolide acetate monthly for at least 1 year; they were compared with 19 healthy controls (55). There was no significant difference between the groups. There was no osteopenia or osteoporosis after therapy.

Since women have a lower initial bone mass than men their fracture risk is higher. Osteoporosis is reversible in premenopausal patients after gonadorelin withdrawal (56). However, the treatment period should be limited to 6 months.

Cross-sectional (57) and longitudinal (58) studies of men with prostate cancer have shown a significant relation between the duration of gonadorelin treatment and bone loss.

Estrogens, etidronate, and parathyroid hormone have been used with partial success to prevent gonadorelin-induced bone loss. In a prospective study of 49 women treated with goserelin and randomized to estradiol plus norethisterone or placebo, bone loss persisted 6 years after stopping therapy, and the hormone replacement therapy had only a minor protective effect (59).

- An 87-year-old man developed progressive proximal limb weakness 1 year after starting leuprolide therapy for prostate cancer (60). Electromyography showed a moderately severe non-inflammatory myopathy without evidence of fiber necrosis or associated biochemical changes. Within 6 months after stopping leuprolide he was able to resume his usual activities.

Three men developed rheumatoid arthritis 1–9 months after starting antiandrogen therapy with either cyproterone acetate or leuprolide acetate (61).

Reproductive system

Ovarian hyperstimulation syndrome (OHSS) affects up to 33% of women undergoing ovulation induction with gonadorelin receptor agonists and gonadotropins given in combination (62), or with gonadotropins alone (63). Gonadotropins are usually withheld if the diagnosis is made before conception (62,64).

OHSS is characterized by cystic ovarian enlargement, increased capillary permeability, and third space fluid accumulation (that is in an extracellular compartment that is not in equilibrium with either the extracellular or intracellular fluid, for example the bowel lumen, subcutaneous tissues, retroperitoneal space, or peritoneal cavity). Risk factors include a previous history of OHSS, age under 30 years (probably because more follicles are available), and polycystic ovary syndrome. Non-pregnant patients usually recover within 14 days with supportive treatment. The severe form (with ascites or pleural effusion and hemoconcentration) occurs in 1–10% of patients (64,65). In critical cases, hypoxemia, renal insufficiency, thromboembolism, and rarely death can occur (66).

- A 29-year-old woman with polycystic ovary syndrome had her first in vitro fertilization cycle of leuprorelin acetate, FSH, and human chorionic gonadotropin (hCG) (67). Within 2 days she complained of abdominal distension, shortness of breath, and abdominal pain. Over the next few days she developed massive ovarian enlargement, ascites, hyponatremia, respiratory failure, and renal insufficiency. This was further complicated by duodenal perforation, probably due to severe physical stress.
- Ovarian hyperstimulation syndrome occurred in a woman with polycystic ovarian syndrome, 3 weeks after an intramuscular injection of leuprorelin acetate for endometriosis (68). She was later given further courses of the drug without this complication.
- A 35-year-old obese woman with a previously undiagnosed pituitary gonadotroph adenoma developed multiple ovarian cysts and abdominal distension after 1 month of leuprolide therapy (69).
- A 32-year-old woman who was not obese developed benign intracranial hypertension in association with ovarian hyperstimulation syndrome after ovulation induction using goserelin, FSH, and hCG (70). The syndrome did not recur during a second pregnancy in which FSH and hCG were not used.

It is unclear which of the hormonal agents used was responsible for this complication in the last case.

Gonadorelin receptor antagonists have been reported to lower the risk of OHSS significantly. A meta-analysis showed that cetrorelix but not ganirelix reduced the incidence of OHSS by 75%, both overall and the severe form (71).

Thromboembolism is a serious complication of OHSS (72–75).

- A previously healthy 34-year-old woman who underwent ovulation induction with leuprorelin acetate and FSH developed abdominal ascites due to OHSS, followed by acute aphasia and right hemiparesis (76). The stroke was caused by a large intracardiac thrombus.

A review identified 54 other reports of thromboembolic disease associated with ovulation induction; 60% were in upper limb veins and two-thirds of the patients had OHSS (77). The mechanism for the increased risk of thrombosis in these patients has not been determined, but hemoconcentration or a hypercoagulable state associated with high estrogen concentrations could be responsible.

One of 66 women randomized to receive goserelin acetate for uterine fibroids withdrew from the study owing to severe pelvic pain (78).

Immunologic

Altered immune function has been reported in several cases associated with gonadorelin agonist therapy. This is possibly related to the initial surge in sex steroids that occurs with these agents, but there is no evidence that this is the mechanism. Cardiac allograft rejection occurred in three men within months of starting gonadorelin therapy for prostate cancer. One died of heart failure, but the other two recovered cardiac function after the gonadorelin agonist was withdrawn (79).

Systemic lupus erythematosus can be exacerbated in the initial gonadotropin-stimulating phase of gonadorelin therapy: in one case this was fatal (80).

Long-Term Effects

Tumorigenicity

Tumor flare occurs in up to 30% of treated patients after the first 4–7 days of gonadorelin therapy, due to an initial surge in gonadotropin concentrations (81). For this reason antiandrogen treatment is often given before gonadorelin in men with prostate cancer. However, despite tumor flare there was no difference in survival in a prospective, multicenter comparison of gonadorelin and surgical oophorectomy in 136 patients (82).

Second-Generation Effects

Pregnancy

Of 34 women who conceived while receiving triptorelin acetate for infertility, five developed gestational diabetes (17%) compared with a background rate of 5% (83). The increased incidence could not be explained by obesity, as only one of these five women had a BMI over 35 kg/m^2; nor could it be explained by polycystic ovary syndrome. Larger studies are required to confirm this finding.

Teratogenicity

Pregnancies have occurred both after low-dose gonadorelin agonist therapy for ovulation induction and after higher-dose therapy for endometriosis or other indications: these have been reviewed in the context of a report of a 36-year-old woman who stopped monthly goserelin injections at 16 weeks of gestation and delivered a healthy girl. Congenital abnormalities have been reported in a few cases, including one child with trisomy 13, one with trisomy 18, and an intrauterine death due to thrombosis; however most pregnancies have had normal outcomes (84).

There was one case of polydactyly with no major defects (3.4%) in the children of 35 women who had

conceived while using triptorelin (78). This was probably coincidental.

Drug Administration

Drug formulations

There is no difference in the adverse effects profiles of long-acting or depot formulations compared with shorter-acting analogues used continuously.

Drug dosage regimens

Intermittent courses of gonadotropin analogues for prostate cancer may reduce the frequency of adverse effects. In 95 patients who received 245 cycles of leuprolide acetate and nilutamide for 8 months, testosterone concentrations recovered during the rest periods (61% of cycles) and sexual function improved (47%) (23).

Drug-Drug Interactions

Oral contraceptives

There were mild increases in serum triglyceride and cholesterol concentrations in 13 hirsute women treated with triptorelin and a triphasic oral contraceptive, in a randomized comparison of triptorelin with flutamide + cyproterone acetate (85). Altered lipid profiles have not been described before in patients receiving gonadorelin agonists and oral contraceptives.

Management of adverse drug reactions

The use of gonadorelin analogues is commonly associated with reduced bone mineral density. In 50 premenopausal women with uterine leiomyomas who received leuprolide acetate depot 3.75 mg every 28 days for 18 cycles with raloxifene 60 mg/day, there was a reduction in leiomyoma size with no significant change in bone mineral density or markers of bone metabolism [86].

References

1. Filicori M. Gonadotrophin-releasing hormone agonists. A guide to use and selection. Drugs 1994;48(1):41–58.
2. Takeuchi H, Kobori H, Kikuchi I, Sato Y, Mitsuhashi N. A prospective randomized study comparing endocrinological and clinical effects of two types of GnRH agonists in cases of uterine leiomyomas or endometriosis. J Obstet Gynaecol Res 2000;26(5):325–31.
3. Potosky AL, Knopf K, Clegg LX, Albertsen PC, Stanford JL, Hamilton AS, Gilliland FD, Eley JW, Stephenson RA, Hoffman RM. Quality-of-life outcomes after primary androgen deprivation therapy: results from the Prostate Cancer Outcomes Study. J Clin Oncol 2001;19(17):3750–7.
4. Gleave ME, Goldenberg SL, Chin JL, Warner J, Saad F, Klotz LH, Jewett M, Kassabian V, Chetner M, Dupont C, Van Rensselaer SCanadian Uro-Oncology Group. Randomized comparative study of 3 versus 8-month

neoadjuvant hormonal therapy before radical prostatectomy: biochemical and pathological effects. J Urol 2001;166(2):500–6.

5. Palomba S, Orio F, Manguso F, Russo T, Falbo A, Lombardi G, Doldo P, Zullo F. Leuprolide acetate treatment with and without coadministration of tibolone in premenopausal women with menstrual cycle-related irritable bowel syndrome. Fertil Steril 2005;83:1012–20.

6. Yim SF, Lau TK, Sahota DS, Chung TK, Chang AM, Haines CJ. Prospective randomized study of the effect of "add-back" hormone replacement on vascular function during treatment with gonadotropin-releasing hormone agonists. Circulation 1998;98(16):1631–5.

7. Azuma T, Kurimoto S, Mikami K, Oshi M. Interstitial pneumonitis related to leuprorelin acetate and flutamide. J Urol 1999;161(1):221.

8. Heinig J, Coenen-Worch V, Cirkel U. Acute exacerbation of chronic maxillary sinusitis during therapy with nafarelin nasal spray. Eur J Obstet Gynecol Reprod Biol 2001;99(2):266–7.

9. Morsi A, Jamal S, Silverberg JD. Pituitary apoplexy after leuprolide administration for carcinoma of the prostate. Clin Endocrinol (Oxf) 1996;44(1):121–4.

10. Foppiani L, Piredda S, Guido R, Spaziante R, Giusti M. Gonadotropin-releasing hormone-induced partial empty sella clinically mimicking pituitary apoplexy in a woman with a suspected non-secreting macroadenoma. J Endocrinol Invest 2000;23(2):118–21.

11. Eaton HJ, Phillips PJ, Hanieh A, Cooper J, Bolt J, Torpy DJ. Rapid onset of pituitary apoplexy after goserelin implant for prostate cancer: need for heightened awareness. Intern Med J 2001;31(5):313–4.

12. Hiroi N, Ichijo T, Shimojo M, Ueshiba H, Tsuboi K, Miyachi Y. Pituitary apoplexy caused by luteinizing hormone-releasing hormone in prolactin-producing adenoma. Intern Med 2001;40(8):747–50.

13. Matsuura I, Saeki N, Kubota M, Murai H, Yamaura A. Infarction followed by hemorrhage in pituitary adenoma due to endocrine stimulation test. Endocr J 2001;48(4):493–8.

14. Minagawa K, Sueoka H. [Seizure exacerbation by the use of leuprorelin acetate for treatment of central precocious puberty in a female patient with symptomatic localization-related epilepsy.]No To Hattatsu 1999;31(5):466–8.

15. Akaboshi S, Takeshita K. A case of atypical absence seizures induced by leuprolide acetate. Pediatr Neurol 2000;23(3):266–8.

16. Stone P, Hardy J, Huddart R, A'Hern R, Richards M. Fatigue in patients with prostate cancer receiving hormone therapy. Eur J Cancer 2000;36(9):1134–41.

17. Fraunfelder FT, Edwards R. Possible ocular adverse effects associated with leuprolide injections. JAMA 1995;273(10):773–4.

18. Warnock JK, Bundren JC, Morris DW. Depressive symptoms associated with gonadotropin-releasing hormone agonists. Depress Anxiety 1998;7(4):171–7.

19. Moghissi KS, Schlaff WD, Olive DL, Skinner MA, Yin H. Goserelin acetate (Zoladex) with or without hormone replacement therapy for the treatment of endometriosis. Fertil Steril 1998;69(6):1056–62.

20. Mahe V, Nartowski J, Montagnon F, Dumaine A, Gluck N. Psychosis associated with gonadorelin agonist administration. Br J Psychiatry 1999;175:290–1.

21. Green HJ, Pakenham KI, Headley BC, Yaxley J, Nicol DL, Mactaggart PN, Swanson C, Watson RB, Gardiner RA. Altered cognitive function in men treated for prostate

cancer with luteinizing hormone-releasing hormone analogues and cyproterone acetate: a randomized controlled trial. BJU Int 2002;90(4):427–32.

22. Heyns CF. Triptorelin in the treatment of prostate cancer. Clinical efficacy and tolerability Am J Cancer 2005;4:169–83.

23. Malone S, Perry G, Segal R, Dahrouge S, Crook J. Long-term side-effects of intermittent androgen suppression therapy in prostate cancer: results of a phase II study. BJU Int 2005;96:514–20.

24. Zinner NR, Bidair M, Ceneno A, Tomera K. Similar frequency of testosterone surge after repeat injections of goserelin (Zoladex) 3.6 mg and 10.8 mg: results of a randomised open-label trial. Urology 2004;64:1177–81.

25. Tanaka T, Niimi H, Matsuo N, Fujieda K, Tachibana K, Ohyama K, Satoh M, Kugu K. Results of long-term follow-up after treatment of central precocious puberty with leuprorelin acetate: evaluation of effectiveness of treatment and recovery of gonadal function. The TAP-144-SR Japanese study group on central precocious puberty. J Clin Endocrinol Metab 2005;90:1371–6.

26. Simons AHM, Roelolofs HJM, Schmoutziguer APE, Roozenburg BJ, van't Hof-van den Brink EP, Schoonderwoerd SA. Early cessation of triptorelin in vitro fertilization: a double-blind, randomized study. Fertil Steril 2005;83:889–96.

27. Freundl G, Godtke K, Gnoth C, Godehardt E, Kienle E. Steroidal "add-back" therapy in patients treated with GnRH agonists. Gynecol Obstet Invest 1998;(45 Suppl 1):22–30discussion 35.

28. Zhao SZ, Kellerman LA, Francisco CA, Wong JM. Impact of nafarelin and leuprolide for endometriosis on quality of life and subjective clinical measures. J Reprod Med 1999;44(12):1000–6.

29. Tahara M, Matsuoka T, Yokoi T, Tasaka K, Kurachi H, Murata Y. Treatment of endometriosis with a decreasing dosage of a gonadotropin-releasing hormone agonist (nafarelin): a pilot study with low-dose agonist therapy ("drawback" therapy). Fertil Steril 2000;73(4):799–804.

30. Morita S, Ueda Y. Graves' disease associated with goserelin acetate. Acta Med Nagasaki 2002;47:79–80.

31. Kasayama S, Miyake S, Samejima Y. Transient thyrotoxicosis and hypothyroidism following administration of the GnRH agonist leuprolide acetate. Endocr J 2000;47(6):783–5.

32. Amino N, Hidaka Y, Takano T, Tatsumi K, Izumi Y, Nakata Y. Possible induction of Graves' disease and painless thyroiditis by gonadotrophin-releasing hormone analogues. Thyroid 2003;8:815–8.

33. Al-Omari WR, Nassir UN, Izzat B. Estrogen "add-back" and lipid profile during GnRH agonist (triptorelin) therapy. Int J Gynaecol Obstet 2001;74(1):61–2.

34. Imai A, Takagi A, Horibe S, Fuseya T, Takagi H, Tamaya T. A gonadotropin-releasing hormone analogue impairs glucose tolerance in a diabetic patient. Eur J Obstet Gynecol Reprod Biol 1998;76(1):121–2.

35. Inaba M, Otani Y, Nishimura K, Takaha N, Okuyama A, Koga M, Azuma J, Kawase I, Kasayama S. Marked hyperglycemia after androgen-deprivation therapy for prostate cancer and usefulness of pioglitazone for its treatment. Metabolism 2005;54(1):55–9.

36. Bogdanos J, Karamanolakis D, Milathianakis C, Repousis P, Tsintavis A, Koutsilieris M. Combined androgen blockade-induced anemia in prostate cancer patients without bone involvement. Anticancer Res 2003;23:1757–62.

37. Strum SB, McDermed JE, Scholz MC, Johnson H, Tisman G. Anaemia associated with androgen deprivation

in patients with prostate cancer receiving combined hormone blockade. Br J Urol 1997;79(6):933–41.

38. Maeda H, Arai Y, Aoki Y, Okubo K, Okada T, Ueda Y. Leuprolide causes pure red cell aplasia. J Urol 1998;160(2):501.

39. Bern MM. Coagulopathy, following medical therapy, for carcinoma of the prostate. Haematology 2005;10(1):65–8.

40. Al-Mondhiry H, Manni A, Owen J, Gordon R. Hemostatic effects of hormonal stimulation in patients with metastatic prostate cancer. Am J Hematol 1988;28:141–5.

41. van Hooren HG, Fischl F, Aboulghar MA, Nicollet B, Behre HM, Van der Ven H, Simon A, Kilani Z, Barri PN, Haberle M, Braat DD, Lambalk NEuropean and Middle East Orgalutran Study Group. Comparable clinical outcome using the GnRH antagonist ganirelix or a long protocol of the GnRH agonist triptorelin for the prevention of premature LH surges in women undergoing ovarian stimulation. Hum Reprod 2001;16(4):644–51.

42. Fluker M, Grifo J, Leader A, Levy M, Meldrum D, Muasher SJ, Rinehart J, Rosenwaks Z, Scott RT Jr, Schoolcraft W, Shapiro DBNorth American Ganirelix Study Group. Efficacy and safety of ganirelix acetate versus leuprolide acetate in women undergoing controlled ovarian hyperstimulation. Fertil Steril 2001;75(1):38–45.

43. Kono T, Ishii M, Taniguchi S. Intranasal buserelin acetate-induced pigmented roseola-like eruption. Br J Dermatol 2000;143(3):658–9.

44. Hirashima N, Shinogi T, Sakashita N, Narisawa Y. A case of cutaneous injury induced by the subcutaneous injection of leuprolide acetate. Nishinihon J Dermatol 2001;63:384–6.

45. Yamano Z, Kusuda Y, Hara S, Shimogaki H, Hamani G. Cutaneous epithelioid granulomas caused by subcutaneous infusion of leuprorelin acetate. A case report. Acta Urol Japan 2004;50:199–202.

46. Yasukawa K, Sawamura D, Sugawara H, Kato N. Leuprorelin acetate granulomas: case reports and review of the literature. Br J Dermatol 2005;152:1045–7.

47. Tonini G, Marioni S, Forleo V, Rustico M. Local reactions to luteinizing hormone releasing hormone analog therapy. J Pediatr 1995;126:159–60.

48. Fogelman I. Gonadotropin-releasing hormone agonists and the skeleton. Fertil Steril 1992;57(4):715–24.

49. Stoch SA, Parker RA, Chen L, Bubley G, Ko YJ, Vincelette A, Greenspan SL. Bone loss in men with prostate cancer treated with gonadotropin-releasing hormone agonists. J Clin Endocrinol Metab 2001;86(6):2787–91.

50. Kiratli BJ, Srinivas S, Perkash I, Terris MK. Progressive decrease in bone density over 10 years of androgen deprivation therapy in patients with prostate cancer. Urology 2001;57(1):127–32.

51. Smith MR, McGovern FJ, Zietman AL, Fallon MA, Hayden DL, Schoenfeld DA, Kantoff PW, Finkelstein JS. Pamidronate to prevent bone loss during androgen-deprivation therapy for prostate cancer. N Engl J Med 2001;345(13):948–55.

52. Diamond TH, Winters J, Smith A, De Souza P, Kersley JH, Lynch WJ, Bryant C. The antiosteoporotic efficacy of intravenous pamidronate in men with prostate carcinoma receiving combined androgen blockade: a double blind, randomized, placebo-controlled crossover study. Cancer 2001;92(6):1444–50.

53. Toussirot E, Wendling D. Fibromyalgia developed after administration of gonadotrophin-releasing hormone analogue. Clin Rheumatol 2001;20(2):150–2.

54. van der Sluis IM, Boot AM, Krenning EP, Drop SL, de Muinck Keizer-Schrama SM. Longitudinal follow-up of bone density and body composition in children with precocious or early puberty before, during and after cessation of GnRH agonist therapy. J Clin Endocrinol Metab 2002;87(2):506–12.

55. Unal O, Berberoglu M, Evliyaoglu O, Adiyaman P, Aycan Z, Ocal G. Effects of bone mineral density of gonadotropin releasing hormone analogs used in the treatment of central precocious puberty. J Pediatr Endocrinol Metab 2003;16:407–11.

56. Paoletti AM, Serra GG, Cagnacci A, Vacca AM, Guerriero S, Solla E, Melis GB. Spontaneous reversibility of bone loss induced by gonadotropin-releasing hormone analogue treatment. Fertil Steril 1996;65(4):707–10.

57. Wei JT, Gross M, Jaffe CA, Gravlin K, Lahaie M, Faerber GJ, Cooney KA. Androgen deprivation therapy for prostate cancer results in significant loss of bone density. Urology 1999;54(4):607–11.

58. Daniell HW, Dunn SR, Ferguson DW, Lomas G, Niazi Z, Stratte PT. Progressive osteoporosis during androgen deprivation therapy for prostate cancer. J Urol 2000;163(1):181–6.

59. Pierce SJ, Gazvani MR, Farquharson RG. Long-term use of gonadotropin-releasing hormone analogues and hormone replacement therapy in the management of endometriosis: a randomized trial with a 6-year follow-up. Fertil Steril 2000;74(5):964–8.

60. Van Gerpen JA, McKinley KL. Leuprolide-induced myopathy. J Am Geriatr Soc 2002;50(10):1746.

61. Pope JE, Joneja M, Hong P. Anti-androgen treatment of prostatic carcinoma may be a risk factor for development of rheumatoid arthritis. J Rheumatol 2002;29(11):2459–62.

62. Whelan JG 3rd, Vlahos NF. The ovarian hyperstimulation syndrome. Fertil Steril 2000;73(5):883–96.

63. Mancini A, Milardi D, Di Pietro ML, Giacchi E, Spagnolo AG, Di Donna V, De Marinis L, Jensen L. A case of forearm amputation after ovarian stimulation for in vitro fertilization–embryo transfer. Fertil Steril 2001;76(1):198–200.

64. Beerendonk CC, van Dop PA, Braat DD, Merkus JM. Ovarian hyperstimulation syndrome: facts and fallacies. Obstet Gynecol Surv 1998;53(7):439–49.

65. Chillik C, Young E, Gogorza S, Estofan D, Neuspiller N, Antunes N Jr, Borges E Jr, Vantman D, Fabres C, Montoya JM, Madero JI, Gutierrez-Najar A, Bronfenmajer S, Kovacs A, Kroeze S, Out HJLatin-American Puregon IVF Study Group. A double-blind clinical trial comparing a fixed daily dose of 150 and 250 IU of recombinant follicle-stimulating hormone in women undergoing in vitro fertilization. Fertil Steril 2001;76(5):950–6.

66. Abramov Y, Elchalal U, Schenker JG. Febrile morbidity in severe and critical ovarian hyperstimulation syndrome: a multicentre study. Hum Reprod 1998;13(11):3128–31.

67. Uhler ML, Budinger GR, Gabram SG, Zinaman MJ. Perforated duodenal ulcer associated with ovarian hyperstimulation syndrome: Case Report. Hum Reprod 2001;16(1):174–6.

68. Jirecek S, Nagele F, Huber JC, Wenzl R. Ovarian hyperstimulation syndrome caused by GnRH-analogue treatment without gonadotropin therapy in a patient with polycystic ovarian syndrome. Acta Obstet Gynecol Scand 1998;77(9):940–1.

69. Castelbaum AJ, Bigdeli H, Post KD, Freedman MF, Snyder PJ. Exacerbation of ovarian hyperstimulation by leuprolide reveals a gonadotroph adenoma. Fertil Steril 2002;78(6):1311–3.
70. Lesny P, Maguiness SD, Hay DM, Robinson J, Clarke CE, Killick SR. Ovarian hyperstimulation syndrome and benign intracranial hypertension in pregnancy after in-vitro fertilization and embryo transfer: case report. Hum Reprod 1999;14(8):1953–5.
71. Ludwig M, Katalinic A, Diedrich K. Use of GnRH antagonists in ovarian stimulation for assisted reproductive technologies compared to the long protocol. Meta-analysis. Arch Gynecol Obstet 2001;265(4):175–82.
72. Ludwig M, Tolg R, Richardt G, Katus HA, Diedrich K. Myocardial infarction associated with ovarian hyperstimulation syndrome. JAMA 1999;282(7):632–3.
73. Belaen B, Geerinckx K, Vergauwe P, Thys J. Internal jugular vein thrombosis after ovarian stimulation. Hum Reprod 2001;16(3):510–2.
74. Loret de Mola JR, Kiwi R, Austin C, Goldfarb JM. Subclavian deep vein thrombosis associated with the use of recombinant follicle-stimulating hormone (Gonal-F) complicating mild ovarian hyperstimulation syndrome. Fertil Steril 2000;73(6):1253–6.
75. Yoshii F, Ooki N, Shinohara Y, Uehara K, Mochimaru F. Multiple cerebral infarctions associated with ovarian hyperstimulation syndrome. Neurology 1999;53(1):225–7.
76. Worrell GA, Wijdicks EF, Eggers SD, Phan T, Damario MA, Mullany CJ. Ovarian hyperstimulation syndrome with ischemic stroke due to an intracardiac thrombus. Neurology 2001;57(7):1342–4.
77. Stewart JA, Hamilton PJ, Murdoch AP. Thromboembolic disease associated with ovarian stimulation and assisted conception techniques. Hum Reprod 1997;12(10):2167–73.
78. Donnez J, Vivancos BH, Kudela M, Audebert A, Jadoul P. A randomised placebo-controlled, dose-ranging trial comparing fulvestrant with goserelin in premenopausal patients with uterine fibroids awaiting hysterectomy. Fertil Steril 2003;79:1380–9.
79. Schofield RS, Hill JA, McGinn CJ, Aranda JM. Hormone therapy in men and risk of cardiac allograft rejection. J Heart Lung Transplant 2002;21(4):493–5.
80. Casoli P, Tumiati B, La Sala G. Fatal exacerbation of systemic lupus erythematosus after induction of ovulation. J Rheumatol 1997;24(8):1639–40.
81. Mahler C. Is disease flare a problem? Cancer 1993;72(Suppl 12):3799–802.
82. Taylor CW, Green S, Dalton WS, Martino S, Rector D, Ingle JN, Robert NJ, Budd GT, Paradelo JC, Natale RB, Bearden JD, Mailliard JA, Osborne CK. Multicenter randomized clinical trial of goserelin versus surgical ovariectomy in premenopausal patients with receptor-positive metastatic breast cancer: an intergroup study. J Clin Oncol 1998;16(3):994–9.
83. Mayer A, Lunenfeld E, Wiznitzer A, Har-vardi I, Bentov Y, Levitas E. Increased prevalence of gestational diabetes mellitus in in vitro fertilization pregnancies inadvertently conceived during treatment with long-acting triptorelin acetate. Fertil Steril 2005;84:789–92.
84. Jimenez-Gordo AM, Espinosa E, Zamora P, Feliu J, Rodriguez-Salas N, Gonzalez-Baron M. Pregnancy in a breast cancer patient treated with a LHRH analogue at ablative doses. Breast 2000;9(2):110–2.
85. Pazos F, Escobar-Morreale HF, Balsa J, Sancho JM, Varela C. Prospective randomized study comparing the long-acting gonadotropin-releasing hormone agonist triptorelin, flutamide, and cyproterone acetate, used in combination with an oral contraceptive, in the treatment of hirsutism. Fertil Steril 1999;71(1):122–8.
86. Palomba S, Orio F Jr, Russo T, Falbo A, Cascella T, Doldo P, Nappi C, Mastrantonio P, Zullo F. Long-term effectiveness and safety of GnRH agonist plus raloxifene administration in women with uterine leiomyomas. Hum Reprod 2004;6:1308–14.

Mitotane

General Information

Mitotane is an inhibitor of intramitochondrial synthesis of pregnenolone and cortisol, used to produce a chemical adrenalectomy in the treatment of adrenal carcinoma and Cushing's disease and syndrome. Its unwanted effects include increased transaminase and alkaline phosphatase activities, reduced leukocyte, platelet and erythrocyte counts, and myasthenia (1).

Organs and Systems

Sensory systems

A pigmentary retinopathy with macular edema and abnormal electroretinography has been attributed to mitotane (2).

Endocrine

Because it inhibits glucocorticoid synthesis, mitotane can cause acute hypoadrenalism (3).

Metabolism

Mitotane 1–5 g daily for 4 weeks was associated with the development of hypercholesterolemia in three cases; the effect had not reverted to normal 3 months later (4).

Hematologic

Pancytopenia has been attributed to mitotane (5).

In six of seven patients with adrenocortical cancer taking mitotane for 1–2 weeks the bleeding time became prolonged; four had platelet aggregation responses compatible with an aspirin-like defect (6).

Liver

All of 10 patients taking mitotane for Cushing's syndrome had rises in either gamma-glutamyl transpeptidase or alanine transaminase, with a maximum increase six times basal value (7). The only variable that correlated with hepatic increase was the body mass index. In contrast, the severity of the disease, alcohol intake, and other biological characteristics did not correlate with transaminase rises.

In six patients with Cushing's syndrome, including one pregnant woman, who took mitotane 0.5 g/week, there was adrenocortical insufficiency requiring hormone replacement in one patient. The only other significant adverse effect was a reversible increase in gamma-glutamyl transpeptidase activity (8).

References

1. Kasperlik-Zaluska AA. Clinical results of the use of mitotane for adrenocortical carcinoma. Braz J Med Biol Res 2000;33(10):1191–6.
2. Ng WT, Toohey MG, Mulhall L, Mackey DA. Pigmentary retinopathy, macular oedema, and abnormal ERG with mitotane treatment. Br J Ophthalmol 2003;87(4):500–1.
3. Pardo C, Boix E, Lopez A, Pico A. Crisis addisoniana secundaria a tratamiento con mitotane. [Adrenal crisis due to mitotane therapy.] Med Clin (Barc) 2002;118(7):278.
4. Vassilopoulou-Sellin R, Samaan NA. Mitotane administration: an unusual cause of hypercholesterolemia. Horm Metab Res 1991;23(12):619–20.
5. Andres E, Vinzio S, Goichot B, Schlienger JL. Mitotane-induced febrile pancytopenia: a first case report in paraneoplastic Cushing's syndrome. Eur J Endocrinol 2001;144(1):81.
6. Haak HR, Caekebeke-Peerlinck KM, van Seters AP, Briet E. Prolonged bleeding time due to mitotane therapy. Eur J Cancer 1991;27(5):638–41.
7. Neuman O, Bruckert E, Chadarevian R, Jacob N, Turpin G. Hepatotoxicité d'un anticortisolique de synthèse: l'op'DDD (Mitotane). [Hepatotoxicity of a synthetic cortisol antagonist: op'DDD (mitotane).] Therapie 2001;56(6):793–7.
8. Knappe G, Gerl H, Ventz M, Rohde W. Langzeit-Therapie des hypothalamisch–hypophysaren Cushing-Syndroms mit Mitotan (o,p'-DDD). [The long-term therapy of hypothalamic–hypophyseal Cushing's syndrome with mitotane (o,p'-DDD).] Dtsch Med Wochenschr 1997;122(28-29):882–6.

Tamoxifen

General Information

Tamoxifen is an estrogen receptor partial agonist with antiestrogenic properties in the breast and estrogenic effects in tissues such as bone and the cardiovascular system. In most cases there is endometrial thickening on ultrasonography, and additional tests, such as hydrosonography or hysteroscopy, are required to confirm the presence of an empty atrophic uterus, as seen in most asymptomatic women taking tamoxifen.

Tamoxifen is commonly used in the treatment of breast carcinoma (1); the overall rates published for adverse effects vary very greatly, between 1 and 60% (2,3). It has also been used as a form of HRT to reduce bone loss and the incidence of fractures in high-risk cases (4). A combination of tamoxifen with ovarian suppression is as effective as the use of cytostatic drugs, and has been claimed to be better tolerated (5–7).

The use of tamoxifen to prevent breast cancer has been reviewed (8). The merits of using tamoxifen to prevent mammary carcinoma in women who have never had the disease but are believed to be at high risk have been disputed (9), but it is clear that it would involve very

long treatment and that one's view of the adverse effects might need to be revised for this class of users. The available data after 5, 10, and 15 years of follow up confirmed an increase in the incidence of endometrial cancer and of thromboembolic complications and suggested ocular toxicity, but these effects were not common and should be more than balanced by the reduced risk of coronary heart disease and osteoporosis (8).

Tamoxifen also has beneficial side effects: it protects the myocardium, reduces the incidence of ischemic heart disease, reduces the loss of bone mineral density, and has beneficial effects on lipids (10). With evidence accumulating from major studies in several countries, there is still considerable optimism regarding the use of tamoxifen or its analogues to prevent breast cancer in high-risk groups, although the results of various studies are not consistent and much detail needs to be filled in (11,12). Chemoprevention with tamoxifen and the newer selective estrogen receptor modulators has to be weighed adequately against possible risks (13). This form of chemoprophylaxis has not been widely adopted; in the population as a whole the proportion of women who stand to benefit is low, and the risks of unnecessary drug treatment in the remainder have to be taken into account. In a survey in North Carolina 10% or less of women in all age groups were potentially eligible for chemoprevention while the maximum proportion of breast cancers prevented in eligible women was estimated at 6.0–8.3% (14). Clearly, the most desirable key to future policy on prophylaxis would be a means of selecting the subgroup at the highest risk, so that drug treatment could be limited to them.

Observational studies

The effect of high-dose tamoxifen as an adjunct to postoperative brain irradiation has been studied for 40 weeks in 12 patients with glioblastoma multiforme, but without controls (15). Two weeks after surgery, the patients were given high-dose oral tamoxifen (120 mg/m^2 bd for 3 months) and 2 weeks later external beam radiotherapy (59.4 Gy, three daily fractions every 6.5 weeks). In one patient tamoxifen was associated with severe vomiting, necessitating dosage reduction and subsequent withdrawal; another patient had bilateral deep venous thrombosis after 51 weeks, but a causal relation was not firmly established. The authors concluded that adjuvant high-dose tamoxifen is relatively well tolerated, although in this series it did not appear to improve the prognosis.

In a small study in the Mayo Clinic the acceptability of using tamoxifen alongside intravenous cisplatin was examined in 15 patients with lung cancer (16). Daily doses in various patients were 160 mg/m^2, 200 mg/m^2, or 250 mg/m^2 for 7 days. Grade 3 anemia occurred in one patient only, at the 200 mg/m^2 dose, while another patient, with an unfavorable cardiovascular history, had an embolic stroke 20 days after completing the course. On the basis of this small trial, the Clinic proposed to continue using high doses of tamoxifen alongside cisplatin in such patients. On present evidence from this and other centers, tamoxifen potentiates the cytostatic effects of cisplatin without clearly increasing the toxicity of the regimen; various mechanisms to explain this apparently useful interaction are being debated.

A short report has been published on the Italian Randomized Trial of Tamoxifen in 2700 women, which is intended to assess the success of the drug set against placebo, used in 2708 women, in preventing breast cancer in a population of hysterectomized post-menopausal women (17). After a median 81 months of follow-up, breast cancers had developed in 34 women in the tamoxifen group and 45 in the placebo group. The effect was highly significant in a subgroup of women considered, in the light of their reproductive and hormonal characteristics, as being at high risk of breast cancer, but was dubious in low-risk women, in whom the risk of cancer may actually have been marginally increased. However, the authors stressed that whatever usefulness the drug proves to have for this purpose must be set against Its adverse effects, such as endometrial cancer and thromboembolic complications. As currently published, the findings did not indicate the incidence of these complications in the study itself.

Comparative studies

One of the many controversies surrounding the use of tamoxifen in elderly women is whether after lumpectomy it should be accompanied by radiotherapy to potentiate the desired effect. It has been suggested that there is not a great deal of merit in adding radiotherapy to tamoxifen, since radiotherapy plus tamoxifen reduces local recurrence of breast cancer in elderly women compared with tamoxifen alone, but survival rates are not improved and benefits are offset by an increase in adverse effects (18).

Tamoxifen versus aromatase inhibitors

While tamoxifen is still widely regarded as the standard adjuvant endocrine treatment for postmenopausal women with localized breast cancer, provided it is hormone receptor positive, there are problems with recurrence and adverse effects. Reservations have recently been expressed about the future place of tamoxifen, and the case has been made that it is time to move from tamoxifen to the oral aromatase inhibitors (19).

There has been a brief report of some of the results of the ATAC trial (part of the CORE study) in 9366 women, which was designed to continue for 5 years, part of which involved directly comparing tamoxifen with the aromatase inhibitor anastrozole (20). The conclusion was that anastrozole should be the preferred treatment in such cases. After a median follow-up of 68 months, anastrozole significantly prolonged disease-free survival (575 events with anastrozole versus 651 with tamoxifen; hazard ratio = 0.87; 95% CI = 0.78, 0.97), prolonged time to recurrence, and significantly reduced distant metastases (324 versus 375) and contralateral breast cancers. There were fewer withdrawals with anastrozole than with tamoxifen, apparently reflecting the fact that anastrozole was also associated with fewer adverse effects (especially gynecological problems and vascular events), although arthralgia and fractures were increased.

The roles of tamoxifen and the aromatase inhibitors as adjuvant therapy for early breast cancer in postmenopausal women have been reviewed, distinguishing three approaches: replacement of tamoxifen as adjuvant therapy for 5 years (early adjuvant therapy); sequencing of tamoxifen before or after an aromatase inhibitor during the first 5 years (early sequential adjuvant therapy); or the use of an aromatase inhibitor after 5 years of tamoxifen (extended adjuvant therapy) (21). Briefly, the conclusions were that at the time of the survey there was little to choose between the three methods in terms of the balance of benefit and harm. However, like others, the authors stressed that agents of this type are proving to be superior to tamoxifen in preventing recurrence of the disease.

There may well be a role for combined therapy with both tamoxifen and an aromatase inhibitor if an optimal benefit to harm balance is to be attained, as suggested by a study of a combination of tamoxifen and exemestane for 8 weeks in 33 postmenopausal women with breast cancer (22). There was a striking absence of endocrine adverse effects.

Others have suggested that patients be treated for a period with tamoxifen and then switched to anastrozole for follow up. A report on the ABCSG 8 trial and the ARNO 95 trial (both of which were prospective open studies) has provided information on this approach (23). Women with hormone-sensitive early breast cancer who had taken adjuvant oral tamoxifen 20 or 30 mg/day for 2 years were randomized to oral anastrozole 1 mg/day (n = 1618) or tamoxifen 20 or 30 mg/day (n = 1606) for the remainder of their adjuvant therapy. At a median follow-up of 28 months, there was a highly significant 40% reduction in the risk of an event with anastrozole compared with tamoxifen (67 versus 110 events; hazard ratio = 0.60; 95% CI = 0.44, 0.81). There were significantly more fractures but significantly fewer case of thrombosis in those who took anastrozole than in those who took tamoxifen. These data lend support to a switch from tamoxifen to anastrozole in patients who have taken adjuvant tamoxifen for 2 years.

The unwanted effects of tamoxifen on the endometrium (including induction of fibroids, polyps, and endometrial cancer) have long been of concern, and attempts are now being made to find ways of preventing or reversing these complications, or finding an alternative treatment that does not involve these risks. Again, promising experience with the aromatase inhibitors features prominently in current recommendations.

In a prospective study in 77 consecutive women with postmenopausal breast cancer scheduled to start endocrine treatment for breast cancer, using either tamoxifen or an aromatase inhibitor tamoxifen treatment significantly increased endometrial thickness and uterine volume after 3 months (24). In additional, tamoxifen induced endometrial cysts and polyps and increased the size of pre-existing fibroids. In contrast, aromatase inhibitors did not stimulate endometrial growth and were not associated with endometrial pathology. Furthermore, they reduced endometrial thickness and uterine volume in patients who had previously taken tamoxifen.

This study has again confirmed that endometrial problems can be induced by tamoxifen early in the course of treatment; and that these problems do not arise with aromatase inhibitors, which may actually reduce the endometrial changes induced by tamoxifen. The idea that the new oral aromatase inhibitors might well replace tamoxifen in breast cancer was tentatively advanced in SEDA-26 (p. 445) and has now been supported by some of the material cited above, as well as by a panel consensus (25). Citing efficacy and safety data on anastrozole, exemestane, and letrozole, the authors concluded that third-generation aromatase inhibitors may be considered first-line therapy of hormone-receptor-positive advanced breast cancer in postmenopausal women and may also be used for preoperative therapy of breast cancer.

Placebo-controlled studies

In the Breast Cancer Prevention Trial (P-1), initiated by the National Surgical Adjuvant Breast and Bowel Project (NSABP) in 1992, more than 13 000 eligible women were randomized to tamoxifen 20 mg/day or placebo for 5 years (26). During 69 months of follow-up tamoxifen reduced the risk of both invasive and non-invasive cancer and reduced fractures of the hip, radius, and spine; however, the rate of endometrial cancer increased (RR = 2.53; 95% CI = 1.35, 4.97), as did the frequency of vascular events.

General adverse effects

The adverse effects of tamoxifen are largely those that one would expect to be associated with a reduction in estrogenic activity, that is hot flushes (which can be severe), dry skin, mental or nervous system effects (such as mild depression, headache, fatigue, nervousness, and tremor), oligomenorrhea and amenorrhea, loss of libido, vaginal discharge, and rare events, such as pruritus, migraine, and edema (SED-12, 1034) (27). Nausea and vomiting are not uncommon. There are also reports of hirsutism, weight gain, rashes, thrombocytopenia, and leukopenia (SED-12, 1034); the hirsutism could reflect a relative dominance of endogenous androgen activity as the degree of estrogenic activity declines. The most specific and dangerous complication of tamoxifen is hypercalcemia, a direct consequence of the successful treatment of mammary carcinoma with bony metastases; the incidence varies greatly. Liver dysfunction and peliosis hepatis have been incidentally reported.

When tamoxifen is used in men (28), common adverse effects have included weight gain (25%), mood alterations (21%), hot flushes (21%), reduced libido (29%), and deep vein thrombosis (4%). The hot flushes respond well to oral clonidine 0.1 mg/day (29).

One expert in the USA (30) has publicly defended the safety of tamoxifen on the grounds that some of its supposed adverse effects may in fact have other causes. It is a difficult argument to follow, since she postulates that several of the unwanted effects referred to are in fact menopausal. However, these are largely likely to be inevitable consequences of the very changes that treatment with tamoxifen is intended to induce, that is suppression of estrogenic effects. Virtually the opposite belief can be derived from a Canadian study, which showed that 25 women taking tamoxifen were diffident about attributing adverse events to the drug, and therefore tended to under-report adverse effects (31). Menopause-like problems with these drugs are clearly likely to persist unless or until more selective SERMs become available, for example substances that act exclusively on the breast tumor.

Organs and Systems

Cardiovascular

Both deep vein thrombosis and pulmonary embolism have been described with tamoxifen.

- Cerebral sinus thrombosis, progressing to hemorrhagic cerebral infarction, occurred in a 52-year-old woman (32).

Although the authors pointed to the absence of risk factors other than the drug, it must be remembered that cerebral venous thrombosis is a recognized complication of various malignancies. In this case the breast tumor had been treated with various cytostatic drugs and stem cell transplantation, and tamoxifen had been given as an adjuvant, and it was believed that the tumor had been eliminated. Nevertheless, in this complex case one should perhaps be hesitant in attributing the complication solely to the drug.

In the light of three further cases of thrombosis, it has been suggested that there may be a particular predisposition to this complication in patients with high circulating concentrations of homocysteine, and that these should be checked for in advance of treatment (33).

Some cases of thrombosis and pulmonary embolism may have been attributable to the primary condition being treated, and the risk must not be over-estimated (34).

An extensive literature survey covering a 7-year period sought to resolve doubts about whether the risk of venous thromboembolism is greater with tamoxifen than with other treatments used to prevent and treat breast cancer, taking careful account of other susceptibility factors that might distort the picture (35). Accurate determination of the rate of thromboembolism was impaired by the lack in most studies of routine assessments to detect asymptomatic cases. However, based on symptomatic cases the risk of thromboembolism was increased two- to three-fold during use of either tamoxifen or raloxifene to prevent breast carcinoma. It is not known whether the risk is increased further in women with inherited hypercoagulable states. In the case of early-stage breast carcinoma, the risk of thromboembolism is increased with both tamoxifen and anastrozole, although the problem appeared to be somewhat less when using anastrozole.

The effect of tamoxifen 20 mg/day on the incidence of venous thromboembolism has been assessed in a placebo-controlled breast cancer prevention trial for 5 years in 5408 hysterectomized women (36). There were 28 incidents of thromboembolism on placebo and 44 on tamoxifen (hazard ratio = 1.63; 95% CI = 1.02, 2.63), 80% of which involved only superficial phlebitis, which accounted for all of the excess due to tamoxifen within 18 months from randomization. Compared with placebo, the risk of venous thromboembolism with tamoxifen was higher in women aged 55 years or older, those with a body mass index of 25 kg/m² or more, those with a raised blood pressure or a total cholesterol of 6.50 mmol/l (250 mg/dl) or greater, current smokers, and those with a family history of coronary heart disease, all familiar risk factors for venous complications. Of the 685 women with a coronary heart disease risk score of 5 or greater, one in the placebo arm and 13 in the tamoxifen arm developed venous thromboembolism. In a multivariate regression analysis, age in excess of 60 years, height of 165 cm or more, and a diastolic blood pressure of 90 mmHg or higher all had independent detrimental effects on the risk of venous thromboembolism during tamoxifen therapy, whereas transdermal estrogen therapy concomitant with tamoxifen was not associated with any excess risk (HR = 0.64; 95% CI = 0.23, 1.82). The authors concluded that the increased risk of venous thromboembolism during the use of tamoxifen was largely associated with the well-known risk factors for this condition, and that this information should be part of pre-treatment counselling.

The risks of venous thromboembolism in women with and without breast cancer have been analysed and are summarized in Table 1 (37). In one case tamoxifen was associated with myocardial infarction (38).

Respiratory

An important synergistic reaction between radiation-related pulmonary fibrosis and tamoxifen has been described in 196 women followed for a minimum of 5 years, with a relative risk of 2.0 (39). However, others have shown that tamoxifen did not increase the pulmonary toxicity of agents such as carmustine and dacarbazine (40).

Nervous system

A short supplementary report on the US NSABP, originally published in 1999, later corrected the original data on adverse effects: among women who had used tamoxifen for an average of 29 months to complement irradiation after lumpectomy for intraductal carcinoma; there were five cases of stroke, compared with only one among the women who had not used tamoxifen (41). In a parallel study of breast cancer prevention there was also a slight but non-significant increase in the incidence of stroke in those taking tamoxifen. It may be wise to regard a history of stroke, transient ischemic attacks, uncontrolled hypertension, diabetes mellitus, or atrial fibrillation as relative contraindications to tamoxifen. On the other hand, other work showed that tamoxifen had precisely the same effect on myoinositol concentrations in the basal ganglia as estrogen replacement therapy did (SEDA-17, 432), which could suggest that there is no risk to brain function.

The effects of estrogen and tamoxifen on positron emission tomography (PET) measures of brain glucose metabolism and magnetic resonance imaging (MRI) have been evaluated as measures of hippocampal atrophy in three groups of postmenopausal women, women taking estrogen, women with breast cancer taking tamoxifen, and women not taking estrogen or tamoxifen (42). In those taking tamoxifen there were widespread areas of hypometabolism in the inferior and dorsal lateral frontal lobes relative to the other two groups. The untreated women had lower metabolism in the inferior frontal cortex and temporal cortex compared with those taking estrogen. Those taking tamoxifen also had significantly lower semantic memory scores than the other two groups. Finally, those taking tamoxifen had smaller right hippocampal volumes than those taking estrogen, an effect that was of borderline significance. Both right and left hippocampal volumes were significantly smaller than in those taking estrogen when a single outlier was removed. Those taking estrogen had hippocampal volumes that were intermediate to the other two groups. The authors

Table 1   Incidences of venous thromboembolism with and without breast cancer taking various treatments (37)

Population	Incidence of venous thromboembolism (per year unless otherwise stated)
General population without cancer	0.12%
Women without cancer	0.08% per year (DVT)
	0.03% per year (PE)
Women without cancer taking tamoxifen	0.12% (DVT)
	0.07% per year (PE)
Women without cancer taking HRT	0.23%
General population	0.6% over 3 years
General population with breast cancer	1.0%
Early-stage breast cancer, no adjuvant treatment	0.8% within 6 weeks after surgery
Early-stage breast cancer, no adjuvant treatment	0.4% over 5 years
Early-stage breast cancer taking tamoxifen	1.7% over 5 years
Early-stage breast cancer, taking adjuvant tamoxifen	1.4% over 5 years
Early-stage breast cancer receiving chemotherapy	2.1% within 6 weeks
Early-stage breast cancer, receiving chemotherapy and taking tamoxifen	11% over 5 years

concluded that these findings provide physiological and anatomical evidence for neuroprotective effects of estrogen. Biochemical changes are difficult to interpret in clinical terms, and there is now an evident need for longer-term controlled work correlating tamoxifen use and cognitive performance.

Sensory systems

There have been repeated reports of ophthalmic complications from tamoxifen, including irreversible retinopathy with seriously reduced visual acuity, refractile opacities, cystoid macular edema, retinal yellow-white dots, and keratopathy (SEDA-6, 356; SEDA-7, 391; SEDA-16, 466).

- Bilateral optic neuritis developed in a woman with breast cancer who was treated for 6 months with tamoxifen (43).

In a prospective study even in low doses (for example 10 mg/day or lower) tamoxifen caused ocular toxicity if given for a sufficiently long period; most of the changes were reversible but they justify very close monitoring (44). A related compound, MER-29 (triparanol), causes cataract and has various other adverse reactions in common with tamoxifen.

Estrogen receptors are present in the retina, and tamoxifen has been stated to affect color vision. In a further study of this phenomenon in 24 middle-aged women who were taking tamoxifen 20 mg/day as adjuvant therapy for early stage breast cancer, visual fields were measured using both short wavelength automated perimetry and frequency doubling perimetry (45). The visual fields were affected, the changes being detectable within 2 years. The effects of tamoxifen were more readily detected with short wavelength automated perimetry, suggesting that it affects some types of visual pathways preferentially, presumably the cone pathways, which are measured with this technique.

Some older work pointed to an increased risk of other ophthalmic complications, including cataract in patients with cancer who took tamoxifen for a longer period. The issue was later examined in Britain using a case-control study design and data collected in the General Practice Research Database relating to women taking tamoxifen for breast cancer, the comparators being women with other cancers who were not taking tamoxifen (46). Current tamoxifen users were not at increased risk of cataract and there was no evidence of an increased risk with increasing cumulative dose (AOR = 1.0, 95%CI = 0.7, 1.4).

Metabolism

Steatosis and adipose tissue distribution has been evaluated using CT scanning in a cross-sectional study of 32 women taking tamoxifen for breast cancer and a similar control group (47). Tamoxifen users generally had more visceral adipose tissue and more liver fat than controls, and had a higher risk of diabetes. It is still unclear whether tamoxifen causes long-term metabolic abnormalities in obese patients, or whether patients with the metabolic syndrome X of obesity are at increased risk of

the complications of tamoxifen. In view of this finding, and earlier results pointing in the same direction, it would be wise in future studies of tamoxifen to monitor metabolic changes in obese women with or without breast cancer.

Tamoxifen has favorable effects on lipid and lipoprotein profiles, reducing concentrations of total and low-density lipoprotein cholesterol. However there is also evidence that it can cause increased serum triglyceride concentrations, which in some cases have risen dangerously. A Taiwan group has sought to determine whether this adverse effect might be avoided by using lower but still effective doses of the drug in women with early breast cancer (48). They found that in 115 patients with breast cancer taking tamoxifen 20 mg bd the serum triglyceride concentration rose significantly after 15 months of therapy, although the increase was only clinically dangerous (400 mg/dl or more) in 14 cases. In these patients the dose was halved to 10 mg/day, and in 10 of the 14 women the triglycerides fell markedly; in the other four they did not, and antilipemic therapy was needed. The authors did not evaluate the efficacy of lower doses, but there is some earlier literature that seems to show that efficacy is attainable at this level.

Hematologic

Thrombosis and pulmonary embolism have been described with tamoxifen (49,50); the number of cases is small, but the association would not be unexpected in view of what is known about the effects of other sex hormones. The primary condition might be responsible, at least in part, for the occurrence of such complications. Tamoxifen does reduce antithrombin III but not to a degree at which a major risk would be expected, and other measurable effects on the coagulation process seem to be slight.

When tamoxifen 20 mg/day was compared with equieffective doses of anastrozole in 668 patients with advanced breast tumors that were hormone receptor-positive or of unknown receptor status, tamoxifen produced too high a rate of thromboembolism and vaginal bleeding to be considered the treatment of choice (51,52).

There is some evidence that one might be able to maintain the therapeutic benefits of tamoxifen in breast cancer at much lower doses (for example 1 mg/day and 5 mg/day) than those generally used (20 mg/day), thus perhaps avoiding the risks associated with thrombogenesis (53). In a non-randomized study, all three doses were studied in 120 women with estrogen receptor-positive breast cancer, comparing the outcome over a 4-week period with that in controls. Expression of the tumor expression marker Ki-67 fell to a similar degree in all three tamoxifen dosage groups, with no difference in the magnitude of reduction among the different dosages. Effects on various blood markers (including insulin-like growth factor-I, sex hormone-binding globulin, low-density lipoprotein cholesterol, ultrasensitive C-reactive protein, fibrinogen, and antithrombin III concentrations) were too variable to draw clear conclusions about whether the lower doses were indeed safer, but they provide a reasonable basis for further examination of the matter (54).

Liver

Liver dysfunction and peliosis hepatis are occasional complications of tamoxifen. There have also been reports of cirrhosis with fatty liver in women taking tamoxifen after surgery for breast cancer (55). The condition is reversible, and liver tests are advisable so that the tamoxifen can be promptly withdrawn if necessary.

- An elderly woman with a history of breast cancer developed multifocal steatohepatitis, but after tamoxifen was withdrawn the CT features improved dramatically, and the hepatic transaminases normalized (56).

The frequency and course of hepatic steatosis due to tamoxifen has been studied using CT scans in 76 patients with breast cancer who took tamoxifen for 5 years (57). In all 29 women developed hepatic steatosis during the first 2 years, four to a severe degree. The liver:spleen ratio returned to normal within a mean of 1.2 years after the end of treatment in 23 of these women. The authors stressed that hepatic dysfunction can occur with tamoxifen, and that it is vital to differentiate the condition from hepatic metastases.

Pancreas

Severe acute pancreatitis has been attributed to tamoxifen (58).

- A woman with hypertriglyceridemia and breast cancer was given tamoxifen and various lipid-regulating agents after mastectomy. She stopped the latter of her own accord after 2 years and had a recurrence of hypertriglyceridemia and pancreatitis.

In this instance there were other possible precipitating factors, particularly hypertriglyceridemia, and it is hard to see why tamoxifen should have been held responsible.

Skin

Tamoxifen has several adverse effects on the skin, including edema, flushing, rashes, hyperhidrosis, urticaria, alopecia, and hypertrichosis. Radiation recall dermatitis, a severe painful inflammatory skin reaction in sites that have previously been exposed to ionized radiation, can occur in patients taking tamoxifen (59). In one case the tamoxifen was withdrawn and the skin healed spontaneously in 7 weeks (60). Toremifene, a tamoxifen analogue, was well tolerated: during 18 months of continuous treatment no signs of radiation recall developed.

Hair

Effects of hormonal or antihormonal products on the hair are reported sporadically.

- A woman taking tamoxifen for metastatic cancer (presumably from the breast) developed alopecia; she

began to lose her hair within 3 months and was entirely bald after 13 months of treatment (61).

The authors did not make it clear whether cytostatic drugs, which can cause alopecia, were also used, but it is striking that there have been several earlier reports of baldness with tamoxifen.

Musculoskeletal

In principle an anti-estrogen might precipitate osteoporosis, but tamoxifen has not been shown to do so; indeed, there is reason to believe that it protects the skeleton against steroid-induced bone loss (62), and in some studies of the state of the bones during treatment with tamoxifen there was actually a higher bone density than in controls.

Sexual function

Tamoxifen can cause loss of libido (63). In 57 patients sexual desire, arousal, and the ability to achieve orgasm were unaffected by tamoxifen (64). There was a 54% incidence of dyspareunia, but this seemed to be a consequence of co-administration of chemotherapy, which can cause vaginal dryness and loss of libido, rather than an effect of tamoxifen.

Reproductive system

Breasts
Tamoxifen can cause a sudden rapid increase in the growth rate of uterine leiomyomas (65).

- A leiomyoma of the breast occurred in a 50-year-old woman taking tamoxifen. It appeared as a discrete mass and had a microscopic pattern akin to leiomyomas at other sites (66).

Ovaries
In premenopausal women, tamoxifen has complex effects on ovarian function, compatible with accelerated development of multiple follicles, with ovarian enlargement and cyst formation (67,68); this might be expected in view of its similarity to clomiphene. Ovarian cysts have also been seen in postmenopausal patients with breast cancer during long-term adjuvant therapy with tamoxifen. Some premenopausal women with breast cancer had very marked increase in estrogen concentrations as a result of increased ovarian estrogen synthesis caused by tamoxifen. All premenopausal women with breast cancer taking tamoxifen should be under close gynecological and ultrasonographic surveillance to detect such effects as soon as they occur.

Dutch workers concluded that patients who were still having a menstrual cycle had a high chance (81%) of developing ovarian cysts during tamoxifen treatment, but that postmenopausal women taking tamoxifen only developed ovarian cysts if their ovaries were able to respond to FSH stimulation, as shown by serum estradiol production (69). Differences in patient populations might explain why some workers (70) still find no association in their patients between tamoxifen and ovarian pathology.

Macroscopically visible cystic endosalpingiosis in the paraovarian region has been described in a woman who had been taking tamoxifen for breast cancer (71).

• A 2.5 cm multicystic lesion was seen on the external surface of the right ovary, and histological examination showed a mass of dilated glands lined by ciliated tubal-type epithelium and set in a fibrovascular stroma. Cystic endosalpingiosis resulting in a tumor-like mass is rarely described and is probably not well recognized by histopathologists.

Although unlikely to be mistaken for malignancy, this kind of lesion can result in diagnostic confusion. The role of tamoxifen in the development of the lesion in this case is not clear, but the estrogenic effects of tamoxifen may have contributed.

In one case, a complex cyst, thought to be due to ovarian hyperstimulation, resolved after monthly administration of a depot gonadorelin (GnRH) receptor agonist without abandoning tamoxifen (72). One might expect some patients to react to tamoxifen with ovarian hyperstimulation, since another non-steroidal antiestrogen (that is clomiphene) is used for ovarian stimulation and also on occasion produces cysts.

In one case reported from Japan, there was torsion of an ovarian cyst (73).

In a study of the mechanism and frequency of this complication, hormone concentrations in 20 premenopausal women taking tamoxifen (20 mg/day) were compared with those in untreated controls (74). Ovarian cysts were found in 80% of the treated patients but only in 8% of controls, and 17-beta-estradiol concentrations were significantly raised.

Uterus

Intermenstrual bleeding is a practical problem during tamoxifen therapy, particularly since it obliges the physician to undertake repeated endometrial investigations to exclude malignancy. Monitoring the uterine cavity in women taking tamoxifen is mandatory, especially when there is postmenopausal bleeding.

Some preliminary but well-designed work has suggested that by inserting a levonorgestrel-releasing intrauterine system it may be possible to limit considerably the problems posed by unscheduled uterine bleeding (75).

Benign thickening of the endometrium is common during tamoxifen treatment, but appears to be fully reversible within a few months of withdrawal (76,77).

The pathology of tamoxifen-associated cases of myometrial adenomyosis has been compared with that in five cases of postmenopausal adenomyosis not associated with tamoxifen. The tumors were not identical: morphological features more often present in the tamoxifen-associated cases were cystic dilatation of glands (which sometimes resulted in grossly visible intramural cystic lesions), fibrosis of the stroma, and various forms of epithelial metaplasia. The proliferative activity in the adenomyosis, as determined by MIB1 staining, was higher in the

tamoxifen group (78), and this could be another mechanism of postmenopausal bleeding among tamoxifen users.

Whether one should routinely screen patients for endometrial changes is disputed; there seems to be no correlation between endometrial thickness and endometrial pathology, and complications could be easily overlooked (79).

The gynecological consequences of antiestrogens (tamoxifen and toremifene) have been evaluated in 167 postmenopausal breast cancer patients in a 3-year prospective study. There was a proliferative endometrium more often in the tamoxifen group than in the toremifene group, but this did not translate into an increase in the rate of endometrial cancer. The authors did not recommend routine surveillance of the endometrium.

Uterine polyps are not uncommon during postmenopausal treatment with tamoxifen (80), and up to 3% can show malignant changes. There has been an attempt to identify risk factors for the development of these polyps, by analysing the histories of 54 women in whom they occurred, as well as the histories of a larger control group without polyps (81). The women who developed polyps had a later menopause, had breast cancer for a longer period, and weighed more.

Endometrial polyps ("basilomas") can become malignant (82,83), perhaps because they lack progesterone receptors and are exposed to unopposed estrogen (84).

The susceptibility factors that predispose to polyps have been sought In 64 patients with polyps (85). The combination of shorter tamoxifen exposure before the diagnosis of primary polyps, lower parity, lower menopausal age at the time of diagnosis of primary polyps, and greater duration of tamoxifen treatment significantly increased the risk of recurrent endometrial polyps. One additional year of tamoxifen treatment increased the risk of recurrent polyps five-fold.

A Japanese study of DNA extracted from endometrial polyps in women treated with tamoxifen showed a three-fold increase in K-ras mutations compared with the incidence in cases of spontaneous endometrial hyperplasia. These findings could support the hypothesis that the endometrial polyps will prove an early indicator for the development of endometrial carcinoma in such patients (86).

Not only can endometrial polyps that arise during tamoxifen treatment undergo malignant degeneration, but in some cases they may be the site of metastases from the original breast cancer. Such polyps must always undergo thorough histological sampling to distinguish the two possibilities. Two cases with metastases from lobular breast carcinoma to a polyp have been described (87).

Tumorigenicity

A variety of uterine tumors have been associated with tamoxifen, Levine et al have now presented what is probably the first report of Tamoxifen-associated uterine liposarcoma has now been observed in a 62-year-old woman (88). The tumor cells were immunoreactive to vimentin, estrogen receptors, and S-100. Surgery was performed, but the tumor recurred 9 months later.

Immunologic

An acute inflammatory polyarthritis resembling rheumatoid arthritis has been reported in three women temporally related to the use of tamoxifen (89).

Long-Term Effects

Tumorigenicity

Several authors (90,91) have described a variety of cases, seven in all, of malignancies secondary to therapeutic dosages of tamoxifen given for 6 months to 10 years.

Uterine fibroids and endometrial polyps (sometimes with bleeding) have been reported in menopausal women who had taken tamoxifen for periods of months or years (SEDA-16, 466) (92,93). In view of this, the question of whether tamoxifen increases the risk of endometrial cancer has been widely discussed. The authors of a 1993 review of the outcome of six major trials tended strongly to the conclusion that tamoxifen can cause both endometrial hyperplasia and endometrial cancer proportional to the total dose (94); the figures pointed to an overall incidence of endometrial cancer of 0.5% in tamoxifen users and 0.1% in controls. Another major review up to 1992 concluded that in the world literature there were 70 cases of uterine malignancies with tamoxifen, including 61 cases of adenocarcinoma of the endometrium and four cases of uterine sarcoma (95).

Six cases of endometrial carcinoma were subsequently reported from France (96), and 36 cases in all had been reported up to that time (97). Although the effect can be caused by tamoxifen alone in women aged over 55, in younger women it is more likely to be an additive one, attributable to use of both tamoxifen and pelvic irradiation in the same subject.

Two distinct patterns of uterine cancer have been shown using magnetic resonance imaging of the tamoxifen-exposed uterus in 35 women (98). Patients with pattern 1 had homogeneous high signal intensity of the endometrium on T2-weighted images and enhancement of the endometrial–myometrial interface and a signal void in the lumen on gadolinium-enhanced images (18 patients). Patients with pattern 2 had heterogeneous endometrial signal intensity on T2-weighted images with enhancement of the endometrial–myometrial interface and lattice-like enhancement traversing the endometrial canal on gadolinium-enhanced images (17 patients).

Although the endometrial cancers associated with tamoxifen are usually pure adenocarcinomas, other types of rare tumors have also been reported. A pure uterine rhabdomyosarcoma has been reported (99), and a mesodermal mixed tumor of the endometrium occurred 5 years after 5 years of tamoxifen therapy (100). The tumor responded only to combined treatment with doxorubicin, cyclophosphamide, 5-fluorouracil, and carboplatin. It is possible that this type of tumor arises later than adenocarcinomas and should be looked for during long-term use of tamoxifen.

- Two well-documented cases of uterine carcinosarcoma have been reported in elderly women after 6 and 7 years of tamoxifen treatment (101). At laparotomy, a heterologous malignant mixed Mullerian tumor with peritoneal spread was found in each case and rapidly proved fatal; large uterine polyps with special histological features may represent an intermediate step in the formation of such tumors (102).

Ten similar cases have been described before.

When assessing the risk of endometrial malignancy in women with breast cancer taking tamoxifen, it is worth taking into account evidence that patients with breast cancer may at the outset have some endometrial pathology. In women with breast cancer scheduled for tamoxifen there were endometrial polyps in 9.3%, endometrial cysts in 16%, and synechiae in 12% at the outset. Tamoxifen significantly increased the incidence of these benign endometrial lesions, usually after less than 1 year of treatment. There were no cases of endometrial carcinoma in 34 patients who had taken tamoxifen for 12–24 months, and only one in 78 patients who had taken it for 5–72 months (103).

The risk that tamoxifen may cause endometrial cancer has been the subject of lively correspondence in the Lancet (104), fired by the paper published in 2000 by Bergman and her colleagues, who had concluded that the endometrial cancers seen with tamoxifen are unusually aggressive (105). Concern was expressed that such a conclusion could lead to even wider hesitation to use tamoxifen in breast cancer, despite the fact that it is already used very selectively, for example in women with positive estrogen receptors. A contradiction between Bergman's results and those of the NSABP P-1 were also highlighted, and doubts expressed whether Bergman's findings justify restricting the use of tamoxifen as a preventive agent. However, a Canadian group adduced its own work to support Bergman's findings, while French workers suggested that her unfavorable results, which were not seen in their own patients, could have been due to selection bias. It was also argued that a progestogen-releasing intrauterine contraceptive device might be used to counter the undesirable effects of tamoxifen on the endometrium. Clearly the issue raised by Bergman is still subject to debate, but it is obvious that physicians who use tamoxifen in advanced breast cancer or as a preventive agent should continue to do so selectively and that ways of protecting the endometrium during tamoxifen therapy need to be found.

The effects of norethisterone on endometrial abnormalities have been studied in 463 postmenopausal women taking tamoxifen or placebo (106). As in other studies, the results showed that any increased risk of endometrial cancer caused by tamoxifen is low and that transvaginal ultrasound screening is probably not justified for asymptomatic women taking tamoxifen. The authors found that 26% of women taking tamoxifen have endometrial thickening of 8 mm or more. It is possible to identify cysts in 7% of these women, polyps in 3%, and both cysts and polyps in 8%. These changes are characteristic of tamoxifen and unlike those seen with estrogen replacement therapy.

Although it has been suggested that tamoxifen-associated endometrial carcinoma has a distinct gene expression profile, this has not been confirmed. There are two types of this cancer, with extremely different molecular profiles, but the distinction is not related to tamoxifen exposure (107). Much other work is being done to determine the characteristics of tamoxifen-associated endometrial tumors, in particular as regards their content of estrogen receptors (ER) and progesterone receptors. The pathological features and expression of ERα, ERβ, and progesterone receptors in these tumors have been compared with matched cases of non-tamoxifen-associated endometrial cancers (108). Compared with spontaneous tumors the drug-associated tumors were characterized by a lower expression of ERα, higher expression of progesterone receptors , and more frequent expression of ERβ. Differential expression of ERα and ERβ may alter the expression of key target genes (such as those induced by AP-1-dependent gene transcription) and contribute to the pathogenesis and clinical behavior of these tumors. Survival was significantly poorer in women with drug-associated tumors than in those with non-drug associated tumors.

The usefulness of transvaginal ultrasound in detecting serious uterine changes in tamoxifen users has been disputed. According to one group it is a dependable diagnostic method (109), whereas others found it disappointing, with a high proportion of false positive results, even when the assessment criteria were chosen so as to exclude mild endometrial thickening (110). Setting these two papers beside one another it seems that one can detect marked endometrial changes but that ultrasound is not a dependable means of determining whether there is malignancy.

Second-Generation Effects

Teratogenicity

Since animal studies suggested the possibility of fetal and neonatal malformations it has for a long time been customary to exclude pregnancy before giving tamoxifen. However, there is currently reason to believe that the risk presented by tamoxifen to the human fetus is very slight or non-existent.

Susceptibility Factors

Genetic factors

Certain women have a genetic predisposition to develop an endometrial malignancy during tamoxifen treatment. There were significant amounts of tamoxifen-DNA adducts in the endometrium in eight of 16 women who took the drug but none at all in others, suggesting that a genotoxic mechanism may be responsible for tamoxifen-induced endometrial cancer (111). However, there is biochemical and histological evidence that tamoxifen-associated endometrial carcinoma is likely to be similar to type I and will therefore have a relatively favorable prognosis (112).

Since tamoxifen is metabolized by CYP450 enzymes, including CYP3A5, and bearing in mind two genetic polymorphisms in CYP3A5 (CYP3A5*3 and CYP3A5*6), it has been suggested that the presence of such polymorphisms in some patients might have an effect on the incidence of adverse effects of tamoxifen. However, a recent study seems to have shown that this is not the case—the metabolism and adverse effects of tamoxifen were the same in subjects with these polymorphisms as in other women (113).

Whether the adverse effects of tamoxifen when used to treat breast cancer recurrence correlate with the quantities of circulating tamoxifen and its metabolites (N-desmethyltamoxifen and 4-hydroxytamoxifen has been studied in 99 women with breast cancer, who had been taking tamoxifen for at least 30 days (114). Women who had at least one tamoxifen-related adverse effect had significantly higher concentrations of tamoxifen than women not did not. Women who reported visual problems had significantly higher concentrations of both tamoxifen and N-desmethyltamoxifen compared with others. However, concentrations of 4-hydroxytamoxifen were negatively associated with vaginal discharge. The authors suggested that that patterns of tamoxifen metabolism and its adverse effects are in some respects related and that studies of the metabolism of tamoxifen could be of value in choosing better tolerated schemes of treatment for individual patients.

Age

There is a very proper reluctance today to interfere with hormonal processes during puberty and adolescence for fear of producing adverse long-term changes. Just as the use of estrogens in rapidly growing girls has largely fallen out of favor in most countries, so the safety of attempts to treat pubertal gynecomastia in boys is being questioned. However, this can be a distressing condition at a sensitive age, and some workers have cautiously used tamoxifen and raloxifene for this purpose. The results of different approaches have been compared in 38 patients with persistent pubertal gynecomastia at an average age of 14 years (115). They received reassurance alone or a 3- to 9-month course of an estrogen receptor modifier (tamoxifen 60 mg/day or raloxifene 10–20 mg bd). There were significant reductions in breast nodule size with both drugs, although the effect was more marked with raloxifene. In these doses, there were no adverse effects. If further work is to be performed it will be important to provide long-term follow-up to detect any unwanted later effects.

Drug–Drug Interactions

Antidepressants

There is an impression, in the light of clinical experience, that antidepressants might reduce the clinical efficacy of tamoxifen (116), but more evidence is needed to confirm or reject this view.

Atracurium dibesilate

Tamoxifen has been associated with prolonged atracurium block in a patient with breast cancer (SEDA-12, 117; 117).

Cytotoxic drugs

An unusual case of rapidly fatal renal failure reported in 1993 could reflect an interaction between tamoxifen and one or more cytostatic agents, with mitomycin C a prime suspect; in a series of breast cancer patients some 10% of those treated both with tamoxifen and a cytostatic agent developed abnormal renal function, progressing towards various stages of hemolytic-uremic syndrome (118).

Diuretics

Many patients who take tamoxifen for breast cancer take other drugs for co-existing illnesses, and the possibility of interactions with these drugs has so far been incompletely studied. In a study of 98 treated women I was shown that co-medication can influence plasma concentrations of tamoxifen and its metabolites (N-desmethyltamoxifen and 4-hydroxytamoxifen) (119). Those taking diuretics had significantly higher plasma concentrations of tamoxifen and N-desmethyltamoxifen than others. Analgesics and anti-inflammatory drugs were negatively associated with plasma tamoxifen concentrations. Chemotherapeutic agents, allergy drugs, antidepressants, and medications for diabetes did not significantly alter plasma concentrations of tamoxifen or its metabolites.

Drug–Procedure Interactions

The use of tamoxifen in combination with radiotherapy appears to increase the risk of breast fibrosis, which is a known effect of irradiation. In a retrospective study of the records of 147 women with breast cancer who had taken part in a major prospective study of tamoxifen 20 mg/day and who had also received adjuvant radiotherapy, 90 were hormone receptor-positive (120). There was a statistically significant difference in terms of mean complication-relapse-free survival rates at 3 years (48% versus 66%) and at 2 years (51% versus 80%) in the tamoxifen and control groups respectively. In each group the mean complication-relapse-free survival rates were significantly lower in patients with low levels of CD8 radiation-induced apoptosis (20%, 66%, and 79% for CD8 < = 16%, 16–24%, and > 24% respectively). There were similar results for the complication-free survival rates. These findings pointed suggest that concomitant use of tamoxifen with irradiation is significantly associated with an increased incidence of grade 2 or higher subcutaneous fibrosis.

Management of adverse drug reactions

Hot flushes/flashes remain a problem when tamoxifen is used to treat breast cancer. In a 4-week study in 22 women with this problem considerable relief was obtained by simultaneous use of oral gabapentin 300 mg tds (121). Occasional side effects were nausea, rash and excessive sleepiness.

References

1. Jaiyesimi IA, Buzdar AU, Decker DA, Hortobagyi GN. Use of tamoxifen for breast cancer: twenty-eight years later. J Clin Oncol 1995;13(2):513–29.
2. Insler V, Lunenfeld B. Anovulation. Contrib Gynecol Obstet 1978;4:6–77.
3. De Muylder X, Neven P. Tamoxifen and potential adverse effects. Cancer J 1993;6:111.
4. Rosenfeld JA. Can the prophylactic use of raloxifene, a selective estrogen-receptor modulator, prevent bone mineral loss and fractures in women with diagnosed osteoporosis or vertebral fractures? West J Med 2000;173(3):186–8.
5. Boccardo F, Rubagotti A, Amoroso D, Mesiti M, Romeo D, Sismondi P, Giai M, Genta F, Pacini P, Distante V, Bolognesi A, Aldrighetti D, Farris A. Cyclophosphamide, methotrexate, and fluorouracil versus tamoxifen plus ovarian suppression as adjuvant treatment of estrogen receptor-positive pre-/perimenopausal breast cancer patients: results of the Italian Breast Cancer Adjuvant Study Group 02 randomized trial. J Clin Oncol 2000;18(14):2718–27.
6. Goldstein SR. Drugs for the gynecologist to prescribe in the prevention of breast cancer: current status and future trends. Am J Obstet Gynecol 2000;182(5):1121–6.
7. Reddy P, Chow MS. Safety and efficacy of antiestrogens for prevention of breast cancer. Am J Health Syst Pharm 2000;57(14):1315–25.
8. Bruzzi P. Tamoxifen for the prevention of breast cancer. Important questions remain unanswered, and existing trials should continue. BMJ 1998;316(7139):1181–2.
9. Kaufman CS, Bear HD. Another view of the tamoxifen trial. J Surg Oncol 1999;72(1):1–8.
10. Baum M. Tamoxifen—the treatment of choice. Why look for alternatives? Br J Cancer 1998;78(Suppl 4):1–4.
11. Cuzick J, Powles T, Veronesi U, Forbes J, Edwards R, Ashley S, Boyle P. Overview of the main outcomes in breast-cancer prevention trials. Lancet 2003;361:296–300.
12. Rastogi P, Vogel VG. Update on breast cancer prevention. Oncology (Huntingdon) 2003;17:799–805.
13. Biglia N, Defabiani E, Ponzone R, Mariani L, Marenco D, Sismondi P. Management of risk of breast carcinoma in postmenopausal women. Endocr Relat Cancer 2004;11:69–83.
14. Lewis CL, Kinsinger LS, Harris RP, Schwartz RJ. Breast cancer in primary care: implications for chemoprevention. Arch Intern Med 2004;164:1897–903.
15. Muanza T, Shenouda G, Souhami L, Leblanc R, Mohr G, Corns R, Langleben A. High dose tamoxifen and radiotherapy in patients with glioblastoma multiforme: a phase IB study. Can J Neurol Sci 2000;27(4):302–6.
16. Perez EA, Gandara DR, Edelman MJ, O'Donnell R, Lauder IJ, DeGregorio M. Phase I trial of high- dose tamoxifen in combination with cisplatin in patients with lung cancer and other advanced malignancies. Cancer Invest 2003;21:1–6.
17. Veronesi U, Maisonneuve P, Rotmensz N, Costa A, Sacchini V, Raviglini R, D'Aiuto G, Lovison F, Gucciardo G, Muraca MG. Pizzichetta MA, Conforti S,

Decensi A, Robertson C, Boyle P, and the Italian Tamoxifen Study Group. Italian randomized trial among women with hysterectomy: tamoxifen and hormone-dependent breast cancer in high-risk women. J Natl Cancer Inst 2003;95:160–5.

18. Anonymous. After lumpectomy, overall survival is similar with tamoxifen alone compared with tamoxifen plus radiotherapy in elderly women with early stage breast cancer, Evid Based Health Care 2005;9:79–80.

19. Fricker J. Letrozole better than tamoxifen in postmenopausal women. Lancet Oncol 2005;6:247.

20. Bradbury J. Results of the ATAC (Arimidex, Tamoxifen, Alone or in Combination) trial after completion of 5 years' adjuvant treatment for breast cancer. Lancet 2005;365:60–2.

21. Mouridsen HT, Robert NJ. The role of aromatase inhibitors as adjuvant therapy for early breast cancer in postmenopausal women. Eur J Cancer 2005;41:1678–89.

22. Love RR, Hutson PR, Havighurst TC, Cleary JF. Endocrine effects of tamoxifen plus exemestane in postmenopausal women with breast cancer. Clin Cancer Res 2005;11:1500–3.

23. Jakesz R, Jonat W, Gnant M, Mittlboeck M, Greil R, Tausch C, Hilfrich J, Kwasny W, Menzel C, Samonigg H, Seifert R, Gademann G, Kaufmann M. Switching of postmenopausal women with endocrine-responsive early breast cancer to anastrozole after 2 years' adjuvant tamoxifen. Combined results of ABCSG trial 8 and the ARNO 95 trial. Lancet 2005;366:455–62.

24. Morales L, Timmerman D, Neven P, Konstantinovic ML, Carbonez A, Van Huffel S, Ameye L, Weltens C, Christiaens MR, Vergote I, Paridaens R. Third generation aromatase inhibitors may prevent endometrial growth and reverse tamoxifen-induced uterine changes in postmenopausal breast cancer patients. Ann Oncol 2005;16:70–4.

25. Joensuu H, Ejlertsen B, Lonning PE, Rutqvist L-E. Aromatase inhibitors in the treatment of early and advanced breast cancer. Acta Oncol 2005;44:23–31.

26. Dunn BK, Ford LG. Prevention of breast cancer. Sem Breast Dis 2000;3:90–9.

27. Sawka CA, Pritchard KI, Paterson AH, Sutherland DJ, Thomson DB, Shelley WE, Myers RE, Mobbs BG, Malkin A, Meakin JW. Role and mechanism of action of tamoxifen in premenopausal women with metastatic breast carcinoma. Cancer Res 1986;46(6):3152–6.

28. Anelli TF, Anelli A, Tran KN, Lebwohl DE, Borgen PI. Tamoxifen administration is associated with a high rate of treatment-limiting symptoms in male breast cancer patients. Cancer 1994;74(1):74–7.

29. Pandya KJ, Raubertas RF, Flynn PJ, Hynes HE, Rosenbluth RJ, Kirshner JJ, Pierce HI, Dragalin V, Morrow GR. Oral clonidine in postmenopausal patients with breast cancer experiencing tamoxifen-induced hot flashes: a University of Rochester Cancer Center Community Clinical Oncology Program study. Ann Intern Med 2000;132(10):788–93.

30. Jones J. Tamoxifen side effects may be attributable to other causes. J Natl Cancer Inst 2001;93(1):11–2.

31. Arnold BJ, Cumming CE, Lees AW, Handman MD, Cumming DC, Urion C. Tamoxifen in breast cancer: symptom reporting. Breast J 2001;7(2):97–100.

32. Finelli PF, Schauer PK. Cerebral sinus thrombosis with tamoxifen. Neurology 2001;56(8):1113–4.

33. Tisman G. Thromboses after estrogen hormone replacement, progesterone or tamoxifen therapy in patients with elevated blood levels of homocysteine. Am J Hematol 2001;68(2):135.

34. Goldhaber SZ. Tamoxifen: preventing breast cancer and placing the risk of deep vein thrombosis in perspective. Circulation 2005;111:539–41.

35. Deitcher SR, Gomes MPV. The risk of venous thromboembolic disease associated with adjuvant hormone therapy for breast carcinoma: a systematic review. Cancer 2004;101:439–49.

36. Decensi A, Maisonneuve P, Rotmensz N, Bettega D, Costa A, Sacchini V, Salvioni A, Travaglini R, Oliviero P, D'Aiuto G, Gulisano M, Gucciardo G, Del Turco MR, Pizzichetta MA, Conforti S, Bonanni B, Boyle P, Veronesi U. Effect of tamoxifen on venous thromboembolic events in a breast cancer prevention trial. Circulation 2005;111:650–6.

37. Decensi A, Maisonneuve P, Rotmensz N, Bettega D, Costa A, Sacchini V, Salvioni A, Travaglini R, Oliviero P, D'Aiuto G, Gulisano M, Gucciardo G, Del Turco MR, Pizzichetta MA, Conforti S, Bonanni B, Boyle P, Veronesi U. Effect of tamoxifen on venous thromboembolic events in a breast cancer prevention trial. Circulation 2005;111:650–6.

38. Ludwig M, Tolg R, Richardt G, Katus HA, Diedrich K. Myocardial infarction associated with ovarian hyperstimulation syndrome. JAMA 1999;282(7):632–3.

39. Bentzen SM, Skoczylas JZ, Overgaard M, Overgaard J. Radiotherapy-related lung fibrosis enhanced by tamoxifen. J Natl Cancer Inst 1996;88(13):918–22.

40. Rusthoven JJ, Quirt IC, Iscoe NA, McCulloch PB, James KW, Lohmann RC, Jensen J, Burdette-Radoux S, Bodurtha AJ, Silver HK, Verma S, Armitage GR, Zee B, Bennett K. Randomized, double-blind, placebo-controlled trial comparing the response rates of carmustine, dacarbazine, and cisplatin with and without tamoxifen in patients with metastatic melanoma. National Cancer Institute of Canada Clinical Trials Group. J Clin Oncol 1996;14(7):2083–90.

41. Dignam JJ, Fisher B. Occurrence of stroke with tamoxifen in NSABP B-24. Lancet 2000;355(9206):848–9.

42. Eberling JL, Wu C, Tong-Turnbeaugh R, Jagust WJ. Estrogen- and tamoxifen-associated effects on brain structure and function. NeuroImage 2004;21:364–71.

43. Pugesgaard T, Von Eyben FE. Bilateral optic neuritis evolved during tamoxifen treatment. Cancer 1986;58(2):383–6.

44. Pavlidis NA, Petris C, Briassoulis E, Klouvas G, Psilas C, Rempapis J, Petroutsos G. Clear evidence that long-term, low-dose tamoxifen treatment can induce ocular toxicity. A prospective study of 63 patients. Cancer 1992;69(12):2961–4.

45. Eisner A, Austin DF, Samples JR. Short wavelength automated perimetry and tamoxifen use. Br J Ophthalmol 2004;88:125–30.

46. Bradbury BD, Lash TL, Kaye JA, Jick SS. Tamoxifen and cataracts: a null association. Breast Cancer Res Treat 2004;87:189–96.

47. Nguyen MC, Stewart RB, Banerji MA, Gordon DH, Kral JG. Relationships between tamoxifen use, liver fat and body fat distribution in women with breast cancer. Int J Obes Relat Metab Disord 2001;25(2):296–8.

48. Liu C-L, Yang T-L. Sequential changes in serum triglyceride levels during adjuvant tamoxifen therapy in breast cancer patients and the effect of dose reduction. Breast Cancer Res Treat 2003;79:11–16.

49. Ferrazzi E, Cartei G, De Besi P, Fornasiero A, Palu G, Paccagnella A, Sperandio P, Fosser V, Grigoletto E, Fiorentino M. Tamoxifen in disseminated breast cancer. Tumori 1977;63(5):463–8.

50. Millward MJ, Cantwell BM, Lien EA, Carmichael J, Harris AL. Intermittent high-dose tamoxifen as a potential modifier of multidrug resistance. Eur J Cancer 1992;28A(4–5):805–10.

51. Bonneterre J, Thurlimann B, Robertson JF, Krzakowski M, Mauriac L, Koralewski P, Vergote I, Webster A, Steinberg M, von Euler M. Anastrozole versus tamoxifen as first-line therapy for advanced breast cancer in 668 postmenopausal women: results of the Tamoxifen or Arimidex Randomized Group Efficacy and Tolerability study. J Clin Oncol 2000;18(22):3748–57.

52. Nabholtz JM, Buzdar A, Pollak M, Harwin W, Burton G, Mangalik A, Steinberg M, Webster A, von Euler MArimidex Study Group. Anastrozole is superior to tamoxifen as first-line therapy for advanced breast cancer in postmenopausal women: results of a North American multicenter randomized trial. J Clin Oncol 2000;18(22):3758–67.

53. Wu K, Brown P. Is low-dose tamoxifen useful for the treatment and prevention of breast cancer? J Natl Cancer Inst 2003;95:766–7.

54. Robertson C, Viale G, Pigatto F, Johansson H, Kisanga ER, Veronesi P, Torrisi R, Cazzaniga M, Mora S, Sandri MT, Pelosi G, Luini A, Goldhirsch A, Lien EA, Veronesi U. A randomized trial of low-dose tamoxifen on breast cancer proliferation and blood estrogenic biomarkers. J Natl Cancer Inst 2003;95:779–90.

55. Oien KA, Moffat D, Curry GW, Dickson J, Habeshaw T, Mills PR, MacSween RN. Cirrhosis with steatohepatitis after adjuvant tamoxifen. Lancet 1999;353(9146):36–7.

56. Cai Q, Bensen M, Greene R, Kirchner J. Tamoxifen-induced transient multifocal hepatic fatty infiltration. Am J Gastroenterol 2000;95(1):277–9.

57. Nishino M, Hayakawa K, Nakamura Y, Morimoto T, Mukaihara S. Effects of tamoxifen on hepatic fat content and the development of hepatic steatosis in patients with breast cancer: high frequency of involvement and rapid reversal after completion of tamoxifen therapy. Am J Radiol 2003;180:129–34.

58. Lin H-H, Hsu CH, Chao YC. Tamoxifen-induced severe acute pancreatitis. Dig Dis Sci 2004;49:997–9.

59. Parry BR. Radiation recall induced by tamoxifen. Lancet 1992;340(8810):49.

60. Bostrom A, Sjolin-Forsberg G, Wilking N, Bergh J. Radiation recall—another call with tamoxifen. Acta Oncol 1999;38(7):955–9.

61. Puglisi F, Aprile G, Sobrero A. Tamoxifen-induced total alopecia. Ann Intern Med 2001;134(12):1154–5.

62. Fentiman IS, Fogelman I. Breast cancer and osteoporosis—a bridge at last. Eur J Cancer 1993;29A(4):485–6.

63. Malinovszky KM, Cameron D, Douglas S, Love C, Leonard T, Dixon JM, Hopwood P, Leonard RC. Breast cancer patients' experiences on endocrine therapy: monitoring with a checklist for patients on endocrine therapy (C-PET). Breast 2004;13(5):363–8.

64. Mortimer JE, Boucher L, Baty J, Knapp DL, Ryan E, Rowland JH. Effect of tamoxifen on sexual functioning in patients with breast cancer. J Clin Oncol 1999;17(5):1488–92.

65. Leo L, Lanza A, Re A, Tessarolo M, Bellino R, Lauricella A, Wierdis T. Leiomyomas in patients receiving tamoxifen. Clin Exp Obstet Gynecol 1994;21(2):94–8.

66. Son EJ, Oh KK, Kim EK, Son HJ, Jung WH, Lee HD. Leiomyoma of the breast in a 50-year-old woman receiving tamoxifen. Am J Roentgenol 1998;171(6):1684–6.

67. Sherman BM, Chapler FK, Crickard K, Wycoff D. Endocrine consequences of continuous antiestrogen therapy with tamoxifen in premenopausal women. J Clin Invest 1979;64(2):398–404.

68. Powles TJ, Jones AL, Ashley SE, O'Brien ME, Tidy VA, Treleavan J, Cosgrove D, Nash AG, Sacks N, Baum M, McKinna JA, Davey JB. The Royal Marsden Hospital pilot tamoxifen chemoprevention trial. Breast Cancer Res Treat 1994;31(1):73–82.

69. Mourits MJ, de Vries EG, Willemse PH, ten Hoor KA, Hollema H, Sluiter WJ, de Bruijn HW, van der Zee AG. Ovarian cysts in women receiving tamoxifen for breast cancer. Br J Cancer 1999;79(11–12):1761–4.

70. McGonigle KF, Vasilev SA, Odom-Maryon T, Simpson JF. Ovarian histopathology in breast cancer patients receiving tamoxifen. Gynecol Oncol 1999;73(3):402–6.

71. McCluggage WG, Weir PE. Paraovarian cystic endosalpingiosis in association with tamoxifen therapy. J Clin Pathol 2000;53(2):161–2.

72. Turan C, Unal O, Dansuk R, Guzelmeric K, Cengizoglu B, Esim E. Successful management of an ovarian enlargement resembling ovarian hyperstimulation in a premenopausal breast cancer patient receiving tamoxifen with cotreatment of GnRH-agonist. Eur J Obstet Gynecol Reprod Biol 2001;97(1):105–7.

73. Nasu K, Miyazaki T, Kiyonaga Y, Kawasaki F, Miyakawa I. Torsion of a functional ovarian cyst in a premenopausal patient receiving tamoxifen. Gynecol Obstet Invest 1999;48(3):200–2.

74. Cohen I, Figer A, Tepper R, Shapira J, Altaras MM, Yigael D, Beyth Y. Ovarian overstimulation and cystic formation in premenopausal tamoxifen exposure: comparison between tamoxifen-treated and nontreated breast cancer patients. Gynecol Oncol 1999;72(2):202–7.

75. Gardner FJ, Konje JC, Abrams KR, Brown LJ, Khanna S, Al-Azzawi F, Bell SC, Taylor DJ. Endometrial protection from tamoxifen-stimulated changes by a levonorgestrel-releasing intrauterine system: a randomised controlled trial. Lancet 2000;356(9243):1711–7.

76. Love CD, Dixon JM. Thickened endometrium caused by tamoxifen returns to normal following tamoxifen cessation. Breast 2000;9(3):156–7.

77. Cohen I, Beyth Y, Azaria R, Flex D, Figer A, Tepper R. Ultrasonographic measurement of endometrial changes following discontinuation of tamoxifen treatment in postmenopausal breast cancer patients. BJOG 2000;107(9):1083–7.

78. McCluggage WG, Desai V, Manek S. Tamoxifen-associated postmenopausal adenomyosis exhibits stromal fibrosis, glandular dilatation and epithelial metaplasias. Histopathology 2000;37(4):340–6.

79. Seoud M, Shamseddine A, Khalil A, Salem Z, Saghir N, Bikhazi K, Bitar N, Azar G, Kaspar H. Tamoxifen and endometrial pathologies: a prospective study. Gynecol Oncol 1999;75(1):15–9.

80. Bakour SH, Khan KS, Newton JR. Evaluation of the endometrium in abnormal uterine bleeding associated with long-term tamoxifen use. Gynaecol Endosc 2000;9:19–22.

81. Cohen I, Azaria R, Bernheim J, Shapira J, Beyth Y. Risk factors of endometrial polyps resected from

postmenopausal patients with breast carcinoma treated with tamoxifen. Cancer 2001;92(5):1151–5.

82. Schlesinger C, Silverberg SG. Tamoxifen-associated polyps (basalomas) arising in multiple endometriotic foci: A case report and review of the literature. Gynecol Oncol 1999;73(2):305–11.

83. Cohen I, Bernheim J, Azaria R, Tepper R, Sharony R, Beyth Y. Malignant endometrial polyps in postmenopausal breast cancer tamoxifen-treated patients. Gynecol Oncol 1999;75(1):136–41.

84. Maia H Jr, Maltez A, Calmon LC, Moreira K, Coutinho EM. Endometrial carcinoma in postmenopausal patients using hormone replacement therapy: a report on four cases. Gynaecol Endosc 1999;8:235–41.

85. Biron-Shental T, Tepper R, Fishman A, Shapira J, Cohen I. Recurrent endometrial polyps in postmenopausal breast cancer patients on tamoxifen. Gynecol Oncol 2003;90:382–6.

86. Hachisuga T, Miyakawa T, Tsujioka H, Horiuchi S, Emoto M, Kawarabayashi T. K-ras mutation in tamoxifen-related endometrial polyps. Cancer 2003;98:1890–7.

87. Houghton JP, Ioffe OB, Silverberg SG, McGrady B, McCluggage WG. Metastatic breast lobular carcinoma involving tamoxifen-associated endometrial polyps: report of two cases and review of tamoxifen-associated polypoid uterine lesions. Mod Pathol 2003;16:395–8.

88. Levine PH, Wei X-J, Gagner J-P, Flax H, Mittal K, Blank SV. Pleomorphic liposarcoma of the uterus. Case report and literature review. Int J Gynecol Pathol 2003;22:407–11.

89. Creamer P, Lim K, George E, Dieppe P. Acute inflammatory polyarthritis in association with tamoxifen. Br J Rheumatol 1994;33(6):583–5.

90. Clement PB, Oliva E, Young RH. Mullerian adenosarcoma of the uterine corpus associated with tamoxifen therapy: a report of six cases and a review of tamoxifen-associated endometrial lesions. Int J Gynecol Pathol 1996;15(3):222–9.

91. Orbo A, Lindal S, Mortensen E. Tamoxifen og endometriecancer. En kasuistikk. [Tamoxifen and endometrial cancer. A case report.] Tidsskr Nor Laegeforen 1996;116(16):1877–8.

92. Boudouris O, Ferrand S, Guillet JL, Madelenat P. Effêts paradoxaux du tamoxifêne sur l'utêrus de la femme. [Paradoxical effects of tamoxifen on the woman's uterus. Apropos of 7 cases of myoma that appeared while under anti-estrogen treatment.] J Gynecol Obstet Biol Reprod (Paris) 1989;18(3):372–8.

93. Nuovo MA, Nuovo GJ, McCaffrey RM, Levine RU, Barron B, Winkler B. Endometrial polyps in postmenopausal patients receiving tamoxifen. Int J Gynecol Pathol 1989;8(2):125–31.

94. Rutqvist LE, Mattsson AThe Stockholm Breast Cancer Study Group. Cardiac and thromboembolic morbidity among postmenopausal women with early-stage breast cancer in a randomized trial of adjuvant tamoxifen. J Natl Cancer Inst 1993;85(17):1398–406.

95. Seoud MA, Johnson J, Weed JC Jr. Gynecologic tumors in tamoxifen-treated women with breast cancer. Obstet Gynecol 1993;82(2):165–9.

96. Treilleux T, Mignotte H, Clement-Chassagne C, Guastalla P, Bailly C. Tamoxifen and malignant epithelial-nonepithelial tumours of the endometrium: report of six cases and review of the literature. Eur J Surg Oncol 1999;25(5):477–82.

97. Ramondetta LM, Sherwood JB, Dunton CJ, Palazzo JP. Endometrial cancer in polyps associated with tamoxifen use. Am J Obstet Gynecol 1999;180(2 Pt 1):340–1.

98. Ascher SM, Johnson JC, Barnes WA, Bae CJ, Patt RH, Zeman RK. MR imaging appearance of the uterus in postmenopausal women receiving tamoxifen therapy for breast cancer: histopathologic correlation. Radiology 1996;200(1):105–10.

99. Okada DH, Rowland JB, Petrovic LM. Uterine pleomorphic rhabdomyosarcoma in a patient receiving tamoxifen therapy. Gynecol Oncol 1999;75(3):509–13.

100. Dumortier J, Freyer G, Sasco AJ, Frappart L, Zenone T, Romestaing P, Trillet-Lenoir V. Endometrial mesodermal mixed tumor occurring after tamoxifen treatment: report on a new case and review of the literature. Ann Oncol 2000;11(3):355–8.

101. Jessop FA, Roberts PF. Mullerian adenosarcoma of the uterus in association with tamoxifen therapy. Histopathology 2000;36(1):91–2.

102. Fotiou S, Hatjieleftheriou G, Kyrousis G, Kokka F, Apostolikas N. Long-term tamoxifen treatment: a possible aetiological factor in the development of uterine carcinosarcoma: two case-reports and review of the literature. Anticancer Res 2000;20(3B):2015–20.

103. Andia D, Lafuente P, Matorras R, Usandizaga JM. Uterine side effects of treatment with tamoxifen. Eur J Obstet Gynecol Reprod Biol 2000;92(2):235–40.

104. Tempfer C, Kubista E, Atkins CD, Narod SA, Pal T, Graham T, Mitchell M, Fyles A, Lasset C, Bonadona V, Mignotte H, Bremond A, Van Leeuwen FE, Bergman L, Beelen MLR, Gallee MPW, Hollema H, Dickson MJ, Pandiarajan T, Kairies P, Marsh F, Mayfield M. Tamoxifen and risk of endometrial cancer. Lancet 2001;357(9249):65–8.

105. Bergman L, Beelen ML, Gallee MP, Hollema H, Benraadt J, van Leeuwen FE. Risk and prognosis of endometrial cancer after tamoxifen for breast cancer. Comprehensive Cancer Centres' ALERT Group. Assessment of Liver and Endometrial cancer Risk following Tamoxifen. Lancet 2000;356(9233):881–7.

106. Powles TJ, Bourne T, Athanasiou S, Chang J, Grubock K, Ashley S, Oakes L, Tidy A, Davey J, Viggers J, Humphries S, Collins W. The effects of norethisterone on endometrial abnormalities identified by transvaginal ultrasound screening of healthy post-menopausal women on tamoxifen or placebo. Br J Cancer 1998;78(2):272–5.

107. Ferguson SE, Olshen AB, Viale A, Awtrey CS, Barakat RR, Boyd J. Gene expression profiling of tamoxifen-associated uterine cancers: evidence for two molecular classes of endometrial carcinoma. Gynecol Oncol 2004;92:719–25.

108. Wilder JL, Shajahan S, Khattar NH, Wilder DM, Yin J, Rushing RS, Beaven R, Kaetzel C, Ueland FR, Van Nagell JR, Kryscio RJ, Lele SM. Tamoxifen-associated malignant endometrial tumors: pathologic features and expression of hormone receptors estrogen-alpha, estrogen-beta and progesterone. A case controlled study. Gynecol Oncol 2004;92:553–8.

109. Strauss HG, Wolters M, Methfessel G, Buchmann J, Koelbl H. Significance of endovaginal ultrasonography in assessing tamoxifen-associated changes of the endometrium. A prospective study. Acta Obstet Gynecol Scand 2000;79(8):697–701.

110. Gerber B, Krause A, Muller H, Reimer T, Kulz T, Makovitzky J, Kundt G, Friese K. Effects of adjuvant tamoxifen on the endometrium in postmenopausal women

with breast cancer: a prospective long-term study using transvaginal ultrasound. J Clin Oncol 2000;18(20):3464–70.

111. Shibutani S, Ravindernath A, Suzuki N, Terashima I, Sugarman SM, Grollman AP, Pearl ML. Identification of tamoxifen-DNA adducts in the endometrium of women treated with tamoxifen. Carcinogenesis 2000;21(8):1461–7.

112. Roy RN, Gerulath AH, Cecutti A, Bhavnani BR. Effect of tamoxifen treatment on the endometrial expression of human insulin-like growth factors and their receptor mRNAs. Mol Cell Endocrinol 2000;165(1–2):173–8.

113. Tucker AN, Tkaczuk KA, Lewis LM, Tomic D, Lim CK, Flaws JA. Management of late intrauterine death using a combination of mifepristone and misoprostol—experience of two regimens. Cancer Lett 2005;217:61–72.

114. Gallicchio L, Lord G, Tkaczuk K, Danton M, Lewis LM, Lim CK, Flaws JA. Association of tamoxifen (TAM) and TAM metabolite concentrations with self-reported side effects of TAM in women with breast cancer. Breast Cancer Res Treat 2004;85:89–97.

115. Lawrence SE, Faught KA, Vethamuthu J, Lawson ML. Beneficial effects of raloxifene and tamoxifen in the treatment of pubertal gynecomastia. J Pediatr 2004;145(1):71–6.

116. Ahmad K. Antidepressants may decrease tamoxifen efficacy. Lancet Oncol 2004;5:6.

117. Naguib M, Gyasi HK. Antiestrogenic drugs and atracurium–a possible interaction? Can Anaesth Soc J 1986;33(5):682–3.

118. Montes A, Powles TJ, O'Brien ME, Ashley SE, Luckit J, Treleaven J. A toxic interaction between mitomycin C and tamoxifen causing the haemolytic uraemic syndrome. Eur J Cancer 1993;29A(13):1854–7.

119. Gallicchio L, Tkaczuk K, Lord G, Danton M, Lewis LM, Lim CK, Flaws JA. Medication use, tamoxifen (TAM), and TAM metabolite concentrations in women with breast cancer. Cancer Lett 2004;211:57–67.

120. Azria D, Gourgou S, Sozzi WJ, Zouhair A, Mirimanoff RO, Kramar A, Lemanski C, Dubois JB, Romieu G, Pelegrin A, Ozsahin M. Concomitant use of tamoxifen with radiotherapy enhances subcutaneous breast fibrosis in hypersensitive patients. Br J Cancer 2004;91:1251–60.

121. Pandya KJ, Thummala AR, Griggs JJ, Rosenblatt JD, Sahasrabudhe DM, Guttuso TJ, Morrow GR, Roscoe JA. Pilot study using gabapentin for tamoxifen-induced hot flashes in women with breast cancer. Breast Cancer Res Treat 2004;83:87–9.

PHOTODYNAMIC THERAPY

General Information

In photodynamic therapy a photosensitizing compound is administered systemically, locally, or topically to a patient with a cancer (1,2,3). After a latent period the cancer is illuminated, with visible light, which, in the presence of oxygen, leads to the generation of cytotoxic species and cell death (4,5). The choice of a photosensitizing compound that is concentrated specifically in the malignant tissue confers selectivity on the technique (6), which has been used to treat skin cancers, (4,7,8), including mycosis fungoides (9), esophageal carcinoma (10),oral and laryngeal cancers (11), bronchogenic carcinomas (12), pleural mesothelioma (13), adenocarcinoma of the stomach and colorectal carcinomas (14), tumors of the bile ducts and pancreas (15), transitional-cell carcinoma of the urinary bladder (16,17), prostate cancer (18), brain tumors (19), and local recurrent breast cancer and gynecological tumors (cervical intraepithelial neoplasia, vulvar intraepithelial neoplasia, and ovarian cancers) (20). It can be combined with anticancer drugs (21) and immunomodulators (22).

Other applications have included hidradenitis suppurativa (23), psoriasis (24), cutaneous Leishmaniasis (25), actinic keratosis (26), actinic cheilitis, sebaceous gland hyperplasia (27), lichen sclerosus, acne vulgaris (28), Barrett's esophagus (29), genital warts (30), and recurrent laryngeal papillomatosis (31,32). Photodynamic therapy with verteporfin has been used in the treatment of age-related macular degeneration (SEDA-30, 545).

The classes of photosensitizers include porphyrin derivatives (33), chlorins and purpurins (34), phthalocyanines (35), porphycenes (36), and fullerenes (37). All have different photochemical and photophysical properties in terms of mechanisms of action and light activation (8). Porphyrins were the first to be used, and the wavelengths of light chosen were based on the absorption spectrum of porphyrins—blue because the largest peak is at 400 nm (the Soret band) and red because it has greater penetration but less absorption at 650 nm (a Q band) (6). Green light at 514 nm has also been used. The molecular mechanisms (38) and the physics, biochemistry, pharmacology, and pathology of the process have been reviewed (3).

Observational Studies

Of 49 patients with advanced esophageal cancer, 22 were given 5-aminolevulinic acid 60 mg/kg orally 6–8 hours before light exposure and 27 were given a hematoporphyrin derivative 2 mg/kg intravenously 48 hours before light exposure (39). There was odynophagia in 9 and 13 patients respectively, fever up to 39.0 °C in the afternoon of the treatment day (n = 5 and 8), and chest pain for 1–2 days (n = 9 and 13) could be observed. After oral administration of 5-aminolevulinic acid dissolved in 250 ml of orange juice all the atients complained of nausea, which was relieved by ondansetron. There were no cases of sunburn.

In a phase II study of the effects of mono-L-aspartyl chlorin e6 in 41 patients with early superficial squamous cell carcinomas of the lung there were no serious adverse effects (40). Photosensitivity was studied by exposure to sunlight for 5 minutes and the results were classified as follows: 0: no reaction; 1: minimum visible erythema; 2: deep clearly defined erythema; 3: intense erythema or edema. Five of 31 patients who were tested at 13 or 14 days after treraqtment had photosensitive reactions; three patients had minimal visible erythema, one had deep clearly defined erythema, and one had blister formation. Of nine patients who were tested at other times from 9–18 days after treatment none had any reactions.

Comparative Studies

In 218 patients with advanced esophageal cancer randomized to photodynamic therapy with porfimer sodium and argon-pumped dye laser or to neodymium:YAG laser therapy, there was equivalent improvement in dysphagia (41). There were more mild to moderate complications after photodynamic therapy, including sunburn in 19%. Perforations from laser treatment or associated dilatation occurred in 1%, after photodynamic therapy and in 7% after neodymium:YAG laser therapy. Ttreatment had to be stopped because of adverse events in 3% of those who were given photodynamic therapy and in 19% after use of the neodymium:YAG laser.

In a partially blinded study in 208 patients with Barrett's esophagus, 138 were treated with porfimer sodium + omeprazole and 70 with omeprazole only (42).The most common adverse events related to porfimer were photosensitivity reactions (69%), esophageal strictures (36%), vomiting (32%), non-cardiac chest pain (20%), pyrexia (20%), dysphagia (19%), constipation (13%), dehydration (12%), nausea (11%), and hiccups (10%). Photosensitivity reactions occurred within 90 days after treatment, typically with sunburn-like reactions especially affecting the face, hands, and neck. Most of the reactions were mild (69%), 24% were moderate, and 7% were severe. Although all resolved, one patient was left with photosensitivity-related keloid scars.

Organs and Systems

Gastrointestinal

Deterioration of esophageal motility can occur after photodynamic therapy for esophageal carcinoma or Barrett's esophagus. Of 23 patients, 13 with esophageal carcinoma and 10 with Barrett's esophagus, 11 had normal motility, six had ineffective esophageal motility, and six had aperistalsis; five of those with aperistalsis had carcinoma (43). Follow-up tracings after photodynamic therapy showed that six had normal motility, seven had ineffective esophageal motility, and 10 had aperistalsis. The authors concluded that photodynamic therapy may worsen esophageal motility in some patients and that dysphagia after photodynamic therapy may be related to underlying esophageal dysmotility and may not always be caused by a stricture or underlying carcinoma.

Of 47 patients referred for endoscopic ablation for Barrett's high grade dysplasia or mucosal carcinoma who were prospectively evaluated with esophageal manometry before and after porfimer sodium, six did not complete the study (44). There was abnormal esophageal motility in 14 patients before photodynamic therapy (three with diffuse esophageal spasm, seven with ineffective esophageal motility, and four with aperistalsis). After photodynamic therapy, three had improved motility and seven worsened. None developed new aperistalsis. Thus, abnormal motility was present in 19 patients after photodynamic therapy. Worsening in function was more likely in patients with longer segment disease.

Skin

The use of hematoporphyrin derivatives is associated with cutaneous photosensitivity, which can persist for up to 3 months (45). Of 180 patients who were given 266 intravenous injections of Photofrin polyporphyrin 0.5–2.0 mg/kg for photodynamic therapy, 20–40% reported some type of phototoxic response. There was an even high incidence in another study, in which 23 patients received a systemic hematoporphyrin derivative and 17 reported cutaneous phototoxicity, including three who had blistering (46). The symptoms lasted for a mean of 6 (range 5–23) weeks. Failure to use photoprotective measures was thought to be the major contributing factor. Other complications included skin hyperpigmentation, ocular discomfort, pruritus, pain at the injection site, and urticaria.

Of 26 patients with recurrent laryngeal papillomatosis who received dihematoporphyrin ether 2.5 mg/kg of intravenously before photodynamic therapy, all had some degree of photosensitivity (47). The reactions included mild erythema and inflammation (88%), swelling (58%), blistering (23%), ocular discomfort (61.5%), pruritus (38%), and hyperpigmentation (46%). The effects lasted for 9 (range 4–17) weeks. The severity of the reactions was mainly determined by how compliant the patient was in following instructions to take precautionary measures.

In 58 patients (29 with lung cancers, five with esophageal cancers, 12 with gastric cancers, 8 with cervical cancers, and 4 with bladder cancers) who were givedn porfimer sodium as part of photodynamic therapy, there was complete remission in 48; there were no serious complications; skin photosensitivity occurred in 13 patients (48).

In 59 Japanese patients with cancers photosensitivity was sutdied by exposure to a slide projector lamp 3 weeks or more after treatment with porfimer sodium (49). Women needed significantly longer recovery periods than men subjects and those with lighter skins were more sensitive.

Newer sensitizers, such as the prophyrin precursor 5-aminolevulinic acid, may cause less phototoxicity. Of 18 patients with colorectal, duodenal, or esophageal tumors who were given 5 aminolaevulinic acid 30–60 mg/kg orally,

followed in 10 cases by a second dose a few weeks later, only two had mild skin photosensitivity reactions; six had transient rises in serum aspartate aminotransferases and five had mild nausea and vomiting (50).

Of 14 healthy men aged 20–26 who were given a single dose of temoporfin 0.100–0.129 mg/kg as part of a pharmacokinetic study and were exposed to a test dose of sunlight 2 weeks later, 12 had no reactions and were told to avoid prolonged exposure to bright sunlight for 3 months (51). Within 48 hours of discharge, 6 of those 12 had developed partial thickness burns on the left forearm and more superficial burns on other body areas (about 1% of the total body surface area) after transient exposure to daylight. Healing was much slower than with conventional thermal injury (28 versus 14 days), and there was prominent scarring in several.

The manufacturers responded that 957 healthy volunteers and patients had been exposed to temoporfin and many had been treated with photodynamic therapy on two or more occasions in clinical studies for a range of different indications (52). In all, 22 serious adverse drug reactions attributable to photosensitivity, including burns, had been reported (2.3% of all subjects), including the six cases described in the report. In clinical studies, there had been 15 serious adverse drug reactions involving burns or photosensitivity reactions in 931 patients (1.6%). They suggested that the reactions had been caused by extravasation of the agent at the site of infusion.

• A 15-year-old girl had a recurrent parietal malignant ependymoma excised followed by photodynamic therapy with poprfimer 0.75 mg/kg intravenously and precautionary use of sunglasses and avoidance of direct sunlight (53). After 48 hours she developed a second-degree burn on a finger to which an oximeter had been attached. The lesion was located on the side of the finger adjacent to the light-emitting diodes.

Light from the pulse oximeter probably activated the photosensitizer.

Urticaria and respiratory distress have been attributed to porfimer sodium (54).

References

1. Kübler AC. Photodynamic therapy. Med Laser Appl 2005;20:37-45.
2. Mitra A, Stables GI. Topical photodynamic therapy for non-cancerous skin conditions. Photodiag Photodyn Ther 2006;3:116-27.
3. Robertson CA, Evans DH, Abrahamse H. Photodynamic therapy (PDT): a short review on cellular mechanisms and cancer research applications for PDT. J Photochem Photobiol B 2009;96(1):1-8.
4. Schuitmaker JJ, Bass P, Van Leengoed HLLM, Van Der Meulen FW, Star WM, Zandwijk N. Photodynamic therapy: a promising new modality for the treatment of cancer. J Photochem Photobiol B Biol 1996;34:3-12.
5. Castano AP, Demidova TN, Hamblin MR. Mechanisms in photodynamic therapy: part two – cellular signalling, cell metabolism and modes of cell death. Photodiag Photodyn Ther 2005;2:1-23.

6. Alexiades-Armenakas M. Laser-mediated photodynamic therapy. Clin Dermatol 2006;24(1):16-25.

7. Brown SB, Brown EA, Walker I. The present and future role of photodynamic therapy in cancer treatment. Lancet Oncol 2004;5(8):497-508.

8. De Rosa FS, Bentley MVLB. Photodynamic therapy of skin cancers: sensitizers, clinical studies and future directives. Pharm Res 2000;17(12):1447-55.

9. Recio ED, Zambrano B, Alonso ML, de Eusebio E, Martín M, Cuevas J, Jaén P. Topical 5-aminolevulinic acid photodynamic therapy for the treatment of unilesional mycosis fungoides: a report of two cases and review of the literature. Int J Dermatol 2008;47(4):410-3.

10. Maier A, Tomaselli F, Matzi V, Rehak P, Pinter H, Smolle-Jüttner FM. Photosensitization with hematoporphyrin derivative compared to 5-aminolaevulinic acid for photodynamic therapy of esophageal carcinoma. Ann Thorac Surg 2001;72(4):1136-40.

11. Biel MA. Photodynamic therapy treatment of early oral and laryngeal cancers. Photochem Photobiol 2007;83(5):1063-8.

12. Savary JF, Monnier P, Fontolliet C, Mizeret J, Wagnières G, Braichotte D, van den Bergh H. Photodynamic therapy for early squamous cell carcinomas of the esophagus, bronchi, and mouth with m-tetra (hydroxyphenyl) chlorin. Arch Otolaryngol Head Neck Surg 1997;123(2):162-8.

13. Ris HB. Photodynamic therapy as an adjunct to surgery for malignant pleural mesothelioma. Lung Cancer 2005;49 Suppl 1:S65-8.

14. Patrice T, Foultier MT, Yactayo S, Adam F, Galmiche JP, Douet MC, Le Bodic L. Endoscopic photodynamic therapy with hematoporphyrin derivative for primary treatment of gastrointestinal neoplasms in inoperable patients. Dig Dis Sci 1990;35(5): 545-52.

15. Wang JB, Liu LX. Use of photodynamic therapy in malignant lesions of stomach, bile duct, pancreas, colon and rectum. Hepatogastroenterology 2007;54(75):718-24.

16. Prout GR Jr, Lin CW, Benson R Jr, Nseyo UO, Daly JJ, Griffin PP, Kinsey J, Tian ME, Lao YH, Mian YZ, et al. Photodynamic therapy with hematoporphyrin derivative in the treatment of superficial transitional-cell carcinoma of the bladder. N Engl J Med 1987;317(20):1251-5.

17. Tian ME. [Photodynamic therapy with hematoporphyrin derivative for transitional-cell carcinoma of the urinary bladder–report of 30 cases.] Zhonghua Zhong Liu Za Zhi 1989;11(4):304-6.

18. Moore CM, Pendse D, Emberton M; Medscape. Photodynamic therapy for prostate cancer—a review of current status and future promise. Nat Clin Pract Urol 2009;6(1):18-30.

19. Eljamel MS. Brain photodiagnosis (PD), fluorescence guided resection (FGR) and photodynamic therapy (PDT): past, present and future. Photodiagnosis Photodyn Ther 2008; 5(1): 29-35.

20. Soergel P, Löning M, Staboulidou I, Schippert C, Hillemanns P. Photodynamic diagnosis and therapy in gynecology. J Environ Pathol Toxicol Oncol 2008;27(4):307-20.

21. Zuluaga MF, Lange N. Combination of photodynamic therapy with anti-cancer agents. Curr Med Chem 2008;15(17):1655-73.

22. Qiang YG, Yow CM, Huang Z. Combination of photodynamic therapy and immunomodulation: current status and future trends. Med Res Rev 2008;28(4):632-44.

23. Rose RF, Stables GI. Topical photodynamic therapy in the treatment of hidradenitis suppurativa. Photodiagnosis Photodyn Ther 2008;5(3):171-5.

24. Tandon YK, Yang MF, Baron ED. Role of photodynamic therapy in psoriasis: a brief review. Photodermatol Photoimmunol Photomed 2008;24(5):222-30.

25. van der Snoek EM, Robinson DJ, van Hellemond JJ, Neumann HA. A review of photodynamic therapy in cutaneous leishmaniasis. J Eur Acad Dermatol Venereol 2008;22(8):918-22.

26. Stritt A, Merk HF, Braathen LR, von Felbert V. Photodynamic therapy in the treatment of actinic keratosis. Photochem Photobiol 2008;84(2):388-98.

27. Richey DF. Aminolevulinic acid photodynamic therapy for sebaceous gland hyperplasia. Dermatol Clin 2007;25(1):59-65.

28. Haedersdal M, Togsverd-Bo K, Wulf HC. Evidence-based review of lasers, light sources and photodynamic therapy in the treatment of acne vulgaris. J Eur Acad Dermatol Venereol 2008;22(3):267-78.

29. Dunn J, Lovat L. Photodynamic therapy using 5-aminolaevulinic acid for the treatment of dysplasia in Barrett's oesophagus. Expert Opin Pharmacother 2008;9(5):851-8.

30. Kacerovska D, Pizinger K, Kumpova M, Cetkovska P. Genital warts treated by photodynamic therapy. Skinmed 2007;6(6):295-7.

31. Abramson AL, Shikowitz MJ, Mullooly VM, Steinberg BM, Amella CA, Rothstein HR. Clinical effects of photodynamic therapy on recurrent laryngeal papillomas.Arch Otolaryngol Head Neck Surg 1992;118(1):25-9.

32. Shikowitz MJ, Abramson AL, Steinberg BM, DeVoti J, Bonagura VR, Mullooly V, Nouri M, Ronn AM, Inglis A, McClay J, Freeman K. Clinical trial of photodynamic therapy with meso-tetra (hydroxyphenyl) chlorin for respiratory papillomatosis. Arch Otolaryngol Head Neck Surg 2005;131(2):99-105.

33. Gorman SA, Brown SB, Griffiths J. An overview of synthetic approaches to porphyrin, phthalocyanine, and phenothiazine photosensitizers for photodynamic therapy. J Environ Pathol Toxicol Oncol 2006;25(1-2):79-108.

34. Kreimer-Birnbaum M. Modified porphyrins, chlorins, phthalocyanines, and purpurins: second-generation photosensitizers for photodynamic therapy. Semin Hematol 1989;26(2):157-73.

35. Miller JD, Baron ED, Scull H, Hsia A, Berlin JC, McCormick T, Colussi V, Kenney ME, Cooper KD, Oleinick NL. Photodynamic therapy with the phthalocyanine photosensitizer Pc 4: the case experience with preclinical mechanistic and early clinical-translational studies. Toxicol Appl Pharmacol 2007;224(3):290-9.

36. Stockert JC, Cañete M, Juarranz A, Villanueva A, Horobin RW, Borrell JI, Teixidó J, Nonell S. Porphycenes: facts and prospects in photodynamic therapy of cancer. Curr Med Chem 2007;14(9):997-1026.

37. Mroz P, Tegos GP, Gali H, Wharton T, Sarna T, Hamblin MR. Photodynamic therapy with fullerenes. Photochem Photobiol Sci 2007;6(11):1139-49.

38. Ortel B, Shea CR, Calzavara-Pinton P. Molecular mechanisms of photodynamic therapy. Front Biosci 2009;14:4157-72.

39. Maier A, Tomaselli F, Matzi V, Rehak P, Pinter H, Smolle-Jüttner FM. Photosensitization with hematoporphyrin derivative compared to 5-aminolaevulinic acid for photodynamic therapy of esophageal carcinoma. Ann Thorac Surg 2001;72(4):1136-40.

40. Kato H, Furukawa K, Sato M, Okunaka T, Kusunoki Y, Kawahara M, Fukuoka M, Miyazawa T, Yana T, Kaoru M, Shiraishi T, Horinouchi H. Phase II clinical study of photodynamic therapy using mono-L-aspartyl chlorin e6 and diode laser for early superficial squamous cell carcinoma of the lung. Lung Cancer 2003;42(1):103-11.

41. Lightdale CJ, Heier SK, Marcon NE, McCaughan JS Jr, Gerdes H, Overholt BF, Sivak MV Jr, Stiegmann GV, Nava HR. Photodynamic therapy with porfimer sodium versus thermal ablation therapy with Nd:YAG laser for palliation of esophageal cancer: a multicenter randomized trial. Gastrointest Endosc 1995;42(6):507-12.

42. Overholt BF, Lightdale CJ, Wang KK, Canto MI, Burdick S, Haggitt RC, Bronner MP, Taylor SL, Grace MG, Depot M; International Photodynamic Group for High-Grade Dysplasia in Barrett's Esophagus. Photodynamic therapy with porfimer sodium for ablation of high-grade dysplasia in Barrett's esophagus: international, partially blinded, randomized phase III trial. Gastrointest Endosc 2005;62(4):488-98; erratum in 2006;63(2):359.

43. Malhi-Chowla N, Wolfsen HC, DeVault KR. Esophageal dysmotility in patients undergoing photodynamic therapy. Mayo Clin Proc 2001;76(10):987-9.

44. Shah AK, Wolfsen HC, Hemminger LL, Shah AA, DeVault KR. Changes in esophageal motility after porfimer sodium photodynamic therapy for Barrett's dysplasia and mucosal carcinoma. Dis Esophagus 2006;19(5):335-9.

45. Dougherty TJ, Cooper MT, Mang TS. Cutaneous phototoxic occurrences in patients receiving Photofrin. Lasers Med Surg 1990;10(5):485–8.

46. Wooten RS, Smith KC, Ahlquist DA, Muller SA, Balm RK. Prospective study of cutaneous phototoxicity after systemic hematoporphyrin derivative. Lasers Surg Med 1988;8(3):294-300.

47. Mullooly VM, Abramson AL, Shikowitz MJ. Dihematoporphyrin ether-induced photosensitivity in laryngeal papilloma patients. Lasers Surg Med 1990;10(4):349-56.

48. Kato H, Horai T, Furuse K, Fukuoka M, Suzuki S, Hiki Y, Ito Y, Mimura S, Tenjin Y, Hisazumi H, et al. Photodynamic therapy for cancers: a clinical trial of porfimer sodium in Japan. Jpn J Cancer Res 1993;84(11):1209-14.

49. Moriwaki SI, Misawa J, Yoshinari Y, Yamada I, Takigawa M, Tokura Y. Analysis of photosensitivity in Japanese cancer-bearing patients receiving photodynamic therapy with porfimer sodium (Photofrin). Photodermatol Photoimmunol Photomed 2001;17(5):241-3.

50. Regula J, MacRobert AJ, Gorchein A, Buonaccorsi GA, Thorpe SM, Spencer GM, Hatfield AR, Bown SG. Photosensitisation and photodynamic therapy of esophaeal, duodenal and colorectal tumors using 5 aminolaevulinic acid induced protoporphyrin IX—a pilot study. Gut 1995;36(1):67–75.

51. Hettiaratchy S, Clarke J. Burns after photodynamic therapy. BMJ 2000;320(7244):1245.

52. Bryce R. Burns after photodynamic therapy. Drug point gives misleading impression of incidence of burns with temoporfin (Foscan). BMJ 2000;320(7251):1731.

53. Farber NE, McNeely J, Rosner D. Skin burn associated with pulse oximetry during perioperative photodynamic therapy. Anesthesiology 1996;84(4):983-5.

54. Karasic DS, Pearson VE. Urticaria and respiratory distress due to porfimer sodium. Ann Pharmacother 2000;34(10):1208-9.

PLATINUM-CONTAINING CYTOSTATIC DRUGS

General Information

Although the main platinum-containing cytotoxic drugs, cisplatin (rINN), carboplatin (rINN), and oxaliplatin (rINN), share some structural similarities, there are marked differences between them in therapeutic uses, pharmacokinetics, and adverse effects profiles (1–4). Compared with cisplatin, carboplatin has inferior efficacy in germ-cell tumors, head and neck cancers, and bladder and esophageal carcinomas, whereas the two drugs appear to have comparable efficacy in ovarian cancer, extensive small-cell lung cancers, and advanced non-small-cell lung cancers (5–7).

Oxaliplatin belongs to the group of diaminocyclohexane (DACH) platinum compounds. It is the first platinum-based drug that has marked efficacy in colorectal cancer when given in combination with 5-fluorouracil and folinic acid (8,9).

Nedaplatin has been registered in Japan, whereas other derivatives, like satraplatin (JM216, which is the only orally available platinum derivative), ZD0473, BBR3464, and SPI-77 (a liposomal formulation of cisplatin), are still under investigation (10–13).

Other platinum-containing compounds under investigation include dexormaplatin, enloplatin, eptaplatin, iproplatin, lobaplatin, miboplatin, miriplatin, ormaplatin, picoplatin, sebriplatin, spiroplatin, and zeniplatin.

The adverse effects of platinum compounds have been reviewed (14).

Mechanism of action

Although the precise mechanism of the cytotoxic action of the platinum-containing compounds has not been fully elucidated, they are thought to act by causing interstrand and intrastrand cross-links in DNA, particularly including two adjacent guanine or two adjacent guanine-adenine bases (15–18). In comparison with cisplatin- or carboplatin-induced DNA lesions, diaminocyclohexane (DACH) platinum DNA adduct formation has been associated with greater cytotoxicity and inhibition of DNA synthesis. In addition, there appears to be a complete lack of cross-resistance between oxaliplatin and cisplatin, which may be related to the bulky DACH carrier ligand of oxaliplatin, hindering DNA repair mechanisms within tumor cells (8,9).

Pharmacokinetics

There are significant pharmacokinetic differences among cisplatin, carboplatin, and oxaliplatin. Cisplatin is the most highly protein-bound (>90%), followed by oxaliplatin (85%) and carboplatin (24–50%).

The negligible nephrotoxicity of oxaliplatin and carboplatin compared with cisplatin may be related to their slower rates of conversion to reactive species. As a result, intensive hydration is not warranted during carboplatin or oxaliplatin infusion, in contrast to cisplatin (1,8–10). In the case of macromolecular platinum-protein complex

formation, decomposition proceeds rather slowly, which may explain why the urinary excretion of total platinum is increased for a long time after treatment, particularly in patients who have been given cisplatin (19,20).

In contrast to cisplatin, carboplatin is primarily eliminated (about 75%) by glomerular filtration, whereas tubular secretion appears to be of minor importance (2–4). It has therefore been recommended that the dose of carboplatin be adjusted according to the individual glomerular filtration rate, in order to avoid high plasma drug concentrations when the dose is calculated according to body surface area (21–23). Individualized carboplatin therapy helps to avoid abnormally high drug concentrations in patients with renal dysfunction and subtherapeutic concentrations in patients with an unexpectedly high glomerular filtration rate (24,25).

Pharmacokinetic-pharmacodynamic correlations between AUC, response rates, and the extent of myelosuppression have been examined retrospectively in patients with advanced ovarian carcinoma (21,24). AUC values below 4 minutes/mg/ml and exceeding 7 minutes/mg/ml cannot be recommended; the former is associated with low response rates and the latter is associated with more pronounced neutropenia and thrombocytopenia without higher response rates. Doses of carboplatin are generally calculated by the Calvert formula (26):

$$\text{Carboplatin dose} = \text{AUC (minutes.mg/ml)} \times (\text{GFR} + 25)$$

However, it is still debatable which method most accurately predicts individual values of glomerular filtration rate or creatinine clearance. Whereas the Cr-EDTA method is the most accurate method of estimating glomerular filtration rate, most clinicians do not use it routinely, and prefer to collect urine for estimation of creatinine clearance. Alternatively, the use of special formulae has been proposed, for example Wright's formula and the formulae of Cockcroft & Gault or Jelliffe (27–29). However, calculation of the glomerular filtration rate or creatinine clearance using such formulae has been associated with some bias in different ranges, regardless of which formula has been used.

After intravenous administration of oxaliplatin, about 33% and 40% of the dose is bound to erythrocytes and plasma proteins. The half-life averages 26 days, which is in accordance with the normal life expectancy of erythrocytes (12–50 days). Oxaliplatin undergoes rapid non-enzymatic biotransformation to form a variety of reactive platinum intermediates, which bind rapidly and extensively to plasma proteins and erythrocytes. The antineoplastic and toxic properties appear to reside in the non-protein bound fraction, whereas platinum bound to plasma proteins or erythrocytes is considered to be pharmacologically inactive. Biotransformation produces DACH-platinum dichloride, 1,2-DACH-platinum dicysteinate, 1,2-DACH-platinum diglutathionate, 1,2-DACH-platinum monoglutathionate, and 1,2-DACH-platinum methionine. The erythrocyte contains only thiol derivatives, whereas all derivatives can be recovered from the plasma.

The platinum-containing metabolites of oxaliplatin are predominantly excreted in the urine (about 50% of the dose within 3 days), whereas drug excretion via the feces is of minor importance (about 5% of the dose after 11 days). The mean total platinum half-life averages 9 days after oxaliplatin administration (130 mg/m^2 intravenously) (8,9). There is a strong negative correlation between the mean plasma concentration of unbound oxaliplatin and renal function; however, moderate renal impairment does not increase the risk of acute toxicity associated with oxaliplatin (30).

General adverse effects

The comparative toxicity and mutagenic effects of platinum anticancer drugs have been reviewed (31).

Of the clinically established platinum compounds, cisplatin has the most toxic effects on organs like the nervous system, the organ of Corti, and the kidneys in a dose-dependent fashion. The dose per cycle has therefore usually been limited to 100–120 mg/m^2 intravenously, in order to avoid drug-induced irreversible organ dysfunction (12,13). The complete spectrum of late or long-term adverse effects of cisplatin in survivors of testicular cancer has been reviewed (32).

In contrast to cisplatin, myelotoxicity represents the most prominent adverse effect of carboplatin. Based on its lower organ toxicity and its better predictable pharmacokinetic behavior, carboplatin has extensively replaced cisplatin in combination chemotherapy for the treatment of ovarian cancer and extensive small cell and non-small cell lung cancer. For other indications, one has to weigh the possibly inferior efficacy of carboplatin against the more pronounced undesirable adverse effects of cisplatin, which may limit its long-term use. Based on its marked organ toxicity, high-dose cisplatin-containing regimens are not feasible, in contrast to carboplatin, which is part of several dose-intensified combination chemotherapy regimens (12,13).

Like carboplatin, oxaliplatin does not usually cause nephrotoxicity. In addition, both drugs are only moderately emetogenic, in contrast to cisplatin. The most important dose-limiting adverse effect of oxaliplatin is a sensory peripheral neuropathy, which has two different forms:

1. a unique acute peripheral sensory (and motor) toxicity that often occurs during or within hours after drug infusion and which is rapidly reversible and aggravated by cold;
2. a peripheral sensory neuropathy related to the cumulative dose, which is generally moderate and slowly reversible, in contrast to the forms that have been described after cisplatin administration.

BBR3464

BBR3464 is the first congener of a novel group of platinum compounds, the so-called cationic trinuclear platins. It binds to DNA more rapidly than cisplatin, which results in long-range interstrand and intrastrand cross-links. It is more potent than cisplatin, and very low dosages were

effective in phase I trials. With a 1-hour intravenous infusion of 1.1 mg/m^2 every 28 days, diarrhea (preceded by abdominal cramps), nausea/vomiting, and neutropenia were the most prominent drug-related adverse effects. There were no signs of drug-related nephrotoxicity, neurotoxicity, or lung dysfunction (12,13,33).

Heptaplatin

Heptaplatin (cis-malonate[(4R,5R)-4,5-bis(aminomethyl)-2-isopropyl-1,3-dioxolane]platinum(II), SKI-2053R, Sunpla) has high antitumor activity against various cancer cell lines, including cisplatin-resistant tumor cells. Preliminary results suggested that it is less nephrotoxic than cisplatin. However, a comparative trial showed that intravenous heptaplatin 400 mg/m^2 was more nephrotoxic than intravenous cisplatin 60 mg/m^2 in terms of uremia and proteinuria, which occurred despite the use of hyperosmolar mannitol and appropriate concomitant hydration (fluid intake at least 3500 ml/day) (34,35).

Nedaplatin

Nedaplatin (cis-diammineglycolatoplatinum, CDGP, 254-S) has some structural similarities to cisplatin and carboplatin. Since 1995 it has been available for therapeutic use in Japan. In phase II trials, it had promising antineoplastic activity in patients with head and neck cancers, non-small cell lung cancers, esophageal cancer, testicular tumors, and cervical cancer. A distinct number of patients with ovarian cancer have responded to nedaplatin (for example 100 mg/m^2 intravenously) even after relapsing following treatment with cisplatin/carboplatin and cyclophosphamide. Its pharmacokinetic behavior is similar to that of carboplatin. It causes less nephrotoxicity than cisplatin, but hematological toxicity is dose-limiting. Other adverse effects include nausea/vomiting and mild peripheral neuropathy (12,13,36). Although nedaplatin is less nephrotoxic than cisplatin, incidental cases of severe nephrotoxicity have occurred. In addition, ototoxicity, similar to that observed after cisplatin, has been documented. Nedaplatin is excreted primarily unchanged by glomerular filtration, and there is a formula for predicting the clearance of unbound platinum after its administration (37).

Satraplatin

Satraplatin (bis-acetato-ammine-dichloro-cyclohexylamine-platinum, JM 216, BMS-182751) is the first oral platinum compound among the third-generation platinum complexes with activity in platinum-sensitive and some platinum-resistant preclinical models. Adverse effects were generally modest (grades I and II), including nausea, fatigue, anorexia, diarrhea, and altered taste. In addition, myelosuppression and rare cases of grades II and III increases in serum creatinine were reported. During phase II trials satraplatin was given in a dose of 120 mg/m^2/day for 5 consecutive days every 3 weeks in untreated patients with lung cancer or 30 mg/m^2/day for 14 consecutive days every 5 weeks in patients with metastatic squamous cell carcinoma. There was no nephrotoxicity or neurotoxicity (38–40). Pharmacokinetic studies showed that very little intact parent compound reached the systemic circulation after oral administration, perhaps because of extensive metabolic biotransformation or rapid reaction of platinum(II) species with DNA or other compounds. One of the intermediate compounds released during biotransformation is JM118, which has a longer half-life than the parent compound. Its particular role in the overall activity of satraplatin is still being investigated (41).

SPI-77

SPI-77 is a stealth liposomal dosage form of cisplatin. One of the main features of stealth liposomes is that they are pegylated on the liposomal surface. Compared with conventional liposomes (for example DaunoXome or Myocet) the half-life of the liposome and its embedded drug in plasma is significantly increased by this modification, because degradation by cells of the mononuclear phagocytic system is impaired; the cells are thereby, as it were, tricked. Liposomal encapsulation of cisplatin has been suggested to reduce systemic drug exposure and may help to increase drug delivery into tumor tissue. Pharmacokinetic studies have shown a slow rate of release of cisplatin from the liposomes, resulting in low systemic exposure to unbound drug. In contrast to conventional cisplatin, the incidence of gastrointestinal toxicity after SPI-77 was low, and so prophylactic antiemetics could be avoided. In addition, renal toxicity has not been observed, which also makes hydration before or after chemotherapy unnecessary. Extensive neurological measurements did not show any adverse effects. In conclusion, the toxicity profile of SPI-77 is encouragin g compared with conventional cisplatin. However, despite its favorable pharmacokinetic behavior, enhanced platinum accumulation in tumor tissue has not yet been detected (42–44).

Tetraplatin

The further development of the third-generation platinum derivative tetraplatin (ormaplatin, trans-D, L-1,2-diaminocyclohexane tetrachloroplatinum) has been abandoned, because drug-induced severe motor and sensory peripheral neuropathy occurred even at low cumulative doses. The high neurotoxic potential of tetraplatin may be associated with its pharmacokinetics: it is rapidly metabolized to 1,2-DACH-platinum dichloride, which was 3.8 times more neurotoxic than oxaliplatin in a neurite outgrowth assay (45).

ZD0473

ZD0473 (formerly AMD473, JM473) was developed in order to overcome acquired or intrinsic (de novo) resistance to cisplatin. Based on the steric bulk of its methyl-substituted pyridine moiety, thiol substitution and drug inactivation is hindered compared with cisplatin. In several in-vitro studies, ZD0473 was active even in cisplatin-refractory tumor cells, whose key mechanism of resistance was based on thiol substitution. In addition, ZD0473 is also active in cisplatin-resistant tumor cells, in which resistance is based on altered drug transport mechanisms or enhanced DNA repair.

Based on encouraging preclinical results, ZD0473 entered clinical phase I/II trials in several solid tumors, including non-small cell lung cancers, mesothelioma, head and neck cancers, and ovarian carcinoma. Its most prominent adverse effects included myelosuppression and nausea/vomiting. Thrombocytopenia and neutropenia were the dose-limiting adverse effects at intravenous doses of 130–150 mg/m^2. In contrast to cisplatin, neurotoxicity, ototoxicity, and renal toxicity have not yet been reported during or after treatment with ZD0473 (12,13,33,36).

Organs and Systems

Cardiovascular

Asymptomatic sinus bradycardia (for example 30–40/minute) is observed within 30 minutes to 2 hours after the start of cisplatin infusion. When cisplatin is withdrawn normal rhythm is restored. Because patients who receive platins are not routinely monitored, drug-induced sinus bradycardia may not be detected in practice. However, several case reports have included heavily pretreated patients, which makes a direct relation between cisplatin administration and the onset of cardiotoxic symptoms much more difficult to assess. In conclusion, no dosage adjustment appears to be warranted in patients with cisplatin-induced sinus bradycardia; however, attention should be paid to patients with resting bradycardia or those using medications known to slow the heart rate (46,47).

- A 60-year-old woman with a squamous cell lung carcinoma developed a paroxysmal supraventricular tachycardia during administration of cisplatin 20 mg/m^2 and etoposide 75 mg/m^2. The dysrhythmia appeared to be related to cisplatin since normal rhythm was restored after cisplatin was withdrawn (48).

Orthostatic hypotension was reported in "several" of 126 patients given cisplatin 50 mg/m^2 on days 1, 8, 29, and 36 as part of treatment for lung cancer in combination with etoposide and chest radiotherapy (49).

There have been 21 reports of life-threatening disease affecting large arteries in patients treated with cisplatin, bleomycin, and vinblastine in combination for germ cell tumors (50,51). Five patients died during or after therapy, three from acute myocardial infarction, one from rectal infarction, and one from cerebral infarction. Other patients who developed major vascular disease, including coronary artery and cerebrovascular disease, have been reported. Symptoms occurred acutely in some (within 48 hours of starting therapy), and after months or years had elapsed in others.

Reduced peripheral circulation, Raynaud's phenomenon, and polyneuropathy have been described after the combined use of cisplatin, bleomycin, and vinblastine for testicular tumors. Of eight cases with polyneuropathy that were investigated, it was not possible to confirm a causative association between Raynaud's phenomenon and the chemotherapy (52).

Platinum compounds have rarely been described to cause phlebitis after intravenous administration (53).

Respiratory

Seven patients died from irreversible respiratory failure after receiving combined cisplatin plus bleomycin chemotherapy; five had raised serum creatinine and all received cisplatin before the bleomycin (54). The authors recommended extreme caution with this combination, and suggested that bleomycin should precede the cisplatin infusion.

Ear, nose, throat

- A 67-year-old white woman with a small cell lung cancer was given six courses of cisplatin and etoposide once every 4 weeks and after the last course developed acute shortness of breath, hoarseness, and stridor, due to bilateral vocal cord paralysis (55).

Nervous system

The neurotoxicity of platinum-containing compounds has been reviewed (56,57), as has the prevention of cisplatin-associated neurotoxicity (58). In experimental measurements of sensory nerve conduction velocity: oxaliplatin caused the most impairment, followed by cisplatin, carboplatin, and satraplatin (JM216) (59). The cumulative incidence of grade 2 peripheral sensory neuropathy with oxaliplatin was 19% (60).

Conventional dosages of carboplatin have been associated with the lowest risk of peripheral neuropathy (for example mild paresthesia) among the approved platinum compounds. It has been estimated that about 4–6% of patients who receive carboplatin develop a peripheral neuropathy. Patients over 65 years of age or patients pretreated with other neurotoxic agents may be at a slightly higher risk (61).

A 47% incidence of peripheral neuropathy of all grades has been reported with cisplatin (62), and a 31% off-therapy deterioration of peripheral neuropathy presenting as muscle cramps and demyelination syndromes has been described (63). Cisplatin causes a well-recognized reversible sensory peripheral neuropathy, starting with depressed deep tendon reflexes and loss of vibration sense, progressing to a sensory ataxia (64). This may be age-related, as the use of high-dose cisplatin in children with neuroblastoma has not been associated with peripheral neuropathy (65). Motor nerves are spared (66). There have also been case reports of cerebral herniation and coma, severe encephalopathy, tonic-clonic seizures with concomitant visual disturbances and changed mental state, insomnia, anxiety, and parkinsonian symptoms. The symptoms generally resolved within several weeks (67–71). In some studies, the nervous system effects were the consequence of cisplatin-induced electrolyte disturbances (for example hyponatremia, hypocalcemia, or hypomagnesemia), rather than a direct action of the platinum derivative in the nervous system (72–74). For example, mental status improved in one patient who was given 3% sodium chloride in order to increase the serum sodium from 118 to 128 mmol/l, whereas diazepam, phenytoin, phenobarbital, and dexamethasone were ineffective (75).

Presentation

In about 90% of patients, oxaliplatin is associated with acute neurosensory toxicity, including dysesthesia and paresthesia. Neurosensory toxicity affects the fingers, toes, perioral and oral regions, and the pharyngolaryngeal tract (in about 1–2% of cases), which is generally induced or aggravated by coldness. As a result, patients should be instructed to avoid exposure to cold. Such symptoms can occur during or shortly after the first course of oxaliplatin. The symptoms are commonly mild and disappear within a few hours or days. Some patients also develop muscle cramps or spasms. The risk of acute neuropathy appears to be lower if oxaliplatin is given in a dosage of 85 mg/m^2 every 2 weeks rather than 130 mg/m^2 every 3 weeks. A further strategy to reduce the risk of acute recurrent pseudolaryngospasm is to increase the infusion duration from 2 to 6 hours during subsequent cycles (76,77). The prophylactic use of infusions containing calcium and magnesium sulfate before and after oxaliplatin can prevent acute neurotoxic symptoms (78).

- A woman developed bilateral blindness and lumbosacral myelopathy within 1 month of having received an autologous bone marrow transplant, cisplatin 55 mg/m^2, carmustine 600 mg/m^2, and cyclophosphamide 1875 mg/m^2 (79).

In addition to the acute neurotoxic symptoms caused by oxaliplatin, about 10–15% of patients develop a moderate neuropathy, particularly after cumulative intravenous doses of 700–800 mg/m^2. The symptoms of cumulative neuropathy include non-cold-related dysesthesia, paresthesia, superficial and deep sensory loss, and eventually sensory ataxia and functional impairment, which persists between treatment cycles. Most of these symptoms usually resolve a few weeks or months after oxaliplatin withdrawal. Lower cumulative doses (for example 510–765 mg/m^2) and higher cumulative doses exceeding 1020 mg/m^2 have been associated with incidences of cumulative grade 3 neurotoxicity of 3.2% and 50% respectively (8,9,76,77). In addition, higher cumulative doses, exceeding 1000 mg/m^2, have been associated with severe, atypical neurotoxic symptoms, such as micturition disturbances and Lhermitte's sign, mimicking cord disease. However, these signs have been observed in only a few patients so far (3.3% in phase 3 trials). Both symptoms appear to be reversible after oxaliplatin withdrawal (80). In some patients oxaliplatin treatment is feasible for as long as 18 months (for example cumulative oxaliplatin dose over 3000 mg/m^2) with no signs of dysesthesia or paresthesia causing functional impairment, indicating high interindividual variability with respect to sensitivity to oxaliplatin-induced cumulative neuropathy (76,77). Whether cumulative sensory neuropathy can occur as a result of accumulation of dichloro-DACH-platinum, a biotransformation product of DACH-platinum, in the axonal and dorsal root ganglia neurons, needs further investigation (45).

Persistent Lhermitte's sign (an electric-like sensation induced by flexion of the neck) suggestive of irreversible spinal cord toxicity has been reported in a patient taking cisplatin and etoposide (81). Of four patients with oxaliplatin neurotoxicity, two presented with Lhermitte's sign, one had urinary retention, and one had both (82). All had received cumulative doses of 1248–2040 mg/m^2, which is more than the generally accepted neurotoxic threshold for oxaliplatin (1000 mg/m^2).

Peripheral paresthesia has been reported 5 years after adjuvant cisplatin-based treatment for stages I and II testicular cancer (83).

Four of eight children developed acute neurological toxicity. Three had seizures and one had transient blindness after high-dose cisplatin (200 mg/m^2) given by continuous infusion over 5 days, followed 10 days later by a further 2 days with 40 mg/m^2/day. These children had the greatest deterioration in renal function, and they may have had impaired clearance of and increased exposure to cisplatin (84).

Peripheral neuropathy with clinical signs and/or symptoms was found in 80% of patients who had received a cumulative dose of 576 mg/m^2 of cisplatin. There was a dose-related reduction in sensory action potential amplitudes (85). The clinical and neurophysiological time progression of the severity of cisplatin polyneuropathy during and after treatment with cisplatin up to a cumulative dose of 600 mg/m^2 has been described (86).

The paraneoplastic neuropathy experienced by women with epithelial ovarian cancer receiving cisplatin has been attributed in certain cases to the drug (87).

- A woman with cancer of the ovary and a man with oat cell carcinoma both developed paresthesia of all four limbs, reduced control of fine movements, and unstable gait after receiving a cumulative dose of 500 mg/m^2 of cisplatin (88). There was distal hypesthesia, with conservation of temperature and pain sensation, areflexia, and sensory ataxia. The woman also had continuous pseudoathetosis. Neurophysiological studies showed absence of peripheral and central sensory potentials and of H-reflexes, normal electromyography, normal motor conduction, and normal mixed silent period.

The target organ in cisplatin neurotoxicity is the dorsal root ganglion. This patient had a syndrome that clinically and neurophysiologically suggested diffuse neuropathic involvement of the dorsal ganglion, in which absence of sensory and H-reflex potentials showed that the small myelinic cells were not altered, consistent with the preservation of pain and temperature sensation.

- A woman developed bilateral blindness and lumbosacral myelopathy within 1 month of having received an autologous bone marrow transplant, cisplatin 55 mg/m^2, carmustine 600 mg/m^2, and cyclophosphamide 1875 mg/m^2 (79).

Encephalopathy has also been reported.

- A 50-year-old woman with carcinoma of the cervix was treated with radiotherapy and six courses of cisplatin (75 mg/m^2 every 3 weeks; total dose 810 mg) (89). The therapy was completed with no obvious acute complications, but 12 weeks after the last course, she developed sudden blindness associated with occipital headache. She had mild global cognitive deficits and intermittent myoclonic jerking of both arms. Her visual acuity was limited to light perception in both eyes; her pupils were symmetrical with no afferent pupillary deficit. Anterior segment examination and dilated fundoscopy were normal; no ocular movements were elicited when a large plain mirror was held in front of her. The rest of the neurological examination was normal. Serum magnesium was reduced to 0.1 mmol/l (reference range 0.7–1.2 mmol/l). Electroencephalography showed diffuse slowing confirming an encephalopathy.

- An 84-year-old woman with adenocarcinoma of the ovary had two fully reversible episodes of non-convulsive encephalopathy, each following a course of cisplatin-based chemotherapy, confirming a causal relation (90). She developed acute confusion, a partial left homonymous hemianopia and a left extinction hemiparesthesia 7 and 10 days after treatment. Brain MRI showed long-standing cerebral microvascular changes and an electroencephalogram showedsided parieto-occipital periodic lateralized epileptiform discharges over a generalized background slowing of activity.

In view of the similarity to posterior leukoencephalopathy, the second case suggests regional endovascular injury rather than direct cerebral toxicity as the initial event in the evolution of encephalopathy.

Strokes have been reported in patients receiving cisplatin.

- A 21-year-old woman with a mixed germ cell tumor of the left ovary was given intravenous chemotherapy including etoposide 100 mg/m^2 on days 1–5, cisplatin 20 mg/m^2 on days 1–5, and bleomycin 30 units on days 2, 8, and 15, all of which she tolerated very well (91). Three weeks later she received a second cycle, which was complicated by an episode of dizziness on day 8. The following day she had an episode of transient dysphasia for 10 minutes. Her third course was uneventful until day 7, when she collapsed with a severesided hemiparesis and dysphasia. Left-sided total anterior circulation infarction was confirmed on MRI scan.

- A 31-year-old man with a seminoma had an orchidectomy, followed by chemotherapy with cisplatin, etoposide, and bleomycin (92). A day after the end of the second course of chemotherapy he became comatose with a heart rate of 150/minute and a systolic blood pressure of 80 mmHg. Cranial angiography showed a thrombosis of the basilar artery and a cranial CT scan showed cerebellar infarction but no brain metastases.

However, the use of other drugs in these patients makes it difficult to assign causality to cisplatin.

Infusions of cisplatin into the axillary artery have led to a bronchial plexopathy rather than the more commonly described lumbosacral nerve plexus lesion (93).

In five patients cerebral herniation followed cisplatin therapy (94). However, all had evidence of an intracerebral tumor with mass effect and the herniation of the brain was thought to be multifactorial rather than directly attributable to cisplatin.

Auditory brainstem responses have been used to detect ototoxicity from cisplatin and carboplatin when used in combination therapy (95).

Mechanism and susceptibility factors

The mechanism of cisplatin-induced neurotoxicity has not been fully explained. Cisplatin appears to affect neurons in the dorsal root ganglia. It has also been suggested that it can act as a calcium channel blocker, altering intracellular calcium homeostasis and leading to apoptosis of exposed neurons, such as those of the dorsal root ganglia. Cisplatin-induced sensory neuropathy is predominantly characterized by symptoms such as numbness and tingling, paresthesia of the upper and lower extremities, reduced deep-tendon reflexes, and leg weakness with gait disturbance. The first symptoms are often observed after a cumulative dose of 300–600 mg/m^2. Risk factors include diabetes mellitus, alcohol consumption, or inherited neuropathies. Advanced age has not been identified as an independent risk factor when there is no co-morbidity (67–70).

The acute neurotoxic effects of oxaliplatin may result from drug-related inhibition of voltage-gated sodium currents (96). It has been suggested that oxalate ions, which are released during oxaliplatin metabolism, might be responsible for the inhibitory effects on the voltage-gated sodium channels, because of their calcium-chelating activity. Whether there are calcium-sensitive, voltage-gated sodium channels that can be affected by oxalate-induced calcium depletion or whether an indirect effect through changes in intracellular calcium-dependent regulatory mechanisms contributes to oxaliplatin-induced sensory neuropathy needs further investigation (97).

The risk of oxaliplatin-induced neurosensory toxicity may be increased after surgery. Of 12 patients with metastatic colorectal cancer, seven reported immediate postoperative aggravation of pre-existing neurotoxicity. Before surgery, they had only acral paresthesia without any functional impairment, whereas after surgery they complained of major worsening of symptoms, including loss of hand grip strength, leading to dependence in dressing, eating, and use of the toilet, or loss of sensitivity, interfering with walking, which could persist for several months (98). The authors speculated that perioperative hemolysis had caused an increase in unconjugated bilirubin and the release of ultrafilterable oxaliplatin, which had previously been confined to the intraerythrocytic compartment. In addition, diffusion of ultrafilterable oxaliplatin out of erythrocytes into the plasma during hemodilution can contribute to the undesirable perioperative increase in unbound oxaliplatin in the plasma.

There is a correlation between the total dose of cisplatin and the vibratory perception threshold of the hand (99).

Dose-relatedness

When three different schedules of cisplatin were evaluated with regard to the drug's neurotoxicity, using the same dose of 450 mg/m^2 for each of the schedules, it was found that cisplatin-induced peripheral neuropathy depended on both total-dose and single-dose intensity (100).

Neurotoxicity in 22 adolescents was related to the prior cumulative dose of cisplatin that had been received; the relative risk increased 3.2-fold up to a dose of 600 mg/m^2, and 4.1-fold up to a dose of 1340 mg/m^2 (101).

By comparing 50 mg/m^2 weekly with 75 mg/m^2 3 times weekly, using detailed neurological and neurophysiological examination, it has been concluded that cisplatin neuropathy is either of sensory or axonal type, and that both are related to total and single doses (102). However, others have suggested that cisplatin-induced peripheral neurotoxicity is related to dose intensity rather than to the total dose received (103).

A 4-year follow-up of comparison of a combination of cyclophosphamide with cisplatin either 50 mg/m^2 or 100 mg/m^2 in ovarian cancer has been reported (104). Peripheral neuropathy was dose-limiting and persistent. Ten of 31 patients had significant toxicity in the high-dose group compared with one of 24 in the low-dose group.

High-dose cisplatin therapy

The use of aggressive hydration using hypertonic saline and sodium thiosulfate, with dose-scheduling, reduces the risks of dose-limiting nephrotoxicity of cisplatin, and this has made possible the use of high-dose cisplatin (over 200 mg/m^2/course). However, such doses can cause severe chronic peripheral neuropathy, ototoxicity, and myelosuppression, although these effects can be reduced by lengthening the infusion time of cisplatin (65). Peripheral neuropathy is the commonest manifestation of cisplatin neurotoxicity; with high-dose administration the incidence and severity increase with the total dose, and it appears to be age-related. It was not seen in 47 children treated with high-dose cisplatin (40 mg/m^2/day for 5 days) for neuroblastoma (105). Autonomic neuropathy, motor neuropathy, and denervation changes in muscles occur occasionally.

In a clinical and electrophysiological study of eight patients treated with high-dose cisplatin (800–1400 mg) plus etoposide and bleomycin, all developed a peripheral sensory neuropathy (106). A reduction in vibratory sensation was the earliest manifestation of the neuropathy and the findings were compatible with primary damage to the dorsal root ganglia with a central-distal axonopathy. No motor nerve abnormalities were detected, apart from one patient with carpal tunnel syndrome, but two patients had prolonged brain-stem auditory-evoked potentials, indicating a central transmission defect. In another clinical and electrophysiological study of seven patients treated with cisplatin, the sensory neuropathy was also axonal, with considerable involvement of proprioception (107). Postmortem study in one case showed degeneration of the posterior columns of the spinal cord and evidence of neuronal loss in the lumbar spinal ganglion.

Eleven patients referred for neurological evaluation after cisplatin infusion into the internal or external iliac arteries for pelvic or lower limb tumors all developed symptoms within 48 hours of nerve or plexus dysfunction within the territory supplied by the cannulated artery (108). The lumbosacral plexus was affected in nine patients, the femoral nerve in one, and the peroneal nerve in one. The doses of cisplatin ranged from 50 to 160 mg/m^2 and they did not correlate with the severity or course of the neuropathy. Small-vessel injury and infarction or a direct toxic effect are likely explanations.

Time-course
In a study of the time-course and prognosis of cisplatin-induced neurotoxicity (for example sural nerve sensory action, conduction velocity, and vibration threshold in the left big toe) in 29 patients with metastatic germ cell tumors, the onset of paresthesia was delayed (109). After completion of chemotherapy (3–4 cycles) only 11% of the patients had neurotoxic symptoms, whereas 3 months later the proportion was 65%. Cisplatin-induced neurological disorders should therefore be evaluated at 1–4 months after the end of weekly cisplatin administration, because during this time the most severe form of cisplatin neurotoxicity is to be expected. There was resolution of symptoms in most of the patients over the next 12 months, suggesting that in some individuals a long period of regeneration is required to restore axonal sensory function. In patients with mild signs of cisplatin-related neuropathy, retreatment is generally feasible after several months (110,111).

Management
Among several thiol compounds, glutathione may provide neuroprotection in patients treated with cisplatin without altering its antineoplastic activity. This protective role may be based on blockade of the accumulation of p53 protein in response to platinum in dorsal root ganglia, thereby hindering platinum-based apoptosis (57,112).

The melanocortin Org 2766, an ACTH analogue, which is not yet available for clinical use, alleviates neurotoxicity due to vinca alkaloids and cisplatin, perhaps by enhancing neural repair. However, whereas preliminary results suggested some neuroprotection in women with ovarian cancer treated with cisplatin, these results were not confirmed in a randomized, multicenter, double-blind, placebo-controlled dose-finding study, even with higher doses of Org 2766 (113).

There is evidence that amifostine can reduce the frequency of cisplatin-induced peripheral neuropathy, allowing higher mean cumulative doses to be used. However, some of the results should be interpreted with caution, because the studies included patients who differed in respect to treatment regimen, disease states, and pretreatment status. The underlying protective effect of amifostine may be based on its capacity to scavenge free radicals

and prevent cisplatin DNA adduct formation in several organs, including the dorsal root ganglia (57).

In a pilot study in 15 patients, subcutaneous amifostine was given 20 minutes before oxaliplatin, in order to counteract oxaliplatin-induced peripheral neurosensory toxicity. In 10 patients, this regimen reduced the severity of cumulative neuropathy without compromising antitumor efficacy; the amifostine was well tolerated (114).

There is increasing evidence that acute oxaliplatin-induced neurotoxicity can be improved by intravenous infusion of calcium gluconate 1000 mg and magnesium sulfate heptahydrate 1000 mg before and after oxaliplatin. It has recently been shown that this strategy could reduce the incidence of acute neurotoxic symptoms, including laryngopharyngeal dysesthesia. Of 101 patients with advanced colorectal cancers who received folinic acid (leucovorin), 5-fluorouracil, and oxaliplatin (85 mg/m^2/2 weeks, 20 patients; 100 mg/m^2/2 weeks, 22 patients; 130 mg/m^2/3 weeks, 59 patients), 63 received infusions of calcium and magnesium (1 g each) before and after oxaliplatin administration (treatment group); 38 patients (control group) did not receive infusions of calcium + magnesium. The median cumulative dose of oxaliplatin was 910 (range 255–2340) mg/m^2 in the calcium/magnesium group and 650 (range 255–1450) mg/m^2 in the control group. At the end of treatment, 27% had neuropathy (any grade) compared with 75% in the control group; 1.6% and 26% had pharyngolaryngeal dysesthesia; and 5% and 24% had grade 3 neuropathy. However, further studies are warranted before this regimen can be generally recommended for reducing the risk of acute neurosensory symptoms associated with oxaliplatin infusion (77,115).

Carbamazepine is a potent sodium channel blocker and has therefore been studied in the prevention of oxaliplatin-induced neuropathy (116). The doses of carbamazepine were adjusted to produce serum concentrations in the range 30–60 µg/ml. None of the patients who took carbamazepine reported symptoms of peripheral neurotoxicity; however, two patients (one who forgot to take carbamazepine and one who stopped taking it because he felt tired) developed grade-1 peripheral sensory neurotoxicity. These symptoms were abolished when carbamazepine was restarted. One can therefore speculate that the concomitant use of carbamazepine may allow the use of a higher cumulative dose of oxaliplatin without the occurrence of grade-4 neuropathy. However, a multicenter trial is warranted to confirm these encouraging preliminary results (117).

In 15 patients with metastatic colorectal cancer who were given gabapentin (100 mg bd or tds) if neuropathic symptoms developed with oxaliplatin, the symptoms disappeared in all patients, even in those who received up to 14 courses of oxaliplatin. Withdrawal of gabapentin resulted in recurrence. However, a controlled trial is required to verify these encouraging preliminary results.

It has been suggested that chronomodulated delivery of oxaliplatin might reduce the incidence of platinum-induced neurotoxicity (118,119). In a randomized, multicenter trial in patients with previously untreated metastases from colorectal cancer, 93 patients were assigned chronotherapy and 93 were assigned constant-rate infusion (120). Chronotherapy reduced the rate of severe mucositis five-fold and halved the rate of functional impairment from peripheral sensitive neuropathy. Median and 3-year survival times were similar in the two groups.

Preliminary results have suggested that glutathione may be neuroprotective in patients receiving oxaliplatin (121).

Sensory systems

Eyes
Ocular effects, including optic neuritis, papilledema, and retrobulbar neuritis, are uncommon adverse effects of cisplatin-containing cancer chemotherapy. The risk of retinal toxicity is restricted to high-dose cisplatin therapy (for example 200 mg/m^2 over 5 days) and can result in blurred vision and altered color perception, which can persist for several months. In contrast to cisplatin, carboplatin is seldom involved in drug-induced visual disturbances. In two cases there was a relation between the administration of carboplatin (800–1200 mg/m^2) and the occurrence of clinical cortical blindness (122). However, both patients had impaired renal function before the start of therapy with carboplatin.

- Ocular toxicity of cisplatin has been reported in a 47-year-old woman who experienced rapid uncontrollable eye movements associated with hypomagnesemia and hypocalcemia in the presence of renal tubular damage (123).

Ears
Cisplatin is ototoxic (95).

Frequency
In serial audiometric testing in 66 patients receiving cisplatin 100 mg/m^2 per course, of 39 evaluable patients, 54% had no or mild hearing loss, 36% developed early hearing loss and 10% had late loss. If early hearing loss occurred and treatment was nevertheless continued, the speech frequencies were eventually affected in 71% of patients (124).

Dose-relatedness
Tinnitus and bilateral high-frequency hearing loss (threshold 3000 Hz) have been observed in up to 31% of patients treated with initial intravenous doses of cisplatin of 50 mg/m^2. There is considerable individual variation in susceptibility to cisplatin-induced ototoxicity, and both peak plasma concentrations and cumulative dose are important. Transient reversible tinnitus occurs commonly, even after low doses, but hearing impairment is more dose-dependent and affected by age, renal function, pre-existing inner ear damage and concomitant loop diuretic and/or aminoglycoside treatment. In in-vitro studies, selective damage to hair cells in the cochlea and in the supporting cells in the cochlear and vestibular parts of the labyrinth has been shown, with arrest of morphogenesis and cytodifferentiation. Morphological changes in the stria vascularis have been noted (125).

An attempt has been made to quantify the ototoxic effects of cisplatin in children by cumulative platinum dose and decibel hearing loss at certain predetermined frequencies. The findings provide useful insight into this toxicity (126). In a study of cisplatin ototoxicity in children it was concluded that 77% experienced ototoxicity with a median cumulative dose of 360 mg/m^2 (127). However, when cisplatin was given by continuous infusion rather than bolus administration in 39 children with germ cell tumors, only one, who had received a total cumulative dose of 500 mg/m^2, had evidence of significant ototoxicity over 6 years after diagnosis (128).

In a series of 154 audiograms, ototoxicity increased with cumulative dosage of cisplatin and low-dose or monthly regimens caused the lowest toxicity (129). Patients who were given high doses over short periods of time, or who developed tinnitus and hearing loss in the speech frequencies, were at the highest risk. In a small series of patients it was confirmed that pretreatment hearing loss does not increase the risk of cisplatin ototoxicity (130). It has been postulated that cisplatin ototoxicity is inversely related to the patient's age (131). A 600 mg/m^2 plateau dose of cisplatin, beyond which hearing loss shows no apparent further deterioration in children and adolescents, has been described (132).

Presentation
Progressive hearing loss develops as a result of repeated administration of cisplatin, until a threshold plateau is reached at 3000–8000 Hz (133). Hearing loss greater than 20 dB with frequency as 5% at 1000 Hz, 31% at 2000 Hz, 59% at 4000 Hz, and 95% at 8000 Hz is described (132). This is the result of damage to the organ of Corti. The ototoxicity is bilateral, symmetrical, progressive, and irreversible. Following one course of cisplatin (150–225 mg/m^2) the mean hearing loss recorded was 27 dB at 8000 Hz, 21 dB at 6000 Hz, and 11 dB at 4000 Hz. Development of hearing loss is independent of pretreatment hearing function (134). Sudden bilateral deafness without tinnitus has been described after a single course of cisplatin at a dose of 120 mg/m^2; the patients showed only slight improvement after 4 weeks (135).

Of 186 women receiving cisplatin 50 mg/m^2 4-weekly for gynecological cancers, 40 developed significant hearing loss of at least 15 dB, but there was no significant loss in the speech frequency range (125). Prior hearing acuity did not influence the incidence or extent of the deterioration.

Susceptibility factors
Susceptibility factors include young age, previous cranial irradiation, pre-existing renal dysfunction or inner ear damage, and the concomitant use of other potentially ototoxic agents, such as aminoglycosides, loop diuretics, or tirapazamine (129,136–142). Previous use of an aminoglycoside increases the risk of ototoxicity. Younger patients and patients who had undergone prior cranial irradiation are more particularly susceptible to audiological changes, which progress in severity with increasing dose (143).

Mechanisms

The mechanisms of cisplatin-induced damage to the outer hairy cells of the cochlea may include the formation of highly reactive oxygen radicals and depletion of glutathione (144). The role of amifostine and glutathione in preventing cisplatin-induced ototoxicity has therefore been studied (145,146). The data are not sufficient to support the use of glutathione in this indication. In contrast, there is some evidence that amifostine may provide protection (147). No ototoxicity developed in 18 patients who received amifostine over 15 minutes, 15–20 minutes before the intravenous administration of cisplatin 50–120 mg/m^2 over 20 minutes. There was transient hearing loss and mild persistent audiometric abnormalities in only 30% of the patients who received cisplatin 150 mg/m^2.

Animal experiments show that cisplatin is only weakly vestibulotoxic (148), and clinical vestibular toxicity is found less often than hearing loss. Of 10 patients who received 80–550 mg cisplatin, clinical features of vestibulotoxicity were analysed in addition to hearing, and patients underwent audiometry, body sway, caloric, and optokinetic and pendular rotation testing (149). Four patients sustained significant hearing loss, five had tinnitus, and three complained of dizziness, giddiness, and/or unsteadiness rather than vertigo. These symptoms were transient, and they occurred usually after several weeks of administration; they were not consistently dose-related. Spontaneous nystagmus was observed in seven and positional nystagmus in six. Caloric and body sway tests were abnormal in the early stages in several patients. The findings were suggestive of a cumulative toxic effect.

In an in-vitro study of the adverse effect of cisplatin on hair cells and other inner ear structures, aimed at determining whether selective damage occurs in inner ear hair cells and whether morphogenesis and cytodifferentiation are influenced by low cisplatin concentrations, even at low cisplatin concentrations (0.1 μg/ml) there was selective damage to hair cells. Incubation at a cisplatin concentration of 1 μg/ml caused morphological damage in the supporting cochlear and vestibular cells, and 10 μg/ml caused total collapse of the membranous labyrinth. Drug exposure arrested morphogenesis as well as cytodifferentiation (150).

Auditory brainstem responses have been used to detect ototoxicity from cisplatin and carboplatin when used in combination therapy (95). The method can detect early high frequency damage due to these drugs up to two or three cycles earlier than conventional audiometry.

The ototoxicity of cisplatin has been studied using distortion-product otoacoustic emissions (DPOAEs) and conventional pure-tone audiometry (151). Cisplatin ototoxicity was detected on average one cycle earlier with DPOAEs than with pure-tone audiometry. The authors suggested that this was because DPOAEs are more sensitive to outer hair cell damage.

Carboplatin and oxaliplatin

In one study only 1.1% of evaluable patients taking carboplatin had ototoxic symptoms, such as tinnitus, or subclinical audiographic changes (152). However, in a series of closely monitored patients there was an incidence of 27% (129). It has also been estimated that 19% of patients receiving carboplatin have significant hearing loss greater than 30 dB; the hearing loss is cumulative and maximum at 8000 Hz; the authors reported two of these patients with hearing loss greater than 10 dB at 1000 Hz. The overall conclusion is that with low-dose, short-schedule, carboplatin therapy, routine audiometry is not justified (152).

After otoacoustic emission testing in 19 children who received cisplatin the authors suggested that this is better at detecting the early cochlear damage associated with cisplatin ototoxicity than traditional pure-tone audiometry, particularly in children, in whom early detection is of the utmost importance (153). In patients who receive high-dose carboplatin, preliminary results suggest that there may be a correlation between the risk of ototoxicity and carboplatin serum concentrations (AUC) during the first course. Patients with high-grade ototoxicity had higher median carboplatin AUCs than patients without any symptoms (122,154).

In another study, carboplatin-induced ototoxicity was reported in 32% of exposed patients. This was similar to cisplatin ototoxicity, although at a lower frequency (4000–8000 Hz) than the often-quoted 6000–8000 Hz for cisplatin. The extent of otic damage was proportional to the dose of carboplatin (155).

Audiological testing has been recommended for patients receiving high-dose carboplatin therapy, following hearing problems in a series of 10 patients with ovarian cancer (156).

There is no evidence that oxaliplatin causes ototoxicity (157).

Smell

About 30% of patients treated with cisplatin have been reported to have some degree of anosmia, which in 1% is severe or complete; the sense of smell returns to normal within 3–4 months of completing cisplatin therapy (158).

Endocrine

The endocrine effects of cisplatin-based chemotherapy were studied in 22 men 9–24 or more months after completion of treatment for germ cell tumors (159). Mean basal FSH and stimulated LH and FSH concentrations were increased but serum testosterone concentrations were similar to untreated controls. Younger patients (under 25 years old) appeared more resistant to these effects of chemotherapy, and the hormonal abnormalities recovered with time.

The long-term effects on Leydig cell function of chemotherapy in 244 patients with germ cell tumors have been studied by measuring concentrations of sex hormone-binding globulin, luteinizing hormone, and follicle-stimulating hormone at least 74 months after chemotherapy (160). The population was divided into groups by cumulative cisplatin exposure (above and below 400 mg/m^2). Low-dose cisplatin exposure had no effect on Leydig cell function, but cumulative high-dose chemotherapy caused persistent impairment.

Metabolism

- Hyperosmolar non-ketotic hyperglycemia occurred in a 61-year-old patient 6 days after a first cycle of cisplatin therapy (161). The patient recovered with conventional conservative management.

Electrolyte balance

Hyponatremia is rare, and persistent hyponatremia very rare in patients taking cisplatin (162). In a detailed description of the biochemical abnormalities that can result from renal tubular dysfunction after cisplatin therapy, it was noted that hypocalciuria is more common than hypomagnesemia, and that there tends to be a state of reduced serum bicarbonate. The most severe renal tubular damage caused by cisplatin is characterized by hypocalciuria, total body magnesium deficiency, and hypokalemic metabolic alkalosis (163).

Other electrolyte disturbances induced by cisplatin include hypocalcemia, hypophosphatemia, hyponatremia, and hypokalemia (164,165). However, these changes are rarely associated with symptoms (166,167).

Metal metabolism

Magnesium

About 75% of patients treated with cisplatin develop hypomagnesemia (serum concentrations below 1.5 mmol/l), which appears to be associated with drug-induced renal tubular damage (168–171). The symptoms include tetany, muscular weakness, tremulousness, dizziness, personality changes, and perioral and peripheral paresthesia (172). Magnesium supplementation is generally recommended during treatment courses with cisplatin (168,170). Sometimes, hypomagnesemia resolves rather slowly and can last several weeks. A significant reduction in serum magnesium and other effects associated with progressive renal dysfunction appear to correlate with high cumulative doses of carboplatin (for example a median cumulative dose of 2590 mg/m^2 in children or in adults undergoing high-dose chemotherapy with peripheral blood stem cell support).

Renal magnesium wasting is the main mechanism responsible for the hypomagnesemia associated with cisplatin (172), and it can be associated with enhanced tubular reabsorption of calcium and consequent hypocalciuria (173). This dissociation in the renal handling of calcium and magnesium is similar to what is found in Bartter's syndrome. The site of the renal tubular defect in these conditions is not known, but there is evidence that active renal tubular transport systems are disrupted.

In a prospective study of 28 patients who received a total of 82 doses of cisplatin, hypomagnesemia occurred in all patients and was associated with significant and prolonged dose-related magnesium wasting. Serum magnesium was 1.8 mg/dl after the fourth dose. Examination of the urine sediment 2–4 days after each dose of cisplatin showed renal tubular epithelial cells, suggesting that cisplatin directly injures the tubules, leading to reduced tubular reabsorption of magnesium, renal magnesium

wasting, and hypomagnesemia (174). In another study, patients receiving cisplatin and concomitant magnesium supplementation developed significantly less renal tubular damage, as assessed by urine N-acetyl-β-D-glucosaminidase (175). No patient developed clinical signs of hypomagnesemia when intravenous or oral supplementation of magnesium was given as soon as the serum magnesium fell to or below 0.45 mmol/l. In patients receiving intracavitary cisplatin in high doses (100–200 mg/m^2), together with intravenous thiosulfate, there was a lower incidence of hypomagnesemia as a result of the thiosulfate; thiosulfate probably inactivated cisplatin before it reached the kidney, by complex formation (176).

Hypomagnesemia secondary to cisplatin administration can be severe enough to present as generalized seizures (172). It more commonly presents with muscular weakness, tremulousness, peripheral paresthesia, tetany, and personality changes. It is dose-related and schedule-related. Loss of magnesium can be prevented by prophylactic magnesium infusion before and during cisplatin administration (177), but this is not universally recommended because of the risk of acute uremia (178).

Zinc

Hyperzincuria and hypozincemia can occur concurrently in patients treated with cisplatin, due to variable excretion of zinc in these cases (179).

Hematologic

Compared with cisplatin and oxaliplatin, carboplatin has the highest myelotoxic potential. Carboplatin-induced myelosuppression is dose-related and results in thrombocytopenia and neutropenia. At conventional doses (AUC 4–7 minutes/μg/ml) about 20–40% of patients develop thrombocytopenia (platelet counts below 50×10^9/l). In contrast, severe neutropenia is less pronounced with conventional doses; about 16–21% of patients develop neutrophil counts less than 1×10^9/l. The lowest leukocyte and platelet counts usually occur at 14–28 days after drug administration. The hemoglobin concentration was below 11 g/dl in 71–91% of patients and below 8 g/dl in 8–21% (155). The severity of drug-induced thrombocytopenia is inversely correlated with the endogenous formation and release of thrombopoietin, which is an important cytokine for de novo platelet formation in the bone marrow. In contrast to conventional dosages, high-dose chemotherapy containing carboplatin is generally associated with severe and life-threatening forms of hematological toxicity, requiring the prophylactic use of recombinant hemopoietic growth factors, such as G-CSF, and peripheral blood stem cell support (180).

Underlying risk factors, which predispose patients to more severe forms of myelosuppression, include lower initial blood cell counts, renal impairment, poor performance status, extensive prior chemotherapy, and advanced age. There is a strong correlation between carboplatin pharmacokinetics and the severity of myelosuppressive adverse effects; an AUC-adapted dosage of carboplatin is therefore highly recommended during conventional dose chemotherapy (22,23,155).

Cisplatin belongs to the most important causative agents for the induction of treatment-related anemia requiring the prophylactic use of erythropoietin or intermittent transfusion of erythrocytes, whereas drug-induced leukopenia and thrombocytopenia are generally mild and transient (180,181). In a pharmacokinetic study, non-protein-bound platinum concentrations in patients with significant falls in hemoglobin (3 g/dl or more) were significantly higher (mean 53 ng/ml) than in patients who did not have significant falls in hemoglobin. The authors suggested that early and simple platinum pharmacokinetic control on the day after first drug administration might be useful in targeting patients who are likely to develop more severe forms of cisplatin-related anemia (182).

Myelosuppression caused by oxaliplatin is generally mild. Grade 3/4 anemia, neutropenia, and thrombocytopenia are observed in only 2–3% of patients. In combination with fluorouracil/folinic acid, the frequency is slightly higher, depending on the dose of fluorouracil (8,9).

Cisplatin causes an increase in erythropoietin, but anemias associated with platinum therapy are independent of this mechanism (183).

Forty patients with lung cancer, treated with a combination of cisplatin, mitomycin, vinblastine, doxorubicin, cyclosphosphamide, and methotrexate, had a significant post-treatment increase in fibrinopeptide A and a fall in fibrinolytic activity, reflected by a fall in functional tissue activator; this appeared to be cumulative, depending on the extent of drug exposure (184).

Gastrointestinal

Of the approved platinum compounds, cisplatin has the greatest emetogenic potential (185). Whereas about 65–94% of patients who receive conventional dosages of carboplatin complain of mild to moderate nausea or vomiting, more than 90% of those who receive cisplatin can have more than 10 vomiting episodes within the first day of administration in the absence of effective antiemetic therapy. An emetogenic episode occurring within 24 hours after drug administration is usually classified as acute emesis; nausea and vomiting that occur thereafter are classified as delayed emesis and may persist over several days. There appears to be a correlation between the time of cisplatin administration and the severity of drug-induced vomiting (186). When cisplatin was given in the morning (0500 hours) vomiting was greater than when it was given in the evening (1700 hours). However, the prophylactic use of a 5-HT$_3$ receptor antagonist reduced the time-of-day dependency. 5-HT$_3$ receptor antagonists, such as dolasetron, granisetron, ondansetron, palonosetron, or tropisetron, particularly in combination with dexamethasone, reduce the severity of acute emesis occurring within the first 24 hours after cisplatin. In contrast, the satisfactory prevention of delayed emesis remains a challenge. There is increasing evidence that the introduction of a novel class of antiemetic agents, the neurokinin-1-receptor antagonists, such as MK869 (aprepitant), may be associated with additional benefit

in combination with a 5-HT$_3$ receptor antagonist in reducing cisplatin-induced nausea and vomiting, both acute and delayed (187).

Nausea, vomiting, and diarrhea are common adverse effects of oxaliplatin and carboplatin, but they are generally mild to moderate, and both are less emetogenic than cisplatin. However, patients who have previously received cisplatin may be at greater risk of vomiting with carboplatin or oxaliplatin (1,8,9).

In an endoscopic study of the acute gastroduodenal toxicity of intravenous cisplatin 10 mg/m^2 and etoposide 107 mg/m^2 (mean dose) given for three doses, a significant number of patients developed gastroduodenal lesions, several of which progressed (188).

Liver

Mild reversible increases in liver function tests can occur in patients who have received platinum compounds (189). However, the platinum compounds are generally not classified as hepatotoxic drugs.

Urinary tract

Cisplatin

Of the approved platinum compounds, cisplatin has the greatest nephrotoxic potential, and the nephrotoxicity is often dose-limiting (190). If dosages exceed 100 mg/m^2 per course or per day, nephrotoxicity is the most severe drug-related adverse effect. It is mainly due to proximal tubular dysfunction (191), with hydropic degeneration, necrosis, and occasional tubular atrophy. Fragments of distal tubular cells have been demonstrated in the urine of patients receiving chemotherapy that included cisplatin (192). The risk is reduced by adequate hydration, which lowers drug concentrations in the renal tubules. Impaired renal function can persist for at least 6 months after treatment has been withdrawn. Indicators of cisplatin-related renal tubular toxicity include changes in creatinine clearance or in urinary alanine aminopeptidase and N-acetyl-β-D-glucosaminidase activities. Blood urea nitrogen and serum creatinine are poor indicators of early renal damage. The nephrotoxicity of cisplatin is primarily tubular, although changes in renal blood flow and glomerular filtration also occur, and hypomagnesemia is common (SEDA-12; 193,194).

The mechanisms of cisplatin-induced nephrotoxicity have not been fully elucidated. Like several nephrotoxic heavy metals (for example mercury), cisplatin can accumulate in the kidney, where it can interact with sulfhydryl compounds, resulting in increased membrane fragility and depletion of intracellular glutathione. There is some evidence that cisplatin can induce apoptosis and necrosis of kidney cells dose-dependently. In vitro studies have suggested that the constitutive expression of antiapoptotic proteins (for example bcl-X) might be inversely correlated with the sensitivity of renal tubular cells (146,195–197).

Cisplatin-induced nephrotoxicity can be detected by a rise in blood urea or by a fall in creatinine clearance. Tubular dysfunction can cause hyponatremia (72), hypokalemia, hypomagnesemia (173), and hypophosphatemia.

Inappropriate ADH secretion may be partly responsible for hyponatremia (191).

In experiments in mice, the trace element selenium, which interacts with heavy metals, reduces the renal, intestinal, hepatic, and hematological toxicity of cisplatin without affecting its antitumor activity (198).

Regarding prolongation of infusion, it has been suggested that there is a correlation between higher plasma platinum concentrations and the risk of cisplatin-induced nephrotoxicity. If platinum concentrations exceed 6 µg/ml, more patients develop nephrotoxicity. These drug concentrations were measured shortly after the end of infusion (for example 5 minutes after intravenous infusions of 100–120 mg/m^2), suggesting that high blood concentrations rather than trough concentrations may be predictively important. As a result, prolongation of cisplatin infusion (for example 6 hours) has been proposed to reduce the risk of cisplatin-induced renal insufficiency (147,199). However, in practice, a 1-hour infusion remains the common standard.

In 35 children who had taken cisplatin for a maximum of 2 years, nephrotoxicity was not related to total dose but was less severe in children who received cisplatin in doses below 40 mg/m^2/day (200). During follow-up for 2 years there was partial but significant recovery of renal function.

The effect of age on nephrotoxicity after treatment with ifosfamide or cisplatin has been studied (201). Children aged 5 years or less had more severe proximal tubular toxicity associated with ifosfamide than older patients. They also had significantly lower plasma phosphate concentrations and a higher fractional excretion of glucose. There was no evidence of glomerular or distal renal tubular damage after ifosfamide and there was no difference between the older and younger children in any other aspect of renal function. In general, age predicts independently the likelihood and severity of genitourinary toxicity caused by cisplatin in combination chemotherapy (202).

Several supportive measures have been proposed in order to circumvent cisplatin-induced nephrotoxicity. These include:

- adequate hydration before and during cisplatin administration and afterwards, in combination with an osmotic diuretic such as mannitol (the current standard method);
- prolongation of the infusion time (for example 6 hours instead of 2 hours);
- fractionation over several days;
- the use of a chronomodulated schedule;
- the use of nephroprotective agents, such as organic thiosulfate compounds.

Sodium thiosulfate protects against cisplatin-induced nephrotoxicity by reacting covalently with cisplatin in the renal tubules. Other protectors include probenecid, orgotein, fosfomycin (203), amifostine (2-[3-aminopropyl) amino]ethylphosphorothioic acid, WR-2721, ethyofos), and anthiol. Experimental study drugs that may be useful in renal protection include BNP7787 (dimesna), selenium, and silibinin (146,204–212). The beneficial role of furosemide is uncertain.

Amifostine is an organic thiophosphate. It is a prodrug, because dephosphorylation by tissue-bound alkaline phosphatase is necessary to form its active metabolite, WR-1065. It protects normal tissues against the toxic effects of radiation, cisplatin, and alkylating agents in animals, perhaps through free radical scavenging, hydrogen ion donation, and the prevention or removal of DNA platinum adducts (213). Amifostine has been used in the pretreatment of patients with metastatic melanoma before administration of cisplatin 60–150 mg/m^2 in an uncontrolled trial of 36 patients (214). There was a response rate of 53% and a low incidence of nephrotoxicity; transient nephrotoxicity occurred in 4% of 82 courses of amifostine given with cisplatin 120 mg/m^2.

In a randomized study, 242 patients with advanced ovarian cancer received intravenous cisplatin 100 mg/m^2 and cyclophosphamide 1000 mg/m^2 once every 3 weeks with or without amifostine 910 mg/m^2. Besides a significant reduction in chemotherapy-induced neutropenia and thrombocytopenia, amifostine produced significant protection against cisplatin-induced nephrotoxicity. Creatinine clearance fell by more than 40% in 60% of the control group compared with 12% of those in the treated group. In addition, the incidence of cisplatin-related hypomagnesemia was less pronounced in the patients who received amifostine.

Dose fractionation over several days has been associated with less kidney damage. The glomerular filtration rate was maintained in patients who received cisplatin 20 mg/m^2/day over 5 consecutive days (215,216). However, patients still had a significant increase in sensitive urinary markers, such as low molecular weight proteins, N-acetyl-β-D-glucosaminidase (NAG), and α–1-microglobulin, showing that conventional approaches can reduce but not completely prevent nephrotoxicity (146,195).

Chronomodulated administration of cisplatin can also reduce drug-induced organ toxicity, for example nephrotoxicity (217,218). Administration of cisplatin in the evening caused markedly less nephrotoxicity and neurotoxicity than morning administration. There is also increasing evidence that all platinum-based anticancer drugs are better tolerated if they are given in the late afternoon or early evening, with less frequent and severe nephrotoxicity, thrombocytopenia, and cumulative peripheral neuropathy after cisplatin, carboplatin, and oxaliplatin. As chronomodulated scheduling appears to affect the adverse effects of all platinum compounds, the mechanism may be based on circadian variation in renal tubular excretion and plasma filtration of platinum compounds, increased plasma protein binding, and reduced tissue susceptibility at about 1600 hours (217–219).

In several studies, intravenous amifostine (910 mg/m^2) preserved glomerular filtration rate when it was co-administered with cisplatin-containing regimens (213). Even after two cycles containing intravenous cisplatin 50 mg/m^2 plus intravenous ifosfamide and etoposide or paclitaxel, glomerular filtration rate can fall by more than 30%, but concomitant use of amifostine prevented this.

Even lower dosages of intravenous amifostine (for example 740 mg/m^2) may be effective (220,221).

Because preclinical results suggested that intracellular glutathione may be involved in the modulation of cisplatin-induced toxicity, several trials (two uncontrolled and two randomized) have been conducted to evaluate the efficacy and tolerability of standard doses of cisplatin with concomitant glutathione. In some studies, glutathione reduced cisplatin-related toxicity without impairing its antineoplastic activity (113). However, a cisplatin dose-escalation study with concomitant administration of glutathione had to be terminated prematurely because of unacceptable ototoxicity. Glutathione has not yet received FDA approval for chemoprotection.

Carboplatin

When carboplatin is used in doses that cause similar hematological toxicity to cisplatin, it has negligible renal, neurological, and auditory toxicity (222,223). In combination with other cytotoxic agents, the maximum tolerated dose is less than normal because of the risk of myelosuppression (224). However, if the dose is increased, as in acute non-lymphocytic leukemia, high-tone hearing loss and renal impairment can occur (225). In this study, all but one patient who developed these adverse effects had also received aminoglycoside antibiotics.

Concomitant intravenous hydration and monitoring is not needed when carboplatin is given in conventional dosages. However, during dose-intensified treatment with carboplatin, the risk of impaired renal function increases. In addition, other nephrotoxic drugs, such as ifosfamide, are often part of those high-dose combination regimens. During a study of the use of high-dose carboplatin (1500 mg/m^2/day or more) on 3 consecutive days, the nephrotoxic profile was comparable to a standard single dose of cisplatin (216).

Ultra-high-dose carboplatin can be safely administered as long as clinicians individualize and adjust the therapy to renal function using ^{51}Cr-EDTA glomerular filtration rate; there was only one death attributed to carboplatin in 31 patients who died of acute renal insufficiency (226).

Mild to moderate reduction in creatinine clearance with rises in serum urea and creatinine were reported in 14% of patients receiving carboplatin in a dose of 400 mg/m^2 for gynecological malignancies. Of the patients who received carboplatin 400 mg/m^2 with vincristine but without hydration for lung cancer, 19% developed renal changes.

During a 2-year follow-up of 23 children receiving carboplatin there were falls in both glomerular filtration rate to 22 ml/minute and serum magnesium concentration to 0.17 mmol/l (166). The authors thought that the fall in glomerular filtration rate, although statistically significant, was not clinically significant, but they were unsure about the long-term clinical effects of the low magnesium.

Intensified carboplatin-containing regimens can predispose patients to drug-induced renal dysfunction when cisplatin has previously been used or when renal function is already impaired (167,227).

In a randomized study of the prophylactic use of amifostine during dose-intensified chemotherapy including carboplatin and ifosfamide, patients in the control arm had a median loss of glomerular filtration rate of 37% compared with baseline after one cycle, and 35% of these patients had glomerular filtration rates below 60 ml/minute on day 10 after treatment. In patients who received amifostine during dose-intensified chemotherapy, the glomerular filtration rate fell only by a median of 10% and no patient developed a glomerular filtration rate below 60 ml/minute by day 10 (228).

Oxaliplatin

Oxaliplatin, when given alone or in combination with fluorouracil, is considered not to be nephrotoxic (166,167,227). There has been a single case of acute tubular necrosis probably caused by oxaliplatin and not related to dehydration or pre-renal insufficiency (229).

Skin

Even in cases of accidental extravasation, the risk of skin ulceration is low. Severe cisplatin-related extravasation injury appears to be primarily restricted to the use of high concentrations (for example 0.75 mg/ml) and infusion over a short time. In such circumstances it is advisable to give a local injection of isotonic thiosulfate solution (0.16 mol/l). Since carboplatin is more slowly activated than cisplatin to active DNA binding moieties and is more water-soluble, there have been no reports of severe carboplatin extravasation and no antidote is necessary (230,231).

- Accidental subcutaneous administration of oxaliplatin resulted in a red-brown painful swelling and sclerosis of the skin within 8 days (232). The symptoms were worst 1 week after extravasation and lasted for about 5 weeks, but the patient, a 52-year-old woman, recovered fully. Acute intervention included local fluid instillation to dilute the extravasation, removal of the cannula, cold packs, and a gel containing aescin and diethylamine salicylate.

Two other cases of oxaliplatin extravasation have been reported (233). Both occurred when the intraport needle disconnected. The initial symptoms were swelling and tenderness at the port site. The patients developed severe inflammation after 3 days. Treatment included local cool packs, diclofenac ointment, and oral indometacin, morphine, or dexamethasone. The authors avoided saline instillation because sodium chloride and oxaliplatin may be incompatible in combination (119). Both patients recovered without any sign of local necrosis and long-term sequelae (233)

Sexual function

Sexual function in men can be compromised by cisplatin + vinblastine + bleomycin chemotherapy. Of 54 patients, 29 had disorders of sexual function 2 years after completion of treatment (234). Ejaculatory dysfunction was tentatively linked to chemotherapy in 30% of those affected. There was reduced libido, usually reversible, in 40 at the time of chemotherapy.

Reproductive system

A cumulative dose–response toxic effect of cisplatin affects gonadal function when the drug is used in children around puberty; this damage is reversible in girls, but not in boys (235).

Immunologic

Cisplatin can cause anaphylactic shock, asthma, or urticaria (236). Hypersensitivity reactions, probably of type I, have also been reported after the administration of cisplatin, carboplatin, and oxaliplatin (237–243). Life-threatening allergy to cisplatin has also been reported after 16 doses of cisplatin 20 mg/m^2/week (244). These allergic reactions can include respiratory dysfunction (for example wheezing, dyspnea), gastrointestinal discomfort (for example abdominal cramps, diarrhea), and rashes (for example pruritus, urticaria, facial erythema, and swelling). The risk of exfoliative dermatitis is very low. In most patients, the first signs of hypersensitivity reactions usually occurred after the administration of multiple intravenous courses containing platinum compounds. Whether patients who are hypersensitive to one platinum compound also react to another cannot be excluded, since some case reports have suggested possible cross-reactions among platinum compounds (245). Sometimes, successful retreatment may be feasible through premedication with glucocorticoids and antihistamines (240).

The frequency of carboplatin-induced hypersensitivity reactions is 2–9%. Of more than 200 patients 16 had allergic reactions to carboplatin (246). According to one retrospective analysis, mild carboplatin-related hypersensitivity reactions, with itching and mild erythema, occurred in 20 of 194 patients, whereas 12 patients developed severe forms of reactions, including diffuse erythroderma, rigor, facial swelling, throat and chest tightness, tachycardia, bronchospasm, and hypertension or hypotension (243). The most important interventive measures in patients with severe forms of hypersensitivity reactions include intravenous adrenaline, glucocorticoids, and antihistamines.

Severe anaphylaxis has been reported in five patients who had already received several cycles (5–12) containing oxaliplatin 100 mg/m^2 every 2 weeks (241). The predominant symptoms included reduced systolic blood pressure, flushing, sweating, headache, tachycardia, and respiratory distress. If retreatment with the causative platinum compound is required in such cases, premedication with a glucocorticoid and antihistamine may prevent recurrence. However, symptoms can occur despite premedication, making drug withdrawal necessary.

There was a 12% incidence rate of hypersensitivity reactions in 205 women who received carboplatin as part of their treatment for gynecological malignancies (247). In trying to characterize these reactions, the authors noted that in about half of the patients, the reaction developed after more than half of their carboplatin had been infused, with a median number of exposures to carboplatin of eight cycles before the reaction.

An effective carboplatin desensitization protocol has been reported in a child with hypersensitivity, allowing additional months of carboplatin treatment (248). After premedication with diphenhydramine, ranitidine, and methylprednisolone, eight dilutions of carboplatin (0.01–50.0 mg) were given intravenously at 15-minute intervals at a rate of 1 mg/minute. Subsequently, carboplatin 600 mg was given as a continuous infusion over 3 hours without adverse effects. Whether desensitization is generally suitable for overcoming allergic adverse events should be tested prospectively (249).

The term "oxaliplatin-induced hypersensitivity reaction" can refer to:

1. acute neurosensory symptoms;
2. a cytokine release syndrome related to increased plasma concentrations of interleukin-6 and tumor necrosis factor alfa;
3. an immunological reaction involving antibody formation and histamine release (238).

In order to prove an underlying allergic disorder, an intradermal skin test with commercial formulations of the platinum compound in different concentrations (for example 0.003–1 mg/ml) can be done (250).

Body temperature

Oxaliplatin is generally well tolerated. Some patients develop fever, which appears to be related to a transient increase in cytokines, particularly interleukin-6 and tumor necrosis factor alfa. In one study the oxaliplatin-induced increase in body temperature correlated with a marked increase in interleukin-6 serum concentrations (peak 133 pg/ml) (251). Interleukin-6 is a proinflammatory cytokine, which stimulates acute phase proteins and B lymphocytes. Premedication with metamizol, dexamethasone, and clarithromycin, which interferes with interleukin-6, did not prevent the fever. The roles of interleukin-6 and tumor necrosis factor alfa in the development of fever is strengthened by the observation that their serum concentrations fell during resolution of the fever (252).

Death

- Fatal acute tumor lysis syndrome has been reported in a 74-year-old woman who received cisplatin (50 mg/m^2 on day 1) and fluorouracil (1000 mg/m^2 by continuous infusion for 5 days) for vulvar carcinoma (253).

Whilst this is a well known complication of chemotherapy, particularly with hematological tumors, it is extremely rare as a complication of neoadjuvant chemotherapy for gynecological tumors.

Long-Term Effects

Tumorigenicity

There is some evidence that platinum compounds are mutagenic in bacteria and can cause chromosomal aberrations in animal cells in tissue culture (254). The risk of secondary leukemia in 28 971 patients with ovarian cancers receiving platinum-based chemotherapy has been evaluated; 96 developed a secondary leukemia (255). The authors concluded that the risk of developing a secondary leukemia while receiving a platinum-based protocol may be increased four-fold. The relative risks for carboplatin and cisplatin were estimated at 6.5 and 3.3 respectively. The relative risks of leukemia after cumulative doses of platinum of less than 500, 500–749, 750–999, and 1000 mg were 1.9, 2.1, 4.1, and 7.6 respectively. The delay between the start of platinum-containing chemotherapy and the occurrence of secondary malignancies was 2.8–7.7 years. In children who received an average cumulative dose of cisplatin of 600 mg/m^2, the estimated incidence of chemotherapy-induced leukemia was 1.5% (256). Concomitant radiation therapy or administration of other carcinogenic agents increases the risk.

Second-Generation Effects

Fertility

There is experimental evidence that several anticancer drugs can cause abnormalities of sperm chromosomes. Preliminary data have suggested that after platinum-containing chemotherapy for testicular cancer, penetration of oocytes can be severely impaired. Cytogenetic study of the spermatozoa has shown that many of the abnormalities correspond to structural aberrations that may not have a pathogenic effect in the production of abortions or children with chromosome abnormalities (257).

In men receiving chemotherapy, the sperm count will return to normal within 2 years of discontinuing chemotherapy in 78% of cases; however, intensive treatment, such as with doses of cisplatin in excess of 500 mg/m^2, reduces the probability of full recovery of normal spermatogenesis (258).

A Danish study group has reported a fertility problem of 53% in patients with unilateral germ cell tumors, but there was no significant difference between orchidectomy and cisplatin-based chemotherapy or subdiaphragmatic irradiation (259). Eight patients remained infertile despite evident recovery of spermatogenesis, and all 22 children conceived post-treatment were born normal and without malformations.

Gonadal function was evaluated in 59 men and 31 women after successful treatment of germ-cell tumors with the POMB/ACE regimen (cisplatin, vincristine, methotrexate, and bleomycin + dactinomycin, cyclophosphamide, and etoposide) (260). Most of the patients recovered fertility; 81% of the men who did not receive para-aortic radiotherapy, whose original tumor bulk was less than 5 cm in diameter, and whose duration of chemotherapy was less than 6 months recovered, compared with 32% who had larger tumors or who received longer courses of chemotherapy, or both. Fertility and pregnancies were undisturbed in 24 women with invasive trophoblastic tumors treated with methotrexate alone, with methotrexate and dactinomycin in combination, or with other combination chemotherapy (261). There were nine subsequent pregnancies, with the birth of eight healthy babies, and one woman requested a termination of pregnancy.

The long-term prognosis for sperm counts after chemotherapy with and without radiation in 71 males treated for non-Hodgkin's lymphoma on the CHOP-Bleomycin combination has been studied (262). Pelvic radiotherapy and cumulative cyclophosphamide dosages of greater than 9.5 g/m^2 are associated independently and in combination with a greater risk of permanent sterility.

Teratogenicity

Cisplatin and related compounds cross the placenta and can therefore cause fetal damage. Cisplatin is teratogenic in mice and embryotoxic in mice and rats. The platins should only be used during pregnancy in life-threatening situations. The patient should be informed of the potential hazard to the fetus (263).

Drug Administration

Drug administration route

There have been several reports of local neurotoxicity after intra-arterial cisplatin. In 63 patients pretreated with low-dose cisplatin given by arterial infusion for head and neck cancer (up to 25 mg/day for 1–10 days), before definitive local treatment, cranial nerve palsies developed on the same side as the cannulated artery in four cases (264). There was ipsilateral involvement of the 9th, 10th, 11th, and 12th cranial nerves in two patients, and the 7th and 12th nerves alone were affected in the other two patients. The palsies appeared at the end of treatment or up to 10 days later and only the 12th nerve palsy in one of the patients with multiple cranial nerve involvement recovered completely. In each patient, no other cause for paresis was found and CT scans showed that the nerves were not infiltrated by tumor. The cumulative dose of cisplatin administered to these four patients was less than that received by the unaffected 59 patients (median 200 mg, range 160–250; compared with 250 mg, range 160–400).

Drug overdose

Irreversible renal insufficiency has been described after accidental overdosage with cisplatin.

- In a 68-year-old woman who received an accidental overdose of cisplatin (480 mg), there was severe vomiting and myelosuppression, irreversible renal insufficiency, and deafness; other effects included seizures, hallucinations, loss of vision, and hepatotoxicity (265).

Drug–Drug Interactions

Antiepileptic drugs

Plasma concentrations of antiepileptic drugs (for example carbamazepine, valproic acid, phenytoin) should be measured more frequently during cisplatin-containing cancer chemotherapy (266,267).

- Cisplatin caused subtherapeutic carbamazepine and valproic acid concentrations in a 38-year-old woman with epilepsy undergoing cytotoxic cancer chemotherapy with doxorubicin and cisplatin, resulting in tonic-clonic seizures; the mechanism was not clear (266).

Etoposide

- A 52-year-old patient with glioblastoma developed severe ocular and orbital toxicity after receiving intracarotid etoposide phosphate and carboplatin (268). Acutely non-pupillary block angle-closure glaucoma developed secondary to uveal effusion in the ipsilateral eye. Four days later, severe orbital inflammation resulted in reduced visual acuity, proptosis, optic neuropathy, and total external ophthalmoplegia.

Fluorouracil

The combination of cisplatin 100 mg/m^2 with 5-fluorouracil 1000 mg/m^2 for 7 days caused angina and ischemic electrocardiographic changes, suggesting synergistic cardiotoxicity (269). There have also been cases of arterial occlusive events (270) and myocardial infarction (271,272), in some cases with evidence of coronary vascular spasm (273,274).

In 39 patients given low-dose continuous fluorouracil and cisplatin 20 mg/m^2/week for 8 weeks, there was a very low incidence of renal toxicity, although electrolyte abnormalities, particularly hyponatremia and hypomagnesemia, were as expected (244).

Irinotecan

The concomitant use of irinotecan as a 1-hour infusion immediately following a 2-hour infusion of oxaliplatin resulted in more severe hypersalivation and abdominal pain than irinotecan monotherapy (275). Acute intervention with atropine alleviated these adverse effects. When the drugs were separated by 1 day, the cholinergic symptoms were not exacerbated. The authors postulated that oxaliplatin might have some acetylcholinesterase inhibitory activity.

Lithium

Some data have suggested that cisplatin-containing chemotherapy can alter lithium clearance through impaired renal function, and lithium therapy should be closely monitored during treatment with cisplatin-containing regimens (276).

Mesna

Platinum agents are combined with ifosfamide in the treatment of cancer. The possibility that mesna may interfere with the anticancer effects of platinum agents has been investigated using cultured malignant glioma cells (277). Mesna protected tumor cell lines from the cytotoxic effect of the platinum agents. This in-vitro study emphasizes the importance of specifying in detail the infusion schedules of mesna and platinum agents.

Methotrexate

A patient with no other risk factors developed irreversible nephrotoxicity after four cycles of carboplatin 300 mg/m^2 and methotrexate 50 mg/m^2 (278). This appears to have been an additive effect of drugs that are not individually nephrotoxic until much higher doses.

Nephrotoxic drugs

Based on its considerable nephrotoxic potential, cisplatin should be given after, rather than before, other anticancer drugs and other drugs with a low therapeutic index (for example aminoglycoside antibiotics or bleomycin) that are primarily excreted in the urine in unchanged form. Concomitant use of potentially nephrotoxic agents (for example conventional amphotericin, tacrolimus) with cisplatin should be avoided (279,280).

Neurotoxic drugs

The concomitant or previous use of potentially neurotoxic drugs (for example paclitaxel, vinca alkaloids, or hexamethylmelamine) can increase the risk of peripheral neuropathy due to platinum compounds (68,69).

Paclitaxel

There is some evidence that there is a clinically significant pharmacokinetic interaction of paclitaxel with cisplatin. When cisplatin was given before paclitaxel, the clearance rate of paclitaxel was 25% less than when the two drugs were given in the opposite sequence. In consequence, neutropenia was more profound with the former schedule (281). In addition, in experimental studies, cytotoxicity increased when human ovarian carcinoma cells were exposed to paclitaxel before cisplatin, whereas the interaction was antagonistic when a 1-hour exposure to cisplatin was followed by a 20-hour exposure to taxol, or when the cells were exposed to cisplatin and taxol for 1 hour concurrently (282). The biochemical basis of this interaction has not been elucidated. The pharmacodynamic interaction may be related to cisplatin-induced alterations in cell-specific and non-specific binding sites for paclitaxel (283). In view of these results, paclitaxel should be given before cisplatin (284). There does not appear to be a similar interaction of paclitaxel with carboplatin (285).

Both cisplatin and paclitaxel are neurotoxic, the toxicity being dose-limiting and cumulative; neurotoxicity due to the combination has been suggested to be synergistic; after five cycles of chemotherapy, 96% of 44 patients had grade 1 toxicity and 52% grade 2 toxicity; 18% with grade 2 or 4 toxicity were withdrawn (286).

In 21 patients with advanced non-small cell lung cancer carboplatin had no effect on the pharmacokinetics of paclitaxel 135–200 mg/m^2 as a 24-hour intravenous infusion(288). Peripheral neuropathy occurred in 13 of 37 patients treated with paclitaxel 175 mg/m^2 and carboplatin(289). The authors concluded that clinically important neurotoxicity increases with every cycle of chemotherapy. The peripheral neuropathy mainly affected sensory fibers without involving motor nerves. The same paclitaxel/carboplatin chemotherapy in 28 women caused no signs of acute central neurotoxicity or neuropsychological deterioration; however, 11 patients had a peripheral neuropathy(290).

Vincristine

In 86 patients treated with cisplatin-based chemotherapy for testicular cancer, cumulative exposure (over 400 mg/m^2) and a previous history of noise exposure were significant susceptibility factors for irreversible ototoxicity; high doses of vincristine (greater than 6 mg/m^2) significantly increased the risk of reversible ototoxicity(287).

References

1. Go RS, Adjei AA. Review of the comparative pharmacology and clinical activity of cisplatin and carboplatin. J Clin Oncol 1999;17(1):409–22.
2. Lipp HP, Bokemeyer C. Clinical pharmacokinetics of cytostatic drugs: efficacy and toxicity (2.2. platinum compounds as anticancer drugs) In: Lipp HP, editor. Anticancer drug toxicity; prevention, management and clinical pharmacokinetics. New York-Basel: Marcel Dekker Inc, 1999:61–81.
3. Woloschuk DM, Pruemer JM, Cluxton RJ Jr. Carboplatin: a new cisplatin analogue. Drug Intell Clin Pharm 1988;22(11):843–9.
4. Calvert AH, Harland SJ, Newell DR, Siddik ZH, Jones AC, McElwain TJ, Raju S, Wiltshaw E, Smith IE, Baker JM, Peckham MJ, Harrap KR. Early clinical studies with cis-diammine-1,1-cyclobutane dicarboxylate platinum II. Cancer Chemother Pharmacol 1982;9(3):140–7.
5. Lokich J, Anderson N. Carboplatin versus cisplatin in solid tumors: an analysis of the literature. Ann Oncol 1998;9(1):13–21.
6. Vermorken JB, ten Bokkel Huinink WW, Eisenhauer EA, Favalli G, Belpomme D, Conte PF, Kaye SB. Advanced ovarian cancer. Carboplatin versus cisplatin. Ann Oncol 1993;4(Suppl 4):41–8.
7. Markman M. Carboplatin and cisplatin: are they equivalent in efficacy in "optimal residual" advanced ovarian cancer? J Cancer Res Clin Oncol 1996;122(8):443–4.
8. Wiseman LR, Adkins JC, Plosker GL, Goa KL. Oxaliplatin: a review of its use in the management of metastatic colorectal cancer. Drugs Aging 1999;14(6):459–75.
9. Culy CR, Clemett D, Wiseman LR. Oxaliplatin. A review of its pharmacological properties and clinical efficacy in metastatic colorectal cancer and its potential in other malignancies. Drugs 2000;60(4):895–924.
10. van Hennik MB, van der Vijgh WJ, Klein I, Elferink F, Vermorken JB, Winograd B, Pinedo HM. Comparative pharmacokinetics of cisplatin and three analogues in mice and humans. Cancer Res 1987;47(23):6297–301.
11. O'Dwyer PJ, Stevenson JP, Johnson SW. Clinical pharmacokinetics and administration of established platinum drugs. Drugs 2000;59(Suppl 4):19–27.
12. Judson I, Kelland LR. New developments and approaches in the platinum arena. Drugs 2000;59(Suppl 4):29–36.
13. Clark DL, Andrews PA, Smith DD, DeGeorge JJ, Justice RL, Beitz JG. Predictive value of preclinical toxicology studies for platinum anticancer drugs. Clin Cancer Res 1999;5(5):1161–7.
14. Zanotti KM, Markman M. Prevention and management of antineoplastic-induced hypersensitivity reactions. Drug Saf 2001;24(10):767–79.
15. Reed E, Yuspa SH, Zwelling LA, Ozols RF, Poirier MC. Quantitation of cis-diamminedichloroplatinum II (cisplatin)- DNA-intrastrand adducts in testicular and ovarian cancer patients receiving cisplatin chemotherapy. J Clin Invest 1986;77(2):545–50.
16. Poirier MC, Reed E, Litterst CL, Katz D, Gupta-Burt S. Persistence of platinum-ammine-DNA adducts in gonads and kidneys of rats and multiple tissues from cancer patients. Cancer Res 1992;52(1):149–53.
17. Poirier MC, Reed E, Zwelling LA, Ozols RF, Litterst CL, Yuspa SH. Polyclonal antibodies to quantitate cis-diamminedichloroplatinum(II)—DNA adducts in cancer patients and animal models. Environ Health Perspect 1985;62:89–94.
18. Knox RJ, Friedlos F, Lydall DA, Roberts JJ. Mechanism of cytotoxicity of anticancer platinum drugs: evidence that cis-diamminedichloroplatinum (II) differ only in the kinetics of their interaction with DNA. Cancer 1986;11:643–5.
19. Gietema JA, Meinardi MT, Messerschmidt J, Gelevert T, Alt F, Uges DR, Sleijfer DT. Circulating plasma platinum more than 10 years after cisplatin treatment for testicular cancer. Lancet 2000;355(9209):1075–6.
20. Schierl R, Rohrer B, Hohnloser J. Long-term platinum excretion in patients treated with cisplatin. Cancer Chemother Pharmacol 1995;36(1):75–8.
21. Jodrell DI, Egorin MJ, Canetta RM, Langenberg P, Goldbloom EP, Burroughs JN, Goodlow JL, Tan S, Wiltshaw E. Relationships between carboplatin exposure and tumor response and toxicity in patients with ovarian cancer. J Clin Oncol 1992;10(4):520–8.
22. Bokemeyer C, Lipp HP. Is there a need for pharmacokinetically guided carboplatin dose schedules? Onkologie 1997;20:343–5.
23. Bergh J. Is pharmacokinetically guided chemotherapy dosage a better way forward? Ann Oncol 2002;13(3):343–4.
24. Jodrell DI. Formula-based dosing for carboplatin. Eur J Cancer 1999;35(9):1299–301.
25. Millward MJ, Webster LK, Toner GC, Bishop JF, Rischin D, Stokes KH, Johnston VK, Hicks R. Carboplatin dosing based on measurement of renal function—experience at the Peter MacCallum Cancer Institute. Aust NZ J Med 1996;26(3):372–9.
26. Calvert AH, Newell DR, Gumbrell LA, O'Reilly S, Burnell M, Boxall FE, Siddik ZH, Judson IR, Gore ME, Wiltshaw E. Carboplatin dosage: prospective evaluation of a simple formula based on renal function. J Clin Oncol 1989;7(11):1748–56.
27. Dooley MJ, Poole SG, Rischin D, Webster LK. Carboplatin dosing: gender bias and inaccurate estimates of glomerular filtration rate. Eur J Cancer 2002;38(1):44–51.
28. Wright JG, Boddy AV, Highley M, Fenwick J, McGill A, Calvert AH. Estimation of glomerular filtration rate in cancer patients. Br J Cancer 2001;84(4):452–9.
29. Wright JG, Calvert AH, Highley MS, Roberts JT, MacGill A, Fenwick J, Boddy AV. Accurate prediction of renal function for carboplatin. Proc Am Assoc Cancer Res 1999;40:25420Abstract.
30. Massari C, Brienza S, Rotarski M, Gastiaburu J, Misset JL, Cupissol D, Alafaci E, Dutertre-Catella H, Bastian G. Pharmacokinetics of oxaliplatin in patients with normal versus impaired renal function. Cancer Chemother Pharmacol 2000;45(2):157–64.
31. Yarema KJ. Comparative toxicities and mutagenics of platinum anticancer drugs. Drug Inf J 1995;29:s1633–44.

32. Vaughn DJ, Gignac GA, Meadows AT. Long-term medical care of testicular cancer survivors. Ann Intern Med 2002;136(6):463–70.

33. Piccart MJ, Lamb H, Vermorken JB. Current and future potential roles of the platinum drugs in the treatment of ovarian cancer. Ann Oncol 2001;12(9):1195–203.

34. Kim NK, Im SA, Kim DW, Lee MH, Jung CW, Cho EK, Lee JT, Ahn JS, Heo DS, Bang YJ. Phase II clinical trial of SKI-2053R, a new platinum analogue, in the treatment of patients with advanced gastric adenocarcinoma. Cancer 1999;86(7):1109–15.

35. Ahn JH, Kang YK, Kim TW, Bahng H, Chang HM, Kang WC, Kim WK, Lee JS, Park JS. Nephrotoxicity of heptaplatin: a randomized comparison with cisplatin in advanced gastric cancer. Cancer Chemother Pharmacol 2002;50(2):104–10.

36. Christian MC. The current status of new platinum analogues. Semin Oncol 1992;19(6):720–33.

37. Ishibashi T, Yano Y, Oguma T. A formula for predicting optimal dosage of nedaplatin based on renal function in adult cancer patients. Cancer Chemother Pharmacol 2002;50(3):230–6.

38. Fokkema E, Groen HJ, Bauer J, Uges DR, Weil C, Smith IE. Phase II study of oral platinum drug JM216 as first-line treatment in patients with small-cell lung cancer. J Clin Oncol 1999;17(12):3822–7.

39. Trudeau M, Stuart G, Hirte H, Drouin P, Plante M, Bessette P, Dulude H, Lebwohl D, Fisher B, Seymour L. A phase II trial of JM-216 in cervical cancer: an NCIC CTG study. Gynecol Oncol 2002;84(2):327–31.

40. Fokkema E, de Vries EG, Meijer S, Groen HJ. Lack of nephrotoxicity of new oral platinum drug JM216 in lung cancer patients. Cancer Chemother Pharmacol 2000;45(1):89–92.

41. Carr JL, Tingle MD, McKeage MJ. Rapid biotransformation of satraplatin by human red blood cells in vitro. Cancer Chemother Pharmacol 2002;50(1):9–15.

42. Meerum Terwogt JM, Groenewegen G, Pluim D, Maliepaard M, Tibben MM, Huisman A, ten Bokkel Huinink WW, Schot M, Welbank H, Voest EE, Beijnen JH, Schellens JM. Phase I and pharmacokinetic study of SPI-77, a liposomal encapsulated dosage form of cisplatin. Cancer Chemother Pharmacol 2002;49(3):201–10.

43. Vail DM, Kurzman ID, Glawe PC, O'Brien MG, Chun R, Garrett LD, Obradovich JE, Fred RM 3rd, Khanna C, Colbern GT, Working PK. STEALTH liposome-encapsulated cisplatin (SPI-77) versus carboplatin as adjuvant therapy for spontaneously arising osteosarcoma (OSA) in the dog: a randomized multicenter clinical trial. Cancer Chemother Pharmacol 2002;50(2):131–6.

44. Schiller JH. Small cell lung cancer: defining a role for emerging platinum drugs. Oncology 2002;63(2):105–14.

45. Luo FR, Wyrick SD, Chaney SG. Comparative neurotoxicity of oxaliplatin, ormaplatin, and their biotransformation products utilizing a rat dorsal root ganglia in vitro explant culture model. Cancer Chemother Pharmacol 1999;44(1):29–38.

46. Tassinari D, Sartori S, Drudi G, Panzini I, Gianni L, Pasquini E, Abbasciano V, Ravaioli A, Iorio D. Cardiac arrhythmias after cisplatin infusion: three case reports and a review of the literature. Ann Oncol 1997;8(12):1263–7.

47. Altundag O, Celik I, Kars A. Recurrent asymptomatic bradycardia episodes after cisplatin infusion. Ann Pharmacother 2001;35(5):641–2.

48. Fassio T, Canobbio L, Gasparini G, Villani F. Paroxysmal supraventricular tachycardia during treatment with cisplatin and etoposide combination. Oncology 1986;43(4):219–20.

49. Albain KS, Rusch VW, Crowley JJ, Rice TW, Turrisi AT 3rd, Weick JK, Lonchyna VA, Presant CA, McKenna RJ, Gandara DR, et al. Concurrent cisplatin/etoposide plus chest radiotherapy followed by surgery for stages IIIA (N2) and IIIB non-small-cell lung cancer: mature results of Southwest Oncology Group phase II study 8805. J Clin Oncol 1995;13(8):1880–92.

50. Samuels BL, Vogelzang NJ, Kennedy BJ. Vascular toxicity following vinblastine, bleomycin, and cisplatin therapy for germ cell tumours. Int J Androl 1987;10(1):363–9.

51. Samuels BL, Vogelzang NJ, Kennedy BJ. Severe vascular toxicity associated with vinblastine, bleomycin, and cisplatin chemotherapy. Cancer Chemother Pharmacol 1987;19(3):253–6.

52. Heier MS, Nilsen T, Graver V, Aass N, Fossa SD. Raynaud's phenomenon after combination chemotherapy of testicular cancer, measured by laser Doppler flowmetry. A pilot study. Br J Cancer 1991;63(4):550–2.

53. Dorr RT. Managing extravasations of vesicant chemotherapy drugs. In: Lipp HP, editor. Anticancer Drug Toxicity; Prevention, Management and Clinical Pharmacokinetics. New York-Basel: Marcel Dekker Inc, 1999:279–318.

54. Rabinowits M, Souhami L, Gil RA, Andrade CA, Paiva HC. Increased pulmonary toxicity with bleomycin and cisplatin chemotherapy combinations. Am J Clin Oncol 1990;13(2):132–8.

55. Taha H, Irfan S, Krishnamurthy M. Cisplatin induced reversible bilateral vocal cord paralysis: an undescribed complication of cisplatin. Head Neck 1999;21(1):78–9.

56. Windebank AJ. Chemotherapeutic neuropathy. Curr Opin Neurol 1999;12(5):565–71.

57. Screnci D, McKeage MJ. Platinum neurotoxicity: clinical profiles, experimental models and neuroprotective approaches. J Inorg Biochem 1999;77(1–2):105–10.

58. Alberts DS, Noel JK. Cisplatin-associated neurotoxicity: can it be prevented? Anticancer Drugs 1995;6(3):369–83.

59. Wilson RH, Lehky T, Thomas RR, Quinn MG, Floeter MK, Grem JL. Acute oxaliplatin-induced peripheral nerve hyper-excitability. J Clin Oncol 2002;20(7):1767–74.

60. Levi F, Zidani R, Brienza S, Dogliotti L, Perpoint B, Rotarski M, Letourneau Y, Llory JF, Chollet P, Le Rol A, Focan C. A multicenter evaluation of intensified, ambulatory, chronomodulated chemotherapy with oxaliplatin, 5-fluorouracil, and leucovorin as initial treatment of patients with metastatic colorectal carcinoma. International Organization for Cancer Chronotherapy. Cancer 1999;85(12):2532–40.

61. Heinzlef O, Lotz JP, Roullet E. Severe neuropathy after high dose carboplatin in three patients receiving multidrug chemotherapy. J Neurol Neurosurg Psychiatry 1998;64(5):667–9.

62. van der Hoop RG, van der Burg ME, ten Bokkel Huinink WW, van Houwelingen C, Neijt JP. Incidence of neuropathy in 395 patients with ovarian cancer treated with or without cisplatin. Cancer 1990;66(8):1697–1702.

63. Siegal T, Haim N. Cisplatin-induced peripheral neuropathy. Frequent off-therapy deterioration, demyelinating syndromes, and muscle cramps. Cancer 1990;66(6):1117–1123.

64. Gessini L, Jandolo B, Pollera C, et al. Neuropatia da cisplatino: un nuovo tipo di polineuropatia assonale ascendente progressiva. Riv Neurobiol 1987;33:75.

65. Holleran WM, DeGregorio MW. Evolution of high-dose cisplatin. Invest New Drugs 1988;6(2):135–42.

66. Riggs JE, Ashraf M, Snyder RD, Gutmann L. Prospective nerve conduction studies in cisplatin therapy. Ann Neurol 1988;23(1):92–4.

67. Mollman JE. Cisplatin neurotoxicity. N Engl J Med 1990;322(2):126–7.

68. Cersosimo RJ. Cisplatin neurotoxicity. Cancer Treat Rev 1989;16(4):195–211.

69. Tuxen MK, Hansen SW. Neurotoxicity secondary to antineoplastic drugs. Cancer Treat Rev 1994;20(2):191–214.

70. Higa GM, Wise TC, Crowell EB. Severe, disabling neurologic toxicity following cisplatin retreatment. Ann Pharmacother 1995;29(2):134–7.

71. Dewar J, Lunt H, Abernethy DA, Dady P, Haas LF. Cisplatin neuropathy with Lhermitte's sign. J Neurol Neurosurg Psychiatry 1986;49(1):96–9.

72. Mariette X, Paule B, Bennet P, Clerc D, Bisson M, Massias P. Cisplatin and hyponatremia. Ann Intern Med 1988;108(5):770–1.

73. Mune T, Yasuda K, Ishii M, Matsunaga T, Miura K. Tetany due to hypomagnesemia induced by cisplatin and doxorubicin treatment for synovial sarcoma. Intern Med 1993;32(5):434–7.

74. Gonzalez C, Villasanta U. Life-threatening hypocalcemia and hypomagnesemia associated with cisplatin chemotherapy. Obstet Gynecol 1982;59(6):732–4.

75. Ritch PS. Cis-dichlorodiammineplatinum II-induced syndrome of inappropriate secretion of antidiuretic hormone. Cancer 1988;61(3):448–50.

76. Cassidy J, Misset JL. Oxaliplatin-related side effects: characteristics and management. Semin Oncol 2002;29(5 Suppl 15):11–20.

77. Gamelin E, Gamelin L, Bossi L, Quasthoff S. Clinical aspects and molecular basis of oxaliplatin neurotoxicity: current management and development of preventive measures. Semin Oncol 2002;29(5 Suppl 15):21–33.

78. Cersosimo RJ. Oxaliplatin-associated neuropathy: a review. Ann Pharmacother 2005;39(1):128–35.

79. Wang MY, Arnold AC, Vinters HV, Glasgow BJ. Bilateral blindness and lumbosacral myelopathy associated with high-dose carmustine and cisplatin therapy. Am J Ophthalmol 2000;130(3):367–8.

80. Taieb S, Trillet-Lenoir V, Rambaud L, Descos L, Freyer G. L'hermitte sign and urinary retention: atypical presentation of oxaliplatin neurotoxicity in four patients. Cancer 2002;94(9):2434–40.

81. List AF, Kummet TD. Spinal cord toxicity complicating treatment with cisplatin and etoposide. Am J Clin Oncol 1990;13(3):256–8.

82. Taieb S, Trillet-Lenoir V, Rambaud L, Descos L, Freyer G. L'hermitte sign and urinary retention: atypical presentation of oxaliplatin neurotoxicity in four patients. Cancer 2002;94(9):2434–40.

83. Nichols CR, Roth BJ, Williams SD, Gill I, Muggia FM, Stablein DM, Weiss RB, Einhorn LH. No evidence of acute cardiovascular complications of chemotherapy for testicular cancer: an analysis of the Testicular Cancer Intergroup Study. J Clin Oncol 1992;10(5):760–5.

84. Highley M, Meller ST, Pinkerton CR. Seizures and cortical dysfunction following high-dose cisplatin administration in children. Med Pediatr Oncol 1992;20(2):143–8.

85. Sghirlanzoni A, Silvani A, Scaioli V, Pareyson D, Marchesan R, Boiardi A. Cisplatin neuropathy in brain tumor chemotherapy. Ital J Neurol Sci 1992;13(4):311–5.

86. LoMonaco M, Milone M, Batocchi AP, Padua L, Restuccia D, Tonali P. Cisplatin neuropathy: clinical course and neurophysiological findings. J Neurol 1992;239(4):199–204.

87. Cavaletti G, Bogliun G, Marzorati L, Marzola M, Pittelli MR, Tredici G. The incidence and course of paraneoplastic neuropathy in women with epithelial ovarian cancer. J Neurol 1991;238(7):371–4.

88. Cano JR, Catalan B, Jara C. Neuronopatia por cisplatino. [Neuronopathy due to cisplatin.] Rev Neurol 1998;27(158):606–10.

89. Al-Tweigeri T, Magliocco AM, DeCoteau JF. Cortical blindness as a manifestation of hypomagnesemia secondary to cisplatin therapy: case report and review of literature. Gynecol Oncol 1999;72(1):120–2.

90. Lyass O, Lossos A, Hubert A, Gips M, Peretz T. Cisplatin-induced non-convulsive encephalopathy. Anticancer Drugs 1998;9(1):100–4.

91. Gamble GE, Tyrrell P. Acute stroke following cisplatin therapy. Clin Oncol (R Coll Radiol) 1998;10(4):274–5.

92. Doehn C, Buttner H, Fornara P, Jocham D. Fatal basilar artery thrombosis after chemotherapy for testicular cancer. Urol Int 2000;65(1):43–5.

93. Kahn CE Jr, Messersmith RN, Samuels BL. Brachial plexopathy as a complication of intraarterial cisplatin chemotherapy. Cardiovasc Intervent Radiol 1989;12(1):47–9.

94. Walker RW, Cairncross JG, Posner JB. Cerebral herniation in patients receiving cisplatin. J Neurooncol 1988;6(1):61–5.

95. De Lauretis A, De Capua B, Barbieri MT, Bellussi L, Passali D. ABR evaluation of ototoxicity in cancer patients receiving cisplatin or carboplatin. Scand Audiol 1999;28(3):139–43.

96. Grolleau F, Gamelin L, Boisdron-Celle M, Lapied B, Pelhate M, Gamelin E. A possible explanation for a neurotoxic effect of the anticancer agent oxaliplatin on neuronal voltage-gated sodium channels. J Neurophysiol 2001;85(5):2293–7.

97. Adelsberger H, Quasthoff S, Grosskreutz J, Lepier A, Eckel F, Lersch C. The chemotherapeutic oxaliplatin alters voltage-gated Na(+) channel kinetics on rat sensory neurons. Eur J Pharmacol 2000;406(1):25–32.

98. Gornet JM, Savier E, Lokiec F, Cvitkovic E, Misset JL, Goldwasser F. Exacerbation of oxaliplatin neurosensory toxicity following surgery. Ann Oncol 2002;13(8):1315–8.

99. Oshita F, Saijo N, Shinkai T, Eguchi K, Sasaki Y, et al. Correlation between total dose of cisplatin and vibratory perception threshold in chemotherapy-induced peripheral neuropathy of cancer patients. Cancer J 1992;5:165–9.

100. Cavaletti G, Marzorati L, Bogliun G, Colombo N, Marzola M, Pittelli MR, Tredici G. Cisplatin-induced peripheral neurotoxicity is dependent on total-dose intensity and single-dose intensity. Cancer 1992;69(1):203–7.

101. Pratt CB, Goren MP, Meyer WH, Singh B, Dodge RK. Ifosfamide neurotoxicity is related to previous cisplatin treatment for pediatric solid tumors. J Clin Oncol 1990;8(8):1399–401.

102. Marzorati L, Bogluin G, Cavaletti G, Tredici G, Pittelli MR. Neurotoxicity of two different cisplatin treatments. Rev Neurobiol 1990;26:459–64.

103. Pollera CF, Pietrangeli A, Giannarelli D. Cisplatin-induced peripheral neurotoxicity: relationship to dose intensity. Ann Oncol 1991;2(3):212.

104. Kaye SB, Paul J, Cassidy J, Lewis CR, Duncan ID, Gordon HK, Kitchener HC, Cruickshank DJ, Atkinson RJ, Soukop M, Rankin EM, Davis JA,

Reed NS, Crawford SM, MacLean A, Parkin D, Sarkar TK, Kennedy J, Symonds RP. Mature results of a randomized trial of two doses of cisplatin for the treatment of ovarian cancer. Scottish Gynecology Cancer Trials Group. J Clin Oncol 1996;14(7):2113–9.

105. Philip T, Ghalie R, Pinkerton R, Zucker JM, Bernard JL, Leverger G, Hartmann O. A phase II study of high-dose cisplatin and VP-16 in neuroblastoma: a report from the Societé Française d'Oncologie Pédiatrique. J Clin Oncol 1987;5(6):941–50.

106. Daugaard GK, Petrera J, Trojaborg W. Electrophysiological study of the peripheral and central neurotoxic effect of cis-platin. Acta Neurol Scand 1987;76(2):86–93.

107. Amiel H, Gherardi R, Giroux C, et al. Neuropathie au cisplatine. Ann Med Interne 1987;138:101.

108. Castellanos AM, Glass JP, Yung WK. Regional nerve injury after intra-arterial chemotherapy. Neurology 1987;37(5):834–7.

109. von Schlippe M, Fowler CJ, Harland SJ. Cisplatin neurotoxicity in the treatment of metastatic germ cell tumour: time course and prognosis. Br J Cancer 2001;85(6):823–6.

110. Quasthoff S, Hartung HP. Chemotherapy-induced peripheral neuropathy. J Neurol 2002;249(1):9–17.

111. van den Bent MJ, van Putten WL, Hilkens PH, de Wit R, van der Burg ME. Retreatment with dose-dense weekly cisplatin after previous cisplatin chemotherapy is not complicated by significant neuro-toxicity. Eur J Cancer 2002;38(3):387–91.

112. Gill JS, Windebank AJ. Cisplatin-induced apoptosis in rat dorsal root ganglion neurons is associated with attempted entry into the cell cycle. J Clin Invest 1998;101(12):2842–50.

113. Cavaletti G, Zanna C. Current status and future prospects for the treatment of chemotherapy-induced peripheral neurotoxicity. Eur J Cancer 2002;38(14):1832–7.

114. Penz M, Kornek GV, Raderer M, Ulrich-Pur H, Fiebiger W, Scheithauer W. Subcutaneous administration of amifostine: a promising therapeutic option in patients with oxaliplatin-related peripheral sensitive neuropathy. Ann Oncol 2001;12(3):421–2.

115. Gamelin E, Gamelin L, Delva R, Guerin-Meyer V, Morel A, Boisdron-Celle M. Prevention of oxaliplatin peripheral sensory neuropathy by Ca+ gluconate/Mg+ chloride infusions: a retrospective study. Proc Am Soc Clin Oncol 2002;21:A624.

116. McLean MJ, Macdonald RL. Carbamazepine and 10,11-epoxycarbamazepine produce use- and voltage-dependent limitation of rapidly firing action potentials of mouse central neurons in cell culture. J Pharmacol Exp Ther 1986;238(2):727–38.

117. Eckel F, Schmelz R, Adelsberger H, Erdmann J, Quasthoff S, Lersch C. Prophylaxe der Oxaliplatin-induzierten Neuropathie mit Carbamazepin. Eine Pilotstudie. [Prevention of oxaliplatin-induced neuropathy by carbamazepine. A pilot study.] Dtsch Med Wochenschr 2002;127(3):78–82.

118. Levi FA, Zidani R, Vannetzel JM, Perpoint B, Focan C, Faggiuolo R, Chollet P, Garufi C, Itzhaki M, Dogliotti L, et al. Chronomodulated versus fixed-infusion-rate delivery of ambulatory chemotherapy with oxaliplatin, fluorouracil, and folinic acid (leucovorin) in patients with colorectal cancer metastases: a randomized multi-institutional trial. J Natl Cancer Inst 1994;86(21):1608–17.

119. Levi F, Metzger G, Massari C, Milano G. Oxaliplatin: pharmacokinetics and chronopharmacological aspects. Clin Pharmacokinet 2000;38(1):1–21.

120. Levi F, Zidani R, Misset JL. Randomised multicentre trial of chronotherapy with oxaliplatin, fluorouracil, and folinic acid in metastatic colorectal cancer. International Organization for Cancer Chronotherapy. Lancet 1997;350(9079):681–6.

121. Cascinu S, Catalano V, Cordella L, Labianca R, Giordani P, Baldelli AM, Beretta GD, Ubiali E, Catalano G. Neuroprotective effect of reduced glutathione on oxaliplatin-based chemotherapy in advanced colorectal cancer: a randomized, double-blind, placebo-controlled trial. J Clin Oncol 2002;20(16):3478–83.

122. McKeage MJ. Comparative adverse effect profiles of platinum drugs. Drug Saf 1995;13(4):228–44.

123. Bachmeyer C, Decroix Y, Medioni J, Dhote R, Benfiguig K, Houillier P, Grateau G. Coma, crise convulsive et troubles de l'oculomotricité hypomagnésémiques et hypocalcémiques aprés chimiothérapie par sels de platine. [Hypomagnesemic and hypocalcemic coma, convulsions and ocular motility disorders after chemotherapy with platinum compounds.] Rev Med Interne 1996;17(6):467–9.

124. Blakley BW, Myers SF. Patterns of hearing loss resulting from cis-platinum therapy. Otolaryngol Head Neck Surg 1993;109(3 Pt 1):385–91.

125. Laurell G, Engstrom B, Hirsch A, Bagger-Sjoback D. Ototoxicity of cisplatin. Int J Androl 1987;10(1):359–62.

126. Cohen BH, Zweidler P, Goldwein JW, Molloy J, Packer RJ. Ototoxic effect of cisplatin in children with brain tumors. Pediatr Neurosurg 1990–91;16(6):292–6.

127. Pasic TR, Dobie RA. Cis-platinum ototoxicity in children. Laryngoscope 1991;101(9):985–91.

128. Gupta AA, Capra M, Papaioannou V, Hall G, Maze R, Dix D, Weitzman S. Low incidence of ototoxicity with continuous infusion of cisplatin in the treatment of pediatric germ cell tumors. J Pediatr Hematol Oncol 2006;28(2):91–4.

129. Waters GS, Ahmad M, Katsarkas A, Stanimir G, McKay J. Ototoxicity due to cis-diamminedichloroplatinum in the treatment of ovarian cancer: influence of dosage and schedule of administration. Ear Hear 1991;12(2):91–102.

130. Durrant JD, Rodgers G, Myers EN, Johnson JT. Hearing loss—risk factor for cisplatin ototoxicity? Observations. Am J Otol 1990;11(5):375–7.

131. Vantrappen G, Rector E, Debruyne F. Cisplatinum ototoxiciteit: klinische studie. [The ototoxicity of cisplatin: a clinical study.] Acta Otorhinolaryngol Belg 1990;44(4):415–21.

132. Skinner R, Pearson AD, Amineddine HA, Mathias DB, Craft AW. Ototoxicity of cisplatinum in children and adolescents. Br J Cancer 1990;61(6):927–31.

133. Kopelman J, Budnick AS, Sessions RB, Kramer MB, Wong GY. Ototoxicity of high-dose cisplatin by bolus administration in patients with advanced cancers and normal hearing. Laryngoscope 1988;98(8 Pt 1):858–64.

134. Laurell G, Borg E. Ototoxicity of cisplatin in gynaecological cancer patients. Scand Audiol 1988;17(4):241–7.

135. Domenech J, Santabarbara P, Carulla M, Traserra J. Sudden hearing loss in an adolescent following a single dose of cisplatin. ORL J Otorhinolaryngol Relat Spec 1988;50(6):405–8.

136. Aguilar-Markulis NV, Beckley S, Priore R, Mettlin C. Auditory toxicity effects of long-term cis-dichlorodiammineplatinum II therapy in genitourinary cancer patients. J Surg Oncol 1981;16(2):111–23.

137. Berg AL, Spitzer JB, Garvin JH Jr. Ototoxic impact of cisplatin in pediatric oncology patients. Laryngoscope 1999;109(11):1806–14.

138. Melamed LB, Selim MA, Schuchman D. Cisplatin ototoxicity in gynecologic cancer patients. A preliminary report. Cancer 1985;55(1):41–3.

139. Hallmark RJ, Snyder JM, Jusenius K, Tamimi HK. Factors influencing ototoxicity in ovarian cancer patients treated with cis-platinum based chemotherapy. Eur J Gynaecol Oncol 1992;13(1):35–44.

140. Chapman P. Rapid onset hearing loss after cisplatinum therapy: case reports and literature review. J Laryngol Otol 1982;96(2):159–62.

141. Cvitkovic E. Cumulative toxicities from cisplatin therapy and current cytoprotective measures. Cancer Treat Rev 1998;24(4):265–81.

142. Laurell G, Beskow C, Frankendal B, Borg E. Cisplatin administration to gynecologic cancer patients. Long-term effects on hearing. Cancer 1996;78(8):1798–804.

143. Weatherly RA, Owens JJ, Catlin FI, Mahoney DH. Cis-platinum ototoxicity in children. Laryngoscope 1991;101(9):917–24.

144. Moroso MJ, Blair RL. A review of cis-platinum ototoxicity. J Otolaryngol 1983;12(6):365–9.

145. Peters U, Preisler-Adams S, Hebeisen A, Hahn M, Seifert E, Lanvers C, Heinecke A, Horst J, Jurgens H, Lamprecht-Dinnesen A. Glutathione S-transferase genetic polymorphisms and individual sensitivity to the ototoxic effect of cisplatin. Anticancer Drugs 2000;11(8):639–43.

146. Kelsen DP, Alcock N, Young CW. Cisplatin nephrotoxicity. Correlation with plasma platinum concentrations. Am J Clin Oncol 1985;8(1):77–80.

147. Foster-Nora JA, Siden R. Amifostine for protection from antineoplastic drug toxicity. Am J Health Syst Pharm 1997;54(7):787–800.

148. Caston J, Doinel L. Comparative vestibular toxicity of dibekacin, habekacin and cisplatin. Acta Otolaryngol 1987;104(3–4):315–21.

149. Kobayashi H, Ohashi N, Watanabe Y, Mizukoshi K. Clinical features of cisplatin vestibulotoxicity and hearing loss. ORL J Otorhinolaryngol Relat Spec 1987;49(2):67–72.

150. Anniko M, Sobin A. Cisplatin: evaluation of its ototoxic potential. Am J Otolaryngol 1986;7(4):276–93.

151. Ozturan O, Jerger J, Lew H, Lynch GR. Monitoring of cisplatin ototoxicity by distortion-product otoacoustic emissions. Auris Nasus Larynx 1996;23:147–51.

152. Kennedy IC, Fitzharris BM, Colls BM, Atkinson CH. Carboplatin is ototoxic. Cancer Chemother Pharmacol 1990;26(3):232–4.

153. Stavroulaki P, Apostolopoulos N, Segas J, Tsakanikos M, Adamopoulos G. Evoked otoacoustic emissions—an approach for monitoring cisplatin induced ototoxicity in children. Int J Pediatr Otorhinolaryngol 2001;59(1):47–57.

154. de Lemos ML. Application of the area under the curve of carboplatin in predicting toxicity and efficacy. Cancer Treat Rev 1998;24(6):407–14.

155. Bauer FP, Westhofen M, Kehrl W. Zur Ototoxizität des Zytostatikums Carboplatin loei Patienten mit Kopf-Hals-Tumoren. [The ototoxicity of the cytostatic drug carboplatin in patients with head-neck tumors.] Laryngorhinootologie 1992;71(8):412–5.

156. Cavaletti G, Bogliun G, Zincone A, Marzorati L, Melzi P, Frattola L, Marzola M, Bonazzi C, Cantu MG, Chiari S, Galli A, Bregni M, Gianni MA. Neuro- and ototoxicity of high-dose carboplatin treatment in poor prognosis ovarian cancer patients. Anticancer Res 1998;18(5B):3797–802.

157. Cavaletti G, Tredici G, Petruccioli MG, Donde E, Tredici P, Marmiroli P, Minoia C, Ronchi A, Bayssas M, Etienne GG. Effects of different schedules of oxaliplatin treatment on the peripheral nervous system of the rat. Eur J Cancer 2001;37(18):2457–63.

158. Soni N, Bajaj B. Toxic effects of cisplatin on olfaction. Pak J Otolaryngol 1991;7:23–5.

159. Bosl GJ, Bajorunas D. Pituitary and testicular hormonal function after treatment for germ cell tumours. Int J Androl 1987;10(1):381–4.

160. Gerl A, Muhlbayer D, Hansmann G, Mraz W, Hiddemann W. The impact of chemotherapy on Leydig cell function in long term survivors of germ cell tumors. Cancer 2001;91(7):1297–303.

161. Sakakura C, Hagiwara A, Kin S, Yamamoto K, Okamoto K, Yamaguchi T, Sawai K, Yamagishi H. A case of hyperosmolar nonketotic coma occurring during chemotherapy using cisplatin for gallbladder cancer. Hepatogastroenterology 1999;46(29):2801–3.

162. Orbo A, Simonsen E. Cisplatin-induced sodium and magnesium wastage. Eur J Cancer 1992;28A(6–7):1294.

163. Bianchetti MG, Kanaka C, Ridolfi-Luthy A, Hirt A, Wagner HP, Oetliker OH. Persisting renotubular sequelae after cisplatin in children and adolescents. Am J Nephrol 1991;11(2):127–30.

164. Blachley JD, Hill JB. Renal and electrolyte disturbances associated with cisplatin. Ann Intern Med 1981;95(5):628–632.

165. Hutchison FN, Perez EA, Gandara DR, Lawrence HJ, Kaysen GA. Renal salt wasting in patients treated with cisplatin. Ann Intern Med 1988;108(1):21–5.

166. English MW, Skinner R, Pearson AD, Price L, Wyllie R, Craft AW. Dose-related nephrotoxicity of carboplatin in children. Br J Cancer 1999;81(2):336–41.

167. Mulder PO, Sleijfer DT, de Vries EG, Uges DR, Mulder NH. Renal dysfunction following high-dose carboplatin treatment. J Cancer Res Clin Oncol 1988;114(2):212–4.

168. Lajer H, Daugaard G. Cisplatin and hypomagnesemia. Cancer Treat Rev 1999;25(1):47–58.

169. Schilsky RL, Barlock A, Ozols RF. Persistent hypomagnesemia following cisplatin chemotherapy for testicular cancer. Cancer Treat Rep 1982;66(9):1767–9.

170. Macaulay VM, Begent RH, Phillips ME, Newlands ES. Prophylaxis against hypomagnesaemia induced by cis-platinum combination chemotherapy. Cancer Chemother Pharmacol 1982;9(3):179–81.

171. Vogelzang NJ, Torkelson JL, Kennedy BJ. Hypomagnesemia, renal dysfunction, and Raynaud's phenomenon in patients treated with cisplatin, vinblastine, and bleomycin. Cancer 1985;56(12):2765–70.

172. Bellin SL, Selim M. Cisplatin-induced hypomagnesemia with seizures: a case report and review of the literature. Gynecol Oncol 1988;30(1):104–13.

173. Mavichak V, Coppin CM, Wong NL, Dirks JH, Walker V, Sutton RA. Renal magnesium wasting and hypocalciuria in chronic cis-platinum nephropathy in man. Clin Sci (Lond) 1988;75(2):203–7.

174. Lam M, Adelstein DJ. Hypomagnesemia and renal magnesium wasting in patients treated with cisplatin. Am J Kidney Dis 1986;8(3):164–9.

175. Willox JC, McAllister EJ, Sangster G, Kaye SB. Effects of magnesium supplementation in testicular cancer patients receiving cis-platin: a randomised trial. Br J Cancer 1986;54(1):19–23.

176. Markman M, Cleary S, Howell SB. Hypomagnesemia following high-dose intracavitary cisplatin with systemically administered sodium thiosulfate. Am J Clin Oncol 1986;9(5):440–3.

177. Kibirige MS, Morris-Jones PH, Addison GM. Prevention of cisplatin-induced hypomagnesemia. Pediatr Hematol Oncol 1988;5(1):1–6.

178. Bauer FP, Westhofen M. Vestibulotoxische Effekte des zytostatikums Carboplatin bei Patienten mit Kopf-Hals-Tumoren. [Vestibulotoxic effects of the cytostatic drug carboplatin in patients with head and neck tumors.] HNO 1992;40(1):19–24.

179. Sweeney JD, Ziegler P, Pruet C, Spaulding MB. Hyperzincuria and hypozincemia in patients treated with cisplatin. Cancer 1989;63(11):2093–5.

180. Kuzur ME, Greco FA. Cisplatin-induced anemia. N Engl J Med 1980;303(2):110–1.

181. Kunikane H, Watanabe K, Fukuoka M, Saijo N, Furuse K, Ikegami H, Ariyoshi Y, Kishimoto S. Double-blind randomized control trial of the effect of recombinant human erythropoietin on chemotherapy-induced anemia in patients with non-small cell lung cancer. Int J Clin Oncol 2001;6(6):296–301.

182. Pivot X, Guardiola E, Etienne M, Thyss A, Foa C, Otto J, Schneider M, Magne N, Bensadoun RJ, Renee N, Milano G. An analysis of potential factors allowing an individual prediction of cisplatin-induced anaemia. Eur J Cancer 2000;36(7):852–7.

183. Hasegawa I, Tanaka K. Serum erythropoietin levels in gynecologic cancer patients during cisplatin combination chemotherapy. Gynecol Oncol 1992;46(1):65–8.

184. Ruiz MA, Marugan I, Estelles A, Navarro I, Espana F, Alberola V, San Juan L, Aznar J, Garcia-Conde J. The influence of chemotherapy on plasma coagulation and fibrinolytic systems in lung cancer patients. Cancer 1989;63(4):643–8.

185. Louvet C, Lorange A, Letendre F, Beaulieu R, Pretty HM, Courchesne Y, Neemeh JA, Monte M, Latreille J. Acute and delayed emesis after cisplatin-based regimen: description and prevention. Oncology 1991;48(5):392–6.

186. Kobayashi M, To H, Tokue A, Fujimura A, Kobayashi E. Cisplatin-induced vomiting depends on circadian timing. Chronobiol Int 2001;18(5):851–63.

187. Campos D, Pereira JR, Reinhardt RR, Carracedo C, Poli S, Vogel C, Martinez-Cedillo J, Erazo A, Wittreich J, Eriksson LO, Carides AD, Gertz BJ. Prevention of cisplatin-induced emesis by the oral neurokinin-1 antagonist, MK-869, in combination with granisetron and dexamethasone or with dexamethasone alone. J Clin Oncol 2001;19(6):1759–67.

188. Sartori S, Nielsen I, Maestri A, Beltrami D, Trevisani L, Pazzi P. Acute gastroduodenal mucosal injury after cisplatin plus etoposide chemotherapy. Clinical and endoscopic study. Oncology 1991;48(5):356–61.

189. Cavalli F, Tschopp L, Sonntag RW, Zimmermann A. A case of liver toxicity following cis-dichlorodiammineplatinum(II) treatment. Cancer Treat Rep 1978;62(12):2125–6.

190. Bergevin P. Nephrotoxicity of cisplatin (cis-diamminedichloroplatinum (II)). Drug Today 1988;24:403.

191. Daugaard G, Abildgaard U, Holstein-Rathlou NH, Bruunshuus I, Bucher D, Leyssac PP. Renal tubular function in patients treated with high-dose cisplatin. Clin Pharmacol Ther 1988;44(2):164–72.

192. Falkenberg FW, Mondorf U, Pierard D, Gauhl C, Mondorf AW, Mai U, Kantwerk G, Meier U, Rindhage A, Rohracker M. Identification of fragments of proximal and distal tubular cells in the urine of patients under cytostatic treatment by immunoelectron microscopy with monoclonal antibodies. Am J Kidney Dis 1987;9(2):129–37.

193. Safirstein R, Wiston J. Cisplatin nephrotoxicity. J UOEH 1987;9(Suppl):216–22.

194. Safirstein R, Winston J, Moel D, Dikman S, Guttenplan J. Cisplatin nephrotoxicity: insights into mechanism. Int J Androl 1987;10(1):325–46.

195. Anand AJ, Bashey B. Newer insights into cisplatin nephrotoxicity. Ann Pharmacother 1993;27(12):1519–25.

196. Tay LK, Bregman CL, Masters BA, Williams PD. Effects of cis-diamminedichloroplatinum(II) on rabbit kidney in vivo and on rabbit renal proximal tubule cells in culture. Cancer Res 1988;48(9):2538–43.

197. Blochl-Daum B, Pehamberger H, Kurz C, Kyrle PA, Wagner O, Muller M, Monitzer B, Eichler HG. Effects of cisplatin on urinary thromboxane B2 excretion. Clin Pharmacol Ther 1995;58(4):418–24.

198. Imura N, Naganuma A, Satoh M, Koyama Y. Depression of toxic effects of anticancer agents by selenium or pretreatment with metallothionein inducers. J UOEH 1987;9(Suppl):223–9.

199. Stewart DJ, Dulberg CS, Mikhael NZ, Redmond MD, Montpetit VA, Goel R. Association of cisplatin nephrotoxicity with patient characteristics and cisplatin administration methods. Cancer Chemother Pharmacol 1997;40(4):293–308.

200. Skinner R, Pearson AD, English MW, Price L, Wyllie RA, Coulthard MG, Craft AW. Cisplatin dose rate as a risk factor for nephrotoxicity in children. Br J Cancer 1998;77(10):1677–82.

201. Skinner R, Pearson AD, Price L, Coulthard MG, Craft AW. The influence of age on nephrotoxicity following chemotherapy in children. Br J Cancer Suppl 1992;18:S30–5.

202. Hargis JB, Anderson JR, Propert KJ, Green MR, Van Echo DA, Weiss RB. Predicting genitourinary toxicity in patients receiving cisplatin-based combination chemotherapy: a Cancer and Leukemia Group B study. Cancer Chemother Pharmacol 1992;30(4):291–6.

203. Saito M, Masaki T, Kato H, Numasaka K. [A clinical evaluation of the protective effect of fosfomycin (FOM) against the cis-diamminedichloroplatinum (CDDP)-induced nephrotoxicity.]Hinyokika Kiyo 1988;34(5):782–9.

204. Pinzani V, Bressolle F, Haug IJ, Galtier M, Blayac JP, Balmes P. Cisplatin-induced renal toxicity and toxicity-modulating strategies: a review. Cancer Chemother Pharmacol 1994;35(1):1–9.

205. Hausheer FH, Kanter P, Cao S, Haridas K, Seetharamulu P, Reddy D, Petluru P, Zhao M, Murali D, Saxe JD, Yao S, Martinez N, Zukowski A, Rustum YM. Modulation of platinum-induced toxicities and therapeutic index: mechanistic insights and first- and second-generation protecting agents. Semin Oncol 1998;25(5):584–99.

206. Bokemeyer C, Fels LM, Dunn T, Voigt W, Gaedeke J, Schmoll HJ, Stolte H, Lentzen H. Silibinin protects against cisplatin-induced nephrotoxicity without compromising cisplatin or ifosfamide anti-tumour activity. Br J Cancer 1996;74(12):2036–41.

207. Markman M, Cleary S, Howell SB. Nephrotoxicity of high-dose intracavitary cisplatin with intravenous thiosulfate protection. Eur J Cancer Clin Oncol 1985;21(9):1015–8.

208. Hayes DM, Cvitkovic E, Golbey RB, Scheiner E, Helson L, Krakoff IH. High dose cis-platinum diammine dichloride: amelioration of renal toxicity by mannitol diuresis. Cancer 1977;39(4):1372–81.

209. Howell SB, Pfeifle CL, Wung WE, Olshen RA, Lucas WE, Yon JL, Green M. Intraperitoneal cisplatin with systemic thiosulfate protection. Ann Intern Med 1982;97(6):845–51.

210. Abe R, Akiyoshi T, Baba T. "Two-route chemotherapy" using cisplatin and its neutralizing agent, sodium thiosulfate, for intraperitoneal cancer. Oncology 1990;47(5):422–6.

211. Leeuwenkamp OR, van der Vijgh WJ, Neijt JP, Pinedo HM. Reaction kinetics of cisplatin and its monoaquated species with the (potential) renal protecting agents (di)mesna and thiosulfate. Estimation of the effect of protecting agents on the plasma and peritoneal AUCs of CDDP. Cancer Chemother Pharmacol 1990;27(2):111–4.

212. Daugaard G, Holstein-Rathlou NH, Leyssac PP. Effect of cisplatin on proximal convoluted and straight segments of the rat kidney. J Pharmacol Exp Ther 1988;244(3):1081–5.

213. Koukourakis MI. Amifostine in clinical oncology: current use and future applications. Anticancer Drugs 2002;13(3):181–209.

214. Glover D, Glick JH, Weiler C, Fox K, Guerry D. WR-2721 and high-dose cisplatin: an active combination in the treatment of metastatic melanoma. J Clin Oncol 1987;5(4):574–578.

215. Hartmann JT, Kollmannsberger C, Kanz L, Bokemeyer C. Platinum organ toxicity and possible prevention in patients with testicular cancer. Int J Cancer 1999;83(6):866–9.

216. Hartmann JT, Fels LM, Franzke A, Knop S, Renn M, Maess B, Panagiotou P, Lampe H, Kanz L, Stolte H, Bokemeyer C. Comparative study of the acute nephrotoxicity from standard dose cisplatin +/− ifosfamide and high-dose chemotherapy with carboplatin and ifosfamide. Anticancer Res 2000;20(5C):3767–73.

217. Hrushesky WJ. Circadian timing of cancer chemotherapy. Science 1985;228(4695):73–5.

218. Hrushesky WJ, Borch R, Levi F. Circadian time dependence of cisplatin urinary kinetics. Clin Pharmacol Ther 1982;32(3):330–9.

219. Levi F, Benavides M, Chevelle C, Le Saunier F, Bailleul F, Misset JL, Regensberg C, Vannetzel JM, Reinberg A, Mathe G. Chemotherapy of advanced ovarian cancer with 4′-O-tetrahydropyranyl doxorubicin and cisplatin: a randomized phase II trial with an evaluation of circadian timing and dose-intensity. J Clin Oncol 1990;8(4):705–14.

220. Hartmann JT, Fels LM, Knop S, Stolt H, Kanz L, Bokemeyer C. A randomized trial comparing the nephrotoxicity of cisplatin/ifosfamide-based combination chemotherapy with or without amifostine in patients with solid tumors. Invest New Drugs 2000;18(3):281–9.

221. Hartmann JT, Knop S, Fels LM, van Vangerow A, Stolte H, Kanz L, Bokemeyer C. The use of reduced doses of amifostine to ameliorate nephrotoxicity of cisplatin/ifosfamide-based chemotherapy in patients with solid tumors. Anticancer Drugs 2000;11(1):1–6.

222. ten Bokkel Huinink WW, van der Burg ME, van Oosterom AT, Neijt JP, George M, Guastalla JP, Veenhof CH, Rotmensz N, Dalesio O, Vermorken JB. Carboplatin in combination therapy for ovarian cancer. Cancer Treat Rev 1988;15(Suppl B):9–15.

223. Anderson H, Wagstaff J, Crowther D, Swindell R, Lind MJ, McGregor J, Timms MS, Brown D, Palmer P. Comparative toxicity of cisplatin, carboplatin (CBDCA) and iproplatin (CHIP) in combination with cyclophosphamide in patients with advanced epithelial ovarian cancer. Eur J Cancer Clin Oncol 1988;24(9):1471–9.

224. Calvert AH, Horwich A, Newlands ES, Begent R, Rustin GJ, Kaye SB, Harris AL, Williams CJ, Slevin ML. Carboplatin or cisplatin? Lancet 1988;2(8610):577–8.

225. Lee EJ, Egorin MJ, Van Echo DA, Cohen AE, Tait N, Schiffer CA. Phase I and pharmacokinetic trial of carboplatin in refractory adult leukemia. J Natl Cancer Inst 1988;80(2):131–5.

226. Lyttelton MP, Newlands ES, Giles C, Bower M, Guimaraes A, O'Reilly S, Rustin GJ, Samson D, Kanfer EJ. High-dose therapy including carboplatin adjusted for renal function in patients with relapsed or refractory germ cell tumour: outcome and prognostic factors. Br J Cancer 1998;77(10):1672–6.

227. Hardy JR, Tan S, Fryatt I, Wiltshaw E. How nephrotoxic is carboplatin? Br J Cancer 1990;61(4):644.

228. Hartmann JT, von Vangerow A, Fels LM, Knop S, Stolte H, Kanz L, Bokemeyer C. A randomized trial of amifostine in patients with high-dose VIC chemotherapy plus autologous blood stem cell transplantation. Br J Cancer 2001;84(3):313–20.

229. Pinotti G, Martinelli B. A case of acute tubular necrosis due to oxaliplatin. Ann Oncol 2002;13(12):1951–2.

230. Marnocha RS, Hutson PR. Intradermal carboplatin and ifosfamide extravasation in the mouse. Cancer 1992;70(4):850–3.

231. Al-Lamki Z, Pearson P, Jaffe N. Localized cisplatin hyperpigmentation induced by pressure. A case report. Cancer 1996;77(8):1578–81.

232. Baur M, Kienzer HR, Rath T, Dittrich C. Extravasation of oxaliplatin (Eloxatin®) – clinical course. Onkologie 2000;23(5):468–71.

233. Kretzschmar A, Thuss-Patience PC, Pink D, Benter T, Jost D, Scholz C, Reichardt P. Extravasations of oxaliplatin. Proc Am Soc Clin Oncol 2002;21:A2900.

234. Nijman JM, Schraffordt Koops H, Oldhoff J, Kremer J, Sleijfer DT. Sexual function after surgery and combination chemotherapy in men with disseminated nonseminomatous testicular cancer. J Surg Oncol 1988;38(3):182–6.

235. Wallace WH, Shalet SM, Crowne EC, Morris-Jones PH, Gattamaneni HR, Price DA. Gonadal dysfunction due to cis-platinum. Med Pediatr Oncol 1989;17(5):409–13.

236. Khan A, Hill JM, Grater W, Loeb E, MacLellan A, Hill N. Atopic hypersensitivity to cis-dichlorodiammineplatinum(II) and other platinum complexes. Cancer Res 1975;35(10):2766–70.

237. Saunders MP, Denton CP, O'Brien ME, Blake P, Gore M, Wiltshaw E. Hypersensitivity reactions to cisplatin and carboplatin—a report on six cases. Ann Oncol 1992;3(7):574–6.

238. Goldberg A, Altaras MM, Mekori YA, Beyth Y, Confino-Cohen R. Anaphylaxis to cisplatin: diagnosis and value of pretreatment in prevention of recurrent allergic reactions. Ann Allergy 1994;73(3):271–2.

239. Rose PG, Fusco N, Fluellen L, Rodriguez M. Carboplatin hypersensitivity reactions in patients with ovarian and peritoneal carcinoma. Int J Gynecol Obstet 1998;8:365–8.

240. Schiavetti A, Varrasso G, Maurizi P, Castello MA. Hypersensitivity to carboplatin in children. Med Pediatr Oncol 1999;32(3):183–5.

241. Tournigand C, Maindrault-Goebel F, Louvet C, de Gramont A, Krulik M. Severe anaphylactic reactions to oxaliplatin. Eur J Cancer 1998;34(8):1297–8.

242. Weidmann B, Mulleneisen N, Bojko P, Niederle N. Hypersensitivity reactions to carboplatin. Report of two patients, review of the literature, and discussion of diagnostic procedures and management. Cancer 1994;73(8):2218–22.

243. Polyzos A, Tsavaris N, Kosmas C, Arnaouti T, Kalahanis N, Tsigris C, Giannopoulos A, Karatzas G, Giannikos L, Sfikakis PP. Hypersensitivity reactions to

carboplatin administration are common but not always severe: a 10-year experience. Oncology 2001;61(2):129–33.

244. Williamson SK, Tangen CM, Maddox AM, Spiridonidis CH, Macdonald JS. Phase II evaluation of low-dose continuous 5-fluorouracil and weekly cisplatin in advanced adenocarcinoma of the stomach. A Southwest Oncology Group study. Am J Clin Oncol 1995;18(6):484–7.

245. Dold F, Hoey D, Carberry M, Musket A, Friedberg V, Mitchell E. Hypersensitivity in patients with metastatic colorectal carcinoma undergoing chemotherapy with oxaliplatin. Proc Am Soc Clin Oncol 2002;21:A1478.

246. Hendrick AM, Simmons D, Cantwell BM. Allergic reactions to carboplatin. Ann Oncol 1992;3(3):239–40.

247. Markman M, Kennedy A, Webster K, Elson P, Peterson G, Kulp B, Belinson J. Clinical features of hypersensitivity reactions to carboplatin. J Clin Oncol 1999;17(4):1141.

248. Sims-McCallum RP. Outpatient carboplatin desensitization in a pediatric patient with bilateral optic glioma. Ann Pharmacother 2000;34(4):477–8.

249. Goldberg A, Confino-Cohen R, Fishman A, Beyth Y, Altaras M. A modified, prolonged desensitization protocol in carboplatin allergy. J Allergy Clin Immunol 1996;98(4):841–3.

250. Meyer L, Zuberbier T, Worm M, Oettle H, Riess H. Hypersensitivity reactions to oxaliplatin: cross-reactivity to carboplatin and the introduction of a desensitization schedule. J Clin Oncol 2002;20(4):1146–7.

251. Ulrich-Pur H, Penz M, Fiebiger WC, Schull B, Kornek GV, Scheithauer W, Raderer M. Oxaliplatin-induced fever and release of IL-6. Oncology 2000;59(3):187–9.

252. Chiche D, Pico JL, Bernaudin JF, Chouaib S, Wollman E, Arnoux A, Denizot Y, Nitenberg G. Pulmonary edema and shock after high-dose aracytine-C for lymphoma; possible role of TNF-alpha and PAF. Eur Cytokine Netw 1993;4(2):147–51.

253. Khalil A, Chammas M, Shamseddine A, Seoud M. Fatal acute tumor lysis syndrome following treatment of vulvar carcinoma: case report. Eur J Gynaecol Oncol 1998;19(4):415–6.

254. Beck DJ, Brubaker RR. Mutagenic properties of cis-plantinum(II)diammino-dichloride in *Escherichia coli*. Mutat Res 1975;27(2):181–9.

255. Travis LB, Holowaty EJ, Bergfeldt K, Lynch CF, Kohler BA, Wiklund T, Curtis RE, Hall P, Andersson M, Pukkala E, Sturgeon J, Stovall M. Risk of leukemia after platinum-based chemotherapy for ovarian cancer. N Engl J Med 1999;340(5):351–7.

256. Duffner PK, Krischer JP, Horowitz ME, Cohen ME, Burger PC, Friedman HS, Kun LE. Second malignancies in young children with primary brain tumors following treatment with prolonged postoperative chemotherapy and delayed irradiation: a Pediatric Oncology Group study. Ann Neurol 1998;44(3):313–6.

257. Pont J, Albrecht W. Fertility after chemotherapy for testicular germ cell cancer. Fertil Steril 1997;68(1):1–5.

258. Meistrich ML, Chawla SP, Da Cunha MF, Johnson SL, Plager C, Papadopoulos NE, Lipshultz LI, Benjamin RS. Recovery of sperm production after chemotherapy for osteosarcoma. Cancer 1989;63(11):2115–23.

259. Hansen PV, Glavind K, Panduro J, Pedersen M. Paternity in patients with testicular germ cell cancer: pretreatment and post-treatment findings. Eur J Cancer 1991;27(11):1385–9.

260. Rustin GJ, Pektasides D, Bagshawe KD, Newlands ES, Begent RH. Fertility after chemotherapy for male and female germ cell tumours. Int J Androl 1987;10(1):389–92.

261. Richter P, Buchholz K, Lotze W. Schwangerschaftsverlauf und Geburt nach zytostatischer Behandlung von Throphoblasttumoren. [Course of pregnancy and labor following cytostatic treatment of trophoblastic tumors.] Zentralbl Gynakol 1987;109(9):586–9.

262. Pryzant RM, Meistrich ML, Wilson G, Brown B, McLaughlin P. Long-term reduction in sperm count after chemotherapy with and without radiation therapy for non-Hodgkin's lymphomas. J Clin Oncol 1993;11(2):239–47.

263. Lamont EB, Schilsky RL. Gonadal toxicity and teratogenicity after cytotoxic chemotherapy. In: Lipp HP, editor. Anticancer Drug Toxicity; Prevention, Management and Clinical Pharmacokinetics. New York-Basel: Marcel Dekker Inc, 1999:491–523.

264. Frustaci S, Barzan L, Comoretto R, Tumolo S, Lo Re G, Monfardini S. Local neurotoxicity after intra-arterial cisplatin in head and neck cancer. Cancer Treat Rep 1987;71(3):257–9.

265. Chu G, Mantin R, Shen YM, Baskett G, Sussman H. Massive cisplatin overdose by accidental substitution for carboplatin. Toxicity and management. Cancer 1993;72(12):3707–14.

266. Neef C, de Voogd-van der Straaten I. An interaction between cytostatic and anticonvulsant drugs. Clin Pharmacol Ther 1988;43(4):372–5.

267. Dofferhoff AS, Berendsen HH, vd Naalt J, Haaxma-Reiche H, Smit EF, Postmus PE. Decreased phenytoin level after carboplatin treatment. Am J Med 1990;89(2):247–8.

268. Lauer AK, Wobig JL, Shults WT, Neuwelt EA, Wilson MW. Severe ocular and orbital toxicity after intra-carotid etoposide phosphate and carboplatin therapy. Am J Ophthalmol 1999;127(2):230–3.

269. Coninx P, Nasca S, Lebrun D, Panis X, Lucas P, Garbe E, Legros M. Sequential trial of initial chemotherapy for advanced cancer of the head and neck. DDP versus DDP + 5-fluorouracil Cancer 1988;62(9):1888–92.

270. Stefenelli T, Kuzmits R, Ulrich W, Glogar D. Acute vascular toxicity after combination chemotherapy with cisplatin, vinblastine, and bleomycin for testicular cancer. Eur Heart J 1988;9(5):552–6.

271. Sasaki M, Suzuki A, Ishihara T. [A case of acute myocardial infarction after treatment with cisplatin.]Gan To Kagaku Ryoho 1989;16(6):2289–91.

272. Tsutsumi I, Ozawa Y, Kawakami A, Fujii H, Asamoto H. [Acute myocardial infarction induced by lung cancer chemotherapy with cisplatin and eto poside.]Gan To Kagaku Ryoho 1990;17(3 Pt 1):413–7.

273. Murin J, Kasper J, Danko J, Cerna M, Bulas J, Uhliar R. Vznik infarktu myokardu u choreho lieceneho 5-fluorouracilom. [The development of myocardial infarct in a patient treated with 5-fluorouracil.] Vnitr Lek 1989;35(10):1020–4.

274. Mazoyer G, Assouline D, Fourchard V, Kalb JC. Cardiotoxicité du 5 fluoro-uracile. A propos d'une observation. [Cardiotoxicity of 5 fluoro-uracil. Apropos of a case.] Rev Mal Respir 1989;6(6):551–3.

275. Dodds HM, Bishop JF, Rivory LP. More about: irinotecan-related cholinergic syndrome induced by coadministration of oxaliplatin. J Natl Cancer Inst 1999;91(1):91–2.

276. Beijnen JH, Vlasveld LT, Wanders J, ten Bokkel Huinink WW, Rodenhuis S. Effect of cisplatin-containing

chemotherapy on lithium serum concentrations. Ann Pharmacother 1992;26(4):488–90.

277. Jäger AH, Bogdahn U, Apfel R, Pfeufer B, Dekant A. In vitro studies on interaction of 4-hydroperoxyifosfamide and 2-mercaptoethanesulphonate in malignant gliomas. J Cancer Res Clin Oncol 1993;119(12):721–6.

278. Dogliotti L, Bertetto O, Berruti A, Clerico M, Fanchini L, Sicora W, Faggiuolo R. Combination chemotherapy with carboplatin and methotrexate in the treatment of advanced urothelial carcinoma. A phase II study. Am J Clin Oncol 1995;18(1):78–82.

279. Haas A, Anderson L, Lad T. The influence of aminoglycosides on the nephrotoxicity of cis-diamminedichloroplatinum in cancer patients. J Infect Dis 1983;147(2):363.

280. Sleijfer S, van der Mark TW, Schraffordt Koops H, Mulder NH. Enhanced effects of bleomycin on pulmonary function disturbances in patients with decreased renal function due to cisplatin. Eur J Cancer 1996;32A(3):550–2.

281. Rowinsky EK, Gilbert MR, McGuire WP, Noe DA, Grochow LB, Forastiere AA, Ettinger DS, Lubejko BG, Clark B, Sartorius SE, et al. Sequences of taxol and cisplatin: a phase I and pharmacologic study. J Clin Oncol 1991;9(9):1692–703.

282. Jekunen AP, Christen RD, Shalinsky DR, Howell SB. Synergistic interaction between cisplatin and taxol in human ovarian carcinoma cells in vitro. Br J Cancer 1994;69(2):299–306.

283. Vanhoefer U, Harstrick A, Wilke H, Schleucher N, Walles H, Schroder J, Seeber S. Schedule-dependent antagonism of paclitaxel and cisplatin in human gastric and ovarian carcinoma cell lines in vitro. Eur J Cancer 1995;31A(1):92–7.

284. Sonnichsen DS, Relling MV. Clinical pharmacokinetics of paclitaxel. Clin Pharmacokinet 1994;27(4):256–69.

285. Baker AF, Dorr RT. Drug interactions with the taxanes: clinical implications. Cancer Treat Rev 2001;27(4):221–33.

286. Wasserheit C, Frazein A, Oratz R, Sorich J, Downey A, Hochster H, Chachoua A, Wernz J, Zeleniuch-Jacquotte A, Blum R, Speyer J. Phase II trial of paclitaxel and cisplatin in women with advanced breast cancer: an active regimen with limiting neurotoxicity. J Clin Oncol 1996;14(7):1993–9Erratum in: J Clin Oncol 1996;14(12):3175.

287. Bokemeyer C, Berger CC, Hartmann JT, Kollmannsberger C, Schmoll HJ, Kuczyk MA, Kanz L. Analysis of risk factors for cisplatin-induced ototoxicity in patients with testicular cancer. Br J Cancer 1998;77(8):1355–62.

288. Kearns CM, Belani CP, Erkmen K, Zuhowski M, Hiponia D, Zacharski D, Engstrom C, Ramanathan R, Trenn MR, Aisner J, et al. Pharmacokinetics of paclitaxel and carboplatin in combination. Semin Oncol 1995;22(5 Suppl 12):1–4discussion 5–7.

289. Mayerhofer K, Bodner-Adler B, Bodner K, Leodolter S, Kainz C. Paclitaxel/carboplatin as first-line chemotherapy in advanced ovarian cancer: efficacy and adverse effects with special consideration of peripheral neurotoxicity. Anticancer Res 2000;20(5C):4047–50.

290. Mayerhofer K, Bodner-Adler B, Bodner K, Saletu B, Schindl M, Kaider A, Hefler L, Leodolter S, Kainz C. A paclitaxel-containing chemotherapy does not cause central nervous adverse effects: a prospective study in patients with ovarian cancer. Anticancer Res 2000;20(5C):4051–5.

RETINOIDS

General Information

Vitamin A (retinol) is a key regulator of epithelial cell proliferation and differentiation. Aberrations in these processes are a feature of many skin diseases, and dermatologists have therefore long taken an interest in vitamin A as a therapeutic agent. However, marginal efficacy and unacceptable adverse effects (Table 1) have minimized the usefulness of vitamin A itself. Therefore, derivatives of vitamin A (retinoids) have been developed.

Tretinoin

Tretinoin (*all-trans*-retinoic acid), a natural metabolite of vitamin A, was the first vitamin A analogue to be used orally, with some success, but its general therapeutic ratio did not differ markedly from that of vitamin A itself.

Tretinoin cream is used extensively for the treatment of acne and photodamaged skin, and local irritant dermatitis is common. With normal use, absorption is minimal and systemic adverse effects are therefore not expected.

Topical tretinoin has also been used as an ophthalmic ointment 0.01% in the treatment of squamous metaplasia associated with dry eyes. In 161 patients with either keratoconjunctivitis sicca or conjunctival cicatricial diseases (Stevens–Johnson syndrome, inactive pemphigoid, radiation-induced dry eye, drug-induced pseudopemphigoid, and toxic epidermal necrolysis) there were no beneficial effects in the former, but significant reversal of conjunctival keratinization in the temporal bulbar site in the latter (1). Adverse effects were limited to blepharoconjunctivitis and resolved on withdrawal.

Tretinoin has been evaluated in 26 patients with histologically confirmed adenocarcinoma of the prostate and manifestations of progressive metastatic disease (2). They received a single oral dose of tretinoin 45 mg/m²/day for 7 days followed by no treatment for 7 days before starting to take tretinoin again. Toxicity was mostly mild. There was cheilosis in eleven patients and vomiting in one. In eight patients there were transient rises in serum triglyceride concentrations up to three times normal, returning

Table 1 Clinical effects of chronic hypervitaminosis A, in order of decreasing frequency (3,4)

Scaling of skin, erythema, pruritus, altered hair growth
Dry mucous membranes, cheilitis, angular stomatitis, gingivitis,glossitis
Pain and tenderness of the bones, restricted movement
Occipital headache
Hyperirritability, sleep disturbances
Papillary edema, diplopia
Anorexia, weight loss
Hepatomegaly, sometimes with splenomegaly
Peripheral edema
Fatigue, lassitude, occasionally somnolence
Hemorrhages, epistaxis, increased menstrual bleeding

to normal within 3–6 weeks, despite continuation of tretinoin. One patient had a severe headache with vomiting on day 1 and required a 30% dosage reduction. No patient withdrew because of toxicity.

Fatal adverse effects have been reported in patients given tretinoin for acute promyelocytic leukemia (5). Of 82 patients with acute promyelocytic leukemia, 35 developed leukocytosis and 22 had fatal adverse effects (15 with the retinoic acid syndrome and 7 with intracranial bleeding). Leukocytosis was a risk factor for fatal adverse effects. The authors suggested that the combination of tretinoin with low-dose harringtonine can reduce the incidence of leukocytosis-related intracranial bleeding and glucocorticoids can reduce mortality from the retinoic acid syndrome.

In another study of 413 patients with acute promyelocytic leukemia treated with tretinoin plus daunorubicin, the retinoic acid syndrome occurred in 64 cases, of which 5 were fatal (6).

Tretinoin 70, 110, 150, 190, or 230 mg/m²/day has been given to 26 patients with advanced potentially hormone-responsive breast cancer taking tamoxifen 20 mg/day (7). At all doses headaches, nausea, skin changes, and bone pain occurred. The headaches were most severe during the first week of treatment, peaking at the end of the first week. They were sometimes associated with nausea and occasionally with vomiting, although there was no other evidence of raised cerebrospinal fluid pressure. Headaches and nausea tended to subside during the weeks when tretinoin was not given and recurred during the weeks of tretinoin reintroduction, although their severity tended to wane with subsequent cycles of treatment. Similarly, skin reactions, such as erythema and desquamation, were dose-related and were most severe during the initial cycles of treatment. Bone pain occurred intermittently. There was life-threatening hypercalcemia in one patient, but it was felt to be due to disease progression. The dose of 230 mg/m²/day produced unacceptable headache and skin toxicity, but doses of up to 190 mg/m²/day were tolerable.

A dry scaling skin rash and cheilitis were the most common adverse effects in 14 patients with prostate cancer treated with tretinoin and 20 patients treated with a combination of *cis*-retinoic acid and interferon α-2a (8). There was anorexia and significant weight loss in under 10% of the patients, but one patient discontinued treatment because of persistent fatigue and anorexia. Hematological toxic effects included leukopenia, neutropenia, anemia, and thrombocytopenia. Two patients with mild urinary hesitancy had acute urinary outlet obstruction within 1 week of starting *cis*-retinoic acid plus interferon. There were mild rises in hepatic transaminases and serum triglycerides in over half of the patients. Most triglyceride concentrations were below 2.3 (reference range 0.6–1.9) mmol/l, but one patient had an extreme rise of triglycerides to 3280 mg/dl. Sensory and mood changes were mild and occurred mostly in those given *cis*-retinoic acid plus interferon. Headaches were the most common neurological abnormality with tretinoin. Pulmonary adverse effects were dyspnea and a non-fatal pulmonary embolism in one patient treated with tretinoin. Other adverse effects included constipation, fever, nausea, vomiting, diarrhea, fatigue, and stomatitis.

In 21 patients with squamous cell carcinomas of the head and neck randomized to tretinoin 45, 50, or 150 mg/m^2 either once daily or as divided doses every 8 hours for 1 year, severe adverse effects included headache in five patients, hypertriglyceridemia in six, mucositis in two, and hyperbilirubinemia, raised alkaline phosphatase, colitis, raised lipase, xerostomia, eczema, and arthritis in one patient each (9). The dose had to be reduced in seven of eight patients with severe toxicity at 90 mg/m^2/day. Three of nine patients taking 45 mg/m^2/day required dose reductions. The plasma AUC of tretinoin did not correlate with the severity or frequency of adverse effects. From these results it can be concluded that 15 mg/m^2/day every 8 hours is a tolerable dose for 1 year in patients with squamous cell carcinomas of the head and neck.

The adverse effects of tretinoin 50 mg/m^2/day for 3 months have been studied in 20 patients with emphysema in a randomized, double-blind, placebo-controlled trial (10). The treatment was well tolerated and associated with only mild adverse effects, including skin changes, such as dry skin and cracking lips in 15 (1 placebo), transient headache in 13 (1), hyperlipidemia in 11 (5), pruritus in 6 (2), muscle/bone pain in 6 (0), generalized fatigue in 6 (2), raised transaminases in 5 (1), a sensation of clogged ears in 3 (2), nausea in 2 (0), hair loss in 2 (0), and blurred vision in 1 (1).

Etretinate and isotretinoin

Since the beginning of the 1980s two synthetic retinoids, etretinate (the ethyl ester of trimethoxymethylphenyl retinoic acid; Tigason; Tegison) and isotretinoin (13-*cis*-retinoic acid; Acutane; Roaccutane), have been successfully administered for a variety of skin disorders, all of which involve disordered epidermal or epithelial cell growth and differentiation as prominent pathogenic features, for example psoriasis, ichthyosis, Darier's disease, lichen planus, and pityriasis rubra pilaris. Isotretinoin has been of great value in the treatment of cystic acne and acne conglobata, with no serious long-term adverse effects (11,12). It has also been used for milder forms of acne (13,14).

Acitretin

In 1990, etretinate (Tigason) was replaced by acitretin (Neo-Tigason), an aromatic retinoid, a carboxylic acid metabolite of etretinate (15). It is effective in pustular psoriasis and psoriatic palmoplantar keratoderma and in combination with PUVA or topical therapy (calcipotriol or glucocorticoids) in the treatment of other forms of psoriasis. It has also been used to treat disorders of keratinization (ichthyosis, palmoplantar keratoderma, Darier's disease) and severe cutaneous forms of lichen planus. It prevents new skin carcinomas in patients with xeroderma pigmentosum and those who are immunosuppressed. The main

advantage of acitretin is its short half-life of 50 hours, compared with over 80 days for etretinate (16).

Adapalene

Topical retinoids and similar drugs, including tretinoin, adapalene, and tazaroten, are the most commonly used topical drugs for acne (17). Adapalene is a synthetic poly-aromatic retinoid and is formulated in a water-based gel (1.0%, Galderma Labs Inc, San Antonio, TX). In a double-blind, multicenter, parallel-group, randomized study the efficacy and adverse effects of 0.1% adapalene gel and 0.1% tretinoin gel in a microsphere formulation were compared over 12 weeks (18). The two drugs had similar effects on the resolution of acne lesions, but tretinoin was significantly more effective in reducing the number of comedones. There were no statistically significant differences between tretinoin and adapalene in the incidences of erythema, burning/stinging, or itching. Most patients had at least one sign of cutaneous irritation over the course of the study (tretinoin 95%, adapalene 91%). The most common adverse effect was erythema (tretinoin 83%, adapalene 66%), followed by peeling (80% and 66%), dryness (67% and 65%), burning/stinging (45% and 36%), and itching (37% and 35%). There were significant differences in the incidence of cutaneous effects in favor of adapalene for dryness at week 8 (tretinoin 34%, adapalene 18%) and week 10 (29% and 12%), and for peeling at week 3 (56% and 39%), week 6 (46% and 26%), week 8 (45% and 17%), and week 10 (35% and 17%). There were no serious adverse events in either group.

In another comparison of the efficacy and adverse effects of adapalene gel 1% or 0.025% tretinoin gel in 150 Chinese patients, similar effects were observed (19). In both groups skin irritation was mild, but it was more pronounced with tretinoin. Burning was the most common unwanted effect in those who used tretinoin compared with adapalene (34 versus 11%). There was dryness of the skin in 34% of those who used tretinoin and in 22% of those who used adapalene. The respective frequencies of scaling were 26 and 15%, and of erythema 26 and 2.7%. Pruritus was the only adverse effect experienced exclusively by those who used adapalene, and it occurred in under 4%. Overall, 46% of those who used tretinoin had some form of irritation, compared with 32% of those who used adapalene.

General adverse effects

Although the various retinoids have similar toxicity profiles, they differ in the extent to which they affect various body systems. Cutaneous and mucous membrane symptoms (up to 70%) are by far the most prominent adverse effects; patients who use isotretinoin have a 50% incidence of conjunctivitis and irritation of the eyes. Musculoskeletal symptoms occur in up to 15% of users. Hypersensitivity reactions are rare and consist of occasional drug rashes. The occurrence of sarcomas in patients treated with isotretinoin may well be a chance finding (SEDA-21, 164); retinoids may prevent or even cure certain malignancies (20). All the retinoids are strongly teratogenic (21–23).

The incidence and time-course of adverse events during a 4-month course of oral isotretinoin (1 mg/kg) for severe acne have been studied prospectively in 189 patients (24). Most of the adverse events were most often reported during the first 3 months of treatment. However, only a few patients were seen every month as scheduled and only 50 of 189 filled in the questionnaire at 4 months.

In a retrospective study, 22 children taking tretinoin (median age 9.3 years, range 1.8–16.3) for a median of 38 (6–138) days were compared with 22 taking conventional therapy (median age 12.3 years, range: 3.2–16.7) (25). Overall, 12 of 22 patients had symptoms associated with tretinoin (Table 2). Three developed the retinoic acid syndrome.

Retinoic acid syndrome
The retinoic acid syndrome is a generalized severe capillary leakage syndrome with leukocyte activation, which results in weight gain, pulmonary infiltrates or pleural effusions with acute respiratory distress, and fever without infection. It occurs in up to 25% of patients. Postmortem reports of patients who have died from this syndrome have shown infiltration of maturing myeloid cells and edema in the lungs (26). The myeloid cells are considered to release various types of cytokines responsible for symptoms such as fever, weight gain, and heart failure. Improvement can be obtained by glucocorticoid treatment, which suppresses the effects of cytokines. Chest CT provides an accurate assessment of the size, number, and distribution of pulmonary opacities associated with the syndrome, as has been demonstrated anecdotally (27).

Of 69 patients with acute promyelocytic leukemia treated with tretinoin for 5 years, 15 developed retinoic acid syndrome (28). The following features were found on chest radiographs: an increased cardiothoracic ratio, an increased pedicle width, pulmonary congestion in 13, pleural effusion in 11, ground-glass opacities, septal lines, and peribronchial cuffing in 9, consolidation and nodules in 7, and an air bronchogram in 5. Three patients had pulmonary hemorrhages and bilateral, diffuse, poorly delineated nodules and ground-glass opacities on radiography. Lung infiltrates cleared completely within 8 days after administration of prednisolone.

- A 69-year-old man developed dyspnea, hypoxia, and heart failure 4 days after starting to take tretinoin 70 mg/day. His highest white blood cell count was $72 \times 109/l$. A plain chest X-ray showed two pulmonary opacities, increased attenuation in the left lower lobe, and bilateral pleural effusions, but a chest CT also showed multiple irregular-shaped opacities localized in the centrilobular and subpleural regions. He improved over 10 days with prednisolone (total dose 5750 mg) and daunorubicin (total dose 360 mg).

The retinoic acid syndrome, its incidence and clinical course, has been investigated in 167 patients taking tretinoin as induction and maintenance therapy for acute promyelocytic leukemia (29). The syndrome did not occur during maintenance therapy. During induction it occurred in 44 patients (26%) at a median of 11 (range 2–47) days. The major manifestations included respiratory distress (84%), fever (81%), pulmonary edema (54%), pulmonary infiltrates (52%), pleural or pericardial effusions (36%), hypotension (18%), bone pain (14%), headache (14%), congestive heart failure (11%), and acute renal insufficiency (11%). The median white blood cell count was $1.45 \times 10^9/l$ at diagnosis and $31 \times 10^9/l$ (range 6.8–$72 \times 10^9/l$) at the time the syndrome developed. Tretinoin was continued in eight of the 44 patients, with subsequent resolution in 7. It was withdrawn in 36 patients and then reintroduced in 19, after which the syndrome recurred in 3, with one death attributable to reintroduction of the drug. Ten of these 36 patients received chemotherapy without further tretinoin, and 8 achieved complete remission. Of seven patients in whom tretinoin was not reintroduced and who were not given chemotherapy, five achieved complete remission and two died. Two deaths were definitely attributable to the syndrome.

Table 2 Features of tretinoin toxicity in 22 patients

Organ system	N (%)	Symptoms	N (%)
Tretinoin-related toxicity	12 (55)	Retinoic acid syndrome	3 (14)
Cardiovascular	5 (23)	Pericardial effusion	1 (5)
		Weight gain	5 (23)
		Arterial hypotension	2 (9)
Respiratory	3 (14)	Adult respiratory distress syndrome	2 (9)
		Pleural effusion	1 (5)
		Pulmonary infiltrates	1 (5)
Nervous system	6 (27)	Headache	6 (27)
		Raised intracranial pressure	1 (5)
Liver and metabolism	12 (55)	Raised transaminases	6 (27)
		Raised bilirubin	1 (5)
		Raised triglycerides	2 (9)
Hematologic	4 (18)	Leukocytosis	4 (18)
Skin andmusculoskeletal	4 (18)	Dry skin	1 (5)
		Itching	1 (5)
		Joint/bone/muscle pain	3 (14)
		Osteonecrosis	1 (5)

In 63 patients with acute promyelocytic leukemia taking tretinoin (60 mg/day) the rates of leukocytosis, intracranial hypertension, and retinoic acid syndrome were 57%, 9.5%, and 3.2% respectively; the death rate was 11% (30). The authors suggested that progressive leukocytosis during tretinoin therapy should be an indication for chemotherapy (for example, with homoharringtonine); if the white cell count exceeds $10 \times 10^9/l$ before treatment, the patient should be given homoharringtonine only; if it is below $5.0 \times 10^9/l$ homoharringtonine plus tretinoin should be used.

A syndrome similar to that of the retinoic acid syndrome occurred after 10 days of tretinoin therapy in a patient with a relapse of acute myeloblastic leukemia (31).

- A 75-year-old woman whose acute myeloblastic leukemia relapsed was treated with one dose of intravenous idarubicin (10 mg/m^2), cytarabine 20 mg subcutaneously for 10 days, and oral tretinoin 45 mg/m^2/day. Ten days later she developed a persistent fever. A chest X-ray and a CT scan showed bilateral pleural effusions and interstitial infiltrates, but no pulmonary embolus. Tretinoin was withdrawn and she was given intravenous dexamethasone 10 mg every 12 hours. Her fever disappeared within 24 hours and her respiratory distress gradually improved during the next 24–48 hours. A chest X-ray 7 days later showed total resolution.

The incidence, clinical features, and outcome of retinoic acid syndrome have been analysed in 413 cases of newly diagnosed acute promyelocytic leukemia (26). Patients under 65 years old with a white blood cell count below 5 x $10^9/l$ were initially randomized to tretinoin followed by chemotherapy or to tretinoin with chemotherapy started on day 3. In patients with white cell counts over $5 \times 10^9/l$ chemotherapy was rapidly added if the white cell count was greater than 6, 10, and $15 \times 10^9/l$ by days 5, 10, and 15 of tretinoin treatment. The retinoic acid syndrome occurred during induction treatment in 64 of 413 patients (15%). Clinical signs developed after a median of 7 (range 0–35) days. In two cases they were present before the start of treatment; in 11 they occurred on recovery from the phase of aplasia due to the addition of chemotherapy. Respiratory distress (98% of patients), fever (81%), pulmonary infiltrates (81%), weight gain (50%), pleural effusion (47%), renal failure (39%), pericardial effusion (19%), cardiac failure (17%), and hypertension (12%) were the main clinical signs. Mechanical ventilation was required in 13 patients and dialysis in 2. A total of 55 patients (86%) who experienced the retinoic acid syndrome achieved complete remission, compared with 94% of patients who had no retinoic acid syndrome, and nine died of the syndrome. None of the patients with complete remission who received tretinoin for maintenance had recurrence of the syndrome. The syndrome was associated with a lower event-free survival and survival at 2 years.

Retinoic acid syndrome has been reported in a patient who developed diffuse alveolar hemorrhage while being treated with tretinoin for acute promyelocytic leukemia (32).

- An 18-year-old woman developed promyelocytic leukemia and was given tretinoin and dexamethasone. At 15 days she developed significant hemoptysis and respiratory failure, requiring mechanical ventilation. Her temperature was 39.1 °C and she had disseminated intravascular coagulation. A lung biopsy showed diffuse interstitial neutrophilic infiltration, interstitial fibrinoid necrosis, and diffuse alveolar hemorrhage; pulmonary capillaritis was diagnosed. She was given intravenous methylprednisolone 1 g/day for 3 days followed by a tapering dose of oral prednisolone. She subsequently completed a full 45-day course of tretinoin.

Organs and Systems

Cardiovascular

An increased risk of thrombotic events, especially coronary thrombosis, has been reported in elderly patients taking retinoids (33). Two patients with acute promyelocytic leukemia developed thrombus in the right ventricle during induction treatment with tretinoin plus idarubicin (34).

- A 51-year-old man with acute promyelocytic leukemia suddenly developed hypoxemia, pulmonary infiltrates, and arterial hypotension, without fever or thoracic pain on day 11 of tretinoin treatment. He was pancytopenic, his coagulation parameters were normal, and cardiological examination was normal. High-dose dexamethasone (10 mg bd) was started, with prompt resolution of the clinical and radiological signs. Eight days later echocardiography showed a 3 cm non-homogeneous mass in the right ventricle. He was given subcutaneous low molecular weight heparin and the thrombus started to get smaller after 17 days. Oral anticoagulant therapy was started, and there was a further reduction of the size of the thrombus over the following year.
- A 32-year-old woman with acute promyelocytic leukemia developed severe retinoic acid syndrome after 3 days, with respiratory failure, fever, and bilateral lung infiltrates. Withdrawal of tretinoin and treatment with dexamethasone and antibiotics rapidly ameliorated the syndrome, and on day 10 tretinoin was restarted. However, routine echocardiography showed a 3 cm pedunculated mass in the right ventricle. There was consistent and stable reduction of the mass after 1 year of oral anticoagulant therapy.

Respiratory

The manufacturers have on record in the USA several pulmonary adverse effects during isotretinoin therapy, including worsening of asthma (SEDA-21, 162), recurrent pneumothorax, pleural effusion, interstitial fibrosis, pulmonary granuloma, and deterioration in lung function tests. Exercise-induced asthma (35) may be caused by a significant reduction in the forced expiratory flow rate (36) and a drying effect of isotretinoin on the mucous membranes of the respiratory tract (37).

Respiratory distress has been attributed to tretinoin.

- A 56-year-old woman with acute promyelocytic leukemia developed a fever of unknown origin, weight gain of 5 kg, and respiratory distress 9 days after the start of treatment with tretinoin 45 mg/m^2 (38). Her white cell count rose to 21×10^9/l despite treatment with cytosine arabinoside and idarubicin. A chest X-ray showed bilateral alveolar opacities. She recovered fully after 5 days of treatment with dexamethasone 10 mg bd.
- A 24-year-old woman with acute promyelocytic leukemia took tretinoin, and 2 days later developed dyspnea and general aching (39). Her total leukocyte count was 5.04×10^9/l, her PaO_2 was 42.5 mmHg, and a chest X-ray showed bilateral parenchymal infiltration consistent with respiratory distress syndrome. She recovered within 3 days of treatment with low-dose cytarabine and glucocorticoids, without withdrawal of the retinoic acid.

Although the retinoic acid syndrome involves the lungs, pulmonary hemorrhage has only rarely been reported. Two patients with acute promyelocytic leukemia developed severe lung hemorrhage during the first 3 weeks of treatment with tretinoin, shortly after the administration of chemotherapy (40).

- A 36-year-old man with acute promyelocytic leukemia was given tretinoin 45 mg/m^2/day, daunorubicin, and cytarabine. A week later his platelet count fell to 10×10^9/l, and the next day he developed dyspnea, hemoptysis, and fever. A chest X-ray showed diffuse bilateral patchy pulmonary infiltrates. Tretinoin was withdrawn, but despite high doses of glucocorticoids and blood products, hemoptysis and respiratory failure continued for 6 weeks, when he improved.
- A 59-year-old man with acute promyelocytic leukemia was given tretinoin 45 mg/m^2/day and chemotherapy. On day 6, his fibrinogen concentration fell to 940 mg/l and he developed a fever (39 °C), dyspnea, and hypotension. A chest X-ray showed a right pleural effusion. Tretinoin was withdrawn and he was given dexamethasone. However, he deteriorated and developed hemoptysis. Despite glucocorticoids and blood products his pulmonary bleeding continued unabated. On day 29 he developed Gram-negative sepsis and died.

Eosinophilic pleural effusion has been attributed to isotretinoin (3).

Pneumonia has also been reported as a possible adverse effect (SEDA-20, 155) (36).

Nervous system

Nervous system disturbances include fatigue, lassitude, vertigo, sweating, hypesthesia, paresthesia, dizziness, fever, amnesia, delirium, flu-like symptoms, somnolence, lethargy, depression (41), and psychological changes. There was a direct correlation between intracranial hypertension and the use of isotretinoin in a retrospective study of spontaneous reports (42).

- An 8-year-old girl with acute promyelocytic leukemia was given cytarabine, etoposide, idarubicin, and tretinoin 25 mg/m^2/day (43). Five days later she developed fever, pleural effusions, and ascites, but the symptoms resolved spontaneously. On day 65 (cumulative dose of tretinoin 1.6 g/m^2) she had nausea and vomiting, severe headache, and diplopia. There was paralysis of the left trochlear nerve bilateral papilledema. A cranial MRI scan was normal. The intracranial pressure was not measured. Tretinoin was withdrawn and she was given glucocorticoids, mannitol, acetazolamide, and pethidine. Her symptoms resolved within 2 days.

A case of multiple mononeuropathies has been attributed to tretinoin (44). The neurological symptoms resembled atypical pseudotumor cerebri with focal neurological signs.

- A 23-year-old woman with acute promyelocytic leukemia was given tretinoin (45 mg/m^2/day) together with daunorubicin and cytarabine. She had a slight headache after the administration of tretinoin. On the 17th day an acute subdural hematoma required operation. Her headache persisted and she complained of diplopia, and burning pain and contact dysesthesia of the back of the left hand and the right foot, with accompanying weakness on day 21. Electrophysiology showed reduced conduction velocity and amplitude in the right peroneal nerve. She also had a right abducens nerve palsy and visual disturbance. There was no papilledema. MRI scan of the brain was normal. On day 51 tretinoin was discontinued. Her symptoms of peripheral neuropathy and the electrophysiological findings gradually improved as did her headache and dry skin, despite continued chemotherapy. The right abducens nerve palsy partly resolved.

The relation between isotretinoin and seizures is still unclear (SEDA-18, 169).

The possible negative effects of short-term oral acitretin 1 mg/kg/day on peripheral nerve function have been assessed in a small prospective study in 13 patients (45). Patients with conditions related to peripheral neuropathy were excluded. There was a fall in the mean amplitude of the sensory action potential of the superficial peroneal nerve after 1 and 3 months of therapy. There was a significant change in one or more neurophysiological parameters in three of 13 patients after 1 month and in nine of 13 patients after 3 months. None of the patients had detectable neurological abnormalities at any time during therapy. Acitretin was withdrawn, and after 6 months three patients gradually improved. Further studies are needed to determine whether neurophysiological evaluation should be routine during treatment with oral retinoids. Peripheral neuropathy has rarely been observed (SEDA-17, 183).

Sensory systems

Eyes

Ocular findings are among the more frequent adverse effects in patients taking isotretinoin (46,47), the most common being blepharoconjunctivitis, which also occurs in those who use tretinoin ophthalmic ointment (1).

Ocular adverse effects secondary to isotretinoin are generally benign in nature and reversible on reduction or withdrawal of therapy. However, papilledema necessitates withdrawal. Corneal opacities should be monitored closely. Although they do not usually interfere with vision, prudence dictates withdrawal of isotretinoin or reduction of the dosage when corneal opacities develop (48). Several cases of cataract have been (unconvincingly) ascribed to isotretinoin (SEDA-19, 157). Etretinate and isotretinoin have caused photophobia and reduced night vision (SEDA-17, 183), and possibly ectropion (SEDA-16, 152).

Corneal opacities after treatment with oral isotretinoin generally disappear after withdrawal. However, in one case they were persistent (49).

- A 39-year-old woman developed corneal opacities while taking oral isotretinoin 1 mg/kg for 6 months. The opacities persisted for at least 6 years after discontinuation of the drug. She had worn soft hydrophilic contact lenses for 10 years before, but without signs of corneal opacity 1 month before treatment was started.

Xerophthalmia, carrying a high risk of blindness, requires the immediate administration of massive doses of vitamin A. An infant who received intramuscular vitamin A for xerophthalmia secondary to cystic fibrosis developed an acute sixth nerve palsy (50).

- A 5-month-old boy with cystic fibrosis and xerophthalmia was given intramuscular vitamin A 50 000 IU (water-miscible retinyl palmitate). After the first dose prominent bulging of the fontanelle developed, but the infant remained alert and was feeding well. Two days later another dose of 50 000 IU was given in two divided doses over 2 days. These doses were well tolerated, with gradual improvement of the bulging fontanelle over 1 week. Five days later, a complete abduction deficit of the left eye developed, in keeping with an acute sixth nerve palsy. There were no other signs of raised intracranial pressure. The sixth nerve palsy resolved fully over the next 2 months. There were no other neurological sequelae. After discharge the infant continued to take oral vitamin A supplements.

In one study, 236 cases of adverse ocular reactions possibly associated with isotretinoin were evaluated (Table 3) (48).

Ears
Unilateral earache has been reported in two patients (SEDA-9, 134). Excessive cerumen production and otitis externa have also been reported.

Taste and smell
Taste and smell can be altered by isotretinoin (SEDA-16, 153) and loss of taste has been attributed to it (SEDA-21, 163).

Psychological, psychiatric

In 1998 depression, psychosis, and suicidal ideation, suicide attempts, and suicide were added to the product label of isotretinoin. Since then the FDA has received increasing number of reports of these problems (53).

Table 3 Adverse ocular effects associated with isotretinoin exposure in 236 patients (51)

Adverse effects	No. of patients
Eyelids	
Blepharoconjunctivitis or meibomianitis (52)	88
Photodermatitis	6
Corneae	
Corneal opacities	12
Dry eyes	47
Contact lens intolerance	19
Optic nerve	
Papilledema or pseudotumor cerebri	18
Optic neuritis	3
Congenital abnormalities	
Microphthalmos	5
Orbital hypertelorism	2
Optic nerve hypoplasia	4
Cortical blindness	1
Others	
Blurred vision	39
Myopia	5
Impaired night vision and dark adaptation (SEDA-10, 25)	3
Ocular inflammation (uveitis, scleritis, retinitis, ophthalmitis, iritis)	7

From the time that isotretinoin was marketed in 1982 up to May 2000 the FDA received 37 reports of patients taking isotretinoin who committed suicide, 110 reports of patients who were hospitalized for depression, suicidal ideation, or suicide attempts, and 284 reports of patients with depression who did not need hospitalization (54). In 62% of the suicide cases a psychiatric history or possible contributing factors were identified, and 69% of patients hospitalized for depression had either a previous psychiatric history of possible contributing factors. Drug withdrawal led to improvement in about one-third of the patients, while in 29% depression persisted after withdrawal. In 24 cases dechallenge and rechallenge were positive. However, since this was a series of spontaneous reports, and since there are no good data on the incidence of depression and suicide among adolescents with acne, a causal relation cannot be concluded.

A change in dreaming pattern has been reported in two patients, occurring within 2–3 weeks after the start of treatment with isotretinoin 40 mg/day for cystic acne (55). One patient also reported increased irritability and bouts of depression. In both patients all the symptoms abated after 4–5 weeks without a change in isotretinoin dosage.

Endocrine

Small reductions in indices of thyroid function have been observed in patients taking etretinate (56). Thyrotoxicosis may have been triggered by isotretinoin in one patient (SEDA-12, 136).

Metabolism

Alterations in lipid metabolism are common and include increases in serum triglyceride and cholesterol concentrations, sometimes persisting after withdrawal of the therapy, and reductions in high-density lipoprotein cholesterol. The incidence of raised serum lipids during therapy with oral isotretinoin 1 mg/kg/day for acne has been reviewed retrospectively in 876 patients, of whom 54 had raised serum cholesterol concentrations (over 5.2 mmol/l) and 45 had triglyceride concentrations above 2.26 mmol/l (57).

Symptoms of hyperlipidemia and the metabolic syndrome have been investigated in a cross-sectional study in young adults who had used isotretinoin for acne for at least 4 weeks (mean dosage 0.56 mg/kg). Those in whom triglyceride concentrations increased by at least 1.0 mmol/l during therapy were termed hyper-responders ($n = 102$), and those in whom triglyceride concentrations changed by 0.1 mmol/l or less were termed non-responders ($n = 100$) (58). Despite similar pretreatment body weights and plasma lipid concentrations, 4 years after completion of isotretinoin therapy the hyper-responders were more likely to have hypertriglyceridemia (OR = 4.8; 95% CI = 1.6, 14), hypercholesterolemia (OR = 9.1; CI = 1.9, 43), truncal obesity (OR = 11.0; CI = 2.0, 59), and hyperinsulinemia (OR = 3.0, CI = 1.6, 5.7) than non-responders. In addition, more hyper-responders had at least one parent with hypertriglyceridemia. Genotypes containing apoE ε2 and apoE ε4 alleles were over-represented among hyper-responders. Although a comparison of hyper-responders with non-responders may lead to overestimation of the risk, these data suggest that those who develop hyperlipidemia while taking isotretinoin are those who are already at risk of hyperlipidemia and the metabolic syndrome.

The consequences of hypertriglyceridemia are not well understood, but there may be an increased risk of cardiovascular disease and pancreatitis (SEDA-13, 123). Patients with an increased tendency to develop hypertriglyceridemia include those with diabetes mellitus, obesity, increased alcohol intake, and a positive family history. With a short course (16 weeks) of isotretinoin it is sufficient to ensure there is no hyperlipidemia before the start of therapy, and to determine the triglyceride response to therapy on one occasion after 4 weeks (59).

Mineral balance

Hypercalcemia has been reported as an adverse effect of systemic retinoid therapy (60).

- A 12-year-old girl with neuroblastoma and normal renal function developed severe hypercalcemia while receiving isotretinoin 160 mg/m^2/day (61). Her hypercalcemia resolved with hydration, diuretic therapy, and temporary withdrawal of isotretinoin. Despite a dosage reduction to 80 mg/m^2/day, severe hypercalcemia recurred during the next treatment cycle. Further treatment with isotretinoin was made tolerable by shortening the duration of the remaining cycles.

- An 11-year-old boy with acute promyelocytic leukemia was given *all-trans*-retinoic acid 47 mg/m^2/day (62). On day 10 he developed headache and nausea. The dose was reduced to 39 mg/m^2/day and he was given glycerol, but his symptoms of pseudotumor cerebri continued. Cranial CT showed neitheroccupying lesions nor brain edema. On day 25, hypercalcemia (3.2 mmol/l) was observed. In spite of conventional therapy the serum calcium concentration continued to rise to 4.0 mmol/l. Tretinoin was withdrawn on day 33. Within 1 week his symptoms resolved. On the second day of a second phase of *all-trans*-retinoic acid therapy, he again developed nausea and headache and the serum calcium concentration gradually increased to 3.3 mmol/l by day 7. Raised concentrations of type 1 cross-linked *N*-telopeptide and deoxypyridinoline suggested increased bone resorption. A bisphosphonate (pamidronate 30 mg) was administered intravenously; the calcium normalized within 2 days and the nausea and headache resolved.

Fluid balance

Generalized edema has been attributed to etretinate (63).

Hematologic

Altered blood clotting due to hypoprothrombinemia, raised erythrocyte sedimentation rate (64), altered red cell count (64), reduced white cell count (64), thrombocytopenia (SEDA-12, 136), and eosinophilia (SEDA-13, 122) have all been observed incidentally (SEDA-17, 184).

Of 31 patients with acute promyelocytic leukemia (15 men and 16 women, median age 43 years) 4 received tretinoin 45 mg/m^2/day and intravenous tranexamic acid 1–2 g for 6 days, 9 received tretinoin, daunorubicin, and cytarabine followed by thioguanine, 15 received chemotherapy, tretinoin, and tranexamic acid, 2 received chemotherapy and tranexamic acid, and 1 received chemotherapy only (65). Three of the four patients who received tretinoin plus tranexamic acid had sudden and rapid deterioration in their condition, leading to early death. At postmortem there were widespread microvascular thromboses in unusual sites (for example the brain and kidneys). The rapid progression to multiorgan failure and the widespread nature of the microthrombi suggests the need for caution in the simultaneous use of tretinoin and tranexamic acid.

Thrombosis during induction treatment with tretinoin, aprotinin, and chemotherapy has been described (66).

Transient polycythemia has been reported during treatment with isotretinoin for severe nodular acne (67).

- A 53-year-old man's hematocrit increased from 0.46 to 0.51 after he had taken isotretinoin for 11 months (180 mg/day for 3 months, 80 mg/day for 6 months, then 20 mg/day). No secondary causes of polycythemia were found and the hematocrit fell to 0.48 3 months after withdrawal of isotretinoin.

The reference range for hematocrit in men is 0.41–0.49, and so the clinical relevance of this observation is unclear.

Attacks of paroxysmal nocturnal hemoglobinuria may possibly be provoked by isotretinoin (SEDA-19, 156).

Extramedullary relapse of acute promyelocytic leukemia, which is rare after chemotherapy alone, was more common after tretinoin, but it is not clear whether it truly increases the risk of extramedullary recurrence and what the risk factors are. In a retrospective analysis of the incidence of extramedullary relapse in patients after prior treatment with tretinoin and in patients previously treated with chemotherapy alone (68) three of the 13 patients who received tretinoin had extramedullary involvement compared with none of the 11 patients previously treated with chemotherapy alone (RR = 2.1; CI = 1.34, 3.29). The retinoic acid syndrome during prior induction treatment was significantly associated with extramedullary relapse (three of five patients with the retinoic acid syndrome versus none of eight without the syndrome (RR = 5.0; CI = 1.4, 17)). Thus, tretinoin may predispose patients with acute promyelocytic leukemia to extramedullary involvement at relapse and the retinoic acid syndrome is a risk factor.

Gastrointestinal

The gastrointestinal adverse effects of retinoids include anorexia, nausea, vomiting, weight loss, stomach pain, thirst, splenomegaly, and acute esophagitis (SEDA-21, 162). Proctosigmoiditis has been reported (SEDA-13, 123).

- Ulcerative colitis occurred in a 17-year-old boy shortly after he had completed a 5-month course of isotretinoin (dose not stated) for acne (69). There was no family history of inflammatory bowel disease.

Although three other cases of inflammatory bowel disease during isotretinoin therapy have been reported (70–72), there have also been reports of the safe use of isotretinoin in patents with a history of inflammatory bowel disease (that is without exacerbation of the inflammatory bowel disease) (70,73,74). Since retinoids are being increasingly used to treat moderately severe acne, larger studies are needed to elucidate the relation between retinoid use and inflammatory bowel disease.

Vasculitis and necrosis of the ileum developed in a patient with acute promyelocytic leukemia treated with *all-trans*-retinoic acid (75).

- A 29-year-old woman with acute promyelocytic leukemia was given tretinoin 45 mg/m^2. On day 20 she developed pain in both hands, wrists, feet, and ankles, with erythema and edema. On day 24 her fever increased to over 38 °C and the white blood cell count was 10.9×10^9/l. She was given dexamethasone (8 mg intravenously on three consecutive days) and all her symptoms quickly resolved, but on day 37 she developed a low-grade fever and polyarthralgia, which persisted. On day 42 she had a profuse bloody stool and her abdominal pain worsened and spread all over the abdomen. At emergency operation there was segmental necrosis in several parts of the ileum, with inflammation invading the serosa. Histology of the ileum showed a

leukocytoclastic vasculitis. After operation tretinoin was withdrawn and she had no fever, edema, arthralgia, or abdominal pain thereafter.

Liver

Hepatomegaly is an adverse effect of retinol and tretinoin. Transient slight rises in liver enzymes, notably aspartate transaminase, alanine transaminase, and alkaline phosphatase, are common, but some cases of hepatotoxicity due to etretinate and acitretin (SEDA-20, 154) have also been reported (76), as has cholestatic jaundice due to etretinate (77). Etretinate may have played a role in a case of liver failure leading to death (76).

The incidence of raised liver enzymes during therapy with oral isotretinoin 1 mg/kg/day for acne has been retrospectively reviewed in 876 patients (57). Liver enzymes (aspartate transaminase, alanine transaminase, and γ-glutamyl transferase) were transiently raised in a minority of patients (number not stated).

Acute liver damage has been attributed to tretinoin (78).

- A 40-year-old man with acute promyelocytic leukemia was given tretinoin 45 mg/m^2/day and intravenous daunorubicin. After 3 weeks his alkaline phosphatase rose to 370 (reference range 82–198) U/l, the gamma-glutamyltranspeptidase to 198 (reference range 7–43) U/l, and the direct bilirubin to 39 (reference range below 10) μmol/l. He had painful hepatomegaly without splenomegaly. Abdominal Doppler ultrasound ruled out biliary tract injury. Percutaneous liver biopsy showed intracellular cholestasis with preservation of hepatic architecture. He was given dexamethasone and tretinoin was withdrawn. After 3 days the symptoms and hepatomegaly abated.

Pancreas

Acute pancreatitis is a rare but serious adverse effect of tretinoin. Three cases associated with isotretinoin-induced hyperglyceridemia have previously been described and two cases associated with tretinoin (79,80).

- A 48-year-old man received tretinoin (45 mg/m^2/day) followed 9 days later by combination chemotherapy for 5 days (81). On day 15 he developed acute epigastric and upper left quadrant pain. He had raised serum lipase (1312 IU/l; reference range 27–208), amylase (509 IU/l; 30–110), and triglycerides (7.77 mmol/l; 0.45–1.82). Abdominal CT showed mild trabeculation of the peripancreatic adipose tissue, but no lithiasis or dilatation of the biliary ducts. Acute pancreatitis caused by hypertriglyceridemia was diagnosed and he was given supportive treatment plus fenofibrate (200 mg/day), without withdrawal of tretinoin. His lipase, amylase, and triglycerides normalized over 10 days.

Urinary tract

Impaired renal function has rarely been caused by isotretinoin (82) and etretinate (83). Abnormalities in urinary proteins, inflammation of the urethral meatus, and nephrolithiasis have rarely occurred. Urethritis may occur more often than has been realized (SEDA-21, 162) (84).

Nephrotic syndrome developed after 4 months treatment with isotretinoin 40 mg/day (85). No other causes were found and the symptoms disappeared within some months with appropriate treatment.

During tretinoin therapy, some patients with retinoic acid syndrome or with a hypercoagulable state develop acute renal insufficiency, usually accompanied by dysfunction of other organs. A patient with acute promyelocytic leukemia developed renal insufficiency alone during tretinoin treatment (86).

- A 72-year-old Japanese man with acute promyelocytic leukemia was given tretinoin 48 mg/m^2 plus idarubicin. On day 17 oliguria occurred and tretinoin was withdrawn on day 20 when the serum creatinine concentration rose to 619 µmol/l (7.0 mg/dl). There were no signs or symptoms of retinoic acid syndrome. A needle biopsy of the left kidney on day 38, when the serum creatinine concentration was 212 µmol/l (2.4 mg/dl), showed granulomatous tubulointerstitial nephritis. The glomeruli were mostly intact and there were no fibrin thrombi or leukemic cell infiltration. After one course of consolidation therapy he was discharged with a normal serum creatinine concentration.

Two cases of bone-marrow transplant nephropathy that developed coincident with retinoid therapy have been reported (87).

- A 3-year-old boy with a neuroblastoma was given cisplatin, adriamycin, and cyclophosphamide for five induction cycles and radiation to sites of residual bony metastases 1 month before autologous bone-marrow transplant, which resulted in an absolute neutrophil count of 500×10^6/l on day 9 and a self-sustaining platelet count over 50×10^{12}/l on day 72. He was randomized to receive retinoids 80 mg/m^2 bd by mouth, beginning on day 100 after bone-marrow transplant. Before beginning *cis*-retinoic acid, his highest serum creatinine concentration was 44 µmol/l on day 8. When *cis*-retinoic acid was begun, his hemoglobin was 9.8 g/dl and his platelet count 97×10^{12}/l. At the end of the second 2-week cycle of retinoic acid he developed a severe headache and diastolic hypertension (BP 120/108 mmHg), a blood urea nitrogen concentration of 4 mmol/l, serum creatinine of 133 µmol/l, hemoglobin of 5.8 g/dl, and platelet count of 57×10^{12}/l. Urinalysis showed erythrocytes and protein. Renal biopsy showed mesangiolysis, wide capillary loops, focal intimal thickening, and vacuolization of glomerular and tubular cells. His hematuria and proteinuria persisted for 4 weeks, and his blood urea nitrogen and serum creatinine gradually improved, as did the hypertension.
- A 5-year-old boy with a neuroblastoma was treated in the same way. On day 105 after bone-marrow transplantation he developed hypertension (BP 140/92 mmHg), hematuria, proteinuria, and a raised serum creatinine. His hemoglobin and platelet count fell. His urine contained protein 800 mg/l, a few hyaline casts, and 25–30 erythrocytes per high-power field. When

nephritis developed, *cis*-retinoid acid was withdrawn. He gradually improved, and his urine cleared of casts, erythrocytes, and protein within 4 weeks.

Skin

Adverse effects of oral retinoids on the skin are common (up to 70%). The symptoms and signs are listed in Table 4. Three cases of scrotal ulceration during *all-trans*-retinoic acid therapy for a microgranular variant of acute promyelocytic leukemia (88,89), together with eight other reported cases (90–92), suggest that this adverse effect is specific for tretinoin. The incidence has been estimated at 12% (88). The pathogenesis is unknown, but it has been suggested to be a manifestation of the retinoic acid syndrome (88). Improvement after the withdrawal of tretinoin and the administration of glucocorticoids supports this assumption. However, activation of neutrophils by superoxide production may also be involved.

Acute febrile neutrophilic dermatosis (Sweet's syndrome) can occur in patients with acute promyelocytic leukemia given a retinoid. Sweet's syndrome is characterized by five cardinal features: fever, neutrophilia, multiple raised painful asymmetric erythematous cutaneous plaques, dermal infiltrates consisting of mature neutrophils, and a rapid response to glucocorticoid therapy. In up to 10–20% of cases it

Table 4 The adverse effects of oral retinoids on the skin and hair

Acne fulminans (SEDA-11, 137)
Angular stomatitis
Balanitis (rare)
Blepharoconjunctivitis
Bullous pemphigoid (SEDA-17, 184)
Cheilitis
Cystic and comedonal acne (SEDA-15, 142)
Dissemination of *Herpes simplex*
Dry mucous membranes
Epistaxis
Eruptive xanthomas (one report)
Erythema multiforme (SEDA-14, 124)
Erythema nodosum (SEDA-21, 163)
Erythroderma
Excess granulation tissue (SEDA-9, 134)
Facial cellulitis (*Staphylococcus aureus*)
Facial dermatitis
Facial erythema
Follicular eczema
Generalized edema
Gingivitis, bleeding gums
Glossitis
Hair curly, possibly due to the combination of
    isotretinoin + azathioprine (SEDA-21, 163)
Hair discoloration (SEDA-19, 157)
Hair growth disturbed
Hair loss
Hair thinning
Hair "unruly" (SEDA-11, 136)
Hirsutism
Hyperhidrosis

(Continued)

Table 4 (Continued)

Hyperpigmentation
Hypopigmentation
Irritant dermatitis
Melasma (SEDA-21, 163)
Mucosal erosions
Mycosis fungoides-like dermatitis (SEDA-10, 125)
Nail deformities (softening, fragility, Beau's lines,
    onycholysis,onychomadesis, onchoschizia, paronychia,
    curly fingernails) (37)
Nail growth reduced
Nasal carriage of *Staphylococcus aureus* (SEDA-12, 131)
Nummular eczema (SEDA-12, 136)
Osteoma cutis exacerbation
Papulopustular palmoplantar eruptions
Pemphigus vulgaris (SEDA-20, 155)
Petechiae
Photoallergy (SEDA-17, 184)
Phototoxicity (SEDA-17, 184)
Pityriasis rosea-like dermatitis
Polyarteritis nodosa (93)
Porokeratosis exacerbation (SEDA-16, 152)
Prurigo nodularis (SEDA-12, 131)
Pruritus
Pseudoporphyria (SEDA-17, 184)
Psoriasis as a Koebner phenomenon (SEDA-13, 123)
Pyogenic granuloma
Rosacea-like eruption
Ruptured striae atrophicae
Sarcoid-like granulomas (SEDA-19, 157)
Scaling of the skin
Scalp folliculitis
Skin fragility and erosions (SEDA-22, 168)
Skin odor abnormal
Skin sticky
Thyroglossal cyst (SEDA-20, 155)
Toxic epidermal necrolysis
Vasculitis (94,95)
Vulvitis
Wound healing delayed
Xeroderma

precedes or coincides with a diagnosis of malignancy, most commonly acute myelogenous leukemia. In cases associated with tretinoin the symptoms come on at 7–34 days and the skin lesions are seen on the face, limbs, and back.

- A 58-year-old woman was given tretinoin 45 mg/m^2/day for acute promyelocytic leukemia and after 9 days she developed symptoms of upper respiratory tract infection and fever (38.2 °C) (96). The next day multiple erythematous and painful cutaneous plaques appeared on her limbs. Her white cell count was 5.71×10^9/l. A skin biopsy showed a normal epidermis with subepidermal edema and dense diffuse perivascular aggregates composed of granulocytes and scattered eosinophils, compatible with Sweet's syndrome. Prednisolone 20 mg/day had no effect, but after 2 days treatment with cytarabine and daunorubicin the rash started to fade and gradually disappeared. Remission was achieved after one course and *all-trans*-retinoic acid was subsequently renewed without complications.

- A 39-year-old man with acute promyelocytic leukemia was given tretinoin 45 mg/m^2 (97). His leukocyte count rose to 34.3×10^9/l on day 11. On day 18 he developed rigors, mild dyspnea, and a fever (39 °C). He had exquisite pain in the right posterior tibial muscle and had several 2-mm erythematous papular and pustular lesions on his limbs and trunk. He was given a cephalosporin and developed painful bilateral nodules in the quadriceps, posterior tibial, and right biceps muscles. An MRI scan showed focal areas of increased T2 signals in the quadriceps muscles bilaterally, in most of the left sartorius and soleus muscles, and in all the compartments of the right leg. There was thickening of the adjacent fascia with subcutaneous edema. Tretinoin was withdrawn and he was given dexamethasone 16 mg/day. The cutaneous lesions improved dramatically and tretinoin 45 mg/m^2 was restarted. The symptoms did not recur.

- A 35-year-old woman with acute promyelocytic leukemia was given tretinoin 45 mg/m^2/day. On day 9 she became febrile (39.5 °C) and had a sore throat with pharyngeal erythema and tender lymphadenopathy. The fever persisted despite cephalosporins, vancomycin, and antibiotics for anaerobic cover. On day 20 she developed severe bilateral anterior leg pain and both anterior tibial muscles were tender. Creatine kinase activity was 348 (reference range 38–176) U/l. Tretinoin was withdrawn and she was given intravenous dexamethasone 10 mg/day. Her fever resolved, her pain abated, and her leg muscles felt softer and less tender. Tretinoin was reintroduced and her symptoms returned.

- A 46-year-old man with promyelocytic leukemia was given tretinoin 45 mg/m^2 plus daunorubicin 60 mg/m^2/day for 3 days and cytarabine 200 mg/m^2/day by continuous infusion for 7 days (98). He became febrile on day 3 and was given cefotaxime and vancomycin. On day 6 he developed non-pruritic, erythematous, violaceous vesicles on the limbs and upper trunk. His temperature rose to 40 °C and he gained 4.5 kg, which was attributed to a mild retinoic acid syndrome. Skin biopsy showed infiltration by neutrophilic granulocytes and marked edema in the dermis, without vasculitis or evidence of leukemic cells, fungi, or herpesvirus. Hepatic enzymes were moderately increased. The clinical presentation and histopathological findings were consistent with Sweet's syndrome. Tretinoin was withdrawn and he was given dexamethasone 40 mg/day for 10 days and then tapering doses of prednisone. He improved, and tretinoin was reintroduced without recurrence.

With topical application of tretinoin, special care should be taken when other drugs are given simultaneously. Dramatic photosensitivity has been associated with the combination of fluorouracil, prochlorperazine, and topical tretinoin (99).

- A 52-year-old woman with a colonic cancer was treated with chemotherapy after surgical resection. She had been applying topical tretinoin (Renova; Ortho Pharmac, Raritan N) cream 0.05% nightly to her face for about 5 years. During that time she had applied a sunscreen while outdoors and had tolerated tretinoin without incident. Her daily oral multivitamin supplement contained 5000 IU of retinol equivalents. About 3 days after her last dose of chemotherapy (leucovorin, fluorouracil, prochlorperazine) she exposed her face to the sun for about 1 hour after applying her usual sunscreen. Shortly afterwards the skin on her face became erythematous and worsened over several days. Her eyes became edematous, itchy, and painful. Within a week the skin on her face had completely desquamated. She stopped using tretinoin. The reaction began to improve and she was pain-free within 1 week. Her appearance returned to normal after about 10 days. During a second cycle of chemotherapy she received the same drugs as during the first, except tretinoin, and reported no significant change in sun exposure or sunscreen application. She tolerated subsequent cycles without adverse skin effects. After completing her monthly chemotherapy cycles, she resumed topical tretinoin without adverse effects.

Leukemia cutis is very rare in acute myelocytic leukemia. Cutaneous relapse in acute promyelocytic leukemia has been reported during a period of complete hematological remission after treatment with tretinoin (100).

- A 51-year-old man with acute promyelocytic leukemia was given induction chemotherapy and tretinoin 45 mg/m^2. After 1 month he developed discrete erythematous papules, although marrow biopsy suggested hematological remission. The papules were disseminated on all his limbs, trunk, and scalp, and were scattered, discrete, and 2–3 mm in diameter. Biopsy showed a moderate perivascular infiltration of medium to large atypical cells, mainly in the upper dermis, suggesting infiltrating promyelocytes. The clinical, histological, and histochemical findings were compatible with leukemia cutis. One week later, a bone-marrow biopsy still showed hematological remission.

Musculoskeletal

Musculoskeletal symptoms occur in 15% of patients who take isotretinoin. These are usually mild and consist of pain, tenderness, and muscle stiffness. Creatine kinase activity can rise, especially in individuals engaging in strenuous physical activity (SEDA-10, 124). Clinical and subclinical muscle damage has been reported from etretinate, acitretin, and isotretinoin (SEDA-21, 162, 163).

Skeletal abnormalities associated with retinoid therapy include Achilles tendonitis (SEDA-17, 185), acute arthritis (SEDA-18, 168; 101), bridging of vertebral bodies, diffuse idiopathic skeletal hyperostosis (DISH), disc narrowing, nasal bone osteophytosis, osteoma cutis, hyperostosis, extraspinal calcifications, costochondritis, enthesiopathy, ossification of tendons and ligamentous insertions, ossification of the posterior longitudinal ligament, periosteal thickening, premature epiphyseal closure, reduced bone density/osteoporosis (102), skeletal aches and pains, slender long bones, and Tietze's syndrome.

Stiff man syndrome has been described 10 days after the start of oral isotretinoin treatment (1 mg/kg/day) and resolved completely within 2 weeks of withdrawal (103). There were no motor or sensory nerve conduction abnormalities. There were no conditions known to be associated with stiff man syndrome, either at the time or during 5 years of follow up.

Adult onset Still's disease occurred after 3 months of oral isotretinoin (104). No other causes were found and the symptoms disappeared with appropriate treatment within some months.

Reproductive system

Breast discharge has been reported (105). Menstrual disturbances occur, and may be under-reported (SEDA-13, 121, 123). Vaginal bleeding in a 64-year-old woman was convincingly ascribed to the daily use of tretinoin cream 0.05% to her face, suggesting a systemic effect (SEDA-16, 159).

Adverse effects of isotretinoin affecting the male reproductive system reported to the manufacturer include gynecomastia, local inflammation/discomfort, potency disorders, reduced fertility, and ejaculatory failure (SEDA-18, 168; 106).

Immunologic

Hypersensitivity reactions to retinoids are rare and consist of occasional drug rashes.

- Immunomodulatory effects of isotretinoin in the treatment of facial acne (40 mg/day for 4 weeks) were blamed for a recurrence of pulmonary alveolar proteinosis in a 16-year-old girl, in whom it had been in spontaneous remission for 2 years (107).

Although the time-course of this effect was suggestive, it should be borne in mind that about 25% of patients with this disease have exacerbations without a clear cause.

Body temperature

An increase in the frequency of attacks of familial Mediterranean fever has been reported after the start of systemic therapy with isotretinoin for nodulocystic acne (108).

- A 32-year-old man with familial Mediterranean fever had one or two attacks per year while taking colchicine twice daily for 10 years. During the first month after starting to take isotretinoin 50 mg/day he had three typical attacks, increasing to one attack a week after dosage increments to 60 mg/day and later 80 mg/day. Isotretinoin was withdrawn and he had no further attacks of familial Mediterranean fever during the following 10 months. Rechallenge was not performed.

Long-Term Effects

Mutagenicity

The reported occurrence of sarcomas in some patients treated with isotretinoin may be a chance finding

(SEDA-21, 164); retinoids may prevent or even cure certain malignancies (20).

Second-Generation Effects

Teratogenicity

Retinoids are strongly teratogenic (21). Pregnancy should be ruled out and an effective form of contraception must be used for at least 1 month before starting therapy, during therapy, and for at least 1 month (isotretinoin) or 2 years (acitretin) after therapy is stopped. Retinoid-induced teratogenicity has been reviewed (22,23).

There are few data about the safety of topical retinoids during pregnancy. The risk of teratogenicity of topical tretinoin, if any, appears to be minimal (SEDA-18, 164; 109). However, there is a case report (110).

- A baby was born missing its right ear and external auditory canal. At 20 months an MRI scan of the brain showed focal atrophy and encephalomalacia of the right parieto-occipital lobe. His mother had used topical tretinoin (Retin A 0.025%) on her face and a large surface of the back before conception and during the first 2–3 months of pregnancy. His father had used oral isotretinoin before conception.

This type of ear abnormality is a typical feature of retinoic acid embryopathy. Given the pattern of malformations in this child, the authors thought that maternal use of topical tretinoin had been responsible. Three other cases of fetal malformations after topical tretinoin use have been reported (111–113).

Multiple congenital anomalies occurred after exposure to isotretinoin in the first trimester (114).

- A neonate whose mother had taken isotretinoin 40 mg/day during the first 2 months of pregnancy had absent auricles, tachypnea, and feeding difficulties. There were signs of heart failure, and echocardiography showed a large subpulmonary ventricular septal defect (Taussig–Bing malformation) and a secundum atrial septal defect. Both great arteries originated from the anterior right ventricle, and there was tricuspid insufficiency. A cranial CT scan showed atresia of the external ear canal, tympanic membrane, middle ear, and antrum. Other ear structures were normal. The child died at home.

Previously published information on outcomes after maternal exposure to topical tretinoin has been limited to three case reports (111–113). A fourth case has been reported (110).

- A boy, born at 41 weeks weighing 4090 g, had no right auricle or external auditory canal. Before conception and during the first months of pregnancy his mother had used topical tretinoin (Retin A 0.025%) on her face and a large area of her back. She had also used vitamins during pregnancy. His father had used oral isotretinoin before conception. At 16 months the baby was babbling. Optokinetic response was diminished and there was no oculovestibular response. At 20 months he was non-verbal and had poor receptive language, compatible with cognitive impairment. A cranial CT scan showed calcification of the right posterior hemisphere and MRI showed reduction in the volume of the right cerebral hemisphere, an infarct in the deep basal ganglia, focal atrophy, and encephalomalacia of the right parieto-occipital lobe. MRA showed marked attenuation of the posterior cerebral artery with poor declination of the more distal cortical, temporal, and occipital branches. A PET scan showed severe hypometabolism of the right posterior parietal, occipital, and temporal lobes, right basal ganglia, and thalamus, and mild hypometabolism of the left cerebellum.

Susceptibility Factors

Renal disease

The concentration of vitamin A is raised in chronic renal insufficiency, because reduced filtration of low molecular proteins results in increased concentrations of retinol binding protein. A retrospective evaluation of 18 liver biopsies in 71 patients on hemodialysis taking therapeutic doses of vitamin A showed hyperplasia of stellate cells in 7, but no evidence of fibrosis (115).

In a patient with renal insufficiency, stellate cell hyperplasia was accompanied by fibrosis (116).

- A 51-year-old man, with a 9-year history of renal insufficiency and an alcohol intake of 4 U/week, underwent transplant nephrectomy. At surgery, ascites and liver cirrhosis were noted. A needle biopsy of the liver 1 month later showed nodular regenerative hyperplasia but no cirrhosis. There were subendothelial vacuolated cells, suggestive of modified stellate cells, and there was adjacent focal perisinusoidal fibrosis. His medications included one multivitamin/mineral supplement per day containing vitamin A 4000 IU. His vitamin A concentration was 1045 (reference range 490–720) ng/ml. Viral and antibody studies were negative.

Drug Administration

Drug formulations

A novel intravenous liposomal formulation of tretinoin (Atragen®, Aronex Pharmaceuticals Inc, The Woodlands, TX), which provides a reliable dose for patients who are unable to swallow or absorb medications, has been evaluated in 69 patients with acute promyelocytic leukemia (117). Liposomal tretinoin (90 mg/m^2) was given every other day until complete remission or a maximum of 56 days. Treatment after complete remission was liposomal tretinoin with or without chemotherapy. Adverse effects (grade 1–2 according to the NCI common toxicity criteria) were the retinoic acid syndrome in 18 patients (grade 3/4 in 10), leukocytosis ($n = 36$), headache ($n = 46$), dry skin ($n = 23$), hypertriglyceridemia ($n = 23$), fever ($n = 18$), nausea ($n = 13$), stomatitis ($n = 11$), vomiting ($n = 10$), cheilitis ($n = 9$), exfoliative dermatitis ($n = 9$), rash ($n = 8$), myalgia ($n = 8$), liver enzyme abnormalities ($n = 7$), bone pain ($n = 6$), arthralgia ($n = 5$), raised LDH activity ($n = 4$), pseudotumor cerebri ($n = 4$; with severe headache, papilledema, increased CSF pressure, and absence of structural cranial lesions by CT or MRI scanning), hypercholesterolemia ($n = 4$), chills ($n = 4$), pruritus ($n = 3$), and diarrhea ($n = 2$).

Drug overdose

The possible symptoms and signs of overdosage are essentially the same as in hypervitaminosis A (see Table 1). The toxicity of overdosage appears to be low, and symptoms are restricted to headache and mucocutaneous adverse effects (118).

Drug–Drug Interactions

Alcohol

Concomitant intake of alcohol induces the transformation of acitretin to etretinate, which has a much longer half-life (84–168 days) (119).

Carbamazepine

No increase in seizure susceptibility was noted in a number of epileptic patients taking concomitant phenytoin, sodium valproate, or carbamazepine. However, it is recommended that carbamazepine concentrations be measured during therapy (12).

Tetracycline

Concurrent use of tetracycline has been considered contraindicated because of the risk of benign intracranial hypertension. However, although either compound alone can provoke this rare adverse effect, there is no evidence of any additive effect (12).

References

1. Soong HK, Martin NF, Wagoner MD, Alfonso E, Mandelbaum SH, Laibson PR, Smith RE, Udell I. Topical retinoid therapy for squamous metaplasia of various ocular surface disorders. A multicenter, placebo-controlled double-masked study. Ophthalmology 1988;95(10):1442–6.
2. Culine S, Kramar A, Droz JP, Theodore C. Phase II study of all-trans retinoic acid administered intermittently for hormone refractory prostate cancer. J Urol 1999;161(1):173–5.
3. Bunker CB, Sheron N, Maurice PD, Kocjan G, Johnson NM, Dowd PM. Isotretinoin and eosinophilic pleural effusion. Lancet 1989;1(8635):435–6.
4. Miller JA, Munro DD. Topical corticosteroids: clinical pharmacology and therapeutic use. Drugs 1980;19(2):119–134.
5. Junjie Y, Zhaoping H, Minfei P. Fatal side-effects of all-trans retinoic acid in the treatment of acute promyelocytic leukemia. Bull Hum Med Univ 1999;24:293–5.
6. Fenaux P, Chastang C, Chevret S, Sanz M, Dombret H, Archimbaud E, Fey M, Rayon C, Huguet F, Sotto JJ, Gardin C, Makhoul PC, Travade P, Solary E, Fegueux N, Bordessoule D, Miguel JS, Link H, Desablens B, Stamatoullas A, Deconinck E, Maloisel F, Castaigne S, Preudhomme C, Degos L. A randomized comparison of all transretinoic acid (ATRA) followed by chemotherapy and ATRA plus chemotherapy and the role of maintenance therapy in newly diagnosed acute promyelocytic leukemia. The European APL Group. Blood 1999;94(4):1192–200.
7. Budd GT, Adamson PC, Gupta M, Homayoun P, Sandstrom SK, Murphy RF, McLain D, Tuason L, Peereboom D, Bukowski RM, Ganapathi R. Phase I/II trial of all-trans retinoic acid and tamoxifen in patients with advanced breast cancer. Clin Cancer Res 1998;4(3):635–42.
8. Kelly WK, Osman I, Reuter VE, Curley T, Heston WD, Nanus DM, Scher HI. The development of biologic end points in patients treated with differentiation agents: an experience of retinoids in prostate cancer. Clin Cancer Res 2000;6(3):838–46.
9. Park SH, Gray WC, Hernandez I, Jacobs M, Ord RA, Sutharalingam M, Smith RG, Van Echo DA, Wu S, Conley BA. Phase I trial of all-trans retinoic acid in patients with treated head and neck squamous carcinoma. Clin Cancer Res 2000;6(3):847–54.
10. Mao JT, Goldin JG, Dermand J, Ibrahim G, Brown MS, Emerick A, McNitt-Gray MF, Gjertson DW, Estrada F, Tashkin DP, Roth MD. A pilot study of all-trans-retinoic acid for the treatment of human emphysema. Am J Respir Crit Care Med 2002;165(5):718–23.
11. Goulden V, Layton AM, Cunliffe WJ. Long-term safety of isotretinoin as a treatment for acne vulgaris. Br J Dermatol 1994;131(3):360–3.
12. Meigel WN. How safe is oral isotretinoin? Dermatology 1997;195(Suppl 1):22–8.
13. Cunliffe WJ, van de Kerkhof PC, Caputo R, Cavicchini S, Cooper A, Fyrand OL, Gollnick H, Layton AM, Leyden JJ, Mascaro JM, Ortonne JP, Shalita A. Roaccutane treatment guidelines: results of an international survey. Dermatology 1997;194(4):351–7.
14. Cunliffe WJ, Stables A. Optimum use of isotretinoin. J Cutan Med Surg 1996;1(Suppl):2–20.
15. Berbis P. Acitretine. [Acitretine.] Ann Dermatol Venereol 2001;128(6–7):737–45.
16. Pilkington T, Brogden RN. Acitretin. A review of its pharmacology and therapeutic use. Drugs 1992;43(4):597–627.
17. Leyden JJ. Therapy for acne vulgaris. N Engl J Med 1997;336(16):1156–62.
18. Nyirady J, Grossman RM, Nighland M, Berger RS, Jorizzo JL, Kim YH, Martin AG, Pandya AG, Schulz KK, Strauss JS. A comparative trial of two retinoids commonly used in the treatment of acne vulgaris. J Dermatolog Treat 2001;12(3):149–57.
19. Tu P, Li GQ, Zhu XJ, Zheng J, Wong WZ. A comparison of adapalene gel 0.1% vs. tretinoin gel 0.025% in the treatment of acne vulgaris in China J Eur Acad Dermatol Venereol 2001;15(Suppl 3):31–6.
20. Peck GL. Therapy and prevention of skin cancer. In: Saurat JH, editor. Retinoids. Basel: S. Karger, 1985:345.
21. Dai WS, LaBraico JM, Stern RS. Epidemiology of isotretinoin exposure during pregnancy. J Am Acad Dermatol 1992;26(4):599–606.
22. Teelmann K. Retinoids: toxicology and teratogenicity to date. Pharmacol Ther 1989;40(1):29–43.
23. Chan A, Hanna M, Abbott M, Keane RJ. Oral retinoids and pregnancy. Med J Aust 1996;165(3):164–7.

24. Hull PR, Demkiw-Bartel C. Isotretinoin use in acne: prospective evaluation of adverse events. J Cutan Med Surg 2000;4(2):66–70.

25. Mann G, Reinhardt D, Ritter J, Hermann J, Schmitt K, Gadner H, Creutzig U. Treatment with all-trans retinoic acid in acute promyelocytic leukemia reduces early deaths in children. Ann Hematol 2001;80(7):417–22.

26. De Botton S, Dombret H, Sanz M, Miguel JS, Caillot D, Zittoun R, Gardembas M, Stamatoulas A, Conde E, Guerci A, Gardin C, Geiser K, Makhoul DC, Reman O, de la Serna J, Lefrere F, Chomienne C, Chastang C, Degos L, Fenaux P. Incidence, clinical features, and outcome of all trans-retinoic acid syndrome in 413 cases of newly diagnosed acute promyelocytic leukemia. The European APL Group. Blood 1998;92(8):2712–2718.

27. Amano Y, Tajika K, Mizuki T, Amano M, Dan K, Kumazaki T. All-trans retinoic acid syndrome: chest CT assessment. Eur Radiol 2001;11(8):1516–7.

28. Jung JI, Choi JE, Hahn ST, Min CK, Kim CC, Park SH. Radiologic features of all-trans-retinoic acid syndrome. Am J Roentgenol 2002;178(2):475–80.

29. Tallman MS, Andersen JW, Schiffer CA, Appelbaum FR, Feusner JH, Ogden A, Shepherd L, Rowe JM, Francois C, Larson RS, Wiernik PH. Clinical description of 44 patients with acute promyelocytic leukemia who developed the retinoic acid syndrome. Blood 2000;95(1):90–5.

30. Han ZP, Lu HB, Shen ZS. [Severe side effects of the treatment of acute promyelocytic leukemia with all-trans retinoic acid.]Hunan Yi Ke Da Xue Xue Bao 2000;25(3):283–4.

31. Lehmann S, Paul C. The retinoic acid syndrome in non-M3 acute myeloid leukaemia: a case report. Br J Haematol 2000;108(1):198–9.

32. Nicolls MR, Terada LS, Tuder RM, Prindiville SA, Schwarz MI. Diffuse alveolar hemorrhage with underlying pulmonary capillaritis in the retinoic acid syndrome. Am J Respir Crit Care Med 1998;158(4):1302–5.

33. Mandelli F, Diverio D, Avvisati G, Luciano A, Barbui T, Bernasconi C, Broccia G, Cerri R, Falda M, Fioritoni G, Leoni F, Liso V, Petti MC, Rodeghiero F, Saglio G, Vegna ML, Visani G, Jehn U, Willemze R, Muus P, Pelicci PG, Biondi A, Lo Coco F. Molecular remission in PML/RAR alpha-positive acute promyelocytic leukemia by combined all-trans retinoic acid and idarubicin (AIDA) therapy. Gruppo Italiano-Malattie Ematologiche Maligne dell'Adulto and Associazione Italiana di Ematologia ed Oncologia Pediatrica Cooperative Groups. Blood 1997;90(3):1014–21.

34. Torromeo C, Latagliata R, Avvisati G, Petti MC, Mandelli F. Intraventricular thrombosis during all-trans retinoic acid treatment in acute promyelocytic leukemia. Leukemia 2001;15(8):1311–3.

35. Fisher DA. Exercise-induced bronchoconstriction related to isotretinoin therapy. J Am Acad Dermatol 1985;13(3):524.

36. Bunker CB, Tomlinson MC, Johnson NM, Dowd PM. Isotretinoin and the lung. Br J Dermatol 1991;125(Suppl 38):29.

37. Sabroe RA, Staughton RC, Bunker CB. Bronchospasm induced by isotretinoin. BMJ 1996;312(7035):886.

38. van de Loosdrecht AA, van Imhoff GW. Images in clinical medicine. All-trans-retinoic acid related pulmonary syndrome in acute promyelocytic leukemia. Neth J Med 1999;54(3):131–2.

39. Kim C, Ki Ko W, Hyun Kwon S, Myung Kang S, Nyun Kim C, Gyoo Yang D, Kyu Kim S, Chang J, Kyu Kim S,

Young Lee W, Ik Yang W. A case of acute respiratory distress syndrome induced by all-trans-retinoic acid. Tuberc Respir Dis 2000;49:93–8.

40. Raanani P, Segal E, Levi I, Bercowicz M, Berkenstat H, Avigdor A, Perel A, Ben-Bassat I. Diffuse alveolar hemorrhage in acute promyelocytic leukemia patients treated with ATRA—a manifestation of the basic disease or the treatment. Leuk Lymphoma 2000;37(5–6):605–10.

41. Byrne A, Hnatko G. Depression associated with isotretinoin therapy. Can J Psychiatry 1995;40(9):567.

42. Fraunfelder FW, Fraunfelder FT, Corbett JJ. Isotretinoin-associated intracranial hypertension. Ophthalmology 2004;111(6):1248–50.

43. Schroeter T, Lanvers C, Herding H, Suttorp M. Pseudotumor cerebri induced by all-trans-retinoic acid in a child treated for acute promyelocytic leukemia. Med Pediatr Oncol 2000;34(4):284–6.

44. Yamaji S, Kanamori H, Mishima A, Fujisawa S, Motomura S, Mohri H. All-trans retinoic acid-induced multiple mononeuropathies. Am J Hematol 1999;60(4):311.

45. Chroni E, Georgiou S, Monastirli A, Paschalis C, Tsambaos D. Effects of short-term oral acitretin therapy on peripheral nerve function: a prospective neurological and neurophysiological study. Acta Dermatol Venereol 2001;81(6):423–5.

46. Lebowitz MA, Berson DS. Ocular effects of oral retinoids. J Am Acad Dermatol 1988;19(1 Pt 2):209–11.

47. Gold JA, Shupack JL, Nemec MA. Ocular side effects of the retinoids. Int J Dermatol 1989;28(4):218–25.

48. Fraunfelder FT, LaBraico JM, Meyer SM. Adverse ocular reactions possibly associated with isotretinoin. Am J Ophthalmol 1985;100(4):534–7.

49. Ellies P, Dighiero P, Legeais JM, Pouliquen YJ, Renard G. Persistent corneal opacity after oral isotretinoin therapy for acne. Cornea 2000;19(2):238–9.

50. Ng EW, Congdon NG, Sommer A. Acute sixth nerve palsy in vitamin A treatment of xerophthalmia. Br J Ophthalmol 2000;84(8):931–2.

51. Parry MF, Rha CK. Pseudomembranous colitis caused by topical clindamycin phosphate. Arch Dermatol 1986;122(5):583–4.

52. Wester RC, Maibach HI. In vivo percutaneous absorption. In: Marzulli FN, Maibach HI, editors. Dermatotoxicology. 2nd ed.. Washington: Hemisphere Publishing Corporation, 1983:131.

53. Wysowski DK, Pitts M, Beitz J. An analysis of reports of depression and suicide in patients treated with isotretinoin. J Am Acad Dermatol 2001;45(4):515–9.

54. Wysowski DK, Pitts M, Beitz J. Depression and suicide in patients treated with isotretinoin. N Engl J Med 2001;344(6):460.

55. Gupta MA, Gupta AK. Isotretinoin use and reports of sustained dreaming. Br J Dermatol 2001;144(4):919–20.

56. Fontan B, Bonafe JL, Moatti JP. Toxic effects of the aromatic retinoid etretinate. Arch Dermatol 1983;119(3):187–8.

57. Alcalay J, Landau M, Zucker A. Analysis of laboratory data in acne patients treated with isotretinoin: is there really a need to perform routine laboratory tests? J Dermatol Treat 2001;12(1):9–12.

58. Rodondi N, Darioli R, Ramelet AA, Hohl D, Lenain V, Perdrix J, Wietlisbach V, Riesen WF, Walther T, Medinger L, Nicod P, Desvergne B, Mooser V. High risk for hyperlipidemia and the metabolic syndrome after an episode of hypertriglyceridemia during 13-cis retinoic acid

therapy for acne: a pharmacogenetic study. Ann Intern Med 2002;136(8):582–9.

59. Barth JH, Macdonald-Hull SP, Mark J, Jones RG, Cunliffe WJ. Isotretinoin therapy for acne vulgaris: a re-evaluation of the need for measurements of plasma lipids and liver function tests. Br J Dermatol 1993;129(6):704–7.

60. Suzumiya J, Asahara F, Katakami H, Kimuran N, Hisano S, Okumura M, Ohno R. Hypercalcaemia caused by all-trans retinoic acid treatment of acute promyelocytic leukaemia: case report. Eur J Haematol 1994;53(2):126–7.

61. Belden TL, Ragucci DP. Hypercalcemia induced by 13-cis-retinoic acid in a patient with neuroblastoma. Pharmacotherapy 2002;22(5):645–8.

62. Sakamoto O, Yoshinari M, Rikiishi T, Fujiwara I, Imaizumi M, Tsuchiya S, Iinuma K. Hypercalcemia due to all-trans retinoic acid therapy for acute promyelocytic leukemia: a case report of effective treatment with bisphosphonate. Pediatr Int 2001;43(6):688–90.

63. Allan S, Christmas T. Severe edema associated with etretinate. J Am Acad Dermatol 1988;19(1 Pt 1):140.

64. Windhorst DB, Nigra T. General clinical toxicology of oral retinoids. J Am Acad Dermatol 1982;6(4 Pt 2 Suppl):675–82.

65. Brown JE, Olujohungbe A, Chang J, Ryder WD, Morganstern GR, Chopra R, Scarffe JH. All-trans retinoic acid (ATRA) and tranexamic acid: a potentially fatal combination in acute promyelocytic leukaemia. Br J Haematol 2000;110(4):1010–2.

66. Kocak U, Gursel T, Ozturk G, Kantarci S. Thrombosis during all-trans-retinoic acid therapy in a child with acute promyelocytic leukemia and factor VQ 506 mutation. Pediatr Hematol Oncol 2000;17(2):177–80.

67. Cakmakci A, Yilmaz AS, Akbulut S, Gul U, Ozyilkan E. Polycythemia in a patient treated with isotretinoin. Ann Pharmacother 2001;35(7–8):964–5.

68. Ko BS, Tang JL, Chen YC, Yao M, Wang CH, Shen MC, Tien HF. Extramedullary relapse after all-trans retinoic acid treatment in acute promyelocytic leukemia—the occurrence of retinoic acid syndrome is a risk factor. Leukemia 1999;13(9):1406–8.

69. Reniers DE, Howard JM. Isotretinoin-induced inflammatory bowel disease in an adolescent. Ann Pharmacother 2001;35(10):1214–6.

70. Godfrey KM, James MP. Treatment of severe acne with isotretinoin in patients with inflammatory bowel disease. Br J Dermatol 1990;123(5):653–5.

71. Martin P, Manley PN, Depew WT, Blakeman JM. Isotretinoin-associated proctosigmoiditis. Gastroenterology 1987;93(3):606–9.

72. Brodin MB. Inflammatory bowel disease and isotretinoin. J Am Acad Dermatol 1986;14(5 Pt 1):843.

73. Schleicher SM. Oral isotretinoin and inflammatory bowel disease. J Am Acad Dermatol 1985;13(5 Pt 1):834–5.

74. Rosen T, Unkefer RP. Treatment of pyoderma faciale with isotretinoin in a patient with ulcerative colitis. Cutis 1999;64(2):107–9.

75. Yamada K, Sugimoto K, Matsumoto T, Narumi K, Oshimi K. All-trans retinoic acid-induced vasculitis and hemonecrosis of the ileum in a patient with acute promyelocytic leukemia. Leukemia 1999;13(4):647–8.

76. Sanchez MR, Ross B, Rotterdam H, Salik J, Brodie R, Freedberg IM. Retinoid hepatitis. J Am Acad Dermatol 1993;28(5 Pt 2):853–8.

77. Gavish D, Katz M, Gottehrer N, Israeli A, Lijovetzky G, Holubar K. Cholestatic jaundice, an unusual side effect of etretinate. J Am Acad Dermatol 1985;13(4):669–70.

78. Perea G, Salar A, Altes A, Brunet S, Sierra J. Acute hepatomegaly with severe liver toxicity due to all-trans-retinoic acid. Haematologica 2000;85(5):551–2.

79. Izumi T, Hatake K, Miura Y. Acute promyelocytic leukemia. N Engl J Med 1994;330(2):141.

80. Yutsudo Y, Imoto S, Ozuru R, Kajimoto K, Itoi H, Koizumi T, Nishimura R, Nakagawa T. Acute pancreatitis after all-trans retinoic acid therapy. Ann Hematol 1997;74(6):295–6.

81. Abou Chacra L, Ghosn M, Ghayad E, Honein K. A case of pancreatitis associated with all-trans-retinoic acid therapy in acute promyelocytic leukemia. Hematol J 2001;2(6):406–7.

82. Pavese P, Kuentz F, Belleville C, Rouge PE, Elsener M. Renal impairment induced by isotretinoin. Nephrol Dial Transplant 1997;12(6):1299.

83. Cribier B, Welsch M, Heid E. Renal impairment probably induced by etretinate. Dermatology 1992;185(4):266–8.

84. Kellock DJ, Parslew R, Mendelsohn SS, O'Mahony CP. Non-specific urethritis—possible association with isotretinoin therapy. Int J STD AIDS 1996;7(2):135–6.

85. van Oers JA, de Leeuw J, van Bommel EF. Nephrotic syndrome associated with isotretinoin. Nephrol Dial Transplant 2000;15(6):923–4.

86. Tomita N, Kanamori H, Fujita H, Maruta A, Naitoh A, Nakamura S, Ota Y, Nozue N, Kihara M, Ishigatsubo Y. Granulomatous tubulointerstitial nephritis induced by all-trans retinoic acid. Anticancer Drugs 2001;12(8):677–80.

87. Turman MA, Hammond S, Grovas A, Rauck AM. Possible association of retinoic acid with bone marrow transplant nephropathy. Pediatr Nephrol 1999;13(9):755–8.

88. Charles KS, Kanaa M, Winfield DA, Reilly JT. Scrotal ulceration during all-trans retinoic (ATRA) therapy for acute promyelocytic leukaemia. Clin Lab Haematol 2000;22(3):171–4.

89. Esser AC, Nossa R, Shoji T, Sapadin AN. All-trans-retinoic acid-induced scrotal ulcerations in a patient with acute promyelocytic leukemia. J Am Acad Dermatol 2000;43(2 Pt 1):316–7.

90. Sun GL. [Treatment of acute promyelocytic leukemia (APL) with all-trans retinoic acid (ATRA): a report of five-year experience.]Zhonghua Zhong Liu Za Zhi 1993;15(2):125–9.

91. Tajima K, Sagae M, Yahagi A, Akiba J, Suzuki K, Hayashi T, Satoh S. [Scrotum exfoliative dermatitis with ulcers associated with treatment of acute promyelocytic leukemia with all-trans retinoic acid.]Rinsho Ketsueki 1998;39(1):48–52.

92. Mori A, Tamura S, Katsuno T, Nishimura Y, Itoh T, Saheki K, Takatsuka H, Wada H, Fujimori Y, Okamoto T, Takemoto Y, Kakishita E. Scrotal ulcer occurring in patients with acute promyelocytic leukemia during treatment with all-trans retinoic acid. Oncol Rep 1999;6(1):55–8.

93. Newman JM, Rindler JM, Bergfeld WF, Brydon JK. Stevens–Johnson syndrome associated with topical nitrogen mustard therapy. J Am Acad Dermatol 1997;36(1):112–4.

94. Reynolds P, Fawcett H, Waldram R, Prouse P. Delayed onset of vasculitis following isotretinoin. Lancet 1989;2(8673):1216.

95. Silverman AK, Ellis CN, Voorhees JJ. Hypervitaminosis A syndrome: a paradigm of retinoid side effects. J Am Acad Dermatol 1987;16(5 Pt 1):1027–39.

96. Levi I, Raanani P, Shalmon B, Schiby-Brilliant R, Ben-Bassat I. Acute neutrophilic dermatosis induced by all-

trans-retinoic acid treatment for acute promyelocytic leukemia. Leuk Lymphoma 1999;34(3–4):401–4.

97. van Der Vliet HJ, Roberson AE, Hogan MC, Morales CE, Crader SC, Letendre L, Pruthi RK. All-trans-retinoic acid-induced myositis: a description of two patients. Am J Hematol 2000;63(2):94–8.

98. Astudillo L, Loche F, Reynish W, Rigal-Huguet F, Lamant L, Pris J. Sweet's syndrome associated with retinoic acid syndrome in a patient with promyelocytic leukemia. Ann Hematol 2002;81(2):111–4.

99. Birner AM, Meyer LP. Photosensitivity associated with fluorouracil, prochlorperazine, and topical tretinoin. Pharmacotherapy 2001;21(2):258–60.

100. Chang SE, Huh J, Choi JH, Sung KJ, Moon KC, Koh JK. Cutaneous relapse in acute promyelocytic leukaemia following treatment with all-trans retinoic acid. Br J Dermatol 1999;141(3):586–7.

101. Hughes RA. Arthritis precipitated by isotretinoin treatment for acne vulgaris. J Rheumatol 1993;20(7):1241–2.

102. DiGiovanna JJ, Sollitto RB, Abangan DL, Steinberg SM, Reynolds JC. Osteoporosis is a toxic effect of long-term etretinate therapy. Arch Dermatol 1995;131(11):1263–7.

103. Chroni E, Sakkis T, Georgiou S, Monastirli A, Pasmatzi E, Paschalis C, Tsambaos D. Stiff-person syndrome associated with oral isotretinoin treatment. Neuromuscul Disord 2002;12(9):886–8.

104. Leibovitch I, Amital H, Levy Y, Langevitz P, Shoenfeld Y. Isotretinoin-induced adult onset Still's disease. Clin Exp Rheumatol 2000;18(5):616–8.

105. Larsen GK. Iatrogenic breast discharge with isotretinoin. Arch Dermatol 1985;121(4):450–1.

106. Coleman R, MacDonald D. Effects of isotretinoin on male reproductive system. Lancet 1994;344(8916):198.

107. Khurshid I, Seymour JF, Nakata K, Downie GH. Recurrent manifestations of idiopathic pulmonary alveolar proteinosis after isotretinoin (Accutane) treatment. Chest 2001;120(Suppl):335.

108. Alli N, Toy GG. Familial Mediterranean fever: attacks during isotretinoin treatment. J Am Acad Dermatol 2002;47(6):967.

109. Jick SS, Terris BZ, Jick H. First trimester topical tretinoin and congenital disorders. Lancet 1993;341(8854):1181–2.

110. Selcen D, Seidman S, Nigro MA. Otocerebral anomalies associated with topical tretinoin use. Brain Dev 2000;22(4):218–20.

111. Camera G, Pregliasco P. Ear malformation in baby born to mother using tretinoin cream. Lancet 1992;339(8794):687.

112. Lipson AH, Collins F, Webster WS. Multiple congenital defects associated with maternal use of topical tretinoin. Lancet 1993;341(8856):1352–3.

113. Navarre-Belhassen C, Blanchet P, Hillaire-Buys D, Sarda P, Blayac JP. Multiple congenital malformations associated with topical tretinoin. Ann Pharmacother 1998;32(4):505–6.

114. Ceviz N, Ozkan B, Eren S, Ors R, Olgunturk R. A case of isotretinoin embryopathy with bilateral anotia and Taussig–Bing malformation. Turk J Pediatr 2000;42(3):239–41.

115. Vannucchi MT, Vannucchi H, Humphreys M. Serum levels of vitamin A and retinol binding protein in chronic renal patients treated by continuous ambulatorial peritoneal dialysis. Int J Vitam Nutr Res 1992;62(2):107–12.

116. Doyle S, Conlon P, Royston D. Vitamin A induced stellate cell hyperplasia and fibrosis in renal failure. Histopathology 2000;36(1):90–1.

117. Douer D, Estey E, Santillana S, Bennett JM, Lopez-Bernstein G, Boehm K, Williams T. Treatment of newly diagnosed and relapsed acute promyelocytic leukemia with intravenous liposomal all-trans retinoic acid. Blood 2001;97(1):73–80.

118. Aubin S, Lorette G, Muller C, Vaillant L. Massive isotretinoin intoxication. Clin Exp Dermatol 1995;20(4):348–50.

119. Larsen FG, Jakobsen P, Knudsen J, Weismann K, Kragballe K, Nielsen-Kudsk F. Conversion of acitretin to etretinate in psoriatic patients is influenced by ethanol. J Invest Dermatol 1993;100(5):623–7.

TAXANES

Docetaxel

General Information

Docetaxel is a taxane that is used in combination with doxorubicin in the treatment of metastatic breast cancer and as a single agent in metastatic lung cancer.

Organs and Systems

Respiratory

Interstitial pneumonitis has been attributed to docetaxel in four cases (1). None of the patients had lung disease and they all had normal liver function. Within 8–14 days of receiving a second cycle of docetaxel (75 mg/m^2 in three cases and 60 mg/m^2 in the other), all developed acute dyspnea and fever, which progressed until they needed ventilation; two died. In contrast, in a study of 33 patients treated with paclitaxel and carboplatin, only one had reduced diffusion capacity for carbon monoxide, with no accompanying clinical or radiological changes (2).

Fluid balance

Fluid retention has previously been reported with docetaxel. Some believe that this effect depends on the dose and the duration of infusion (3,4) and that high concentrations of M4, the cyclized oxazolidinedione metabolite of docetaxel, cause more pronounced fluid retention.

Hematologic

In 46 chemotherapy-naive patients, docetaxel had an important but reversible non-specific lymphopenic effect, thought to be associated with an increased risk of non-neutropenic infections (5).

Gastrointestinal

Three of 14 patients in a phase 1 study of docetaxel plus vinorelbine for metastatic breast cancer developed colitis (6). A further three patients were identified in other studies of docetaxel.

Skin

Of 99 patients who received low-dose docetaxel (60 mg/m^2 every 3 or 4 weeks), 25 had skin toxicity, mainly erythema and nail changes (7). Of a subset of 25 patients who received irradiation before docetaxel, four had recall dermatitis during their first infusion of docetaxel. All had previously received doxorubicin, which may in part have explained some of the toxicity.

Maculopapular eruptions and desquamation of hands and/or feet occurred in 35% of patients with non-small cell lung cancers given docetaxel (8).

Four cases of fixed plaques of erythrodysesthesia have been attributed to intravenous docetaxel (9). There had been no extravasation or previous skin injury. While this was a new presentation, the authors did not explain why the lesions were not just late presentations of small-volume extravasation injuries.

Nails

Onycholysis has been reported in patients receiving docetaxel (10).

Immunologic

A 25% incidence of grade 2 or more severe immunological reactions to docetaxel has been reported after the use of oral prednisone (100 mg orally before treatment and 50 mg once on the morning of treatment and the following 2 days) in 20 patients with non-small-cell lung cancers (8). No other premedications were given routinely. If infusion-related symptoms occurred, the infusion was interrupted and diphenhydramine was given. On subsequent cycles those patients then were routinely premedicated with diphenhydramine 25 or 50 mg intravenously and cimetidine 300 mg intravenously.

References

1. Read WL, Mortimer JE, Picus J. Severe interstitial pneumonitis associated with docetaxel administration. Cancer 2002;94(3):847–53.
2. Dimopoulou I, Galani H, Dafni U, Samakovii A, Roussos C, Dimopoulos MA. A prospective study of pulmonary function in patients treated with paclitaxel and carboplatin. Cancer 2002;94(2):452–8.
3. Shin E, Ishitobi M, Hiraoia M, Kazumasa F, Hideyuki M, Nishisho I, Toshiro S, Yasunori H, Tosimasa T. Phase I study of docetaxel administered by bi-weekly infusion to patients with metastatic breast cancer. Anticancer Res 2000;20(6C):4721–6.
4. Rosing H, Lustig V, van Warmerdam LJ, Huizing MT, ten Bokkel Huinink WW, Schellens JH, Rodenhuis S, Bult A, Beijnen JH. Pharmacokinetics and metabolism of docetaxel administered as a 1-h intravenous infusion. Cancer Chemother Pharmacol 2000;45(3):213–8.
5. Kotsakis A, Sarra E, Peraki M, Koukourakis M, Apostolaki S, Souglakos J, Mavromanomakis E, Vlachonikolis J, Georgoulias V. Docetaxel-induced lymphopenia in patients with solid tumors: a prospective phenotypic analysis. Cancer 2000;89(6):1380–6.
6. Ibrahim NK, Sahin AA, Dubrow RA, Lynch PM, Boehnke-Michaud L, Valero V, Buzdar AU, Hortobagyi GN. Colitis associated with docetaxel-based chemotherapy in patients with metastatic breast cancer. Lancet 2000;355(9200):281–3.
7. Ando M, Watanabe T, Nagata K, Narabayashi M, Adachi I, Katsumata N. Efficacy of docetaxel 60 mg/m^2 in patients with metastatic breast cancer according to the status of anthracycline resistance J Clin Oncol 2001;19(2):336–42.
8. Miller VA, Rigas JR, Francis PA, Grant SC, Pisters KM, Venkatraman ES, Woolley K, Heelan RT, Kris MG. Phase II trial of a 75-mg/m^2 dose of docetaxel with prednisone

premedication for patients with advanced non-small cell lung cancer. Cancer 1995;75(4):968–72.

9. Chu CY, Yang CH, Yang CY, Hsiao GH, Chiu HC. Fixed erythrodysaesthesia plaque due to intravenous injection of docetaxel. Br J Dermatol 2000;142(4):808–11.

10. Correia O, Azevedo C, Pinto Ferreira E, Braga Cruz F, Polonia J. Nail changes secondary to docetaxel (Taxotere). Dermatology 1999;198(3):288–90.

Paclitaxel

General Information

Paclitaxel is a complex plant product derived from the bark of the yew tree, *Taxus brevifolia*. It has been used for the treatment of metastatic carcinoma of the ovary and breast. It has also been investigated in the treatment of other carcinomas, including non-small-cell lung cancer, malignant melanoma, head and neck cancers, acute leukemias, and Kaposi's sarcoma. The recommended dosage for the treatment of ovarian and breast carcinoma is 175 mg/m^2 given intravenously over 3 hours every 3 weeks. However, various dosage and administration schedules have been investigated.

Mechanism of action

Paclitaxel acts by enhancing microtubule assembly and stabilizing microtubules (1,2). Microtubules consist of polymers of tubulin in dynamic equilibrium with tubulin heterodimers. Their principal function is the formation of the mitotic spindle during cell division, but they are also active in many interphase functions, such as cellular motility, intracellular transport, and signal transmission. Paclitaxel inhibits the depolymerization of tubulin, and the microtubules formed in the presence of paclitaxel are extremely stable and dysfunctional. This stabilization impairs the essential assembly and disassembly required for dynamic cellular processes, and death of the cell results through disruption of the normal microtubular dynamics required for interphase processes and cell division. In tumor cells, cytotoxicity is represented by the appearance of abnormal microtubular bundles, which accumulate during G2 and mitosis, blocking the cell cycle (3).

Pharmacokinetics

Paclitaxel has non-linear kinetics: peak plasma concentrations and drug exposure increase disproportionately with increasing doses and the pharmacokinetics depend on the schedule of administration. Saturation is reached with high-dose short infusions (4). Paclitaxel has been reported to follow both biphasic (5) and triphasic models (6). The half-life has been estimated at 6–13 hours after intravenous administration (7).

After intravenous administration, paclitaxel is extensively distributed, despite extensive binding to plasma proteins (89%), presumably albumin (2). Its routes of elimination have not been fully elucidated, but renal clearance accounts for an insignificant proportion of total systemic clearance, suggesting that metabolism, biliary excretion, or excretion via other routes are responsible for elimination (6). High concentrations of paclitaxel and its hydroxylated metabolites have been found in rat and human bile, suggesting hepatic metabolism (8). In all, 11 metabolites of paclitaxel have been identified, and paclitaxel metabolism to 6-α-hydroxypaclitaxel is an important detoxification pathway (6,9).

The effects of renal and hepatic dysfunction on paclitaxel elimination have not been studied extensively. Since renal clearance accounts for a small proportion of total clearance, dosage modifications are not considered necessary in patients with renal dysfunction.

One study has shown that patients with existing liver dysfunction have a reduced total body clearance of paclitaxel and require dosage reductions (10). A dosage reduction of 50% has been suggested in patients with moderate or severe hyperbilirubinemia or increased serum transaminases (4).

Paclitaxel is formulated in a mixture of ethanol and Cremophor EL (polyethoxylated castor oil). Cremophor reduced the electrophoretic mobility of serum lipoproteins along with the appearance of a lipoprotein dissociation product. After serum was exposed to Cremophor in vitro or in vivo there was substantial binding of paclitaxel to the lipoprotein dissociation product(s), and this could represent an important factor in the distribution of paclitaxel (11).

General adverse effects

A summary of the incidences of the adverse effects of paclitaxel in single-agent studies in 402 patients is given in Table 1 (12).

Organs and Systems

Cardiovascular

Paclitaxel causes disturbances in cardiac rhythm, but the relevance of these effects has not been fully elucidated. Originally, all patients in trials of paclitaxel were under continuous cardiac monitoring, owing to the risk of hypersensitivity reactions, and cardiac disturbances were therefore more likely to be detected. Many trials limited eligibility to patients without a history of cardiac abnormalities and to those who were not taking medications likely to alter cardiac conduction. The incidence of cardiac dysrhythmias in the population under study not treated with paclitaxel is unknown, and it is therefore not always possible to attribute dysrhythmias to paclitaxel in these patients. The Cremophor EL vehicle does not appear to be implicated in the incidence of dysrhythmias, although hypotension associated with hypersensitivity reactions may occur (13).

The most common effect of paclitaxel is asymptomatic bradycardia, which occurred in 29% of patients in one phase 2 trial (14) and in 9% of patients in a further assessment of 402 patients in phase 2 trials (15). One

Table 1 Incidences of adverse effects of paclitaxel

Adverse effect	Incidence (%)
Cardiovascular	
Bradycardia during infusion	10
Hypotension during infusion	23
Severe cardiovascular events	1
Abnormal electrocardiogram (all patients)	30
Abnormal electrocardiogram (patients with normal baseline)	19
Nervous system	
Peripheral neuropathy	
Any symptoms	62
Severe symptoms	4
Hematologic	
Neutropenia $<2 \times 10^9/l$	92
Neutropenia $<0.5 \times 10^9/l$	67
Leukopenia $<4 \times 10^9/l$	93
Leukopenia $<1 \times 10^9/l$	26
Thrombocytopenia $<100 \times 10^9/l$	27
Thrombocytopenia $<50 \times 10^9/l$	10
Anemia <11 g/dl	90
Anemia <8 g/dl	24
Liver	
Bilirubin raised	8
Alkaline phosphatase activity raised	23
Aspartate transaminase (AsT) activity raised	16
Gastrointestinal	
Nausea and vomiting	59
Diarrhea	43
Mucositis	39
Hair	
Alopecia	82
Musculoskeletal	
Myalgia/arthralgia	
Any symptoms	55
Severe symptoms	4
Immunologic reactions (with premedication)	
Any	41
Severe	2

phase 1 trial showed no significant cardiac dysrhythmias (16), while another reported cardiac toxicity in 14% of patients, 74% of these being due to asymptomatic bradycardia (17). Bradycardia is not an indication for discontinuation of treatment, unless it is associated with atrioventricular conduction disturbances or clinically significant effects (for example symptomatic hypotension). More significant bradydysrhythmias and atrioventricular conduction disturbances have been reported during clinical trials, including Mobitz I (Wenckebach syndrome) and Mobitz II atrioventricular block (14,18).

One patient died in heart failure 7 days after receiving paclitaxel by infusion; this patient had no prior history of cardiac problems, apart from mild hypertension (19).

The authors of a review of the cardiac toxicity associated with paclitaxel in a number of studies concluded that the overall incidence of serious cardiac events is low (0.1%) (20). Heart block and conduction abnormalities occurred infrequently and were often asymptomatic. Sinus bradycardia was the most frequent, occurring in 30% of patients. The causal relation of paclitaxel to atrial and ventricular dysrhythmias and cardiac ischemia was not entirely clear. There did not appear to be any evidence of cumulative toxicity or augmentation of acute cardiac effects of the anthracyclines.

In an attempt to clarify further the cardiotoxicity of paclitaxel, its effect on cardiovascular autonomic regulation has been investigated in 14 women (21). The authors concluded that autonomic modulation of heart rate is impaired by paclitaxel, but they were unable to say whether it would return to normal on withdrawal. They also investigated the effect of docetaxel on neural cardiovascular regulation in women with breast cancer, previously treated with anthracyclines (22). They concluded that docetaxel did not impair vagal cardiac control. The changes that they observed in blood pressure suggest that docetaxel changes sympathetic vascular control, although these changes seemed to be related to altered cardiovascular homeostasis rather than peripheral sympathetic neuropathy.

Continuous cardiac monitoring is recommended for patients with serious conduction abnormalities; however, routine cardiac monitoring is considered unnecessary in patients without a history of cardiac conduction abnormalities (7). Further studies are needed to determine the risk in patients treated with paclitaxel with predisposing cardiac risk factors.

Respiratory

Effects of paclitaxel on the respiratory system are generally related to hypersensitivity reactions. One case of pneumonitis was possibly due to a hypersensitivity reaction to either paclitaxel or its vehicle Cremophor EL; treatment with corticosteroids resulted in improvement (23). One patient developed tachypnea and cyanosis and subsequently died of pulmonary edema 7 days after receiving an infusion of paclitaxel (19).

Nervous system

The most common nervous system effect is peripheral neuropathy, although one patient developed tonic-clonic seizures whilst receiving paclitaxel and required treatment with benzodiazepines and barbiturates (14). Motor weakness has occasionally been reported (24).

Neurotoxicity associated with paclitaxel is dose-dependent, cumulative, and characterized principally by a sensory and motor peripheral neuropathy. Neuropathy appears to be related to axonal degeneration and demyelination (25). Neurological toxicity is usually reversible after termination of therapy, and although it rarely requires withdrawal of therapy, it has been the dose-limiting adverse effect in some phase 1 trials (5,26). This effect became more apparent as higher doses of paclitaxel were used, particularly in combination with growth factors, which allow escalating doses of paclitaxel to be administered. A high-dose study has shown dose-related toxicity, with a dose-limiting ceiling at 775 mg/m^2, when paresthesia occurs (27). Patients with co-existing medical illnesses associated with peripheral neuropathy, such as diabetes mellitus and alcohol abuse, may be more prone to develop peripheral neuropathy.

Peripheral neuropathy presents as numbness, burning, and tingling in a glove-and-stocking distribution. Symptoms usually begin 24–72 hours after treatment with paclitaxel, with a symmetrical distal loss of sensation. Most cases occur at doses over 200 mg/m^2 and particularly after multiple courses (24–26). Mild to moderate sensory neuropathy has occurred in 52% of patients treated with doses of 175 mg/m^2, while only 36% experienced neuropathy at doses of at least 135 mg/m^2 (17,24,28,29). At the lower dose of 135 mg/m^2, the effects are usually limited to a mild sensory neuropathy (17,29).

The incidence of peripheral neuropathy increases substantially at doses above 250 mg/m^2 (14,16,18–20, 25,29–32). Neuropathy was the dose-limiting adverse effect in one phase 1 trial with doses of 275 mg/m^2, and patients experienced grade 2–3 neurotoxicity 1–3 days after treatment (5). The symptoms generally subsided within several weeks to months. A study of adverse effects in patients in phase 2 trials showed that peripheral neuropathy occurred in 62% of 402 patients (15). Of patients receiving higher doses (190 mg/m^2 or more), 80% had symptoms that were mild or moderate. In severe cases of peripheral neuropathy a dose reduction of 20% is recommended for subsequent courses (7).

Previous treatment with other neurotoxic agents may compound the problem. In one study symptoms of neurotoxicity were observed in one patient who received concomitant cisplatin with paclitaxel (33). However, signs and symptoms of neurotoxicity have been insignificant in combination treatments of cisplatin and paclitaxel in other trials (1). Pre-existing neuropathy as a result of previous therapy is not a contraindication to paclitaxel (7).

Tricyclic antidepressants, in particular amitriptyline, and venlafaxine are helpful in relieving symptoms of paclitaxel-induced peripheral neuropathy (1,26,33,34).

Sensory systems

Transient scintillating scotomata have been observed in the visual fields of both eyes in nine patients receiving paclitaxel infusions in doses of 175 and 225 mg/m^2 (35). Involvement of the optic nerve was confirmed, and this is likely to have been related to optic nerve conduction abnormalities associated with the neurological effects of paclitaxel. The abnormalities were not progressive and there was some degree of recovery, although one patient sustained a permanent reduction in vision.

Hematologic

Bone marrow suppression is a dose-limiting adverse effect often encountered with paclitaxel. Neutropenia occurs most commonly 8–10 days after treatment, and recovery usually occurs on days 15–21. Paclitaxel is relatively platelet-sparing, and thrombocytopenia and anemia are rare (26). There is no evidence that neutropenia is cumulative, suggesting that paclitaxel may not irreversibly damage hemopoietic stem cells (1).

Neutropenia is dose- and schedule-related and is less common with shorter infusion schedules. At doses of 110–250 mg/m^2 over 24 hours, neutropenia is usually severe, and grade 4 neutropenia develops in a large proportion of patients. Paclitaxel given as a 3-hour infusion causes less severe neutropenia (17,24,29). An analysis of patients receiving either a 3-hour or 24-hour infusion of 175 or 135 mg/m^2 showed that severe neutropenia was more common with the 24-hour infusions: 75% of patients developed severe neutropenia (absolute neutrophil count below 500 × 10^6/l) and episodes of fever (29). Doses of 200–250 mg/m^2 also cause severe neutropenia when paclitaxel was given as a 24-hour infusion, but recovery of neutrophil count was fairly rapid (13,14,26,33,36,37).

The duration of neutropenia is usually brief and treatment delays for unresolved adverse hematological effects at day 21 are rare. Paclitaxel-induced neutropenia does not always lead to infectious complications, and therefore a dosage reduction for neutropenia alone is not considered necessary (14,16,18–20,29,30).

Prior myelotoxic chemotherapy and/or radiotherapy appear to be major risk factors in determining the severity of neutropenia (1,13). Doses of 200 and 250 mg/m^2 over short infusion times induce minimal myelosuppression in patients who have had minimal prior therapy (26,30); however, seven patients (1.6%) died because of toxicity in another trial in patients with ovarian cancer who had received extensive previous chemotherapy; deaths were due to sepsis or severe neutropenia (13).

Other data suggest that neutropenia may be related to pharmacological exposure, and phase 1 studies have shown that the severity of paclitaxel-induced neutropenia correlates with the area under the paclitaxel concentration–time curve (36).

The incidence of neutropenia has also been investigated in combination schedules. Patients receiving paclitaxel in combination with cyclophosphamide have severe neutropenia more often than with single treatment (72% of patients). Paclitaxel given as a 24-hour infusion before cyclophosphamide is more likely to cause severe neutropenia compared with patients who receive cyclophosphamide first (31).

Attempts to overcome neutropenia include the use of human granulocyte colony stimulating factor (GCSF). The absolute neutrophil counts are generally higher and the duration of severe neutropenia is shorter when GCSF is given 24 hours after paclitaxel and continued until there is recovery of the neutrophil count. When paclitaxel is given in combination with GCSF, doses of 250 mg/m^2 given over 24 hours every 3 weeks are possible without inducing dose-limiting neutropenia (16). Three-hour infusion schedules have also been successful using doses of 250 mg/m^2 in combination with GCSF and doxorubicin (32). Other dose-limiting adverse effects tend to predominate when paclitaxel is given in higher doses in combination with GCSF.

Recommendations currently specify that patients should not be retreated with paclitaxel until the neutrophil count recovers to $2.5 \times 10^9/1$ and the platelet count recovers to over $100 \times 10^9/1$ (7).

Gastrointestinal

Severe nausea, vomiting, and diarrhea are uncommon with paclitaxel (1). Although about half of the patients in one study had vomiting or diarrhea, under 5% were severe events (15). In another phase 2 trial, there were 11 episodes of nausea and vomiting in 281 courses (14). Four patients developed diarrhea, but this was not clinically significant. Generally, symptoms of nausea, vomiting, and diarrhea associated with paclitaxel therapy are mild.

Mucositis and stomatitis have been reported with paclitaxel. Mucositis is characterized by ulceration of the lips, pharynx, and oral cavity, occurring 3–7 days after paclitaxel treatment (1,13,14,17,24,26,29,33,36–38). Mucositis appears to be more common during treatment of acute leukemias rather than solid tumors, when doses above 390 mg/m^2 are used (24). Severe mucositis occurred during second and third courses, suggesting a cumulative effect, and was more severe if treatment was given at 15 days or less after previous

courses. Patients with hematological malignancies are more prone to breakdown of the mucosal barrier, and this may account for the increased incidence of mucositis. Narcotic analgesics are effective in controlling the pain associated with mucositis (1).

Severe abdominal pain occurred in 25 patients treated with intraperitoneal paclitaxel in doses over 175 mg/m^2 (39).

Transient paralytic ileus occurred in two patients in one study (29). Both patients were diabetic, and these symptoms may have been an additional manifestation of autonomic neuropathy.

Postmortem examinations of patients treated with paclitaxel have shown mucosal ulceration of the esophagus, stomach, small intestine, and colon (40). Changes associated with epithelial necrosis and mitotic arrest were most prominent in patients who had recently been treated with paclitaxel. These findings suggest that paclitaxel causes transient mitotic arrest associated with cell necrosis.

Urinary tract

Reversible renal insufficiency has been reported in one patient who was treated with paclitaxel by the intraperitoneal route (39).

Skin

Local venous effects, including erythema, tenderness, and discomfort, can occur at the injection site during paclitaxel infusion (13). Inflammation is evident within hours and usually resolves within 21 days. Inflammation occurs in areas of drug extravasation along with prolonged soft tissue injuries, and necrotic changes have been reported in one patient at the site of extravasation (41). Inflammation is most likely to be due to the drug, but the Cremophor EL vehicle may be implicated, as it produces mild inflammation in animals (41).

There is little information on the treatment of extravasation of paclitaxel, as it has not been common during clinical trials. However, a soft-tissue injury occurred in one patient at the site of previous extravasation after treatment with paclitaxel in a different limb (42). This resolved within 7 days.

Radiation dermatitis has been reported in a patient who received a single infusion of paclitaxel (43). This was attributed to the potentiation of radiation effects by paclitaxel because of the close time relation between the radiotherapy and paclitaxel therapy.

Hair

Alopecia occurs in nearly all patients who receive paclitaxel, but it has unique characteristics. Hair loss is sudden and complete, and many patients often experience loss of all body hair, including axillary and pubic hair, eyelashes, and eyebrows (28,44). The loss of body hair often occurs with cumulative therapy and is more severe after longer infusion times.

Nails

Onycholysis occurred in five of 21 patients who received more than six doses of paclitaxel 100 mg/m^2/week (45). The authors also provided a useful review of onycholysis caused by other chemotherapy.

Musculoskeletal

An arthralgia/myalgia syndrome occurs 2–5 days after chemotherapy in about 20–30% of patients receiving paclitaxel and is possibly dose-related (1). It commonly occurs at doses above 170 mg/m^2 (29). Symptoms of myalgia usually involve the shoulder and paraspinal muscles, while arthralgia is common in the large joints of the arms and legs (1,13). Symptoms can be controlled by non-steroidal anti-inflammatory drugs (13) and perhaps gabapentin (46). The incidence of arthralgia and myalgia is also increased in patients who receive GCSF, with symptoms occurring more frequently in 86% of patients compared with patients who receive similar doses without growth factor support (28%) (16).

The severity of myalgia and arthralgia correlated significantly with the total cumulative dose of paclitaxel 210 mg/m^2/cycle by 3-hour infusion in 247 patients with a median cumulative dose of 630 mg/m^2 (47).

Immunologic

Acute hypersensitivity reactions were common during phase 1 trials of paclitaxel, and this caused delays in the completion of many trials. Reactions were mild to severe and consisted of cutaneous flushing, bronchospasm, bradycardia, and hypotension; the reactions occurred after either the first or second dose (48). The mechanism of these reactions is uncertain, but they are thought to be non-immunologically mediated, and direct histamine release by mast cells is probably responsible. A large dose of Cremophor EL is used in the formulation of paclitaxel, and this may play an important part in these hypersensitivity reactions; Cremophor EL induces similar reactions in dogs by direct release of histamine (4).

In a study of 32 patients, 84% of those who received paclitaxel developed hypersensitivity reactions characterized by hypotension, respiratory distress, and urticaria (35). These symptoms further confirm that histamine is likely to be the cause of the reaction. The majority of reactions (53%) occurred within 2–3 minutes after the administration of paclitaxel and 78% within 10 minutes. There was one fatal reaction, characterized by hypotension and asystole. Most reactions to paclitaxel occurred after the first or second dose, and hypersensitivity reactions were more common with shorter infusion schedules. Since the duration of the infusion affected the incidence of hypersensitivity reactions, an extension of the infusion duration was investigated. Longer infusion schedules were associated with a reduced incidence of hypersensitivity reactions, the frequency of severe reactions being reduced from 12% or more to 5% with longer infusion times (5,15,49).

Premedication regimens of glucocorticoids and histamine H$_1$ and H$_2$ receptor antagonists have been used in an attempt to prevent hypersensitivity reactions in other

phase 1 trials. These trials were successfully completed using infusion schedules of 1–120 hours and doses of 135–390 mg/m^2, with a lower incidence of hypersensitivity reactions (15,17,28,29,37,44,48). However, the use of premedication did not completely prevent such reactions. There were incidences of 16, 13, and 7% with 3-hour, 6-hour, and 24-hour infusion schedules respectively, despite premedication (48), while only 1.5% of patients developed reactions in a trial with doses of 125–250 mg/m^2 over 24 hours with glucocorticoids and histamine receptor antagonists (29). Only one patient out of 26 developed a hypersensitivity reaction with doses of 150–250 mg/m^2 over 24 hours (26). The relative merits of longer infusion times and premedication are not entirely clear.

In one study of infusion of doses of 175–275 mg/m^2 over 6 hours without premedication, there was only one hypersensitivity reaction in 32 patients (49), while patients who received paclitaxel administered over 1 hour with premedication developed no serious hypersensitivity reactions (37). There were no hypersensitivity reactions in 40 patients who received fractionated doses of paclitaxel administered over 3–5 days, with cumulative doses of 120–250 mg/m^2 (36). In a randomized comparison of two doses of paclitaxel given by 3-hour or 24-hour infusions, premedication alone was sufficient to prevent hypersensitivity reactions with either infusion duration (29).

Premedication, consisting of dexamethasone 20 mg intravenously, 12 and 6 hours before the infusion, and diphenhydramine 50 mg and cimetidine 300 mg, intravenously 30 minutes before the infusion, are now routinely given before patients are treated with paclitaxel, and this, as well as a recommended infusion time of 3 hours, has reduced the incidence and severity of hypersensitivity reactions. A single dose of dexamethasone 16 mg given 30 minutes before paclitaxel was effective in preventing hypersensitivity reactions in 43 patients (38); however, whether a single dose of a glucocorticoid is sufficient for prophylaxis is controversial.

About 2% of all patients who receive paclitaxel with preventive premedication will develop a severe hypersensitivity reaction, characterized by dyspnea, hypotension, angioedema, and urticaria, and requiring treatment. Minor reactions occur in 39% of patients but do not require therapeutic intervention (7).

There was a 9% incidence of clinically important hypersensitivity reactions to paclitaxel in 450 women with gynecological malignancies treated with paclitaxel either alone or in combination regimens (50). There was a significant association between bee sting or animal allergy and paclitaxel hypersensitivity in 57 patients with a variety of tumors (51).

Drug–Drug Interactions

General

Drug interactions with paclitaxel have been reviewed (52). The most important of these are the pharmacodynamic interactions with other cytostatic drugs, but pharmacokinetic interactions have also been described.

Paclitaxel is metabolized by the cytochrome P_{450} isoenzymes CYP2C and CYP3A4 (53), and drugs that inhibit or induce these isozymes would be expected to alter the metabolism of paclitaxel. In vitro ranitidine, diphenhydramine, vincristine, vinblastine, and doxorubicin had little or no effect on the metabolism of paclitaxel, but barbiturates stimulated hydroxylation of the side-chain by induction of CYP3A isoforms (53).

Anthracyclines

The combination of doxorubicin plus paclitaxel is cardiotoxic. Various authors have suggested that after a median cumulative dose of 480 mg/m^2, 50% of patients will have a reduced left ventricular ejection fraction and 20% will develop congestive heart failure.

In 36 women with previously untreated metastatic breast cancer, paclitaxel dose-dependently increased the plasma concentrations of doxorubicin and its metabolite doxorubicinol; this was attributed to competition for biliary excretion of taxanes and anthracyclines mediated by P-glycoprotein (54).

Two studies of the combination of epirubicin plus paclitaxel have shown less reduction in left ventricular ejection fraction and no clinical evidence of cardiac failure (55,56).

Ketoconazole

In patients with ovarian cancer, ketoconazole, 100–1600 mg as a single oral dose 3 hours after paclitaxel 175 mg/m^2 as a 3-hour continuous intravenous infusion, did not alter plasma concentrations of paclitaxel or its principal metabolite, 6-alpha-hydroxypaclitaxel (57).

Platinum-containing cytotoxic drugs

In 21 patients with advanced non-small cell lung cancer carboplatin had no effect on the pharmacokinetics of paclitaxel 135–200 mg/m^2 as a 24-hour intravenous infusion (58). Peripheral neuropathy occurred in 13 of 37 patients treated with paclitaxel 175 mg/m^2 and carboplatin (59). The authors concluded that clinically important neurotoxicity increases with every cycle of chemotherapy. The peripheral neuropathy mainly affected sensory fibers without involving motor nerves. The same paclitaxel/carboplatin chemotherapy in 28 women caused no signs of acute central neurotoxicity or neuropsychological deterioration; however, 11 patients had a peripheral neuropathy (60).

There is some evidence that there is a clinically significant pharmacokinetic interaction of paclitaxel with cisplatin. When cisplatin was given before paclitaxel, the clearance rate of paclitaxel was 25% less than when the two drugs were given in the opposite sequence. In consequence, neutropenia was more profound with the former schedule (62). In addition, in experimental studies, cytotoxicity increased when human ovarian carcinoma cells were exposed to paclitaxel before cisplatin, whereas the interaction was antagonistic when a 1-hour exposure to cisplatin was followed by a 20-hour exposure to taxol, or when the cells were exposed to cisplatin and taxol for 1 hour concurrently (63). The biochemical basis of this interaction has not been elucidated. The pharmacodynamic interaction may be related to cisplatin-induced alterations in cell-specific and non-specific binding sites for paclitaxel (64). In view of these results, paclitaxel should be given before cisplatin (65). There does not appear to be a similar interaction of paclitaxel with carboplatin (66).

Both cisplatin and paclitaxel are neurotoxic, the toxicity being dose-limiting and cumulative; neurotoxicity due to the combination has been suggested to be synergistic; after five cycles of chemotherapy, 96% of 44 patients had grade 1 toxicity and 52% grade 2 toxicity; 18% with grade 2 or 4 toxicity were withdrawn (67).

Trastuzumab

In primates, trastuzumab clearance was reduced when it was administered with paclitaxel (61).

References

1. Rowinsky EK, Cazenave LA, Donehower RC. Taxol: a novel investigational antimicrotubule agent. J Natl Cancer Inst 1990;82(15):1247–59.
2. Rowinsky EK, Onetto N, Canetta RM, Arbuck SG. Taxol: the first of the taxanes, an important new class of antitumor agents. Semin Oncol 1992;19(6):646–62.
3. Horwitz SB, Cohen D, Rao S, Ringel I, Shen HJ, Yang CP. Taxol: mechanisms of action and resistance. J Natl Cancer Inst Monogr 1993;(15):55–61.
4. Rowinsky EK, Donehower RC. Paclitaxel (taxol). N Engl J Med 1995;332(15):1004–14.
5. Wiernik PH, Schwartz EL, Strauman JJ, Dutcher JP, Lipton RB, Paietta E. Phase I clinical and pharmacokinetic study of taxol. Cancer Res 1987;47(9):2486–93.
6. Huizing MT, Keung AC, Rosing H, van der Kuij V, ten Bokkel Huinink WW, Mandjes IM, Dubbelman AC, Pinedo HM, Beijnen JH. Pharmacokinetics of paclitaxel and metabolites in a randomized comparative study in platinum-pretreated ovarian cancer patients. J Clin Oncol 1993;11(11):2127–35.
7. Bristol-Myers Squibb Pharmaceuticals. Taxol (paclitaxel). ABPI Data Sheet Compendium. 1995.
8. Monsarrat B, Alvinerie P, Wright M, Dubois J, Gueritte-Voegelein F, Guenard D, Donehower RC, Rowinsky EK. Hepatic metabolism and biliary excretion of Taxol in rats and humans. J Natl Cancer Inst Monogr 1993;(15):39–46.
9. Gianni L, Kearns CM, Giani A, Capri G, Vigano L, Lacatelli A, Bonadonna G, Egorin MJ. Nonlinear pharmacokinetics and metabolism of paclitaxel and its pharmacokinetic/pharmacodynamic relationships in humans. J Clin Oncol 1995;13(1):180–90.
10. Wilson W, Berg S, Kang K. Phase I/II study of Taxol. 96 hour infusion in refractory lymphoma and breast cancer: pharmacodynamics and analysis of multi drug resistance (mdr-1). Proc Am Soc Clin Oncol 1993;335:134.
11. Sykes E, Woodburn K, Decker D, Kessel D. Effects of Cremophor EL on distribution of Taxol to serum lipoproteins. Br J Cancer 1994;70(3):401–4.
12. Abrams JS, Moore TD, Friedman M. New chemotherapeutic agents for breast cancer. Cancer 1994;74(Suppl 3):1164–76.

13. Rowinsky EK, Eisenhauer EA, Chaudhry V, Arbuck SG, Donehower RC. Clinical toxicities encountered with paclitaxel (Taxol). Semin Oncol 1993;20(4 Suppl 3):1–15.

14. McGuire WP, Rowinsky EK, Rosenshein NB, Grumbine FC, Ettinger DS, Armstrong DK, Donehower RC. Taxol: a unique antineoplastic agent with significant activity in advanced ovarian epithelial neoplasms. Ann Intern Med 1989;111(4):273–9.

15. Onetto N, Canetta R, Winograd B, Catane R, Dougan M, Grechko J, Burroughs J, Rozencweig M. Overview of Taxol safety. J Natl Cancer Inst Monogr 1993;(15):131–9.

16. Schiller JH, Storer B, Tutsch K, Arzoomanian R, Alberti D, Feierabend C, Spriggs D. Phase I trial of 3-hour infusion of paclitaxel with or without granulocyte colony-stimulating factor in patients with advanced cancer. J Clin Oncol 1994;12(2):241–8.

17. Trimble EL, Adams JD, Vena D, Hawkins MJ, Friedman MA, Fisherman JS, Christian MC, Canetta R, Onetto N, Hayn R, Arbuck S. Paclitaxel for platinum-refractory ovarian cancer: results from the first 1,000 patients registered to National Cancer Institute Treatment Referral Center 9103. J Clin Oncol 1993;11(12):2405–10.

18. Rowinsky EK, McGuire WP, Guarnieri T, Fisherman JS, Christian MC, Donehower RC. Cardiac disturbances during the administration of taxol. J Clin Oncol 1991;9(9):1704–12.

19. Alagaratnam TT. Sudden death 7 days after paclitaxel infusion for breast cancer. Lancet 1993;342(8881):1232–3.

20. Arbuck SG, Strauss H, Rowinsky E, Christian M, Suffness M, Adams J, Oakes M, McGuire W, Reed E, Gibbs H, Greenfield R, Montello M. A reassessment of cardiac toxicity associated with Taxol. J Natl Cancer Inst Monogr 1993;(15):117–30.

21. Ekholm EM, Salminen EK, Huikuri HV, Jalonen J, Antila KJ, Salmi TA, Rantanen VT. Impairment of heart rate variability during paclitaxel therapy. Cancer 2000;88(9):2149–53.

22. Ekholm E, Rantanen V, Bergman M, Vesalainen R, Antila K, Salminen E. Docetaxel and autonomic cardiovascular control in anthracycline treated breast cancer patients. Anticancer Res 2000;20(3B):2045–8.

23. Goldberg HL, Vannice SB. Pneumonitis related to treatment with paclitaxel. J Clin Oncol 1995;13(2):534–5.

24. Rowinsky EK, Burke PJ, Karp JE, Tucker RW, Ettinger DS, Donehower RC. Phase I and pharmacodynamic study of taxol in refractory acute leukemias. Cancer Res 1989;49(16):4640–7.

25. Lipton RB, Apfel SC, Dutcher JP, Rosenberg R, Kaplan J, Berger A, Einzig AI, Wiernik P, Schaumburg HH. Taxol produces a predominantly sensory neuropathy. Neurology 1989;39(3):368–73.

26. Wiernik PH, Schwartz EL, Einzig A, Strauman JJ, Lipton RB, Dutcher JP. Phase I trial of taxol given as a 24-hour infusion every 21 days: responses observed in metastatic melanoma. J Clin Oncol 1987;5(8):1232–9.

27. Somlo G, Doroshow JH, Synold T, Longmate J, Reardon D, Chow W, Forman SJ, Leong LA, Margolin KA, Morgan RJ Jr, Raschko JW, Shibata SI, Tetef ML, Yen Y, Kogut N, Schriber J, Alvarnas J. High-dose paclitaxel in combination with doxorubicin, cyclophosphamide and peripheral blood progenitor cell rescue in patients with high-risk primary and responding metastatic breast carcinoma: toxicity profile, relationship to paclitaxel pharmacokinetics and short-term outcome. Br J Cancer 2001;84(12):1591–8.

28. Gore ME, Levy V, Rustin G, Perren T, Calvert AH, Earl H, Thompson JM. Paclitaxel (Taxol) in relapsed and refractory ovarian cancer: the UK and Eire experience. Br J Cancer 1995;72(4):1016–9.

29. Eisenhauer EA, ten Bokkel Huinink WW, Swenerton KD, Gianni L, Myles J, van der Burg ME, Kerr I, Vermorken JB, Buser K, Colombo N, Bacon M, Santabarbara P, Onetto N, Winograd B, Canetta R. European–Canadian randomized trial of paclitaxel in relapsed ovarian cancer: high-dose versus low-dose and long versus short infusion. J Clin Oncol 1994;12(12):2654–66.

30. Holmes FA, Walters RS, Theriault RL, Forman AD, Newton LK, Raber MN, Buzdar AU, Frye DK, Hortobagyi GN. Phase II trial of taxol, an active drug in the treatment of metastatic breast cancer. J Natl Cancer Inst 1991;83(24):1797–805.

31. Kennedy MJ, Donehower RC, Rowinsky EK. Treatment of metastatic breast cancer with combination paclitaxel/cyclophosphamide. Semin Oncol 1995;22(4 Suppl 8):23–7.

32. Fisherman JS, McCabe M, Noone M, Ognibene FP, Goldspiel B, Venzon DJ, Cowan KH, O'Shaughnessy JA. Phase I study of Taxol, doxorubicin, plus granulocyte-colony stimulating factor in patients with metastatic breast cancer. J Natl Cancer Inst Monogr 1993;(15):189–94.

33. Freilich RJ, Seidman AD. Pruritis caused by 3-hour infusion of high-dose paclitaxel and improvement with tricyclic antidepressants. J Natl Cancer Inst 1995;87(12):933–4.

34. Durand JP, Goldwasser F. Dramatic recovery of paclitaxel-disabling neurosensory toxicity following treatment with venlafaxine. Anticancer Drugs 2002;13(7):777–80.

35. Capri G, Munzone E, Tarenzi E, Fulfaro F, Gianni L, Caraceni A, Martini C, Scaioli V. Optic nerve disturbances: a new form of paclitaxel neurotoxicity. J Natl Cancer Inst 1994;86(14):1099–101.

36. Lokich J, Anderson N, Bern M, Coco F, Dow E, Moore C, Zipoli T, Gonzalves L. Multi-day fractionated administration schedule for paclitaxel. Ann Oncol 1995;6(9):883–5.

37. Hainsworth JD, Greco FA. Paclitaxel administered by 1-hour infusion. Preliminary results of a phase I/II trial comparing two schedules. Cancer 1994;74(4):1377–82.

38. Parikh B, Khanolkar S, Advani SH, Dhabhar B, Chandra M. Safety profile of single-dose dexamethasone premedication for paclitaxel. J Clin Oncol 1996;14(7):2189–90.

39. Markman M, Rowinsky E, Hakes T, Reichman B, Jones W, Lewis JL Jr, Rubin S, Curtin J, Barakat R, Phillips M, Hurowitz L, Almadrones L, Hoskins W. Phase I trial of intraperitoneal taxol: a Gynecoloic Oncology Group study. J Clin Oncol 1992;10(9):1485–91.

40. Hruban RH, Yardley JH, Donehower RC, Boitnott JK. Taxol toxicity. Epithelial necrosis in the gastrointestinal tract associated with polymerized microtubule accumulation and mitotic arrest. Cancer 1989;63(10):1944–50.

41. Ajani JA, Dodd LG, Daugherty K, Warkentin D, Ilson DH. Taxol-induced soft-tissue injury secondary to extravasation: characterization by histopathology and clinical course. J Natl Cancer Inst 1994;86(1):51–3.

42. Shapiro J, Richardson GE. Paclitaxel-induced "recall" soft tissue injury occurring at the site of previous extravasation with subsequent intravenous treatment in a different limb. J Clin Oncol 1994;12(10):2237–8.

43. Raghavan VT, Bloomer WD, Merkel DE. Taxol and radiation recall dermatitis. Lancet 1993;341(8856):1354.

44. Peereboom DM, Donehower RC, Eisenhauer EA, McGuire WP, Onetto N, Hubbard JL, Piccart M, Gianni L, Rowinsky EK. Successful re-treatment with taxol after major hypersensitivity reactions. J Clin Oncol 1993;11(5):885–90.

45. Hussain S, Anderson DN, Salvatti ME, Adamson B, McManus M, Braverman AS. Onycholysis as a complication of systemic chemotherapy: report of five cases associated

with prolonged weekly paclitaxel therapy and review of the literature. Cancer 2000;88(10):2367–71.

46. Nguyen VH, Lawrence HJ. Use of gabapentin in the prevention of taxane-induced arthralgias and myalgias. J Clin Oncol 2004;22(9):1767–9.

47. Kunitoh H, Saijo N, Furuse K, Noda K, Ogawa M. Neuromuscular toxicities of paclitaxel 210 mg m(-2) by 3-hour infusion Br J Cancer 1998;77(10):1686–8.

48. Weiss RB, Donehower RC, Wiernik PH, Ohnuma T, Gralla RJ, Trump DL, Baker JR Jr, Van Echo DA, Von Hoff DD, Leyland-Jones B. Hypersensitivity reactions from taxol. J Clin Oncol 1990;8(7):1263–8.

49. Brown T, Havlin K, Weiss G, Cagnola J, Koeller J, Kuhn J, Rizzo J, Craig J, Phillips J, Von Hoff D. A phase I trial of taxol given by a 6-hour intravenous infusion. J Clin Oncol 1991;9(7):1261–7.

50. Markman M, Kennedy A, Webster K, Kulp B, Peterson G, Belinson J. Paclitaxel-associated hypersensitivity reactions: experience of the gynecologic oncology program of the Cleveland Clinic Cancer Center. J Clin Oncol 2000;18(1):102–5.

51. Grosen E, Siitari E, Larrison E, Tiggelaar C, Roecker E. Paclitaxel hypersensitivity reactions related to bee-sting allergy. Lancet 2000;355(9200):288–9.

52. Baker SD. Drug interactions with the taxanes. Pharmacotherapy 1997;17(5 Pt 2):S126–32.

53. Monsarrat B, Royer I, Wright M, Cresteil T. Biotransformation of taxoids by human cytochromes P450: structure–activity relationship. Bull Cancer 1997;84(2):125–33.

54. Gianni L, Vigano L, Locatelli A, Capri G, Giani A, Tarenzi E, Bonadonna G. Human pharmacokinetic characterization and in vitro study of the interaction between doxorubicin and paclitaxel in patients with breast cancer. J Clin Oncol 1997;15(5):1906–15.

55. Rischin D, Smith J, Millward M, Lewis C, Boyer M, Richardson G, Toner G, Gurney H, McKendrick J. A phase II trial of paclitaxel and epirubicin in advanced breast cancer. Br J Cancer 2000;83(4):438–42.

56. Lalisang RI, Voest EE, Wils JA, Nortier JW, Erdkamp FL, Hillen HF, Wals J, Schouten HC, Blijham GH. Dose-dense epirubicin and paclitaxel with G-CSF: a study of decreasing intervals in metastatic breast cancer. Br J Cancer 2000;82(12):1914–9.

57. Jamis-Dow CA, Pearl ML, Watkins PB, Blake DS, Klecker RW, Collins JM. Predicting drug interactions in vivo from experiments in vitro. Human studies with paclitaxel and ketoconazole. Am J Clin Oncol 1997;20(6):592–9.

58. Kearns CM, Belani CP, Erkmen K, Zuhowski M, Hiponia D, Zacharski D, Engstrom C, Ramanathan R, Trenn MR, Aisner J, et al. Pharmacokinetics of paclitaxel and carboplatin in combination. Semin Oncol 1995;22(5 Suppl 12):1–4discussion 5–7.

59. Mayerhofer K, Bodner-Adler B, Bodner K, Leodolter S, Kainz C. Paclitaxel/carboplatin as first-line chemotherapy in advanced ovarian cancer: efficacy and adverse effects with special consideration of peripheral neurotoxicity. Anticancer Res 2000;20(5C):4047–50.

60. Mayerhofer K, Bodner-Adler B, Bodner K, Saletu B, Schindl M, Kaider A, Hefler L, Leodolter S, Kainz C. A paclitaxel-containing chemotherapy does not cause central nervous adverse effects: a prospective study in patients with ovarian cancer. Anticancer Res 2000;20(5C):4051–5.

61. McKeage K, Perry CM. Trastuzumab: a review of its use in the treatment of metastatic breast cancer overexpressing HER2. Drugs 2002;62(1):209–43.

62. Rowinsky EK, Gilbert MR, McGuire WP, Noe DA, Grochow LB, Forastiere AA, Ettinger DS, Lubejko BG, Clark B, Sartorius SE, et al. Sequences of taxol and cisplatin: a phase I and pharmacologic study. J Clin Oncol 1991;9(9):1692–703.

63. Jekunen AP, Christen RD, Shalinsky DR, Howell SB. Synergistic interaction between cisplatin and taxol in human ovarian carcinoma cells in vitro. Br J Cancer 1994;69(2):299–306.

64. Vanhoefer U, Harstrick A, Wilke H, Schleucher N, Walles H, Schroder J, Seeber S. Schedule-dependent antagonism of paclitaxel and cisplatin in human gastric and ovarian carcinoma cell lines in vitro. Eur J Cancer 1995;31A(1):92–7.

65. Sonnichsen DS, Relling MV. Clinical pharmacokinetics of paclitaxel. Clin Pharmacokinet 1994;27(4):256–69.

66. Baker AF, Dorr RT. Drug interactions with the taxanes: clinical implications. Cancer Treat Rev 2001;27(4):221–33.

67. Wasserheit C, Frazein A, Oratz R, Sorich J, Downey A, Hochster H, Chachoua A, Wernz J, Zeleniuch-Jacquotte A, Blum R, Speyer J. Phase II trial of paclitaxel and cisplatin in women with advanced breast cancer: an active regimen with limiting neurotoxicity. J Clin Oncol 1996;14(7):1993–9. Erratum in: J Clin Oncol 1996;14(12):3175.

TOPOISOMERASE INHIBITORS

General Information

Inhibitors of topoisomerase I and topoisomerase II are the most commonly used anticancer drugs. The camptothecins—topotecan and irinotecan (CPT-11)—interact with the enzyme topoisomerase I; the podophyllotoxins—etoposide and teniposide—target topoisomerase II. They cause various forms of single- and double-strand breaks in DNA (1–7). Other drugs inhibit both enzymes simultaneously (8) (see below).

The anthracyclines and related compounds, such as mitoxantrone and amsacrine (9), also exert their cytotoxic effects via inhibition of topoisomerase II. However, they differ from the camptothecins and podophyllotoxins in respect to DNA intercalation and have a different pattern of cardiac toxicity.

Inhibitors of topoisomerase I

Camptothecins were originally isolated from the wood, bark, and fruit of the oriental tree *Camptotheca acuminata* ("tree of joy"). Why the tree produces these highly toxic alkaloids is not known, but the most likely reason is that the toxins are part of a survival strategy in combating herbivores. Among a lot of isolated plant constituents, the naturally occurring alkaloid camptothecin (CAM, NSC94600) was identified as a highly potent inhibitor of topoisomerase I, which is overexpressed in many cancers. The water-soluble salt CAM-sodium, which was introduced in early preclinical trials in the 1960s, was highly toxic in animals. Hemorrhagic cystitis, leukopenia, and thrombocytopenia were its dose-limiting toxic effects. In addition, sterile hemorrhagic cystitis, myelosuppression, and gastrointestinal toxic effects were common in patients during phase I studies. Clinical testing of CAM-sodium was therefore discontinued in the 1970s. However, the semisynthetic derivatives irinotecan and topotecan are highly active in several malignancies and do not cause hemorrhagic cystitis, because of their greater physicochemical stability and solubility at lower pH values. However, the drugs differ from each other in approved therapeutic uses, recommended doses, toxicity profiles, and pharmacokinetics (1–5).

Several camptothecin analogues are currently being investigated. The water-soluble derivatives lurtotecan (GI147211) and exatecan (DX-8951-f) and the poorly water-soluble analogues 9-aminocamptothecin and 9-nitrocamptothecin, which can be given orally, are in various stages of development (3,10–13).

Exatecan is a novel synthetic camptothecin derivative with a unique hexacyclic structure. It does not require metabolic activation, whereas irinotecan does. In vitro experiments in various cell lines have suggested that exatecan may be 6 and 28 times more active than SN-38 (7-ethyl-10-hydroxycamptothecin, the active metabolite of irinotecan) and topotecan respectively. Furthermore, it has a 2–10 times higher therapeutic index than irinotecan and topotecan. In addition, exatecan may even be active in P-glycoprotein-mediated multidrug-resistant tumor cells.

Its dose-limiting adverse effects are neutropenia and liver dysfunction. The recommended dosages of exatecan for phase II trials are 0.5 mg/m^2/day or 0.3 mg/m^2/day as a 30-minute infusion on 5 consecutive days for minimally pretreated and heavily pretreated patients respectively (14,15).

Current clinical investigations with topoisomerase I inhibitors include the feasibility of oral administration of topotecan and irinotecan, the use of a liposomal lurtotecan formulation (NX211), and the use of a pegylated derivative of the naturally occurring camptothecin, which is soluble in aqueous solutions even at low pH values (3,10).

Inhibitors of topoisomerase II

Etoposide and teniposide are semisynthetic derivatives of podophyllin, which was originally isolated from the root of the Indian podophyllum plant. After extensive isolation procedures, the most effective "antileukemic" factor was identified as 4'-demethylepipodophyllin benzylidiene glucoside (DEPBG). Etoposide, its water-soluble derivative etoposide phosphate, and teniposide are semisynthetic analogues of DEPBG with increased antineoplastic activity. Etoposide is active in testicular tumors, non-Hodgkin's lymphoma, Hodgkin's disease, other lymphomas, ovarian carcinoma, gastric carcinoma, breast cancer, small-cell and non-small-cell lung cancers, and cancers of unknown origin. The major indications for teniposide include lymphoma, bladder cancer, acute lymphoblastic leukemia, and glioblastoma (6,7).

Dual inhibitors of topoisomerases I and II

Intoplicin is one of the first congeners of the so-called dual inhibitors of topoisomerases I and II (16). These new antitumor drugs interact with both topoisomerase I and II simultaneously. This mechanism of action appears to be advantageous, because selective inhibition of topoisomerase I has been reported to increase topoisomerase II enzyme activity and vice versa, which may be important for the development of drug resistance (17–20). Intoplicin may overcome this limitation. In phase I trials, intoplicin has been reported to cause dose-limiting liver toxicity; other adverse effects were sporadic and mild (16).

Another dual inhibitor of topoisomerase I and topoisomerase II is XR 5000 (N-2-[(dimethylamino)ethyl]acridine-4-carboxamine). Its cytotoxicity was not affected by the presence of P-glycoprotein, and it seems to be a promising candidate, even in highly resistant tumor cells. However, neither complete nor partial remission was observed during a phase II trial in 20 patients with advanced or metastatic colorectal cancer (21).

A novel pentafluorinated epipodophylloid characterized by marked antitumor activity in vivo is F11872. It is a dual inhibitor of the catalytic activity of both topoisomerases I and II, with markedly superior activity in vivo compared with other dual inhibitors, such as intoplicin, TAS-103, and others (22).

Mechanisms of action

Topoisomerase I is the target enzyme for the inhibitory effects of camptothecins. It modulates the topological structure of DNA by inducing transient DNA breaks. Single-strand breaks help to remove excessive positive and negative DNA supercoils, which arise during DNA replication and transcription. The interaction between the camptothecins and the enzyme results in the formation of a topoisomerase-I-DNA complex (23).

Etoposide and teniposide interact with topoisomerase II within the tumor cell. This nuclear enzyme catalyses the passage of DNA across adjacent strands during cell division and is most active during the late S and G2 phases of the cell cycle. If the tumor cell is exposed to etoposide during this stage, stabilization of the enzyme-DNA complex results in double- and single-strand breaks in DNA as well as cell-cycle arrest. Several studies have shown that the activity of etoposide is schedule dependent, which means that its antiproliferative effect on tumor cells is greater when it is given over several consecutive days rather than on a single day. At higher dosages, podophyllotoxins may also act as spindle poisons (24).

In contrast to topoisomerase II, cellular concentrations of topoisomerase I are relatively independent of the cell-cycle phase in normal tissues. Thus, topoisomerase I activity is only slightly increased in cells and tissues under conditions of proliferation. However, higher constitutive activities of this enzyme can be detected in several tumor tissues (for example adenocarcinoma of the colon and rectum) compared with healthy tissues (25).

Pharmacokinetics

Camptothecins

Both irinotecan and topotecan contain lactone structures, which can be hydrolysed non-enzymatically into the open-ring form. Under acidic conditions, the equilibrium between the biologically active lactone form and the less active carboxylated form is generally shifted to the lactone form, whereas at physiological or higher values of pH, the lactone form is unstable, because hydrolysis to the open form is favored. In addition, owing to preferential binding of the salt form to serum albumin, the affinity of the carboxylated form for human serum albumin is estimated to be 100 times higher than that of the lactone form. In consequence, when irinotecan is given intravenously, more than 95% of the dose is bound to serum albumin as inactive drug, and is therefore at least transiently unavailable to exert its antineoplastic activity (26–29). Novel camptothecin derivatives, such as exatecan or lurtotecan, are more resistant to rapid hydrolysis because of structural modifications, for example the removal of the 20-OH group (3,10,14,15).

Irinotecan

Irinotecan has been approved for first-line and second-line treatment of advanced colorectal cancer. Conventional dosages range from 350 mg/m^2 intravenously every 3 weeks to 100–125 mg/m^2 intravenously weekly when it is given as a single agent, and 80–180 mg/m^2 intravenously when it is given in combination with 5-fluorouracil and folinic acid weekly (the AIO regimen) or every 14 days (the De Gramont regimen) (4,30).

In contrast to the structurally related topotecan, irinotecan is a prodrug, which has to be converted to its active form, SN-38 (4,30). Cleavage of the side-chain, a bulky piperidino moiety, at the C10 position is rapidly catalysed by carboxylesterases after intravenous administration. SN-38 (7-ethyl-10-hydroxy-camptothecin) is 1000 times more potent than the parent compound. There is an equilibrium between the active lactone and the inactive carboxylated forms in a pH- and protein-dependent manner for both irinotecan and SN-38 (31,32).

The SN-38 is inactivated by conjugation, catalysed by isoforms of uridine diphosphate glucuronosyltransferase, principally UGT 1A7 (33–35). Pharmacogenetic defects in glucuronidation (for example Gilbert's syndrome and Crigler–Najjar syndrome type I) result in impaired glucuronidation. The incidence of Gilbert's syndrome is 0.5–15% in different ethnic groups, and there is significant variability of UGT 1A activity in human livers, with a 17-fold difference between minimum and maximum rates of SN-38 glucuronidation. Patients with Gilbert's syndrome are at increased risk of irinotecan-induced gastrointestinal toxicity and leukopenia if conventional dosages are used (36–40). Paracetamol is a poor predictor of SN-38 glucuronidation capacity based on metabolism by another isozyme (UGT 1A6). However, genotype screening is increasingly becoming feasible. Thus, empirical irinotecan dosage modification or the selection of another anticancer drug is appropriate in patients with poor glucuronidation capacity (36–40).

Both irinotecan and SN-38 are primarily excreted into the bile by the canalicular multispecific organic anion transporter (cMOAT), a member of the ATP cassette of transporters. Therefore, inhibitors of cMOAT, such as ciclosporin, can reduce the clearance of irinotecan and SN-38 (41,42).

The SN-38 glucuronide can be deconjugated in the gut to active SN-38 by bacterial glucuronidases. This enterohepatic circulation of SN-38 results in a further plasma peak, and SN-38 released within the gut lumen has been suggested to be an important cause of delayed intestinal toxicity; in animal experiments constitutive bacterial beta-glucuronidase activity correlated with irinotecan-induced cecal damage. In contrast, the prophylactic use of oral antibiotics (for example aminoglycosides or quinolones) or specific glucuronidase inhibitors resulted in attenuation of intestinal toxicity (43).

Aminopentane-carboxylic acid (APC) is a second major metabolite of irinotecan; it is formed by oxidation of the terminal piperidine ring, catalysed by CYP3A4. APC itself is not hydrolysed to SN-38 and is only a weak inhibitor of topoisomerase I (44–48). However, potent CYP3A4 inducers (for example St. John's wort, carbamazepine, and phenytoin) or inhibitors (for example itraconazole) alter irinotecan pharmacokinetics (49–54). Other identified metabolites include NPC (7-ethyl-10-(4-amino-1-piperidono)carbonyloxycamptothecin), 5-hydroxyirinotecan, and RPR112526 (a decarboxylated product of the acid form of the irinotecan lactone).

Further drug interactions occur if constitutive SN-38 glucuronidation capacity is modified. For example, phenobarbital may induce UGT 1A activity, whereas valproic acid may inhibit it. Thus, co-administration can alter the clearance of irinotecan.

A half-life of 5–14 hours has been reported after intravenous infusion of irinotecan over 30 and 90 minutes. The half-life of the active metabolite SN-38 (total) is 6–14 hours. However, continuous 5-day intravenous infusion schedules result in prolonged half-lives (about 27 hours and 30 hours for irinotecan and SN-38 respectively). In general, the C_{max} of SN-38 is more than 100 times lower than the corresponding value for irinotecan. Plasma concentrations of SN-38 glucuronide were higher than the corresponding concentrations of SN-38: the AUC of SN-38 glucuronide was at least 10 times higher than that of SN-38 (44–47).

Because of the importance of hepatic metabolism in SN-38 elimination by glucuronidation, the biliary clearance of irinotecan and its metabolites is delayed in patients with impaired hepatic function (55–57), and there is a negative correlation between serum bilirubin concentrations and the total body clearance of irinotecan. In a patient with moderately impaired liver function, it was necessary to reduce the dose to 100 mg/m^2 instead of 350 mg/m^2 intravenously thrice-weekly, in order to achieve half-lives and C_{max} values of irinotecan and SN-38 comparable to those observed in patients with normal liver function (55). However, the corresponding AUCs were still significantly increased, resulting in more severe leukopenia and delayed diarrhea. The authors concluded that to improve tolerance, exposure to the drug in a patient of this kind should not exceed 30 mg/m^2 intravenously.

Detailed studies of irinotecan dose modification in patients with liver dysfunction are warranted. According to the results of pharmacokinetic studies, thrice-weekly intravenous doses of irinotecan have been recommended: 350 mg/m^2 in patients with bilirubin concentrations up to 1.5 times the upper limit of the reference range and 200 mg/m^2 in patients with bilirubin concentrations 1.5–3.0 times the upper limit of the reference range (56).

The systemic availability of oral irinotecan is low and variable (10–20%). Transintestinal transport of irinotecan and SN-38 by P-glycoprotein and cytochrome P_{450}-mediated first-pass removal in the intestine accounts for the low absolute availability of irinotecan.

Topotecan

Topotecan has been approved for the treatment of advanced pretreated ovarian and small-cell lung cancer in several countries. After intravenous administration of conventional dosages (for example 1.5 mg/m^2/day for 5 consecutive days) its half-life is 2–4 hours. Prolonged infusion for 3, 5, or 21 days increases drug exposure without affecting the disposition of topotecan (29).

The ratio of the AUCs of the lactone and total topotecan appears to be relatively constant and averages about 0.3, which means that only 30% of the total drug concentration in the plasma represents the closed-ring lactone form. The distribution volume at steady state is 25–75 l/m^2, indicating extensive binding to tissues. Erythrocytes act as a depot for topotecan (lactone), with steady-state concentrations almost 1.7 times those obtained in plasma.

Topotecan is primarily excreted unchanged in the urine. About 49% of the intravenous dose is recovered in the urine as parent drug and 18% in the feces (58). Despite high urinary concentrations, topotecan does not cause urinary toxicity, because of its high water solubility (58,59). Dosage modification is warranted in patients with impaired renal function (60). Reduced doses of 0.75 mg/m^2/day and 0.5 mg/m^2/day have been recommended in untreated and extensively pretreated patients with reduced creatinine clearance (20–40 ml/minute). It has also been suggested that dosage adjustment may even be required if the creatinine clearance is 40–60 ml/minute (61). The recommended starting dose should be 1.2 mg/m^2/day intravenously on five consecutive days, in order to reduce the risk of severe myelosuppression. Because there is no information about topotecan in patients with severe renal insufficiency (creatinine clearance below 20 ml/minute), topotecan should not be given to them (60). There is some evidence that topotecan is hemodialysable (62).

Hepatic metabolism of topotecan, mediated by cytochrome P_{450} isozymes, is of minor quantitative importance (26–29,58). Metabolic pathways include N-dealkylation (producing N-demethyltopotecan) and glucuronidation. There is some evidence that potent inhibitors or inducers of CYP3A4 alter the clearance of topotecan (58).

After conventional intravenous dosages of topotecan (for example 1.5 mg/m^2 as a 30-minute infusion on days 1–5) the mean half-life, plasma clearance, and volume of distribution are respectively 2.7 hours, 1.1 ml/minute, and 170 litres. The plasma protein binding of topotecan is low (7–35%). In contrast to many other anticancer drugs, topotecan can penetrate the central nervous system. If the blood–brain barrier is intact, more than 30% of the plasma concentration can be recovered in the cerebrospinal fluid (26–29,58). Nevertheless, based on case reports and experimental data, intrathecal drug administration has been suggested to be advantageous, in order to achieve higher drug concentrations in the cerebrospinal fluid and to avoid systemic toxicity (63,64).

The systemic availability of oral topotecan is about 30%. Dose-limiting toxicity was reached at a dose of 0.6 mg/m^2 bd and consisted of diarrhea, which started from day 12 to day 20. Other toxic effects, including leukopenia and thrombocytopenia, were mild. The recommended dose for phase II trials was 0.5 mg/m^2 bd for 21 days (65–67).

Podophyllotoxins
Etoposide

At low doses of oral etoposide (for example 50–100 mg), the systemic availability averages 66%, and at higher dosages (100 mg/m^2 and over) 47%. If etoposide phosphate is used, the values are higher (range 66–84%) (68–73).

After intravenous administration of etoposide 150 mg/m^2, the peak plasma concentration averages 20 micrograms/ml and the half-life 7.1 hours. Drug clearance and distribution volume are about 16 ml/minute/m^2 and 17 l/m^2 (6,7,74). With respect to plasma concentrations of etoposide, intravenous etoposide phosphate is equivalent to intravenous etoposide with conventional or intensified dose schedules (75–79). After intravenous administration, the prodrug etoposide phosphate undergoes rapid hydrolysis catalysed by alkaline phosphatase; this conversion is linear even at high intravenous doses of 1200 mg/m^2 infused over 2 hours on days 1 and 2.

About 96% of the dose of etoposide is bound to plasma proteins, the fraction 4% being unbound (80–83). There is a higher risk of myelotoxicity when the unbound fraction is increased by factors such as hyperbilirubinemia or hypoalbuminemia, which is common in patients with hepatic dysfunction or cachexia-inducing tumors (84,85). The variability in unbound drug concentrations has been suggested to be important in the setting of intravenous high-dose etoposide and reinfusion of autologous peripheral blood stem cells. If drug concentrations persist over a longer period of time, the success of engraftment may be severely impaired. Thus, plasma concentration monitoring has been suggested, in order to identify patients at increased risk (86,87).

The renal clearance of etoposide is about 30–40% of the total plasma clearance. Even in patients with nearly normal creatinine concentrations (100–130 μmol/l), there is a slight but significant increase in the AUC, but without more pronounced hematological toxicity. Hepatic etoposide metabolism is mediated by CYP3A4, and results in the production of catechol metabolites. Although these catechols contribute relatively little to the metabolism of etoposide, they may contribute to its late adverse effects, for example secondary malignancies. Further metabolic pathways include glucuronidation and hydroxyacid formation (88). Dosage reductions of 33 and 50% have been recommended for patients with creatinine clearances of 15–25 ml/minute and under 15 ml/minute respectively. In patients with obstructive jaundice and a reduced glomerular filtration rate, a 50% dosage reduction has been recommended empirically (6,7,88,89).

In patients with very severe forms of renal insufficiency, only moderate amounts of etoposide can be eliminated by hemodialysis (90). In patients with brain metastases, high intravenous dosages of etoposide may be needed in order to achieve adequate drug concentrations in the cerebrospinal fluid. In such patients, intrathecal drug administration may be an alternative, in order to reduce systemic toxicity associated with dose-intensive chemotherapy. However, this mode of etoposide administration has not been established (91,92).

There is large interindividual variability in etoposide plasma concentrations with conventional dosages, and some authors have suggested that plasma concentration monitoring would reduce the pharmacokinetic variability and optimize outcomes (93,94).

Teniposide

Teniposide undergoes more extensive metabolic degradation than etoposide, resulting in the catechol derivative 4′-demethyldeoxy-podophyllotoxin. The aglycone and the *trans/cis*-hydroxy acids appear to be formed by pH-dependent hydrolysis reactions (7,95,96).

Plasma concentration monitoring has been proposed to be beneficial in patients receiving teniposide. For example, in one study, maintaining steady-state concentrations above 12 micrograms/ml appeared to be important for clinical responses in patients with recurrent leukemia, lymphoma, or neuroblastoma (95). In 10 patients, whose steady-state concentrations were maintained above 12 micrograms/ml, there was shrinkage of the tumor, whereas only five of 13 patients with lower steady-state concentrations had a response. Teniposide has been used as a continuous infusion over 72 hours in intravenous doses of 300–750 mg/m^2.

The mean systemic availability of teniposide after oral administration is about 42% (range 20–71%). Teniposide capsules 50 mg have been suggested to be useful, but no oral formulation has been approved so far (96).

General adverse effects

The dose-limiting adverse effects of irinotecan depend largely on the dosage schedule. Myelosuppression, particularly leukopenia and neutropenia and rarely thrombocytopenia and anemia, have been observed. Gastrointestinal toxicity (that is, diarrhea) is also common and can be acute or subacute. The most dose-limiting adverse effect of topotecan is myelosuppression, which correlates with individual drug exposure. In contrast, gastrointestinal toxicity is generally mild (97–99).

Common adverse effects of etoposide and teniposide (100) include dose-limiting myelosuppression (causing neutropenia more often than thrombocytopenia), dose-dependent nausea or vomiting, and alopecia. Mucositis can be dose limiting, particularly in patients receiving high doses of etoposide. Hypersensitivity reactions are more common with etoposide and teniposide than with etoposide phosphate, because the formulations of the former contain sensitizing solubilizers. Both drugs have been associated with acute myelogenous leukemia.

Organs and Systems

Cardiovascular

There are reports of myocardial infarction in patients who have received combination chemotherapy containing etoposide. The mechanisms have not been clearly elucidated.

- A 28-year-old man with a non-seminomatous retroperitoneal germ-cell cancer received etoposide (180 mg/day intravenously on days 1–5), bleomycin, and cisplatin (101). He had no cardiac risk factors and no history of cardiac symptoms. On day 3, during infusion of bleomycin, he developed chest pain and dyspnea. The infusion was discontinued and he was given glyceryl trinitrate and diazepam; his symptoms resolved. On day 4 he was given etoposide as scheduled, but four hours later developed severe angina. The electrocardiogram and raised cardiac enzymes were consistent with an acute posterolateral myocardial infarction. He was given heparin, aspirin, and nitrates, and the chemotherapy was discontinued. Within 20 hours his chest pain completely disappeared and his electrocardiogram became normal.

If hypotension occurs during drug administration, it usually subsides when the infusion ends and intravenous fluids or other supportive agents are given. Elderly patients may be particularly susceptible to etoposide-induced hypotension. During a phase I trial of etoposide by continuous infusion, 17 patients were given 75 mg/m^2/day for 5 days and later courses of 100 mg/m^2/day and 150 mg/m^2/day (102). Two patients with pre-existing cardiovascular disease developed myocardial infarctions, one at the 100 mg/m^2/day dose and the other at the 150 mg/m^2/day dose. Another patient developed congestive heart failure at the end of the 5-day infusion and died on day 8; however, this patient also received a saline load of 1500 ml/day for 5 days during etoposide administration and had had previous episodes of congestive cardiac failure. The authors concluded that in patients with underlying cardiovascular disease etoposide must be administered cautiously and that extensive saline loading should be avoided in patients with a history of previous congestive heart failure.

Nervous system

Fatigue is a frequent adverse effect of topotecan and occurs in up to 70% of patients when they receive 1.5 mg/m^2/day (30-minute infusions) for 5 days repeated at day 22; however, only 10% have severe symptoms (4). Topotecan causes headache in some patients.

Rare cases of peripheral neuropathy have been reported after intravenous topotecan, but a causal relation is uncertain.

Neurotoxicity occurs in under 1% of patients who receive teniposide or etoposide, and is more common after high dosages. Adverse nervous system effects, including headache, transient mental confusion, and vertigo, may be related to the blood alcohol concentration, since teniposide and etoposide formulations contain alcohol (103).

Acute neurological dysfunction with exacerbation of pre-existing neurological disorders has been reported after treatment with high-dose etoposide (over 800 mg/m^2/day) given with autologous bone marrow transplantation (104). This happened 9–10 days after the start of treatment, and it abated without sequelae after prompt steroid therapy. Changes in intracranial pressure may explain this acute disturbance.

Peripheral neuropathy, mainly mild and infrequent, has been observed after conventional dosages of etoposide and teniposide. However, during combination therapy with etoposide and vinca alkaloids, more serious forms of peripheral neuropathy have been reported. Of 142 patients with autologous bone marrow transplantation given high-dose etoposide (for example 60 mg/kg combined with melphalan), six developed grade 2–3 polyneuropathy starting 2–8 weeks after transplantation.

About 76% of patients given irinotecan complained of weakness. Grade 3 and 4 weakness has been described in 12–15% with weekly or thrice-weekly administration and during the administration of combination regimens containing fluorouracil.

Hematologic

Myelosuppression, neutropenia, and to a lesser extent thrombocytopenia, are dose-limiting toxic effects of topotecan. Reversible non-cumulative neutropenia usually occurs

at between days 8 and 15 after an intravenous dosage of 1.5 mg/m^2 on five consecutive days. The nadir of the neutrophil count occurs on day 11, with recovery on day 21. Neutropenia, with cell counts less than 1.5×10^9/l (grade 2) and 0.5×10^9/l (grade 4), is observed in 70–97% of patients. In addition, 4–33% of patients treated with conventional dosages of topotecan develop neutropenic fever (97–99).

Thrombocytopenia, with platelet counts under 50×10^9/l (grade 3) and 25×10^9/l (grade 4), occurs in 25–77% of patients, with a nadir on day 15 and recovery on day 21. Platelet transfusions are needed in 4–27% of patients. Anemia, defined as a fall in hemoglobin below 8 g/dl (grade 3) or 6.5 g/dl (grade 4), has been reported in 21–41% of patients; erythrocyte transfusions were required in about 25% of treatment courses. More extensive myelosuppression can occur in patients who have been pretreated with cytotoxic drugs. The extent of myelosuppression correlates significantly with both the total topotecan AUC and the topotecan lactone AUC. When prophylactic G-CSF is given, thrombocytopenia is the dose-limiting myelotoxic effect (97–99).

Leukopenia is a dose-limiting adverse effect of irinotecan. Weekly intravenous doses (for example 100–125 mg/m^2) appear to produce a slightly greater incidence of grade 3–4 neutropenia compared with 3-weekly schedules (350 mg/m^2) (16–28 versus 14–22%). The median leukocyte nadir occurs on day 21 (15–27) and recovers 8 days later. Severe anemia (hemoglobin concentrations below 8 g/dl) and severe thrombocytopenia (platelet count below 50×10^9/l) occur in 15 and 2% of patients respectively. There is eosinophilia in up to one-third of patients (2,3).

Myelosuppression is a dose-limiting adverse effect of etoposide and teniposide. Leukopenia is the most common adverse effect associated with oral and intravenous etoposide. Nadirs in neutrophil counts generally occur within 7–14 days. Severe forms following conventional etoposide doses can be expected in about 17% of patients. Thrombocytopenia occurs in 23% of etoposide-treated patients and about 9% are severe (counts below 50×10^9/l). Leukopenia and thrombocytopenia occur respectively in 65 and 80% of patients after administration of teniposide (6,7).

Gastrointestinal

Anorexia, nausea and vomiting, and diarrhea are generally mild after the administration of conventional doses of etoposide and teniposide. Stomatitis is uncommon and mucositis starts to be more severe in patients who receive intravenous doses of etoposide up to 1000 mg/m^2. Gastrointestinal toxicity after topotecan is generally mild to moderate. Under 10% of patients complain of grade 3/4 nausea and vomiting, diarrhea or constipation, abdominal pain, or stomatitis. Mucositis is uncommon and mild after intravenous topotecan.

Besides leukopenia, diarrhea is the major dose-limiting adverse effect of irinotecan (105,106). There are two different forms. The acute form occurs very early and is due to inhibition of acetylcholinesterase. The delayed-onset form occurs simultaneously with the leukocyte nadir and depends on the concentration of the active compound SN-38 in the plasma and bowel.

The acute form of diarrhea is short-lived and can be effectively prevented or rapidly suppressed by concomitant atropine. The cholinergic symptoms are accompanied by abdominal cramps (36%), sweating (57%), salivation (11%), visual disturbances (15%), lacrimation (12%), and piloerection (3%). The recommended dose of atropine is 0.25 mg intravenously for prevention or 0.25–1.0 mg for acute treatment of patients with early cholinergic symptoms. As cholinergic symptoms have not been observed with other camptothecin derivatives, it can be speculated that these adverse effects are restricted to irinotecan, whose piperidino group bears some structural similarity to the potent nicotine receptor stimulant dimethylphenylpiperazinium (106).

Delayed-onset diarrhea of all grades of severity occurs in nearly 90% of patients during the first three treatment cycles with irinotecan. It can resemble a cholera-like syndrome, which occurs several days after completion of the infusion. There is grade 3/4 diarrhea (grade 3 being at least 7–9 stools per day, incontinence, or severe cramps; grade 4 being 10 stools or more per day, grossly bloody stools, or a need for total parenteral nutrition) in 31–37% of patients treated weekly and in 35–39% of patients treated with 3-weekly regimens. The median day of occurrence was day 6 (range days 2–12). Of the four major pathophysiological mechanisms of diarrhea (osmotic, secretory, altered motility, and exudative), irinotecan-induced watery diarrhea appears to be secretory, defined by abnormal ion transport in intestinal epithelial cells (105).

There is increasing evidence that the extent and severity of gastrointestinal toxicity correlates with concentrations of the active compound SN-38 in the plasma and bowel. The role of plasma pharmacokinetics in predicting the severity of irinotecan-induced diarrhea has been highlighted by the introduction of a biliary index, which is the product of the relative area ratio of SN-38 to SN-38 glucuronide and the total AUC. According to preliminary evidence, preventive measures should be considered when the biliary index exceeds 3.484 hours.micrograms/ml (107,108).

Because SN-38 glucuronide undergoes deconjugation by bacteria-derived beta-glucuronidase in the bowel after biliary excretion, a strategy for reducing irinotecan-induced subacute diarrhea has been proposed: inhibition of intestinal microflora by a broad-spectrum antibiotic. In one study, this ameliorated subacute diarrhea in subsequent cycles; in six of seven patients, the prophylactic oral use of neomycin resulted in less severe forms of diarrhea compared with controls (43). About 30% of irinotecan is excreted via the bile unchanged and may be directly converted to SN-38 in the bowel by intestinal carboxyesterases; however, specific non-absorbable inhibitors of intestinal carboxyesterases for oral use are not yet available.

Because the equilibrium between the active lactone form and the ring-opened carboxylate form is pH dependent, oral alkalinization with a mixture consisting of sodium bicarbonate (2.0 g/day), magnesium oxide (2.0–4.0 g/day), water (pH over 7.2, 1.5–2 l/day), and ursodeoxycholic acid (300 mg/day), combined with "controlled" defecation was used in a phase II trial to reduce subacute gastrointestinal toxicity. Anticancer activity was maintained and the incidences of diarrhea and myelosuppression were significantly reduced compared with a non-randomized control group (109–111).

The efficacy of symptomatic antidiarrheal treatment with several drugs, including loperamide, octreotide, racecadodril, and budesonide, has been assessed (105,112,113). Loperamide is recommended when the first signs of subacute, late-onset diarrhea occur; the dose is 4 mg at the start, followed by 2 mg every 2 hours, continued until the diarrhea has stopped for at least 12 hours. Premedication with loperamide is not indicated. Some authors also recommend dosage modification in subsequent cycles. If loperamide alone is insufficient, racecadodril (acetorphane, Tiorfan) 100 mg tds can be added. Racecadodril belongs to a group of drugs that block cAMP-mediated hypersecretion in the gut by inhibiting the intestinal enzyme enkephalinase. The somatostatin analogue octreotide is effective in loperamide-refractory patients with severe diarrhea despite loperamide and/or acetorphane. Subcutaneous doses of 100 micrograms tds up to 500 micrograms every 8 hours for 48–96 hours have produced improvement in diarrhea by one WHO toxicity grade or even more (105).

Oral budesonide has also been proposed to be beneficial in patients with subacute diarrhea. It has 90% first-pass removal in the liver, and so its systemic activity is low. Budesonide controls symptoms of diarrhea in most patients with inflammatory bowel disease. Preliminary data have suggested that the use of budesonide in patients with irinotecan-induced diarrhea could reduce the severity of symptoms. In addition, in a phase III trial budesonide 3 mg tds prevented irinotecan-induced diarrhea to a moderate extent. Budesonide is an option in patients who do not respond to high-dose oral loperamide (113).

The use of oral immunomodulators (for example interleukin-15 and Kampo medicines) has been suggested in order to reduce irinotecan-related diarrhea; however, randomized clinical trials are required, to assess efficacy (42).

Liver

Etoposide has been associated with increased liver enzymes, but a causal relation has not been established (114).

Urinary tract

Camptothecin can cause hemorrhagic cystitis (115), which has not been reported with semisynthetic camptothecin derivatives, supposedly because they are highly soluble in aqueous solutions even at low pH values. However, in a study of the use of camptothecin conjugated to a water-soluble polymer, two of three patients who received 80 mg/m^2/week developed hemorrhagic cystitis (grade 1/3 dysuria and grade 2/3 hematuria) during the second and third cycles; at 120 mg/m^2/week there was grade 1 bladder toxicity in two of three patients (116).

Skin

Skin rashes involving the trunk, scalp, and limbs have been reported in 17–25% of patients receiving topotecan as a short-term infusion, whereas continuous drug infusion appears to be very rarely associated with rashes. These skin reactions typically appear on days 4–8 and resolve on day 15.

- A 45-year-old woman received topotecan and colony-stimulating factor for ovarian cancer and developed erythematous and slightly pruritic plaques on the upper and lower limbs and ear lobes about one week later (117). The lesions subsided spontaneously in about 10 days and recurred after the next dose. A skin biopsy showed neutrophilic eccrine hidradenitis; all skin cultures were negative.

Skin rashes due to podophyllotoxin derivatives may be hypersensitivity reactions and can be related to the drug itself or more commonly to the vehicles used. Dose-related, non-IgE-mediated hypersensitivity has been reported in 16 children receiving teniposide (118). Other published reports of hypersensitivity or anaphylactoid reactions to teniposide include degranulation of basophils (119,120), and eight anaphylactic reactions in children, all associated with the use of intravenous teniposide 150 mg/m^2 (121).

There has been a single report of etoposide-induced hand–foot syndrome (122).

Hair

Reversible alopecia is very common at standard doses of podophyllotoxin derivatives, starting at doses of 500 mg/m^2 of etoposide. It is also common even with low, continuous oral doses of etoposide (for example 50 mg/m^2/day). Partial or complete alopecia occurs in 12–70% of patients taking topotecan or irinotecan (123).

Immunologic

The epipodophyllotoxins etoposide and teniposide can cause hypersensitivity reactions, which appear to be of type I (124). In a review of 93 cases, the characteristic features of the hypersensitivity reactions that occurred after intravenous etoposide included bronchospasm, facial flushing, rashes, dyspnea, fever, chills, tachycardia, chest tightness, cyanosis, and changes in blood pressure (hypotension and hypertension) (125).

Hypersensitivity to etoposide or tenoposide has been reported in 50 of a series of 108 patients. The risk is related to the cumulative dose, reaching a maximum at 1500–2000 mg/m^2 in the case of tenoposide and 2000–3000 mg/m^2 for etoposide (126). Acute hypersensitivity reactions, characterized by hypotension, bronchospasm, and facial flushing, have been associated with etoposide (127,128). Rechallenge with appropriate prophylactic cover supported the association.

Very severe forms of hypersensitivity reactions, such as Stevens–Johnson syndrome, are very rare (129). Anaphylactic-like reactions have occurred in 0.7–2% of patients after etoposide administration. Some data suggest that the overall frequency of hypersensitivity reactions to teniposide may be as high as 50% if all forms of hypersensitivity are considered. With very few exceptions,

patients recover quickly when the drug infusion is stopped immediately (124).

Hypersensitivity reactions to etoposide or teniposide usually occur within minutes after intravenous administration, and are probably related to release of vasoactive substances by basophils and/or mast cells. Several reports have suggested that premedication with an antihistamine and/or a corticosteroid may prevent further hypersensitivity reactions, even in patients with a history of previous reactions. However, this strategy should not be followed when patients have had severe hypersensitivity reactions, such as long-lasting bronchospasm or severe hypotension (130,131). Etoposide was successfully restarted in 78% of patients who had had a hypersensitivity reaction, especially when the drug was infused at a slower rate after premedication with an antihistamine and/or a glucocorticoid (132).

Hypersensitivity reactions to etoposide and teniposide occur in 33–51% of patients (123,124) and are primarily related to adjuvants in the parenteral formulations rather than the drugs themselves. In the case of teniposide, the solubilizing adjuvant polyethoxylated castor oil (Cremophor EL) has been implicated. However, in nine children who had facial edema and flushing after receiving teniposide, the drug alone degranulated basophils in vitro, causing histamine release, while Cremophor did not (119). In addition, etoposide formulations for parenteral use contain several adjuvants, including polysorbate 80, benzyl alcohol, and polyethylene glycol, because it is sparingly soluble in aqueous solutions, and these may contribute to hypersensitivity reactions. Polysorbate 80 may also be implicated in rare cases of hypotension and metabolic acidosis, particularly with high dosages (133).

In contrast, the structurally related etoposide phosphate is highly soluble in aqueous solutions and no solubilizing adjuvants are necessary. Preliminary data suggest that the incidence of hypersensitivity reactions is lower with etoposide phosphate than with etoposide, strengthening the hypothesis that adjuvants have a major role in the development of allergic reactions (123,124). In one case, a patient who had a type I hypersensitivity reaction to etoposide was successfully retreated with etoposide phosphate (134).

On the other hand, cross-reactivity to etoposide has been observed in patients with hypersensitivity reactions to teniposide, suggesting that allergic reactions are not exclusively restricted to the use of the solvents. In addition, hypersensitivity reactions have also been reported after oral etoposide (123,124).

- Hypotension, bronchospasm, and facial flushing occurred in a 38-year-old man with advanced testicular cancer associated with an intravenous infusion of etoposide (127). The reaction began within 3 minutes after the start of the infusion and resolved with intravenous fluids and diphenhydramine. Later, he was given four doses of etoposide after pretreatment with diphenhydramine and dexamethasone, without incident.

Successful rechallenge has been reported after a reaction to etoposide in a 19-year-old man, who was successfully re-treated with etoposide phosphate with only antiemetic doses of glucocorticoids as cover (134). This case tends to support the old assumption that etoposide hypersensitivity is due to the excipients in the formulation.

Long-Term Effects

Mutagenicity

Etoposide and teniposide are mutagenic in various bacterial and mammalian genotoxicity tests (135).

Tumorigenicity

Based on animal experiments, etoposide and teniposide should be classified as potential carcinogens (136).

Exposure to etoposide and teniposide has been reported to be an important risk factor for the development of secondary acute myelogenous leukemia (137–143). Etoposide has been suggested to have considerable leukemogenic activity. Of 119 patients with advanced non-small-cell lung cancers, 24 survived for more than 1 year after treatment with etoposide and cisplatin with or without vindesine (144). Of these 24 patients, four developed secondary acute myelogenous leukemia at 13, 19, 28, and 35 months from the start of treatment, having received a twofold greater cumulative dose of etoposide (6.8 versus 3.0 g/m^2). Podophyllotoxin-related secondary acute myelogenous leukemia has a rather short latent period (2–3 years), and differs from malignancies caused by other drugs (for example alkylating agents) by its unique molecular marker, a balanced translocation involving the mixed-lineage leukemia (MLL) gene on chromosome 11 ("11q23 abnormalities") (145). Southern blot analysis of enzyme-digested DNA from etoposide-treated cell lines and from peripheral blood cells after treatment with etoposide showed frequent rearrangements of MLL, but not of other genes (146). There are differences between the chromosomal abnormalities and the subsequent acute myeloid leukemia associated with the alkylating agents and those following topoisomerase inhibition by podophyllotoxins (147). The alkylating agents cause abnormalities of chromosomes 5 and 7, singly or together, and the podophyllotoxins damage the 11q23 chromosome locus (145).

- A 15-year-old white girl with stage II Hodgkin's disease, who was treated with a combination of vincristine, doxorubicin, bleomycin, and etoposide (total dose 2000 mg/m^2) over 4 months followed by radiotherapy, developed secondary acute myelogenous leukemia 16 months after the initial diagnosis (142).
- An 11-year-old boy with virus-associated hemophagocytic syndrome was treated with intravenous and oral etoposide (0.3 g and 2.8 g/m^2 respectively) and developed acute myelogenous leukemia 26 months after the diagnosis (142).

These reports and others confirm that even conventional doses of etoposide can be associated with a risk of secondary acute myelogenous leukemia. The risk appears to be related to both the schedule and the cumulative dose, and it can be aggravated by addition of alkylating agents and/or radiotherapy (148,149).

Two of 21 adults with Hodgkin's disease developed secondary acute myelogenous leukemia after receiving a regimen that included a cumulative dose of etoposide of 945–3640 mg/m^2 given over 3–6 months (141). Both patients also received MOPP after primary treatment failure, and the disease itself is associated with a high risk of secondary malignancies; however, the short latency period before the development of acute myelogenous leukemia (17–32 months) was thought to be typical of podophyllotoxin-associated disease. Altogether the etoposide-related incidence of secondary acute myelogenous leukemia in three retrospective case series was 0.4–8.1%. Secondary leukemia developed 9–68 months after the diagnosis of the first cancer.

Teniposide is about 10 times more potent than etoposide in causing DNA damage in vitro and in vivo. In 21 of 733 children with acute lymphoblastic leukemia in remission, who received maintenance therapy with teniposide once or twice weekly in combination with other anticancer drugs, the risk of secondary acute myelogenous leukemia was about 12 times higher than in patients who had been treated with less intensive schedules (for example a short course of teniposide for induction chemotherapy) (149).

In conclusion, podophyllotoxin-containing regimens carry a small but significant risk of secondary acute myelogenous leukemia. The risk may be increased by higher total cumulative doses (for example etoposide over 2 g/m^2), weekly or twice-weekly schedules, the concomitant administration of drugs that inhibit DNA repair, concomitant radiotherapy, or the use of high doses of cisplatin. It has therefore been recommended that etoposide be used cautiously in low-risk diseases.

Second-Generation Effects

Fertility

The effects on fertility of inhibitors of topoisomerases I and II have not yet been fully elucidated. However, ovarian failure, amenorrhea, anovulatory cycles, and hypomenorrhea have been described in women receiving etoposide (150).

Teratogenicity

Anticancer drugs can be classified as potentially teratogenic and embryocidal, and can cause embryonic resorption, spinal defects, decreased fetal weight, and fetal abnormalities. However, there are no controlled studies of the use of these drugs in pregnant women, and women of childbearing potential should be advised to avoid pregnancy while they are receiving chemotherapy and should be informed about the potential hazards to the fetus (151).

Drug Administration

Drug administration route

The safe intraventricular administration of etoposide has been reported (152).

Drug–Drug Interactions

Ciclosporin

The coadministration of etoposide and high-dose ciclosporin resulted in increased etoposide serum concentrations (153). Lower doses of etoposide were therefore recommended when combined with high-dose ciclosporin.

Cisplatin

Co-administration of cisplatin before topotecan has a sequence-dependent effect on the disposition of topotecan. Cisplatin-related acute changes in glomerular filtration rate can temporarily alter topotecan clearance, causing more severe myelosuppression. Nevertheless, this sequence has been recommended in clinical trials, based on its high antineoplastic efficacy. Patients therefore have to be monitored closely when the two agents are given together (154).

Docetaxel

Topotecan reduced docetaxel clearance by 50% and increased the severity of neutropenia when given over three consecutive days before the combination (155). The underlying reason for this interaction has not been elucidated; however, when combination therapy is used, docetaxel should be scheduled on day 1 and topotecan on days 1–4.

Enzyme inducers

Etoposide and teniposide are substrates of CYP3A4, and their clearance rate is increased by inducers such as carbamazepine, phenobarbital, phenytoin, rifampicin, and St. John's wort (49,51–54,156).

Enzyme inhibitors

Potent inhibitors of CYP3A4, such as ketoconazole or itraconazole, reduce the formation of inactive aminopentane-carboxylic acid from irinotecan, resulting in higher concentrations of the active metabolite SN-38. In seven patients who received irinotecan 350 mg/m^2 alone intravenously for 90 minutes and followed 3 weeks later by irinotecan 100 mg/m^2 in combination with ketoconazole 200 mg orally for 2 days, ketoconazole reduced the formation of aminopentane-carboxylic acid by 87% and increased the formation of SN-38 by 109%; irinotecan clearance and the formation of SN-38 glucuronide were not affected (50).

Fluorouracil

If irinotecan is combined with 5-fluorouracil and calcium folinate, an infusion regimen of fluorouracil rather than bolus administration is associated with a lower incidence of severe toxicity (leukopenia and life-threatening sepsis) (157).

Neomycin

Diarrhea ameliorated in six of seven patients treated with irinotecan in combination with oral neomycin at 1000 mg

tds (43). Neomycin had no effect on the pharmacokinetics of irinotecan and its major metabolites.

Oxaliplatin

Irinotecan (80 mg/m^2 intravenously) given as a 1-hour infusion immediately after oxaliplatin (85 mg/m^2 intravenously) was associated with hypersalivation and abdominal pain (158,159). These symptoms disappeared after an injection of atropine but recurred when irinotecan was given as a single agent or when the two drugs were separated by 24 hours. However, restarting the original schedule once more resulted in extended cholinergic symptoms. It has been postulated that oxaliplatin potentiates the direct inhibitory effect of irinotecan on acetylcholinesterase.

St. John's wort

St. John's wort (300 mg tds, starting 14 days before administration) reduced the AUC of the active metabolite of irinotecan, SN-38, by 42% and the severity of expected myelosuppression (51). Leukocyte and neutrophil counts were reduced by 8.6% and 4.3% after St. John's wort co-administration in contrast to monotherapy (reductions of 56% and 63%). In addition, the AUC of aminopentane-carboxylic acid was reduced by 28%. Whether the concomitant use of dexamethasone had some effect on this interaction has not been elucidated.

Valspodar

Valspodar significantly increased the AUC and half-life of etoposide, and dosage reductions of up to 66% are required to minimize toxicity when these drugs are used together.

References

1. Potmesil M. Camptothecins: from bench research to hospital wards. Cancer Res 1994;54(6):1431–9.
2. Iyer L, Ratain MJ. Clinical pharmacology of camptothecins. Cancer Chemother Pharmacol 1998;42(Suppl):S31–43.
3. Garcia-Carbonero R, Supko JG. Current perspectives on the clinical experience, pharmacology, and continued development of the camptothecins. Clin Cancer Res 2002;8(3):641–61.
4. Rothenberg ML. Topoisomerase I inhibitors: review and update. Ann Oncol 1997;8(9):837–55.
5. Dennis MJ, Beijnen JH, Grochow LB, van Warmerdam LJ. An overview of the clinical pharmacology of topotecan. Semin Oncol 1997;24(1 Suppl 5):S5–S12-5–18.
6. Joel S. The clinical pharmacology of etoposide: an update. Cancer Treat Rev 1996;22(3):179–221.
7. Clark PI, Slevin ML. The clinical pharmacology of etoposide and teniposide. Clin Pharmacokinet 1987;12(4):223–52.
8. Minderman H, Wrzosek C, Cao S, Utsugi T, Kobunai T, Yamada Y, Rustum YM. Mechanism of action of the dual topoisomerase-I and -II inhibitor TAS-103 and activity against (multi)drug resistant cells. Cancer Chemother Pharmacol 2000;45(1):78–84.

9. Rene B, Fosse P, Khelifa T, Jacquemin-Sablon A, Bailly C. Cytotoxicité et interaction de dérivés de l'amsacrine avec l'ADN topo-isomerase II: role du substituant en position 1′du noyau aniline. [Cytotoxicity and interaction of amsacrine derivatives with topoisomerase II: role of the 1′substitute on the aniline nucleus.] Bull Cancer 1997;84(10):941–8.

10. Bailly C. Homocamptothecins: potent topoisomerase I inhibitors and promising anticancer drugs. Crit Rev Oncol Hematol 2003;45(1):91–108.

11. de Jonge MJ, Verweij J, Loos WJ, Dallaire BK, Sparreboom A. Clinical pharmacokinetics of encapsulated oral 9-aminocamptothecin in plasma and saliva. Clin Pharmacol Ther 1999;65(5):491–9.

12. Ellerhorst JA, Bedikian AY, Smith TM, Papadopoulos NE, Plager C, Eton O. Phase II trial of 9-nitrocamptothecin (RFS 2000) for patients with metastatic cutaneous or uveal melanoma. Anticancer Drugs 2002;13(2):169–72.

13. Rowinsky EK, Rizzo J, Ochoa L, Takimoto CH, Forouzesh B, Schwartz G, Hammond LA, Patnaik A, Kwiatek J, Goetz A, Denis L, McGuire J, Tolcher AW. A phase I and pharmacokinetic study of pegylated camptothecin as a 1-hour infusion every 3 weeks in patients with advanced solid malignancies. J Clin Oncol 2003;21(1):148–157.

14. Minami H, Fujii H, Igarashi T, Itoh K, Tamanoi K, Oguma T, Sasaki Y. Phase I and pharmacological study of a new camptothecin derivative, exatecan mesylate (DX-8951f), infused over 30 minutes every three weeks. Clin Cancer Res 2001;7(10):3056–64.

15. Rowinsky EK, Johnson TR, Geyer CE Jr, Hammond LA, Eckhardt SG, Drengler R, Smetzer L, Coyle J, Rizzo J, Schwartz G, Tolcher A, Von Hoff DD, De Jager RL. DX-8951f, a hexacyclic camptothecin analogue, on a daily-times-five schedule: a phase I and pharmacokinetic study in patients with advanced solid malignancies. J Clin Oncol 2000;18(17):3151–63.

16. van Gijn R, ten Bokkel Huinink WW, Rodenhuis S, Vermorken JB, van Tellingen O, Rosing H, van Warmerdam LJ, Beijnen JH. Topoisomerase I/II inhibitor intoplicine administered as a 24 h infusion: phase I and pharmacologic study Anticancer Drugs 1999;10(1):17–23.

17. Whitacre CM, Zborowska E, Gordon NH, Mackay W, Berger NA. Topotecan increases topoisomerase IIalpha levels and sensitivity to treatment with etoposide in schedule-dependent process. Cancer Res 1997;57(8):1425–8.

18. Bonner JA, Kozelsky TF. The significance of the sequence of administration of topotecan and etoposide. Cancer Chemother Pharmacol 1996;39(1–2):109–12.

19. Dowlati A, Levitan N, Gordon NH, Hoppel CL, Gosky DM, Remick SC, Ingalls ST, Berger SJ, Berger NA. Phase II and pharmacokinetic/pharmacodynamic trial of sequential topoisomerase I and II inhibition with topotecan and etoposide in advanced non-small-cell lung cancer. Cancer Chemother Pharmacol 2001;47(2):141–8.

20. Hammond LA, Eckardt JR, Ganapathi R, Burris HA, Rodriguez GA, Eckhardt SG, Rothenberg ML, Weiss GR, Kuhn JG, Hodges S, Von Hoff DD, Rowinsky EK. A phase I and translational study of sequential administration of the topoisomerase I and II inhibitors topotecan and etoposide. Clin Cancer Res 1998;4(6):1459–67.

21. Caponigro F, Dittrich C, Sorensen JB, Schellens JH, Duffaud F, Paz Ares L, Lacombe D, de Balincourt C, Fumoleau P. Phase II study of XR 5000, an inhibitor of topoisomerases I and II, in advanced colorectal cancer. Eur J Cancer 2002;38(1):70–4.

22. Etievant C, Kruczynski A, Barret JM, Perrin D, van Hille B, Guminski Y, Hill BT. F 11782, a dual inhibitor of topoisomerases I and II with an original mechanism of action in vitro, and markedly superior in vivo antitumour activity, relative to three other dual topoisomerase inhibitors, intoplicin, aclarubicin and TAS-103. Cancer Chemother Pharmacol 2000;46(2):101–13.

23. Malonne H, Atassi G. DNA topoisomerase targeting drugs: mechanisms of action and perspectives. Anticancer Drugs 1997;8(9):811–22.

24. Long BH. Mechanisms of action of teniposide (VM-26) and comparison with etoposide (VP-16). Semin Oncol 1992;19(2 Suppl 6):3–19.

25. Husain I, Mohler JL, Seigler HF, Besterman JM. Elevation of topoisomerase I messenger RNA, protein, and catalytic activity in human tumors: demonstration of tumor-type specificity and implications for cancer chemotherapy. Cancer Res 1994;54(2):539–46.

26. Kollmannsberger C, Mross K, Jakob A, Kanz L, Bokemeyer C. Topotecan—a novel topoisomerase I inhibitor: pharmacology and clinical experience. Oncology 1999;56(1):1–12.

27. Von Pawel J. Topotecan (Hycamtin): potent cytostatic action by selective topoisomerase I inhibition. Onkologie 1997;20:380–6.

28. O'Reilly S. Topotecan: what dose, what schedule, what route? Clin Cancer Res 1999;5(1):3–5.

29. Grochow LB, Rowinsky EK, Johnson R, Ludeman S, Kaufmann SH, McCabe FL, Smith BR, Hurowitz L, DeLisa A, Donehower RC, Noe D. Pharmacokinetics and pharmacodynamics of topotecan in patients with advanced cancer. Drug Metab Dispos 1992;20(5):706–13.

30. Rothenberg ML, Cox JV, DeVore RF, Hainsworth JD, Pazdur R, Rivkin SE, Macdonald JS, Geyer CE Jr, Sandbach J, Wolf DL, Mohrland JS, Elfring GL, Miller LL, Von Hoff DD. A multicenter, phase II trial of weekly irinotecan (CPT-11) in patients with previously treated colorectal carcinoma. Cancer 1999;85(4):786–95.

31. Guemei AA, Cottrell J, Band R, Hehman H, Prudhomme M, Pavlov MV, Grem JL, Ismail AS, Bowen D, Taylor RE, Takimoto CH. Human plasma carboxylesterase and butyrylcholinesterase enzyme activity: correlations with SN-38 pharmacokinetics during a prolonged infusion of irinotecan. Cancer Chemother Pharmacol 2001;47(4):283–90.

32. Hennebelle I, Terret C, Chatelut E, Bugat R, Canal P, Guichard S. Characterization of CPT-11 converting carboxylesterase activity in colon tumor and normal tissues: comparison with p-nitro-phenylacetate converting carboxylesterase activity. Anticancer Drugs 2000;11(6):465–470.

33. Gupta E, Mick R, Ramirez J, Wang X, Lestingi TM, Vokes EE, Ratain MJ. Pharmacokinetic and pharmacodynamic evaluation of the topoisomerase inhibitor irinotecan in cancer patients. J Clin Oncol 1997;15(4):1502–10.

34. Ratain MJ. Insights into the pharmacokinetics and pharmacodynamics of irinotecan. Clin Cancer Res 2000;6(9):3393–4.

35. Lokiec F, Canal P, Gay C, Chatelut E, Armand JP, Roche H, Bugat R, Goncalves E, Mathieu-Boue A. Pharmacokinetics of irinotecan and its metabolites in human blood, bile, and urine. Cancer Chemother Pharmacol 1995;36(1):79–82.

36. Innocenti F, Iyer L, Ratain MJ. Pharmacogenetics of anticancer agents: lessons from amonafide and irinotecan. Drug Metab Dispos 2001;29(4 Pt 2):596–600.

37. Iyer L, King CD, Whitington PF, Green MD, Roy SK, Tephly TR, Coffman BL, Ratain MJ. Genetic predisposition to the metabolism of irinotecan (CPT-11). Role of uridine diphosphate glucuronosyltransferase isoform 1A1 in the glucuronidation of its active metabolite (SN-38) in human liver microsomes. J Clin Invest 1998;101(4):847–54.

38. Kraemer D, Scheurlen M. Morbus Gilbert und Crigler–Najjar-Syndrom Typ I und II beruhen auf mutationen im selben genlocus UGT1A1. [Gilbert disease and type I and II Crigler–Najjar syndrome due to mutations in the same UGT1A1 gene locus.] Med Klin (Munich) 2002;97(9):528–32.

39. Ando Y, Saka H, Asai G, Sugiura S, Shimokata K, Kamataki T. UGT1A1 genotypes and glucuronidation of SN-38, the active metabolite of irinotecan. Ann Oncol 1998;9(8):845–7.

40. Innocenti F, Undevia SD, Iyer L, Das S, Karrison T, Janish L, Ramirez J, Rudin CM, Vokes EE, Ratain MJ. UT1A1*28 polymorphism is a predictor of neutropenia in irinotecan chemotherapy. Proc ASCO 2003;22:A495.

41. Yamamoto W, Verweij J, de Bruijn P, de Jonge MJ, Takano H, Nishiyama M, Kurihara M, Sparreboom A. Active transepithelial transport of irinotecan (CPT-11) and its metabolites by human intestinal Caco-2 cells. Anticancer Drugs 2001;12(5):419–32.

42. Xu Y, Villalona-Calero MA. Irinotecan: mechanisms of tumor resistance and novel strategies for modulating its activity. Ann Oncol 2002;13(12):1841–51.

43. Kehrer DF, Sparreboom A, Verweij J, de Bruijn P, Nierop CA, van de Schraaf J, Ruijgrok EJ, de Jonge MJ. Modulation of irinotecan-induced diarrhea by cotreatment with neomycin in cancer patients. Clin Cancer Res 2001;7(5):1136–41.

44. Slatter JG, Schaaf LJ, Sams JP, Feenstra KL, Johnson MG, Bombardt PA, Cathcart KS, Verburg MT, Pearson LK, Compton LD, Miller LL, Baker DS, Pesheck CV, Lord RS 3rd. Pharmacokinetics, metabolism, and excretion of irinotecan (CPT-11) following I.V. infusion of [(14)C]CPT-11 in cancer patients Drug Metab Dispos 2000;28(4):423–33.

45. Sparreboom A, de Jonge MJ, de Bruijn P, Brouwer E, Nooter K, Loos WJ, van Alphen RJ, Mathijssen RH, Stoter G, Verweij J. Irinotecan (CPT-11) metabolism and disposition in cancer patients. Clin Cancer Res 1998;4(11):2747–54.

46. Dodds HM, Clarke SJ, Findlay M, Bishop JF, Robert J, Rivory LP. Clinical pharmacokinetics of the irinotecan metabolite 4-piperidinopiperidine and its possible clinical importance. Cancer Chemother Pharmacol 2000;45(1):9–14.

47. Santos A, Zanetta S, Cresteil T, Deroussent A, Pein F, Raymond E, Vernillet L, Risse ML, Boige V, Gouyette A, Vassal G. Metabolism of irinotecan (CPT-11) by CYP3A4 and CYP3A5 in humans. Clin Cancer Res 2000;6(5):2012–20.

48. Sai K, Kaniwa N, Ozawa S, Sawada JI. A new metabolite of irinotecan in which formation is mediated by human hepatic cytochrome P-450 3A4. Drug Metab Dispos 2001;29(11):1505–13.

49. Mansky PJ, Straus SE. St. John's wort: more implications for cancer patients. J Natl Cancer Inst 2002;94(16):1187–8.

50. Kehrer DF, Mathijssen RH, Verweij J, de Bruijn P, Sparreboom A. Modulation of irinotecan metabolism by ketoconazole. J Clin Oncol 2002;20(14):3122–9.

51. Mathijssen RH, Verweij J, de Bruijn P, Loos WJ, Sparreboom A. Effects of St. John's wort on irinotecan metabolism. J Natl Cancer Inst 2002;94(16):1247–9.

52. Murry DJ, Cherrick I, Salama V, Berg S, Bernstein M, Kuttesch N, Blaney SM. Influence of phenytoin on the disposition of irinotecan: a case report. J Pediatr Hematol Oncol 2002;24(2):130–3.

53. Mathijssen RH, Sparreboom A, Dumez H, van Oosterom AT, de Bruijn EA. Altered irinotecan metabolism in a patient receiving phenytoin. Anticancer Drugs 2002;13(2):139–40.

54. Crews KR, Stewart CF, Jones-Wallace D, Thompson SJ, Houghton PJ, Heideman RL, Fouladi M, Bowers DC, Chintagumpala MM, Gajjar A. Altered irinotecan pharmacokinetics in pediatric high-grade glioma patients receiving enzyme-inducing anticonvulsant therapy. Clin Cancer Res 2002;8(7):2202–9.

55. van Groeningen CJ, Van der Vijgh WJ, Baars JJ, Stieltjes H, Huibregtse K, Pinedo HM. Altered pharmacokinetics and metabolism of CPT-11 in liver dysfunction: a need for guidelines. Clin Cancer Res 2000;6(4):1342–6.

56. Raymond E, Boige V, Faivre S, Sanderink GJ, Rixe O, Vernillet L, Jacques C, Gatineau M, Ducreux M, Armand JP. Dosage adjustment and pharmacokinetic profile of irinotecan in cancer patients with hepatic dysfunction. J Clin Oncol 2002;20(21):4303–12.

57. Ong SY, Clarke SJ, Bishop J, Dodds HM, Rivory LP. Toxicity of irinotecan (CPT-11) and hepato-renal dysfunction. Anticancer Drugs 2001;12(7):619–25.

58. Herben VM, Schoemaker E, Rosing H, van Zomeren DM, ten Bokkel Huinink WW, Dubbelman R, Hearn S, Schellens JH, Beijnen JH. Urinary and fecal excretion of topotecan in patients with malignant solid tumours. Cancer Chemother Pharmacol 2002;50(1):59–64.

59. Loos WJ, Gelderblom HJ, Verweij J, Brouwer E, de Jonge MJ, Sparreboom A. Gender-dependent pharmacokinetics of topotecan in adult patients. Anticancer Drugs 2000;11(9):673–80.

60. O'Reilly S, Rowinsky EK, Slichenmyer W, Donehower RC, Forastiere AA, Ettinger DS, Chen TL, Sartorius S, Grochow LB. Phase I and pharmacologic study of topotecan in patients with impaired renal function. J Clin Oncol 1996;14(12):3062–73.

61. Montazeri A, Culine S, Laguerre B, Pinguet F, Lokiec F, Albin N, Goupil A, Deporte-Fety R, Bugat R, Canal P, Chatelut E. Individual adaptive dosing of topotecan in ovarian cancer. Clin Cancer Res 2002;8(2):394–9.

62. Herrington JD, Figueroa JA, Kirstein MN, Zamboni WC, Stewart CF. Effect of hemodialysis on topotecan disposition in a patient with severe renal dysfunction. Cancer Chemother Pharmacol 2001;47(1):89–93.

63. Blaney SM, Cole DE, Godwin K, Sung C, Poplack DG, Balis FM. Intrathecal administration of topotecan in nonhuman primates. Cancer Chemother Pharmacol 1995;36(2):121–4.

64. Blaney SM, Heideman R, Berg S, Adamson P, Gillespie A, Geyer JR, Packer R, Matthay K, Jaeckle K, Cole D, Kuttesch N, Poplack DG, Balis FM. Phase I clinical trial of intrathecal topotecan in patients with neoplastic meningitis. J Clin Oncol 2003;21(1):143–7.

65. von Pawel J, Gatzemeier U, Pujol JL, Moreau L, Bildat S, Ranson M, Richardson G, Steppert C, Riviere A, Camlett I, Lane S, Ross G. Phase II comparator study of oral versus intravenous topotecan in patients with chemosensitive small-cell lung cancer. J Clin Oncol 2001;19(6):1743–9.

66. Creemers GJ, Gerrits CJ, Eckardt JR, Schellens JH, Burris HA, Planting AS, Rodriguez GI, Loos WJ, Hudson I, Broom C, Verweij J, Von Hoff DD. Phase I and pharmacologic study of oral topotecan administered twice daily for 21 days to adult patients with solid tumors. J Clin Oncol 1997;15(3):1087–93.

67. Gore M, Oza A, Rustin G, Malfetano J, Calvert H, Clarke-Pearson D, Carmichael J, Ross G, Beckman RA, Fields SZ. A randomised trial of oral versus intravenous topotecan in patients with relapsed epithelial ovarian cancer. Eur J Cancer 2002;38(1):57–63.

68. Jagodic M, Cufer T, Zakotnik B, Cervek J. Selection of candidates for oral etoposide salvage chemotherapy in heavily pretreated breast cancer patients. Anticancer Drugs 2001;12(3):199–204.

69. Harvey VJ, Slevin ML, Joel SP, Johnston A, Wrigley PF. The effect of dose on the bioavailability of oral etoposide. Cancer Chemother Pharmacol 1986;16(2):178–81.

70. Aita P, Robieux I, Sorio R, Tumolo S, Corona G, Cannizzaro R, Colussi AM, Boiocchi M, Toffoli G. Pharmacokinetics of oral etoposide in patients with hepatocellular carcinoma. Cancer Chemother Pharmacol 1999;43(4):287–94.

71. Hande KR, Krozely MG, Greco FA, Hainsworth JD, Johnson DH. Bioavailability of low-dose oral etoposide. Clin Oncol 1993;11(2):374–7.

72. Millward MJ, Newell DR, Yuen K, Matthews JP, Balmanno K, Charlton CJ, Gumbrell L, Lind MJ, Chapman F, Proctor M, Simmonds D, Cantwell BMJ, Calvert AH. Pharmacokinetics and pharmacodynamics of prolonged oral etoposide in women with metastatic breast cancer. Cancer Chemother Pharmacol 1995;37(1–2):161–7.

73. Chabot GG, Armand JP, Terret C, de Forni M, Abigerges D, Winograd B, Igwemezie L, Schacter L, Kaul S, Ropers J, Bonnay M. Etoposide bioavailability after oral administration of the prodrug etoposide phosphate in cancer patients during a phase I study. J Clin Oncol 1996;14(7):2020–30.

74. Hande KR. Etoposide: four decades of development of a topoisomerase II inhibitor. Eur J Cancer 1998;34(10):1514–21.

75. Schacter LP, Igwemezie LN, Seyedsadr M, Morgenthien E, Randolph J, Albert E, Santabarbara P. Clinical and pharmacokinetic overview of parenteral etoposide phosphate. Cancer Chemother Pharmacol 1994;34(Suppl):S58–63.

76. Kaul S, Igwemezie LN, Stewart DJ, Fields SZ, Kosty M, Levithan N, Bukowski R, Gandara D, Goss G, O'Dwyer P, Schacter LP, Barbhaiya RH. Pharmacokinetics and bioequivalence of etoposide following intravenous administration of etoposide phosphate and etoposide in patients with solid tumors. J Clin Oncol 1995;13(11):2835–41.

77. Budman DR, Igwemezie LN, Kaul S, Behr J, Lichtman S, Schulman P, Vinciguerra V, Allen SL, Kolitz J, Hock K, O'Neill K, Schacter L, Barbhaiya RH. Phase I evaluation of a water-soluble etoposide prodrug, etoposide phosphate, given as a 5-minute infusion on days 1, 3, and 5 in patients with solid tumors. J Clin Oncol 1994;12(9):1902–9.

78. Reif S, Kingreen D, Kloft C, Grimm J, Siegert W, Schunack W, Jaehde U. Bioequivalence investigation of high-dose etoposide and etoposide phosphate in lymphoma patients. Cancer Chemother Pharmacol 2001;48(2):134–40.

79. Kreis W, Budman DR, Vinciguerra V, Hock K, Baer J, Ingram R, Schacter LP, Fields SZ. Pharmacokinetic evaluation of high-dose etoposide phosphate after a 2-hour infusion in patients with solid tumors. Cancer Chemother Pharmacol 1996;38(4):378–84.

80. Joel SP, Shah R, Slevin ML. Etoposide dosage and pharmacodynamics. Cancer Chemother Pharmacol 1994;34(Suppl):S69–75.

81. Joel SP, Shah R, Clark PI, Slevin ML. Predicting etoposide toxicity: relationship to organ function and protein binding. J Clin Oncol 1996;14(1):257–67.

82. Liu B, Earl HM, Poole CJ, Dunn J, Kerr DJ. Etoposide protein binding in cancer patients. Cancer Chemother Pharmacol 1995;36(6):506–12.

83. Nguyen L, Chatelut E, Chevreau C, Tranchand B, Lochon I, Bachaud JM, Pujol A, Houin G, Bugat R, Canal P. Population pharmacokinetics of total and unbound etoposide. Cancer Chemother Pharmacol 1998;41(2):125–32.

84. D'Incalci M, Rossi C, Zucchetti M, Urso R, Cavalli F, Mangioni C, Willems Y, Sessa C. Pharmacokinetics of etoposide in patients with abnormal renal and hepatic function. Cancer Res 1986;46(5):2566–71.

85. Stewart CF, Arbuck SG, Fleming RA, Evans WE. Changes in the clearance of total and unbound etoposide in patients with liver dysfunction. J Clin Oncol 1990;8(11):1874–9.

86. Mross K, Bewermeier P, Kruger W, Stockschlader M, Zander A, Hossfeld DK. Pharmacokinetics of undiluted or diluted high-dose etoposide with or without busulfan administered to patients with hematologic malignancies. J Clin Oncol 1994;12(7):1468–74.

87. Schwinghammer TL, Fleming RA, Rosenfeld CS, Przepiorka D, Shadduck RK, Bloom EJ, Stewart CF. Disposition of total and unbound etoposide following high-dose therapy. Cancer Chemother Pharmacol 1993;32(4):273–8.

88. Relling MV, Nemec J, Schuetz EG, Schuetz JD, Gonzalez FJ, Korzekwa KR. O-demethylation of epipodophyllotoxins is catalyzed by human cytochrome P450 3A4. Mol Pharmacol 1994;45(2):352–8.

89. Hande KR, Wolff SN, Greco FA, Hainsworth JD, Reed G, Johnson DH. Etoposide kinetics in patients with obstructive jaundice. J Clin Oncol 1990;8(6):1101–7.

90. Holthuis JJ, Van de Vyver FL, van Oort WJ, Verleun H, Bakaert AB, De Broe ME. Pharmacokinetic evaluation of increasing dosages of etoposide in a chronic hemodialysis patient. Cancer Treat Rep 1985;69(11):1279–82.

91. Kiya K, Uozumi T, Ogasawara H, Sugiyama K, Hotta T, Mikami T, Kurisu K. Penetration of etoposide into human malignant brain tumors after intravenous and oral administration. Cancer Chemother Pharmacol 1992;29(5):339–42.

92. van der Gaast A, Sonneveld P, Mans DR, Splinter TA. Intrathecal administration of etoposide in the treatment of malignant meningitis: feasibility and pharmacokinetic data. Cancer Chemother Pharmacol 1992;29(4):335–7.

93. Minami H, Ratain MJ, Ando Y, Shimokata K. Pharmacodynamic modeling of prolonged administration of etoposide. Cancer Chemother Pharmacol 1996;39(1–2):61–6.

94. Hande K, Messenger M, Wagner J, Krozely M, Kaul S. Inter- and intrapatient variability in etoposide kinetics with oral and intravenous drug administration. Clin Cancer Res 1999;5(10):2742–7.

95. Rodman JH, Abromowitch M, Sinkule JA, Hayes FA, Rivera GK, Evans WE. Clinical pharmacodynamics of continuous infusion teniposide: systemic exposure as a determinant of response in a phase I trial. J Clin Oncol 1987;5(7):1007–14.

96. Splinter TA, Holthuis JJ, Kok TC, Post MH. Absolute bioavailability and pharmacokinetics of oral teniposide. Semin Oncol 1992;19(2 Suppl 6):28–34.

97. Breidenbach M, Rein DT, Schondorf T, Schmidt T, Konig E, Valter M, Kurbacher CM. Hematological side-effect profiles of individualized chemotherapy regimen for recurrent ovarian cancer. Anticancer Drugs 2003;14(5):341–6.

98. Rowinsky EK, Grochow LB, Sartorius SE, Bowling MK, Kaufmann SH, Peereboom D, Donehower RC. Phase I and pharmacologic study of high doses of the topoisomerase I inhibitor topotecan with granulocyte colony-stimulating factor in patients with solid tumors. J Clin Oncol 1996;14(4):1224–35.

99. Saltz L, Sirott M, Young C, Tong W, Niedzwiecki D, Tzy-Jyun Y, Tao Y, Trochanowski B, Wright P, Barbosa K, et al. Phase I clinical and pharmacology study of topotecan given daily for 5 consecutive days to patients with advanced solid tumors, with attempt at dose intensification using recombinant granulocyte colony-stimulating factor. J Natl Cancer Inst 1993;85(18):1499–507.

100. Hande KR. Topoisomerase II inhibitors. In: Giaccone G, Schilsky R, Sondel P, editors. Cancer Chemotherapy and Biological Response Modifiers. Amsterdam: Elsevier, 2003:103–25.

101. Schwarzer S, Eber B, Greinix H, Lind P. Non-Q-wave myocardial infarction associated with bleomycin and etoposide chemotherapy. Eur Heart J 1991;12(6):748–50.

102. Aisner J, Van Echo DA, Whitacre M, Wiernik PH. A phase I trial of continuous infusion VP16–213 (etoposide). Cancer Chemother Pharmacol 1982;7(2–3):157–60.

103. Imrie KR, Couture F, Turner CC, Sutcliffe SB, Keating A. Peripheral neuropathy following high-dose etoposide and autologous bone marrow transplantation. Bone Marrow Transplant 1994;13(1):77–9.

104. Leff RS, Thompson JM, Daly MB, Johnson DB, Harden EA, Mercier RJ, Messerschmidt GL. Acute neurologic dysfunction after high-dose etoposide therapy for malignant glioma. Cancer 1988;62(1):32–5.

105. Saliba F, Hagipantelli R, Misset JL, Bastian G, Vassal G, Bonnay M, Herait P, Cote C, Mahjoubi M, Mignard D, Cvitkovic E. Pathophysiology and therapy of irinotecan-induced delayed-onset diarrhea in patients with advanced colorectal cancer: a prospective assessment. J Clin Oncol 1998;16(8):2745–51.

106. Gandia D, Abigerges D, Armand JP, Chabot G, Da Costa L, De Forni M, Mathieu-Boue A, Herait P. CPT-11-induced cholinergic effects in cancer patients. J Clin Oncol 1993;11(1):196–7.

107. Gupta E, Lestingi TM, Mick R, Ramirez J, Vokes EE, Ratain MJ. Metabolic fate of irinotecan in humans: correlation of glucuronidation with diarrhea. Cancer Res 1994;54(14):3723–5.

108. Castellanos C, Aldaz A, Zufia L, Gurpide A, Navarro V, Quero C, Martin-Algarra S. Biliary index accurately predict the severity of irinotecn-induced delayed diarrea in colorectal cancer patients. Proc ASCO 2003;22:A648.

109. Ikegami T, Ha L, Arimori K, Latham P, Kobayashi K, Ceryak S, Matsuzaki Y, Bouscarel B. Intestinal alkalization as a possible preventive mechanism in irinotecan (CPT-11)-induced diarrhea. Cancer Res 2002;62(1):179–87.

110. Takeda Y, Kobayashi K, Akiyama Y, Soma T, Handa S, Kudoh S, Kudo K. Prevention of irinotecan (CPT-11)-induced diarrhea by oral alkalization combined with control of defecation in cancer patients. Int J Cancer 2001;92(2):269–75.

111. Takasuna K, Hagiwara T, Hirohashi M, Kato M, Nomura M, Nagai E, Yokoi T, Kamataki T. Inhibition of intestinal microflora beta-glucuronidase modifies the distribution of the active metabolite of the antitumor agent, irinotecan hydrochloride (CPT-11) in rats. Cancer Chemother Pharmacol 1998;42(4):280–6.

112. Barbounis V, Koumakis G, Vassilomanolakis M, Demiri M, Efremidis AP. Control of irinotecan-induced diarrhea by octreotide after loperamide failure. Support Care Cancer 2001;9(4):258–60.

113. Karthaus M, Ballo H, Steinmetz T, Geer T, Schimke J, Braumann D, Behrens R, Kindler M, Greinwald R, Kleeberg U. Budesonide for prevention of CPT-11-induced diarrhea. Results of a double-blind placebo-controlled multicenter randomised phase III study in patients with advanced colorectal cancer. Proc ASCO 2003;22:A2935.

114. Mitchell RB, Wagner JE, Karp JE, Watson AJ, Brusilow SW, Przepiorka D, Storb R, Santos GW, Burke PJ, Saral R. Syndrome of idiopathic hyperammonemia after high-dose chemotherapy: review of nine cases. Am J Med 1988;85(5):662–7.

115. Rivory LP, Robert J. Pharmacologie de la camptothécine et de ses dérivés. [Pharmacology of camptothecin and its derivatives.] Bull Cancer 1995;82(4):265–85.

116. Wachters FM, Groen HJ, Maring JG, Gietema JA, Porro M, Dumez H, de Vries EG, van Oosterom AT. A phase I study with MAG-camptothecin intravenously administered weekly for 3 weeks in a 4-week cycle in adult patients with solid tumours. Br J Cancer 2004;90(12):2261–7.

117. Marini M, Wright D, Ropolo M, Abbruzzese M, Casas G. Neutrophilic eccrine hidradenitis secondary to topotecan. J Dermatolog Treat 2002;13(1):35–7.

118. Carstensen H, Nolte H, Hertz H. Teniposide-induced hypersensitivity reactions in children. Lancet 1989;2(8653):55.

119. Nolte H, Carstensen H, Hertz H. VM-26 (teniposide)-induced hypersensitivity and degranulation of basophils in children. Am J Pediatr Hematol Oncol 1988;10(4):308–12.

120. van de Kerkhof PC, de Vaan GA, Holland R. Pyoderma gangrenosum in acute myeloid leukaemia during immunosuppression. Eur J Pediatr 1988;148(1):34–6.

121. Siddall SJ, Martin J, Nunn AJ. Anaphylactic reactions to teniposide. Lancet 1989;1(8634):394.

122. Schey SA, Cooper J, Summerhayes M. The "handfoot syndrome" occurring with chronic administration of etoposide. Eur J Haematol 1992;48(2):118–9.

123. Alley E, Green R, Schuchter L. Cutaneous toxicities of cancer therapy. Curr Opin Oncol 2002;14(2):212–6.

124. Weiss RB. Hypersensitivity reactions. Semin Oncol 1992;19(5):458–77.

125. Hoetelmans RM, Schornagel JH, ten Bokkel Huinink WW, Beijnen JH, Da Camara C, Dion P. Hypersensitivity reactions to etoposide. Ann Pharmacother 1996;30(4):367–71.

126. Kellie SJ, Crist WM, Pui CH, Crone ME, Fairclough DL, Rodman JH, Rivera GK. Hypersensitivity reactions to epipodophyllotoxins in children with acute lymphoblastic leukemia. Cancer 1991;67(4):1070–5.

127. Cersosimo RJ, Calarese P, Karp DD. Acute hypotensive reaction to etoposide with successful rechallenge: case report and review of the literature. DICP 1989;23(11):876–7.

128. Tester WJ, Cohn JB, Fleekop PD, Rabinowitz MS, Lieberman JS. Successful rechallenge to etoposide after an acute vasomotor response. J Clin Oncol 1990;8(9):1600–1.

129. Jameson CH, Solanki DL. Stevens–Johnson syndrome associated with etoposide therapy. Cancer Treat Rep 1983;67(11):1050–1.

130. Ogle KM, Kennedy BJ. Hypersensitivity reactions to etoposide. A case report and review of the literature. Am J Clin Oncol 1988;11(6):663–5.

131. Bernstein BJ, Troner MB. Successful rechallenge with etoposide phosphate after an acute hypersensitivity reaction to etoposide. Pharmacotherapy 1999;19(8):989–91.

132. Hudson MM, Weinstein HJ, Donaldson SS, Greenwald C, Kun L, Tarbell NJ, Humphrey WA, Rupp C, Marina NM, Wilimas J, Link MP. Acute hypersensitivity reactions to etoposide in a VEPA regimen for Hodgkin's disease. J Clin Oncol 1993;11(6):1080–4.

133. McLeod HL, Baker DK Jr, Pui CH, Rodman JH. Somnolence, hypotension, and metabolic acidosis following high-dose teniposide treatment in children with leukemia. Cancer Chemother Pharmacol 1991;29(2):150–4.

134. Siderov J, Prasad P, De Boer R, Desai J. Safe administration of etoposide phosphate after hypersensitivity reaction to intravenous etoposide. Br J Cancer 2002;86(1):12–3.

135. Nakanomyo H, Hiraoka M, Shiraya M. [Mutagenicity tests of etoposide and teniposide.]J Toxicol Sci 1986;11(Suppl 1):301–10.

136. Anderson RD, Berger NA. International Commission for Protection Against Environmental Mutagens and Carcinogens. Mutagenicity and carcinogenicity of topoisomerase-interactive agents. Mutat Res 1994;309(1):109–42.

137. Kollmannsberger C, Beyer J, Droz JP, Harstrick A, Hartmann JT, Biron P, Flechon A, Schoffski P, Kuczyk M, Schmoll HJ, Kanz L, Bokemeyer C. Secondary leukemia following high cumulative doses of etoposide in patients treated for advanced germ cell tumors. J Clin Oncol 1998;16(10):3386–91.

138. Duffner PK, Krischer JP, Horowitz ME, Cohen ME, Burger PC, Friedman HS, Kun LE. Second malignancies in young children with primary brain tumors following treatment with prolonged postoperative chemotherapy and delayed irradiation: a Pediatric Oncology Group study. Ann Neurol 1998;44(3):313–6.

139. Horibe K, Matsushita T, Numata S, Miyajima Y, Katayama I, Kitabayashi T, Yanai M, Sekiguchi N, Egi S. Acute promyelocytic leukemia with t(15;17) abnormality after chemotherapy containing etoposide for Langerhans cell histiocytosis. Cancer 1993;72(12):3723–6.

140. Relling MV, Yanishevski Y, Nemec J, Evans WE, Boyett JM, Behm FG, Pui CH. Etoposide and antimetabolite pharmacology in patients who develop secondary acute myeloid leukemia. Leukemia 1998;12(3):346–52.

141. Zulian GB, Selby P, Milan S, Nandi A, Gore M, Forgeson G, Perren TJ, McElwain TJ. High dose melphalan, BCNU and etoposide with autologous bone marrow transplantation for Hodgkin's disease. Br J Cancer 1989;59(4):631–5.

142. Stine KC, Saylors RL, Sawyer JR, Becton DL. Secondary acute myelogenous leukemia following safe exposure to etoposide. J Clin Oncol 1997;15(4):1583–6.

143. Houck W, Einhorn LH. Secondary leukemias in germ cell tumor patients undergoing autologous stem cell transplantation utilizing high-dose etoposide. Proc ASCO 2003;22:A1566.

144. Ratain MJ, Kaminer LS, Bitran JD, Larson RA, Le Beau MM, Skosey C, Purl S, Hoffman PC, Wade J, Vardiman JW, et al. Acute nonlymphocytic leukemia following etoposide and cisplatin combination chemotherapy for advanced non-small-cell carcinoma of the lung. Blood 1987;70(5):1412–7.

145. Rubin CM, Arthur DC, Woods WG, Lange BJ, Nowell PC, Rowley JD, Nachman J, Bostrom B, Baum ES, Suarez CR, et al. Therapy-related myelodysplastic syndrome and acute myeloid leukemia in children: correlation between chromosomal abnormalities and prior therapy. Blood 1991;78(11):2982–8.

146. Pui CH, Relling MV. Topoisomerase II inhibitor-related acute myeloid leukaemia. Br J Haematol 2000;109(1):13–23.

147. Pedersen-Bjergaard J, Philip P. Two different classes of therapy-related and de-novo acute myeloid leukemia? Cancer Genet Cytogenet 1991;55(1):119–24.

148. Hawkins MM, Wilson LM, Stovall MA, Marsden HB, Potok MH, Kingston JE, Chessells JM. Epipodophyllotoxins, alkylating agents, and radiation and risk of secondary leukaemia after childhood cancer. BMJ 1992;304(6832):951–8.

149. Pui CH, Ribeiro RC, Hancock ML, Rivera GK, Evans WE, Raimondi SC, Head DR, Behm FG, Mahmoud MH, Sandlund JT, Crist W. Acute myeloid leukemia in children treated with epipodophyllotoxins for acute lymphoblastic leukemia. N Engl J Med 1991;325(24):1682–7.

150. Lamont EB, Schilsky RL. Gonadal toxicity and teratogenicity after cytotoxic chemotherapy. In: Lipp HP, editor. Anticancer Drug Toxicity: Prevention, Management and Clinical Pharmacokinetics. New York–Basel: Marcel Dekker Inc, 1999:491–523.

151. Matsui H, Iitsuka Y, Seki K, Sekiya S. Pregnancy outcome after treatment with etoposide (VP-16) for low-risk gestational trophoblastic tumor. Int J Gynecol Cancer 1999;9(2):166–9.

152. Fleischhack G, Reif S, Hasan C, Jaehde U, Hettmer S, Bode U. Feasibility of intraventricular administration of etoposide in patients with metastatic brain tumours. Br J Cancer 2001;84(11):1453–9.

153. Lum BL, Kaubisch S, Yahanda AM, Adler KM, Jew L, Ehsan MN, Brophy NA, Halsey J, Gosland MP, Sikic BI. Alteration of etoposide pharmacokinetics and pharmacodynamics by cyclosporine in a phase I trial to modulate multidrug resistance. J Clin Oncol 1992;10(10):1635–42.

154. Rowinsky EK, Kaufmann SH, Baker SD, Grochow LB, Chen TL, Peereboom D, Bowling MK, Sartorius SE, Ettinger DS, Forastiere AA, Donehower RC. Sequences of topotecan and cisplatin: phase I, pharmacologic, and in vitro studies to examine sequence dependence. J Clin Oncol 1996;14(12):3074–84.

155. Zamboni WC, Egorin MJ, Van Echo DA, Day RS, Meisenberg BR, Brooks SE, Doyle LA, Nemieboka NN, Dobson JM, Tait NS, Tkaczuk KH. Pharmacokinetic and pharmacodynamic study of the combination of docetaxel and topotecan in patients with solid tumors. J Clin Oncol 2000;18(18):3288–94.

156. Baker DK, Relling MV, Pui CH, Christensen ML, Evans WE, Rodman JH. Increased teniposide clearance with concomitant anticonvulsant therapy. J Clin Oncol 1992;10(2):311–5.

157. Kohne CH, Van Cutsem E, Wils JA, Bokemeyer C, El-Serafi M, Lutz M, Lorenz M, Anak O, Genicot B, Nordlinger Bthe EORTC GI Group. Irinotecan improves the activity of the AIO regimen in metastatic colorectal cancer: results of EORTC GI-group study 40986. Proc Am Soc Clin Oncol 2003;22:A1018.

158. Dodds HM, Bishop JF, Rivory LP. More about: irinotecan-related cholinergic syndrome induced by coadministration of oxaliplatin. J Natl Cancer Inst 1999;91(1):91–2.

159. Wasserman E, Cuvier C, Lokiec F, Goldwasser F, Kalla S, Mery-Mignard D, Ouldkaci M, Besmaine A, Dupont-Andre G, Mahjoubi M, Marty M, Misset JL, Cvitkovic E. Combination of oxaliplatin plus irinotecan in patients with gastrointestinal tumors: results of two independent phase I studies with pharmacokinetics. J Clin Oncol 1999;17(6):1751–9.

TYROSINE KINASE INHIBITORS

General Information

Tyrosine kinase inhibitors are effective in the targeted treatment of various malignancies. Imatinib was the first to be introduced into clinical oncology, and it was followed by drugs such as dasatinib, gefitinib, erlotinib, sorafenib, and sunitinib. Although they share the same mechanism of action, namely competitive ATP inhibition at the catalytic binding site of tyrosine kinase, they differ from each other in the spectrum of targeted kinases, their pharmacokinetics, and their adverse effects (1).

Organs and Systems

Skin and hair

With variations from drug to drug, tyrosine kinase inhibitors cause skin toxicity, including folliculitis, in more than 50% of patients (2). Among the tyrosine kinase inhibitors that are so far commercially available, the agents that target EGFR, erlotinib and gefitinib, have the broadest spectrum of adverse effects on the skin and hair, including folliculitis, paronychia, facial hair growth, facial erythema, and varying forms of frontal alopecia. In contrast, folliculitis is not common during administration of sorafenib and sunitinib, which target VEGFR, PDGFR, FLT3, and others, whereas both agents have been associated with subungual splinter hemorrhages. Periorbital edema is a common adverse effect of imatinib (2).

References

1. Maitland ML, Ratain MJ. Terminal ballistics of kinase inhibitors: there are no magic bullets. Ann Intern Med 2006;145:702-3.
2. Robert C, Soria JC, Spatz A, Le Cesne A, Malka D, Pautier P, Wechsler J, Lhomme C, Escudier B, Boige V, Armand JP, Le Chevalier T. Cutaneous side-effects of kinase inhibitors and blocking antibodies. Lancet Oncol 2005;6:491-500.

Dasatinib

General Information

Dasatinib (BMS-354825), a thiazole carboximide derivative, is structurally related to imatinib. It targets src kinase and imatinib-resistant bcr-abl kinase and has impressive activity in patients with chronic myeloid leukemia or Philadelphia chromosome-positive acute lymphoblastic leukemia (1,2).

Although dasatinib has been approved for these indications in a dosage of 70 mg bd, the search for the optimal dose regimen continues (3). Preliminary data suggest that 100 mg/day may offer a more favorable benefit to harm balance in patients with chronic myeloid leukemia that is resistant to imatinib or in whom imatinib causes unacceptable adverse effects. Compared with conventional twice daily dosing, intermittent tyrosine kinase inhibition produces clinical remissions with improved safety, with the lowest incidence of pleural effusion (all grades), neutropenia (grades 3–4), and thrombocytopenia (grades 3–4). In addition, the use of dasatinib 100 mg/day makes dosage reductions less necessary than dosage schedules based on 50 mg bd (4), 140 mg/day, or 70 mg bd. However, the accelerated phase or blast crisis makes doses of up to 100 mg bd necessary.

The main adverse effects of dasatinib include grade 3/4 hematological toxicity (for example neutropenia and thrombocytopenia), liver abnormalities, diarrhea, headache, peripheral edema, and hypocalcemia. In addition, pleural effusion is of clinical concern and may need treatment with diuretics and thoracentesis or pleurodesis.

Pharmacokinetics

Dasatinib is well absorbed from the gastrointestinal tract (2). However, its solubility is pH dependent, and the AUC of dasatinib can be reduced significantly when antacids or famotidine are used concomitantly (by 55% and 61% respectively). Dasatinib undergoes extensive metabolism by CYP3A4 and has an active metabolite. Further enzymes involved in the metabolism of dasatinib include FMO-3 and UGT isozymes. Exposure to the active metabolite, which is equipotent with the parent compound, represents about 5% of the AUC of dasatinib. Dasatinib and its metabolites are primarily excreted via the feces. The half-life of the parent compound is 3–5 hours.

Organs and Systems

Skin

The difference in targets between imatinib and dasatinib may explain the observed risk of panniculitis with the latter.

- A 55-year old woman with chronic myeloid leukemia did not have a major cytogenetic response to imatinib mesylate, even in a dose of 800 mg/day, because of the activation-loop mutation H396R (5). When she was given dasatinib (70 mg bd) for 4 weeks she developed a fever (38.1°C) and painful subcutaneous nodules with overlying erythema on her thighs. After withdrawal of dasatinib the rash resolved within 1 week. However, her symptoms recurred when dasatinib was restarted, with manifestations on the arms, legs, and vulva. Biopsy of the skin lesions showed a lobular panniculitis, with massive infiltration by polymorphonuclear leukocytes. Withdrawal and reintroduction together with prednisone 50 mg/day) successfully controlled the panniculitis.

References

1. O'Hare T, Walters DK, Stoffregen EP, Jia T, Manley PW, Mestan J, Cowan-Jacob SW, Lee FY, Heinrich MC, Deininger MW, Druker BJ. In vitro activity of Ber-Abl inhibitors AMN107 and BMS-354825 against clinically relevant imatinib resistant Abl kinase domain mutants. Cancer Res 2005;65:4500-5.
2. Talpaz M, Shah NP, Kantarjian H, Donato N, Nicoll J, Paquette R, Cortes J, O'Brien S, Nicaise C, Bleickardt E, Blackwood-Chirchir MA, Iyer V, Chen TT, Huang F, Decillis AP, Sawyers CL. Dasatinib in imatinib-resistant Philadelphia chromosome-positive leukemias. N Engl J Med 2006;354:2531-41.
3. Soverini S, Martinelli G, Colarossi S, Gnani A, Rondoni M, Castagnetti F, Paolini S, Rosti G, Baccarani M. Second-line treatment with dasatinib in patients resistant to imatinib can select novel inhibitor-specific BCR-ABL mutants in Ph+ ALL. Lancet Oncol 2007;8:273-74.
4. Shah NP, Kim DW, Kantarjian HM, Rousselot P, Dorlhiac-Llacer PE, Milone JH, Bleickardt E, Francis S, Hochhaus A. Dasatinib 50 mg or 70 mg bid compared to 100 mg or 140 mg qd in patients with CML in chronic phase (CP) who are resistant or intolerant to imatinib: one-year result of CA180034. ASCO Annual Meeting Proceedings. J Clin Oncol 2007;25 (June 20 Suppl):7004.
5. Assouline S, Laneuville P, Gambacorti-Passerini C. Panniculitis during dasatinib therapy for imatinib-resistant chronic myelogenous leukemia. N Engl J Med 2006;354:2623-4.

Erlotinib

General Information

Erlotinib is the second inhibitor EGFR tyrosine kinase to have been approved for the treatment of locally advanced non-small-cell lung cancer after failure of at least one prior cytotoxic drug regimen (1). It has also been approved for the first-line treatment of metastatic pancreatic cancer in combination with gemcitabine (2).

Erlotinib should be taken in a dosage of 150 mg/day on an empty stomach at least 1 hour before or 2 hours after a meal.

The most common adverse effects of erlotinib include grade 3/4 rashes and diarrhea, which occur in 9% and 6% of patients respectively, and which warrant drug withdrawal in 1% of patients. Sun protection is generally recommended, because inhibition of EGFR in the skin potentiates the harmful effects of ultraviolet radiation. In patients with lower constitutive concentrations of melanin in the skin, for example Fitzpatrick skin phototypes I and II, higher sensitivity to ultraviolet radiation and a higher probability of more severely graded rash are expected (3). Withdrawal of erlotinib has been recommended when signs of new or progressive unexplained pulmonary symptoms are observed, such as dyspnea, cough, and fever, in order to reduce the risk of interstitial lung disease.

Pharmacokinetics

The absolute systemic availability of erlotinib averages 59% and is significantly increased by a meal. Antacids, proton pump inhibitors, and histamine H2 receptor antagonists impair the absorption of erlotinib, because its solubility is reduced at pH values exceeding 5.0. More than 90% of a dose is metabolized in the liver, primarily by CYP3A4 and CYP1A2. OSI-420, the major metabolite, has antineoplastic activity. Excretion is mainly via the feces. The half-life averages 36 hours, and steady-state concentrations are reached within 7–8 days.

Organs and Systems

Skin

In 42 patients with either unresectable or metastatic biliary cancer, erlotinib 150 mg/day orally produced mild (grade 1/2) rashes in all those who responded; three had grade 2/3 rashes, which required dosage reductions (4).

Drug-Drug Interactions

In a small study in patients with gliomas, the median plasma AUC of erlotinib was significantly reduced by enzyme-inducing antiepileptic drugs, although the dose of erlotinib had been doubled beforehand from 450 mg/day to 900 mg/day (5). In contrast, the AUC of the active metabolite OSI-420 increased about threefold, which may have compensated for the reduction in exposure to the parent compound. Drug concentrations in the cerebrospinal fluid were 1–3% of the peak plasma concentrations.

Erlotinib is a potent inhibitor of CYP1A1 and UGT1A1 and a moderate inhibitor of CYP3A4 and CYP2C8. However, the relevance of these in vitro data to clinical practice has not been elucidated.

References

1. Shepherd FA, Rodrigues Pereira J, Ciuleanu T, Tan EH, Hirsh V, Thongprasert S, Campos D, Maoleekoonpiroj S, Smylie M, Martins R, van Kooten M, Dediu M, Findlay B, Tu D, Johnston D, Bezjak A, Clark G, Santabrbara P, Seymour L; National Cancer Institute of Canada Clinical Trials Group. Erlotinib in previously treated non-small-cell lung cancer. N Engl J Med 2005;353:123-32.
2. Moore MJ, Goldstein D, Hamm J, Figer A, Hecht JR, Gallinger S, Au HJ, Murawa P, Walde D, Wolff RA, Campos D, Lim R, Ding K, Clark G, Voskoglou-Nomikos T, Ptasynski M, Parulekar W; National Cancer Institute of Canada Clinical Trials Group. Erlotinib plus gemcitabine compared of gemcitabine alone in patients with advanced pancreatic cancer. A phase III trial of the National Cancer Institute of Canada Clinical Trials Group (NCIC-CTG). J Clin Oncol 2007;25:1960-6.
3. Lai SE, Minnelli L, O'Keeffe P, Rademaker A, Patel J, Bennett CL, Lacouture ME. Influence of skin color in the development of erlotinib-induced rash: a report from the SERIES Clinic. ASCO Annual Meeting Proceedings. J Clin Oncol 2007;25 (June 20 Suppl):9127.

4. Philip PA, Mahoney MR, Allmer C, Thomas J, Pitot HC, Kim G, Donehower RC, Fitch T, Picus J, Erlichman C. Phase II study of erlotinib in patients with advanced biliary cancer. J Clin Oncol 2006;24:3069-74.

5. Buie LW, Lindley C, Shih T, Ewend M, Smith JK, Skelton M, Kwock L, Morris D, Tucker C, Collichio F. Plasma pharmacokinetics and cerebrospinal fluid concentrations of erlotinib in high-grade gliomas: a novel, phase I, dose escalation study. ASCO Annual Meeting Proceedings. J Clin Oncol 2007; 25(June 20 Suppl):2054.

Gefitinib

General Information

Gefitinib is an anilinoquinazoline derivative, the first agent to have been introduced as a potent inhibitor of EGFR tyrosine kinase for the treatment of advanced non-small-cell lung cancer refractory or resistant to cytotoxic chemotherapy. Case series have shown significant radiographic regression and improvement of symptoms. A history of never smoking cigarettes and bronchoalveolar histology are significant predictors of a radiographic response to gefitinib. In addition, there are higher response rates in Japanese versus non-Japanese subjects, in those of performance status 0 to 1, in women, and in those with adenocarcinoma histology and prior immunotherapy or hormonal therapy. If several of these characteristics are present simultaneously, higher response rates and a longer median survival time with gefitinib, or the structurally related erlotinib, can be expected (1).

The recommended dose of gefitinib is 250 mg/day, and 500 mg/day causes increased toxicity without additional efficacy.

Pharmacokinetics

The mean absolute systemic availability after oral administration averages 60% (2). Gefitinib probably crosses the blood-brain barrier, which is favorable in patients with metastatic disease (3). Its half-life is about 48 hours, and steady-state concentrations are achieved within 10 days. Hepatic metabolism via CYP3A4 and biliary excretion are the major routes of elimination, and renal excretion is of minor importance.

Organs and Systems

Respiratory

The most serious adverse effect of gefitinib is lung toxicity, including rapidly progressive dyspnea with a risk of severe hypoxemia and bilateral ground-glass attenuation on chest CT.

Of 110 patients with non-small-cell lung cancer who took gefitinib over 3 months, 12 developed significant lung toxicity and five died from progressive complications, including chronic pulmonary fibrosis. The mechanism may involve impairment of healing of epithelium,

since EGF is needed to regenerate damaged alveolar epithelial cells. Thus, any underlying lung damage (for example pre-existing pulmonary fibrosis) may predispose to lung toxicity (4,5).

• A 70-year-old woman with a long history of smoking developed a non-small-cell lung cancer, stage IV (6). She was given radiotherapy and chemotherapy consisting of cisplatin and gemcitabine. However, she developed hemolytic–uremic syndrome, with raised LDH activity, hypoalbuminemia, reticulocytosis, and a high blood urea nitrogen concentration. When the disease progressed she was given gefitinib 250 mg/day, which resulted in improvement in tumor-related bone pain after several days. However, she developed a characteristic drug-related acneoid reaction and after 2 months developed progressive dyspnea and a dry cough, which gradually worsened. She had interstitial infiltrates in both lungs. Despite high-dose glucocorticoids, her condition worsened and she needed mechanical ventilation. She then developed hemodynamic instability and died.

Gastrointestinal

During treatment with efitinib 250 mg/day about 40% of patients develop diarrhea grade 2, which can be successfully controlled in most cases by symptomatic treatment with loperamide. Patients are advised to take loperamide 4 mg immediately, followed by 2 mg after every loose bowel movement (up to a maximum of 10 mg/day). If the is response inadequate, withdrawal of gefitinib may be warranted (7).

Skin

Gefitinib-associated skin reactions correlate with an increased likelihood of radiographic tumor response and symptomatic improvement, similar to the structurally related erlotinib and the monoclonal antibody cetuximab. However, durable radiographic regression and improvement of symptoms have also been observed in patients with only mild forms of rash and diarrhea.

The combination of clindamycin 1% and benzoylperoxide 5% gel has been used with some success for the treatment of inflammatory pustular lesions. If gel formulations are not well tolerated, oral minocycline 100 mg bd can be used instead. The roles of topical retinoids, topical or systemic corticosteroids, or topical pimecrolimus creams have not been clearly elucidated. In patients with very dry skin, Eucerin cream, Cetaphil cream, Aquaphor healing ointment, or Big Balm can be helpful in treating fissures on the palms and soles (7).

EGFR ligands (for example TGFα, EGF, HB-EGF) are cytokines that are excreted by keratinocytes during wound healing. It is therefore possible that wound healing may be impaired during the administration of EGFR tyrosine kinase inhibitors. However, in contrast to some preclinical results, no interference with would healing was seen with gefitinib in a series of patients who underwent laparotomy with concomitant lysis of adhesions and skin incisions (8).

- A 72-year-old man with a history of metastatic non-small-cell lung cancer required internal fixation for bone metastasis 2 months after he started to take gefitinib. A 4 cm skin incision on the left forearm was made for the procedure. He continued to take gefitinib until the day before surgery and resumed 24 hours after surgery. His skin wound healing was unremarkable.

Hair

EGFR tyrosine kinase inhibitors can cause a folliculitis, with a median time to onset of 7–10 days. Follicular papules and pustules rarely reach grade 3/4 severity, including the facial area, the forehead, and the upper chest and back. In contrast to juvenile acne, bacterial cultures of the initial primary lesions are usually negative (9). The mechanism has not been clearly elucidated but it may involve disordered regulation of keratinocyte biology and homeostasis of hair follicles related to EGFR inhibition. A further mechanism may be increased expression of p27Kip1 in basal and follicular keratinocytes and modified chemokine expression, resulting in greater skin inflammation. Withdrawal usually leads to rapid improvement and in some cases spontaneous reduction of symptoms has been observed in spite of continued treatment (10).

Inhibitors of EGFR tyrosine kinase can change scalp hair, slow hair growth, and cause frontal alopecia. In contrast, facial hair and eyelashes can grow progressively, particularly in women. It has been speculated that modification of the interaction between the EGFR-dependent and androgen-dependent signalling pathways may be the underlying mechanism (10).

Nails

Inhibitors of EGFR tyrosine kinase can cause paronychial inflammation with symptoms such as erythema, painful lateral fingernails or toenails and pyogenic granuloma-like lesions. These can resolve spontaneously and commonly disappear after treatment is withdrawn. Topical glucocorticoids, local antiseptics, avoiding cutting nails too short, and avoiding the use of shoes that are too tight have been advised to minimize paronychial inflammation (7).

Management of Adverse Drug Reactions

Increased thromboxane B2 and sP-selectin has been observed in patients taking gefitinib. In one study there were fewer adverse effects in 12 patients who took low-dose aspirin with gefitinib than in 28 who took gefitinib alone (11). The addition of reduced the frequencies of rash and diarrhea while therapeutic efficacy was not affected. The authors suggested that some gefitinib-related adverse effects may be due to platelet activation.

References

1. Cersosimo RJ. Gefitinib: a new antineoplastic for advanced non-small-cell lung cancer. Am J Health-Syst Pharm 2004;61:889–98.
2. Baselga J, Rischin D, Ranson M, Calvert H, Raymond E, Kieback DG, Kaye SB, Gianni L, Harris A, Bjork T, Averbuch SD, Feyereislova A, Swaisland H, Rojo F, Albanell J. Phase I safety, pharmacokinetic, and pharmacodynamic trial of ZD 1839, a selective oral epidermal growth factor receptor tyrosine kinase inhibitor, in patients with five selected solid tumor types. J Clin Oncol 2002;20:4292–302.
3. Villano JL, Mauer AM, Vokes EE. A case study documenting the anticancer activity of ZD1839 (Iressa) in the brain. Ann Oncol 2003;14:656–8.
4. Inomata S, Takahashi H, Nagata M, Yamada G, Shiratori M, Tanaka H, Satoh M, Saitoh T, Sato T, Abe S. Acute lung injury as an adverse event of gefitinib. Anticancer Drugs 2004;15:461–7.
5. Inoue A, Saijo Y, Maemondo M, Gomi K, Tokue Y, Kimura Y, Ebina M, Kikuchi T, Moriya T, Nukiwa T. Severe acute interstitial pneumonia and gefitinib. Lancet 2003;361:137–39.
6. Rabinowits G, Herchenhorn D, Rabinowits M, Weatge D, Torres W. Fatal pulmonary toxicity in a patient treated with gefitinib for non-small cell lung cancer after previous hemolytic–uremic syndrome due to gemcitabine. Anticancer Drugs 2003;14:665–8.
7. Shah NT, Kris MG, Pao W, Tyson LB, Pizzo BM, Heinemann MH, Ben-Porat L, Sachs DL, Heelan RT, Miller VA. Practical management of patients with non-small-cell lung cancer treated with gefitinib. J Clin Oncol 2005;23:165–74.
8. Govindan R, Behnken D, Read W, McLeod H. Wound healing is not impaired by the epidermal growth factor receptor-tyrosine kinase inhibitor gefitinib. Ann Oncol 2003;14:1330–1.
9. Veronese ML, Mosenkis A, Flaherty KT, Gallagher M, Stevenson JP, Townsend RR, O'Dwyer PJ. Mechanisms of hypertension associated with BAY 43-9006. J Clin Oncol 2006;24:1363–9.
10. Robert C, Soria JC, Spatz A, Le Cesne A, Malka D, Pautier P, Wechsler J, Lhomme C, Escudier B, Boige V, Armand JP, Le Chevalier T. Cutaneous side-effects of kinase inhibitors and blocking antibodies. Lancet Oncol 2005;6:491–500.
11. Kanazawa S, Yamaguchi K, Kinoshita Y, Muramatsu M, Komiyama Y, Nomura S. Aspirin reduces adverse effects of gefitinib. Anticancer Drugs 2006;17:423–7.

Imatinib mesylate

General Information

Imatinib (STI571), an inhibitor of bcr-abl tyrosine kinase, has become the first-line agent in the treatment of the chronic phase of chronic myeloid leukaemia and of locally advanced and metastatic gastrointestinal stromal tumors (GISTs) that express the CD117 antigen. The recommended dosage is 400 mg/day for patients with chronic myeloid leukaemia and for GIST and 600 mg/day in the accelerated phase or blast crisis of chronic myeloid leukaemia. The dose should be taken once a day with a meal and a large glass of water.

Pharmacokinetics

The mean absolute systemic availability of imatinib is about 98% (1). CYP3A4 plays a pivotal role in imatinib metabolism; N-demethylated imatinib is the main metabolite and is active (2). The plasma AUC for this metabolite is about 15% of the AUC of imatinib. Drug elimination is primarily mediated via the feces (3,4). The half-lives of imatinib and N-demethylimatinib are 18–27 hours and 40–74 hours respectively. The peak concentrations average 3340 ng/ml and 781 ng/ml, and trough concentrations 1540 ng/ml and 508 ng/ml respectively (5). These values were not changed significantly in patients with end-stage renal disease or on hemodialysis. Dosage adjustment is not therefore necessary in patients with renal impairment (6). Imatinib can also be used in patients with even severely impaired hepatic function (7).

- A 58-year-old patient with decompensated alcoholic liver cirrhosis developed a well-differentiated hepatocellular carcinoma (8). Because of in vitro sensitivity of the cells to antibodies against c-kit and cytokeratin 7, imatinib was given in a dosage of 100 mg bd based on increased transaminases and cholestasis. A year later the tumor mass had disappeared as assessed by histology, perhaps because of tumor necrosis.

Imatinib is generally well tolerated. Besides mild to moderate hematological toxicity, its adverse effects include fluid retention, edema, nausea, and some skin disorders (9,10). There have also been case reports of hepatitis.

Organs and Systems

Cardiovascular

It has been suggested that imatinib may have caused severe heart failure and left ventricular dysfunction in 10 patients with pre-existing conditions such as hypertension, diabetes mellitus, and coronary heart disease (11). Experimental studies have shown that imatinib induces apoptosis in isolated cardiac myocytes (11). Several trials and a database of six registration trials have therefore been reviewed.

- The Italian Cooperative Study Group—four consecutive studies of imatinib therapy in 833 patients with Philadelphia chromosome-positive chronic myeloid leukemia, observed for a median of 19–64 months (12). The overall cardiac mortality rate was 0.3%.
- The MD Anderson experience—clinical trials of imatinib from July 1998 to July 2006, with median follow-up of 5 years (13). In all the imatinib protocols, standard research monitoring procedures were conducted before treatment and at regular intervals. Electrocardiography, echocardiography, and chest radiography were conducted routinely before treatment and as clinically indicated during follow-up. The eligibility criteria excluded patients with cardiac problems (NYHA classes III and

IV). After reviewing all reported adverse events, particularly those that could be considered as having a cardiac origin, 22 patients (1.8%) were identified as having symptoms that could be attributed to congestive heart failure, of whom 12 had previously received interferon and three had received anthracyclines. They included nine patients reported elsewhere (11). Their median age was 70 (range 49–83) years. The median time from the start of imatinib therapy to a cardiac adverse event was 162 (range 2–2045) days. Eighteen patients had previous medical conditions that predisposed them to cardiac disease: congestive heart failure (n = 6), diabetes mellitus (n = 6), hypertension (n = 10), coronary artery disease (n = 8), dysrhythmias (n = 3), and cardiomyopathy (n = 1). Of the 22 patients, 15 underwent echocardiography or multiple gated acquisition (MUGA) scanning at the time of the event: nine of these 15 patients had low ejection fractions, and six of these nine had significant conditions that predisposed them to cardiac disease (three had coronary artery disease, two congestive heart failure, and one a cardiomyopathy). Of the 22 patients with symptoms of congestive heart failure, 11 continued to take imatinib with dosage adjustments and management of congestive heart failure without further complications. However, with the host of confounding factors involved in these patients, the occurrence of congestive heart failure related to the use of imatinib was reasonably unambiguous in only seven of the 1276 patients reviewed (0.5%).

- Novartis clinical database—six registration trials comprising 2327 patients who took imatinib as monotherapy. These trials represented 5595 patient-years of exposure to imatinib (average exposure 2.4 years). Twelve cases of congestive heart failure (0.5%) were considered to be incident cases (with no previous history of congestive heart failure or left ventricular dysfunction) with a possible or probable relation to imatinib. If these cases are related to the 5595 patients-years of imatinib exposure the incidence of congestive heart failure is 0.2% per year across all trials
- In the largest international, randomized phase III study reported to date, 1106 patients with newly diagnosed chronic myeloid leukemia were randomized to either initial therapy with imatinib or the previous standard treatment of interferon plus cytosine arabinoside (14). Both regimens were examined for cardiac safety according to an analysis of adverse events as described above. The incident cases of cardiac failure and left ventricular dysfunction, possibly or probably related to exposure to the study medication, was 0.04% per year (1 case in 2309 patient-years) for patients taking imatinib versus 0.75% per year (four cases in 536 patient-years of exposure) in patients taking interferon + cytosine arabinoside.

Imatinib therapy as a cause of congestive heart failure seems to be rare. When it occurs, the symptoms most commonly occur in elderly patients with pre-existing cardiac conditions and may often reflect predisposing cardiac compromise compounded by some element of fluid retention. Patients with a previous cardiac history should be monitored closely and treated aggressively with diuretics if they develop fluid retention.

Sensory systems

Imatinib often causes facial edema. In some patients, intense eyelid edema can result in ophthalmologic symptoms, including ptosis, blepharoconjunctivitis, visual obstruction, or even retinal edema. Inhibition of PDGFR leads to dysregulation of the tension between endothelial cells and the extracellular matrix. Severe periorbital edema may need surgical debulking of excess skin, fat, and edema of the lower eyelids, and can produce immediate improvement in visual function. In one case there was no recurrence 6 months after surgery (15).

Mineral metabolism

In a retrospective analysis imatinib caused hypophosphatemia more often than expected. Hypophosphatemia was more pronounced in younger patients, who had taken higher doses imatinib. The underlying mechanism may include reduced activity of PDGFR. Impairment of bone turnover and osteomalacia may therefore be expected during imatinib therapy. Whether phosphate and vitamin D concentrations should be measured routinely during imatinib therapy, with the aim of prescribing phosphate if necessary, is a matter of current debate (16).

Hematologic

Patients can develop myelosuppression during imatinib therapy, perhaps because of inhibition of c-kit, a cytokine that is involved in early hemopoiesis, inhibition of which can result in more than expected suppression of normal progenitors. It has not yet been elucidated why patients with hypereosinophilic syndrome or atypical chronic myelomonocytic leukemia experience imatinib-related neutropenia very rarely compared with patients with advanced chronic myeloid leukemia. However, there is some evidence that the more severe the myelosuppression with imatinib, the larger the response, suggesting that this adverse effect is a prognostic factor. It has therefore been proposed that imatinib-related myelosuppression may be a therapeutic effect on Philadelphia chromosome-positive clones rather than inhibition of normal hemopoiesis. Whereas empirical interruption of treatment or dosage modification may affect the outcome in chronic myeloid leukemia, some authors have suggested the use of G-CSF (for example filgrastim 300 micrograms subcutaneously 2 or 3 times a week) in patients who have myelosuppression at doses of imatinib of 300 mg/day (17).

Liver

There have been a few case reports of hepatotoxicity in patients taking imatinib, so far exclusively in women. It has been proposed that high drug concentrations of imatinib may predispose to an increased risk of liver damage; however, it is not clear whether immunological

idiosyncrasy (i.e. a hypersusceptibility reaction) or a metabolic disorder is the underlying reason.

- A 40-year-old woman with chronic myeloid leukemia in the chronic phase took imatinib mesylate because of resistance to interferon (18). She achieved a complete clinical remission after 3 months but the molecular response was incomplete. Six months later she developed hepatitis without any evidence of active viral infection. Serum concentrations of imatinib were markedly raised (8107 ng/ml), although she had stopped taking it 6 days before. At that stage there was a complete molecular response. Several weeks later her hepatic function had recovered and she had a normal blood count with a normal differential count. Rechallenge with imatinib was not performed.

Skin

There is some evidence that the severity of skin reactions due to imatinib is dose-related in the therapeutic range of doses (i.e. collateral effects, see page xxix). Mild forms are common at doses of 200–600 mg/day, whereas severe eruptions have been described in patients taking higher doses (600–1000 mg/day) (19). Re-exposure to higher doses resulted in relapse of skin eruptions, which highlights the need for adequate dosage reduction in affected patients. In case series, imatinib mesylate has been reported to cause reversible hypopigmentation of the skin, which may be dose-related in the therapeutic range (20,21). This benign adverse effect occurred within the first month of treatment. The underlying mechanism may involve a regulatory disorder in melanocyte development and survival, which depends on KIT and SCF.

- A 60-year-old white woman with a GIST took imatinib 400 mg/day for 2 months with lansoprazole 15 mg/day (22). She developed bilateral palpebral edema with hyperemic conjunctivae and labial edema. After withdrawal and reintroduction of both drugs, she developed generalized skin reactions, even at a low dose of imatinib and a concomitant glucocorticoid plus lansoprazole. When imatinib and lansoprazole were withdrawn, the skin toxicity did not progress.

The authors suggested that the skin effect may have result from (1) the well-known drug-related adverse effects of imatinib and lansoprazole on the skin and (2) inhibition of lansoprazole clearance by imatinib.

Drug-Drug Interactions

Imatinib is an inhibitor of some cytochrome P450 isozymes, such as CYP3A4, CYP2C9, and CYP2D6, and may affect the pharmacokinetics of substrates such as ciclosporin, warfarin, and some tricyclic antidepressants (23).

Management of Adverse Drug Reactions

Supportive management of common imatinib-related adverse effects has been described (24). Severe nausea may require antiemetics (for example a $5HT_3$ receptor antagonist or prochlorperazine). Diarrhea can be controlled by loperamide. Rashes may need topical or systemic steroids. Muscle cramps may need electrolyte substitution with magnesium and calcium. Bone aches may be alleviated with coxibs.

References

1. Beumer JH, Natale JJ, Lagattuta TF, Raptis A, Egorin MJ. Disposition of imatinib and its metabolite CGP74588 in patients with chronic myelogenous leukemia and short-bowel syndrome. Pharmacotherapy 2006;26:903–7.
2. Dutreix C, Peng B, Mehring G, Hayes M, Capdeville R, Pokorny R, Seiberling M. Pharmacokinetic interaction between ketoconazole and imatinib mesylate (Glivec) in healthy subjects. Cancer Chemother Pharmacol 2004;54:290–4.
3. Fausel CA. Novel treatment strategies for chronic myeloid leukaemia. Am J Health-Syst Pharm 2006;63:S15–S20.
4. Garcia-Manero G, Faderl S, O'Brien S, Cortes J, Talpaz M, Kantarjian HM. Chronic myelogenous leukemia: a review and update of therapeutic strategies. Cancer 2003;98:437–57.
5. Schleyer E, Ottmann O-G, Illmer T, Pursche S, Leopold T, Bonin M, Freiberg-Richter J, Jenke1A, Platzbecker U, Bornhäuser M, Ehninger G, le Coutre P. Pharmakokinetik von Imatinib (STI571) und seinem Hauptmetaboliten N-Desmethyl-Imatinib. Tumordiagn Ther 2004;25:192–6.
6. Pappas P, Karavasilis V, Briasoulis E, Pavlidis N, Marselos M. Pharmacokinetics of imatinib mesylate in end stage renal disease. A case study. Cancer Chemother Pharmacol 2005;56:358–60.
7. Bauer S, Hagen V, Pielken HJ, Bojko P, Seeber S, Schütte J. Imatinib mesylate therapy in patients with gastrointestinal stromal tumors and impaired liver function. Anticancer Drugs 2002;13:847–9.
8. Ramadori G, Füzesi L, Grabbe E, Pieler T, Armbrust T. Successful treatment on hepatocellular carcinoma with the tyrosine kinase inhibitor imatinib in a patient with liver cirrhosis. Anticancer Drugs 2004;15:405–9.
9. De Arriba JJ, Nerín C, García E, Gómez-Aldaraví L, Vila B. Severe hemolytic anemia and skin reaction in a patient treated with imatinib. Ann Oncol 2003;14:962.
10. van Oosterom AT, Judson I, Verweij J, Stroobants S, Donato di Paola E, Dimitrijevic S, Martens M, Webb A, Sciot R, Van Glabbeke M, Silberman S, Nielsen OS; European Organisation for Research and Treatment of Cancer Soft Tissue and Bone Sarcoma Group. Safety and efficacy of imatinib (STI571) in metastatic gastrointestinal stroma tumours: a phase I study. Lancet 2001;358:1421–3.
11. Kerkelä R, Grazette L, Yacobi R, Iliescu E, Patten R, Beahm C, Walters B, Shevtsov S, Pesant S, Clubb FJ, Rosenzweig A, Salomon RN, Van Etten RA, Alroy J, Durand JB, Force T. Cardiotoxicity of the cancer therapeutic agent imatinib mesylate. Nat Med 2006;12:908–16.
12. Rosti G, Martinelli G, Baccarani M. In reply to "Cardiotoxicity of the cancer therapeutic agent imatinib mesylate" Nat Med 2007;13:15–16.
13. Atallah E, Kantarjian H, Cortes J. In reply to "Cardiotoxicity of the cancer therapeutic agent imatinib mesylate". Nat Med 2007;13:14–16.
14. Hatfield A, Owen S, Pilot PR. In reply to "Cardiotoxicity of the cancer therapeutic agent imatinib mesylate". Nat Med 2007;13:13–16.
15. Esmaeli B, Prieto VG, Butler CE, Kim SK, Ahmadi MA, Kantarjian HM, Talpaz M. Severe periorbital edema secondary to STI571 (Gleevec). Cancer 2002;95:881–7.
16. Berman E, Nicolaides M, Maki RG, Fleisher M, Chanel S, Scheu K, Wilson BA, Heller G, Sauter NP. Altered bone and mineral metabolism in patients receiving imatinib mesylate. N Engl J Med 2006;354:2006–13.
17. Sneed TB, Kantarjian HM, Talpaz M, O'Brien S, Rios MB, Bekele BN, Zhou X, Resta D, Wierda W, Faderl S, Giles F, Cortes JE. The significance of myelosuppression during therapy with imatinib mesylate in patients with chronic myelogenous leukemia in chronic phase. Cancer 2004;100:116–21.
18. Kikuchi S, Muroi K, Takahashi S, Kawano-Yamamoto C, Takatoku M, Miyazato A, Nagai T, Mori M, Komatsu N, Ozawa K. Severe hepatitis and complete molecular response caused by imatinib mesylate: possible association of its serum concentration with clinical outcomes. Leukemia Lymphoma 2004;45:2349–51.
19. Brouard M, Saurat JH. Cutaneous reactions to STI571. N Engl J Med 2001;345:618–9.
20. Tsao AS, Kantarjian H, Cortes J, et al. Imatinib mesylate causes hypopigmentation in the skin. Cancer 2003;98:2483–7.
21. Ugurel S, Hildenbrand R, Dippel E, Hochhaus A, Schadendorf D. Dose-dependent severe cutaneous reactions to imatinib. Br J Cancer 2003;88:1157–9.
22. Sessa C, Viganò L, Grasselli G, Trigo J, Marimon I, Lladò A, Locatelli A, Ielmini N, Marsoni S, Gianni L. Phase I clinical and pharmacological evaluation of the multi-tyrosine kinase inhibitor SU006668 by chronic oral dosing. Eur J Cancer 2006;42:171–8.
23. Kajita T, Higashi Y, Imamura M, Maida C, Fujii Y, Yamamoto I, Miyamoto E. Effect of imatinib mesilate on the disposition kinetics of ciclosporin in rats. J Pharm Pharmacol 2006;58:997–1000.
24. Elliott M, Mesa RA, Tefferi A. Adverse events after imatinib mesylate therapy. N Engl J Med 2002;9:712–3.

Lapatinib

General Information

Lapatinib, a 4-anilinoquinazoline derivative, is the first dual tyrosine kinase inhibitor. In contrast to erlotinib and gefitinib, it inhibits both the ErbB1/HER1 (EGFR) tyrosine kinase and the ErbB2/HER 2 tyrosine kinase simultaneously. It is used in patients with advanced metastatic breast cancer who are refractory to anthracyclines or taxanes together with trastuzumab (1). It is given orally in a dose of 1.25 g/day on days 1–14 every 21 days) together with capecitabine (1.0 g/m» bd on days 1–14 every 21 days).

Lapatinib is generally well tolerated. Grade 3 diarrhea is dose-limiting, whereas adverse effects such as acneiform rash, nausea, and fatigue are moderate (grades 1–2).

Pharmacokinetics

Lapatinib peak concentrations are reached after 3–4 hours (2). Absorption is increased about three-fold when it is given with a meal, and administration on an empty stomach has been recommended, in contrast to the co-administered capecitabine, which should be taken with food. The half-life of lapatinib increases significantly from about 11 hours to 24 hours during repeated administration, probably because of inhibition of CYP3A4. Lapatinib crosses the blood–brain barrier, which may help in the treatment of brain metastases, which are of concern in about one-third of women with ErbB2 over-expression. Elimination is primarily by hepatic metabolism and biliary excretion; renal excretion is minor. Recovery of lapatinib in the feces accounts for about 27% (3–67%) of an oral dose.

Organs and Systems

Cardiovascular

The incidence of cardiac toxicity with lapatinib appears to be low; in one study only 37 of 2812 women (1.3%) had a fall in left ventricular ejection fraction (LVEF) of at least 20% from baseline (2). The onset of reduced LVEF occurred within 9 weeks of treatment in 68% of cases and was rarely symptomatic and generally reversible and non-progressive. The duration of reduction in LVEF averaged 42 days.

Drug-Drug Interactions

Lapatinib is a substrate of CYP3A4, and successive increases in dose may be necessary up to 4.5 g/day in patients who take inducing agents, such as carbamazepine 200 mg bd, which reduced the AUC of lapatinib by about 72% (3).

Lapatinib may inhibit the metabolism of other CYP3A4 substrates, including SN38, resulting in a significant increase in AUC and Cmax (4).

References

1. Nelson MH, Dolder CR. Lapatinib: a novel dual tyrosine kinase inhibitor with activity in solid tumors. Ann Pharmacother 2006;40: 61–9.
2. Terkola R. Lapatinib ditosylate (Tykerb). Eur J Oncol Pharm 2007;1:13–17.
3. GlaxoSmithKline. Tykerb. http://us.gsk.com/products/assets/us_tykerb.pdf.
4. Midgley R, Flaherty KT, Haller DG, Versola MJ, Smith DA, Koch KM, Pandite L, Kerr DJ, O'Dwyer PJ, Middleton MR. Phase I study of lapatinib, a dual kinase inhibitor, in combination with irinotecan 5-fluorouracil and leucovorin. ASCO Annual Meeting Proceedings. J Clin Oncol 2005;23 (June 1 Suppl):3086.

Nilotinib

General Information

Nilotinib (AMN 107) is a second-generation tyrosine kinase inhibitors with structural similarity to imatinib. It does not affect src kinase at therapeutic doses. Nilotinib is 20–50 times more potent than imatinib, which may encourage its use in patients who are refractory to imatinib. Nilotinib is generally well tolerated, as has been shown in recent phase II studies (1,2). The most frequent grade 3/4 laboratory abnormalities in 316 patients included thrombocytopenia (29%), neutropenia (28%), and asymptomatic increases in lipase activity (15%). Pleural and pericardial effusions and pulmonary edema were rare (under 1%). Growth factors or platelet transfusions were required very rarely.

References

1. Kantarjian H, Giles F, Wunderle L, Bhalla K, O'Brien S, Wassmann B, Tanaka C, Manley P, Rae P, Mietlowski W, Bochinski K, Hochhaus A, Griffin JD, Hoelzer D, Albitar M, Dugan M, Cortes J, Alland L, Ottmann OG. Nilotinib in imatinib-resistant CML and Philadelphia chromosome-positive ALL. N Engl J Med 2006;354:2542-51.
2. Rosti G, le Coutre P, Bhalla K, Giles F, Ossenkoppele G, Hochhaus A, Gattermann N, Haque A, Weitzman A, Baccarani M, Kantarjian H. A phase II study of nilotinib administered to imatinib resistant and intolerant patients with chronic myelogenous leukemia (CML) in chronic phase (CP). ASCO Annual Meeting Proceedings. J Clin Oncol 2007;25 (June 20 Suppl):7007.

Pazopanib

General Information

Pazopanib is a potent, selective, broad-spectrum, multi-targeted inhibitor of receptor tyrosine kinases, including VEGFR-1, VEGFR-2, VEGFR-3, PDGFR-α/β, and c-kit. It is still under clinical investigation. Total disease control in patients with advanced renal cell carcinoma was 82%. The most common adverse events included rises in transaminases, diarrhea, fatigue, nausea, hair depigmentation, and hypertension. According to a recent interim analysis, adverse effects led to drug withdrawal in 5% of patients. Preliminary data suggest additional activity of the drug in ovarian cancer, with a comparable spectrum of adverse effects (1,2).

References

1. Friedlander M, Hancock KC, Benigno B, Rischin D, Messing M, Stringer CA, Tay EH, Kathman S, Matthys G, Lager JJ. Pazopanib (GW786034) is active in women with advanced epithelial ovarian fallopian tube and peritoneal cancers: initial results of a phase II study. ASCO Annual Meeting Proceedings. J Clin Oncol 2007;25 (June 20 Suppl):5561.
2. Hutson TE, Davis ID, Machiels JP, de Souza PL, Hong BF, Rottey S, Baker KL, Crofts T, Pandite L, Figlin R. Pazopanib (GW786034) is active in metastatic renal cell carcinoma (RCC): interim results of a phase II randomized discontinuation trial (RDT). ASCO Annual Meeting Proceedings. J Clin Oncol 2007;25 (June 20 Suppl):5031.

Sorafenib

General Information

Sorafenib (BAY 43-9006) is a multi-targeted inhibitor of tyrosine kinase that inhibits c-RAF and b-RAF kinases as well as VEGFR-2, VEGFR-3, FLT-3, c-kit, and the PDGFR tyrosine kinase in vitro (1). Sorafenib is effective in pretreated renal cell carcinoma and advanced Child A hepatocellular carcinoma.

The incidence of treatment-related grade 3/4 adverse events in phase I studies with sorafenib (n = 179) included hand–foot skin reactions (8%), hypertension (4%), diarrhea (2%), reduced hemoglobin concentration (3%), and fatigue (5%). There is some evidence that grade 2–3 hand–foot syndrome and/or diarrhea correlates with the increase of time to progression compared with patients without such signs of toxicity (2).

Pharmacokinetics

The recommended oral dose, 400 mg bd, should not be taken with a fat-rich meal, because of reduced absorption by about 38–49% compared to intake on an empty stomach. Sorafenib is metabolized to some extent by CYP3A4, resulting in a pyridine-N-oxide derivative with similar antineoplastic activity to the parent compound. Elimination is primarily via the feces, about 51% of the dose being excreted as unchanged drug (1,3).

Organs and Systems

Cardiovascular

Grade 3 hypertension is very common in patients taking sorafenib. The median time of onset in patients taking the anti-VEGF antibody bevacizumab was 131 (range 7–316) days. Twelve of 20 patients who took with sorafenib had a rise in systolic blood pressure of at least 20 mmHg compared with baseline, with a median change of 21 mmHg after 3 weeks (4). There as a significant inverse relation between increased systolic blood pressure and a reduction in catecholamines, suggesting a secondary response to the increase in blood pressure.

Tyrosine kinase inhibitors of the VEGF and PDGF receptor pathways may target the VHL hypoxia-inducible gene pathway, which results in inhibition of hypoxia-inducible factor (HIF)-induced gene products. The latter mediate physiological responses of the myocardium to ischemia, including myocardial remodelling, peri-infarct vascularization, and vascular permeability.

Tyrosine kinase inhibitor-induced inhibition of HIF may be associated with more severe myocardial damage than previously expected. Of 73 patients with advanced renal cell carcinoma and normal creatine kinase MB fraction and cardiac troponin T at baseline, 23% had a significant increase in creatine kinase and troponin T after 2–32 weeks, with symptoms in seven (5). One patient had an acute coronary artery occlusion and myocardial infarction. Electrocardiographic changes and biochemical

markers are important indicators, and both should be measured regularly irrespective of whether sunitinib or sorafenib is used.

Endocrine

Patients with metastatic renal cell carcinoma commonly develop mild biochemical thyroid function test abnormalities while taking sorafenib. However, compared with sunitinib, which is associated with a high incidence of thyroid dysfunction, making routine monitoring necessary, patients taking sorafenib need thyroid function monitoring only if clinically indicated (6).

Drug-Drug Interactions

Theoretically, important drug interactions can be expected during the co-administration of potent CYP3A4 inducing agents (for example rifamycins, St. John's wort, phenytoin, carbamazepine) and CYP3A4 inhibitors (for example triazole antifungal drugs). However, the co-administration of ketoconazole 400 mg/day with sorafenib 50 mg/day did not result in changes in sorafenib pharmacokinetics, perhaps because sorafenib is a low-clearance drug (7). It is also possible that reduced N-oxide formation may be compensated by a small increase in UGT1A9-mediated glucuronidation. Therefore, no dose adjustment appears to be warranted during co-administration of sorafenib with ketoconazole and probably structurally related triazole antifungal drugs.

In vitro, sorafenib inhibits some other CYP isozymes, such as CYP2C9, CYP2B6, CYPC8, and some UGT isozymes, such as UGT1A1 and UGT1A9 (3). Co-administration of sorafenib with CPT-11, paclitaxel, or propofol is therefore not recommended until further data are available.

References

1. Larkin J, Eisen T. Kinase inhibitors in the treatment of renal cell carcinoma. Crit Rev Oncol Hematol 2006;60:216-26.
2. Strumberg D, Awada A, Hirte H, Clark JW, Seeber S, Piccart P, Hofstra E, Voliotis D, Christensen O, Brueckner A, Schwartz B. Pooled safety analysis of BAY 43-9006 (sorafenib) monotherapy in patients with advanced solid tumours: is rash associated with treatment outcome? Eur J Cancer 2006;42:548-56.
3. Hahn O, Stadler W. Sorafenib. Curr Opin Oncol 2006;18:615-21.
4. Veronese ML, Mosenkis A, Flaherty KT, Gallagher M, Stevenson JP, Townsend RR, O'Dwyer PJ. Mechanisms of hypertension associated with BAY 43-9006. J Clin Oncol 2006;24:1363-9.
5. Schmidinger M, Vogl UM, Schukro C, Bojic A, Bojic M, Schmidinger H, Zielinski CC. Cardiac involvement in patients with sorafenib or sunitinib treatment for metastatic renal cell carcinoma. ASCO Annual Meeting Proceedings. J Clin Oncol 2007;25 (June 20 Suppl):5110.
6. Tamaskar IR, Unnithan J, Garcia JA, Dreicer R, Wood L, Iochimescu A, Bukowski R, Rini B. Thyroid function test (TFT) abnormalities in patients (pts) with metastatic renal cell carcinoma (RCC) treated with sorafenib. ASCO Annual Meeting Proceedings. J Clin Oncol 2007;25 (June 20 Suppl):5048.

7. Lathia C, Lettieri J, Cihon F, Gallentine M, Radtke M, Sundaresan P. Lack of effect of ketoconazole-mediated CYP3A inhibition on sorafenib clinical pharmacokinetics. Cancer Chemother Pharmacol 2006;57:685-92.

Sunitinib

General Information

Sunitinib (SU 11248) is a multi-targeted tyrosine kinase inhibitor which is highly active in patients with advanced renal cell carcinoma and gastrointestinal stromal tumors (GIST) (1). The recommended dose is 50 mg/day, in a schedule of 4 weeks on treatment followed by 2 weeks off (2,3,4,5). An alternative is continuous dosing with 37.5 mg/day.

The most commonly reported grade 3 adverse effects related to sunitinib include fatigue, stomatitis, hypertension, dermatitis, depigmentation of the hair and skin (probably due to the yellow color of the drug itself), subungual splinter hemorrhages, bleeding events (for example epistaxis), and gastrointestinal discomfort, (for example nausea and diarrhea). Grade 3/4 laboratory abnormalities include neutropenia, thrombocytopenia, anaemia, and raised plasma lipase activity. Dosage modifications (for example from 50 to 37.5 or 25 mg/day) were primarily based on severe forms of fatigue or increased amylase and lipase activities (1).

Pharmacokinetics

Oral sunitinib is well absorbed from the gastrointestinal tract. Drug exposure is slightly increased after food, but administration is generally feasible with or without food (6).

Sunitinib is mainly metabolized by CYP3A4, producing a major metabolite with comparable antineoplastic activity and comprising 23–37% of total exposure. The active metabolite and other CYP3A4-mediated biotransformation products are mostly excreted via the feces; the renal route accounts for less than 20% of the dose. The half-lives of sunitinib and its major metabolite are 40–60 hours and 80–110 hours respectively. Accumulation of the parent compound and its active metabolite occurred during repeated daily administration up to 3- to 4-fold and 7- to 10-fold respectively. Steady-state concentrations are commonly achieved after 10–14 days (5,6).

The AUC of sunitinib and total drug exposure correlated significantly with the probability of a partial response in cytokine-refractory patients with renal cell carcinoma and with the time to progression and overall survival, according to pharmacokinetic and efficacy data from three studies. These data suggest that there is an association between increased exposure to the active drug in the plasma and the probability of clinical benefit.

Organs and Systems

Endocrine

Sunitinib has been related to an increasing frequency of hypothyroidism. Screening for signs of hypothyroidism is recommended, with frequent measurements of TSH concentrations every 2–3 months in order to start levothyroxine in time.

In a prospective, observational cohort study in a tertiary-care hospital, there were abnormal serum TSH concentrations in 26 of 42 patients) who took sunitinib for renal cell carcinoma or GIST. Persistent primary hypothyroidism, isolated TSH suppression, and transient mild rises in TSH were found in 36%, 10%, and 17% of patients respectively. There appears to be a correlation between the duration of use of sunitinib and suppressed TSH concentrations as well as a risk of hypothyroidism. Whether sunitinib induces destructive thyroiditis through follicular cell apoptosis has not been fully elucidated (7,8,9).

Drug-Drug Interactions

Sunitinib and its major metabolite do not appear to cause clinically important drug–drug interactions. However, the concomitant use of potent inducers of CYP3A4 (for example rifampicin) or inhibitors of CYP3A4 (e.g. ketoconazole) may warrant an increase in dosage to a maximum of 87.5 mg/day or a dosage reduction to a minimum of 37.5 mg/day. The concomitant use of St. John's wort is generally not recommended because of unpredictable drug concentrations (1).

References

1. Larkin J, Eisen T. Kinase inhibitors in the treatment of renal cell carcinoma. Crit Rev Oncol Hematol 2006;60:216-26.
2. Motzer RJ, Hoosen S, Bello CL, Christensen JG. Sunitinib maleate for the treatment of solid tumours: a review of current clinical data. Expert Opin Investig Drugs 2006;15:553-61.
3. Motzer RJ, Hutson TE, Tomczak P, Michaelson MD, Bukowski RM, Rixe O, Oudard S, Negrier S, Szczylik C, Kim ST, Chen I, Bycott PW, Baum CM, Figlin RA. Sunitinib versus interferon alfa in metastatic renal-cell carcinoma. N Engl J Med 2007;356:115-24.
4. Motzer RJ, Michaelson MD, Redman BG, Hudes GR, Wilding G, Figlin RA, Ginsberg MS, Kim ST, Baum CM, DePrimo SE, Li JZ, Bello CL, Theuer CP, George DJ, Rini BI. Activity of SU11248, a multitargeted inhibitor of vascular endothelial growth factor receptor and platelet-derived growth factor receptor, in patients with metastatic renal cell carcinoma. J Clin Oncol 2006;24:16-24.
5. Motzer RJ, Rini BI, Bukowski RM, Curti BD, George DJ, Hudes GR, Redman BG, Margolin KA, Merchan JR, Wilding G, Ginsberg MS, Bacik J, Kim ST, Baum CM, Michaelson MD. Sunitinib in patients with metastatic renal cell carcinoma. JAMA 2006;295:2516-24.
6. Bello CL, Sherman L, Zhou J, Verkh L, Smeraglia J, Mount J, Klamerus KJ. Effect of food on the pharmacokinetics of

sunitinib malate (SU11248), a multi-targeted receptor tyrosine kinase inhibitor: results from a phase I study in healthy subjects. Anticancer Drugs 2006;17:353-8.

7. Desai J, Yassa L, Marqusee E, George S, Frates MC, Chen MH, Morgan JA, Dychter SS, Larsen PR, Demetri GD, Alexander EK. Hypothyroidism after sunitinib treatment for patients with gastrointestinal stromal tumors. Ann Intern Med 2006;145:660-4.

8. de Groot JW, Links TP, van der Graaf WT. Tyrosine kinase inhibitors causing hypothyroidism in a patient on levothyroxine. Ann Oncol 2006;17:1719-20.

9. Rini BI, Tamaskar I, Shaheen P, Salas R, Garcia J, Wood L, Reddy S, Dreicer R, Bukowski RM. Hypothyroidism in patients with metastatic renal cell carcinoma treated with sunitinib. J Natl Cancer Inst 2007;99:81-3.

VINCA ALKALOIDS

General Information

From among nearly 30 different alkaloids that have been isolated from the periwinkle *Catharanthus roseus* (Apocynaceae), vincristine and vinblastine have been assessed to have the highest antitumor activity. Both have a large dimeric asymmetric structure composed of a dihydroindole nucleus (vindoline ring) and an indole nucleus, linked by a carbon–carbon bond. In contrast, the derivatives vindesine (deacetyl vinblastine amide sulfate (DVAS)) and vinorelbine are semisynthetic (1–3). Finally, vinflunine, the latest semisynthetic vinca alkaloid, is a fluorinated derivative that is still under clinical investigation and has a different inhibitory action than other vinca alkaloids. Preliminary results suggest that this congener may be less toxic on the peripheral and autonomic nervous systems (4).

Vincristine

Vincristine is part of many chemotherapeutic regimens, based on its lack of myelosuppressive toxicity. It is used, for example, in the treatment of acute lymphocytic leukemia (ALL), acute myeloid leukemia (AML), lymphomas, neuroblastoma, brain tumors, and Wilms' tumor. The generally recommended dose in adults is 1.4 mg/m^2/week intravenously (5). Some clinicians have recommended an absolute upper limit of 2 mg, but this limitation is still a matter of debate (6). The usual pediatric dosage is $1.5–2$ mg/m^2, but for children weighing 10 kg or less or who have a body surface area less than 1 m^2, the manufacturers recommend that treatment should be begun at 0.05 mg/kg once a week (5).

Vinblastine

Vinblastine is used in combination with other cytotoxic agents for the treatment of disseminated Hodgkin's disease stages III and IV, non-Hodgkin's lymphoma, histiocytic lymphoma, and advanced carcinoma of the testis. It has also been used for the treatment of bladder cancer, melanoma, and renal cell cancer. The usual adult dosage is $3–6$ mg/m^2 intravenously for the treatment of testicular germ cell tumors and Hodgkin's disease (1,2).

Vindesine

Vindesine (DVAS) was the first semi-synthetic vinca alkaloid derivative introduced into clinical oncology. It differs solely from vinblastine in the nature of the substituted functional group attached to the vindoline ring. Vindesine has been most extensively studied in the treatment of non-small cell lung cancers. A randomized study has shown that vindesine (3 mg/m^2 intravenously) was substantially better than vincristine (1.4 mg/m^2 intravenously) both given weekly for 4 weeks, then every 2 weeks for 1 month, then monthly. However, another study showed that vindesine may be inferior to the structurally related vinorelbine in the treatment of advanced non-small cell lung cancers with overall response rates of 9 and 29%, respectively. Vindesine has also been used in patients with advanced malignant melanomas. Potential indications that have been studied with vindesine include head and neck cancer, ALL, lymphomas, and breast cancer. However, its precise role and clinically relevant advantages to other available vinca alkaloids needs further investigation (7–10).

Vinorelbine

Vinorelbine has become a pivotal agent for treating adjuvant non-small cell lung cancer (stages IB-III) and the palliative treatment of non-small cell lung cancer (stages IIIB and IV), often in combination with drugs like cisplatin. In addition, vinorelbine plays an important part in the treatment of advanced and metastatic breast cancer. Its role in the treatment of advanced cervical cancer is still under investigation. The usual intravenous dosage is $20–30$ mg/m^2 (vinorelbine base) given once a week. In contrast to the other congeners, vinorelbine can also be taken orally based on its absolute systemic availability of about 44% after administration as a capsule. Oral dosages of 60 and 80 mg/m^2 have been said to be pharmacokinetically and clinically equivalent to intravenous dosages of 25 and 30 mg/m^2 respectively (2,11).

Mechanism of action

All four vinca alkaloids block mitosis with metaphase arrest. Their antitumor activity is based on their high binding affinity to intracellular tubulin, which is the protein subunit of the spindle microtubules. The binding constants of vincristine, vinblastine, and vindesine for tubulin are 8, 6, and 3.3 nmol/l respectively (9,10). The formation of complexes between the vinca alkaloids and tubulin prevents the polymerization of the tubulin subunits to microtubules, which results in depolymerization of microtubules and inhibition of microtubule assembly. Based on the fact that microtubule assemblies also play a pivotal role in the movement of neurotransmitter substances along neuronal axons, vinca alkaloids can cause neurotoxicity, particularly at higher concentrations (9,10).

Pharmacokinetics

After intravenous administration, plasma concentrations of vinca alkaloids fall triphasically, with an initial rapid phase. All four congeners are extensively distributed into peripheral compartments, but passage across the blood–brain barrier is limited (11,12). In addition to tissue binding, vinca alkaloids bind to blood constituents like human platelets and lymphocytes. Binding to plasma proteins has been estimated to be from about 80% to more than 90%, with an unbound fraction of about 0.10–0.20. Binding to whole blood is usually higher than in serum, which reflects substantial binding to platelets (11,12).

All four congeners are extensively metabolized in the liver and excreted in the bile (13). Their metabolic biotransformation is primarily mediated by CYP3A. Deacetylvinorelbine, the primary metabolite of vinorelbine, has remarkable antitumor activity; however, the amounts detected in blood after conventional doses of vinorelbine are very low, which suggests that this metabolite does not contribute significantly to the overall antitumor activity of vinorelbine (14,15). Based on the pivotal role of CYP3A isozymes during the catabolism of vinca alkaloids, care is warranted when using concomitant drugs that inhibit these isozymes (16,17).

The half-lives of vinblastine, vindesine, and vinorelbine are all about 24 hours; vincristine has a much longer half-life of about 3.5 days (5). Because biliary and fecal drug excretion is of major quantitative importance during the elimination of vinca alkaloids, patients with impaired hepatic clearance and increased bilirubin concentrations may need dosage modification in order to avoid critical drug accumulation. CYP3A4 activity measurement (for example by the monoethylglycinexylidide test) might be the most appropriate method to estimate individual capacity to metabolize drugs like vinorelbine; however, such methods have not yet been routinely established in most cancer centers. Empirically, it is prudent to reduce doses by about 50% in patients with liver volume replacement by tumor that exceeds 75% (18).

Vinorelbine is the only vinca congener that can also be used orally. Its oral availability averages 43% and is not affected by food (19). The interpatient variability in blood concentrations is in the same range as after intravenous administration (15).

General adverse effects

The most important adverse effects of vinca alkaloids include nervous system disorders, hematological effects, and gastrointestinal discomfort. Respiratory and cardiovascular adverse effects have to be particularly considered during combination chemotherapy. All the vinca alkaloids are tissue irritants, and extravasation without any adequate supportive management can result in severe local ulceration (1,2,5,8,20).

Vinca alkaloids are primarily metabolized by CYP3A4, inducers, inhibitors of which can significantly change their pharmacokinetics (16,17,21).

Organs and Systems

Cardiovascular

Vinca alkaloid-associated myocardial infarction, angina pectoris, and transient electrocardiographic changes related to coronary ischemia are limited to case reports (22–24). In addition, patients with these adverse effects received combination cancer chemotherapy, containing drugs such as bleomycin and cisplatin, which both have been suggested to cause cardiovascular adverse effects.

- A 64-year-old Japanese man developed chest pain with concomitant lateral ST segment depression after treatment with intravenous cisplatin 70 mg/m^2, vincristine 1.2 mg/m^2, and bleomycin 12 U/m^2. There was no history of predisposing factors and the symptoms disappeared quickly with glyceryl trinitrate. During the following cycle, containing cisplatin and verapamil as an antianginal agent, chest pain did not reoccur (23).
- A 46-year-old man developed a Q-wave inferior and a right ventricular myocardial infarct with postinfarction angina after the third cycle of vincristine + doxorubicin for multiple myeloma. The patient had no risk factors for ischemic heart disease, except for a positive smoking history, nor for hyperviscosity (24).

There is some evidence that both vincristine and doxorubicin are more often associated with ischemic heart disease than other cancer chemotherapeutic agents. Whether drug-induced platelet activation, altered clotting, or endovascular damage are responsible for vascular toxicity is still unclear. The risk of ischemic heart disease must therefore be kept in mind when patients receive a combination of doxorubicin and vincristine, especially when potential risk factors have been identified. Whether the structural similarity between vinca alkaloids and ergot alkaloids, which are vasospastic, is relevant is highly speculative.

After administration of vinorelbine, chest pain occurs in up to 5% of patients. However, subsequent analysis showed that most patients had underlying cardiovascular disease or a tumor in the chest, making interpretation difficult (2,20). Three patients developed acute cardiopulmonary toxicity after vinorelbine therapy (25). The symptoms mimicked acute cardiac ischemia, but with no electrocardiographic changes or raised cardiac enzymes. In two patients, tachypnea, râles, wheezing, and severe dyspnea responded to inhaled salbutamol. One patient developed pulmonary edema and bilateral pleural effusions, which contained no malignant cells when drained.

Venous discomfort and venous chemical phlebitis have been reported with vinorelbine 30 mg/m^2, with an incidence of up to 31% (26,27). The risk is increased in obesity (27). Pain along the vein occurred in five of 43 patients receiving vinorelbine 30 mg/m^2/week; none developed extravasation, but their symptoms were very similar (28). A similar rate of toxicity, 4.5%, has been reported in a review of the use of vinorelbine in 321 patient2s with breast cancer (29).

Respiratory

Acute shortness of breath and bronchospasm have been reported after the administration of vinca alkaloids, for example vinblastine and vindesine (30–34). The respiratory effects, including abrupt onset of progressive dyspnea, non-productive cough, pleuritic chest pain, profound wheezing, and diffuse basal crackles, were more common when mitomycin was used concomitantly. The onset of symptoms can be rapid (for example a few minutes to 1–5 hours after administration) or subacute (for example up to 2 weeks). If patients have pre-existing pulmonary dysfunction, intensified treatment, including glucocorticoids, may be indicated. Most case reports with vinca alkaloid-associated pulmonary toxicity included vinblastine, usually in combination with other known pneumotoxic agents, or thoracic irradiation. Patients receiving combination chemotherapy including vinca alkaloids should be monitored carefully for pulmonary symptoms. The underlying mechanism of vinca alkaloid pulmonary toxicity is unclear, but may involve a hypersensitivity reaction.

Nervous system

The most commonly reported dose-limiting toxic effect of vinca alkaloids is a mixed sensorimotor polyneuropathy (35). Vincristine has been associated with highest incidence, followed by vindesine and vinblastine; vinorelbine causes less neurotoxicity than the other congeners (2,5,8,36). The neurotoxic effects of vinca alkaloids are reversible (5).

The vinca alkaloids may have synergistic effects on the nervous system. Amongst 17 patients with metastatic breast cancer given the four-drug combination, vincristine + vinblastine + doxorubicin + cyclophosphamide, there was a high incidence of acute neurotoxicity at half the usual therapeutic dose of vincristine and vinblastine (37).

Nerve palsies

Cranial nerve palsies can occur with the vinca alkaloids (38–42).

There have been several reports of isolated vincristine-induced recurrent laryngeal nerve paralysis (38,43–47).

Peripheral neuropathy

The features of vinca alkaloid-induced polyneuropathy include early loss of tendon reflexes at the ankles and distal paresthesia, followed by loss of touch, pain, and vibration sensations. Other symptoms include headache, malaise, weakness, dizziness, severe face and jaw pain, and vocal cord paralysis. The first symptoms usually occur a few days after drug administration (36). Gastrointestinal discomfort, particularly constipation, abdominal pain, and adynamic ileus, can occur through an autonomic neuropathy (5,48).

Higher drug concentrations during monotherapy (possibly related to impaired drug excretion in patients with hepatic dysfunction) or prolonged periods of treatment are important predisposing factors for more severe forms of neurotoxicity. The same is true of concomitant use of potent CYP3A inhibitors, such as erythromycin, itraconazole, or quinupristin/dalfopristin, which can increase plasma vinca alkaloid drug concentrations (5).

Of 22 patients given vindesine 2 mg/m^2 on 2 consecutive days weekly, four developed a peripheral neuropathy with paresthesia, and five developed muscle weakness with loss of deep tendon reflexes (49). Neuropathies were pronounced at sites of pre-existing nerve damage. If a tumor had previously damaged peripheral nerves, or if a chordotomy had been performed, the paresthesia that developed

at that site was often painful. Neurotoxicity was reversible, and the longest interval to full recovery was 3 months.

In 40 patients, orofacial pain developed as a manifestation of neuropathy about 3 days after vincristine administration, lasting for a mean duration of 2 days. Half of the patients were affected in the first week, and pain was commonest in young patients and in smokers (50).

With vinorelbine, incidence rates of 1.3% for peripheral neuropathies (mainly loss of deep tendon reflexes) and 4.1% for autonomic neuropathies (manifested by constipation) have been reported from a European overview of 321 patients (29).

The pathogenesis of vincristine-induced neuropathy has not been fully elucidated, but very probably altered axoplasmic transport processes are of major importance, since neurons treated with vincristine lose portions of their axonal microtubules (35). There is marked interindividual variability in sensitivity to this toxic effect, partially based on different predisposing factors, for example diabetes mellitus, pretreatment with other potentially neurotoxic agents (such as cisplatin and taxanes), or familial disorders (such as Charcot–Marie–Tooth syndrome) 37,51,52.

Several drugs have been proposed to be neuroprotective, including folinic acid, vitamin B_1, vitamin B_6, glutamic acid, Org 2766, insulin-like growth factor (IGF-1), and nerve growth factor. However, most drugs have been studied in experimental systems and there are only a few case reports suggesting clinical benefit. In contrast, folinic acid, vitamins B_1, B_{16}, and B_{12}, which were promising in experimental systems, failed to provide protection from vincristine-induced neuropathy in clinical studies. In the case of L-glutamic acid, which can be given orally, there was some neuroprotective activity; however, more information is needed to exclude any impairment of vincristine-induced antineoplastic activity, when both agents are used together on the same day (5).

The ACTH analogue Org 2766 was studied in a randomized, double-blind, placebo-controlled trial as a neuroprotective agent in patients receiving vincristine (53). In spite of positive results, the study design was later criticized because of a significantly higher number of younger patients in the Org 2766 group. In addition, there are contradictory results on the potential effect of Org 2766 on the overall antineoplastic activity of vincristine.

In a prospective, double-blind, placebo-controlled study, concurrent oral administration of 500 mg glutamic acid tds with vincristine reduced the incidence of subjective and objective signs of vincristine neurotoxicity (54). There were no differences in constipation, weakness, or loss of knee reflexes. There were no severe gastrointestinal adverse effects.

During recent years, more attention has been paid to nerve growth factor as a neuroprotective agent, since it may induce microtubule assembly, especially during neurite outgrowth. For instance, patients with a sensory neuropathy related to the use of cancer chemotherapy including paclitaxel, vincristine, or cisplatin had a significant reduction in plasma nerve growth factor concentrations (5). Acetyl-L-carnitine has been considered for neuroprotection because it increases nerve growth factor expression. However, as in the case of L-glutamine or Org 2766, more information is needed to evaluate any potential effect on vincristine antitumor efficacy.

Pre-existing neurological disease can predispose to severe vincristine neuropathy (55). For example, Charcot–Marie–Tooth disease is regarded as a contraindication to the use of vincristine (56). There have been four cases of vincristine-induced neuropathy in Charcot–Marie–Tooth disease; one was fatal, and in the other three there was severe quadriplegia, which resolved. A predisposition to vincristine neuropathy has been described in a patient with pre-existing Friedreich's ataxia (56). When vincristine 0.625 mg/m²/week was given to 264 patients for a maximum of 10 weeks, the incidence of grade 3/4 neuropathy rate was 7%, suggesting that dose intensity rather than total dose may be important for determining the severity of this toxic effect. The rate of grade 1–4 neuropathy was 56% (57).

Finally, the aminothiol amifostine has been proposed to be effective in preventing vincristine-induced neurotoxicity; however, clinical data are still lacking to assess its role as a neuroprotective agent in terms of vinca alkaloids (5).

Myeloencephalopathy

Central nervous system toxicity is unusual with vinca alkaloids, because they do not readily cross the blood–brain barrier. However, fatal myeloencephalopathy can occur a few hours after accidental intrathecal drug administration (58,59), with severe bilateral leg pain, and over the next 36 hours progressive leg weakness, urinary retention, meningism, fever, and somnolence. Other effects include absence of deep tendon and gag reflexes and disappearance of rectal tone. In spite of high-dose folinic acid rescue, patients became comatose, for example by the fourth day after injection, with loss of brain stem function a few days later.

Seizures

Seizures associated with intravenous use of vinca alkaloids are very rare (60–62). Some cases may have been due to SIADH-associated hyponatremia. Other forms include tumor-related effects, nervous system infections, or cerebral hemorrhage, which often make direct causal relations between drug exposure and nervous system adverse effects very difficult.

- An 8-year-old girl with leukemia had tonic-clonic convulsions and life-threatening encephalopathy after intravenous vincristine. After the second dose (1.5 mg/m² in combination with prednisone) she developed seizures and bilateral translucencies in the CT scan. When vincristine was withdrawn in subsequent cycles, the symptoms disappeared (61).

Four of 350 patients without a history of seizures developed generalized seizures 5–6 days after the first, second, and eleventh doses of intravenous vincristine. However, seizures did not recur in later cycles. It is difficult to implicate vincristine as a cause of these adverse effects (62). Tonic-clonic seizures were only reported in four patients 7 days after vindesine administration. All

patients had pre-existing cerebral deposits of melanoma, possibly mimicking nervous system adverse effects (8).

Sensory systems

Eyes

Reversible visual damage has been attributed to vincristine.

- An 18-year-old man with lymphocytic leukemia became completely blind for 6 months after a fifth 10-day cycle of therapy with vincristine 2 mg intravenously followed by cyclophosphamide 600 mg orally for 5 days with prednisolone 100 mg orally for 5 days (63).
- A 15-year-old girl developed bilateral optic atrophy after treatment with weekly vincristine, posterior craniectomy, and whole neuraxis radiation therapy (64). Withdrawal resulted in recovery of visual function.

In 50 patients, ptosis and diplopia related to vincristine occurred in 16 (64). The exact pathomechanism of this adverse effect has not been elucidated.

Studies on monkeys have demonstrated visual loss and optic atrophy with intravitreous injection of vincristine. Clinical reports of postvincristine optic atrophy are rare. Most are irreversible, progressing to permanent blindness. There is commonly coexistent peripheral or cranial neuropathy (65). It is possible that certain patients are predisposed to vincristine-induced optic atrophy. Optic neuropathy after a single small dose of vincristine has been reported in a single case; the dose of vincristine was small (1275 mg), and the latent period before onset of visual loss was brief (6–8 weeks) (66). Previously reported cases have had multiple injections of vincristine and the latent period was longer than 3 months.

Ears

Vinca alkaloids can have ototoxic effects, such as tinnitus and transient hearing loss. In addition, vestibular disorders can cause dizziness, nystagmus, and vertigo (67,68).

- A 29-year-old man with recurrent Hodgkin's disease was treated with the ABVD regimen (doxorubicin, bleomycin, vinblastine, and dacarbazine) (69). He complained of tinnitus after each treatment cycle, with an onset of about 6 hours and a duration of 7–10 days. These symptoms interfered with reading, watching television, and general concentration. Based on audiography before and several hours after several cycles, there was evidence of mild sensorineural hearing loss in the high-decibel range 48 and 72 hours after drug administration. Six months after the completion of cancer chemotherapy, there was still some mild high-frequency sensorineural hearing loss in the left ear.

The authors concluded that vinblastine may have been responsible, because the other agents have not yet been associated with ototoxicity and because vincristine can cause ototoxicity too. The mechanism of this adverse effect is unclear but it may involve vinca alkaloid-associated damage to the eighth cranial nerve. This means that care should be taken when vinca alkaloids are used together with platinum compounds, especially cisplatin.

Endocrine

A rare but well-known adverse effect of vinca alkaloids, including vinorelbine, is the syndrome of inappropriate secretion of antidiuretic hormone (SIADH) (70–72). The diagnosis is usually based on clinical and laboratory findings. There are falls in plasma sodium (below 120 mmol/l), chloride (below 90 mmol/l), and osmolality (below 230 mosm/kg). Further features include lethargy, anorexia, nausea, listlessness, and rarely coma, particularly when serum sodium falls below 110 mmol/l. Treatment is based on withdrawal of the causative agent and the administration of 0.9% saline and potassium (for example 40 mmol/l) at an infusion rate of 200 ml/hour. Further treatment strategies include demeclocycline (for example 300 mg bd), which can be continued for the duration of further vinca alkaloid-containing cycles. In one case demeclocycline prevented SIADH during further courses of vinorelbine (72).

Asian patients have been proposed to be at higher risk of SIADH during treatment with vincristine. Between 1983 and 1999, 76 cases of hyponatremia and/or SIADH related to the use of vincristine were reported to the global adverse event database of Eli Lilly and Company. The average age of the patients was 36 years (range 2 weeks to 86 years) and 62% were male. Most of the patients had received vincristine for leukemia or lymphomas. Of the 76 reports, 39 included background information on race: 35 patients were Asian, three were Caucasian, and one was black. The authors concluded that there may be a correlation between race and vinca alkaloid-associated SIADH/hyponatremia; however, the reasons are still unclear (73).

Hematologic

The most frequent adverse effect of vinblastine, vindesine, and vinorelbine is hematological toxicity (1,2,5,7,8). Leukopenia, particularly neutropenia, occurs more often than thrombocytopenia or anemia. The nadir in the leukocyte count after vinblastine occurs 4–10 days after administration, with recovery within another 7–14 days. Blood counts should generally be measured weekly and before the administration of each dose, in order to avoid severe forms of myelosuppression, neutropenic fever, or infections (20).

Oral vinorelbine is also associated with neutropenia. In one small study in patients with breast cancer treated with 50–160 mg/week, the incidence of grade 3–4 neutropenia was 32% (14). The incidence of severe neutropenia is higher with vinorelbine than the other vinca alkaloids. However, mean recovery (about 9- days) appears to be somewhat shorter with vinorelbine than with compounds vinblastine and vindesine (average 14–21 days) (1,2).

Gastrointestinal

Constipation is common when vinca alkaloids cause an autonomic neuropathy. Laxatives such as lactulose or polyethylene glycol-containing solutions can prevent adynamic subileus during treatment courses containing vinca alkaloids (48,74).

In contrast to constipation, nausea and vomiting are neither frequent nor dose-limiting adverse effects of vinca alkaloids. The regular use of antiemetics, such as 5-HT$_3$ receptor antagonists in combination with dexamethasone, is not recommended. However, oral vinorelbine has been associated with more severe forms of nausea and vomiting, with a frequency that is higher than after intravenous administration; in these patients and in particular those with predisposing factors for nausea and vomiting, metoclopramide and 5-HT$_3$ receptor antagonists are justified (75).

Skin

Vinca alkaloids are potential vesicants (76–78) and accidental drug extravasation can cause severe soft tissue ulceration. The initial symptoms include marked pain, erythema, and local swelling for several hours up to a day; later effects include blisters and severe painful skin ulcers, several days and 3 weeks after extravasation respectively. The lesions usually heal very slowly and sometimes require surgical intervention. Because vinca alkaloid extravasation can have severe effects, the use of antidotes is highly recommended when extravasation is suspected. In addition, venous irritation can be worsened if the vinca alkaloid is infused over at least 20–30 minutes rather than 6–10 minutes.

Among several antidotes for the treatment of vinca alkaloid extravasation, hyaluronidase is the most effective (79). Seven patients with extravasation of vincristine, vinblastine, or vinorelbine received hyaluronidase 250 units diluted in 6 ml of 0.9% saline, through the indwelling needle or, when the needle had been already removed, as six subcutaneous injections around the extravasation site. None developed skin necrosis. Local mild skin warming in order to produce local vasodilatation may have an additional beneficial effect, but should be avoided when simultaneous extravasation of a vinca alkaloid and an anthracycline is suspected, because local warming can worsen the anthracycline-associated local reaction, whereas local cooling, which is generally beneficial in anthracycline-related extravasation alone, can worsen skin necrosis due to vinca alkaloids (76).

Hair

Vinca alkaloids are associated with a low incidence of alopecia. In about 10% of patients, there can be gradual thinning of hair, but very few patients develop total hair loss (1,5,7).

Reproductive system

Based on comparative studies of the relative gonadal toxicity of several antineoplastic agents in experimental models and humans, the vinca alkaloids vinblastine and vincristine have negligible potency for killing stem cells. Permanent recovery of sperm counts and preserved ovarian function, depending on the patient's age at the time of treatment and the total cumulative dose, can be expected after treatment with vinca alkaloids (80–82).

Body temperature

Nine of 31 Japanese children receiving maintenance vincristine chemotherapy for either leukemia or lymphoma developed a fever over 38°C (83). An allergic mechanism was proposed. Concurrent glucocorticoids as part of the regimen appeared to be protective. Younger children were at greater risk. Peak temperatures occurred within 24 hours of vincristine administration. The pyrexia lasted from 6 hours to 4 days and the condition was self-limiting.

Long-Term Effects

Drug tolerance

Resistance to vinca alkaloids can be mediated by glycoprotein B, a transmembrane pump that is part of the multidrug resistance (MDR) phenotype (5).

Mutagenicity

Vinca alkaloids are less mutagenic than other cytotoxic agents like the N-Lost derivatives or bleomycin. Positive or negative results in mutagenicity tests depend on the test system used. For instance, vinorelbine significantly increased the frequencies of micronuclei in binucleate lymphocytes (84). In Chinese hamster ovary cells vinorelbine arrested cells at the first metaphase and caused an increase in abnormal anaphases, containing chiefly lagging chromosomes and multipolar spindles (85). These results suggest that vinorelbine does not directly damage DNA, but acts on spindle microtubules, altering chromosome movement and causing aneuploidy. However, it has no mutagenic effects in the Ames test.

Tumorigenicity

In the International Agency for Research and Treatment of Cancer (IARC), the vinca alkaloids were classified in group 3, which means that they cannot yet be classified in group 1 (proven human carcinogens), 2A (probably carcinogenic), or 2B (possibly carcinogenic) (86,87).

Second-Generation Effects

Teratogenicity

There is evidence that vinca alkaloids are teratogenic. Vinblastine caused malformations after first trimester administration (88–90). However, since vinca alkaloids are often combined with other cytotoxic drugs, it is difficult to relate any teratogenic effect to the vinca alkaloid alone (88). In mice and rabbits, vinblastine was embryotoxic and fetotoxic (89). However, it is unclear whether vinca alkaloids can cross the placenta because of their high molecular weights (about 1000 g/mol).

- Two pregnant women with breast cancer received two or three courses of intravenous vinorelbine 20–30 mg/m^2 and fluorouracil 500–750 mg/m^2 at 24, 28, and 29 weeks

of gestation; there were no adverse effects in the two newborns (90). A third patient also had epirubicin and cyclophosphamide and her infant, who had been exposed to the four-drug regimen, developed transient anemia at 21 days of age which resolved spontaneously. All three infants were developing normally at 2–3 years of age.

According to the FDA classification, the potential therapeutic benefits of vinca alkaloids have to be outweighed with the potential teratogenic risks (FDA classification D). All women of childbearing potential should be advised to avoid becoming pregnant while receiving cytotoxic cancer chemotherapy (80).

Drug Administration

Drug administration route

In seven patients (median age 7 years), limb and jaw muscle pain, starting at days 3–5 of an intravenous infusion of vincristine and requiring opiate analgesia, was the most pronounced adverse effect (68).

Guidance on the safe administration of intrathecal chemotherapy has been issued in the UK (91), following a case in which vincristine was fatally injected into the cerebrospinal fluid (92).

Drug–Drug Interactions

Asparaginase

Asparaginase and vincristine should not be used together on the same day, since simultaneous administration can cause increased vincristine toxicity. It has been suggested that this is due to a deleterious effect of asparaginase on hepatic function, reducing the metabolism of vincristine (5).

Carbamazepine

In a small pharmacokinetic study the clearance of vincristine was 65% greater than in patients who were not taking carbamazepine and the half-life and AUC of vincristine were reduced by 35 and 43% respectively (93).

Erythromycin

Toward the end of a phase I study of vinblastine plus oral ciclosporin to reverse multidrug resistance, three patients also received erythromycin to raise their ciclosporin concentrations; all developed severe toxicity consistent with a much higher dose of vinblastine than was actually given (94).

Itraconazole

The concomitant use of itraconazole with vincristine increased the incidence of neurotoxicity in children and adults with acute lymphoblastic leukemia (95,96).

- A 19-year-old woman developed severe abdominal pain and constipation 28 days after starting to take itraconazole as antifungal prophylaxis when receiving vincristine for acute lymphoblastic leukemia. She had hypertension, marked abdominal distension and tenderness, and absent bowel sounds. Withdrawal of itraconazole resulted in resolution of symptoms and vincristine was continued (96).

- A 72-year-old patient developed painful oral mucositis and constipation 3 days after being given vinorelbine and itraconazole (97). Further complications included neutropenia and hypoxia and he died.

Concomitant use of itraconazole 2.5 mg/kg/day and vincristine in five children receiving vincristine resulted in hypertension, paralytic ileus, and SIADH (95).

Enhanced and potentially life-threatening neurotoxicity of vinca alkaloids through concomitant therapy with itraconazole has been the subject of several compelling reports (98–101). Enhancement of vincristine neurotoxicity results in polyneuropathy and paralytic ileus (106,102,103). The interaction is reversible, and readministration of vinca alkaloids may be safe after a prolonged washout (98). The mechanism has not been formally elucidated, but may be either competition for oxidative metabolism, leading to increased systemic exposure (104), or inhibition of the transmembrane P glycoprotein efflux pump (105), leading to increased intracellular concentrations of vinca alkaloids (105). The concomitant use of itraconazole and vinca alkaloids is therefore contraindicated.

Two adults with acute lymphoblastic leukemia developed unusually severe neurotoxicity caused by vincristine, which was probably the result of an interaction with itraconazole suspension (102).

Phenytoin

In a small pharmacokinetic study, the clearance of vincristine was 65% greater than in patients who were not taking phenytoin and the half-life and AUC of vincristine were reduced by 35 and 43% respectively (93).

References

1. Zhou XJ, Rahmani R. Preclinical and clinical pharmacology of vinca alkaloids. Drugs 1992;44(Suppl 4):1–16.
2. Budman DR. New vinca alkaloids and related compounds. Semin Oncol 1992;19(6):639–45.
3. Malawista SE, Sato H, Bensch KG. Vinblastine and griseofulvin reversibly disrupt the living mitotic spindle. Science 1968;160(829):770–2.
4. Kruczynski A, Hill BT. Vinflunine, the latest vinca alkaloid in clinical development. A review of its preclinical anticancer properties. Crit Rev Oncol Hematol 2001;40(2):159–73.
5. Gidding CE, Kellie SJ, Kamps WA, de Graaf SS. Vincristine revisited. Crit Rev Oncol Hematol 1999;29(3):267–87.
6. McCune JS, Lindley C. Appropriateness of maximum-dose guidelines for vincristine. Am J Health Syst Pharm 1997;54(15):1755–8.
7. Cersosimo RJ, Bromer R, Licciardello JT, Hong WK. Pharmacology, clinical efficacy and adverse effects of vindesine sulfate, a new vinca alkaloid. Pharmacotherapy 1983;3(5):259–74.
8. Summerhayes M. Vindesine: ten years in the pharmacy. EHP 1996;2:214–21.
9. Jordan MA, Himes RH, Wilson L. Comparison of the effects of vinblastine, vincristine, vindesine, and vinepidine on microtubule dynamics and cell proliferation in vitro. Cancer Res 1985;45(6):2741–7.
10. Singer WD, Himes RH. Cellular uptake and tubulin binding properties of four vinca alkaloids. Biochem Pharmacol 1992;43(3):545–51.
11. Rahmani R, Gueritte F, Martin M, Just S, Cano JP, Barbet J. Comparative pharmacokinetics of antitumor vinca alkaloids: intravenous bolus injections of Navelbine and related alkaloids to cancer patients and rats. Cancer Chemother Pharmacol 1986;16(3):223–8.
12. Nelson RL, Dyke RW, Root MA. Comparative pharmacokinetics of vindesine, vincristine and vinblastine in patients with cancer. Cancer Treat Rev 1980;7(Suppl 1):17–24.
13. Jackson DV Jr, Castle MC, Bender RA. Biliary excretion of vincristine. Clin Pharmacol Ther 1978;24(1):101–7.
14. Deporte-Fety R, Simon N, Fumoleau P, Campone M, Kerbrat P, Bonneterre J, Fargeot P, Urien S. Population pharmacokinetics of short intravenous vinorelbine infusions in patients with metastatic breast cancer. Cancer Chemother Pharmacol 2004;53(3):233–8.
15. Variol P, Nguyen L, Tranchand B, Puozzo C. A simultaneous oral/intravenous population pharmacokinetic model for vinorelbine. Eur J Clin Pharmacol 2002;58(7):467–76.
16. Zhou-Pan XR, Seree E, Zhou XJ, Placidi M, Maurel P, Barra Y, Rahmani R. Involvement of human liver cytochrome P450 3A in vinblastine metabolism: drug interactions. Cancer Res 1993;53(21):5121–6.
17. Kajita J, Kuwabara T, Kobayashi H, Kobayashi S. CYP3A4 is mainly responsibile for the metabolism of a new vinca alkaloid, vinorelbine, in human liver microsomes. Drug Metab Dispos 2000;28(9):1121–7.
18. Robieux I, Sorio R, Borsatti E, Cannizzaro R, Vitali V, Aita P, Freschi A, Galligioni E, Monfardini S. Pharmacokinetics of vinorelbine in patients with liver metastases. Clin Pharmacol Ther 1996;59(1):32–40.
19. Rowinsky EK, Lucas VS, Hsieh AL, Wargin WA, Hohneker JA, Lubejko B, Sartorius SE, Donehower RC. The effects of food and divided dosing on the bioavailability of oral vinorelbine. Cancer Chemother Pharmacol 1996;39(1–2):9–16.
20. Furuse K, Kubota K, Kawahara M, Takada M, Kimura I, Fujii M, Ohta M, Hasegawa K, Yoshida K, Nakajima S, Ogura T, Niitani HJapan Lung Cancer Vinorelbine Study Group. Phase II study of vinorelbine in heavily previously treated small cell lung cancer. Oncology 1996;53(2):169–72.
21. Chan JD. Pharmacokinetic drug interactions of vinca alkaloids: summary of case reports. Pharmacotherapy 1998;18(6):1304–7.
22. Cargill RI, Boyter AC, Lipworth BJ. Reversible myocardial ischaemia following vincristine containing chemotherapy. Respir Med 1994;88(9):709–10.
23. Dixon A, Nakamura JM, Oishi N, Wachi DH, Fukuyama O. Angina pectoris and therapy with cisplatin, vincristine, and bleomycin. Ann Intern Med 1989;111(4):342–3.
24. Calvo-Romero JM, Fernandez-Soria-Pantoja R, Arrebola-Garcia JD, Gil-Cubero M. Ischemic heart disease associated with vincristine and doxorubicin chemotherapy. Ann Pharmacother 2001;35(11):1403–5.
25. Karminsky N, Merimsky O, Kovner F, Inbar M. Vinorelbine-related acute cardiopulmonary toxicity. Cancer Chemother Pharmacol 1999;43(2):180–2.
26. Feun LG, Savaraj N, Hurley J, Marini A, Lai S. A clinical trial of intravenous vinorelbine tartrate plus tamoxifen in the treatment of patients with advanced malignant melanoma. Cancer 2000;88(3):584–8.
27. Yoh K, Niho S, Goto K, Ohmatsu H, Kubota K, Kakinuma R, Nishiwaki Y. High body mass index

correlates with increased risk of venous irritation by vinorelbine infusion. Jpn J Clin Oncol 2004;34(4):206–9.

28. Frasci G, Comella G, Comella P, Salzano F, Cremone L, Della Volpe N, Imbriani A, Persico G. Mitoxantrone plus vinorelbine with granulocyte-colony stimulating factor (G-CSF) support in advanced breast cancer patients. A dose and schedule finding study. Breast Cancer Res Treat 1995;35(2):147–56.

29. Fumoleau P, Delozier T, Extra JM, Canobbio L, Delgado FM, Hurteloup P. Vinorelbine (Navelbine) in the treatment of breast cancer: the European experience. Semin Oncol 1995;22(2 Suppl 5):22–8.

30. Luedke D, McLaughlin TT, Daughaday C, Luedke S, Harrison B, Reed G, Martello O. Mitomycin C and vindesine associated pulmonary toxicity with variable clinical expression. Cancer 1985;55(3):542–5.

31. Kris MG, Pablo D, Gralla RJ, Burke MT, Prestifilippo J, Lewin D. Dyspnea following vinblastine or vindesine administration in patients receiving mitomycin plus vinca alkaloid combination therapy. Cancer Treat Rep 1984;68(7–8):1029–31.

32. Konits PH, Aisner J, Sutherland JC, Wiernik PH. Possible pulmonary toxicity secondary to vinblastine. Cancer 1982;50(12):2771–4.

33. Ballen KK, Weiss ST. Fatal acute respiratory failure following vinblastine and mitomycin administration for breast cancer. Am J Med Sci 1988;295(6):558–60.

34. Hoelzer KL, Harrison BR, Luedke SW, Luedke DW. Vinblastine-associated pulmonary toxicity in patients receiving combination therapy with mitomycin and cisplatin. Drug Intell Clin Pharm 1986;20(4):287–9.

35. Legha SS. Vincristine neurotoxicity. Pathophysiology and management. Med Toxicol 1986;1(6):421–7.

36. Chauncey TR, Showel JL, Fox JH. Vincristine neurotoxicity. JAMA 1985;254(4):507.

37. Stewart DJ, Maroun JA, Lefebvre B, Heringer R. Neurotoxicity and efficacy of combined vinca alkaloids in breast cancer. Cancer Treat Rep 1986;70(5):571–3.

38. Manelis G, Aderka D, Manelis J, Horn I. [Recurrent laryngeal nerve palsy and dysphagia for liquids due to vincristine.]Harefuah 1976;91(3–4):84–5.

39. Toker E, Yenice O, Ogut MS. Isolated abducens nerve palsy induced by vincristine therapy. J AAPOS 2004;8(1):69–71.

40. Lash SC, Williams CP, Marsh CS, Critchley C, Hodgkins PR, Mackie EJ. Acute sixth-nerve palsy after vincristine therapy. J AAPOS 2004;8(1):67–8.

41. Fujishita M, Tamura A, Yamada M, Uemura Y, Niiya K, Yoshimoto S, Kubonishi I, Taguchi H, Yoshino T, Ohtsuki Y, et al. [Quadriplegia and cranial nerve palsy during treatment by vincristine in blastic crisis of chronic myelocytic leukemia: report of an autopsy case.]Rinsho Ketsueki 1986;27(8):1437–42.

42. Mahajan SL, Ikeda Y, Myers TJ, Baldini MG. Acute acoustic nerve palsy associated with vincristine therapy. Cancer 1981;47(10):2404–6.

43. Annino DJ Jr, MacArthur CJ, Friedman EM. Vincristine-induced recurrent laryngeal nerve paralysis. Laryngoscope 1992;102(11):1260–2.

44. Nunez E, Solano D, Arreita A, Franco-Vicario R, Miguel F. Paralisis recurrencial inducida por vincristina. [Vincristine-induced recurrent laryngeal nerve paralysis.] Rev Clin Esp 1992;190(4):214–5.

45. Tobias JD, Bozeman PM. Vincristine-induced recurrent laryngeal nerve paralysis in children. Intensive Care Med 1991;17(5):304–5.

46. Delaney P. Vincristine-induced laryngeal nerve paralysis. Neurology 1982;32(11):1285–8.

47. Whittaker JA, Griffith IP. Recurrent laryngeal nerve paralysis in patients receiving vincristine and vinblastine. BMJ 1977;1(6071):1251–2.

48. Raphaelson MI, Stevens JC, Newman RP. Vincristine neuropathy with bowel and bladder atony, mimicking spinal cord compression. Cancer Treat Rep 1983;67(6):604–5.

49. Rhomberg WU. Vindesine for recurrent and metastatic cancer of the uterine cervix: a phase II study. Cancer Treat Rep 1986;70(12):1455–7.

50. McCarthy GM, Skillings JR. Jaw and other orofacial pain in patients receiving vincristine for the treatment of cancer. Oral Surg Oral Med Oral Pathol 1992;74(3):299–304.

51. Parimoo D, Jeffers S, Muggia FM. Severe neurotoxicity from vinorelbine–paclitaxel combinations. J Natl Cancer Inst 1996;88(15):1079–80.

52. Hogan-Dann CM, Fellmeth WG, McGuire SA, Kiley VA. Polyneuropathy following vincristine therapy in two patients with Charcot–Marie–Tooth syndrome. JAMA 1984;252(20):2862–3.

53. van Kooten B, van Diemen HA, Groenhout KM, Huijgens PC, Ossenkoppele GJ, Nauta JJ, Heimans JJ. A pilot study on the influence of a corticotropin (4–9) analogue on vinca alkaloid-induced neuropathy. Arch Neurol 1992;49(10):1027–31.

54. Jackson DV, Wells HB, Atkins JN, Zekan PJ, White DR, Richards F 2nd, Cruz JM, Muss HB. Amelioration of vincristine neurotoxicity by glutamic acid. Am J Med 1988;84(6):1016–22.

55. Thoumie P, Diverrez JR, Guidet B. Polynevrite aiguë a la vincristine préscrite pour un cancer du sein chez une patiente atteinte de maladie de Friedreich. Sem Hop Paris 1989;65:30.

56. Griffiths JD, Stark RJ, Ding JC, Cooper IA. Vincristine neurotoxicity in Charcot-Marie-Tooth syndrome. Med J Aust 1985;143(7):305–6.

57. Budd GT, Green S, O'Bryan RM, Martino S, Abeloff MD, Rinehart JJ, Hahn R, Harris J, Tormey D, O'Sullivan J, et al. Short-course FAC-M versus 1 year of CMFVP in node-positive, hormone receptor-negative breast cancer: an intergroup study. J Clin Oncol 1995;13(4):831–9.

58. Zaragoza MR, Ritchey ML, Walter A. Neurourologic consequences of accidental intrathecal vincristine: a case report. Med Pediatr Oncol 1995;24(1):61–2.

59. Dettmeyer R, Driever F, Becker A, Wiestler OD, Madea B. Fatal myeloencephalopathy due to accidental intrathecal vincristin administration: a report of two cases. Forensic Sci Int 2001;122(1):60–4.

60. Johnson FL, Bernstein ID, Hartmann JR, Chard RL Jr. Seizures associated with vincristine sulfate therapy. J Pediatr 1973;82(4):699–702.

61. Hurwitz RL, Mahoney DH Jr, Armstrong DL, Browder TM. Reversible encephalopathy and seizures as a result of conventional vincristine administration. Med Pediatr Oncol 1988;16(3):216–9.

62. Murphy JA, Ross LM, Gibson BE. Vincristine toxicity in five children with acute lymphoblastic leukaemia. Lancet 1995;346(8972):443.

63. Awidi AS. Blindness and vincristine. Ann Intern Med 1980;93(5):781.

64. Shurin SB, Rekate HL, Annable W. Optic atrophy induced by vincristine. Pediatrics 1982;70(2):288–91.

65. Pinkerton CR, McDermott B, Philip T, Biron P, Ardiet C, Vandenberg H, Brunat-Mentigny M. Continuous vincristine infusion as part of a high dose chemoradiotherapy regimen: drug kinetics and toxicity. Cancer Chemother Pharmacol 1988;22(3):271–4.

66. Teichmann KD, Dabbagh N. Severe visual loss after a single dose of vincristine in a patient with spinal cord astrocytoma. J Ocul Pharmacol 1988;4(2):117–21.

67. Schweitzer VG. Ototoxicity of chemotherapeutic agents. Otolaryngol Clin North Am 1993;26(5):759–89.

68. Lugassy G, Shapira A. A prospective cohort study of the effect of vincristine on audition. Anticancer Drugs 1996;7(5):525–6.

69. Moss PE, Hickman S, Harrison BR. Ototoxicity associated with vinblastine. Ann Pharmacother 1999;33(4):423–5.

70. Cutting HO. Inappropriate secretion of antidiuretic hormone secondary to vincristine therapy. Am J Med 1971;51(2):269–71.

71. Stahel RA, Oelz O. Syndrome of inappropriate ADH secretion secondary to vinblastine. Cancer Chemother Pharmacol 1982;8(2):253–4.

72. Garrett CA, Simpson TA Jr. Syndrome of inappropriate antidiuretic hormone associated with vinorelbine therapy. Ann Pharmacother 1998;32(12):1306–9.

73. Hammond IW, Ferguson JA, Kwong K, Muniz E, Delisle F. Hyponatremia and syndrome of inappropriate anti-diuretic hormone reported with the use of vincristine: an over-representation of Asians? Pharmacoepidemiol Drug Saf 2002;11(3):229–34.

74. Tomomasa T, Miyazawa R, Kato M, Hoshino M, Tabata M, Kaneko H, Suzuki M, Kobayashi T, Morikawa A. Prolonged gastrointestinal dysmotility in a patient with hemophagocytic lymphohistiocytosis treated with vincristine. Dig Dis Sci 1999;44(9):1755–7.

75. Jassem J, Ramlau R, Karnicka-Mlodkowska H, Krawczyk K, Krzakowski M, Zatloukal P, Lemarie E, Hartmann W, Novakova L, O'Brien M, Depierr A. A multicenter randomized phase II study of oral vs. intravenous vinorelbine in advanced non-small-cell lung cancer patients. Ann Oncol 2001;12(10):1375–81.

76. Dorr RT. Managing extravasation of vesicant chemotherapy drugs. In: Lipp HP, editor. Anticancer Drug Toxicity; Prevention, Management and Clinical Pharmacokinetics. New York–Basel: Marcel Dekker Inc, 1999:279–318.

77. Bellone JD. Treatment of vincristine extravasation. JAMA 1981;245(4):343.

78. Rittenberg CN, Gralla RJ, Rehmeyer TA. Assessing and managing venous irritation associated with vinorelbine tartrate (Navelbine). Oncol Nurs Forum 1995;22(4):707–10.

79. Bertelli G, Dini D, Forno GB, Gozza A, Silvestro S, Venturini M, Rosso R, Pronzato P. Hyaluronidase as an antidote to extravasation of vinca alkaloids: clinical results. J Cancer Res Clin Oncol 1994;120(8):505–6.

80. Lamont EB, Schilsky RL. Gonadal toxicity and teratogenicity after cytotoxic chemotherapy. In: Lipp HP, editor. Anticancer Drug Toxicity. Prevention, Management and Clinical Pharmacokinetics. New York–Basel: Marcel Dekker Inc, 1999:491–523.

81. Meistrich ML. Effects of chemotherapy and radiotherapy on spermatogenesis. Eur Urol 1993;23(1):136–42.

82. .Rautonen J, Koskimies AI, Siimes MA. Vincristine is associated with the risk of azoospermia in adult male survivors of childhood malignancies. Eur J Cancer 1992;28A(11):1837–41.

83. Ishii E, Hara T, Mizuno Y, Ueda K. [Vincristine-induced fever in children with leukaemia and lymphoma.]Saishin Igaku 1988;6:1341.

84. Gonzalez-Cid M, Cuello MT, Larripa I. Comparison of the aneugenic effect of vinorelbine and vincristine in cultured human lymphocytes. Mutagenesis 1999;14(1):63–6.

85. Gonzalez-Cid M, Cuello MT, Larripa I. Mitotic arrest and anaphase aberrations induced by vinorelbine in hamster cells in vitro. Anticancer Drugs 1997;8(5):529–32.

86. Bokemeyer C, Kollmannsberger C. Secondary malignancies. In: Lipp HP, editor. Anticancer Drug Toxicity. Prevention, Management and Clinical Pharmacokinetics. New York-Basel: Marcel Dekker Inc, 1999:525–47.

87. Boivin JF. Second cancers and other late side effects of cancer treatment. A review. Cancer 1990;65(Suppl 3):770–5.

88. Lacher MJ. Use of vinblastine sulfate to treat Hodgkin's disease during pregnancy. Ann Intern Med 1964;61:113–5.

89. Product information. NavelbineGlaxo Wellcome;. 1999.

90. Cuvier C, Espie M, Extra JM, Marty M. Vinorelbine in pregnancy. Eur J Cancer 1997;33(1):168–9.

91. Toft B. Toft Report. External enquiry into the adverse incident that occurred at Queen's Medical Centre, Nottingham, 4 March, 2001. London: Department of Health;. 2001.

92. NHS Executive. National guidance on the safe administration of intrathecal chemotherapy. HSC 2000;022.

93. Villikka K, Kivisto KT, Maenpaa H, Joensuu H, Neuvonen PJ. Cytochrome P450-inducing antiepileptics increase the clearance of vincristine in patients with brain tumors. Clin Pharmacol Ther 1999;66(6):589–93.

94. Tobe SW, Siu LL, Jamal SA, Skorecki KL, Murphy GF, Warner E. Vinblastine and erythromycin: an unrecognized serious drug interaction. Cancer Chemother Pharmacol 1995;35(3):188–90.

95. Bohme A, Ganser A, Hoelzer D. Aggravation of vincristine-induced neurotoxicity by itraconazole in the treatment of adult ALL. Ann Hematol 1995;71(6):311–2.

96. Gillies J, Hung KA, Fitzsimons E, Soutar R. Severe vincristine toxicity in combination with itraconazole. Clin Lab Haematol 1998;20(2):123–4.

97. Bosque E. Possible drug interaction between itraconazole and vinorelbine tartrate leading to death after one dose of chemotherapy. Ann Intern Med 2001;134(5):427.

98. Jeng MR, Feusner J. Itraconazole-enhanced vincristine neurotoxicity in a child with acute lymphoblastic leukemia. Pediatr Hematol Oncol 2001;18(2):137–42.

99. Bosque E. Possible drug interaction between itraconazole and vinorelbine tartrate leading to death after one dose of chemotherapy. Ann Intern Med 2001;134(5):427.

100. Kamaluddin M, McNally P, Breatnach F, O'Marcaigh A, Webb D, O'Dell E, Scanlon P, Butler K, O'Meara A. Potentiation of vincristine toxicity by itraconazole in children with lymphoid malignancies. Acta Paediatr 2001;90(10):1204–7.

101. Sathiapalan RK, El-Solh H. Enhanced vincristine neurotoxicity from drug interactions: case report and review of literature. Pediatr Hematol Oncol 2001;18(8):543–6.

102. Gillies J, Hung KA, Fitzsimons E, Soutar R. Severe vincristine toxicity in combination with itraconazole. Clin Lab Haematol 1998;20(2):123–4.

103. Bohme A, Ganser A, Hoelzer D. Aggravation of vincristine-induced neurotoxicity by itraconazole in the treatment of adult ALL. Ann Hematol 1995;71(6):311–2.

104. Zhou-Pan XR, Seree E, Zhou XJ, Placidi M, Maurel P, Barra Y, Rahmani R. Involvement of human liver cytochrome P450 3A in vinblastine metabolism: drug interactions. Cancer Res 1993;53(21):5121–6.

105. Gupta S, Kim J, Gollapudi S. Reversal of daunorubicin resistance in P388/ADR cells by itraconazole. J Clin Invest 1991;87(4):1467–9.

106. Woodland C, Ito S, Koren G. A model for the prediction of digoxin–drug interactions at the renal tubular cell level. Ther Drug Monit 1998;20(2):134–8.

OTHER ANTICANCER DRUGS

Asparaginase

General Information

Asparaginase is an enzyme that acts by breaking down the amino acid L-asparagine to aspartic acid and ammonia. It interferes with the growth of malignant cells that cannot synthesize L-asparagine. Its action is reportedly specific for the G_1 phase of the cell cycle. It is used mainly for the induction of remissions in acute lymphoblastic leukemia.

Nomenclature

Colaspase and crisantaspase are the British Approved Names of asparaginase obtained from cultures of *Escherichia coli* and *Erwinia carotovora* respectively.

Organs and Systems

Nervous system

In a review of 28 central nervous system thrombotic or hemorrhagic events and eight peripheral thromboses related to L-asparaginase, the median time from initial treatment to adverse reaction was 16–17 days (1). Most patients recovered completely, although five cases had residual neurological deficits and one died from superior sagittal sinus thrombosis. Five patients with cerebral thrombosis complicating asparaginase/prednisone/vincristine induction therapy for acute lymphoblastic leukemia were found to have a reduced platelet count after the event and, in three of them, sequential changes in von Willebrand factor multimer pattern (2). The other two patients were only studied at presentation and their multimer pattern was not appreciably different to pooled plasma from seven controls without thromboses. The findings were consistent with thrombotic complications caused by platelet agglutination by plasma Von Willebrand factor.

Metabolism

Asparaginase can reduce insulin production (3) and precipitate diabetic ketoacidosis (4,5).

Hematologic

Thrombosis and hemorrhage are well-recognized complications in 1–2% of patients receiving asparaginase. This is due to a coagulopathy, which has been variously attributed to reduced concentrations of fibrinogen, factors IX, XI, VIII complex, antithrombin III, and plasminogen (6).

In one study, 12 children in complete remission treated with daily asparaginase alone were investigated for platelet and clotting abnormalities (7). Changes in prothrombin time, partial thromboplastin time, and fibrinogen remained close to the reference range, and platelet function was normal. There were reduced concentrations of physiological inhibitors of coagulation (protein C and antithrombin III). Thrombosis was uncommon. These results are consistent with those of another study of asparaginase as a single agent in 14 children with acute lymphoblastic leukemia (8). There was severe deficiency of antithrombin III and protein C, with co-existing hypocoagulability; equilibrium between the two partly explained the lack of thromboembolic phenomena. The hypocoagulability was due to hypofibrinogenemia and reduced concentrations of vitamin K-dependent factors.

Three patients developed bilateral venous sinus thromboses after receiving asparaginase; the diagnosis and follow-up of this complication have been succinctly reviewed (9). In another patient receiving asparaginase, central nervous system thrombosis was associated with a transient acquired type II pattern of von Willebrand's disease (10).

Mouth

Acute parotitis has been attributed to L–asparaginase in association with hyperglycemia (11).

Liver

Most patients who receive asparaginase develop liver function abnormalities, which can be fatal (12). This adverse effect is of major concern in patients who are also taking other hepatotoxic drugs, such as methotrexate and mercaptopurine. Jaundice and increased serum bilirubin and transaminases occur often, and hepatomegaly and fatty deposits occur occasionally.

Pancreas

Pancreatitis has been reported in up to 16% of children receiving asparaginase for a variety of neoplasms (13). Pseudocyst formation has been described (14).

Immunologic

Asparaginase can cause allergic reactions (15), which increase with the number of doses within a cycle and the number of exposures, irrespective of drug-free intervals. There is a pegylated formulation (PEG-ASNase; Oncaspar™) with a prolonged half-life and different allergenic properties from conventional asparaginase-containing formulations. These claims have been investigated, and the authors concluded that although the hypersensitivity rate was lower, it was still significant; furthermore, there was no cross-sensitivity in previously treated patients (16). There were no allergic reactions to pegylated asparaginase compared with 30% with non-pegylated asparaginase in 70 children with acute lymphoblastic leukemia or non-Hodgkin's lymphoma, and other toxic effects were also less common (17).

References

1. Ott N, Ramsay NK, Priest JR, Lipton M, Pui CH, Steinherz P, Nesbit ME Jr. Sequelae of thrombotic or hemorrhagic complications following L-asparaginase therapy for childhood lymphoblastic leukemia. Am J Pediatr Hematol Oncol 1988;10(3):191–5.
2. Pui CH, Jackson CW, Chesney CM, Abildgaard CF. Involvement of von Willebrand factor in thrombosis following asparaginase–prednisone–vincristine therapy for leukemia. Am J Hematol 1987;25(3):291–8.
3. Meschi F, di Natale B, Rondanini GF, Uderzo C, Jankovic M, Masera G, Chiumello G. Pancreatic endocrine function in leukemic children treated with L-asparaginase. Horm Res 1981;15(4):237–41.
4. Rovira A, Cordido F, Vecilla C, Bernacer M, Valverde I, Herrera Pombo JL. Study of beta-cell function and erythrocyte insulin receptors in a patient with diabetic ketoacidosis associated with L-asparaginase therapy. Acta Paediatr Scand 1986;75(4):670–1.
5. Hsu YJ, Chen YC, Ho CL, Kao WY, Chao TY. Diabetic ketoacidosis and persistent hyperglycemia as long-term complications of L-asparaginase-induced pancreatitis. Zhonghua Yi Xue Za Zhi (Taipei) 2002;65(9):441–5.
6. O'Meara A, Daly M, Hallinan FH. Increased antithrombin III concentration in children with acute lymphatic leukaemia receiving L-asparaginase therapy. Med Pediatr Oncol 1988;16(3):169–74.
7. Homans AC, Rybak ME, Baglini RL, Tiarks C, Steiner ME, Forman EN. Effect of L-asparaginase administration on coagulation and platelet function in children with leukemia. J Clin Oncol 1987;5(5):811–7.
8. Mielot F, Danel P, Boyer C, Coulombel L, Dommergues JP, Tchernia G, Larrieu MJ. Déficits acquis en antithrombine III et en proteine C au cours due traitement par la L-asparaginase. [Acquired deficiencies in antithrombin III and C protein during treatment with L-asparaginase.] Arch Fr Pediatr 1987;44(3):161–5.
9. Schick RM, Jolesz F, Barnes PD, Macklis JD. MR diagnosis of dural venous sinus thrombosis complicating L-asparaginase therapy. Comput Med Imaging Graph 1989;13(4):319–27.
10. Shapiro AD, Clarke SL, Christian JM, Odom LF, Hathaway WE. Thrombosis in children receiving L-asparaginase. Determining patients at risk. Am J Pediatr Hematol Oncol 1993;15(4):400–5.
11. Uysal K, Uguz A, Olgun N, Sarialioglu F, Buyukgebiz A. Hyperglycemia and acute parotitis related to L-asparaginase therapy. J Pediatr Endocrinol Metab 1996;9(6):627–9.
12. Sahoo S, Hart J. Histopathological features of L-asparaginase-induced liver disease. Semin Liver Dis 2003;23(3):295–9.
13. Sadoff J, Hwang S, Rosenfeld D, Ettinger L, Spigland N. Surgical pancreatic complications induced by L-Asparaginase. J Pediatr Surg 1997;32(6):860–3.
14. Bertolone SJ, Fuenfer MM, Groff DB, Patel CC. Delayed pancreatic pseudocyst formations. Long-term complication of L-asparaginase treatment. Cancer 1982;50(12):2964–6.
15. Korholz D, Wahn U, Jurgens H, Wahn V. Allergische Reaktionen unter der Behandlung mit L-Asparaginase. Bedeutung spezifischer IgE-Antikorper. [Allergic reactions in treatment with L-asparaginase. Significance of specific IgE antibodies.] Monatsschr Kinderheilkd 1990;138(1):23–5.
16. Vieira Pinheiro JP, Muller HJ, Schwabe D, Gunkel M, Casimiro da Palma J, Henze G, von Schutz V, Winkelhorst M, Wurthwein G, Boos J. Drug monitoring of low-dose PEG-asparaginase (Oncaspar) in children with relapsed acute lymphoblastic leukaemia. Br J Haematol 2001;113(1):115–9.
17. Muller HJ, Loning L, Horn A, Schwabe D, Gunkel M, Schrappe M, von Schutz V, Henze G, Casimiro da Palma J, Ritter J, Pinheiro JP, Winkelhorst M, Boos J. Pegylated asparaginase (Oncaspar) in children with ALL: drug monitoring in reinduction according to the ALL/NHL-BFM 95 protocols. Br J Haematol 2000;110(2):379–84.

Hydroxycarbamide

General Information

Hydroxycarbamide (hydroxyurea) is used to treat a variety of cancers, myeloproliferative disorders, and sickle cell disease, and has been studied in patients with HIV infection (1). It inhibits ribonucleotide reductase and increases concentrations of iron nitrosyl hemoglobin, nitrite, and nitrate, suggesting in vivo metabolism of hydroxycarbamide to nitric oxide (2).

Organs and Systems

Hematologic

Concern about the toxicity of hydroxycarbamide, expressed in a report from the AIDS Clinical Trials Group (ACTG 5025 report), has led to a retrospective study of the antiviral activity, immunological effects, and tolerability of hydroxycarbamide in combination with didanosine (3). Hematological adverse events were the most frequent and involved 37 of the 65 patients. Neutropenia was the commonest adverse event (26 patients) and it was occasionally accompanied by anemia or thrombocytopenia. However, these effects normalized spontaneously, despite continued therapy.

Of 16 children receiving hydroxycarbamide in combination with nucleoside analogues, 4 developed neutropenia (below $1.5 \times 10^9/l$) by weeks 2 or 4 (4). Hydroxycarbamide was temporarily withdrawn and then reintroduced without further ill effects after the neutrophil count had returned to normal.

Mouth and teeth

In a retrospective study of the antiviral activity, immunological effects, and tolerability of hydroxycarbamide in combination with didanosine, mouth ulceration was recorded in eight of the 65 patients and this led to discontinuation in one patient (3).

Pancreas

In a retrospective study of the antiviral activity, immunological effects, and tolerability of hydroxycarbamide in combination with didanosine, there was increased serum amylase activity in 15 of the 65 patients; although asymptomatic, it occasioned withdrawal of therapy in four patients (3).

Skin

The incidence of skin lesions in patients taking hydroxycarbamide is 10–35%. They usually occur after several years of maintenance therapy. However, one patient developed lichen planus-like dermatitis on his hands after just 15 days of treatment (5).

Hydroxycarbamide can cause hyperpigmentation of the nails and palmar creases and leg ulcers (6,7). Leg ulcers occurred in 41 patients taking hydroxycarbamide (8). They had a mean age of 67 years and mean therapy duration of 5 years, and none had any underlying vascular disease. There were megaloblastic erythrocytes trapped in the capillary beds, causing local tissue anoxia, and the authors postulated that the megaloblastic erythrocytes had resulted from hydroxycarbamide and that the ulcers were due to consequent impaired circulation and cutaneous atrophy; they also commented that there was no major vascular disease that could have accounted for the leg ulcers. The degeneration of lichen planus-like skin lesions into full-blown ulcers has been described in 14 patients who developed extremely painful leg ulcers, most commonly on the malleoli. The patients had been taking hydroxycarbamide for an average of 6 years and nine had multiple ulcers (9).

Acral erythema, dermatomyositis-like changes on the backs of the hands, squamous cell neoplasms on sun-exposed sites, and ulcers on the legs, genitalia, and oral mucosae have also been reported (10).

Immunologic

Hydroxycarbamide has been associated with Behçet's syndrome (11).

Body temperature

- A 64-year-old woman with essential thrombocythemia developed a fever after 3 weeks of treatment with hydroxycarbamide 1000 mg/day; the fever subsided on withdrawal and recurred on rechallenge (12).

Drug–Drug Interactions

Busulfan

During long-term follow-up of patients treated with busulfan and hydroxycarbamide for essential thrombocythemia, seven patients (13%) taking hydroxycarbamide developed secondary acute leukemia, myelodysplasia, or solid tumors, compared with only one of the control group; none of the 20 patients who had never been treated with chemotherapy developed secondary malignancies compared with three of the 77 given hydroxycarbamide only and five of the 15 given busulfan plus hydroxycarbamide. This suggests that the combination of busulfan plus hydroxycarbamide causes a significantly increased risk of secondary malignancies (13).

References

1. Gibbs MA, Sorensen SJ. Hydroxyurea in the treatment of HIV-1. Ann Pharmacother 2000;34(1):89–93.
2. King SB. The nitric oxide producing reactions of hydroxyurea. Curr Med Chem 2003;10(6):437–52.
3. Biron F, Ponceau B, Bouhour D, Boibieux A, Verrier B, Peyramond D. Long-term safety and antiretroviral activity of hydroxyurea and didanosine in HIV-infected patients. J Acquir Immune Defic Syndr 2000;25(4):329–36.
4. Kline MW, Calles NR, Simon C, Schwarzwald H. Pilot study of hydroxyurea in human immunodeficiency virus-infected children receiving didanosine and/or stavudine. Pediatr Infect Dis J 2000;19(11):1083–6.
5. Radaelli F, Calori R, Faccini P, Maiolo AT. Early cutaneous lesions secondary to hydroxyurea therapy. Am J Hematol 1998;58(1):82–3.
6. O'Branski EE, Ware RE, Prose NS, Kinney TR. Skin and nail changes in children with sickle cell anemia receiving hydroxyurea therapy. J Am Acad Dermatol 2001;44(5):859–61.
7. Chaine B, Neonato MG, Girot R, Aractingi S. Cutaneous adverse reactions to hydroxyurea in patients with sickle cell disease. Arch Dermatol 2001;137(4):467–70.
8. Sirieix ME, Debure C, Baudot N, Dubertret L, Roux ME, Morel P, Frances C, Loubeyres S, Beylot C, Lambert D, Humbert P, Gauthier O, Dandurand M, Guillot B, Vaillant L, Lorette G, Bonnetblanc JM, Lok C, Denoeux JP. Leg ulcers and hydroxyurea: forty-one cases. Arch Dermatol 1999;135(7):818–20.
9. Best PJ, Daoud MS, Pittelkow MR, Petitt RM. Hydroxyurea-induced leg ulceration in 14 patients. Ann Intern Med 1998;128(1):29–32.
10. Vassallo C, Passamonti F, Merante S, Ardigo M, Nolli G, Mangiacavalli S, Borroni G. Muco-cutaneous changes during long-term therapy with hydroxyurea in chronic myeloid leukaemia. Clin Exp Dermatol 2001;26(2):141–8.
11. Vaiopoulos G, Terpos E, Viniou N, Nodaros K, Rombos J, Loukopoulos D. Behçet's disease in a patient with chronic myelogenous leukemia under hydroxyurea treatment: a case report and review of the literature. Am J Hematol 2001;66(1):57–8.
12. Braester A, Quitt M. Hydroxyurea as a cause of drug fever. Acta Haematol 2000;104(1):50–1.
13. Finazzi G, Ruggeri M, Rodeghiero F, Barbui T. Second malignancies in patients with essential thrombocythaemia treated with busulphan and hydroxyurea: long-term follow-up of a randomized clinical trial. Br J Haematol 2000;110(3):577–83.

CORTICOSTEROIDS AND PROSTAGLANDINS

Corticosteroids—glucocorticoids

General Information

Nomenclature

The two main classes of adrenal corticosteroids are properly known as glucocorticoids and mineralocorticosteroids. The former are often known by shorter names and are commonly referred to as "glucocorticoids", "corticosteroids", "corticoids", or even simply "steroids"; the latter are often referred to as "mineralocorticoids". Here we shall use the terms "glucocorticoids" and "mineralocorticoids". When referring to both we shall use the term "corticosteroids".

Relative potencies

The main human anti-inflammatory corticosteroid, the glucocorticoid cortisol (hydrocortisone), as secreted by the adrenal gland, has generally been replaced by related glucocorticoids of synthetic origin for therapeutic purposes. These Δ^1-dehydrated glucocorticoids are designed to imitate the physiological hormone. They have marked glucocorticoid potency but only minor effects on sodium retention and potassium excretion; the relative glucocorticoid and mineralocorticoid potencies of the best-known compounds, insofar as these potencies are agreed, are compared in Table 1.

Over many years, a great deal of research has been devoted to producing better glucocorticoids for therapeutic use. Those endeavors have succeeded only in part; from the start the mineralocorticoid effects were sufficiently minor to be nonproblematic; the fact that successive synthetic glucocorticoids had an increasing potency in terms of weight was not of direct therapeutic significance; and the most hoped-for aim, that of dissociating wanted from unwanted glucocorticoid effects has not been achieved (1). Most untoward effects, such as those due to the catabolic and gluconeogenic activities of the glucocorticoid family, probably cannot be dissociated entirely from the anti-inflammatory activity (2) it is possible that myopathy and muscle wasting are actually more common when triamcinolone or dexamethasone are used, but this may merely reflect overdosage of these potent

drugs. However, some progress in achieving a dissociation of effects has been made. Beclomethasone does have a relatively greater local than systemic effect. Deflazacort, one of the few new glucocorticoids to have been developed in recent years, originally promised reduced intensity of adverse effects, for example on bone mineral density, but the early promise has not held up (SEDA-18, 389). Cloprednol seems to affect the hypothalamic–pituitary–adrenal axis much less than other glucocorticoids, and to cause less excretion of nitrogen and calcium (3).

Uses

Most patients who are treated therapeutically with glucocorticoids do not have glucocorticoid deficiency. Adverse reactions to glucocorticoids depend very largely on the ways in which, and the purposes for which, they are used. There are four groups of uses.

(1) Substitution therapy is used in cases of primary and secondary adrenocortical insufficiency; the aim is to provide glucocorticoids and mineralocorticoids in physiological amounts, and the better the dosage regimen is adapted to the individual's needs, the less the chance of adverse effects (1).

(2) Anti-inflammatory and immunosuppressive therapy exploits the immunosuppressive, anti-allergic, anti-inflammatory, anti-exudative, and anti-proliferative effects of the glucocorticoids (2). The desired pharmacodynamic effects reflect a general influence of these substances on the mesenchyme, where they suppress reactions that result in the symptoms of inflammation, exudation, and proliferation; the non-specific effects of glucocorticoids on the mesenchyme are part of their physiological actions, but they can only be obtained to a clinically useful extent by using dosages at which the more specific (and unwanted) physiological effects also occur. High doses sufficient to suppress immune reactions are used in patients who have undergone organ transplantation.

(3) Hormone suppression therapy can be used, for example, to inhibit the adrenogenital syndrome (3). Higher doses are used. The treatment of the adrenogenital syndrome is only partly substitutive and has to be adapted to the individual case, but doses are needed

Table 1 Relative potencies of glucocorticoids

Compound	Glucocorticoid potency relative to hydrocortisone	Mineralocorticoid potency	Equivalent doses (mg)
Cortisone	0.8	++	25
Hydrocortisone	1.0	++	20
Prednisone	4	+	5
Prednisolone	4	+	5
Methylprednisolone	5	0	4
Triamcinolone	5	0	4
Paramethasone	10	0	2
Fluprednisolone	10	0	1.5
Dexamethasone	30	0	0.75
Betamethasone	30	0	0.6

at which various hormonal effects of the glucocorticoids and mineralocorticoids are likely to become troublesome.

(4) Massive doses of glucocorticoids, far exceeding physiological amounts, are given in the immediate management of anaphylaxis, although their beneficial effects are delayed for several hours. This is because, in severely ill patients, early administration of hydrocortisone 100–300 mg as the sodium succinate salt can gradually enhance the actions of adrenaline (4). Glucocorticoids have been used as an adjunct to the use of inotropic and vasopressor drugs for septic shock. Their efficacy, as well as their proposed mechanisms of action, is controversial; inhibition of complement-mediated aggregation and resultant endothelial injury, and inhibition of the release of beta-endorphin are current theories of their mechanism of action. However, controlled studies have not indicated a beneficial effect of high-dose glucocorticoid therapy in treating septic shock (5,6). Hence, there is no established role for glucocorticoids in the treatment of shock, except shock caused by adrenal insufficiency.

Routes of administration

Glucocorticoids can be given by the following routes:

- oral
- rectal
- intravenous
- intramuscular
- inhalation
- nasal
- topical (skin, eyes, ears)
- intradermal
- intra-articular and periarticular
- intraspinal (epidural, intrathecal)
- intracapsular (breast)

All of these routes are covered in this monograph, except the inhalation route, which is the subject of a separate monograph.

Observational studies

A study has been undertaken to clarify whether glucocorticoid excess affects endothelium-dependent vascular relaxation in glucocorticoid treated patients and whether dexamethasone alters the production of hydrogen peroxide and the formation of peroxynitrite, a reactive molecule between nitric oxide and superoxide, in cultured human umbilical endothelial cells (7). Glucocorticoid excess impaired endothelium-dependent vascular relaxation in vivo and enhanced the production of reactive oxygen species to cause increased production of peroxynitrite in vitro. Glucocorticoid-induced reduction in nitric oxide availability may cause vascular endothelial dysfunction, leading to hypertension and atherosclerosis.

Comparative studies

In another randomized trial, the effects and adverse effects of early dexamethasone on the incidence of chronic lung disease have been evaluated in 50 high-risk preterm infants (8). The treated infants received dexamethasone intravenously from the fourth day of life for 7 days (0.5 mg/kg/day for the first 3 days, 0.25 mg/kg/day for the next 3 days, and 0.125 mg/kg/day on the seventh day). The incidence of chronic lung disease at 28 days of life and at 36 weeks of postconceptional age was significantly lower in the infants who were given dexamethasone, who also remained intubated and required oxygen therapy for a shorter period. Hyperglycemia, hypertension, growth failure, and left ventricular hypertrophy were the transient adverse effects associated with early glucocorticoid administration. Early dexamethasone administration may be useful in preventing chronic lung disease, but its use should be restricted to preterm high-risk infants.

Placebo-controlled studies

Patients taking glucocorticoids have an increased risk of infections, including those produced by opportunistic and rare pathogens. However, it has been suggested that glucocorticoid administration in severe community-acquired pneumonia could attenuate systemic inflammation and lead to earlier resolution of pneumonia and a reduction in sepsis-related complications. In a placebo-controlled study in 46 patients with severe community-acquired pneumonia who received protocol-guided antibiotic treatment hydrocortisone (intravenous 200 mg bolus followed by infusion at a rate of 10 mg/hour) for 7 days produced significant clinical improvement (9). Adverse effects were not described.

Although there have been several trials of early dexamethasone to determine whether it would reduce mortality and chronic lung disease in infants with respiratory distress, the optimal duration and adverse effects of such therapy are unknown. The purpose of one study was: (a) to determine if a 3-day course of early dexamethasone therapy would reduce chronic lung disease and increase survival without chronic lung disease in neonates who received surfactant therapy for respiratory distress syndrome and (b) to determine the associated adverse effects (10). This was a prospective, placebo-controlled, multicenter, randomized study of a 3-day course of early dexamethasone therapy, beginning at 24–48 hours of life in 241 neonates, who weighed 500–1500 g, had received surfactant therapy, and were at significant risk of chronic lung disease or death. Infants randomized to dexamethasone received a 3-day tapering course (total dose 1.35 mg/kg) given in six doses at 12-hour intervals. Chronic lung disease was defined by the need for supplementary oxygen at a gestational age of 36 weeks. Neonates randomized to early dexamethasone were more likely to survive without chronic lung disease (RR = 1.3; CI = 1.0, 1.7) and were less likely to develop chronic lung disease (RR = 0.6; CI = 0.3, 0.98). Mortality rates were not significantly different. Subsequent dexamethasone therapy was less in early dexamethasone-treated neonates (RR = 0.8; CI = 0.70, 0.96). Very early (before 7 days of life) intestinal perforations were more common among dexamethasone-treated neonates (8 versus 1%). The authors concluded that an early 3-day course of dexamethasone increases survival without chronic lung disease, reduces chronic lung disease, and reduces late dexamethasone therapy in high-risk, low birthweight infants who receive surfactant therapy for respiratory distress syndrome. The potential benefits of early dexamethasone therapy in the regimen used in this trial need to be weighed against the risk of early intestinal perforation.

Although dexamethasone is commonly associated with transient adverse effects, several randomized trials have shown that it rapidly reduces oxygen requirements and shortens the duration of ventilation. A randomized study was designed to evaluate the effects of two different dexamethasone courses on growth in preterm infants (11). The first phase included 30 preterm infants at high risk of chronic lung disease, of whom 15 (8 boys) were given dexamethasone for 14 days, from the tenth day of life; they received a total dose of 4.75 mg/kg; 15 babies were assigned to the control group (8 boys). The second phase included 30 preterm infants at high risk of chronic lung disease, of whom 15 babies (7 boys) were treated with dexamethasone for 7 days, from the fourth day of life; they received a total dose of 2.38 mg/kg; 15 babies were assigned to the control group (9 boys). Infants given dexamethasone had significantly less weight gain than controls, but they caught up soon after the end of treatment. At 30 days of life, the gains in weight and length in each group were similar to those in control infants, but those given dexamethasone had significantly less head growth. There were no differences between the groups at discharge. The longer-term impact of postnatal dexamethasone on mortality and morbidity is less clear. Better data, from larger clinical trials with longer follow-up, will determine whether this kind of treatment enhances lives, makes little difference, causes significant harm, or does several of these things (12).

Systematic reviews

A systematic review of glucocorticoid adjunctive therapy in adults with acute bacterial meningitis has been published (13). Five trials involving 623 patients were included (pneumococcal meningitis = 234, meningococcal meningitis = 232, others = 127, unknown = 30). Treatment with glucocorticoids was associated with a significant reduction in mortality (RR = 0.6; 95% CI = 0.4, 0.8) and in neurological sequelae (RR = 0.6; 95% CI = 0.4, 1), and with a reduction in case-fatality in pneumococcal meningitis of 21% (RR = 0.5; 95% CI = 0.3, 0.8). In meningococcal meningitis, mortality (RR = 0.9; 95% CI = 0.3, 2.1) and neurological sequelae (RR = 0.5; 95% CI = 0.1, 1.7) were both reduced, but not significantly. Adverse events were similar in the treatment and placebo groups (RR = 1; CI = 0.5, 2), with gastrointestinal bleeding in 1% of glucocorticoid-treated patients and 4% of

the rest. The authors recommended the early use of glucocorticoid therapy in adults in whom acute community-acquired bacterial meningitis is suspected.

A systematic review of randomized controlled trials has been performed to determine whether dexamethasone therapy in the first 15 days of life prevents chronic lung disease in premature infants (14). Studies were identified by a literature search using Medline (1970–97) supplemented by a search of the Cochrane Library (1998, Issue 4). Inclusion criteria were: (a) prospective randomized design with initiation of dexamethasone therapy within the first 15 days of life; (b) report of the outcome of interest; and (c) less than 20% crossover between the treatment and control groups during the study period. The primary outcomes were mortality at hospital discharge and the development of chronic lung disease at 28 days of life and 36 weeks postconceptional age. The secondary outcomes were the presence of a patent ductus arteriosus and treatment adverse effects. Dexamethasone reduced the incidence of chronic lung disease by 26% at 28 days (RR = 0.74; CI = 0.57, 0.96) and 48% at 36 weeks postconceptional age (RR = 0.52; CI = 0.33, 0.81). These reductions were more significant when dexamethasone was started in the first 72 hours of life. The 24% relative risk reduction of deaths was marginally significant (RR = 0.76; CI = 0.56, 1.04). The 27% reduction in patent ductus arteriosus and the 11% increase in infections were not statistically significant, nor were any other changes. The conclusion from this meta-analysis was that systemic dexamethasone given to at-risk infants soon after birth may reduce the incidence of chronic lung disease. There was no evidence of significant short-term adverse effects.

General adverse effects

The incidence and severity of adverse reactions to glucocorticoids depend on the dose and duration of treatment. Even the very high single doses of glucocorticoids, such as methylprednisolone, which are sometimes used, do not cause serious adverse effects, whereas an equivalent dose given over a long period of time can cause many long-term effects.

The two major risks of long-term glucocorticoid therapy are adrenal suppression and Cushingoid changes. During prolonged treatment with anti-inflammatory doses, glucose intolerance, osteoporosis, acne vulgaris, and a greater or lesser degree of mineralocorticoid-induced changes can occur. In children, growth can be retarded, and adults who take high doses can have mental changes. There may be a risk of gastroduodenal ulceration, although this is much less certain than was once thought. Infections and abdominal crises can be masked. Some of these effects reflect the catabolic properties of the glucocorticoids, that is their ability to accelerate tissue breakdown and impair healing. Allergic reactions can occur.

Anyone who prescribes long-term glucocorticoids should have a checklist in mind of the undesired effects that they can exert, both during treatment and on

Table 2 Risks of long-term glucocorticoid therapy

1. Exogenous hypercorticalism with Cushing's syndrome
Moon face (facial rounding)
Central obesity
Striae
Hirsutism
Acne vulgaris
Ecchymoses
Hypertension
Osteoporosis
Proximal myopathy
Disorders of sexual function
Diabetes mellitus
Hyperlipidemia
Disorders of mineral and fluid balance (depending on the type of glucocorticoid)
2. Adrenal insufficiency
Insufficient or absent stress reaction
Withdrawal effects
3. Unwanted results accompanying desired effects
Increased risk of infection
Impaired wound healing
Peptic ulceration, bleeding, and perforation
Growth retardation
4. Other adverse effects
Mental disturbances
Encephalopathy
Increased risk of thrombosis
Posterior cataract
Increased intraocular pressure and glaucoma
Aseptic necrosis of bone

withdrawal, so that any harm that occurs can be promptly detected and countered. The main groups of risks arising from long-term treatment with glucocorticoids are summarized in Table 2.

The adverse reactions that were reported in a study of 213 children are listed in Table 3 (15).

Drug interactions that affect the efficacy of glucocorticoids have been reviewed (16).

Table 3 Adverse reactions in 213 children given intravenous methylprednisolone

Adverse effect	Number
Behavioral changes	21
Abdominal disorders	11
Pruritus	9
Urticaria	5
Hypertension	5
Bone pain	3
Dizziness	3
Fatigue	2
Fractures	2
Hypotension	2
Lethargy	2
Tachycardia	2
Anaphylactoid reaction	1
"Grey appearance"	1

Organs and Systems

Cardiovascular

The considerable body of evidence that glucocorticoids can cause increased rates of vascular mortality and the underlying mechanisms (increased blood pressure, impaired glucose tolerance, dyslipidemia, hypercoagulability, and increased fibrinogen production) have been reviewed (17). In view of their adverse cardiovascular effects, the therapeutic options should be carefully considered before long-term glucocorticoids are begun; although they can be life-saving, dosages should be regularly reviewed during long-term therapy, in order to minimize complications.

The benefit of glucocorticoid therapy is often limited by several adverse reactions, including cardiovascular disorders such as hypertension and atherosclerosis. Plasma volume expansion due to sodium retention plays a minor role, but increased peripheral vascular resistance, due in part to an increased pressor response to catecholamines and angiotensin II, plays a major role in the pathogenesis of hypertension induced by glucocorticoid excess. However, the molecular mechanism remains unclear.

Long-term systemic administration of glucocorticoids might be expected, because of their effects on vascular fragility and wound healing, to increase the risk of vascular complications during percutaneous coronary intervention. To assess the potential risk of long-term glucocorticoid use in the setting of coronary angioplasty, 114 of 12 883 consecutively treated patients who were taking long-term glucocorticoids were compared with those who were not. Glucocorticoid use was not associated with an increased risk of composite events of major ischemia but was associated with a threefold risk of major vascular complications and a three- to fourfold risk of coronary perforation (18).

Hypertension

The secondary mineralocorticoid activity of glucocorticoids can lead to salt and water retention, which can cause hypertension. Although the detailed mechanisms are as yet uncertain, glucocorticoid-induced hypertension often occurs in elderly patients and is more common in patients with total serum calcium concentrations below the reference range and/or in those with a family history of essential hypertension (SEDA-20, 368; 19).

Hemangioma is the most common tumor of infancy, with a natural history of spontaneous involution. Some hemangiomas, however, as a result of their proximity to vital structures, destruction of facial anatomy, or excessive bleeding, can be successfully treated with systemic glucocorticoids between other therapies. The risk of hypertension is poorly documented in this setting. In one prospective study of 37 infants (7 boys, 17 girls; mean age 3.5 months, range 1.5–10) with rapidly growing complicated hemangiomas treated with oral prednisone 1–5 mg/kg/day, blood pressure increased in seven cases (20). Cardiac ultrasound examination in five showed two cases of myocardial hypertrophy, which was unrelated to the hypertension and which regressed after withdrawal of the prednisone.

Myocardial ischemia

Cortisone-induced cardiac lesions are sometimes reported and electrocardiographic changes have been seen in patients taking glucocorticoids (21). Whereas abnormal myocardial hypertrophy in children has perhaps been associated more readily with corticotropin, it has been seen on occasion during treatment with high dosages of glucocorticoids, with normalization after dosage reduction and withdrawal.

Fatal myocardial infarction occurred after intravenous methylprednisolone for an episode of ulcerative colitis (22).

- A day after a dose of intravenous methylprednisolone 60 mg a 79-year-old woman developed acute thoracic pain and collapsed. An electrocardiogram showed signs of a myocardial infarction and her cardiac enzyme activities were raised. She died within several hours. Autopsy showed an anterior transmural myocardial infarction and mild atheromatous lesions in the coronary arteries.

This report highlights the risk of cardiovascular adverse effects with short courses of glucocorticoid therapy in elderly patients with inflammatory bowel disease, even with rather low-dosage regimens. Acute myocardial infarction occurred in an old man with coronary insufficiency and giant cell arteritis after treatment with prednisolone (SEDA-10, 343) but could well have been coincidental.

Myocardial ischemia has been reportedly precipitated by intramuscular administration of betamethasone

(SEDA-21, 413; 23). It has been suggested that long-term glucocorticoid therapy accelerates atherosclerosis and the formation of aortic aneurysms, with a high risk of rupture (SEDA-20, 369; 24).

Patients with seropositive rheumatoid arthritis taking long-term systemic glucocorticoids are at risk of accelerated cardiac rupture in the setting of transmural acute myocardial infarction treated with thrombolytic drugs (25).

- Two women and one man, aged 53–74 years, died after they received thrombolytic therapy for acute myocardial infarction. All three had a long history of seropositive rheumatoid arthritis treated with prednisone 5–20 mg/day for many years.

Cardiomyopathy

Postnatal exposure to glucocorticoids has been associated with hypertrophic cardiomyopathy in neonates. Such an effect has not previously been described in infants born to mothers who received antenatal glucocorticoids. Three neonates (gestational ages 36, 29, and 34 weeks), whose mothers had been treated with betamethasone prenatally in doses of 12 mg twice weekly for 16 doses, 8 doses, and 5 doses respectively, developed various degrees of hypertrophic cardiomyopathy diagnosed by echocardiography (26). There was no maternal evidence of diabetes, except for one infant whose mother had a normal fasting and postprandial blood glucose before glucocorticoid therapy, but an abnormal 1-hour postprandial glucose after 8 weeks of betamethasone therapy, with a normal HbA$_{1C}$ concentration. There was no family history of hypertrophic cardiomyopathy, no history of maternal intake of other relevant medications, no hypertension, and none of the infants received glucocorticoids postnatally. Follow-up echocardiography showed complete resolution in all infants. The authors suggested that repeated antenatal maternal glucocorticoids might cause hypertrophic cardiomyopathy in neonates. These changes appear to be dose- and duration-related and are mostly reversible.

Transient hypertrophic cardiomyopathy is a rare sequel of the concurrent administration of glucocorticoid and insulin excess (SEDA-21, 412; 27). The heart is also almost certainly a site for myopathic changes analogous to those that affect other muscles.

Transient hypertrophic cardiomyopathy has been attributed to systemic glucocorticoid administration for a craniofacial hemangioma (28).

- A 69-day-old white child presented with a rapidly growing 2.5 × 1.5 cm hemangioma of the external left nasal side wall. He was normotensive and there was no family history of cardiomyopathy or maternal gestational diabetes. Because of nasal obstruction and possible visual obstruction, he was given prednisolone 3 mg/kg/day. After 10 weeks his weight had fallen from 7.6 to 7.1 kg and 2 weeks later he became tachypneic with a respiratory rate of 40/minutes. A chest X-ray showed cardiomegaly and pulmonary venous congestion. An echocardiogram showed hypertrophic cardiomyopathy. The left ventricular posterior wall thickness was 10 mm (normal under 4 mm), and the peak left ventricular outflow gradient was 64 mmHg. He was given a beta-blocker and a diuretic and the glucocorticoid dose was tapered. The cardiomyopathy eventually resolved.

Dilated cardiomyopathy caused by occult pheochromocytoma has been described infrequently.

- A 34-year-old woman had acute congestive heart failure 12 hours after administration of dexamethasone 16 mg for an atypical migraine (29). The authors postulated that the acute episode had been induced by the dexamethasone, which increased the production of adrenaline, causing beta$_2$-adrenoceptor stimulation, peripheral vasodilatation, and congestive heart failure.

In an addendum the authors reported another similar case.

Obstructive cardiomyopathy has been attributed to a glucocorticoid in a child with subglottal stenosis (30).

- A 4-month-old boy (weight 4 kg) developed fever, nasal secretions, and stridor due to a subglottal granuloma. Dexamethasone 1 mg/kg/day was started and tapered over 1 week. The mass shrank to 25% of its original size but the symptoms recurred 2 weeks later. The granuloma was excised and dexamethasone 1 mg/kg/day was restarted. After 5 days he developed a tachycardia (140/minute) and a new systolic murmur. Echocardiography showed severe ventricular hypertrophy with dynamic left ventricular outflow tract obstruction. The dexamethasone was weaned over several days. Over the next 3 weeks several echocardiograms showed rapid resolution of the outflow tract obstruction and gradual improvement of the cardiac hypertrophy. After 8 months there was no further problem.

Cardiac dysrhythmias

Serious cardiac dysrhythmias and sudden death have been reported with pulsed methylprednisolone. Oral methylprednisolone has been implicated in a case of sinus bradycardia (31).

- A 14-year-old boy received an intravenous dose of methylprednisolone 30 mg/kg for progressive glomerulonephritis. After 5 hours, his heart rate had fallen to 50/minute and an electrocardiogram showed sinus bradycardia. His heart rate then fell to 40/minutes and a temporary transvenous pacemaker was inserted and methylprednisolone was withdrawn. His heart rate increased to 80/minutes over 3 days. After a further 3 days, he was treated with oral methylprednisolone 60 mg/m^2/day and his heart rate fell to 40/minutes in 5 days. Oral methylprednisolone was stopped on day 8 of treatment and his heart rate normalized.

Hypokalemia, secondary to mineralocorticoid effects, can cause cardiac dysrhythmias and cardiac arrest.

Recurrent cardiocirculatory arrest has been reported (32).

- A 60-year-old white man was admitted for kidney transplantation. Immediately after reperfusion and intravenous methylprednisolone 500 mg, he developed severe bradycardia with hypotension and then cardiac arrest. After resuscitation, his clinical state improved quickly, but on the morning of the first postoperative day

directly after the intravenous administration of methylprednisolone 250 mg, he had another episode of severe bradycardia, hypotension, and successful cardiopulmonary resuscitation. A third episode occurred 24 hours later after intravenous methylprednisolone 100 mg, again followed by rapid recovery after resuscitation. Two weeks later, during a bout of acute rejection, he was given intravenous methylprednisolone 500 mg, after which he collapsed and no heartbeat or breathing was detectable; after cardiopulmonary resuscitation he was transferred to the intensive care unit, where he died a few hours later.

If patients at risk are identified, glucocorticoid bolus therapy should be avoided or, if that is not possible, should only be done under close monitoring.

Pericarditis

- Disseminated *Varicella* and staphylococcal pericarditis developed in a previously healthy girl after a single application of triamcinolone cream 0.1% to relieve pruritus associated with *Varicella* skin lesions (SEDA-22, 443; 33).

Vasculitis

Long-term treatment with glucocorticoids can cause arteritis, but patients with rheumatoid arthritis have a special susceptibility to vascular reactions, and cases of periarteritis nodosa after withdrawal of long-term glucocorticoids have been reported (34).

Respiratory

Local adverse effects are common in patients with asthma who use inhaled glucocorticoids, as suggested by a survey of the prevalence of throat and voice symptoms in patients with asthma using glucocorticoids by metered-dose pressurized aerosol (SEDA-20, 369; 35).

There have been no reports of an increased frequency of lower respiratory tract infections. However, patients with aspiration of gastric material who were treated with glucocorticoids did not have improved survival but had a higher incidence of pneumonia (SED-12, 982).

In cases of pneumothorax with closed thoracotomy tube drainage, chronic glucocorticoid treatment has been reported to delay and impede re-expansion of the lung (SED-8, 820).

Hiccup is a rare complication of glucocorticoid therapy; five cases have been published at various times (36).

- A 59-year-old man had intractable hiccups during treatment with dexamethasone for multiple myeloma (37).
- Persistent hiccupping has been described in a 30-year-old man after the administration of a single intravenous dose of dexamethasone (16 mg) (38). The symptom was resistant to metoclopramide and resolved spontaneously after 4 days. On rechallenge, the hiccups recurred within 2 hours and disappeared after 36 hours.

Low-dose metoclopramide can be effective and may allow a patient to continue beneficial therapy without the discomfort and exhaustion that can accompany intractable hiccups.

Ear, nose, throat

Atrophic changes and fungal and other infections can alter the nasal mucosa after aerosol treatment (39), and since most systematic published documentation on these intranasal products is limited to 1–2 years of experience (although they have been in use for a far longer period), some reserve is warranted with respect to their long-term safety and the wisdom of continual use.

Nervous system

Cerebral venous thrombosis associated with glucocorticoid treatment has rarely been reported. A relation between glucocorticoids and venous thrombosis has already been suggested but has never been clearly understood. Three young patients, two women (aged 28 and 45) and one man (aged 38 years), developed cerebral venous thrombosis after intravenous high-dose glucocorticoids (40). All presented with probable multiple sclerosis according to clinical, CSF, and MRI criteria. All had a lumbar puncture and were then treated with methylprednisolone 1 g/day for 5 days. All the usual causes of cerebral venous thrombosis were systematically excluded. The authors proposed that glucocorticoids interfere with blood coagulation and suggested that the administration of glucocorticoids after a lumbar puncture carries a particular risk of complications.

Dexamethasone is widely used for the prevention and treatment of chronic lung disease in premature infants, in whom follow-up studies have raised the possibility of an association with alterations in neuromotor function and somatic growth. In 159 survivors (mean age 53 months) of a previous placebo-controlled study, the children who had received dexamethasone had a significantly higher incidence of cerebral palsy (39/80 versus 12/79; OR = 4.62; 95% CI = 2.38, 8.98) (41). The most common form of cerebral palsy was spastic diplegia. Developmental delay was more frequent in the dexamethasone group (44/80 versus 23/79; OR = 2.9; CI = 1.5, 5.4). In a systematic review the authors concluded that postnatal dexamethasone at currently recommended doses should be avoided because of long-term neurological adverse effects (42). Lower doses of dexamethasone or inhaled glucocorticoids might be indicated for ill ventilator-dependent infants with chronic lung disease after the age of 2 weeks.

In 146 children who participated in a placebo-controlled trial of early postnatal dexamethasone therapy for the prevention of the chronic lung disease of prematurity, follow-up at school age (mean age 8 years old) showed that the children who had received dexamethasone were significantly shorter than the controls (mean height 122.8 cm versus 126.4 cm for boys and 121.3 cm versus 124.7 cm for girls) and had a significantly smaller head circumference (49.8 cm versus 50.6 cm) (43). They also had significantly poorer motor skills, motor coordination, and visuomotor integration. Compared with the controls, the children who had received dexamethasone had significantly lower IQ scores, including full scores

(mean 78.2 versus 84.4), verbal scores (84.1 versus 88.4), and performance scores (76.5 versus 84.5). The frequency of clinically significant disabilities was higher among the children who had received dexamethasone than among the controls (39% versus 22%). The authors did not recommend the routine use of dexamethasone therapy for the prevention or treatment of chronic lung disease.

Long-term treatment with glucocorticoids can cause cerebral atrophy (44).

Severe organic brain syndrome has been seen in six patients taking long-term glucocorticoids (SEDA-3, 304). The manifestations included confusion, disorientation, apathy, confabulation, irrelevant speech, and slow thinking; the symptoms occurred abruptly.

Latent epilepsy can be made manifest by glucocorticoid treatment. Seizures in patients with lung transplants were related to glucocorticoids, which had been used in high dosages to prevent organ rejection. There was an increased risk of seizures in younger patients (under 25 years) and with intravenous methylprednisolone (SEDA-21, 413) (45).

Long-term glucocorticoid treatment can result in papilledema and increased intracranial pressure (the syndrome of pseudotumor cerebri or so-called "benign intracranial hypertension"), particularly in children.

- Benign intracranial hypertension occurred in a 7-month-old child after withdrawal of topical betamethasone ointment and in a 7-year-old boy treated with a 1% cortisol ointment in large amounts.
- A 6-year-old girl, who had taken prednisone for 2.5 years for nephrotic syndrome with seven relapses in 3 years, developed symptoms of benign intracranial hypertension after oral glucocorticoid dosage reduction over 10 months from 30 mg/day to 2.5 mg/every other day (46). Laboratory studies and head CT scan were normal, but there was bilateral papilledema and the cerebrospinal fluid pressure was increased. She was given prednisone 1 mg/kg/day initially, with acetazolamide, and 25 ml of cerebrospinal fluid was removed. All her symptoms resolved and treatment was gradually withdrawn. She developed no further visual failure.

The symptoms can simulate those of an intracranial tumor. All patients taking large doses of glucocorticoids who complain of headache or blurred vision, particularly after a reduction in dosage, should have an ophthalmoscopic examination to exclude this complication. Paradoxically, cerebral edema occurring during a surgical procedure can be partly prevented by glucocorticoids (47).

An encephalopathy can occur at any age (SEDA-18, 387), not necessarily in association with intracranial hypertension.

There have been repeated reports of epidural lipomatosis, which can lead to spinal cord compression (48,49) or spinal fracture (50); in one instance, the excised lipomata contained brown fat, a phenomenon that may prove to be not unusual in glucocorticoid-induced lipomata (SEDA-16, 451).

- A 40-year-old woman with ulcerative colitis took cortisone 20 mg/day and developed progressive paraplegia

(50). There was kyphosis of the thoracic spine from T7 to T9, with pathological fractures. An MRI scan showed massive epidural fat extending from T1 to T9. She recovered 3 months after surgical removal of the epidural fat.

- A 78-year-old man was given methylprednisolone (60 mg/day reducing to 8 mg/day) for temporal arteritis (51). After 4 months, he developed numbness and paresis of the legs and hyperalgesia at dermatomes T3 and T4. After 10 months he had marked disturbance of proprioception combined with spinal ataxia and an increasing loss of motor bladder control. There was an intraspinal epidural lipoma in the dorsal part of the spine from T1-10. The fat was removed surgically and within 4 weeks his gait disturbance and proprioception improved, the sensory deficit abated, and the bladder disorder disappeared completely.

- A 57-year-old man took prednisone 20–30 mg/day for 13 years for rheumatoid arthritis (52). He had been treated unsuccessfully with gold, azathioprine, hydroxychloroquine, and sulfasalazine; tapering his glucocorticoid dosage had been unsuccessful. He developed worsening back pain in his thoracic spine and lateral leg weakness. He was unable to walk. He was Cushingoid and had marked thoracic kyphosis associated with multiple vertebral body fractures in T5-8. An MRI scan at T5-6 showed displacement and compression of the spinal cord by high-signal epidural fat, which had caused anterior thecal displacement and total effacement of cerebrospinal fluid.

The authors of the last report commented on the high dose of prednisone used.

Glucocorticoid-induced spinal epidural lipomatosis is not very common in children. Spinal magnetic resonance imaging was performed in 125 children with renal diseases (68 boys); they either had back pain or numbness, were obese, or had taken a cumulative dose of prednisone of more than 500 mg/kg; there was lipomatosis in five patients (53).

In the past there was reason to think that glucocorticoids might precipitate multiple sclerosis. However, this has not been confirmed, and there is evidence that a special glucocorticoid regimen can actually be capable of retarding deterioration in multiple sclerosis (SEDA-18, 387).

A Guillain–Barré-like syndrome occurred in a patient receiving high-dose intravenous glucocorticoid therapy (SEDA-16, 449). Although glucocorticoids have been used successfully to treat weakness due to chronic inflammatory demyelinating sensorimotor neuropathy, other types of acquired chronic demyelinating neuropathies can be impaired by these drugs.

- In four patients with a pure motor demyelinating neuropathy treated with oral prednisolone (60 mg/day) motor function rapidly deteriorated within 4 weeks of starting prednisolone (SEDA-19, 375; 54). Intravenous immunoglobulin some months later in two of them produced clear improvement in strength and motor nerve conduction.

Sensory systems

The eye can be involved in generalized adverse reactions to systemically administered glucocorticoids. For example, conjunctivitis can occur as part of an allergic reaction and infections of the eye can be masked as a result of anti-inflammatory and analgesic effects. Ophthalmoplegia can occur as one of the consequences of glucocorticoid myopathy (SEDA-16, 450). Two complications that require special discussion are cataract and glaucoma.

Cataract

Oral glucocorticoid treatment is a risk factor for the development of posterior subcapsular cataract. A review of nine studies including 343 asthmatics treated with oral glucocorticoids showed a prevalence of posterior subcapsular cataracts of 0–54% with a mean value of 9% (55). In a 1993 study in children taking low-dose prednisone there were cataracts in seven of 23 cases (56). Some studies have shown a clear correlation with the duration of treatment and total dosage, others have not (SEDA-17, 449). The use of inhaled glucocorticoids was associated with a dose-dependent increased risk of posterior subcapsular and nuclear cataracts in 3654 patients aged 49–97 years (SEDA-22, 446; 57). Data on glucocorticoid use were available for 3313 of these patients; glucocorticoid use was classified as none in 2784 patients, inhaled only in 241, systemic only in 177, and both inhaled and systemic in 111. Compared with nonuse, current or prior use of inhaled glucocorticoids was associated with a significant increase in the prevalence of nuclear cataracts (adjusted relative prevalence = 1.5; 95% CI = 1.2, 1.9) and posterior subcapsular cataracts (1.9; 1.3, 2.8), but not cortical cataracts. The increased prevalence of posterior subcapsular cataracts was significantly associated with current use of inhaled glucocorticoids (2.6; 1.7, 4.0); there was no association with past use. Current use of inhaled glucocorticoids was also associated with an increased prevalence of cortical cataracts (1.4; 1.1, 1.7). The highest prevalences of posterior subcapsular and grade 4 or 5 nuclear cataracts were found in patients who had taken a cumulative dose of beclomethasone over 2000 mg.

It has been suggested that the risk of cataract is higher in patients with rheumatoid arthritis than in patients with bronchial asthma, and it is also higher in children. The reversibility of the lenticular changes has often been discussed (58,59), but even without glucocorticoid withdrawal regression has been found in children taking long-term treatment (60). Nevertheless, some 7% of the patients who develop cataract caused by glucocorticoid treatment have to be operated on. A change in permeability of the lens capsule, followed by altered electrolyte concentrations in the lens and a change in the mucopolysaccharides in the lens have been advanced as reasons for the development of cataract.

Increased intraocular pressure and glaucoma

Ocular hypertension and open-angle glaucoma are well-known adverse effects of ophthalmic administration of glucocorticoids (SEDA-17, 449).

Frequency

A total of 113 patients with angiographically proven subretinal neovascularization were enrolled into a prospective study of the effects of intravitreal triamcinolone (61). About 30% developed a significant rise in intraocular pressure (at least 5 mmHg) above baseline during the first 3 months.

A large case-control study, in which 9793 elderly patients with ocular hypertension or open-angle glaucoma were compared with 38 325 controls, has shown an increased risk of these complications with oral glucocorticoids (SEDA-22, 446; 62). The risk of ocular hypertension or open-angle glaucoma increased with increasing dose and duration of use of the oral glucocorticoid. There was no significant increase in the risk of ocular hypertension or open-angle glaucoma in patients who had stopped taking oral glucocorticoids 15–45 days before. The authors estimated that the excess risk of ocular hypertension or open-angle glaucoma with current oral glucocorticoid use is 43 additional cases per 10 000 patients per year. However, in patients taking over 80 mg/day of hydrocortisone equivalents, the excess risk is 93 additional cases per 10 000 patients per year. Monitoring of intraocular pressure may be justified in long-term users of oral glucocorticoids, as it is in long-term users of topical glucocorticoids.

Prolonged use of high doses of inhaled glucocorticoids also increases the risk of ocular hypertension and open-angle glaucoma (SEDA-22, 446; 63). In a case-control study of the records of 9793 elderly patients with ocular hypertension or open-angle glaucoma over a 6-year period, there was a significantly increased risk of ocular hypertension and open-angle glaucoma in patients who had taken high doses of inhaled glucocorticoids (1500–1600 micrograms) for 3 months or longer (OR = 1.44; 95% CI = 1.01, 2.06). Both a high dosage of inhaled glucocorticoid and prolonged continuous duration of therapy had to be present to increase the risk.

Glaucoma and ocular hypertension have been reported after dermal application of glucocorticoids for facial atopic eczema (SEDA-19, 376) (64), and after treatment with beclomethasone by nasal spray and inhalation (SEDA-20, 373; 65).

The effects of topical dexamethasone on intraocular pressure have been compared with those of fluorometholone (SEDA-22, 446; 66). The ocular hypertensive response to topical dexamethasone in children occurs more often, more severely, and more rapidly than that reported in adults. It should be avoided in children if possible and it is desirable to monitor the intraocular pressure when it is being used. Fluorometholone may be more acceptable.

Pathogenesis

The pathogenesis of glucocorticoid-induced glaucoma is still unknown, but there is reduced outflow, and excessive accumulation of mucopolysaccharides may be a major factor. An association with cataract and papilledema has often been observed. The rise in intraocular pressure is variable: in the pediatric study of low dose cited above there was a reversible effect in only two of 23 subjects

compared with controls, but in other studies serious increases in pressure have occurred, with a risk of blindness.

There is almost certainly a genetic predisposition to glucocorticoid-induced glaucoma, as there is to glaucoma in general.

Susceptibility factors

Children have more frequent, more severe, and more rapid ocular hypertensive responses to topical dexamethasone than adults. In one case a systemic glucocorticoid caused significant but asymptomatic ocular hypertension in a child (67).

- A 9-year-old girl with acute lymphoblastic leukemia received a 5-week course of oral prednisolone 60 mg/day (2.3 mg/kg/day). She did not receive any other systemic medications that have a known effect on intraocular pressure. Her baseline pressures in the right and left eyes were 16 and 17 mmHg with visual acuities of 20/20 and 20/15 respectively. The cup-to-disk ratio was 0.5 in both eyes, with normal visual fields. She was not myopic and had no family history of glaucoma or glucocorticoid responsiveness. After 8 days of systemic glucocorticoid therapy, her intraocular pressures increased to 39 mmHg and 38 mmHg in the right and left eyes respectively. Gonioscopy confirmed an open drainage angle in both eyes. She was given topical betaxolol 0.25% and dorzolamide 2% bd. However, her intraocular pressure continued to increase to 52 mmHg in the right eye and 47 mm Hg in the left eye on day 10. Topical latanoprost 0.001% od and brimonidine 0.2% bd were added, and the intraocular pressures fell to 38 mmHg and 36 mmHg. Two days after withdrawal of the prednisolone, the intraocular pressure returned rapidly to 17 mm Hg in both eyes. Over the next 6 weeks, this was maintained despite stepwise withdrawal of all glaucoma medications. Four months later, she was given a 4-week course of oral dexamethasone 10 mg/day and had similar patterns of changes in intraocular pressure. Oral acetazolamide was prescribed. She remained largely asymptomatic throughout, except for one episode of reduced visual acuity from 20/20 to 20/40 in the right eye when the intraocular pressure reached 52 mmHg.

Chorioretinopathy

Systemic glucocorticoid treatment can cause severe exacerbation of bullous exudative retinal detachment and lasting visual loss in some patients with idiopathic central serous chorioretinopathy (SEDA-20, 374; 68). The atypical presentation of this condition can include peripheral retinal capillary nonperfusion and retinal neovascularization. The treatment of choice in patients with idiopathic central serous chorioretinopathy is laser photocoagulation.

In a prospective, case-control study 38 consecutive patients (28 men and 10 women), aged 28–63 years with central serous chorioretinopathy, were compared with 38 age- and sex-matched controls (28 men and 10 women) aged 27–65 years (69). Eleven patients (29%; eight men and three women) with central serous chorioretinopathy were taking glucocorticoids, compared with two patients (5.2%; one man and one woman) in the control group (OR = 7.33, 95% CI = 1.49, 36).

Subtenon local injection of a glucocorticoid is effective in the treatment of certain forms of uveitis. Central serous chorioretinopathy, confirmed by optical coherence tomography, developed after a single local subtenon glucocorticoid injection to treat HLA-B27-associated iritis (70).

- A healthy 37-year-old man developed progressive blurred vision, photophobia, and floaters in the left eye. Best-corrected visual acuity was 20/20 in the right eye and 20/50 in the left eye. The intraocular pressures were 21 mmHg in the right eye and 16 mmHg in the left eye. The anterior and posterior segments of the right eye were normal, but the anterior segment of the left eye showed 2+ conjunctival injection and mild keratitic precipitates. There was a 2+ anterior chamber cellular reaction with a 1 mm hypopyon, engorged iris vessels, and fibrinous iris posterior synechiae that were released after pupillary dilatation. Binocular and indirect ophthalmoscopy of the left eye showed a normal optic nerve, macula, retinal vasculature, and periphery. There was no evidence of retinal or vitreous inflammation, vasculitis, or cystoid macular edema. The fovea was well visualized after pupillary dilatation, with a normal and distinct foveal reflex. HLA-B27 iritis was suspected and subsequently confirmed with positive serotyping. He was given prednisolone acetate 1% every hour, cycloplegic eye drops, and a 1.0 ml periocular injection of triamcinolone acetonide (40 mg/ml) into the subtenon space of the left eye. Within 1 week, there was a marked therapeutic response, with complete resolution of the hypopyon and fibrin deposition and partial improvement in acuity to 20/40 in the left eye. There were only occasional residual anterior chamber inflammatory cells. Macular biomicroscopy showed the new development of subretinal fluid and serous pigment epithelial detachment at the fovea. Fluorescein angiography confirmed an enlarging pinpoint spot of hyperfluorescence. Optical coherence tomography confirmed the subretinal location of this fluid collection, consistent with a diagnosis of central serous chorioretinopathy. The topical glucocorticoid drops were rapidly tapered and withdrawn over 5 days. There was progressive reduction in subretinal fluid and gradual improvement in visual acuity. By 12 weeks the fluid had resolved and visual acuity recovered to 20/20 in the left eye.

Endophthalmitis

Intravitreal triamcinolone injection is safe and effective for cystoid macular edema caused by uveitis, diabetic maculopathy, and central retinal vein occlusion, and for pseudophakic cystoid macular edema. Potential risks include glaucoma, cataract, retinal detachment, and endophthalmitis. Infectious endophthalmitis is extremely rare when appropriate sterile technique is practised. Seven patients developed a clinical picture simulating endophthalmitis after intravitreal injection of triamcinolone (71). The authors believed that this effect was a toxic

reaction to the injected material and explained that the differential diagnosis of infectious endophthalmitis in eyes that have been injected with triamcinolone under sterile conditions includes a sterile toxic endophthalmitis that requires careful monitoring, perhaps every 8-12 hours, in order to determine whether the inflammation is worsening or improving. Resolution occurs spontaneously, and in the absence of eye pain unnecessary intervention can be avoided.

Hypopyon associated with non-infectious endophthalmitis after intravitreal injection of triamcinolone has been described previously (72). Pseudohypopyon and sterile endophthalmitis after intravitreal injection of triamcinolone for pseudophakic cystoid macular edema has been reported (73).

- An 88-year-old woman underwent phacoemulsification surgery, which was complicated by posterior capsule rupture. Anterior vitrectomy was performed, with implantation of a silicone intraocular lens into the sulcus. Postoperatively, she developed cystoid macular edema, which failed to respond to topical dexamethasone, topical ketorolac, and posterior subtenon injection of triamcinolone, limiting visual acuity to 6/24 at 7 months after the surgery. An intravitreal injection of triamcinolone acetonide (4 mg in 0.1 ml) (Kenalog®, Bristol-Myers Squibb, Middlesex, UK) was administered through the pars plana with a 30-gauge needle using a sterile technique. Three days later she reported painless loss of vision, which had developed immediately after the injection. Visual acuity was reduced to perception of hand movements. There was minimal conjunctival injection and the cornea was clear. A 3 mm pseudohypopyon, consisting of refractile crystalline particles, was visible in the anterior chamber, associated with 3+ anterior chamber cells (or particles). Severe vitreous haze prevented visualization of the retina. Because infectious endophthalmitis could not be excluded, she was treated with intravitreal injections of ceftazidime and vancomycin. Vitreous and aqueous taps were performed and the pseudohypopyon was completely aspirated from the anterior chamber. The next day a 2 mm pseudohypopyon had reformed. The position of the pseudohypopyon depended on gravity and shifted with changes in head position. Aqueous and vitreous cultures were negative. Microscopy of the aspirated pseudohypopyon showed triamcinolone particles with no cells. The pseudohypopyon, vitreous haze, and cystoid macular edema (as demonstrated on optical coherence tomography) resolved spontaneously over 6 weeks and visual acuity recovered to 6/12.

The pseudohypopyon was a unique feature of this case and was due to the presence of a posterior capsule defect enabling the passage of triamcinolone from the vitreous cavity into the anterior chamber. The authors commented that presumably the triamcinolone crystals had been carried into the anterior chamber by currents generated by saccadic eye movements in the partially vitrectomized vitreous cavity. In this case the pseudohypopyon was distinguishable from an infective or inflammatory hypopyon by its ground glass appearance, the presence of refractile particles, and its shifting position, which depended on the patient's head position. The absence of ocular pain, photophobia, ciliary injection, or iris vessel dilatation suggested a non-inflammatory response and perhaps it would be appropriate to monitor such patients closely rather than administering intravitreal antibiotics.

Keratopathy and keratitis

Band-shaped keratopathy is caused by the deposition of calcium salts in the basement membrane of the corneal epithelium and superficial stroma. It is typically a chronic process that develops over a period of months and years, and is associated with chronic corneal or intraocular inflammation.

- Infectious crystalline keratopathy developed in a 73-year-old woman with noninsulin-dependent diabetes mellitus after the use of topical prednisolone 1% eye-drops, for conjunctival injection over 12 months (SEDA-20, 372; 74).
- Acute-onset calcific band keratopathy has been reported in a woman using topical prednisolone (SEDA-20, 372; 75).

Patients with severe keratoconjunctivitis sicca are at definite risk of this complication, and the addition of phosphate-containing eye-drops tilted the precariously balanced situation toward precipitation of calcium in the cornea and bandage contact lens. Acetate-containing rather than phosphate-containing glucocorticoid eye drops may be a safer alternative in patients with such predisposing factors.

Bacterial keratitis is one of the most frequent ophthalmic infections. In a meta-analysis of publications from 1950 to 2000, the use of a topical glucocorticoid before the diagnosis of bacterial keratitis significantly predisposed to ulcerative keratitis in eyes with pre-existing corneal disease (OR = 2.63; 95% CI = 1.41, 4.91). Previous glucocorticoid use significantly increased the risk of antibiotic failure or other infectious complications (OR = 3.75; 95% CI = 2.52, 5.58). The use of glucocorticoids with an antibiotic for the treatment of bacterial keratitis did not increase the risk of complications, but neither did it improve the outcome of treatment.

Retinal damage

An apparent association between severe retinopathy of prematurity and dexamethasone therapy has been shown in a retrospective study (SEDA-20, 372; 76). Infants treated with dexamethasone required longer periods of mechanical ventilation (44 versus 26 days), had a longer duration of supplemental oxygen (57 versus 29 days), had a higher incidence of patent ductus arteriosus (28/38 versus 18/52), and required surfactant therapy more often for respiratory distress syndrome (17/38 versus 11/52). Prospective, randomized, controlled studies are needed to correct for differences in severity of cardiorespiratory disease. Until such studies are available, careful consideration must be given to indications, dosage, time of

initiation, and duration of treatment with dexamethasone in infants of extremely low birthweight.

Retinal hemorrhage occurred in four women after they had received epidural methylprednisolone for chronic back and hip pain (SEDA-20, 373; 77). Retinal and choroidal vascular occlusions are a serious and sometimes lasting complication of periocular and facial injections of glucocorticoids (SEDA-21, 416).

Toxic optic neuropathy

Toxic optic neuropathy can occur and may underlie various reports of sudden blindness in patients taking glucocorticoids. In one case, transient visual loss occurred on several occasions, each time after administration of a glucocorticoid (SEDA-17, 447). In another case, blindness occurred suddenly and paradoxically after glucocorticoid injections into the nasal turbinates (78). Although glucocorticoids are sometimes used successfully to relieve pre-existing optic neuritis, a number of such patients react adversely with increased episodes of visual loss.

Exophthalmos

Exophthalmos has been described incidentally as a complication of long-term glucocorticoid therapy and there has been a series of 21 cases (79).

Psychological

The psychostimulant effects of the glucocorticoids are well known (80), and their dose dependency is recognized (SED-11, 817); they may amount to little more than euphoria or comprise severe mental derangement, for example mania in an adult with no previous psychiatric history (SEDA-17, 446) or catatonic stupor demanding electroconvulsive therapy (81). In their mildest form, and especially in children, the mental changes may be detectable only by specific tests of mental function (82). Mental effects can occur in patients treated with fairly low doses; they can also occur after withdrawal or omission of treatment, apparently because of adrenal suppression (83,84).

- A 32-year-old woman developed irritability, anger, and insomnia after taking oral prednisone (60 mg/day) for a relapse of ileal Crohn's disease (85). The prednisone was withdrawn and replaced by budesonide (9 mg/day), and the psychiatric adverse effects were relieved after 3 days. A good clinical response was maintained, with no relapse after 2 months of budesonide therapy.

Seventeen patients taking long-term glucocorticoid therapy (16 women, mean age 47 years, mean prednisone dose 16 mg, mean length of current treatment 92 months) and 15 matched controls were assessed with magnetic resonance imaging and proton magnetic resonance spectroscopy, neurocognitive tests (including the Rey Auditory Verbal Learning Test, Stroop Colour Word Test, Trail Making Test, and estimated overall intelligent quotient), and psychiatric scales (including the Hamilton Rating Scale for Depression, Young Mania Rating Scale, and Brief Psychiatric Rating Scale) (86). Glucocorticoid-treated patients had smaller hippocampal volumes and lower N-acetylaspartate ratios than controls. They had lower scores on the Rey Auditory Verbal Learning Test and Stroop Colour Word Test (declarative memory deficit) and higher scores on the Hamilton Rating Scale for Depression and the Brief Psychiatric Rating Scale (depression). These findings support the idea that chronic glucocorticoid exposure is associated with changes in hippocampal structure and function.

Development

Dexamethasone has been used in ventilator-dependent preterm infants to reduce the risk and severity of chronic lung disease. Usually it is given in a tapering course over a long period (42 days). The effects of dexamethasone on developmental outcome at 1 year of age has been evaluated in 118 infants of very low birthweights (47 boys and 71 girls, aged 15–25 days), who were not weaning from assisted ventilation (87). They were randomly assigned double-blind to receive placebo or dexamethasone (initial dose 0.25 mg/kg) tapered over 42 days. A neurological examination, including ultrasonography, was done at 1 year of age. Survival was 88% with dexamethasone and 74% with placebo. Both groups obtained similar scores in mental and psychomotor developmental indexes. More dexamethasone-treated infants had major intracranial abnormalities (21 versus 11%), cerebral palsy (25 versus 7%; OR = 5.3; CI = 1.3, 21), and unspecified neurological abnormalities (45 versus 16%; OR = 3.6; CI = 1.2, 11). Although the authors suggested an adverse effect, they added other possible explanations for these increased risks (improved survival in those with neurological injuries or at increased risk of such injuries).

Behavioral disorders

Children have marked increases in behavioral problems during treatment with high-dose prednisone for relapse of nephrotic syndrome, according to the results of a study conducted in the USA (88). Ten children aged 2.9–15 years (mean 8.2 years) received prednisone 2 mg/kg/day, tapering at the time of remission, which was at week 2 in seven patients. At baseline, eight children had normal behavioral patterns and two had anxious/depressed and aggressive behavior using the Child Behaviour Checklist (CBCL). During high-dose prednisone therapy, five of the eight children with normal baseline scores had CBCL scores for anxiety, depression, and aggressive behavior above the 95th percentile for age. The two children with high baseline CBCL scores had worsening behavioral problems during high-dose prednisone. Behavioral problems occurred almost exclusively in the children who received over 1 mg/kg every 48 hours. Regression analysis showed that prednisone dosage was a strong predictor of increased aggressive behaviour.

Intravenous methylprednisolone was associated with a spectrum of adverse reactions, most frequently behavioral disorders, in 213 children with rheumatic disease, according to the results of a US study (12). However, intravenous methylprednisolone was generally well tolerated. The children received their first dose of intravenous methylprednisolone 30 mg/kg over at least 60 minutes, and if the first dose was well tolerated they were given

further infusions at home under the supervision of a nurse. There was at least one adverse reaction in 46 children (22%) of whom 18 had an adverse reaction within the first three doses. The most commonly reported adverse reactions were behavioral disorders (21 children), including mood changes, hyperactivity, hallucinations, disorientation, and sleep disorders. Several children had serious acute reactions, which were readily controlled. Most of them were able to continue methylprednisolone therapy with premedication or were given an alternative glucocorticoid. The researchers emphasized the need to monitor treatment closely and to have appropriate drugs readily available to treat adverse reactions.

Large doses are most likely to cause the more serious behavioral and personality changes, ranging from extreme nervousness, severe insomnia, or mood swings to psychotic episodes, which can include both manic and depressive states, paranoid states, and acute toxic psychoses. A history of emotional disorders does not necessarily preclude glucocorticoid treatment, but existing emotional instability or psychotic tendencies can be aggravated by glucocorticoids. Such patients as these should be carefully and continuously observed for signs of mental changes, including alterations in the sleep pattern. Aggravation of psychiatric symptoms can occur not only during high-dose oral treatment, but also after any increase in dosage during long-term maintenance therapy; it can also occur with inhalation therapy (89). The psychomotor stimulant effect is said to be most pronounced with dexamethasone and to be much less with methylprednisolone, but this concept of a differential psychotropic effect still has to be confirmed.

Memory

The effects of prednisone on memory have been assessed (SEDA-21, 413; 90). Glucocorticoid-treated patients performed worse than controls in tests of explicit memory. Pulsed intravenous methylprednisolone (2.5 g over 5 days, 5 g over 7 days, or 10 g over 5 days) caused impaired memory in patients with relapsing-remitting multiple sclerosis, but this effect is reversible, according to the results of an Italian study (91). Compared with ten control patients, there was marked selective impairment of explicit memory in 14 patients with relapsing-remitting multiple sclerosis treated with pulsed intravenous methylprednisolone. However, this memory impairment completely resolved 60 days after methylprednisolone treatment.

Glucocorticoids can regulate hippocampal metabolism, physiological functions, and memory. Despite evidence of memory loss during glucocorticoid treatment (SEDA-23, 428), and correlations between memory and cortisol concentrations in certain diseases, it is unclear whether exposure to the endogenous glucocorticoid cortisol in amounts seen during physical and psychological stress in humans can inhibit memory performance in otherwise healthy individuals. In an elegant experiment on the effect of cortisol on memory, 51 young healthy volunteers (24 men and 27 women) participated in a double-blind, randomized, crossover, placebo-controlled trial of cortisol 40 mg/day or 160 mg/day for 4 days (92). The lower dose of cortisol was equivalent to the cortisol delivered during a mild stress and the higher dose to major stress. Cognitive performance and plasma cortisol were evaluated before and until 10 days after drug administration. Cortisol produced a dose-related reversible reduction in verbal declarative memory without effects on nonverbal memory, sustained or selective attention, or executive function. Exposure to cortisol at doses and plasma concentrations associated with physical and psychological stress in humans can reversibly reduce some elements of memory performance.

Prednisone, 10 mg/day for 1 year, has been evaluated in 136 patients with probable Alzheimer's disease in a double-blind, randomized, placebo-controlled trial (93). There were no differences in the primary measures of efficacy (cognitive subscale of the Alzheimer Disease Assessment Scale), but those treated with prednisone had significantly greater memory impairment (Clinical Dementia sum of boxes), and agitation and hostility/suspicion (Brief Psychiatric Rating Scale). Other adverse effects in those who took prednisone were reduced bone density and a small rise in intraocular pressure.

In healthy individuals undergoing acute stress, there was specifically impaired retrieval of declarative long-term memory for a word list, suggesting that cortisol-induced impairment of retrieval may add significantly to the memory deficits caused by prolonged treatment (94).

In 52 renal transplant recipients (mean age 45 years, 34 men and 18 women) taking prednisone (100 mg/day for 3 days followed by 10 mg/day for as long as needed; mean dose 11 mg/day) there was a major reduction in immediate recall but not delayed recall (95). However, there was a significant correlation between mean prednisone dose and delayed recall. In animals, phenytoin pretreatment blocks the effects of stress on memory and hippocampal histology.

In a double blind, randomized, placebo-controlled trial 39 patients (mean age 44 years, 8 men) with allergies or pulmonary or rheumatological illnesses who were taking prednisone (mean dose 40 mg/day) were randomized to either phenytoin (300 mg/day) or placebo for 7 days (96). Those who took phenytoin had significantly smaller increases in a mania self-report scale. There was no effect on memory. Thus, phenytoin blocked the hypomanic effects of prednisone, but not the effects on declarative memory.

Sleep

The effects of acute systemic dexamethasone administration on sleep structure have been investigated. Dexamethasone caused significant increases in REM latency, the percentage time spent awake, and the percentage time spent in slow-wave sleep. There were also significant reductions in the percentage time spent in REM sleep and the number of REM periods (SEDA-21, 413; 97).

Psychiatric

Use of glucocorticoids is associated with adverse psychiatric effects, including mild euphoria, emotional lability,

panic attacks, psychosis, and delirium. Although high doses increase the risks, psychiatric effects can occur after low doses and different routes of administration. Of 92 patients with systemic lupus erythematosus (78 women, mean age 34 years) followed between 1999 and 2000, psychiatric events occurred in six of those who were treated with glucocorticoids for the first time or who received an augmented dose, an overall 4.8% incidence (98). The psychiatric events were mood disorders with manic features (delusions of grandiosity) ($n = 3$) and psychosis (auditory hallucinations, paranoid delusions, and persecutory ideas) ($n = 3$). Three patients were first time users (daily prednisone dose 30–45 mg/day) and three had mean increases in daily prednisone dose from baseline of 26 (range 15–33) mg. All were hypoalbuminemic and none had neuropsychiatric symptoms before glucocorticoid treatment. All the events occurred within 3 weeks of glucocorticoid administration. In five of the six episodes, the symptoms resolved completely after dosage reduction (from 40 mg to 18 mg) but in one patient an additional 8-week course of a phenothiazine was given. In a multivariate regression analysis, only hypoalbuminemia was an independent predictor of psychiatric events (HR = 0.8, 95% CI = 0.60, 0.97).

Although mood changes are common during short-term, high-dose, glucocorticoid therapy, there are virtually no data on the mood effects of long-term glucocorticoid therapy. Mood has been evaluated in 20 outpatients (2 men, 18 women), aged 18–65 years taking at least 7.5 mg/day of prednisone for 6 months (mean current dose 19 mg/day; mean duration of current prednisone treatment 129 months) and 14 age-matched controls (1 man, 13 women), using standard clinician-rated measures of mania (Young Mania Rating Scale, YMRS), depression (Hamilton Rating Scale for Depression, HRSD), and global psychiatric symptoms (Brief Psychiatric Rating Scale, BPRS, and the patient-rated Internal State Scale, ISS) (99). Syndromal diagnoses were evaluated using a structured clinical interview. The results showed that symptoms and disorders are common in glucocorticoid-dependent patients. Unlike short-term prednisone therapy, long-term therapy is more associated with depressive than manic symptoms, based on the clinician-rated assessments. The Internal State Scale may be more sensitive to mood symptoms than clinician-rated scales.

Psychoses

Mania has been attributed to glucocorticoids (100).

- A 46-year-old man, with an 8-year history of cluster headaches and some episodes of endogenous depression, took glucocorticoids 120 mg/day for a week and then a tapering dosage at the start of his latest cluster episode. His headaches stopped but then recurred after 10 days. He was treated prophylactically with verapamil, but a few days later, while the dose of glucocorticoid was being tapered, he developed symptoms of mania. The glucocorticoids were withdrawn, he was given valproic acid, and his mania resolved after 10 days. Verapamil prophylaxis was restarted and he had no more cluster headaches.

The authors commented that the manic symptoms had probably been caused by glucocorticoids or glucocorticoid withdrawal. They concluded that patients with cluster headache and a history of affective disorder should not be treated with glucocorticoids, but with valproate or lithium, which are effective in both conditions. Lamotrigine, an anticonvulsive drug with mood-stabilizing effects, may prevent glucocorticoid-induced mania in patients for whom valproate or lithium are not possible (101).

Glucocorticoids can cause neuropsychiatric adverse effects that dictate a reduction in dose and sometimes withdrawal of treatment. Of 32 patients with asthma (mean age 47 years) who took prednisone in a mean dosage of 42 mg/day for a mean duration of 5 days, those with past or current symptoms of depression had a significant reduction in depressive symptoms during prednisone therapy compared with those without depression (102). After 3–7 days of therapy there was a significant increase in the risk of mania, with return to baseline after withdrawal.

The management of a psychotic reaction in an Addisonian patient taking a glucocorticoid needs special care (SED-8, 820). Psychotic reactions that do not abate promptly when the glucocorticoid dosage is reduced to the lowest effective value (or withdrawn) may need to be treated with neuroleptic drugs; occasionally these fail and antidepressants are needed (SEDA-18, 387). However, in other cases, antidepressants appear to aggravate the symptoms.

- Two patients with prednisolone-induced psychosis improved on giving the drug in three divided daily doses. Recurrence was avoided by switching to enteric-coated tablets.

This suggests that in susceptible patients the margin of safety may be quite narrow (SED-12, 982). It is possible that reduced absorption accounted for the improvement in this case, but attention should perhaps be focused on peak plasma concentrations rather than average steady-state concentrations.

Two women developed secondary bipolar disorder associated with glucocorticoid treatment and deteriorated to depressive–catatonic states without overt hallucinations and delusions (103).

- A 21-year-old woman, who had taken prednisolone 60 mg/day for dermatomyositis for 1 year developed a depressed mood, pessimistic thought, irritability, poor concentration, diminished interest, and insomnia. Although the dose of prednisolone was tapered and she was treated with sulpiride, a benzamide with mild antidepressant action, she never completely recovered. After 5 months she had an exacerbation of her dermatomyositis and received two courses of methylprednisolone pulse therapy. Two weeks after the second course, while taking prednisolone 50 mg/day, she became hypomanic and euphoric. She improved substantially with neuroleptic medication and continued to take

prednisolone 5 mg/day. About 9 months later she developed depressive stupor without any significant psychological stressor or changes in prednisolone dosage. She had mutism, reduction in contact and reactivity, immobility, and depressed mood. Manic or mixed state and psychotic symptoms were not observed. She was initially treated with intravenous clomipramine 25 mg/day followed by oral clomipramine and lithium carbonate. She improved markedly within 2 weeks with a combination of clomipramine 100 mg/day and lithium carbonate 300 mg/day. Prednisolone was maintained at 5 mg/day.

- A 23-year-old woman with ulcerative colitis and no previous psychiatric disorders developed emotional lability, euphoria, persecutory delusions, irritability, and increased motor and verbal activity 3 weeks after starting to take betamethasone 4 mg/day. She improved within a few weeks with bromperidol 3 mg/day. After 10 months she became unable to speak and eat, was mute, depressive, and sorrowful, and responded poorly to questions. There were no neurological signs and betamethasone had been withdrawn 10 months before. She was treated with intravenous clomipramine 25 mg/day and became able to speak. Intravenous clomipramine caused dizziness due to hypotension, and amoxapine 150 mg/day was substituted after 6 days. All of her symptoms improved within 10 days. Risperidone was added for mood lability and mild persecutory ideation.

In one case, glucocorticoid-induced catatonic psychosis unexpectedly responded to etomidate (104).

- A 27-year-old woman with myasthenia gravis taking prednisolone 100 mg/day became unresponsive and had respiratory difficulties. She was given etomidate 20 mg intravenously to facilitate endotracheal intubation. One minute later she became alert and oriented, with normal muscle strength, and became very emotional. Eight hours later she again became catatonic and had a similar response to etomidate 10 mg. Glucocorticoid-induced catatonia was diagnosed, her glucocorticoid dosage was reduced, and she left hospital uneventfully 4 days later.

The effect of etomidate on catatonia, similar to that of amobarbital, was thought to be due to enhanced GABA receptor function in patients with an overactive reticular system.

A case report has suggested that risperidone, an atypical neuroleptic drug, can be useful in treating adolescents with glucocorticoid-induced psychosis and may hasten its resolution (105).

- A 14-year-old African-American girl with acute lymphocytic leukemia was treated with dexamethasone 24 mg/day for 25 days. Four days after starting to taper the dose she had a psychotic reaction with visual hallucinations, disorientation, agitation, and attempts to leave the floor. Her mother refused treatment with haloperidol. Steroids were withdrawn and lorazepam was given as needed. Nine days later the symptoms had not improved. She was given risperidone 1 mg/day; within 3 days the psychotic reaction began to improve and by 3 weeks the symptoms had completely resolved.

Obsessive-compulsive disorder

Obsessive-compulsive behavior after oral cortisone has been described (106).

- A 75-year-old white man, without a history of psychiatric disorders, took cortisone 50 mg/day for 6 weeks for pulmonary fibrosis and developed severe obsessive-compulsive behavior without affective or psychotic symptoms. He was given risperidone without any beneficial effect. The dose of cortisone was tapered over 18 days. An MRI scan showed no signs of organic brain disease and an electroencephalogram was normal. His symptoms improved 16 days after withdrawal and resolved completely after 24 days. Risperidone was withdrawn without recurrence.

Endocrine

The endocrine effects of the glucocorticoids variously involve the pituitary–adrenal axis, the ovaries and testes, the parathyroid glands, and the thyroid gland.

Pituitary gland

Empty sella syndrome occurred in a boy who developed hypopituitarism after long-term pulse therapy with prednisone for nephrotic syndrome (107).

- A 16-year-old Japanese boy's growth and development was normal until the age of 2 years. He then developed nephrotic syndrome and was treated with pulsed glucocorticoid therapy nine times over the next 14 years. After the age of 3 years, his rate of growth had fallen. At 16 years, when he was taking prednisone 60 mg/m^2/day he was given prednisone on alternate days and the dose was gradually tapered. The secretion of pituitary hormones, except antidiuretic hormone, was impaired and an MRI scan of his brain showed an empty sella and atrophy of the pituitary gland.

When markedly impaired growth is noted in patients treated with glucocorticoids long-term or in pulses, it is necessary to assess pituitary function and the anatomy of the pituitary gland. Children who receive glucocorticoid pulse therapy may develop an empty sella more frequently than is usually recognized.

Pituitary–adrenal axis

Raised glucocorticoid plasma concentrations usually result, after 2 weeks, in the first signs of iatrogenic Cushing's syndrome. The characteristic symptoms can occur individually or in combination. Whereas in Cushing's disease or corticotropin–induced Cushing's syndrome, the predominant symptoms are in part determined by hyperandrogenicity and tend to comprise hypertension, acne, impaired sight, disorders of sexual function, hirsutism or virilism, striae of the skin, and plethora, Cushing's syndrome due to glucocorticoid therapy is likely to cause benign intracranial hypertension, glaucoma, subcapsular cataract, pancreatitis, aseptic necrosis of the bones, and panniculitis. Obesity, facial rounding, psychiatric symptoms, edema, and delayed wound healing are common to these different forms of Cushing's syndrome.

It has been said that Cushing-like effects are to be expected if the function of the adrenal cortex is suppressed by daily doses of more than 50 mg hydrocortisone or its equivalent. However, pituitary–adrenal suppression has been described at lower dosage equivalents, for example during prolonged intermittent therapy with dexamethasone (108). The secondary adrenal insufficiency caused by therapeutically effective doses can be observed even after giving prednisone 5 mg tds for only 1 week; after withdrawal, adrenal suppression lasts for some days. If one continues this treatment for about 20 weeks, maximal atrophy of the adrenal cortex results, and lasts for some months. This effect begins with inhibition of the hypothalamus, and culminates in true atrophy of the adrenal cortex. It can occur even with glucocorticoids given by inhalation (109). Inhaled fluticasone is associated with at least a twofold greater suppression of adrenal function than inhaled budesonide microgram for microgram, according to the results of a crossover study (SEDA-21, 415; 110). Patients with liver disease may experience adrenal suppression with lower doses of glucocorticoids (111). It is advisable to use alternate-day therapy to avoid suppression of corticotropin secretion in patients who will need long-term therapy; it will produce the same therapeutic effect as daily dosage. It can be helpful to measure the degree of suppression of corticotropin secretion during long-term glucocorticoid treatment of asthmatic children, as a means of optimizing therapy and avoiding excessive dosage (112). The period of time during which the patient should be considered at risk of adrenal insufficiency after withdrawal of oral prednisolone treatment in childhood nephrotic syndrome is still controversial. A study in such patients has suggested that adrenal insufficiency may occur up to 9 months after treatment has ended (SEDA-19, 376; 113).

Many protocols for treating children with early B cell acute lymphoblastic leukemia involve 28 consecutive days of high-dose glucocorticoids during induction. The effect of this therapy on adrenal function has been prospectively evaluated (114) in 10 children by tetracosactide stimulation before the start of dexamethasone therapy and every 4 weeks thereafter until adrenal function returned to normal. All had normal adrenal function before dexamethasone treatment and impaired adrenal responses 24 hours after completing therapy. Each child felt ill for 2–4 weeks after completing therapy. Seven patients recovered normal adrenal function after 4 weeks, but three did not have normal adrenal function until 8 weeks after withdrawal. Thus, high-dose dexamethasone therapy can cause adrenal insufficiency lasting more than 4 weeks after the end of treatment. This problem might be avoided by tapering doses of glucocorticoids and providing supplementary glucocorticoids during periods of increased stress.

Tolerance to glucocorticoids in this, as in some other respects, varies from individual to individual; some patients tolerate 30 mg of prednisone for a long time without developing Cushing's syndrome, while others develop symptoms at 7.5 mg; the doses recommended today to avoid Cushing's syndrome in most patients are usually equivalent to hydrocortisone 20 mg. Cushing's syndrome and other systemic adverse effects can occur not only from oral and injected glucocorticoids, but also from topical and intranasal treatment (115) and intrapulmonary or epidural administration (SEDA-19, 376; SEDA-20, 370; 116,117).

- Two patients developed hypopituitarism and empty sella syndrome during glucocorticoid pulse therapy for nephrotic syndrome (SEDA-22, 444; 118).

Glucocorticoid-treated patients with inadequate adrenal function who have an intercurrent illness or are due to undergo surgery will have an inadequate reaction to the resulting stress and need to be temporarily protected by additional glucocorticoid (119).

Iatrogenic Cushing's syndrome after a single low dose is exceptional (120).

- A 45-year-old woman was given a single-dose of intramuscular triamcinolone acetonide 40 mg for acute laryngitis and 1 month later was noted to have a cushingoid appearance. Endocrinological tests confirmed hypothalamic–pituitary–adrenal (HPA) axis suppression. Eight months later, the cushingoid appearance had completely disappeared and HPA function had spontaneously recovered.

Pseudohyperaldosteronism has been reported even after intranasal application of 9-alpha-fluoroprednisolone (SEDA-11, 340).

Parathyroid function

There is antagonism between the parathyroid hormone and glucocorticoids (121). Latent hyperparathyroidism can be unmasked by glucocorticoids (122).

Thyroid function

Even a single dose of corticotropin briefly inhibits the secretion of thyrotrophic hormone. The uptake of radioactive iodine is also suppressed by corticotropin and by glucocorticoids, but this has no clinical relevance. Pathological changes in thyroid function induced by glucocorticoid treatment are reportedly rare.

Metabolism

Glucose metabolism

All glucocorticoids increase gluconeogenesis. The turnover of glucose is increased, more being metabolized to fat, and blood glucose concentration is increased by 10–20%. Glucose tolerance and sensitivity to insulin are reduced, but provided pancreatic islet function is normal, carbohydrate metabolism will not be noticeably altered. So-called "steroid diabetes," a benign diabetes without a tendency to ketosis, but with a low sensitivity to insulin and a low renal threshold to glucose, only develops in one-fifth of patients treated with high glucocorticoid dosages. Even in patients with diabetes, ketosis is not to be expected, since glucocorticoids have antiketotic

activity, presumably through suppression of growth hormone secretion.

Glucocorticoid treatment of known diabetics normally leads to deregulation, but this can be compensated for by adjusting the dose of insulin. The increased gluconeogenesis induced by glucocorticoids mainly takes place in the liver, but glucocorticoid treatment is especially likely to disturb carbohydrate metabolism in liver disease.

When hyperglycemic coma occurs it is almost always of the hyperosmolar nonketotic type. After termination of glucocorticoid treatment, steroid diabetes normally disappears. An apparent exception to these findings is provided by the case of a patient in whom glucocorticoid treatment was followed by severe diabetes with diabetic nephropathy, but this was a seriously ill individual who had already undergone renal transplantation (SEDA-17, 449). Gestational diabetes mellitus was more common in women who had received glucocorticoids with or without beta-adrenoceptor agonists for threatened preterm delivery compared with controls (SEDA-22, 445; 123).

Glucocorticoids probably have more than one effect on carbohydrate metabolism. An increase in fasting glucagon concentration has been observed in volunteers given prednisolone 40 mg/day for 4 days, and this effect may be involved, alongside gluconeogenesis, in glucocorticoid-induced hyperglycemia. Some newer glucocorticoids have been claimed to have smaller effects on blood glucose (as well as less salt and water retention), but further studies are needed to confirm whether this interesting therapeutic approach has been successful (SEDA-13, 353).

Deflazacort, an oxazoline derivative of prednisolone, was introduced as a potential substitute for conventional glucocorticoids in order to ameliorate glucose intolerance. In a randomized study in kidney transplant recipients with pre- or post-transplantation diabetes mellitus, 42 patients who switched from prednisone to deflazacort (in the ratio 5:6 mg) were prospectively compared with 40 patients who continued to take prednisone (SEDA-22, 445; 124). During the mean follow-up period of 13 months, neither graft dysfunction nor acute rejection developed in the conversion group, and there was improvement in blood glucose control. When the conversion group was stratified into those with pre- or post-transplantation diabetes, there were promising effects in the patients with post-transplantation diabetes. More than a 50% dosage reduction of hypoglycemic drugs was possible in 42% of those with post-transplantation diabetes.

The risk of hyperglycemia requiring treatment in patients receiving oral glucocorticoids has been quantified in a case-control study of 11 855 patients, 35 years of age or older, with newly initiated treatment with a hypoglycemic drug (SEDA-19, 375; 125). The risk for initiating hypoglycemic therapy increased with the recent use of a glucocorticoid. The risk grew with increasing average daily glucocorticoid dosage (in mg of hydrocortisone equivalents): 1.77 for 1–39 mg/day, 3.02 for 40–79 mg/day, 5.82 for 80–119 mg/day, and 10.34 for 120 mg/day or more.

Lipid metabolism

High-dose glucocorticoid therapy can cause marked hypertriglyceridemia, with milky plasma (SEDA-15, 421; SEDA-16, 450). It has been suggested that this is caused by abnormal accumulation of dietary fat, reduced post-heparin lipolytic activity, and glucose intolerance (126). An association between glucocorticoid exposure and hypercholesterolemia has been found in several studies (127) and can contribute to an increased risk of atherosclerotic vascular disease.

Most premature neonates need intravenous lipids during the first few weeks of life to acquire adequate energy intake and prevent essential fatty acid deficiency before they can tolerate all nutrition via enteral feeds. Dexamethasone is associated with multiple adverse effects in neonates, including poor weight gain and impairment of glucose and protein metabolism. In ten neonates (four boys, mean age 17.3 days) taking dexamethasone for bronchopulmonary dysplasia, intravenous lipids (3 g/kg/day) caused hypertriglyceridemia in the presence of hyperinsulinemia and increased free fatty acid concentrations (128). Because of concomitant hyperinsulinemia, the authors speculated that dexamethasone reduced fatty acid oxidation, explaining poor weight gain.

Altered fat deposition has been repeatedly reported. Fat can be deposited epidurally and at other sites. Adiposis dolora, which involves the symmetrical appearance of multiple painful fat deposits in the subcutaneous tissues, has on one occasion been attributed to glucocorticoids (SEDA-16, 451).

Tumor lysis syndrome

Acute tumor lysis syndrome is a life-threatening metabolic emergency that results from rapid massive necrosis of tumor cells. There have been repeated reports of an acute tumor lysis syndrome when glucocorticoids are administered in patients with pre-existing lymphoid tumors (129).

- A 60-year-old woman took dexamethasone 4 mg 8-hourly for dyspnea due to a precursor T lymphoblastic lymphoma-leukemia with bilateral pleural effusions and a large mass in the anterior mediastinum (130). She developed acute renal insufficiency and laboratory evidence of the metabolic effects of massive cytolysis. She received vigorous hydration, a diuretic, allopurinol, and hemodialysis. She recovered within 2 weeks and then underwent six courses of CHOP chemotherapy. The mediastinal mass regressed completely. She remained asymptomatic until she developed full-blown acute lymphoblastic leukemia, which was resistant to treatment.

Electrolyte balance

The severity of potassium loss due to glucocorticoids depends partly on the amount of sodium in the diet; the most widely used synthetic glucocorticoids cause less potassium excretion than natural hydrocortisone does. Prednisone and prednisolone have a glucocorticoid activity 4–5 times that of hydrocortisone, but their mineralocorticoid activity is less (see Table 1); even at high

dosages they do not cause noteworthy sodium and water retention. Of the major synthetic glucocorticoids, dexamethasone has the strongest anti-inflammatory, hyperglycemic, and corticotropin-inhibitory activity; sodium retention is completely absent; the degree of glucocorticoid-induced metabolic alkalosis may also be less with dexamethasone than with hydrocortisone or methylprednisolone (SEDA-10, 343).

Mineral balance

There can be increases in calcium and phosphorus loss because of effects on both the kidney and the bowel, with increased excretion and reduced resorption (131). Tetany, which has been seen in patients receiving high-dose long-term intravenous glucocorticoids, has been explained as being due to hypocalcemia, and there are also effects on bone. Tetany has also been reported in a patient with latent hyperparathyroidism after the administration of a glucocorticoid (122).

Hypocalcemic encephalopathy occurred in a 35-year-old woman with hypoparathyroidism. It was believed that the administration of methylprednisolone intramuscularly had precipitated severe hypocalcemia, which had led to a metabolic encephalopathy (SEDA-20, 371; 132).

The administration of large doses of glucocorticoids to patients with major burns presenting with low cardiac output has been reported to produce a reversible drop in serum zinc, which might lead to impaired tissue repair (SED-8, 824), but it is not clear whether this has clinical effects.

Metal metabolism

Glucocorticoids increase chromium losses and glucocorticoid-induced diabetes can be reversed by chromium supplementation (133). Doses of hypoglycemic drugs were also reduced by 50% in all patients when they were given supplementary chromium.

Hematologic

Erythrocytes

Polycythemia is a symptom of Cushing's syndrome, and conversely anemia correlates with Addison's disease, but polycythemia is not generally encountered as a consequence of treatment with glucocorticoids, perhaps because there is no increased secretion of androgens; an increase in hemoglobin was nevertheless the most frequent adverse effect observed in a study over 8 years of 77 patients treated for hyperergic-allergic reactions. At the beginning of treatment more than 40% (and during continuous therapy more than 70%) of patients showed this change in erythrocytes (134). There was leukocytosis in more than 60% in the early phases and in more than 40% later (134). Thrombocytosis occurred in 5–10% during continuous treatment. This report agrees fairly well with some older publications, but it has been noted in the past that in the long run very high-dose glucocorticoid treatment can result in suppression of the activity of the bone marrow with fatty infiltration replacing hemopoietic tissue.

Leukocytes

Not all classes of leukocytes are affected by glucocorticoids in the same way. The total leukocyte count is increased, but the number of eosinophilic leukocytes falls, as does the lymphocyte count. The number of monocytes is reduced, as is their capacity to perform phagocytosis.

In children, a leukemoid reaction has been induced by betamethasone treatment (135); this possibility must always be borne in mind, since glucocorticoids can actually be used to treat leukemia or its complications. A case of very high white blood cell count with neutrophilia in a preterm infant whose mother had received two doses of betamethasone prenatally to enhance fetal lung maturation is one of a short list of leukemoid reactions possibly attributable to antenatal glucocorticoid treatment (136).

It is possible that in children with acute lymphoblastic leukemia, glucocorticoid therapy adversely affects the duration of remissions, and it has therefore been suggested that leukemia should be ruled out in children before starting long-term therapy with glucocorticoids (SEDA-11, 340). Depression of the lymphocyte count seems to be a general and direct action of the glucocorticoids (137), but the mechanism is still incompletely understood; certainly, lymphocytolysis seems to be increased by glucocorticoids. Studies of lymphocyte subpopulations show a preferential reduction in T cells, while B cells are constant or slightly reduced. B lymphocyte function (measured as immunoglobulin synthesis) falls, suppressor T lymphocyte activity is suppressed, and helper T lymphocyte function is unaffected by glucocorticoids (SEDA-3, 308) (138).

- Fever and leukopenia with methylprednisolone and prednisolone has been reported in a 29-year-old woman with systemic lupus erythematosus (139).

The authors commented that fever associated with glucocorticoids occurs frequently, whereas leukopenia is rare. Fever and leukopenia are important signs of an exacerbation of systemic lupus erythematosus, and it would be difficult to distinguish between an exacerbation of the disease and an adverse effect of glucocorticoids.

Platelets and coagulation

In heart transplant recipients, intramuscular glucocorticoids can impair fibrinolysis, producing susceptibility to thrombotic disease (SEDA-22, 443; 140). They can also increase the platelet count. In one patient the blue toe syndrome occurred repeatedly when glucocorticoids were used to increase the platelet count (SEDA-16, 451).

Mouth

Oral candidiasis is seen in some 5–10% of patients who use inhaled glucocorticoids, particularly when oral hygiene is poor, but is rarely symptomatic. The risk can be reduced by the use of a large-volume spacer (141,142).

Hypertrophy of the tongue has been attributed to inhaled beclomethasone and may have been related to edema of the buccal mucosa and tongue from direct contact with the glucocorticoid, infection, glossitis caused by glucocorticoid therapy, a direct effect of glucocorticoids on the tongue muscle, or excess localized deposition of fat, as is seen in patients given systemic glucocorticoids (SEDA-20, 371; 143).

Gastrointestinal

Peptic ulceration

It is no longer seriously believed that glucocorticoid treatment in adults markedly increases the risk of peptic ulceration (144,145). However, the symptoms of an existing peptic ulcer can certainly be masked. There may also be a genuine risk of ulcerative disorders in premature children. The issue has often been complicated by the simultaneous (sometimes unrecorded) use of ulcerogenic non-steroidal anti-inflammatory agents. A meta-analysis of whether glucocorticoid therapy caused peptic ulcer and other putative complications of glucocorticoid therapy was negative: peptic ulcers occurred in nine of 3267 patients in the placebo group (0.03%) and 13 of 3335 patients in the glucocorticoid group (0.04%).

Peptic ulcer should not be considered a contraindication when glucocorticoid therapy is indicated (SEDA-19, 376; 146). However, the risk of a fatal outcome due to ulcer complications was increased about fourfold in a previous case-control study. Gastrointestinal hemorrhage occurred more often in glucocorticoid-treated patients (2.25%) than in controls (1.6%) (147). The frequency of gastrointestinal bleeding in these studies compares well with earlier observations in the Boston Collaborative Surveillance Program's 1978 report, according to which 0.5% of a large series of medical inpatients taking glucocorticoids had gastrointestinal bleeding sufficiently severe to require transfusions and 28% had minor bleeding (SED-12, 986).

- A 47-year-old woman developed a gastrocolic fistula during treatment with aspirin (dosage and duration of therapy not stated) and prednisone for chronic rheumatoid arthritis (148).

The author commented that 50–75% of gastrocolic fistulas are related to benign gastric ulcers secondary to the use of NSAIDs. The use of aspirin plus prednisone, as in this patient, increases the risk of complication of peptic ulcer disease two- to fourfold.

The mechanism of whatever harm glucocorticoids may do to the stomach is not clear; cortisol neither consistently increases acid or pepsinogen secretion, nor reduces the protective production of mucin by the gastric mucosa. Serum gastrin concentrations are raised in Cushing's syndrome and in patients taking prolonged glucocorticoid treatment. On the other hand, the secretion of prostaglandin E_2 in gastric juice in response to pentagastrin was impaired during glucocorticoid therapy in children. Since PGE_2 has a cytoprotective effect on the gastric mucosa, impaired secretion in response to increased acid secretion during glucocorticoid therapy may be related to the development of peptic ulcer (SEDA-19, 376; 149).

Some reports suggest that people with hepatic cirrhosis or nephrotic syndrome are particularly at risk. Whatever the degree of risk, patients taking long-term glucocorticoids should be regularly checked to detect peptic ulcers, which can bleed and even perforate without producing pain. There do not seem to be differences in gastric tolerance between the various synthetic glucocorticoids.

Regional ileitis

While glucocorticoids may have a beneficial effect on regional ileitis, perforation of the ileum, lymphatic dilatation, and microscopic fistulae have been observed after treatment.

Ischemic colitis

Glucocorticoids should be used with caution in progressive systemic sclerosis, and concomitant administration of anticoagulants to prevent ischemic colitis is recommended when administering glucocorticoids in high doses, especially by pulse therapy (SEDA-21, 415; 150).

Ulcerative colitis

A possible risk of glucocorticoid treatment of ulcerative colitis is the development of toxic megacolon or colonic perforation. A change from ulcerative colitis to Crohn's disease may have been induced by prolonged treatment with glucocorticoids (SEDA-19, 376; 151). This case provides further evidence for the view that ulcerative colitis and Crohn's disease may represent a continuous spectrum of inflammatory bowel disease and raises the possibility that reduced polymorphonuclear leukocyte function caused by glucocorticoids may have provoked the development of granulomata.

Diverticular disease

Existing diverticula can perforate during glucocorticoid therapy (SEDA-18, 387). Abdominal tenderness is the most common and often the only early sign of perforated diverticula in patients taking glucocorticoids. However, in some cases, even abdominal tenderness is absent (SEDA-22, 445; 152).

- Perforation of the sigmoid colon occurred in a 61-year-old Caucasian man with colonic diverticular disease and rheumatoid arthritis treated with pulses of methylprednisolone 1 g (153).

The authors suggested that methylprednisolone pulses should be used carefully in patients over 50 years of age and/or people with demonstrated or suspected diverticular disease.

The importance of treatment with glucocorticoids and NSAIDs in the development of sigmoid diverticular abscess perforation has been the subject of a case-control study in 64 patients (38 women), median age 70 years (range 39–91) and 320 age- and sex-matched controls (154). Independently of rheumatic diagnosis glucocorticoid treatment was strongly associated with sigmoid diverticular abscess perforation (OR = 32; 95% CI = 6.4, 159).

Liver

The process of gluconeogenesis, which is promoted by glucocorticoids, takes place mainly in the liver. The glycolytic enzymes of the liver are also activated by these glucocorticoids. The synthesis of ribonucleic acid and of enzymes involved in protein catabolism is increased, but the process of protein catabolism takes place outside the liver as well, for example in the muscles. There is experimental evidence for glucocorticoid-induced enhancement of hepatic lipid synthesis (SEDA-3, 308), but the main effect of glucocorticoids in this connection is lipid mobilization from adipose tissue. The influence of long-term glucocorticoid treatment on liver function is still unknown. If pathological changes are diagnosed, the possible influence of the disease which is being treated has to be borne in mind.

Liver damage from glucocorticoids is rarely severe, but fatal liver failure has been reported.

- A 71-year-old white woman with a compressive optic neuropathy was given five cycles of intravenous methylprednisolone 1 g/day for 3 days followed by tapering oral cortisone for 10–14 days (155). The intervals between cycles were 14 days to 6 weeks. She was otherwise healthy and had no history of liver disease. Her liver function tests were normal or only slightly raised during the first five cycles. She then developed raised liver enzymes, a prolonged prothrombin time, and fatal liver failure. Postmortem examination showed necrosis of the liver parenchyma. Hepatitis serology (A, B, and C) was negative as was in situ hybridization for immunohistochemical proof of hepatitis Bs and Bc or delta virus antibodies in the liver.

- A 53-year-old woman who took prednisolone 20 mg/day for systemic lupus erythematosus for 38 days developed increased aspartate transaminase and alanine transaminase activities (175 and 144 IU/l respectively on day 38 and 871 and 658 IU/l on day 69) (156). She denied taking hepatotoxic drugs. Serological tests for hepatitis viruses were all negative. Autoantibodies against mitochondria and smooth muscle were not detected. Ultrasound and CT scan were consistent with fatty infiltration. Histology showed macrovesicular fat infiltration, periportal cell infiltration with fibrosis, and a few Mallory bodies. The glucocorticoid was gradually tapered and the transaminases gradually fell.

- A 67-year-old teetotaler was given intravenous prednisolone 25 mg tds for primary dermatomyositis and 8 days later developed painless icteric hepatitis, with daily progressive marked deterioration of liver biochemistry (157). She had not taken any other hepatotoxic drugs, and serological tests for hepatitis and hepatotropic viruses were all negative. Antinuclear, antimitochondrial, and smooth muscle autoantibodies were negative. Ultrasound and CT scan of the upper abdomen showed liver fatty infiltration. Prednisolone was tapered gradually, and she gradually improved. However, on day 26 she developed pneumonia and died 6 days later.

Glucocorticoid treatment in the early phase of acute viral hepatitis carries the risk of transition to chronic active hepatitis (SEDA-3, 308).

Three children developed hepatomegaly and raised liver enzymes after receiving high-dose dexamethasone therapy (0.66–1.09 mg/kg/day) (158).

There has been a report of seven cases of acute severe liver damage associated with intravenous glucocorticoid pulse therapy in patients with Grave's ophthalmopathy (159).

Pancreas

Pancreatitis and altered pancreatic secretion can occur at any time during long-term glucocorticoid treatment (SED-12, 986; SEDA-14, 339; 160). Necrosis of the pancreas during glucocorticoid treatment has been described and can be lethal. Impairment of pancreatic function can predispose to glucocorticoid-induced pancreatitis. Two other cases of glucocorticoid-induced pancreatitis have been reported (161).

- A 74-year-old woman with seronegative rheumatoid arthritis was given sulfasalazine followed by methotrexate, both of which were withdrawn because of adverse effects. She also took prednisone 10 mg/day. She developed acute abdominal pain and fever (38.7°C) with no chills. Her serum amylase was 269 IU/l, serum lipase 300 IU/l, and urinary amylase 2895 IU/l. There was no evidence of tumor, hypertriglyceridemia, or lithiasis. In addition to prednisone, she was taking amlodipine, bromazepam, and omeprazole, none of which have been reported to cause pancreatitis. A marked improvement was noted after prednisone withdrawal.
- A 68-year-old woman who had taken prednisone 30 mg/day for polymyalgia rheumatica for 6 months developed sharp stabbing abdominal pain, fever (39°C), and vomiting. Her serum amylase was 310 IU/l, serum lipase 340 IU/l, and urinary amylase 1560 IU/l. Other causes of pancreatitis were ruled out. She had been taking a thiazide diuretic therapy for the past 10 years. Her symptoms improved noticeably after prednisone withdrawal.

Although the literature suggests a causal relation between glucocorticoid therapy and these various pancreatic complications there is still no certainty; glucocorticoid treatment is, after all, often given simultaneously with other forms of therapy which can cause pancreatitis (SED-11, 82). The strongest evidence that there is a causal relation is provided by a Japanese report on 52 autopsies, which showed marked changes in pancreatic histology in glucocorticoid-treated patients compared with controls (SEDA-17, 449).

Acute pancreatitis after rechallenge provides direct evidence that hydrocortisone can cause acute pancreatitis in a patient with ulcerative colitis (162).

- An 18-year old youth was admitted with a history of large bowel diarrhea off and on for 6 months before admission. There was a history of passage of blood mixed with stools for the same duration. There was no history of fever, arthralgias, jaundice, or red eyes. At the time of admission he was passing 10-12 stools in 24

hours, and 6-7 of them contained blood. His pulse rate was 100/minute and there was pallor and minimal pedal edema. He was tender in the flanks with exaggerated bowel sounds. Sigmoidoscopy showed ulceration, erythema, friability, and loss of vascular pattern in the rectum and sigmoid colon, suggestive of ulcerative colitis. A rectal biopsy showed crypt atrophy, crypt abscesses, a mixed cellular infiltrate, goblet cell depletion, and submucosal edema. He was given intravenous fluids and injectable hydrocortisone 100 mg six times an hour. Injections of ofloxacin and metronidazole were added later, because his leukocyte count was $15.6 \times 10^9/l$. On the second day of treatment he developed epigastric pain radiating to the back. The pain was continuous, associated with vomiting, and relieved by sitting in the knee-chest position. Acute pancreatitis was corroborated by a serum lipase activity of 650 units/l and high serum amylase activity (550 units/l). Ultrasonography showed a bulky, heterogeneous pancreas with ill defined margins, suggestive of pancreatitis. There were no gallstones. Hydrocortisone was withdrawn and the rest of the treatment continued. Mesalazine was added after 1 day. The pancreatitis resolved in 48 hours, as did the diarrhea. After 1 month the patient was readmitted with a relapse of ulcerative colitis. This time his stool frequency was 4–5 stools in 24 hours, and most contained some blood. There was no fever and his total leukocyte count was normal. He was given mesalazine enemas and injectable hydrocortisone. On the second day after admission, he had a similar bout of acute pancreatitis. Hydrocortisone was withdrawn and he recovered.

Urinary tract

Urinary calculi are more likely during glucocorticoid treatment because of increased excretion of calcium and phosphate (131).

Prednisolone can cause an abrupt rise in proteinuria in patients with nephrotic syndrome. A placebo-controlled study in 26 patients aged 18–68 years with nephrotic syndrome has clarified the mechanisms responsible for this (163). Systemic and renal hemodynamics and urinary protein excretion were measured after prednisolone (125 mg or 150 mg when body weight exceeded 75 kg) and after placebo. Prednisolone increased proteinuria by changing the size–selective barrier of the glomerular capillaries. Neither the renin–angiotensin axis nor prostaglandins were involved in these effects of prednisolone on proteinuria.

Changes resembling diabetic nodular glomerular sclerosis have been seen in glucocorticoid-treated nephrosis.

Treatment with glucocorticoids can result in minor increases in the urinary content of leukocytes and erythrocytes without clear renal injury (164).

The use of high doses of glucocorticoids to counter rejection of renal transplants is still a matter of intensive study; the optimal dose to ensure an effect without undue risk of complications has yet to be agreed on (165).

Vasopressin-resistant polyuria induced by intravenous administration of a therapeutic dose of dexamethasone has been reported (SEDA-20, 370; 166) and nocturia is fairly common during glucocorticoid treatment (167).

The administration of glucocorticoids should be undertaken with caution in progressive systemic sclerosis and the concomitant administration of anticoagulants to prevent scleroderma renal crisis is recommended when administering glucocorticoids in high doses, especially by pulse therapy (SEDA-21, 415; 150).

Skin

Acne is common during treatment, particularly after topical application, and is said to be correlated with the use of compounds that have a particularly strong local effect (168), although this is not proven.

Leukoderma can occur, accompanied by normal melanocyte function but reduced phagocytic activity of the keratinocytes to eliminate the melanosomes (169). Depigmentation can occur at the site of injection of glucocorticoids.

Three cases of severe lipoatrophy, one also with leukoderma, occurring within the same family after intramuscular injection of triamcinolone, suggested genetic susceptibility to this adverse effect (SEDA-3, 303).

Inhibition of the function of the sebaceous glands in the skin is caused by glucocorticoids whilst androgens stimulate their function (170).

A delayed hypersensitivity reaction, characterized by a skin rash, due to dexamethasone has been reported (171). These kinds of reactions to systemic glucocorticoids are rarely reported.

- A 59-year-old woman, who had not used glucocorticoids before, developed an exfoliative rash on her face, upper chest, and skin folds after 3 days treatment with oral dexamethasone (dosage not stated) for an acute episode of encephalomyelitis disseminata. Dexamethasone was immediately withdrawn and her skin lesions resolved over several days. Patch tests were positive to dexamethasone, betamethasone, and clobetasol, but negative to other glucocorticoids, including prednisolone, hydrocortisone butyrate, methylprednisolone, and triamcinolone. Prick tests with all of these glucocorticoids were negative. She tolerated oral methylprednisolone without adverse effects.

Reduced skin thickness and bruising

The glucocorticoids reduce subcutaneous collagen and cause atrophic changes in the skin (172). Subcutaneous atrophy after intramuscular and intra-articular injection has often been reported. Ecchymosis and paper-thin skin folds recall those seen in old people. An increased incidence of subcutaneous ecchymosis in older women has been observed during treatment with triamcinolone acetate (173). Purpura has been observed during glucocorticoid treatment and an increased fragility of the capillaries is thought to occur in about 60% of these patients. There have been reports of cutaneous bruising after the use of high doses of inhaled glucocorticoids (budesonide and

beclomethasone), suggesting systemic absorption (SEDA-21, 416; 174).

Prednicarbate is a topical glucocorticoid that seems to have an improved benefit–harm balance, as has been shown in 24 healthy volunteers (7 men, 17 women, aged 25–49 years) in a double-blind, randomized, placebo-controlled study of the effects of prednicarbate, mometasone furoate, and betamethasone 17-valerate on total skin thickness over 6 weeks (175). On day 36, total skin thickness was reduced by a mean of 1% in test fields treated with vehicle; the relative reductions were 13, 17, and 24% for prednicarbate, mometasone furoate, and betamethasone 17-valerate respectively. There were visible signs of atrophy or telangiectasia in two subjects each with betamethasone 17-valerate and mometasone furoate, but not with prednicarbate or its vehicle.

Contact allergy

Topical glucocorticoids are well-known contact sensitizers. Immediate allergic or allergic-like reactions to systemic glucocorticoids also occur, but less often. Two atopic patients developed urticaria, possibly IgE-mediated, from a hydrocortisone injection or infusion (176) and other reactions have been reported.

- A 50-year-old woman developed contact dermatitis on her legs after she applied hydrocortisone aceponate cream (Efficort) to psoriatic lesions on her lower back (177). Similar lesions also occurred on her legs after she used topical betamethasone cream (Diprosone). However, no eczema developed on or around the site of application. Patch tests were negative to a range of glucocorticoids, including Efficort and Diprosone creams. However, a repeated open application test was positive with Efficort cream, hydrocortisone aceponate 0.127% in petroleum, and tixocortol pivalate 1% in petroleum.
- A 42-year-old woman developed a nonpigmented fixed drug eruption after skin testing and an intra-articular injection of triamcinolone acetonide, which has not been previously reported (178).

Contact allergy to glucocorticoids was evaluated in 7238 patients in a multicenter multinational study of five drugs: budesonide, betamethasone-17-valerate, clobetasol-17-propionate, hydrocortisone-17-butyrate, and tixocortol-21-pivalate. There was a positive patch-test reaction to at least one of the glucocorticoids in 189 patients (2.6%). The incidence ranged from 0.4% in Spain to 6.4% in Belgium. Positive reactions were more frequent with budesonide (100 results) and tixocortol (98 reactions) (SEDA-21, 415; 179). Contact allergic reactions to intranasal budesonide and fluticasone propionate have been described. Many of these cases were characterized by perinasal eczema, often with vesicles, and edema as the initial symptoms. Lesions sometimes spread to the upper lip, cheeks, and eyelids. For fluticasone propionate, analysis of data on adverse events from the Spontaneous Reporting System of the US FDA Division of Epidemiology and Surveillance showed that, in the first 5 months after its introduction into the USA in 1995, 46 patients reported 89 adverse events suspected to be caused by fluticasone propionate intranasal spray. Central nervous system symptoms occurred in 46%, cardiac symptoms in 28%, dermatological symptoms in 39%, and epistaxis in 6.5%. These numbers may underestimate the problem, since no cases reported by the drug manufacturer were included. These results suggest that safety issues may differentiate budesonide and fluticasone propionate from other intranasal glucocorticoids, such as beclomethasone dipropionate (SEDA-21, 415; 180).

Budesonide is advocated as a marker molecule for glucocorticoid contact allergy. When patch testing glucocorticoids, one must consider both their sensitizing potential and their anti-inflammatory properties, as well as the possibility of different time courses of such properties. The dose–response relation for budesonide has therefore been investigated with regard to dose, occlusion time, and reading time in 10 patients (ages not stated) who were patch tested with budesonide in ethanol in serial dilutions from 2.0% down to 0.0002%, with occlusion times of 48, 24, and 5 hours (181). Readings were on days 2, 4, and 7. The 48-hour occlusion detected most positive reactors (8/10) at a reading time of 4 days and 0.002% detected most contact allergies. The "edge effect" (reactions with a peripheral ring due to suppression of the allergic reaction under the patch because of the intrinsic anti-inflammatory effect of the glucocorticoid itself) was noted with several concentrations at early readings. That lower concentrations can detect budesonide allergy better at early readings and that patients with an "edge reaction" can have positive reactions to lower concentrations can be explained by individual glucocorticoid reactivity, the dose–response relation, and the time-courses of the elicitation and the anti-inflammatory capacity.

- A 36-year-old man, who had a long history of atopic dermatitis of the neck, chest, and arms, developed allergic contact dermatitis after topical administration of clobetasone ointment 0.05% (Kindavate) and prednisolone ointment 0.3% (Lidomex) (182). Patch tests with both ointments showed a positive reaction only to Kindavate. Further testing with the separate ingredients of Kindavate showed positive reactions to 0.05, 0.01, and 0.005% clobetasone on day 7.
- A 40-year-old woman had a flare-up of her eczema (183). She had had previous negative patch tests 10 years before. She had taken topical glucocorticoids and emollients for a few months, but had not used budesonide. Patch testing with the European standard series showed a positive reaction to budesonide 0.1% at 3 days. All other allergens were negative. The only antecedent exposure was that she had three children with asthma, all of whom regularly used inhaled budesonide and occasionally nebulizers. She had not used the inhaler but had helped her children to manage the devices. A subsequent patch test with powdered budesonide from the inhaler was positive.
- A 14-year-old girl with newly diagnosed systemic lupus erythematosus developed a pruritic bullous eruption while taking prednisone 20 mg/day (184). She was given a single daily dose of intravenous

methylprednisolone 60 mg with rapid improvement. In preparation for discharge, the glucocorticoid was changed to oral prednisone 60 mg/day, to which she developed a pruritic bullous eruption consistent with erythema multiforme. She underwent immediate and delayed hypersensitivity tests. Intradermal and patch tests to liquid prednisone were positive. She was given oral methylprednisolone 48 mg/day and has not had recurrence of the skin lesions.
- A 27-year-old woman, a pharmacist, had dermatitis on three separate occasions a few hours after she started to take oral deflazacort 6 mg for vesicular hand eczema (185). On each occasion, her symptoms included a widespread macular rash mainly on the inner aspects of her arms and legs and buttocks. She also had severe scaling, fever, nausea, vomiting, malaise, and hypotension. A skin biopsy was consistent with erythema multiforme, and direct immunofluorescence showed granular deposits at the dermoepidermal junction. Patch tests to the commercial formulation of deflazacort 6 mg (1% aqueous solution) and to pure deflazacort (1% aqueous solution) were positive, but there were no cross-reactions to other glucocorticoids.

The author of the last report commented that the patient probably developed hypersensitivity to deflazacort as a result of occupational exposure.

Other cases of erythema multiforme-like contact dermatitis after topical budesonide have been reported (SEDA-21, 415; 186). In a large case-control study, potential cases of severe forms of erythema multiforme, toxic epidermal necrolysis and Stevens–Johnson syndrome, were collected in four European countries (France, Portugal, Italy, and Germany) (SEDA-20, 371; 187). There was a significant relation with glucocorticoid use in the preceding week (multivariate analysis relative risk = 4.4; 95% CI = 1.9, 10), or when prescribed for long-term therapy (crude relative risk for use less than 2 months = 54; 95% CI = 23, 124). The estimates of excess risks associated with glucocorticoids or sulfonamides (which are well-known to cause these syndromes), expressed as the number of cases attributable to the drug per million users in 1 week, were 1.5 and 4.5 respectively.

Cross-reactivity between glucocorticoids and progestogens has been described (188).

- A 68-year-old woman, with a prolonged history of pityriasis lichenoides chronica treated with topical glucocorticoids, including hydrocortisone, took a formulation containing conjugated estrogens 0.625 mg and hydroxyprogesterone acetate 5 mg (frequency of administration not stated) for late menopausal syndrome. Years later she started to have pruritus, a maculopapular rash, and flu-like symptoms for several days before menstruation. On this occasion, she presented with a severe, pruritic, papulovesicular eruption on her chest, back, abdomen, and legs. The eruption had developed after treatment for 7 days with the estrogen–progestogen formulation; she had developed similar symptoms on several previous occasions after taking the same medication. She was treated with antihistamines and her skin eruption resolved within a few days. Patch tests were positive to

17-OH-progesterone, tixocortol pivalate, and budesonide.

The authors hypothesized that this patient, who had taken topical glucocorticoids for several years, had become sensitive and that the recurrent episodes of autoimmune progestogen dermatitis were related to endogenous progestogen sensitivity following cross-sensitivity to glucocorticoids. This hypothesis was supported by the development of recurrent eczema several times after she took an estrogen–progestogen preparation.

Musculoskeletal

Osteoporosis

The use of glucocorticoids is associated with reduced bone mineral density, bone loss, osteoporosis, and fractures. This has been described during the long-term use of glucocorticoid by any route of administration (SEDA-19, 377; SEDA-20, 374). The effects of glucocorticoids on bone have been reviewed (SEDA-21, 417; 189). Biochemical markers of bone mineral density are listed in Table 4. In patients with secondary hypoadrenalism, hydrocortisone 30 mg/day for replacement produced a significant fall in osteocalcin, indicating bone loss. Lower doses of hydrocortisone (10 mg and 20 mg) produced similar efficacy in terms of quality of life but smaller effects on osteocalcin concentrations and therefore a reduction in bone loss (190). Three studies add evidence of the deleterious effects of oral glucocorticoids and high doses of inhaled glucocorticoids on bone mineral density (191) and the risk of fractures (192,193).

The fluorinated glucocorticoids are said to have relatively more catabolic activity than others and might have a greater effect on the skeleton but such impressions may merely reflect the general potency of some newer glucocorticoids and a tendency to use them in inappropriate doses. A relatively new glucocorticoid, deflazacort, has been proposed to have less effect on bone metabolism, but a double-blind study has failed to show an advantage compared with prednisolone (SEDA-21, 417; 194).

Osteoporosis induced by chronic glucocorticoid therapy has been reviewed in patients with obstructive lung diseases (195) and patients with skin diseases (196).

Table 4 Biochemical markers of bone mineral density

Bone formation
Blood
Alkaline phosphatase (bone-specific)
Osteocalcin
Procollagen type I carboxy-terminal propeptide (PICP)
Procollagen type I amino-terminal propeptide (PINP)
Procollagen type III amino-terminal propeptide (PIIINP)
Bone resorption
Blood
Acid phosphatase (acid-resistant)
Type I collagen carboxy-terminal telopeptide (ICTP)
Urine
Calcium
Hydroxyproline
Cross-linked peptides (pyridinium and deoxypyridinoline)

Presentation

Of the effects of glucocorticoids on the skeleton, osteoporosis is the most important clinically; manifestations can include vertebral compression fractures, scoliosis resulting in respiratory embarrassment, and fractures of the long bones. The risk of vertebral fractures is not different in patients taking or not taking glucocorticoids in whom bone mineral density is similar (197).

Glucocorticoids can even cause osteoporosis when they are used for long-term replacement therapy in the Addison's disease, as has been shown by a study of 91 patients who had taken glucocorticoids for a mean of 10.6 years, in whom bone mineral density was reduced by 32% compared with age-matched controls (SEDA-19, 377; 198). However, these results contrasted with the results of a Spanish study in patients with Addison's disease, in which no direct relation was found between replacement therapy and either bone density or biochemical markers of bone turnover of calcium metabolism (alkaline phosphatase, osteocalcin, procollagen I type, parathormone, and 1,25-dihydroxycolecalciferol) (SEDA-19, 377; 199).

Atraumatic posterior pelvic ring fractures that simulate the form of presentation of metastatic diseases can be produced by glucocorticoid administration (SEDA-19, 377; 200).

Accelerated bone loss, with an increased risk of first hip fracture, occurred in elderly women taking oral glucocorticoids (201). At baseline, 122 (1.5%) women were taking inhaled glucocorticoids only (median dose equivalent to inhaled beclomethasone 168 micrograms/day), 228 (2.8%) were taking oral glucocorticoids (median dose equivalent to prednisone 5 mg/day) with or without inhaled glucocorticoids, and 7718 were not taking any glucocorticoids. The women who were taking oral glucocorticoids had lower mean bone mineral density at 3.6 years than nonusers, with an interim fall that was twice as fast. First hip fracture occurred in 4.8% of the women who were taking oral glucocorticoids and in 2.8% of the women who were not (RR = 2.1; CI = 1.0, 4.4). The researchers said that the power of the study was not sufficient to determine the relative risk of hip fracture in women taking inhaled glucocorticoids.

A reduction in bone mineral density has been described in 23 patients (19 men) with chronic fatigue syndrome taking low-dose glucocorticoids in a double-blind, randomized, placebo-controlled study (202). The patients took hydrocortisone 25–35 mg/day or matched placebo for 3 months. Mean bone mineral density in the spine fell by 2% with hydrocortisone and increased by 1% with placebo.

A group of 367 patients with lung disease taking oral glucocorticoids (177 women, mean age 68 years, 190 men, mean age 70 years) and 734 matched controls completed a questionnaire about lifestyle, fractures, and other possible adverse effects of glucocorticoids (203). The cumulative incidence of fractures from the time of diagnosis was 23% in patients taking oral glucocorticoids and 15% in the controls (OR = 1.8; 95% CI = 1.3, 2.6). Fractures of the vertebrae were more likely (OR = 10; 95% CI = 2.9, 35). The adverse effects were dose-related, with a higher risk of all fractures (OR = 2.22; 95% CI = 1.04, 4.8) and vertebral fractures (OR = 9.2; 95% CI = 2.4, 36) in those who took the highest compared with the lowest cumulative doses (61 versus 5 g).

Systemic glucocorticoids are often prescribed for rheumatoid arthritis. Even in low doses they can have clinical benefits and can inhibit joint damage, but they can cause osteoporotic fractures. In a 2-year double-blind, randomized, placebo-controlled trial in 81 patients (29 men, mean age 62 years) with early active rheumatoid arthritis who had not been treated with disease-modifying antirheumatic drugs, 41 were assigned to oral prednisone 10 mg/day and 40 to placebo. NSAIDs were allowed in both groups and after 6 months, sulfasalazine (2 g/day) could be prescribed as rescue medication. Those who took prednisone had more clinical improvement with less use of concomitant drugs. After month 6, radiological scores had progressed significantly less in those who took prednisone. After 24 months, seven patients had new vertebral fractures, five in the prednisone group and two in the placebo group (204).

Mechanisms

There have been reviews of the mechanisms and adverse effects of glucocorticoids in rheumatoid arthritis (205) and the pathogenesis, diagnosis, and treatment of glucocorticoid-induced osteoporosis in patients with pulmonary diseases (206). Several mechanisms underlie the effect of glucocorticoids on bone, both biochemical and cellular. Effects on calcium are:

(a) increased excretion of calcium into the bowel and inhibition of its absorption;
(b) inhibition of the tubular re-absorption of calcium in the kidney;
(c) increased mobilization of calcium from the skeleton.

When calcium homeostasis cannot be maintained, the resulting hypocalcemia can have serious consequences (SEDA-18, 388) (207,208). This so-called "glucocorticoid hyperparathyroidism" was the explanation traditionally most prominently advanced for glucocorticoid osteoporosis, but it is not the only one and may not be the most central. Other biochemical effects include:

(a) a catabolic effect on protein metabolism, causing a reduction in the bone matrix;
(b) altered vitamin D metabolism, with reduced concentrations of vitamin D metabolites (209);
(c) a dose-dependent reduction of serum osteocalcin, a bone matrix protein that appears to correlate with bone formation.

Measurement of serum osteocalcin is a useful marker for glucocorticoid-induced osteoporosis, and can be used alongside other measures noted below.

Various cellular mechanisms are involved in the production of glucocorticoid-induced osteoporosis (SEDA-20, 375) (210). The major change is a reduction in osteoblast activity that results in a reduced working rate (mean appositional rate), and a reduced active life-span of osteoblasts. The cellular mechanism seems to be related to diminished production of cytokines and other locally acting factors. Increased bone resorption and reduced calcium absorption have also been described. A sophisticated mathematical

model has been used to describe changes in calcium kinetics in patients treated with glucocorticoids (SEDA-20, 375) (211). Plasma calcium concentrations were higher than in controls, with a marked reduction in calcium flow into the irreversible stable bone compartment in glucocorticoid-treated patients. The authors concluded that prednisone has direct effects on osteoblast function.

Osteoprotegerin (osteoclastogenesis inhibitory factor, OCIF) has been identified as a novelly secreted cytokine receptor that plays an important role in the negative regulation of osteoclastic bone resorption. There are reports that suggest that glucocorticoids promote osteoclastogenesis by inhibiting osteoprotegerin production in vitro, thereby enhancing bone resorption. However, there are only a few clinical reports in which the regulatory functions of osteoprotegerin have been explored. In order to clarify the potential role of osteoprotegerin in the pathogenesis of glucocorticoid-induced osteoporosis, Japanese investigators have measured serum osteoprotegerin and other markers of bone metabolism before and after glucocorticoid therapy in patients with various renal diseases (212). The findings suggested that short-term administration of glucocorticoids significantly suppresses serum osteoprotegerin and osteocalcin. This might be relevant to the development of glucocorticoid-induced osteoporosis via enhancement of bone resorption and suppression of bone formation. Further long-term studies are needed to elucidate the mechanism of the glucocorticoid-induced reduction in circulating osteoprotegerin and its participation in the pathogenesis of osteoporosis.

Although glucocorticoids can cause changes in trabecular microarchitecture, loss of bone (reduced bone density) seems to be the major determinant of osteoporosis (213). Bone resorption seems to involve the receptor of the activator of the nucleus factor KB ligand (RANK-L) and osteoprotegerin. RANK-L binds to a specific receptor in osteoclasts, and in the presence of the macrophage colony stimulating factor (M-CSF) it induces osteoclastogenesis (the development of mature osteoclasts) and suppression of normal osteoclast apoptosis. Osteoprotegerin is a soluble decoy receptor that binds to and neutralizes RANK-L and so reduces osteoclastogenesis. Glucocorticoids increase the expression of RANK-L and M-CSF and reduce osteoprotegerin production by osteoblasts. The net result is enhanced osteoclastic activity. Other inflammatory mediators, such as tumor necrosis factor-alfa and interleukin-6, have similar biological actions to glucocorticoids. Glucocorticoids reduce osteoblast numbers and function by reducing the replication and differentiation of osteoblasts and by increasing apoptosis in mature osteoblasts. Glucocorticoids inhibit osteoblastic synthesis of type I collagen, the major component of bone extracellular matrix. They can induce apoptosis of osteocytes, and this could be the mechanism of osteonecrosis. Two other factors are involved in bone loss: firstly, glucocorticoids increase renal calcium elimination and reduce intestinal calcium absorption, leading to a negative calcium balance, which can lead to secondary hyperparathyroidism; secondly, glucocorticoids reduce the production of gonadal hormones. The histological effects of glucocorticoids are a reduced rate of bone formation, reduced trabecular wall thickness, and apoptosis of bone cells. These effects lead to osteoporosis and fractures.

Although glucocorticoid use seems to be an important factor for low mineral density, sex hormones have also been suggested as an important determinant of bone mineral content. Bone mineral density and sex hormone status have been studied in 99 men with rheumatoid arthritis and 68 age-matched controls (SEDA-20, 375) (214). There were significant reductions in lumbar and femoral density, and salivary testosterone, androstenedione, and dehydroepiandrosterone in the patients. Salivary testosterone correlated with femoral density. By multiple regression analysis, weight, serum testosterone concentrations, and cumulative dose of glucocorticoid were significant predictors of lumbar bone density. Weight, age, androstenedione concentrations, and cumulative dose of glucocorticoids were significant predictors of femoral bone density.

Dose relation
Dose is an important factor, but these adverse effects have been described after low doses. The risk of hip fracture associated with glucocorticoid use has been studied in Denmark in a population-based case-control study in 6660 subjects with hip fractures and 33 272 age-matched population controls (215). Data on prescriptions for glucocorticoid within the last 5 years before the index date were retrieved from a population-based prescription database. Doses were recalculated to prednisolone equivalents. Cases and controls were grouped according to cumulative glucocorticoid dose:

1. not used;
2. under 130 mg (equivalent to prednisolone 30 mg/day for 4 days given for an acute exacerbation of asthma);
3. 130–499 mg (equivalent to a short course of prednisolone of 450 mg) for acute asthma;
4. 500–1499 mg (equivalent to prednisolone 7.5 mg/day for 6 months or 800 micrograms/day of inhaled budesonide for 1 year);
5. 1500 mg or more (equivalent to more than 4.1 mg day for 1 year, a long-term high dose).

A conditional logistic regression was used and adjusted for potential confounders including sex, redeemed prescriptions for hormone replacement therapy, antiosteoporotic, anxiolytic, antipsychotic, and antidepressant drugs. Compared with never users, there was an increased risk of hip fracture in glucocorticoid users, with increasing cumulative doses of any type of drug used during the preceding 5 years. For doses of prednisolone under 130 mg, the adjusted risk (OR) was 0.96 (95% CI = 0.89, 1.04); for 130-499 mg the OR was 1.17 (1.01, 1.35); for 500-1499 mg the OR was 1.36 (1.19, 1.56); and for 1500 mg or more the OR was 1.65 (1.43, 1.92). There was an also increased risk when the study population was stratified according to sex, age, and type of glucocorticoid (systemic or topical). This study showed that even a limited daily dose of glucocorticoids (more than an average dose of prednisolone of about 71 micrograms/day) was associated with an increased risk of hip fracture.

Doses of prednisone of 7.5 mg/day can cause premature or exaggerated osteoporosis. However, it is unclear whether a dose of 5 mg/day has the same effect. In a double-blind, randomized, placebo-controlled, 8-week trial 50 healthy postmenopausal women (mean age 57 years) were randomly assigned to prednisone 5 mg/day or matching placebo for 6 weeks, followed by a 2-week recovery phase (216). Prednisone rapidly and significantly decreased serum concentrations of propeptide of type I N-terminal procollagen, propeptide of type I C-terminal procollagen, and osteocalcin, and free urinary deoxypyridinoline compared with placebo. These changes were largely reversed during the recovery period. In conclusion, low-dose prednisone significantly reduced indices of bone formation and bone resorption in postmenopausal women.

Lumbar spine bone mineral density has been assessed in 76 prepubertal asthmatics (mean age 7.7 years, 26 girls) using glucocorticoids (217). After stratification for dose and route of administration, the children who used over 800 micrograms/day of inhaled glucocorticoids, with or without intermittent oral glucocorticoids, had a significant lower weight-adjusted bone density than children who used 400–800 micrograms/day of inhaled glucocorticoids (mean difference -0.05 g/cm^2; 95% CI = -0.02, -0.09). Bone mass was similar in children who did not use inhaled glucocorticoids and those who used 400–800 micrograms/day.

In kidney transplant recipients, lumbar bone loss was significantly higher in 20 patients who took daily prednisone (5.9%, mean dosage 0.19 mg/kg/day) than in 27 patients who used alternate-day prednisone (1.1%, mean dosage 0.15 mg/kg/day) (218).

Time course
The loss of bone mineral after organ and tissue transplant associated with immunosuppressive therapy follows a delayed time course. The long-term effects of immunosuppressive therapy on bone density have been determined in 25 cardiac transplant patients (SEDA-20, 375) (219). As expected, there was bone loss in the spine during the first year, but this was not maintained during the second and third years after transplantation, despite continuing maintenance immunosuppression with prednisolone. Only four patients, all of whom were hypogonadal, continued to lose bone.

Susceptibility factors
The overall effect of glucocorticoids on bone mineral content differs between patients on comparable treatments, which suggests that some patients are more predisposed than others (SEDA-3, 306), and probably also that the standards of evaluation used in different clinics are not comparable. This variability and the wide range of products and dosage schemes used mean that one does not have a clear impression of what constitutes a safe regimen as far as the skeleton is concerned (SEDA-20, 374), or whether any regimen is safe in this respect. Certainly, in a series of men with rheumatoid arthritis, even a very low dose of glucocorticoids (for example 10 mg or less of prednisolone daily) has proved to have

a significant effect on bone mineral density (220); other work has provided similar results (SEDA-20, 374; 221). In another published study, patients who took 1–4 mg/day had the same density as those who were not taking glucocorticoids. Patients who took 5–9 mg/day and those who took more than 10 mg/day had significantly lower bone density (84 and 81% of control values respectively) (SEDA-20, 374; 222).

Glucocorticoid-related complications have been described in 748 adult kidney transplant recipients, followed for at least 1 year. For bone/joint complications, the multivariate analysis showed that the only significant variable was the cumulative duration of glucocorticoid therapy. For avascular necrosis, no variables were significant (SEDA-19, 377; 223).

In a similar study of 65 renal transplant patients treated with immunosuppressive drugs for at least 6 months, multivariate analysis showed that cumulative glucocorticoid dose and female sex were the major predictors of low vertebral bone density (SEDA-19, 377; 224).

In another study, the loss of bone density correlated with the cumulative dose of prednisolone (21 g total dose at 11.4 mg/day) and renal function (SEDA-21, 417; 225).

In a review of renal transplantation during 1974–94, 166 patients were classified into those with osteonecrosis of the femoral head (22 patients) and those without (47 patients) (SEDA-21, 417; 226). The total dose of methyl-prednisolone was higher in those with osteonecrosis. All five patients who had received intravenous pulse doses over 2000 mg had osteonecrosis.

The risk of vertebral deformity is increased by the combination of an oral glucocorticoid and advanced age, according to the findings in 229 patients (69% women) taking long-term oral glucocorticoids (prednisone equivalents of 5 mg/day or more) and 286 untreated controls (227). The duration of treatment was 0.5–37 (median 4.8) years. More than 60% of the treatment group were aged over 60 years, and most (62%) had been treated for rheumatoid arthritis. Bone mineral density data were analysed in 194 patients. The researchers identified at least one vertebral deformity (defined as a more than 20% reduction in anterior, middle, or posterior vertebral height) in 65 (28%) of the patients in the treatment group, and two or more fractures were identified in 25 (11%). In the treatment group, vertebral deformities were significantly more common in men than in women, and the prevalence of deformities increased with age. Compared with patients aged under 60 years, glucocorticoid-treated patients aged 70–79 years had a five-fold increased risk of vertebral deformity (OR = 5.1; 95% CI = 2.0, 13). The prevalence of vertebral deformities increased significantly with age in the glucocorticoid group. While the mean spine and femoral bone mineral density scores were lower in the glucocorticoid group, logistic regression analysis showed that bone mineral density was only a modest predictor of deformity. Age is an important independent risk factor, with very high prevalence rates in those over 70 years. Increasing duration of glucocorticoid use may increase the risk of fracture.

Osteoporosis is common in Crohn's disease, often because of glucocorticoids. Budesonide as controlled-release capsules is a locally acting glucocorticoid with low systemic availability. In a randomized study in 272 patients with Crohn's disease involving the ileum and/or ascending colon, budesonide and prednisolone were compared for 2 years in doses adapted to disease activity (228). There was active disease in 181, of whom 98 were glucocorticoid-naive; 90 had quiescent disease and were corticosteroid-dependent. Efficacy was similar in the two groups, but treatment-related adverse effects were less frequent with budesonide. The glucocorticoid-naive patients who took budesonide had smaller reductions in bone mineral density than those who took prednisolone (mean –1.04% versus –3.84%).

Comparisons of glucocorticoids

Bone loss induced by glucocorticoids has been assessed in three different populations. A group of 374 subjects (mean age 35 years, 55% women) with mild asthma taking beta-adrenoceptor agonists only, were randomized to inhaled glucocorticoids (budesonide or beclomethasone) or non-glucocorticoid treatment for 2 years (229). Bone mineral density was measured blind after 6, 12, and 24 months. Mean doses of budesonide and beclomethasone were 389 micrograms/day and 499 micrograms/day, respectively. At the end of follow-up, the subjects who had used glucocorticoids had better asthma control. The mean changes in bone density over 2 years in the budesonide, beclomethasone, and control groups were 0.1%, –0.4%, and 0.4% for the lumbar spine and –0.9%, –0.9%, and –0.4% for the neck of the femur. The daily dose of inhaled glucocorticoid was related to the reduction in bone mineral density only at the lumbar spine. Low to moderate doses of inhaled glucocorticoids caused little change in bone mineral density over 2 years and provided better asthma control.

Diagnosis

Several techniques are used to measure bone density. Cortical bone can be assessed in peripheral sites by single-photon absorptiometry and a combination of cortical and trabecular bone in central sites by dual X-ray absorptiometry. Trabecular bone can be assessed by quantitative computer tomography scanning of the lumbar spine. Since single-photon absorptiometry and dual X-ray absorptiometry give a negligible dose of radiation, they are useful for population screening. However, these two techniques are not sensitive enough to show subtle changes in bone density over short periods of time. Quantitative computed tomography gives a significant dose of radiation (of the order of one-tenth of a lateral X-ray of the spine) but can focus on trabecular bone, which has a tenfold greater turnover, compared with cortical bone. Quantitative computed tomography is more sensitive to changing bone density over time.

Other methods, such as the fasting urinary hydroxyproline/creatinine ratio, alkaline phosphatase activity, dual-absorption photometry of the hip, and serum osteocalcin measurements, can also be used, depending on an individual clinic's equipment and experience (SEDA-17, 447).

Management

The prevention and treatment of glucocorticoid bone loss in patients with skin diseases have been reviewed (196). Strategies for the management of this problem have been discussed (SEDA-22, 213) and the clinical implications of trials in the management of glucocorticoid-induced osteoporosis have been reviewed (230). Provided no fractures have occurred, loss of bone mineral density seems to be reversible when treatment is withdrawn (SEDA-18, 389). The management of glucocorticoid-induced osteoporosis has been revised by the UK Consensus Group Meeting on Osteoporosis (SEDA-20, 376; 212) and by the American College of Rheumatology (SEDA-21, 417; 231).

Guidelines for the prevention and treatment of glucocorticoid-induced osteoporosis have been published (232). Although there are several consensus statements and recommendations for prophylactic measures against glucocorticoid-induced osteoporosis in patients with rheumatoid arthritis, prophylaxis is commonly underprescribed. In two recent studies of 191 and 92 patients taking long-term glucocorticoids, relatively few were taking primary prevention, although some were taking vitamin D and calcium tablets. Around 65–68% of all those who qualified for prophylaxis for glucocorticoid-induced osteoporosis did not receive therapy, and only 9% of those in one study and 21% in the other were taking bisphosphonates (233,234).

Low availability compounds

Bone loss in patients taking oral budesonide has been evaluated in a longitudinal study in which bone mineral density was measured annually for 2 years in 138 patients (67 men, mean age 36 years old) with quiescent Crohn's disease (235). They took budesonide (8.5 mg/day; $n = 48$), prednisone (10.5 mg/day, $n = 45$), or non-steroidal drugs ($n = 45$). After 1 year, the bone mineral density in the lumbar spine fell by 2.36% in those who took budesonide, by 0.61% in those who took prednisone, and by 0.09% in those who took non-steroidal drugs. In the second year, the largest fall occurred in those who took budesonide (1.97%), but the differences between the groups were not significant. After 2 years, bone mineral density in the femoral neck fell by 2.94% with budesonide, 0.36% with prednisone, and 1.05% with the non-steroidal drugs. These results suggest that budesonide can cause bone loss, but the non-randomized design of the study limits conclusions about the comparison between budesonide and prednisone.

Pulse administration

The administration of glucocorticoids in sporadic pulses has been shown not to reduce bone density in patients with multiple sclerosis. In a prospective study, 30 patients were given 1000 mg/day of methylprednisolone intravenously for 3 days, followed by oral prednisone in tapering dosage for 2 weeks. Bone density was determined in the lumbar spine and femoral neck before and at 2, 4, and 6

months after therapy. At baseline, the patients had a reduced bone mass compared with controls; this reduction did not correlate with previous exposure to glucocorticoids. Ambulant patients during follow-up after glucocorticoid pulse therapy had an increase in lumbar bone density (+1.7% at 6 months). Average femoral density did not change; however, in patients who required a walking stick or other aid, femoral density fell (–1.6%), while in those with better ambulation it increased (+2.9%). These results suggest that inactivity is the main factor causing bone loss in patients treated with sporadic pulses of glucocorticoids (SEDA-21, 417; 236).

Calcium and vitamin D analogues

Infusion of ionic calcium has sometimes been used to counteract the malabsorption of calcium in patients taking long-term glucocorticoids, particularly in patients who develop secondary hypoparathyroidism (SEDA-3, 306). There is also evidence that in amenorrheic or menopausal women requiring glucocorticoids, the adverse effects on the vertebrae can be countered by hormonal replacement therapy with estrogen and progesterone (237); progestogens similarly seem to have a promising effect in men, and while they cause a fall in serum testosterone they apparently do not undermine the desired effects of glucocorticoids (SEDA-16, 449).

The administration of calcium and vitamin D3 can prevent bone loss induced by glucocorticoids, and trials have confirmed its efficacy when given for 2 years. Patients taking prednisone and placebo lost bone density in the lumbar spine at a rate of 2% per year. Those taking prednisone and calcium plus vitamin D3 gained bone mineral density at a rate of 0.72% per year. Calcium plus vitamin D3 did not improve bone mineral density in patients who were not taking prednisone (SEDA-21, 417; 238).

In a similar randomized double-blind study, the effects of vitamin D (50 000 units/week) and calcium (1000 mg/day) were evaluated in 62 patients with different rheumatic diseases treated with prednisone (10–100 mg/day) (SEDA-21, 418; 239). The primary outcome was bone mineral density in the lumbar spine at 36 months. Patients taking placebo had reductions of 4.1, 3.8, and 1.5% at 12, 24, and 36 months respectively. Patients taking calcium and vitamin D had reductions of 2.6, 3.7, and 2.2% respectively. The results suggested that preventive therapy could be beneficial early in the prevention of glucocorticoid-induced bone loss, but there was no evidence of long-term beneficial effects. In kidney transplant patients, the preventive administration of 25-hydroxycolecalciferol and calcium reduced bone loss in the spine and femoral neck and the number of new vertebral crush fractures (SEDA-21, 418; 240). In children with rheumatic diseases taking glucocorticoids, calcium and vitamin D supplementation improved spinal bone density, although osteocalcin concentrations remained low (SEDA-19, 378; 241).

A meta-analysis has shown that alfacalcidol and calcitriol prevent bone loss induced by glucocorticoid (effect size = 0.43) but not fractures (242).

Alfacalcidol and vitamin D_3 have been compared in patients with established glucocorticoid-induced osteoporosis with or without vertebral fractures (243). Patients taking long-term glucocorticoids were included as matched pairs to receive randomly either alfacalcidol 1 microgram/day plus calcium 500 mg/day (n = 103) or vitamin D_3 1000 IU/day plus calcium 500 mg/day (n = 101). The two groups were well matched in terms of mean age, sex ratio, mean height and weight, daily dosage and duration of glucocorticoid therapy, and the percentages of the three underlying diseases (chronic obstructive pulmonary disease, rheumatoid arthritis, and polymyalgia rheumatica). The baseline mean bone mineral density values (expressed as T scores, the number of standard deviations from the mean of the healthy population) at the lumbar spine were −3.26 (alfacalcidol) and −3.25 (vitamin D_3) and at the femoral neck −2.81 and −2.84 respectively. The prevalence rates of vertebral and non-vertebral fractures did not differ. During the 3-year study, the median percentage bone mineral density increased at the lumbar spine by 2.4% with alfacalcidol and decreased by 0.8% with vitamin D_3. There also was a significantly larger median increase at the femoral neck with alfacalcidol (1.2%) than with vitamin D_3 (0.8%). The 3-year rates of patients with at least one new vertebral fracture were 9.7% with alfacalcidol and 25% with vitamin D_3 (RR = 0.61; 95% CI = 0.24, 0.81). The 3-year rates of patients with at least one new non-vertebral fracture were 15% with alfacalcidol and 25% with vitamin D_3 (RR = 0.41; 95% CI = 0.06, 0.68). The 3-year rates of patients with at least one new fracture of any kind were 19% with alfacalcidol and 41% with vitamin D_3 (RR = 0.52; 95% CI = 0.25, 0.71). Those who took alfacalcidol had a substantially larger reduction in back pain than those who took vitamin D_3. Generally, adverse effects in both groups were mild, and only three patients taking alfacalcidol and two taking vitamin D_3 had moderate hypercalcemia. The authors concluded that alfacalcidol plus calcium is greatly superior to vitamin D_3 plus calcium in the treatment of established glucocorticoid-induced osteoporosis.

Calcitonin

Less clear are the results observed after the administration of salmon calcitonin. The usefulness of intranasally administered salmon calcitonin for 2 years has been evaluated in 44 glucocorticoid-dependent asthmatics (SEDA-19, 378; 244). All were taking calcium supplements (1000 mg/day), but one group also took calcitonin (100 IU every other day). Calcitonin increased spinal bone mass during first year of treatment, and maintained bone mass in a steady state during the second year. However, the rate of vertebral fractures was similar in the two groups. The addition of salmon calcitonin did not increase the efficacy of calcium plus vitamin D in the prevention of bone loss in 48 newly diagnosed patients taking glucocorticoids for temporal arteritis and polymyalgia rheumatica in a double-blind, randomized, placebo-controlled trial (SEDA-21, 418; 245). However, salmon calcitonin nasal spray prevented bone loss in the lumbar spine of 31 patients treated with prednisone for polymyalgia rheumatica (SEDA-22, 448; 246). They were randomized to salmon calcitonin nasal spray (200 IU/day) or matched placebo for 1 year. Both groups were treated with calcium supplements if their dietary intake was below 800 mg/day. With calcitonin, the mean bone mineral density in the lumbar spine fell by 1.3% and with placebo by 5% after 1 year. There were no differences in the hip, including the femoral neck and trochanter, or in total body bone density.

Bisphosphonates

There have been several studies of the use of bisphosphonates in preventing glucocorticoid-induced osteoporosis.

Intermittent cyclical etidronate prevented bone loss induced by prednisone in 10 postmenopausal women with temporal arteritis (SEDA-19, 378; 247). Cyclical etidronate (400 mg/day for 2 weeks every 3 months) plus ergocalciferol (0.5 mg/week) was given to 15 postmenopausal women (mean age 63 years) starting glucocorticoid therapy (prednisone 5–20 mg/day). A control group of 11 postmenopausal women (mean age 60 years) with glucocorticoid-induced osteoporosis were treated with calcium supplements only (1 g/day). During the first year, the cyclical regimen significantly increased lumbar and femoral neck bone density compared with placebo (7 and 2.5% for spine and femur respectively). After the second year of cyclical therapy, femoral neck bone density continued to increase while lumbar spine density remained stable (SEDA-20, 376; 248). The effect of intermittent cyclical therapy with etidronate has been investigated in the prevention of bone loss in 117 patients taking high-dose glucocorticoid therapy (a mean daily dose of at least 7.5 mg for 90 days followed by at least 2.5 mg/day for at least 12 months) (249). The patients were randomized to oral etidronate 400 mg/day or placebo for 14 days, followed by 76 days of oral calcium carbonate (500 mg elemental calcium), cycled over 12 months. The mean lumbar spine bone density changed 0.30% and −2.79% in the etidronate and placebo groups respectively. The mean difference between the groups after 1 year (3.0%) was significant. The changes in the femoral neck and greater trochanter were not different between the groups. There was a reduction in pyridinium cross-links, significant from baseline at both 6 and 12 months, in the etidronate group. Osteocalcin increased in the placebo group, and the differences between the groups at 6 and 12 months were −25% and −35% respectively. There was no significant difference between the groups in the number of adverse events, including gastrointestinal disorders. In a placebo-controlled study of the effects of 104 weeks of intermittent cyclical etidronate therapy in 49 patients, the same dose and cycles were used as in the previous study, but calcium (97 mg/day) was given with vitamin D (400 IU) (250). Intermittent cyclical etidronate therapy with vitamin D supplementation significantly increased lumbar spine bone mineral density by 4.5 in patients with osteoporosis resulting from long-term treatment with glucocorticoids.

Intermittent etidronate has been evaluated in a randomized controlled trial in 102 Japanese patients who had taken over 7.5 mg/day of prednisolone for at least 90 days (251). They were randomized to etidronate disodium 200 mg/day for 2 weeks plus calcium lactate 3.0 g/day and alfacalcidol 0.75 micrograms/day) or control (calcium lactate 3.0 g and alfacalcidol 0.75 micrograms/day). Bone mineral density in the lumbar spine and the rate of new vertebral fractures at 48 and 144 weeks were evaluated. With etidronate the mean lumbar spine bone mineral density increased by 3.7% and 4.8% at 48 and 144 weeks respectively. In the control group, the mean lumbar spine bone mineral density increased by 1.5% and 0.4% at 48 and 144 weeks respectively. Of three subgroups, men, premenopausal women, and postmenopausal women, the postmenopausal women had the greatest benefit. Two control patients had new vertebral fractures, whereas there were no fractures with etidronate.

Clodronate 100 mg by intramuscular route once a week was effective in the prevention of glucocorticoid-induced bone loss and fractures in patients with arthritis compared with calcium 1000 mg/day and vitamin D 800 mg/day (252).

Ibandronate can be given intravenously every 3 months. Its efficacy has been demonstrated in men and women with established glucocorticoid-induced osteoporosis in 115 subjects who were randomly assigned to daily calcium supplements (500 mg) plus either ibandronate injections 2 mg every 3 months or daily oral alfacalcidol 1 microgram for up to 3 years (253,254). After 3 years, intermittent intravenous ibandronate produced significantly greater increases than daily oral alfacalcidol in mean bone mineral density in the lumbar spine (13% versus 2.6%), and femoral neck (5.2% versus 1.9%). However, there were no differences between the groups with respect to fractures.

Pamidronate disodium has been compared with calcium supplementation in an open trial of primary prevention of glucocorticoid-induced osteoporosis in 27 patients with different rheumatic conditions, randomly assigned to pamidronate (90 mg intravenously every 3 months) plus calcium (800 mg calcium carbonate) or calcium only for 1 year (SEDA-22, 448; 255). The glucocorticoids were given in a starting dosage of 10–80 mg/day. With pamidronate there was a significant increase in bone density (3.6% lumbar, 2.2% femoral neck), but there was a significant reduction with calcium (–5.3% in both spine and femoral neck).

The effects of risedronate on bone density and vertebral fracture have been studied in 518 patients (mean age 59 years, 40% with rheumatoid arthritis, 56% men, 64% of the women postmenopausal) taking moderate to high doses of oral glucocorticoids (equivalent to prednisone 7.5 mg/day or more) (256). The patients were randomized double-blind to placebo, or risedronate 2.5 or 5 mg/day for 1 year. All took elemental calcium 1000 mg/day and vitamin D 400 IU/day. The mean density of the lumbar spine fell by 1% in the placebo group and increased by 1.3% and 1.9% with risedronate 2.5 and 5 mg respectively. There was a significant reduction of 70% in the risk of vertebral fracture with risedronate 5 mg compared

with placebo. There were similar incidences of adverse effects in all the groups.

Similar results have been reported in a clinical trial in 290 patients (38% men, 55% of the women postmenopausal) taking high-dose glucocorticoid therapy (prednisone over 7.5 mg/day or equivalent) (257). The subjects were randomized to receive placebo or risedronate 2.5 or 5 mg/day for 1 year. All took elemental calcium 1000 mg/day and vitamin D 400 IU/day. Risedronate 5 mg increased bone mineral density at 1 year by a mean of 2.9% in the lumbar spine, 1.8% in the femoral neck, and 2.4% in the trochanter. The values for placebo were 0.4%, –0.3%, and 1.0% respectively. The results for risedronate 2.5 mg were positive but not significant compared with placebo. The incidence of spinal fractures was reduced by 70% in the combined risedronate treatment groups compared with placebo. Risedronate and placebo caused similar adverse effects.

In a 1-year extension of a previous double-blind, randomized, placebo-controlled study, two doses of alendronate (5 and 10 mg/day) were compared in 66 men and 142 women taking glucocorticoids (at least 7.5 mg/day of prednisone or equivalent) (258). The extension was also double-blind, but those who had taken alendronate 2.5 mg/day in the previous study were given 10 mg/day. All the patients took supplementary calcium and vitamin D. The primary end-point was the mean percentage change in lumbar spine bone mineral density from baseline to 2 years. In those who took alendronate 5, 10, and 2.5/10 mg/day, bone mineral density increased significantly by 2.8, 3.9, and 3.7% respectively, and fell by –0.8% with placebo. There were significantly fewer patients with new vertebral fractures in the alendronate group compared with placebo (0.7 versus 6.8%). Adverse events were similar across the groups.

No data are available about the effects on bone mineral density of withdrawing bisphosphonates. Of 183 patients who participated in a randomized, placebo-controlled trial of the efficacy of alendronate 5 and 10 mg/day on the prevention and treatment of glucocorticoid-induced osteoporosis during 1 year 90 participated in a follow-up study for 3.3-4.6 years (259). In the subgroup that continued to take a glucocorticoid (more than 6 mg/day of prednisone or equivalent for more than 1 year) and took alendronate for less than 90 days ($n = 11$), there was bone loss after the end of the trial (–5.1% at the lumbar spine to –9.2% at the femoral neck). In the subgroup that continued to take glucocorticoids and alendronate for more than 300 days ($n = 31$), there was a small gain in the lumbar spine (+0.1%) and no significant loss in the femoral neck (–0.1%). Although the study had limitations, particularly loss to follow-up of a considerable number of patients, the results suggested that sustained treatment with alendronate maintains bone mineral density, and that patients who discontinue alendronate and continue to take glucocorticoids lose bone mass in the femoral neck and lumbar spine.

Parathyroid hormone

Parathyroid hormone (parathormone) is an anabolic osteotrophic agent. Randomized controlled trials have shown the efficacy of human parathormone, hPTH (1-34), in improving bone mass and reducing the risk of fractures in postmenopausal osteoporosis. In 51 women who had been postmenopausal for at least 3 years and who had taken both glucocorticoids (mean dose of prednisone 5-20 mg/day or equivalent for at least 1 year) and hormone replacement therapy (HRT; Premarin 0.625 mg/day or equivalent) were randomized to either HRT + parathormone 40 micrograms/day for 1 year or HRT only (260). Vertebral cross-sectional area increased by 4.8%, and 1 year after treatment was withdrawn it was still 2.6% higher than at baseline. In the control group there was no change. In addition, estimated vertebral compressive strength increased by more than 200% over baseline with parathormone and there was no change in the control group.

Fluoride

Fluoride is a potent stimulator of trabecular bone formation. Sodium monofluorophosphate was given to 48 patients with osteoporosis due to glucocorticoids (more than 10 mg of prednisone equivalents/day). Patients were randomly allocated to 1 g of calcium carbonate (control) or 200 mg of sodium monofluorophosphate plus 1 g of calcium carbonate for 18 months. At the end of the study lumbar spine bone density had increased by 7.8% in the fluoride group versus 3.3% in the controls. There were no changes in femoral neck density (SEDA-20, 376; 261).

Growth hormone

Growth hormone is a potent anabolic agent that stimulates protein synthesis, cell growth, and osteoblast activity. Recombinant human growth hormone has been used in patients taking long-term glucocorticoid treatment with suppressed endogenous growth hormone responses to GH-releasing hormone (SEDA-20, 376; 262). A single daily dose of 0.1 IU/kg of human growth hormone was given subcutaneously to nine nonobese patients. There was a significant increase in nitrogen balance, osteocalcin, carboxy-terminal propeptide of type I procollagen, and carboxy-terminal telopeptide of type I collagen. Growth hormone also lowered total high density lipoprotein, and low density lipoprotein cholesterol. These preliminary data suggest that growth hormone could ameliorate some adverse effects induced by long-term glucocorticoids.

Others

Other agents are effective in special populations. Vitamin K prevented bone loss in 20 patients with chronic glomerulonephritis treated with prednisolone (263) and ciclosporin 4.8 mg/kg/day prevented glucocorticoid-induced osteopenia in 52 patients taking prednisone 10 mg/day after kidney transplantation (264).

Avascular necrosis

Avascular aseptic necrosis of bone (SEDA-19, 377) (265,266) is a well-recognized adverse effect related to high-dose glucocorticoid therapy (equivalent to more than 4000 mg of prednisone) for extended periods (3 months or longer) but can occur after short-term glucocorticoid therapy. It occurs in a wide range of patients with many different disorders and is particularly likely to involve the femoral and humeral heads. The first lesions are often localized small osteolytic areas in the subchondral bone, where they can be diagnosed early by X-radiography. Magnetic resonance imaging (MRI) is one of the more sensitive techniques to diagnose avascular necrosis of the femoral head. The development and changes in avascular necrosis of the femoral head had been studied by MRI in patients with systemic lupus erythematosus treated with long-term prednisolone administration (SEDA-19, 377; SEDA-19, 164). MRI abnormalities could be detected soon after the start of glucocorticoid therapy or were associated with increased dosages for treating exacerbation of the disease. Normal hips are rarely involved in avascular osteonecrosis. However, aseptic osteonecrosis of the femoral head is often seen in young patients; the lunate, capitate, and patella are their locations. Usually only one joint is involved, although lesions can be multiple. Whether intra-articular injections of glucocorticoids can cause necrosis of bone is still uncertain.

Femoral head necrosis in kidney transplant recipients who receive postoperative immunosuppression with prednisone can be prevented, at least to some extent, by minimizing the dosage of prednisone whenever feasible (267). Of 750 patients (445 men and 305 women) who had undergone kidney transplantation in 1968–95, 374 had received an average of 12.5 g of prednisone during the first year after surgery (high-dose prednisone group) and 276 had received an average of 6.5 g during this time (low-dose prednisone group) plus ciclosporin. Femoral head necrosis occurred in 42/374 patients (11%) in the high-dose prednisone group, an average of 26 months after transplantation. In contrast, femoral head necrosis occurred in only 19/376 patients (5.1%) in the low-dose group an average of 21 months after transplantation. The difference between the high- and low-dose groups was highly significant.

The risk of avascular necrosis has been assessed in a nested case-control study using computer records (268). There were 31 cases during 720 000 person-years Avascular necrosis was strongly associated with glucocorticoid exposure (RR = 16). When total prednisone exposure over 35 months was stratified into three levels (under 440 mg, 440–1290 mg, and over 1290 mg), there was no excess risk for cumulative doses of up to 440 mg (RR = 0; 95% CI = 0, 5). The relative risk was increased for doses between 440 and 1290 mg (RR = 6; CI = 1, 43) and indeterminately increased at doses over 1290 mg (CI = 26, infinity).

In 15 men with osteonecrosis of the femoral head after short-term therapy the mean duration of therapy was 21 (range 7–39) days and the mean dose in milligram equivalents of prednisone was 850 (range 290–3300) mg (269). The time from administration of glucocorticoids to hip pain was 17 (range 6–33) months. A new case of bilateral avascular necrosis of the femoral heads after high-dose short-term dexamethasone therapy as an antiemetic in cancer chemotherapy has been reported (270).

Myopathy

The presence of physiological amounts of glucocorticoids is necessary for the normal functioning of muscle. Excessive glucocorticoid concentrations, in contrast, result in protein catabolism and a reduced rate of muscle protein synthesis (271), and hence in muscle atrophy and fibrosis. The molecular and biochemical basis of myopathy has been widely studied, and the mechanism has been attributed to impairment of glycogen synthesis. Muscle glycogen synthase protein content and activity was measured in samples from 14 patients taking glucocorticoids after kidney transplantation and from 20 healthy subjects (SEDA-21, 418; 272). The patients had impaired activation of glycogen synthase and reduced enzyme activity. Muscular weakness can of course also result from glucocorticoid-induced hypokalemia. In spontaneous Cushing's syndrome, there is muscle involvement in some 50% of cases (273).

Among reports of myopathy in patients taking glucocorticoids, involvement of the respiratory muscles is often mentioned (274,275), possibly because this is particularly likely to have clinical consequences. Patients on mechanically assisted ventilation may be particularly at risk of myopathy (SEDA-18, 390). However, any muscle can be affected; one often sees weakness and atrophy of the hip muscles and (in about half the cases) the shoulder muscles and the proximal muscles of the limbs.

The myopathy usually develops gradually, without pain, and symmetrically. However, a single epidural injection of a glucocorticoid for lumbar radicular pain has caused Cushing's syndrome and myopathy (SEDA-20, 370; 97).

There is a suggestion that the incidence of myopathy is greatest during treatment with compounds that are fluorinated at the 9-alpha position, such as triamcinolone, but this may simply reflect its general potency. In children, the risk of effects on muscles is relatively high.

Biopsy is not justified as a routine, but it is useful as a diagnostic tool in distinguishing suspected corticoid myopathy from diseases of the muscles or vascular system with inflammation that may have been the indication for giving glucocorticoids in the first place; electromyographic measurements cannot confirm the diagnosis.

After termination of treatment the myopathy normally improves over a period of several months.

Damage to tendons and fascia

Tendons can be injured by glucocorticoids and can rupture (276). Ten cases of Achilles tendon rupture were seen in a single clinic over a 10-year period (SEDA-17, 448). The risk seems to be greater if local (for example intra-articular) injections are used.

Rupture of the plantar fascia induced by glucocorticoids has usually been reported in athletes. However, a case of spontaneous degenerative rupture has been reported in a 72-year-old man who had received four glucocorticoid injections over 1 year for plantar fasciitis (SEDA-21, 418) (277).

- A 69-year-old man with newly diagnosed giant cell arteritis was given prednisone 30 mg bd, and 2 weeks later developed severe pain along his Achilles tendons bilaterally; 1 week later the left tendon ruptured (278). Despite immobilization his pain worsened. The prednisone was gradually tapered and the symptoms abated, with complete recovery.

In the previous literature this adverse reaction was described in patients taking glucocorticoids for from 4 months to several years.

Joints

Among the adverse effects of pulse glucocorticoid therapy, joint manifestations are rare. A woman with systemic lupus erythematosus and nephritis developed transient bilateral knee effusions during pulse therapy with high doses of glucocorticoids (279).

- A 62-year old woman was admitted to hospital with lupus nephritis. A kidney biopsy showed a mesangioproliferative glomerulonephritis (WHO class III). After 4 months of inadequate response to traditional treatment, she started monthly pulse glucocorticoid therapy (methylprednisolone 1 g for 3 days) before immunosuppressive drugs. After 2 days of pulse glucocorticoid therapy she complained of pain and flexion discomfort in both knees, which were swollen. At arthrocentesis synovial fluid was aspirated (5 ml from the right knee and 6 ml from the left). The fluid was colorless, with a high viscosity and excellent mucin clot formation. There was only 1 mononuclear cell/mm^3 in the right knee synovial fluid and no cells in the left. There were no crystals. Inflammatory laboratory measurements carried out simultaneously were unchanged. X-rays of the affected joints were normal. The effusion resolved with arthrocentesis and did not recur.

The author proposed that raised arterial pressure, which is an adverse effect of high dose glucocorticoid treatment, and low oncotic pressure due to a low protein plasma concentration in a patient with nephrotic syndrome, could have increased trans-synovial fluid flow at a lower arterial pressure than normal.

Growth in children

The possibility that inhaled glucocorticoids may impair growth in children is of concern, but difficult to assess, as severe chronic asthma can impair growth. If not adequately controlled, asthma modifies the prepubertal growth spurt, the pubertal growth spurt, and the catch-up phase, which allows the child to attain adult height. There is a wide range of individual responses and some children have adverse effects with relatively small doses of glucocorticoids. It is still not clear whether this is a transient phenomenon, causing a slowing of growth and maturational delay with no adverse effect on adult height, or whether growth can be permanently impaired. Ideally studies should establish the effect of asthma treatments on final adult height (compared with predicted values for sex and parental height). Such studies pose considerable logistic problems. For this reason most studies have measured growth over shorter time spans. Outcome measures have been expressed as the height velocity or growth rate, that is changes in height over a defined time. Alternatively height is measured and compared with that of age- and sex-matched controls. Such relatively short-term studies do not necessarily predict the effects of treatment on eventual adult height.

The growth-inhibiting effects of glucocorticoids in children are related not only to inhibition of growth hormone secretion, but also to the sensitivity of the peripheral tissues to the effects of growth hormone. By means of overnight profile analysis it was shown that glucocorticoid treatment reduces the amplitude but not the number of pulses of the physiological growth hormone secretion (SEDA-14, 335; 280).

Effects on growth occur early in treatment: with sensitive testing methods they can be detected in growing children within a few weeks of starting therapy. The effects can be produced by any route of administration, including even inhalation therapy (at least with dexamethasone) (SEDA-18, 391). Comparisons of attained heights with expected heights in children who have used inhaled or oral glucocorticoids have been summarized in a meta-analysis (SEDA-19, 375; 281). There was a significant but small tendency for glucocorticoid therapy in general to be associated with reduced final height. However, this effect varied according to the route of administration. As expected, there was significant impairment of growth with prednisone and other oral glucocorticoids. On the other hand, inhaled beclomethasone dipropionate was associated with normal stature, even when it was used in higher dosages, for longer durations, or in patients with more severe asthma. In another study in 94 children aged 7–9 years, beclomethasone in a dosage taken by many children with mild asthma (400 micrograms/day) significantly reduced growth (SEDA-20, 369; 282). In children with growth suppression during therapy with inhaled beclomethasone or budesonide (200–400 micrograms/day) there was catch-up growth when they switched to equipotent dosages of inhaled fluticasone (100–200 micrograms/day) (SEDA-21, 414; 283). However, in six children with severe asthma, treatment with inhaled high-dosage fluticasone 1000 micrograms/day was associated with growth retardation and adrenal insufficiency (SEDA-21, 414; 284). In one child, growth rate and adrenal function normalized 9 months after the fluticasone dosage was reduced to 500 micrograms/day.

It is generally agreed that the use of single doses of prednisone on alternate mornings minimizes growth retardation but does not avoid it; in children it has been shown that biochemical markers of growth are lower in patients receiving daily glucocorticoid therapy than in patients treated with an alternate-day regimen or not receiving glucocorticoids (SED-12, 988; 285).

It has long been thought by some physicians that the impairment of growth caused by glucocorticoids can be lessened by switching to corticotropin, but this is uncertain. Compensatory treatment with anabolic hormones is definitely not recommended today, since they do not stimulate growth but actually impede it by promoting closure of the epiphyses. Recombinant growth hormone (rGH) treatment of poorly growing children with glucocorticoid-dependent renal disease has often been observed to improve linear growth. However, the dosage of prednisone has been reported to be a critical factor in determining the efficacy of rGH therapy in glucocorticoid-dependent children (SEDA-19, 375; 286). When the dose of prednisone was greater than 0.35 mg/kg/day, rGH did not increase the linear growth rate. At lower doses, the response was inversely related to the amount of prednisone.

Provided glucocorticoid treatment is terminated before the end of puberty, total growth may catch up with the physiological norm (SEDA-17, 448). Concern has been expressed that fear of growth retardation can result in unjustifiable denial of glucocorticoid therapy. It does, however, seem highly advisable to keep doses as low as possible and to switch to a therapeutic regimen that excludes glucocorticoids as children approach the expected onset of puberty (SEDA-14, 335).

Serum osteocalcin determinations appear to be a helpful marker to evaluate the effects of glucocorticoids on growth in children.

One unanswered question is whether the growth suppression that occurs in children during glucocorticoid treatment persists after treatment is withdrawn and affects final adult height. In an attempt to answer this question, growth 6–7 years after withdrawal of alternate-day prednisone has been evaluated in children (aged 6–14 years) with cystic fibrosis who had participated in a multicenter trial from 1986 to 1991 (287). Of 224 children, 161 had been randomized to prednisone (1 or 2 mg/kg) and 73 to placebo. At the time of the study, 68% were aged 18 years or more. Height fell during prednisone therapy, but catch-up growth began 2 years after withdrawal. However, the heights of the boys treated with prednisone remained significantly lower by 4 cm than those who took placebo. In contrast, in the girls there were no differences in height at 2–3 years after prednisone withdrawal.

Reproductive system

Reduced sperm count and motility and inhibition of the secretory function of the testicles during glucocorticoid treatment have been reported and discussed in relation to the suppression of adrenal androgen production. These reports still await confirmation.

Since amenorrhea is a symptom of Cushing's syndrome, disorders of menstruation are common in fertile women taking higher doses of glucocorticoids (SEDA-3, 305). On the other hand, plasma cortisol concentrations in normally menstruating women have marked circadian variation, the extent of which can reach 200% or more (288), with the peak of the cortisol plasma concentrations at mid-cycle and near its end. Inhibition of ovulation by triamcinolone 25 mg has been reported when the drug is given on day 1 or 2 of the cycle. How glucocorticoids interfere with the hormonal control of the menstrual cycle is still unknown (289).

Women should be warned about the possibility of menstrual disorders after local triamcinolone injections (290). When premenopausal women received their first injection of triamcinolone intra-articularly ($n = 46$), injected into soft tissue ($n = 24$), or epidurally ($n = 7$) they were specifically asked to report flushing or menstrual irregularities during a mean follow-up period of 6 weeks. Of the 77 women in the study, 39 reported menstrual disorders. The onset of menstruation was later than expected in ten women and earlier in 16 women. There was reduced loss of blood and/or a shorter duration of menstruation in four women and increased loss of blood and/or a longer duration of menstruation in 18. Also, 22 women had flushing. Menstrual disorders occurred significantly less often in women who were taking oral contraceptives.

Immunologic

Since the glucocorticoids have immunosuppressive and anti-inflammatory properties, one would not expect allergic reactions to be a problem, except when excipients act as allergens. Nevertheless, allergic reactions to glucocorticoids themselves have been reported (SEDA-21, 419; 291). Immunological reactions to glucocorticoids have been reviewed (292). Reactions can be of types I, III, or IV. Immediate reactions usually occur in patients with asthma and in those who have to use glucocorticoids repeatedly. Other susceptibility factors include female sex and hypersensitivity to acetylsalicylic acid. Often excipients are implicated (succinates, sulfites, and carboxymethylcellulose). Cross-reactivity does not necessarily occur; patients with immediate reactions to hydrocortisone and methylprednisolone can often tolerate prednisone and prednisolone and second-generation compounds, such as dexamethasone and betamethasone. Urticaria after glucocorticoid treatment has been explained as a reaction of the mesenchyme. Also, an increase in eosinophilic leukocytes (which normally are diminished by glucocorticoids) has been reported as a first reaction to treatment with glucocorticoids.

Class I reactions

To date, there have been about 100 published reports of immediate hypersensitivity reactions after oral and parenteral administration of glucocorticoids. Although there is evidence that glucocorticoids themselves can cause these reactions, there is debate about the mechanism. Anaphylactic shock has been described after intranasal

hydrocortisone acetate, intramuscular methylprednisolone (SEDA-21, 419; 293), intravenous methylprednisolone (SEDA-22, 448; 294), intramuscular dexamethasone (SEDA-22, 448; 295), and intra-articular methylprednisolone (SEDA-22, 449; 296). A life-threatening anaphylactic-like reaction to intravenous hydrocortisone has been described in patients with asthma (297). Acute laryngeal obstruction has been described after the intravenous administration of hydrocortisone (SEDA-22, 449; 298). There is some reason to believe that sodium succinate esters are more likely to cause hypersensitivity reactions (SEDA-17, 449), but unconjugated glucocorticoids can definitely produce allergy in some cases (SEDA-16, 452).

- A 64-year-old woman with a history of bronchial asthma developed increasing shortness of breath after an upper respiratory tract infection (299). Her medication included inhaled salbutamol as necessary, theophylline 300 mg bd, and aspirin 325 mg/day. She was given nebulized salbutamol and ipratropium and hydrocortisone 200 mg intravenously. Within 30 minutes, she developed a generalized rash, fever (38.3°C), and respiratory distress. She was promptly intubated and mechanical ventilation was started. No further doses of glucocorticoid were given. Skin testing with various parenteral formulations of glucocorticoids produced a 5 mm wheal at the site of hydrocortisone and methylprednisolone injections. She was subsequently given a challenge dose of triamcinolone using a metered-dose inhaler with no reaction, and was therefore continued on this medication.

- An anaphylactoid reaction (angioedema, generalized urticaria, worsening bronchospasm, and marked hypotension) occurred in a 35-year-old man with multiple sclerosis who became allergic to methylprednisolone (dose not stated) after starting treatment with interferon beta-1b (300). He had previously been treated with different courses of methylprednisolone. Clinicians should be aware that the complexity of the effects of interferon beta-1b on the immune system can lead to unexpected outcomes. It is uncertain whether the sequence of events here was due to an effect of interferon beta-1b or to coincidence.

- A 17-year-old boy, with an 11-year history of asthma, had anaphylaxis with respiratory distress shortly after he received intravenous methylprednisolone for an exacerbation of asthma while taking a tapering course of oral prednisone 15 mg/day (301). He had been glucocorticoid-dependent for at least 1 year. He reported having received intravenous glucocorticoids previously. He was treated with inhaled salbutamol and then intravenous methylprednisolone 125 mg over 15–30 seconds, and 3–4 minutes later became flushed and dyspneic, and developed diffuse urticarial lesions on his trunk and face and an undetectable blood pressure. He was treated with adrenaline, but required intubation. Sinus bradycardia developed and then asystole. He was successfully resuscitated and a 10–15 seconds period of generalized tonic-clonic activity was treated with diazepam. He remained unresponsive to stimulation for 30 minutes. However, he awoke 1 hour after his respiratory arrest and was extubated and discharged the following day taking a tapering dosage of prednisone.

- An anaphylactoid reaction occurred in a 68-year-old woman after treatment with intravenous methylprednisolone for asthma. She had developed urticaria with methylprednisolone 1 year earlier, but the reaction had been thought to be related to the solvent in the formulation (302).
- Forty minutes after a first dose of prednisone 25 mg, a 17-year-old girl with a history of aspirin intolerance had generalized flushing, hives, hypogastric pain, and abdominal cramps, followed by vomiting and diarrhea (303). She lost consciousness and developed arterial hypotension. She responded to intravenous diphenhydramine and hydrocortisone. Intradermal skin tests were positive for prednisone and negative for methylprednisolone and hydrocortisone. An oral challenge test with prednisone led to flushing, nausea, dizziness, tachycardia, and hypotension and responded to intravenous diphenhydramine and hydrocortisone. Challenge tests with intravenous methylprednisolone and hydrocortisone were negative.
- A 75-year-old man developed triamcinolone-induced anaphylaxis and dose-related positive prick skin tests to triamcinolone, suggesting that an IgE-mediated hypersensitivity mechanism may have played a part (304).
- A 30-year-old man with recurrent atopic eczema of the head and neck, generalized xerosis, keratosis pilaris of the arms, and a history of dyshidrosis was initially treated with prednisolone-21-acetate ointment (305). His skin eruption became worse. He was given oral prednisolone 25 mg, and 5 hours after the first dose developed intense generalized pruritus with erythema and swelling of the face. After 24 hours there was generalized erythema with disseminated partly follicular papules. There was an eosinophilia ($1.1 \times 10^9/l$). Total IgE was not raised. Patch tests showed delayed reactions to hydrocortisone 1%, prednisolone 1%, prednisolone-21-acetate ointment, and prednisolone 2.5%. Prick and intradermal tests with methylprednisolone succinate, hydrocortisone succinate, betamethasone, and triamcinolone acetonide in concentrations up to 1 : 10 were negative at 15 minutes. However, 4 hours after intradermal testing, generalized pruritus developed and 24 hours later there was a disseminated partly follicular eczematous reaction with involvement of the flexural areas. Biopsy of the eruptions caused by prednisolone and of the positive skin reaction to methylprednisolone succinate showed superficial dermatitis with a perivascular infiltration consisting predominantly of CD4+ cells and some eosinophils. Immunofluorescence showed increased expression of HLA-DR molecules on the CD4+ and CD8+ cells. During the exanthema caused by prednisolone, interleukin-5 (14 pg/ml), interleukin-6 (38 pg/ml), and interleukin-10 (26 pg/ml) were detected in the blood; 2 months after recovery these cytokines were not detectable.

The authors of the last report commented that generalized delayed type hypersensitivity to systemic administration of a glucocorticoid is rare. Despite the potent immunosuppressive effect of glucocorticoids on immunocompetent cells, the clinical features, the skin biopsy specimen, and the positive delayed skin test reactions strongly suggested an immunological mechanism: T cells were clearly involved and the high concentrations of interleukins 5, 6, and 10 were consistent with a T helper type 2 reaction. The raised concentrations of interleukin-5 were probably responsible for the blood and tissue eosinophilia.

Skin prick tests and intradermal tests to hydrocortisone and methylprednisolone, intradermal tests to betamethasone and dexamethasone, and oral challenge tests to betamethasone and deflazacort were performed in 10 patients with adverse reactions to systemic hemisuccinate esters of hydrocortisone and methylprednisolone (306). The skin prick tests and intradermal tests results suggested the possibility of an IgE-mediated mechanism for allergic reactions to hydrocortisone and methylprednisolone. The authors hypothesized that this mechanism is probably due, at least in part, to a glucocorticoid-glyoxal compound, a degradation product of cortisol, which in aqueous solution may be responsible for presenting steroid carbon rings to the immune system. They suggested that betamethasone and deflazacort could be reserved for emergency use in patients with adverse reactions to other glucocorticoids.

Budesonide has been marketed in oral form for intestinal inflammatory disease. An non-IgE-mediated anaphylactic reaction has been associated with oral budesonide (307).

- A 32-year-old woman with Crohn's disease, who had taken prednisone 20 mg/day and azathioprine 150 mg/day, switched to budesonide 9 mg/day because of weight gain, and 5 minutes after the first capsule her tongue and throat swelled, accompanied by wheeziness and diarrhea. She was given clemastine and recovered after 4 ays. Intracutaneous tests with diluted budesonide suggested a non-IgE-mediated reaction. She had a previous history of a similar reaction to mesalazine. One year later her tongue and throat swelled after intravenous dexamethasone.

Urticaria with angioedema has been described in a patient taking deflazacort (308).

- A 64-year-old woman with allergic alveolitis caused by parakeet feathers improved with intravenous methylprednisolone, and was given oral deflazacort 60 mg/day, to be reduced progressively. After 30 days she developed generalized itchy blotches and lip edema. At that time she was mistakenly taking deflazacort in a dose of 120 mg/day. She was given an antihistamine, without any improvement. Deflazacort was then replaced by prednisolone and her symptoms disappeared immediately. Skin tests (a prick test and an epicutaneous test) were positive with deflazacort. Oral provocation with deflazacort 30 mg was positive, with the immediate appearance of the same symptoms as in the initial episode.

Class III reactions

Allergy to topical glucocorticoids in inflammatory bowel disease has been reported (309).

- A 57-year old Caucasian man with inflammatory bowel disease was given prednisolone metasulfobenzoate sodium enemas twice daily and oral mesalazine 800 mg tds for about 5 months, without improvement. He stopped using the prednisolone enemas but continued to take mesalazine. Within 48 hours of stopping prednisolone his symptoms resolved completely. The theoretical possibility of contact allergy was entertained. Patch tests with a standard battery of contact allergens, including tixocortol pivalate and budesonide, were ++ positive with budesonide. At follow up 3 months later he was symptom free.

The authors advised that allergy to topical glucocorticoids should be considered in patients using rectal steroids whose condition unexpectedly fails to improve or in whom there is unexpected deterioration.

Vasculitis

Exacerbation of giant cell arteritis, with clinical signs of an evolving vertebrobasilar stroke, has been attributed to prednisolone (310).

- A 64-year-old man with giant cell arteritis was given prednisolone 60 mg/day. Within 5 days he developed double vision and agitation and became drowsy and confused. A cranial MRI scan showed recent cerebral lesions and a Doppler scan showed high-resistant blood flow in both vertebral arteries. He had an episode of complete loss of vision and was given dexamethasone and intravenous heparin followed by warfarin. He gradually improved over the next few weeks but was left with cognitive and memory deficits.

Immunosuppression

Glucocorticoids inhibit the formation of antibodies. Of 111 consecutive heart transplant recipients taking oral prednisone (mean 13.8 months), 57% developed hypogammaglobulinemia (IgG below 7 g/l) (311). Those with severe hypogammaglobulinemia (IgG below 3.5 g/l) were at increased risk of opportunistic infections compared with those with IgG concentrations over 3.5 g/l (55 versus 5%, OR = 23). Parenteral glucocorticoid pulse therapy was associated with a significantly increased risk of severe hypogammaglobulinemia (OR = 15).

With long-term treatment, IgG subclass deficiencies can become marked (312). There is suppression of the antigen–antibody reaction, and since this reaction itself normally results in liberation of kinins, the latter is also suppressed. Failure of kinin liberation leads in turn to inhibition of invasion of sensitized leukocytes and reduced production and maturation of phagocytes. Undoubtedly, it is true that using minimal effective doses will avoid the most serious consequences, but the problem cannot be fully circumvented, since the anti-inflammatory effects themselves involve some inhibition of the migration of leukocytes and phagocytosis.

Dexamethasone significantly affected the antibody response of preterm infants with chronic lung disease to immunization against *Haemophilus influenzae* (313). Serum samples were obtained before and after immunization from an unselected cohort of 59 preterm infants (30 boys; gestational age 175–208 days). *Haemophilus influenzae* antibodies were measured using ELISA. IgG antibody concentrations in 16 infants who received no dexamethasone were 0.16 and 4.63 microgram/ml before and after immunization respectively. The corresponding values for those who received dexamethasone were 0.10 and 0.51 microgram/ml.

Infection risk

The consequence of this interference with immune responses can be multiplication of bacteria and an increased risk of bacterial intoxication when infection does occur; hence, the frequency and severity of clinical infections tend to increase during glucocorticoid therapy. Aggravation of existing tuberculosis and reactivation of completely quiescent cases of this infection are classic consequences demanding prophylactic measures; atypical mycobacteria have also caused tissue infections (SEDA-17, 449). Other bacterial infections, some severe and proceeding to sepsis, have followed glucocorticoid treatment. There is little evidence that glucocorticoids, even in high dosages and early in the course of infection, significantly alter the ultimate outcome (314). Use of glucocorticoids in the treatment of septic shock is not recommended in the absence of adrenal suppression.

It has been suggested that there are some differences between drugs. The use of fluticasone nasal spray to control polyp recurrence after functional endoscopic sphenoethmoidectomy should be viewed with caution, as it has been said to be associated with a high incidence of severe postoperative infection compared with beclomethasone (SEDA-21, 375; 315).

Acute generalized exanthematous pustulosis due to a glucocorticoid has been reported (SEDA-21, 416; 316).

In a retrospective study, postoperative infectious complications were evaluated in 159 patients with inflammatory bowel disease undergoing elective surgery (317). Immunosuppression consisted of glucocorticoid monotherapy (n = 56), a glucocorticoid + azathioprine or mercaptopurine (n = 52), and neither a glucocorticoid nor azathioprine or mercaptopurine (n = 51). The adjusted odds ratios for any infection and major infections in patients who took glucocorticoid were 3.69 and 5.54 respectively, and in patients who took azathioprine or mercaptopurine 1.68 and 1.20. Thus, preoperative use of glucocorticoid in patients with inflammatory bowel disease increased the risk of postoperative infectious complications.

Bacterial infections

Infections with *Clostridium difficile*, *Pseudomonas aeruginosa*, and *Listeria monocytogenes* (SEDA-22, 450; 318) have occasionally been precipitated or aggravated by glucocorticoids, as has tuberculous peritonitis (SEDA-20, 377; 319).

The cumulative and mean daily dosages of glucocorticoids in patients with systemic lupus erythematosus, inflammatory myopathy, overlap syndrome, or mixed connective tissue disease were the most important risk factors for the development of tuberculosis, according to a study conducted in Korea (320). Records were analysed from 269 patients who had been hospitalized during a 5-year period. In 21 patients active tuberculosis developed after a mean duration of 27 months from diagnosis of their rheumatic disease, an incidence rate of 20 cases per 1000 patient-years. The mean cumulative and daily dosages of prednisolone during the follow-up period were 31 594 and 25 mg respectively in patients who developed tuberculosis, compared with 17 043 and 18 mg in patients who did not. Glucocorticoid pulse therapy was a risk factor for the development of tuberculosis.

- A 43-year-old woman developed cavitary lung tuberculosis after she received methotrexate and glucocorticoid pulse therapy for rheumatoid arthritis (321).

The authors commented that the onset of the lung infection appeared to be closely related to methotrexate and glucocorticoid pulse therapy, because of the interval between drug administration and the onset of tuberculosis, and the lack of other risk factors for opportunistic infections.

In a retrospective study, the use of glucocorticoids during *Pneumocystis jiroveci* pneumonia (mean total dose methylprednisolone 420 mg, mean treatment duration 12 days) did not increase the risk of development or relapse of tuberculosis or other AIDS-related diseases (SEDA-20, 377; 322). The study included 129 patients (72 who took glucocorticoids and 57 who did not) who were followed up at 6, 12, 18, and 24 months of glucocorticoid therapy. The rates of infections were similar in both groups, and the cumulative rate of tuberculosis at 2 years was 12–13%.

Mycobacterium avium septic arthritis has been reported in two patients with pre-existing rheumatic disease (scleroderma and polymyositis) who were taking prednisolone and azathioprine; the infection was in the left shoulder in one patient and in the knee in the other (323).

The use of glucocorticoids in patients with hematological diseases is a factor that facilitates the occurrence of *Legionella pneumophila* pneumonia, and 10 episodes of this infection were possibly related to glucocorticoids in a series of 67 cases of Legionnaires' disease diagnosed in a single institution during 2.5 years (324).

Viral infections

Infections such as chickenpox can have serious consequences, including death, in patients taking systemic glucocorticoids (SEDA-19, 378; SEDA-20, 377; 325,326). It has been suggested that *Varicella zoster* immunoglobulin should be given to patients in contact with chickenpox if they have taken glucocorticoids in dosages over 0.5 mg/kg/day

during the preceding 3 months, in the context of near-fatal chickenpox in a child receiving prednisolone (SEDA-20, 377; 327). Smallpox vaccination has in the past resulted in vaccinia gangrenosum in patients taking glucocorticoids, and the current type of *Varicella* vaccine is much more likely to produce rashes in children who are already taking glucocorticoids than in controls (SEDA-16, 452).

Herpes simplex virus encephalitis after myxedema coma has been described in an 81-year-old man treated with hydrocortisone (100 mg 8-hourly) and levothyroxine (328). In renal transplantation, two cases of death from *Herpes simplex* as a result of glucocorticoid treatment are on record (SED-8, 827; SEDA-17, 449).

Fungal and yeast infections

Fungal and yeast infections (including cases of fulminant fungal pericarditis, mucormycosis, *Aspergillus fumigatus* infection, and cutaneous alternariosis) can be precipitated or aggravated by glucocorticoid treatment (SEDA-17, 449; SEDA-18, 390; SEDA-20, 377; SEDA-21, 418; SEDA-22, 449; 329–332).

Primary esophageal histoplasmosis must be considered in patients who have a history of gastroesophageal reflux disease and are immunosuppressed by long-term glucocorticoids (SEDA-22, 450; 333). Oropharyngeal candidiasis is a well-described adverse effect of inhaled glucocorticoids. However, few cases of esophageal candidiasis have been reported (SEDA-22, 179).

Invasive pulmonary aspergillosis with cerebromeningeal involvement has been described after short-term intravenous administration of methylprednisolone (SEDA-22, 449; 334). Of 473 HIV-infected children, 7 (1.5%) developed invasive aspergillosis during the study period (1987–95) (SEDA-22, 449; 335). Sustained neutropenia or glucocorticoid therapy as predisposing factors for invasive aspergillosis were found in only two patients.

- Fatal pulmonary infection with *Aspergillus fumigatus* and *Nocardia asteroides* has been described in a patient who took prednisone 1 mg/kg/day for 1 month for bronchiolitis obliterans (336).
- Fatal *Aspergillus* myocarditis, probably related to short-term administration of glucocorticoids, has been described in a 58-year-old man, who had an acute exacerbation of his chronic obstructive pulmonary disease and received oxygen, bronchodilators, omeprazole, co-amoxiclav, and intravenous methylprednisolone 40 mg 8-hourly; he died 5 days later and postmortem examination showed a fungal myocarditis (337).
- Fatal aspergillosis with a thyroid gland abscess occurred in a 74-year-old man after treatment with prednisolone for polymyalgia rheumatica (338).
- *Cryptoccocus neoformans* meningitis occurred in a 15-year old child with acute lymphoblastic leukemia (339). The clinical signs, headache, and a sixth nerve palsy on the right side, occurred at the end of the maintenance therapy when complete remission had been obtained (after 100 weeks of maintenance therapy, including multiple intermittent doses of dexamethasone). Culture of the cerebrospinal fluid confirmed

cryptoccocal meningitis, and antifungal therapy produced a complete clinical response.

- *Scedosporium apiospermum* infection occurred in the left forearm of an 81-year-old man who was taking chronic oral prednisone (increased to 40 mg/day 1 month before presentation) for lung fibrosis (340).

Cutaneous alternariosis (infection with *Alternaria alternata*) has been described in a 78-year-old farmer with idiopathic pulmonary fibrosis taking oral prednisone 20 mg/day (341).

The effect of dexamethasone has been assessed in a retrospective chart review study in neonates weighing less than 1200 g, both with ($n = 65$) and without ($n = 269$) *Candida* sepsis; dexamethasone therapy and prolonged antibiotic therapy were associated with *Candida* infection (342).

In a retrospective study that included 163 consecutive recipients of allogenic hemopoietic stem cell transplants with invasive fungal infections, the possible role of glucocorticoid therapy was evaluated. The administration of high-dose glucocorticoids (2 mg/kg/day or more) was associated with an increased risk of mold infection ($HR = 4.0$, 95% $CI = 1.7$, 9.6) and an increased risk of mold infection-related death (1 year survival 11% compared with 44% when patients took doses less than 2 mg/kg/day) (343).

Fatal cerebral involvement in systemic aspergillosis has been described in a 25-year old woman with severe thrombocytopenia (platelet count $10 \times 10^9/l$) and mild intermittent leukopenia (granulocytes $0.375–3 \times 10^9/l$) who was taking prednisone 1–1.5 mg/kg/day and azathioprine 100–200 mg/day (344).

Helminth infections

Strongyloidiasis (SEDA-20, 377; SEDA-21, 419; SEDA-22, 449; 345–347) has been precipitated or aggravated by glucocorticoids.

Protozoal infections

Toxoplasmosis has been precipitated by glucocorticoids (348,349).

Pneumocystis jiroveci pneumonia has been precipitated or aggravated by glucocorticoids (SEDA-20, 377; SEDA-22, 450; 272,350,351). There is some concern about the use of glucocorticoids as adjunctive therapy in patients with AIDS who develop *Pneumocystis jiroveci* pneumonia. The immunosuppressant properties of glucocorticoids have been reported to enhance the risk of tuberculosis

and other AIDS-related diseases (for example Kaposi's sarcoma or cytomegalovirus infection).

Amebic dysentery has been precipitated by glucocorticoids (352).

Death

Mortality associated with glucocorticoid has been retrospectively studied in 556 patients with chronic obstructive pulmonary disease admitted to a rehabilitation center (353). Median survival was 38 months and 280 patients died during follow-up. On multivariate analysis, oral glucocorticoid use at a prednisone equivalent of 10 mg/day without inhaled glucocorticoid was associated with an increased risk of death ($RR = 2.34$; 95% $CI = 1.24$, 4.44), and 15 mg/day increased the risk further ($RR = 4.03$; 95% $CI = 1.99$, 8.15). The risk of death was not increased in those using 5 mg/day or when patients used any oral dose in combination with inhaled glucocorticoids.

Long-Term Effects

Drug withdrawal

Suppression of adrenocortical function is one of the consequences of repeated administration of glucocorticoids; after termination of treatment a withdrawal syndrome can occur. In many cases this is unpleasant rather than acutely dangerous; in such instances the patients may have headache, nausea, dizziness, anorexia, weakness, emotional changes, lethargy, and perhaps fever; in some cases severe mental disorders occur and there are repeated reports of benign intracranial hypertension (354). The glucocorticoid withdrawal syndrome also seems to underlie the "glucocorticoid pseudorheumatism" that can occur when the drugs are withdrawn in rheumatic patients.

Withdrawal symptoms disappear if the glucocorticoid is resumed, but as a rule they will in any case vanish spontaneously within a few days. More serious consequences can ensue, however, in certain types of cases and if adrenal cortical atrophy is severe. In patients treated with corticoids for the nephrotic syndrome and apparently cured, the syndrome is particularly likely to relapse on withdrawal of therapy if the adrenal cortex is atrophic (SEDA-3, 305). In some cases, acute adrenocortical insufficiency after glucocorticoid treatment has actually proved fatal. It is advisable to withdraw long-term glucocorticoid therapy gradually so that the cortex has sufficient opportunity to recover. Table 5 lists methods of

Table 5 Suggested methods of withdrawing prednisolone

Circumstances	Change in daily dose
The problem has resolved and treatment has been given for only a few weeks	Reduce by 2.5 mg every 3 or 4 days down to 7.5 mg/day; then reduce more slowly, for example by 2.5 mg every week, fortnight, or month
There is uncertainty about disease resolution and/or therapy has been given for many weeks	Reduce by 2.5 mg every fortnight or month down to 7.5 mg/day then reduce by 1 mg every month
Symptoms of the disease are likely to recur on withdrawal (for example rheumatoid arthritis)	Reduce by 1 mg every month

withdrawing prednisolone after long-term therapy in different circumstances (355).

Anorexia nervosa has been precipitated by withdrawal of oral prednisolone for asthma (SEDA-21, 414; 356).

A case of papilledema as a manifestation of raised intracranial pressure has been reported following withdrawal of topical glucocorticoids (SEDA-3, 305).

Panniculitis, which causes erythematous, firm, warm subcutaneous nodules, can occur within 2 weeks of withdrawal of large doses of glucocorticoids, but case reports confirm that resolution without scarring is the rule and that reintroduction of glucocorticoids is not necessary for improvement (357).

Churg–Strauss syndrome has come into prominence with the introduction of the leukotriene receptor antagonists, because they allow glucocorticoid-dependent asthmatics to discontinue their oral prednisolone. Five patients developed Churg–Strauss syndrome when their oral glucocorticoids were withdrawn (358). The duration of oral glucocorticoid therapy was 3–216 months and the dosage of prednisolone was 2.5–25.5 mg/day. The diagnosis of Churg–Strauss syndrome was made from 6 to 83 months after withdrawal of the oral glucocorticoids. These case reports support the hypothesis that it is the withdrawal of glucocorticoids that unmasks the underlying systemic vasculitis in these patients with asthma, rather than an effect of the new therapeutic agents that permits the reduction (and withdrawal) of prednisolone. Case-control studies are needed to determine the respective roles of the new therapeutic agents, prednisolone withdrawal, or other factors in the emergence of Churg–Strauss syndrome in these asthmatic patients

Tumorigenicity

Direct tumor-inducing effects of the glucocorticoids are not known, but the particular risk that malignancies in patients undergoing immunosuppression with these or other drugs will spread more rapidly is a well-recognized problem.

- Progressive endometrial carcinoma associated with azathioprine and prednisone therapy has been reported (359).
- Rapid progression of Kaposi's sarcoma 10 weeks after combined treatment with glucocorticoids and cyclophosphamide has been described; marked improvement of the skin lesions was noted after discontinuation of prednisone therapy (360).

Patients (mean age 39 years, $n = 1862$) who underwent 1924 renal transplantations from March 1995 to May 1997 were followed for 3–150 months. They received one of the following regimens: prednisolone plus azathioprine (group 1; $n = 100$); prednisolone plus azathioprine plus ciclosporin (group 2; $n = 1464$); and the same therapy as group 2 plus either muromonab-CD3 or antithymocyte globulin as induction or antirejection therapy (group 3; $n = 298$). The mean time to appearance of neoplasia after renal transplantation was 48 months. Malignancies developed earlier in group 3 patients (mean time to appearance 31 months) than in group 2 (39 months) and in group 1 (90 months). Seven of the patients who developed malignancies had also

received pulse methylprednisolone for acute rejection. The authors concluded that the treatment of acute rejection with pulsed methylprednisolone and the use of muromonab-CD3 and antithymocyte globulin may lead to an increased incidence of malignancies after renal transplantation. They recommended that strategies be implemented for the early detection of malignancy (361)

In seven patients, accelerated growth of Kaposi's sarcoma lesions during glucocorticoid therapy suggested that glucocorticoids can alter the biological behavior of this malignant disease (362). Hydrocortisone accelerates the growth of cell lines derived from Kaposi's sarcoma cells cultured in vitro and this may partially explain these findings. Reports continue to point to the reversibility of the condition when glucocorticoids are withdrawn (363).

Kaposi's sarcoma has been associated with prednisolone therapy in two elderly women (364).

- An 84-year-old woman with polymyalgia rheumatica and a 79-year-old woman with undifferentiated connective tissue disease and leukocytoclastic vasculitis were given prednisolone 20 mg/day with subsequent dosage reductions. The first patient developed a raised purpuric rash and lymphedema of the left leg within 5 months and the second developed large purple nodules on the soles of her feet and the backs of her hands accompanied by periorbital and peripheral edema. Skin biopsies showed Kaposi's sarcoma, and both patients had raised IgG antibody titers to human herpesvirus-8.

Prior infection with herpesvirus-8 is a requisite for the development of Kaposi's sarcoma. The question arises as to how glucocorticoid treatment alone can lead to the emergence of this malignancy. In vitro evidence supports the hypothesis that glucocorticoids have a direct role in stimulating tumor development and the activation of herpesvirus-8.

A possible relation between systemic glucocorticoid use and a risk of esophageal cancer has been described in a population-based study in Denmark, in which the prescriptions database and the Danish cancer registry were linked (365). There was an increase in the number of cases observed ($n = 36$) compared with the number expected ($n = 19$), with a standardized incidence ratio of 1.92 (95% CI = 1.34, 2.65).

Second-Generation Effects

Pregnancy

A single course of a glucocorticoid given to women at risk of preterm delivery promotes fetal lung maturation, reduces the incidence of respiratory distress syndrome, and reduces neonatal morbidity and mortality. In a retrospective analysis of 306 infants of gestational age under 34 weeks, there was an association between glucocorticoid use and gastroesophageal reflux (366). In this series, 71% of the neonates (216/306) received antenatal glucocorticoids. More babies who received antenatal glucocorticoids had clinical evidence of gastroesophageal reflux (27% versus 12%). There was a significant increase in the incidence of gastroesophageal reflux with increasing courses of antenatal steroids: no course 12%, one course 25%, and two or more courses 32%.

However, there is still controversy about the use of single or repeat courses. It seems that betamethasone is more active in reducing neonatal deaths and produces fewer adverse effects than dexamethasone (367).

In a statement, the American Academy of Pediatrics and the Canadian Paediatric Society did not recommend the routine use of systemic dexamethasone for the prevention or treatment of chronic lung disease in infants with very low birthweights, because it does not reduce overall mortality and is associated with impaired growth and neurodevelopment delay (368,369).

In an analysis of 595 preterm infants born at 26–32 weeks gestation during a randomized controlled trial for the prevention of lung disease, glucocorticoids given to women at risk of preterm delivery promoted fetal lung maturation, reduced the incidence of respiratory distress syndrome, and reduced neonatal morbidity and mortality (370). Dexamethasone was given as either two doses of 12 mg 24 hours apart or four doses of 6 mg every 6 hours. Mortality was 9.2% after three or more courses, compared with 4.8% after one or two courses. This association was not explained by other factors (maternal or other common preterm morbidities).

The effects of glucocorticoids on uterine activity and preterm labor in high-order multiple gestations have been retrospectively reviewed (SEDA-20, 377; 371). In 15 women with triplet or quadruplet pregnancies, 17 out of 57 courses of betamethasone were associated with episodes of significant contractions requiring tocolytic intervention; 11 of these episodes were associated with cervical change and four resulted in premature delivery. The authors did not recommend the use of glucocorticoids if patients have more than 3.5 contractions per hour.

Prenatal glucocorticoid therapy to enhance fetal lung maturation reduces neonatal morbidity and mortality. However, adverse effects of serial courses of betamethasone on mother and fetus can occur.

For example, single versus multiple courses of antenatal glucocorticoids have been compared retrospectively in 704 pregnancies that resulted in pre-term births at 24–32 weeks. There three groups: 294 neonates whose mothers had not received glucocorticoids, 257 who had received a single dose, and 153 who had received multiple doses. Multiple doses compared with a single dose was associated with increased positive maternal cultures (44% versus 31%), small for gestational age infants (35% versus 21%), and intraventricular haemorrhage (45% versus 34%) (372).

In a retrospective study of the use of betamethasone every 12 hours versus 24 hours for anticipated preterm delivery in 909 pregnancies, three groups were identified: those who had not received antenatal glucocorticoids, those who had received betamethasone 12 hours apart, and those who received 24-hour dosing (373). There was significantly more maternal antibiotic use (90% versus 84%) and more neonatal surfactant use (40% versus 26%) in the 12-hour group compared with the 24-hour group. For all other outcomes there was no clinically significant difference.

Endocrine

Maternal hyperadrenalism occurred after five courses of betamethasone to enhance fetal lung maturation (374).

- A 26-year-old woman was given intravenous salbutamol 0.3 mg/hour for preterm labor, and intramuscular betamethasone 12 mg/day for 2 days. Daily oral tocolysis (salbutamol 2 mg every 6 hours plus nicardipine 50 mg every 12 hours) and betamethasone every week were continued at home for 3 weeks. The mother developed amyotrophy, acne on the face and trunk, moon face, hirsutism with whiskers, and thin skin. Free urinary cortisol was less than 5 micrograms/day (reference range 25–90), plasma cortisol was less than 10 ng/ml (100–200), and the salivary cortisol was less than 0.6 ng/ml (2.3–4.7). One hour after intramuscular tetracosactide 250 micrograms, her plasma cortisol was 102 ng/ml (reference range over 210) and the salivary cortisol was 3.1 ng/ml (13–25), indicating no adrenocortical response. She was given hydrocortisone 20 mg/day, and 2 months later adrenocortical insufficiency persisted, with a plasma cortisol of 152 ng/ml after corticotropin stimulation. One year later, she still required hydrocortisone 10 mg/day.

Hyperadrenalism has never otherwise been reported after the sequential use of glucocorticoids for fetal lung maturation.

A study in 10 women has been conducted to determine whether betamethasone administered at risk of preterm delivery causes adrenal suppression (375). After adrenal stimulation with corticotropin 1 microgram at 24–25 weeks, each woman received two intramuscular doses of betamethasone 12 mg 24 hours apart; 1 week later, another corticotropin test was followed by another two doses of betamethasone; a third corticotropin stimulation test was carried out 1 week later. All the women had normal baseline and stimulated cortisol concentrations during the first corticotropin stimulation test. Mean baseline serum cortisol concentrations fell with each corticotropin stimulation test (from 700 nmol/l (254 micrograms/l) before betamethasone to 120 nmol/l (43 micrograms/l) 1 week after the second course of betamethasone). The mean stimulated cortisol concentrations also fell significantly, from 910 nmol/l (330 micrograms/l) to 326 nmol/l (118 micrograms/l). There was evidence of adrenal suppression in four patients after the first course of betamethasone and in seven patients after the second course. There was no evidence of Addisonian crisis antepartum or intrapartum.

Musculoskeletal

Osteonecrosis of the femoral head can occur with glucocorticoids in nonpregnant individuals, but has not previously been reported in pregnancy (376).

- A 37-year-old white woman was given betamethasone, two doses of 12 mg over a day, at 24 weeks of a twin pregnancy, because of a history of growth restriction in her first pregnancy. At 25 weeks Doppler of the umbilical vessels suggested a reduction in end-diastolic flow in one twin. Betamethasone was prescribed again and was repeated weekly to a total of six courses because of the high risk of preterm delivery. At 30 weeks she complained of pain in the right hip exacerbated by weight bearing, which increased over the following 7 days until standing was impossible. An MRI scan showed avascular necrosis of the femoral head.

Infection risk

The use of betamethasone for the treatment of premature rupture of membranes during pregnancy is associated with an increased prevalence of maternal and neonatal infections. Two reports have described the risk of infections associated with the use of glucocorticoids during pregnancy. Of 374 patients with preterm premature rupture of membranes, 99 received a single course of glucocorticoids, 72 received multiple courses, and 203 were not treated with glucocorticoids (377). Only multiple courses of betamethasone increased the incidence of early-onset neonatal sepsis, chorioamnionitis, and endometritis in mothers. A single course of glucocorticoid was not significantly associated with any maternal or neonatal infectious complications. The incidence of maternal infections in 37 patients who received three or more courses of betamethasone (median 6, range 3–10) because of the risk of preterm delivery has been evaluated, with 70 healthy pregnant women as controls (378). Of those treated with betamethasone, 65% developed infectious diseases compared with 18% of controls. Symptomatic lower urinary tract infections (35 versus 2.7%) and serious bacterial infections (24 versus 0%) were more frequent in treated mothers. Eight of nine serious infections occurred in patients exposed to five or more courses of glucocorticoids.

Singleton pregnancies delivered at 24–34 weeks after antenatal betamethasone exposure have been prospectively analysed, in order to study the incidence of perinatal infection (379). There were 453 patients, 267 of whom took a single course of betamethasone (two doses of 12 mg in 24 hours), and 186 of whom took a multiple course (more than two doses in the 24 hours after the initial course). Multiple courses were significantly associated with early-onset neonatal sepsis (OR = 5.0; 95% CI = 1.0, 23), neonatal death (OR = 2.9; CI = 1.3, 6.9), chorioamnionitis (OR = 10; CI = 2.1, 65), and endometritis (OR = 3.6; CI = 1.7, 8.1). Respiratory distress and intraventricular hemorrhage were similar in the two groups. Although the study was non-randomized the results suggest an increased risk of neonatal infection and death after multiple courses of dexamethasone during pregnancy.

In a retrospective study in 609 mothers and their 713 infants who were treated with 1–12 courses of antenatal glucocorticoids, data from 369 singleton preterm infants born at 34 weeks or later, 210 multiple gestations, and 134 infants delivered at 35 weeks or later were analysed (380). The incidence of respiratory distress syndrome was 45% for single courses and 35% for multiple courses of glucocorticoids (OR = 0.44; 95% CI = 0.25, 0.79). The multiple-course group also had significantly less cases of patent ductus arteriosus (20 versus 13%). The incidences of death before discharge and other neonatal morbidities

were similar. The multiple-course group had a significant reduction of 0.46 cm in head circumference at birth when adjusted for gestational age and pre-eclampsia. The two groups had similar birthweights. Infants born at more than 35 weeks, multiple-gestation infants, and infants who were born more than 7 days after the last dose of glucocorticoid had similar outcomes, regardless of the number of courses they had received. Mothers treated with multiple courses compared with a single course had a significantly higher incidence of postpartum endometritis, even though they had a lower incidence of prolonged rupture of membranes (24 versus 33%) and similar cesarean delivery rates. In conclusion, antenatal exposure to multiple courses of glucocorticoids compared with a single course resulted in a significant reduction in the incidence of respiratory distress syndrome in singleton preterm infants delivered within a week of the last glucocorticoid dose. This was associated with a reduction in head circumference at birth and an increased incidence of maternal endometritis. Whether the potential benefits of repeated therapy outweigh the risks will ultimately be determined in randomized controlled trials.

In a retrospective study of the benefits and risks of multiple courses of glucocorticoids in patients with preterm premature rupture of membranes, 170 preterm singleton infants were evaluated (381). They were divided into three groups: non-use ($n = 50$), single courses ($n = 76$), and multiple courses ($n = 44$). There was a higher incidence of chorioamnionitis those who had received multiple courses.

Teratogenicity

Teratogenic effects of glucocorticoids, which have been demonstrated in animal experiments since 1950, have not generally been confirmed in man. The question whether a disease that has had to be treated with glucocorticoids in pregnancy or the glucocorticoid treatment itself may have caused congenital anomalies reported anecdotally usually cannot be answered in any individual case. Dexamethasone, for instance, given in a suppressive dosage, seems to have been therapeutically effective in endocrine abnormal pregnancy with congenital adrenogenital syndrome (382); how is one to distinguish cause and effect here? Cleft lip and palate, seen in animal studies, have not been encountered more often in the offspring of glucocorticoid-treated women than in those of untreated women. In several small series of patients in whom glucocorticoids were used before and during pregnancy, no congenital abnormalities were seen on follow-up, but material on which to base a firm judgement is lacking. Certainly, the evidence to date does not suggest that on teratological grounds one should hesitate to administer glucocorticoids for therapeutic reasons during pregnancy (SEDA-3, 306).

However, first trimester in utero exposure to a glucocorticoid was associated with a small risk of major neonatal malformations, according to the results of a Canadian meta-analysis (383). Six cohort studies and one case-control study were analysed, and the results showed that women who had taken long-term glucocorticoid therapy during pregnancy were more likely to have a baby with a major malformation than women who had not (OR = 2.46; 95% CI = 1.41, 4.29).

Glucocorticoids have been used in cases of hyperemesis gravidarum when standard antiemetics are ineffective. In an observational comparison of women with complicated hyperemesis gravidarum and weight loss, over 5% of pre-pregnant weight treated with (n = 30) or without (n = 25) glucocorticoids, gestational evolution and singleton birth-weights were not different in the two groups (384).

A hydatidiform mole during pregnancy may have been due to the glucocorticoids used in an immunosuppressive regimen (385).

- A 33-year-old woman took immunosuppressive therapy after renal transplantation: ciclosporin (dosage adjusted to achieve blood concentrations of 120–160 ng/ml), azathioprine 1 mg/kg (frequency of administration not sta-ted), and methylprednisolone 40 mg/day from day 1 after transplantation, tapered weekly by 4–8 mg/day. Because of rejection symptoms at weeks 1, 4, and 7, she received three cycles of intravenous methylprednisolone 250 mg/day, each cycle lasting 5–7 days; she also received a bolus dose of methylprednisolone 500 mg on day 0. Pregnancy was diagnosed on day 12 after transplantation (9 weeks after conception). At week 6 after transplantation she had a missed abortion. Curettage was performed and a partial hydatidiform mole was detected. She was discharged at week 10 and immunosuppressive therapy was tapered.

The teratogenic effects of prednisone have been evalu-ated in a placebo-controlled study in 372 women and a meta-analysis (386). There was no statistical difference in the rate of major anomalies between the glucocorticoid-exposed women and the controls. The meta-analysis included 10 studies (six cohort and four case-control stu-dies), with data from 535 exposed and 50 845 nonexposed women. The odds ratios for major malformations were 1.5 (95% CI = 0.8, 2.6) for the cohort studies and 3.4 (CI = 2.0, 5.7) for the case-control studies. The results suggest that although prednisone does not represent a major teratogenic risk in humans in therapeutic doses, it does increase the risk of oral cleft defects by an order of 3.4-fold.

Fetotoxicity

The effect of prolonged antenatal betamethasone (three or more weekly administrations) has been studied in 414 fetuses (387). Multidose betamethasone was not associated with higher risks of antenatal maternal fever, chorioamnionitis, reduced birthweight, neonatal adrenal suppression, neonatal sepsis, or neonatal death.

The effects of antenatal dexamethasone on birthweight have been studied in 961 infants and matched controls (388). Dexamethasone-treated infants had significantly lower birthweights (after adjustment for week of gesta-tion). The average differences from controls were 12 g at 24–26 weeks, 63 g at 27–29 weeks, 161 g at 30–32 weeks, and 80 g at 33–34 weeks. In the case of preterm rupture of membranes, the data were not conclusive.

Betamethasone, two doses of 12 mg a day apart, in 40 pregnant women (27–34 weeks) caused important changes in fetal physiology (389). Fetal breathing (the number of breathing episodes and the total breathing time in 30 minutes) fell by 83% and fetal limb and trunk movements fell by 53% and 49% respectively. These changes were transient and returned to the range of nor-mality 96 hours after administration. There were no changes in Doppler velocimetry of the umbilical and mid-dle cerebral arteries. Awareness of these effects may pre-vent unnecessary iatrogenic delivery of preterm infants who present abnormal biophysical profile scores 2 days after glucocorticoid exposure.

Retardation of intrauterine growth by glucocorticoids has been reported not only in animals but also in man. In a 1990 case from France, dwarfism (as well as Cushing's syndrome) was recorded in a child whose mother had received high-dose glucocorticoids during pregnancy.

It has been suggested that the risk of stillbirth may be increased by glucocorticoid treatment; the figures are suggestive, but the possibility that the disorder that led to the use of the glucocorticoid was itself responsible for the less favorable outcome cannot be excluded (390).

Prevention of the respiratory distress syndrome in antici-pated prematurity has become a widely accepted (though not uncontroversial) indication for glucocorticoids in late pregnancy, the compound most often used being dexa-methasone. The timing of such treatment in late pregnancy seems to be of crucial importance (SEDA-3, 306); the pos-sible adverse effects on the mother and child are still being discussed. The issue has been extensively reviewed (SEDA-17, 445). A meta-analysis of 15 trials, involving 1780 patients treated with glucocorticoids and 1780 controls, has shown a lower risk of the syndrome, and a substantial reduction in neonatal mortality (OR = 0.60; 95% CI = 0.48, 0.76), with-out a higher risk of infection in the mother or maternal pulmonary edema (SEDA-20, 377; 391). In the mother, labor can be delayed by such glucocorticoid therapy (SEDA-3, 306); the combination of this treatment with sympathomimetic drugs may put the mother at risk of fluid retention with pulmonary edema (SED-12, 990), although it is not clear whether this problem only occurs when both drugs are used.

As far as the child is concerned, there may be only moderate adrenal suppression (392), although in some cases substitution treatment with glucocorticoids can be necessary in such babies; short-term treatment with beta-methasone shortly before birth generally does not inhibit the infant's adrenal capacity to react to corticotropin (393). A single case of a leukemoid reaction in a preterm infant has been observed, after the mother was given betamethasone shortly before delivery (SEDA-3, 306).

On the other hand, there are many reports of hyperten-sion (394), and electrocardiographic and other studies have often confirmed the presence of a disproportionately serious and bilateral hypertrophic obstructive cardiomyo-pathy, which unless it proves fatal is, in general, reversible once the glucocorticoids are withdrawn (SEDA-18, 386). Although the issue is confounded by the possibility that infants with bronchopulmonary dysplasia may be innately hypertensive, there seems no doubt as to the effect.

Most babies treated with glucocorticoids for lung dys-plasia also show an appreciable rise in blood urea nitrogen, due almost entirely to an increase in structural protein catabolism (395). Serious gastrointestinal complications can occur. In one typical series of premature neonates treated in this way there were three such instances (perforated duodenal ulcer, perforated gastric ulcer, and upper gastrointestinal hemorrhage, the last two proving fatal) (396); the symptoms are apparently not masked by the glucocorticoid, as one would expect in adults. Treated infants also tend to have a low pH, which is unusual in premature babies (SEDA-18, 445).

In 534 individuals aged 30 years, whose mothers had participated in a double-blind, randomized, placebo-controlled trial of antenatal betamethasone (two intra-muscular doses 24 hours apart) for the prevention of neonatal respiratory distress syndrome, there were no differences between those exposed to betamethasone and placebo in body size, blood lipids, blood pressure, plasma cortisol, prevalence of diabetes, or history of cardiovascular disease (397). After the oral glucose tolerance test, those who had been exposed to betamethasone had higher plasma insulin concentrations at 30 minutes (61 versus 52 mIU/l) and lower glucose concentrations at 120 minutes (4.8 versus 5.1 mmol/l) than did those exposed to placebo. Antenatal exposure to betamethasone might result in insulin resistance in adult offspring, but has no effect on cardiovascular risk factors at 30 years of age.

In an Italian prospective study, 201 preterm singleton infants received one or more antenatal courses of a glucocorticoid (398). Neurodevelopment was evaluated at 2 years; 138 subjects received at least one complete course of betamethasone (37 multiple) and 63 patients received dexamethasone (33 multiple). The prevalence of infant leukomalacia was 26% after a complete course of glucocorticoid, 40% after one additional course, 42% after two additional courses, and 44% after more than two additional courses. The corresponding prevalences of 2-year infant neurodevelopmental abnormalities, considering the same categories of glucocorticoid exposure, were 18%, 21%, 29%, and 35% respectively. However, most of the risk was related to dexamethasone administration. Compared with betamethasone, exposure to multiple doses of dexamethasone was associated with an increased risk of leukomalacia (OR = 3.21; 95% CI = 1.07, 9.77) and overall 2-year infant neurodevelopmental abnormalities (OR = 3.63; 95% CI = 1.03, 14).

In an Australian cohort study, 541 very preterm infants were followed for physical, cognitive, and psychological assessment up to 6 years after administration of glucocorticoids during pregnancy (399). Although increasing numbers of antenatal glucocorticoid courses (two intramuscular doses of betamethasone 11.4 mg) were associated with a reduction in the rate of cerebral palsy, three or more courses were also associated with increased rates of aggressive/destructive, distractible, and hyperkinetic behavior, and these effects were present at ages 3 and 6 years. Intelligence quotients were unaffected by antenatal use of a glucocorticoid.

In 192 adult offspring (mean age 31 years) of mothers who had taken part in a randomized controlled trial of antenatal betamethasone for the prevention of neonatal respiratory distress syndrome (87 exposed to betamethasone two doses 24 hours apart, and 105 exposed to placebo) there were no alterations in cognitive functioning, working memory and attention, psychiatric morbidity, handedness, or health-related quality-of-life in adulthood (400).

The effects of a single antenatal dose of a glucocorticoid on prostanoids have been evaluated in 43 singleton pregnancies in women who were taking betamethasone or not (401). Betamethasone (dose not described) reduced maternal PGE_2 concentrations, with concomitant increases in the fetoplacental compartment. Umbilical cord thromboxane B_2 concentrations in the treated group were significantly lower than the non-treated group, resulting in a higher ratio of 6-keto$PGF_{1\alpha}$ to thromboxane B2. Considering the regulatory role of PGE_2 and PGI_2 in fetal lung development and neonatal transition homeostasis, these results suggest a mechanism, at least in part, for the beneficial effects of antenatal glucocorticoids on fetal lung maturation and neonatal cardiopulmonary homeostasis at birth.

Clearly, the duration of such treatment after delivery should be as brief as possible, but there is no reason for such concern as would lead to withholding therapy; one Dutch study with a 10-year follow-up detected no problems with exposed children's intellectual, motor, or social functioning compared with controls (135).

A meta-analysis, including 15 controlled trials and involving more than 1400 women, has shown that antenatal glucocorticoids in women with ruptured membranes may be beneficial in reducing the risks of neonatal death (RR = 0.68; 95% CI = 0.43, 1.07) and respiratory distress syndrome (RR = 0.56; CI = 0.46, 0.70), with no increase in the risk of infection in either the mother (RR = 0.88; CI = 0.61, 1.20) or baby (RR = 1.05; CI = 0.66, 1.68) (402).

A reduction in fetal response to vibroacoustic stimulation (vibroacoustic startle reflex) has been reported during 48 hours after the administration to pregnant women of two doses of betamethasone (12 mg 2 days apart) (403). The authors recommended that this test should not be used to evaluate well-being in fetuses exposed to glucocorticoids.

Susceptibility Factors

Genetic factors

Significant differences in the pharmacokinetics of methylprednisolone have been described in black and white renal transplant patients. Black patients had a slower clearance rate and a lower apparent volume of distribution. They had higher cortisol concentrations throughout the day, with higher nadir concentrations. Some of them had glucocorticoid-associated diabetes, and no white patients did. Further studies are needed to define the differences between the races (SEDA-20, 377; 404).

Age

Children

Inhaled glucocorticoids are recommended as first-line therapy for persistent asthma in children, to reduce both asthma symptoms and inflammatory markers. Treatment should be begun early in the course of the disease, because inhaled glucocorticoids can preserve airway function and prevent airway remodelling and subsequent irreversible airway obstruction (405). Because asthma is a chronic disease requiring long-term treatment, it is very important to balance the safety and efficacy of inhaled glucocorticoids to achieve optimal long-term results. Major safety concerns in children are the potential adverse effects on growth, adrenal function, and bone mass. Overall, the benefits of inhaled glucocorticoids clearly outweigh their potential adverse effects and the risks of poor asthma control. However, high doses of inhaled glucocorticoids in children are still of concern (406). It is of utmost importance to use the lowest effective dose, to limit systemic availability by selecting drugs with high first-pass hepatic inactivation, and to instruct patients on proper inhalation technique. Moreover, the use of adjuvant asthma medications acting by different mechanisms can help to reduce inhaled glucocorticoid dosages (405,406). These add-on therapies include leukotriene modifiers, long-acting beta$_2$-agonists, cromoglicate and nedocromil, and in selected cases theophylline. These agents should be added to, but should not in any case replace, inhaled glucocorticoid therapy (405,406).

The use of postnatal glucocorticoids in very premature infants is controversial; although dexamethasone reduces bronchopulmonary dysplasia, it has been associated with severe adverse effects (407). In 220 infants with a birth-weight of 501–1000 g randomized to placebo or dexamethasone (0.15 mg/kg/day for 3 days and tapering over a period of 7 days) the relative risk of death or chronic lung disease compared with controls was 0.9 (95% CI = 0.8–1.1) at 36 weeks of gestational age (353). Infants treated with dexamethasone were less likely to need supplementary oxygen. Dexamethasone was associated with increased risks of hypertension (RR = 7.4; 95% CI = 2.7, 20.2), hyperglycemia (RR = 2.0; 95% CI = 1.1, 3.6), spontaneous gastrointestinal perforation (13 versus 4%), lower weight, and a smaller head circumference.

Elderly people

Prolonged use of glucocorticoids in elderly people can exacerbate diabetes, hypertension, congestive heart failure, and osteoporosis, or cause depression. In a retrospective, controlled study, the risks of high-dose intravenous or oral glucocorticoid therapy were assessed in 55 patients with Crohn's disease who were over the age of 50 years (408). They had a higher risk of developing hypertension, hypokalemia, and changes in mental state.

Hepatic disease

In patients with acute hepatitis and active hepatitis, protein binding of the glucocorticoids will be reduced and peak concentrations of administered glucocorticoids increased. Conversion of prednisone to prednisolone has been reported to be impaired in chronic active liver disease (409). However, although plasma prednisolone concentrations were more predictable after the administration of prednisolone than of prednisone to a group of healthy subjects (410), there was no difference in patients with chronic active hepatitis. There was also impaired elimination of prednisolone in these patients. In a review of the pharmacokinetics of prednisone and prednisolone it was concluded that fear of inadequate conversion of prednisone into prednisolone was not justified (411). Patients with hepatic disease suffer adrenal suppression more readily (111).

Other features of the patient

Menopause

Significant differences in the pharmacokinetics of prednisolone amongst menopausal women have been described (SEDA-21, 419; 412). The postmenopausal women had reduced unbound clearance (30%), reduced total clearance, and an increased half-life. Similar results are seen in the postmenopausal women who took estrogen or estrogen–progestogen therapy.

Protein binding

The association between low serum albumin concentrations and complications of prednisone has been long recognized, and it is an elementary pharmacokinetic principle that concentrations of unbound drug in plasma (the fraction that can reach the tissues) will be increased when binding of a drug to serum albumin is reduced (413).

Systemic lupus erythematosus

In 539 patients with systemic lupus erythematosus, organ damage was associated with glucocorticoid therapy compared with controls (414). Oral prednisone 10 mg/day for 10 years (cumulative dose 36.6 g) was significantly associated with osteoporotic fractures (RR = 2.5; 95% CI = 1.7, 3.7), symptomatic coronary artery disease (RR = 1.7; CI = 1.1, 2.5), and cataracts (RR = 1.7; CI = 1.4, 2.5). Avascular necrosis was associated with high-dose prednisone (at least 60 mg/day for at least 2 months; RR = 1.2; CI = 1.1, 1.4). Intravenous pulses of methylprednisolone (1000 mg for 1–3 days) were associated with a small increase in the risk of osteoporotic fractures (RR = 1.3; CI = 1.0, 1.8).

Drug Administration

Drug formulations

The development of adverse effects has been evaluated after switching from conventional glucocorticoids to a pH-modified release formulation, Eudragit L-coated budesonide, in 178 patients with Crohn's disease who had taken 5–30 mg/day of prednisolone equivalents for at least 2 weeks (415). The percentage of patients with glucocorticoid-related adverse effects fell from 65% at entry to 43% at the end of the study. The total number of glucocorticoid-related adverse effects fell significantly from 269 to 90. In conclusion, switching from conventional glucocorticoids to budesonide leads to a significant reduction in glucocorticoid-related adverse effects in patients with Crohn's disease without causing rapid deterioration of the disease.

Drug contamination

Unregulated Chinese herbal products adulterated with glucocorticoids have been detected (416). Dexamethasone was present in eight of 11 Chinese herbal creams analysed by UK dermatologists. The creams contained dexamethasone in concentrations inappropriate for use on the face or in children (64–1500 micrograms/g). The cream with the highest concentration of dexamethasone was prescribed to treat facial eczema in a 4-month-old baby. In all cases, it had been assumed that the creams did not contain glucocorticoids. The authors were concerned that these patients received both unlabelled and unlicensed topical glucocorticoids. They wrote that "greater regulation and restriction needs to be imposed on herbalists, and continuous monitoring of side effects of these medications is necessary."

Drug dosage regimens

Daily or alternate-day administration

The unwanted effects of the glucocorticoids can be reduced to some extent by altering the dosage routine, for example by giving them on alternate days or giving the total daily dose every morning.

Because of circadian variation in endogenous glucocorticoid secretion, the pituitary–adrenal axis is suppressed more easily in the night than during the day (417). Thus, administration of the total dose as a single dose in the morning is preferable to twice daily dosing or administration in the evening alone.

Alternate-day therapy (giving twice the daily dose on alternate days) can in some cases maintain the therapeutic efficacy of oral glucocorticoids, while reducing their adverse effects (418–420).

Use in fixed combinations

Fixed combinations of oral glucocorticoids with nonsteroidal anti-inflammatory analgesics or broncholytic drugs that have to be given repeatedly during the day are undesirable, since their pattern of administration is determined in part by the demands of the other components; the glucocorticoid is thus likely to be given in such a way that it alters the circadian rhythm of endogenous glucocorticoids.

Pulse or megadose therapy

Extremely large intravenous doses of glucocorticoids given at longer intervals can sometimes be effective when a patient does not respond to conventional high doses. Systemic lupus erythematosus, various rheumatic diseases, and the treatment of renal graft rejection are indications for this type of use (SEDA-6, 331). High doses of glucocorticoids also have an antiemetic effect in patients with cancers.

No adverse effects are to be expected after a single injection of a high dose of a glucocorticoid, but some serious complications have been observed with repeated use, including both infections and the known direct adverse effects of glucocorticoids. Cases of ventricular dysrhythmias and atrial fibrillation have been reported (SEDA-18, 391). With pulse therapy, the nature of the injected glucocorticoid seems to be important; for example, hydrocortisone, which is more rapidly metabolized, seems to be better tolerated than dexamethasone (SEDA-6, 331).

Pulsed glucocorticoid therapy for moderately severe ulcerative colitis, given on an out-patient basis, can induce remission more quickly than conventional oral glucocorticoid therapy (421). There were no serious adverse effects in 11 patients given pulsed glucocorticoids or in eight treated conventionally. The two regimens were equally efficacious.

Drug administration route

Most knowledge of the adverse effects of glucocorticoids has been acquired in connection with their use as oral products. However, various other routes of administration have been developed, sometimes specifically in the hope of securing a local therapeutic effect while avoiding systemic adverse reactions. Although experience has shown that the latter cannot be eliminated in this way, they can be diminished in some cases. In other cases, new problems arise. Administration by inhalation is covered in the monograph on inhaled glucocorticoids.

Topical administration to the skin

For a list of the local effects of topical glucocorticoids see separate monograph. The percutaneous absorption of high-potency topical glucocorticoids has been documented, but hypothalamic–pituitary–adrenal axis suppression, leading to clinically significant adrenal insufficiency or Cushing's syndrome, is infrequent. In most cases in which systemic adverse effects occur, misuse of a product can be blamed. For example, a 4-month old boy developed iatrogenic Cushing's syndrome, which occurred when his mother used excessive amounts of clobetasol 17-propionate and hydrocortisone 17-butyrate cream for 2 months to treat a diaper rash (422). Two patients developed adrenal suppression after the unregulated use of betamethasone dipropionate 0.05% ointment (about 80 g/week) or clobetasol 0.05% ointment (up to 100 g/week), obtained without prescription to treat psoriasis (423).

Although glucocorticoids are used to treat eczema, they can sometimes cause or exacerbate it.

- A 74-year-old man developed worsening eczema 24 hours after he applied clobetasol (Decloban) to treat chronic eczema of his external ear (424). Twelve years earlier he had noted exacerbation of a cutaneous lesion after he had applied a topical glucocorticoid. He had also had generalized erythema after an intra-articular injection of paramethasone. Patch tests to a series of glucocorticoids were positive for all drugs except flupametasone, fluocortine, and tixocortol. In addition, intradermal tests were positive to hydrocortisone and prednisolone, despite negative patch tests.

The authors commented that most glucocorticoid-sensitized patients react to several of the same group and less frequently of different groups. No case of hypersensitivity to glucocorticoids of all four classes has previously been reported.

- Chronic lichenified eczema has been attributed to prolonged use of topical methylprednisolone aceponate and budesonide (strength and duration of therapy not stated) in a 26-year-old woman (425). Patch tests were positive for methylprednisolone aceponate and budesonide cream, but negative for all other topical glucocorticoids.
- An 18-year-old woman presented with a pruritic eczematous eruption that developed after topically applying an ointment containing hydrocortisone acetate, neomycin sulfate, and *Centella asiatica* (426). She was positive to all three ingredients of the ointment.

Two patients developed central serous chorioretinopathy after prolonged treatment with glucocorticoids applied locally to the skin (427).

- A 32-year-old man complained of reduced vision and metamorphopsia in the right eye. Best-corrected visual acuity was 20/25 in right eye and 20/20 in left eye. The left fundus was normal but in the right eye there was a well-circumscribed, shallow, serous detachment of the sensory retina. The clinical appearance was consistent with central serous chorioretinopathy, and the diagnosis was confirmed by fluorescein angiography, which showed a leakage point at the superior macula, spreading slowly in an inkblot configuration into the subretinal space. He had seborrheic dermatitis involving the central face, eyebrows, eyelids, and scalp for 2 years treated with topical hydrocortisone acetate cream 1%. After the initial prescription, he used the cream without further medical consultation when his symptoms got worse and used it for 4 weeks, 3–4 times a day before developing central serous chorioretinopathy.
- A 37-year-old man developed blurred vision in the left eye. He had central serous chorioretinopathy in the contralateral eye 5 years before, for which he had been treated with laser photocoagulation. Best-corrected visual acuity was 20/20 in each eye. There were scars from previous laser photocoagulation at the superior macula in the right eye. In the left eye there was a well-delineated area of serous detachment temporal to the fovea and small yellowish precipitates at the posterior aspect of the detached retina. Fluorescein angiography showed a leakage point at the upper pole of the detachment. He had pityriasis versicolor, for which he had used local diflucortolone valerate cream 0.1% in combination with isoconazole nitrate 1%. He had used the cream occasionally but had used it for 3 weeks before the onset of symptoms. He also used diflucortolone valerate cream 0.1% during the first episode of central serous chorioretinopathy.

The effects of exposure to topical glucocorticoids during pregnancy have been evaluated in a population-based follow-up study in 363 primigravida exposed to topical glucocorticoids during pregnancy and 9263 controls who received no prescriptions at all (428). The prevalence of malformations was 2.9% among 170 infants exposed to glucocorticoids during the first trimester and 3.6% among the controls. There were no increases in the risks of low birthweight, malformations, or preterm delivery in the offspring of women who were exposed to topical glucocorticoids during pregnancy.

Topical administration to the eye

Glucocorticoids that have been used for local ophthalmic treatment include medrysone, fluorometholone, tetrahydroxytriamcinolone, and clobetasone. Loteprednol etabonate 0.5% increases intraocular pressure less than dexamethasone. Studies on animal models of uveitis and two randomized double-masked trials showed that loteprednol etabonate 0.5% was less potent than dexamethasone, prednisolone acetate 1%, or fluorometholone, which may partly explain the improved toxicity profile of loteprednol etabonate (429).

Clinicians should not prescribe glucocorticoid-containing eye-drops unless they have performed a slit-lamp examination with tonometry, have assurance of appropriate follow-up, and understand the differential diagnosis, evaluation, and treatment. Unless clearly indicated, prescribing volumes larger than 5 ml or providing refillable prescriptions should be avoided. It should be stressed that excessive use of glucocorticoids can result in corneal Herpes infection and mycosis.

Since glucocorticoids reduce the immunological defences of the body to most types of infection, their use in the eyes should be monitored carefully. When long-term use is necessary, even with oral or inhalation therapy, eye examination should be performed every 6 months. The ophthalmological follow-up of patients using topical glucocorticoids should include tonometry at least twice a year, careful slit-lamp examination for early signs of herpetic or fungal keratitis and for changes in the equatorial and posterior subcapsular portions of the lens, examination of pupillary size and lid position, and staining of the cornea to detect possible punctate keratitis. Blood glucose concentrations should be checked if there are symptoms that suggest hyperglycemia.

Sensory systems

Ocular adverse effects of local or systemic administration of glucocorticoids include cataracts, glaucoma, papilledema, pseudotumor cerebri, activation of corneal infections, superficial keratitis, ptosis, pupillary dilatation, conjunctival palpebral petechiae, uveitis, and scleromalacia. Topical ocular application and facial application can cause high glucocorticoid concentrations in the anterior compartment of the eye. Serious visual loss can occur owing to the development of cataract in patients using glucocorticoid creams.

Glucocorticoid creams applied topically to the skin are routinely used in the treatment of many skin disorders, and their use on the face in severe atopic eczema is relatively common. Three patients developed advanced glaucoma while using topical facial glucocorticoids. Two other patients developed ocular hypertension secondary to topical facial glucocorticoids (430).

The use of a combination of a glucocorticoid with an antimicrobial drug is illogical and should generally be avoided because of the possibility of the emergence of resistant bacterial strains. It would be highly preferable if prescriptions for these drugs were issued by ophthalmologists only, at least in those parts of the world where adequate medical services are available.

Three vision-threatening complications have been described due to the indiscriminate use of glucocorticoid-containing eyedrops (431).

- A 31-year-old man noted a blind spot in his right eye. He had worn contact lenses for 10 years to correct his myopia. He had applied Tobradex ointment (tobramycin 0.3% and dexamethasone 0.1%) to each eye every evening for the past 4 years because of irritation due to contact lenses, and continuous refills of this prescription were obtained through an acquaintance who was employed in a pharmacy. With spectacle correction his visual acuity was 20/25 in each eye. The intraocular pressure was 52 mmHg in his right eye and 37 mmHg in his left eye. The optic discs showed glaucomatous cupping in each eye. Automated visual field testing showed superior and inferior arcuate defects typical of glaucoma in both eyes. Slit-lamp biomicroscopy showed mild papillary conjunctivitis bilaterally due to contact lenses. The antibiotic + glucocorticoid ointment was withdrawn and his bilateral glucocorticoid-induced open-angle glaucoma was treated with antiglaucomatous drugs.
- A 15-year-old boy felt a foreign body sensation in his right eye after he had been raking hay. His local physician prescribed a suspension of tobramycin 0.3% + dexamethasone 0.1% tds, but 6 days later referred him for evaluation of a suspected fungal keratitis. He had a corneal epithelial defect with an underlying dense inflammatory infiltrate. Corneal scrapings contained fungal hyphae and *Fusarium* species was identified. Natamycin 5% was administered topically every hour, the infection resolved, and his visual acuity returned to 20/20 despite a dense corneal scar.
- A 56-year-old woman had bilateral primary open-angle glaucoma without visual field loss, which was well controlled with a long-term topical beta-blocker in each eye. She underwent a left dacryocystorhinostomy for nasolacrimal duct obstruction, but developed persistent tearing and irritation of the left eye several months postoperatively. A suspension of tobramycin 0.3% + dexamethasone 0.1% was prescribed, which she continued to use as needed for 6 months. Pain and reduced vision persisted in her left eye. Corrected visual acuity was 20/20 in her right eye and 20/60 in her left eye. The intraocular pressures were 18 mmHg in her right eye and 68 mmHg in her left eye. Automated visual field testing showed a normal field in her right eye, but only a central island and a crescent of temporal visual field in her left eye. External examination showed persistent nasolacrimal duct obstruction on the left side with mild conjunctival injection. The diagnosis was primary open-angle glaucoma in both eyes, which was exacerbated by topically applied

glucocorticoids in her left eye. The antibiotic + glucocorticoid suspension was withdrawn, and a topical ocular hypotensive therapeutic regimen was initiated in her left eye.

Susceptibility factors

Local and systemic adverse effects of ophthalmic glucocorticoids occur in children more often, more severely, and more rapidly than in adults, for unknown reasons. It could be that children have relatively immature chamber angles, giving rise to a rapidly increasing intraocular pressure (432).

Glaucoma has been reported after the use of a glucocorticoid ointment in a young boy (432).

- A 6-year-old boy underwent a resection of levator palpebrae superioris for congenital blepharoptosis. Postoperatively, an ointment containing 0.1% dexamethasone and neomycin (Maxitrol) was applied to the operated eyelid three times a day to reduce lid edema. Four days later the surgical correction was satisfactory and there were no symptoms, but the intraocular pressure was raised to 44 mmHg in the operated eye, although normal in the other eye. The glucocorticoid was withdrawn and topical ocular hypotensive agents were prescribed. The intraocular pressure returned to normal the next day, and the antiglaucoma treatments were maintained for 1 week and tapered over the next 2 weeks. Subsequent follow-up confirmed normal intraocular pressure and no glaucomatous damage.

The ocular hypertensive response in this case could have been due to systemic absorption of glucocorticoid through the skin of the eyelid, especially when there was a surgical wound. Alternatively, a sufficient amount of ointment could have seeped over the eyelid margins, causing the rise in intraocular pressure, similar to the application of eye-drops, as has been reported in another child, who also had Cushing's syndrome, a rare result of ophthalmic glucocorticoids (433).

- An 11-year-old boy with iridocyclitis developed Cushing's syndrome, a posterior subcapsular cataract, and increased intraocular pressure in both eyes after the topical administration of prednisolone acetate 1% eye-drops bilaterally for 6 months. The Cushing's syndrome was aggravated when periocular methylprednisolone acetate was started while bilateral posterior subtenon injections of 80 mg of suspension were continued every 6 weeks for 6 months. He had not used systemic glucocorticoids before.

Topical administration to the nose

The safety of nasal glucocorticoids in the treatment of allergic rhinitis has been reviewed (434,435). The local application of glucocorticoids for seasonal or perennial rhinitis often results in systemic adverse effects. The use of nasal sprays containing a glucocorticoid that has specific topical activity (such as beclomethasone dipropionate or flunisolide) seems to reduce the systemic adverse effects, but they can nevertheless occur, even to the extent of suppression of basal adrenal function in children (436). Local adverse effects include *Candida* infection, nasal stinging, epistaxis, throat irritation (437), and, exceptionally, anosmia (438).

Nervous system
Benign intracranial hypertension with nasal glucocorticoids has been reported (439).

- A 13-year-old boy with Crohn's disease in remission, who had taken fluticasone aqueous nasal spray 50 micrograms to each nostril od regularly for 5 days, gave a 10-day history of head and back pain. He had a right sixth nerve palsy with bilateral swelling of his optic discs. An unenhanced computer tomogram was normal and magnetic resonance imaging excluded cavernous sinus thrombosis. The cerebrospinal fluid was clear with no cells, and protein and glucose concentrations were normal.

Although there was no clear temporal relation between the onset of the symptoms and the regular use of fluticasone, the authors proposed that the fluticasone was responsible, because the symptoms resolved after drug withdrawal. The association remains unproven but it does highlight the possibility of an association.

Sensory systems
Nasal budesonide or beclomethasone 100 micrograms bd for 3–9 months had no effect on the eyes in 26 patients who had undergone endoscopic sinus surgery (440). Ophthalmologic examination, tonometry, visual field testing, and biomicroscopic studies showed no evidence of ocular hypertension or posterior subcapsular cataract.

Ear, nose, and throat
The use of intranasal glucocorticoids in the treatment of allergic and vasomotor rhinitis in Sweden has doubled over a period of 5 years, and the number of reported cases of nasal septum perforation increased over the same time (441). The most common risk factor in 32 patients with nasal septum perforation (21 women, 11 men) was glucocorticoid treatment. Information from the Swedish Drug Agency showed that 38 cases of glucocorticoid-induced perforation had been reported over 10 years. The number of adverse effects per million Defined Daily Doses averaged 0.21. The risk of perforation was greatest during the first 12 months of treatment and most cases were in young women.

Endocrine
Aqueous nasal triamcinolone spray 220 or 440 micrograms od for the treatment of allergic rhinitis reportedly had no measurable adverse effects on adrenocortical function in 80 children (aged 6–12 years) in a placebo-controlled, double-blind study (442). Plasma triamcinolone concentrations measured over 6 hours fell rapidly and there was little or no accumulation during 6 weeks.

There have been reports of Cushing's syndrome after prolonged use of intranasal betamethasone 0.1% for chronic catarrh in two boys (443) and from an interaction of nasal fluticasone with ritonavir (444).

- A 30-year-old man who was using an intranasal formulation of fluticasone (therapeutic indication not stated), developed Cushing's syndrome about 5 months after starting ritonavir 600 mg bd, zidovudine, and lamivudine for HIV infection. His plasma cortisol concentrations were undetectable, his corticotrophin was low (under 2 pmol/l), and his 24-hours urinary cortisol excretion was under 30 nmol/l. Further investigations were consistent with secondary adrenal failure or with glucocorticoid use. He admitted to having used a topical glucocorticoid cream for 2 months. However, 6 weeks after he stopped using this cream, his plasma cortisol concentrations were still undetectable. It was then established that he had used nasal fluticasone propionate 200 micrograms/day for about 1 year before starting ritonavir. Ritonavir was replaced by nevirapine, and he continued to use fluticasone nasal spray. Three weeks later, his plasma cortisol concentration had increased to 290 nmol/l. Ritonavir was then added and his plasma cortisol concentration fell rapidly. Ritonavir was stopped again and his cortisol concentration normalized and his Cushingoid facies improved.

The authors thought it likely that inhibition of cytochrome P-450 by ritonavir increased the systemic availability of fluticasone and thus caused Cushing's syndrome in this patient.

Musculoskeletal
Osteonecrosis of the femoral head after the use of a glucocorticoid nasal spray has been reported (445).

- A 48-year-old man taking losartan, low-dose amitriptyline, and triamcinolone acetonide nasal spray developed pain in the abdomen and hips. Radiography and magnetic resonance imaging showed rapidly progressive bilateral osteonecrosis of the femoral heads. He had used excessive amounts of nasal glucocorticoids, and during the previous 12 months had used triamcinolone acetonide 110 micrograms qds in each nostril.

Intralesional injection
Intralesional triamcinolone acetonide has been used extensively for the treatment of hypertrophic and keloid scars. Complications are few, usually being local skin color changes, prominent vascular markings, or subcutaneous atrophy. Cushing's syndrome after intralesional administration of triamcinolone acetate has been described in two adults and two children (aged 10 years and 21 months) after treatment of hypertrophic burn scars with intralesional triamcinolone acetonide (SEDA-21, 419) (408). These two children may have had a form of hypersensitivity to triamcinolone acetonide, as Cushing's syndrome was not the result of overdosage.

- Acute anaphylaxis occurred in an 18-year-old man after the third course of intradermal injections of triamcinolone suspension ("Kenalog" 10 mg per treatment) for alopecia areata (446). Subsequent rechallenge with intradermal triamcinolone 1 ml resulted in the same anaphylactic reaction as before and his serum IgE concentration was increased.

Immediate hypersensitivity reactions to paramethasone acetate, causing widespread eruptions, have been described in at least four cases. Delayed allergic reactions are less common.

- A woman had received intralesional paramethasone and other topical glucocorticoids several times for alopecia between the ages of 7 and 18 years (447). When she was 30 she was again treated with intralesional paramethasone for a relapse of alopecia. She developed pruritus after the first intralesional injection and erythema, edema, and vesicles 6–8 hours later. A biopsy showed spongiform lymphocytic folliculitis with spongiosis and exocytosis in the sweat gland ducts and in the pilosebaceous unit. She was treated with triamcinolone cream and her skin lesions resolved. Patch tests were positive for paramethasone, with cross-reactivity to tixocortol pivalate, hydrocortisone, and hydrocortisone butyrate.

Intraspinal injection
Intrathecal
The effects of intrathecal administration, both wanted and unwanted, are still much debated (448). The question as to whether oral glucocorticoid therapy should be preferred to intrathecal injections is raised by the harmful effects that have sometimes occurred after the latter, although some of these may have been caused by irritative substances in the injection fluid (SEDA-6, 331). The same local glucocorticoid concentrations can probably be attained with fewer problems with oral administration. Epidural injection of glucocorticoids seems to be safer than intrathecal injection, but injection of high doses can cause the same systemic adverse effects as seen with oral treatment. Facial flushing and erythema after lumbar epidural glucocorticoid administration have been reported (SEDA-20, 378; 449).

Glucocorticoids given intrathecally can cause a rise in cerebrospinal fluid protein and carry the risk of arachnoiditis (SED-8, 820). Chemical meningitis has been reported after two intrathecal injections of methylprednisolone acetate (450) and after lumbar facet joint block (SEDA-17, 450). Intraspinal injections of hydrocortisone for multiple sclerosis apparently led in one case to a cauda equina syndrome, with subsequent ulceromutilating acropathy (SEDA-17, 450). Intra-discal injections of triamcinolone acetonide in a number of French cases led to disk or epidural calcification, sometimes symptomless (SEDA-17, 450).

Postlumbar puncture syndrome with abducent nerve palsy followed the use of intrathecal prednisolone for the treatment of low back pain and sciatica (451).

- A 38-year-old woman received intrathecal prednisolone 3 ml (strength not stated) and 1 day later developed a postural headache, nausea, and dizziness. She was treated with intravenous fluids and analgesics. Eight days later she suddenly developed a complete palsy of the right abducent nerve. An MRI brain scan showed contrast meningeal enhancement typical of postlumbar puncture syndrome. She was treated with oral

glucocorticoids and blood patching was performed. Her headache began to resolve a week later. Four months later she had almost completely recovered function of her abducent nerve and a repeat MRI scan was normal.

Epidural
The indications, rationale, techniques, alternatives, contraindications, complications, and efficacy of lumbar and caudal epidural glucocorticoid injections have been reviewed (SEDA-21, 420; 452).

Bilateral posterior subcapsular cataracts have been reported after treatment with epidural methylprednisolone for low back pain secondary to degenerative joint disease and disk protrusion (453).

- A 42-year-old man had received 15 epidural injections of methylprednisolone 80 mg over 10 years. About 6 weeks after his last injection, he developed progressively worsening cloudy vision. He had bilateral posterior subcapsular cataracts and subsequently underwent bilateral cataract removal.

The authors commented that it is possible that multiple epidural glucocorticoid injections had contributed to cataract formation. The patient also had several other risk factors for cataracts (cigarette smoking, alcohol consumption, exposure to ultraviolet radiation, low socioeconomic class, and low intake of antioxidant vitamins). However, the role of these other risk factors was speculative.

Symptoms consistent with complex regional pain syndrome have been reported after a cervical epidural glucocorticoid injection (SEDA-22, 451; 454).

Spinal epidural lipomatosis secondary to exogenous administration of glucocorticoids is a rare condition that has been reported almost exclusively in association with systemic treatment. However, local epidural administration has also been implicated (455).

One case of *Staphylococcus aureus* meningitis, a rare complication of epidural analgesia, has been published. The same patient developed a cauda equina syndrome of uncertain etiology, although neural ischemia as a result of meningitis secondary to immunosuppression was possible (SEDA-21, 420; 456). A unique case of transient profound paralysis after epidural glucocorticoid injection (acute paraplegia) has now been reported (SEDA-22, 451; 457). Diplopia associated with the peridural or intrathecal infiltration of prednisolone have not been previously reported (SEDA-22, 451; 458).

Of 31 patients who received 1 ml (40 mg) of methylprednisolone epidurally at the end of microdiscectomy, three developed epidural abscesses (459). These results were compared with a historical series of 400 patients not taking glucocorticoids, who had no deep infection. Although the data were limited, epidural glucocorticoids after discectomy should not be recommended.

Cervical epidural glucocorticoid injection is often used for the treatment of cervical radiculopathy. Subjective patient satisfaction has been reported, but controlled trials have not yet delineated the effectiveness of this procedure. Three cases of severe pain consistent with nerve injury have been reported immediately after cervical epidural glucocorticoid injection, bringing into question the benefit–harm balance of this technique (460).

Intra-articular and periarticular administration

Local injections of glucocorticoids into and around the joints can have a dramatic therapeutic effect, but the catabolic effect can have serious consequences, including adverse effects on joint structure (461) and on local tendons, subcutaneous atrophy, and possibly osteonecrosis. Provided the state of the joint is carefully inspected before any new injection is given, and the interval between the injections is not less than 4 weeks, the risk seems to be small enough to justify treatment in invalidating cases (SEDA-3, 307).

Respiratory

Hiccups have been reported after intra-articular administration (462).

- A 38-year-old man had an intra-articular injection of betamethasone dipropionate (dose not stated) into his right ankle, and the day after had hiccups that lasted for 24 hours and then resolved without treatment. Some months later, because of persistent arthritis, he received a further injection of betamethasone dipropionate into his right ankle. Once again, he had hiccups the following day. On this occasion, the hiccups resolved after 2 weeks, following treatment with levomepromazine.

Psychiatric

Neuropsychiatric effects of glucocorticoids, like hallucinations, can result from intra-articular administration (SEDA-22, 444) (463).

Endocrine

An acute adrenal crisis occurred in a woman who received an intra-articular glucocorticoid for pseudogout of the knee (464).

- An 87-year-old woman received intra-articular betamethasone (Diprophos) 7 mg on three occasions for painful knee joints over 6 months. Six weeks after the last injection she developed diffuse pain and contractures in the legs, fatigue, nausea, abdominal pain, and weight loss of 6 kg. Both knee joints were tender but there was no effusion. Her serum sodium concentration was 123 mmol/l, serum osmolality 254 mosmol/kg, urine sodium 136 mmol/l, and urinary osmolality 373 mosmol/kg. The syndrome of inappropriate antidiuretic hormone secretion was diagnosed, but despite treatment she remained drowsy and hyponatremic. About a week later, she developed hypotension and symptoms of an acute abdomen. Further investigations showed that her basal cortisol concentration was low (36 nmol/l) but it increased to 481 nmol/l after a short tetracosactide test, consistent with acute adrenal crisis. She recovered rapidly after treatment with oral hydrocortisone, but still required glucocorticoid substitution several months later.

Skin

An erythema multiforme-like eruption has been reported after intra-articular triamcinolone in the right knee, with cross-sensitivity to budesonide (465).

- A 70-year-old man had received three intra-articular injections of triamcinolone (dose not stated) into the same knee over 3 months without any allergic reactions. However, 12–24 hours after the last injection he developed pruritus and erythema at the injection site. This eruption was treated with topical budesonide, but within the next few hours, acute eczema developed. The lesions spread to his legs and abdomen, and were erythematous, edematous, and resembled erythema multiforme. He was treated with boric acid solution dressings, emollients, and oral antihistamines. His lesions gradually resolved and did not recur during 8 months of follow-up. A month after the lesions had resolved, he underwent patch testing, which was positive to triamcinolone 1% and budesonide 1% in petrolatum, but negative to other glucocorticoids.

Musculoskeletal

An arthropathy induced by glucocorticoid crystals has been reported (466).

- A 65-year-old man with bilateral osteoarthritis of the knees developed an effusion in the left knee. The swollen joint was treated with an intra-articular injection of triamcinolone hexacetonide 40 mg. The next day, he developed acute arthritis in the injected knee; the joint was swollen and tender and he was unable to walk. Examination of the joint fluid showed 35 ml of a thick, turbid, yellowish synovial fluid with a leukocyte count of 13×10^6/l (95% neutrophils). Gram and acridine orange stains were negative. Wet preparations of the specimen with polarizing compensated microscopy showed numerous birefringent, pleomorphic intra- and extracellular crystals of glucocorticoid. He underwent joint lavage with 1 l of isotonic saline and recovered, completely within one day.

The conclusive diagnosis in this case was triamcinolone hexacetonide crystal-induced arthropathy.

Osteomyelitis after three glucocorticoid injections for tennis elbow has been reported; the second injection was given 3 months after the first and the third 2 days later (467). This case illustrates the need for vigilance, even after common procedures, and that exacerbation of symptoms after local glucocorticoid injections should prompt the doctor to review the diagnosis and consider the need for further investigation.

Anaphylaxis occurred in two women after intra-articular administration of paramethasone plus mepivacaine 2% (468).

- A 44-year-old woman developed generalized pruritus 10 minutes after intra-articular paramethasone and mepivacaine and 30 minutes later developed generalized urticaria, tachycardia, and dyspnea. She received emergency treatment and her condition initially improved. However, her symptoms recurred after 6 hours and she was treated again and then discharged taking oral dexchlorphenira-mine. She had a history of allergic contact dermatitis due to nickel sulfate sensitization, and 7 years before had had generalized urticaria and dyspnea after intra-articular administration of a glucocorticoid.

- A 31-year-old woman developed generalized pruritus and urticaria, facial edema, and dyspnea 2 hours after the intra-articular administration of paramethasone and mepivacaine. She was treated with an intramuscular glucocorticoid and antihistamines, with worsening of her symptoms. She received intravenous fluids and dex-chlorpheniramine, but her symptoms recurred after 1 hour, when she was given subcutaneous adrenaline, intravenous fluids and dexchlorpheniramine. She was later discharged taking oral diphenhydramine. She had a history of a systemic reaction after the administration of a glucocorticoid and a local anesthetic.

Skin prick tests were positive for isolated paramethasone in both patients, but negative for mepivacaine. There has only been one previous report of anaphylaxis in associa-tion with paramethasone.

Inadvertent intra-arterial injection

Particularly when injecting glucocorticoids locally, for example to relieve arthritis of the wrist, accidental injec-tion into an artery is possible. Severe local ischemia can result (SEDA-17, 450).

Intracapsular injection

The use of implants for augmentation of the breast can lead to capsular contracture. Patients with intractable capsular contracture are treated with intracapsular injec-tion of triamcinolone. Major complications included three cases of major atrophy requiring surgical correction. This problem appeared to have been eliminated by reduction of the dose of triamcinolone from 50 to 25 mg. There was one implant puncture (SEDA-19, 379; 469).

Rectal administration

Systemic absorption of glucocorticoids can occur after rectal administration.

- A 48-year-old woman developed avascular necrosis 9 months after she had completed a 3-month course of hydrocortisone 100 mg retention enemas once or twice daily for ulcerative proctitis (470). An MRI scan showed multiple bony infarcts in her distal femora, proximal tibiae, and posterior proximal right fibular head, extending from the diaphysis to the epiphysis, consistent with avascular necrosis.
- Cushing's syndrome occurred in a 65-year-old woman with ulcerative colitis who received a daily betametha-sone enema (471).

The authors of the second report reported the pharmaco-kinetics of betamethasone after rectal dosing, with plasma concentrations of betamethasone high enough to cause Cushing's syndrome. Suppression of the hypothalamic–pituitary–adrenal axis disappeared after the dosage sche-dule was changed from daily to three times a week. These

findings suggest that a considerable amount of beta-methasone is absorbed after rectal dosing.

Occupational exposure

Occupational exposure to glucocorticoids can cause adverse effects. Facial plethora has been found in workers manufacturing synthetic glucocorticoids, some of them having grossly abnormal responses to tetracosactide.

- A 58-year-old woman, who had been involved in the manufacturing of glucocorticoid creams and ointments for over 10 years, developed occupational contact sen-sitization to topical glucocorticoids (472). Patch tests were positive to hydrocortisone, hydrocortisone buty-rate, and tixocortol pivalate. Intradermal tests were positive to hydrocortisone succinate, methylpredniso-lone, and prednisolone. An oral challenge with beta-methasone 0.75 mg, 2.5 mg, and 8 mg on three consecutive days resulted in no adverse reactions.

It has been recommended that all workers manufacturing potent glucocorticoids should be screened regularly for glucocorticoid overdosage and should be moved regularly to units processing other drugs (473).

Drug overdose

High doses of glucocorticoids in patients with cancers can increase the risk of metastases, for example in breast cancer; this has been attributed in some cases to immu-nosuppression (474). These hormones should therefore only be used in patients with those types of tumors for which they are known to improve the efficacy of the cancer treatment.

A curious reaction to intravenous high-dose dexa-methasone, used as an antiemetic agent in cancer che-motherapy or for other purposes, is sudden severe itching, burning, and constrictive pain in the perineal region, which has been described in several published reports (SEDA-11, 336; 475).

Drug–Drug Interactions

Albendazole

Dexamethasone reduced the clearance of albendazole and increased its half-life; plasma concentrations almost doubled (SEDA-22, 450; 476).

Amiodarone

Budesonide for collagenous colitis caused Cushing's syn-drome in a patient with chronic renal insufficiency taking amiodarone for paroxysmal atrial fibrillation (477).

- An 81-year-old man with persistent diarrhea was given oral budesonide 9 mg/day, following unsuccessful treat-ment with mesalazine and prednisone. He was also taking amiodarone 100 mg/day. His diarrhea resolved within 6 weeks, and attempts to reduce the dosage of bzudesonide resulted in recurrent diarrhea. After 11 months he developed Cushing's syndrome, which persisted despite a reduction in dosage to 3 mg/day. His mild diarrhea recurred and the dosage of budesonide was increased to 6 mg/day with worsening of Cushing's syndrome; the dosage was reduced to 3 mg/day. Four weeks later amiodarone was withdrawn. The symptoms of Cushing's syndrome resolved within 4 weeks.

The authors suggested that the development of Cushing's syndrome and its persistence at a low dosage of budesonide was caused by inhibition of the metabolism of budesonide by amiodarone.

Anticoagulants

Intravenous methylprednisolone (1 g/day for 3 days) has been reported to inhibit the metabolism of oral anticoagulants (acenocoumarol and fluindione) in 10 patients, increasing the INR by 8 (range 5–20) (478).

Glucocorticoids can also alter the response to anticoagulants. A raised tolerance to heparin has been reported and a fall in fibrinolytic activity has been seen during glucocorticoid treatment (SED-8, 816). The entire clotting mechanism and particularly the prothrombin time should therefore be checked periodically in patients taking glucocorticoids concomitantly with anticoagulants, particularly if the glucocorticoid dose is changed. In addition there is an increased risk of gastric bleeding in patients taking both glucocorticoids and anticoagulants.

Antifungal azoles

Itraconazole 200 mg/day markedly increased plasma methylprednisolone concentrations and reduced morning plasma cortisol concentrations by over 80% in 10 healthy volunteers (479). The C_{max}, AUC, and half-life of methylprednisolone were increased 1.9, 3.9, and 2.4 times respectively.

Itraconazole 200 mg/day orally for 4 days markedly reduced the clearance and increased the half-life of intravenous methylprednisolone from 2.1 to 4.8 hours in a double-blind, randomized, two-phase, crossover study in nine healthy volunteers (SEDA-23, 430; 480). The volume of distribution was not affected. The mean morning plasma cortisol concentration during the itraconazole phase, measured 24 hours after methylprednisolone, was only 9% of that during the placebo phase (11 versus 117 ng/ml).

The authors of these two reports recommended that care be taken when methylprednisolone is prescribed in combination with itraconazole or other potent inhibitors of CYP3A4.

Itraconazole, given orally increased oral prednisolone concentrations by only 24% (481) but increased intravenous dexamethasone concentrations 3.3-fold and oral dexamethasone 3.7-fold (482).

In another study, ketoconazole was given orally as 200 mg od for 4 days, following a single oral dose of budesonide 3 mg either at the same time as ketoconazole or 12 hours before (483). Ketoconazole increased budesonide concentrations (C_{max} and AUC) 6.8- to 7.6-fold when the two drugs were co-administered; with a 12-hour

separation, budesonide concentrations increased only 1.7- to 2.1-fold.

Aprepitant

Aprepitant is a neurokinin-1 receptor antagonist that, in combination with a glucocorticoid and a $5HT_3$ receptor antagonist, is very effective in preventing chemotherapy-induced nausea and vomiting. At therapeutic doses it is also a moderate inhibitor of CYP3A4. Coadministration of aprepitant with dexamethasone or methylprednisolone resulted in increased plasma glucocorticoid concentrations (484). These findings suggest that the dose of these glucocorticoids should be adjusted when aprepitant is given.

Calcium channel blockers

Methylprednisolone concentrations increased with the coadministration of diltiazem (2.6-fold) and mibefradil (3.8-fold) (485).

Ciclosporin

Glucocorticoids cause additive immunosuppression when they are given with other immunosuppressants, such as ciclosporin (SEDA-22, 451; 486).

The AUC of plasma prednisolone has been studied in patients with stable renal transplants (487). The prednisolone AUC was significantly higher in women and in those who took ciclosporin. The highest AUC was in women taking estrogen supplements and ciclosporin. A significantly higher proportion of patients taking ciclosporin + azathioprine + prednisolone had glucocorticoid adverse effects compared with those taking azathioprine + prednisolone. Furthermore, more women than men had adverse effects and the prednisone AUC was greater in those with adverse effects than without. Ciclosporin was thought to have increased the systemic availability of prednisolone, most probably by inhibiting P glycoprotein. Because the major contributor to AUC is the maximum post-dose concentration, it may be possible to use single-point monitoring (2 hours after the dose) for routine clinical studies.

Clarithromycin

Clarithromycin inhibits CYP3A4, which is responsible for the metabolic clearance of prednisolone, the biologically active metabolite of prednisone. Clarithromycin (500 mg bd for 2 days) reduced the clearance of methylprednisolone by 65% and significantly increased its plasma concentrations; clarithromycin did not influence the clearance or plasma concentrations of prednisone (488). Acute mania has been reported to be related to inhibition of the metabolic clearance of prednisone by clarithromycin (SEDA-22, 444; 489).

Cyclophosphamide

The effect of prednisone 1 mg/kg on the pharmacokinetics of cyclophosphamide and its initial metabolites 4-hydroxycyclophosphamide and aldophosphamide (the acyclic tautomer of 4-hydroxycyclophosphamide) has been studied between the first and sixth cycles in seven patients (two men) with systemic vasculitis receiving intravenous cyclophosphamide 0.6 g/m² as a 1-hour intravenous infusion every 3 weeks for six cycles (490). Prednisone reduced the clearance of cyclophosphamide from 5.8 to 4.0 l/hour, reducing the amount of initial metabolites formed. Although the clinical significance of this interaction is unclear, 4-hydroxycyclophosphamide and aldophosphamide are probably responsible for the cytotoxic activity of cyclophosphamide, and increased cyclophosphamide dosages should be considered in patients taking prednisone.

Diuretics

Glucocorticoids with mineralocorticoid activity potentiate potassium loss when they are given with potassium-wasting diuretics (491).

Globulin

A case report with a review of 27 cases of thromboembolic events after the administration of intravenous globulin with or without glucocorticoids has been published (492). The authors suggested that this combined therapy should be administered with caution because of its potential synergistic thrombotic risk.

Grapefruit juice

Methylprednisolone concentrations increased with the co-administration of grapefruit juice (1.75-fold) (493).

Leukotriene receptor antagonists

In a probable pharmacodynamic interaction, severe peripheral edema followed treatment with montelukast and prednisone for asthma (494).

- A 23-year-old man, with a history of asthma, house dust mite allergy, and rhinoconjunctivitis, presented with acute respiratory symptoms. He was given oral cetirizine, inhaled salmeterol, and fluticasone propionate, and oral prednisone 40 mg/day for 1 week and 20 mg/day for 1 week. His asthma recurred when prednisone was withdrawn and he took oral prednisone 60 mg/day for 1 week and 40 mg/day for 1 week. He also took montelukast 10 mg/day. He then developed severe peripheral edema with a gain in weight of 13 kg. Prednisone was withdrawn and his edema resolved. Montelukast was continued.

The author commented that the patient had tolerated prednisone without montelukast and montelukast without prednisone. However, he had severe edema when both drugs were used together. Montelukast may have potentiated glucocorticoid-induced renal tubular sodium and fluid retention. Both have been associated with edema.

Oral contraceptives

Oral contraceptives increased budesonide concentrations by only 22%, but prednisolone concentrations increased by 131%, suggesting a clinically important interaction (495).

Phenobarbital

Phenobarbital increases the metabolism of glucocorticoids, reducing the half-life by some 50% (496).

Phenytoin

Phenytoin increases the metabolism of glucocorticoids, reducing the half-life by some 50% (496).

Rifampicin

Rifampicin and other drugs that induce liver enzymes increase the metabolism of glucocorticoids (497), sufficient to reduce their therapeutic effects, for example in asthma (498).

Salicylates

Glucocorticoids reduce the plasma concentrations of salicylates (499). If they are given with aspirin or other anti-inflammatory drugs, there may be an additive effect on the gastric wall, leading to an increased risk of bleeding and ulceration (500–502).

Diagnosis of adverse drug reactions

The short Synacthen (tetracosactide) test is the most commonly used test for assessing adrenal suppression. The potential of a simpler and more cost-effective procedure, the morning salivary cortisol concentration, as an out-patient screening tool to detect adrenal suppression in patients using topical intranasal glucocorticoids for rhinosinusitis has been investigated in 48 patients who were using topical glucocorticoids (503). The morning salivary cortisol measurement was a useful screening tool for adrenal suppression in this setting.

Osteoporosis and osteopenia are usually evaluated by measuring bone density using dual-energy X-ray absorptiometry (DXA). However, there is increased interest in measuring not only bone density but also some structural properties of the bone, such as elasticity and trabecular stiffness and connectivity, which are more closely related to bone strength. Quantitative ultrasound could theoretically provide information on bone structure, as has been suggested by a prospective study in patients with glucocorticoid-induced osteoporosis (504), but further studies are needed to define the role of quantitative ultrasonography in the prediction of fracture and in the clinical management of glucocorticoid-induced osteoporosis.

Management of adverse drug reactions

Mood stabilizers, such as lithium, lamotrigine, and carbamazepine, may be effective in treating glucocorticoid-induced mood symptoms. In an open trial, 12 patients with glucocorticoid-induced manic or mixed symptoms were treated with olanzapine 2.5 mg/day initially, increasing to a maximum of 20 mg/day; 11 of the 12 patients had significant improvement (505).

References

1. Kaiser H. Cortisone derivate in Klinik und PraxisStuttgart-New York: Thieme;. 1987.

2. Labhart A. Adrenal cortex. In: Labhart A, editor. Clinical Endocrinology. Berlin-Heidelberg-New York: Springer, 1985:373.

3. Medici TC, Ruegsegger P. Does alternate-day cloprednol therapy prevent bone loss? A longitudinal double-blind, controlled clinical study. Clin Pharmacol Ther 1990;48(4):455–66.

4. Iwasaki E, Baba M. [Pharmacokinetics and pharmacodynamics of hydrocortisone in asthmatic children.]Arerugi 1993;42(10):1555–62.

5. Bone RC, Fisher CJ Jr, Clemmer TP, Slotman GJ, Metz CA, Balk RA. A controlled clinical trial of high-dose methylprednisolone in the treatment of severe sepsis and septic shock. N Engl J Med 1987;317(11):653–8.

6. The Veterans Administration Systemic Sepsis Cooperative Study Group. Effect of high-dose glucocorticoid therapy on mortality in patients with clinical signs of systemic sepsis. N Engl J Med 1987;317(11):659–65.

7. Iuchi T, Akaike M, Mitsui T, Ohshima Y, Shintani Y, Azuma H, Matsumoto T. Glucocorticoid excess induces superoxide production in vascular endothelial cells and elicits vascular endothelial dysfunction. Circ Res 2003; 92: 81–7.

8. Romagnoli C, Zecca E, Vento G, De Carolis MP, Papacci P, Tortorolo G. Early postnatal dexamethasone for the prevention of chronic lung disease in high-risk preterm infants. Intensive Care Med 1999;25(7):717–21.

9. Confalonieri M, Urbino R, Potena A, Piattella M, Parigi P, Puccio G, Della Porta R, Giorgio C, Blasi F, Umberger R, Meduri GU. Hydrocortisone infusion for severe community-acquired pneumonia: a preliminary randomized study. Am J Respir Crit Care Med 2005;171(3):242–8.

10. Garland JS, Alex CP, Pauly TH, Whitehead VL, Brand J, Winston JF, Samuels DP, McAuliffe TL. A three-day course of dexamethasone therapy to prevent chronic lung disease in ventilated neonates: a randomized trial. Pediatrics 1999;104(1 Part 1):91–9.

11. Romagnoli C, Zecca E, Vento G, Maggio L, Papacci P, Tortorolo G. Effect on growth of two different dexamethasone courses for preterm infants at risk of chronic lung disease. A randomized trial. Pharmacology 1999;59(5):266–74.

12. Tarnow-Mordi W, Mitra A. Postnatal dexamethasone in preterm infants is potentially lifesaving, but follow up studies are urgently needed. BMJ 1999;319(7222):1385–6.

13. van de Beek D, de Gans J, McIntyre P, Prasad K. Steroids in adults with acute bacterial meningitis: a systematic review. Lancet Infect Dis 2004; 4: 139–43.

14. Arias-Camison JM, Lau J, Cole CH, Frantz ID 3rd. Meta-analysis of dexamethasone therapy started in the first 15 days of life for prevention of chronic lung disease in premature infants. Pediatr Pulmonol 1999;28(3):167–74.

15. Klein-Gitelman MS, Pachman LM. Intravenous corticosteroids: adverse reactions are more variable than expected in children. J Rheumatol 1998;25(10):1995–2002.

16. Feldweg AM, Leddy JP. Drug interactions affecting the efficacy of corticosteroid therapy. A brief review with an illustrative case. J Clin Rheumatol 1999;5:143–50.

17. Maxwell SR, Moots RJ, Kendall MJ. Corticosteroids: do they damage the cardiovascular system? Postgrad Med J 1994;70(830):863–70.

18. Ellis SG, Semenec T, Lander K, Franco I, Raymond R, Whitlow PL. Effects of long-term prednisone (> = 5 mg) use on outcomes and complications of percutaneous coronary intervention. Am J Cardiol 2004; 93: 1389–90.

19. Sato A, Funder JW, Okubo M, Kubota E, Saruta T. Glucocorticoid-induced hypertension in the elderly. Relation to serum calcium and family history of essential hypertension. Am J Hypertens 1995;8(8):823–8.

20. Thedenat B, Leaute-Labreze C, Boralevi F, Roul S, Labbe L, Marliere V, Taieb A. Surveillance tensionnelle des nourrissons traites par corticotherapie generale pour un hemangiome. [Blood pressure monitoring in infants with hemangiomas treated with corticosteroids.] Ann Dermatol Venereol 2002;129(2):183–5.

21. Stewart IM, Marks JSECG. Abnormalities in steroid-treated rheumatoid patients. Lancet 1977;2(8050):1237–8.

22. Baty V, Blain H, Saadi L, Jeandel C, Canton P. Fatal myocardial infarction in an elderly woman with severe ulcerative colitis. what is the role of steroids? Am J Gastroenterol 1998;93(10):2000–1.

23. Machiels JP, Jacques JM, de Meester A. Coronary artery spasm during anaphylaxis. Ann Emerg Med 1996;27(5):674–5.

24. Sato O, Takagi A, Miyata T, Takayama Y. Aortic aneurysms in patients with autoimmune disorders treated with corticosteroids. Eur J Vasc Endovasc Surg 1995;10(3):366–9.

25. Kotha P, McGreevy MJ, Kotha A, Look M, Weisman MH. Early deaths with thrombolytic therapy for acute myocardial infarction in corticosteroid-dependent rheumatoid arthritis. Clin Cardiol 1998;21(11):853–6.

26. Yunis KA, Bitar FF, Hayek P, Mroueh SM, Mikati M. Transient hypertrophic cardiomyopathy in the newborn following multiple doses of antenatal corticosteroids. Am J Perinatol 1999;16(1):17–21.

27. Gill AW, Warner G, Bull L. Iatrogenic neonatal hypertrophic cardiomyopathy. Pediatr Cardiol 1996;17(5):335–9.

28. Pokorny JJ, Roth F, Balfour I, Rinehart G. An unusual complication of the treatment of a hemangioma. Ann Plast Surg 2002;48(1):83–7.

29. Kothari SN, Kisken WA. Dexamethasone-induced congestive heart failure in a patient with dilated cardiomyopathy caused by occult pheochromocytoma. Surgery 1998;123(1):102–5.

30. Balys R, Manoukian J, Zalai C. Left ventricular hypertrophy with outflow tract obstruction-a complication of dexamethasone treatment for subglottic stenosis. Int J Pediatr Otorhinolaryngol 2005;69(2):271–3.

31. Kucukosmanoglu O, Karabay A, Ozbarlas N, Noyan A, Anarat A. Marked bradycardia due to pulsed and oral methylprednisolone therapy in a patient with rapidly progressive glomerulonephritis. Nephron 1998;80(4):484.

32. Schult M, Lohmann D, Knitsch W, Kuse ER, Nashan B. Recurrent cardiocirculatory arrest after kidney transplantation related to intravenous methylprednisolone bolus therapy. Transplantation 1999;67(11):1497–8.

33. Brumund MR, Truemper EJ, Lutin WA, Pearson-Shaver AL. Disseminated varicella and staphylococcal pericarditis after topical steroids. J Pediatr 1997;131(1 Part 1):162–3.

34. Kaiser H. Cortisonderivate in Klink und Praxis. 7th edn.. Stuttgart: G.Thieme;. 1977.

35. Williamson IJ, Matusiewicz SP, Brown PH, Greening AP, Crompton GK. Frequency of voice problems and cough in patients using pressurized aerosol inhaled steroid preparations. Eur Respir J 1995;8(4):590–2.

36. Lim BS, Choi WY, Choi JW. A case of steroid-induced intractable hiccup. Tuberc Respir Dis 1991;38:304–7.

37. Cersosimo RJ, Brophy MT. Hiccups with high dose dexamethasone administration: a case report. Cancer 1998;82(2):412–4.

38. Ross J, Eledrisi M, Casner P. Persistent hiccups induced by dexamethasone. West J Med 1999;170(1):51–2.

39. Poynter D. Beclomethasone dipropionate aerosol and nasal mucosa. Br J Clin Pharmacol 1977;4(Suppl 3):S295–301.

40. Albucher JF, Vuillemin-Azais C, Manelfe C, Clanet M, Guiraud-Chaumeil B, Chollet F. Cerebral thrombophlebitis in three patients with probable multiple sclerosis. Role of lumbar puncture or intravenous corticosteroid treatment. Cerebrovasc Dis 1999;9(5):298–303.

41. Shinwell ES, Karplus M, Reich D, Weintraub Z, Blazer S, Bader D, Yurman S, Dolfin T, Kogan A, Dollberg S, Arbel E, Goldberg M, Gur I, Naor N, Sirota L, Mogilner S, Zaritsky A, Barak M, Gottfried E. Early postnatal dexamethasone treatment and increased incidence of cerebral palsy. Arch Dis Child Fetal Neonatal Ed 2000;83(3):F177–81.

42. Halliday HL. Postnatal steroids and chronic lung disease in the newborn. Paediatr Respir Rev 2004; 5 Suppl A: S245–8.

43. Yeh TF, Lin YJ, Lin HC, Huang CC, Hsieh WS, Lin CH, Tsai CH. Outcomes at school age after postnatal dexamethasone therapy for lung disease of prematurity. N Engl J Med 2004;350:1304–13.

44. Bentson J, Reza M, Winter J, Wilson G. Steroids and apparent cerebral atrophy on computed tomography scans. J Comput Assist Tomogr 1978;2(1):16–23.

45. Vaughn BV, Ali II, Olivier KN, Lackner RP, Robertson KR, Messenheimer JA, Paradowski LJ, Egan TM. Seizures in lung transplant recipients. Epilepsia 1996;37(12):1175–9.

46. Lorrot M, Bader-Meunier B, Sebire G, Dommergues JP. Hypertension intracranienne benigne: une complication meconnue de la corticotherapie. [Benign intracranial hypertension: an unrecognized complication of corticosteroid therapy.] Arch Pediatr 1999;6(1):40–2.

47. Kalapurakal JA, Silverman CL, Akhtar N, Laske DW, Braitman LE, Boyko OB, Thomas PR. Intracranial meningiomas: factors that influence the development of cerebral edema after stereotactic radiosurgery and radiation therapy. Radiology 1997;204(2):461–5.

48. Laroche F, Chemouilli R, Carlier P. Efficacy of conservative treatment in a patient with spinal cord compression due to corticosteroid-induced epidural lipomatosis. Rev Rheum (English Edn) 1993;30:729–31.

49. Roy-Camille R, Mazel C, Husson JL, Saillant G. Symptomatic spinal epidural lipomatosis induced by a long-term steroid treatment. Review of the literature and report of two additional cases. Spine 1991;16(12):1365–71.

50. Andress HJ, Schurmann M, Heuck A, Schmand J, Lob G. A rare case of osteoporotic spine fracture associated with epidural lipomatosis causing paraplegia following long-term cortisone therapy. Arch Orthop Trauma Surg 2000;120(7–8):484–6.

51. Pinsker MO, Kinzel D, Lumenta CB. Epidural thoracic lipomatosis induced by long-term steroid treatment case illustration. Acta Neurochir (Wien) 1998;140(9):991–2.

52. Parker CT, Jarek MJ, Finger DR. Corticosteroid-associated epidural lipomatosis. J Clin Rheumatol 1999;5:141–2.

53. Kano K, Kyo K, Ito S, Nishikura K, Ando T, Yamada Y, Arisaka O. Spinal epidural lipomatosis in children with renal diseases receiving steroid therapy. Pediatr Nephrol 2005;20(2):184–9.

54. Donaghy M, Mills KR, Boniface SJ, Simmons J, Wright I, Gregson N, Jacobs J. Pure motor demyelinating neuropathy: deterioration after steroid treatment and improvement with intravenous immunoglobulin. J Neurol Neurosurg Psychiatry 1994;57(7):778–83.

55. Urban RC Jr, Cotlier E. Corticosteroid-induced cataracts. Surv Ophthalmol 1986;31(2):102–10.

56. Kaye LD, Kalenak JW, Price RL, Cunningham R. Ocular implications of long-term prednisone therapy in children. J Pediatr Ophthalmol Strabismus 1993;30(3):142–4.

57. Cumming RG, Mitchell P, Leeder SR. Use of inhaled corticosteroids and the risk of cataracts. N Engl J Med 1997;337(1):8–14.

58. Abramson HA. May corticosteroid cataracts be reversible. J Asthma Res 1977;14(3):vii–viii.

59. Lubkin VL. Steroid cataract – a review and a conclusion. J Asthma Res 1977;14(2):55–9.

60. Forman AR, Loreto JA, Tina LU. Reversibility of corticosteroid-associated cataracts in children with the nephrotic syndrome. Am J Ophthalmol 1977;84(1):75–8.

61. Wingate RJ, Beaumont PE. Intravitreal triamcinolone and elevated intraocular pressure. Aust NZ J Ophthalmol 1999;27(6):431–2.

62. Garbe E, LeLorier J, Boivin JF, Suissa S. Risk of ocular hypertension or open-angle glaucoma in elderly patients on oral glucocorticoids. Lancet 1997;350(9083):979–82.

63. Garbe E, LeLorier J, Boivin JF, Suissa S. Inhaled and nasal glucocorticoids and the risks of ocular hypertension or open-angle glaucoma. JAMA 1997;277(9):722–7.

64. Novack GD. Ocular toxicology. Curr Opin Ophthalmol 1994;5(6):110–4.

65. Opatowsky I, Feldman RM, Gross R, Feldman ST. Intraocular pressure elevation associated with inhalation and nasal corticosteroids. Ophthalmology 1995;102(2):177–9.

66. Kwok AK, Lam DS, Ng JS, Fan DS, Chew SJ, Tso MO. Ocular-hypertensive response to topical steroids in children. Ophthalmology 1997;104(12):2112–6.

67. Tham CCY, Ng JSK, Li RTH, Chik KW, Lam DSC. Intraocular pressure profile of a child on a systemic corticosteroid. Am J Ophthalmol 2004;137:198–201.

68. Gass JD, Little H. Bilateral bullous exudative retinal detachment complicating idiopathic central serous chorioretinopathy during systemic corticosteroid therapy. Ophthalmology 1995;102(5):737–47.

69. Karadimas P, Bouzas EA. Glucocorticoid use represents a risk factor for central serous chorioretinopathy: a prospective, case-control study. Graefe's Arch Clin Exp Ophthalmol 2004;242:800–2.

70. Baumal CR, Martidis A, Truong SN. Central serous chorioretinopathy associated with periocular corticosteroid injection treatment for HLA-B27-associated iritis. Arch Ophthalmol 2004;122:926–8.

71. Roth DB, Chieh J, Spirn MJ, Green SN, Yarian DL, Chaudhry NA. Noninfectious endophthalmitis associated with intravitreal triamcinolone injection. Arch Ophthalmol 2003;121:1279–82.

72. Roth DB, Chieh J, Spirn MJ, Green SN, Yarian DL, Chaudhry NA. Noninfectious endophthalmitis associated with intravitreal triamcinolone injection. Arch Ophthalmol 2003;121:1279–82.

73. Chen SDM, Lochhead J, McDonald B, Patel CK. Pseudohypopyon after intravitreal triamcinolone injection for the treatment of pseudophakic cystoid macular oedema. Br J Ophthalmol 2004;88:843–4.

74. Apel A, Campbell I, Rootman DS. Infectious crystalline keratopathy following trabeculectomy and low-dose topical steroids. Cornea 1995;14(3):321–3.

75. Rao GP, O'Brien C, Hicky-Dwyer M, Patterson A. Rapid onset bilateral calcific band keratopathy associated with phosphate-containing steroid eye drops. Eur J Implant Refractive Surg 1995;7:251–2.

76. Ramanathan R, Siassi B, deLemos RA. Severe retinopathy of prematurity in extremely low birth weight infants after short-term dexamethasone therapy. J Perinatol 1995;15(3):178–82.

77. Kushner FH, Olson JC. Retinal hemorrhage as a consequence of epidural steroid injection. Arch Ophthalmol 1995;113(3):309–13.

78. Byers B. Blindness secondary to steroid injections into the nasal turbinates. Arch Ophthalmol 1979;97(1):79–80.

79. Van Dalen JT, Sherman MD. Corticosteroid-induced exophthalmos. Doc Ophthalmol 1989;72(3–4):273–7.

80. Klein JF. Adverse psychiatric effects of systemic glucocorticoid therapy. Am Fam Physician 1992;46(5):1469–74.

81. Doherty M, Garstin I, McClelland RJ, Rowlands BJ, Collins BJ. A steroid stupor in a surgical ward. Br J Psychiatry 1991;158:125–7.

82. Satel SL. Mental status changes in children receiving glucocorticoids. Review of the literature. Clin Pediatr (Phila) 1990;29(7):383–8.

83. Alpert E, Seigerman C. Steroid withdrawal psychosis in a patient with closed head injury. Arch Phys Med Rehabil 1986;67(10):766–9.

84. Hassanyeh F, Murray RB, Rodgers H. Adrenocortical suppression presenting with agitated depression, morbid jealousy, and a dementia-like state. Br J Psychiatry 1991;159:870–2.

85. Nahon S, Pisanté L, Delas N. A successful switch from prednisone to budesonide for neuropsychiatric adverse effects in a patient with ileal Crohn's disease. Am J Gastroenterol 2001;96(1):1953–4.

86. Brown ES, J Woolston D, Frol A, Bobadilla L, Khan DA, Hanczyc M, Rush AJ, Fleckenstein J, Babcock E, Cullum CM. Hippocampal volume, spectroscopy, cognition, and mood in patients receiving corticosteroid therapy. Biol Psychiatry 2004;55:538–45.

87. O'Shea TM, Kothadia JM, Klinepeter KL, Goldstein DJ, Jackson BG, Weaver RG III, Dillard RG. Randomized placebo-controlled trial of a 42-day tapering course of dexamethasone to reduce the duration of ventilator dependency in very low birth weight infants: outcome of study participants at 1-year adjusted age. Pediatrics 1999;104(1 Part 1):15–21.

88. Soliday E, Grey S, Lande MB. Behavioral effects of corticosteroids in steroid–sensitive nephrotic syndrome. Pediatrics 1999;104(4):e51.

89. Kaiser H. Psychische Storungen nach Beclomethasondipropionat-Inhalation?. [Mental disorders following beclomethasone dipropionate inhalation?.] Med Klin 1978;73(38):1334.

90. Keenan PA, Jacobson MW, Soleymani RM, Mayes MD, Stress ME, Yaldoo DT. The effect on memory of chronic prednisone treatment in patients with systemic disease. Neurology 1996;47(6):1396–402.

91. Oliveri RL, Sibilia G, Valentino P, Russo C, Romeo N, Quattrone A. Pulsed methylprednisolone induces a reversible impairment of memory in patients with relapsing-remitting multiple sclerosis. Acta Neurol Scand 1998;97(6):366–9.

92. Newcomer JW, Selke G, Melson AK, Hershey I, Craft S, Richards K, Alderson AL. Decreased memory performance in healthy humans induced by stress-level cortisol treatment. Arch Gen Psychiatry 1999;56(6): 527–533.

93. Aisen PS, Davis KL, Berg JD, Schafer K, Campbell K, Thomas RG, Weiner MF, Farlow MR, Sano M, Grundman M, Thal LJ. A randomized controlled trial of prednisone in Alzheimer's disease. Alzheimer's Dis Cooperative Study. Neurology 2000;54(3):588–93.

94. de Quervain DJ, Roozendaal B, Nitsch RM, McGaugh JL, Hock C. Acute cortisone administration impairs retrieval of long-term declarative memory in humans. Nat Neurosci 2000;3(4):313–4.

95. Bermond B, Surachno S, Lok A, ten Berge IJ, Plasmans B, Kox C, Schuller E, Schellekens PT, Hamel R. Memory functions in prednisone-treated kidney transplant patients. Clin Transplant 2005;19(4):512–7.

96. Brown ES, Stuard G, Liggin JD, Hukovic N, Frol A, Dhanani N, Khan DA, Jeffress J, Larkin GL, McEwen BS, Rosenblatt R, Mageto Y, Hanczyc M, Cullum CM. Effect of phenytoin on mood and declarative memory during prescription corticosteroid therapy. Biol Psychiatry 2005;57(5):543–8.

97. Moser NJ, Phillips BA, Guthrie G, Barnett G. Effects of dexamethasone on sleep. Pharmacol Toxicol 1996;79(2):100–2.

98. Chau SY, Mok CC. Factors predictive of corticosteroid psychosis in patients with systemic lupus erythematosus. Neurology 2003;61:104–7.

99. Bolanos SH, Khan DA, Hanczyc M, Bauer MS, Dhanani N, Brown ES. Assessment of mood states in patients receiving long-term corticosteroid therapy and in controls with patient-rated and clinician-rated scales. Ann Allergy Asthma Immunol 2004;92:500–5.

100. Preda A, Fazeli A, McKay BG, Bowers MB Jr, Mazure CM. Lamotrigine as prophylaxis against steroid-induced mania. J Clin Psychiatry 1999;60(10):708–9.

101. Preda A, Fazeli A, McKay BG, Bowers MB Jr, Mazure CM. Lamotrigine of prophylaxis against steroid-induced mania. J. Clin Psychiatry 1999;60(10):708–9.

102. Brown ES, Suppes T, Khan DA, Carmody TJ 3rd. Mood changes during prednisone bursts in outpatients with asthma. J Clin Psychopharmacol 2002;22(1):55–61.

103. Wada K, Suzuki H, Taira T, Akiyama K, Kuroda S. Successful use of intravenous clomipramine in depressive–catatonic state associated with corticosteroid treatment. Int J Psych Clin Pract 2004;8:131–3.

104. Ilbeigi MS, Davidson ML, Yarmush JM. An unexpected arousal effect of etomidate in a patient on high-dose steroids. Anesthesiology 1998;89(6):1587–9.

105. Kramer TM, Cottingham EM. Risperidone in the treatment of steroid-induced psychosis. J Child Adolesc Psychopharmacol 1999;9(4):315–6.

106. Scheschonka A, Bleich S, Buchwald AB, Ruther E, Wiltfang J. Development of obsessive-compulsive behaviour following cortisone treatment. Pharmacopsychiatry 2002;35(2):72–4.

107. Kamoda T, Nakahara C, Matsui A. A case of empty sella after steroid pulse therapy for nephrotic syndrome. J Rheumatol 1998;25(4):822–3.

108. Rabhan NB. Pituitary-adrenal suppression and Cushing's syndrome after intermittent dexamethasone therapy. Ann Intern Med 1968;69(6):1141–8.

109. Zwaan CM, Odink RJ, Delemarre-van de Waal HA, Dankert-Roelse JE, Bokma JA. Acute adrenal insufficiency after discontinuation of inhaled corticosteroid therapy. Lancet 1992;340(8830):1289–90.

110. Clark DJ, Grove A, Cargill RI, Lipworth BJ. Comparative adrenal suppression with inhaled budesonide and

fluticasone propionate in adult asthmatic patients. Thorax 1996;51(3):262–6.

111. Marazzi MG, Agnese G, Gremmo M, Cotellessa M, Garibaldi L. Problemi relativi alla funzionalita surrenalica in corso di terapia cortisonica protratta in soggetti con epatite cronica: nota preliminare. [Problems concerning adrenal function during prolonged corticoid treatment in patients with chronic hepatitis. Preliminary note.] Minerva Pediatr 1978;30(11):937–44.

112. Dutau G, Rochiccioli P. Exploration corticotrope au cours des traitements prolongés par le dipropionate de béclométhasone chez l'enfant. [Corticotropic testing during long-term beclomethasone dipropionate treatment asthmatic children.] Poumon Coeur 1978;34(4):247–53.

113. Sumboonnanonda A, Vongjirad A, Suntornpoch V, Petrarat S. Adrenal function after prednisolone treatment in childhood nephrotic syndrome. J Med Assoc Thai 1994;77(3):126–9.

114. Felner EI, Thompson MT, Ratliff AF, White PC, Dickson BA. Time course of recovery of adrenal function in children treated for leukemia. J Pediatr 2000;137(1):21–4.

115. Reiner M, Galeazzi RL, Studer H. Cushing-Syndrom und Nebennierenrinden-Suppression durch intranasale Anwendung von Dexamethasonpraparaten. [Cushing's syndrome and adrenal suppression by means of intranasal use of dexamethasone preparations.] Schweiz Med Wochenschr 1977;107(49):1836–7.

116. Kay J, Findling JW, Raff H. Epidural triamcinolone suppresses the pituitary–adrenal axis in human subjects. Anesth Analg 1994;79(3):501–5.

117. Boonen S, Van Distel G, Westhovens R, Dequeker J. Steroid myopathy induced by epidural triamcinolone injection. Br J Rheumatol 1995;34(4):385–6.

118. Kobayashi S, Warabi H, Hashimoto H. Hypopituitarism with empty sella after steroid pulse therapy. J Rheumatol 1997;24(1):236–8.

119. Grabner W. Zur induzierten NNR-Insuffizienz bei chirurgischen Eingriffen. [Problems of corticosteroid-induced adrenal insufficiency in surgery.] Fortschr Med 1977;95(30):1866–8.

120. Iglesias P, González J, Díez JJ. Acute and persistent iatrogenic Cushing's syndrome after a single dose of triamcinolone acetonide. J Endocrinol Invest 2005;28(11):1019–23.

121. Mukai T. [Antagonism between parathyroid hormone and glucocorticoids in calcium and phosphorus metabolism.]Nippon Naibunpi Gakkai Zasshi 1965;41(8):950–9.

122. Kahn A, Snapper I, Drucker A. Corticosteroid-induced tetany in latent hypoparathyroidism. Arch Intern Med 1964;114:434–8.

123. Fisher JE, Smith RS, Lagrandeur R, Lorenz RP. Gestational diabetes mellitus in women receiving beta-adrenergics and corticosteroids for threatened preterm delivery. Obstet Gynecol 1997;90(6):880–3.

124. Kim YS, Kim MS, Kim SI, Lim SK, Lee HY, Han DS, Park K. Post-transplantation diabetes is better controlled after conversion from prednisone to deflazacort: a prospective trial in renal transplants. Transpl Int 1997;10(3):197–201.

125. Gurwitz JH, Bohn RL, Glynn RJ, Monane M, Mogun H, Avorn J. Glucocorticoids and the risk for initiation of hypoglycemic therapy. Arch Intern Med 1994;154(1):97–101.

126. Bagdade JD, Porte D Jr, Bierman EL. Steroid-induced lipemia. A complication of high-dosage corticosteroid therapy. Arch Intern Med 1970;125(1):129–34.

127. Ettinger WH Jr, Hazzard WR. Elevated apolipoprotein-B levels in corticosteroid-treated patients with systemic lupus erythematosus. J Clin Endocrinol Metab 1988;67(3):425–8.

128. Amin SB, Sinkin RA, McDermott MP, Kendig JW. Lipid intolerance in neonates receiving dexamethasone for bronchopulmonary dysplasia. Arch Pediatr Adolesc Med 1999;153(8):795–800.

129. Tiley C, Grimwade D, Findlay M, Treleaven J, Height S, Catalano J, Powles R. Tumour lysis following hydrocortisone prior to a blood product transfusion in T-cell acute lymphoblastic leukaemia. Leuk Lymphoma 1992;8(1–2):143–6.

130. Lerza R, Botta M, Barsotti B, Schenone E, Mencoboni M, Bogliolo G, Pannacciulli I, Arboscello E. Dexamethasone-induced acute tumor lysis syndrome in a T-cell malignant lymphoma. Leuk Lymphoma 2002;43(5):1129–32.

131. Balli F, Benatti C. Terapia corticosteroidea protratta e metabolismo fosfo-calcico. II. Modificazioni del metabolismo fosfo-calcico in soggetti nefrosici sottoposti a terapia carticosteroidea protratta. [Prolonged corticosteroid therapy and phospho-calcic metabolism. II. Changes of phospho-calcic metabolism in nephrotic subjects subjected to prolonged corticoid therapy.] Minerva Pediatr 1968;20(45):2315–25.

132. Handa R, Wali JP, Singh RI, Aggarwal P. Corticosteroids precipitating hypocalcemic encephalopathy in hypoparathyroidism. Ann Emerg Med 1995;26(2):241–2.

133. Ravina A, Slezak L, Mirsky N, Bryden NA, Anderson RA. Reversal of corticosteroid-induced diabetes mellitus with supplemental chromium. Diabet Med 1999;16(2):164–7.

134. Schneider J, Burmeister H, Ruiz-Torres A. Langzeitstudien uber die Wirksamkeit der Dauertherapie bei hyperergisch-allergischen Erkrankungen mit Prednisolon. [Longitudinal study about the efficacy of long term prednisolone therapy in hyperergic-allergic diseases.] Verh Dtsch Ges Inn Med 1977;83:1785–8.

135. Schmand B, Neuvel J, Smolders-de Haas H, Hoeks J, Treffers PE, Koppe JG. Psychological development of children who were treated antenatally with corticosteroids to prevent respiratory distress syndrome. Pediatrics 1990;86(1):58–64.

136. Bielawski D, Hiatt IM, Hegyi T. Betamethasone-induced leukaemoid reaction in pre-term infant. Lancet 1978;1(8057):218–9.

137. Craddock CG. Corticosteroid-induced lymphopenia, immunosuppression, and body defense. Ann Intern Med 1978;88(4):564–6.

138. Saxon A, Stevens RH, Ramer SJ, Clements PJ, Yu DT. Glucocorticoids administered in vivo inhibit human suppressor T lymphocyte function and diminish B lymphocyte responsiveness in in vitro immunoglobulin synthesis. J Clin Invest 1978;61(4):922–30.

139. Maeshima E, Yamada Y, Yukawa S. Fever and leucopenia with steroids. Lancet 2000;355(9199):198.

140. Patrassi GM, Sartori MT, Livi U, Casonato A, Danesin C, Vettore S, Girolami A. Impairment of fibrinolytic poten-

tial in long-term steroid treatment after heart transplantation. Transplantation 1997;64(11):1610–4.

141. The British Thoracic and Tuberculosis Association. Inhaled corticosteroids compared with oral prednisone in patients starting long-term corticosteroid therapy for asthma. Lancet 1975;2(7933):469–73.

142. Salzman GA, Pyszczynski DR. Oropharyngeal candidiasis in patients treated with beclomethasone dipropionate delivered by metered-dose inhaler alone and with Aerochamber. J Allergy Clin Immunol 1988;81(2):424–8.

143. Linder N, Kuint J, German B, Lubin D, Loewenthal R. Hypertrophy of the tongue associated with inhaled corticosteroid therapy in premature infants. J Pediatr 1995;127(4):651–3.

144. Spiro HM. Is the steroid ulcer a myth? N Engl J Med 1983;309(1):45–7.

145. Messer J, Reitman D, Sacks HS, Smith H Jr, Chalmers TC. Association of adrenocorticosteroid therapy and peptic-ulcer disease. N Engl J Med 1983;309(1):21–4.

146. Conn HO, Poynard T. Corticosteroids and peptic ulcer: meta-analysis of adverse events during steroid therapy. J Intern Med 1994;236(6):619–32.

147. Henry DA, Johnston N, Dobson A, Duggan J. Fatal peptic ulcer complications and the use of non-steroidal antiinflammatory drugs, aspirin, and corticosteroids. BMJ (Clin Res Ed) 1987;295:1227.

148. Suazo-Barahona J, Gallegos J, Carmona-Sanchez R, Martinez R, Robles-Diaz G. Nonsteroidal anti-inflammatory drugs and gastrocolic fistula. J Clin Gastroenterol 1998;26(4):343–5.

149. Shimizu T, Yamashiro Y, Yabuta K. Impaired increase of prostaglandin E2 in gastric juice during steroid therapy in children. J Paediatr Child Health 1994;30(2):169–72.

150. Yamanishi Y, Yamana S, Ishioka S, Yamakido M. Development of ischemic colitis and scleroderma renal crisis following methylprednisolone pulse therapy for progressive systemic sclerosis. Intern Med 1996;35(7):583–6.

151. Dwarakanath AD, Nash J, Rhodes JM. "Conversion" from ulcerative colitis to Crohn's disease associated with corticosteroid treatment. Gut 1994;35(8):1141–4.

152. Sharma R, Gupta KL, Ammon RH, Gambert SR. Atypical presentation of colon perforation related to corticosteroid use. Geriatrics 1997;52(5):88–90.

153. Candelas G, Jover JA, Fernandez B, Rodriguez-Olaverri JC, Calatayud J. Perforation of the sigmoid colon in a rheumatoid arthritis patient treated with methylprednisolone pulses. Scand J Rheumatol 1998;27(2):152–3.

154. Mpofu S, Mpofu CMA, Hutchinson D, Maier AE, Dodd SR, Moots RJ. Steroids, non-steroidal anti-inflammatory drugs, and sigmoid diverticular abscess perforation in rheumatic conditions. Ann Rheum Dis 2004;63:588–90.

155. Weissel M, Hauff W. Fatal liver failure after high-dose glucocorticoid pulse therapy in a patient with severe thyroid eye disease. Thyroid 2000;10(6):521.

156. Nanki T, Koike R, Miyasaka N. Subacute severe steatohepatitis during prednisolone therapy for systemic lupus erythematosis. Am J Gastroenterol 1999;94(11):3379.

157. Dourakis SP, Sevastianos VA, Kaliopi P. Acute severe steatohepatitis related to prednisolone therapy. Am J Gastroenterol 2002;97(4):1074–5.

158. Verrips A, Rotteveel JJ, Lippens R. Dexamethasone-induced hepatomegaly in three children. Pediatr Neurol 1998;19(5):388–91.

159. Marinò M, Morabito E, Brunetto MR, Bartalena L, Pinchera A, Marocci C. Acute and severe liver damage associated with intravenous glucocorticoid pulse therapy in patients with Graves' ophthalmopathy. Thyroid 2004;14:403–6.

160. Hamed I, Lindeman RD, Czerwinski AW. Case report: acute pancreatitis following corticosteroid and azathioprine therapy. Am J Med Sci 1978;276(2):211–9.

161. Di Fazano CS, Messica O, Quennesson S, Quennesson ER, Inaoui R, Vergne P, Bonnet C, Bertin P, Treves R. Two new cases of glucocorticoid-induced pancreatitis. Rev Rhum Engl Ed 1999;66(4):235.

162. Khanna S, Kumar A. Acute pancreatitis due to hydrocortisone in a patient with ulcerative colitis. J Gastroenterol Hepatol 2003;18:1010–1.

163. Reichert LJ, Koene RA, Wetzels JF. Acute haemodynamic and proteinuric effects of prednisolone in patients with a nephrotic syndrome. Nephrol Dial Transplant 1999;14(1):91–7.

164. Charpin J, Arnaud A, Boutin C, Aubert J, Murisasco A, Gotte G. Long-term corticosteroid therapy and its effect on the kidney. Acta Allergol 1969;24(1):49–56.

165. Gray D, Shepherd H, Daar A, Oliver DO, Morris PJ. Oral versus intravenous high-dose steroid treatment of renal allograft rejection. The big shot or not? Lancet 1978;1(8056):117–8.

166. Toftegaard M, Knudsen F. Massive vasopressin-resistant polyuria induced by dexamethasone. Intensive Care Med 1995;21(3):238–40.

167. Editorial. Nocturia during steroid therapy. BMJ 1970;4(729):193–4.

168. Wendt H. Klinisch-pharmakologische Untersuchungen zur akneinduzierenden Wirkung von Fluorcortinbutylester. [Clinico-pharmacological studies on the acne-inducing action of fluocortin butylester.] Arzneimittelforschung 1977;27(11a):2245–6.

169. Bioulac P, Beylot C. Etude ultrastructurale d'une leuco-dermie secondaire a une injection intraarticulaire de corti-coides. [Ultrastructural study of a leukoderma secondary to an intra-articular injection of corticoids.] Ann Dermatol Venereol 1977;104(12):883–5.

170. Bondy PhK. Disorders of the adrenal cortex. In: Wilson JD, Foster DW, editors. Williams' Textbook of Endocrinology. 7th edn. Philadelphia: Saunders, 1985:816.

171. Reinhold K, Schneider L, Hunzelmann N, Krieg T, Scharffetter-Kochanek K. Delayed-type allergy to systemic corticosteroids. Allergy 2000;55(11):1095–6.

172. Shuster S, Raffle EJ, Bottoms E. Skin collagen in rheumatoid arthritis and the effect of corticosteroids. Lancet 1967;2:525.

173. Mathov E, Grad P, Scaglia H. Provocación de hemorragias uterinas anormales y hematomas subcutáneos por el uso de la acetonida de la triamcinoona en pacientes alérgicas. [Provocation of uterine hemorrhages and subcutaneous hematomas by the use of triamcinolone acetonide in allergic patients.] Prensa Med Argent 1971;58(16):826–9.

174. Roy A, Leblanc C, Paquette L, Ghezzo H, Cote J, Cartier A, Malo JL. Skin bruising in asthmatic subjects treated with high doses of inhaled steroids: frequency and association with adrenal function. Eur Respir J 1996;9(2):226–31.

175. Korting HC, Unholzer A, Schafer-Korting M, Tausch I, Gassmueller J, Nietsch KH. Different skin thinning potential of equipotent medium-strength glucocorticoids. Skin Pharmacol Appl Skin Physiol 2002;15(2):85–91.

176. Sener O, Caliskaner Z, Yazicioglu K, Karaayvaz M, Ozanguc N. Nonpigmenting solitary fixed drug eruption after skin testing and intra-articular injection of

triamcinolone acetonide. Ann Allergy Asthma Immunol 2001;86(3):335–6.

177. Weber F, Barbaud A, Reichert-Penetrat S, Danchin A, Schmutz JL. Unusual clinical presentation in a case of contact dermatitis due to corticosteroids diagnosed by ROAT. Contact Dermatitis 2001;44(2):105–6.

178. Sener O, Caliskaner Z, Yazicioglu K, Karaayvaz M, Ozanguc N. Nonpigmenting solitary fixed drug eruption after skin testing and intra-articular injection of triamcinolone acetonide. Ann Allergy Asthma Immunol 2001;86(3):335–6.

179. Dooms-Goossens A, Andersen KE, Brandao FM, Bruynzeel D, Burrows D, Camarasa J, Ducombs G, Frosch P, Hannuksela M, Lachapelle JM, Lahti A, Menne T, Wahlberg JE, Wilkinson JD. Corticosteroid contact allergy: an EECDRG multicentre study. Contact Dermatitis 1996;35(1):40–4.

180. Quintiliani R. Hypersensitivity and adverse reactions associated with the use of newer intranasal corticosteroids for allergic rhinitis. Curr Ther Res Clin Exp 1996;57:478–88.

181. Isaksson M, Bruze M, Goossens A, Lepoittevin JP. Patch testing with budesonide in serial dilutions. the significance of dose, occlusion time and reading time. Contact Dermatitis 1999;40(1):24–31.

182. Murata T, Tanaka M, Dekio I, Tanikawa A, Nishikawa T. Allergic contact dermatitis due to clobetasone butyrate. Contact Dermatitis 2000;42(5):305.

183. O'Hagan AH, Corbett JR. Contact allergy to budesonide in a breath-actuated inhaler. Contact Dermatitis 1999;41(1):53.

184. Lew DB, Higgins GC, Skinner RB, Snider MD, Myers LK. Adverse reaction to prednisone in a patient with systemic lupus erythematosus. Pediatr Dermatol 1999;16(2):146–50.

185. Garcia-Bravo B, Repiso JB, Camacho F. Systemic contact dermatitis due to deflazacort. Contact Dermatitis 2000;43(6):359–60.

186. Stingeni L, Caraffini S, Assalve D, Lapomarda V, Lisi P. Erythema-multiforme-like contact dermatitis from budesonide. Contact Dermatitis 1996;34(2):154–5.

187. Roujeau JC, Kelly JP, Naldi L, Rzany B, Stern RS, Anderson T, Auquier A, Bastuji-Garin S, Correia O, Locati F, Mockenhaupt M, Paoletti C, Shapiro S, Shear N, Schüpf E, Kaufman DW. Medication use and the risk of Stevens–Johnson syndrome or toxic epidermal necrolysis. N Engl J Med 1995;333(24):1600–7.

188. Ingber A, Trattner A, David M. Hypersensitivity to an oestrogen–progesterone preparation and possible relationship to autoimmune progesterone dermatitis and corticosteroid hypersensitivity. J Dermatol Treat 1999;10:139–40.

189. Picado C, Luengo M. Corticosteroid-induced bone loss. Prevention and management. Drug Saf 1996;15(5):347–59.

190. Wichers M, Springer W, Bidlingmaier F, Klingmuller D. The influence of hydrocortisone substitution on the quality of life and parameters of bone metabolism in patients with secondary hypocortisolism. Clin Endocrinol (Oxf) 1999;50(6):759–65.

191. Langhammer A, Norjavaara E, de Verdier MG, Johnsen R, Bjermer L. Use of inhaled corticosteroids and bone mineral density in a population based study: the Nord–Trondelag Health Study (the HUNT Study). Pharmacoepidemiol Drug Saf 2004;13:569–79.

192. Suissa S, Baltzan M, Kremer R, Ernst P. Inhaled and nasal corticosteroid use and the risk of fracture. Am J Respir Crit Care Med 2004;169:83–8.

193. Steinbuch M, Youket TE, Cohen S. Oral glucocorticoid use is associated with an increased risk of fracture. Osteoporos Int 2004;15:323–8.

194. Krogsgaard MR, Thamsborg G, Lund B. Changes in bone mass during low dose corticosteroid treatment in patients with polymyalgia rheumatica. a double blind, prospective comparison between prednisolone and deflazacort. Ann Rheum Dis 1996;55(2):143–6.

195. Goldstein MF, Fallon JJ Jr, Harning R. Chronic glucocorticoid therapy-induced osteoporosis in patients with obstructive lung disease. Chest 1999;116(6):1733–49.

196. Yosipovitch G, Hoon TS, Leok GC. Suggested rationale for prevention and treatment of glucocorticoid-induced bone loss in dermatologic patients. Arch Dermatol 2001;137(4):477–81.

197. Selby PL, Halsey JP, Adams KR, Klimiuk P, Knight SM, Pal B, Stewart IM, Swinson DR. Corticosteroids do not alter the threshold for vertebral fracture. J Bone Miner Res 2000;15(5):952–6.

198. Zelissen PM, Croughs RJ, van Rijk PP, Raymakers JA. Effect of glucocorticoid replacement therapy on bone mineral density in patients with Addison disease. Ann Intern Med 1994;120(3):207–10.

199. Valero MA, Leon M, Ruiz Valdepenas MP, Larrodera L, Lopez MB, Papapietro K, Jara A, Hawkins F. Bone density and turnover in Addison's disease: effect of glucocorticoid treatment. Bone Miner 1994;26(1):9–17.

200. Heiner JP, Joyce MJ, Carter JR, Makley JT. Atraumatic posterior pelvic ring fractures simulating metastatic disease in patients with metabolic bone disease. Orthopedics 1994;17(3):285–9.

201. Baltzan MA, Suissa S, Bauer DC, Cummings SR. Hip fractures attributable to corticosteroid use. Study Osteoporotic Fractures Group. Lancet 1999;353(9161):1327.

202. McKenzie R, Reynolds JC, O'Fallon A, Dale J, Deloria M, Blackwelder W, Straus SE. Decreased bone mineral density during low dose glucocorticoid administration in a randomized, placebo controlled trial. J Rheumatol 2000;27(9):2222–6.

203. Walsh LJ, Wong CA, Oborne J, Cooper S, Lewis SA, Pringle M, Hubbard R, Tattersfield AE. Adverse effects of oral corticosteroids in relation to dose in patients with lung disease. Thorax 2001;56(4):279–84.

204. van Everdingen AA, Jacobs JW, Siewertsz Van Reesema DR, Bijlsma JW. Low-dose prednisone therapy for patients with early active rheumatoid arthritis: clinical efficacy, disease-modifying properties, and side effects: a randomized, double-blind, placebo-controlled clinical trial. Ann Intern Med 2002;136(1):1–12.

205. Townsend HB, Saag KG. Glucocorticoid use in rheumatoid arthritis: benefits, mechanisms, and risks. Clin Exp Rheumatol 2004;22(Suppl 35):S77–82.

206. Gluck O, Colice G. Recognizing and treating glucocorticoid-induced osteoporosis in patients with pulmonary diseases. Chest 2004;125:1859–76.

207. Lukert BP, Adams JS. Calcium and phosphorus homeostasis in man. Effect Corticosteroids. Arch Intern Med 1976;136(11):1249–53.

208. Hahn TJ. Corticosteroid-induced osteopenia. Arch Intern Med 1978;138(Spec No):882–5.

209. Chesney RW, Mazess RB, Hamstra AJ, DeLuca HF, O'Reagan S. Reduction of serum-1, 25-dihydroxyvitamin-D3 in children receiving glucocorticoids. Lancet 1978;2(8100):1123–5.

210. Eastell R. Management of corticosteroid-induced osteoporosis. UK Consensus Group Meeting on Osteoporosis. J Intern Med 1995;237(5):439–47.

211. Goans RE, Weiss GH, Abrams SA, Perez MD, Yergey AL. Calcium tracer kinetics show decreased irreversible flow to bone in glucocorticoid treated patients. Calcif Tissue Int 1995;56(6):533–5.

212. Sasaki N, Kusano E, Ando Y, Yano K, Tsuda E, Asano Y. Glucocorticoid decreases circulating osteoprotegerin (OPG): possible mechanism for glucocorticoid induced osteoporosis. Nephrol Dial Transplant 2001;16(3):479–82.

213. Lespessailles E, Siroux V, Poupon S, Andriambelosoa N, Pothuaud L, Harba R, Benhamou CL. Long-term corticosteroid therapy induces mild changes in trabecular bone texture. J Bone Miner Res 2000;15(4):747–53.

214. Mateo L, Nolla JM, Bonnin MR, Navarro MA, Roig-Escofet D. Sex hormone status and bone mineral density in men with rheumatoid arthritis. J Rheumatol 1995;22(8):1455–60.

215. Vestergaard P, Olsen ML, Paaske Johnsen S, Rejnmark L, Sorensen HT, Mosekilde L. Corticosteroid use and risk of hip fracture: a population-based case-control study in Denmark. J Intern Med 2003;254:486–93.

216. Ton FN, Gunawardene SC, Lee H, Neer RM. J. Effects of low-dose prednisone on bone metabolism. Bone Miner Res 2005;20(3):464–70.

217. Harris M, Hauser S, Nguyen TV, Kelly PJ, Rodda C, Morton J, Freezer N, Strauss BJ, Eisman JA, Walker JL. Bone mineral density in prepubertal asthmatics receiving corticosteroid treatment. J Paediatr Child Health 2001;37(1):67–71.

218. Lane NE. An update on glucocorticoid-induced osteoporosis. Rheum Dis Clin North Am 2001;27(1):235–53.

219. Henderson NK, Sambrook PN, Kelly PJ, Macdonald P, Keogh AM, Spratt P, Eisman JA. Bone mineral loss and recovery after cardiac transplantation. Lancet 1995;346(8979):905.

220. Garton MJ, Reid DM. Bone mineral density of the hip and of the anteroposterior and lateral dimensions of the spine in men with rheumatoid arthritis. Effects of low-dose corticosteroids. Arthritis Rheum 1993;36(2):222–8.

221. Saito JK, Davis JW, Wasnich RD, Ross PD. Users of low-dose glucocorticoids have increased bone loss rates: a longitudinal study. Calcif Tissue Int 1995;57(2):115–9.

222. Buckley LM, Leib ES, Cartularo KS, Vacek PM, Cooper SM. Effects of low dose corticosteroids on the bone mineral density of patients with rheumatoid arthritis. J Rheumatol 1995;22(6):1055–9.

223. Fryer JP, Granger DK, Leventhal JR, Gillingham K, Najarian JS, Matas AJ. Steroid-related complications in the cyclosporine era. Clin Transplant 1994;8(3 Part 1):224–9.

224. Wolpaw T, Deal CL, Fleming-Brooks S, Bartucci MR, Schulak JA, Hricik DE. Factors influencing vertebral bone density after renal transplantation. Transplantation 1994;58(11):1186–9.

225. Yun YS, Kim BJ, Hong SP, Lee TW, Lim CG, Kim MJ. Changes of bone metabolism indices in patients receiving immunosuppressive therapy including low doses of steroids after renal transplantation. Transplant Proc 1996;28(3):1561–4.

226. Saisu T, Sakamoto K, Yamada K, Kashiwabara H, Yokoyama T, Iida S, Harada Y, Ikenoue S, Sakamoto M, Moriya H. High incidence of osteonecrosis of femoral head in patients receiving more than 2 g of intravenous methylprednisolone after renal transplantation Transplant Proc 1996;28(3):1559–60.

227. Naganathan V, Jones G, Nash P, Nicholson G, Eisman J, Sambrook PN. Vertebral fracture risk with long-term corticosteroid therapy: prevalence and relation to age, bone density, and corticosteroid use. Arch Intern Med 2000;160(19):2917–22.

228. Schoon EJ, Bollani S, Mills PR, Israeli E, Felsenberg D, Ljunghall S, Persson T, Haptén-White L, Graffner H, Bianchi Porro G, Vatn M, Stockbrügger RW; Matrix Study Group. Bone mineral density in relation to efficacy and side effects of budesonide and prednisolone in Crohn's disease. Clin Gastroenterol Hepatol 2005;3(2):113–21.

229. Tattersfield AE, Town GI, Johnell O, Picado C, Aubier M, Braillon P, Karlstrom R. Bone mineral density in subjects with mild asthma randomized to treatment with inhaled corticosteroids or non-corticosteroid treatment for two years. Thorax 2001;56(4):272–8.

230. Sambrook PN. Corticosteroid osteoporosis: practical implications of recent trials. J Bone Miner Res 2000;15(9):1645–9.

231. American College of Rheumatology Task Force on Osteoporosis Guidelines. Recommendations for the prevention and treatment of glucocorticoid-induced osteoporosis. Arthritis Rheum 1996;39(11):1791–801.

232. Bone and Tooth Society. National Osteoporosis Society, Royal College of Physicians. Glucocorticoid-induced Osteoporosis. Guidelines for Prevention and TreatmentLondon: Royal College of Physicians;. 2002.

233. Hart SR, Green B. Osteoporosis prophylaxis during corticosteroid treatment: failure to prescribe. Postgrad Med J 2002;78(918):242–3.

234. Gudbjornsson B, Juliusson UI, Gudjonsson FV. Prevalence of long term steroid treatment and the frequency of decision making to prevent steroid induced osteoporosis in daily clinical practice. Ann Rheum Dis 2002;61(1):32–6.

235. Cino M, Greenberg GR. Bone mineral density in Crohn's disease: a longitudinal study of budesonide, prednisone, and nonsteroid therapy. Am J Gastroenterol 2002;97(4):915–21.

236. Schwid SR, Goodman AD, Puzas JE, McDermott MP, Mattson DH. Sporadic corticosteroid pulses and osteoporosis in multiple sclerosis. Arch Neurol 1996;53(8):753–7.

237. Lukert BP, Johnson BE, Robinson RG. Estrogen and progesterone replacement therapy reduces glucocorticoid-induced bone loss. J Bone Miner Res 1992;7(9):1063–9.

238. Buckley LM, Leib ES, Cartularo KS, Vacek PM, Cooper SM. Calcium and vitamin D3 supplementation prevents bone loss in the spine secondary to low-dose corticosteroids in patients with rheumatoid arthritis. A randomized, double-blind, placebo-controlled trial. Ann Intern Med 1996;125(12):961–8.

239. Adachi JD, Bensen WG, Bianchi F, Cividino A, Pillersdorf S, Sebaldt RJ, Tugwell P, Gordon M, Steele M, Webber C, Goldsmith CH. Vitamin D and calcium in the prevention of corticosteroid induced osteoporosis: a 3 year followup. J Rheumatol 1996;23(6):995–1000.

240. Talalaj M, Gradowska L, Marcinowska-Suchowierska E, Durlik M, Gaciong Z, Lao M. Efficiency of preventive treatment of glucocorticoid-induced osteoporosis with 25-hydroxyvitamin D3 and calcium in kidney transplant patients. Transplant Proc 1996;28(6):3485–7.

241. Warady BD, Lindsley CB, Robinson FG, Lukert BP. Effects of nutritional supplementation on bone mineral

status of children with rheumatic diseases receiving corticosteroid therapy. J Rheumatol 1994;21(3):530–5.

242. Richy F, Ethgen O, Bruyere O, Reginster JY. Efficacy of alphacalcidol and calcitriol in primary and corticosteroid-induced osteoporosis: a meta-analysis of their effects on bone mineral density and fracture rate. Osteoporos Int 2004;15:301–10.

243. Ringe JD, Dorst A, Faber H, Schacht E, Rahlfs VW. Superiority of alfacalcidol over plain vitamin D in the treatment of glucocorticoid-induced osteoporosis. Rheumatol Int 2004;24:63–70.

244. Luengo M, Pons F, Martinez de Osaba MJ, Picado C. Prevention of further bone mass loss by nasal calcitonin in patients on long term glucocorticoid therapy for asthma: a two year follow up study. Thorax 1994;49(11):1099–102.

245. Healey JH, Paget SA, Williams-Russo P, Szatrowski TP, Schneider R, Spiera H, Mitnick H, Ales K, Schwartzberg P. A randomized controlled trial of salmon calcitonin to prevent bone loss in corticosteroid-treated temporal arteritis and polymyalgia rheumatica. Calcif Tissue Int 1996;58(2):73–80.

246. Adachi JD, Bensen WG, Bell MJ, Bianchi FA, Cividino AA, Craig GL, Sturtridge WC, Sebaldt RJ, Steele M, Gordon M, Themeles E, Tugwell P, Roberts R, Gent M. Salmon calcitonin nasal spray in the prevention of corticosteroid-induced osteoporosis. Br J Rheumatol 1997;36(2):255–9.

247. Mulder H, Struys A. Intermittent cyclical etidronate in the prevention of corticosteroid-induced bone loss. Br J Rheumatol 1994;33(4):348–50.

248. Diamond T, McGuigan L, Barbagallo S, Bryant C. Cyclical etidronate plus ergocalciferol prevents glucocorticoid-induced bone loss in postmenopausal women. Am J Med 1995;98(5):459–63.

249. Roux C, Oriente P, Laan R, Hughes RA, Ittner J, Goemaere S, Di Munno O, Pouilles JM, Horlait S, Cortet B. Randomized trial of effect of cyclical etidronate in the prevention of corticosteroid-induced bone loss. Ciblos Study Group. J Clin Endocrinol Metab 1998;83(4):1128–33.

250. Pitt P, Li F, Todd P, Webber D, Pack S, Moniz C. A double blind placebo controlled study to determine the effects of intermittent cyclical etidronate on bone mineral density in patients on long-term oral corticosteroid treatment. Thorax 1998;53(5):351–6.

251. Sato S, Ohosone Y, Suwa A, Yasuoka H, Nojima T, Fujii T, Kuwana M, Nakamura K, Mimori T, Hirakata M. Effect of intermittent cyclical etidronate therapy on corticosteroid induced osteoporosis in Japanese patients with connective tissue disease: 3 year follow up. J Rheumatol 2003;30: 2673–9.

252. Frediani B, Falsetti P, Baldi F, Acciai C, Filippou G, Marcolongo R. Effects of 4-year treatment with once-weekly clodronate on prevention of corticosteroid-induced bone loss and fractures in patients with arthritis: evaluation with dual-energy X-ray absorptiometry and quantitative ultrasound. Bone 2003;33:575–81.

253. Ringe JD, Dorst A, Faber H, Ibach K, Preuss J. Three-monthly ibandronate bolus injection offers favorable tolerability and sustained efficacy advantage over two years in established corticosteroid-induced osteoporosis. Rheumatol (Oxf) 2003;42:743–9.

254. Ringe JD, Dorst A, Faber H, Ibach K, Sorenson F. Intermittent intravenous ibandronate injections reduce vertebral fracture risk in corticosteroid-induced

osteoporosis: results from a long-term comparative study. Osteoporos Int 2003;14:801–7.

255. Boutsen Y, Jamart J, Esselinckx W, Stoffel M, Devogelaer JP. Primary prevention of glucocorticoid-induced osteoporosis with intermittent intravenous pamidronate: a randomized trial. Calcif Tissue Int 1997;61(4):266–71.

256. Wallach S, Cohen S, Reid DM, Hughes RA, Hosking DJ, Laan RF, Doherty SM, Maricic M, Rosen C, Brown J, Barton I, Chines AA. Effects of risedronate treatment on bone density and vertebral fracture in patients on corticosteroid therapy. Calcif Tissue Int 2000;67(4):277–85.

257. Reid DM, Hughes RA, Laan RF, Sacco-Gibson NA, Wenderoth DH, Adami S, Eusebio RA, Devogelaer JP. Efficacy and safety of daily risedronate in the treatment of corticosteroid-induced osteoporosis in men and women: a randomized trial. European Corticosteroid-Induced Osteoporosis Treatment Study. J Bone Miner Res 2000;15(6):1006–13.

258. Adachi JD, Saag KG, Delmas PD, Liberman UA, Emkey RD, Seeman E, Lane NE, Kaufman JM, Poubelle PE, Hawkins F, Correa-Rotter R, Menkes CJ, Rodriguez-Portales JA, Schnitzer TJ, Block JA, Wing J, McIlwain HH, Westhovens R, Brown J, Melo-Gomes JA, Gruber BL, Yanover MJ, Leite MO, Siminoski KG, Nevitt MC, Sharp JT, Malice MP, Dumortier T, Czachur M, Carofano W, Daifotis A. Two-year effects of alendronate on bone mineral density and vertebral fracture in patients receiving glucocorticoids: a randomized, double-blind, placebo-controlled extension trial. Arthritis Rheum 2001;44(1):202–11.

259. Emkey R, Delmas PD, Goemaere S, Liberman UA, Poubelle PE, Daifotis AG, Verbruggen N, Lombardi A, Czachur M. Changes in bone mineral density following discontinuation or continuation of alendronate therapy in glucocorticoid-treated patients: a retrospective, observational study. Arthritis Rheum 2003;48:1102–8.

260. Rehman Q, Lang TF, Arnaud CD, Modin GW, Lane NE. Daily treatment with parathyroid hormone is associated with an increase in vertebral cross-sectional area in post-menopausal women with glucocorticoid-induced osteoporosis. Osteoporos Int 2003;14:77–81.

261. Rizzoli R, Chevalley T, Slosman DO, Bonjour JP. Sodium monofluorophosphate increases vertebral bone mineral density in patients with corticosteroid-induced osteoporosis. Osteoporos Int 1995;5(1):39–46.

262. Giustina A, Bussi AR, Jacobello C, Wehrenberg WB. Effects of recombinant human growth hormone (GH) on bone and intermediary metabolism in patients receiving chronic glucocorticoid treatment with suppressed endogenous GH response to GH-releasing hormone. J Clin Endocrinol Metab 1995;80(1):122–9.

263. Yonemura K, Kimura M, Miyaji T, Hishida A. Short-term effect of vitamin K administration on prednisolone-induced loss of bone mineral density in patients with chronic glomerulonephritis. Calcif Tissue Int 2000;66(2):123–8.

264. Westeel FP, Mazouz H, Ezaitouni F, Hottelart C, Ivan C, Fardellone P, Brazier M, El Esper I, Petit J, Achard JM, Pruna A, Fournier A. Cyclosporine bone remodeling effect prevents steroid osteopenia after kidney transplantation. Kidney Int 2000;58(4):1788–96.

265. Abe H, Sako H, Okino K, Nakane Y, Kodama M, Park KI, Inoue H, Kim CJ, Tomoyoshi T. Clinical study of aseptic

necrosis of bone after renal transplantation. Transplant Proc 1994;26(4):1987.

266. Alarcon GS, Mikhail I, Jaffe KA, Bradley LA, Bailey WC. Hip osteonecrosis secondary to the administration of corticosteroids for feigned bronchial asthma. The clinical spectrum of the factitious disorders. Arthritis Rheum 1994;37(1):139–41.

267. Lausten GS, Lemser T, Jensen PK, Egfjord M. Necrosis of the femoral head after kidney transplantation. Clin Transplant 1998;12(6):572–4.

268. Bauer M, Thabault P, Estok D, Chrinstiansen C, Platt R. Low-dose corticosteroids and avascular necrosis of the hip and knee. Pharmacoepidemiol Drug Saf 2000;9:187–91.

269. McKee MD, Waddell JP, Kudo PA, Schemitsch EH, Richards RR. Osteonecrosis of the femoral head in men following short-course corticosteroid therapy: a report of 15 cases. CMAJ 2001;164(2):205–6.

270. Virik K, Karapetis C, Droufakou S, Harper P. Avascular necrosis of bone: the hidden risk of glucocorticoids used as antiemetics in cancer chemotherapy. Int J Clin Pract 2001;55(5):344–5.

271. Gibson JN, Poyser NL, Morrison WL, Scrimgeour CM, Rennie MJ. Muscle protein synthesis in patients with rheumatoid arthritis: effect of chronic corticosteroid therapy on prostaglandin F2 alpha availability. Eur J Clin Invest 1991;21(4):406–12.

272. Ekstrand A, Schalin-Jantti C, Lofman M, Parkkonen M, Widen E, Franssila-Kallunki A, Saloranta C, Koivisto V, Groop L. The effect of (steroid) immunosuppression on skeletal muscle glycogen metabolism in patients after kidney transplantation. Transplantation 1996;61(6):889–93.

273. Anonymous. Corticosteroid myopathy. Lancet 1970;2:1118.

274. Janssens S, Decramer M. Corticosteroid-induced myopathy and the respiratory muscles. Report of two cases. Chest 1989;95(5):1160–2.

275. Weiner P, Azgad Y, Weiner M. The effect of corticosteroids on inspiratory muscle performance in humans. Chest 1993;104(6):1788–91.

276. Halpern AA, Horowitz BG, Nagel DA. Tendon ruptures associated with corticosteroid therapy. West J Med 1977;127(5):378–82.

277. Pai VS. Rupture of the plantar fascia. J Foot Ankle Surg 1996;35(1):39–40.

278. Bunch TJ, Welsh GA, Miller DV, Swaroop VS. Acute spontaneous Achilles tendon rupture in a patient with giant cell arteritis. Ann Clin Lab Sci 2003;33:326–8.

279. Schiavon F. Transient joint effusion: a forgotten side effect of high dose corticosteroid treatment. Ann Rheum Dis 2003;62:491–2.

280. Motson RW, Glass DN, Smith DA, Daly JR. The effect of short- and long-term corticosteroid treatment on sleep-associated growth hormone secretion. Clin Endocrinol (Oxf) 1978;8(4):315–26.

281. Allen DB, Mullen M, Mullen B. A meta-analysis of the effect of oral and inhaled corticosteroids on growth. J Allergy Clin Immunol 1994;93(6):967–76.

282. Doull IJ, Freezer NJ, Holgate ST. Growth of prepubertal children with mild asthma treated with inhaled beclomethasone dipropionate. Am J Respir Crit Care Med 1995;151(6):1715–9.

283. Whitaker K, Webb J, Barnes J, Barnes ND. Effect of fluticasone on growth in children with asthma. Lancet 1996;348(9019):63–4.

284. Todd G, Dunlop K, McNaboe J, Ryan MF, Carson D, Shields MD. Growth and adrenal suppression in asthmatic children treated with high-dose fluticasone propionate. Lancet 1996;348(9019):27–9.

285. Travis LB, Chesney R, McEnery P, Moel D, Pennisi A, Potter D, Talwalkar YB, Wolff E. Growth and glucocorticoids in children with kidney disease. Kidney Int 1978;14(4):365–8.

286. Rivkees SA, Danon M, Herrin J. Prednisone dose limitation of growth hormone treatment of steroid-induced growth failure. J Pediatr 1994;125(2):322–5.

287. Lai HC, FitzSimmons SC, Allen DB, Kosorok MR, Rosenstein BJ, Campbell PW, Farrell PM. Risk of persistent growth impairment after alternate-day prednisone treatment in children with cystic fibrosis. N Engl J Med 2000;342(12):851–9.

288. Diczfalusy E, Landgren BM. Hormonal changes in the menstrual cycle. In: Diczfalusy D, editor. Regulation of Human Fertility. Copenhagen: Scriptor, 1977:21.

289. Cunningham GR, Goldzieher JW, de la Pena A, Oliver M. The mechanism of ovulation inhibition by triamcinolone acetonide. J Clin Endocrinol Metab 1978;46(1):8–14.

290. Mens JM, Niço de Wolf A, Berkhout BJ, Stam HJ. Disturbance of the menstrual pattern after local injection with triamcinolone acetonide. Ann Rheum Dis 1998;57(11):700.

291. Lopez-Serrano MC, Moreno-Ancillo A, Contreras J, Ortega N, Cabanas R, Barranco P, Munoz-Pereira M. Two cases of specific adverse reactions to systemic corticosteroids. J Invest Allergol Clin Immunol 1996;6(5):324–7.

292. Ventura MT, Muratore L, Calogiuri GF, Dagnello M, Buquicchio R, Nicoletti A, Altamura M, Sabba C, Tursi A. Allergic and pseudoallergic reactions induced by glucocorticoids: a review. Curr Pharm Des 2003;9:1956–64.

293. Moreno-Ancillo A, Martin-Munoz F, Martin-Barroso JA, Diaz-Pena JM, Ojeda JA. Anaphylaxis to 6-alpha-methylprednisolone in an eight-year-old child. J Allergy Clin Immunol 1996;97(5):1169–71.

294. van den Berg JS, van Eikema Hommes OR, Wuis EW, Stapel S, van der Valk PG. Anaphylactoid reaction to intravenous methylprednisolone in a patient with multiple sclerosis. J Neurol Neurosurg Psychiatry 1997;63(6):813–4.

295. Figueredo E, Cuesta-Herranz JI, De Las Heras M, Lluch-Bernal M, Umpierrez A, Sastre J. Anaphylaxis to dexamethasone. Allergy 1997;52(8):877.

296. Mace S, Vadas P, Pruzanski W. Anaphylactic shock induced by intraarticular injection of methylprednisolone acetate. J Rheumatol 1997;24(6):1191–4.

297. Hayhurst M, Braude A, Benatar SR. Anaphylactic-like reaction to hydrocortisone. S Afr Med J 1978;53(7):259–60.

298. Srinivasan V, Lanham PR. Acute laryngeal obstruction – reaction to intravenous hydrocortisone? Eur J Anaesthesiol 1997;14(3):342.

299. Vaghjimal A, Rosenstreich D, Hudes G. Fever, rash and worsening of asthma in response to intravenous hydrocortisone. Int J Clin Pract 1999;53(7):567–8.

300. Clear D. Anaphylactoid reaction to methyl prednisolone developing after starting treatment with interferon beta-1b. J Neurol Neurosurg Psychiatry 1999;66(5):690.

301. Schonwald S. Methylprednisolone anaphylaxis. Am J Emerg Med 1999;17(6):583–5.

302. Vanpee D, Gillet JB. Allergic reaction to intravenous methylprednisolone in a woman with asthma. Ann Emerg Med 1998;32(6):754.

303. Polosa R, Prosperini G, Pintaldi L, Rey JP, Colombrita R. Anaphylaxis after prednisone. Allergy 1998;53(3):330–1.

304. Karsh J, Yang WH. An anaphylactic reaction to intra-articular triamcinolone: a case report and review of the literature. Ann Allergy Asthma Immunol 2003;90:254–8.

305. Yawalkar N, Hari Y, Helbing A, von Greyerz S, Kappeler A, Baathen LR, Pichler WJ. Elevated serum levels of interleukins 5, 6, and 10 in a patient with drug-induced exanthem caused by systemic corticosteroids. J Am Acad Dermatol 1998;39(5 Part 1):790–3.

306. Ventura MT, Calogiuri GF, Matino MG, Dagnello M, Buquicchio R, Foti C, Di Corato R. Alternative glucocorticoids for use in cases of adverse reaction to systemic glucocorticoids: a study on 10 patients. Br J Dematol 2003;148:139–41.

307. Heeringa M, Zweers P, de Man RA, de Groot H. Drug Points: Anaphylactic-like reaction associated with oral budesonide. BMJ 2000;321(7266):927.

308. Gomez CM, Higuero NC, Moral de Gregorio A, Quiles MH, Nunez Aceves AB, Lara MJ, Sanchez CS. Urticaria–angioedema by deflazacort. Allergy 2002;57(4):370–1.

309. Monk BE, Skipper D. Allergy to topical corticosteroids in inflammatory bowel disease. Gut 2003;52:597.

310. Staunton H, Stafford F, Leader M, O'Riordain D. Deterioration of giant cell arteritis with corticosteroid therapy. Arch Neurol 2000;57(4):581–4.

311. Schols AM, Wesseling G, Kester AD, de Vries G, Mostert R, Slangen J, Wouters EF. Dose dependent increased mortality risk in COPD patients treated with oral glucocorticoids. Eur Respir J 2001;17(3):337–42.

312. Klaustermeyer WB, Gianos ME, Kurohara ML, Dao HT, Heiner DC. IgG subclass deficiency associated with corticosteroids in obstructive lung disease. Chest 1992;102(4):1137–42.

313. Robinson MJ, Campbell F, Powell P, Sims D, Thornton C. Antibody response to accelerated Hib immunisation in preterm infants receiving dexamethasone for chronic lung disease. Arch Dis Child Fetal Neonatal Ed 1999;80(1):F69–71.

314. Sprung CL, Caralis PV, Marcial EH, Pierce M, Gelbard MA, Long WM, Duncan RC, Tendler MD, Karpf M. The effects of high-dose corticosteroids in patients with septic shock. A prospective, controlled study. N Engl J Med 1984;311(18):1137–43.

315. Mostafa BE. Fluticasone propionate is associated with severe infection after endoscopic polypectomy. Arch Otolaryngol Head Neck Surg 1996;122(7):729–31.

316. Demitsu T, Kosuge A, Yamada T, Usui K, Katayama H, Yaoita H. Acute generalized exanthematous pustulosis induced by dexamethasone injection. Dermatology 1996;193(1):56–8.

317. Aberra FN, Lewis JD, Hass D, Rombeau JL, Osborne B, Lichtenstein GR. Corticosteroids and immunomodulators: postoperative infectious complication risk in inflammatory bowel disease patients. Gastroenterology 2003;125:320–7.

318. Hedderwick SA, Bonilla HF, Bradley SF, Kauffman CA. Opportunistic infections in patients with temporal arteritis treated with corticosteroids. J Am Geriatr Soc 1997;45(3):334–7.

319. Korula J. Tuberculous peritonitis complicating corticosteroid therapy for acute alcoholic hepatitis. Dig Dis Sci 1995;40(10):2119–20.

320. Kim HA, Yoo CD, Baek HJ, Lee EB, Ahn C, Han JS, Kim S, Lee JS, Choe KW, Song YW. *Mycobacterium tuberculosis* infection in a corticosteroid-treated rheumatic disease patient population. Clin Exp Rheumatol 1998;16(1):9–13.

321. di Girolamo C, Pappone N, Melillo E, Rengo C, Giuliano F, Melillo G. Cavitary lung tuberculosis in a rheumatoid arthritis patient treated with low-dose methotrexate and steroid pulse therapy. Br J Rheumatol 1998;37(10):1136–7.

322. Martos A, Podzamczer D, Martinez-Lacasa J, Rufi G, Santin M, Gudiol F. Steroids do not enhance the risk of developing tuberculosis or other AIDS-related diseases in HIV-infected patients treated for *Pneumocystis carinii* pneumonia. AIDS 1995;9(9):1037–41.

323. Bridges MJ, McGarry F. Two cases of *Mycobacterium avium* septic arthritis. Ann Rheum Dis 2002;61(2):186–7.

324. Fernandez-Aviles F, Batlle M, Ribera JM, Matas L, Sabria M, Feliu E. *Legionella* sp pneumonia in patients with hematologic diseases. A study of 10 episodes from a series of 67 cases of pneumonia. Haematologica 1999;84(5):474–5.

325. Rice P, Simmons K, Carr R, Banatvala J. Near fatal chickenpox during prednisolone treatment. BMJ 1994;309(6961):1069–70.

326. Choong K, Zwaigenbaum L, Onyett H. Severe varicella after low dose inhaled corticosteroids. Pediatr Infect Dis J 1995;14(9):809–11.

327. Burnett I. Severe chickenpox during treatment with corticosteroids. Immunoglobulin should be given if steroid dosage was > or = 0.5 mg/kg/day in preceding three months BMJ 1995;310(6975):327Erratum in BMJ 1995;310(6978):534.

328. Doherty MJ, Baxter AB, Longstreth WT Jr. Herpes simplex virus encephalitis complicating myxedema coma treated with corticosteroids. Neurology 2001;56(8):1114–5.

329. Pingleton WW, Bone RC, Kerby GR, Ruth WE. Oropharyngeal candidiasis in patients treated with triamcinolone acetonide aerosol. J Allergy Clin Immunol 1977;60(4):254–8.

330. Nenoff P, Horn LC, Mierzwa M, Leonhardt R, Weidenbach H, Lehmann I, Haustein UF. Peracute disseminated fatal *Aspergillus fumigatus* sepsis as a complication of corticoid-treated systemic lupus erythematosus. Mycoses 1995;38(11–12):467–71.

331. Wald A, Leisenring W, van Burik JA, Bowden RA. Epidemiology of *Aspergillus infections* in a large cohort of patients undergoing bone marrow transplantation. J Infect Dis 1997;175(6):1459–66.

332. Machet L, Jan V, Machet MC, Vaillant L, Lorette G. Cutaneous alternariosis: role of corticosteroid-induced cutaneous fragility. Dermatology 1996;193(4):342–4.

333. Fucci JC, Nightengale ML. Primary esophageal histoplasmosis. Am J Gastroenterol 1997;92(3):530–1.

334. Monlun E, de Blay F, Berton C, Gasser B, Jaeger A, Pauli G. Invasive pulmonary aspergillosis with cerebromeningeal involvement after short-term intravenous corticosteroid therapy in a patient with asthma. Respir Med 1997;91(7):435–7.

335. Shetty D, Giri N, Gonzalez CE, Pizzo PA, Walsh TJ. Invasive aspergillosis in human immunodeficiency virus-infected children. Pediatr Infect Dis J 1997;16(2):216–21.

336. Fernandez JM, Sanchez E, Polo FJ, Saez L. Infección pulmonar por *Aspergillus fumigatus* y *Nocardia asteroides* como complicación del tratamiento con glucocorticoides. Med Clin (Barc) 2000;114:358.

337. Carrascosa Porras M, Herreras Martinez R, Corral Mones J, Ares Ares M, Zabaleta Murguiondo M, Ruchel R. Fatal *Aspergillus* myocarditis following short-term corticosteroid therapy for chronic obstructive pulmonary disease. Scand J Infect Dis 2002;34(3):224–7.

338. Vogeser M, Haas A, Ruckdeschel G, von Scheidt W. Steroid-induced invasive aspergillosis with thyroid gland abscess and positive blood cultures. Eur J Clin Microbiol Infect Dis 1998;17(3):215–6.

339. Mavinkurve-Groothuis AMC, Bokkerink JPM, Verweij PE, Veerman AJP, Hoogerbrugge PM. Cryptococcal meningitis in a child with acute lymphoblastic leukemia. Pediatr Infect Dis J 2003;22:576.

340. Bower CP, Oxley JD, Campbell CK, Archer CB. Cutaneous *Scedosporium apiospermum* infection in an immunocompromised patient. J Clin Pathol 1999;52(11):846–8.

341. Ioannidou DJ, Stefanidou MP, Maraki SG, Panayiotides JG, Tosca AD. Cutaneous alternariosis in a patient with idiopathic pulmonary fibrosis. Int J Dermatol 2000;39(4):293–5.

342. Pera A, Byun A, Gribar S, Schwartz R, Kumar D, Parimi P. Dexamethasone therapy and *Candida* sepsis in neonates less than 1250 grams. J Perinatol 2002;22(3):204–8.

343. Fukuda T, Boeckh M, Carter RA, Sandmaier BM, Maris MB, Maloney DG, Martin PJ, Storb RF, Marr KA. Risks and outcomes of invasive fungal infections in recipients of allogenic hematopoietic stem cell transplants after nonmyeloablative conditioning. Blood 2003;102:827–33.

344. Buchheidt D, Hummel M, Diehl S, Hehlmann R. Fatal cerebral involvement in systemic aspergillosis: a rare complication of steroid-treated autoimmune bicytopenia. Eur J Haematol 2004;72:375–6.

345. Sen P, Gil C, Estrellas B, Middleton JR. Corticosteroid-induced asthma: a manifestation of limited hyperinfection syndrome due to *Strongyloides stercoralis*. South Med J 1995;88(9):923–7.

346. Mariotta S, Pallone G, Li Bianchi E, Gilardi G, Bisetti A. *Strongyloides stercoralis* hyperinfection in a case of idiopathic pulmonary fibrosis. Panminerva Med 1996;38(1):45–7.

347. Leung VK, Liew CT, Sung JJ. Fatal strongyloidiasis in a patient with ulcerative colitis after corticosteroid therapy. Am J Gastroenterol 1997;92(8):1383–4.

348. Schipperijn AJM. Flare-up of toxoplasmosis due to corticosteroid therapy in pulmonary sarcoidosis. Ned T Geneesk 1970;114:1710.

349. Cohen SN. Toxoplasmosis in patients receiving immunosuppressive therapy. JAMA 1970;211(4):657–60.

350. Sy ML, Chin TW, Nussbaum E. *Pneumocystis carinii* pneumonia associated with inhaled corticosteroids in an immunocompetent child with asthma. J Pediatr 1995;127(6):1000–2.

351. Bachelez H, Schremmer B, Cadranel J, Mouly F, Sarfati C, Agbalika F, Schlemmer B, Mayaud CM, Dubertret L. Fulminant *Pneumocystis carinii* pneumonia in 4 patients with dermatomyositis. Arch Intern Med 1997;157(13):1501–3.

352. Kanani SR, Knight R. Amoebic dysentery precipitated by corticosteroids. BMJ 1969;3(662):114.

353. Stark AR, Carlo WA, Tyson JE, Papile LA, Wright LL, Shankaran S, Donovan EF, Oh W, Bauer CR, Saha S, Poole WK, Stoll BJ. National Institute of Child Health and Human Development Neonatal Research Network. Adverse effects of early dexamethasone in extremely-low-birth-weight infants. National Institute of Child Health and Human Development Neonatal Research Network. N Engl J Med 2001;344(2):95–101.

354. Lucas A, Coll J, Salinas I, Sanmarti A. Hipertensión intracraneal benigna tras suspensión de corticoterapia en una paciente previaments intervenida por enfermedad de Cushing. [Benign intracranial hypertension following the suspension of corticotherapy in a female patient previously operated on for Cushing's disease.] Med Clin (Barc) 1991;97(12):473.

355. Richards D, Aronson J. The Oxford Handbook of Practical Drug TherapyOxford: Oxford University Press;. 2004.

356. Morgan J, Lacey JH. Anorexia nervosa and steroid withdrawal. Int J Eat Disord 1996;19(2):213–5.

357. Silverman RA, Newman AJ, LeVine MJ, Kaplan B. Poststeroid panniculitis: a case report. Pediatr Dermatol 1988;5(2):92–3.

358. Le Gall C, Pham S, Vignes S, Garcia G, Nunes H, Fichet D, Simonneau G, Duroux P, Humbert M. Inhaled corticosteroids and Churg–Strauss syndrome: a report of five cases. Eur Respir J 2000;15(5):978–81.

359. Hodgkinson DJ, Williams TJ. Endometrial carcinoma associated with azathioprine and cortisone therapy. A case report. Gynecol Oncol 1977;5(3):308–12.

360. Erban SB, Sokas RK. Kaposi's sarcoma in an elderly man with Wegener's granulomatosis treated with cyclophosphamide and corticosteroids. Arch Intern Med 1988;148(5):1201–3.

361. Thiagarajan CM, Divakar D, Thomas SJ. Malignancies in renal transplant recipients. Transplant Proc 1998;30(7):3154–5.

362. Gill PS, Loureiro C, Bernstein-Singer M, Rarick MU, Sattler F, Levine AM. Clinical effect of glucocorticoids on Kaposi sarcoma related to the acquired immunodeficiency syndrome (AIDS). Ann Intern Med 1989;110(11):937–40.

363. Tebbe B, Mayer-da-Silva A, Garbe C, von Keyserlingk HJ, Orfanos CE. Genetically determined coincidence of Kaposi sarcoma and psoriasis in an HIV-negative patient after prednisolone treatment. Spontaneous regression 8 months after discontinuing therapy. Int J Dermatol 1991;30(2):114–20.

364. Vincent T, Moss K, Colaco B, Venables PJ. Kaposi's sarcoma in two patients following low-dose corticosteroid treatment for rheumatological disease. Rheumatology (Oxford) 2000;39(11):1294–6.

365. Sorensen HT, Mellemkjaer L, Friis S, Olsen JH. Use of systemic corticosteroids and risk of esophageal cancer. Epidemiology 2002;13(2):240–1.

366. Chin S-OS, Brodsky NL, Bhandari V. Antenatal steroid use is associated with increased gastroesophageal reflux in neonates. Am J Perinatol 2003;20:205–13.

367. Jobe AH, Soll RF. Choice and dose of corticosteroid for antenatal treatments. Am J Obstet Gynecol 2004;190: 878–81.

368. Committee on Fetus and Newborn. Postnatal corticosteroids to treat or prevent chronic lung disease in preterm infants. Pediatrics 2002;109(2):330–8.

369. Canadian Paediatric Society and American Academy of Pediatrics. Postnatal corticosteroids to treat or prevent chronic lung disease in preterm infants. Pediatr Child Health 2002;7:20–8.

370. Banks BA, Macones G, Cnaan A, Merrill JD, Ballard PL, Ballard RA. North American TRH Study Group. Multiple courses of antenatal corticosteroids are associated with early severe lung disease in preterm neonates. J Perinatol 2002;22(2):101–7.

371. Elliott JP, Radin TG. The effect of corticosteroid administration on uterine activity and preterm labor in high-order multiple gestations. Obstet Gynecol 1995;85(2):250–4.

372. Ogunyemi D. A comparison of the effectiveness of single-dose vs multi-dose antenatal corticosteroids in pre-term neonates. Obstet Gynaecol 2005;25(8):756–60.

373. Haas DM, McCullough W, Olsen CH, Shiau DT, Richard J, Fry EA, McNamara MF. Neonatal outcomes with different betamethasone dosing regimens: a comparison. J Reprod Med 2005;50(12):915–22.

374. Schmitz T, Goffinet F, Barrande G, Cabrol D. Maternal hypercorticism from serial courses of betamethasone. Obstet Gynecol 1999;94(5 Part 2):849.

375. Helal KJ, Gordon MC, Lightner CR, Barth WH Jr. Adrenal suppression induced by betamethasone in women at risk for premature delivery. Obstet Gynecol 2000;96(2):287–90.

376. Spencer C, Smith P, Rafla N, Weatherell R. Corticosteroids in pregnancy and osteonecrosis of the femoral head. Obstet Gynecol 1999;94(5 Part 2):848.

377. Vermillion ST, Soper DE, Chasedunn-Roark J. Neonatal sepsis after betamethasone administration to patients with preterm premature rupture of membranes. Am J Obstet Gynecol 1999;181(2):320–7.

378. Rotmensch S, Vishne TH, Celentano C, Dan M, Ben-Rafael Z. Maternal infectious morbidity following multiple courses of betamethasone. J Infect 1999;39(1):49–54.

379. Vermillion ST, Soper DE, Newman RB. Neonatal sepsis and death after multiple courses of antenatal betamethasone therapy. Am J Obstet Gynecol 2000;183(4):810–4.

380. Abbasi S, Hirsch D, Davis J, Tolosa J, Stouffer N, Debbs R, Gerdes JS. Effect of single versus multiple courses of antenatal corticosteroids on maternal and neonatal outcome. Am J Obstet Gynecol 2000;182(5):1243–9.

381. Yang SH, Choi SJ, Roh CR, Kim JH. Multiple courses of antenatal corticosteroid therapy in patients with preterm premature rupture of membranes. J Perinat Med 2004;32:42–8.

382. Stockli A, Keller M. Kongenitales adrenogenitales Syndrom und Schwangerschaft. [Congenital adrenogenital syndrome and pregnancy.] Schweiz Med Wochenschr 1969;99(4):126–8.

383. Beique LC, Friesen MH, Park LY, Diaz-Citrin O, Koren G, Einarson TR. Major malformations associated with corticosteroid exposure during the first trimester: a meta-analysis. Can J Hosp Pharm 1998;51:83.

384. Moran P, Taylor R. Management of hyperemesis gravidarum: the importance of weight loss as a criterion for steroid therapy. QJM 2002;95(3):153–8.

385. Markert UR, Klemm A, Flossmann E, Werner W, Sperschneider H, Funfstuck R. Renal transplantation in early pregnancy with acute graft rejection and development of a hydatidiform mole. Clin Nephrol 1998;49(6):391–2.

386. Park-Wyllie L, Mazzotta P, Pastuszak A, Moretti ME, Beique L, Hunnisett L, Friesen MH, Jacobson S, Kasapinovic S, Chang D, Diav-Citrin O, Chitayat D, Nulman I, Einarson TR, Koren G. Birth defects after maternal exposure to corticosteroids: prospective cohort study and meta-analysis of epidemiological studies. Teratology 2000;62(6):385–92.

387. Harding JE, Pang J, Knight DB, Liggins GC. Do antenatal corticosteroids help in the setting of preterm rupture of membranes? Am J Obstet Gynecol 2001;184(2):131–9.

388. Bloom SL, Sheffield JS, McIntire DD, Leveno KJ. Antenatal dexamethasone and decreased birth weight. Obstet Gynecol 2001;97(4):485–90.

389. Rotmensch S, Liberati M, Celentano C, Efrat Z, Bar-Hava I, Kovo M, Golan A, Moravski G, Ben-Rafael Z. The effect of betamethasone on fetal biophysical activities and Doppler velocimetry of umbilical and middle cerebral arteries. Acta Obstet Gynecol Scand 1999;78(9):768–73.

390. Warrell DW, Taylor R. Outcome for the foetus of mothers receiving prednisolone during pregnancy. Lancet 1968;1(7534):117–8.

391. Crowley PA. Antenatal corticosteroid therapy: a meta-analysis of the randomized trials, 1972–94. Am J Obstet Gynecol 1995;173(1):322–35.

392. Kairalla AB. Hypothalamic–pituitary–adrenal axis function in premature neonates after extensive prenatal treatment with betamethasone: a case history. Am J Perinatol 1992;9(5–6):428–30.

393. Ohrlander S, Gennser G, Nilsson KO, Eneroth P. ACTH test to neonates after administration of corticosteroids during gestation. Obstet Gynecol 1977;49(6):691–4.

394. Ohlsson A, Calvert SA, Hosking M, Shennan AT. Randomized controlled trial of dexamethasone treatment in very-low-birth-weight infants with ventilator-dependent chronic lung disease. Acta Paediatr 1992;81(10):751–6.

395. Brownlee KG, Ng PC, Henderson MJ, Smith M, Green JH, Dear PR. Catabolic effect of dexamethasone in the preterm baby. Arch Dis Child 1992;67(1 Spec No):1–4.

396. O'Neil EA, Chwals WJ, O'Shea MD, Turner CS. Dexamethasone treatment during ventilator dependency: possible life threatening gastrointestinal complications. Arch Dis Child 1992;67(1 Spec No):10–1.

397. Dalziel SR, Walker NK, Parag V, Mantell C, Rea HH, Rodgers A, Harding JE. Cardiovascular risk factors after antenatal exposure to betamethasone: 30-year follow-up of a randomised controlled trial. Lancet 2005;365(9474):1856–62.

398. Spinillo A, Viazzo F, Colleoni R, Chiara A, Maria Cerbo R, Fazzi E. Two-year infant neurodevelopmental outcome after single or multiple antenatal courses of corticosteroids to prevent complications of prematurity. Am J Obstet Gynecol 2004;191:217–24.

399. French NP, Hagan R, Evans SF, Mullan A, Newnham JP. Repeated antenatal corticosteroids: effects on cerebral palsy and childhood behavior. Am J Obstet Gynecol 2004; 190: 588–95.

400. Dalziel SR, Lim VK, Lambert A, McCarthy D, Parag V, Rodgers A, Harding JE. Antenatal exposure to betamethasone: psychological functioning and health related quality of life 31 years after inclusion in randomised controlled trial. BMJ 2005;331(7518):665.

401. Cho S, Beharry KD, Valencia AM, Guajardo L, Nageotte MP, Modanlou HD. Maternal and feto-placental prostanoid responses to a single course of antenatal betamethasone. Prostaglandins Other Lipid Mediat 2005;78(1-4):139–59.

402. Harding JE, Pang J, Knight DB, Liggins GC. Do antenatal corticosteroids help in the setting of preterm rupture of membranes? Am J Obstet Gynecol 2001;184(2):131–9.

403. Rotmensch S, Celentano C, Liberati M, Sadan O, Glezerman M. The effect of antenatal steroid administration on the fetal response to vibroacoustic stimulation. Acta Obstet Gynecol Scand 1999;78(10):847–51.

404. Tornatore KM, Biocevich DM, Reed K, Tousley K, Singh JP, Venuto RC. Methylprednisolone pharmacokinetics, cortisol response, and adverse effects in black and white renal transplant recipients. Transplantation 1995;59(5):729–36.

405. Skoner DP. Balancing safety and efficacy in pediatric asthma management. Pediatrics 2002;109(Suppl 2):381–92.

406. Allen DB. Safety of inhaled corticosteroids in children. Pediatr Pulmonol 2002;33(3):208–20.

407. Thebaud B, Lacaze-Masmonteil T, Watterberg K. Postnatal glucocorticoids in very preterm infants: "the good, the bad, and the ugly"? Pediatrics 2001;107(2):413–5.

408. Akerkar GA, Peppercorn MA, Hamel MB, Parker RA. Corticosteroid-associated complications in elderly Crohn's disease patients. Am J Gastroenterol 1997;92(3):461–4.

409. Powell LW, Axelsen E. Corticosteroids in liver disease: studies on the biological conversion of prednisone to prednisolone and plasma protein binding. Gut 1972;13(9):690–6.

410. Davis M, Williams R, Chakraborty J, English J, Marks V, Ideo G, Tempini S. Prednisone or prednisolone for the treatment of chronic active hepatitis? A comparison of plasma availability. Br J Clin Pharmacol 1978;5(6):501–5.

411. Frey BM, Frey FJ. Clinical pharmacokinetics of prednisone and prednisolone. Clin Pharmacokinet 1990;19(2):126–46.

412. Harris RZ, Tsunoda SM, Mroczkowski P, Wong H, Benet LZ. The effects of menopause and hormone replacement therapies on prednisolone and erythromycin pharmacokinetics. Clin Pharmacol Ther 1996;59(4):429–35.

413. Lewis GP, Jusko WJ, Graves L, Burke CW. Prednisone side-effects and serum-protein levels. A collaborative study. Lancet 1971;2(7728):778–80.

414. Zonana-Nacach A, Barr SG, Magder LS, Petri M. Damage in systemic lupus erythematosus and its association with corticosteroids. Arthritis Rheum 2000;43(8):1801–8.

415. Andus T, Gross V, Caesar I, Schulz HJ, Lochs H, Strohm WD, Gierend M, Weber A, Ewe K, Scholmerich J; German/Austrian Budesonide Study Group. Replacement of conventional glucocorticoids by oral pH-modified release budesonide in active and inactive Crohn's disease: results of an open, prospective, multicenter trial. Dig Dis Sci 2003;48:373–8.

416. Keane FM, Munn SE, du Vivier AW, Taylor NF, Higgins EM. Analysis of Chinese herbal creams prescribed for dermatological conditions. BMJ 1999;318(7183):563–4.

417. Reinberg AE. Chronopharmacology of corticosteroids and ACTH. In: Lammer B, editor. Chronopharmacology. Cellular and Biochemical Interactions. New York and Basel: Marcel Dekker Inc, 1989:137–67.

418. Kimura Y, Fieldston E, Devries-Vandervlugt B, Li S, Imundo L. High dose, alternate day corticosteroids for systemic onset juvenile rheumatoid arthritis. J Rheumatol 2000;27(8):2018–24.

419. Kaiser BA, Polinsky MS, Palmer JA, Dunn S, Mochon M, Flynn JT, Baluarte HJ. Growth after conversion to alternate-day corticosteroids in children with renal transplants: a single-center study. Pediatr Nephrol 1994;8(3):320–5.

420. Blair GP, Light RW. Treatment of chronic obstructive pulmonary disease with corticosteroids. Comparison of daily vs alternate-day therapy. Chest 1984;86(4):524–8.

421. Oshitani N, Kamata N, Ooiso R, Kawashima D, Inagawa M, Sogawa M, Iimuro M, Jinno Y, Watanabe K, Higuchi K, Matsumoto T, Arakawa T. Outpatient treatment of moderately severe active ulcerative colitis with pulsed steroid therapy and conventional steroid therapy. Dig Dis Sci 2003;4:1002–5.

422. Ermis B, Ors R, Tastekin A, Ozkan B. Cushing's syndrome secondary to topical corticosteroids abuse. Clin Endocrinol 2003;58:795–7.

423. Gilbertson EO, Spellman MC, Piacquadio DJ, Mulford MI. Super potent topical corticosteroid use associated with adrenal suppression: clinical considerations. J Am Acad Dermatol 1998;38(2 Part 2):318–21.

424. Marcos C, Allegue F, Luna I, Gonzalez R. An unusual case of allergic contact dermatitis from corticosteroids. Contact Dermatitis 1999;41(4):237–8.

425. Corazza M, Virgili A. Allergic contact dermatitis from 6alpha-methylprednisolone aceponate and budesonide. Contact Dermatitis 1998;38(6):356–7.

426. Oh C, Lee J. Contact allergy to various ingredients of topical medicaments. Contact Dermatitis 2003;49:49–50.

427. Karadimas P, Kapetanios A, Bouzas EA. Central serous chorioretinopathy after local application of glucocorticoids for skin disorders. Arch Ophthalmol 2004; 122: 784–6.

428. Mygind H, Thulstrup AM, Pedersen L, Larsen H. Risk of intrauterine growth retardation, malformations and other birth outcomes in children after topical use of corticosteroid in pregnancy. Acta Obstet Gynecol Scand 2002;81(3):234–9.

429. Whitcup SM, Ferris FL 3rd. New corticosteroids for the treatment of ocular inflammation. Am J Ophthalmol 1999;127(5):597–9.

430. Aggarwal RK, Potamitis T, Chong NH, Guarro M, Shah P, Kheterpal S. Extensive visual loss with topical facial steroids. Eye 1993;7(5):664–6.

431. Baratz KH, Hattenhauer MG. Indiscriminate use of corticosteroid-containing eyedrops. Mayo Clin Proc 1999;74(4):362–6.

432. Chua JK, Fan DS, Leung AT, Lam DS. Accelerated ocular hypertensive response after application of corticosteroid ointment to a child's eyelid. Mayo Clin Proc 2000;75(5):539.

433. Ozerdem U, Levi L, Cheng L, Song MK, Scher C, Freeman WR. Systemic toxicity of topical and periocular corticosteroid therapy in an 11-year-old male with posterior uveitis. Am J Ophthalmol 2000;130(2):240–1.

434. Mehle ME. Are nasal steroids safe? Curr Opin Otolaryngol Head Neck Surg 2003;11:201–5.

435. Salib RJ, Howarth PH. Safety and tolerability profiles of intranasal antihistamines and intranasal corticosteroids in the treatment of allergic rhinitis. Drug Saf 2003;26:863–93.

436. Priftis K, Everard ML, Milner AD. Unexpected side-effects of inhaled steroids: a case report. Eur J Pediatr 1991;150(6):448–9.

437. Stead RJ, Cooke NJ. Adverse effects of inhaled corticosteroids. BMJ 1989;298(6671):403–4.

438. Whittet HB, Shinkwin C, Freeland AP. Anosmia due to nasal administration of corticosteroid. BMJ 1991;303(6803):651.

439. Bond DW, Charlton CP, Gregson RM. Benign intracranial hypertension secondary to nasal fluticasone propionate. BMJ 2001;322(7291):897.

440. Ozturk F, Yuceturk AV, Kurt E, Unlu HH, Ilker SS. Evaluation of intraocular pressure and cataract formation following the long-term use of nasal corticosteroids. Ear Nose Throat J 1998;77(10):846–51.

441. Cervin A, Andersson M. Intranasal steroids and septum perforation – an overlooked complication? A description of the course of events and a discussion of the causes. Rhinology 1998;36(3):128–32.

442. Nayak AS, Ellis MH, Gross GN, Mendelson LM, Schenkel EJ, Lanier BQ, Simpson B, Mullin ME, Smith JA. The effects of triamcinolone acetonide aqueous nasal spray on adrenocortical function in children with allergic rhinitis. J Allergy Clin Immunol 1998;101(2 Part 1):157–62.

443. Findlay CA, Macdonald JF, Wallace AM, Geddes N, Donaldson MD. Childhood Cushing's syndrome induced by betamethasone nose drops, and repeat prescriptions. BMJ 1998;317(7160):739–40.

444. Hillebrand-Haverkort ME, Prummel MF, ten Veen JH. Ritonavir-induced Cushing's syndrome in a patient treated with nasal fluticasone. AIDS 1999;13(13):1803.

445. Mistlin A, Gibson T. Osteonecrosis of the femoral head resulting from excessive corticosteroid nasal spray use. J Clin Rheumatol 2004;10:45–6.

446. Downs AM, Lear JT, Kennedy CT. Anaphylaxis to intradermal triamcinolone acetonide. Arch Dermatol 1998;134(9):1163–4.

447. Miranda-Romero A, Bajo-del Pozo C, Sanchez-Sambucety P, Martinez-Fernandez M, Garcia-Munoz M. Delayed local allergic reaction to intralesional parametha-sone acetate. Contact Dermatitis 1998;39(1):31–2.

448. Wilkinson HA. Intrathecal Depo-Medrol: a literature review. Clin J Pain 1992;8(1):49–56.

449. DeSio JM, Kahn CH, Warfield CA. Facial flushing and/or generalized erythema after epidural steroid injection. Anesth Analg 1995;80(3):617–9.

450. Plumb VJ, Dismukes WE. Chemical meningitis related to intrathecal corticosteroid therapy. South Med J 1977;70(10):1241–3.

451. Dumont D, Hariz H, Meynieu P, Salama J, Dreyfus P, Boissier MC. Abducens palsy after an intrathecal gluco-corticoid injection. Evidence for a role of intracranial hypotension. Rev Rhum Engl Ed 1998;65(5):352–4.

452. Spaccarelli KC. Lumbar and caudal epidural corticosteroid injections. Mayo Clin Proc 1996;71(2):169–78.

453. Chen YC, Gajraj NM, Clavo A, Joshi GP. Posterior sub-capsular cataract formation associated with multiple lumbar epidural corticosteroid injections. Anesth Analg 1998;86(5):1054–5.

454. Siegfried RN. Development of complex regional pain syndrome after a cervical epidural steroid injection. Anesthesiology 1997;86(6):1394–6.

455. Sandberg DI, Lavyne MH. Symptomatic spinal epidural lipomatosis after local epidural corticosteroid injections: case report. Neurosurgery 1999;45(1):162–5.

456. Cooper AB, Sharpe MD. Bacterial meningitis and cauda equina syndrome after epidural steroid injections. Can J Anaesth 1996;43(5 Part 1):471–4.

457. McLain RF, Fry M, Hecht ST. Transient paralysis associated with epidural steroid injection. J Spinal Disord 1997;10(5):441–4.

458. Brocq O, Breuil V, Grisot C, Flory P, Ziegler G, Euller-Ziegler L. Diplopie après infiltrations peridurale et intra-durale de prédnisolone. Deux observations. [Diplopia after peridural and intradural infiltrations of prednisolone. 2 cases.] Presse Méd 1997;26(6):271.

459. Lowell TD, Errico TJ, Eskenazi MS. Use of epidural steroids after discectomy may predispose to infection. Spine 2000;25(4):516–9.

460. Field J, Rathmell JP, Stephenson JH, Katz NP. Neuropathic pain following cervical epidural steroid injection. Anesthesiology 2000;93(3):885–8.

461. Sparling M, Malleson P, Wood B, Petty R. Radiographic followup of joints injected with triamcinolone hexaceto-nide for the management of childhood arthritis. Arthritis Rheum 1990;33(6):821–6.

462. Gutierrez-Urena S, Ramos-Remus C. Persistent hiccups associated with intraarticular corticosteroid injection. J Rheumatol 1999;26(3):760.

463. Daragon A, Vittecoq O, Le Loet X. Visual hallucinations induced by intraarticular injection of steroids. J Rheumatol 1997;24(2):411.

464. Wicki J, Droz M, Cirafici L, Vallotton MB. Acute adrenal crisis in a patient treated with intraarticular steroid therapy. J Rheumatol 2000;27(2):510–1.

465. Valsecchi R, Reseghetti A, Leghissa P, Cologni L, Cortinovis R. Erythema-multiforme-like lesions from triam-cinolone acetonide. Contact Dermatitis 1998;38(6):362–3.

466. Selvi E, De Stefano R, Lorenzini S, Marcolongo R. Arthritis induced by corticosteroid crystals. J Rheumatol 2004;31:622.

467. Jawed S, Allard SA. Osteomyelitis of the humerus following steroid injections for tennis elbow. Rheumatology (Oxford) 2000;39(8):923–4.

468. Montoro J, Valero A, Serra-Baldrich E, Amat P, Lluch M, Malet A. Anaphylaxis to parametasone with tolerance to other corticosteroids. Allergy 2000;55(2):197–8.

469. Caffee HH. Intracapsular injection of triamcinolone for intractable capsule contracture. Plast Reconstr Surg 1994;94(6):824–8.

470. Braverman DL, Lachmann EA, Nagler W. Avascular necrosis of bilateral knees secondary to corticosteroid enemas. Arch Phys Med Rehabil 1998;79(4):449–52.

471. Tsuruoka S, Sugimoto K, Fujimura A. Drug-induced Cushing syndrome in a patient with ulcerative colitis after betamethasone enema: evaluation of plasma drug concentration. Ther Drug Monit 1998;20(4):387–9.

472. Lauerma AI. Occupational contact sensitization to corti-costeroids. Contact Dermatitis 1998;39(6):328–9.

473. Newton RW, Browning MC, Iqbal J, Piercy N, Adamson DG. Adrenocortical suppression in workers manufacturing synthetic glucocorticoids. BMJ 1978;1(6105):73–4.

474. Nixon DW, Shlaer SM. Fulminant lung metastases from cancer of the breast. Med Pediatr Oncol 1981;9(4):381–5.

475. Klygis LM. Dexamethasone-induced perineal irritation in head injury. Am J Emerg Med 1992;10(3):268.

476. Takayanagui OM, Lanchote VL, Marques MP, Bonato PS. Therapy for neurocysticercosis: pharmacokinetic interaction of albendazole sulfoxide with dexamethasone. Ther Drug Monit 1997;19(1):51–5.

477. Ahle GB, Blum AL, Martinek J, Oneta CM, Dorta G. Cushing's syndrome in an 81-year-old patient treated with budesonide and amiodarone. Eur J Gastroenterol Hepatol 2000;12(9):1041–2.

478. Costedoat-Chalumeau N, Amoura Z, Aymard G, Sevin O, Wechsler B, Du Cacoub PLT, Diquet B, Ankri A, Piette JC. Potentiation of vitamin K antagonists by high-dose intravenous methylprednisolone. Ann Intern Med 2000;132(8):631–5.

479. Varis T, Kaukonen KM, Kivisto KT, Neuvonen PJ. Plasma concentrations and effects of oral methylprednisolone are considerably increased by itraconazole. Clin Pharmacol Ther 1998;64(4):363–8.

480. Varis T, Kivisto KT, Backman JT, Neuvonen PJ. Itraconazole decreases the clearance and enhances the effects of intravenously administered methylprednisolone in healthy volunteers. Pharmacol Toxicol 1999;85(1):29–32.

481. Varis T, Kivisto KT, Neuvonen PJ. The effect of itracona-zole on the pharmacokinetics and pharmacodynamics of oral prednisolone. Eur J Clin Pharmacol 2000;56(1):57–60.

482. Varis T, Kivisto KT, Backman JT, Neuvonen PJ. The cytochrome P450 3A4 inhibitor itraconazole markedly increases the plasma concentrations of dexamethasone and enhances its adrenal-suppressant effect. Clin Pharmacol Ther 2000;68(5):487–94.

483. Seidegard J. Reduction of the inhibitory effect of ketoconazole on budesonide pharmacokinetics by separation of their time of administration. Clin Pharmacol Ther 2000;68(1):13–7.

484. McCrea JB, Majumdar AK, Goldberg MR, Iwamoto M, Gargano C, Panebianco DL, Hesney M, Lines CR, Petty KJ, Deutsch PJ, Murphy MG, Gottesdiener KM, Goldwater DR, Blum RA. Effects of the neurokinin1 receptor antagonist aprepitant on the pharmacokinetics of dexamethasone and methylprednisolone. Clin Pharmacol Ther 2003;74:17–24.

485. Varis T, Backman JT, Kivisto KT, Neuvonen PJ. Diltiazem and mibefradil increase the plasma concentrations and greatly enhance the adrenal-suppressant effect of oral methylprednisolone. Clin Pharmacol Ther 2000;67(3):215–21.

486. Quan VA, Saunders BP, Hicks BH, Sladen GE. Cyclosporin treatment for ulcerative colitis complicated by fatal *Pneumocystis carinii* pneumonia. BMJ 1997;314(7077):363–4.

487. Potter JM, McWhinney BC, Sampson L, Hickman PE. Area-under-the-curve monitoring of prednisolone for dose optimization in a stable renal transplant population. Ther Drug Monit 2004;26:408–14.

488. Fost DA, Leung DY, Martin RJ, Brown EE, Szefler SJ, Spahn JD. Inhibition of methylprednisolone elimination in the presence of clarithromycin therapy. J Allergy Clin Immunol 1999;103(6):1031–5.

489. Finkenbine R, Gill HS. Case of mania due to prednisone-clarithromycin interaction. Can J Psychiatry 1997;42(7):778.

490. Belfayol-Pisante L, Guillevin L, Tod M, Fauvelle F. Possible influence of prednisone on the pharmacokinetics of cyclophosphamide in systemic vasculitis. Clin Drug Invest 1999;18:225–31.

491. Manchon ND, Bercoff E, Lemarchand P, Chassagne P, Senant J, Bourreille J. Frequence et gravité des interactions médicamenteuses dans une population agée: étude prospective concernant 639 malades. [Incidence and severity of drug interactions in the elderly. a prospective study of 639 patients.] Rev Med Interne 1989;10(6):521–5.

492. Feuillet L, Guedj E, Laksiri N, Philip E, Habib G, Pelletier J, Cherif AA. Deep vein thrombosis after intravenous immunoglobulins associated with methylprednisolone. Thromb Haemost 2004;92:662–5.

493. Varis T, Kivisto KT, Neuvonen PJ. Grapefruit juice can increase the plasma concentrations of oral methylprednisolone. Eur J Clin Pharmacol 2000;56(6–7):489–93.

494. Geller M. Marked peripheral edema associated with montelukast and prednisone. Ann Intern Med 2000;132(11):924.

495. Seidegard J, Simonsson M, Edsbacker S. Effect of an oral contraceptive on the plasma levels of budesonide and prednisolone and the influence on plasma cortisol. Clin Pharmacol Ther 2000;67(4):373–81.

496. Schönhofer PS. Interaktionen antirheumatisch wirksamer Substanzen. [Interactions of antirheumatic agents.] Internist (Berl) 1979;20(9):433–8.

497. Strayhorn VA, Baciewicz AM, Self TH. Update on rifampin drug interactions III. Arch Intern Med 1997;157(21):2453–8.

498. Dhanoa J, Natu M, Massey S. Worsening of steroid depending bronchial asthma following rifampicin administration. J Assoc Physicians India 1998;46(2):242.

499. Edelman J, Potter JM, Hackett LP. The effect of intra-articular steroids on plasma salicylate concentrations. Br J Clin Pharmacol 1986;21(3):301–7.

500. Nielsen GL, Sorensen HT, Mellemkjoer L, Blot WJ, McLaughlin JK, Tage-Jensen U, Olsen JH. Risk of hospitalization resulting from upper gastrointestinal bleeding among patients taking corticosteroids: a register-based cohort study. Am J Med 2001;111(7):541–5.

501. Garcia Rodriguez LA, Hernandez-Diaz S. The risk of upper gastrointestinal complications associated with non-steroidal anti-inflammatory drugs, glucocorticoids, acetaminophen, and combinations of these agents. Arthritis Res 2001;3(2):98–101.

502. Weil J, Langman MJ, Wainwright P, Lawson DH, Rawlins M, Logan RF, Brown TP, Vessey MP, Murphy M, Colin-Jones DG. Peptic ulcer bleeding: accessory risk factors and interactions with nonsteroidal anti-inflammatory drugs. Gut 2000;46(1):27–31.

503. Patel RS, Shaw SR, McIntyre HE, McGarry GW, Wallace AM. Morning salivary cortisol versus short Synacthen test as a test of adrenal suppression. Ann Clin Biochem 2004;41:408–10.

504. Cepollaro C, Gonnelli S, Rottoli P, Montagnani A, Caffarelli C, Bruni D, Nikiforakis N, Fossi A, Rossi S, Nuti R. Bone ultrasonography in glucocorticoid-induced osteoporosis. Osteoporos Int 2005;16(8):743–8.

505. Brown ES, Chamberlain W, Dhanani N, Paranjpe P, Carmody TJ, Sargeant M. An open-label trial of olanzapine for corticosteroid-induced mood symptoms. J Affect Disord 2004;83(2–3):277–81.

Corticosteroids—glucocorticoids, inhaled

General Information

Treatment with inhaled glucocorticoids reduces the need for oral glucocorticoids in the treatment of severe asthma. The compounds used for inhalation have high local activity and low systemic availability when delivered to the lung. However, if sufficient amounts of glucocorticoids reach the bronchioles be absorbed, systemic effects will occur. Furthermore, a proportion of the dose intended for inhalation is actually swallowed and is absorbed from the gastrointestinal tract. The consequence is that if sufficiently high doses are used, enough drug will be absorbed from the respiratory and gastrointestinal surfaces to result in systemic effects.

Systemic availability of inhaled glucocorticoids can be reduced in two ways. First, by using esters that reduced local absorption; in the case of beclomethasone the dipropionate is used. Secondly, by using glucocorticoids that are extensively metabolized in the liver after absorption from the gut, such as fluticasone and budesonide. These strategies can be combined: fluticasone is given as the ester fluticasone propionate.

When a patient switches from oral or parenteral therapy to inhalation therapy, the systemic effect is reduced, just as if the dose of systemic glucocorticoid is reduced, and precautions should be taken to avoid withdrawal symptoms.

Systemic availability of inhaled glucocorticoids

The systemic availability of an inhaled glucocorticoid represents the additive and complex combination of pulmonary and gastrointestinal drug absorption. Absorption is influenced by many factors, including delivery device, the use of a spacer, the particle size of the inhaled drug, and the absorption and metabolism of the swallowed drug (1).

In healthy volunteers, high doses of both budesonide and fluticasone were readily absorbed after inhalation from a metered-dose aerosol (2). Fluticasone is extensively metabolized by the liver, so measurable concentrations of parent drug in the systemic circulation reflect efficient absorption across the lung. Lower doses of these inhaled glucocorticoids also result in some systemic absorption, reflected in effects on the hypothalamic–pituitary–adrenal axis (3).

The extent of absorption of inhaled glucocorticoids tends to be less in asthmatic subjects than in healthy volunteers. In a study of fluticasone (500 micrograms via a dry powder device) in asthmatic patients with a wide range of severity, there was a highly significant linear correlation between lung function (expressed as percentage predicted FEV_1) and the absolute magnitude of adrenal suppression (4). In 11 patients with moderately severe asthma (mean FEV_1 54% predicted), who took fluticasone 1000 micrograms/day via a metered-dose inhaler with a spacer, the systemic availability of fluticasone was significantly less (10%) than in 13 healthy controls (21%). The plasma fluticasone concentrations (expressed as AUC) correlated positively with gas transfer (5). In contrast, there was no difference in plasma concentrations of fluticasone and budesonide between 15 mild asthmatics (mean FEV_1 81% predicted) and healthy volunteers after inhalation of 1000 micrograms of either drug with single or repeated dosing (6). Taken together, these studies suggest that patients with severe asthma are protected from the systemic adverse effects of high doses of inhaled glucocorticoids, owing to airways obstruction and reduced lung availability. However, as their lung function improves with continued use of the inhaled glucocorticoids, it is likely that the lung availability of inhaled glucocorticoid will increase. This likely outcome is a compelling argument for reducing the dose of inhaled glucocorticoids to a lowest dose that maintains optimal control of asthma and optimal lung function.

Plasma concentrations have been measured in 13 healthy subjects and eight patients with mild asthma using inhaled fluticasone propionate 1000 micrograms bd via Diskus or pressurized metered-dose inhaler and of budesonide 1000 micrograms bd daily via Turbuhaler for 7 days. Twenty-four-hour plasma cortisol concentrations were determined to assess the systemic activity of fluticasone propionate and budesonide. At steady state, the systemic availability of budesonide via Turbuhaler (39%) was significantly higher than that of fluticasone propionate via Diskus (13%) or inhaler (21%). Fluticasone propionate had a larger distribution volume and slower rates of absorption and clearance. Despite a significantly higher pulmonary availability of budesonide via Turbuhaler, plasma cortisol suppression was less than that of fluticasone propionate via inhaler and similar to that of fluticasone propionate via Diskus. There were no differences between healthy subjects and patients with mild asthma in subgroup analyses. However, this study had some limitations as the doses of fluticasone propionate and budesonide were not equipotent, fluticasone being twice as potent as budesonide (7).

The effects of fluticasone 1500 micrograms/day and budesonide 1600 micrograms/day, both by dry powder inhalation, on three systemic markers (urinary concentrations of total cortisol metabolites, morning serum cortisol, and osteocalcin concentrations) have been investigated in 46 healthy and 31 asthmatic subjects (8). Urinary total cortisol metabolite concentrations represented the most sensitive marker of the systemic effects of inhaled glucocorticoids, and were lower in healthy subjects treated with fluticasone than in asthmatic patients, suggesting greater systemic availability of fluticasone in healthy subjects. A similar correlation was not found for budesonide. Fluticasone impaired the hypothalamic–pituitary–adrenal axis more than budesonide, while budesonide significantly lowered serum osteocalcin concentrations, which reflect osteoblastic activity. The authors suggested that different inhaled glucocorticoids have different effects on the hypothalamic–pituitary–adrenal axis and bone metabolism. This study also had its limitations given that the fluticasone and budesonide doses were not equipotent (9).

The safety and efficacy of fluticasone, beclomethasone dipropionate, and budesonide have been compared in a randomized trial in 133 patients with chronic severe asthma who required at least 1750 micrograms/day of beclomethasone/budesonide (10). The patients were randomized to their regular beclomethasone/budesonide or to fluticasone at about half the dose for 6 months. The patients who used fluticasone had a better safety profile, especially with regard to adrenocortical function and bone turnover, while maintaining asthma control. There were significant increases in morning serum cortisol concentrations, the urine cortisol:creatinine ratio, serum osteocalcin, and the serum (deoxy)-pyridinoline:creatinine ratio only with fluticasone, suggesting less suppression of the hypothalamic–pituitary–adrenal axis. The 2:1 potency ratio for clinical efficacy of fluticasone and budesonide/beclomethasone seems to be maintained even at doses of 2000 micrograms/day or higher.

Since many patients with allergic asthma also have rhinitis, they may be taking both inhaled glucocorticoids for their asthma and intranasal formulations for their hay fever. The total systemic availability of glucocorticoids has been studied after the addition of intranasal therapy in patients already taking inhaled glucocorticoids (11) in 12 moderately severe asthmatic subjects (mean FEV_1 84% predicted), who were randomized in a placebo-controlled, two-way, crossover comparison of inhaled fluticasone (880 micrograms bd) plus intranasal fluticasone (200 micrograms od), inhaled triamcinolone (800 micrograms bd) plus intranasal triamcinolone (220 micrograms od), and respective placebos. Both the inhaled glucocorticoids caused significant suppression of adrenocorticoid activity, although the addition of intranasal formulations did not produce further significant suppression. There were more individual subjects with abnormally low cortisol values when intranasal fluticasone was added. These findings suggest that the dose of intranasal glucocorticoids should be taken into account (particularly if used in the long term) when considering the systemic availability of glucocorticoids used in the treatment of asthma and hay fever.

The concept of the L:T ratio in inhalation therapy is a useful one, where L represents the local or lung availability of an inhaled drug and T the total systemic availability. This ratio will be affected by differences in first-pass metabolism. Another important variable that determines the L:T ratio is the inhalation device. The L:T ratio for budesonide is 0.66–0.85, depending on the method of inhalation (12).

Another way of describing the L:T ratio concept is that of "pulmonary targeting." Drug properties that improve pulmonary targeting include slow absorption from the lungs, low oral systemic availability, and rapid systemic clearance.

budesonide = beclomethasone dipropionate > triamcinolone acetonide = flunisolide. Potency differences can be overcome by giving a larger dose of the less potent drug. However, comparisons between glucocorticoids must measure the systemic effects as well as the lung effect of each dose (13).

Inhalation devices

The importance of the inhalation device has been shown in studies of beclomethasone. Pressurized metered-dose inhalers containing chlorofluorocarbons produce relatively large particles that deposit less than 10% of the delivered dose in the lungs, primarily in the large airways, more than 90% being deposited in the oropharynx. A hydrofluoroalkane beclomethasone multidose aerosol (Qvar 3M Pharmaceuticals) delivers a smaller particle size. More than 50% is deposited in the lungs in animal and mechanical models. This has been confirmed using radiolabelled Qvar in patients with asthma and in healthy volunteers. In these subjects, 50–60% of the dose is deposited throughout the airways and about 30% in the oropharynx. The breath-activated Autohaler provides lung deposition equivalent to an optimally used Qvar inhaler, by automatically delivering drug early in the inhalation. Neither of these devices is improved by the addition of a spacer (14).

Both inhaled and swallowed fractions cause significant systemic activity, the degree of which depends on the inhaler device used. In one study, systemic activity was greater using a dry power inhaler (52%) than a pressurized metered-dose inhaler with a large volume spacer

(28%) (15). It was recommended that when high-dose beclomethasone is used, a pressurized metered-dose inhaler with a large volume spacer would help in limiting potential adverse effects.

The systemic availability of inhaled budesonide has been measured in 15 healthy volunteers, using an open crossover design. Each subject was given three treatments, intravenous budesonide 0.5 mg, inhaled budesonide (from a metered-dose inhaler with a Nebuhaler) 1 mg (200 micrograms × 5) plus oral charcoal, and inhaled budesonide 1 mg without oral charcoal. The treatment order was randomized. The mean systemic availability of inhaled budesonide compared with intravenous budesonide was 36% with charcoal and 35% without charcoal, indicating that the absorption of budesonide from the gastrointestinal tract did not contribute to its systemic availability. Pulmonary deposition was 36% with charcoal and 34% without. When the inhaler was used incorrectly, that is, the canister was shaken only before the first of the five inhalations, systemic availability fell by 50%. This shows that the performance of each inhaler is very dependent on proper use (16).

The available studies suggest that fluticasone is more effective than beclomethasone, triamcinolone, or budesonide. However, budesonide delivered by Turbuhaler has equivalent efficacy to fluticasone delivered by metered-dose inhaler or Diskhaler, and is more effective than beclomethasone. When comparative safety is considered, budesonide and triamcinolone delivered by metered-dose inhaler have less systemic activity than fluticasone. Beclomethasone and fluticasone delivered by metered-dose inhaler are equivalent. Budesonide delivered by Turbuhaler has less systemic activity than fluticasone delivered by Diskhaler (17).

The equivalence of inhaled glucocorticoids based on equipotent (cortisol suppression) effects has been studied by the Asthma Clinical Research Network (ACRN). Six different inhaled glucocorticoids and matched placebos (beclomethasone chlorofluorocarbon, budesonide dry powder inhaler, fluticasone dry powder inhaler, fluticasone chlorofluorocarbon metered-dose inhaler, flunisolide chlorofluorocarbon, and triamcinolone chlorofluorocarbon) were compared by measuring their systemic effects (18). Glucocorticoid-naïve patients with asthma ($n = 156$) were enrolled at six centers and a one-week doubling dose design was used for each of the six inhaled glucocorticoids and matched placebos to a total of four doses. The best outcome variable for the reliable assessment of a systemic effect was the 12-hour AUC of the hourly overnight plasma cortisol measurements from 8 p.m. to 8 a.m. Microgram comparisons of the glucocorticoids could only be performed at 10% cortisol suppression, because fluticasone did not cause higher suppression. The following equipotent doses (that is, doses producing equal systemic cortisol suppression) were found: flunisolide 936 micrograms; triamcinolone 787 micrograms; beclomethasone 548 micrograms; fluticasone dry powder: 445 micrograms; budesonide 268 micrograms; and fluticasone metered-dose inhaler 111 micrograms. The ranking of systemic effects was very similar to that found earlier in a large meta-analysis (19).

Dry powder inhaler and pressurized metered-dose inhaler for administration of low-dose budesonide (400 micrograms/day) have been compared (20). Only the dry powder caused suppression of the hypothalamic–pituitary–adrenal axis. As effective inhaled glucocorticoid therapy is expected to cause detectable reductions in the physiological secretion of cortisol (1), low-dose budesonide by pressurized metered-dose inhaler is probably not effective. In another study, budesonide inhalation suspension, developed for nebulization to meet the specific needs of infants and young children, did not cause significant suppression of hypothalamic–pituitary–adrenal axis function (basal plasma cortisol concentrations and corticotropin test) in doses from 0.25 to 1.0 mg (21). However, inhaled fluticasone propionate by pressurized metered-dose inhaler with a spacer in 62 children resulted in abnormal morning cortisol concentrations in 36% (17 using a low dose of 176 micrograms/day; 43 using a high dose, over 880 micrograms/day) (22).

In a randomized, double-blind study, adult asthmatic patients took budesonide 800 micrograms/day over 12 weeks either by Easyhaler ($n = 103$) or by Turbuhaler ($n = 58$) dry powder inhaler. The Easyhaler was equivalent to the Turbuhaler with regard to safety and efficacy, but was more acceptable to the patients (23).

Therapeutic studies

Budesonide

Inhaled budesonide has been studied in the management of moderately severe, acute asthma in children (24). After treatment with nebulized terbutaline, 11 children were randomly allocated to receive one dose of either budesonide 1600 micrograms by Turbuhaler or prednisolone 2 mg/kg. There was no significant difference in the improvement of the pulmonary index score or peak expiratory flow rate. Children treated with budesonide had an earlier clinical response than those given prednisolone. Prednisolone caused a fall in serum cortisol concentration. The authors concluded that children with moderately severe asthma attacks could be effectively treated with a short-term course of inhaled budesonide, starting with a high dose and reducing over the following week.

In 81 patients with acute asthma, mean age 38 years, inhaled budesonide 1600 micrograms bd via Turbuhaler was compared with oral prednisolone (40 mg on day 1, reducing to 5 mg by day 7) in a randomized, double-blind, parallel-group design (25). The mean increase in FEV_1 from baseline to day 7 was 17% with budesonide and 18% with prednisolone. Mean values of morning peak expiratory flow rate increased from day 1 to day 7 by 67 l/second with budesonide and by 57 l/second with prednisolone. There were no statistically significant differences between the groups in either symptoms or the number of doses of rescue medication. The authors concluded that high-dose inhaled budesonide may be a substitute for oral therapy in the treatment of an acute attack of asthma.

The effect of supplementary inhaled budesonide in acute asthma has been evaluated in a randomized, double-blind comparison with standard treatment in 44 children aged 6 months to 18 years with a moderate to severe exacerbation of asthma (26). Prednisone 1 mg/kg orally and nebulized salbutamol (0.15 mg/kg) every 30 minutes for three doses and then every hour for 4 hours were given to all children. In addition, each child was given 2 mg of nebulized budesonide or nebulized isotonic saline. There was a more rapid discharge rate in the budesonide group. There were no adverse effects. The authors concluded that nebulized budesonide may be an effective adjunct to oral prednisone in the management of moderate to severe exacerbations of asthma.

Fluticasone

Inhaled fluticasone 500 micrograms bd from a pressurized metered-dose inhaler for 6 months has been compared with placebo in a randomized, double-blind trial in 280 patients with COPD, aged 50–75 years (27). There was no significant difference in the number of patients who suffered one or more exacerbations. Moderate or severe exacerbations occurred significantly more often with placebo than with fluticasone. Diary-card scores, morning peak expiratory flow rate, clinic FEV_1, FVC, and mid-expiratory flow all improved significantly with fluticasone. Scores for median daily cough and sputum volume were significantly lower with fluticasone than with placebo. At the end of treatment, patients using fluticasone had increased their 6-minute walking distance significantly more than those using placebo. Fluticasone propionate was tolerated, as well as placebo, with few adverse effects and no clinically important effect on mean serum cortisol concentration. The authors suggested that inhaled glucocorticoids may have an important place in the long-term management of patients with COPD.

Local adverse effects

The local adverse effects of inhaled glucocorticoids have been studied in a prospective, cross-sectional, cohort study in 639 asthmatic children using beclomethasone (721 micrograms/day) or budesonide (835 micrograms/day) for at least one month (28). The local adverse effects included cough (40%), thirst (22%), hoarseness (14%), dysphonia (11%), oral candidiasis (11%), perioral dermatitis (2.9%), and tongue hypertrophy (0.1%). A spacer doubled the incidence of coughing.

Potent glucocorticoids in high local doses increase the risk of local infection and even promote atrophy of the bronchial mucosa. The latter effect has not proved clinically important, but there is an increased incidence of oropharyngeal candidiasis. The incidence varies depending on the population studied and the criteria used to make the diagnosis; candidiasis can affect 13–71% of patients, the highest incidence being seen with doses up to 0.8 mg. Candidiasis rarely requires treatment or withdrawal of the drug. Local measures, such as gargling immediately after inhalation of the aerosol, and the use of a large-volume spacer are effective in reducing the incidence of this complication. However, candidiasis can result in dysphonia.

A local myopathy caused by inhaled glucocorticoids can also cause dysphonia. However, patients with asthma have more dysphonia and vocal fold pathology than healthy controls and inhaled glucocorticoids can improve the voice in some patients (SEDA-21, 188).

In some patients, the propellant used in certain aerosols can cause acute bronchoconstriction (SEDA-6, 332).

Organs and Systems

Sensory systems

Cataract

In a population-based cross-sectional study of vision and common eye diseases in 3654 people, 49–97 years of age, inhaled glucocorticoid use was reported by 370 subjects, of whom 164 reported current use and 206 previous use. Subjects who reported using inhaled glucocorticoids had a higher prevalence of nuclear cataracts (OR = 1.5; CI = 1.2, 1.9) and posterior subcapsular cataracts (OR = 1.9; CI = 1.3, 2.8). The highest prevalence (27%) was in patients whose lifetime dose was more than 2000 mg (relative prevalence 5.5) (SEDA-22, 187).

In 3677 patients undergoing cataract extraction over 2 years compared with a matched control group of 21 868 people, the patients were more likely to undergo cataract extraction if they had used inhaled glucocorticoids for more than 3 years (OR = 3.06; CI = 1.53, 6.13). This risk was not significant in patients who used low to medium doses (1000 micrograms/day or less) when the OR was 1.63 (CI = 0.85, 3.13) after 2 years. The OR was higher in patients using average daily doses of beclomethasone dipropionate or budesonide (over 1000 micrograms) (OR = 3.40; CI = 1.49, 7.76) after more than 2 years of treatment (29).

In a nested case-control analysis based on a retrospective, observational, cohort study, 103 289 asthmatic patients using inhaled glucocorticoids were identified from the UK General Practice Database and were compared with 98 527 asthmatic patients with no history of glucocorticoid use (30). There was a slightly increased risk of cataract in those who used inhaled glucocorticoids (RR = 1.3; 95% CI = 1.1, 1.5). The relative risk of cataract was 2.0 in oral glucocorticoid users relative to glucocorticoid non-users (95% CI = 1.5, 2.2). The risk ratio increased with extensive use of inhaled glucocorticoids, but not with moderate use. The association of extensive use with cataract was most pronounced in those aged 70 years and over, and there was no effect in those aged under 40. The increased risk of cataract in patients aged 70 years and over persisted after controlling for cataract risk factors, such as smoking, diabetes mellitus, hypertension, and sex.

In another study, treatment for 2 years with fluticasone propionate (500 micrograms bd) had no significant effect on ophthalmic parameters (glaucoma and posterior subcapsular cataracts) (31). Slit lamp examinations were carried out in 157 asthmatic children treated with inhaled budesonide at a mean daily dose of 504 (range 189–1322) micrograms for 3–6 years (mean 4.4 years). Posterior subcapsular cataract due to budesonide was not detected (32).

Glaucoma

A case-control study compared 9793 patients with open-angle glaucoma or ocular hypertension to 38 325 randomly selected controls (33). There was no association between the use of inhaled or intranasal glucocorticoids and the risk of open-angle glaucoma or ocular hypertension. In patients who were currently using high doses, there was a small but significant increase in risk (OR = 1.44; CI = 1.01, 2.06).

Psychological

High doses of oral glucocorticoids can cause adverse psychiatric effects, including mild euphoria, emotional lability, panic attacks, psychosis, and delirium. There have been sporadic case reports of similar reactions in patients using inhaled glucocorticoids. Of 60 preschool children with a recent diagnosis of asthma taking inhaled budesonide 100–200 micrograms/day, nine had suspected psychological adverse events after 18 months, according to their parents (34). The symptoms reported were irritability, depression, aggressiveness, excitability, and hyperactivity. These adverse events disappeared when the medication was terminated or reduced and recurred when budesonide was restarted at higher doses. Most of the symptoms occurred within 2 days from starting the high dose (200 micrograms 2–4 times a day).

Endocrine

Hypothalamic–pituitary–adrenal axis function provides one of the most sensitive markers of the systemic activity of inhaled glucocorticoids (35), and suppression can be used as a surrogate marker for adverse effects of inhaled glucocorticoids in other tissues.

The different methods of assessing hypothalamic–pituitary–adrenal axis activity in patients using inhaled glucocorticoids have been compared (36). The AUC of serum cortisol concentrations was the most reliable method. There were significant positive correlations between AUC and the 8 a.m. serum and salivary cortisol concentrations. The authors favored the non-invasive method of salivary concentration measurement. However, 24-hour urine collection is not recommended, as it correlated only moderately well. This finding is consistent with the results of other studies. Urinary free-cortisol estimation based on immunoassay after inhaled glucocorticoids may be an unreliable surrogate marker of adrenal suppression, and studies using this method should be interpreted with caution (37).

A review of the literature from 1 January 1966 to 31 July 1998 identified 27 studies in which the effects of inhaled glucocorticoids on adrenal function were measured. A meta-regression of adrenal suppression in these 27 studies showed that adrenal suppression occurred with high doses of inhaled glucocorticoids (above 1500 micrograms/day; 750 micrograms/day for fluticasone propionate). However, there is a considerable degree of interindividual susceptibility. Meta-analysis showed significantly greater potency for dose-related adrenal suppression with fluticasone propionate compared with beclomethasone dipropionate, budesonide, or triamcinolone acetonide. Prednisolone and fluticasone propionate were approximately equivalent in a dose ratio of 10:1 (19).

Beclomethasone

Adrenal function has been assessed by low-dose adreno-corticotropin (ACTH) stimulation in 12 adult asthmatic patients using inhaled beclomethasone (200–900 micrograms/day) before and after switching to inhaled fluticasone (200–600 micrograms/day) (38). Switching from beclomethasone to fluticasone led to a 40% reduction in corticosteroid dosage, improved lung function, and caused a significant rise in the adrenal gland response to ACTH. The reduced risk of adrenal gland suppression associated with fluticasone was most notably due to a lower overall dose of inhaled glucocorticoids.

Budesonide

The effects of budesonide aqueous nasal spray (64 micrograms/day) on adrenal function were studied in a 6-week double-blind, placebo-controlled study in 78 patients with allergic rhinitis aged 2–5 years (39). Adrenal function, evaluated by the mean change in morning plasma cortisol concentration after cosyntropin stimulation, was not suppressed. This dose of budesonide by nasal spray is unlikely to have significant systemic activity.

Ciclesonide

The effect of inhaled ciclesonide on adrenal function has been analysed in 164 asthmatic adults in a double-blind, randomized, placebo-controlled study (40). The patients used ciclesonide 320 micrograms once daily, ciclesonide 320 micrograms twice daily, or fluticasone propionate 440 micrograms twice daily for 12 weeks. Adrenal function was significantly suppressed by fluticasone propionate but not by ciclesonide. Oral candidiasis was reported in 2.4% of patients on ciclesonide versus 22% of patients on fluticasone propionate. Even high daily doses of ciclesonide up to 1280 micrograms did not suppress adrenal function, as measured by 24-hour urinary cortisol excretion (41). This is in accordance with other studies in asthmatic subjects, in which serum or 24-hour urinary cortisol concentrations were unchanged by ciclesonide (42–48).

A pharmacokinetic–pharmacodynamic modelling analysis pooled data from 635 adults and children using ciclesonide in daily doses of 40–2880 micrograms to study the effect of ciclesonide on endogenous cortisol release (49). Using an E_{max} model, less than 1% of all observed desisobutyrylciclesonide concentrations were higher than the EC_{50} for cortisol suppression, indicating negligible changes in cortisol concentrations at therapeutically relevant doses. Systemic availability was estimated to be about 50% in patients with impaired liver function, compared with healthy individuals, but this was unlikely to be clinically significant.

In general, ciclesonide in daily doses of up to 640 micrograms can be considered to be safe with respect to adrenal function. Its long-term safety profile is similarly advantageous, and administration in daily doses up to 1280 micrograms over 52 weeks was not associated with systemic or local adverse effects in patients with persistent asthma (50).

Fluticasone

While suppression of adrenal gland function is associated with daily doses of fluticasone above 750 micrograms, the impact of concurrent moderate-dose fluticasone and oral steroids on adrenal response is unknown. Adult patients using intranasal steroids, low-dose fluticasone (440 micrograms/day), or high-dose fluticasone (880 micrograms/day) underwent a low-dose co-syntropin stimulation test to assess adrenal response before and 2 days after oral prednisone 60 mg/day (51). One of 31 control patients and one of 13 patients using moderate-dose fluticasone had suppressed adrenal gland function on the second day of oral prednisone, which normalized by the second week of treatment. However, 14 of 19 patients using high-dose fluticasone had suppressed adrenal gland function on day 2 with recovery in 10 of the 19 patients within 4 weeks. In conclusion, concurrent standard-dose oral prednisone burst and moderate-dose fluticasone transiently suppress adrenal gland function, while concurrent high-dose fluticasone leads to prolonged impairment. Patients using high-dose fluticasone should be closely monitored.

Six patients with pre-existing HIV-lipodystrophy developed symptomatic Cushing's syndrome when treated with inhaled fluticasone at varying doses for asthma while concurrently taking low-dose ritonavir-boosted protease inhibitor antiretroviral regimens for HIV infection (52). Stimulation studies showed evidence of adrenal suppression in all patients. After withdrawal of inhaled fluticasone, four patients developed symptomatic hypoadrenalism, and three required oral glucocorticoid support for several months. Other complications included evidence of osteoporosis (n = 3), crush fractures (n = 1), and exacerbation of pre-existing type 2 diabetes mellitus (n = 1).

In a randomized, placebo-controlled study, the activity of the hypothalamic–pituitary–adrenal axis was assessed at baseline and after 21 days by determining 22-hour time-integrated serum cortisol concentrations, 24-hour urinary cortisol (corrected for creatinine), and morning salivary cortisol concentrations in 153 patients with mild to moderate asthma, randomly assigned to either inhaled flunisolide (500 or 1000 micrograms bd), inhaled fluticasone (110, 220, 330, or 440 micrograms bd), oral prednisone (7.5 mg/day), or placebo (19). Flunisolide and fluticasone caused dose-dependent suppression of the hypothalamic–pituitary–adrenal axis, and fluticasone was significantly more potent. However, the lowest fluticasone dose (110 micrograms/day) had no effect. These findings are consistent with those of a previous meta-analysis, which showed that fluticasone caused a greater dose-related suppression of the hypothalamic–pituitary–adrenal axis than other inhaled glucocorticoids (53). Fluticasone is more lipophilic than flunisolide and therefore has a larger volume of distribution and a longer half-life (35), but it is not clear how this might be associated with the larger effect described here.

The effect of fluticasone aqueous nasal spray on the hypothalamic–pituitary–adrenal axis has been compared with that of oral prednisone and placebo, using a 6-hour tetracosactide infusion test in a 4-week, randomized, double-blind, placebo-controlled study in 105 adults with allergic rhinitis randomly assigned to receive fluticasone 200 micrograms od, fluticasone 400 micrograms bd, oral prednisone 7.5 mg od, oral prednisone 15 mg od, or placebo (54). Fluticasone 400 micrograms bd and both doses of prednisone caused a significant reduction in the morning plasma cortisol concentration. The two fluticasone treatments produced no significant change in the hypothalamic–pituitary–adrenal axis response to co-syntropin. This contrasted with oral prednisone 7.5 or 15 mg od, which significantly reduced both plasma cortisol concentrations after co-syntropin and 24-hour urinary cortisol excretion.

Mometasone

The effect of increasing doses of mometasone furoate and fluticasone propionate by dry powder inhaler on adrenal function was studied by using overnight urinary cortisol in 21 patients with asthma (55). Patients were randomized in a crossover fashion to receive 2-weekly consecutive doubling doses of either fluticasone propionate (500, 1000, and 2000 micrograms/day) or mometasone furoate (400, 800, and 1600 micrograms/day). Both treatments were associated with significant suppression of adrenal function at high and medium doses.

Adrenal suppression with DPI formulations of mometasone furoate and fluticasone propionate has been studied in 21 asthmatic patients in a randomized crossover study (56). Every 2 weeks the patients used consecutive doubling incremental doses of either mometasone furoate via Twisthaler™ (400, 800, and 1600 micrograms/day) or fluticasone propionate via Accuhaler™ (500, 1000, and 2000 micrograms/day). There was significant suppression of adrenal function with both mometasone furoate and fluticasone propionate at high and medium doses.

Triamcinolone

The effect of inhaled triamcinolone on adrenal response has been assessed in 221 patients with chronic obstructive airway disease in a randomized placebo-controlled trial (57). The patients received either inhaled triamcinolone 1200 micrograms/day or placebo for 3 years. Basal cortisol concentrations were significantly lower with triamcinolone than placebo after 1 and 3 years. Cortisol concentrations were not suppressed at 30 minutes and 60 minutes after co-syntropin injection. The authors concluded that triamcinolone is safe in chronic obstructive airway disease patients at the tested dose with respect to adrenal gland response.

Adrenal suppression by inhaled glucocorticoids in children

Inhaled glucocorticoids are being prescribed more and more in younger children at an earlier stage of their disease and for longer periods; children with severe asthma are also treated with larger doses than licensed. Therefore, considerations of their systemic effects are of importance. Symptomatic adrenal insufficiency has been reported in children after various regimens of inhaled glucocorticoids.

- Four boys 4–8 years old with symptomatic adrenal insufficiency had all used consistent high doses of fluticasone propionate 1000–1500 micrograms/day over extended periods (16 months to 5 years) (58). They presented with acute hypoglycemia secondary to iatrogenic adrenal suppression, with abnormal corticotropin tests, although none had Cushingoid features.
- A 33-year-old man and three children (two girls, one boy, 7–9 years) presented with symptomatic adrenal insufficiency (59). All three children had seizures because of hypoglycemia, and the man had a low blood pressure, nausea, and fatigue. In all cases, corticotropin tests were abnormal, showing adrenal insufficiency. The children had used fluticasone propionate 500–2000 micrograms/day and the man had recently switched from fluticasone propionate 1000–2000 micrograms/day to budesonide dry powder inhaler 800 micrograms/day. Only one of the children had used oral glucocorticoids in the previous year.
- A 21-month-old boy had a hypoglycemia-induced seizure in the setting of adrenal suppression (60). He had been given increasing doses of budesonide up to 2000 micrograms qds and oral glucocorticoids until the age of 15 months.
- A 32-month-old girl developed hypoglycemic seizures (61). She had been given fluticasone propionate 440–880 micrograms/day and up to 5 months before the incident oral glucocorticoids.
- Two girls aged 11 and 16 years, one boy aged 12 years, and one woman aged 54 years developed hypothalamic–pituitary–adrenal axis suppression during treatment with inhaled fluticasone propionate 220–880 micrograms bd for long-term control of asthma; however, two of the patients also took oral prednisone or prednisolone (62). Because of poor growth, an 8-year-old girl's asthma medication was changed from budesonide to fluticasone propionate 250 micrograms/day (63). However, 5 months later she had developed a round face. Her early morning cortisol concentration was less than 30 nmol/l (reference range 140–720) and her growth had been no more than 0.5 cm during the past 5 months. Fluticasone propionate was discontinued. After 1 month, her Cushingoid features had resolved and her fasting morning cortisol concentration was 310 nmol/l.
- A 32-year-old woman's asthma regimen was changed from budesonide to fluticasone propionate 500 micrograms/day and salmeterol (44). Eight months later, she was evaluated because of excessive bodyweight gain; her serum cortisol concentration was 16 nmol/l. Fluticasone propionate was replaced with nedocromil and 1 month later her serum cortisol concentration had normalized.

In addition to these case reports, there has been a survey of symptomatic adrenal suppression associated with inhaled glucocorticoids in the UK (64). Only 24% of the questionnaires were returned (709 responses), and there were 28 cases of symptomatic adrenal suppression reported in children and five in adults (including the 10 cases discussed above). The children presented mostly with hypoglycemia and coma, whereas the adults mainly had lethargy and nausea. No obvious precipitating cause was found in 65% of the cases. In four children, diagnosis was delayed by 3 months to 2 years. All but three patients had been treated with fluticasone propionate alone, but at high daily doses (children 500–2000 micrograms, adults 1000–2000 micrograms). One child had used both fluticasone propionate and budesonide, and one adult and one child used beclomethasone dipropionate.

A series of cases has illustrated the unexpected occurrence of symptomatic adrenal insufficiency in eight asthmatic children using inhaled glucocorticoids (65). The authors concluded that therapeutic doses of inhaled glucocorticoids can provoke paradoxical symptoms of adrenal insufficiency. Very high doses (calculated according to body surface area) may partly explain marked suppression of the hypothalamic–pituitary–adrenal axis. The need to taper inhaled glucocorticoid doses and to recognize the possibility of life-threatening acute adrenal insufficiency is of utmost importance.

In a double-blind, randomized pilot study of the efficacy and adverse effects of inhaled fluticasone in 25 newborn preterm infants who required mechanical ventilation for treatment of respiratory distress syndrome, the infants were randomized to receive inhaled fluticasone 1000 micrograms/day or placebo (66). The hypothalamic–pituitary–adrenal axis was assessed by the response to corticotropin-releasing factor. All basal and post-stimulation plasma corticotropin and serum cortisol concentrations were significantly less with inhaled fluticasone than placebo. Cumulative high-dose inhaled glucocorticoids caused moderately severe suppression of both the pituitary and the adrenal glands. This systemic activity is probably associated with pulmonary vascular absorption that avoids hepatic first-pass metabolism.

Chronic inhalation of beclomethasone dipropionate (up to 1000 micrograms/day) can produce adrenal suppression in some children. This effect is reduced by the attachment of a large volume spacer to the aerosol (SEDA-21, 188). Budesonide inhaled from the Turbuhaler, at doses of 800 or 1600 micrograms/day), did not produce any statistically significant suppression of the hypothalamic–pituitary–adrenal axis compared with placebo. The reduction was significant only after 3200 micrograms/day of budesonide when suppression equivalent to 10 mg/day oral prednisone was seen (67). Fluticasone propionate powder, 500 micrograms bd, given using a Diskhaler, for 104 weeks caused only minimal changes in the hypothalamic–pituitary–adrenal axis (31). Inhaled fluticasone propionate 400 micrograms/day for 8 weeks did not cause adrenal suppression in asthmatic children. In children, the benefit/risk ratio generally decreases at doses above 400 micrograms/day of fluticasone propionate (68). Hypothalamic–pituitary–adrenal axis suppression has been reported with inhaled fluticasone propionate at doses in excess of 1000 micrograms/day (SEDA-21, 188).

Endocrine effects of budesonide have been assessed in 29 asthmatic children aged 6 months to 3 years by measuring fasting plasma cortisol concentrations and performing an ACTH stimulation test in a double-blind, randomized, placebo-controlled study (69). The patients received budesonide either 2 mg followed by a stepwise reduction of 25% every second day or 0.5 mg/day or placebo for 8 days. Neither fasting nor 1-hour post-stimulation plasma cortisol concentrations differed in any group.

Adrenal function was suppressed by high-dose inhaled budesonide (400–900 micrograms/m^2/day) in a dose-related manner in 19 children aged 5–12 years (70). Baseline assessments showed significantly less adrenal suppression with budesonide than beclomethasone at comparable doses. In a subsequent randomized, double-blind, placebo-controlled study in 404 asthmatic children aged 6–18 years, inhaled budesonide at a daily dose of up to 800 micrograms for 12 weeks was associated with adrenal suppression in 12%, but adrenal suppression was not clinically apparent in any of the children (71). In a case-control study, 21% of asthmatic children using therapeutic doses of budesonide had signs and symptoms of adrenal suppression (72), but these were not clinically important. Current data suggest individual idiosyncratic sensitivity of some children to inhaled glucocorticoids: eight cases of symptomatic adrenal insufficiency have been identified with therapeutic doses of budesonide (73).

The long-term effects of budesonide on adrenal function have been assessed in 63 asthmatic children using budesonide 400 micrograms/day, nedocromil 16 mg/day, or placebo over 3 years (74). There were no differences in serum cortisol concentrations after ACTH stimulation between the three treatment groups, regardless of the time after ACTH administration or months of follow-up. Cumulative inhaled glucocorticoid exposure did not affect the serum cortisol response to ACTH or urinary free cortisol excretion at 3 years.

Short-term lower-leg growth rate and adrenal function was assessed in 24 children aged 6–12 years using increasing doses of ciclesonide (40, 80, and 160 micrograms) in a randomized, double-blind, placebo-controlled, crossover study (75). Ciclesonide had no effect on lower-leg growth rate or adrenal function.

In a cross-sectional study, adrenal function was assessed in 50 asthmatic children and adolescents using high-dose inhaled fluticasone, by measuring early morning serum cortisol and tetracosactrin stimulation (76). The mean fluticasone daily dose was 925 micrograms for a mean duration of 2 years. In 36 patients with morning serum cortisol concentration less than 400 nmol/l a tetracosactrin stimulation test showed that six had a pathological response. Biochemical evidence of impaired adrenal gland function was thus found in 12% of the patients, suggesting that high-dose fluticasone can be associated with dose-dependent adrenocortical suppression.

Different inhaled glucocorticoids have been compared for their suppressing effects on the hypothalamic–pituitary–adrenal axis (18). In a large meta-analysis, budesonide or beclomethasone dipropionate in doses of over 1500 micrograms/day was associated with adrenal suppression in adults (19). In children, fluticasone propionate 200 micrograms/day or budesonide 400 micrograms/day caused detectable adrenal gland suppression (77). For interpretation of the different studies, it is very important to distinguish between detectable indicators for systemic drug action (that is, reduced morning cortisol) and true suppression of the hypothalamic–pituitary–adrenal axis, as determined by adrenal function tests (standard-dose or low-dose corticotropin test), which are more predictive of possible systemic adverse effects (1).

The fact that fluticasone propionate is involved in the vast majority of the published cases should be discussed further. The systemic concentration of an inhaled glucocorticoid depends on the absorbed fraction of the drug in the gut and in the lung. Swallowed fluticasone propionate is almost completely metabolized in the liver by CYP3A4 (first-pass effect over 99.9%) before reaching the systemic circulation; however, its metabolic clearance can be altered in patients with low CYP3A4 expression and activity (78). Pulmonary absorbed fluticasone propionate is very potent; because of its pronounced lipophilicity, it binds with higher affinity to glucocorticoid receptors and has a larger distribution volume and a longer half-life than other inhaled glucocorticoids (79). These characteristics give it the potential of accumulating with multiple doses.

Other factors that determine the absorbed fraction of inhaled glucocorticoids include the age of the child, as lung deposition of inhaled drugs increases with age (80). Therefore, the minimum effective dose may fall as the child becomes older. Moreover, it is reasonable to hypothesize that systemic absorption will increase once asthma control is established (81). Furthermore, patient adherence and inhaler technique are two factors that can have a large influence on the amount of glucocorticoid inhaled and absorbed.

However, the most important factor is the dose. The safety and efficacy of fluticasone propionate in children in daily doses of 100–200 micrograms have been demonstrated in many studies (82). The doses in the case reports of symptomatic adrenal suppression have to be considered as being excessively high. These reports reflect excessive dosing of inhaled glucocorticoids, and in some cases a residual effect of previous oral glucocorticoid treatment cannot be excluded. The use of excessive doses is empirical and not supported by the literature. All inhaled glucocorticoids have a flat dose–response curve (83). Extensive clinical experience with inhaled glucocorticoids over the past 20 years has suggested that the risk of adrenal insufficiency with inhaled glucocorticoids alone is very low when recommended doses are used (84). To avoid symptomatic adrenal suppression, the lowest effective dose should always be used. Before automatically increasing the dose in refractory patients, the diagnosis should be reconsidered. Furthermore, a reduction in the dosage of inhaled glucocorticoid can also be achieved with the addition of adjuvant therapies, such as leukotriene receptor antagonists and long-acting β_2-adrenoceptor agonists (85).

Monitoring children using inhaled glucocorticoids has been discussed (1). Children using low to moderate doses of inhaled glucocorticoids (up to 200 micrograms of fluticasone propionate or budesonide) do not require routine hypothalamic–pituitary–adrenal axis measurement. In children using consistently higher doses (up to 400 micrograms of fluticasone propionate or budesonide) or using glucocorticoids by other routes, morning plasma cortisol should be monitored periodically because of the increased risk of clinically significant adrenal suppression. If cortisol concentrations are below 276 μmol/l (100 ng/ml), functional testing of the hypothalamic–pituitary–adrenal axis should be considered.

Metabolism

Impaired diabetic control has been reported with high doses of inhaled glucocorticoids.

- A 67-year-old man with asthma and non-insulin-dependent diabetes mellitus, taking glibenclamide 5 mg/day and metformin 1700 mg/day, had glycated hemoglobin concentrations of 7.0–7.3% (86). For asthma, he used nebulized ipratropium bromide 0.5 mg and salbutamol 5 mg qds. He was given inhaled fluticasone propionate 2000 micrograms/day by metered-dose inhaler through a Volumatic spacer device, with beneficial effect. In the third week he developed persistent glycosuria and the dose of fluticasone was reduced stepwise to 500 micrograms/day. He was then rechallenged by increasing his daily dose of fluticasone from 500 to 1000 micrograms. Within a week he had glycosuria, which again resolved on reduction of the dose of fluticasone. His glycated hemoglobin concentration rose to 7.8% after 1000 micrograms/day and to 8.2% after 2000 micrograms/day.
- Deterioration in glucose control occurred in a 64-year-old man with non-insulin-dependent diabetes mellitus (87). High doses of both fluticasone (2000 micrograms/day) and budesonide (2000 micrograms/day) had produced glycosuria despite treatment with glibenclamide and metformin 1700 mg/day. On reducing the dose of budesonide, there was a commensurate fall in glycosylated hemoglobin and glycosuria. There was no glycosuria at a daily maintenance dose of 800 micrograms and the glycosylated hemoglobin fell from 8.2 to 7.2%.

The association between inhaled glucocorticoids and the risk of diabetes mellitus in elderly people (over 65 years) has been investigated in two Canadian studies. In a nested case-control study of the association between current use of inhaled glucocorticoids and the risk of using antidiabetic drugs among 21 645 subjects the risk of diabetes was not statistically significant (88). Moreover, there was no statistically significant increase in risk among users of high-dose beclomethasone compared with non-users. In a retrospective population-based cohort study using administrative databases, the association between oral and inhaled glucocorticoid use and the onset of diabetes mellitus in the elderly was quantified (89). Users of proton pump inhibitors ($n = 53\ 845$) were the controls. Relative to controls, oral glucocorticoid users ($n = 31\ 864$) were more likely to develop diabetes mellitus, but there was no association between the use of inhaled glucocorticoids ($n = 38\ 441$) and diabetes mellitus. These results suggest that the use of inhaled glucocorticoids in elderly people does not significantly increase the risk of diabetes mellitus.

Skin

Reduced skin thickness

Skin thickness (measured with ultrasound) was not significantly different from controls in patients taking low-dose beclomethasone dipropionate (200–800 micrograms/day). There was a reduction in skin thickness of 15–19% in patients using high dose beclomethasone dipropionate (1000–2500 micrograms/day), and 28–33% in patients using long-term oral prednisolone (5–20 mg/day). Bruising occurred in 12% of controls, 33% of patients using low-dose beclomethasone dipropionate, 48% of patients using high-dose beclomethasone dipropionate, and 80% of patients using oral prednisolone (90). Other workers have concluded that patients using beclomethasone dipropionate who report bruising are older (61 versus 52 years), take higher daily doses (1388 versus 1067 micrograms), and have been on treatment longer (55 versus 43 months) (91). The number of bruises seems to be inversely related to the concentration of urinary cortisol (SEDA-21, 188). In children using budesonide (189–1322 micrograms/day) for 3–6 years, there was no increase in bruising (32).

The effect of long-term inhaled glucocorticoids (800–1000 micrograms/day of either budesonide or beclomethasone) on skin collagen synthesis and thickness has been prospectively investigated in 27 consecutive new asthmatic patients (92). Asthma was treated with a moderate dosage of inhaled glucocorticoids. Skin thickness was measured before treatment and at 3 and 6 months using ultrasound on the abdomen and the upper right arm. Suction blisters were induced on the abdominal skin using a disposable suction blister device. Blister fluid was collected and kept frozen for radioimmunoassay of PINP and PIIINP. Skin punch biopsies were taken from the abdominal wall for the determination of skin hydroxyproline. After 1–2 years, 20 subjects attended for a further measurement of skin thickness. Control data were obtained in 14 healthy women who were followed for 6 months. PINP and PIIINP concentrations in blister fluid were followed in eight male volunteers for 1 year. There was no significant change in abdominal skin thickness after 6 months of inhaled glucocorticoids. In the upper arm there was a small, significant reduction from 1.64 to 1.50 mm after 6 months. After 1–2 years the skin thickness in the abdomen and upper arm was unchanged in 14 subjects who had used only inhaled glucocorticoids, but in six patients who had taken supplementary oral glucocorticoids for one to several weeks there was thinning of the skin in the upper arm but not the abdomen. The procollagen propeptides were markedly reduced in blister fluid at 3 and 6 months. There was no significant change in skin collagen expressed as hydroxyproline. Thus, despite evidence of a reduction in collagen synthesis, skin thickness and collagen did not change, possibly because the degradation and turnover of collagen slowed down. However, in the six patients who subsequently used oral glucocorticoids, skin thickness decreased.

Bruising

Since the original observation of the association between high-dose glucocorticoids and purpura and dermal thinning, easy bruising of the skin has become recognized as a systemic adverse effect of inhaled glucocorticoids (90). In a double-blind crossover study 69 asthmatic subjects received either the usual dose of beclomethasone dipropionate or fluticasone (at half the dose of beclomethasone) both for 4 months (93). The frequency and severity of skin bruising were assessed by questionnaire, and the numbers of bruises were assessed by direct examination. The dose of fluticasone was selected on the basis of previous studies that showed that it had comparable efficacy when given in half the dose of beclomethasone. This dose of fluticasone had comparable efficacy with respect to the control of asthma, but there was no skin bruising. These findings suggest that the systemic availability of equieffective doses of fluticasone is less than that of beclomethasone.

Contact allergy

Nasal glucocorticoids and inhaled glucocorticoids can have adverse effects on the nose and mouth, including pruritus, burning, dryness, erythema, edema, dry cough, and odynophagia; less commonly, they can cause eczema and urticaria, particularly on the face. Contact dermatitis to glucocorticoids can be facilitated by impaired epithelial barriers, and has been found in 4.7% of patients receiving topical hydrocortisone (94). Inhaled glucocorticoids can cause hypersensitivity reactions, especially in patients with chronic eczema who have been sensitized to local glucocorticoids.

Tixocortol pivalate is a marker for glucocorticoid contact allergy, as a positive patch test suggests established contact allergy to hydrocortisone, prednisolone, and their derivatives (95). A literature search via Medline from 1966 to May 2000 revealed only one patient hypersensitive to tixocortol pivalate and budesonide in a pilot study in 34 patients (10 with asthma, 13 with rhinitis, 11 with both) (96). From case reports, the prevalence of glucocorticoid-induced contact allergy has been estimated at 2.9–5%.

Based on these observations it has been concluded that patients who use inhaled glucocorticoids and develop unprecedented skin reactions during therapy should be tested for glucocorticoid-related contact allergy (97). Switching from one of the four main glucocorticoid groups to another might prove successful in these cases.

Two cases of perioral dermatitis have been associated with the use of inhaled glucocorticoids (98).

- A 38-year-old woman who had used inhaled beclomethasone daily (dosage not stated) during the winter for the past 5 years for mild asthma, developed a perioral rash with numerous small pustules and papules. She stopped using beclomethasone and was treated with oral erythromycin and topical tretinoin. Her rash resolved within 4 weeks. One year later, she restarted beclomethasone and her rash reappeared after 2 weeks. There was no recurrence of her perioral dermatitis during subsequent treatment with monthly intramuscular injections of betamethasone.
- A 46-year-old woman, who had used inhaled budesonide (dosage not stated) for 8 years for vasomotor rhinitis, developed a recurrent perioral rash, which responded to treatment with oral erythromycin 1 g/day for 6 weeks. One year later, she had a recurrence, which resolved with oral erythromycin. She continued to use inhaled budesonide.

As cross-reactivity within glucocorticoid groups may be clinically relevant, skin patch testing has been proposed in cases of suspected glucocorticoid allergy, to identify the substances that can be safely administered (99). The prevalence of glucocorticoid allergy has been studied by skin patch testing in 30 patients using inhaled or intranasal glucocorticoids (100). Four patients had a positive patch test (three allergic reactions and one irritant reaction). Eight different glucocorticoids were used, but allergic reactions occurred only with budesonide. The authors therefore suggested that budesonide is more likely to cause contact hypersensitivity, but also referred to the possible relevance of allergic or irritant reactions to preservatives.

Contact allergy to glucocorticoids is not rare in patients with atopic dermatitis. In patients with known contact allergy to budesonide, allergic skin reactions can also occur when inhaled forms of the drug are used, as shown by a randomized, double-blind, placebo-controlled study in 15 non-asthmatic patients with budesonide hypersensitivity on patch testing (101). In four of seven patients who used inhaled budesonide, there was reactivation of the 6-week-old patch test sites and they had new distant skin lesions. No flare-up reactions were observed in the other 11 patients (three had used inhaled budesonide and eight placebo for 1 week). None of the patients developed respiratory symptoms; spirometry and peak expiratory flow rates remained normal.

Musculoskeletal

Bone

Studies of the effects of inhaled glucocorticoids have used biochemical markers of bone function and imaging techniques to assess bone mineral density. Some of the biochemical markers are summarized in Table 1. Initial, short-term studies caused concern about the effect of inhaled glucocorticoids on bone metabolism. Beclomethasone dipropionate 2000 micrograms/day reduced serum osteocalcin concentrations at 1 and 2 weeks, and they returned to normal at 1 and 2 weeks after withdrawal. Nebulized budesonide (2000 micrograms bd) produced a similar increase in FEV_1 to oral prednisolone 30 mg/day given over 5 days. Serum osteocalcin was significantly higher: 2.3 (0.9–3.7) ng/ml with budesonide compared with 0.6 (0–1.2) ng/ml with prednisolone. The 24-hour urinary calcium to creatinine ratio was significantly lower in patients treated with nebulized budesonide (SEDA-22, 183). After 4 weeks on beclomethasone dipropionate or budesonide 800 micrograms/day, there were significant but paradoxical changes in osteocalcin and PICP (both markers of bone formation). Osteocalcin concentrations fell, but PICP concentrations rose. Patients on beclomethasone dipropionate 800 micrograms/day followed for 30 months showed no change in markers of resorption (ICTP) or formation (PICP) (SEDA-22, 183).

While biochemical markers of bone metabolism may be sensitive to the effects of glucocorticoids in the short term, the relation between changes in these markers and intermediate measures, such as bone mineral density, and the more important clinical outcomes of fractures, is unknown. In a random stratified sample of 3222 women in the perimenopausal age range (47–56 years), including 119 women with asthma, bone mineral density was measured to determine whether asthma was a risk factor of osteoporosis and to investigate the effect of inhaled glucocorticoids (102). The subjects had predominantly adult-onset asthma, as the age at diagnosis was over 40 years. There were 26 patients who were treated mainly with inhaled glucocorticoids (average daily dose 1000 micrograms). The asthmatic women in this general perimenopausal population had slightly reduced spinal and femoral neck bone mineral density compared with non-asthmatic women. These differences were more prominent in women who were not taking hormone replacement therapy. The reduction in bone mineral density may be due to

Table 1 Biochemical markers of bone mineral density

Bone formation	Bone resorption
Blood	*Blood*
Alkaline phosphatase (bone-specific)	Acid phosphatase (acid-resistant)
Osteocalcin	Type I collagen carboxy-terminal telopeptide (ICTP)
Procollagen type I carboxy-terminal propeptide (PICP)	*Urine*
Procollagen type I amino-terminal propeptide (PINP)	Calcium
Procollagen type III amino-terminal propeptide (PIIINP)	Hydroxyproline Cross-linked peptides (pyridinium and deoxypyridinoline)

glucocorticoids, and hormone replacement therapy appears to be protective against bone loss in asthmatics as well as healthy subjects. Cross-sectional studies such as this provide information about association but do not imply causality, for which longitudinal studies are required. Studies of the effects of inhaled glucocorticoids on markers of bone mineral density have provided conflicting data (103).

Effects on bone mineral density

Bone mineral density has been measured in a 3-year prospective study in 109 premenopausal asthmatic women, aged 18–45 years, all of whom used inhaled triamcinolone acetonide (104). They were grouped according to their inhaled glucocorticoid use at base line (no glucocorticoids and triamcinolone less than 800 micrograms/day or more than 800 micrograms/day). Therapy with triamcinolone was associated with a dose-related fall in bone mineral density at the hip overall and the trochanter. There was no effect at the femoral neck or the spine. None of the measured serum or urinary markers of bone turnover predicted the degree of bone loss. The dose-related loss of bone mineral density was suggested to be clinically related to prolonged treatment with inhaled glucocorticoids, and periodic bone mineral density assessment in patients taking high-dose inhaled glucocorticoids was proposed.

The effect of beclomethasone on bone mineral density has been examined over 1 year in 36 premenopausal and early postmenopausal women with asthma using inhaled glucocorticoids (beclomethasone at a mean dose of 542 micrograms/day) compared with 45 healthy matched controls (105). In early postmenopausal asthmatic women using beclomethasone, bone mineral density was significantly lower than in the controls, but not in premenopausal asthmatic women using inhaled beclomethasone. Serum osteocalcin concentrations were lower in the early postmenopausal asthmatic women using inhaled glucocorticoids than in the healthy controls, suggesting reduced bone formation, which leads to more pronounced bone loss. Ovarian hormones were suggested to offset the bone-depleting effects of inhaled beclomethasone in premenopausal women by maintaining or stimulating osteoblastic function.

There were significant reductions in bone mineral density in the lumbar spine and femur in 32 asthmatic women taking long-term inhaled beclomethasone (750–1500 micrograms/day) compared with 26 healthy controls (106). Control subjects and asthmatic patients were matched for age, sex, menopausal status, body-mass index, calcium intake, and physical activity. Loss of bone mass was more pronounced in the postmenopausal women. The authors identified several risk factors for accelerated bone loss in the lumbar spine, including postmenopausal status, low body-mass index, long duration of disease, long-term inhaled glucocorticoid therapy, and higher average daily and cumulative inhaled glucocorticoid doses.

The effects of inhaled budesonide 800 micrograms/day and fluticasone 400 micrograms/day on bone metabolism,

morning cortisol concentrations, and clinical parameters have been studied in eight asthmatic patients (107). There were no changes in serum and bone alkaline phosphatase, osteocalcin, carboxyterminal propeptide of type 1 procollagen, and urinary calcium and deoxypyridinoline concentrations over 6 months. The authors concluded that fluticasone is as effective as twice the dose of budesonide in controlling asthmatic symptoms, without adverse effects on bone metabolism.

In a prospective comparison of the changes in bone mineral density in adults with mild asthma, 374 subjects with mild asthma (mean FEV_1 86% predicted; mean age 35 years; 55% women) were randomized to receive inhaled budesonide, inhaled beclomethasone, or non-glucocorticoid treatment (the control group) for 2 years (108). Bone mineral density was measured blind after 6, 12, and 24 months. The median daily doses of budesonide (87 subjects) and beclomethasone (74 subjects) were 389 and 499 micrograms respectively. The mean changes in bone density over 2 years in the budesonide, beclomethasone, and control groups were 0.1, −0.4, and 0.4% in the lumbar spine and −0.9, −0.9, and −0.4% in the neck of the femur. The mean daily dose of inhaled glucocorticoid was related to the reduction in bone mineral density only in the lumbar spine. Low to moderate doses of inhaled glucocorticoids caused little change in bone mineral density over 2 years and provided better asthma control.

In a retrospective cohort comparison of patients using inhaled glucocorticoids or bronchodilators with controls, there was an increased risk of fractures, particularly at the hip and spine, in those using inhaled glucocorticoids. There were no differences in relative fracture risks with different drugs, for example fluticasone, budesonide, beclomethasone (109). In an earlier retrospective study, there was a dose-dependent increase in bone fracture risk with oral glucocorticoids (110).

The effects of inhaled glucocorticoids on bone mineral density (measured using dual X-ray absorptiometry of the spine and hip) and biochemical parameters were followed over 18 months. Mean serum osteocalcin concentrations were significantly lower in patients taking beclomethasone dipropionate or budesonide at doses of 800 micrograms/day and more. However, bone mineral density of the lumbar spine and hip was not affected. The normal advancement of bone mineral density expected in growing children was not affected by inhaled glucocorticoids taken for 7–16 months (SEDA-22, 184).

Treatment with beclomethasone dipropionate 1500 micrograms/day for 6 weeks significantly reduced markers of bone formation (osteocalcin and PICP), whereas fluticasone propionate 750 micrograms/day had no effect. Neither drug affected biochemical markers of bone resorption. There was no significant change in bone density (SEDA-22, 183).

Effects on bone mineral density in children

A cross-sectional study in children (111) showed no significant difference in total and anteroposterior spine bone mineral density between children with asthma treated with long-term budesonide (200–800 micrograms for at least 6 months; $n = 52$) and asthmatic children who had never used inhaled glucocorticoids ($n = 22$). These results are in agreement with those of a larger cross-sectional study of the effects of long-term treatment (3–6 years, mean 4.5 years) with inhaled budesonide on total bone mineral density in children with asthma ($n = 157$). The results provided evidence that long-term treatment with inhaled glucocorticoids in moderate dosages is unlikely to affect bone mineral density adversely in children with asthma (112). However, a study of the association of clinical risk factors and bone density with fractures in 324 prepubertal children, of whom 32 had a fracture, suggested that for total fracture risk bone mineral density may be less important than clinical risk factors (113). In a multivariate model incorporating age, weight, height, breast-feeding history, sports participation, and the use of inhaled glucocorticoids, these factors accounted for 10% of the variability in the risk of fracture. Surprisingly, bone mineral density in the lumbar spine, femoral neck, and total body bone did not differ between those with and without fractures.

In a small cross-sectional study, bone mineral density was studied in 20 prepubertal asthmatic patients treated with moderate to high doses of inhaled glucocorticoids (under 400 micrograms/day beclomethasone or budesonide or over 200 micrograms/day fluticasone) (114). Volumetric trabecular bone mineral density of the lumbar spine and distal radius were measured using dual energy X-ray absorptiometry and were within the reference ranges.

Bone mineral density (measured by dual X-ray absorptiometry) did not change significantly in asthmatic children treated for 3–6 years with a mean daily dose of 504 micrograms (189–1322 micrograms) budesonide (112).

In 23 children, randomized to either fluticasone 100 micrograms bd or beclomethasone 200 micrograms bd for 20 months, there was a significant increase in bone mineral density in the lumbar spine with time, following the normal growth pattern (115).

Comparisons with placebo

More data on the effect of inhaled glucocorticoids on bone mineral density in adults have been generated by the large randomized, multicenter, double-blind, placebo-controlled EUROSCOPE (European Respiratory Society Study on Chronic Obstructive Pulmonary Disease) study of 912 patients with chronic obstructive pulmonary disease randomly assigned to treatment for 3 years with budesonide 800 micrograms/day or placebo (116). There were no significant differences in bone mineral density at L2–4 vertebrae, the femoral neck, trochanter, or Ward's triangle; nor did the fracture rate between budesonide-treated and placebo-treated patients differ. These findings are in contrast to recent data from the Lung Health Study, which showed that triamcinolone 1200 micrograms/day for 4 years was associated with a statistically significant 2% reduction in bone mineral density in the femoral neck compared with placebo (117).

Comparisons of glucocorticoids

In a 12-month, multicenter comparison of fluticasone propionate 250–500 micrograms/day with beclomethasone dipropionate 500–1000 micrograms/day, the two drugs had an equal therapeutic effect. Fluticasone propionate treatment resulted in a higher bone mineral density (assessed at the hip) and higher serum osteocalcin concentrations.

In a prospective randomized comparison of the effects of fluticasone propionate 1000 micrograms/day and budesonide 1600 micrograms/day, over 1 year, bone mineral density measured in the spine was normal at the start of the study and increased slightly with time in both groups, as did serum osteocalcin concentration.

Fluticasone propionate 1000 micrograms/day or beclomethasone dipropionate 2000 micrograms/day taken for 2 years caused no change in biochemical markers of bone metabolism. Bone mineral density, measured by dual X-ray absorptiometry or single-photon absorptiometry, showed no consistent change. However, when bone mineral density was measured using quantitative computed tomography of the lumbar spine, beclomethasone dipropionate was associated with a small fall in bone mineral density, which stabilized by 24 months. It is doubtful that a small fall in bone density seen only on quantitative computed tomography is clinically relevant (SEDA-22, 184).

The efficacy and safety of fluticasone 750 micrograms/day and beclomethasone 1500 micrograms/day delivered by a spacer device have been compared in 30 asthmatic children in a 12-week, randomized, double-blind, crossover study (118). All of the children had persistent asthma requiring 1000–2000 micrograms/day of inhaled glucocorticoids before the trial. There was no significant difference in efficacy, as judged by daytime and nighttime symptom scores and PEFR. There was a minimal reduction in serum cortisol in both groups. Both groups had identical height gain velocities. At the doses used in this trial, the authors were unable to show a safety advantage of fluticasone over beclomethasone, as assessed by cortisol concentrations.

In a 1-year prospective, randomized, open comparison of inhaled fluticasone 500 micrograms bd with budesonide 800 micrograms bd delivered by metered-dose inhaler and large volume spacer, bone mineral density was measured in 29 patients in the lumbar spine and femoral neck (119). Bone mineral density in the spine increased slightly in both groups over the 12 months. Serum osteocalcin concentrations increased from baseline in both treatment groups (fluticasone +17%, budesonide +14%). The percentage change from baseline in bone mineral density of the spine correlated with the increase in serum osteocalcin. Mean serum cortisol concentrations remained in the reference range after both inhaled glucocorticoids.

It can be hypothesized that different glucocorticoids have different systemic effects, and therefore different effects on bone metabolism. An alternative hypothesis is that these effects are dose dependent (85), support for which comes from a population-based case-control study of 16 341 older patients with hip fractures (mean age 79 years) and 29 889 controls; recent use of an inhaled glucocorticoid was associated with a small dose-dependent increase in the risk of hip fracture (120).

Comparisons with other drugs

Bone mineral density was measured after 7.4 months in 49 asthmatic children, 38 of whom took inhaled beclomethasone, average daily dose 276 micrograms, and 11 sodium cromoglicate, average daily dose 30 mg (121). Children who had used beclomethasone had grown as much as those who used sodium cromoglicate. Trabecular and cortical bone mineral density in the proximal forearm and lumbar spine increased to the same extent in both groups.

The effects of fluticasone 50 micrograms bd or sodium cromoglicate 20 mg qds on growth over 12 months have been studied in 122 asthmatic children aged 4–10 years (122). The mean height velocity was 6 cm/year with fluticasone and 6.5 cm/year with sodium cromoglicate. There was no significant treatment difference in the mean 24-hour urinary-free cortisol concentrations at 6 or 12 months. Mean predicted peak expiratory flow rate improved over 1 year in both groups, but to a greater extent with fluticasone. The authors concluded that growth was normal in mildly asthmatic children using fluticasone (50 micrograms bd) for 1 year. Fluticasone was more effective than sodium cromoglicate, with fewer withdrawals and greater improvement in lung function.

Dose relation

Current evidence suggests that the changes in bone mineral density in asthmatic patients who take inhaled glucocorticoids occur within the high therapeutic range of doses. In patients with mild asthma who are well maintained on low doses of inhaled glucocorticoids, the benefits derived from good control of the asthma appear to outweigh any concerns about minor changes in bone mineral density. The picture is less clear in patients with other risk factors, such as estrogen deficiency and advancing years.

No adverse effect on bone has been shown with beclomethasone dipropionate or budesonide at doses less than 1000 micrograms/day or fluticasone propionate less than 500 micrograms/day. Most patients obtain a good therapeutic response at these doses. Higher doses may be required in some patients. Aerosols delivering doses of beclomethasone dipropionate 250 and 500 micrograms, budesonide 400 micrograms and fluticasone propionate 250 and 500 micrograms should be reserved for patients in whom the requirement for a high dose has been demonstrated in an adequate trial of therapy.

In an uncontrolled study, 56 women with asthma taking long-term inhaled glucocorticoids had bone mineral density measurements of the lumbar spine and hip (123). Women who had taken more than three short courses of systemic glucocorticoids per year over the preceding 3 years were excluded. Data on duration of use and dose of inhaled glucocorticoids were obtained from the patients' medical records. Doses of inhaled

glucocorticoids were arbitrarily classified as low (under 500 micrograms/day), medium (500–1000 micrograms/day), and high (over 1000 micrograms/day). More than half the women (61%) had reduced bone mineral density at either the hip or lumbar spine. Amongst the postmenopausal women in the study, 17% of those aged under 65 years had osteoporosis compared with 43% of those aged over 65 years. These figures exceeded those from a national sample of estrogen-deficient women, in which 5.7% under the age of 65 and 29% over the age of 65 years had osteoporosis. Bone mineral density loss increased with higher doses of inhaled glucocorticoids, from 5% in the low-dose group to 50% in the high-dose group. Whilst this is a potentially important finding in women at risk of osteoporosis because of the menopause, there are some aspects of the design of the study that limit the applicability of the findings. There was no appropriate age- and ethnicity-matched control group, and the contribution of nasal glucocorticoids was not accurately assessed.

In a large cross-sectional study, patients aged 20–40 years with asthma who had taken inhaled glucocorticoids for a median of 6 years were studied (124). Patients were excluded if they had taken a course of oral or parenteral glucocorticoids in the past 6 months or more than two courses ever, or if they had had more than 10 inhalers of nasal glucocorticoids or more than 10 prescriptions of a dermal glucocorticoid. Computerized records of general practices were used to identify patients for the study. Bone mineral density was measured at the lumbar spine (L2–L4) and the left femur (neck, Ward's triangle, trochanter). The cumulative dose of inhaled glucocorticoid was expressed as a product of the mean daily dose and time (mg days). This information was obtained from a patient questionnaire and validated against general practice computer and paper records. More than half of the patients (119/196) were women and the median cumulative dose of inhaled glucocorticoid was 876 mg (range 88–4380 mg). There was a significant inverse relation between the cumulative dose of inhaled glucocorticoid and bone mineral density at the spine and hip in both men and women. A doubling of cumulative dose was associated with a 0.16 times SD reduction in bone mineral density. Extrapolation from cross-sectional data such as these requires confirmation in longitudinal studies, since bone loss with oral glucocorticoids is more rapid in the first 12–24 months of therapy.

Bone mineral density has been measured at 3-year intervals in 51 patients taking inhaled glucocorticoids for asthma (125). The patients were divided into a high-dose group taking over 800 micrograms/day of beclomethasone or budesonide (n = 28, mean dose 983 micrograms/day) and a control group taking no inhaled glucocorticoid or less than 500 micrograms/day (n = 23, mean dose 309 micrograms/day). Whilst there were statistically significant reductions in bone markers, such as serum calcium and phosphorus and osteocalcin, over the 3-year period in each group, there was no significant reduction in bone mineral density in either group of asthmatic patients. Although the change in bone mineral density in the high-dose group was small over the 3-year period and not statistically significant, there was a correlation between bone loss and the daily dose of inhaled glucocorticoids. There was no significant correlation between the changes in bone density and either the initial bone density or biomarkers of bone turnover for the level of physical activity. This longitudinal study has shown the unreliability of biomarkers of bone turnover in predicting changes in bone density (and presumably relevant clinical outcomes, such as risk of fracture) and shows the need for measurement of bone mineral density in asthmatic patients who are deemed to be at risk of bone loss. Such patients include those taking oral glucocorticoids, perimenopausal women not taking hormone replacement therapy, and patients who need high doses of inhaled glucocorticoids. Whilst patients in this study did not have significant changes in bone mineral density over 3 years, the effects of higher doses remain uncertain, so it would be prudent to measure bone mineral density in patients who need higher doses.

Time course

The time course of changes in bone mineral density with inhaled glucocorticoids has yet to be determined. Longitudinal studies will be required to determine whether bone loss is most rapid in the first 12–24 months after initiating inhaled glucocorticoid therapy, as is the case with oral glucocorticoids (126) and whether the risk of fracture falls towards baseline after withdrawal of treatment, as was suggested by the GPRD (General Practice Research Database) study (114).

In older women with asthma, who have an increased risk of osteoporosis, there was no significant change in bone mineral density after 1 year of treatment with beclomethasone dipropionate 1000 micrograms/day (127).

Bone mineral density, bone turnover markers, and adrenal glucocorticoid hormones have been measured in 53 patients (34 women, 19 men) with chronic bronchial asthma who took either inhaled beclomethasone or budesonide in doses of at least 1500 micrograms/day for at least 12 months (128). The patients were divided into those who had taken oral glucocorticoids for more than 1 month and those who had not. Bone mineral density was measured at the lumbar spine and the proximal femur. The values were about one standard deviation lower in men and women taking oral glucocorticoids or very high doses of inhaled glucocorticoids. The reduction in bone mineral density was enough to a double the risk of fracture at these sites. There was suppression of both endogenous glucocorticoid and adrenal androgen production in all subjects. Adrenal androgen suppression may increase the susceptibility of postmenopausal women treated with an oral glucocorticoid to bone loss.

Risk of fracture

Although studies in which biochemical markers of bone turnover are measured for periods of 1–2 months do not predict the development of bone thinning, osteoporosis, or fracture, they can be useful in comparing the potential effects on bone of different glucocorticoids. Studies of bone mineral density over longer time periods relate more directly to osteoporosis and fracture risk.

Whilst there have been several studies of the effects of inhaled glucocorticoids on bone mineral density, there are few data on the effects of inhaled glucocorticoids on the risk of fracture. In a retrospective cohort study the risk of fracture was established by examining the General Practice Research Database (GPRD), which is run by the Medicines Control Agency in the UK (114). Users of inhaled glucocorticoids were defined as permanently registered patients aged 18 years or more who received one or more prescriptions for inhaled glucocorticoids during the time from enrolment in the GPRD until the end of data collection. Patients who received a prescription for oral glucocorticoids for a period of 6 months before to 91 days after the last prescription for an inhaled glucocorticoid were excluded. There were two comparison groups: a bronchodilator group, which included adults who received prescriptions for non-systemic glucocorticoids and bronchodilators, and a second control group who received non-systemic glucocorticoids but never inhaled systemic glucocorticoids or bronchodilators. The database included over 440 000 patients and all patients who had fractures were identified from their medical records during the follow-up period, which was 91 days after the last prescription for an inhaled glucocorticoid. The relative rates of non-vertebral, hip, and vertebral fractures during inhaled glucocorticoid treatment compared with controls were 1.15 (95% CI = 1.10, 1.20), 1.22 (CI = 1.04, 1.43), and 1.51 (CI = 1.22, 1.85) respectively. There were no differences between inhaled glucocorticoids and bronchodilators (non-vertebral fracture relative rate = 1). The authors concluded that users of inhaled glucocorticoids may have an increased risk of fracture, particularly at the hip and spine, but that this excess risk may be related more to the underlying respiratory disease than to the inhaled glucocorticoids.

There were no major differences between the three groups in baseline fracture history. About 1% in each cohort recorded a history of non-vertebral fractures in the year before baseline. During the follow-up, the incidence of non-vertebral fractures was 1.4 fractures per 100 persons with inhaled glucocorticoids, 1.4 with bronchodilators, and 1.1 in the control group. Comparing inhaled glucocorticoid users with a control group, there was a dose response for hip and vertebral fractures. For a standardized daily dose of under 300 micrograms/day of budesonide, hip fracture was 0.95, rising to 1.06 at doses of 300–700 micrograms/day and 1.77 at doses of 700 micrograms/day or more. There was no consistent trend in the rate of fractures amongst users of inhaled glucocorticoid compared with bronchodilators.

This is a noteworthy study because it has examined the most important clinical outcome of change in bone mineral density: the risk of fracture. The results point to an increased risk of fracture, especially at the hip and the vertebral bodies, amongst patients who use inhaled glucocorticoids as well as those using bronchodilators, when compared with patients not using these drugs. Fracture risk tended to fall after withdrawal of inhaled glucocorticoids or bronchodilators. These findings suggest that low-dose inhaled glucocorticoids are not associated with an increased risk of fracture and that patients with chronic respiratory disease who use any inhaled therapy are at risk compared with a control population. There were no differences in fracture risk between the various types of bronchodilators, suggesting that the underlying lung disease itself was the basis of risk rather than any particular type of bronchodilator. The authors noted that 1.9% of patients were using doses of budesonide equivalents of over 1500 micrograms/day and that the possibility of a more pronounced increased fracture risk at these high doses cannot be excluded. The age- and sex-specific incidence of fracture in the control group was similar to that of the general population in the GPRD.

Estimates of the important outcome of bone fracture have shown a small increased risk with inhaled glucocorticoids, but this may well be a feature of the disease rather than the therapy, because comparisons with treatment with bronchodilator drugs show no difference between risk factors in patients taking glucocorticoids or bronchodilators.

Prevention of osteoporosis with bisphosphonates
The effect of high-dose inhaled glucocorticoids and antiresorptive therapy with sodium etidronate has been studied for 18 months in 38 Chinese patients (24 men and 14 premenopausal women aged 30–50 years), of whom 28 were asthmatics who had already been treated for at least 12 months with high-dose inhaled glucocorticoids (beclomethasone or budesonide over 1.5 mg/day), and 10 healthy controls (129). The patients were randomly allocated to (1) no supplement, (2) a calcium supplement 1000 mg/day, or (3) cyclical sodium etidronate 400 mg/day for 14 days followed by calcium 1000 mg/day for 76 days. All three groups continued to take inhaled glucocorticoids. Bone mineral density was measured at the lumbar spine and hip. Bone mineral density in the group one patients fell by about 1% over 18 months and rose by about 1.5% in the healthy controls, neither change being significant. In groups 2 and 3 bone mineral density rose significantly at 12 and 18 months by 2 and 3% respectively. Serum osteocalcin concentrations fell significantly in all three groups of asthmatic patients but not in the controls. There were no significant changes in serum alkaline phosphatase or parathyroid hormone. In the patients taking calcium, with or without etidronate, mean serum calcium increased. The authors suggested that calcium supplementation and cyclical etidronate work by reducing bone resorption, and hence reduced bone turnover, rather than by increasing bone formation. This is consistent with the fall in serum osteocalcin.

The efficacy of clodronate in treating glucocorticoid-induced bone loss in asthmatic subjects has been evaluated in a double-blind study in 74 adults (41 women and 33 men, mean age 57 years) with a long history (mean 8.1 years) of oral and inhaled glucocorticoid use, randomized to clodronate 800, 1600, or 2400 mg/day or placebo (130). There was no increase in bone mineral density with placebo or clodronate 800 mg/day, but a significant dose-related increase with clodronate 1600 and 2400 mg/day.

The most common adverse effect was gastric irritation in the patients who took the highest dose of clodronate.

Growth
Oral glucocorticoids inhibit growth by blunting pulsatile growth hormone secretion, by decreasing insulin-like growth factor-1 activity, and by directly inhibiting collagen synthesis (131). Although inhalation reduces systemic exposure, concerns have been raised regarding the potential effects on growth and final height in children, especially when inhaled glucocorticoids are used for long periods.

Uninterrupted administration of moderate-dose inhaled glucocorticoids (for example 400 micrograms/day of budesonide equivalents) has been associated with a suppressed growth rate in some children with asthma. Budesonide reduced the growth by 1 and 1.4 cm over 7 and 12 months, respectively (132). Consequently, in the USA, a class label warning for inhaled glucocorticoids about growth retardation in children was introduced in 1998, when the FDA decided to alter the class labeling for all inhaled and nasal glucocorticoids in children, to indicate that the use of recommended doses might be associated with a reduction in growth velocity (19). However, the available studies suggest that in children, the major advantages of adequate asthma control with inhaled glucocorticoids outweigh any potential adverse effects on growth.

However, results from trials in asthmatic children can be flawed by confounding variables. Severe asthma can itself have a negative effect on growth and adversely affect adult height, as with any chronic disease. Even in well-controlled asthma, children typically show retardation in pubertal growth spurt and attain normal adult height later. As growth in children is non-linear over time, trials over short periods are likely to capture short-term effects of inhaled glucocorticoids rather than the long-term outcome. Furthermore, the growth-retarding effect of inhaled glucocorticoids is more pronounced at the start of treatment.

Long-term studies have suggested that a temporary short-term or medium-term reduction in growth velocity is normally compensated for later on, and individuals attain normal adult height (133,134). The effects of inhaled glucocorticoids on growth rate over weeks and months are dose-dependent, and dose-response curves of pulmonary and adverse systemic effects differ widely, so that individual titration of the inhaled glucocorticoid dose according to the severity of the disease is strongly recommended, and the lowest dose of inhaled glucocorticoids that controls the disease should always be preferred. In conclusion, accumulating evidence shows that children with asthma, even when treated with inhaled glucocorticoids for years, attain normal adult height. However, close growth monitoring during inhaled glucocorticoid therapy is recommended, as idiosyncratic responses can occur, probably owing to individual glucocorticoid receptor polymorphism (135).

A two-part review was published in 2002, addressing the difficulties of assessing the effects of asthma therapy on childhood growth and reviewing the published literature based on the authors' recommendations (136,137). In the first part (136), a simple classification system for growth studies was developed:

- comparisons with placebo (type 1 studies);
- comparisons with non-steroidal asthma therapy (type 2 studies);
- comparisons with another inhaled glucocorticoid (type 3 studies);
- comparisons with "real life" asthma therapy (type 4 studies).

In the context of these different study types, the authors also discussed the choice of end-point, key trial design issues, the selection and numbers of subjects in the active and control groups, the duration of assessments, and methods for measuring height and data analysis. They also elaborated specific recommendations regarding study duration, age/sexual maturity of the patients, exclusion criteria for height and growth velocity, permitted therapy during the study, the protocol for height measurement, the numbers of patients for adequate statistical power, and methods for statistical analysis (136).

In the second part, they selected 18 growth studies that included minimal criteria, such as selected control group, measured height by stadiometry, and at least a 12-month duration; they compared the design attributes of these studies with the described recommendations (137). Of the 18 selected studies, 17 were susceptible to one or more important confounding factors; nevertheless, the outcomes of all 18 studies were considered to be consistent. In summary, impaired growth velocity was found with budesonide and beclomethasone dipropionate compared with placebo, non-steroidal treatment, and fluticasone propionate during 1–2 years of therapy, but none of the inhaled glucocorticoids appeared to affect final height (137). Growth in children treated with low-dose fluticasone propionate (up to 200 micrograms/day) for 1 year is similar to growth in those treated with placebo or non-steroidal therapy. Standard pediatric doses of inhaled glucocorticoids (less than 800 micrograms of budesonide and less than 400 micrograms of budesonide or fluticasone) are considered not to affect growth adversely (84,138). The risk of growth suppression depends on the dose, the administration regimen, and the delivery device.

An important confounding factor is the influence of non-adherence to inhaled glucocorticoid treatment (139). Sensitive and reliable measures of adherence should be applied when evaluating long-term effects on height.

The time of dosing can influence the effect of inhaled glucocorticoids on growth suppression in the prepubertal child, since growth hormone secretion is generally confined to nighttime. Therefore, once-daily morning dosing could be advantageous (140).

For clinical practice, the lowest effective dose should be achieved, and all children using inhaled glucocorticoids should have their growth measured every 6 months, as this is a sensitive method of detecting significant systemic effects (84,140).

These results apply to children over 4 years of age; for younger children only assumptions can be entertained and age-specific studies are needed (140).

Dose relation

Lumbar spine bone mineral density has been assessed in 76 prepubertal asthmatics (mean age 7.7 years, 26 girls) using glucocorticoids (141). After stratification for dose and route of administration, the children who used over 800 micrograms/day of inhaled glucocorticoids, with or without intermittent oral glucocorticoids, had a significant lower weight-adjusted bone density than children who used 400–800 micrograms/day of inhaled glucocorticoids (mean difference -0.05 g/cm^2; 95% CI = -0.02, -0.09). Bone mass was similar in children who did not use inhaled glucocorticoids and those who used 400–800 micrograms/day.

The authors of a review concluded, from short-term and intermediate-term growth studies, that there are no clinically significant adverse effects on growth with inhaled glucocorticoids at normal pediatric doses (100–200 micrograms/day budesonide equivalents), but that growth retardation can occur with all inhaled glucocorticoids at higher doses (142). Individual idiosyncratic adverse reactions are rare. Long-term studies and studies that have examined the effect on final adult height have been consistent in showing significantly reduced growth rates during the first months and up to 2 years of treatment with inhaled glucocorticoids. However, children treated with inhaled glucocorticoids attain their predicted adult height to the same extent as their healthy peers. It is important to note that changes in growth rate during the first year of inhaled glucocorticoid treatment cannot be used to predict final adult height.

Growth velocity measured over a 12-month period in prepubertal children with asthma was reduced by prior treatment with inhaled glucocorticoids for an average of 2.7 years. However, measurement of biochemical markers (Table 1) gave conflicting results. Osteocalcin concentrations were reduced, but alkaline phosphatase did not change. PINP and PIIINP were reduced, but PICP increased. ICTP, a marker for collagen I degradation, fell.

Comparisons of glucocorticoids

Fluticasone propionate 400 micrograms/day or budesonide 800 micrograms/day were administered for 20 weeks to children with moderate to severe asthma aged 4–12 years. Fluticasone propionate was superior to budesonide in improving peak expiratory flow and comparable in controlling symptoms. Growth was reduced with budesonide treatment compared with fluticasone propionate treatment mean difference, 6.2 mm (CI = 2.9, 9.6). There was no difference in serum cortisol suppression (143).

Comparisons with other drugs

Beclomethasone dipropionate 400 micrograms/day and salmeterol 50 micrograms bd were compared in asthmatic children treated for 12 months. Beclomethasone dipropionate treatment resulted in better overall asthma control. Over 12 months, linear growth was 3.96 cm/year in the children using beclomethasone dipropionate, compared with 5.40 cm/year in those who used salmeterol and 5.04 cm/year in a placebo group (SEDA-22, 186).

The long-term effects of inhaled glucocorticoids on growth in children have been recently assessed. In the so-called CaAMP Study (144), children aged 5–12 years with mild to moderate asthma were randomized to budesonide 200 micrograms bd ($n = 311$), nedocromil 8 mg bd ($n = 312$), or placebo ($n = 418$). At the end of the 4–6 year treatment period, the mean increase in height in the budesonide group was 1.1 cm less than in the placebo group. The difference between budesonide and placebo in the rate of growth was evident primarily within the first year but did not increase thereafter, and all the groups had similar growth velocity by the end of the treatment period.

Comparisons with oral glucocorticoids

A meta-analysis of 21 studies in which 810 asthmatic children were treated with oral prednisolone (8 trials) and/or beclomethasone dipropionate, dosage range 200–900 micrograms/day (12 trials) has been reported. Significant suppression of growth occurred with oral glucocorticoids but not with beclomethasone dipropionate (145).

Reversibility

Growth data obtained in 50 children who used beclomethasone dipropionate over 7 months suggested that any growth suppression is temporary and that growth velocity recovers during continuing treatment. Growth velocity fell most in the first 6 weeks of treatment, from 0.140 to 0.073 mm/week (0.067 mm/week; 95% CI = 0.015, 0.120). There were similar reductions at 12 and 18 weeks. After this, growth velocity increased to rates seen before treatment began: 0.138 mm/week at 24 weeks and 0.120 mm/week at 30 weeks (146).

Long-term use of beclomethasone dipropionate 400–600 micrograms/day was reported to delay the onset of puberty. However, subsequent catch-up growth was unaffected and subjects reached their normal predicted adult height (147).

Children taking budesonide (mean daily dose 412 micrograms, range 110–877 micrograms) for periods of 3–13 years have been followed to adulthood to determine their final height (134). These 142 budesonide-treated children were compared with 18 control patients with asthma who had never taken inhaled glucocorticoids and 51 healthy siblings of the patients in the budesonide group. These children, who had taken long-term inhaled glucocorticoids, attained normal adult height. There was no evidence of a dose–response relation between the mean daily dose of budesonide, the cumulative dose, or the duration of treatment with budesonide and the difference between the measured and target adult heights.

These studies are important, because several previous reports of growth during a period of 1 year after beginning treatment with inhaled glucocorticoids (in daily doses of about 400 micrograms of budesonide) identified growth retardation of about 1.5 cm. The mechanism for the termination after 1 year of the effects on growth is uncertain.

Immunologic

Hypersensitivity to inhaled glucocorticoids is rare.

- An asthmatic patient using inhaled budesonide and salbutamol developed an acute asthma attack. Despite emergency treatment the patient deteriorated, requiring endotracheal intubation and assisted ventilation, and there was no improvement until the glucocorticoid was withdrawn, after which there was steady improvement. Skin prick tests with prednisolone, sodium hemisuccinate, and 6-methylprednisolone-sodium hemisuccinate were positive. Thirty minutes after intradermal 6-methylprednisolone-sodium hemisuccinate 4 mg, the patient developed a dry cough, dyspnea, and wheezing and a 17% fall in FEV_1.

- A 37-year-old woman who was pregnant developed Churg–Strauss syndrome after withdrawal of her usual high-dose inhaled glucocorticoid therapy (drug not stated) that she had used for 3 years for bronchial asthma (148).

The authors of the second report commented that activated eosinophils and their cytotoxic products, such as eosinophil catatonic protein, may play a part in the pathogenesis of Churg–Strauss syndrome. Measuring serum concentrations of eosinophil catatonic protein may be useful in monitoring disease activity, since concentrations were increased before treatment and normalized afterwards.

Infection risk

Inhaled or topical immunosuppressive and anti-inflammatory glucocorticoids increase the risk of oral candidiasis (149). Patients who harbor oral *Candida* before they use inhaled glucocorticoids may have an increased risk. The location and degree of oral candidiasis seems to be related to dosage, administration frequency, and inhalation technique. Preventive measures include using a spacer, lowering the dosage, and rinsing the mouth after use.

The frequency of oral candidiasis has been studied in 143 asthmatic patients using inhaled glucocorticoids (96 fluticasone and 47 beclomethasone dipropionate), 11 asthmatic patients not using inhaled glucocorticoids, and 86 healthy volunteers (150). Quantitative fungal cultures were performed by aseptically obtaining a retropharyngeal wall swab. The growth of *Candida* species was significantly greater in asthmatic patients taking inhaled glucocorticoids. The presence of *Candida* was also significantly greater in patients with oral symptoms than in asymptomatic patients, and in patients using fluticasone (26%) compared with those using beclomethasone (11%). The presence of *Candida* correlated with the dose of fluticasone but not with the inhaled dose of beclomethasone. *Candida* species were rarely found in asthmatic patients not using glucocorticoids or in healthy volunteers. Gargling with Invasive aspergillosis occurred after high-dose inhaled fluticasone (440 micrograms qds) and zafirlukast 20 mg/day in a 44-year old man with moderately severe asthma; this is the first report of invasive pulmonary aspergillosis associated with an inhaled glucocorticoid (151).

Second-Generation Effects

Teratogenicity

Congenital malformations that may be associated with inhaled budesonide in pregnancy have been evaluated using the Swedish Medical Birth Registry (152). Of 2014 infants whose mothers started to use inhaled budesonide in early pregnancy, 75 (3.7%) had a congenital malformation; the corresponding rate among all infants born in 1995–97 was 3.5%. Five infants had chromosomal anomalies that were unlikely to have been caused by drugs. This study did not identify teratogenic properties of inhaled budesonide.

Drug–Drug Interactions

HIV protease inhibitors

Cushing's syndrome can be caused by the co-administration of a glucocorticoid and inhibitors of CYP3A4, such as HIV protease inhibitors, resulting in increased plasma glucocorticoid concentrations.

- Cushing's syndrome occurred in a 44-year-old HIV-positive patient who used inhaled fluticasone (500 micrograms qds) for severe asthma for 2 years (153). Stavudine and nevirapine were replaced by abacavir and ritonavir + lopinavir and 2 months later he developed the typical features of Cushing syndrome.

In this case an interaction of ritonavir + lopinavir with fluticasone was suspected, because fluticasone is metabolized by CYP3A4, which ritonavir inhibits.

Itraconazole

Interactions with other drugs can increase plasma concentrations of inhaled glucocorticoids. Itraconazole, a potent inhibitor of CYP3A4, markedly increased plasma concentrations of inhaled budesonide (154).

Cushing's syndrome of rapid onset occurred during combined treatment with inhaled budesonide and itraconazole (155).

- A 4-year old boy with cystic fibrosis developed persistent bronchospasm. Allergic bronchopulmonary aspergillosis was suspected and he was given oral itraconazole 100 mg bd, inhaled formoterol 12 micrograms/day, and inhaled budesonide 200 micrograms bd. After 2 weeks his respiratory symptoms had improved but he had a moon face and swollen abdomen, his blood pressure was 121/75 mmHg, and his weight had increased by 1.5 kg. A morning sample showed low cortisol concentrations (under 3 ng/ml) and a reduced plasma ACTH (12 pg/ml). Itraconazole was withdrawn and budesonide was reduced and withdrawn after 2 weeks. He was given hydrocortisone to prevent acute adrenal insufficiency. He recovered over the next 3 months.

This adverse effect could have been due to inhibition of the metabolism of budesonide by itraconazole.

Cushing's syndrome has been attributed to the combination of itraconazole and inhaled budesonide (156).

- A 70-year-old white woman taking inhaled budesonide 400 micrograms tds developed multiple, small, purple, non-tender nodules in the subcutaneous tissues of her left leg. Biopsy of a nodule showed fungal hyphae, and *Scedosporium apiospermum* was isolated. She was treated with itraconazole suspension 200 mg bd, with complete clinical resolution after 4 weeks. Within 8 weeks after starting itraconazole, she developed swollen ankles, shortness of breath, fatigue, lethargy, and progressive severe leg weakness. Her doctor attributed her increased breathlessness to worsening asthma and increased the dose of inhaled budesonide to 800 micrograms bd. She had a Cushingoid appearance, her skin was thin, with multiple bruises over her body, her blood pressure was 170/90 mmHg, and she had proximal muscle weakness in the legs. The plasma cortisol concentration was below 2 (reference range 50–250) µg/l and tetracosactide 250 micrograms produced a rise to 11 µg/l after 60 minutes. The adrenocorticotropic hormone (ACTH) concentration was below 6.8 (9–52) ng/l and the 24-hour urine free cortisol was below 73 (350–1100) µg/l. Itraconazole and inhaled budesonide were withdrawn, and the secondary adrenal insufficiency was treated with hydrocortisone replacement. Inhaled beclomethasone 250 micrograms bd was given by metered-dose inhaler and 4 weeks later she developed a local recurrence of the *S. apiospermum* infection, which was treated with voriconazole 200 mg bd for 3 months, with complete resolution.

Voriconazole is predominantly metabolized by CYP2C19, and although it is an inhibitor of CYP3A4 its inhibitory effects are much less than those of itraconazole, as shown in this case, in which it appeared not to interact with beclomethasone, while itraconazole did.

Ritonavir

Ritonavir is a potent inhibitor of CYP3A4. In healthy volunteers a low dose of ritonavir increases the plasma concentrations of fluticasone and reduces cortisol concentrations, probably due to increased systemic availability of fluticasone. Ritonavir has also caused Cushing's syndrome in a patient using fluticasone propionate 1000 micrograms/day (157). Five cases of iatrogenic Cushing's syndrome with osteoporosis and secondary adrenal failure have been described in patients with HIV taking oral ritonavir and inhaled glucocorticoids (four fluticasone and one budesonide) (158).

References

1. Allen DB. Sense and sensitivity: assessing inhaled corticosteroid effects on the hypothalamic–pituitary–adrenal axis. Ann Allergy Asthma Immunol 2002;89(6):537–9.
2. Minto C, Li B, Tattam B, Brown K, Seale JP, Donnelly R. Pharmacokinetics of epimeric budesonide and fluticasone

propionate after repeat dose inhalation—intersubject variability in systemic absorption from the lung. Br J Clin Pharmacol 2000;50(2):116–24.

3. Donnelly R, Williams KM, Baker AB, Badcock CA, Day RO, Seale JP. Effects of budesonide and fluticasone on 24-hour plasma cortisol. A dose-response study. Am J Respir Crit Care Med 1997;156(6):1746–51.

4. Weiner P, Berar-Yanay N, Davidovich A, Magadle R. Nocturnal cortisol secretion in asthmatic patients after inhalation of fluticasone propionate. Chest 1999;116(4):931–4.

5. Brutsche MH, Brutsche IC, Munawar M, Langley SJ, Masterson CM, Daley-Yates PT, Brown R, Custovic A, Woodcock A. Comparison of pharmacokinetics and systemic effects of inhaled fluticasone propionate in patients with asthma and healthy volunteers: a randomised crossover study. Lancet 2000;356(9229):556–61.

6. Lofdahl CG, Thorsson L. No difference between asthmatic patients and healthy subjects in lung uptake of fluticasone propionate. Eur Respir J 1999;14:466S.

7. Harrison TW, Wisniewski A, Honour J, Tattersfield AE. Comparison of the systemic effects of fluticasone propionate and budesonide given by dry powder inhaler in healthy and asthmatic subjects. Thorax 2001;56(3):186–91.

8. Fabbri L, Melara R. Systemic effects of inhaled corticosteroids are milder in asthmatic patients than in normal subjects. Thorax 2001;56(3):165–6.

9. Berend N, Kellett B, Kent N, Sly PD, Bowler S, Burdon J, Dennis C, Gibson P, James A, Jenkins C. Collaborative Study Group of the Australian Lung Foundation. Improved safety with equivalent asthma control in adults with chronic severe asthma on high-dose fluticasone propionate. Respirology 2001;6(3):237–46.

10. Dubus JC, Marguet C, Deschildre A, Mely L, Le Roux P, Brouard J, Huiart L. Reseau de Recherche Clinique en Pneumonologie Pédiatrique. Local side-effects of inhaled corticosteroids in asthmatic children: influence of drug, dose, age, and device. Allergy 2001;56(10):944–8.

11. Wilson AM, Lipworth BJ. 24 hour and fractionated profiles of adrenocortical activity in asthmatic patients receiving inhaled and intranasal corticosteroids. Thorax 1999;54(1):20–6.

12. Borgstrom L. Local versus total systemic bioavailability as a means to compare different inhaled formulations of the same substance. J Aerosol Med 1998;11(1):55–63.

13. Kelly HW. Establishing a therapeutic index for the inhaled corticosteroids. Part I. Pharmacokinetic/pharmacodynamic comparison of the inhaled corticosteroids. J Allergy Clin Immunol 1998;102(4 Pt 2):S36–51.

14. Leach C. Targeting inhaled steroids. Int J Clin Pract Suppl 1998;96:23–7.

15. Trescoli C, Ward MJ. Systemic activity of inhaled and swallowed beclomethasone dipropionate and the effect of different inhaler devices. Postgrad Med J 1998;74(877):675–7.

16. Thorsson L, Edsbacker S. Lung deposition of budesonide from a pressurized metered-dose inhaler attached to a spacer. Eur Respir J 1998;12(6):1340–5.

17. O'Byrne PM, Pedersen S. Measuring efficacy and safety of different inhaled corticosteroid preparations. J Allergy Clin Immunol 1998;102(6 Pt 1):879–86.

18. Martin RJ, Szefler SJ, Chinchilli VM, Kraft M, Dolovich M, Boushey HA, Cherniack RM, Craig TJ, Drazen JM, Fagan JK, Fahy JV, Fish JE, Ford JG, Israel E, Kunselman SJ, Lazarus SC, Lemanske RF Jr, Peters SP, Sorkness CA. Systemic effect comparisons of six inhaled corticosteroid preparations. Am J Respir Crit Care Med 2002;165(10):1377–83.

19. Lipworth BJ. Systemic adverse effects of inhaled corticosteroid therapy: A systematic review and meta-analysis. Arch Intern Med 1999;159(9):941–55.

20. Goldberg S, Einot T, Algur N, Schwartz S, Greenberg AC, Picard E, Virgilis D, Kerem E. Adrenal suppression in asthmatic children receiving low-dose inhaled budesonide: comparison between dry powder inhaler and pressurized metered-dose inhaler attached to a spacer. Ann Allergy Asthma Immunol 2002;89(6):566–71.

21. Irani AM, Cruz-Rivera M, Fitzpatrick S, Hoag J, Smith JA. Effects of budesonide inhalation suspension on hypothalamic–pituitary–adrenal-axis function in infants and young children with persistent asthma. Ann Allergy Asthma Immunol 2002;88(3):306–12.

22. Eid N, Morton R, Olds B, Clark P, Sheikh S, Looney S. Decreased morning serum cortisol levels in children with asthma treated with inhaled fluticasone propionate. Pediatrics 2002;109(2):217–21.

23. Tukiainen H, Rytila P, Hamalainen KM, Silvasti MS, Keski-Karhu J. Finnish Study Group. Safety, tolerability and acceptability of two dry powder inhalers in the administration of budesonide in steroid-treated asthmatic patients. Respir Med 2002;96(4):221–9.

24. Volovitz B, Bentur L, Finkelstein Y, Mansour Y, Shalitin S, Nussinovitch M, Varsano I. Effectiveness and safety of inhaled corticosteroids in controlling acute asthma attacks in children who were treated in the emergency department: a controlled comparative study with oral prednisolone. J Allergy Clin Immunol 1998;102(4 Pt 1):605–9.

25. Nana A, Youngchaiyud P, Charoenratanakul S, Boe J, Lofdahl CG, Selroos O, Stahl E. High-dose inhaled budesonide may substitute for oral therapy after an acute asthma attack. J Asthma 1998;35(8):647–55.

26. Sung L, Osmond MH, Klassen TP. Randomized, controlled trial of inhaled budesonide as an adjunct to oral prednisone in acute asthma. Acad Emerg Med 1998;5(3):209–13.

27. Paggiaro PL, Dahle R, Bakran I, Frith L, Hollingworth K, Efthimiou J. Multicentre randomised placebo-controlled trial of inhaled fluticasone propionate in patients with chronic obstructive pulmonary disease. International COPD Study Group. Lancet 1998;351(9105):773–80Erratum in: Lancet 1998;351(9120):1968.

28. Jick SS, Vasilakis-Scaramozza C, Maier WC. The risk of cataract among users of inhaled steroids. Epidemiology 2001;12(2):229–34.

29. Garbe E, Suissa S, LeLorier J. Association of inhaled corticosteroid use with cataract extraction in elderly patients. JAMA 1998;280(6):539–43Erratum in: JAMA 1998;280(21):1830.

30. Kennedy L, Rusch VW, Strange C, Ginsberg RJ, Sahn SA. Pleurodesis using talc slurry. Chest 1994;106(2):342–6.

31. Li JT, Ford LB, Chervinsky P, Weisberg SC, Kellerman DJ, Faulkner KG, Herje NE, Hamedani A, Harding SM, Shah T. Fluticasone propionate powder and lack of clinically significant effects on hypothalamic–pituitary–adrenal axis and bone mineral density over 2 years in adults with mild asthma. J Allergy Clin Immunol 1999;103(6):1062–8.

32. Agertoft L, Larsen FE, Pedersen S. Posterior subcapsular cataracts, bruises and hoarseness in children with asthma receiving long-term treatment with inhaled budesonide. Eur Respir J 1998;12(1):130–5.

33. Garbe E, LeLorier J, Boivin JF, Suissa S. Inhaled and nasal glucocorticoids and the risks of ocular hypertension or open-angle glaucoma. JAMA 1997;277(9):722–7.

34. Hederos CA. Neuropsychologic changes and inhaled corticosteroids. J Allergy Clin Immunol 2004;114:451–2.

35. Casale TB, Nelson HS, Stricker WE, Raff H, Newman KB. Suppression of hypothalamic–pituitary–adrenal axis activity with inhaled flunisolide and fluticasone propionate in adult asthma patients. Ann Allergy Asthma Immunol 2001;87(5):379–85.

36. Nelson HS, Stricker W, Casale TB, Raff H, Fourre JA, Aron DC, Newman KB. A comparison of methods for assessing hypothalamic–pituitary–adrenal HPA axis activity in asthma patients treated with inhaled corticosteroids. J Clin Pharmacol 2002;42(3):319–26.

37. Fink RS, Pierre LN, Daley-Yates PT, Richards DH, Gibson A, Honour JW. Hypothalamic–pituitary–adrenal axis function after inhaled corticosteroids: unreliability of urinary free cortisol estimation. J Clin Endocrinol Metab 2002;87(10):4541–6.

38. Niitsuma T, Okita M, Sakurai K, Morita S, Tsuyuguchi M, Matsumura Y, Hayashi T, Koshishi T, Oka K, Homma M. Adrenal function as assessed by low-dose adrenocorticotropin hormone test before and after switching from inhaled beclomethasone dipropionate to inhaled fluticasone propionate. J Asthma 2003;40:515–22.

39. Kim KT, Rabinovitch N, Uryniak T, Simpson B, O'Dowd L, Casty F. Effect of budesonide aqueous nasal spray on hypothalamic–pituitary–adrenal axis function in children with allergic rhinitis. Ann Allergy Asthma Immunol 2004;93:61–7.

40. Lipworth BJ, Kaliner MA, LaForce CF, Baker JW, Kaiser HB, Amin D, Kundu S, Williams JE, Engelstaetter R, Banerji DD. Effect of ciclesonide and fluticasone on hypothalamic–pituitary–adrenal axis function in adults with mild-to-moderate persistent asthma. Ann Allergy Asthma Immunol 2005;94:465–72.

41. Szefler SJ, Rohatagi S, Williams JE, Lloyd M, Kundu S, Banerji D. Ciclesonide, a novel inhaled steroid, does not affect hypothalamic–pituitary–adrenal axis function in patients with moderate-to-severe persistent asthma. Chest 2005;128(3):1104–14.

42. Derom E, Van DV, V, Marissens S, Engelstatter R, Vincken W, Pauwels R. Effects of inhaled ciclesonide and fluticasone propionate on cortisol secretion and airway responsiveness to adenosine 5'monophosphate in asthmatic patients. Pulm Pharmacol Ther 2005;18:328–36.

43. Langdon CG, Adler M, Mehra S, Alexander M, Drollmann A. Once-daily ciclesonide 80 or 320 microg for 12 weeks is safe and effective in patients with persistent asthma. Respir Med 2005;99:1275–85.

44. Pearlman DS, Berger WE, Kerwin E, LaForce C, Kundu S, Banerji D. Once-daily ciclesonide improves lung function and is well tolerated by patients with mild-to-moderate persistent asthma. J Allergy Clin Immunol 2005;116:1206–12.

45. Postma DS, Sevette C, Martinat Y, Schlosser N, Aumann J, Kafe H. Treatment of asthma by the inhaled corticosteroid ciclesonide given either in the morning or evening. Eur Respir J 2001;17:1083–8.

46. Szefler S, Rohatagi S, Williams J, Lloyd M, Kundu S, Banerji D. Ciclesonide, a novel inhaled steroid, does not affect hypothalamic–pituitary–adrenal axis function in patients with moderate-to-severe persistent asthma. Chest 2005;128:1104–14.

47. Weinbrenner A, Huneke D, Zschiesche M, Engel G, Timmer W, Steinijans VW, Bethke T, Wurst W, Drollmann A, Kaatz HJ, Siegmund W. Circadian rhythm of serum cortisol after repeated inhalation of the new topical steroid ciclesonide. J Clin Endocrinol Metab 2002;87:2160–3.

48. Lee DK, Fardon TC, Bates CE, Haggart K, McFarlane LC, Lipworth BJ. Airway and systemic effects of hydrofluoroalkane formulations of high-dose ciclesonide and fluticasone in moderate persistent asthma. Chest 2005;127:851–60.

49. Rohatagi S, Krishnaswami S, Pfister M, Sahasranaman S. Model-based covariate pharmacokinetic analysis and lack of cortisol suppression by the new inhaled corticosteroid ciclesonide using a novel cortisol release model. Am J Ther 2005;12:385–97.

50. Chapman KR, Boulet LP, D'Urzo AD. Long-term administration of ciclesonide is safe and well tolerated in patients with persistent asthma. 4th Triennial World Asthma Meeting (WAM). February 16–19, Bangkok, Thailand, 2004:61.

51. Nguyen KL, Lauver D, Kim I, Aresery M. The effect of a steroid "burst" and long-term, inhaled fluticasone propionate on adrenal reserve. Ann Allergy Asthma Immunol 2003;91:38–43.

52. Samaras K, Pett S, Gowers A, McMurchie M, Cooper DA. Iatrogenic Cushing's syndrome with osteoporosis and secondary adrenal failure in human immunodeficiency virus-infected patients receiving inhaled corticosteroids and ritonavir-boosted protease inhibitors: six cases. J Clin Endocrinol Metab 2005;90(7):4394–8.

53. Patel L, Wales JK, Kibirige MS, Massarano AA, Couriel JM, Clayton PE. Symptomatic adrenal insufficiency during inhaled corticosteroid treatment. Arch Dis Child 2001;85(4):330–4.

54. Vargas R, Dockhorn RJ, Findlay SR, Korenblat PE, Field EA, Kral KM. Effect of fluticasone propionate aqueous nasal spray versus oral prednisone on the hypothalamic–pituitary–adrenal axis. J Allergy Clin Immunol 1998;102(2):191–7.

55. Fardon TC, Lee DK, Haggart K, McFarlane LC, Lipworth BJ. Adrenal suppression with dry powder formulations of fluticasone propionate and mometasone furoate. Am J Respir Crit Care Med 2004;170:960–6.

56. Fardon TC, Lee DK, Haggart K, McFarlane LC, Lipworth BJ. Adrenal suppression with dry powder formulations of fluticasone propionate and mometasone furoate. Am J Respir Crit Care Med 2004;170:960–6.

57. Eichenhorn MS, Wise RA, Madhok TC, Gerald LB, Bailey WC, Tashkin DP, Scanlon PD. Lack of long-term adverse adrenal effects from inhaled triamcinolone. Lung Health Study II. Chest 2003;124:57–62.

58. Drake AJ, Howells RJ, Shield JP, Prendiville A, Ward PS, Crowne EC. Symptomatic adrenal insufficiency presenting with hypoglycaemia in children with asthma receiving high dose inhaled fluticasone propionate. BMJ 2002;324(7345):1081–2.

59. Todd GR, Acerini CL, Buck JJ, Murphy NP, Ross-Russell R, Warner JT, McCance DR. Acute adrenal crisis in asthmatics treated with high-dose fluticasone propionate. Eur Respir J 2002;19(6):1207–9.

60. Dunlop KA, Carson DJ, Shields MD. Hypoglycemia due to adrenal suppression secondary to high-dose nebulized corticosteroid. Pediatr Pulmonol 2002;34(1):85–6.

61. Kennedy MJ, Carpenter JM, Lozano RA, Castile RG. Impaired recovery of hypothalamic–pituitary–adrenal axis

function and hypoglycemic seizures after high-dose inhaled corticosteroid therapy in a toddler. Ann Allergy Asthma Immunol 2002;88(5):523–6.

62. Duplantier JE, Nelson RP Jr, Morelli AR, Good RA, Kornfeld SJ. Hypothalamic–pituitary–adrenal axis suppression associated with the use of inhaled fluticasone propionate. J Allergy Clin Immunol 1998;102(4 Pt 1):699–700.

63. Zimmerman B, Gold M, Wherrett D, Hanna AK. Adrenal suppression in two patients with asthma treated with low doses of the inhaled steroid fluticasone propionate. J Allergy Clin Immunol 1998;101(3):425–6.

64. Todd GR, Acerini CL, Ross-Russell R, Zahra S, Warner JT, McCance D. Survey of adrenal crisis associated with inhaled corticosteroids in the United Kingdom. Arch Dis Child 2002;87(6):457–61.

65. Wilkinson SM, Cartwright PH, English JS. Hydrocortisone: an important cutaneous allergen. Lancet 1991;337(8744):761–2.

66. Ng PC, Fok TF, Wong GW, Lam CW, Lee CH, Wong MY, Lam K, Ma KC. Pituitary–adrenal suppression in preterm, very low birth weight infants after inhaled fluticasone propionate treatment. J Clin Endocrinol Metab 1998;83(7):2390–3.

67. Aaronson D, Kaiser H, Dockhorn R, Findlay S, Korenblat P, Thorsson L, Kallen A. Effects of budesonide by means of the Turbuhaler on the hypothalmic–pituitary–adrenal axis in asthmatic subjects: a dose-response study. J Allergy Clin Immunol 1998;101(3):312–9.

68. Lipworth BJ. Airway and systemic effects of inhaled corticosteroids in asthma: dose response relationship. Pulm Pharmacol 1996;9(1):19–27.

69. Volovitz B, Nussinovitch M. Effect of high starting dose of budesonide inhalation suspension on serum cortisol concentration in young children with recurrent wheezing episodes. J Asthma 2003;40:625–9.

70. Yiallouros PK, Milner AD, Conway E, Honour JW. Adrenal function and high dose inhaled corticosteroids for asthma. Arch Dis Child 1997;76:405–10.

71. Shapiro G, Bronsky EA, LaForce CF, Mendelson L, Pearlman D, Schwartz RH, Szefler SJ. Dose-related efficacy of budesonide administered via a dry powder inhaler in the treatment of children with moderate to severe persistent asthma. J Pediatr 1998;132:976–82.

72. Priftis KN, Papadimitriou A, Gatsopoulou E, Yiallouros PK, Fretzayas A, Nicolaidou P. The effect of inhaled budesonide on adrenal and growth suppression in asthmatic children. Eur Respir J 2006;27:316–20.

73. Patel L, Wales JK, Kibirige MS, Massarano AA, Couriel JM, Clayton PE. Symptomatic adrenal insufficiency during inhaled corticosteroid treatment. Arch Dis Child 2001;85:330–4.

74. Bacharier LB, Raissy HH, Wilson L, McWilliams B, Strunk RC, Kelly HW. Long-term effect of budesonide on hypothalamic–pituitary–adrenal axis function in children with mild to moderate asthma. Pediatrics 2004;113:1693–9.

75. Agertoft L, Pedersen S. Short-term lower-leg growth rate and urine cortisol excretion in children treated with ciclesonide. J Allergy Clin Immunol 2005;115:940–5.

76. Sim D, Griffiths A, Armstrong D, Clarke C, Rodda C, Freezer N. Adrenal suppression from high-dose inhaled fluticasone propionate in children with asthma. Eur Respir J 2003;21:633–6.

77. Kannisto S, Korppi M, Remes K, Voutilainen R. Adrenal suppression, evaluated by a low dose adrenocorticotropin test, and growth in asthmatic children treated with inhaled steroids. J Clin Endocrinol Metab 2000;85(2):652–7.

78. Shimada T, Yamazaki H, Mimura M, Inui Y, Guengerich FP. Interindividual variations in human liver cytochrome P-450 enzymes involved in the oxidation of drugs, carcinogens and toxic chemicals: studies with liver microsomes of 30 Japanese and 30 Caucasians. J Pharmacol Exp Ther 1994;270(1):414–23.

79. Derendorf H, Hochhaus G, Meibohm B, Mollmann H, Barth J. Pharmacokinetics and pharmacodynamics of inhaled corticosteroids. J Allergy Clin Immunol 1998;101(4 Pt 2):S440–6.

80. Onhoj J, Thorsson L, Bisgaard H. Lung deposition of inhaled drugs increases with age. Am J Respir Crit Care Med 2000;162(5):1819–22.

81. Russell G. Inhaled corticosteroids and adrenal insufficiency. Arch Dis Child 2002;87(6):455–6.

82. Russell G. Fluticasone propionate in children. Respir Med 1994;88(Suppl A):25–9.

83. Bousquet J, Ben-Joseph R, Messonnier M, Alemao E, Gould AL. A meta-analysis of the dose-response relationship of inhaled corticosteroids in adolescents and adults with mild to moderate persistent asthma. Clin Ther 2002;24(1):1–20.

84. Sizonenko PC. Effects of inhaled or nasal glucocorticosteroids on adrenal function and growth. J Pediatr Endocrinol Metab 2002;15(1):5–26.

85. Allen DB. Safety of inhaled corticosteroids in children. Pediatr Pulmonol 2002;33(3):208–20.

86. Faul JL, Tormey W, Tormey V, Burke C. High dose inhaled corticosteroids and dose dependent loss of diabetic control. BMJ 1998;317(7171):1491.

87. Faul JL, Cormican LJ, Tormey VJ, Tormey WP, Burke CM. Deteriorating diabetic control associated with high-dose inhaled budesonide. Eur Respir J 1999;14(1):242–3.

88. Dendukuri N, Blais L, LeLorier J. Inhaled corticosteroids and the risk of diabetes among the elderly. Br J Clin Pharmacol 2002;54(1):59–64.

89. Blackburn D, Hux J, Mamdani M. Quantification of the risk of corticosteroid-induced diabetes mellitus among the elderly. J Gen Intern Med 2002;17(9):717–20.

90. Capewell S, Reynolds S, Shuttleworth D, Edwards C, Finlay AY. Purpura and dermal thinning associated with high dose inhaled corticosteroids. BMJ 1990;300(6739):1548–51.

91. Mak VH, Melchor R, Spiro SG. Easy bruising as a side-effect of inhaled corticosteroids. Eur Respir J 1992;5(9):1068–74.

92. Haapasaari K, Rossi O, Risteli J, Oikarinen A. Effects of long-term inhaled corticosteroids on skin collagen synthesis and thickness in asthmatic patients. Eur Respir J 1998;11(1):139–43.

93. Malo JL, Cartier A, Ghezzo H, Mark S, Brown J, Laviolette M, Boulet LP. Skin bruising, adrenal function and markers of bone metabolism in asthmatics using inhaled beclomethasone and fluticasone. Eur Respir J 1999;13(5):993–8.

94. Dooms-Goossens A. Allergy to inhaled corticosteroids: a review. Am J Contact Dermatitis 1995;6:1–3.

95. Isaksson M, Bruze M, Hornblad Y, Svenonius E, Wihl JA. Contact allergy to corticosteroids in asthma/rhinitis patients. Contact Dermatitis 1999;40(6):327–8.

96. Isaksson M. Skin reactions to inhaled corticosteroids. Drug Saf 2001;24(5):369–73.

97. Israel E, Banerjee TR, Garrett MPH, Fitzmaurice GM, Kotlov TV, LaHive K, LeBoff MS. Effects of inhaled glucocorticoids on bone density in premenopausal women. N Engl J Med 2001;345(13):941–7.

98. Shiri J, Amichai B. Perioral dermatitis induced by inhaled corticosteroids. J Dermatol Treat 1998;9:259–60.

99. Ellepola AN, Samaranayake LP. Inhalational and topical steroids, and oral candidosis: a mini review. Oral Dis 2001;7(4):211–6.

100. National Asthma Education Program, National Institutes of Health. Guidelines for the Diagnosis and Management of Asthma. Publication No 91–3042 Bethesda: United States Department of Health and Human Services;. 1991.

101. Isaksson M, Bruze M. Allergic contact dermatitis in response to budesonide reactivated by inhalation of the allergen. J Am Acad Dermatol 2002;46(6):880–5.

102. Laatikainen AK, Kroger HP, Tukiainen HO, Honkanen RJ, Saarikoski SV. Bone mineral density in perimenopausal women with asthma: a population-based cross-sectional study. Am J Respir Crit Care Med 1999;159(4 Pt 1):1179–85.

103. Wong CA, Subakumar G, Casey PM. Effects of asthma and asthma therapies on bone mineral density. Curr Opin Pulm Med 2002;8(1):39–44.

104. Fujita K, Kasayama S, Hashimoto J, Nagasaka Y, Nakano N, Morimoto Y, Barnes PJ, Miyatake A. Inhaled corticosteroids reduce bone mineral density in early post-menopausal but not premenopausal asthmatic women. J Bone Miner Res 2001;16(4):782–7.

105. Sivri A, Coplu L. Effect of the long-term use of inhaled corticosteroids on bone mineral density in asthmatic women. Respirology 2001;6(2):131–4.

106. Harmanci E, Colak O, Metintas M, Alatas O, Yurdasiper A. Fluticasone propionate and budesonide do not influence bone metabolism in the long term treatment of asthma. Allergol Immunopathol (Madr) 2001;29(1):22–7.

107. Reilly SM, Hambleton G, Adams JE, Mughal MZ. Bone density in asthmatic children treated with inhaled corticosteroids. Arch Dis Child 2001;84(2):183–4.

108. Tattersfield AE, Town GI, Johnell O, Picado C, Aubier M, Braillon P, Karlstrom R. Bone mineral density in subjects with mild asthma randomised to treatment with inhaled corticosteroids or non-corticosteroid treatment for two years. Thorax 2001;56(4):272–8.

109. Poon E, Fewings JM. Generalized eczematous reaction to budesonide in a nasal spray with cross-reactivity to triamcinolone. Australas J Dermatol 2001;42(1):36–7.

110. Bennett ML, Fountain JM, McCarty MA, Sherertz EF. Contact allergy to corticosteroids in patients using inhaled or intranasal corticosteroids for allergic rhinitis or asthma. Am J Contact Dermat 2001;12(4):193–6.

111. Bahceciler NN, Sezgin G, Nursoy MA, Barlan IB, Basaran MM. Inhaled corticosteroids and bone density of children with asthma. J Asthma 2002;39(2):151–7.

112. Agertoft L, Pedersen S. Bone mineral density in children with asthma receiving long-term treatment with inhaled budesonide. Am J Respir Crit Care Med 1998;157(1):178–83.

113. Ma DQ, Jones G. Clinical risk factors but not bone density are associated with prevalent fractures in prepubertal children. J Paediatr Child Health 2002;38(5):497–500.

114. van Staa TP, Leufkens HG, Cooper C. Use of inhaled corticosteroids and risk of fractures. J Bone Miner Res 2001;16(3):581–8.

115. Gregson RK, Rao R, Murrills AJ, Taylor PA, Warner JO. Effect of inhaled corticosteroids on bone mineral density in childhood asthma: comparison of fluticasone propionate with beclomethasone dipropionate. Osteoporos Int 1998;8(5):418–22.

116. Johnell O, Pauwels R, Lofdahl CG, Laitinen LA, Postma DS, Pride NB, Ohlsson SV. Bone mineral density in patients with chronic obstructive pulmonary disease treated with budesonide Turbuhaler. Eur Respir J 2002;19(6):1058–63.

117. Lung Health Study Research Group. Effect of inhaled triamcinolone on the decline in pulmonary function in chronic obstructive pulmonary disease. N Engl J Med 2000;343(26):1902–9.

118. Fitzgerald D, Van Asperen P, Mellis C, Honner M, Smith L, Ambler G. Fluticasone propionate 750 micrograms/day versus beclomethasone dipropionate 1500 micrograms/day: comparison of efficacy and adrenal function in paediatric asthma. Thorax 1998;53(8):656–61.

119. Hughes JA, Conry BG, Male SM, Eastell R. One year prospective open study of the effect of high dose inhaled steroids, fluticasone propionate, and budesonide on bone markers and bone mineral density. Thorax 1999;54(3):223–9.

120. Hubbard RB, Smith CJ, Smeeth L, Harrison TW, Tattersfield AE. Inhaled corticosteroids and hip fracture: a population-based case-control study. Am J Respir Crit Care Med 2002;166(12 Pt 1):1563–6.

121. Martinati LC, Bertoldo F, Gasperi E, Fortunati P, Lo Cascio V, Boner AL. Longitudinal evaluation of bone mass in asthmatic children treated with inhaled beclomethasone dipropionate or cromolyn sodium. Allergy 1998;53(7):705–8.

122. Price JF, Russell G, Hindmarsh PC, Weller P, Heaf DP, Williams J. Growth during one year of treatment with fluticasone propionate or sodium cromoglycate in children with asthma. Pediatr Pulmonol 1997;24(3):178–86.

123. Bonala SB, Reddy BM, Silverman BA, Bassett CW, Rao YA, Amara S, Schneider AT. Bone mineral density in women with asthma on long-term inhaled corticosteroid therapy. Ann Allergy Asthma Immunol 2000;85(6 Pt 1): 495–500.

124. Wong CA, Walsh LJ, Smith CJ, Wisniewski AF, Lewis SA, Hubbard R, Cawte S, Green DJ, Pringle M, Tattersfield AE. Inhaled corticosteroid use and bone-mineral density in patients with asthma. Lancet 2000;355(9213):1399–403.

125. Boulet LP, Milot J, Gagnon L, Poubelle PE, Brown J. Long-term influence of inhaled corticosteroids on bone metabolism and density. Are biological markers predictors of bone loss? Am J Respir Crit Care Med 1999;159(3):838–44.

126. Sambrook P, Birmingham J, Kempler S, Kelly P, Eberl S, Pocock N, Yeates M, Eisman J. Corticosteroid effects on proximal femur bone loss. J Bone Miner Res 1990;5(12):1211–6.

127. Herrala J, Puolijoki H, Impivaara O, Liippo K, Tala E, Nieminen MM. Bone mineral density in asthmatic women on high-dose inhaled beclomethasone dipropionate. Bone 1994;15(6):621–3.

128. Ebeling PR, Erbas B, Hopper JL, Wark JD, Rubinfeld AR. Bone mineral density and bone turnover in asthmatics treated with long-term inhaled or oral gluco-corticoids. J Bone Miner Res 1998;13(8):1283–9.

129. Wang WQ, Ip MS, Tsang KW, Lam KS. Antiresorptive therapy in asthmatic patients receiving high-dose inhaled steroids: a prospective study for 18 months. J Allergy Clin Immunol 1998;101(4 Pt 1):445–50.

130. Herrala J, Puolijoki H, Liippo K, Raitio M, Impivaara O, Tala E, Nieminen MM. Clodronate is effective in preventing corticosteroid-induced bone loss among asthmatic patients. Bone 1998;22(5):577–82.

131. Lo Cascio V, Bonucci E, Imbimbo B, Ballanti P, Adami S, Milani S, Tartarotti D, DellaRocca C. Bone loss in response to long-term glucocorticoid therapy. Bone Miner 1990;8(1):39–51.

132. Allen DB. Influence of inhaled corticosteroids on growth: a pediatric endocrinologist's perspective. Acta Paediatr 1998;87(2):123–9.

133. Norjavaara E, Gerhardsson De Verdier M, Lindmark B. Reduced height in swedish men with asthma at the age of conscription for military service. J Pediatr 2000;137(1): 25–29.

134. Agertoft L, Pedersen S. Effect of long-term treatment with inhaled budesonide on adult height in children with asthma. N Engl J Med 2000;343(15):1064–9.

135. Brand PL. Inhaled corticosteroids reduce growth. Or do they? Eur Respir J 2001;17(2):287–94.

136. Price J, Hindmarsh P, Hughes S, Effthimiou J. Evaluating the effects of asthma therapy on childhood growth: principles of study design. Eur Respir J 2002;19(6):1167–78.

137. Price J, Hindmarsh P, Hughes S, Efthimiou J. Evaluating the effects of asthma therapy on childhood growth: what can be learnt from the published literature? Eur Respir J 2002;19(6):1179–93.

138. Wolthers OD. Growth problems in children with asthma. Horm Res 2002;57(Suppl 2):83–7.

139. Wolthers OD, Allen DB. Inhaled corticosteroids, growth, and compliance. N Engl J Med 2002;347(15):1210–1.

140. Allen DB. Inhaled corticosteroid therapy for asthma in preschool children: growth issues. Pediatrics 2002;109(Suppl 2):373–80.

141. Pedersen S. Do inhaled corticosteroids inhibit growth in children? Am J Respir Crit Care Med 2001;164(4):521–35.

142. Thorsson L, Edsbacker S, Kallen A, Lofdahl CG. Pharmacokinetics and systemic activity of fluticasone via Diskus and pMDI, and of budesonide via Turbuhaler. Br J Clin Pharmacol 2001;52(5):529–38.

143. Ferguson AC, Spier S, Manjra A, Versteegh FG, Mark S, Zhang P. Efficacy and safety of high-dose inhaled steroids in children with asthma: a comparison of fluticasone propionate with budesonide. J Pediatr 1999;134(4):422–7.

144. The Childhood Asthma Management Program Research Group. Long-term effects of budesonide or nedocromil in children with asthma. N Engl J Med 2000;343(15):1054–63.

145. Allen DB, Mullen M, Mullen B. A meta-analysis of the effect of oral and inhaled corticosteroids on growth. J Allergy Clin Immunol 1994;93(6):967–76.

146. Doull IJ, Campbell MJ, Holgate ST. Duration of growth suppressive effects of regular inhaled corticosteroids. Arch Dis Child 1998;78(2):172–3.

147. Balfour-Lynn L. Growth and childhood asthma. Arch Dis Child 1986;61(11):1049–55.

148. Priori R, Tomassini M, Magrini L, Conti F, Valesini G. Churg–Strauss syndrome during pregnancy after steroid withdrawal. Lancet 1998;352(9140):1599–600.

149. Sears MR, Taylor DR. The beta 2-agonist controversy. Observations, explanations and relationship to asthma epidemiology. Drug Saf 1994;11(4):259–83.

150. Fukushima C, Matsuse H, Tomari S, Obase Y, Miyazaki Y, Shimoda T, Kohno S. Oral candidiasis associated with inhaled corticosteroid use: comparison of fluticasone and

beclomethasone. Ann Allergy Asthma Immunol 2003;90:646–51.

151. Leav BA, Fanburg B, Hadley S. Invasive pulmonary aspergillosis associated with high-dose inhaled fluticasone. N Engl J Med 2000;343(8):586.

152. Kallen B, Rydhstroem H, Aberg A. Congenital malformations after the use of inhaled budesonide in early pregnancy. Obstet Gynecol 1999;93(3):392–5.

153. Rouanet I, Peyriere H, Mauboussin JM, Vincent D. Cushing's syndrome in a patient treated by ritonavir/lopinavir and inhaled fluticasone. HIV Med 2003;4:149–50.

154. Raaska K, Niemi M, Neuvonen M, Neuvonen PJ, Kivisto KT. Plasma concentrations of inhaled budesonide and its effects on plasma cortisol are increased by the cytochrome P4503A4 inhibitor itraconazole. Clin Pharmacol Ther 2002;72(4):362–9.

155. De Wachter E, Vanbesien J, De Schutter I, Malfroot A, De Schepper J. Rapidly developing Cushing syndrome in a 4-year-old patient during combined treatment with itraconazole and inhaled budesonide. Eur J Pediatr 2003;162:488–9.

156. Bolland MJ, Bagg W, Thomas MG, Lucas JA, Ticehurst R, Black PN. Cushing's syndrome due to interaction between inhaled corticosteroids and itraconazole. Ann Pharmacother 2004;38:46–9.

157. Clevenbergh P, Corcostegui M, Gerard D, Hieronimus S, Mondain V, Chichmanian RM, Sadoul JL, Dellamonica P. Iatrogenic Cushing's syndrome in an HIV-infected patient treated with inhaled corticosteroids (fluticasone propionate) and low dose ritonavir enhanced PI containing regimen. J Infect 2002;44(3):194–5.

158. Samaras K, Pett S, Gowers A, McMurchie M, Cooper DA. Iatrogenic Cushing's syndrome with osteoporosis and secondary adrenal failure in human immunodeficiency virus-infected patients receiving inhaled corticosteroids and ritonavir-boosted protease inhibitors: six cases. J Clin Endocrinol Metab 2005;90(7):4394–8.

Prostaglandins

General Information

Eicosanoids are the oxygenated metabolites of 20-carbon unsaturated fatty acids found in the phospholipids of cell membranes (Greek eikosi = 20). The eicosanoids include the prostaglandins, thromboxanes, and leukotrienes. Precursor fatty acids include arachidonic acid C20:4n–6 (for 2-series prostaglandins and thromboxane and 4-series leukotrienes), dihomogammalinolenic acid C20:3n–6 (for PGE$_1$), and eicosapentaenoic acid C20:5n–3 (for 3-series prostaglandins and 5-series leukotrienes). Naturally occurring eicosanoids are predominantly metabolites of arachidonic acid, reflecting the dominance of n–6 fatty acids in the terrestrial food chain.

The principal biologically active, naturally occurring prostaglandins are prostaglandin E$_1$ (PGE$_1$), prostaglandin E$_2$ (PGE$_2$), prostaglandin F$_{2\alpha}$ (PGF$_{2\alpha}$), prostacyclin

Table 1 Indications for prostaglandin therapy

In obstetrics
   First- and second-trimester abortion
   Cervical reopening
   Induction of labor
   Augmentation of labor
   Postpartum hemorrhage
   Ectopic pregnancy
   Lactation suppression
In gastrointestinal disease
   Peptic ulceration
   Liver transplantation
   Chemotherapy-induced mucosal lesions
In cardiovascular disease
   Congenital cardiac malformations
   Raynaud's syndrome
   Chronic obstructive pulmonary disease
   Adult respiratory distress syndrome
   Pulmonary hypertension
   Arterial occlusive disease
   Extracorporeal circulation
In urology
   Erectile dysfunction
   Cystitis after radiation or chemotherapy
In ophthalmology
   Glaucoma

(PGI_2), and thromboxane (TXA_2). These agents have various, sometimes opposed, biological actions (1). Their half-lives are short, owing to their rapid breakdown (a few minutes for PGE_2 and $PGF_{2\alpha}$, a few seconds for PGI_2) (2). Prostaglandins thus have principally local biological actions. Analogues (mostly methyl derivatives) have been synthesized and are more slowly inactivated. The adverse reactions encountered when prostaglandins are used therapeutically will depend on the indications (see Table 1), since these will determine the dose and route of administration and hence the type of reaction likely to occur. Many of the problems experienced are attributable to their main pharmacological effects (Table 2).

Nomenclature

The names of prostaglandins are generally abbreviated to a three-letter abbreviation with a subscripted number. The first two letters are always PG; the third is E, F, or I. The recommended International Non-proprietary Names (rINNs) of various prostaglandins are given in Table 3. The convention is that, for example, PGE_1 is the name given to the endogenous prostaglandin and alprostadil is the name given to the same compound available for exogenous administration.

Synthetic analogues of PGE_1, PGE_2, PGF_1, $PGF_{2\alpha}$, and PGI_2

Synthetic analogues of prostaglandins are listed in Table 4. Their use allows reduction of dosages and adverse effects. In general, they cause fewer adverse effects than their naturally occurring counterparts, although this depends on the method of administration.

Newer analogues (3) and oral forms (4) are in development.

General adverse effects

The most prominent and frequent adverse effects of prostaglandins are those on the gastrointestinal tract. However, the most dangerous are likely to be the cardiovascular effects, which in predisposed patients can sometimes cause life-threatening collapse and heart failure. Hyperthermia and headache are frequent nervous system effects. Epileptiform convulsions occur rarely. When used for termination of pregnancy, uterine hyperstimulation and, less often, uterine rupture can occur (5). Hypersensitivity to prostaglandins can cause skin reactions, bronchospasm (also seen as a direct pharmacological effect), and occasionally anaphylaxis. Tumor-inducing effects have not been reported. There have been a few reports of infants with limb deformities with and without Möbius sequence after exposure to misoprostol (a PGE_1 analogue) in the first trimester.

Prostaglandins in cardiovascular disease

Maintenance of the ductus arteriosus
PGE_1 and PGE_2 are effective in maintaining the patency of the ductus arteriosus in the initial management of congenital cardiac malformations (6,7). The most frequent adverse effects during prolonged treatment are diarrhea, necrotizing enterocolitis, cortical hyperostosis (8–10), fever, respiratory depression and apnea, and seizure-like activity (11). The frequency of adverse effects is not necessarily reduced with low-dose intravenous or oral administration (12). Maternal/fetal hyperglycemia due to reduced insulin secretion is rare, except in the infants of diabetic mothers (13). Less common adverse effects include gastric outlet obstruction due to antral hyperplasia (14).

Raynaud's phenomenon and digital ischemia
Studies of PGE_1 infusion for treatment of Raynaud's syndrome have shown variable changes in frequency of attacks and of healing ischemic digital ulcers (15–18). Prostacyclin infusion (using PGI_2 or its synthetic analogue iloprost) appears to have beneficial effects, both in reducing the severity and frequency of attacks and healing ischemic digital ulcers. Adverse effects are common and include headache, flushing, jaw pain, nausea, vomiting, diarrhea, and inflammation and pain at the injection site (19,20). Iloprost has also been used effectively in the treatment of local gangrene secondary to chemotherapy (21). Application of a PGE_2 analogue to the skin produced both subjective and objective improvement in patients with Raynaud's syndrome and produced only minor self-limiting adverse effects (headache, flushing, and diarrhea) (22).

Peripheral vascular disease
Synthetic PGI_2 has been used in arterial occlusive disease as an anti-aggregatory drug (23–28). Adverse effects are common (85%). Headache, fever, nausea, anorexia, diarrhea, pain at the infusion site, and arthralgia are the most prominent. A single study has suggested an increased risk

Table 2 Actions of prostaglandins

Prostaglandin E series
  Increased hormone secretion
    Growth hormone, corticotropin, thyrotropin, luteinizing hormone, thyroid hormone, insulin, glucocorticoids, progesterone, erythropoietin, renin
  Increased body temperature
  Sensitization of pain-mediating nerve fibers
  Increased force of myocardial contraction
  Increased blood flow in gastric mucosa, liver, kidney, and placenta
  Increased renal secretion of sodium, potassium, and water
  Antagonistic action against antidiuretic hormone
  Increased intraocular pressure
  Increased permeability of blood capillaries
  Increased gastrointestinal motility
  Reduced gastrointestinal secretions
  Reduced blood pressure
  Bronchodilatation
  Inhibition of bronchial secretions
  Sedation
  Contraction of the non-pregnant uterus
  Induction of abortion and labor
Prostaglandin F series
  Bronchial constriction, especially in patients with asthma
  Reduced pulmonary blood flow and increased pulmonary blood pressure
  Increased erythropoietin secretion
  Increased neurotransmission at sympathetic nerve endings
  Increased gastrointestinal motility
  Reduced blood pressure
  Sedation (effects on the central nervous system)
  Luteolytic effects in mammalian species (except man)
  Induction of abortion and labor
Prostaglandin I series
  Reduced platelet aggregation
  Reduced mean arterial pressure
  Reduced total peripheral and pulmonary resistances
  Increased heart rate
  Increased renal secretion of sodium (tubular effect)

Table 3 Recommended International Non-proprietary Names (rINNs) and chemical names of the major prostaglandins

Prostaglandin	rINN	Chemical name (omitting stereochemical information)
PGE_1	Alprostadil	11,15-dihydroxy-9-oxoprosta-13-en-1-oic acid
PGE_2	Dinoprostone	11,15-dihydroxy-9-oxoprosta-5,13-dien-1-oic acid
$PGF_{2\alpha}$	Dinoprost	9,11,15-trihydroxyprosta-5,13-dien-1-oic acid
PGI_2 (PGX, prostacyclin)	Epoprostenol	6,9-epoxy-11,15-dihydroxyprosta-5,13-dien-1-oic acid

of thromboembolism after the use of iloprost in peripheral vascular disease (29).

Beraprost, an epoprostenol (PGI_2) analogue, has been studied in intermittent claudication. Adverse events include gastrointestinal disorders, headaches, skin disorders, and fever (30).

Primary pulmonary hypertension
Initial studies of continuous intravenous prostacyclin infusion in patients with primary pulmonary hypertension have shown sustained improvement in pulmonary artery pressure, exercise capacity, and survival compared with historical controls (31,32). Minor complications (diarrhea, jaw pain, flushing, photosensitivity, and headache) were dose-related. Serious complications were related to problems with the drug delivery system, including catheter thrombosis, sepsis, and temporary interruption of the infusion, resulting in abrupt deterioration (31).

Table 4 Synthetic analogues of prostaglandins (rINNs except where stated)

PGE₁ analogues
   Enisoprost
   Limaprost
   Mexiprostil
   Misoprostol
   Ornoprostil
   Rioprostil
   Rosaprostol
PGE₂ analogues
   Arbaprostil
   Enprostil
   Gemeprost
   Meteneprost
   Nocloprost
   Sulprostone
   Trimoprostol
   Viprostol
PGF₁ analogues
   Prostalene (pINN)
PGF₂ₐ analogues
   Alfaprostol
   Bimatoprost
   Carboprost
   Cloprostenol
   Fenprostalene
   Fluprostenol
   Latanoprost
   Luprostiol
   Tiaprost
   Travoprost
   Unoprostone
PGI₂ analogues
   Beraprost
   Cicaprost
   Ciprostene
   Iloprost

Regulation of pulmonary vascular perfusion in advanced respiratory disease

PGE_1 significantly reduces right ventricular pulmonary after-load in patients with pulmonary hypertension due to chronic obstructive airways disease (33). PGE_1 can also be useful in the treatment of adult respiratory distress syndrome (34). Preliminary studies using aerosolized prostacyclin showed a reduction in pulmonary artery pressure and improved arterial oxygenation with reduction in intrapulmonary shunt in ventilated patients with adult respiratory distress syndrome (35) and severe community-acquired pneumonia (36). However, ventilated patients with severe community-acquired pneumonia and pre-existing fibrosis required much higher doses, with a reduction in systemic vascular resistance and an increase in intrapulmonary shunting (36). A single report described improved oxygenation, mainly due to reduction of intrapulmonary shunting, in two neonates with pulmonary hypertension treated with aerosolized prostacyclin (37).

Other uses

PGI_2 has been used to reduce the re-stenosis rate during transluminal coronary angioplasty (38).

Prostacyclin infusion (using PGI_2 or its synthetic analogue, iloprost) has been used during extracorporeal circulation to prevent blood clotting in the dialyser coil (39). The risk of severe hypotension can be avoided by carefully controlling the infusion rate.

Prostaglandins in gastrointestinal disease

Peptic ulceration and NSAID-induced gastropathy

Prostaglandins of the E series (misoprostol, enprostil) have antiulcer activity in the upper gastrointestinal tract (40). They inhibit gastric acid secretion at modest doses and provide mucosal protection against noxious agents, including non-steroidal anti-inflammatory drugs, smoking, alcohol, and chemotherapy. They have been used to prevent NSAID-induced gastroduodenal lesions (41,42). They may also be effective in preventing NSAID-induced renal impairment (43).

The cure rate for gastric and duodenal ulcers is comparable to the results with H_2-receptor antagonists (44–46). Relapses appear to be fewer with prostaglandin therapy (44,45). Healing of duodenal ulcers refractory to H_2-receptor antagonists has been described.

Diarrhea (4–38%), abdominal pain or cramp, flatulence, and nausea or vomiting account for most of the adverse effects reported. No biochemical or hematological adverse effects have been noted.

These agents are contraindicated in women of childbearing age, unless they are using adequate contraceptive measures, because of uncertain abortifacient effects. They have been used as illegal abortifacients in some countries (47).

Prostaglandins in liver disease

Liver failure and transplant dysfunction

Prostaglandins of the E series (both intravenous and oral formulations) have been used to treat fulminant hepatic failure, primary non-function following orthotopic liver transplantation, and recurrent hepatitis B infection after orthotopic liver transplantation in open trials (48–50). Adverse effects are almost universal. They include gastrointestinal symptoms (abdominal pain and cramping, watery diarrhea), which affect 33–100% and are more common with oral formulations and possibly amongst those with raised blood glucose concentrations. Cardiovascular effects, which affect about 33%, include migraine, hypotension, peripheral edema, and myocardial infarction (in those with pre-existing risk factors). Painful clubbing and cortical hyperostosis (92–100%) developed 10–60 days after the start of intravenous or oral therapy. Arthritis/arthralgia developed in 8% of those receiving intravenous and 92% of those taking oral PGE_1 or PGE_2. All adverse reactions appear to be dose-related and resolve with reductions in dose. Two patients developed calcium oxalate stones after 1 year of oral therapy (51).

Prostaglandins in urology

Prostacyclin infusion in men with persistent pain associated with Peyronie's disease was of little value but produced marked adverse effects (bradycardia, hypotension, nausea, flushing) (52).

A single dose of PGE_1 into the corpus cavernosum is highly effective in inducing artificial penile erection in cases of erectile dysfunction. The reported adverse effects include pain and a burning sensation, prolonged penile erection, and local fibrosis. The incidence of pain was high (75%) in older studies (53), while later data improved to 13–44% (54–57). Pain is cited as a prominent factor in non-adherence to therapy and in the dropout rate of patients from self-injection programs, although the incidence may fall with time (57). An alprostadil sterile powder formulation had a lower incidence of pain after penile injection (6.6%), attributed to lower doses and the lack of alcohol in the formulation (58). Burning and pain can be reduced by using a lower initial dose, with incremental increases until a satisfactory erection is produced (59).

Although the incidence of priapism varies in different studies, depending on its definition (erection lasting anywhere from 2 to 11 hours), an analysis of 48 studies in 8090 patients showed an overall incidence of 1% (55).

Prolonged erections induced by PGE_1 usually require drainage and phenylephrine irrigation, although a small percentage can be managed with oral terbutaline or oral pseudoephedrine if treated within 3 hours of PGE_1 injection (56). Local fibrosis is infrequent, occurring in 2% at 6 months and in 8% at 18 months (60). A single case of Peyronie's-like plaque and penile curvature deformity has been reported after repeated PGE_1 use (61).

Complications of alprostadil injections include hematoma and ecchymoses (8%) and systemic effects (6%), which mostly occur in the urogenital system (testicular pain and swelling, scrotal pain and edema, changes in urinary frequency, hematuria, and pelvic pain) (62). In 1% there were symptoms related to hypotension.

Massive diffuse hemorrhage due to cyclophosphamide-induced or radiation cystitis has been treated successfully with intravesicular PGE_1, PGE_2, and carboprost. Febrile reactions and severe bladder spasm are dose-dependent (63–65).

Prostaglandins in ophthalmology

Topical PGE_2 and $PGF_{2\alpha}$ significantly reduce intraocular pressure for at least 24 hours and are used in the treatment of glaucoma. Derivatives of the isopropyl ester of $PGF_{2\alpha}$ appear to be the most effective. Transient ocular adverse effects include conjunctival hyperemia, local irritation, intermittent photophobia, and pain in the eye (66–68). Newer derivatives, such as latanoprost, travoprost, and bimatoprost, appear to be better tolerated, with less severe and less frequent adverse effects (69). They reduce intraocular pressure by increasing uveoscleral outflow. The ocular pressure-lowering effect of latanoprost appears to be additive with timolol, with mild transient hyperemia in 50% of those treated with latanoprost alone (70).

Latanoprost, travoprost, and bimatoprost cause increased pigmentation of the iris in some patients after prolonged treatment (3.0–4.5 months) (71). Most data have been obtained with latanoprost, and it appears that there is a predisposition to iris pigmentation in patients with eyes of hazel or heterochromic color. As latanoprost and travoprost are selective agonists at $PGF_{2\alpha}$ receptors, it is likely that the phenomenon is mediated by these receptors. Latanoprost stimulates melanogenesis in iris melanocytes, and transcription of the tyrosinase gene is upregulated. No evidence of harmful consequences of this adverse effect has been found, and the only disadvantage appears to be potential heterochromia between the eyes in unilaterally treated patients: the heterochromia is likely to be permanent, or very slowly reversible (72–74).

The adverse effects of travoprost include gradual darkening of the color of the iris and the eyelid skin, increased thickness, number, and darkness of the eyelashes, conjunctival hyperemia, and ocular pruritus (75).

Cystoid macular edema, iritis, *Herpes simplex* keratitis, periocular skin darkening, and headaches have been described in patients treated with prostaglandin analogues. These adverse effects occur rarely, and cystoid macular edema, iritis and *H. simplex* keratitis occur in eyes with risk factors. Repeated rechallenge with masked controls is required to establish a causal relation. However, even without firm establishment of a causal relation, caution is advised with the use of prostaglandin analogues in the eyes of patients with risk factors for macular edema, iritis, and *H. simplex* keratitis (76).

The ocular adverse effects of latanoprost include conjunctival hyperemia, iris pigmentation, periocular skin color changes, anterior uveitis, and cystoid macular edema in pseudophakic patients (77,78). *H. simplex* dendritic keratitis has been reported after treatment with latanoprost (79). In patients with uveitic glaucoma, latanoprost can cause increased intraocular pressure and recurrence of inflammation (80).

Exacerbation of angina pectoris has been described in association with latanoprost (81). $PGF_{2\alpha}$ is a vasoconstrictor, and systemic absorption of topical latanoprost can cause vasoconstriction in coronary arteries.

Three patients had new-onset migraine after using latanoprost, perhaps through activation of the trigeminal vascular system (82).

Prostaglandins in obstetrics

Prostaglandins of the E and F series are widely used in obstetrics for ripening the uterine cervix and stimulating uterine contraction at any stage of pregnancy. They are used in first- and second-trimester abortions, cervical priming, the induction and augmentation of labor, and postpartum hemorrhage (83–89). The route of administration can be vaginal, cervical, extra-amniotic, intra-amniotic, oral, intramuscular, or intravenous, and varies according to indication. Mifepristone (RU 486), a synthetic 19-norsteroid and progesterone antagonist, has been used in combination with synthetic prostaglandins in the induction of abortion.

A less well-established use involves intratubal injection of $PGF_{2\alpha}$ for ectopic pregnancy (90,91). Oral PGE_2 can be used to suppress lactation, for which it is as effective as bromocriptine, and causes less breast tenderness (92).

Organs and Systems

Cardiovascular

Both PGE_2 and $PGF_{2\alpha}$ commonly cause a fall in blood pressure and a degree of bradycardia (1,93). PGE_2 can cause vasodilatation of small vessels and $PGF_{2\alpha}$ can cause vasoconstriction (94). These changes are common but often mild. However, angina pectoris and myocardial infarction have been reported with prostaglandins of all types, particularly after inadvertent intramyometrial injection (95–98). A single case of pulmonary edema after the infusion of PGE_1 has been reported (99). In patients with pre-existing cardiovascular disease, the risk of serious aggravation is very real, and both pre-existing hypertension and states of shock can be worsened. A severe rise in maternal blood pressure occurred in a few cases in which fetal death was associated with unresolved pre-eclampsia.

Respiratory

People with asthma are more sensitive than healthy subjects to bronchoconstriction induced by $PGF_{2\alpha}$ (100,101).

Nervous system

Increased body temperature, pyrexia (both intra- and postpartum), and chills are thought to result from central stimulation of temperature regulatory centers by prostaglandins (102,103). Headache and migraine are the most common adverse effects on the central nervous system (5,104).

Prostaglandin therapy can cause electroencephalographic abnormalities (105). Convulsions, which occur occasionally, are a particular risk in epileptic patients (5,104,105). The combination of prostaglandins and oxytocin can be complicated by tonic-clonic seizures (106).

Enhancement of the pain sensation may reflect a direct effect on nerve fibers. The presence of pain correlates well with the effect on the uterus.

Sensory systems

Increased intraocular pressure and miosis have been reported (5,104).

Mouth and teeth

Gingivitis has been associated with obstetric prostaglandins (5).

Gastrointestinal

Nausea, vomiting, diarrhea, and abdominal pain (107) occur in about 90% of all patients given prostaglandins systemically. The frequency and duration of these adverse effects depend on the mode of application, the dosage, and the molecule used, and are very variable (108).

Reproductive system

Uterine hypertonia and hyperstimulation are well-recognized adverse effects of induction of abortion and labor with prostaglandins. Cervical rupture and uterine rupture have been reported with every prostaglandin and analogue, even in previously unscarred uteri (5,109–116). The risks can be minimized by using lower doses (0.5 mg intracervically or 3 mg intravaginally), by allowing longer intervals between re-applications, and by avoiding combination with oxytocin, which has a potentiating effect. However, there is a single case report of uterine rupture in a multiparous woman with unscarred uterus following low-dose (1.5 mg) intravaginal PGE_2 (117). In the event of uterine hyperstimulation, beta$_2$-adrenoceptor agonists may reduce uterine contractility. Intensive monitoring of uterine activity and fetal condition is mandatory, since the rate of absorption of PGE_2 after intravaginal or cervical administration is unpredictable.

Second-Generation Effects

Teratogenicity

Seven Brazilian infants were born with limb deficiencies both with and without Möbius sequence after exposure to misoprostol in the first trimester during unsuccessful abortion attempts (118).

Fetotoxicity

Like oxytocin, prostaglandins have been responsible rarely for fetal distress and even fetal death (119,120). The risk of fetal death underlines the importance of cardiotocography during prostaglandin (pre)induction. Prostaglandins should be used with extreme caution if there is a risk of placental insufficiency (120).

The incidence of neonatal jaundice was not increased after induction of labor with prostaglandins (47).

Susceptibility Factors

When PGE_2 and $PGF_{2\alpha}$ are used for induction of labor and abortion, the following contraindications must be respected and (until proven otherwise) also apply to the methyl analogues of these two prostaglandins:

- previous cesarean section or hysterotomy (because of the risk of rupture) (110);
- previous major abdominal surgery;
- prior abnormal delivery;
- a history of severe abdominal inflammation and/or infection;

- a predisposition to uterine cramps or tetanus uteri.

However, uneventful vaginal deliveries have been reported in patients with two previous cesarean sections in whom labor was induced with vaginal PGE_2 (121). Women with a history of six or more deliveries and anomalies of the fetus (for example hydrocephalus causing cephalopelvic disproportion) must also be excluded.

Predispositions to glaucoma, epilepsy, pre-eclampsia, hypertension, asthma, and ischemic heart disease are relative contraindications.

Drug Administration

Drug administration route

Intrauterine infusion
Intrauterine infusion (intra-amniotic or extra-amniotic) has been reported to be associated with fewer gastrointestinal symptoms and less fever than parenteral or intravaginal administration (122). In intra-amniotic use, the puncture must be guided by ultrasonography, and before injection a control aspiration of some amniotic fluid is required in order to avoid intrauterine or intravascular injection. Uterine rupture has been described with intra-amniotic treatment.

Intramuscular or intradermal injection
Inflammation and pain are common at the site of injection when prostaglandins are given intramuscularly or intradermally (123,124).

Intravenous injection
Prostaglandins have been used intravenously, both for induction of mid-trimester abortion and for induction of labor in cases of intrauterine death. The same adverse effects as described above occur, and are usually very pronounced. Routine premedication with an antiemetic and an antidiarrheal agent significantly reduces gastrointestinal adverse effects.

Inhalation
Intravenous epoprostenol increases exercise tolerance, improves pulmonary hemodynamics, and improves survival in patients with primary pulmonary hypertension. However, there are limitations to intravenous administration, and a significant proportion of patients develop catheter-related problems, such as thrombosis, pump failure, and catheter-related sepsis. In an attempt to improve delivery, several trials of aerosolized prostacyclin have been undertaken, primarily in patients with primary pulmonary hypertension.

There has been a sequential comparison of inhaled nitric oxide 40 ppm with aerosolized iloprost 14–17 micrograms in 35 adults with primary pulmonary hypertension (125). Five of the patients had minor headache and facial flushing during inhalation of iloprost, but these symptoms were short-lived and abated a few minutes after the inhalation ended. One patient had mild jaw pain after aerosolized iloprost, but again this was short-lived. There was an unexpected increase in pulmonary artery pressure in 10 patients and vascular resistance in six patients who received nitric oxide. The authors were uncertain of the cause of this increase, as nitric oxide generally behaves as a vasodilator, but they noted that nitric oxide is a vasoconstrictor in certain conditions, such as the presence of hemolysate (126).

There has been a trial of aerosolized iloprost in 24 patients with primary pulmonary hypertension and New York Heart Association class III or IV disability, who were refractory to conventional medical treatment (127). They were given aerosolized iloprost in a total daily dose of 100–150 micrograms (in 6–8 divided doses, given every 2–3 hours while awake) over 12 months. The treatment was generally well tolerated, except for coughing during inhalation, which was common initially but resolved spontaneously in all patients within the first 4 weeks. Five patients reported symptoms of flushing, headache, and jaw pain at the end of inhalation, but all rated the symptoms as mild and none discontinued treatment because of adverse effects. There was an asymptomatic but significant fall in systemic arterial pressure (from 98 to 90 mmHg) and vascular resistance at 3 and 12 months compared with baseline.

The effects of aerosolized iloprost have been reported in three patients with severe pulmonary hypertension (mean pulmonary artery pressure 50 mmHg or more) who were already being treated with intravenous epoprostenol (10–16 micrograms/kg/minute) (128). The aim of the study was to replace continuous intravenous epoprostenol with intermittent aerosolized iloprost (150–300 micrograms/day in 6–18 divided doses). All three patients had gradual weaning of intravenous epoprostenol (1 micrograms/kg/minute every 3–10 hours) under close supervision and hemodynamic monitoring in intensive care. All three had initial falls in pulmonary arterial pressure and improved right ventricular function with inhaled iloprost. The first could not be fully weaned from epoprostenol, because of right ventricular failure with dyspnea and hypoxemia, accompanied by a three-fold increase in serum bilirubin and lactate dehydrogenase and echocardiographically demonstrated right ventricular failure. The second and third patients both tolerated complete withdrawal of epoprostenol. However, one developed right ventricular failure within 2 hours of withdrawal. The third was successfully discharged from hospital taking aerosolized therapy, but presented 2 weeks later with severe right ventricular failure. Thus, caution should be taken in patients who have been previously maintained on intravenous prostacyclin when trying to convert to aerosolized therapy, as there appears to be a high chance of treatment failure, which can occur abruptly.

Platelet function after inhaled prostacyclin has been measured in a randomized, double-blind study in 28 patients undergoing elective cardiothoracic surgery (129). They were given aerosolized prostacyclin (5 or 10 micrograms) for 6 hours postoperatively. All the patients, regardless of dose, had a lower rate of platelet aggregation in response to adenosine diphosphate (ADP) than controls. There were no differences in clinically significant indices, such as chest tube drainage or bleeding time. This study has shown that prostacyclin, given as an aerosol, can cause measurable alterations in platelet function, with a possibly higher risk of bleeding.

References

1. Dusting GJ, Moncada S, Vane JR. Prostaglandins, their intermediates and precursors: cardiovascular actions and regulatory roles in normal and abnormal circulatory systems. Prog Cardiovasc Dis 1979;21(6):405–30.
2. Nakano J. General pharmacology of prostaglandins. In: Cuthbert MF, editor. The Prostaglandins: Pharmacological and Therapeutic Advances. Philadelphia: JB Lippincott, 1973:23–124.
3. Hattori R, Yui Y, Shirotani M, Kawai C. A stable prostacyclin analogue, 9B methylcarbacyclin (U-61, 431F). Cardiovasc Drug Rev 1992;10:233–42.
4. Hildebrand M, Pfeffer M, Mahler M, Staks T, Windt-Hanke F, Schutt A. Oral iloprost in healthy volunteers. Eicosanoids 1991;4(3):149–54.
5. Karim SMM. Prostaglandin—physiological basis of practical applications. In: Proceedings 6th Asia and Oceania Congress in Endocrinology 1978;.
6. Momma K, Takao A, Sone K, Tashiro M. Prostaglandin E1 treatment of ductus-dependent infants with congenital heart disease. Int Angiol 1984;3:33.
7. van der Sijp JR, Rohmer J. Prostaglandinetherapie bij pasgeborenen met een ductus Botalli-afhankeliijke circulatie. [Prostaglandin therapy in newborn infants with a Botalli duct-dependent circulation.] Tijdschr Kindergeneeskd 1985;53(1):20–5.
8. Woo K, Emery J, Peabody J. Cortical hyperostosis: a complication of prolonged prostaglandin infusion in infants awaiting cardiac transplantation. Pediatrics 1994;93(3):417–20.
9. Letts M, Pang E, Simons J. Prostaglandin-induced neonatal periostitis. J Pediatr Orthop 1994;14(6):809–13.
10. Kaufman MB, El-Chaar GM. Bone and tissue changes following prostaglandin therapy in neonates. Ann Pharmacother 1996;30(3):269–77.
11. Lewis AB, Freed MD, Heymann MA, Roehl SL, Kensey RC. Side effects of therapy with prostaglandin E1 in infants with critical congenital heart disease. Circulation 1981;64(5):893–8.
12. Singh GK, Fong LV, Salmon AP, Keeton BR. Study of low dosage prostaglandin—usages and complications. Eur Heart J 1994;15(3):377–81.
13. Cohen MH, Nihill MR. Postoperative ketotic hyperglycemia during prostaglandin E1 infusion in infancy. Pediatrics 1983;71(5):842–4.
14. Peled N, Dagan O, Babyn P, Silver MM, Barker G, Hellmann J, Scolnik D, Koren G. Gastric-outlet obstruction induced by prostaglandin therapy in neonates. N Engl J Med 1992;327(8):505–10.
15. Gryglewski RJ. Prostacyclin: pharmacology and clinical trials. Int Angiol 1984;3:89.
16. Katoh K, Kawai T, Narita M, Uemura J, Tani K, Okubo T. Use of prostaglandin E1 (lipo-PGE1) to treat Raynaud's phenomenon associated with connective tissue disease: thermographic and subjective assessment. J Pharm Pharmacol 1992;44(5):442–4.
17. Langevitz P, Buskila D, Lee P, Urowitz MB. Treatment of refractory ischemic skin ulcers in patients with Raynaud's phenomenon with PGE1 infusions. J Rheumatol 1989;16(11):1433–5.
18. Mohrland JS, Porter JM, Smith EA, Belch J, Simms MH. A multiclinic, placebo-controlled, double-blind study of prostaglandin E1 in Raynaud's syndrome. Ann Rheum Dis 1985;44(11):754–60.
19. Wigley FM, Wise RA, Seibold JR, McCloskey DA, Kujala G, Medsger TA Jr, Steen VD, Varga J, Jimenez S, Mayes M, Clements PJ, Weiner SR, Porter J, Ellman M, Wise C, Kaufman LD, Williams J, Dole W. Intravenous iloprost infusion in patients with Raynaud phenomenon secondary to systemic sclerosis. A multicenter, placebo-controlled, double-blind study. Ann Intern Med 1994;120(3):199–206.
20. Belch JJ, Newman P, Drury JK, McKenzie F, Capell H, Leiberman P, Forbes CD, Prentice CR. Intermittent epoprostenol (prostacyclin) infusion in patients with Raynaud's syndrome. A double-blind controlled trial. Lancet 1983;1(8320):313–5.
21. Vowden P, Wilkinson D, Kester RC. Treatment of digital ischaemia associated with chemotherapy using the prostacyclin analogue iloprost. Eur J Vasc Surg 1991;5(5):593–5.
22. Belch JJ, Madhok R, Shaw B, Sturrock RD, Forbes CD. Double-blind trial of CL115,347, a transdermally absorbed prostaglandin E2 analogue, in treatment of Raynaud's phenomenon. Lancet 1985;1(8439):1180–3.
23. Gruss JD, Vargas-Montano H, Bartels D, et al. Use of prostaglandins in arterial occlusion diseases. Int Angiol 1984;3:7.
24. Shionoya S. Clinical experience with prostaglandin E1 in occlusive arterial disease. Int Angiol 1984;3:99.
25. Tanabe T, Mishima Y, Shionoya Y, Katsumara T, Kusaba A. Effect of intravenous drip infusion of prostaglandin E1 on peripheral vascular reconstruction. Int Angiol 1984;3(Suppl):63.
26. Nizankowski R, Krolikowski W, Bielatowicz J, Szczeklik A. Prostacyclin for ischemic ulcers in peripheral arterial disease. A random assignment, placebo controlled study. Thromb Res 1985;37(1):21–8.
27. Telles GS, Campbell WB, Wood RF, Collin J, Baird RN, Morris PJ. Prostaglandin E1 in severe lower limb ischaemia: a double-blind controlled trial. Br J Surg 1984;71(7):506–8.
28. Staben P, Albring M. Treatment of patients with peripheral arterial occlusive disease Fontaine stage III and IV with intravenous iloprost: an open study in 900 patients. Prostaglandins Leukot Essent Fatty Acids 1996;54(5):327–33.
29. Kovacs IB, Mayou SC, Kirby JD. Infusion of a stable prostacyclin analogue, iloprost, to patients with peripheral vascular disease: lack of antiplatelet effect but risk of thromboembolism. Am J Med 1991;90(1):41–6.
30. Lievre M, Azoulay S, Lion L, Morand S, Girre JP, Boissel JP. A dose-effect study of beraprost sodium in intermittent claudication. J Cardiovasc Pharmacol 1996;27(6):788–93.
31. Barst RJ, Rubin LJ, McGoon MD, Caldwell EJ, Long WA, Levy PS. Survival in primary pulmonary hypertension with long-term continuous intravenous prostacyclin. Ann Intern Med 1994;121(6):409–15.
32. Higenbottam TW, Spiegelhalter D, Scott JP, Fuster V, Dinh-Xuan AT, Caine N, Wallwork J. Prostacyclin (epoprostenol) and heart-lung transplantation as treatments for severe pulmonary hypertension. Br Heart J 1993;70(4):366–70.
33. Gassner A, Sommer G, Fridrich L, Magometschnigg D, Priol A. Der Einfluss von Prostaglandin E1

(Alprostadil) auf die pulmonale Hypertonie bei Patienten mit chronisch obstructiven Atemwegserkrankungen (COPD). [Effect of prostaglandin El (alprostadil) on pulmonary hypertension in patients with chronic obstructive respiratory tract diseases (COPD).] Prax Klin Pneumol 1988;42(7):521–4.

34. Sinzinger H, Fitscha P. Leberfunktionsparameter und Fibrinogen bei i.a. und i.v. PGE1-infusion. [Liver function parameters and fibrinogen in intra-arterial and intravenous PGE1 infusion.] Wien Klin Wochenschr 1988;100(14):488–90.

35. Walmrath D, Schneider T, Pilch J, Grimminger F, Seeger W. Aerosolised prostacyclin in adult respiratory distress syndrome. Lancet 1993;342(8877):961–2.

36. Walmrath D, Schneider T, Pilch J, Schermuly R, Grimminger F, Seeger W. Effects of aerosolized prostacyclin in severe pneumonia. Impact of fibrosis. Am J Respir Crit Care Med 1995;151(3 Pt 1):724–30.

37. Bindl L, Fahnenstich H, Peukert U. Aerosolised prostacyclin for pulmonary hypertension in neonates. Arch Dis Child Fetal Neonatal Ed 1994;71(3):F214–6.

38. Darius H, Nixdorff U, Zander J, Rupprecht HJ, Erbel R, Meyer J. Effects of ciprostene on restenosis rate during therapeutic transluminal coronary angioplasty. Agents Actions Suppl 1992;37:305–11.

39. Zusman RM, Rubin RH, Cato AE, Cocchetto DM, Crow JW, Tolkoff-Rubin N. Hemodialysis using prostacyclin instead of heparin as the sole antithrombotic agent. N Engl J Med 1981;304(16):934–9.

40. O'Keefe SJ, Spitaels JM, Mannion G, Naiker N. Misoprostol, a synthetic prostaglandin E1 analogue, in the treatment of duodenal ulcers. A double-blind, cimetidine-controlled trial. S Afr Med J 1985;67(9):321–4.

41. Graham DY, White RH, Moreland LW, Schubert TT, Katz R, Jaszewski R, Tindall E, Triadafilopoulos G, Stromatt SC, Teoh LS. Duodenal and gastric ulcer prevention with misoprostol in arthritis patients taking NSAIDs. Misoprostol Study Group. Ann Intern Med 1993;119(4):257–62.

42. Grazioli I, Avossa M, Bogliolo A, Broggini M, Carcassi A, Carcassi U, Cecconami L, Ligniere GC, Colombo B, Consoli G, et al. Multicenter study of the safety/efficacy of misoprostol in the prevention and treatment of NSAID-induced gastroduodenal lesions. Clin Exp Rheumatol 1993;11(3):289–94.

43. Wilkie ME, Davies GR, Marsh FP, Rampton DS. Effects of indomethacin and misoprostol on renal function in healthy volunteers. Clin Nephrol 1992;38(6):334–7.

44. Goldin E, Fich A, Eliakim R, Zimmerman J, Ligumsky M, Rachmilewitz D. Comparison of misoprostol and ranitidine in the treatment of duodenal ulcer. Isr J Med Sci 1988;24(6):282–5.

45. Wilson DE. Misoprostol and gastroduodenal mucosal protection (cytoprotection). Postgrad Med J 1988;64(Suppl 1):7–11.

46. Watkinson G, Hopkins A, Akbar FA. The therapeutic efficacy of misoprostol in peptic ulcer disease. Postgrad Med J 1988;64(Suppl 1):60–77.

47. Lange AP, Secher NJ, Westergaard JG, Skovgard I. Neonatal jaundice after labour induced or stimulated by prostaglandin E2 or oxytocin. Lancet 1982;1(8279):991–4.

48. Greig PD, Woolf GM, Sinclair SB, Abecassis M, Strasberg SM, Taylor BR, Blendis LM, Superina RA, Glynn MF, Langer B, Levy GA. Treatment of primary liver graft nonfunction with prostaglandin E1. Transplantation 1989;48(3):447–53.

49. Flowers M, Sherker A, Sinclair SB, Greig PD, Cameron R, Phillips MJ, Blendis L, Chung SW, Levy GA. Prostaglandin E in the treatment of recurrent hepatitis B infection after orthotopic liver transplantation. Transplantation 1994;58(2):183–92.

50. Tancharoen S, Jones RM, Angus PW, Michell ID, McNicol L, Hardy KJ. Prostaglandin E1 therapy in orthotopic liver transplantation recipients: indications and outcome. Transplant Proc 1992;24(5):2248–9.

51. Cattral MS, Altraif I, Greig PD, Blendis L, Levy GA. Toxic effects of intravenous and oral prostaglandin E therapy in patients with liver disease. Am J Med 1994;97(4):369–73.

52. Strachan JR, Pryor JP. Prostacyclin in the treatment of painful Peyronie's disease. Br J Urol 1988;61(6):516–7.

53. Waldhauser M, Schramek P. Efficiency and side effects of prostaglandin E1 in the treatment of erectile dysfunction. J Urol 1988;140(3):525–7.

54. Derouet H, Weirauch A, Bewermeier H. Prostaglandin E1 (PGE1) in der Diagnostik und Langzeittherapie der erektilen Dysfunktion. [Prostaglandin E1 (PGE1) in diagnosis and long-term therapy of erectile dysfunction.] Urologe A 1996;35(1):62–7.

55. Lea AP, Bryson HM, Balfour JA. Intracavernous alprostadil. A review of its pharmacodynamic and pharmacokinetic properties and therapeutic potential in erectile dysfunction. Drugs Aging 1996;8(1):56–74.

56. Canale D, Giorgi PM, Lencioni R, Morelli G, Gasperi M, Macchia E. Long-term intracavernous self-injection with prostaglandin E1 for the treatment of erectile dysfunction. Int J Androl 1996;19(1):28–32.

57. The European Alprostadil Study Group. The long-term safety of alprostadil (prostaglandin-E1) in patients with erectile dysfunction. Br J Urol 1998;82(4):538–43.

58. Colli E, Calabro A, Gentile V, Mirone V, Soli M. Alprostadil sterile powder formulation for intracavernous treatment of erectile dysfunction. Eur Urol 1996;29(1):59–62.

59. Chen J, Godschalk M, Katz PG, Mulligan T. The lowest effective dose of prostaglandin E1 as treatment for erectile dysfunction. J Urol 1995;153(1):80–1.

60. Lowe FC, Jarow JP. Placebo-controlled study of oral terbutaline and pseudoephedrine in management of prostaglandin E1-induced prolonged erections. Urology 1993;42(1):51–4.

61. Chen J, Godschalk M, Katz PG, Mulligan T. Peyronie's-like plaque after penile injection of prostaglandin E1. J Urol 1994;152(3):961–2.

62. Linet OI, Ogrinc FG. Efficacy and safety of intracavernosal alprostadil in men with erectile dysfunction. The Alprostadil Study Group. N Engl J Med 1996;334(14):873–7.

63. Hemal AK, Vaidyanathan S, Sankaranarayanan A, Ayyagari S, Sharma PL. Control of massive vesical hemorrhage due to radiation cystitis with intravesical instillation of 15 (s) 15-methyl prostaglandin F2-alpha. Int J Clin Pharmacol Ther Toxicol 1988;26(10):477–8.

64. Levine LA, Jarrard DF. Treatment of cyclophosphamide-induced hemorrhagic cystitis with intravesical carboprost tromethamine. J Urol 1993;149(4):719–23.

65. Trigg ME, O'Reilly J, Rumelhart S, Morgan D, Holida M, de Alarcon P. Prostaglandin E1 bladder instillations to

control severe hemorrhagic cystitis J Urol 1990;143(1):92–4.

66. Flach AJ, Eliason JA. Topical prostaglandin E2 effects on normal human intraocular pressure. J Ocul Pharmacol 1988;4(1):13–8.

67. Lee PY, Shao H, Xu LA, Qu CK. The effect of prostaglandin F2 alpha on intraocular pressure in normotensive human subjects. Invest Ophthalmol Vis Sci 1988;29(10):1474–7.

68. Patel SS, Spencer CM. Latanoprost. A review of its pharmacological properties, clinical efficacy and tolerability in the management of primary open-angle glaucoma and ocular hypertension. Drugs Aging 1996;9(5):363–78.

69. Serle JB. Pharmacological advances in the treatment of glaucoma. Drugs Aging 1994;5(3):156–70.

70. Rulo AH, Greve EL, Hoyng PF. Additive effect of latanoprost, a prostaglandin F2 alpha analogue, and timolol in patients with elevated intraocular pressure. Br J Ophthalmol 1994;78(12):899–902.

71. Stjernschantz JW, Albert DM, Hu DN, Drago F, Wistrand PJ. Mechanism and clinical significance of prostaglandin-induced iris pigmentation. Surv Ophthalmol 2002;47(Suppl 1):S162–75.

72. Fristrom B. A 6-month, randomized, double-masked comparison of latanoprost with timolol in patients with open angle glaucoma or ocular hypertension. Acta Ophthalmol Scand 1996;74(2):140–4.

73. Watson P, Stjernschantz J. A six-month, randomized, double-masked study comparing latanoprost with timolol in open-angle glaucoma and ocular hypertension. The Latanoprost Study Group. Ophthalmology 1996;103(1):126–37.

74. Camras CB. Comparison of latanoprost and timolol in patients with ocular hypertension and glaucoma: a six-month masked, multicenter trial in the United States. The United States Latanoprost Study Group. Ophthalmology 1996;103(1):138–47.

75. Chernin T. The eyes have it. FDA clears several ophthalmic drops for glaucoma in a row. Drug Topics 2001;145:20.

76. Schumer RA, Camras CB, Mandahl AK. Putative side effects of prostaglandin analogues. Surv Ophthalmol 2002;47(Suppl 1):S219.

77. Linden C. Therapeutic potential of prostaglandin analogues in glaucoma. Expert Opin Investig Drugs 2001;10(4):679–94.

78. Wand M, Ritch R, Isbey EK Jr, Zimmerman TJ. Latanoprost and periocular skin color changes. Arch Ophthalmol 2001;119(4):614–5.

79. Ekatomatis P. *Herpes simplex* dendritic keratitis after treatment with latanoprost for primary open angle glaucoma. Br J Ophthalmol 2001;85(8):1008–9.

80. Sacca S, Pascotto A, Siniscalchi C, Rolando M. Ocular complications of latanoprost in uveitic glaucoma: three case reports. J Ocul Pharmacol Ther 2001;17(2):107–13.

81. Mitra M, Chang B, James T. Drug points. Exacerbation of angina associated with latanoprost. BMJ 2001;323(7316):783.

82. Weston BC. Migraine headache associated with latanoprost. Arch Ophthalmol 2001;119(2):300–1.

83. Hayashi RH, Castillo MS, Noah ML. Management of severe postpartum hemorrhage due to uterine atony using an analogue of prostaglandin F2 alpha. Obstet Gynecol 1981;58(4):426–9.

84. Pulkkinen MO, Kajanoja P, Kivikoski A, Saastamoinen J, Selander K, Tuimala R. Abortion with sulprostone, a prostaglandin E2 derivative. Int J Gynaecol Obstet 1980;18(1):40–3.

85. Robins J, Surrago EJ. Alternatives in midtrimester abortion induction. Obstet Gynecol 1980;56(6):716–22.

86. Thong KJ, Robertson AJ, Baird DT. A retrospective study of 932 second trimester terminations using gemeprost (16,16 dimethyl-trans delta 2 PGE1 methyl ester). Prostaglandins 1992;44(1):65–74.

87. Hill NCW, Selinger M, Ferguson J, MacKenzie IZ. Management of intra-uterine fetal death with vaginal administration of gemeprost or prostaglandin E2: a random allocation controlled trial. J Obstet Gynaecol 1991;11:422–6.

88. Poulsen HK, Moller LK, Westergaard JG, Thomsen SG, Giersson RT, Arngrimsson R. Open randomized comparison of prostaglandin E2 given by intracervical gel or vagitory for preinduction cervical ripening and induction of labor. Acta Obstet Gynecol Scand 1991;70(7–8):549–53.

89. Jaschevatzky OE, Dascalu S, Noy Y, Rosenberg RP, Anderman S, Ballas S. Intrauterine PGF2 alpha infusion for termination of pregnancies with second-trimester rupture of membranes. Obstet Gynecol 1992;79(1):32–4.

90. Egarter C, Husslein P. Treatment of tubal pregnancy by prostaglandins. Lancet 1988;1(8594):1104–5.

91. Eckford S, Fox R. Intratubal injection of prostaglandin in ectopic pregnancy. Lancet 1993;342(8874):803.

92. England MJ, Tjallinks A, Hofmeyr J, Harber J. Suppression of lactation. A comparison of bromocriptine and prostaglandin E2. J Reprod Med 1988;33(7):630–2.

93. Lee JB. Cardiovascular–renal effects of prostaglandins: the antihypertensive, natriuretic renal "endocrine" function. Arch Intern Med 1974;133(1):56–76.

94. Olsson AG, Carlson LA. Clinical, hemodynamic and metabolic effects of intraarterial infusions of prostaglandin E1 in patients with peripheral vascular disease. Adv Prostaglandin Thromboxane Res 1976;1:429–32.

95. Bugiardini R, Galvani M, Ferrini D, Gridelli C, Tollemeto D, Mari L, Puddu P, Lenzi S. Myocardial ischemia induced by prostacyclin and iloprost. Clin Pharmacol Ther 1985;38(1):101–8.

96. Fliers E, Duren DR, van Zwieten PA. A prostaglandin analogue as a probable cause of myocardial infarction in a young woman. BMJ 1991;302(6773):416.

97. Lennox CE, Martin J. Cardiac arrest following intramyometrial prostaglandin E2. J Obstet Gynaecol 1991;11:263–4.

98. Meyer WJ, Benton SL, Hoon TJ, Gauthier DW, Whiteman VE. Acute myocardial infarction associated with prostaglandin E2. Am J Obstet Gynecol 1991;165(2):359–60.

99. White JL, Fleming NW, Burke TA, Katz NM, Moront MG, Kim YD. Pulmonary edema after PGE1 infusion. J Cardiothorac Anesth 1990;4(6):744–7.

100. Smith AP, Cuthbert MF. The response of normal and asthmatic subjects to prostaglandins E2 and F2alpha by different routes, and their significance in asthma. Adv Prostaglandin Thromboxane Res 1976;1:449–59.

101. Fishburne JI Jr, Brenner WE, Braaksma JT, Hendricks CH. Bronchospasm complicating intravenous prostaglandin F 2a for therapeutic abortion. Obstet Gynecol 1972;39(6):892–6.

102. Milton AS. Modern views on the pathogenesis of fever and the mode of action of antipyretic drugs. J Pharm Pharmacol 1976;28(Suppl 4):393–9.

103. Callen PJ, de Louvois J, Hurley R, Trudinger BJ. Intrapartum and postpartum pyrexia and infection after induction with extra-amniotic prostaglandin E2 in tylose. Br J Obstet Gynaecol 1980;87(6):513–8.

104. Haller U, Kubli R. Klinische Nebenwirkungen und Komplikationen der Prostaglandine bei Abortinduktion. Gynekologie 1978;11:39.

105. Lyneham RC, Low PA, McLeod JC, Shearman RP, Smith ID, Korda AR. Convulsions and electroencephalogram abnormalities after intra-amniotic prostaglandin F2a. Lancet 1973;2(7836):1003–5.

106. Sederberg-Olsen J, Olsen CE. Prostaglandin–oxytocin induction of mid-trimester abortion complicated by grand mal-like seizures. Acta Obstet Gynecol Scand 1983;62(1):79–81.

107. Rachmilewitz D. Prostaglandins and diarrhea. Dig Dis Sci 1980;25(12):897–9.

108. Kirton KT, Kimball FA, Porteus SE. Reproductive physiology: prostaglandin-associated events. Adv Prostaglandin Thromboxane Res 1976;2:621–5.

109. Cederqvist LL, Birnbaum SJ. Rupture of the uterus after midtrimester prostaglandin abortion. J Reprod Med 1980;25(3):136–8.

110. Bromham DR, Anderson RS. Uterine scar rupture in labour induced with vaginal prostaglandin E2. Lancet 1980;2(8192):485–6.

111. El-Etriby EK, Daw E. Rupture of the cervix during prostaglandin termination of pregnancy. Postgrad Med J 1981;57(666):265–6.

112. Sawyer MM, Lipshitz J, Anderson GD, Dilts PV Jr. Third-trimester uterine rupture associated with vaginal prostaglandin E2. Am J Obstet Gynecol 1981;140(6):710–1.

113. Geirsson RT. Uterine rupture following induction of labour with prostaglandin E2 pessaries, an oxytocin infusion and epidural analgesia. J Obstet Gynecol 1981;2:76.

114. Thavarasah AS, Achanna KS. Uterine rupture with the use of Cervagem (prostaglandin E1) for induction of labour on account of intrauterine death. Singapore Med J 1988;29(4):351–2.

115. Maymon R, Shulman A, Pomeranz M, Holtzinger M, Haimovich L, Bahary C. Uterine rupture at term pregnancy with the use of intracervical prostaglandin E2 gel for induction of labor. Am J Obstet Gynecol 1991;165(2):368–70.

116. Maymon R, Haimovich L, Shulman A, Pomeranz M, Holtzinger M, Bahary C. Third-trimester uterine rupture after prostaglandin E2 use for labor induction. J Reprod Med 1992;37(5):449–52.

117. Azem F, Jaffa A, Lessing JB, Peyser MR. Uterine rupture with the use of a low-dose vaginal PGE2 tablet. Acta Obstet Gynecol Scand 1993;72(4):316–7.

118. Gonzalez CH, Vargas FR, Perez AB, Kim CA, Brunoni D, Marques-Dias MJ, Leone CR, Correa Neto J, Llerena Junior JC, de Almeida JC. Limb deficiency with or without Mobius sequence in seven Brazilian children associated with misoprostol use in the first trimester of pregnancy. Am J Med Genet 1993;47(1):59–64.

119. Quinn MA, Murphy AJ. Fetal death following extra-amniotic prostaglandin gel. Report of two cases. Br J Obstet Gynaecol 1981;88(6):650–1.

120. Beck I, Clayton JK. Hazards of prostaglandin pessaries in postmaturity. Lancet 1982;2(8290):161.

121. Chattopadhyay SK, Sherbeeni MM, Anokute CC. Planned vaginal delivery after two previous caesarean sections. Br J Obstet Gynaecol 1994;101(6):498–500.

122. Quinn MA, Shekleton PA, Wein R, Kloss M. Single dose extra-amniotic prostaglandin gel for midtrimester termination of pregnancy. Aust NZ J Obstet Gynaecol 1980;20(2):77–9.

123. Moncada S, Ferreira SH, Vane JR. Sensitization of pain receptors of dog knee joint by prostaglandins. In: Robinson HJ, Vane JR, editors. Prostaglandin Synthetase Inhibitors. New York: Raven Press, 1974:189.

124. Ferreira SH, Moncada S, Vane JR. Prostaglandins and signs and symptoms of inflammation. In: Robinson HJ, Vane JR, editors. Prostaglandin Synthetase Inhibitors. New York: Raven Press, 1974:175.

125. Hoeper MM, Olschewski H, Ghofrani HA, Wilkens H, Winkler J, Borst MM, Niedermeyer J, Fabel H, Seeger W, Grimminger F, et al. A comparison of the acute hemodynamic effects of inhaled nitric oxide and aerosolized iloprost in primary pulmonary hypertension. German PPH study group. J Am Coll Cardiol 2000;35(1):176–82.

126. Voelkel NF, Lobel K, Westcott JY, Burke TJ. Nitric oxide-related vasoconstriction in lungs perfused with red cell lysate. FASEB J 1995;9(5):379–86.

127. Hoeper MM, Schwarze M, Ehlerding S, Adler-Schuermeyer A, Spiekerkoetter E, Niedermeyer J, Hamm M, Fabel H. Long-term treatment of primary pulmonary hypertension with aerosolized iloprost, a prostacyclin analogue. N Engl J Med 2000;342(25):1866–70.

128. Schenk P, Petkov V, Madl C, Kramer L, Kneussl M, Ziesche R, Lang I. Aerosolized iloprost therapy could not replace long-term IV epoprostenol (prostacyclin) administration in severe pulmonary hypertension. Chest 2001;119(1):296–300.

129. Haraldsson A, Kieler-Jensen N, Wadenvik H, Ricksten SE. Inhaled prostacyclin and platelet function after cardiac surgery and cardiopulmonary bypass. Intensive Care Med 2000;26(2):188–94.

Alprostadil

General Information

Alprostadil is PGE_1 available for exogenous administration. Alprostadil is widely used in neonates with cyanotic congenital heart disease to maintain the patency of the ductus arteriosus. Reported adverse effects include fever, apnea, flushing, bradycardia, and hyperostosis. Continuous chronic infusion of alprostadil via a portable pump and neuromuscular electrical stimulation help to improve the quality of life in patients with severe chronic heart failure waiting for a donor heart, as both treatments can be performed at home.

Of 15 neonates with hypoplastic left heart syndrome (nine boys and six girls; median weight 3123 g) included in a cardiac transplant program between January 1993 and August 1996, who received continuous perfusion of alprostadil from the time of diagnosis of the cardiomyo-pathy, 13 received transplants and 6 died in the operating room (1). All had short-term adverse effects from the continuous perfusion of alprostadil, including slight fever and irritability. However, none had apneic pauses. Cortical hyperostosis occurred in 13 and antral hyperpla-sia in 12, but in all transplanted cases regression of the antral hyperplasia was seen after 6 months and regression of the cortical hyperostosis was seen after 12 months.

Organs and Systems

Cardiovascular

Moderate or severe phlebitis can occur at the site of venepuncture in some patients who receive alprostadil by infusion. It is sometimes severe enough to necessitate withdrawal of therapy. The frequency and severity of phlebitis has been investigated in 18 men, mean age 63 (range 47–78) years, with peripheral vascular disease who received a 2-hour infusion twice daily (2). Although it is usual to dissolve 60 micrograms of alprostadil in 500 ml of fluid to avoid phlebitis, in this study 200 ml was used to prevent volume overload. The solution was neutralized to pH 7.4 with 4 ml of 7% sodium bicarbonate. Two patients had grade 0, four grade 1, 11 grade 2, and one grade 3 phlebitis (by Dinley's criteria (3)). Age correlated nega-tively with the severity of phlebitis. Usually, alprostadil infusion therapy is stopped when phlebitis reaches grade 4 or more, but there were no such cases in this study.

Respiratory

Bilateral pleural effusions have been associated with alprostadil (4).

- After surgery to re-attach an amputated hand, a 75-year-old man was given urokinase 240 000 U/day and heparin 20 000 U/day, each for 6 days, and alprostadil 120 micrograms/day for 12 days. From day 7 he started to have respiratory distress, which progressed gradually. A chest X-ray and CT on day 12 showed bilateral pleural effusions and a pericardial effusion. There was mild peripheral edema. The total protein was 52 g/l, albumin 22 g/l, and hemoglobin 7.6 g/dl. Analysis of the pleural fluid showed that it was an exudate, with a positive Rivalta reaction, carcinoembryonic antigen 1.7 ng/ml, glucose 6.3 mmol/l; total protein 29 g/l, lac-tate dehydrogenase 129 U/l, total cholesterol 0.8 mmol/l, and no acid-fast bacilli. Alprostadil was withdrawn, and after 8 days the pleural effusion disappeared and the respiratory distress improved.

The mechanism of pleural effusion in the present case was suspected to be increased capillary permeability due to alprostadil; hypoalbuminemia probably also contributed.

Hematologic

Investigators from the Department of Pediatrics in Johns Hopkins Hospital, after seeing a neonate who had marked leukocytosis temporally related to alprostadil, conducted a retrospective study of neonatal leukocytosis induced by

alprostadil in 45 neonates (5). They concluded that alprostadil infusion is a predictable cause of leukocytosis in neonates with congenital heart disease. Alprostadil-induced leukocytosis was especially prominent in three patients with splenic disorders associated with the hetero-taxy syndrome. Many of the other adverse effects of alprostadil, including respiratory depression, hypoten-sion, fever, and lethargy, were also associated with sepsis. The authors considered that it is reasonable to look for sepsis in infants receiving alprostadil, but that it is equally reasonable to withdraw empirical therapy once infection has been ruled out. Leukocytosis associated with alpros-tadil infusion has not been previously reported and is not listed in the alprostadil package insert.

Skin

Penile shaft lichen sclerosus has been reported in a 63-year-old man in association with alprostadil intracaver-nous injection for erectile dysfunction (6). The authors suggested that the lichen sclerosus had been caused by (1) an isomorphic response to the trauma of repeated needle injection; (2) a local cutaneous response to alprostadil-induced collagen synthesis or alprostadil-induced fibro-blast production of IL-6, with secondary paracrine/auto-crine-induced collagen synthesis by improper skin exposure by direct injection to the skin or by retrograde flow of alprostadil through the needle puncture tract; or (3) a random occurrence of separate events.

A neonate with transposition of the great vessels devel-oped urticaria during treatment with alprostadil (7). While flushing and peripheral edema are well recognized, urticaria has not been described before.

Allergic contact dermatitis has been attributed to lata-noprost (8).

- An 85-year-old man with glaucoma developed tearing, red eyes, and pruritic, edematous, eczematous eyelids. Treatment for presumed ocular rosacea and seborrhea with oral tetracyclines, topical glucocorticoids, and metro-nidazole gel was unhelpful. He was using topical carbox-ymethylcellulose sodium 1%, propylmethylcellulose 0.3%, polyvinyl alcohol 1.4%, latanoprost, and levobuno-lol. Patch-testing with a standard 64-antigen patch elicited a strong reaction only to balsam of Peru. However, repeated open application of levobunolol and latanoprost for 4 days elicited a strong positive reaction to latanoprost.

The harlequin color change is an unusual cutaneous phenomenon observed in neonates as transient benign episodes of sharply demarcated erythema on half of the infant, with simultaneous contralateral blanching. This self-resolving phenomenon usually occurs in the setting of hypoxia, as seen in prematurity or congenital heart disease. Two neonates with congenital heart anomalies demonstrated the harlequin color change (9). In one the skin showed a course related to the dose of systemic prostaglandin E_1, suggesting a possible association.

- A full-term girl with transposition of the great vessels and an intact intraventricular septum developed a migratory macular erythema on the tenth day of life. The color change was blanchable, with no surface changes, and distributed mostly on the head and neck, with a few patches on the trunk and midline demarcation. There was no correlation between the color change and the position of the child. The event lasted several hours and resolved spontaneously with no skin sequelae. Intravenous diphenhydramine had no effect. At the time of this episode, the child was clinically stable and mechanically ventilated, with normal vital signs and acid-base balance. Medications consisted of PGE_1 by continuous infusion, furosemide, midazolam, morphine, and pancuronium (doses not stated). One day later, arterial switch surgery was performed and PGE_1 was withdrawn. No further color change or rash occurred after withdrawal of PGE_1.

- A full-term girl with pulmonary atresia and an intact intraventricular septum had balloon dilatation of the pulmonary valve performed on the third day of life. Eight days later she developed a macular blanchable erythema involving several areas of the head and neck and on one-half of the trunk with sharp demarcation along the midline. The color change did not respond to intravenous diphenhydramine. The episode lasted 30 minutes and resolved spontaneously. Medications at the time were PGE_1 by continuous infusion, furosemide, propranolol, midazolam, morphine, and pancuronium (doses not stated). On the same day as the initial episode of color change, she developed cardiovascular instability with low oxygen saturation. After she had been intubated and ventilated, a bolus of PGE_1 was administered (dose not stated). The color change recurred, showing prominent macular erythema in a migratory pattern over the face and neck, and on either side of the truncal midline. The erythema was brighter and more extensive than in the previous episode, and was not affected by position. The colour change was not responsive to intravenous diphenhydramine or topical hydrocortisone. This second episode recurred intermittently over the next 8 days, becoming significantly less prominent as PGE_1 was gradually weaned. After the withdrawal of PGE_1, no further color change was noted.

As this adverse effect is not serious, PGE_1 should be continued until surgical correction is performed. Recognition of the association between systemic PGE_1 infusion and the harlequin color change may assist the clinician to manage neonates with cyanotic heart disease and to avoid unnecessary exposure to pharmacological agents given to treat the rash.

Musculoskeletal

Alprostadil infusion can produce bone cortical hyperostosis. Periosteal changes have been described in 15 neonates after the administration of alprostadil for more than 1 week (10). Serum alkaline phosphatase activity was significantly raised. The long bones and clavicles were most commonly involved and symmetrically affected. The scapula was involved in two cases and the ribs in seven. The involvement of clavicles has not been previously reported.

Hypertrophic osteoarthropathy has been reported in a woman with severe chronic heart failure who was referred for cardiac rehabilitation (11).

- A 56-year-old woman with muscle weakness and severe chronic heart failure (NYHA Class III) caused by aortic coarctation received an intravenous infusion of alprostadil 5 nanograms/kg/minute. Although her hemodynamics improved, her muscle weakness and exercise intolerance persisted. Neuromuscular electrical stimulation of both thigh muscles was begun. However, during simultaneous continuous intravenous infusion of alprostadil, she developed pain in her knees and elbows. The overlying skin was warm and dusky red and the subcutaneous tissues were swollen. The discomfort was aggravated by motion. There were signs of non-inflammatory synovial effusions and X-rays showed symmetric bilateral periosteal bone deposition in the distal humerus and synovial effusions in both knees. The bone scintigram showed increased bilateral symmetrical tracer uptake in both knees, ankles, wrists, and carpal bones, and increased radionuclide uptake in periarticular regions. Secondary hypertrophic osteoarthropathy caused by continuous intravenous infusion of alprostadil was diagnosed. The dosage of alprostadil was reduced to 2.5 nanograms/kg/minute, and the signs of osteoarthropathy disappeared within 5 days.

Sexual function

Intracavernosal alprostadil was effective and well tolerated in the treatment of erectile dysfunction, according to the results of a 6-month study (funded by Pharmacia & Upjohn) in 848 men (mean age 52 years) with at least a 4-month history of erectile dysfunction (12). This is provided that the individual dose is established by titration and patients receive training in injection techniques and periodic supervision during treatment. An initial dose was established for each patient and the patients then administered the alprostadil themselves at home. Of 727 evaluable patients, 682 (94%) had at least one erectile response after the injection of alprostadil, and 88% of injections lead to a satisfactory sexual response. The most commonly reported adverse event was penile pain, reported by 44% of patients, but only after 8% of injections. In just over half of the patients who had penile pain, the condition was reported as mild. Prolonged erection, penile fibrosis, and priapism occurred in 8, 4, and 0.9% of patients respectively. Treatment was withdrawn because of medical events in 4% of patients, and drug-related events accounted for treatment withdrawal in 2% of patients.

There is a high dropout rate from self-injection therapy for erectile dysfunction. Of 86 patients aged 36–76 years who had been using home treatment for at least 3 months, 17 had discontinued treatment (13). The patients were evaluated by interview and clinical examination. Patients still in the program used one injection every 2 weeks, and those who had given up treatment had used one injection in 3 weeks. They were in the program for 39 and 16 months respectively, and had used a mean of 50 versus 12 injections respectively. There was no difference in the number of injections that produced unsatisfactory penile rigidity, prolonged erections, hematomas at the injection site, corporeal fibrosis, secondary penile deviation, or mean estimated duration of a drug-induced erection. Patient satisfaction, estimated partner satisfaction, increase in self-esteem, and negligible effort in performing injections were all significantly better for those still in the program. The authors commented that the reasons for dropout from self-injection therapy were not based on objective adverse effects and discomfort. Patients who leave the program are less motivated, less satisfied with the quality of drug-induced sexuality, consider the effort of giving the injections to be substantial, and have not achieved improved self-esteem.

There has been a report of a long-term follow-up program for treatment of erectile dysfunction in 32 patients who used alprostadil for a minimum of 5 years under standardized protocol conditions (14). All the patients had organic erectile dysfunction, and their mean age was 59 years. The period of observation was on average 75 months, and the mean dose of alprostadil was 14 µg. In all, 6799 injections were registered. The average number of injections was 213 per patient, 2.8 injections per month per patient. As regards adverse effects, hematomas occurred in 1.9% of the patients and there were five cases of prolonged erection (0.07%) caused by unauthorized redosing. Three patients developed reversible penile nodules. In 10 patients, the initial dosage had to be increased. Five patients dropped out after 5 years, none of them because of treatment complications.

The impact of treatment with transurethral alprostadil for erectile dysfunction on the quality of life of 249 men and their partners has been evaluated (15). The men had organic erectile dysfunction of more than 3 months' duration and self-administered transurethral alprostadil in an open, dose-escalating, outpatient study. Patients with a sufficient response ($n = 159$) were randomly assigned double-blind to either active medication or placebo for 3 months at home. Drug-related urogenital pain was reported by 12% of patients during outpatient dosing. However, this pain was usually mild, and only five patients (2%) discontinued treatment. One patient reported minor urethral bleeding/spotting. The transurethral administration of alprostadil was associated with minimal or no discomfort in 83–88% of patients. In the outpatient study, dizziness occurred in one patient and hypotension in one patient. During home treatment, drug-related urogenital pain was reported by 11 patients (14%), minor urethral bleeding/spotting by one (1.3%), and dizziness by 2 (2.6%). One patient reported prolonged erections on two occasions during home treatment, each lasting less than 5 hours.

The incidence of priapism after intracorporeal administration of alprostadil is 1%. Priapism after medicated urethral system for erection (MUSE) has been reported (16).

- A 57-year-old man with erectile impotence, who had previously been treated with intracorporeal injections of papaverine and alprostadil, resulting in recurrent episodes of priapism necessitating aspiration, decided to try intraurethral alprostadil (MUSE). The dose needed to achieve a full erection in the clinic was titrated to 1 µg, but after 5 months this was found to

be inadequate unless supplemented by a hot bath before MUSE administration. The patient stated that with MUSE alone the erection lasted for 5–10 minutes but on the two previous occasions when he had had a hot bath for 20 minutes and then used MUSE, the erection had lasted 3–4 hours. However, on the third occasion, priapism lasted 20 hours and necessitated corporeal aspiration for detumescence.

Immunologic

When latanoprost was applied for 4 months to the eyes in 14 patients, there was an increase in HLA-DR expression (17). Since HLA-DR is a marker of ocular surface inflammation, these results suggested a subclinical inflammatory reaction to latanoprost. However, the clinical significance of HLA-DR expression is not clear.

References

1. Caballero S, Torre I, Arias B, Blanco D, Zabala JI, Sanchez Luna M. Efectos secundarios de la prostaglandina E1 en el manejo del sindrome de corazon izquierdo hipoplastico en espera de trasplante cardiaco. [Secondary effects of prostaglandin E1 on the management of hypoplastic left heart syndrome while waiting for heart transplantation.] An Esp Pediatr 1998;48(5):505–9.
2. Fujita M, Hatori N, Shimizu M, Yoshizu H, Segawa D, Kimura T, Iizuka Y, Tanaka S. Neutralization of prostaglandin E1 intravenous solution reduces infusion phlebitis. Angiology 2000;51(9):719–23.
3. Lewis GB, Hecker JF. Infusion thrombophlebitis. Br J Anaesth 1985;57(2):220–33.
4. Watanabe H, Anayama S, Horiuchi T, Sato E, Hamada Y, Ishihara H. Pleural effusion caused by prostaglandin E_1 preparation. Chest 2003; 123: 952–3.
5. Arav-Boger R, Baggett HC, Spevak PJ, Willoughby RE. Leukocytosis caused by prostaglandin E1 in neonates. J Pediatr 2001;138(2):263–5.
6. English JC 3rd, King DH, Foley JP. Penile shaft hypopigmentation: lichen sclerosus occurring after the initiation of alprostadil intracavernous injections for erectile dysfunction. J Am Acad Dermatol 1998;39(5 Pt 1):801–3.
7. Carter EL, Garzon MC. Neonatal urticaria due to prostaglandin E1. Pediatr Dermatol 2000;17(1):58–61.
8. Jerstad KM, Warshaw E. Allergic contact dermatitis to latanoprost. Am J Contact Dermat 2002;13(1):39–41.
9. Rao J, Campbell ME, Krol A. The harlequin color change and association with prostaglandin E_1. Pediatr Dermatol 2004; 21: 573–6.
10. Nadroo AM, Shringari S, Garg M, al-Sowailem AM. Prostaglandin induced cortical hyperostosis in neonates with cyanotic heart disease. J Perinat Med 2000;28(6):447–52.
11. Crevenna R, Quittan M, Hulsmann M, Wiesinger GF, Keilani MY, Kainberger F, Leitha T, Fialka-Moser V, Pacher R. Hypertrophic osteoarthropathy caused by PGE1 in a patient with congestive heart failure during cardiac rehabilitation. Wien Klin Wochenschr 2002;114(3):115–8.
12. Alvarez E, Andrianne R, Arvis G, Boezaart F, Buvat J, Czyzyk A, et al. The long-term safety of alprostadil (prostaglandin-E1) in patients with erectile dysfunction. The European Alprostadil Study Group. Br J Urol 1998;82(4):538–43.

13. Lehmann K, Casella R, Blochlinger A, Gasser TC. Reasons for discontinuing intracavernous injection therapy with prostaglandin E1 (alprostadil). Urology 1999;53(2):397–400.
14. Hauck EW, Altinkilic BM, Schroeder-Printzen I, Rudnick J, Weidner W. Prostaglandin E1 long-term self-injection programme for treatment of erectile dysfunction—a follow-up of at least 5 years. Andrologia 1999;31(Suppl 1):99–103.
15. Williams G, Abbou CC, Amar ET, Desvaux P, Flam TA, Lycklama a Nijeholt GA, Lynch SF, Morgan RJ, Muller SC, Porst H, Pryor JP, Ryan P, Witzsch UK, Hall MM, Place VA, Spivack AP, Todd LK, Gesundheit N. The effect of transurethral alprostadil on the quality of life of men with erectile dysfunction, and their partners. MUSE Study Group. Br J Urol 1998;82(6):847–54.
16. Bettocchi C, Ashford L, Pryor JP, Ralph DJ. Priapism after transurethral alprostadil. Br J Urol 1998;81(6):926.
17. Guglielminetti E, Barabino S, Monaco M, Mantero S, Rolando M. HLA-DR expression in conjunctival cells after latanoprost. J Ocul Pharmacol Ther 2002;18(1):1–9.

Beraprost

General Information

Beraprost is a stable, orally active analogue of PGI_2. It has been tested in patients with intermittent claudication in a randomized, placebo-controlled trial (1). Beraprost improved walking distance more often than placebo. It also reduced the incidence of critical cardiovascular events, but the trial was not powered for statistical validation of this effect. As with iloprost, headache and flushing were the most common adverse effects.

Reference

1. Lievre M, Morand S, Besse B, Fiessinger JN, Boissel JP. Oral Beraprost sodium, a prostaglandin I(2) analogue, for intermittent claudication: a double-blind, randomized, multicenter controlled trial. Beraprost et Claudication Intermittente (BERCI) Research Group. Circulation 2000;102(4):426–31.

Bimatoprost

General Information

Bimatoprost is an analogue of $PGF_{2\alpha}$, used to treat glaucoma. It is believed to lower intraocular pressure by increasing the outflow of aqueous humor through both the trabecular meshwork and uveoscleral routes.

Organs and Systems

Sensory systems

Bimatoprost can cause gradual darkening of the color of the eyes and the eyelid skin, increased thickness, numbers and darkness of eyelashes, conjunctival hyperemia, and ocular pruritus (1). Darkening of the iris occurs in 1.1% of patients (2).

Hair

Eyelash growth was reported in 36–48% of patients after 6 months of using bimatoprost (2).

References

1. Cantor LB. Bimatoprost: a member of a new class of agents, the prostamides, for glaucoma management. Expert Opin Investig Drugs 2001;10(4):721–31.
2. Sherwood M, Brandt J. Bimatoprost Study Groups 1 and 2. Six-month comparison of bimatoprost once-daily and twice-daily with timolol twice-daily in patients with elevated intraocular pressure. Surv Ophthalmol 2001;45(Suppl 4):S361–8.

Carboprost

General Information

Carboprost is a 15-methylated analogue of $PGF_{2\alpha}$. It is used in termination of pregnancy, in the management of labor, and to treat postpartum hemorrhage and uterine atony.

Organs and Systems

Respiratory

Pulmonary edema has been attributed to carboprost (1).

- An 18-year-old woman at 37 weeks gestation was given prostaglandin E_2 gel for cervical ripening followed by oxytocin. After delivery by cesarean section uterine atony, which did not respond to oxytocin and methylergometrine maleate, was treated with intramyometrial 15-methyl-prostaglandin $F_{2\alpha}$ 0.25 mg. After 5 minutes, her SpO_2 fell to 89 and she had dyspnea and sinus tachycardia due to acute pulmonary edema.

Gastrointestinal

Vomiting is a common adverse effect of $PGF_{2\alpha}$ (2).

Reproductive system

Uterine rupture has been reported after intramuscular injection of carboprost to terminate a mid-trimester pregnancy (3).

Drug Administration

Drug overdose

A neonate was accidentally given a large dose of carboprost and recovered (4).

- A full-term neonate was accidentally given carboprost 250 µg intramuscularly in an error for hepatitis vaccine. Within 15 minutes, he became tachypneic and hypertensive and then developed bronchospasm and dystonic movements and/or seizure activity in the arms. He was hyperthermic and had diarrhea. He recovered within 18 hours.

References

1. Rodriguez de la Torre MR, Gallego Alonso JI, Gil Fernandez M. Edema pulmonar en una cesarea relacionado con la administracion de 15-metil prostaglandina F2 alpha. [Pulmonary edema related to administration of 15-methyl-prostaglandin F2 alpha during a cesarean section.] Rev Esp Anestesiol Reanim 2004;51(2):104–7.
2. Biswas A, Roy S. A comparative study of the efficacy and safety of synthetic prostaglandin E2 derivative and 15-methyl prostaglandin F2 alpha in the termination of midtrimester pregnancy. J Indian Med Assoc 1996;94(8):292–3.
3. Tripathy SN. Uterine rupture following intramuscular injection of carboprost in midtrimester pregnancy termination. J Indian Med Assoc 1985;83(9):328.
4. Mrvos R, Kerr FJ, Krenzelok EP. Carboprost exposure in a newborn with recovery. J Toxicol Clin Toxicol 1999;37(7):865–7.

Dinoprostone

General Information

Dinoprostone is PGE_2 available for exogenous administration.

Organs and Systems

Reproductive system

Uterine rupture occurred after labor had been induced with dinoprostone at 10 days after term; the baby was born dead (1).

- A 26-year-old woman, whose first child had been delivered by elective cesarean section at 38 weeks of gestation because of a breech presentation, was given two doses of dinoprostone vaginal gel 1 mg 6 hours apart; 8 hours after the second dose her cervix was soft, fully effaced, and dilated to 3 cm. Since her uterine contractions were only mild and irregular, she underwent amniotomy and an infusion of oxytocin was begun. Fetal tachycardia occurred 4 hours later,

with recurrent decelerations. Prolonged deceleration of the fetal heart then occurred and there was fresh vaginal bleeding. Uterine rupture was suspected and the neonate was delivered by emergency cesarean section, but could not be resuscitated. The mother required a blood transfusion, but subsequently made a good recovery.

The authors commented that induction with prostaglandins in women with a previous lower segment cesarean scar is associated with a risk of symptomatic scar rupture no greater than 0.6%, and the vaginal delivery rate is about 75%, that is similar to rates quoted for spontaneous labor in women with a cesarean scar. At present, faced with the lack of comparative evidence, clinicians can only provide women with the best estimate of risk based on uncontrolled observational data.

Reference

1. Vause S, Macintosh M. Evidence based case report: use of prostaglandins to induce labour in women with a caesarean section scar. BMJ 1999;318(7190):1056–8.

Enprostil

General Information

Enprostil is a synthetic analogue of PGE_2.

Organs and Systems

Gastrointestinal

Even in doses insufficient to control ulcer symptoms, enprostil has a higher incidence of adverse effects than the H_2-receptor antagonists. In a randomized, double-blind, endoscopically controlled study, 98 patients with gastric ulcers were treated with either enprostil 70 micrograms bd or ranitidine 150 mg bd (1). The healing rates at 4, 8, and 12 weeks were similar. After ulcer healing, half the patients were followed for 1 year without treatment and the others were given enprostil 70 micrograms/day. Diarrhea was a common adverse effect of enprostil, and seven patients withdrew because of diarrhea or abdominal pain.

Reference

1. Morgan AG, Pacsoo C, Taylor P, McAdam WA. A comparison between enprostil and ranitidine in the management of gastric ulceration. Aliment Pharmacol Ther 1990;4(6):635–641.

Epoprostenol

General Information

Epoprostenol is PGI_2 available for exogenous administration. It has become the preferred long-term treatment for patients with primary pulmonary hypertension who continue to have symptoms in spite of conventional therapy. However, tolerance, which always occurs, has made dosing uncertain. The effectiveness of epoprostenol given according to an aggressive dosing strategy for longer than 1 year has been investigated in these patients (1). The dose of epoprostenol was increased by 2.4 nanograms/kg/minute each month to the maximum tolerated dose. Adverse effects were common and included diarrhea, jaw pain, headaches, and flushing in all patients.

Organs and Systems

Respiratory

Pulmonary veno-occlusive disease is a rare form of pulmonary hypertension associated with fibrotic occlusion of the smaller pulmonary veins. Although vasodilator therapy is effective in many patients with primary pulmonary hypertension, the role of vasodilators in veno-occlusive disease is unclear, because of concerns about precipitating pulmonary edema. There have been reports of successful therapy with oral vasodilators or intravenous prostacyclin. In contrast, there has been a description of a patient who developed acute pulmonary edema and respiratory failure 15 minutes after the start of a low-dose prostacyclin infusion 2 nanograms/kg/minute, leading to death an hour later (2). This case has several important implications for the management of patients with pulmonary hypertension. Although previous reports suggested that prostacyclin may be safe in patients with pulmonary veno-occlusive disease, the experience reported here suggests that even in very low doses prostacyclin can produce acute decompensation. Thus, consideration must be given to the diagnosis of pulmonary veno-occlusive disease in all patients with suspected primary pulmonary hypertension.

Further cases of pulmonary edema have been reported during continuous intravenous epoprostenol in patients with severe pulmonary hypertension and pulmonary capillary hemangiomatosis, a rare condition characterized by proliferation of thin-walled microvessels in the alveolar walls (3). This report suggests that epoprostenol should not be used in such patients.

- A 66-year-old woman with scleroderma and severe pulmonary hypertension was given continuous intravenous epoprostenol 2 and then 4 nanograms/kg/minute (total duration 48 hours) (4). Two weeks later her dyspnea had improved, but her leg was swollen and her oxygen saturation had fallen. Her dosage of epoprostenol was increased to 5 nanograms/kg/minute. One month later she developed increasing dyspnea, a non-productive cough, severe edema of her legs, and severe hypoxemia.

She had gained 5 kg in weight and there were new bibasal lung crackles. A chest X-ray showed bilateral air-space opacities and bilateral effusions. Her PaO_2 was 5.7 kPa, $PaCO_2$ 3.9 kPa, and the arterial pH 7.51. Pulmonary veno-occlusive disease was diagnosed and the infusion of epoprostenol was gradually tapered over the next 48 hours. She died 6 days later withsided heart failure. At autopsy, histological examination showed thickening of the alveolar septa by proliferation of dilated capillaries on both sides of the alveolar walls, consistent with pulmonary capillary hemangiomatosis.

- A 61-year-old woman developed pulmonary edema during treatment with epoprostenol for severe pulmonary hypertension associated with limited scleroderma (5). She received an infusion of epoprostenol 1 nanogram/kg/minute, and the dosage was increased by 1–2 nanograms/kg/minute every 15 minutes. At a dosage of 6 nanograms/kg/minute, her pulmonary vascular resistance had fallen by 60% and her cardiac output had increased by 55%. However, at this dosage, she became acutely dyspneic. Epoprostenol was withdrawn, she was treated with furosemide and high-flow oxygen, and her symptoms resolved. Because no other therapy was available, she agreed to restart epoprostenol therapy the next day, 1 nanogram/kg/minute, increasing by 1 nanogram/kg/minute every 24 hours to 3 nanograms/kg/minute at discharge. Over the next 6 months, the dosage of epoprostenol was gradually increased to 20 nanograms/kg/minute. She had a significant improvement in her exercise tolerance and there was no evidence of pulmonary edema. However, after about 7 months of marked clinical improvement, she developed right ventricular decompensation. Increased doses of epoprostenol were ineffective and she died. Autopsy showed severe obliterative and plexogenic pulmonary arteriopathy.

This is the first case in which epoprostenol has been successfully restarted. The authors commented that pulmonary edema during acute infusion of epoprostenol is considered a contraindication to its further use. They theorized that the pulmonary edema could have occurred secondary to the dramatic increase in pulmonary perfusion at 6 nanograms/kg/minute of epoprostenol and subsequent rapid shifts in vascular hydrostatic pressure. The slow increase in dosage during reinstitution may have averted the dramatic increase in pulmonary perfusion.

Interstitial pneumonia has been reported in a patient taking epoprostenol for primary pulmonary hypertension (6).

- A 25-year-old woman with primary pulmonary hypertension, dyspnea, and exacerbation of edema was given an infusion of epoprostenol 0.5 ng/kg/minute with incremental increases of 0.5 ng/kg/minute every 12 hours. After 5 days she was receiving 4.5 ng/kg/minute. Her chest X-ray showed rapid changes in bilateral infiltrates and her respiration gradually deteriorated so that she required tracheal intubation and inhaled nitric oxide 10–20 ppm. Despite intensive antibiotic therapy, her oxygenation did not improve. The flow rate of nitric oxide was increased and she was given methylprednisolone 500 mg/day for 3 days and then weaned to oral prednisolone 40 mg/day. Her oxygenation improved and the dose of prednisolone was reduced to 20 mg/day. Ten days after intubation, she had massive bleeding from a gastric ulcer, which required a blood transfusion and endoscopic hemostasis. Prednisolone was withdrawn. One week later, her chest X-ray began to show bilateral infiltrates and a CT scan showed diffuse nodular interstitial changes, consistent with interstitial pneumonia. She was given methylprednisolone 500 mg/day for 3 days followed by prednisolone 40 mg/day, which resulted in significant improvement. Because the cause of her respiratory failure was unknown a lymphocyte stimulation test was conducted with epoprostenol and was positive (273% compared with control). She was given prostaglandin E_1 (PGE_1) instead of epoprostenol, after which her oxygenation, chest X-ray, and CT scan became stable.

Hematologic

Patients with end-stage liver failure, portal hypertension, and associated pulmonary artery hypertension (portopulmonary hypertension) have a high mortality when undergoing liver transplantation. Successful transplantation in these patients may depend on efforts to reduce pulmonary artery pressure. To this end, some centers are using a continuous intravenous infusion of epoprostenol, which has been shown to improve symptoms, extend life span, and reduce pulmonary artery pressure in patients with primary pulmonary hypertension. There have been four cases in which treatment of portopulmonary hypertension with continuous intravenous epoprostenol was followed by the development of progressive splenomegaly, with worsening thrombocytopenia and leukopenia (7). This finding may limit the usefulness of epoprostenol in portopulmonary hypertension and influence the timing of transplantation in such patients.

Skin

Common dose-limiting adverse effects of epoprostenol (including flushing) are attributed to vasodilatation. However, patients can develop a persistent rash distinct from the flushing associated with epoprostenol. The clinical and pathological findings have been described in 12 patients who developed a persistent rash while receiving long-term epoprostenol for pulmonary arterial hypertension (8).

Drug-drug interactions

Anticoagulants

Anticoagulants and continuous intravenous infusion of epoprostenol are the standard treatments for primary pulmonary hypertension. However, their combined use increases the likelihood of hemorrhagic complications, as demonstrated in a retrospective study of 31 consecutive patients with primary pulmonary hypertension (mean

age, 29 years, 10 men, 21 women), nine of whom had 11 bleeding episodes; nine episodes were cases of alveolar hemorrhage and two patients had severe respiratory distress (9). The mean dose of epoprostenol at the time of the first bleeding episode was 89 ng/kg/minute. More of the patients who had a bleeding episode died (67% versus 41%).

Management of adverse drug reactions

Long-term therapy with epoprostenol, a potent prostacyclin and short-acting vasodilator, improves hemodynamics, exercise capacity, and survival in adults and children with pulmonary hypertension. However, epoprostenol has several inherent drawbacks (SEDA-24, 463). Bosentan, a dual endothelin receptor antagonist, lowers pulmonary artery pressure and resistance and improves exercise tolerance in adults with pulmonary arterial hypertension. Based on a case series that suggested that epoprostenol can be withdrawn from a select group of adults with normal pulmonary pressures, it has been shown that bosentan facilitates the reduction of epoprostenol dosages and the severity of its associated adverse effects, without adversely affecting hemodynamic parameters in selected children (10). Further randomized studies are required to determine if use of bosentan concomitantly with epoprostenol improves hemodynamics and may allow safe weaning or discontinuation of epoprostenol.

In a double-blind, placebo-controlled study, the Bosentan Randomized trial of Endothelin Antagonist Therapy for Pulmonary Arterial Hypertension (BREATHE-2), 33 patients took epoprostenol (2 ng/kg/min initially, increasing to a mean dosage of 14 ng/kg/min at week 16) and were then randomized for 16 weeks in a 2:1 ratio to bosentan (62.5 mg bd for 4 weeks then 125 mg bd) or placebo (11). There was a non-significant trend towards hemodynamic and clinical improvement with to the combination. There were several early and late major complications (four withdrawals with bosentan + epoprostenol: two deaths due to cardiopulmonary failure, one clinical worsening, and one increase in hepatic transaminases; and one withdrawal due to increased hepatic transaminases with placebo + epoprostenol. Power was the major limitation of this study, in which only 33 patients were enrolled, and the results should be interpreted with caution. Additional information is needed to evaluate the benefit to harm balance of combined bosentan + epoprostenol therapy in pulmonary arterial hypertension.

References

1. McLaughlin VV, Genthner DE, Panella MM, Rich S. Reduction in pulmonary vascular resistance with long-term epoprostenol (prostacyclin) therapy in primary pulmonary hypertension. N Engl J Med 1998;338(5):273–7.
2. Palmer SM, Robinson LJ, Wang A, Gossage JR, Bashore T, Tapson VF. Massive pulmonary edema and death after

prostacyclin infusion in a patient with pulmonary veno-occlusive disease. Chest 1998;113(1):237–40.

3. Humbert M, Maitre S, Capron F, Rain B, Musset D, Simonneau G. Pulmonary edema complicating continuous intravenous prostacyclin in pulmonary capillary hemangio-matosis. Am J Respir Crit Care Med 1998;157(5 Pt 1):1681–1685.

4. Gugnani MK, Pierson C, Vanderheide R, Girgis RE. Pulmonary edema complicating prostacyclin therapy in pulmonary hypertension associated with scleroderma: a case of pulmonary capillary hemangiomatosis. Arthritis Rheum 2000;43(3):699–703.

5. Farber HW, Graven KK, Kokolski G, Korn JH. Pulmonary edema during acute infusion of epoprostenol in a patient with pulmonary hypertension and limited scleroderma. J Rheumatol 1999;26(5):1195–6.

6. Morimatsu H, Goto K, Matsusaki T, Katayama H, Matsubara H, Ohe T, Morita K. Rapid development of severe interstitial pneumonia caused by epoprostenol in a patient with primary pulmonary hypertension. Anesth Analg 2004; 99: 1205–7.

7. Findlay JY, Plevak DJ, Krowka MJ, Sack EM, Porayko MK. Progressive splenomegaly after epoprostenol therapy in portopulmonary hypertension. Liver Transpl Surg 1999;5(5):362–5.

8. Myers SA, Ahearn GS, Selim MA, Tapson VF. Cutaneous findings in patients with pulmonary arterial hypertension receiving long-term epoprostenol therapy. J Am Acad Dermatol 2004; 51: 98–102.

9. Ogawa A, Matsubara H, Fujio H, Miyaji K, Nakamura K, Morita H, Saito H, Kusano KF, Emori T, Date H, Ohe T. Risk of alveolar hemorrhage in patients with primary pulmonary hypertension—anticoagulation and epoprostenol therapy. Circ J 2005; 69(2): 216–20.

10. Ivy DD, Doran A, Clausen L, Bingaman D, Yetman A. Weaning and discontinuation of epoprostenol in children with idiopathic pulmonary arterial hypertension receiving concomitant bosentan. Am J Cardiol 2004; 93: 943–6.

11. Humbert M, Barst RJ, Robbins IM, Channick RN, Galie N, Boonstra A, Rubin LJ, Horn EM, Manes A, Simonneau G. Combination of bosentan with epoprostenol in pulmonary arterial hypertension: BREATHE-2. Eur Respir J 2004; 24: 353–9.

Gemeprost

General Information

Gemeprost is an analogue of PGE_2. Vaginal gemeprost is effective in inducing first and second trimester abortion and in cervical priming before vacuum aspiration. Pyrexia, vomiting, and diarrhea were experienced in 20% of patients (1).

In a double-blind, randomized, controlled trial, 896 healthy women requesting a medical abortion (57–63 days gestation, mean age 25 years) were randomized to a single oral dose of mifepristone 200 or 600 mg, both followed in 48 hours by gemeprost 1 mg vaginally (2). The complete abortion rates were similar with the lower and higher doses of mifepristone (92 versus 92%). The incidences of adverse effects were similar, with the exception of nausea at 1 week, which was less frequent in the low-dose group (3.6 versus 7.6%).

Organs and Systems

Cardiovascular

Two women developed myocardial ischemia during treatment with gemeprost for termination of pregnancy (3).

- A 29-year-old woman, a smoker with a history of renal insufficiency, obesity, hypertension, hypercholesterolemia, and cardiac dysrhythmias, underwent termination of pregnancy at 10 weeks with a pessary of gemeprost 1 mg and 5 hours later dilatation and evacuation, followed by tubal ligation. After surgery, her blood pressure became unmeasurable, her heart rate dropped to 40/minute, and she developed ventricular fibrillation. She was given streptokinase and intravenous heparin for suspected pulmonary embolism; her blood pressure rose and was maintained with adrenaline and noradrenaline. Angiography showed an 80% stenosis of her right coronary artery and complete occlusion of the anterior interventricular branch. Blood flow was re-established by coronary angioplasty.

- A 32-year-old woman, a smoker, had an evacuation after the death of her fetus at 18 weeks. Two pessaries of gemeprost 1 mg were inserted 7.25 hours apart, and about 90 minutes later she became unconscious, apneic, and cyanotic, and had dilated pupils and no detectable blood pressure or pulse. She was given 100% oxygen, intravenous adrenaline and dobutamine, and a crystalloid infusion. Her systolic pressure rose to 100 mmHg. Coronary angiography showed left and circumflex coronary artery spasm.

The author commented that the myocardial ischemia experienced by both of these patients was thought to be due to prostaglandin-induced coronary spasm. It would be prudent to monitor every woman treated with gemeprost during the course of an abortion.

Skin

Toxic epidermal necrolysis has been attributed to mifepristone/gemeprost (4).

References

1. Thong KJ, Robertson AJ, Baird DT. A retrospective study of 932 second trimester terminations using gemeprost (16,16 dimethyl-trans delta 2 PGE1 methyl ester). Prostaglandins 1992;44(1):65–74.

2. Weston BC. Migraine headache associated with latanoprost. Arch Ophthalmol 2001;119(2):300–1.

3. Schulte-Sasse U. Life threatening myocardial ischaemia associated with the use of prostaglandin E1 to induce abortion. BJOG 2000;107(5):700–2.

4. Lecorvaisier-Pieto C, Joly P, Thomine E, Tanasescu S, Noblet C, Lauret P. Toxic epidermal necrolysis after mifepristone/gemeprost-induced abortion. J Am Acad Dermatol 1996;35(1):112.

Iloprost

General Information

Iloprost is an analogue of prostacyclin (PGI_2), the pharmacodynamic properties of which it mimics, namely inhibition of platelet aggregation, vasodilatation, and cytoprotection (as yet ill-defined). Iloprost has greater chemical stability than prostacyclin, which facilitates its clinical use (1).

Iloprost is mainly used in patients with chronic critical leg ischemia due to atherosclerosis or Buerger's disease. Episodic digital ischemia in patients with systemic sclerosis or related disorders is another use. The most frequently observed adverse effects, facial flushing and headache, are caused by profound vasodilatation.

Most clinical experience with iloprost has been gained in patients with critical leg ischemia. An intermittent intravenous infusion of up to 2 nanograms/kg/minute for 2–4 weeks reduced rest pain and improved ulcer healing in roughly half of the patients with critical leg ischemia, including diabetics. Compared with placebo, the improvement obtained with iloprost was significant in most but not all individual clinical trials. In addition, a meta-analysis showed a 15% reduction in major amputation rate compared with placebo (2).

Observational studies

The use of iloprost has been proposed in patients with systemic sclerosis, a disease that is often characterized by pulmonary hypertension and Raynaud's phenomenon. Three patients with systemic sclerosis who were treated with iloprost developed acute thrombotic events (3). In one case, intestinal infarction occurred 1 day after infusion of iloprost. In another patient the left kidney was not perfused 22 days after the last infusion of iloprost because of thrombosis of the left renal artery. The last patient, 9 months after the start of treatment with iloprost, and 5 days after the last infusion, had an anterolateral myocardial infarction. The authors commented that their observations did not allow them to conclude that there is a direct relation between infusion of iloprost and thrombotic events. However, they said that this possibility should be considered, and they suggested that risk factors for thromboembolism should be carefully evaluated in each patient with systemic sclerosis who is receiving iloprost.

Inhalation of aerosolized iloprost is being tested in patients with severe primary or secondary pulmonary hypertension refractory to conventional therapy. The aim is to produce predominantly pulmonary vasodilatation without significant systemic effects. In an uncontrolled series of 19 patients, the most common adverse effects of inhaled iloprost were coughing, nausea, edema, and thoracic pain (4). In most patients, these effects were transient and rarely required a change in therapy.

Comparative studies

In a randomized, controlled study of cyclic iloprost or nifedipine in 46 patients with systemic sclerosis, the predictable adverse effects of iloprost (headache, nausea and vomiting, and diarrhea) were common but quickly resolved after the end of the infusion (5). They rarely required a temporary dose reduction. Hypotension occurred less often than with nifedipine.

The effects of PGE_1 and iloprost on microcirculation have been investigated in a randomized crossover study in 36 patients with peripheral arterial occlusive disease stage III and IV according to Fontaine (6). They received PGE_1 and iloprost by single 3-hour intravenous infusions on two different days at doses recommended by the manufacturers or as have been used in previous studies (PGE_1: first hour 20 micrograms, next 2 hours 30 micrograms each; iloprost: first hour 0.5 ng/kg/minute, next 2 hours 1.0 ng/kg/minute). Adverse effects occurred in 19% (PGE_1) and 31% (iloprost). Dosage reduction was required in three patients receiving iloprost (hypotension, nausea, irritation of the infused vein), and in none in those receiving PGE_1.

Placebo-controlled studies

A multicenter, randomized, parallel-group comparison of two different doses of oral iloprost and placebo has been conducted, to identify the optimal dose of oral iloprost on the basis of efficacy and tolerability in patients with Raynaud's phenomenon secondary to systemic sclerosis (7). A total of 103 patients were given total daily doses of iloprost of 100 micrograms ($n = 33$) or 200 micrograms ($n = 35$) or placebo ($n = 35$) for 6 weeks. The mean percentage reductions in the frequency, total daily duration, and severity of attacks of Raynaud's phenomenon were greater in the iloprost groups at the end of treatment and at the end of follow-up. Adverse effects were reported by 80% of patients taking placebo, 85% taking oral iloprost 100 micrograms/day, and 97% taking oral iloprost 100 micrograms/day. There were significant differences in the frequency of five types of adverse events. Headache, flushing, nausea, and trismus were all more common with increasing iloprost dose, while flu-like illnesses were most commonly reported in the placebo group. Treatment was prematurely discontinued in 9, 30, and 51% respectively, and discontinuation was precipitated by adverse events in 6, 27, and 51%.

General adverse effects

The adverse effects of iloprost occur within or above the usual dosage range and are predictable from its pharmacological effects. Minor vascular reactions during infusion (characterized by facial flushing and headache) are so common as to make double-blind trials impossible. Gastrointestinal effects become more prevalent at higher dosages, and include nausea, vomiting, abdominal cramps, and diarrhea. Less common adverse effects include restlessness, sweating, local erythema along the infusion line, wheals, fatigue, and muscle pain. Clinically significant hypotension is rare with the doses tested. The untoward effects resolve rapidly after the infusion is discontinued.

Therapy with iloprost is usually started with a dosage of 0.5 nanogram/kg/minute and increased in increments until either minor vascular reactions occur or a dosage of 2 nanograms/kg/minute has been reached. The optimal total dose remains to be established.

Organs and Systems

Cardiovascular

Myocardial ischemia is unusual during infusion of iloprost. It mainly occurs in patients with pre-existing coronary disease, when it is ascribed to a steal phenomenon detrimental to the subendocardial tissue. As a rule it is transient and exceptionally proceeds to infarction. However, such an event has now been reported in a patient with systemic sclerosis (8).

- A 57-year-old man with a 1-year history of systemic sclerosis and ischemia of several digits received a first infusion of iloprost using the recommended stepwise increasing dosage scheme; he developed sudden chest pain, with inferior ST segment elevation. Emergency coronary angiography showed an occlusion of the circumflex coronary artery, for which a stent was inserted. At angiography 3 years earlier his coronary arteries had been normal. He died 5 months later from cardiogenic pulmonary edema.

Musculoskeletal

Four women with CREST syndrome or systemic sclerosis had pain and eventually contracture of the masseter muscles during infusion of iloprost for severe attacks of Raynaud's phenomenon (9). The adverse effect was quickly reversed by reducing the infusion rate. There were no electrocardiographic or cardiac enzyme changes. The mechanism of this effect is obscure.

Drug Administration

Drug administration route

An oral formulation has been investigated in patients with Raynaud's phenomenon secondary to systemic sclerosis and in patients with severe ischemia due to Buerger's disease or to atherosclerosis. The first reports were not particularly encouraging in terms of efficacy. Tolerance is acceptable: 6% of patients discontinued iloprost compared with 2% with placebo (10,11).

References

1. England MJ, Tjallinks A, Hofmeyr J, Harber J. Suppression of lactation. A comparison of bromocriptine and prostaglandin E2. J Reprod Med 1988;33(7):630–2.
2. Lee JB. Cardiovascular-renal effects of prostaglandins: the antihypertensive, natriuretic renal "endocrine" function. Arch Intern Med 1974;133(1):56–76.
3. Tedeschi A, Meroni PL, Del Papa N, Salmaso C, Boschetti C, Miadonna A. Thrombotic events in patients with systemic sclerosis treated with iloprost. Arthritis Rheum 1998;41(3):559–60.
4. Olschewski H, Ghofrani HA, Schmehl T, Winkler J, Wilkens H, Hoper MM, Behr J, Kleber FX, Seeger W. Inhaled iloprost to treat severe pulmonary hypertension. An uncontrolled trial. German PPH Study Group. Ann Intern Med 2000;132(6):435–43.
5. Pfeiffer N, Grierson I, Goldsmith H, Hochgesand D, Winkgen-Bohres A, Appleton P. Histological effects in the iris after 3 months of latanoprost therapy: the Mainz 1 study. Arch Ophthalmol 2001;119(2):191–6.
6. Schellong S, Altmann E, Von Bilderling P, Rudofsky G, Waldhausen P, Rogatti W. Microcirculation and tolerability following i.v. infusion of PGE1 and iloprost: a randomized cross-over study in patients with critical limb ischemia. Prostaglandins Leukot Essent Fatty Acids 2004; 70: 503–9.
7. Black CM, Halkier-Sorensen L, Belch JJ, Ullman S, Madhok R, Smit AJ, Banga JD, Watson HR. Oral iloprost in Raynaud's phenomenon secondary to systemic sclerosis: a multicentre, placebo-controlled, dose-comparison study. Br J Rheumatol 1998;37(9):952–60.
8. Marroun I, Fialip J, Deleveaux I, Andre M, Lamaison D, Cabane J, Piette JC, Eschalier A, Aumaitre O. Infarctus du myocarde sous iloprost chez un patient atteint de sclérodermie. [Myocardial infarction and iloprost in a patient with scleroderma.] Therapie 2001;56(5):630–2.
9. Boubakri C, Bouchou K, Guy C, Roy M, Cathebras P. Douleurs masseterines: un effet indésirable méconnu de l'iloprost. [Masseter pain: aé little known, undesirable effect of iloprost.] Presse Méd 2000;29(35):1935–6.
10. Olsson AG, Carlson LA. Clinical, hemodynamic and metabolic effects of intraarterial infusions of prostaglandin E1 in patients with peripheral vascular disease. Adv Prostaglandin Thromboxane Res 1976;1:429–32.
11. Bugiardini R, Galvani M, Ferrini D, Gridelli C, Tollemeto D, Mari L, Puddu P, Lenzi S. Myocardial ischemia induced by prostacyclin and iloprost. Clin Pharmacol Ther 1985;38(1):101–8.

Latanoprost

General Information

Latanoprost is an analogue of $PGF_{2\alpha}$, used to treat glaucoma. The use of latanoprost and unoprostone in the treatment of open-angle glaucoma and ocular hypertension has been reviewed (1). More data on safety are needed to calculate its benefit-to-harm balance.

Latanoprost caused reduced intraocular pressure by 20–40% in adults with open-angle glaucoma or ocular hypertension, but its efficacy and safety in children have not been widely reported. Most children reported so far gained little benefit on intraocular pressure from latanoprost, but older children and those with juvenile-onset open-angle glaucoma do gain a significant ocular hypotensive effect. Systemic and ocular adverse effects in children using latanoprost are infrequent (2).

Organs and Systems

Cardiovascular

Two patients in their seventies developed hypertension during treatment with topical latanoprost (dosage not stated) for open-angle glaucoma; both were also taking tocopherol (vitamin E) supplements. Neither had a previous history of hypertension (3). The authors commented that it is likely that systemic absorption of topical latanoprost could cause hypertension. Self-medication with vitamin E has been reported to aggravate or precipitate hypertension.

Coronary spasm has been attributed to latanoprost (4).

- A 58-year-old man with stable angina pectoris started to use latanoprost eye drops and over the next few days his angina worsened and occurred at rest. After 15 days, he had syncope during physical exercise. Angiography showed coronary spasm.

Respiratory

Latanoprost rarely causes systemic effects. However, it aggravated respiratory symptoms in a patient with chronic bronchitis and emphysema, with improvement after latanoprost was withdrawn (5).

Nervous system

Three cases of headache after latanoprost have been described (6).

- A 65-year-old man with primary open-angle glaucoma intolerant of dipivefrin and beta-blockers used latanoprost in both eyes at bedtime. He had no prior history of migraine, but he began to have headaches, the frequency and severity of which increased until they were occurring daily. The pain was not relieved by over-the-counter or narcotic analgesics, and he was virtually incapacitated. Latanoprost was discontinued and he had almost immediate relief, with only one migraine during the following week, and he was headache-free for the next 10 months. He then agreed to rechallenge. After the second night of latanoprost therapy his headache recurred, and therapy was withdrawn 2 days later when he had incapacitating pain. Headache did not recur within 4 months of follow-up.
- A 65-year-old man with primary open-angle glaucoma, using levobunolol hydrochloride 0.5%, was given a nighttime dose of latanoprost. The next morning he awoke with a severe bifrontal throbbing headache, photophobia, and slight blurring of vision. The headache intensified, and 4 days later a CT scan was normal. On the sixth day he stopped using latanoprost. His headache disappeared within 24 hours and did not recur during follow-up for 1 year.
- A 54-year-old woman with primary open-angle glaucoma, using betaxolol hydrochloride 0.5%, had mild progression of visual field loss in her left eye. Latanoprost was added nightly to her left eye. A few hours after the first dose she was awakened by a severe unilateral pounding headache extending from the left

eye and brow to the left cranium. There were no associated neurological symptoms. The headache resolved spontaneously the next day, but recurred on three nights after instillation of latanoprost. On the fourth night the headache did not occur. She continued to use latanoprost, and the headache did not return.

Sensory systems

Corneal damage

Four patients treated with latanoprost developed dendritiform epitheliopathy, a sign of corneal toxicity; the lesions reversed in 1–4 weeks after latanoprost withdrawal (7).

Three cases of *Herpes simplex* keratitis developed during latanoprost therapy (8).

- One patient, with a history of *H. simplex* keratitis, had recurrence with latanoprost (4 months); the infection resolved on withdrawal but recurred on rechallenge.
- The second patient, with a history of *H. simplex* keratitis, had bilateral recurrence with latanoprost (1 month); antiviral therapy did not eradicate the infection until latanoprost was withdrawn.
- The third patient developed the infection after 1 month; the keratitis cleared on withdrawal of latanoprost and antiviral therapy; reinstitution of latanoprost with prophylactic antiviral medication (valaciclovir) kept the cornea clear, but as soon as the antiviral drug was discontinued, *H. simplex* virus keratitis reappeared.

Although the mechanism is unclear, it is known that inhibitors of prostaglandin synthesis reduce recurrence of epithelial *H. simplex* infections and prostaglandins may stimulate their occurrence.

Iris pigmentation

Latanoprost can produce darkening of the iris in 10–25% of patients treated for 0.5–2 years. The incidence of iris pigmentation differs between eyes with differently colored irises: green–brown, yellow–brown, and blue–brown eyes, in that order, have the highest incidences, whereas eyes with uniformly blue, grey, or green irises are much less affected, even after 2 years of treatment. About 60% of eyes with an initial green–brown iris will have increased pigmentation within 1 year. The corresponding figure for initially blue–brown eyes is about 20%. All patients who have developed increased pigmentation of the iris have been withdrawn from studies, and during follow-up for up to almost 3 years the change in iris pigmentation has been stable without signs of reversibility or further increase. Nevi and freckles have not changed color or size. Apart from the change in color the iris looks normal and pigmentation dispersion has not been observed. No cell proliferation is involved and the change in color is due to melanogenesis. It has been concluded that the change in iris pigmentation is unlikely to cause any long-term consequence besides the cosmetic one. The possibility of late loss of pigment and induction of a pigmentary glaucoma also seems unlikely; melanocytes in the iris are continent and do not release melanin (9).

In an observational cohort study of 43 patients, 30 had a definite acquired iris anisochromia (10).

The time of onset of the changes in iris pigmentation can be as early as 3 months. The earliest reported change in iris color occurred in a 78-year-old woman, whose iris color changed from blue–green to brown–green within 4 weeks (11). The pigmentation is irreversible. In a 50-year-old man with peripheral iris darkening after latanoprost treatment, the darkening did not change appreciably for several years after withdrawal (12).

The fine structure of an iridectomy specimen from a 65-year-old woman treated with latanoprost has been reported (13). She received latanoprost for 13.5 months and the drug was withdrawn because of iris color change. She underwent cataract surgery 16 months after stopping the drug and a sector iridectomy was obtained. The authors found some melanocytes with atypical features, including nuclear chromatin margination, prominent nucleoli, and invagination of the nucleoli. These characteristics are also seen in precancerous lesions, in the normal ageing iris, and in patients with glaucoma.

The effects of latanoprost on iris structure were assessed in 17 patients with bilateral primary open-angle glaucoma. In each case an iridectomy was performed in one eye, which served as a control. The other eye was then treated with latanoprost for 6 months followed by iridectomy. Light and electronic microscopy showed no evidence of early ultrastructural changes in the latanoprost-treated eyes (14).

The long-term safety of topical latanoprost in the long-term treatment of open-angle glaucoma has been assessed in two studies. To investigate the possible appearance of trabecular pigmentation, 50 subjects who used latanoprost were evaluated by gonioscopic photography of the inferior quadrant at baseline and every 3 months during the first year and every 6 months during the second and third years (15). In all 41 subjects (79 eyes) completed the 3-year follow-up and none had any increase in the grade of trabecular pigmentation, including 10 subjects (20 eyes) in whom iris pigment increased. The safety of latanoprost after 5 years of treatment has been reported in 380 subjects, of whom 353 were evaluated at 4 years and 344 completed the 5th year (16). In 127 (33%) there was increased iris pigmentation in one or both eyes after 5 years. Of the patients who developed iris pigmentation, 89% had a baseline eye color known to be susceptible to color change (mixed-color irises containing brown areas). Patient with blue-grey eyes and no brown pigment did not develop increased iris pigmentation. In the 127 patients who developed iris pigmentation, it occurred during the first 8 months of the study in 94, during the first 12 months in 103, and during the first 24 months in 103. All developed the condition after 36 months. There was hypertrichosis in 14%.

Seven patients using different topical prostaglandin F_{2a} analogues developed bilateral poliosis, which appeared at 1.5–6 months after the start of therapy (17). Four used latanoprost, two used bimatoprost, and one used travaprost.

The mechanism of iris pigmentation due to latanoprost is unknown. In an in vitro experiment using uveal melanocytes, the addition of latanoprost increased melanin content, melanin production, and tyrosinase activity (18). Alpha-methyl-para-tyrosine, an inhibitor of tyrosinase (the enzyme that transforms tyrosine to levodopa), completely prevented the latanoprost-induced stimulation of melanogenesis.

Of 17 patients requiring filtering surgery for primary open-angle glaucoma randomized to receive latanoprost ($n = 8$) or alternative medications ($n = 9$) for 3 months before surgery, all had peripheral iridectomy specimens, and there were color changes in one case (19). No morphological changes or cellular proliferation were found in any specimen.

Iris cyst associated with latanoprost has been described in a 76-year-old woman (20). Latanoprost was given for 5 weeks, and during a re-examination a large iris cyst was observed in her right eye. The cyst disappeared 3 weeks after latanoprost withdrawal.

Uveitis

In four patients with complicated open-angle glaucoma, in whom anterior uveitis appeared to be associated with latanoprost, the uveitis was unilateral and occurred only in the eye receiving latanoprost in three patients. In one patient, latanoprost was used in both eyes, and the uveitis was bilateral (21). Four of five eyes had a history of prior inflammation and/or prior incisional surgery. All patients were rechallenged. The uveitis improved after withdrawal and recurred after rechallenge in all eyes. The authors concluded that topical prostaglandin analogues may be relatively contraindicated in patients with a history of uveitis or prior ocular surgery. There may also be a risk in eyes that have not had previous uveitis or incisional surgery.

Optic disc and macular edema

A case of bilateral optic disc edema has been described (22).

- A 64-year-old woman was included in a randomized, double-blind trial of drugs used in the treatment of ocular hypertension. After 3 months, examination of the optic nerve showed bilateral edema. She had been using latanoprost 0.0005% eye-drops at night to both eyes. Latanoprost was withdrawn and the disc edema resolved at 1 week.

Cystoid macular edema developed in two patients treated with topical latanoprost for glaucoma (23). Latanoprost was withdrawn, and the cystoid macular edema was treated with topical corticosteroids and ketorolac, with improvement in visual acuity. The macular edema resolved in both cases.

Cystoid macular edema has been reported in four other patients shortly after they started to use latanoprost (24) and other reports have appeared (25–29). A possible explanation is enhanced disruption of the blood–aqueous barrier induced by latanoprost (28).

A review of the published literature (28 eyes in 25 patients) has shown that in all cases there were other associated risk factors, so that a definitive conclusion about a causal relation cannot be reached (30). Nevertheless, latanoprost should be used with caution in patients with risk factors for cystoid macular edema and special surveillance is necessary.

Choroidal detachment

The use of latanoprost after trabeculectomy can cause choroidal detachment (31).

- A 36-year-old man with juvenile open-angle glaucoma in both eyes and traumatic glaucoma in the left eye had extensive iridodialysis and angle recession of about 180° in the left eye. He was treated with topical timolol 0.5% bd and later daily latanoprost 0.005% to both eyes. Immediately after surgery for cataract extraction and intraocular lens implantation combined with trabeculectomy he had a large fall in intraocular pressure and 2 days later developed severe pain, gross impairment of vision, and intense congestion in the left eye. Indirect ophthalmoscopy showed an inferior choroidal detachment. Topical latanoprost was immediately stopped in the left eye and systemic prednisolone 1.5 mg/kg/day was continued. Within 7 days, the choroidal detachment settled.

The authors suggested that the drastic fall in intraocular pressure after trabeculectomy had resulted from an unusually large increase in uveoscleral outflow because of latanoprost. This was because of the additive effect of two factors: trabeculectomy-associated ciliary body detachment and the pre-existing cleft between the ciliary body stroma and the sclera, evidenced by extensive angle recession. The latter was perhaps responsible for the large fall in intraocular pressure (from 32 to 16 mmHg) when latanoprost was first introduced. Although the patient did not have uveitis, prostaglandin-mediated damage to the blood retinal barrier could also have contributed to choroidal detachment. They cautioned against the use of latanoprost as an adjunctive pressure-lowering agent after glaucoma filtration surgery.

Iris cyst

An iris cyst has been attributed to latanoprost (32).

- A 67-year old woman with advanced chronic angle-closure glaucoma was treated with laser iridotomy on both eyes followed by pilocarpine 2% and a beta-blocker. Later she used latanoprost instead, and intraocular pressures were maintained at 12-15 mmHg. There were no abnormal responses except mild hyperemia of the conjunctivae. After about 9 months she developed an iris pigment epithelial cyst on the posterior iris surface. Latanoprost was withdrawn and dorzolamide and a beta-blocker used instead. The iris cyst gradually shrank and completely disappeared from the pupil margin within 5 months. During follow-up for 4 months there was no recurrence.

Skin

Hyperpigmentation of the eyelids can occur during latanoprost therapy.

- A 62-year old Korean woman treated with latanoprost for 4 months developed eyelid pigmentation in both

upper and lower eyelids of both eyes (33). There was no increase in iris pigmentation. The eyelid pigmentation gradually diminished after withdrawal, but minimal brownish coloration remained along the lower eyelid folds in both eyes at 4 months.

- A 75-year-old woman with open-angle glaucoma who had used latanoprost for 15 months reported that the skin around her eyes was much darker than on the rest of her face (34). The darkening had occurred gradually. Latanoprost was withdrawn; 1 month later there was a discernible lightening of the periocular skin and 2 months after withdrawal the skin was significantly lighter.

Hair

Eyelashes

Latanoprost causes growth of lashes and ancillary hairs around the eyelids, with greater thickness and length of lashes, additional rows of lashes, and conversion of vellus to terminal hairs in canthal areas and regions adjacent to lashes. As well as increased growth, there is also increased pigmentation. Vellus hairs on the lower eyelids also undergo increased growth and pigmentation. Latanoprost caused changes in eyelashes in 26% of 194 patients over 12 months; the changes included increased length, thickness, density, and color (19).

Latanoprost therapy for 2–17 days can cause changes comparable to chronic therapy. The increased number and length of visible lashes are consistent with the ability of latanoprost to induce and prolong anagen growth in telogen (resting) follicles while producing hypertrophic changes in the involved follicles. Laboratory studies suggest that the initiation and completion of the effects of latanoprost on hair growth occur very early in the anagen phase and that the likely target is the dermal papilla.

Latanoprost can even reverse alopecia of the eyelashes (35).

- A 53-year-old woman, with glaucoma and loss of the eyelashes secondary to alopecia following an allergic response to ibuprofen was given latanoprost (36). After 3 weeks her eyelashes were noticeable and 2 months later full growth had occurred.
- Quantitative analysis of eyelash lengthening in 17 patients treated with latanoprost showed a significant increase in eyelash length in the treated eyes (37).

Increased pigmentation of the eyelashes has been reported in a patient treated with latanoprost (38).

Sweat glands

Heavy sweating occurred in a 6-year-old boy with aniridia and glaucoma during treatment with latanoprost eye-drops (39). Other combinations of drugs for glaucoma had been ineffective in reducing the intraocular pressure. He was given latanoprost eye-drops (dose not stated) at night in combination with a beta-blocker during the day. However, at night he had very heavy sweating. His pyjamas had to be changed regularly about 1–2 hours after he went to sleep. When latanoprost was withdrawn, the heavy sweating resolved. When it was restarted, the heavy sweating recurred.

The author commented that systemic absorption occurred for the most part through the mucous membranes of the nose and throat, since the sweating was less severe when the boy's lacrymal points were compressed for 10 minutes after the administration of latanoprost.

- A 55-year-old woman with primary chronic angle glaucoma was given latanoprost ophthalmic solution (0.005%, 1 drop/day) (40). After 3 days, 1–2 hours after administration, she reported severe sweating involving the entire body and drenching all her clothes. The excessive sweating disappeared on withdrawal of latanoprost and did not occur when she was given bimatoprost. One month later, latanoprost was restarted and the severe sweating recurred on the first day of therapy. Latanoprost was withdrawn and bimatoprost was started again.

Infection risk

Two cases of *H. simplex* virus dermatitis of the periocular skin have been reported in patients using latanoprost (41). Cases of *H. simplex* keratitis are mentioned above, under sensory systems.

Second-Generation Effects

Teratogenicity

Latanoprost exposure has been reported in 11 pregnancies (42). All the women used latanoprost in the first trimester, and embryo exposure lasted from a minimum of 4 days to a maximum of 70 days. There was complete follow-up in 10 cases: nine women delivered normal fetuses without malformations and one pregnancy was complicated by early spontaneous abortion 2 weeks after treatment was completed in a 46-year-old primigravida. The children were considered normal at follow-up within 2 years.

Drug-drug interactions

Non-steroidal anti-inflammatory drugs

Latanoprost induces the formation of endogenous prostaglandins including prostaglandin E_2 (dinoprostone), which could affect extracellular matrix metabolism in ciliary smooth muscle cells. It has therefore been hypothesized that latanoprost ophthalmic solution may reduce intraocular pressure by either direct signal transduction through prostaglandin $F_{2\alpha}$ receptors and by an indirect action through induced endogenous prostaglandins. Non-steroidal anti-inflammatory drugs (NSAIDs) inhibit the induction of endogenous prostaglandins by suppressing the activity of cyclo-oxygenases. Moreover, recent studies have shown that some NSAIDs also inhibit the formation of latanoprost-induced endogenous prostaglandins. Thus, NSAIDs may oppose intraocular pressure reduction by latanoprost. In a prospective observer

masked study of the effects of bromfenac sodium hydrate eye-drops on latanoprost-induced intraocular pressure reduction in 13 volunteers (43). Latanoprost significantly reduced intraocular pressure by about 5.7 mmHg, and this effect was attenuated by about 1.5 mmHg by co-administration of bromfenac. Bromfenac on its own did not affect intraocular pressure.

References

1. Eisenberg DL, Camras CB. A preliminary risk-benefit assessment of latanoprost and unoprostone in open-angle glaucoma and ocular hypertension. Drug Saf 1999;20(6):505–14.
2. Enyedi LB, Freedman SF. Latanoprost for the treatment of pediatric glaucoma. Surv Ophthalmol 2002;47(Suppl 1):S129–32.
3. Peak AS, Sutton BM. Systemic adverse effects associated with topically applied latanoprost. Ann Pharmacother 1998;32(4):504–5.
4. Marti V, Guindo J, Valles E, Domínguez de Rozas JM. Angina variante asociada con latanoprost. Med Clin (Barc) 2005; 125(6): 238–9.
5. Veyrac G, Chiffoleau A, Cellerin L, Larousse C, Bourin M. Latanoprost (Xalatan) et effect systémique respiratoire? A propos d'un cas. [Latanoprost (Xalatan) and a systemic respiratory effect? Apropos of a case.] Therapie 1999;54(4):494–6.
6. Weston BC. Migraine headache associated with latanoprost. Arch Ophthalmol 2001;119(2):300–1.
7. Sudesh S, Cohen EJ, Rapuano CJ, Wilson RP. Corneal toxicity associated with latanoprost. Arch Ophthalmol 1999;117(4):539–40.
8. Wand M, Gilbert CM, Liesegang TJ. Latanoprost and *Herpes simplex* keratitis. Am J Ophthalmol 1999;127(5):602–4.
9. Alm A. Prostaglandin derivates as ocular hypotensive agents. Prog Retin Eye Res 1998;17(3):291–312.
10. Teus MA, Arranz-Marquez E, Lucea-Suescun P. Incidence of iris colour change in latanoprost treated eyes. Br J Ophthalmol 2002;86(10):1085–8.
11. Pappas RM, Pusin S, Higginbotham EJ. Evidence of early change in iris color with latanoprost use. Arch Ophthalmol 1998;116(8):1115–6.
12. Camras CB, Neely DG, Weiss EL. Latanoprost-induced iris color darkening: a case report with long-term follow-up. J Glaucoma 2000;9(1):95–8.
13. Grierson I, Lee WR, Albert DM. The fine structure of an iridectomy specimen from a patient with latanoprost-induced eye color change. Arch Ophthalmol 1999;117(3):394–6.
14. Pfeiffer N, Grierson I, Goldsmith H, Appleton P, Hochgesand D, Winkgen A. Fine structural evaluation of the iris after unilateral treatment with latanoprost in patients undergoing bilateral trabeculectomy (the Mainz II study). Arch Ophthalmol 2003; 121: 23–31.
15. Nakamura Y, Nakamura Y, Morine-Shinjo S, Sakai H, Sawaguchi S. Assessment of chamber angle pigmentation during longterm latanoprost treatment for open-angle glaucoma. Acta Ophthalmol Scand 2004; 82: 158–60.
16. Alm A, Schoenfelder J, McDermott J. A 5-year, multicenter, open-label, safety study of adjunctive latanoprost therapy for glaucoma. Arch Ophthalmol 2004; 122: 957–65.
17. Chen CS, Wells J, Craig JE. Topical prostaglandin F(2alpha) analog induced poliosis. Am J Ophthalmol 2004; 137: 965–6.

18. Drago F, Marino A, La Manna C. Alpha-methyl-p-tyrosine inhibits latanoprost-induced melanogenesis in vitro. Exp Eye Res 1999;68(1):85–90.

19. Netland PA, Landry T, Sullivan EK, Andrew R, Silver L, Weiner A, Mallick S, Dickerson J, Bergamini MV, Robertson SM, Davis AA. Travoprost Study Group. Travoprost compared with latanoprost and timolol in patients with open-angle glaucoma or ocular hypertension. Am J Ophthalmol 2001;132(4):472–84.

20. Krohn J, Hove VK. Iris cyst associated with topical administration of latanoprost. Am J Ophthalmol 1999;127(1):91–3.

21. Fechtner RD, Khouri AS, Zimmerman TJ, Bullock J, Feldman R, Kulkarni P, Michael AJ, Realini T, Warwar R. Anterior uveitis associated with latanoprost. Am J Ophthalmol 1998;126(1):37–41.

22. Stewart O, Walsh L, Pande M. Bilateral optic disc oedema associated with latanoprost. Br J Ophthalmol 1999;83(9):1092–3.

23. Callanan D, Fellman RL, Savage JA. Latanoprost-associated cystoid macular edema. Am J Ophthalmol 1998;126(1):134–5.

24. Ayyala RS, Cruz DA, Margo CE, Harman LE, Pautler SE, Misch DM, Mines JA, Richards DW. Cystoid macular edema associated with latanoprost in aphakic and pseudophakic eyes. Am J Ophthalmol 1998;126(4):602–4.

25. Avakian A, Renier SA, Butler PJ. Adverse effects of latanoprost on patients with medically resistant glaucoma. Arch Ophthalmol 1998;116(5):679–80.

26. Gaddie IB, Bennett DW. Cystoid macular edema associated with the use of latanoprost. J Am Optom Assoc 1998;69(2):122–8.

27. Heier JS, Steinert RF, Frederick AR Jr. Cystoid macular edema associated with latanoprost use. Arch Ophthalmol 1998;116(5):680–2.

28. Miyake K, Ota I, Maekubo K, Ichihashi S, Miyake S. Latanoprost accelerates disruption of the blood–aqueous barrier and the incidence of angiographic cystoid macular edema in early postoperative pseudophakias. Arch Ophthalmol 1999;117(1):34–40.

29. Moroi SE, Gottfredsdottir MS, Schteingart MT, Elner SG, Lee CM, Schertzer RM, Abrams GW, Johnson MW. Cystoid macular edema associated with latanoprost therapy in a case series of patients with glaucoma and ocular hypertension. Ophthalmology 1999;106(5):1024–9.

30. Schumer RA, Camras CB, Mandahl AK. Latanoprost and cystoid macular edema: is there a causal relation? Curr Opin Ophthalmol 2000;11(2):94–100.

31. Sodhi PK, Sachdev MS, Gupta A, Verma LK, Ratan SK. Choroidal detachment with topical latanoprost after glaucoma filtration surgery. Ann Pharmacother 2004; 38: 510–1.

32. Lai IC, Kuo MT, Teng IMC. Iris pigment epithelial cyst induced by topical administration of latanoprost. Br J Ophthalmol 2003; 87: 366.

33. Kook MS, Lee K. Increased eyelid pigmentation associated with use of latanoprost. Am J Ophthalmol 2000;129(6):804–6.

34. Wand M, Ritch R, Isbey EK Jr, Zimmerman TJ. Latanoprost and periocular skin color changes. Arch Ophthalmol 2001;119(4):614–5.

35. Johnstone MA, Albert DM. Prostaglandin-induced hair growth. Surv Ophthalmol 2002;47(Suppl 1):S185–202.

36. Mansberger SL, Cioffi GA. Eyelash formation secondary to latanoprost treatment in a patient with alopecia. Arch Ophthalmol 2000;118(5):718–9.

37. Sugimoto M, Sugimoto M, Uji Y. Quantitative analysis of eyelash lengthening following topical latanoprost therapy. Can J Ophthalmol 2002;37(6):342–5.

38. Reynolds A, Murray PI, Colloby PS. Darkening of eyelashes in a patient treated with latanoprost. Eye 1998;12(Pt 4):741–3.

39. Schmidtborn F. Systemische Nebenwirkung von Latanoprost bei einem Kind mit Aniridie und Glaukom. [Systemic side-effects of latanoprost in a child with aniridia and glaucoma.] Ophthalmologe 1998;95(9):633–4.

40. Kumar H, Sony P, Gupta V. Profound sweating episodes and latanoprost. Clin Experiment Ophthalmol 2005; 33(6): 675.

41. Morales J, Shihab ZM, Brown SM, Hodges MR. *Herpes simplex* virus dermatitis in patients using latanoprost. Am J Ophthalmol 2001;132(1):114–6.

42. De Santis M, Lucchese A, Carducci B, Cavaliere AF, De Santis L, Merola A, Straface G, Caruso A. Latanoprost exposure in pregnancy. Am J Ophthalmol 2004; 138: 305–6.

43. Kashiwagi K., Tsukahara S. Effect of non-steroidal anti-inflammatory ophthalmic solution on intraocular pressure reduction by latanoprost. Br J Ophthalmol 2003; 87: 297–301.

Misoprostol

General Information

Misoprostol, an analogue of PGE_1, is licensed for use in the management of gastroduodenal ulceration. It is an effective myometrial stimulant of the pregnant uterus and is used for the induction of labor and as abortifacient, both alone and in combination with other substances (for example mifepristone). It provides an effective alternative to gemeprost, the most widely used prostaglandin pessaries in combination with mifepristone.

Vaginal misoprostol is more effective and better tolerated than oral misoprostol for induction of first and second trimester abortions after the administration of mifepristone (1,2). It is more effective than either gemeprost or sulprostone combined with mifepristone for induction of first trimester abortion, although uterine rupture has been reported (3).

Intramuscular methotrexate 50 mg/m^2 followed by intravaginal misoprostol was effective in the induction of first trimester abortion. Adverse events following the administration of misoprostol included nausea (12%), vomiting (8.1%), diarrhea (7.4%), and fevers/chills (3.4%) (4).

Observational studies

A single intravaginal dose of misoprostol 800 micrograms can obtain an abortion. The success rate has been assessed in 102 pregnant patients with amenorrhea for less than 42 weeks (5). After 1 day and 3 days of administration the abortion rates were 72 and 87% respectively. A second dose 7 days later increased the cumulative rate to 92%. The main complaints were pain (85%), nausea (21%), and headache (18%). Similar results were obtained in 2295 pregnant women (up to 56 days of gestation), who took a single oral dose of mifepristone (200 mg) and were randomized to self-administer misoprostol 800 micrograms/day at home for 1, 2, or 3 days (6). Complete abortion rates were 98, 98, and 96% among those who took misoprostol for 1, 2, and 3 days respectively. There were similar frequencies of adverse effects in all groups (cramping, nausea, fever/chills, dizziness, vomiting, headache, and diarrhea).

Misoprostol has been used to induce abortions in 150 adolescents (age range 12–17 years) at gestations of 63–84 days (7). They received vaginal misoprostol 800 micrograms/day to a maximum of three doses. Complete abortion occurred in 84%. Adverse effects were more frequent in these adolescents than in adult women, and included nausea (31%), vomiting (41%), diarrhea (48%), dizziness (19%), headache (17%), a subjective feeling of fever (26%), flushing (16%), and chills (49%).

The efficacy and tolerability of sublingual misoprostol has been evaluated in an uncontrolled trial in China in 50 women who requested medical abortions at up to 12 weeks of gestation (8). All received three doses of misoprostol 600 micrograms sublingually 3-hourly, and two more doses of 600 micrograms sublingually if an abortion did not occur. The overall complete abortion rate was 86% and the mean number of doses of misoprostol required was four. There was no significant change in hemoglobin concentration and the median duration of vaginal bleeding was 15 days. Lower abdominal pain, fatigue, diarrhea, fever, and chills were the most common adverse effects, and they occurred more often (from 70 to 100%) than in studies in which repeated doses of vaginal misoprostol were used.

In a retrospective study in patients with pre-eclampsia undergoing cervical ripening the complications associated with vaginal misoprostol (n = 95) and dinoprostone (n = 108) vaginal inserts before induction of labor have been reported (9). The incidence of uterine hyperstimulation requiring emergency cesarean section because of fetal heart rate abnormalities was significantly higher among patients who received misoprostol (18% versus 8.3%). The overall incidence of abruptio placenta was also significantly higher among those who received misoprostol (14% versus 1.9%).

Comparative studies

Different prostaglandins

Extra-amniotic dinoprost ($PGF_{2\alpha}$) and intracervical misoprostol have been compared for termination of pregnancy in 40 women at 16–24 weeks of gestation (10). All the women given dinoprost aborted within 28 hours and 16 within 20 hours; termination of pregnancy was complete in 13 cases. With misoprostol, all the women aborted within 20 hours, 18 within 13 hours; termination of pregnancy was complete in 17 cases. The mean time to induction of abortion was 16 hours for extra-amniotic dinoprost and 10 hours for intracervical misoprostol (significantly quicker). The incidence of prostaglandin-associated pyrexia, vomiting, and diarrhea was significantly higher with dinoprost. Abdominal pain was similar in the two groups.

Oxytocin

Misoprostol and oxytocin have been compared in three trials during vaginal and cesarean delivery. The first trial included 663 women (mean age 25 years, mean parity 2) with uncomplicated vaginal deliveries (11). They were randomized to receive two tablets of misoprostol (total dose 400 micrograms, dissolved in saline 5 ml and given as a micro-enema) or oxytocin (10 IU intramuscularly), with a double-dummy technique. There were no significant differences between the groups in mean hemoglobin and hematocrit, volume of blood loss, or duration of third-stage labor. Shivering (38 versus 15%) and an increased mean temperature were significantly more common among those who received misoprostol.

The second trial included 60 women who were randomized to oral misoprostol (400 micrograms) or intravenous oxytocin (10 IU) during cesarean section (12). Estimated blood loss was 545 ml (95% CI = 476, 614) in those given misoprostol and 533 ml (95% CI = 427, 639) in those given oxytocin. The hemoglobin concentration and hematocrit were similar in the two groups.

The third trial included 2058 patients (mean age 28 years, 53% nulliparous) with a singleton pregnancy, a low risk of postpartum hemorrhage, and vaginal delivery (13). They were randomly assigned to either intramuscular Syntometrine 1 ml (oxytocin 5 units plus ergometrine 0.5 mg) or oral misoprostol 600 micrograms. There were no significant differences between the two groups in mean blood loss, the incidence of postpartum hemorrhage, or the fall in hemoglobin concentration. The need for oxytocic medication was higher with misoprostol, but manual removal of the placenta was required more often. Shivering (30 versus 9.9%) and transient pyrexia (temperature over 38°C, 8.5 versus 1.3%) were more common with misoprostol. Misoprostol could be an alternative to oxytocic drugs in reducing postpartum blood loss.

Placebo-controlled studies

Oral misoprostol 400 micrograms has been compared with placebo in the routine management of the third-stage of labor. In this study shivering was a specific adverse effect of oral misoprostol in the puerperium (19 versus 5%; RR = 3.69; 95% CI = 2.05, 6.64) (14).

The adverse effects of misoprostol have been evaluated in a large double-blind randomized placebo-controlled trial sponsored by the WHO in 15 clinics in 11 countries in 2219 healthy pregnant women requesting medical abortion after up to 63 days of amenorrhea (15). They were given oral mifepristone 200 mg on day 1, followed by 800 micrograms either orally or vaginally on day 3. The oral group and one of the vaginal groups continued taking oral misoprostol 400 micrograms bd for 7 days and the vaginal-only group took oral placebo. Pregnancy-related symptoms abated in all the groups after misoprostol and breast tenderness was reduced by mifepristone. Oral misoprostol was associated with a higher frequency of nausea and vomiting than vaginal administration at 1 hour after administration. With oral misoprostol, diarrhea was more frequent at 1, 2, and 3 hours after administration. Misoprostol caused *fever* during at least 3 hours after administration in up to 6% of the women, the peak being slightly higher and later with vaginal administration. Lower abdominal pain peaked at 1 and 2 hours after oral misoprostol and at 2 and 3 hours after vaginal misoprostol. In the two groups of women who continued to take misoprostol, 27% had diarrhea between the misoprostol visit and the 2-week follow up visit, compared with 9% in the placebo group.

Systematic reviews

A systematic review of the use of misoprostol for induction of labor has been published (16). The meta-analysis included all randomized clinical trials registered in the Cochrane Pregnancy and Childbirth Group. Vaginal misoprostol was associated with increased uterine hyperstimulation, both without fetal heart changes (RR = 1.67; CI = 1.30, 2.14) and with associated fetal heart rate changes (RR = 1.45; CI = 1.04, 2.04). There was also an increase in meconium-stained amniotic fluid (RR = 1.38; CI = 1.06, 1.79).

General adverse effects

The most common adverse effects during misoprostol use in labor include pyrexia (temperature over 38°C), shivering, postpartum hemorrhage, nausea, vomiting, diarrhea, hot flushes, headache, and vertigo. When it is used in the first or second trimesters for pregnancy termination, its adverse effects include fever, chills, vomiting, diarrhea, moderate and severe abdominal pain, profuse bleeding, dysfunctional uterine bleeding, dizziness, and headache.

Organs and Systems

Reproductive system

The effects of vaginal misoprostol for third trimester cervical ripening or induction of labor has been reviewed (17).

Several cases of uterine rupture due to misoprostol after second trimester have been reported. However, unexpectedly, administration of misoprostol for cervical ripening before surgical evacuation of a missed abortion reportedly produced *uterine rupture* in the first trimester (18).

- A 30-year-old woman with amenorrhea for 8 weeks had vaginal bleeding probably secondary to a missed abortion. Transvaginal ultrasonography showed a single fetus of 6 weeks without cardiac activity. She was scheduled for dilatation and evacuation but 1 hour after a single oral dose of misoprostol 400 micrograms she developed severe abdominal pain, hypotension (70/40 mmHg), and abdominal distension and rebound tenderness. The hemoglobin concentration was 6.5 g/l. Emergency laparoscopy showed a 1.5 cm rupture of the left uterine horn.

She had had a previous cesarean section, but it is very unlikely that that contributed, because the uterine rupture occurred at a different site to the caesarean incision (low-flap transverse section).

Infection risk

There were four deaths in previously healthy women due to endometritis and toxic shock syndrome within 1 week after medically induced abortions with oral mifepristone 200 mg and vaginal misoprostol 800 micrograms; in two cases *Clostridium sordellii* was found (19). Another similar case was reported in Canada in 2001. Endometritis and toxic shock syndrome associated with *C. sordellii* are rare. Of 10 cases identified by authors in the previous literature, eight occurred after the delivery of live-born infants, one after a medical abortion, and one was not associated with pregnancy. The cases produced an FDA alert with a "Dear Health Care Provider" letter from the manufacturer and publication of a "Dispatch" in the Morbidity and Mortality Weekly Report (20).

Body temperature

Severe hyperthermia has been reported after misoprostol (21).

- A 31-year primigravida had a missed abortion after 12 weeks of amenorrhea and was admitted for evacuation of the uterus. Preoperative cervical priming was done with intravaginal misoprostol 600 micrograms. Within 30 minutes of insertion of the misoprostol tablets she had chills and rigors, felt unwell, and started to have lower abdominal cramps. She was febrile (39.5°C) and her pulse rate was 90/minute. The undissolved misoprostol tablets were removed digitally and her vagina was douched. Ice sponging lowered her temperature. A rectal suppository of diclofenac 25 mg and an intramuscular injection of promethazine 25 mg were given. Her temperature remained high at 38°C for 3 hours and normalized after 5 hours.

Second-Generation Effects

Pregnancy

Cervical laceration associated with misoprostol has been reported in a 33-year-old woman who received four doses of vaginal misoprostol (total dose 100 micrograms) for labor induction. Uterine rupture has occurred during induction of labor with misoprostol, usually in women who have had a previous cesarean section (22,23). Uterine dehiscence occurred in one and uterine rupture in three of 48 women with prior cesarean sections treated with intravaginal misoprostol 50 micrograms for cervical ripening (24). In comparison, uterine rupture occurred in one of 89 women who had an oxytocin infusion and none of 24 patients who received intravaginal alprostadil.

- Transvaginal misoprostol for induction of labor caused uterine rupture in a 26-year-old woman with a previous low transverse cesarean delivery (25).
- In two cases, disruption of prior uterine incisions occurred after misoprostol (26).

- In two cases, uterine rupture occurred after inappropriate use (27). In one case the dose of 200 micrograms was too high. In the other case oxytocin was started 5 hours after the second misoprostol tablet, while the usual recommendation is to wait at least 12 hours. One patient had also had a previous dilatation and curettage for spontaneous abortion, which is a predisposing factor for uterine rupture in labor.

Seven pregnant women who had uterine rupture after intravaginal administration of misoprostol for induction of labor (SEDA-23, 436) had all undergone cesarean section in previous pregnancies (28).

- The first four women (aged 26–36 years) underwent induction of labor at 37–40 weeks of gestation. They received 1–2 doses of intravaginal misoprostol 25 micrograms; three of the women then received intravenous oxytocin. Soon after the first woman began pushing, there was fetal heart rate deceleration and the fetal head could not be palpated in the vagina. Emergency laparotomy showed that the baby was free in the abdominal cavity and the woman had a bladder defect. The bladder and uterine defects were repaired successfully and the mother received a transfusion of packed erythrocytes.
- In the second case, there was sudden fetal bradycardia. Laparotomy showed a large clot overlying the previous uterine incision. Dissection through the hematoma showed complete separation of the uterine incision. After delivery, the uterine rupture site and a cervical laceration were successfully repaired.
- The third woman had sudden-onset severe abdominal pain and fetal decelerations were detected. Emergency laparotomy showed complete separation of the uterine scar; both the fetus and the placenta were free in the abdominal cavity. The uterine defect was repaired and the woman recovered. However, the baby subsequently died.
- The fourth woman began to have extreme pain and fetal bradycardia then occurred. Uterine rupture from the previous incision was found at emergency cesarean section, with the baby's arm extending through the lacerated area. The uterine defect was successfully repaired.
- Uterine rupture also occurred in another three women (ages not stated) after misoprostol (dosages not stated) was used to induce labor. One underwent cesarean section because labor did not progress. During the procedure, the fetal hand and head were outside the uterine cavity (maternal and fetal outcome not stated).
- The other two women underwent emergency cesarean deliveries because of fetal bradycardia. Both had complete uterine wall separation; one had a stellate laceration involving the previous incision, and the other had a hematoma associated with the scar disruption. Outcomes were good in both cases.

In view of these cases, the authors recommended that there be a moratorium on the use of misoprostol in the setting of a scarred uterus until the relative risks have been thoroughly investigated in appropriately controlled trials.

Uterine rupture has also been associated with misoprostol (200 micrograms vaginally) during second trimester termination of pregnancy. Occasionally, uterine rupture can occur in women who have not had a previous cesarean section, as happened in two women, one of whom had a normal delivery and the other curettage after abortion (29).

Misoprostol is not approved by the FDA for any obstetric indication. In 2000, the manufacturers GD Searle distributed a "Dear Health Care Provider" letter in the USA, emphasizing the fact that misoprostol, by any route of administration, is not intended for the induction of labor or as a cervical ripening agent before termination of pregnancy (30). Searle has become aware of instances in which misoprostol was used for such purposes, in spite of its being specifically contraindicated for use during pregnancy. The following serious adverse events have been reported after such off-label use: maternal or fetal death; uterine hyperstimulation; uterine rupture or perforation requiring surgical repair, hysterectomy, or salpingo-oophorectomy; amniotic fluid embolism; severe vaginal bleeding; retained placenta; shock; fetal bradycardia; and pelvic pain. Searle does not intend to study or support the use of misoprostol for pregnancy termination or labor induction. The company is therefore unable to provide complete risk information for misoprostol when it is used for such purposes. Furthermore, the effects of misoprostol on the later growth, development, and functional maturation of children who are exposed to it during induction of labor have not been established.

Teratogenicity

The common phenotypical effects of exposure of the fetus to misoprostol in utero have been defined in 42 infants who were exposed to misoprostol during the first 3 months of gestation, and then born with congenital abnormalities (31). Equinovarus with cranial nerve defects occurred in 17 infants. Ten children had equinovarus as part of more extensive arthrogryposis. The most distinctive phenotypes were arthrogryposis confined to the legs (five cases) and terminal transverse limb defects (nine cases), with or without Möbius' syndrome. The most common dose of misoprostol was 800 (range 200–16 000) micrograms. Deformities attributed to vascular disruption were found in these children. The authors suggested that the uterine contractions induced by misoprostol cause vascular disruption in the fetus, including brainstem ischemia. Information on the effects of taking misoprostol during pregnancy should be made more widely available, to dissuade women from misusing the drug. Additional information on the risk associated with continuing a pregnancy to term after a failure of mifepristone and prostaglandin has been provided (32).

Data from Brazil, where misoprostol has been used orally and vaginally as an abortifacient, have suggested a relation between the use of misoprostol by women in an unsuccessful attempt to terminate pregnancy and Möbius' syndrome (congenital facial paralysis) in their infants (33). The frequencies of misoprostol use during the first trimester by mothers of infants in whom Möbius' syndrome was diagnosed and mothers of infants with neural-tube defects have been compared. There were 96 infants with Möbius' syndrome and 96 with neural-tube defects. The mean age at the time of the diagnosis of Möbius' syndrome was 16 (range 0.5–78) months and the diagnosis of neural-tube defects was made within 1 week of birth in most cases. Of the mothers of the infants with Möbius' syndrome, 47 had used misoprostol in the first trimester of pregnancy, compared with three of the mothers of the infants with neural-tube defects (OR = 30; 95% CI = 12, 76). Of the mothers of the infants with Möbius' syndrome, 20 had taken misoprostol only orally (OR = 39; CI = 9.5, 159), 20 had taken misoprostol both orally and vaginally, three had taken it vaginally, and four did not report how they had taken it. The authors concluded that attempted abortion with misoprostol is associated with an increased risk of Möbius' syndrome in infants.

In another case-control study in Brazil, 93 cases of prenatal exposure to misoprostol and 279 controls were recruited (34). Vascular disruption defects (transverse terminal limb reductions, Möbius and/or Poland sequences, hypoglossia–hypodactyly sequence, arthrogryposis, intestinal atresia, hemifacial microsomia, microtia, and porencephalic cyst) were identified in 32 exposed infants compared with only 12 controls.

In another case-control study in Brazil, congenital anomalies were compared in 34 misoprostol-exposed children and 4639 unexposed controls (35). Misoprostol exposure significantly increased the risk of arthrogryposis (OR = 8.5; 95% CI = 2, 37), hydrocephalus (OR = 4.2; CI = 1.5, 12), terminal transverse limb reduction (OR = 12; CI = 3.5, 41), and limb constriction ring or skin scars (OR = 40; CI = 11, 153). There were 13 different defects not previously described in the misoprostol-exposed cases, but only holoprosencephaly and bladder exstrophy significantly exceeded the expected number.

Mothers who used misoprostol during pregnancy as an abortifacient had an increased risk of having a baby with congenital anomalies (OR = 2.4; 95% CI = 1.0, 6.2), as reported in a case-control study in Fortaleza, Brazil (36). Multiple malformations have been described associated with the use of misoprostol (37).

• A 23-year-old woman took oral misoprostol 600 micrograms/day twice when she was 7 weeks pregnant to induce an abortion. At 12 weeks she developed a *Varicella* infection. At 15 weeks, ultrasound showed a fetus of 14.5 weeks size with several abnormalities. After amniocentesis at 17 weeks, an elective abortion was performed. The fetus had amputation deformities at the proximal interphalangeal joints of four fingers, with distal fusion of the proximal finger stumps by thin strands of tissue; the index finger was normal. The left leg had an amputation deformity at the mid-tibial/fibular level. There was an omphalocele. Histological examination of the placenta showed an absence of amnion on the chorionic surface, with reactive changes in the superficial chorionic stroma and "vernix granulomas" on the chorionic surface. These findings are diagnostic of early amnion rupture. There were no features of *Varicella* embryopathy.

Möbius' syndrome in association with congenital central alveolar hypoventilation has been described in Brazil (38).

Misoprostol-induced arthrogryposis has been reported in 15 Brazilian patients (39).

Drug Administration

Drug administration route

In a randomized controlled trial, 74 primigravidae who were undergoing surgical abortion were randomly assigned to misoprostol 400 micrograms sublingually or vaginally 2–4 hours before surgery (40). Efficacy was similar in the two groups. Women who took sublingual misoprostol had significantly more *nausea* (63% versus 32%), vomiting (29% versus 6%), diarrhea (6% versus 0%), and unpleasant taste in the mouth (39% versus 3%) compared with the women who used vaginal misoprostol.

In another study, 100 pregnant women who opted for termination of pregnancy at 6–12 weeks gestation were randomly allocated to misoprostol 400 micrograms sublingually or vaginally 2 hours before suction evacuation (41). There was a significant difference between the sublingual and vaginal misoprostol groups with respect to mean cervical dilatation (8.6 mm versus 6.8 mm). However, the durations of the procedures (3.03 versus 3.16 minutes) and the amounts of blood loss (29 versus 31.2 ml) were not different. The women who used sublingual misoprostol had significantly more shivering and preoperative vaginal bleeding (68% versus 56%). Sublingual misoprostol is an effective alternative to vaginal administration for cervical priming before surgical abortion, despite a higher incidence of adverse effects.

The pharmacokinetics of misoprostol 600 mg after oral and rectal administration have been compared in 20 women after delivery (42). After rectal administration there was a higher AUC, but lower C_{max} and a later t_{max}; these findings are consistent with a slower speed but a greater extent of absorption. In 275 women randomized to oral misoprostol 600 micrograms or rectal misoprostol 400 or 600 micrograms after delivery, shivering was reported by 76% of the patients given oral misoprostol and 55% of those given rectal misoprostol. Thus, rectal misoprostol is associated with less toxicity than oral misoprostol.

References

1. el-Refaey H, Rajasekar D, Abdalla M, Calder L, Templeton A. Induction of abortion with mifepristone (RU 486) and oral or vaginal misoprostol. N Engl J Med 1995;332(15):983–7.
2. Jain JK, Mishell DR Jr. A comparison of misoprostol with and without laminaria tents for induction of second-trimester abortion. Am J Obstet Gynecol 1996;175(1):173–7.
3. Phillips K, Berry C, Mathers AM. Uterine rupture during second trimester termination of pregnancy using

mifepristone and a prostaglandin. Eur J Obstet Gynecol Reprod Biol 1996;65(2):175–6.

4. Creinin MD, Vittinghoff E, Keder L, Darney PD, Tiller G. Methotrexate and misoprostol for early abortion: a multi-center trial. I. Safety and efficacy. Contraception 1996;53(6):321–7.

5. Bugalho A, Mocumbi S, Faundes A, David E. Termination of pregnancies of <6 weeks gestation with a single dose of 800 microg of vaginal misoprostol. Contraception 2000;61(1):47–50.

6. Schaff EA, Fielding SL, Westhoff C, Ellertson C, Eisinger SH, Stadalius LS, Fuller L. Vaginal misoprostol administered 1, 2, or 3 days after mifepristone for early medical abortion: A randomized trial. JAMA 2000;284(15):1948–53.

7. Acharya G, Al-Sammarai MT, Patel N, Al-Habib A, Kiserud T. A randomized, controlled trial comparing effect of oral misoprostol and intravenous syntocinon on intra-operative blood loss during cesarean section. Acta Obstet Gynecol Scand 2001;80(3):245–50.

8. Tang OS, Miao BY, Lee SW, Ho PC. Pilot study on the use of repeated doses of sublingual misoprostol in termination of pregnancy up to 12 weeks gestation: efficacy and accept-ability. Hum Reprod 2002;17(3):654–8.

9. Fontenot MT, Lewis DF, Barton CB, Jones EM, Moore JA, Evans AT. Abruptio placentae associated with misoprostol use in women with preeclampsia. J Reprod Med 2005; 50(9): 653–8.

10. Ghorab MN, El Helw BA. Second-trimester termination of pregnancy by extra-amniotic prostaglandin F2alpha or endocervical misoprostol. A comparative study. Acta Obstet Gynecol Scand 1998;77(4):429–32.

11. Ng PS, Chan AS, Sin WK, Tang LC, Cheung KB, Yuen PM. A multicentre randomized controlled trial of oral misopros-tol and i.m. syntometrine in the management of the third stage of labour Hum Reprod 2001;16(1):31–5.

12. Oyelese Y, Landy HJ, Collea JV. Cervical laceration asso-ciated with misoprostol induction. Int J Gynaecol Obstet 2001;73(2):161–2.

13. Al-Hussaini TK. Uterine rupture in second trimester abor-tion in a grand multiparous woman. A complication of mis-oprostol and oxytocin. Eur J Obstet Gynecol Reprod Biol 2001;96(2):218–9.

14. Hofmeyr GJ, Nikodem VC, de Jager M, Gelbart BR. A randomised placebo controlled trial of oral misoprostol in the third stage of labour. Br J Obstet Gynecol 1998;105(9):971–5.

15. Honkanen H, Piaggio G, Hertzen H, Bartfai G, Erdenetungalag R, Gemzell-Danielsson K, Gopalan S, Horga M, Jerve F, Mittal S, Thi Nhu Ngoc N, Peregoudov A, Prasad RN, Pretnar-Darovec A, Shah RS, Song S, Tang OS, Wu SC; WHO Research Group on Post-Ovulatory Methods for Fertility Regulation. WHO multinational study of three misoprostol regimens after mifepristone for early medical abortion. BJOG 2004; 111: 715–25.

16. Hofmeyr GJ, Gulmezoglu AM, Alfirevic Z. Misoprostol for induction of labour: a systematic review. Br J Obstet Gynecol 1999;106(8):798–803.

17. Hofmeyr GJ, Gulmezoglu AM. Vaginal misoprostol for cervical ripening and induction of labour. Cochrane Database Syst Rev 2003; (1): CD000941.

18. Kim JO, Han JY, Choi JS, Ahn HK, Yang JH, Kang IS, Song MJ, Nava-Ocampo AA. Oral misoprostol and uterine rupture in the first trimester of pregnancy: a case report. Reprod Toxicol 2005; 20(4): 575–7.

19. Fischer M, Bhatnagar J, Guarner J, Reagan S, Hacker JK, Van Meter SH, Poukens V, Whiteman DB, Iton A, Cheung M,

Dassey DE, Shieh WJ, Zaki SR. Fatal toxic shock syndrome associated with Clostridium sordellii after medical abortion. N Engl J Med 2005; 353(22): 2352–60.

20. Centers for Disease Control and Prevention. Clostridium sordellii toxic shock syndrome after medical abortion with mifepristone and intravaginal misoprostol—United States and Canada, 2001–2005. MMWR Morb Mortal Wkl Rep 2005; 54: 724.

21. Fong YF, Singh K, Prasad RN. Severe hyperthermia follow-ing use of vaginal misoprostol for pre-operative cervical priming. Int J Gynaecol Obstet 1999;64(1):73–4.

22. Gherman RB, McBrayer S, Browning J. Uterine rupture associated with vaginal birth after cesarean section: a com-plication of intravaginal misoprostol? Gynecol Obstet Invest 2000;50(3):212–3.

23. Jwarah E, Greenhalf JO. Rupture of the uterus after 800 micrograms misoprostol given vaginally for termination of pregnancy. BJOG 2000;107(6):807.

24. Hill DA, Chez RA, Quinlan J, Fuentes A, LaCombe J. Uterine rupture and dehiscence associated with intravaginal misopros-tol cervical ripening. J Reprod Med 2000;45(10):823–6.

25. Sciscione AC, Nguyen L, Manley JS, Shlossman PA, Colmorgen GH. Uterine rupture during preinduction cervi-cal ripening with misoprostol in a patient with a previous Caesarean delivery. Aust NZ J Obstet Gynaecol 1998;38(1):96–7.

26. Wing DA, Lovett K, Paul RH. Disruption of prior uterine incision following misoprostol for labor induction in women with previous cesarean delivery. Obstet Gynecol 1998;91(5 Pt 2):828–30.

27. Fletcher H, McCaw-Binns A. Rupture of the uterus with misoprostol (prostaglandin El) used for induction of labour. J Obstet Gynaecol 1998;18(2):184–5.

28. Plaut MM, Schwartz ML, Lubarsky SL. Uterine rupture associated with the use of misoprostol in the gravid patient with a previous cesarean section. Am J Obstet Gynecol 1999;180(6 Pt 1):1535–42.

29. Mathews JE, Mathai M, George A. Uterine rupture in a multiparous woman during labor induction with oral mis-oprostol. Int J Gynaecol Obstet 2000;68(1):43–4.

30. Searle GD. Important drug warning concerning unapproved use of intravaginal or oral misoprostol in pregnant women for induction of labor or abortion. Media Release 23 August 2000.

31. Gonzalez CH, Marques-Dias MJ, Kim CA, Sugayama SM, Da Paz JA, Huson SM, Holmes LB. Congenital abnormalities in Brazilian children associated with misoprostol misuse in first trimester of pregnancy. Lancet 1998;351(9116):1624–7.

32. Sitruk-Ware R, Davey A, Sakiz E. Fetal malformation and failed medical termination of pregnancy. Lancet 1998;352(9124):323.

33. Pastuszak AL, Schuler L, Speck-Martins CE, Coelho KE, Cordello SM, Vargas F, Brunoni D, Schwarz IV, Larrandaburu M, Safattle H, Meloni VF, Koren G. Use of misoprostol during pregnancy and Möbius' syndrome in infants. N Engl J Med 1998;338(26):1881–5.

34. Vargas FR, Schuler-Faccini L, Brunoni D, Kim C, Meloni VF, Sugayama SM, Albano L, Llerena JC Jr, Almeida JC, Duarte A, Cavalcanti DP, Goloni-Bertollo E, Conte A, Koren G, Addis A. Prenatal exposure to miso-prostol and vascular disruption defects: a case-control study. Am J Med Genet 2000;95(4):302–6.

35. Orioli IM, Castilla EE. Epidemiological assessment of mis-oprostol teratogenicity. BJOG 2000;107(4):519–23.

36. Brasil R, Coelho HL, D'Avanzo B, La Vecchia C. Misoprostol and congenital anomalies. Pharmacoepidemiol Drug Saf 2000;9:401–3.

37. Genest DR, Di Salvo D, Rosenblatt MJ, Holmes LB. Terminal transverse limb defects with tethering and omphalocele in a 17 week fetus following first trimester misoprostol exposure. Clin Dysmorphol 1999;8(1):53–8.

38. Nunes ML, Friedrich MA, Loch LF. Association of misoprostol, Moebius syndrome and congenital central alveolar hypoventilation. Case report. Arq Neuropsiquiatr 1999;57(1):88–91.

39. Coelho KE, Sarmento MF, Veiga CM, Speck-Martins CE, Safatle HP, Castro CV, Niikawa N. Misoprostol embryotoxicity: clinical evaluation of fifteen patients with arthrogryposis. Am J Med Genet 2000;95(4):297–301.

40. Hamoda H, Ashok PW, Flett GM, Templeton A. A randomized controlled comparison of sublingual and vaginal administration of misoprostol for cervical priming before first-trimester surgical abortion. Am J Obstet Gynecol 2004; 190: 55–9.

41. Vimala N, Mittal S, Kumar S, Dadhwal V, Sharma Y. A randomized comparison of sublingual and vaginal misoprostol for cervical priming before suction termination of first-trimester pregnancy. Contraception 2004; 70: 117–20.

42. Khan RU, El-Refaey H. Pharmacokinetics and adverse-effect profile of rectally administered misoprostol in the third stage of labor. Obstet Gynecol 2003; 101: 968–74.

Sulprostone

General Information

Sulprostone is a synthetic prostaglandin analogue of PGE_2 used for inducing uterine contraction.

In large series, sulprostone has had good tolerability with a very low complication rate. The most severe complication is myocardial infarction secondary to coronary spasm, with a frequency of one in 20 000, usually in smokers and women over 35 years of age with cardiovascular disease (SEDA-23, 436).

Organs and Systems

Cardiovascular

Several experimental studies have provided support for the hypothesis that coronary spasm plays a major role in the pathophysiology of myocardial infarction during the administration of sulprostone. However, the possibility of myocardial infarction is not mentioned in the product information.

- Two cases of myocardial infarction (one fatal) have been reported in patients receiving sulprostone with mifepristone (1,2).
- Myocardial infarction has been reported in a woman aged 35 years with normal coronary arteries and good left ventricular function (3).
- A 30-year-old woman developed uterine atony and bleeding after induced abortion because of fetal death at 17 weeks of gestation (4). Sulprostone was given intravenously at a rate of 500 micrograms/hour.

When additional sulprostone was injected into the uterine cervix, the patient sustained a myocardial infarction, with ventricular fibrillation and cardiocirculatory arrest, most probably due to coronary artery spasm. She was resuscitated and recovered completely.

Sulprostone should be used with care, particularly in patients with cardiac risk factors, and only in settings equipped to manage complications.

Cardiac dysrhythmias have been reported after the administration of misoprostol.

- A 38-year-old woman developed complete heart block, ventricular fibrillation, and subsequent asystole about 7 minutes after intravenous sulprostone 30 micrograms over 5 minutes, after she had previously been given a total dose of intramyometrial sulprostone 500 micrograms at seven different points for postpartum hemorrhage after cesarean section (5).

The time-course suggested that the most likely cause of the arrest was the intravenous sulprostone. Contributory causes may have been hemorrhagic shock, electrolyte abnormalities, and hypothermia (from massive blood transfusion).

- Cardiac arrest occurred in a 39-year-old woman 3.5 hours after the administration of sulprostone 250 micrograms directly into the uterine wall for postpartum hemorrhage after manual removal of the placenta (6). She had specific contraindications to sulprostone, as formulated by the French authorities: age over 35 years, heavy cigarette smoking, and cardiovascular risk factors.

In the Netherlands, sulprostone is registered for intravenous administration only. The authors strongly advised against administration directly into the uterine wall.

Nervous system

Seizures have been described during pregnancy termination induced by sulprostone (7).

Liver

Sulprostone has been associated with minor abnormalities of liver function (8).

Urinary tract

Sulprostone has been associated with minor abnormalities of kidney function (8).

Reproductive system

Sulprostone can cause rupture of the uterine cervix (9).

- A 43-year-old woman, who had previously had a first trimester miscarriage that required evacuation of the uterus and a normal vaginal delivery at term 4 years before, was admitted for an abortion at 16 weeks. Ripening of the cervix was started with a pessary of gemeprost 1 mg. After 3 hours, when the cervix was 1 cm dilated, an intramuscular injection of sulprostone

500 mg was given. After 30 minutes she developed persistent abdominal pain, which became a continuous cramping and then a shooting pain; a male fetus of 170 g was aborted. There was a 3 cm longitudinal cervical rupture located posteriorly that reached the posterior fornix.

References

1. Anonymous. A death associated with mifeprostone/sulprostone. Lancet 1991;337:969–70.
2. Ulmann A, Silvestre L, Chemama L, Rezvani Y, Renault M, Aguillaume CJ, Baulieu EE. Medical termination of early pregnancy with mifepristone (RU 486) followed by a prostaglandin analogue. Study in 16,369 women. Acta Obstet Gynecol Scand 1992;71(4):278–83.
3. Feenstra J, Borst F, Huige MC, Oei SG, Stricker BH. Acuut myocardinfarct na toediening van sulproston. [Acute myocardial infarct following sulproston administration.] Ned Tijdschr Geneeskd 1998;142(4):192–5.
4. Kulka PJ, Quent P, Wiebalck A, Jager D, Strumpf M. Myocardial infarction after sulprostone therapy for uterine atony and bleeding: a case report. Geburtshilfe Frauenheilk 1999;59:634–7.
5. Chen FG, Koh KF, Chong YS. Cardiac arrest associated with sulprostone use during caesarean section. Anaesth Intensive Care 1998;26(3):298–301.
6. Beerendonk CC, Massuger LF, Lucassen AM, Lerou JG, van den Berg PP. Circulatiestilstand na gebruik van sulproston bij fluxus post partum. [Circulatory arrest following sulprostone administration in postpartum hemorrhage.] Ned Tijdschr Geneeskd 1998;142(4):195–7.
7.. Brandenburg H, Jahoda MG, Wladimiroff JW, Los FJ, Lindhout D. Convulsions in epileptic women after administration of prostaglandin E2 derivative. Lancet 1990;336(8723):1138.
8. Ranjan V, Hingorani V, Kinra G, Agarwal N, Pande Y. Evaluation of sulprostone for second trimester abortions and its effects on liver and kidney function. Contraception 1982;25(2):175–84.
9. Corrado F, D'Anna R, Cannata ML. Rupture of the cervix in a sulprostone induced abortion in the second trimester. Arch Gynecol Obstet 2000;264(3):162–3.

Travoprost

General Information

Travoprost is a derivative of fluprostenol and $PGF_{2\alpha}$ and has intraocular pressure-lowering activity.

Organs and Systems

Sensory systems

Travoprost causes changes in iris pigmentation (3.1–5.0%) and changes in eyelash characteristics, including length, thickness, density, and color (44–57%), similar to those described with latanoprost, after 12 months (1).

Gastrointestinal

Abdominal cramp has been attributed to travoprost (2).

- A 34-year-old woman with primary open-angle glaucoma began topical application of travoprost ophthalmic solution (0.004%, 1 drop/day) and 30 minutes later developed abdominal cramp that lasted for 2 hours. The same symptoms appeared on 3 days after drug administration. The pain disappeared after travoprost withdrawal.

In order to investigate this adverse effect, a series of single-blind trials were carried out with the informed consent of the patient (including rechallenge with travoprost and other prostaglandin analogues and dechallenges). Abdominal cramp did not develop after substitution of travoprost with latanoprost or isotonic saline, but recurred on rechallenge with travoprost.

References

1. Netland PA, Landry T, Sullivan EK, Andrew R, Silver L, Weiner A, Mallick S, Dickerson J, Bergamini MV, Robertson SM, Davis AATravoprost Study Group. Travoprost compared with latanoprost and timolol in patients with open-angle glaucoma or ocular hypertension. Am J Ophthalmol 2001;132(4):472–84.
2. Lee YC. Abdominal cramp as an adverse effect of travoprost. Am J Ophthalmol 2005; 139(1): 202–3.

Unoprostone

General Information

Unoprostone is a synthetic prostaglandin analogue of $PGF_{2\alpha}$ used in the treatment of glaucoma. Its mechanism of action is believed to be by enhancing uveoscleral outflow, like latanoprost.

Organs and Systems

Sensory systems

The use of unoprostone in the treatment of open-angle glaucoma and ocular hypertension has been reviewed (1). Most of the literature is in Japanese. The adverse effects of unoprostone are similar to those of latanoprost: conjunctival hyperemia, iris pigmentation, hypertrichosis and hyperpigmentation of eyelashes, and rarely systemic effects (1).

Reference

1. Eisenberg DL, Camras CB. A preliminary risk-benefit assessment of latanoprost and unoprostone in open-angle glaucoma and ocular hypertension. Drug Saf 1999;20(6):505–14.

INTERFERONS

General Information

The interferons, first described in 1957, include at least five natural human glycoproteins (alfa, beta, gamma, omega, and tau). Only the first three types are currently used, and they differ both structurally and antigenically. Interferon alfa is produced by macrophages, B cells, and null lymphocytes, interferon beta by fibroblasts, epithelial cells, and macrophages, and interferon gamma from T lymphocytes and macrophages after antigenic or mitogenic stimulation. The interferons share 30–40% of sequence homology and have antiviral and antiproliferative actions. Interferon gamma, produced by activated T cells and natural killer cells, is recognized by a different receptor and acts primarily as an immunoregulatory cytokine.

Uses

The uses of interferons are listed in Table 1.

Two authoritative reviews have outlined the therapeutic potential of interferons (1,2). A wide range of viral diseases or cancers are other candidates for interferon therapy (3–5).

Mechanisms of action

On binding to surface receptors, interferon alfa results in activation of cytoplasmic enzymes affecting messenger RNA translation and protein synthesis (6). The antiviral state takes hours to develop but can persist for days.

Besides broad antiviral activity, interferons are of major importance in regulating immunological functions.

General adverse effects

The adverse effects of interferon are multifarious and the natural products seem to be less toxic than the pure synthetic compounds. Influenza-like symptoms with fever, chills, fatigue, myalgia, arthralgia, nausea, and lethargy, starting within 1 week after the start of treatment and lasting 1–7 days, seem to be very common (7,8). Adverse effects also include neurotoxicity (paresthesia, polyneuropathy), hepatic toxicity, renal toxicity, and an increase in eyelash growth (9–13). Neutralizing antibodies can lead to resistance in patients with hairy cell leukemia and chronic myeloid leukemia (14,15). The route of administration influences the provocation of an antibody response, and recombinant interferon beta is more likely to be immunogenic when given subcutaneously or intramuscularly than when given intravenously (16). Raynaud's phenomenon has been described after treatment with interferon alfa (17), and exacerbation of multiple sclerosis has been observed after treatment with interferon gamma.

The most common adverse effects reported in two large multicenter studies were fever (60%), leukopenia (43%), increased serum aspartate transaminase activity (30%), anorexia (30%), thrombocytopenia (25%), fatigue (21%), nausea, and vomiting (17%) (18,19). Compared with subcutaneous administration, intravenous interferon

Table 1 Names of different types of interferons and their indications

Generic name and trade name	Indications
Interferon alfa Human natural leukocyte interferon alfa (IFN alfa-n3; Alferon) Lymphoblastoid interferon alfa (IFN alfa-n1; Welferon) Recombinant interferon alfa-2a (rIFN alfa-2a; Roferon) Recombinant interferon alfa-2b (rIFN alfa-2b; Intron A) Recombinant interferon alfa-2c (rIFN alfa,2c; Berofor)	Malignant diseases: hairy cell leukemia, chronic myelogenous leukemia, cutaneous T cell lymphoma, follicular lymphoma, multiple myeloma, Kaposi's sarcoma, diffuse melanoma, renal cell carcinoma, carcinoid tumors Viral diseases: condylomata acuminata, chronic active hepatitis B and C
Interferon beta Natural fibroblast (Fiblaferon) Recombinant interferon beta (rIFN beta; Avonex) Recombinant interferon beta-1b (rIFN beta-1b; Betaseron)	Multiple sclerosis
Interferon gamma Recombinant interferon gamma-1b (rIFN gamma-1b; Actimmune)	Chronic granulomatous disease

alfa is associated with similar adverse effects of greater severity and frequency (20,21).

References

1. Galvani D, Griffiths SD, Cawley JC. Interferon for treatment: the dust settles. BMJ (Clin Res Ed) 1988;296(6636):1554–6.

2. Merigan TC. Human interferon as a therapeutic agent: a decade passes. N Engl J Med 1988;318(22):1458–60.

3. Agarwala SS, Kirkwood JM. Interferons in the therapy of solid tumors. Oncology 1994;51(2):129–36.

4. Urabe A. Interferons for the treatment of hematological malignancies. Oncology 1994;51(2):137–41.

5. Dorr RT. Interferon-alpha in malignant and viral diseases. A review. Drugs 1993;45(2):177–211.

6. Stiehm ER, Kronenberg LH, Rosenblatt HM, Bryson Y, Merigan TC. UCLA conference. Interferon: immunobiology and clinical significance. Ann Intern Med 1982;96(1):80–93.

7. Alexander GJ, Brahm J, Fagan EA, Smith HM, Daniels HM, Eddleston AL, Williams R. Loss of HBsAg with interferon therapy in chronic hepatitis B virus infection. Lancet 1987;2(8550):66–9.

8. Giles FJ, Singer CR, Gray AG, Yong KL, Brozovic M, Davies SC, Grant IR, Hoffbrand AV, Machin SJ, Mehta AB, et al. Alpha-interferon therapy for essential thrombocythaemia. Lancet 1988;2(8602):70–2.

9. Korenman J, Baker B, Waggoner J, Everhart JE, Di Bisceglie AM, Hoofnagle JH. Long-term remission of chronic hepatitis B after alpha-interferon therapy. Ann Intern Med 1991;114(8):629–34.

10. Scott GM, Ward RJ, Wright DJ, Robinson JA, Onwubalili JK, Gauci CL. Effects of cloned interferon alpha 2 in normal volunteers: febrile reactions and changes in circulating corticosteroids and trace metals. Antimicrob Agents Chemother 1983;23(4):589–92.

11. Ingimarsson S, Cantell K, Strander H. Side effects of long-term treatment with human leukocyte interferon. J Infect Dis 1979;140(4):560–3.

12. Cheeseman SH, Rubin RH, Stewart JA, Tolkoff-Rubin NE, Cosimi AB, Cantell K, Gilbert J, Winkle S, Herrin JT, Black PH, Russell PS, Hirsch MS. Controlled clinical trial of prophylactic human-leukocyte interferon in renal transplantation. Effects on cytomegalovirus and herpes simplex virus infections. N Engl J Med 1979;300(24):1345–9.

13. Smedley H, Katrak M, Sikora K, Wheeler T. Neurological effects of recombinant human interferon. BMJ (Clin Res Ed) 1983;286(6361):262–4.

14. Inglada L, Porres JC, La Banda F, Mora I, Carreno V. Anti-IFN-alpha titres during interferon therapy. Lancet 1987;2(8574):1521.

15. Steis RG, Smith JW 2nd, Urba WJ, Clark JW, Itri LM, Evans LM, Schoenberger C, Longo DL. Resistance to recombinant interferon alfa-2a in hairy-cell leukemia associated with neutralizing anti-interferon antibodies. N Engl J Med 1988;318(22):1409–13.

16. Konrad MW, Childs AL, Merigan TC, Borden EC. Assessment of the antigenic response in humans to a recombinant mutant interferon beta. J Clin Immunol 1987;7(5):365–75.

17. Roy V, Newland AC. Raynaud's phenomenon and cryoglobulinaemia associated with the use of recombinant human alpha-interferon. Lancet 1988;1(8591):944–5.

18. Taguchi T. Clinical studies of recombinant interferon alfa-2a (Roferon-A) in cancer patients. Cancer 1986;57(Suppl 8):1705–8.

19. Umeda T, Niijima T. Phase II study of alpha interferon on renal cell carcinoma. Summary of three collaborative trials. Cancer 1986;58(6):1231–5.

20. Mirro J, Dow LW, Kalwinsky DK, Dahl GV, Weck P, Whisnant J, Murphy SB. Phase I-II study of continuous-infusion high-dose human lymphoblastoid interferon and the in vitro sensitivity of leukemic progenitors in non-lymphocytic leukemia. Cancer Treat Rep 1986;70(3):363–367.

21. Muss HB, Costanzi JJ, Leavitt R, Williams RD, Kempf RA, Pollard R, Ozer H, Zekan PJ, Grunberg SM, Mitchell MS, et al. Recombinant alfa interferon in renal cell carcinoma: a randomized trial of two routes of administration. J Clin Oncol 1987;5(2):286–91.

Interferon alfa

General Information

Interferon alfa is used as purified natural leukocyte or lymphoblastoid human interferon, or as a recombinant DNA preparation. Work to assign the most frequently observed amino acids at each position has led to a so-called consensus interferon alfa (1). Relatively low doses (3–10 MU three times a week) are now being used in most indications, except in AIDS-related Kaposi's sarcoma (up to 30 MU/day). Although the half-life is only 4–5 hours, its biological effects persist for 2–3 days.

Observational studies

Considerable efforts have been made to improve the efficacy of interferon alfa in patients with chronic hepatitis C. Currently used regimens, including long-term interferon alfa alone or in combination with ribavirin, produce a sustained response rate of 40–50%. Other possibly effective strategies include a longer duration of treatment, higher fixed doses, and high-dose induction (2). A longer duration of treatment has been evaluated in patients with chronic hepatitis B. In 118 patients, treatment for 32 rather than 16 weeks enhanced the virological response to hepatitis B without increasing the severity of adverse effects, except for hair loss, which was more frequent during prolonged therapy (3).

A wide range of persistent symptoms has been reported during interferon alfa treatment for chronic hepatitis C. An analysis of 222 patients from the USA and France, enrolled in a multicenter trial, suggested that pretreatment symptoms were an important predictor of moderate or severe (defined as debilitating) adverse effects during treatment with interferon alfa (4). Compared with baseline, the incidences of moderate and severe fatigue, myalgia, arthralgia, headache, dry eyes, and dry mouth increased significantly after 6 months. In each case, the development of these debilitating adverse effects was associated with the presence of that symptom at baseline. They were more often reported in patients who received interferon alfa daily than three times weekly, and in US than French patients, suggesting possible differences in cultural attitudes toward illness. There was also increased use of antidepressants during the 6-month survey.

Low daily doses of interferon alfa have been used with small doses of cytarabine in the treatment of early chronic myelogenous leukemia (5). With doses sufficient to obtain a good cytogenetic response (for example 3.7 MU/m^2/day plus cytarabine 7.5 mg/day) toxicity was considered acceptable. There was significant fatigue in 43% of cases, significant neurological changes in 27%, weight loss in 19%, and oral ulcers in 4%.

Comparative studies

Interferon alfa, in combination with ribavirin, is currently first-line therapy for patients with chronic hepatitis C and compensated liver disease, and its use has been extensively reviewed (6). A meta-analysis of trials in patients who were previously non-responsive to interferon alfa alone showed that treatment withdrawal for an adverse event was more frequent in patients who received combination therapy (8.8%) compared with interferon alfa monotherapy (4%) (7). However, treatment withdrawal is more frequent in practice. In a retrospective analysis of 441 consecutive patients treated with interferon alfa and ribavirin, 25% of patients discontinued treatment because of adverse effects (8). The study identified female sex, a dose of interferon alfa above 15 MU/week, and naive patients as independent susceptibility factors for premature withdrawal.

Comparisons of different forms of interferon alfa

In a randomized comparison of recombinant interferon alfa-2b and interferon alfa n-3 (9 MU/week for 1 year) in 168 naive patients with chronic hepatitis C, there was no significant difference in clinical outcomes and the incidence or type of adverse effects between the groups (9). There was a non-significant trend toward more severe leukopenia and a higher incidence of severe thyroid disorders in patients who received recombinant interferon alfa-2b.

Pegylated interferon alfa-2a is a modified form of interferon alfa; it produces higher serum concentrations and has greater efficacy. In 1530 patients with chronic hepatitis C, pegylated interferon alfa-2b had a similar profile of adverse effects to unmodified interferon alfa-2b, but with more frequent dose-limiting neutropenia (10). Two other studies have shown that peginterferon alfa-2a once weekly is more effective than unmodified interferon alfa-2a three times weekly in patients with chronic hepatitis C (11,12). The frequency and severity of adverse effects with the two treatments were very similar and were consistent with the known adverse effects of interferon alfa. In one study, a neutrophil count below 0.5×10^9/l was more frequent with peginterferon alfa than with unmodified interferon alfa (12/265 versus 4/261), but none of these patients required treatment withdrawal or had serious infections in relation to neutropenia (12). In the other study, the proportion of patients who required dosage modification because of

thrombocytopenia was also higher with peginterferon alfa (18 versus 6%), but no patients had clinically significant bleeding disorders (11). Taken together, these studies suggest that pegylated interferon alfa may produce more frequent or more severe hemotoxic effects than unmodified interferon alfa.

In 1530 patients with chronic hepatitis C, pegylated interferon alfa-2b had a similar profile of adverse effects to unmodified interferon alfa-2b, but with more frequent dose-limiting neutropenia (10). No particular adverse effect has emerged since the use of this new formulation.

General adverse effects

The adverse effects of interferon alfa have mostly been reported after systemic administration, as intranasal use was not associated with more frequent adverse effects than placebo (13). Almost all patients treated with interferon alfa have experienced adverse effects, most of which are mild to moderate in intensity and easily manageable without withdrawal of treatment (14). The incidence and profile of adverse effects reported with the available types of interferon alfa are very similar (SEDA-21, 369; SEDA-22, 399), but they differ with the dose, schedule of administration, and the disease. At least 4–5% of patients with chronic hepatitis C had to discontinue treatment because of adverse effects, and dosage reduction was required in 9–22% of those receiving 9–15 MU/week (15). In a large retrospective evaluation of 11 241 patients with chronic viral hepatitis, the incidence of fatal or life-threatening adverse effects related to interferon alfa was one in 1000; events included irreversible liver failure, severe bone marrow depression, and attempted suicide (16). Overall, severe adverse effects were observed in 1% of patients, and comprised mostly thyroid disorders, neuropsychiatric manifestations, and cutaneous adverse effects. In other studies in patients with chronic hepatitis, the incidence of major adverse effects was 25% in 659 patients (17); in Japan, dosage reduction or withdrawal was necessary in 31% of 987 patients receiving relatively high dosages of interferon alfa (18–70 MU weekly) (18). The safety of interferon alfa in children appears to be similar to that in adults (19). The pathogenesis of most adverse effects observed with interferon alfa is poorly understood, but two main mechanisms are commonly postulated, namely a direct toxic effect or an indirect immune-mediated effect.

During the first days of treatment, virtually all patients have a flu-like syndrome with fever, chills, tachycardia, malaise, headache, arthralgias and myalgias, but tachyphylaxis usually develops after 1–2 weeks of treatment (20). Late febrile reactions are rarely noted (21). Although the severity increases with the dose, the flu-like syndrome is rarely treatment-limiting and it can be partly prevented by the prophylactic administration of paracetamol (acetaminophen). The acute release of fever-promoting factors, for example the eicosanoids, IL-1, and TNF alfa, secondary to interferon alfa is the suggested mechanism.

Although the adverse effects profiles of the currently available formulations of interferon alfa are very similar, patients who have adverse effects with one formulation can be successfully re-treated with another type of interferon alfa. This has been shown in 22 patients in whom lymphoblastoid interferon alfa was withdrawn because of severe adverse effects (leukopenia, thrombocytopenia, thyroid disorders, and psychiatric disturbances) and were successfully re-treated with similar dosages of leukocyte interferon alfa (22). Only one of these patients had severe leukopenia again.

Organs and Systems

Cardiovascular

Hypotension or hypertension, benign sinus or supraventricular tachycardia, and rarely distal cyanosis, have been reported within the first days of treatment in 5–15% of patients receiving high-dose interferon alfa (20). These adverse effects are usually benign, except in high-risk patients with a previous history of dysrhythmias, coronary disease, or cardiac dysfunction.

Cardiac complications
Severe or life-threatening cardiotoxicity is infrequent and mostly reported in the form of a subacute complication in patients with cancer, and in those with pre-existing heart disease or receiving high-dose interferon alfa. Atrioventricular block, life-threatening ventricular dysrhythmias, pericarditis, dilated cardiomyopathy, cardiogenic shock, asymptomatic or symptomatic myocardial ischemia or even infarction, and sudden death have been observed (SED-13, 1091) (SEDA-20, 326) (SEDA-22, 369) (23). The combination of high-dose interleukin-2 (IL-2) with interferon alfa enhanced cardiovascular complications, namely cardiac ischemia and ventricular dysfunction (24).

Cardiomyopathy has been attributed to interferon alfa in an infant (25).

- A 3-month-old boy was given interferon alfa (2.5–5.5 MU/m^2) for chronic myelogenous leukemia. After 7.5 months he developed progressive respiratory distress, with anorexia, irritability, and nocturnal sweating. A chest X-ray showed cardiomegaly, an echocardiogram showed a markedly dilated left ventricle, and an electrocardiogram showed left ventricular hypertrophy with abnormal repolarization. Viral cultures and serology for cytomegalovirus, parvovirus B19, and enterovirus were negative. Infectious diseases and metabolic disturbances were excluded. Interferon alfa was withdrawn and digoxin, furosemide, and an angiotensin-converting enzyme inhibitor were given. One year later, he was asymptomatic without further cardiac treatment.

Similar, but anecdotal reports were also described in patients without evidence of previous cardiac disease and receiving low-dose interferon alfa (SEDA-20, 326). In chronic viral hepatitis, only seven of 11 241 patients had severe cardiac adverse effects (16). The exact risk of such cardiovascular adverse effects is unknown. In patients with chronic viral hepatitis, cardiovascular test

results were not modified when patients were re-examined after at least 6 months of treatment, even where there was an earlier cardiac history (26), but there was a potentially critical reversible reduction in left ventricular ejection of more than 10% in another prospective study (27).

Myocardial dysfunction can completely reverse after withdrawal of interferon alfa and does not exclude further treatment with lower doses (28).

- A 47-year-old man with renal cancer and no previous history of cardiovascular disease developed gradually worsening exertional dyspnea after he had received interferon alfa in a total dose of 990 MU over 5 years. Echocardiography and a myocardial CT scan confirmed a dilated cardiomyopathy, with left ventricle dilatation and diffuse heterogeneous perfusion at rest. He improved after interferon alfa withdrawal and treatment with furosemide, quinapril, and digoxin. Myocardial scintigraphy confirmed normal perfusion. He restarted low-dose interferon alfa (6 MU/week) 1 year later and had no recurrence of congestive heart failure after a 1-year follow-up period.

Patients with pre-existing cardiac disease are more likely to develop cardiovascular toxicity while receiving interferon alfa, but these complications are rare. Among 89 patients with chronic hepatitis C, 12-lead electrocardiography monthly during a 12-month treatment period and follow-up for 6-months showed only minimal and nonspecific abnormalities in five patients (two had right bundle branch block, one left anterior hemiblock, and two unifocal ventricular extra beats) (29). None of these disorders required treatment withdrawal, and complete noninvasive cardiovascular assessment was normal. Overall, the role of interferon alfa was uncertain and the 5.6% incidence of electrocardiographic abnormalities was suggested to be similar to that expected in the general population. Nevertheless, severe cardiac dysrhythmias are still possible in isolated cases, as illustrated by the development of third-degree atrioventricular block, reversible on withdrawal, in a 57-year-old man with lower limb arteritis but no other cardiovascular disorder (30).

Peripheral vascular complications
Raynaud's phenomenon
Raynaud's phenomenon can occur, particularly in patients with chronic myelogenous leukemia (SEDA-20, 326) (31), and severe cases were complicated by digital necrosis (SEDA-20, 326) (SEDA-21, 369).

In 24 cases of Raynaud's syndrome, interferon alfa was the causative agent in 14, interferon beta in 3, and interferon gamma in 5 (32). There was no consistent delay in onset and the duration of treatment before the occurrence of symptoms ranged from 2 weeks to more than 4 years. The most severe cases were complicated by digital artery occlusion and necrosis requiring amputation. Few patients had other ischemic symptoms, such as myocardial, ophthalmic, central nervous system, or muscular manifestations. Severe Raynaud's phenomenon was also reported in a 5-year-old girl with hepatitis C (33).

Cryoglobulinemia

Although most patients with mild-to-moderate clinical manifestations of hepatitis C virus-associated mixed cryoglobulinemia improved during treatment with interferon alfa, acute worsening of ischemic lesions has been reported in three patients who had prominent cryoglobulinemia-related ischemic manifestations (34). All three had acute progression of pre-existing peripheral ischemia or leg ulcers within the first month of treatment, and transmetatarsal or right toe amputations were required in two. The lesions healed after interferon alfa withdrawal. It was therefore suggested that the anti-angiogenic activity of interferon alfa may also impair revascularization and healing of ischemic lesions in patients with initially severe ischemic manifestations.

Venous thrombosis

Whereas clinically insignificant coagulation abnormalities have been documented in patients receiving high-dose continuous interferon alfa (35), isolated cases of venous thrombosis have been observed (SEDA-20, 329) (36). Interferon alfa can also induce the production of antiphospholipid antibodies (SEDA-20, 329) (SEDA-21, 371). In one study, antiphospholipid antibodies were found in five of 12 patients with melanoma treated with interferon alfa alone or with interferon alfa plus interleukin-2; deep venous thrombosis occurred in four patients with antiphospholipid antibodies (37). Although the underlying neoplasia undoubtedly played a role in the further development of venous thrombosis, the causative role of interferon alfa was suggested by the absence of antiphospholipid antibodies and venous thrombosis in eight patients treated with interleukin-2 alone.

Other vascular complications

Other anecdotal reports included acrocyanosis and peripheral arterial occlusion (SED-13, 1095) (SEDA-22, 400). Although the causal relation is unclear, interferon alfa was considered as a possible cause in the triggering of acute cerebrovascular hemorrhage or ischemic neurological symptoms in few patients (SEDA-21, 370) (SEDA-22, 400). The pathogenic mechanisms of these vascular effects are still unclear; vasculitis, hypercoagulability, vasospasm, a paradoxical anginal effect of interferon alfa, or an underlying cardiovascular disease have all been suggested as underlying processes.

Respiratory

The respiratory adverse effects of interferon alfa include interstitial pneumonitis (38), which is rare. Since the first description of interstitial pneumonitis associated with interferon alfa in Japanese patients who also used the popular "Sho-saiko-t" herbal formulation, similar cases have been described in Western patients, suggesting that interferon alfa can be the sole cause in some patients (SED-13, 1091) (SEDA-20, 326) (SEDA-21, 370) (39,40). Interferon alfa was also suspected to be involved in one case of biopsy-proven bronchiolitis obliterans-organizing pneumonia (41). Clinical symptoms of pneumonitis appeared 3–12 weeks after the onset of interferon alfa

therapy, and after withdrawal of treatment they usually completely resolved, either spontaneously or after a short course of glucocorticoid treatment. Immune-mediated pulmonary toxicity involving the activation of T cells was considered as a likely mechanism. The uncommon features of bronchiolitis obliterans-organizing pneumonia have been reported in three other patients who received interferon alfa together with ribavirin or cytosine arabinoside (42,43).

In four patients with hematological malignancies who developed symptoms suggestive of pneumonitis (that is a dry cough and dyspnea) after 1 week to 38 months of interferon alfa treatment, there was a marked reduction in carbon monoxide diffusion capacity in all cases, whereas there were pathological findings in ordinary chest X-rays in only two (44). What the authors called ultracardiography and high-resolution CT scanning were suggested to have higher sensitivity in evaluating pulmonary symptoms. In three patients, complete reversal was obtained after interferon alfa withdrawal, either spontaneously or after corticosteroid treatment, although one patient required long-term glucocorticoid treatment.

In a retrospective review of 70 patients with hepatitis C enrolled in four clinical trials, there were four cases of significant pulmonary toxicity (two of bronchiolitis obliterans and two of interstitial pneumonitis) (45). Three recovered completely, but one still required glucocorticoids for exertional dyspnea that persisted 17 months after interferon alfa withdrawal. The authors suggested that there was an increased risk with high-dose interferon, because three of these patients received high doses (5 MU/day) or pegylated interferon alfa. In contrast, they were unaware of any significant pulmonary toxicity in any of their approximately 500 patients with hepatitis C.

Interferon alfa can cause exacerbation of asthma (SED-14, 1248).

- Acute exacerbation of asthma has been reported in two men aged 27 and 57 years with a previous history of mild asthma (46). They developed progressive aggravation of asthma within 8–10 weeks of treatment for chronic hepatitis C, and finally required emergency treatment with systemic glucocorticoids and inhaled beta$_2$ adrenoceptor agonists. Severe asthma recurred 2–3 weeks after interferon alfa rechallenge in both patients.

Although these cases are anecdotal, they strongly suggest that interferon alfa should be regarded as a possible cause of asthma exacerbation in predisposed patients.

- Sustained and isolated dry cough has been attributed to interferon alfa in a 49-year-old woman (47). The symptoms disappeared after withdrawal, recurred on readministration, and again resolved after withdrawal. No other cause was found after thorough investigation.

Pleural effusion has been attributed to interferon alfa (48).

- A 54-year-old man received interferon alfa-2a, 9 MU/day, for chronic hepatitis C. He developed an asymptomatic right pleural effusion after 14 days. Although his serum titer of antinuclear antibodies was slightly increased, a more complete screening for autoimmune disease was negative. An infectious origin was also ruled out. The pleural effusion spontaneously disappeared after interferon alfa withdrawal and did not recur.

Although the mechanism of this adverse effect was purely speculative, it was suggested that interferon alfa might have induced a reaction similar to the immunopathological mechanism involved in serositis associated with systemic lupus erythematosus.

Pulmonary artery hypertension has been attributed to interferon alfa (49).

- A 23-year-old man taking hydroxycarbamide 1.5 g/day and interferon alfa-2b (less than 10 MU/day) for chronic lymphocytic leukemia had progressive dyspnea and a non-productive cough after about 5 months. The electrocardiogram showed axis deviation, incomplete right bundle-branch block, and right ventricular hypertrophy. The estimated pulmonary artery pressure by echocardiography was 80 mmHg and there were signs of right heart failure. Respiratory function tests showed a restrictive defect, and the chest X-ray showed pulmonary congestion without infiltrates. The patient's clinical status and respiratory function tests improved rapidly after withdrawal of interferon alfa while hydroxycarbamide was continued, and a mean pulmonary artery pressure of 34 mmHg was measured by right heart catheterization 1 month later. At 6 months, the systolic pulmonary artery pressure estimated by echocardiography had fallen to 35 mmHg and the electrocardiogram returned to normal after 1 year.

The authors mentioned that intravenous interferon alfa in sheep had caused an increase in pulmonary artery pressure.

Nervous system

Peripheral neuropathy

Dose-related distal paresthesia occurred in as many as 7% of patients (20), but new onset or worsening of neuropathy has rarely been attributed to interferon alfa. A sensorimotor polyneuropathy was the most frequent presentation (50). The symptoms usually developed after 2–28 weeks of treatment. Such reports were mostly described in patients who received high cumulative doses of interferon alfa, but induction or exacerbation of peripheral sensorimotor axonal neuropathy, particularly in patients with chronic hepatitis C and mixed cryoglobulinemia, was also observed after long-term or low-dose treatment (SED-13, 1092; SEDA-20, 327; SEDA-21, 370; 51). Nerve biopsy showed necrotizing vasculitis or axonal degeneration. Most patients stabilized or improved slowly over several months after interferon alfa withdrawal and/or treatment with corticosteroids. Several patients also required plasmapheresis or cyclophosphamide. Although several authors have suggested an autoimmune process, the underlying pathogenic mechanism is unclear.

Other rare forms of neuropathy (SED-13, 1092) include mononeuropathy multiplex (52), acute axonal

polyneuropathy (53), anterior ischemic optic neuropathy (54), trigeminal sensory neuropathy (55), bilateral neuralgic amyotrophy (56), brachial plexopathy (57), and symptoms suggestive of leukoencephalopathy (58).

Cranial nerve palsies

There have been reports of interferon alfa-induced cranial nerve palsies, including Bell's palsy.

Two patients, one of whom also received ribavirin, had facial nerve palsy after 5 and 8 months of interferon alfa therapy (59). The palsy resolved completely in one patient after withdrawal and the administration of prednisolone; however, in the other case, the palsy resolved without drug withdrawal, suggesting coincidence.

Two other cases of Bell's palsy, which reversed after interferon alfa withdrawal, have been reported (60). Although the delay in onset (7.5 and 8 weeks) suggested that interferon alfa might be the cause, one patient had no recurrence after rechallenge. A coincidental adverse event cannot therefore be completely ruled out.

Demyelination

Various forms of interferon alfa-induced neuropathy have been reported (SED-14, 1249), but chronic inflammatory demyelinating polyneuropathy has seldom been described (61,62).

- In two patients with chronic hepatitis C or malignant melanoma, paresthesia and tiredness occurred after 6 weeks and 9 months of treatment respectively. Despite withdrawal of interferon alfa, the neurological symptoms worsened initially and a diagnosis of chronic inflammatory demyelinating polyneuropathy was finally confirmed several weeks later. One patient improved after an extended course of plasma exchange and the other required immunoglobulins and prednisolone. Mild to moderate neurological abnormalities persisted at follow-up in both patients.

Multiple sclerosis has been attributed to interferon alfa (63).

- A 29-year-old woman received interferon alfa-2b (6–10 MU/day) for chronic myeloid leukemia, and about 3 years later developed headaches, back pain, progressive visual disturbance, and a sensory deficit in the legs. MRI scans of the brain and spinal cord suggested a first episode of multiple sclerosis. In addition, the myelin basic protein concentration was slightly raised, and perimetry showed bilateral optic neuritis. Most of her neurological symptoms, except central vision impairment, improved after interferon alfa withdrawal and treatment with high-dose methylprednisolone. As a major partial cytogenetic response had been obtained with interferon, she was given natural interferon alfa (3 MU/day) 2 months later. After 2 days of treatment, she complained of transient but severe pain in the back and the legs, and developed acute paraplegia and loss of micturition desire. Again, interferon was withdrawn and she was given high-dose methylprednisolone. There was no further neurological deterioration at follow-up.

This account is reminiscent of the various autoimmune diseases that can be unmasked or exacerbated by interferon alfa.

Extrapyramidal effects

Extrapyramidal effects have been occasionally reported as a manifestation of persistent neurotoxicity induced by interferon alfa. This issue has been addressed in a report of severe refractory akathisia (64).

- A 28-year-old man received interferon alfa (5 MU/day for 28 days) for chronic hepatitis B. At the end of treatment he developed a slight parkinsonian gait, and 8 days later had a fever with vomiting, insomnia, restlessness, and raised serum creatine kinase activity (4946 IU/l). He had severe akathisia with psychomotor excitement and parkinsonism. Despite treatment with clonazepam, thioridazine, propranolol, trihexyphenidyl, and bromocriptine, his condition progressively worsened. He was finally given intravenous levodopa for 8 days and recovered dramatically within the next few days.

This report, together with previous experimental data, suggests that levodopa might be useful in alleviating some of the manifestations of persistent interferon alfa-induced neurotoxicity.

In two other patients, akathisia occurred shortly after they had started to take interferon alfa; one improved after the frequency of injections was reduced (65). Unfortunately, this report did not provide sufficient convincing evidence for a causal relation; the development of akathisia may have been coincidental.

Chorea is a very rare manifestation of interferon alfa neurotoxicity (SEDA-20, 327).

- A 68-year-old woman developed progressive personality changes and 2 months later permanent choreic movements of the four limbs (66). She had taken interferon alfa-2b (3 MU/day) and hydroxyurea 50 mg/kg/day for chronic myeloid leukemia for 2 years and had no history of psychiatric disorders. Neuropsychological testing showed frontal subcortical dysfunction. There were no abnormalities in the Huntington disease gene. She progressively worsened over the next 6 months. The electroencephalogram was disorganized, with diffuse slow waves, and she was bedridden. Interferon alfa was withdrawn. The chorea ceased 1 month later and she completely recovered cognitive function. Electroencephalography was normal 6 and 12 months later.

The authors attributed these events to antidopaminergic effects of interferon alfa.

Seizures

Although generalized tonic-clonic seizures have occasionally been described during trials of high doses of interferon alfa, they have also been reported after the use of intermediate or even low doses (67–69). There was a 1.3% incidence of generalized seizures in a retrospective study of 311 patients treated with low doses for chronic viral

hepatitis (70). In another study, tonic-clonic seizures were identified in 4% of children treated for chronic hepatitis B (71). As seizures occurred only in children under 5 years of age with fever or potential perinatal nervous system injury, immaturity of the nervous system was suggested to be an additional factor for interferon alfa-induced neurotoxicity in children.

- In three patients, seizures occurred after a cumulative dose of 266–900 MU (72,73). Two were retreated with a lower dose and remained free of seizures, so that the strength of the causal relation was debatable (72). However, a dose-related effect was still possible.
- Another patient with a history of bipolar mood disorder experienced had his first four episodes of seizures with a prolonged delirious state 1 week after withdrawal of interferon alfa (73).

Reversible photosensitive seizures have also been reported (74).

- A 62-year-old man without a personal or family history of epilepsy received interferon alfa (3 MU three times a week) for 2 years for multiple myeloma. He had frequent episodes of myoclonic jerks in the face, especially when the sun was shining while driving his car. He also had one generalized seizure. Electroencephalography showed a paroxysmal response to intermittent photic stimulation and magnetic resonance imaging was normal. The seizures disappeared and his electroencephalogram normalized after interferon alfa withdrawal.

In this case, the possible role of interferon alfa was suspected only late during treatment, indicating that patients should be regularly questioned about neurological symptoms, because more severe complications might have occurred.

In a prospective study of the effect of interferon alfa (56 MU/day for 4 weeks then 27 MU/week for 20 weeks) in 56 patients with chronic hepatitis C, there was diffuse electroencephalographic slowing at 2 and 4 weeks of treatment, suggesting mild encephalopathy (75). These changes completely reversed after withdrawal. However, the dosage used in this Japanese study was relatively high compared with the dosages currently used in Western countries. In addition, the clinical relevance of these electroencephalographic changes was not investigated.

Neuromuscular function

A number of reports have confirmed that interferon alfa can induce or unmask underlying silent myasthenia gravis (SED-13, 1097; SEDA-20, 327; SEDA-21, 370). The diagnostic criteria for myasthenia gravis were clearly fulfilled in these reports, and an autoimmune reaction was the most likely mechanism, as each patient had positive serum anti-acetylcholine receptor antibodies and required permanent anticholinesterase drugs long after interferon alfa withdrawal. Myasthenia gravis developed in two patients treated with interferon alfa-2b for chronic hepatitis C, one of whom also took ribavirin (76,77). Both had an increase in acetylcholine receptor antibody titers and required permanent pyridostigmine and immunosuppressant treatment. These findings suggest that interferon alfa does not cause myasthenia gravis but unmasks it.

Sensory systems

Eyes

Ophthalmic disorders can occur during interferon alfa treatment (78–84) and some of the literature has been reviewed (85). Retinopathy consisting of cotton-wool spots and/or superficial retinal hemorrhages has been reported with a variable incidence (18–86%), and the available data suggest that the increased incidence can be influenced by an initial high dose of interferon alfa. Whereas diabetes mellitus and systemic hypertension have been identified as possible susceptibility factors, the incidence of retinopathy was not significantly increased in 19 patients with chronic renal insufficiency, compared with 17 patients without chronic renal insufficiency (86). However, it was felt that renal insufficiency may be associated with the most severe cases, that is those requiring dosage reductions.

In one study, in which prospective ophthalmic examinations were made before and at regular 2-week intervals after the beginning and end of treatment, 28 of 81 patients who received a uniform total dose of natural interferon alfa (478 MU) for chronic hepatitis C developed the typical findings of interferon-induced asymptomatic retinopathy (cotton-wool spots and/or retinal hemorrhages) (84). In contrast, there were no lesions in the 25 patients with chronic hepatitis C who did not receive interferon alfa or in the 20 with diabetes mellitus and/or hypertension but without chronic hepatitis C. Most of the cases were observed within 4 months of treatment, and the lesions always abated after withdrawal or even despite continuation, suggesting that treatment can be continued unless patients develop symptoms. Indeed, most patients with retinopathy associated with interferon alfa remained asymptomatic.

The pathogenesis of retinopathy associated with interferon alfa is unclear. In 45 patients with chronic hepatitis C (25 treated with interferon) there was an association between retinal hemorrhages caused by interferon alfa (six patients) and a concomitant significant increase in plasma-activated complement (C5a), compared with baseline C5a serum concentrations (87). However, the signification and contribution of raised C5a concentrations in the pathogenesis of ocular complications needs to be clarified, although it has been suggested that retinal hemorrhage could be predicted on the basis of raised C5a concentrations (88).

Although most patients with interferon alfa retinopathy remain asymptomatic, ocular complications, such as reduced vision or complete visual loss due to occlusive vasculitis, central retinal artery occlusion, or anterior ischemic optic neuropathy, continue to be reported in a very few patients (SED-13, 1096) (82,85,89–93). However, subclinical but eventually long-lasting or even irreversible abnormally long visual evoked responses have been identified in 24% of patients (SEDA-22, 403). Regular ophthalmological monitoring to detect retinal changes, even though the patient is still asymptomatic, is therefore strongly recommended in patients receiving interferon alfa.

Other isolated reports of ophthalmic abnormalities refer to optic neuritis with blurring of vision, cortical blindness with fatal encephalopathy, mononeural abducent nerve paralysis, and complete but reversible bilateral oculomotor nerve paralysis (SED-13, 1096; 94–97).

- A 60-year-old smoker was treated with interferon alfa (100 MU/week for 2 months and 9 MU/week for 15 weeks) for cutaneous melanoma. Ocular examination was normal before treatment, but he developed acute loss of peripheral vision in his left eye after 23 weeks. Examination was consistent with anterior ischemic optic neuropathy, and there was optic disc edema, a pupillary defect, and circular visual field constriction in the left eye. There was renal artery constriction in both eyes. Despite treatment with aspirin, high-dose dexamethasone, heparin, and finally withdrawal of interferon alfa, loss of visual function progressed and affected both eyes. Ciclosporin was started, but he was considered to have irreversible loss of visual function.

This report shows that interferon alfa can be a potent precipitator of extremely severe ocular disorders and also argues for careful ocular surveillance in patients receiving adjuvant interferon alfa for high-risk resected melanoma.

Of 57 patients treated with interferon for renal cell carcinoma, two developed multiple retinal exudates associated with visual disturbance; both had taken vinblastine concurrently. The precise role of interferon in this reaction is unknown (98).

Ears

In 49 patients, there was reversible otological impairment with tinnitus, mild-to-moderate hearing loss or both in respectively 8, 16, and 20% of patients after interferon alfa or interferon beta administration (SEDA-19, 336). These disorders tended to occur more frequently in patients on high cumulative doses, but led to withdrawal of treatment in only two patients. Complete but reversible hearing loss, and acute unilateral vestibular dysfunction with spontaneous vertigo and nystagmus have each been reported in one patient receiving interferon alfa (SEDA-21, 372).

Sudden hearing loss has been reported (SEDA-21, 372) and in one case of promptly reversible hearing loss on interferon alfa withdrawal, the presence of anti-endothelial cell antibodies was suggested to have played a role in the development of autoimmune microvascular damage (99).

Smell

Patients treated with interferon alfa sometimes complain of transient taste or smell alterations, but anosmia has been reported (SEDA-22, 403; 100).

- A 37-year-old man received interferon alfa for chronic hepatitis C. After 2 weeks he complained of smelling difficulties and subsequently developed complete anosmia. There were no other neurological symptoms and complete neurological examination was normal. Anosmia still persisted 13 months after drug withdrawal.

- In both patients, the persistence of anosmia late after interferon alfa was resumed indicates that a causal relation to treatment is purely speculative.

Psychological, psychiatric

Neuropsychiatric complications of interferon alfa were recognized in the early 1980s and represent one of the most disturbing adverse effects of interferon alfa (SED-13, 1091; SEDA-20, 327; SEDA-22, 400). Reviews have provided comprehensive analysis of the large amount of experimental and clinical data that have accumulated since 1979 (101,102).

> DoTS classification (BMJ 2003; 327:1222–5)
> Dose-relation: collateral effect
> Time-course: intermediate or delayed
> Susceptibility factors: pre-existing psychiatric disorders, organic brain injury, or addictive behavior

Presentation

Within a large spectrum of symptoms, complications are classified as acute, subacute, or chronic.

Acute neuropsychological disturbances are usually associated with the flu-like syndrome and include headache, fatigue, and weakness, drowsiness, somnolence, subtle impairment of memory or concentration, and lack of initiative (20). This pattern of cognitive impairment is similar to changes observed during influenza and has also been described in healthy patients who have received a single dose of interferon alfa (103). More severe acute manifestations (for example, marked somnolence or lethargy, frank encephalopathy with visual hallucinations, dementia or delirium, and sometimes coma) have been almost exclusively described in patients receiving more than 20–50 MU (20); vertigo, cramps, apraxia, tremor and dizziness were also reported.

The subacute or chronic neuropsychiatric effects of long-term therapy are usually non-specific, with cognitive impairment (for example visuospatial disorientation, attentional deficits, memory disturbances, slurred speech, difficulties in reading and writing), changes in emotion, mood, and behavior (for example psychomotor slowing, hypersomnia, loss of interest, affective disorders, irritability, agitation, delirium, paranoia, aggressiveness, and murderous impulses). Post-traumatic stress symptoms have also been reported (SEDA-22, 400). As a result, severe psychic distress can be observed during long-lasting treatment or in patients who are otherwise not severely affected (20,104). The most severe psychiatric complications of interferon alfa include rare cases of homicidal ideation, suicidal ideation, and attempted suicide (105).

The clinical features of mania have been described in four patients with malignant melanoma, with a detailed review of nine other published cases (106). Although seven suffered from depression during treatment, the onset of mania or hypomania was often associated with interferon alfa dosage fluctuation (withdrawal or dose reduction) or introduction of an antidepressant for interferon alfa-induced depression. In these patients, the risk of mood fluctuations persisted for several months after interferon alfa withdrawal, and low-dose gabapentin was considered useful in treating manic disorders and in preventing mood fluctuations. Interferon alfa was suggested as a possible cause of persistent manic-depressive illness for more than 4 years in a 40-year-old man (107). Although the manic episodes may have been coincidental, the negative history and the age of onset are in keeping with a possible role of interferon alfa treatment.

The clinical features, management, and prognosis of psychiatric symptoms in patients with chronic hepatitis C have been reviewed using data from 943 patients treated with interferon alfa (85%) or interferon beta (15%) for 24 weeks (108). Interferon-induced psychiatric symptoms were identified in 40 patients (4.2%) of those referred for psychiatric examination. They were classified in three groups according to the clinical profile: 13 cases of generalized anxiety disorder (group A), 21 cases of mood disorders with depressive features (group B), and six cases of other psychiatric disorders, including psychotic disorders with delusions/hallucinations ($n = 4$), mood disorders with manic features ($n = 1$), and delirium ($n = 1$) (group C). The time to onset of the symptoms differed significantly between the three groups: 2 weeks in group A, 5 weeks in group B, and 11 weeks in group C. Women were more often affected than men. There was no difference in the incidence or nature of the disorder according to the type of interferon used. Whereas most patients who required psychotropic drugs were able to complete treatment, 10 had to discontinue interferon treatment because of severe psychiatric symptoms, 5 from group B and five from group C. Twelve patients still required psychiatric treatment for more than 6 months after interferon withdrawal. In addition, residual symptoms (anxiety, insomnia, and mild hypothymia) were still present at the end of the survey in seven patients. Delayed recovery was mostly observed in patients in group C and in patients treated with interferon beta. Although several patients with a previous history of psychiatric disorders are sometimes successfully treated with interferon alfa, severe decompensation with persistent psychosis should be regarded as a major possible complication (109).

The neuropsychological adverse effects of long-term treatment have been assessed in 14 patients with myeloproliferative disorders using a battery of psychometric and electroneurological tests before and after 3, 6, 9, and 12 months of treatment (median dose 25 MU/week) (110). In contrast to several previous studies, there was no significant impairment of neurological function, and attention and short-term memory improved during treatment. Despite the small number of patients, these results suggest that prolonged interferon alfa treatment did not cause severe cognitive dysfunction, at least in patients with cancer.

Diagnosis

Electroencephalographic (EEG) findings show reversible cerebral changes with slowing of dominant alpha wave activity, and occasional appearance of one and two activity in the frontal lobes, suggesting a direct effect on fronto-subcortical functions. Marked electroencephalographic abnormalities are sometimes observed in asymptomatic patients. The pattern of changes is identical whatever the dose, but the severity of symptoms is dose- and schedule-related. Most patients improve or recover after dosage reduction or withdrawal, and protracted toxicity, with impaired memory, deficits in motor coordination, persistent frontal lobe executive functions, Parkinson-like tremor, and mild dementia, have been occasionally reported (111).

In a study of 67 patients with chronic viral hepatitis, the self-administered Minnesota Multiphasic Personality Inventory (MMPI), which determines the patient's psychological profile, significantly correlated with the clinical evaluation and was a sensitive and reliable tool for identifying patients at risk of depressive symptoms before the start of interferon alfa therapy (112). It was also successfully used to monitor patients during treatment.

Frequency

The most typical psychiatric symptoms reported by patients taking interferon alfa are depressive symptoms, at rates of 10–40% in most studies (113–116). In four clinical studies in a total of 210 patients with chronic hepatitis C, the rate of major depressive disorders during interferon alfa treatment was 23–41% (117–120).

Suicidal ideation or suicidal attempts have been reported in 1.3–1.4% of patients during interferon alfa treatment for chronic viral hepatitis or even within the 6 months after withdrawal (121,122), but the excess risk related to interferon alfa is not known.

Time-course

Subacute or chronic neuropsychiatric manifestations are more typically identified after several weeks of treatment and are among the most frequent treatment-limiting adverse effects (104,115,123–125). The onset can be insidious in patients treated with low doses, or subacute in those who receive high doses. Most patients develop severe depressive symptoms within the first 3 months of treatment (117–120).

Although psychiatric manifestations usually appear during interferon alfa therapy, delayed reactions can occur.

- A 37-year-old man without a previous psychiatric history developed major depression with severe psychotic features within days after the discontinuation of a 1-year course of interferon alfa-2b (126).

In 10 patients with melanoma and no previous psychiatric disorders, depression scores measured on the Montgomery-Asberg Depression Rating Scale were significantly increased after 4 weeks of high-dose interferon alfa (127). Patients whose scores were higher before treatment developed the worst symptoms of depression during treatment. This positive correlation provides striking evidence that baseline and regular assessment of mood and cognitive functions are necessary to detect disorders as early as possible.

Mechanisms

Although very few studies have specifically investigated the role of the underlying disease, the findings of significant neuropsychiatric deterioration during interferon alfa treatment compared with placebo or no treatment in chronic hepatitis C, chronic myelogenous leukemia, or amyotrophic lateral disease strongly suggested a causal role of interferon alfa (128–130).

The mechanism by which the systemic administration of interferon alfa produces neurotoxicity is unclear, and might result from a complex of direct and indirect effects involving the brain vasculature, neuroendocrine system, neurotransmitters and the secondary cytokine cascade with cytokines which exert effects on the nervous system, for example interleukin-1, interleukin-2, or tumor necrosis factor alfa (131). Whether a clinical effect is directly mediated through the action of a given cytokine or results from a secondary pathway through the induction of other cytokines or second messengers is difficult to determine.

A study in 18 patients treated with interferon alfa for chronic hepatitis C has given insights into the possible pathophysiological mechanism of depression (132). Depression rating scales, plasma tryptophan concentrations, and serum kynurenine and serotonin concentrations were measured at baseline and after 2, 4, 16, and 24 weeks of treatment with interferon alfa 3–6 MU 3–6 times weekly. During treatment, tryptophan and serotonin concentrations fell significantly, while kynurenine concentrations rose significantly. Depression rating scales also rose from baseline after the first month of treatment, with continued increases thereafter. In addition, there was a relation between increased scores of depression and changes in serum kynurenine and serotonin concentrations. These changes suggested a predominant role of the serotonergic system in the pathophysiological mechanisms of interferon alfa-associated depression. Accordingly, 35 of 42 patients included in three open trials of antidepressant treatment responded to a selective serotonin reuptake inhibitor drug, such as citalopram or paroxetine, and were able to complete interferon treatment (119,133,134).

Susceptibility factors

Various possible susceptibility factors have been analysed in several studies (118–120,135). Sex, the dose or type of interferon alfa (natural or recombinant), a prior personal history of psychiatric disease, substance abuse, the extent of education, the duration and severity of the underlying chronic hepatitis, and scores of depression before interferon alfa treatment were not significantly different between patients with and without interferon alfa-induced depression. Advanced age was suggested to be a risk factor in only one study (120). Although a worsening of psychiatric symptoms was noted during treatment in 11 patients receiving psychiatric treatment before starting interferon, only one was unable to complete the expected 6-month course of interferon alfa and ribavirin therapy (118).

Of 91 patients treated with interferon alfa-2b and low-dose cytarabine for chronic myelogenous leukemia, 22 developed severe neuropsychiatric toxicity (136). Their symptoms consisted mostly of severe depression or psychotic behavior, which resolved on withdrawal in all patients. The time to toxicity ranged from as early as 2 weeks to as long as 184 weeks after the start of treatment. Five of six patients had recurrent or worse symptoms after re-administration of both drugs. Several baseline factors were analysed, but only a pretreatment history of neurological or psychiatric disorders was considered to be a reliable risk factor. Severe neuropsychiatric toxicity developed during treatment in 63% of patients with previous neuropsychiatric disorders compared with 10% in patients without. It is unlikely that the combination of interferon alfa-2b with low-dose cytarabine potentiated the neuropsychiatric adverse effects of interferon alfa in this study. Indeed, previous experience with this combination, but after exclusion of patients with a psychiatric history, was not associated with such a high incidence of neuropsychiatric toxicity or any significant difference in toxicity between interferon alfa alone and interferon alfa plus low-dose cytarabine.

Patients receiving high doses of interferon alfa or long-term treatment are more likely to develop pronounced symptoms (123). A previous history of psychiatric disorders, organic brain injury, or addictive behavior are among potential susceptibility factors, but worsening of an underlying psychiatric disease is not the rule, provided that strict psychiatric surveillance and continuation of psychotropic drugs are maintained (137). Other putative susceptibility factors include the intraventricular administration of interferon alfa, previous or concomitant cranial irradiation, asymptomatic brain metastases, and pre-existing intracerebral ateriosclerosis (SED-13, 1092; 115,138–142). Despite early findings, co-infection with HIV has not been confirmed to be a susceptibility factor (SEDA-20, 327).

The occurrence of psychiatric disorders has been prospectively investigated in 63 patients who received a 6-month course of interferon alfa (9 MU/week) for hepatitis C (143). All were assessed at baseline with the Structured Clinical Interview for DSM-III-R (SCID) and monitored monthly with the Hopkins Symptoms Checklist (SCL-90). Most had a history of alcohol or polysubstance dependence, and 12 had a lifetime diagnosis of major depression. There were no significant changes in the SCL-90 scores during the 6-month period of survey in the 49 patients who completed the study, even in those who had a lifetime history of major depression. At 6 months, there was probable minor depression in eight patients and major depression in one; none had attempted suicide.

In a prospective study, 50 patients with chronic hepatitis B or C who received 18–30 MU/week of natural or recombinant interferon alfa were followed for 12 months (144). The SCID before starting interferon alfa identified 16 patients with a current psychiatric diagnosis and eight with a previous psychiatric disorder; 26 patients free of any psychiatric history constituted the control group. Psychiatric manifestations during treatment occurred in 11 patients (five from the control group), major depression in five, depressive disorders in three, severe dysphoria in two, and generalized anxiety disorder in one. Most of them were successfully treated with psychological support and drug therapy. Overall, 20 patients interrupted interferon alfa (10 in each group), including three for psychiatric adverse effects, but patients with a pre-existing or recent psychiatric diagnosis were no more likely to withdraw from treatment than the controls.

Of 33 patients with chronic hepatitis C treated with interferon alfa, 9 MU/week for 3–12 months, prospectively evaluated using the Montgomery-Asberg Depression Rating Scale (MADRS) before and after 12 weeks of treatment, eight developed depressive symptoms, of whom four had major depression without a previous psychiatric history (145). All four recovered after treatment with antidepressants. This study confirmed that a high baseline MADRS is significantly associated with the occurrence of depressive symptoms.

These studies have confirmed that previous psychiatric disorders are not necessarily a contraindication to a potentially effective treatment. However, patients with depressive symptoms immediately before treatment are still regarded at risk of severe psychiatric deterioration with treatment (113).

Management

The management of the psychiatric complications of interferon alfa has not been carefully investigated, but multiple approaches are theoretically possible. Various pharmacological and non-pharmacological interventions have been discussed (146), and prompt intervention should be carefully considered in every patient who develops significant neuropsychiatric adverse effects while receiving interferon alfa. Depending on the clinical manifestations, proposed treatment options include antidepressants, psychostimulants, or antipsychotic drugs.

Based on a possible reduction in central dopaminergic activity mediated by the binding of interferon alfa to opioid receptors, naltrexone has been proposed as a means of improving cognitive dysfunction (123).

Selective serotonin re-uptake inhibitors have been advocated as the drugs of choice to allow completion of interferon alfa treatment (113), but that was based on very limited experience and the unproven assumption that SSRIs are safe in patients with underlying liver disease. The preliminary results of a double-blind, placebo-controlled study showed that 2 weeks of pretreatment with paroxetine significantly reduced the occurrence of major depression in 16 patients on high-dose interferon alfa for malignant melanoma (147). In a placebo-controlled trial, the preventive effects of paroxetine (mean maximal dose of 31 mg) were studied in 40 patients with high-risk malignant melanoma and interferon alfa-induced depression (148). Treatment started 2 weeks before adjuvant high-dose interferon alfa. Paroxetine significantly reduced the incidence of major depression (45% in the placebo group and 11% in the paroxetine group) and the rate of interferon alfa withdrawal (35 versus 5%). Although the number of patients was small and the duration of the survey short (12 weeks), this suggests that paroxetine effectively prevents the risk of depressive disorders in patients eligible for high-dose interferon alfa. However, these results are limited, because patients with melanoma who receive adjuvant high-dose interferon alfa are particularly likely to develop depression. The safety of prophylaxis with paroxetine also requires additional data, because three patients taking paroxetine developed retinal hemorrhages, including one with irreversible loss of vision.

- In contrast to this study, a 31-year-old woman with major depressive disorder, which responded to paroxetine and trazodone, had progressive recurrence of mood disorders after the introduction of interferon alfa for essential thrombocythemia (149).

This suggests that interferon alfa can also reverse the response to antidepressants.

Endocrine

Pituitary

Interferon alfa can stimulate the hypothalamic–pituitary–adrenal axis, with a marked increase in cortisol and adrenocorticotrophic hormone secretion after acute administration (SED-13, 1093). No further stimulation was observed after several weeks of treatment, pointing to possible down-regulation of the ACTH secretory system. As a result, long-term treatment with interferon alfa is not thought to influence pituitary hormones significantly, and the concentration of several hormones, for example calcitonin, LH, FSH, prolactin, growth hormone, ACTH, cortisol, testosterone, and estradiol, were not modified by prolonged interferon alfa treatment (150,151). No clinical endocrinopathies attributable to such disorders in the regulation of these hormones have yet been reported.

Although the rate of growth was significantly lower than predicted in 35% of children receiving long-term treatment for recurrent respiratory papillomatosis (152), only one case of growth retardation has been reported in other settings (SEDA-19, 335). A significant reduction in weight and nutritional status was observed during treatment with interferon alfa for 6 months for chronic viral hepatitis in children aged 4–16 years, but this was transient and not associated with growth impairment (153).

Reversible hypopituitarism with antibodies to pituitary GH3 cells and exacerbation of Sheehan's syndrome have been reported (SED-13, 1093) (SEDA-21, 371).

A syndrome resembling inappropriate antidiuretic hormone secretion has been described in a few patients receiving high-dose interferon alfa (SED-13, 1093) (154).

Thyroid

Since the original 1988 report of hypothyroidism in patients with breast cancer receiving leukocyte-derived interferon alfa (155), numerous investigators have provided clear clinical and biological data on thyroid disorders induced by different forms of interferon in patients with various diseases (21,156–159). Two of these reports also mentioned associated adverse effects that developed concomitantly, namely myelosuppression and severe proximal myopathy (Hoffmann's syndrome).

Presentation and outcomes

The spectrum of interferon alfa-induced thyroid disorders ranges from asymptomatic appearance or increase in antithyroid autoantibody titers to moderate or severe clinical features of hypothyroidism, hyperthyroidism, and acute biphasic thyroiditis. Antithyroid hormone antibodies have also been found in one patient, and this could have been the cause of erroneously raised thyroid hormone concentrations (160).

The clinical, biochemical, and thyroid imaging characteristics of thyrotoxicosis resulting from interferon alfa treatment have been retrospectively analysed from data on 10 of 321 patients with chronic hepatitis (75 with chronic hepatitis B and 246 with chronic hepatitis C) who developed biochemical thyrotoxicosis (161). Seven patients had symptomatic disorders, but none had ocular symptoms or a palpable goiter. Six had features of Graves' disease that required interferon alfa withdrawal in four and prolonged treatment with antithyroid drugs in all six. Three presented with transient thyrotoxicosis that subsequently progressed to hypothyroidism and required interferon withdrawal in one and thyroxine treatment in all three.

Although much work on thyroid autoimmunity associated with interferon alfa has accumulated, little is known about the very long-term outcome of this disorder. In 114 patients with chronic hepatitis C and no previous thyroid disease who were treated with interferon alfa-2a for 12 months, data on thyroid status were retrospectively obtained at the end of treatment, 6 months after withdrawal, and after a median of 6.2 years (162). Among 36 patients who had thyroid autoantibodies at the end of treatment, the authors identified three groups according to the long-term outcome: 16 had persistent thyroiditis, 10 had remitting/relapsing thyroiditis (that is antibodies became negative after 6 months of therapy and were again positive thereafter), and 10 had transient thyroiditis. Therefore, 72% of these patients had chronic thyroid autoimmunity at the end of follow-up and 12 developed subclinical hypothyroidism. In contrast, only one of 78 patients negative for thyroid autoantibodies developed thyroid autoantibodies. Although none of the patients had clinical thyroid dysfunction, this study suggests that long-term surveillance of thyroid disorders is useful in patients who have high autoantibody titers at the end of treatment with interferon alfa.

Although thyroid disorders in patients treated with interferon alfa generally follows a benign course after interferon alfa withdrawal or specific treatment, severe long-lasting ophthalmopathy resulting from Graves' disease has been described in a 49-year-old woman (163).

Time-course

Clinical symptoms usually occur after 2–6 months of treatment and occasionally after interferon alfa withdrawal.

- A middle-aged woman developed subacute thyroiditis by the sixth month of treatment with interferon alfa (164). She also had the classic symptoms of hyperthyroidism, although it is clear that these could easily have been mistaken for adverse effects of interferon alfa itself, for example weakness, weight loss, and palpitation.

After 6 months of treatment, 12% of patients with chronic hepatitis C had thyroid disorders, compared with 3% of patients with chronic hepatitis B. This study also suggested a possible relation between low free triiodothyronine serum concentrations before treatment and the subsequent occurrence of thyroid dysfunction. After a follow-up of 6 months after the end of interferon alfa treatment, 60% of affected patients with chronic hepatitis C still had persistent thyroid dysfunction; all had been positive for thyroid peroxidase antibodies before treatment. Long-term surveillance is therefore needed in these patients.

Frequency

In a prospective study, the overall incidence of biochemical thyroid disorders was 12% in 254 patients with chronic hepatitis C randomized to receive ribavirin plus high-dose interferon alfa (6 MU/day for 4 weeks then 9 MU/week for 22 weeks) or conventional treatment (9 MU/week for 26 weeks) (165). There was no difference in the incidence or the time to occurrence of thyroid disorders between the groups. Of the 30 affected patients, 11 (37%) had positive thyroid peroxidase autoantibodies (compared with 1% of patients without thyroid dysfunction), nine developed symptomatic thyroid dysfunction, and only three had to discontinue treatment. There was no correlation between the viral response and the occurrence of thyroid disorders, and only female sex and Asian origin were independent predictors of thyroid disorders.

Data on the incidence of thyroid disorders in interferon alfa-treated patients vary, largely because the follow-up duration, the nature of the study (prospective or retrospective), biological monitoring, diagnostic criteria, and the underlying disease differ from study to study (156). The incidence of clinical or subclinical thyroid abnormalities is generally 5–12% in large prospective studies in patients with chronic hepatitis C treated for 6–12 months, but it reached 34% in one study (21,166). The incidence was far lower in patients with chronic hepatitis B, at 1–3%. A wider range in incidence was found in patients with cancer, with no clinical thyroid disorders in 54 patients treated during a mean of 16 months for hematological malignancies (167), whereas in many other studies there was a 10–45% incidence (156). Even more impressive was the escalating incidence of thyroid disorders in patients with cancer receiving both interferon alfa and interleukin-2 (qv).

Mechanisms

Possible mechanisms need to be clarified. Since thyroid autoantibodies are detected in most patients who develop thyroid disorders, the induction or exacerbation of pre-existing latent thyroid autoimmunity is the most attractive hypothesis. This is in accordance with the relatively frequent occurrence of other autoantibodies or clinical auto-immune disorders in patients who develop thyroid disorders (168). However, 20–30% of patients who develop thyroid diseases have no thyroid antibodies, and it is thus not yet proven that autoimmunity is the universal or primary mechanism. In fact, there were subtle and reversible defects in the intrathyroidal organification of iodine in 22% of antithyroid antibody-negative patients treated with interferon alfa (169). In addition, the acute systemic administration of interferon alfa in volunteers or chronic hepatitis patients reduces TSH concentrations (SED-13, 1093) (170), and in vitro studies have suggested that interferon alfa directly inhibits thyrocyte function (SED-13, 1093) (171). Finally, the thyroid autoantibody pattern in patients who developed thyroid dysfunction during cytokine treatment was not different from that of patients without thyroid dysfunction, but differed significantly from that of patients suffering from various forms of spontaneous autoimmune thyroid disease (172).

Susceptibility factors

In addition to the underlying disease, there are many potential susceptibility factors (21,173). There is as yet no definitive evidence that age, sex, dose, and duration of treatment play an important role in the development of thyroid disorders. However, patients with previous thyroid abnormalities are predisposed to develop more severe thyroid disease (SEDA-20, 328). The incidence of thyroid disease was not different between natural and recombinant interferon alfa. Although this should be taken into account, a previous familial or personal history of thyroid disease was generally not considered a major risk factor. Finally, only pre-treatment positivity or the development of thyroid antibodies during treatment seem to be strongly associated with the occurrence of thyroid dysfunction.

In 175 patients with hepatitis B or C virus infections, women with chronic hepatitis C and patients with previously high titers of antithyroid autoantibodies were more likely to develop thyroid disorders (174).

The immunological predisposition to thyroid disorders has been studied in 17 of 439 Japanese patients who had symptomatic autoimmune thyroid disorders during interferon alfa treatment (175). There was a significantly higher incidence of the human leukocyte antigen (HLA)-A2 haplotype compared with the general Japanese population (88 versus 41%), suggesting that HLA-A2 is a possible additional risk factor for the development of interferon alfa-induced autoimmune thyroid disease.

Among other potential predisposing factors, treatment with iodine for 2 months in 21 patients with chronic hepatitis C receiving interferon alfa did not increase the likelihood of thyroid abnormalities compared with eight patients who received iodine alone, but abnormal thyroid tests were more frequent compared with 27 patients who received interferon alfa alone (176). This suggests that excess iodine had no synergistic effects on the occurrence of thyroid dysfunction induced by interferon alfa.

The occurrence of thyroid dysfunction in 72 patients treated with interferon alfa plus ribavirin (1.0–1.2 g/day) has been compared with that of 75 age- and sex-matched patients treated with interferon alfa alone for chronic hepatitis C (177). Of the former, 42 patients, and of the latter, 40 patients had received previous treatment with interferon alfa alone. There was no difference in the rate of thyroid autoimmunity (antithyroglobulin, antithyroid peroxidase, and thyroid-stimulating hormone receptor antibodies) between the two groups, but the patients who received interferon alfa plus ribavirin developed subclinical or overt hypothyroidism more often (15 versus 4%). Similarly, the incidence of hypothyroidism increased to 19% in patients who underwent a second treatment with interferon alfa plus ribavirin compared with 4.8% after the first treatment with interferon alfa alone, while the incidence remained essentially the same in patients who had two consecutive treatments with interferon alfa alone (4.7 and 7.1% respectively). Furthermore, there was no higher incidence of thyroid autoimmunity or clinical disorders after a second course of interferon alfa whether alone or combined with ribavirin in patients who had no thyroid autoantibodies at the end of a first course of interferon alfa alone, suggesting that these patients are relatively protected against the development of thyroid autoimmunity.

Management

The management of clinical thyroid dysfunction depends on the expected benefit of interferon alfa. Assay of thyroid antibodies before treatment, and regular assessment of TSH concentrations in treated patients, even after interferon alfa withdrawal, are useful as a means of predicting and detecting the risk of thyroid disorders. Complete recovery of normal thyroid function is usually observed after thyroxine replacement but sometimes requires interferon alfa withdrawal. Sustained hypothyroidism requiring long-term substitution treatment has occasionally been observed (SED-13, 1092) (178), and is more likely in patients with initially severe hypothyroidism and raised thyroid antibody titers (179). By contrast, hyperthyroidism generally requires the prompt withdrawal of interferon alfa, and severe forms may require radical radioiodine therapy. Although not enough data are available on the long-term consequences of interferon alfa-induced thyroid dysfunction, the recurrence of thyroid abnormalities after the administration of pharmacological doses of iodine should be borne in mind (180).

Parathyroid

Exacerbation of secondary hyperparathyroidism occurred in a 20-year-old renal transplant patient who also developed psoriasis during interferon alfa treatment (181). Both disorders resolved after withdrawal.

Adrenal

Of 62 initially autoantibody-negative patients treated with interferon alfa for chronic hepatitis C for a mean of 8 months, three developed antibodies to 21b-hydroxylase, a sensitive assay of adrenocortical autoimmunity (182). However, there were no cases of Addison's disease or subclinical adrenal insufficiency. This study suggested that the adrenal cortex is another potential target organ of autoimmune effects of interferon alfa, along with thyroid and pancreatic islet cells.

Metabolism

Diabetes mellitus

The development or worsening of insulin-dependent diabetes mellitus is limited to isolated case reports in patients treated with interferon alfa or interferon alfa plus interleukin-2 (SEDA-20, 328; SEDA-21, 371). In chronic hepatitis, diabetes mellitus was noted in only 10 of 11 241 treated patients (16). Although a relation between chronic hepatitis C and the occurrence of glucose metabolism disorders is possible (183), reports of diabetes mellitus in patients treated with interferon alfa were probably more than coincidental. Indeed, there have been reports of prompt amelioration or complete recovery after interferon alfa withdrawal (SED-13, 1092; 184–186) and of successive episodes of diabetes after each course of interferon alfa (SEDA-21, 371).

- In three middle-aged patients, diabetes was diagnosed after 3–7 months of treatment with interferon alfa-2b and ribavirin, and two presented with severe ketoacidosis (187,188). There was a family history of diabetes in one patient and two had high titers of glutamic acid decarboxylase antibodies before treatment. One patient never had diabetes-related serum autoantibodies before or after interferon alfa therapy. All three required permanent insulin treatment despite withdrawal of interferon alfa.

- Insulin-dependent diabetes mellitus has been reported after 2 weeks to 6 months of treatment with interferon alfa in four patients with chronic hepatitis C (189). All discontinued interferon alfa, and one woman who restarted treatment had a subsequent increase in insulin requirements.

A 75 g oral glucose tolerance test was performed before and after 3 months of interferon alfa treatment in 32 patients with chronic hepatitis C, of whom 15 also had an intravenous glucose test (190). Baseline evaluation showed that five patients had mild diabetes mellitus, three had impaired glucose tolerance, and 24 were normal. After 3 months of treatment, two patients with diabetes mellitus shifted to impaired glucose tolerance, and all patients with impaired glucose tolerance had normal glucose tolerance. Only three initially normal patients developed impaired glucose tolerance and none had newly diagnosed diabetes mellitus. From these results, and in contrast to previous reports (SED-14, 1250), it appears that interferon alfa did not have any adverse effects on insulin sensitivity and glucose tolerance after 3 months of treatment.

Interferon alfa may produce more severe changes than interferon beta (191).

- A 39-year-old man with diabetes, stabilized with insulin 22 U/day for 13 years, received interferon beta (6 MU/day) for chronic hepatitis C. His diabetes progressively worsened, necessitating insulin 50 U/day. After 4 weeks, interferon beta was replaced by interferon alfa (10 MU/day). Shortly afterwards he developed severe diabetic ketoacidosis and shock, which reversed after hemodynamic support and continuous hemodiafiltration.

Mechanisms

Autoimmunity was suggested as a likely mechanism, with HLA-DR4 haplotype and/or islet cell antibody (ICA) positivity at the time of diagnosis in several patients. Because the induction of ICA antibodies in patients treated with interferon alfa has never been otherwise demonstrated (21), the triggering, rather than the induction, of a latent autoimmune phenomenon in patients with a genetic susceptibility is probable (192).

More direct interference with glucose metabolism cannot be excluded. Interferon alfa can reduce the sensitivity of peripheral tissues or liver to insulin and accelerate the destruction of stimulated pancreatic beta-cells (193,194); this could be a possible mechanism in patients not exhibiting islet cell antibodies. This is also in keeping with rare instances of induction or exacerbation of type II non-insulin dependent diabetes mellitus (SEDA-19, 335).

Insulin antibodies were also found in six of 58 patients treated for chronic viral hepatitis (195) and that was associated with signs of insulin allergy in one patient (SEDA-19, 335).

Susceptibility factors

Patients with obesity and a family or previous history of glucose intolerance should be considered more predisposed to interferon alfa-induced diabetes, but the association is not consistently found (SEDA-20, 328).

Dyslipidemia

Interferon alfa often affects lipid metabolism and produces a reversible reduction in cholesterol and, more consistently, increases in triglyceride concentrations (SEDA-20, 328; SEDA-21, 371). Meticulous blood lipid investigation showed a significant rise in serum triglyceride and lipoprotein(a) concentrations and reductions in total cholesterol, HDL cholesterol, LDL cholesterol, and apoprotein A1.

Marked hypertriglyceridemia (10–20 µg/ml), which abates when treatment is withdrawn, has sometimes been observed (SED-13, 1093; 196,197). Inhibitory effects of interferon alfa on lipoprotein lipase and triglyceride lipase or increased hepatic lipogenesis have been suggested (198,199). Diet and lipid-lowering drugs have been proposed as means of maintaining acceptable triglyceride concentrations during long-term interferon alfa

therapy. Although the possibility of pancreatic or cardiovascular complications should be borne in mind, no secondary clinical consequences of interferon alfa-induced blood lipid disorders have been so far reported.

In a prospective study of lipid changes in 36 patients with chronic hepatitis C treated with interferon alfa for 6 months, the most prominent findings included increases in triglycerides, VLDL cholesterol, and apolipoprotein B, and falls in HLD cholesterol and apolipoprotein A1 (200). Three patients also developed chylomicronemia and two of those had severe hypertriglyceridemia. All three patients had triglycerides over 2 µg/ml before treatment, suggesting that patients with abnormal serum triglyceride concentrations at baseline are more likely to develop marked hypertriglyceridemia.

Porphyria

- A severe acute flare of porphyria cutanea tarda has been reported in a 61-year-old man after 4 months of treatment with interferon alfa-2b plus ribavirin for chronic hepatitis C (201). No further relapse was observed after chloroquine treatment, despite continuation of the antiviral drugs.

This patient had previously had episodes of small blisters that spontaneously resolved, and hereditary porphyria cutanea tarda was demonstrated by chromatographic and mutation analysis.

Hematologic

Hematological toxicity due to interferon alfa commonly includes dose-related leukopenia, neutropenia, and thrombocytopenia, whereas anemia is rare and usually moderate (202).

Reductions in platelet count and leukocyte count were usually in the range of 30–50% compared with baseline, but severe and reversible thrombocytopenia ($<49 \times 10^9$/l) or neutropenia ($<0.9 \times 10^9$/l) were noted in 10 and 20% of patients (203). However, life-threatening neutropenia or thrombocytopenia were reported in only six of 11 241 patients with chronic viral hepatitis (16), and reports of Coombs'-negative hemolytic anemia or complete agranulocytosis are sparse (SED-13, 1094; SEDA-20, 329).

In a retrospective study of 158 patients with chronic viral hepatitis treated for 6–12 months, lymphoblastoid interferon alfa produced the largest fall in leukocyte and platelet counts (−38 and −32% versus baseline values), recombinant interferon alfa was associated with intermediate toxicity (−32 and −26%), and leukocyte interferon alfa produced the smallest reduction (−27 and −22%) (204). The lowest mean values were observed after an average of 4–5 months. However, the clinical relevance of these differences is probably minimal, because the overall reduction in leukocyte and platelet numbers was small, and no patients developed clinical symptoms of cytopenia.

Mechanisms

Interferon alfa has direct myelosuppressive effects and can also cause hematological disorders by immune blood cell destruction, as suggested by reports of immune-mediated thrombocytopenia, immune hemolytic anemia (205,206), or a positive direct Coombs' test, with or without hemolysis (207–209).

The kinetics of the hemotoxic effects of interferon alfa have been studied in 76 patients with chronic hepatitis C (210). There were significant falls in white blood cell count and platelet count within 12 hours after the first injection, and a second fall in platelet count after 2 weeks, but not further thereafter. This rapid time-course suggests that liver or spleen sequestration of blood cells, rather than direct bone marrow suppression or immune-mediated hematological toxicity, is the most likely explanation for this acute hemotoxic effect, which does not preclude continuation of treatment.

Susceptibility factors

Susceptibility factors for severe hematological toxicity include cirrhosis and hypersplenism.

Prior interferon alfa treatment lasting for more than 6 months and withdrawn for 2–3 months was also one of the most significant factors to explain a reduced yield of peripheral blood stem cells in 88 previously autografted patients with myeloma undergoing G-CSF stimulation for future autotransplantation (211). As suggested by this study, the myelosuppressive effects of interferon alfa may be prolonged to such an extent that a minimum delay of more than 2–3 months after interferon alfa withdrawal should be considered before harvesting bone marrow cells.

Pancytopenia or aplasia, sometimes fatal, have been reported only in patients who had received previous chemotherapy, as has severe and even fatal erythrocytosis in patients with hairy cell leukemia (SED-13, 1094) (212–216).

Anemia

Isolated anemia is not a common feature of the hemotoxic effects of interferon alfa, and pure red cell aplasia has been reported in two patients with chronic leukemia for several months (217,218). Both patients improved progressively after replacement of interferon alfa by hydroxyurea. However, one required erythrocyte transfusions for 14 months.

- Pernicious anemia with a low vitamin B_{12} concentration and positive intrinsic factor antibodies has been reported in a 54-year-old woman who was receiving interferon alfa as a maintenance treatment for relapsing chronic hepatitis C (219).

Rapid exacerbation (1–21 days) or delayed (3–38 months) de novo appearance of immune hemolytic anemia has been reported after initiation of interferon alfa treatment in nine patients with lymphoproliferative disorders (220). However, this rare event was identified in only 1% of 581 patients receiving interferon alfa alone or as part of a chemotherapeutic regimen for chronic myelogenous leukemia (221). A mechanism close to that observed with alpha-methyldopa has been thought to be involved (208). The direct antiglobulin test was positive in 32% of 28

chronic myeloid leukemia patients after a median of 1 year of treatment with interferon alfa (222).

Interferon alfa can also induce multiple antibody formation to transfused blood cell antigens, with subsequent massive hemolysis (223).

- A 33-year-old man developed a delayed hemolytic reaction 7 days after red cell transfusion (224). Additional investigations showed the presence of an anti-M antibody, the production of which was supposedly caused by chemoimmunotherapy (interferon alfa, interleukin-2, and 5-fluorouracil) which was begun 24 hours after transfusion.

Leukopenia

The dose of interferon alfa is usually halved when the neutrophil count falls below 0.75×10^9/l or the drug is permanently withdrawn when it falls below 0.5×10^9/l. However, this issue has recently been challenged by a retrospective analysis of 11 patients with compensated cirrhosis, four of whom had severe neutropenia (that is 0.4 to 0.67×10^9/l) during the first 2 months of treatment (225). They remained asymptomatic and the neutropenia spontaneously reversed despite continued treatment.

In one study in 119 patients treated with interferon alfa and ribavirin for chronic hepatitis C, in whom neutropenia was not considered as a cause for exclusion or dosage modification, the neutrophil count fell by an average of 34% (31–74%) (226). During the course of treatment, 32 patients had at least one neutrophil count below 1×10^9/l, 11 had a neutrophil count below 0.75×10^9/l, and 2 had a neutrophil count below 0.5×10^9/l; however, none of these patients required dosage modification because of neutropenia. None of the 22 patients who developed documented or suspected bacterial infections during or immediately after treatment withdrawal had concomitant neutropenia. The three black patients with constitutional neutropenia (pretreatment neutrophil counts below 1.5×10^9/l) had only minimal changes in their neutrophil counts during treatment and no infection, suggesting that these patients can be safely treated.

Thrombocytopenia

Although inhibition of stem-cell proliferation is the most likely mechanism of hematological toxicity, increased platelet hepatic uptake has been suggested to account for thrombocytopenia (227). Raised serum thrombopoietin concentrations were found in patients with interferon alfa-induced thrombocytopenia (228). However, there is evidence that serum thrombopoietin concentrations in patients who have had thrombocytopenia during interferon alfa treatment for chronic viral hepatitis C either do not increase (in patients with compensated cirrhosis) or increase only moderately and less than expected (in non-cirrhotic patients) (229). The authors proposed that interferon alfa impairs liver production of thrombopoietin, raising the possibility of testing thrombopoietin administration in patients with severe thrombocytopenia before or during treatment with interferon alfa (230).

- In a 45-year-old man treated with pegylated interferon alfa-2b for relapsing chronic hepatitis C, thrombocytopenia recovered over 2 months, despite initial treatment with glucocorticoids and immunoglobulin (231).

Interferon alfa-induced immune-mediated thrombocytopenia shares many features with idiopathic thrombocytopenic purpuras and may be therefore coincidental (SED-13, 1094; SEDA-20, 328; SEDA-21, 371), but recurrence of thrombocytopenia on interferon alfa readministration strongly supports a causal role of interferon alfa (232). Cross reaction with interferon beta was not found in an isolated report (SEDA-20, 329). Even though severe and even fatal worsening of idiopathic thrombocytopenic purpura has been observed after administration of interferon alfa (SED-13, 1094; SEDA-20, 328), interferon alfa was not considered harmful in patients with chronic hepatitis C who were previously positive for platelet- associated immunoglobulin G (233).

Thrombotic thrombocytopenic purpura is a possible complication of interferon alfa in patients with chronic myelogenous leukemia, and can develop even after a successful prolonged (2–3 years) treatment (234). Complete recovery is expected after prompt medical management with plasma exchange and glucocorticoids.

Platelet aggregation
The effects of interferon alfa-2b on platelet aggregation have been studied in 29 patients with melanoma who received a low-dose regimen (9 MU/week in five patients) or a high-dose regimen (100 MU/m^2/week intravenously for 4 weeks, then 30 MU/m^2/week subcutaneously for 48 weeks in 24 patients) (235). Compared with pretreatment values and healthy controls, there was significant inhibition of platelet aggregation in the high-dose group, while the effects were minimal in the low-dose group. In the high-dose group, the inhibition was more prominent during the subcutaneous maintenance dose and was still detectable 8 weeks after interferon alfa withdrawal in 60% of the tested samples. An increased risk of bleeding should therefore be anticipated in patients who receive high-dose interferon alfa.

Clotting factors
Clotting disorders due to interferon alfa have rarely been reported.

- Asymptomatic prolongation of the activated partial thromboplastin time associated with lupus anticoagulant and a reduction in the coagulation activity of factors IX, XI, and XII occurred after 10 weeks of interferon alfa-2b and ribavirin in a 60-year-old woman with chronic hepatitis C (236). There were no arguments in favor of an antiphospholipid syndrome, and all the abnormalities normalized after withdrawal.

Interferon alfa was suspected of having induced the development of anti-factor VIII autoantibodies in one patient with hemophilia who survived and one without hemophilia who subsequently died from acute hemorrhage (SED-13, 1094; 237,238).

- There was significant bleeding with hematomas in association with an inhibitor of factor VIII in a 58-year-old man who took interferon alfa for 1 year for chronic myelogenous leukemia (239). The factor VIII inhibitor, which was markedly raised, disappeared within 6 weeks of interferon alfa withdrawal and prednisone treatment.

By contrast, in a small uncontrolled study, there was no increase in antifactor VIII antibodies in patients with hemophilia A treated with interferon alfa (240).

Gastrointestinal

Mild and transient gastrointestinal disorders, namely nausea, vomiting, diarrhea or anorexia, were observed in 30–40% of patients, and their severity is typically dose-related (20). Dryness or inflammation of the oropharynx, and moderate stomatitis were sometimes noted, but severe painful oral ulcers recurring after interferon alfa re-administration have been reported (241). More severe forms of digestive disease have been described in isolated case histories with microscopic colitis and the occurrence or the exacerbation of ulcerative colitis (SED-13, 1094; SEDA-21, 372).

Celiac disease
Celiac disease was observed after 2–3 months of interferon alfa treatment in two patients with chronic hepatitis C aged 34 and 38 years (242). Both had total villous atrophy on distal duodenal biopsy, were positive for antiendomysial antibodies, and responded to a gluten-free diet. Three other cases were reported after 1–5 months of treatment for chronic hepatitis C (37,243). The diagnosis was confirmed in all three patients, based on the presence of total villous atrophy on distal duodenal biopsy, positivity of antiendomysial antibodies, and recovery with a gluten-free diet. Pretreatment antiendomysial antibodies were positive in the two patients tested. As suggested in one patient, interferon alfa can be safely continued providing that a gluten-free diet is strictly respected.

Enteritis
Eosinophilic enteritis has been attributed to interferon alfa (244).

- A 23-year-old man with no previous history of digestive disorders took interferon alfa for chronic hepatitis C. After 2 weeks of treatment, he had severe abdominal pain and diarrhea. The absolute eosinophil count was 7.5×10^9/l, with 40% eosinophils on bone marrow aspiration and a markedly high IgE concentration. Radiological examination showed diffuse jejunal and ileal wall thickening and gross ascites with numerous eosinophils. Complete resolution was obtained after interferon alfa withdrawal and prednisolone treatment. There was no recurrence after prednisolone was withdrawn.
- A 23-year-old man with no previous history of digestive disorders took interferon alfa for chronic hepatitis C. After 2 weeks of treatment, he had severe abdominal pain and diarrhea. The absolute eosinophil count was

$7.5 \times 10^9/l$, with 40% eosinophils on bone marrow aspiration and a markedly high IgE concentration. Radiological examination showed diffuse jejunal and ileal wall thickening and gross ascites with numerous eosinophils. Complete resolution was obtained after interferon alfa withdrawal and prednisolone treatment. There was no recurrence after prednisolone was withdrawn.

Colitis

Microscopic colitis and new or worsened ulcerative colitis have been attributed to interferon alfa (SED-13, 1094; SEDA-21, 372). Ischemic colitis has been reported in two of 280 patients treated for chronic hepatitis C (245).

Liver

Asymptomatic and reversible rises in serum transaminases have been reported in 25–30% of patients receiving high-dose interferon alfa (20). Although direct hepatotoxicity has been suspected in isolated and unexplained cases of severe liver failure (SED-13, 1094), most data favored exacerbation of chronic viral hepatitis or latent autoimmuine hepatitis.

Exacerbation of chronic viral hepatitis

In the treatment of chronic hepatitis B, HBe seroconversion was sometimes preceded by transient and moderate worsening of serum transaminases, but severe exacerbation of chronic hepatitis B infection and fatal liver failure can occur. Such fatalities were reported in under 0.5% of patients with hepatitis B (246). Patients with active cirrhosis or a previous history of decompensated cirrhosis are particularly susceptible to these complications (247).

Acute exacerbation of hepatitis is an extremely rare complication of chronic hepatitis C treatment. An exaggerated immune response to hepatitis virus was supposedly the cause of acute icteric hepatitis in two patients (SEDA-21, 372) (248).

- A 43-year-old man had a moderate rise in hepatic transaminase activities after 4 weeks of interferon alfa treatment. His liver tests normalized after withdrawal, but the aspartate transaminase activity increased dramatically shortly after treatment was restarted. His condition rapidly deteriorated, with a diagnosis of hepatorenal failure, and he finally required liver transplantation. Histological examination of the liver showed advanced micronodular cirrhosis, a feature not found on pretreatment liver biopsy.

In another study, only four of 11 241 patients treated with interferon alfa died of fulminant liver failure (16).

Autoimmune hepatitis

More disturbing are reports of interferon alfa-induced acute exacerbation of latent autoimmune hepatitis (SED-13, 1094) (249–256). Further analysis showed that these patients were initially misdiagnosed as having hepatitis C, and autoimmune hepatitis reversible by glucocorticoid treatment was later proven to be the correct diagnosis. It was later found that latent chronic autoimmune hepatitis can be present in patients with unequivocal serological evidence of chronic hepatitis C (249,257). The co-existence of serological markers of autoimmune hepatitis and confirmed hepatitis C before treatment with interferon alfa in the same patient is very disturbing, because the distinction cannot readily be made on the basis of biological and histological data. As glucocorticoids can increase the extent of viremia, and since in addition interferon alfa can acutely exacerbate latent autoimmune liver disease, this has raised the question of how to deal with these patients. In those without serological markers of autoimmune liver disease, only close monitoring of liver function to detect any sudden increase in alanine transaminase activity is helpful, because the systematic detection of autoantibodies proves unable to predict the risk of overt autoimmune hepatitis (257). In those with both hepatitis C virus and autoantibodies, there is as yet no consensus on the therapeutic management. Glucocorticoids may actually increase the extent of viremia, while interferon alfa may exacerbate autoimmune hepatitis. As a result, controversies have emerged, with several investigators advocating glucocorticoids as first line treatment and providing a safe option in patients with high antibody titers, whereas others have found interferon alfa to be more appropriate (SED-13, 1094; SEDA-20, 329; SEDA-21, 372).

De novo induction rather than exacerbation of autoimmune hepatitis is still possible, as indicated by anecdotal reports in patients with cancer or chronic viral hepatitis (SED-13, 1094; SEDA-22, 402). Such a very rare event is in keeping with the usual absence of autoantibody specific for autoimmune liver disease after interferon alfa treatment.

Positive serological markers of autoimmune hepatitis before treatment in patients with concomitant chronic hepatitis C are sometimes associated with further exacerbation of an underlying autoimmune liver disease during interferon alfa treatment. Of three patients with raised antimitochondrial antibodies (over 1:160), only the two patients with M2 (with or without M4 or M8) subtypes had biochemical exacerbation of cholestasis and an unfavorable response to interferon alfa (255). Although very few patients were investigated, determination of antibodies against submitochondrial particles may help to identify patients who are likely to have no benefit and even exacerbation of liver disease with interferon alfa.

In 25 children with chronic hepatitis C, pretreatment positivity for liver/kidney microsomal type 1 (LKM-1) antibodies was associated with more frequent treatment-limiting increases in serum alanine transaminase activity (256). Withdrawal of interferon alfa-2b because of hypertransaminasemia was required in three of four LKM-1 positive children compared with two of the 21 LKM-1 negative children. Although none developed features of autoimmune hepatitis, careful surveillance of hepatic function is recommended in LKM-1-positive patients.

Other complications

Interferon alfa-associated macrovesicular steatosis has been reported (258).

- A 50-year-old woman without a history of liver disease, dyslipidemia, diabetes, obesity, or alcoholism started taking interferon alfa (7.5 MU/day) for chronic myelogenous leukemia together with allopurinol and hydroxyurea for 2 weeks. Her liver tests were normal before treatment but transaminase activities were greatly increased after 2 weeks. Serological tests for hepatitis B and C and HIV were negative, as was screening for serum antitissue antibodies. Liver biopsy showed severe macrovesicular steatosis (80% of hepatocytes) without steatohepatitis. Liver tests completely normalized on interferon alfa withdrawal. A few weeks after interferon alfa was restarted in a lower dose (3–5 MU/day), she again had a rise in liver enzymes, and a second liver biopsy showed unchanged findings. Liver tests remained stable despite treatment continuation.

Other adverse liver effects reported with interferon alfa include primary biliary cirrhosis (SEDA-20, 329) and granulomatous hepatitis (SEDA-20, 329; SEDA-21, 372) (259).

Pancreas

Asymptomatic rises in pancreatic enzymes and reversible acute pancreatitis have been reported in isolated patients, with no mention of hypertriglyceridemia (SEDA-19, 336).

- A 54-year-old man developed abdominal pain from the beginning of interferon alfa treatment (260). Two weeks later his serum amylase and lipase peaked at about three times the upper limit of normal. Careful radiological investigations ruled out pancreatic calcification and biliary or pancreatic lithiasis and showed only pancreatic enlargement. Complete improvement occurred after treatment withdrawal. As in the very few previous cases, there was no hypertriglyceridemia in this patient.

A definite case of pancreatitis proven by positive rechallenge was also briefly cited in a review of drug-associated pancreatitis spontaneously reported to the Dutch adverse drug reactions system (261).

Two cases of interferon alfa-induced acute pancreatitis in patients with chronic hepatitis C were particularly convincing, because other causes were carefully ruled out and clinical symptoms or biological abnormalities recurred after rechallenge in both patients (262). Although one patient also took ribavirin, recurrence was observed after re-administration of interferon alfa alone. Lipid disorders were not found in these patients, confirming that interferon alfa-induced pancreatitis is not due to hypertriglyceridemia.

Urinary tract

Mild and usually asymptomatic proteinuria, leukocyturia, microscopic hematuria, or moderate increases in serum creatinine were observed in 15–25% of patients (20). There was moderate deterioration of glomerular and tubular renal function in most interferon alfa-treated patients assessed prospectively with a number of renal function markers (263).

In patients receiving high-dose interferon alfa, severe proteinuria and nephrotic syndrome have sometimes been noted (264).

- A 57-year-old woman developed severe nephrotic syndrome after 3 months of interferon alfa re-treatment, and renal biopsy showed minimal change nephrotic syndrome with T cell-predominant interstitial nephritis (265). Proteinuria persisted despite interferon alfa withdrawal and resolved only after glucocorticoid treatment.
- A 55-year-old woman was treated with interferon alfa and ribavirin for 1 year and developed asymptomatic nephrotic syndrome with focal segmental glomerulosclerosis on renal biopsy (266). Proteinuria slowly improved over the next 21 months.

Interferon alfa-induced acute renal insufficiency is rare and has mostly been reported in patients with underlying renal disease, in those receiving high dosages, or in those with varied malignancies (SED-13; 1095; SEDA-20, 329; SEDA-21, 372; 267,268). Very few cases have been described in patients with chronic hepatitis (SEDA-21, 372; SEDA-22, 402). It has also been reported after intravesical administration (SEDA-21, 372). When available, pathological findings have pointed variously to nephrotic syndrome with minimal-change nephropathy and acute tubulointerstitial nephritis, nephrotic syndrome with severe glomerular changes, membranoproliferative glomerulonephritis, extracapillary glomerulonephritis with crescents, focal segmental glomerulosclerosis, and acute tubular necrosis. Renal dysfunction usually resolves after withdrawal of interferon alfa, but irreversible alteration or incomplete resolution of renal function have occasionally been noted.

A review of 15 other available reports of renal insufficiency and proteinuria in patients with chronic myeloid leukemia or other malignancies confirmed that the histological spectrum of renal lesions associated with interferon alfa is varied, and includes membranous glomerulonephritis, minimal change glomerulonephritis, acute interstitial nephritis, hemolytic–uremic syndrome, and thrombotic microangiopathy. Renal complications were reversible in nine patients; three patients had persistent proteinuria, and four had persistent renal dysfunction, of whom three required chronic hemodialysis. Two-thirds of the patients developed renal complications within 1 month of treatment with interferon alfa, and one-third had received a relatively low dosage of interferon alfa (9–15 MU/week).

The mechanism of interferon alfa nephrotoxicity is probably multifactorial and may involve a direct nephrotoxic effect with a possible additive effect of concomitant NSAID therapy, a T cell-mediated immune effect, immune-complex renal disease, or an autoimmune etiology (SED-13, 1095; 269–274).

Acute renal insufficiency has also occurred as a consequence of interferon alfa-induced hemolytic–uremic syndrome, thrombotic thrombocytopenic purpura, or renal thrombotic microangiopathy (SED-13, 1095; 234,275–278). The diagnosis was made after 7 months to 10 years of treatment (median 50 months) with weekly doses of 15–70 MU. This rare but extremely severe complication has almost exclusively been reported in patients treated for chronic myelogenous leukemia, so that the respective roles of interferon alfa and the underlying hematological malignancy are undetermined. However, at least one case has been reported in a patient with hepatitis C (SEDA-22, 402). From a total of 15 cases, renal prognosis was poor, with early deaths in four patients, chronic hemodialysis in eight, and chronic renal insufficiency in three.

To determine the characteristics of thrombotic microangiopathy associated with interferon alfa, data from eight patients were carefully examined (279). All had chronic myeloid leukemia and had received high-dose interferon alfa (mean 39 MU/week) for a long time (mean 32 months) before diagnosis. Severe arterial hypertension was the most common sign before diagnosis. Five patients had distal ischemic lesions that required amputation in one, and all had typical lesions of renal thrombotic microangiopathy involving both glomeruli and small arterioles. After interferon alfa withdrawal, two recovered normal renal function, three had persistent renal insufficiency, one relapsed 17 months after treatment withdrawal, and two required chronic dialysis. One patient had already had reversible renal insufficiency during a previous course of interferon alfa. From a review of 21 other previously published similar cases, the authors confirmed that interferon alfa-induced thrombotic microangiopathy mostly occurred in patients with chronic myeloid leukemia, whereas only two cases were reported in patients with chronic hepatitis C and one in a patient with hairy cell leukemia. The delayed occurrence of renal toxicity was also suggested to be highly predictive of histological thrombotic microangiopathy.

Possible deleterious effects of interferon alfa on renal graft function are repeatedly reported (280).

- A 43-year-old man with stable renal graft function, taking ciclosporin, methylprednisolone, and azathioprine, developed chronic myelogenous leukemia and received interferon alfa (3 MU/day). Seven weeks later, he became tired and had increased proteinuria and a raised serum creatinine concentration (574 μmol/l). Interferon alfa was withdrawn and he received high-dose methylprednisolone for suspected acute graft rejection. This was unsuccessful and a first renal biopsy showed widespread interstitial edema that could not be correctly interpreted. Hemodialysis was restarted, and he finally developed a catheter infection and died from sepsis. Histology of the explanted renal graft showed severe, predominantly acute, vascular rejection.

The rapid occurrence of renal dysfunction after interferon alfa in this case suggested a causal relation.

Skin

A wide range of skin lesions has been reported, and most include skin dryness, rash, diffuse erythema, or urticaria, occurring in 5–12% of patients (20,281). However, severe dermatological complications are rare. In a prospective survey of 120 patients treated during 6–18 months for chronic viral hepatitis, only three developed lichen planus and one relapsing aphthous stomatitis (282).

Injection site reactions
Subcutaneous interferon alfa sometimes causes local erythema and skin induration, which can be prevented by regularly changing the site of injection. Isolated reports have described more severe local reactions, with inflammatory painful nodules, purpuric papules and vasculitis, local ulceration, and injection site necrosis (SED-13; 1095; SEDA-20, 330; SEDA-21, 372; SEDA-22, 402). Despite previous findings, even patients receiving low-dose interferon alfa can have severe injection site reactions. A localized intradermal bullous eruption, which recurred following each interferon alfa injection, was also reported (283).

Severe injection site reactions have been extensively detailed in six patients who had local cutaneous necrosis or indurated erythema after 1–10 months of treatment with low-dose interferon alfa (284). Four patients had concomitant risk factors known to reduce microcirculation, that is beta-blockers, dihydroergotamine, and cigarette smoking. The lesions healed after medical treatment in five patients, but one required surgical excision. The ulcers healed slowly and full recovery occurred only after a mean of 16 weeks after drug withdrawal. The lesions did not recur after interferon alfa re-administration at the other injection sites.

As with interferon alfa, pegylated interferon alfa has been associated with injection site skin necrosis (285). Severe local reactions after subcutaneous injections mostly consist of ulceration and skin necrosis, but a variety of reactions have been described. Prominent suppuration and granulomatous dermatitis at the injection sites of interferon alfa have been reported in two patients (286). Three patients who had severe rashes while receiving pegylated interferon alfa-2a or 2b had positive intracutaneous tests to both pegylated forms of interferon alfa but not to standard interferon alfa-2a or 2b (287). One of these patients subsequently tolerated standard interferon alfa. Cutaneous ulcers have also been reported in patients treated with peginterferon alfa-2b (288,289). In the latter case, the lesions healed under local therapy and the same dose of interferon was maintained.

Lichen planus
The new occurrence or exacerbation of lichen planus is a well-known complication of interferon alfa, but this has been a source of a considerable debate (SED-13, 1095; SEDA-20, 330; SEDA-22, 402). Indeed, most patients have received interferon alfa for chronic hepatitis C, an underlying disease that is controversially thought to be associated with a spontaneously higher incidence of lichen planus (290). In addition, complete reversibility of previous lichen planus was sometimes observed in patients treated with interferon alfa (SEDA-20, 330). Whatever the truth of the matter, the recurrence of lesions after interferon alfa re-administration or reports of lichen

planus in patients with cancer (291–293) argues strongly for a direct causal link with interferon alfa. Local treatment and PUVA were sometimes sufficient to alleviate symptoms, but withdrawal of interferon alfa was required in the most severe cases (SED-13, 1095).

Pemphigus and pemphigoid
Bullous pemphigus and pemphigoid with circulating pemphigus-like autoantibodies, pemphigus foliaceus with anti-intercellular IgG antibodies, and paraneoplastic pemphigus due to interferon alfa have rarely been reported (SED-13, 1095), as has extensive oral pemphigus (294).

- A 28-year-old woman developed oral ulcers after a 5-month course of interferon alfa-2a for chronic hepatitis C. She had multiple erosions on both lips, the tongue, the floor of the mouth, the soft palate, the pharyngeal walls, and the laryngeal mucosa, but there were no skin or genital lesions. Raised double-stranded DNA antibody titers were found. Histology showed pemphigus vulgaris, and complete resolution was obtained by withdrawal of interferon alfa and immunosuppressive and local treatment.

This case was thought to have been due to the immunomodulatory effects of interferon alfa.

Psoriasis
The first reports of psoriasis in cancer patients treated with high-dose interferon alfa were followed by a controversial debate (295,296). However, numerous cases have confirmed that interferon alfa can either induce typical psoriasis or worsen pre-existing psoriasis (SED-13, 1095; 297), an observation that is compatible with interferon alfa-induced imbalance toward an increased Th1 response. This was particularly exemplified by the reversibility of the lesions after withdrawal of treatment and the prompt recurrence of symptoms after interferon alfa re-administration. Exacerbation of psoriasis usually occurred within the first month, whereas a minimum of 2–3 months of treatment was required in patients without a past history of psoriasis (297). Psoriatic lesions at the sites of injection were suggested to be potential indicators for further generalization of psoriasis. In more severe cases, there was concomitant development of monoarticular or polyarticular joint symptoms (SED-13, 1095; SEDA-21, 372). Pustular psoriasis with balanitis and erosive monoarthritis, suggesting incomplete Reiter's syndrome, was also reported in one patient with HLA-B27 (298).

Vitiligo
Vitiligo has sometimes been reported in patients with malignant melanoma, for example in 17–25% of patients receiving interferon alfa alone (SEDA-21, 372). There have also been a few reports of vitiligo in patients with chronic hepatitis C (SEDA-20, 330), and one patient had both scleroderma and vitiligo (SEDA-19, 336).

Other complications
A spectrum of cutaneous lesions has been described distant from sites of interferon alfa injection. The clinical and histological characteristics of inflammatory skin lesions that occurred away from injection sites have been investigated in 20 patients treated with interferon alfa-2a or 2b plus ribavirin for chronic hepatitis C (299). Cutaneous lesions developed between 2 weeks and 4 months and consisted of pruritic papular erythematous eruptions with occasional vesicles. These eczema-like skin lesions predominated on the distal limbs, the head, and the neck. Photosensitivity was also noted in four patients and mucous lesions in two. Skin biopsy mostly showed non-specific mononuclear infiltrates. The skin lesions were promptly reversible in 10 patients who required treatment withdrawal, while others improved after symptomatic treatment. Two of the three patients who again received the same or another type of interferon alfa had recurrence of their lesions. Skin tests performed in six patients were negative, including the two patients who relapsed after rechallenge with interferon alfa, and were therefore considered unhelpful.

- Radiation recall dermatitis developed in a 29-year-old woman after high-dose intravenous interferon alfa-2b was given 5 days after the completion of radiotherapy for malignant melanoma (300).

The authors suggested that interferon alfa can trigger an inflammatory reaction in patients whose inflammatory response threshold has been lowered by irradiation.

- A 46-year-old woman developed transient facial erythema with telangiectasia after each injection of interferon alfa, resolving within 1–2 days, and completely disappearing after definitive withdrawal of treatment 7 months later (301).
- Two patients treated with pegylated interferon alfa-2b and ribavirin developed cutaneous thrombotic microangiopathy (302).
- A 54-year-old woman had small bullous lesions mainly on the backs of her hands and feet after 6 months of treatment with pegylated interferon alfa-2b plus ribavirin for chronic hepatitis C. The lesions lasted 48 hours and healed rapidly after rupture of the bullae.
- A 62-year-old woman developed generalized pruritus and excoriated lesions after 5 months of treatment with pegylated interferon alfa-2b plus ribavirin. The lesions were maximal on the backs of her hands and feet after 8 months of treatment, but there were no bullae.

Skin biopsies in the last two patients showed microthrombi of the dermal capillaries and a necrotic epidermis. Immunofluorescence showed only fibrinogen. Some bullous lesions were still present 1 month after withdrawal in the first patient, while the second patient responded to local corticosteroids and a reduced dose of pegylated interferon alfa, but continued to have episodes of severe pruritus.

Other dermatological complications have in most instances been reported as single case histories, so that any causal relation with interferon alfa awaits confirmation. These reports have included worsening of lichen myxedematosus, injection site pyoderma gangrenosum, a polymorphous light eruption (SEDA-22, 372), and a fatal case of histiocytic cytophagic panniculitis (SEDA-20, 330).

- Meyerson's phenomenon, multiple focal and transient eczematous eruptions around melanocytic nevi, has been reported in a 24-year-old man when the dosage of interferon alfa for Behçet's disease was doubled (303).
- Bullous lesions with specific infiltrates of mycosis fungoides have been reported in a 67-year-old woman who took interferon alfa for 2 months for mycosis fungoides (304).

Although in the second case the syndrome could not be definitely attributed to interferon alfa, the authors noted that bullous mycosis fungoides is an extremely rare variant of this disease and withdrawal of interferon alfa led to healing of the blisters without further recurrence.

Hair

Moderate and reversible alopecia secondary to telogen effluvium is common (7–30%), and sometimes recedes despite continued treatment (305). Alopecia areata has very occasionally been described (306).

- Injection-site alopecia has been reported in three patients, affecting the thighs in two patients and the abdomen in one (307). A reversible focal telogen effluvium secondary to high local concentrations of interferon alfa was the most likely cause, indicating that rotating injection sites are needed to prevent this adverse effect.
- Alopecia areata after 7 months of interferon alfa, slowly reversible on withdrawal, has also been reported in a 36-year-old woman (308).

In two patients with previously natural curly hairs, the combination of interferon alfa plus ribavirin was suggested to have triggered a rapid change in hair texture, with diffuse straightening hairs, eyelashes, and eyebrow hypertrichosis (309). In one patient, a causal role of treatment was supported by the spontaneous recovery of hair abnormalities after withdrawal and the recurrence of similar abnormalities on rechallenge.

Excessive growth of eyelashes and nail damage due to *Tinea unguium* have been occasionally reported in patients receiving interferon alfa (SED-13, 1095; SEDA-21, 372). Hypertrichosis of the eyelashes (trichomegaly) developed in two of 36 patients with chronic viral hepatitis who were examined for ocular complications during treatment with high-dose interferon alfa (18–30 MU/week) (86). These two patients had received the highest dose of interferon alfa.

Musculoskeletal

Arthralgia, myalgias, and muscle weakness are typically observed during the early influenza-like reaction (20). Direct muscle toxicity of interferon alfa can result in acute rhabdomyolysis, in some cases fatal after the dose of interferon alfa was increased (SEDA-19, 330; SEDA-21, 372).

- A 26-year-old man with a malignant melanoma had two episodes of acute severe rhabdomyolysis after each exposure to a chemotherapy regimen containing interferon alfa and dacarbazine (310). As a few cases of rhabdomyolysis have been previously reported after interferon alfa alone (SEDA-19, 336; SEDA-20, 330; SEDA-22, 403), interferon alfa was suggested as the most likely cause.
- Acute rhabdomyolysis occurred in a 34-year-old woman with a melanoma treated with interferon alfa 20 MU/m^2/day (311). There was no recurrence on retreatment with a lower dose (down to 6.6 MU/m^2/day), suggesting that this was a dose-related complication.
- A 34-year-old man with scleromyxedema had flu-like symptoms and muscle pain after the first injection of interferon alfa 6 MU (312). After three additional injections at 2-day intervals, his muscle symptoms worsened and were associated with mild quadriparesis, reduced deep tendon reflexes, dark urine, confusion, and agitation. Biological findings were consistent with acute rhabdomyolysis, and electromyography showed rare denervation potentials. His symptoms resolved and the laboratory findings normalized within 15 days.

Delayed muscular adverse effects have been occasionally reported including the clinical exacerbation of a latent myopathy (SEDA-19, 336), delayed and severe myopathic changes (313), myositis, polymyositis, and a Lambert–Eaton-like syndrome (SEDA-19, 336; SEDA-20, 330; SEDA-22, 403).

- Three patients developed unilateral or bilateral avascular necrosis of the femoral head after 3–54 months of treatment with interferon alfa for chronic myelogenous leukemia (314). One required bilateral hip replacement and two significantly improved after interferon alfa withdrawal. One patient received further interferon alfa without exacerbation.

Although there were risk factors for avascular necrosis in two of the patients (a short course of methylprednisolone and moderate alcohol consumption), the authors did not consider them to be significant. They identified seven other reported cases of avascular necrosis in patients with chronic myeloid leukemia, including two patients who were taking interferon alfa at the time of the complication. One patient with pre-existing avascular necrosis had an acute exacerbation within 1 month of interferon alfa and required hip replacement. Although any causal relation with treatment remains purely speculative, the authors argued that the known antiangiogenic effects of interferon alfa could have predisposed patients to avascular necrosis.

Sexual function

Sexual complaints attributed to interferon alfa, namely decreased libido, impotence, or erectile failure, are usually concomitant to other neuropsychiatric symptoms, and cases of reversible impotence are anecdotal (315). The mechanisms accounting for these adverse effects are unclear, and changes in sex hormone concentrations have not been consistently reported. In one study in healthy women, interferon alfa produced falls in serum progesterone and estradiol concentrations (316), but neither impairment of libido nor impairment of fertility has apparently been reported in women. No evidence of gonadal toxicity or sexual dysfunction was found in 43 men with hairy cell leukemia who received interferon alfa for 2–12 months compared with 33 patients who received no systemic therapy (317). Finally, sexual complaints reported during interferon alfa treatment of chronic hepatitis C were presumably related to fatigue, anxiety, or psychological disorders rather than to endocrinological changes (SEDA-21, 373).

Immunologic

Hypersensitivity reactions

No IgE-mediated immediate-type allergic reactions to interferon alfa have ever been conclusively documented. A recurrent non-IgE-mediated anaphylactic reaction, possibly due to mast cell degranulation, has been described in a patient with mastocytosis (318).

- A 64-year-old man with no history of allergy had progressive fatigue, loss of appetite, and facial edema after 6 months of interferon alfa-2b treatment for chronic hepatitis C (319). Angioedema was diagnosed and it resolved after withdrawal of interferon alfa and a short course of prednisolone. Serum immunoglobulin E and plasma bradykinin concentrations were raised, but the C1 esterase inhibitor and serum complement concentrations were normal.
- A 47-year-old man, who had previously received a 2-month course of interferon alfacon-1 for chronic hepatitis C, started interferon alfa-2b 8 months later (320). He developed mild generalized pruritus the day after the second injection, and dyspnea with diffuse urticaria within a few hours after the third injection. Skin tests were not performed, and IgG but not IgE antibodies to interferon alfa were found.

These cases do not formally show a causal relation with interferon alfa, and at best they suggest that an IgE-mediated reaction is probably not the cause of hypersensitivity reactions to interferon alfa. In the first case, the mechanism may have been similar to that observed with angiotensin-converting enzyme inhibitors.

Cases of contact dermatitis have suggested that interferon alfa-2c can cause cell-mediated delayed hypersensitivity (321,322).

Interferon alfa antibodies

Both binding and neutralizing antibodies to interferon alfa can be detected in interferon alfa-treated patients, and the incidence or clinical significance of these antibodies is the subject of continuous controversy, which has been addressed in a number of studies or general reviews (SED-13, 1096; SEDA-20, 330; SEDA-21, 373; 156,323–325).

In various studies, the incidence of antibody formation has ranged from zero to more than 50% of patients. However, any comparison between studies is difficult, because the underlying treated disease, the type of interferon used, the route of administration, the dosage regimen, the schedule of treatment, and the method of assay have differed from one investigation to another. Antibodies to interferon alfa have been reported to be more frequent in patients receiving long-term, instead of short-term, treatment, in patients receiving subcutaneous rather than intravenous interferon alfa, and in patients receiving low rather than high doses (156). Complete disappearance of interferon alfa antibodies was usually observed after withdrawal. Interferon alfa formulations also differ in antigenicity. Using the same anti-interferon alfa antibody assay, a higher frequency of antibodies to recombinant interferon alfa-2a has repeatedly been reported compared with other recombinant or natural interferon alfa formulations in patients treated by the same route and with the same treatment schedule. In 296 patients with chronic hepatitis, binding and neutralizing antibodies were found in 45 and 20% respectively of patients receiving recombinant interferon alfa-2a compared with 15 and 6.9% of those receiving recombinant interferon alfa-2b, and 9.4 and 1.2% of those receiving interferon alfa-n1 (326,327). There were similar differences in the immunogenic potential of the two recombinant interferon alfa formulations in 159 patients with chronic myelogenous leukemia (328). Overall, the incidence of binding antibodies is in the range of 20–50% for recombinant interferon alfa-2a, 6–10% for recombinant interferon alfa-2b, and 1–6% for interferon alfa-n1 (324).

The clinical significance of binding antibodies appears to be limited to a possible change in interferon alfa pharmacokinetics. By contrast, neutralizing antibodies, which are usually detected within 2–4 months of treatment, can theoretically reduce the clinical response to interferon alfa and cause interpatient variability in response to treatment, but this is still debated (323–325). Although several studies have failed to detect any loss of therapeutic response, response failure or the reversal of an initial clinical response, simultaneously with (or soon after) the appearance of neutralizing antibodies, have been reported. In large-scale studies, the clinical response to recombinant interferon alfa was significantly less in patients with neutralizing antibodies, and it has therefore been suggested that the appearance of neutralizing antibodies provides the prime explanation for those instances in which there is a relapse or a breakthrough of the disease before the completion of treatment (329–335). In addition, in patients who cease to respond therapeutically after recombinant interferon alfa antibody formation, a change to natural interferon alfa has proved successful in restoring the response in some cases (335–338). This has led to the suggestion that the formation of neutralizing antibodies represents a specific immune response to the recombinant preparations, and that natural interferon alfa can overcome the neutralizing activity of antibodies to recombinant interferon alfa. On the other hand, neutralizing antibodies were not associated with immune complex-associated diseases or hypersensitivity reactions, and exerted no influence on interferon alfa-associated adverse effects. They can even be accompanied by improvement in the flu-like syndrome.

Autoantibodies

Collectively, several antibodies (mostly antinuclear, antithyroid, parietal cell, liver/kidney microsome, and smooth muscle antibodies, and rheumatoid factor) can be detected before interferon alfa treatment in about one-third of patients. Increased titers or the occurrence of various autoantibodies were observed in 4–30% of previously autoantibody-negative patients (21,156). These autoantibodies do not affect the response to interferon alfa treatment (339–341). Although it was initially felt that interferon alfa might facilitate the development of autoimmune disease in patients previously positive for non-organ-specific autoantibodies, the evidence is still limited and the clinical consequences of such autoantibodies are unclear. Except for thyroiditis, large studies in patients with chronic viral hepatitis C receiving interferon alfa did not show a significant increase in overt autoimmune diseases, despite the pre-existence or further positivity of several autoantibodies (SED-13, 1096; SEDA-20, 330; SEDA-21, 373; SEDA-22, 405). However, in 83 patients with chronic hepatitis C there were one or more pre-existing autoantibodies (mostly low-titer antinuclear antibodies) in 35 patients (group I), of whom seven had clinical evidence of immune-mediated disorders, whereas five of 48 patients without pre-existing autoantibodies (group II) had similar disorders (342). After 12–48 weeks of treatment with interferon alfa in 44 patients, there were new immune-mediated disorders in six of the 20 patients in group I (thyroid disorders in three, arthropathy in two, and psoriasis in one), but none in the 24 patients in group II. Patients who are positive for autoantibodies before interferon alfa may therefore be much more likely to develop autoimmune diseases, particularly thyroid disorders, during interferon alfa treatment.

As a result, there is no clear consensus about the management of patients previously positive for non-organ specific autoantibodies, but it is usually considered that low autoantibody titers or the absence of concomitant symptoms suggestive of autoimmune disease is not a contraindication to treatment.

Autoimmune disorders

The possibility of autoimmune disorders during interferon alfa treatment has been addressed by many authors. The spectrum of interferon alfa-induced immune diseases includes organ-specific and systemic autoimmune diseases, such as thyroiditis, diabetes, hematological disorders, systemic lupus erythematosus, rheumatoid arthritis, dermatological disease, and myasthenia gravis (156). Several have been discussed in appropriate sections elsewhere in this monograph. The exact role of interferon alfa is usually difficult to ascertain, because the underlying disease, that is chronic hepatitis C, can also be associated with immune-mediated disease.

Two studies have provided insights into the incidence and risk factors of the immune-mediated complications of interferon alfa in patients with chronic myeloid leukemia. In the first study, 13 of 46 patients had autoimmune manifestations consisting of a combination of autoimmune thyroiditis in four, a direct antiglobulin test without hemolysis in eight, cryoagglutinins in one, Raynaud's phenomenon in two, and chronic autoimmune hepatitis in one (343). Overall, six patients had clinically symptomatic manifestations after a median of 15 months of treatment. In the second study, there were autoimmune diseases in seven of 76 patients after a median of 19 months of treatment, including hypothyroidism in one, immune-mediated hemolysis in two, systemic lupus erythematosus in two, Raynaud's phenomenon in one, and mixed connective tissue disease in one (344). In both studies there was a strong association with female sex and it was confirmed that patients who developed clinical autoimmune complications had had relatively long exposures to interferon alfa.

The management of patients with chronic hepatitis C and associated features of autoimmune disease carries the risk of exacerbating the underlying disease. Different treatment strategies, including interferon alfa alone or combined with ribavirin or glucocorticoids, or no treatment, have been discussed (345).

Behçet's disease

Characteristic features of Behçet's disease or isolated positive skin tests were found in one study of patients with chronic myelogenous leukemia treated with interferon alfa (346). No other reports confirmed these findings.

Dermatomyositis

Occasional reports have suggested that interferon alfa can cause dermatomyositis (347).

- A 57-year-old woman received adjuvant high-dose interferon alfa 16 months after removal of a malignant melanoma. About 6 weeks later, she developed hand swelling, fatigue, myalgia, arthralgia, and weakness. Interferon alfa was withdrawn. She had multiple joint involvement, and radiological imaging showed bilateral interstitial pulmonary infiltrates. Anti-Jo antibodies were positive but other autoantibodies were negative. She also had violet eyelid discoloration with edema, tenderness in various muscle groups, and reduced strength in the shoulders. The muscle biopsy showed scattered necrotic fibers and basophilic regenerative fibers. She gradually recovered with methotrexate and corticosteroids, and the titer of anti-Jo antibodies fell dramatically.

Polyarteritis nodosa

Severe polyarteritis nodosa-like systemic vasculitis has been reported (SEDA-20, 330) and cutaneous polyarteritis nodosa has been attributed to interferon alfa (348).

- A 50-year-old woman was given interferon alfa for chronic hepatitis C and primary biliary cirrhosis, and within 2 months became febrile and developed a diffuse nodular erythematous rash. The skin biopsy showed typical features of necrotizing angiitis, and cutaneous periarteritis nodosa was diagnosed. Full recovery was obtained after interferon alfa withdrawal and prednisolone treatment.

According to the authors, it is not known whether this complication was directly due to interferon alfa, represented the triggering of latent periarteritis nodosa in a patient with primary biliary cirrhosis, or whether it was a coincidental adverse event.

Polymyositis

- Polymyositis has very rarely been associated with interferon alfa, but has been reported together with autoimmune thyroiditis in a 48-year-old woman after treatment for 5 months for malignant melanoma (349).

There have been two reports of polymyositis in association with interferon alfa treatment for hematological malignancies (123,350). In both cases, clinical and/or electrophysiological recovery occurred after drug withdrawal, spontaneously or after a short course of glucocorticoids.

Sarcoidosis

The early impression that interferon alfa, alone or in combination with ribavirin, could reactivate or cause new subcutaneous sarcoid nodules and pulmonary or generalized sarcoidosis, has been confirmed by several reports, with prompt recovery after interferon alfa withdrawal (SED-13, 1097; SEDA-20, 330; SEDA-22, 404). The incidence may have been underestimated; in one series, 3 patients out of 60 who received interferon alfa alone or combined with ribavirin developed pulmonary sarcoidosis (351). In a review of 27 cases, the time to onset was 15 days to 30 months, and there were dermatological signs in 50% (352). Five patients had also taken ribavirin, but an enhanced T cell immune reaction from the combination of interferon alfa plus ribavirin is speculative. However. the association of cutaneous or systemic sarcoidosis with interferon alfa, alone or in association with ribavirin, has been exemplified by various reports (353,354), including one patient whose sarcoidosis resolved with prednisone despite continued interferon alfa treatment (355).

- A 60-year-old woman receiving interferon alfa developed cutaneous sarcoid foreign body granulomas at the sites of a previously childhood skin injury (356).

This suggests that interferon alfa may facilitate the development of cutaneous sarcoid granuloma from particulate foreign matter.

De novo sarcoidosis has been reported in six patients (357–361) and reactivation of pre-existing disease in one (362). One of these patients had chronic hepatitis B, suggesting that interferon alfa treatment rather than the underlying disease was the most probable triggering factor. Remission was observed in all patients after withdrawal, either spontaneously or after glucocorticoid treatment.

Sjögren's syndrome

One report of Sjögren's syndrome in a patient taking interferon alfa should be regarded with caution (SEDA-20, 330).

Systemic lupus erythematosus and rheumatoid arthritis

The possible role of interferon alfa in the development of rheumatoid arthritis or systemic lupus erythematosus has been described in isolated cases (363,364), and confirmed cases of systemic lupus erythematosus have very occasionally been reported (SED-13, 1096; SEDA-20, 330). In most of these cases, the predominance of young patients and female sex, the presence of renal or skin involvement, the findings of positive antibodies to double-stranded DNA, and the rapid onset after the start of treatment, as well as persistence of symptoms after interferon alfa withdrawal, are more in keeping with unmasking by interferon alfa of idiopathic lupus rather than with a new drug-induced illness. The reactivation or appearance of inflammatory rheumatological disorders consistent with rheumatoid arthritis or lupus-like polyarthritis were also consistently reported (SEDA-20, 330; 365,366). In a review of 37 published cases of interferon alfa-induced arthritis, symmetrical polyarthritis was the most common feature, and antinuclear antibodies or rheumatoid factor were found in 72 and 34%, respectively (367). Although spontaneous improvement was sometimes observed after withdrawal of interferon alfa, more severe cases required anti-inflammatory, antimalarial, or immunosuppressive drugs. In five of eight patients rechallenged with interferon alfa, there was recurrence of arthritis.

There was an unexpectedly high incidence of rheumatoid and lupus-like symptoms (27 of 137 patients), namely arthralgia, arthritis, myalgia, and Raynaud's phenomenon, in patients with myeloproliferative disorders taking interferon alfa alone or combined with interferon gamma (365). However, only a minority of affected patients fulfilled the diagnostic criteria for systemic lupus erythematosus. By contrast, systemic autoimmune diseases appeared to be genuine but very rare complications of interferon alfa in chronic hepatitis C, with only one case of lupus-like syndrome and two cases of polyarthritis in a survey of 677 patients (18).

Other reports included seronegative polyarthritis, acute seronegative monoarthritis of the hip, and seropositive monoarthritis of the metatarsophalangeal of the right foot (SED-13, 1097).

Systemic lupus erythematosus has been reported in two patients given interferon alfa for chronic hepatitis C (363,368). However, it is not known whether this complication was coincidental or treatment-related.

Systemic sclerosis

Systemic sclerosis has been attributed to interferon alfa-2a (369).

- A 52-year-old woman received interferon alfa-2a for chronic myeloid leukemia and after about 2 years developed fever, dyspnea, and limb edema. The erythrocyte sedimentation rate was 50 mm/hour and pulmonary imaging showed pulmonary vascular congestion. She improved after interferon alfa withdrawal and administration of diuretics, but similar symptoms recurred 3 months later. She also had progressive thickening of the skin on the hands and wrists. There was diffuse parenchymal and interstitial fibrosis of the lungs, absence of peristalsis on esophagogastroduodenoscopy, renal impairment, and positive antisclero-70 antibodies. Capillaroscopy showed typical features of scleroderma. Based on these findings, a diagnosis of systemic sclerosis was suggested and she slowly improved over the next months with cyclophosphamide, prednisone, iloprost, and hydroxyurea.

This patient had the HLA-DR11 haplotype, which is associated with systemic sclerosis, and this suggests that interferon alfa may have triggered the autoimmune phenomenon.

Vasculitis with cryoglobulinemia

Interferon alfa can sometimes aggravate hepatitis C-related cryoglobulinemia.

- A fatal exacerbation of hepatitis C-related cryoglobulinemia, preceded by rapid deterioration of neurological status, massive upper gastrointestinal bleeding, and diffuse hemorrhagic gastritis with vasculitic changes on gastroscopy, has been reported within the first 3 weeks of interferon alfa treatment in a 51-year-old woman (370).

However, cryoglobulin-associated vasculitis is a recognized manifestation of hepatitis C infection. Reports of vasculitis in interferon alfa-treated patients should therefore be interpreted with caution (SED-13, 1095) (371). In addition, several isolated reports suggested that exacerbation of cryoglobulinemia might also be the result of interferon alfa treatment (SEDA-19, 337).

Interferon alfa and transplantation

A possibly deleterious effect of pre- or post-transplant interferon alfa therapy in transplant recipients has been emphasized by several studies and case reports. These point to a higher incidence or greater severity of graft-versus-host reactions in patients who have received an allogeneic bone marrow transplant (SED-13, 1097; 372,373), significant deterioration of renal function or an increased risk of glucocorticoid-resistant rejection in renal transplant patients (SED-13, 1097; 374), and a possibly increased risk of acute or chronic rejection in liver transplant patients (375,376). These findings are still the subject of debate, as the available data consist mainly of retrospective or poorly controlled studies with a limited number of patients (377,378). In addition, several other investigators have failed to identify any deleterious influence of interferon alfa treatment in transplant recipients (SEDA-21, 373; SEDA-22, 403). This issue warrants further large scale, prospective, controlled studies.

Immunosuppressive effects

Isolated reports of *Candida* esophagitis or *Pneumocystis jiroveci* (*Pneumocystis carinii*) infections in immunocompetent patients and the possible decrease in CD4+ T cells with or without opportunistic infections in several HIV-infected patients (SED-13, 1097; 379) suggest that unexpected immunosuppressive effects of interferon alfa can occur. An autoimmune destruction of CD4 cells in patients with a particular HLA haplotype has been proposed as a possible mechanism (380). One patient also had an acute and fatal acute precipitation of infection with *Entamoeba histolytica* (SEDA-22, 403). However, the available evidence is still very limited and no firm conclusion can be drawn on a possible association between interferon alfa treatment and a fall in CD4 cell count or an immunosuppressive effect.

Two patients aged 38 and 54 years with hemodialysis-dependent end-stage renal insufficiency developed severe bacterial infections, osteomyelitis, and prostatitis, within 3 months of interferon alfa-2b treatment for hepatitis C virus infection (381).

Possible exacerbation of latent parasitic infection by interferon alfa has been reported (SEDA-22, 403).

- Two patients receiving interferon alfa plus ribavirin for chronic hepatitis C developed symptomatic strongyloidiasis within 2–3 weeks of treatment (382).

Because both drugs have immunomodulatory effects, it was not determined which one was the more likely cause.

Graft-versus-host disease

There are still uncertainties about the possible relation between interferon alfa and an increased incidence or severity of acute graft-versus-host disease after bone marrow transplantation. Late-onset, severe, atypical chronic graft-versus-host disease has been attributed to interferon alfa (383).

- A 44-year-old woman received interferon alfa 6 MU/day for relapse of chronic myeloid leukemia 7 years after successful bone marrow transplantation. About 2 years later, interferon alfa was withdrawn because of diffuse erythematous skin lesions with discoid lupus erythematosus on skin biopsy and severe dysphagia with esophagitis and pseudomembranes at endoscopy. Fever, bilateral pulmonary infiltrates, and respiratory distress syndrome subsequently developed, and she required mechanical ventilation. An open lung biopsy showed features of chronic pulmonary graft-versus-host disease. All her symptoms completely resolved with ciclosporin and corticosteroids. An infectious cause was ruled out.

In this case, the clinical presentation was compatible with typical chronic graft-versus-host disease. Whether interferon alfa induced or aggravated chronic graft-versus-host disease in this patient was an open question.

Death

There is a debate as to whether previous interferon alfa adversely affects the outcome of bone marrow transplantation in chronic myelogenous leukemia.

In a retrospective study of 153 patients who underwent bone-marrow transplantation for chronic myelogenous leukemia, pretransplant interferon alfa treatment for more than 12 months was associated with a significant increase in transplant-related mortality during the first 2 years when compared with patients who received pre-transplant interferon alfa for less than 12 months (28 of 46 patients versus nine of 38) (384). This adverse outcome was also more frequent in patients who discontinued treatment less than 3 months before transplantation.

Of eight studies, five showed no harmful effect and three suggested an increased risk of post-transplant complications or mortality (SEDA-22, 403; SEDA-23, 395).

The outcome of bone marrow transplantation in 152 patients (86 on interferon alfa, 66 on chemotherapy) included in two consecutive randomized trials, has been analysed prospectively (385). Whereas the duration of interferon alfa treatment did not influence the outcome of transplantation, there was a significant reduction in survival: the 5-year survival was 45% in the 50 patients who were still receiving interferon alfa within 3 months before bone marrow transplantation and 71% in the 36 patients who were not. According to the authors, interferon alfa should not be prescribed in patients who are likely candidates for early bone marrow transplantation.

Long-Term Effects

Tumorigenicity

Compared with untreated patients and patients treated with busulfan or hydroxyurea, interferon alfa produced a significantly higher frequency of clonal aberrant cytogenetic abnormalities and chronic clonal evolution in patients with chronic myeloid leukemia (386). However, the possible role of interferon alfa in the secondary occurrence of hematological malignancies is purely speculative. Only isolated cases of myeloproliferative syndrome, leukemia, or lymphoma have been attributed to interferon alfa (SED-13, 1098; SEDA-20, 331; SEDA-21, 373). There was no increased incidence of second cancers in patients treated for hairy cell leukemia (SEDA-20, 331).

Second-Generation Effects

Teratogenicity

In experimental models there has been no evidence of mutagenic or teratogenic effects of interferon alfa, and placental transfer is unlikely or very low (387). Immediately after delivery, interferon alfa concentrations in the breast milk or in the sera of two newborns were very low compared with maternal serum concentrations (388). Uncomplicated and successful pregnancies have been detailed in several patients treated for hematological malignancies or chronic hepatitis C, with interferon alfa exposure during the first trimester or even the whole of pregnancy (SED-13, 1098; SEDA-20, 331; 389–392). In only three cases have premature delivery or moderate intrauterine growth retardation been observed, and any direct causal relation to interferon alfa treatment is doubtful. One report mentioned transient and moderate

thrombocytopenia in a neonate born to a woman who had received interferon alfa throughout pregnancy (391).

Although no long-term follow-up is as yet available, clinical examination performed up to 2–3 years after delivery in at least seven babies has proved normal. Despite these reassuring data, the safety of interferon alfa during pregnancy still awaits further documentation, and it is advisable to delay therapy of non-life-threatening disease in pregnant women, especially during the first trimester.

Susceptibility Factors

Age

There is little information on the use of interferon alfa in children with chronic hepatitis C. In a review of 19 studies published between 1990 and 2000, there were data on only 366 treated children (105 untreated) and they suggested a higher rate of sustained response than in adults (393). Besides flu-like symptoms, reversible weight loss, neutropenia, and alopecia were the most commonly reported adverse events, but adverse events were not systematically recorded in these studies.

Although the anti-angiogenic effects of interferon alfa have been successfully used to treat severe hemangiomas in infants, the possibility of spastic diplegia is a matter of concern (SEDA-22, 404). Spastic diplegia developed in five of 26 infants during treatment, with possibly significant functional sequelae (394), and in one of 53 infants treated for a median of 51 weeks (395). Persistent, severe, spastic diplegia occurred after 1 year of treatment in a 5-month-old boy (396). Because the immature central nervous system of infants may be more susceptible to interferon alfa toxicity, it has been stressed that this treatment should be reserved for infants with life-threatening hemangiomas (397). That interferon alfa can play a role in the occurrence of this acute neurological complication has been further substantiated by the finding of abnormally high interferon serum concentrations in 45% of neonates with spontaneous cerebral palsy compared with control children (398).

Renal disease

High daily dosage or serum concentrations of interferon alfa may be associated with more frequent and more severe adverse effects during the treatment of chronic hepatitis C in hemodialysis patients. In one study, three of 10 hemodialysis patients had severe neurological adverse effects (generalized seizures or posterior leukoencephalopathy) (399). In another study, three of six patients receiving daily injections had to discontinue treatment because of depression, loss of consciousness, and persistent high-grade fever, while no serious adverse effects were reported in three other patients who received interferon alfa three times a week (400). In both studies, there were significant changes in interferon alfa pharmacokinetics (higher C_{max}, AUC, and half-life) in hemodialysis patients compared with patients with normal renal function, consistent with altered clearance of interferon alfa.

Drug Administration

Drug formulations

The FDA has expanded the indications for a combination product to include patients with chronic hepatitis C who have not been treated with interferon alfa. This product, Rebetron Combination Therapy (Schering), contains recombinant interferon alfa-2b for injection (Intron A) plus ribavirin (Rebetol) in capsules, and was previously only approved for patients who had relapsed after treatment with interferon alone (401). Serious adverse effects, such as depression, suicidal ideation, and suicide, have occurred with this regimen and patients should be closely monitored.

Drug administration route

The use of intraspinal interferon alfa (1 MU three times a week for 4 weeks) in 22 patients with neoplastic meningitis was associated with frequent adverse effects that mostly manifested as chronic fatigue syndrome in 91% of patients (severe in 45%) and arachnoiditis in 73% (severe in 9%) (402). Interferon alfa-induced immune dysregulation in an immunologically predisposed patient was suggested to account for this complication.

Drug–Drug Interactions

Alcohol

Even moderate but continuing alcohol consumption needs to be taken seriously in patients receiving interferon alfa, and exacerbation of previous acute alcohol hepatitis has been reported in two patients with chronic hepatitis C, despite reduced alcohol consumption (403). Liver transaminases subsequently normalized after withdrawal of interferon alfa in both patients.

Angiotensin-converting enzyme inhibitors

An increased risk of severe and early but reversible neutropenia has been found in patients taking angiotensin-converting enzyme inhibitors (enalapril and captopril) with interferon alfa (404).

Carmustine

Owing to its antineoplastic properties, interferon alfa is sometimes used with cytostatic drugs. In 275 patients randomized to receive radiation and carmustine either alone or with interferon alfa for high-grade glioma, there was no significant improvement in the overall survival and time to disease progression in those given interferon alfa, but a higher incidence of adverse effects, namely fever, chills, myalgia, lethargy, headache, and seizures (405).

13-Cisretinoic acid

The combination of interferon alfa with 13-cis-retinoic acid may have potentiated the occurrence of fatal radiation pneumonitis (SEDA-21, 374).

Clozapine

Agranulocytosis was observed when interferon alfa was given to a patient taking long-term clozapine (SEDA-22, 404), but this is a known risk of the latter. In one case, agranulocytosis occurred after 7 weeks of combined therapy in a 29-year-old patient who had been taking clozapine for more than 5 years without developing hematological abnormalities (423). Even so, it was not clear in these cases whether the agranulocytosis was due to the combination of clozapine with interferon-alfa or the clozapine alone.

Coumarin anticoagulants

There have been two reports of increased prothrombin time in patients taking warfarin or acenocoumarol (SEDA-19, 337; SEDA-22, 374).

Cyclophosphamide

Depending on the timing of exposure, interferon alfa may adversely affect the pharmacokinetic and hematological effects of cyclophosphamide. In 10 patients with multiple myeloma, interferon alfa given 2 hours before cyclophosphamide infusion significantly reduced cyclophosphamide clearance and produced less exposure to its metabolite 4-hydroxycyclophosphamide compared with interferon administration 24 hours after cyclophosphamide (406). This resulted in a significantly greater fall in white blood cell count in patients who received interferon alfa after cyclophosphamide.

Erythropoietin

Reduced efficacy of human erythropoietin, requiring increased erythropoietin dosages, has been clearly documented in several patients receiving interferon alfa (407–409), an effect that is probably mediated by interferon alfa-induced suppression of erythropoiesis.

5-Fluorouracil

One would expect drugs with myelosuppressive effects to exacerbate the hematological toxicity of interferon alfa. However, even though interferon alfa is increasingly used with other cytotoxic drugs, no specific and unexpected adverse effects have been reported, except for the combination of interferon alfa with 5-fluorouracil, which produced increased serum concentrations of fluorouracil and a significantly higher incidence of severe adverse effects, namely gastrointestinal and myelosuppressive adverse effects (410,411).

Melphalan

Interferon-induced fever has been thought to increase the cytotoxicity of melphalan (412).

Oral hypoglycemic drugs

There has been one report of hypoglycemia in a patient treated with metformin and chlorpropamide (SEDA-21, 374).

Paroxetine

It has been suggested that concomitant treatment with paroxetine may be a susceptibility factor for retinal damage by interferon alfa (82).

Phenazone (antipyrine)

Interferon alfa inhibits several hepatic microsomal cytochrome P_{450} enzymes in vitro and in vivo (SED-13, 1099; 20,413). However, repeated injections of interferon alfa produced conflicting results, with no change in salivary phenazone clearance (SED-13, 1099; 414).

Ribavirin

The combination of interferon alfa with ribavirin is one of the most promising treatments for chronic hepatitis C. However, two patients developed rapid and particularly severe anemia within 4 and 6 weeks of combined treatment (415). One patient required erythrocyte transfusions, and both recovered after withdrawal. The combination of pure red cell aplasia due to interferon alfa and hemolytic anemia due to ribavirin was suggested to have accounted for this possible interaction.

There was an increased incidence of adverse skin effects, mostly eczema, malar erythema, and lichenoid eruptions, in 33 patients who received combination of interferon alfa with ribavirin compared with 35 patients treated with interferon alfa alone (416).

Thalidomide

In 13 patients with metastatic renal cell carcinoma, the combination of interferon alfa-2a (27 MU/week) and thalidomide produced severe neurological toxicity in four patients, an incidence that was considered to be far greater than would be expected with either drug alone (417).

Theophylline

Interferon alfa inhibits several hepatic microsomal cytochrome P_{450} enzymes in vitro and in vivo (20) and reduces theophylline clearance (SED-13, 1099; 418–420).

Zidovudine

Synergistic hemotoxicity has sometimes resulted from the combination of interferon alfa with zidovudine in AIDS-associated Kaposi's sarcoma, but this regimen is considered to be relatively safe (421,422).

References

1. Keeffe EB, Hollinger FBConsensus Interferon Study Group. Therapy of hepatitis C: consensus interferon trials. Hepatology 1997;26(3 Suppl 1):S101–7.
2. Davis GL. New schedules of interferon for chronic hepatitis C. J Hepatol 1999;31(Suppl 1):227–31.
3. Janssen HL, Gerken G, Carreno V, Marcellin P, Naoumov NV, Craxi A, Ring-Larsen H, Kitis G, van Hattum J, de Vries RA, Michielsen PP, ten Kate FJ, Hop WC, Heijtink RA, Honkoop P, Schalm SW. Interferon alfa for chronic hepatitis B infection: increased efficacy of prolonged treatment. The European Concerted Action on Viral Hepatitis (EUROHEP). Hepatology 1999;30(1):238–43.
4. Cotler SJ, Wartelle CF, Larson AM, Gretch DR, Jensen DM, Carithers RL Jr. Pretreatment symptoms and dosing regimen predict side-effects of interferon therapy for hepatitis C. J Viral Hepat 2000;7(3):211–7.
5. Kantarjian HM, O'Brien S, Smith TL, Rios MB, Cortes J, Beran M, Koller C, Giles FJ, Andreeff M, Kornblau S, Giralt S, Keating MJ, Talpaz M. Treatment of Philadelphia chromosome-positive early chronic phase chronic myelogenous leukemia with daily doses of interferon alpha and low-dose cytarabine. J Clin Oncol 1999;17(1):284–92.
6. Scott LJ, Perry CM. Interferon-alpha-2b plus ribavirin: a review of its use in the management of chronic hepatitis C. Drugs 2002;62(3):507–56.
7. San Miguel R, Guillen F, Cabases JM, Buti M. Meta-analysis: combination therapy with interferon-alpha 2a/2b and ribavirin for patients with chronic hepatitis C previously non-responsive to interferon. Aliment Pharmacol Ther 2002;16(9):1611–21.
8. Gaeta GB, Precone DF, Felaco FM, Bruno R, Spadaro A, Stornaiuolo G, Stanzione M, Ascione T, De Sena R, Campanone A, Filice G, Piccinino F. Premature discontinuation of interferon plus ribavirin for adverse effects: a multicentre survey in "real world" patients with chronic hepatitis C. Aliment Pharmacol Ther 2002;16(9):1633–9.
9. Ascione A, De Luca M, Di Costanzo GG, Picciotto FP, Lanza AG, Canestrini C, Morisco F, Tuccillo C, Caporaso N. Incidence of side effects during therapy with different types of alpha interferon: a randomised controlled trial comparing recombinant alpha 2b versus leukocyte interferon in the therapy of naive patients with chronic hepatitis C. Curr Pharm Des 2002;8(11):977–80.
10. Manns MP, McHutchison JG, Gordon SC, Rustgi VK, Shiffman M, Reindollar R, Goodman ZD, Koury K, Ling M, Albrecht JK. Peginterferon alfa-2b plus ribavirin compared with interferon alfa-2b plus ribavirin for initial treatment of chronic hepatitis C: a randomised trial. Lancet 2001;358(9286):958–65.
11. Heathcote EJ, Shiffman ML, Cooksley WG, Dusheiko GM, Lee SS, Balart L, Reindollar R, Reddy RK, Wright TL, Lin A, Hoffman J, De Pamphilis J. Peginterferon alfa-2a in patients with chronic hepatitis C and cirrhosis. N Engl J Med 2000;343(23):1673–80.
12. Zeuzem S, Feinman SV, Rasenack J, Heathcote EJ, Lai MY, Gane E, O'Grady J, Reichen J, Diago M, Lin A, Hoffman J, Brunda MJ. Peginterferon alfa-2a in patients with chronic hepatitis C. N Engl J Med 2000;343(23):1666–72.
13. Wiselka MJ, Nicholson KG, Kent J, Cookson JB, Tyrrell DA. Prophylactic intranasal alpha 2 interferon and viral exacerbations of chronic respiratory disease. Thorax 1991;46(10):706–11.
14. Saracco G, Rizzetto M. A practical guide to the use of interferons in the management of hepatitis virus infections. Drugs 1997;53(1):74–85.
15. Poynard T, Leroy V, Cohard M, Thevenot T, Mathurin P, Opolon P, Zarski JP. Meta-analysis of interferon randomized trials in the treatment of viral hepatitis C: effects of dose and duration. Hepatology 1996;24(4):778–89.

16. Fattovich G, Giustina G, Favarato S, Ruol A. A survey of adverse events in 11,241 patients with chronic viral hepatitis treated with alfa interferon. J Hepatol 1996;24(1):38–47.

17. De Sanctis GM, D'Errico DAF, Leonetti G, et al. Occurrence of major side effects in patients with chronic viral liver disease treated with interferons. Mediter J Infect Parasit Dis 1995;10:225–30.

18. Okanoue T, Sakamoto S, Itoh Y, Minami M, Yasui K, Sakamoto M, Nishioji K, Katagishi T, Nakagawa Y, Tada H, Sawa Y, Mizuno M, Kagawa K, Kashima K. Side effects of high-dose interferon therapy for chronic hepatitis C. J Hepatol 1996;25(3):283–91.

19. Iorio R, Pensati P, Botta S, Moschella S, Impagliazzo N, Vajro P, Vegnente A. Side effects of alpha-interferon therapy and impact on health-related quality of life in children with chronic viral hepatitis. Pediatr Infect Dis J 1997;16(10):984–90.

20. Vial T, Descotes J. Clinical toxicity of the interferons. Drug Saf 1994;10(2):115–50.

21. Vial T, Bailly F, Descotes J, Trepo C. Effets secondaires de l'interféron alpha. [Side effects of interferon-alpha.] Gastroenterol Clin Biol 1996;20(5):462–89.

22. Cacopardo B, Benanti F, Brancati G, Romano F, Nunnari A. Leucocyte interferon-alpha retreatment for chronic hepatitis C patients previously intolerant to other interferons. J Viral Hepat 1998;5(5):333–9.

23. Sonnenblick M, Rosin A. Cardiotoxicity of interferon. A review of 44 cases. Chest 1991;99(3):557–61.

24. Kruit WH, Punt KJ, Goey SH, de Mulder PH, van Hoogenhuyze DC, Henzen-Logmans SC, Stoter G. Cardiotoxicity as a dose-limiting factor in a schedule of high dose bolus therapy with interleukin-2 and alpha-interferon. An unexpectedly frequent complication. Cancer 1994;74(10):2850–6.

25. Angulo MP, Navajas A, Galdeano JM, Astigarraga I, Fernandez-Teijeiro A. Reversible cardiomyopathy secondary to alpha-interferon in an infant. Pediatr Cardiol 1999;20(4):293–4.

26. Kadayifci A, Aytemir K, Arslan M, Aksoyek S, Sivri B, Kabakci G. Interferon-alpha does not cause significant cardiac dysfunction in patients with chronic active hepatitis. Liver 1997;17(2):99–102.

27. Sartori M, Andorno S, La Terra G, Pozzoli G, Rudoni M, Sacchetti GM, Inglese E, Aglietta M. Assessment of interferon cardiotoxicity with quantitative radionuclide angiocardiography. Eur J Clin Invest 1995;25(1):68–70.

28. Kuwata A, Ohashi M, Sugiyama M, Ueda R, Dohi Y. A case of reversible dilated cardiomyopathy after alpha-interferon therapy in a patient with renal cell carcinoma. Am J Med Sci 2002;324(6):331–4.

29. Colivicchi F, Magnanimi S, Sebastiani F, Silvestri R, Magnanimi R. Incidence of electrocardiographic abnormalities during treatment with human leukocyte interferon-alfa in patients with chronic hepatitis C but without pre-existing cardiovascular disease. Curr Ther Res Clin Exp 1998;59:692–6.

30. Parrens E, Chevalier JM, Rougier M, Douard H, Labbe L, Quiniou G, Broustet A, Broustet JP. Apparition d'un bloc auriculo-ventriculaire du troisième degré sous interféron alpha: à propos d'un cas. [Third degree atrio-ventricular block induced by interferon alpha. Report of a case.] Arch Mal Coeur Vaiss 1999;92(1):53–6.

31. Creutzig A, Caspary L, Freund M. The Raynaud phenomenon and interferon therapy. Ann Intern Med 1996;125(5):423.

32. Schapira D, Nahir AM, Hadad N. Interferon-induced Raynaud's syndrome. Semin Arthritis Rheum 2002;32(3):157–62.

33. Iorio R, Spagnuolo MI, Sepe A, Zoccali S, Alessio M, Vegnente A. Severe Raynaud's phenomenon with chronic hepatis C disease treated with interferon. Pediatr Infect Dis J 2003;22(2):195–7.

34. Cid MC, Hernandez-Rodriguez J, Robert J, del Rio A, Casademont J, Coll-Vinent B, Grau JM, Kleinman HK, Urbano-Marquez A, Cardellach F. Interferon-alpha may exacerbate cryoblobulinemia-related ischemic manifestations: an adverse effect potentially related to its anti-angiogenic activity. Arthritis Rheum 1999;42(5):1051–5.

35. Mirro J Jr, Kalwinsky D, Whisnant J, Weck P, Chesney C, Murphy S. Coagulopathy induced by continuous infusion of high doses of human lymphoblastoid interferon. Cancer Treat Rep 1985;69(3):315–7.

36. Durand JM, Quiles N, Kaplanski G, Soubeyrand J. Thrombosis and recombinant interferon-alpha. Am J Med 1993;95(1):115–6.

37. Becker JC, Winkler B, Klingert S, Brocker EB. Antiphospholipid syndrome associated with immunotherapy for patients with melanoma. Cancer 1994;73(6):1621–4.

38. Karim A, Ahmed S, Khan A, Steinberg H, Mattana J. Interstitial pneumonitis in a patient treated with alpha-interferon and ribavirin for hepatitis C infection. Am J Med Sci 2001;322(4):233–5.

39. Chin K, Tabata C, Sataka N, Nagai S, Moriyasu F, Kuno K. Pneumonitis associated with natural and recombinant interferon alfa therapy for chronic hepatitis C. Chest 1994;105(3):939–41.

40. Ishizaki T, Sasaki F, Ameshima S, Shiozaki K, Takahashi H, Abe Y, Ito S, Kuriyama M, Nakai T, Kitagawa M. Pneumonitis during interferon and/or herbal drug therapy in patients with chronic active hepatitis. Eur Respir J 1996;9(12):2691–6.

41. Ogata K, Koga T, Yagawa K. Interferon-related bronchiolitis obliterans organizing pneumonia. Chest 1994;106(2):612–3.

42. Kumar AS, Russo MW, Esposito S, Borczuk A, Jacobson I, Brown M, Brown RS. Severe pulmonary toxicity of interferon and ribavirin therapy in chronic hepatitis C. Am J Gastroenterol 2001;96(Suppl):127.

43. Patel M, Ezzat W, Pauw KL, Lowsky R. Bronchiolitis obliterans organizing pneumonia in a patient with chronic myelogenous leukemia developing after initiation of interferon and cytosine arabinoside. Eur J Haematol 2001;67(5–6):318–21.

44. Anderson P, Hoglund M, Rodjer S. Pulmonary side effects of interferon-alpha therapy in patients with hematological malignancies. Am J Hematol 2003;73(1):54–8.

45. Kumar KS, Russo MW, Borczuk AC, Brown M, Esposito SP, Lobritto SJ, Jacobson IM, Brown RS Jr. Significant pulmonary toxicity associated with interferon and ribavirin therapy for hepatitis C. Am J Gastroenterol 2002;97(9):2432–40.

46. Bini EJ, Weinshel EH. Severe exacerbation of asthma: a new side effect of interferon-alpha in patients with asthma and chronic hepatitis C. Mayo Clin Proc 1999;74(4):367–370.

47. Pileire G, Leclerc P, Hermant P, Meeus E, Camus P. Toux chronique isolée pendant un traitement par interféron. [Isolated chronic cough during interferon therapy.] Presse Méd 1999;28(17):913.

48. Takeda A, Ikegame K, Kimura Y, Ogawa H, Kanazawa S, Nakamura H. Pleural effusion during interferon treatment

for chronic hepatitis C. Hepatogastroenterology 2000;47(35):1431–5.

49. Fruehauf S, Steiger S, Topaly J, Ho AD. Pulmonary artery hypertension during interferon-alpha therapy for chronic myelogenous leukemia. Ann Hematol 2001;80(5):308–10.

50. Boonyapisit K, Katirji B. Severe exacerbation of hepatitis C-associated vasculitic neuropathy following treatment with interferon alpha: a case report and literature review. Muscle Nerve 2002;25(6):909–13.

51. Tambini R, Quattrini A, Fracassetti O, Nemni R. Axonal neuropathy in a patient receiving interferon-alpha therapy for chronic hepatitis C. J Rheumatol 1997;24(8):1656–7.

52. Maeda M, Ohkoshi N, Hisahara S, Mizusawa H, Shoji S. [Mononeuropathy multiplex in a patient receiving interferon alpha therapy for chronic hepatitis C.]Rinsho Shinkeigaku 1995;35(9):1048–50.

53. Jaubert D, Hauteville D, Pelissier JF, Muzellec Y. Neuropathie periphérique au cours d'un traitement par interféron alpha. [Peripheral neuropathy during interferon alpha therapy.] Presse Méd 1991;20(5):221–2.

54. Purvin VA. Anterior ischemic optic neuropathy secondary to interferon alfa. Arch Ophthalmol 1995;113(8):1041–4.

55. Read SJ, Crawford DH, Pender MP. Trigeminal sensory neuropathy induced by interferon-alpha therapy. Aust NZ J Med 1995;25(1):54.

56. Bernsen PL, Wong Chung RE, Vingerhoets HM, Janssen JT. Bilateral neuralgic amyotrophy induced by interferon treatment. Arch Neurol 1988;45(4):449–51.

57. Loh FL, Herskovitz S, Berger AR, Swerdlow ML. Brachial plexopathy associated with interleukin-2 therapy. Neurology 1992;42(2):462–3.

58. Merimsky O, Reider I, Merimsky E, Chaitchik S. Interferon-related leukoencephalopathy in a patient with renal cell carcinoma. Tumori 1991;77(4):361–2.

59. Ogundipe O, Smith M. Bell's palsy during interferon therapy for chronic hepatitis C infection in patients with haemorrhagic disorders. Haemophilia 2000;6(2):110–2.

60. Hwang I, Calvit TB, Cash BD, Holtzmuller KC. Bell's palsy. A rare complication of interferon therapy for hepatitis C. Am J Gastroenterol 2002;87(Suppl):207–8.

61. Anthoney DA, Bone I, Evans TR. Inflammatory demyelinating polyneuropathy: a complication of immunotherapy in malignant melanoma. Ann Oncol 2000;11(9):1197–200.

62. Meriggioli MN, Rowin J. Chronic inflammatory demyelinating polyneuropathy after treatment with interferon-alpha. Muscle Nerve 2000;23(3):433–5.

63. Kataoka I, Shinagawa K, Shiro Y, Okamoto S, Watanabe R, Mori T, Ito D, Harada M. Multiple sclerosis associated with interferon-alpha therapy for chronic myelogenous leukemia. Am J Hematol 2002;70(2):149–53.

64. Sunami M, Nishikawa T, Yorogi A, Shimoda M. Intravenous administration of levodopa ameliorated a refractory akathisia case induced by interferon-alpha. Clin Neuropharmacol 2000;23(1):59–61.

65. Horikawa N, Yamazaki T, Sagawa M, Nagata T. A case of akathisia during interferon-alpha therapy for chronic hepatitis type C. Gen Hosp Psychiatry 1999;21(2):134–5.

66. Moulignier A, Allo S, Zittoun R, Gout O. Recombinant interferon-alpha-induced chorea and frontal subcortical dementia. Neurology 2002;58(2):328–30.

67. Hibi H, Itoh K, Kamiya T, Yamada Y, Shimoji T. [Grand mal like attack by interferon injection in case of renal cell carcinoma.]Hinyokika Kiyo 1991;37(1):69–72.

68. Janssen HL, Berk L, Vermeulen M, Schalm SW. Seizures associated with low-dose alpha-interferon. Lancet 1990;336(8730):1580.

69. Miller VS, Zwiener RJ, Fielman BA. Interferon-associated refractory status epilepticus. Pediatrics 1994;93(3):511–2.

70. Shakil AO, Di Bisceglie AM, Hoofnagle JH. Seizures during alpha interferon therapy. J Hepatol 1996;24(1):48–51.

71. Woynarowski M, Socha J. Seizures in children during interferon alpha therapy. J Hepatol 1997;26(4):956–7.

72. Ameen M, Russell-Jones R. Seizures associated with interferon-alpha treatment of cutaneous malignancies. Br J Dermatol 1999;141(2):386–7.

73. Seno H, Inagaki T, Itoga M, Miyaoka T, Ishino H. A case of seizures 1 week after the cessation of interferon-alpha therapy. Psychiatry Clin Neurosci 1999;53(3):417–20.

74. Brouwers PJ, Bosker RJ, Schaafsma MR, Wilts G, Neef C. Photosensitive seizures associated with interferon alfa-2a. Ann Pharmacother 1999;33(1):113–4.

75. Kamei S, Tanaka N, Mastuura M, Arakawa Y, Kojima T, Matsukawa Y, Takasu T, Moriyama M. Blinded, prospective, and serial evaluation by quantitative-EEG in interferon-alpha-treated hepatitis-C. Acta Neurol Scand 1999;100(1):25–33.

76. Borgia G, Reynaud L, Gentile I, Cerini R, Ciampi R, Dello Russo M, Piazza M. Myasthenia gravis during low-dose IFN-alpha therapy for chronic hepatitis C. J Interferon Cytokine Res 2001;21(7):469–70.

77. Weegink CJ, Chamuleau RA, Reesink HW, Molenaar DS. Development of myasthenia gravis during treatment of chronic hepatitis C with interferon-alpha and ribavirin. J Gastroenterol 2001;36(10):723–4.

78. Guyer DR, Tiedeman J, Yannuzzi LA, Slakter JS, Parke D, Kelley J, Tang RA, Marmor M, Abrams G, Miller JW, et al. Interferon-associated retinopathy. Arch Ophthalmol 1993;111(3):350–6.

79. Hayasaka S, Fujii M, Yamamoto Y, Noda S, Kurome H, Sasaki M. Retinopathy and subconjunctival haemorrhage in patients with chronic viral hepatitis receiving interferon alfa. Br J Ophthalmol 1995;79(2):150–2.

80. Kawano T, Shigehira M, Uto H, Nakama T, Kato J, Hayashi K, Maruyama T, Kuribayashi T, Chuman T, Futami T, Tsubouchi H. Retinal complications during interferon therapy for chronic hepatitis C. Am J Gastroenterol 1996;91(2):309–13.

81. Soushi S, Kobayashi F, Obazawa H, Kigasawa K, Shiraishi K, Itakura M, Matsuzaki S. [Evaluation of risk factors of interferon-associated retinopathy in patients with type C chronic active hepatitis.]Nippon Ganka Gakkai Zasshi 1996;100(1):69–76.

82. Hejny C, Sternberg P, Lawson DH, Greiner K, Aaberg TM Jr. Retinopathy associated with high-dose interferon alfa-2b therapy. Am J Ophthalmol 2001;131(6):782–7.

83. Jain K, Lam WC, Waheeb S, Thai Q, Heathcote J. Retinopathy in chronic hepatitis C patients during interferon treatment with ribavirin. Br J Ophthalmol 2001;85(10):1171–3.

84. Saito H, Ebinuma H, Nagata H, Inagaki Y, Saito Y, Wakabayashi K, Takagi T, Nakamura M, Katsura H, Oguchi Y, Ishii H. Interferon-associated retinopathy in a uniform regimen of natural interferon-alpha therapy for chronic hepatitis C. Liver 2001;21(3):192–7.

85. Hayasaka S, Nagaki Y, Matsumoto M, Sato S. Interferon associated retinopathy. Br J Ophthalmol 1998;82(3):323–5.

86. Kadayifcilar S, Boyacioglu S, Kart H, Gursoy M, Aydin P. Ocular complications with high-dose interferon alpha in chronic active hepatitis. Eye 1999;13(Pt 2):241–6.

87. Sugano S, Suzuki T, Watanabe M, Ohe K, Ishii K, Okajima T. Retinal complications and plasma C5a levels

during interferon alpha therapy for chronic hepatitis C. Am J Gastroenterol 1998;93(12):2441–4.

88. Sugano S, Yanagimoto M, Suzuki T, Sato M, Onmura H, Aizawa H, Makino H. Retinal complications with elevated circulating plasma C5a associated with interferon-alpha therapy for chronic active hepatitis C. Am J Gastroenterol 1994;89(11):2054–6.

89. Ene L, Gehenot M, Horsmans Y, Detry-Morel M, Geubel AP. Transient blurred vision after interferon for chronic hepatitis C. Lancet 1994;344(8925):827–8.

90. Yamada H, Mizobuchi K, Isogai Y. Acute onset of ocular complications with interferon. Lancet 1994;343(8902):914.

91. Lohmann CP, Kroher G, Bogenrieder T, Spiegel D, Preuner J. Severe loss of vision during adjuvant interferon alfa-2b treatment for malignant melanoma. Lancet 1999;353(9161):1326.

92. Perlemuter G, Bodaghi B, Le Hoang P, Izem C, Buffet C, Wechsler B, Piette JC, Cacoub P. Visual loss during interferon-alpha therapy in hepatitis C virus infection. J Hepatol 2002;37(5):701–2.

93. Gupta R, Singh S, Tang R, Blackwell TA, Schiffman JS. Anterior ischemic optic neuropathy caused by interferon alpha therapy. Am J Med 2002;112(8):683–4.

94. Manesis EK, Petrou C, Brouzas D, Hadziyannis S. Optic tract neuropathy complicating low-dose interferon treatment. J Hepatol 1994;21(3):474–7.

95. Merimsky O, Nisipeanu P, Loewenstein A, Reider-Groswasser I, Chaitchik S. Interferon-related cortical blindness. Cancer Chemother Pharmacol 1992;29(4):329–30.

96. Fukumoto Y, Shigemitsu T, Kajii N, Omura R, Harada T, Okita K. Abducent nerve paralysis during interferon alpha-2a therapy in a case of chronic active hepatitis C. Intern Med 1994;33(10):637–40.

97. Bauherz G, Soeur M, Lustman F. Oculomotor nerve paralysis induced by alpha II-interferon. Acta Neurol Belg 1990;90(2):111–4.

98. Fossa SD. Is interferon with or without vinblastine the "treatment of choice" in metastatic renal cell carcinoma? The Norwegian Radium Hospital's experience 1983–1986. Semin Surg Oncol 1988;4(3):178–83.

99. Cadoni G, Marinelli L, De Santis A, Romito A, Manna R, Ottaviani F. Sudden hearing loss in a patient hepatitis C virus (HCV) positive on therapy with alpha-interferon: a possible autoimmune-microvascular pathogenesis. J Laryngol Otol 1998;112(10):962–3.

100. Kraus I, Vitezic D. Anosmia induced with alpha interferon in a patient with chronic hepatitis C. Int J Clin Pharmacol Ther 2000;38(7):360–1.

101. Schaefer M, Engelbrecht MA, Gut O, Fiebich BL, Bauer J, Schmidt F, Grunze H, Lieb K. Interferon alpha (IFNalpha) and psychiatric syndromes: a review. Prog Neuropsychopharmacol Biol Psychiatry 2002;26(4):731–46.

102. Van Gool AR, Kruit WH, Engels FK, Stoter G, Bannink M, Eggermont AM. Neuropsychiatric side effects of interferon-alfa therapy. Pharm World Sci 2003;25(1):11–20.

103. Smith A, Tyrrell D, Coyle K, Higgins P. Effects of interferon alpha on performance in man: a preliminary report. Psychopharmacology (Berl) 1988;96(3):414–6.

104. Meyers CA, Valentine AD. Neurological and psychiatric adverse effects of immunological therapy. CNS Drugs 1995;3:56–68.

105. James CW, Savini CJ. Homicidal ideation secondary to interferon. Ann Pharmacother 2001;35(7–8):962–3.

106. Greenberg DB, Jonasch E, Gadd MA, Ryan BF, Everett JR, Sober AJ, Mihm MA, Tanabe KK, Ott M, Haluska FG. Adjuvant therapy of melanoma with interferon-alpha-2b is associated with mania and bipolar syndromes. Cancer 2000;89(2):356–62.

107. Monji A, Yoshida I, Tashiro K, Hayashi Y, Tashiro N. A case of persistent manic depressive illness induced by interferon-alfa in the treatment of chronic hepatitis C. Psychosomatics 1998;39(6):562–4.

108. Hosoda S, Takimura H, Shibayama M, Kanamura H, Ikeda K, Kumada H. Psychiatric symptoms related to interferon therapy for chronic hepatitis C: clinical features and prognosis. Psychiatry Clin Neurosci 2000;54(5):565–72.

109. Schafer M, Boetsch T, Laakmann G. Psychosis in a methadone-substituted patient during interferon-alpha treatment of hepatitis C. Addiction 2000;95(7):1101–4.

110. Mayr N, Zeitlhofer J, Deecke L, Fritz E, Ludwig H, Gisslinger H. Neurological function during long-term therapy with recombinant interferon alpha. J Neuropsychiatry Clin Neurosci 1999;11(3):343–8.

111. Rohatiner AZ, Prior PF, Burton AC, Smith AT, Balkwill FR, Lister TA. Central nervous system toxicity of interferon. Br J Cancer 1983;47(3):419–22.

112. Scalori A, Apale P, Panizzuti F, Mascoli N, Pioltelli P, Pozzi M, Redaelli A, Roffi L, Mancia G. Depression during interferon therapy for chronic viral hepatitis: early identification of patients at risk by means of a computerized test. Eur J Gastroenterol Hepatol 2000;12(5):505–9.

113. Dieperink E, Willenbring M, Ho SB. Neuropsychiatric symptoms associated with hepatitis C and interferon alpha: A review. Am J Psychiatry 2000;157(6):867–76.

114. Zdilar D, Franco-Bronson K, Buchler N, Locala JA, Younossi ZM. Hepatitis C, interferon alfa, and depression. Hepatology 2000;31(6):1207–11.

115. Renault PF, Hoofnagle JH, Park Y, Mullen KD, Peters M, Jones DB, Rustgi V, Jones EA. Psychiatric complications of long-term interferon alfa therapy. Arch Intern Med 1987;147(9):1577–80.

116. Prasad S, Waters B, Hill PB, et al. Psychiatric side effects of interferon alpha-2b in patients treated for hepatitis C. Clin Res 1992;40:840A.

117. Bonaccorso S, Marino V, Biondi M, Grimaldi F, Ippoliti F, Maes M. Depression induced by treatment with interferon-alpha in patients affected by hepatitis C virus. J Affect Disord 2002;72(3):237–41.

118. Dieperink E, Ho SB, Thuras P, Willenbring ML. A prospective study of neuropsychiatric symptoms associated with interferon-alpha-2b and ribavirin therapy for patients with chronic hepatitis C. Psychosomatics 2003; 44(2):104–112.

119. Hauser P, Khosla J, Aurora H, Laurin J, Kling MA, Hill J, Gulati M, Thornton AJ, Schultz RL, Valentine AD, Meyers CA, Howell CD. A prospective study of the incidence and open-label treatment of interferon-induced major depressive disorder in patients with hepatitis C. Mol Psychiatry 2002;7(9):942–7.

120. Horikawa N, Yamazaki T, Izumi N, Uchihara M. Incidence and clinical course of major depression in patients with chronic hepatitis type C undergoing interferon-alpha therapy: a prospective study. Gen Hosp Psychiatry 2003;25(1):34–8.

121. Janssen HL, Brouwer JT, van der Mast RC, Schalm SW. Suicide associated with alfa-interferon therapy for chronic viral hepatitis. J Hepatol 1994;21(2):241–3.

122. Rifflet H, Vuillemin E, Oberti F, Duverger P, Laine P, Garre JB, Cales P. Pulsions suicidaires chez des malades atteints d'hépatite chronique C au cours ou au décours du

traitement par l'interféron alpha. [Suicidal impulses in patients with chronic viral hepatitis C during or after therapy with interferon alpha.] Gastroenterol Clin Biol 1998;22(3):353–7.

123. Valentine AD, Meyers CA, Kling MA, Richelson E, Hauser P. Mood and cognitive side effects of interferon-alpha therapy. Semin Oncol 1998;25(1 Suppl 1):39–47.

124. Adams F, Quesada JR, Gutterman JU. Neuropsychiatric manifestations of human leukocyte interferon therapy in patients with cancer. JAMA 1984;252(7):938–41.

125. Bocci V. Central nervous system toxicity of interferons and other cytokines. J Biol Regul Homeost Agents 1988;2(3):107–18.

126. Prior TI, Chue PS. Psychotic depression occurring after stopping interferon-alpha. J Clin Psychopharmacol 1999;19(4):385–6.

127. Capuron L, Ravaud A. Prediction of the depressive effects of interferon alfa therapy by the patient's initial affective state. N Engl J Med 1999;340(17):1370.

128. McDonald EM, Mann AH, Thomas HC. Interferons as mediators of psychiatric morbidity. An investigation in a trial of recombinant alpha-interferon in hepatitis-B carriers. Lancet 1987;2(8569):1175–8.

129. Pavol MA, Meyers CA, Rexer JL, Valentine AD, Mattis PJ, Talpaz M. Pattern of neurobehavioral deficits associated with interferon alfa therapy for leukemia. Neurology 1995;45(5):947–50.

130. Poutiainen E, Hokkanen L, Niemi ML, Farkkila M. Reversible cognitive decline during high-dose alpha-interferon treatment. Pharmacol Biochem Behav 1994;47(4):901–5.

131. Licinio J, Kling MA, Hauser P. Cytokines and brain function: relevance to interferon-alpha-induced mood and cognitive changes. Semin Oncol 1998;25(1 Suppl 1):30–8.

132. Bonaccorso S, Marino V, Puzella A, Pasquini M, Biondi M, Artini M, Almerighi C, Verkerk R, Meltzer H, Maes M. Increased depressive ratings in patients with hepatitis C receiving interferon-alpha-based immunotherapy are related to interferon-alpha-induced changes in the serotonergic system. J Clin Psychopharmacol 2002;22(1):86–90.

133. Gleason OC, Yates WR, Isbell MD, Philipsen MA. An open-label trial of citalopram for major depression in patients with hepatitis C. J Clin Psychiatry 2002;63(3):194–8.

134. Kraus MR, Schafer A, Faller H, Csef H, Scheurlen M. Paroxetine for the treatment of interferon-alpha-induced depression in chronic hepatitis C. Aliment Pharmacol Ther 2002;16(6):1091–9.

135. Pariante CM, Landau S, Carpiniello BCagliari Group. Interferon alfa-induced adverse effects in patients with a psychiatric diagnosis. N Engl J Med 2002;347(2):148–9.

136. Hensley ML, Peterson B, Silver RT, Larson RA, Schiffer CA, Szatrowski TP. Risk factors for severe neuropsychiatric toxicity in patients receiving interferon alfa-2b and low-dose cytarabine for chronic myelogenous leukemia: analysis of Cancer and Leukemia Group B 9013. J Clin Oncol 2000;18(6):1301–8.

137. Van Thiel DH, Friedlander L, Molloy PJ, Fagiuoli S, Kania RJ, Caraceni P. Interferon-alpha can be used successfully in patients with hepatitis C virus-positive chronic hepatitis who have a psychiatric illness. Eur J Gastroenterol Hepatol 1995;7(2):165–8.

138. Adams F, Fernandez F, Mavligit G. Interferon-induced organic mental disorders associated with unsuspected pre-existing neurologic abnormalities. J Neurooncol 1988;6(4):355–9.

139. Meyers CA, Obbens EA, Scheibel RS, Moser RP. Neurotoxicity of intraventricularly administered alpha-interferon for leptomeningeal disease. Cancer 1991;68(1):88–92.

140. Hagberg H, Blomkvist E, Ponten U, Persson L, Muhr C, Eriksson B, Oberg K, Olsson Y, Lilja A. Does alpha-interferon in conjunction with radiotherapy increase the risk of complications in the central nervous system? Ann Oncol 1990;1(6):449.

141. Laaksonen R, Niiranen A, Iivanainen M, Mattson K, Holsti L, Farkkila M, Cantell K. Dementia-like, largely reversible syndrome after cranial irradiation and prolonged interferon treatment. Ann Clin Res 1988;20(3):201–3.

142. Mitsuyama Y, Hashiguchi H, Murayama T, Koono M, Nishi S. An autopsied case of interferon encephalopathy. Jpn J Psychiatry Neurol 1992;46(3):741–8.

143. Mulder RT, Ang M, Chapman B, Ross A, Stevens IF, Edgar C. Interferon treatment is not associated with a worsening of psychiatric symptoms in patients with hepatitis C. J Gastroenterol Hepatol 2000;15(3):300–3.

144. Pariante CM, Orru MG, Baita A, Farci MG, Carpiniello B. Treatment with interferon-alpha in patients with chronic hepatitis and mood or anxiety disorders. Lancet 1999;354(9173):131–2.

145. Castera L, Zigante F, Bastie A, Buffet C, Dhumeaux D, Hardy P. Incidence of interferon alfa-induced depression in patients with chronic hepatitis C. Hepatology 2002;35(4):978–9.

146. Valentine AD. Managing the neuropsychiatric adverse effects of interferon treatment. BioDrugs 1999;11:229–37.

147. Miller A, Musselman D, Pena S, Su C, Pearce B, Nemeroff C. Pretreatment with the antidepressant paroxetine, prevents cytokine-induced depression during IFN-alpha therapy for malignant melanoma. Neuroimmunomodulation 1999;6:237.

148. Musselman DL, Lawson DH, Gumnick JF, Manatunga AK, Penna S, Goodkin RS, Greiner K, Nemeroff CB, Miller AH. Paroxetine for the prevention of depression induced by high-dose interferon alfa. N Engl J Med 2001;344(13):961–6.

149. McAllister-Williams RH, Young AH, Menkes DB. Antidepressant response reversed by interferon. Br J Psychiatry 2000;176:93.

150. Del Monte P, Bernasconi D, De Conca V, Randazzo M, Meozzi M, Badaracco B, Mesiti S, Marugo M. Endocrine evaluation in patients treated with interferon-alpha for chronic hepatitis C. Horm Res 1995;44(3):105–9.

151. Muller H, Hiemke C, Hammes E, Hess G. Sub-acute effects of interferon-alpha 2 on adrenocorticotrophic hormone, cortisol, growth hormone and prolactin in humans. Psychoneuroendocrinology 1992;17(5):459–65.

152. Crockett DM, McCabe BF, Lusk RP, Mixon JH. Side effects and toxicity of interferon in the treatment of recurrent respiratory papillomatosis. Ann Otol Rhinol Laryngol 1987;96(5):601–7.

153. Gottrand F, Michaud L, Guimber D, Ategbo S, Dubar G, Turck D, Farriaux JP. Influence of recombinant interferon alpha on nutritional status and growth pattern in children with chronic viral hepatitis. Eur J Pediatr 1996;155(12):1031–4.

154. Farkkila AM, Iivanainen MV, Farkkila MA. Disturbance of the water and electrolyte balance during

high-dose interferon treatment. J Interferon Res 1990;10(2):221–7.

155. Fentiman IS, Balkwill FR, Thomas BS, Russell MJ, Todd I, Bottazzo GF. An autoimmune aetiology for hypothyroidism following interferon therapy for breast cancer. Eur J Cancer Clin Oncol 1988;24(8):1299–303.

156. Vial T, Descotes J. Immune-mediated side-effects of cytokines in humans. Toxicology 1995;105(1):31–57.

157. Fortis A, Christopoulos C, Chrysadakou E, Anevlavis E. De Quervain's thyroiditis associated with interferon-alpha-2b therapy for non-Hodgkin's lymphoma. Clin Drug Invest 1998;16:473–5.

158. Ghilardi G, Gonvers JJ, So A. Hypothyroid myopathy as a complication of interferon alpha therapy for chronic hepatitis C virus infection. Br J Rheumatol 1998;37(12):1349–51.

159. Schmitt K, Hompesch BC, Oeland K, von Staehr WG, Thurmann PA. Autoimmune thyroiditis and myelosuppression following treatment with interferon-alpha for hepatitis C. Int J Clin Pharmacol Ther 1999;37(4):165–7.

160. Papo T, Oksenhendler E, Izembart M, Leger A, Clauvel JP. Antithyroid hormone antibodies induced by interferon-alpha. J Clin Endocrinol Metab 1992;75(6):1484–6.

161. Wong V, Fu AX, George J, Cheung NW. Thyrotoxicosis induced by alpha-interferon therapy in chronic viral hepatitis. Clin Endocrinol (Oxf) 2002;56(6):793–8.

162. Carella C, Mazziotti G, Morisco F, Manganella G, Rotondi M, Tuccillo C, Sorvillo F, Caporaso N, Amato G. Long-term outcome of interferon-alpha-induced thyroid autoimmunity and prognostic influence of thyroid autoantibody pattern at the end of treatment. J Clin Endocrinol Metab 2001;86(5):1925–9.

163. Binaghi M, Levy C, Douvin C, Guittard M, Soubrane G, Coscas G. Ophtalmopathie de Basedow sévère liée a l'interféron alpha. [Severe thyroid ophthalmopathy related to interferon alpha therapy.] J Fr Ophtalmol 2002;25(4):412–5.

164. Sunbul M, Kahraman H, Eroglu C, Leblebicioglu H, Cinar T. Subacute thyroiditis in a patient with chronic hepatitis C during interferon treatment: a case report. Ondokuz Mayis Univ Tip Derg 1999;16:62–6.

165. Dalgard O, Bjoro K, Hellum K, Myrvang B, Bjoro T, Haug E, Bell H. Thyroid dysfunction during treatment of chronic hepatitis C with interferon alpha: no association with either interferon dosage or efficacy of therapy. J Intern Med 2002;251(5):400–6.

166. Preziati D, La Rosa L, Covini G, Marcelli R, Rescalli S, Persani L, Del Ninno E, Meroni PL, Colombo M, Beck-Peccoz P. Autoimmunity and thyroid function in patients with chronic active hepatitis treated with recombinant interferon alpha-2a. Eur J Endocrinol 1995;132(5):587–93.

167. Vallisa D, Cavanna L, Berte R, Merli F, Ghisoni F, Buscarini L. Autoimmune thyroid dysfunctions in hematologic malignancies treated with alpha-interferon. Acta Haematol 1995;93(1):31–5.

168. Marazuela M, Garcia-Buey L, Gonzalez-Fernandez B, Garcia-Monzon C, Arranz A, Borque MJ, Moreno-Otero R. Thyroid autoimmune disorders in patients with chronic hepatitis C before and during interferon-alpha therapy. Clin Endocrinol (Oxf) 1996;44(6):635–42.

169. Roti E, Minelli R, Giuberti T, Marchelli S, Schianchi C, Gardini E, Salvi M, Fiaccadori F, Ugolotti G, Neri TM, Braverman LE. Multiple changes in thyroid function in patients with chronic active HCV hepatitis treated with recombinant interferon-alpha. Am J Med 1996;101(5):482–7.

170. Barreca T, Picciotto A, Franceschini R, et al. Effects of acute administration of recombinant interferon alpha 2b on pituitary hormone secretion in patients with chronic active hepatitis. Curr Ther Res 1992;52:695–701.

171. Yamazaki K, Kanaji Y, Shizume K, Yamakawa Y, Demura H, Kanaji Y, Obara T, Sato K. Reversible inhibition by interferons alpha and beta of ^{125}I incorporation and thyroid hormone release by human thyroid follicles in vitro. J Clin Endocrinol Metab 1993;77(5):1439–41.

172. Schuppert F, Rambusch E, Kirchner H, Atzpodien J, Kohn LD, von zur Muhlen A. Patients treated with interferon-alpha, interferon-beta, and interleukin-2 have a different thyroid autoantibody pattern than patients suffering from endogenous autoimmune thyroid disease. Thyroid 1997;7(6):837–42.

173. Watanabe U, Hashimoto E, Hisamitsu T, Obata H, Hayashi N. The risk factor for development of thyroid disease during interferon-alpha therapy for chronic hepatitis C. Am J Gastroenterol 1994;89(3):399–403.

174. Fernandez-Soto L, Gonzalez A, Escobar-Jimenez F, Vazquez R, Ocete E, Olea N, Salmeron J. Increased risk of autoimmune thyroid disease in hepatitis C vs hepatitis B before, during, and after discontinuing interferon therapy. Arch Intern Med 1998;158(13):1445–8.

175. Kakizaki S, Takagi H, Murakami M, Takayama H, Mori M. HLA antigens in patients with interferon-alpha-induced autoimmune thyroid disorders in chronic hepatitis C. J Hepatol 1999;30(5):794–800.

176. Minelli R, Braverman LE, Valli MA, Schianchi C, Pedrazzoni M, Fiaccadori F, Salvi M, Magotti MG, Roti E. Recombinant interferon alpha (rIFN-alpha) does not potentiate the effect of iodine excess on the development of thyroid abnormalities in patients with HCV chronic active hepatitis. Clin Endocrinol (Oxf) 1999;50(1):95–100.

177. Carella C, Mazziotti G, Morisco F, Rotondi M, Cioffi M, Tuccillo C, Sorvillo F, Caporaso N, Amato G. The addition of ribavirin to interferon-alpha therapy in patients with hepatitis C virus-related chronic hepatitis does not modify the thyroid autoantibody pattern but increases the risk of developing hypothyroidism. Eur J Endocrinol 2002;146(6):743–9.

178. Marcellin P, Pouteau M, Renard P, Grynblat JM, Colas Linhart N, Bardet P, Bok B, Benhamou JP. Sustained hypothyroidism induced by recombinant alpha interferon in patients with chronic hepatitis C. Gut 1992;33(6):855–6.

179. Mekkakia-Benhabib C, Marcellin P, Colas-Linhart N, Castel-Nau C, Buyck D, Erlinger S, Bok B. Histoire naturelle des dysthyroïdies survenant sous interféron dans le traitement des hépatites chroniques C. [Natural history of dysthyroidism during interferon treatment of chronic hepatitis C.] Ann Endocrinol (Paris) 1996;57(5):419–27.

180. Minelli R, Braverman LE, Giuberti T, Schianchi C, Gardini E, Salvi M, Fiaccadori F, Ugolotti G, Roti E. Effects of excess iodine administration on thyroid function in euthyroid patients with a previous episode of thyroid dysfunction induced by interferon-alpha treatment. Clin Endocrinol (Oxf) 1997;47(3):357–61.

181. Calvino J, Romero R, Suarez-Penaranda JM, Arcocha V, Lens XM, Mardaras J, Novoa D, Sanchez-Guisande D. Secondary hyperparathyroidism exacerbation: a rare side-effect of interferon-alpha? Clin Nephrol 1999;51(4):248–51.

182. Wesche B, Jaeckel E, Trautwein C, Wedemeyer H, Falorni A, Frank H, von zur Muhlen A, Manns MP, Brabant G. Induction of autoantibodies to the adrenal cortex and pancreatic islet cells by interferon alpha therapy for chronic hepatitis C. Gut 2001;48(3):378–83.

183. Fraser GM, Harman I, Meller N, Niv Y, Porath A. Diabetes mellitus is associated with chronic hepatitis C but not chronic hepatitis B infection. Isr J Med Sci 1996;32(7):526–30.

184. Gori A, Caredda F, Franzetti F, Ridolfo A, Rusconi S, Moroni M. Reversible diabetes in patient with AIDS-related Kaposi's sarcoma treated with interferon alpha-2a. Lancet 1995;345(8962):1438–9.

185. Guerci AP, Guerci B, Levy-Marchal C, Ongagna J, Ziegler O, Candiloros H, Guerci O, Drouin P. Onset of insulin-dependent diabetes mellitus after interferon-alfa therapy for hairy cell leukaemia. Lancet 1994;343(8906):1167–8.

186. Mathieu E, Fain O, Sitbon M, Thomas M. Diabète autoimmun après traitement par interféron alpha. [Autoimmune diabetes after treatment with interferon-alpha.] Presse Méd 1995;24(4):238.

187. Eibl N, Gschwantler M, Ferenci P, Eibl MM, Weiss W, Schernthaner G. Development of insulin-dependent diabetes mellitus in a patient with chronic hepatitis C during therapy with interferon-alpha. Eur J Gastroenterol Hepatol 2001;13(3):295–8.

188. Recasens M, Aguilera E, Ampurdanes S, Sanchez Tapias JM, Simo O, Casamitjana R, Conget I. Abrupt onset of diabetes during interferon-alpha therapy in patients with chronic hepatitis C. Diabet Med 2001;18(9):764–7.

189. Mofredj A, Howaizi M, Grasset D, Licht H, Loison S, Devergie B, Demontis R, Cadranel JF. Diabetes mellitus during interferon therapy for chronic viral hepatitis. Dig Dis Sci 2002;47(7):1649–54.

190. Ito Y, Takeda N, Ishimori M, Akai A, Miura K, Yasuda K. Effects of long-term interferon-alpha treatment on glucose tolerance in patients with chronic hepatitis C. J Hepatol 1999;31(2):215–20.

191. Hayakawa M, Gando S, Morimoto Y, Kemmotsu O. Development of severe diabetic keto-acidosis with shock after changing interferon-beta into interferon-alpha for chronic hepatitis C. Intensive Care Med 2000;26(7):1008.

192. Fabris P, Betterle C, Greggio NA, Zanchetta R, Bosi E, Biasin MR, de Lalla F. Insulin-dependent diabetes mellitus during alpha-interferon therapy for chronic viral hepatitis. J Hepatol 1998;28(3):514–7.

193. Koivisto VA, Pelkonen R, Cantell K. Effect of interferon on glucose tolerance and insulin sensitivity. Diabetes 1989;38(5):641–7.

194. Imano E, Kanda T, Ishigami Y, Kubota M, Ikeda M, Matsuhisa M, Kawamori R, Yamasaki Y. Interferon induces insulin resistance in patients with chronic active hepatitis C. J Hepatol 1998;28(2):189–93.

195. di Cesare E, Previti M, Russo F, Brancatelli S, Ingemi MC, Scoglio R, Mazzu N, Cucinotta D, Raimondo G. Interferon-alpha therapy may induce insulin autoantibody development in patients with chronic viral hepatitis. Dig Dis Sci 1996;41(8):1672–7.

196. Elisaf M, Tsianos EV. Severe hypertriglyceridaemia in a non-diabetic patient after alpha-interferon. Eur J Gastroenterol Hepatol 1999;11(4):463.

197. Junghans V, Runger TM. Hypertriglyceridaemia following adjuvant interferon-alpha treatment in two patients with malignant melanoma. Br J Dermatol 1999;140(1):183–4.

198. Shinohara E, Yamashita S, Kihara S, Hirano K, Ishigami M, Arai T, Nozaki S, Kameda-Takemura K, Kawata S, Matsuzawa Y. Interferon alpha induces disorder of lipid metabolism by lowering postheparin lipases and cholesteryl ester transfer protein activities in patients with chronic hepatitis C. Hepatology 1997;25(6):1502–6.

199. Yamagishi S, Abe T, Sawada T. Human recombinant interferon alpha-2a (r IFN alpha-2a) therapy suppresses hepatic triglyceride lipase, leading to severe hypertriglyceridemia in a diabetic patient. Am J Gastroenterol 1994;89(12):2280.

200. Fernandez-Miranda C, Castellano G, Guijarro C, Fernandez I, Schoebel N, Larumbe S, Gomez-Izquierdo T, del Palacio A. Lipoprotein changes in patients with chronic hepatitis C treated with interferon-alpha. Am J Gastroenterol 1998;93(10):1901–4.

201. Jessner W, Der-Petrossian M, Christiansen L, Maier H, Steindl-Munda P, Gangl A, Ferenci P. Porphyria cutanea tarda during interferon/ribavirin therapy for chronic hepatitis C. Hepatology 2002;36(5):1301–2.

202. Ernstoff MS, Kirkwood JM. Changes in the bone marrow of cancer patients treated with recombinant interferon alpha-2. Am J Med 1984;76(4):593–6.

203. Poynard T, Bedossa P, Chevallier M, Mathurin P, Lemonnier C, Trepo C, Couzigou P, Payen JL, Sajus M, Costa JMMulticenter Study Group. A comparison of three interferon alfa-2b regimens for the long-term treatment of chronic non-A, non-B hepatitis. N Engl J Med 1995;332(22):1457–62.

204. Toccaceli F, Rosati S, Scuderi M, Iacomi F, Picconi R, Laghi V. Leukocyte and platelet lowering by some interferon types during viral hepatitis treatment. Hepatogastroenterology 1998;45(23):1748–52.

205. de-la-Serna-Higuera C, Barcena-Marugan R, Sanz-de-Villalobos E. Hemolytic anemia secondary to alpha-interferon treatment in a patient with chronic C hepatitis. J Clin Gastroenterol 1999;28(4):358–9.

206. Landau A, Castera L, Buffet C, Tertian G, Tchernia G. Acute autoimmune hemolytic anemia during interferon-alpha therapy for chronic hepatitis C. Dig Dis Sci 1999;44(7):1366–7.

207. Akard LP, Hoffman R, Elias L, Saiers JH. Alpha-interferon and immune hemolytic anemia. Ann Intern Med 1986;105(2):306.

208. Barbolla L, Paniagua C, Outeirino J, Prieto E, Sanchez Fayos J. Haemolytic anaemia to the alpha-interferon treatment: a proposed mechanism. Vox Sang 1993;65(2):156–7.

209. Braathen LR, Stavem P. Autoimmune haemolytic anaemia associated with interferon alfa-2a in a patient with mycosis fungoides. BMJ 1989;298(6689):1713.

210. Dormann H, Krebs S, Muth-Selbach U, Brune K, Schuppan D, Hahn EG, Schneider HT. Rapid onset of hematotoxic effects after interferon alpha in hepatitis C. J Hepatol 2000;32(6):1041–2.

211. Singhal S, Mehta J, Desikan K, Siegel D, Singh J, Munshi N, Spoon D, Anaissie E, Ayers D, Barlogie B. Collection of peripheral blood stem cells after a preceding autograft: unfavorable effect of prior interferon-alpha therapy. Bone Marrow Transplant 1999;24(1):13–7.

212. Harousseau JL, Milpied N, Bourhis JH, Guimbretiere L, Talmant P. Aplasie fatale après traitement par interféron alpha d'une leucémie myéloïde chronique après greffe de moelle osseuse allogénique. [Lethal aplasia after treatment with alpha-interferon of recurrent chronic myeloid leukemia following allogeneic bone marrow graft.] Presse Méd 1988;17(2):80–1.

213. Hoffmann A, Kirn E, Krueger GR, Fischer R. Bone marrow hypoplasia and fibrosis following interferon treatment. In Vivo 1994;8(4):605–12.

214. Shepherd PC, Richards S, Allan NC. Severe cytopenias associated with the sequential use of busulphan and interferon-alpha in chronic myeloid leukaemia. Br J Haematol 1994;86(1):92–6.

215. Talpaz M, Kantarjian H, Kurzrock R, Gutterman JU. Bone marrow hypoplasia and aplasia complicating interferon therapy for chronic myelogenous leukemia. Cancer 1992;69(2):410–2.

216. Steis RG, VanderMolen LA, Lawrence J, Sing G, Ruscetti F, Smith JW 2nd, Urba WJ, Clark J, Longo DL. Erythrocytosis in hairy cell leukaemia following therapy with interferon alpha. Br J Haematol 1990;75(1):133–5.

217. Hirri HM, Green PJ. Pure red cell aplasia in a patient with chronic granulocytic leukaemia treated with interferon-alpha. Clin Lab Haematol 2000;22(1):53–4.

218. Tomita N, Motomura S, Ishigatsubo Y. Interferon-alpha-induced pure red cell aplasia following chronic myelogenous leukemia. Anticancer Drugs 2001;12(1):7–8.

219. Willson RA. Interferon alfa-induced pernicious anemia in chronic hepatitis C infection. J Clin Gastroenterol 2001;33(5):426–7.

220. Andriani A, Bibas M, Callea V, De Renzo A, Chiurazzi F, Marceno R, Musto P, Rotoli B. Autoimmune hemolytic anemia during alpha interferon treatment in nine patients with hematological diseases. Haematologica 1996;81(3):258–60.

221. Sacchi S, Kantarjian H, O'Brien S, Cohen PR, Pierce S, Talpaz M. Immune-mediated and unusual complications during interferon alfa therapy in chronic myelogenous leukemia. J Clin Oncol 1995;13(9):2401–7.

222. Steegmann JL, Pinilla I, Requena MJ, de la Camara R, Granados E, Fernandez Villalta MJ, Fernandez-Ranada JM. The direct antiglobulin test is frequently positive in chronic myeloid leukemia patients treated with interferon-alpha. Transfusion 1997;37(4):446–7.

223. McNair ANB, Jacyna MR, Thomas HC. Severe haemolytic transfusion reaction occurring during alpha-interferon therapy for chronic hepatitis. Eur J Gastroenterol Hepatol 1991;3:193–4.

224. Parry-Jones N, Gore ME, Taylor J, Treleaven JG. Delayed haemolytic transfusion reaction caused by anti-M antibody in a patient receiving interleukin-2 and interferon for metastatic renal cell cancer. Clin Lab Haematol 1999;21(6):407–8.

225. Renou C, Harafa A, Bouabdallah R, Demattei C, Cummins C, Rifflet H, Muller P, Ville E, Bertrand J, Benderitter T, Halfon P. Severe neutropenia and posthepatitis C cirrhosis treatment: is interferon dose adaptation at once necessary? Am J Gastroenterol 2002;97(5):1260–3.

226. Soza A, Everhart JE, Ghany MG, Doo E, Heller T, Promrat K, Park Y, Liang TJ, Hoofnagle JH. Neutropenia during combination therapy of interferon alfa and ribavirin for chronic hepatitis C. Hepatology 2002;36(5):1273–9.

227. Sata M, Yano Y, Yoshiyama Y, Ide T, Kumashiro R, Suzuki H, Tanikawa K. Mechanisms of thrombocytopenia induced by interferon therapy for chronic hepatitis B. J Gastroenterol 1997;32(2):206–10.

228. Shiota G, Okubo M, Kawasaki H, Tahara T. Interferon increases serum thrombopoietin in patients with chronic hepatitis C. Br J Haematol 1997;97(2):340–2.

229. Peck-Radosavljevic M, Wichlas M, Pidlich J, Sims P, Meng G, Zacherl J, Garg S, Datz C, Gangl A, Ferenci P. Blunted thrombopoietin response to interferon alfa-induced thrombocytopenia during treatment for hepatitis C. Hepatology 1998;28(5):1424–9.

230. Martin TG, Shuman MA. Interferon-induced thrombocytopenia: is it time for thrombopoietin. Hepatology 1998;28(5):1430–2.

231. Sagir A, Wettstein M, Heintges T, Haussinger D. Autoimmune thrombocytopenia induced by PEG-IFN-alpha2b plus ribavirin in hepatitis C. Dig Dis Sci 2002;47(3):562–3.

232. Zuffa E, Vianelli N, Martinelli G, Tazzari P, Cavo M, Tura S. Autoimmune mediated thrombocytopenia associated with the use of interferon-alpha in chronic myeloid leukemia. Haematologica 1996;81(6):533–5.

233. Taliani G, Duca F, Clementi C, De Bac C. Platelet-associated immunoglobulin G, thrombocytopenia and response to interferon treatment in chronic hepatitis C. J Hepatol 1996;25(6):999.

234. Rachmani R, Avigdor A, Youkla M, Raanani P, Zilber M, Ravid M, Ben-Bassat I. Thrombotic thrombocytopenic purpura complicating chronic myelogenous leukemia treated with interferon-alpha. A report of two successfully treated patients. Acta Haematol 1998;100(4):204–6.

235. Gutman H, Schachter J, Stopel E, Gutman R, Lahav J. Impaired platelet aggregation in melanoma patients treated with interferon-alpha-2b adjuvant therapy. Cancer 2002;94(3):780–5.

236. Carmona-Soria I, Jimenez-Saenz M, Gonzalez-Vilches J, Herrerias-Gutierrez JM. Development of lupic anticoagulant during combination therapy in a patient with chronic hepatitis C. J Hepatol 2001;34(6):965–7.

237. Castenskiold EC, Colvin BT, Kelsey SM. Acquired factor VIII inhibitor associated with chronic interferon-alpha therapy in a patient with haemophilia A. Br J Haematol 1994;87(2):434–6.

238. Stricker RB, Barlogie B, Kiprov DD. Acquired factor VIII inhibitor associated with chronic interferon-alpha therapy. J Rheumatol 1994;21(2):350–2.

239. English KE, Brien WF, Howson-Jan K, Kovacs MJ. Acquired factor VIII inhibitor in a patient with chronic myelogenous leukemia receiving interferon-alfa therapy. Ann Pharmacother 2000;34(6):737–9.

240. Mauser-Bunschoten EP, Damen M, Reesink HW, Roosendaal G, Chamuleau RA, van den Berg HM. Formation of antibodies to factor VIII in patients with hemophilia A who are treated with interferon for chronic hepatitis C. Ann Intern Med 1996;125(4):297–9.

241. Qaseem T, Jafri W, Abid S, Hamid S, Khan H. A case report of painful oral ulcerations associated with the use of alpha interferon in a patient with chronic hepatitis due to non-A non-B non-C virus. Mil Med 1993;158(2):126–7.

242. Bardella MT, Marino R, Meroni PL. Celiac disease during interferon treatment. Ann Intern Med 1999;131(2):157–8.

243. Cammarota G, Cuoco L, Cianci R, Pandolfi F, Gasbarrini G. Onset of coeliac disease during treatment with interferon for chronic hepatitis C. Lancet 2000;356(9240):1494–5.

244. Kakumitsu S, Shijo H, Akiyoshi N, Seo M, Okada M. Eosinophilic enteritis observed during alpha-interferon therapy for chronic hepatitis C. J Gastroenterol 2000;35(7):548–51.

245. Tada H, Saitoh S, Nakagawa Y, Hirana H, Morimoto M, Shima T, Shimamoto K, Okanoue T, Kashima K. Ischemic

colitis during interferon-alpha treatment for chronic active hepatitis C. J Gastroenterol 1996;31(4):582–4.

246. Janssen HL, Brouwer JT, Nevens F, Sanchez-Tapias JM, Craxi A, Hadziyannis S. Fatal hepatic decompensation associated with interferon alfa. European concerted action on viral hepatitis (Eurohep). BMJ 1993;306(6870):107–8.

247. Krogsgaard K, Marcellin P, Trepo C, Berthelot P, Sanchez-Tapias JM, Bassendine M, Tran A, Ouzan D, Ring-Larsen H, Lindberg J, Enriquez J, Benhamou JP, Bindslev N. Prednisolone withdrawal therapy enhances the effect of human lymphoblastoid interferon in chronic hepatitis B. INTERPRED Trial Group. J Hepatol 1996;25(6):803–13.

248. Lock G, Reng CM, Graeb C, Anthuber M, Wiedmann KH. Interferon-induced hepatic failure in a patient with hepatitis C. Am J Gastroenterol 1999;94(9):2570–1.

249. Farhat BA, Johnson PJ, Williams R. Hazards of interferon treatment in patients with autoimmune chronic active hepatitis. J Hepatol 1994;20(4):560–1.

250. Papo T, Marcellin P, Bernuau J, Durand F, Poynard T, Benhamou JP. Autoimmune chronic hepatitis exacerbated by alpha-interferon. Ann Intern Med 1992;116(1):51–3.

251. Payen JL, Rabbia I, Combis M, Voigt JJ, Vinel P, Pascal JP. Révélation d'une hépatite auto-immune par l'interféron. [Disclosure of autoimmune hepatitis by interferon.] Gastroenterol Clin Biol 1993;17(5):404–5.

252. Ruiz-Moreno M, Rua MJ, Carreno V, Quiroga JA, Manns M, Meyer zum Buschenfelde KH. Autoimmune chronic hepatitis type 2 manifested during interferon therapy in children. J Hepatol 1991;12(2):265–6.

253. Tran A, Beusnel C, Montoya ML, Lussiez V, Hebuterne X, Rampal P. Hépatite autoimmune de typ 1 révélée par un traitement par interféron. [Autoimmune hepatitis type 1 revealed during treatment with interferon.] Gastroenterol Clin Biol 1992;16(8–9):722–3.

254. Vento S, Di Perri G, Garofano T, Cosco L, Concia E, Ferraro T, Bassetti D. Hazards of interferon therapy for HBV-seronegative chronic hepatitis. Lancet 1989;2(8668):926.

255. Garrido Palma G, Sanchez Cuenca JM, Olaso V, Pina R, Urquijo JJ, Lopez Viedma B, Bustamante M, Berenguer M, Berenguer J. Response to treatment with interferon-alfa in patients with chronic hepatitis C and high titers of -M2, -M4 and -M8 antimitochondrial antibodies. Rev Esp Enferm Dig 1999;91(3):168–81.

256. Iorio R, Giannattasio A, Vespere G, Vegnente A. LKM1 antibody and interferon therapy in children with chronic hepatitis C. J Hepatol 2001;35(5):685–7.

257. Garcia-Buey L, Garcia-Monzon C, Rodriguez S, Borque MJ, Garcia-Sanchez A, Iglesias R, DeCastro M, Mateos FG, Vicario JL, Balas A, et al. Latent autoimmune hepatitis triggered during interferon therapy in patients with chronic hepatitis C. Gastroenterology 1995;108(6):1770–7.

258. Castera L, Kalinsky E, Bedossa P, Tertian G, Buffet C. Macrovesicular steatosis induced by interferon alfa therapy for chronic myelogenous leukaemia. Liver 1999;19(3):259–60.

259. Ryan BM, McDonald GS, Pilkington R, Kelleher D. The development of hepatic granulomas following interferon-alpha2b therapy for chronic hepatitis C infection. Eur J Gastroenterol Hepatol 1998;10(4):349–51.

260. Sevenet F, Sevenet C, Capron D, Descombes P. Pancréatite aiguë et interféron. [Acute pancreatitis and interferon.] Gastroenterol Clin Biol 1999;23(11):1256.

261. Eland IA, van Puijenbroek EP, Sturkenboom MJ, Wilson JH, Stricker BH. Drug-associated acute pancreatitis: twenty-one years of spontaneous reporting in The Netherlands. Am J Gastroenterol 1999;94(9):2417–22.

262. Eland IA, Rasch MC, Sturkenboom MJ, Bekkering FC, Brouwer JT, Delwaide J, Belaiche J, Houbiers G, Stricker BH. Acute pancreatitis attributed to the use of interferon alfa-2b. Gastroenterology 2000;119(1):230–3.

263. Kurschel E, Metz-Kurschel U, Niederle N, Aulbert E. Investigations on the subclinical and clinical nephrotoxicity of interferon alpha-2B in patients with myeloproliferative syndromes. Ren Fail 1991;13(2–3):87–93.

264. Selby P, Kohn J, Raymond J, Judson I, McElwain T. Nephrotic syndrome during treatment with interferon. BMJ (Clin Res Ed) 1985;290(6476):1180.

265. Nishimura S, Miura H, Yamada H, Shinoda T, Kitamura S, Miura Y. Acute onset of nephrotic syndrome during interferon-alpha retreatment for chronic active hepatitis C. J Gastroenterol 2002;37(10):854–8.

266. Willson RA. Nephrotoxicity of interferon alfa–ribavirin therapy for chronic hepatitis C. J Clin Gastroenterol 2002;35(1):89–92.

267. Nassar GM, Pedro P, Remmers RE, Mohanty LB, Smith W. Reversible renal failure in a patient with the hypereosinophilia syndrome during therapy with alpha interferon. Am J Kidney Dis 1998;31(1):121–6.

268. Dimitrov Y, Heibel F, Marcellin L, Chantrel F, Moulin B, Hannedouche T. Acute renal failure and nephrotic syndrome with alpha interferon therapy. Nephrol Dial Transplant 1997;12(1):200–3.

269. Averbuch SD, Austin HA 3rd, Sherwin SA, Antonovych T, Bunn PA Jr, Longo DL. Acute interstitial nephritis with the nephrotic syndrome following recombinant leukocyte a interferon therapy for mycosis fungoides. N Engl J Med 1984;310(1):32–5.

270. Kimmel PL, Abraham AA, Phillips TM. Membranoproliferative glomerulonephritis in a patient treated with interferon-alpha for human immunodeficiency virus infection. Am J Kidney Dis 1994;24(5):858–63.

271. Traynor A, Kuzel T, Samuelson E, Kanwar Y. Minimal-change glomerulopathy and glomerular visceral epithelial hyperplasia associated with alpha-interferon therapy for cutaneous T cell lymphoma. Nephron 1994;67(1):94–100.

272. Fahal IH, Murry N, Chu P, Bell GM. Acute renal failure during interferon treatment. BMJ 1993;306(6883):973.

273. Lederer E, Truong L. Unusual glomerular lesion in a patient receiving long-term interferon alpha. Am J Kidney Dis 1992;20(5):516–8.

274. Durand JM, Retornaz F, Cretel E, et al. Glomérulonéphrite extracapillaire au cours d'un traitement par interféron alpha. Rev Med Interne 1993;14:1138.

275. Jadoul M. Interferon-alpha-associated focal segmental glomerulosclerosis with massive proteinuria in patients with chronic myeloid leukemia following high dose chemotherapy. Cancer 1999;85(12):2669–70.

276. Honda K, Ando A, Endo M, Shimizu K, Higashihara M, Nitta K, Nihei H. Thrombotic microangiopathy associated with alpha-interferon therapy for chronic myelocytic leukemia. Am J Kidney Dis 1997;30(1):123–30.

277. Ravandi-Kashani F, Cortes J, Talpaz M, Kantarjian HM. Thrombotic microangiopathy associated with interferon therapy for patients with chronic myelogenous leukemia: coincidence or true side effect? Cancer 1999;85(12):2583–8.

278. Vacher-Coponat H, Opris A, Daniel L, Harle JR, Veit V, Olmer M. Thrombotic microangiopathy in a patient with

chronic myelocytic leukaemia treated with alpha-interferon. Nephrol Dial Transplant 1999;14(10):2469–71.

279. Zuber J, Martinez F, Droz D, Oksenhendler E, Legendre CGroupe D'Etude Des Nephrologues D'Ile-de-France (GENIF). Alpha-interferon-associated thrombotic microangiopathy: a clinicopathologic study of 8 patients and review of the literature. Medicine (Baltimore) 2002;81(4):321–31.

280. Bren A, Kandus A, Ferluga D. Rapidly progressive renal graft failure associated with interferon-alpha treatment in a patient with chronic myelogenous leukemia. Clin Nephrol 1998;50(4):266–7.

281. Asnis LA, Gaspari AA. Cutaneous reactions to recombinant cytokine therapy. J Am Acad Dermatol 1995;33(3):393–410.

282. Dalekos GN, Hatzis J, Tsianos EV. Dermatologic disease during interferon-alpha therapy for chronic viral hepatitis. Ann Intern Med 1998;128(5):409–10.

283. Andry P, Weber-Buisset MJ, Fraitag S, Brechot C, De Prost Y. Toxidermie bulleuse à l'Introna. [Bullous drug eruption caused by Introna.] Ann Dermatol Venereol 1993;120(11):843–5.

284. Sparsa A, Loustaud-Ratti V, Liozon E, Denes E, Soria P, Bouyssou-Gauthier ML, Le Brun V, Boulinguez S, Bedane C, Scribbe-Outtas M, Outtas O, Labrousse F, Bonnetblanc JM, Bordessoule D, Vidal E. Réactions cutanées ou nécrose à l'interféron alpha: peut-on reprendre l'interféron? A propos de six cas. [Cutaneous reactions or necrosis from interferon alpha: can interferon be reintroduced after healing? Six case reports.] Rev Med Interne 2000;21(9):756–63.

285. Kurzen H, Petzoldt D, Hartschuh W, Jappe U. Cutaneous necrosis after subcutaneous injection of polyethylene-glycol-modified interferon alpha. Acta Dermatol Venereol 2002;82(4):310–2.

286. Sanders S, Busam K, Tahan SR, Johnson RA, Sachs D. Granulomatous and suppurative dermatitis at interferon alfa injection sites: report of 2 cases. J Am Acad Dermatol 2002;46(4):611–6.

287. Jessner W, Kinaciyan T, Formann E, Steindl-Munda P, Ferenci P. Severe skin reactions during therapy for chronic hepatitis C associated with delayed hypersensitivity to pegylated interferons. Hepatology 2002;36:361.

288. Heinzerling L, Dummer R, Wildberger H, Burg G. Cutaneous ulceration after injection of polyethylene-glycol-modified interferon alpha associated with visual disturbances in a melanoma patient. Dermatology 2000;201(2):154–7.

289. Bessis D, Charron A, Rouzier-Panis R, Blatiere V, Guilhou JJ, Reynes J. Necrotizing cutaneous lesions complicating treatment with pegylated-interferon alfa in an HIV-infected patient. Eur J Dermatol 2002;12(1):99–102.

290. Cribier B, Garnier C, Laustriat D, Heid E. Lichen planus and hepatitis C virus infection: an epidemiologic study. J Am Acad Dermatol 1994;31(6):1070–2.

291. Dupin N, Chosidow O, Frances C, et al. Lichen planus after alpha-interferon therapy for chronic hepatitis C. Eur J Dermatol 1994;4:535–6.

292. Strumia R, Venturini D, Boccia S, Gamberini S, Gullini S. UVA and interferon-alfa therapy in a patient with lichen planus and chronic hepatitis C. Int J Dermatol 1993;32(5):386.

293. Aubin F, Bourezane Y, Blanc D, Voltz JM, Faivre B, Humbert PH. Severe lichen planus-like eruption induced by interferon-alpha therapy. Eur J Dermatol 1995;5:296–9.

294. Marinho RT, Johnson NW, Fatela NM, Serejo FS, Gloria H, Raimundo MO, Velosa JF, Ramalho FJ,

Moura MC. Oropharyngeal pemphigus in a patient with chronic hepatitis C during interferon alpha-2a therapy. Eur J Gastroenterol Hepatol 2001;13(7):869–72.

295. Quesada JR, Gutterman JU. Psoriasis and alpha-interferon. Lancet 1986;1(8496):1466–8.

296. Harrison PV, Peat MJ. Effect of interferon on psoriasis. Lancet 1986;2(8504):457–8.

297. Nguyen C, Misery L, Tigaud JD, Petiot A, Fiere D, Faure M, Claudy A. Psoriasis induit par l'interféron alpha. A propos d'une observation. [Psoriasis induced by interferon-alpha. Apropos of a case.] Ann Med Interne (Paris) 1996;147(7):519–21.

298. Cleveland MG, Mallory SB. Incomplete Reiter's syndrome induced by systemic interferon alpha treatment. J Am Acad Dermatol 1993;29(5 Pt 1):788–9.

299. Dereure O, Raison-Peyron N, Larrey D, Blanc F, Guilhou JJ. Diffuse inflammatory lesions in patients treated with interferon alfa and ribavirin for hepatitis C: a series of 20 patients. Br J Dermatol 2002;147(6):1142–6.

300. Thomas R, Stea B. Radiation recall dermatitis from high-dose interferon alfa-2b. J Clin Oncol 2002;20(1):355–7.

301. Tursen U, Kaya TI, Ikizoglu G. Interferon-alpha 2b induced facial erythema in a woman with chronic hepatitis C infection. J Eur Acad Dermatol Venereol 2002;16(3):285–6.

302. Creput C, Auffret N, Samuel D, Jian R, Hill G, Nochy D. Cutaneous thrombotic microangiopathy during treatment with alpha-interferon for chronic hepatitis C. J Hepatol 2002;37(6):871–2.

303. Krischer J, Pechere M, Salomon D, Harms M, Chavaz P, Saurat JH. Interferon alfa-2b-induced Meyerson's nevi in a patient with dysplastic nevus syndrome. J Am Acad Dermatol 1999;40(1):105–6.

304. Pfohler C, Ugurel S, Seiter S, Wagner A, Tilgen W, Reinhold U. Interferon-alpha-associated development of bullous lesions in mycosis fungoides. Dermatology 2000;200(1):51–3.

305. Tosti A, Misciali C, Bardazzi F, Fanti PA, Varotti C. Telogen effluvium due to recombinant interferon alpha-2b. Dermatology 1992;184(2):124–5.

306. Agesta N, Zabala R, Diaz-Perez JL. Alopecia areata during interferon alpha-2b/ribavirin therapy. Dermatology 2002;205(3):300–1.

307. Lang AM, Norland AM, Schuneman RL, Tope WD. Localized interferon alfa-2b-induced alopecia. Arch Dermatol 1999;135(9):1126–8.

308. Kernland KH, Hunziker T. Alopecia areata induced by interferon alpha? Dermatology 1999;198(4):418–9.

309. Bessis D, Luong MS, Blanc P, Chapoutot C, Larrey D, Guilhou JJ, Guillot B. Straight hair associated with interferon-alfa plus ribavirin in hepatitis C infection. Br J Dermatol 2002;147(2):392–3.

310. Hauschild A, Moller M, Lischner S, Christophers E. Repeatable acute rhabdomyolysis with multiple organ dysfunction because of interferon alpha and dacarbazine treatment in metastatic melanoma. Br J Dermatol 2001;144(1):215–6.

311. van Londen GJ, Mascarenhas B, Kirkwood JM. Rhabdomyolysis, when observed with high-dose interferon-alfa (HDI) therapy, does not always exclude resumption of HDI. J Clin Oncol 2001;19(17):3794.

312. Ozdag F, Akar A, Eroglu E, Erbil H. Acute rhabdomyolysis during the treatment of scleromyxedema with interferon alfa. J Dermatolog Treat 2001;12(3):167–9.

313. Dippel E, Zouboulis CC, Tebbe B, Orfanos CE. Myopathic syndrome associated with long-term

recombinant interferon alfa treatment in 4 patients with skin disorders. Arch Dermatol 1998;134(7):880–1.

314. Kozuch P, Talpaz M, Faderl S, O'Brien S, Freireich EJ, Kantarjian H. Avascular necrosis of the femoral head in chronic myeloid leukemia patients treated with interferon-alpha: a synergistic correlation? Cancer 2000;89(7):1482–9.

315. Alvarez JS, Sacristan JA, Alsar MJ. Interferon alpha-2a-induced impotence. Ann Pharmacother 1991;25:1397.

316. Kauppila A, Cantell K, Janne O, Kokko E, Vihko R. Serum sex steroid and peptide hormone concentrations, and endometrial estrogen and progestin receptor levels during administration of human leukocyte interferon. Int J Cancer 1982;29(3):291–4.

317. Schilsky RL, Davidson HS, Magid D, Daiter S, Golomb HM. Gonadal and sexual function in male patients with hairy cell leukemia: lack of adverse effects of recombinant alpha 2-interferon treatment. Cancer Treat Rep 1987;71(2):179–81.

318. Pardini S, Bosincu L, Bonfigli S, Dore F, Longinotti M. Anaphylactic-like syndrome in systemic mastocytosis treated with alpha-2-interferon. Acta Haematol 1991;85(4):220.

319. Ohmoto K, Yamamoto S. Angioedema after interferon therapy for chronic hepatitis C. Am J Gastroenterol 2001;96(4):1311–2.

320. Beckman DB, Mathisen TL, Harris KE, Boxer MB, Grammer LC. Hypersensitivity to IFN-alpha. Allergy 2001;56(8):806–7.

321. Detmar U, Agathos M, Nerl C. Allergy of delayed type to recombinant interferon alpha 2c. Contact Dermatitis 1989;20(2):149–50.

322. Pigatto PD, Bigardi A, Legori A, Altomare GF, Riboldi A. Allergic contact dermatitis from beta-interferon in eye-drops. Contact Dermatitis 1991;25(3):199–200.

323. Antonelli G. In vivo development of antibody to interferons: an update to 1996. J Interferon Cytokine Res 1997;17(Suppl 1):S39–46.

324. McKenna RM, Oberg KE. Antibodies to interferon-alpha in treated cancer patients: incidence and significance. J Interferon Cytokine Res 1997;17(3):141–3.

325. Bonino F, Baldi M, Negro F, Oliveri F, Colombatto P, Bellati G, Brunetto MR. Clinical relevance of anti-interferon antibodies in the serum of chronic hepatitis C patients treated with interferon-alpha. J Interferon Cytokine Res 1997;17(Suppl 1):S35–8.

326. Antonelli G, Currenti M, Turriziani O, Dianzani F. Neutralizing antibodies to interferon-alpha: relative frequency in patients treated with different interferon preparations. J Infect Dis 1991;163(4):882–5.

327. Antonelli G, Currenti M, Turriziani O, Riva E, Dianzani F. Relative frequency of nonneutralizing antibodies to interferon (IFN) in hepatitis patients treated with different IFN-alpha preparations. J Infect Dis 1992;165(3):593–4.

328. Von Wussow P, Hehlmann R, Hochhaus T, Jakschies D, Nolte KU, Prummer O, Ansari H, Hasford J, Heimpel H, Deicher H. Roferon (rIFN-alpha 2a) is more immunogenic than intron A (rIFN-alpha 2b) in patients with chronic myelogenous leukemia. J Interferon Res 1994;14(4):217–9.

329. Milella M, Antonelli G, Santantonio T, Currenti M, Monno L, Mariano N, Angarano G, Dianzani F, Pastore G. Neutralizing antibodies to recombinant alpha-interferon and response to therapy in chronic hepatitis C virus infection. Liver 1993;13(3):146–50.

330. Antonelli G, Giannelli G, Currenti M, Simeoni E, Del Vecchio S, Maggi F, Pistello M, Roffi L, Pastore G,

Chemello L, Dianzani F. Antibodies to interferon (IFN) in hepatitis C patients relapsing while continuing recombinant IFN-alpha2 therapy. Clin Exp Immunol 1996;104(3):384–7.

331. Hanley JP, Jarvis LM, Simmonds P, Ludlam CA. Development of anti-interferon antibodies and break-through hepatitis during treatment for HCV infection in haemophiliacs. Br J Haematol 1996;94(3):551–6.

332. Roffi L, Mels GC, Antonelli G, Bellati G, Panizzuti F, Piperno A, Pozzi M, Ravizza D, Angeli G, Dianzani F, et al. Breakthrough during recombinant interferon alfa therapy in patients with chronic hepatitis C virus infection: prevalence, etiology, and management. Hepatology 1995;21(3):645–9.

333. Rajan GP, Seifert B, Prummer O, Joller-Jemelka HI, Burg G, Dummer R. Incidence and in-vivo relevance of anti-interferon antibodies during treatment of low-grade cutaneous T-cell lymphomas with interferon alpha-2a combined with acitretin or PUVA. Arch Dermatol Res 1996;288(9):543–8.

334. Tefferi A, Grendahl DC. Natural leukocyte interferon-alpha therapy in patients with chronic granulocytic leukemia who have antibody-mediated resistance to treatment with recombinant interferon-alpha. Am J Hematol 1996;52(3):231–3.

335. Russo D, Candoni A, Zuffa E, Minisini R, Silvestri F, Fanin R, Zaja F, Martinelli G, Tura S, Botta G, Baccarani M. Neutralizing anti-interferon-alpha antibodies and response to treatment in patients with Ph+ chronic myeloid leukaemia sequentially treated with recombinant (alpha 2a) and lymphoblastoid interferon-alpha. Br J Haematol 1996;94(2):300–5.

336. Milella M, Antonelli G, Santantonio T, Giannelli G, Currenti M, Monno L, Turriziani O, Pastore G, Dianzani F. Treatment with natural IFN of hepatitis C patients with or without antibodies to recombinant IFN. Hepatogastroenterology 1995;42(3):201–4.

337. Wussow PV, Jakschies D, Freund M, Hehlmann R, Brockhaus F, Hochkeppel H, Horisberger M, Deicher H. Treatment of anti-recombinant interferon-alpha 2 antibody positive CML patients with natural interferon-alpha. Br J Haematol 1991;78(2):210–6.

338. von Wussow P, Pralle H, Hochkeppel HK, Jakschies D, Sonnen S, Schmidt H, Muller-Rosenau D, Franke M, Haferlach T, Zwingers T, et al. Effective natural interferon-alpha therapy in recombinant interferon-alpha-resistant patients with hairy cell leukemia. Blood 1991;78(1):38–43.

339. Wada M, Kang KB, Kinugasa A, Shintani S, Sawada K, Nishigami T, Shimoyama T. Does the presence of serum autoantibodies influence the responsiveness to interferon-alpha 2a treatment in chronic hepatitis C? Intern Med 1997;36(4):248–54.

340. Cassani F, Cataleta M, Valentini P, Muratori P, Giostra F, Francesconi R, Muratori L, Lenzi M, Bianchi G, Zauli D, Bianchi FB. Serum autoantibodies in chronic hepatitis C: comparison with autoimmune hepatitis and impact on the disease profile. Hepatology 1997;26(3):561–6.

341. Noda K, Enomoto N, Arai K, Masuda E, Yamada Y, Suzuki K, Tanaka M, Yoshihara H. Induction of antinuclear antibody after interferon therapy in patients with type-C chronic hepatitis: its relation to the efficacy of therapy. Scand J Gastroenterol 1996;31(7):716–22.

342. Bell TM, Bansal AS, Shorthouse C, Sandford N, Powell EE. Low-titre auto-antibodies predict autoimmune disease during interferon-alpha treatment of chronic hepatitis C. J Gastroenterol Hepatol 1999;14(5):419–22.

343. Steegmann JL, Requena MJ, Martin-Regueira P, De La Camara R, Casado F, Salvanes FR, Fernandez Ranada JM. High incidence of autoimmune alterations in chronic myeloid leukemia patients treated with interferon-alpha. Am J Hematol 2003;72(3):170–6.

344. Tothova E, Kafkova A, Stecova N, Fricova M, Guman T, Svorcova E. Immune-mediated complications during interferon alpha therapy in chronic myelogenous leukemia. Neoplasma 2002;49(2):91–4.

345. Lunel F, Cacoub P. Treatment of autoimmune and extrahepatic manifestations of hepatitis C virus infection. J Hepatol 1999;31(Suppl 1):210–6.

346. Budak-Alpdogan T, Demircay Z, Alpdogan O, Direskeneli H, Ergun T, Bayik M, Akoglu T. Behçet's disease in patients with chronic myelogenous leukemia: possible role of interferon-alpha treatment in the occurrence of Behçet's symptoms. Ann Hematol 1997;74(1):45–48.

347. Dietrich LL, Bridges AJ, Albertini MR. Dermatomyositis after interferon alpha treatment. Med Oncol 2000;17(1):64–9.

348. Dohmen K, Miyamoto Y, Irie K, Takeshita T, Ishibashi H. Manifestation of cutaneous polyarteritis nodosa during interferon therapy for chronic hepatitis C associated with primary biliary cirrhosis. J Gastroenterol 2000;35(10):789–793.

349. Cirigliano G, Della Rossa A, Tavoni A, Viacava P, Bombardieri S. Polymyositis occurring during alpha-interferon treatment for malignant melanoma: a case report and review of the literature. Rheumatol Int 1999;19(1–2):65–7.

350. Hengstman GJ, Vogels OJ, ter Laak HJ, de Witte T, van Engelen BG. Myositis during long-term interferon-alpha treatment. Neurology 2000;54(11):2186.

351. Hoffmann RM, Jung MC, Motz R, Gossl C, Emslander HP, Zachoval R, Pape GR. Sarcoidosis associated with interferon-alpha therapy for chronic hepatitis C. J Hepatol 1998;28(6):1058–63.

352. Cogrel O, Doutre MS, Marliere V, Beylot-Barry M, Couzigou P, Beylot C. Cutaneous sarcoidosis during interferon alfa and ribavirin treatment of hepatitis C virus infection: two cases. Br J Dermatol 2002;146(2):320–4.

353. Savoye G, Goria O, Herve S, Riachi G, Noblesse I, Bastien L, Courville P, Lerebours E. Probable sarcoïdose cutanée après bi-thérapie associant ribavirine et interferon-alpha pour une hépatite chronique virale C. [Probable cutaneous sarcoidosis associated with combined ribavirin and interferon-alpha therapy for chronic hepatitis C.] Gastroenterol Clin Biol 2000;24(6–7):679.

354. Vander Els NJ, Gerdes H. Sarcoidosis and IFN-alpha treatment. Chest 2000;117(1):294.

355. Fiorani C, Sacchi S, Bonacorsi G, Cosenza M. Systemic sarcoidosis associated with interferon-alpha treatment for chronic myelogenous leukemia. Haematologica 2000;85(9):1006–7.

356. Eberlein-Konig B, Hein R, Abeck D, Engst R, Ring J. Cutaneous sarcoid foreign body granulomas developing in sites of previous skin injury after systemic interferon-alpha treatment for chronic hepatitis C. Br J Dermatol 1999;140(2):370–2.

357. Gitlin N. Manifestation of sarcoidosis during interferon and ribavirin therapy for chronic hepatitis C: a report of two cases. Eur J Gastroenterol Hepatol 2002;14(8):883–5.

358. Husa P, Klusakova J, Jancikova J, Husova L, Horalek F. Sarcoidosis associated with interferon-alpha therapy for chronic hepatitis B. Eur J Intern Med 2002;13(2):129–31.

359. Nawras A, Alsolaiman MM, Mehboob S, Bartholomew C, Maliakkal B. Systemic sarcoidosis presenting as a granulomatous tattoo reaction secondary to interferon-alpha treatment for chronic hepatitis C and review of the literature. Dig Dis Sci 2002;47(7):1627–31.

360. Noguchi K, Enjoji M, Nakamuta M, Sugimoto R, Kotoh K, Nawata H. Various sarcoid lesions in a patient induced by interferon therapy for chronic hepatitis C. J Clin Gastroenterol 2002;35(3):282–4.

361. Tahan V, Ozseker F, Guneylioglu D, Baran A, Ozaras R, Mert A, Ucisik AC, Cagatay T, Yilmazbayhan D, Senturk H. Sarcoidosis after use of interferon for chronic hepatitis C: report of a case and review of the literature. Dig Dis Sci 2003;48(1):169–73.

362. Li SD, Yong S, Srinivas D, Van Thiel DH. Reactivation of sarcoidosis during interferon therapy. J Gastroenterol 2002;37(1):50–4.

363. Boonen A, Stockbrugger RW, van der Linden S. Pericarditis after therapy with interferon-alpha for chronic hepatitis C. Clin Rheumatol 1999;18(2):177–9.

364. Johnson DM, Hayat SQ, Burton GV. Rheumatoid arthritis complicating adjuvant interferon-alpha therapy for malignant melanoma. J Rheumatol 1999;26(4):1009–10.

365. Wandl UB, Nagel-Hiemke M, May D, Kreuzfelder E, Kloke O, Kranzhoff M, Seeber S, Niederle N. Lupus-like autoimmune disease induced by interferon therapy for myeloproliferative disorders. Clin Immunol Immunopathol 1992;65(1):70–4.

366. Conlon KC, Urba WJ, Smith JW 2nd, Steis RG, Longo DL, Clark JW. Exacerbation of symptoms of autoimmune disease in patients receiving alpha-interferon therapy. Cancer 1990;65(10):2237–42.

367. Nesher G, Ruchlemer R. Alpha-interferon-induced arthritis: clinical presentation treatment, and prevention. Semin Arthritis Rheum 1998;27(6):360–5.

368. Fukuyama S, Kajiwara E, Suzuki N, Miyazaki N, Sadoshima S, Onoyama K. Systemic lupus erythematosus after alpha-interferon therapy for chronic hepatitis C: a case report and review of the literature. Am J Gastroenterol 2000;95(1):310–2.

369. Beretta L, Caronni M, Vanoli M, Scorza R. Systemic sclerosis after interferon-alfa therapy for myeloproliferative disorders. Br J Dermatol 2002;147(2):385–6.

370. Friedman G, Mehta S, Sherker AH. Fatal exacerbation of hepatitis C-related cryoglobulinemia with interferon-alpha therapy. Dig Dis Sci 1999;44(7):1364–5.

371. Pateron D, Fain O, Sehonnou J, Trinchet JC, Beaugrand M. Severe necroziting vasculitis in a patient with hepatitis C virus infection treated by interferon. Clin Exp Rheumatol 1996;14(1):79–81.

372. Samson D, Volin L, Schanz U, Bosi A, Gahrtron G. Feasibility and toxicity of interferon maintenance therapy after allogeneic BMT for multiple myeloma: a pilot study of the EBMT. Bone Marrow Transplant 1996;17(5):759–762.

373. Morton AJ, Gooley T, Hansen JA, Appelbaum FR, Bruemmer B, Bjerke JW, Clift R, Martin PJ, Petersdorf EW, Sanders JE, Storb R, Sullivan KM, Woolfrey A, Anasetti C. Association between pretransplant interferon-alpha and outcome after unrelated donor marrow transplantation for chronic myelogenous leukemia in chronic phase. Blood 1998;92(2):394–401.

374. Rostaing L, Izopet J, Baron E, Duffaut M, Puel J, Durand D. Treatment of chronic hepatitis C with recombinant interferon alpha in kidney transplant recipients. Transplantation 1995;59(10):1426–31.

375. Dousset B, Conti F, Houssin D, Calmus Y. Acute vanishing bile duct syndrome after interferon therapy for recurrent HCV infection in liver-transplant recipients. N Engl J Med 1994;330(16):1160–1.

376. Féray C, Samuel D, Gigou M, Paradis V, David MF, Lemonnier C, Reynes M, Bismuth H. An open trial of interferon alfa recombinant for hepatitis C after liver transplantation: antiviral effects and risk of rejection. Hepatology 1995;22(4 Pt 1):1084–9.

377. Pohanka E, Kovarik J. Is treatment with interferon-alpha in renal transplant recipients still justified? Nephrol Dial Transplant 1996;11(6):1191–2.

378. Min AD, Bodenheimer HC Jr. Does interferon precipitate rejection of liver allografts? Hepatology 1995;22(4 Pt 1):1333–5.

379. Soriano V, Bravo R, Samaniego JG, Gonzalez J, Odriozola PM, Arroyo E, Vicario JL, Castro A, Colmenero M, Carballo E, et alHIV-Hepatitis Spanish Study Group. CD4+ T-lymphocytopenia in HIV-infected patients receiving interferon therapy for chronic hepatitis C. AIDS 1994;8(11):1621–2.

380. Vento S, Di Perri G, Cruciani M, Garofano T, Concia E, Bassetti D. Rapid decline of CD4+ cells after IFN alpha treatment in HIV-1 infection. Lancet 1993;341(8850):958–959.

381. Marten D, Holtzmuller K, Julia F. Bacterial infections complicating hepatitis C infected hemodialysis dependent patients treated with interferon alfa. Am J Gastroenterol 2002;97(Suppl):163–4.

382. Parana R, Portugal M, Vitvitski L, Cotrim H, Lyra L, Trepo C. Severe strongyloidiasis during interferon plus ribavirin therapy for chronic HCV infection. Eur J Gastroenterol Hepatol 2000;12(2):245–6.

383. Serrano J, Prieto E, Mazarbeitia F, Roman A, Llamas P, Tomas JF. Atypical chronic graft-versus-host disease following interferon therapy for chronic myeloid leukaemia relapsing after allogeneic BMT. Bone Marrow Transplant 2001;27(1):85–7.

384. Beelen DW, Elmaagacli AH, Schaefer UW. The adverse influence of pretransplant interferon-alpha (IFN-alpha) on transplant outcome after marrow transplantation for chronic phrase chronic myelogenous leukemia increases with the duration of IFN-alpha exposure. Blood 1999;93(5):1779–810.

385. Hehlmann R, Hochhaus A, Kolb HJ, Hasford J, Gratwohl A, Heimpel H, Siegert W, Finke J, Ehninger G, Holler E, Berger U, Pfirrmann M, Muth A, Zander A, Fauser AA, Heyll A, Nerl C, Hossfeld DK, Loffler H, Pralle H, Queisser W, Tobler A. Interferon-alpha before allogeneic bone marrow transplantation in chronic myelogenous leukemia does not affect outcome adversely, provided it is discontinued at least 90 days before the procedure. Blood 1999;94(11):3668–77.

386. Johansson B, Fioretos T, Billstrom R, Mitelman F. Abberant cytogenetic evolution pattern of Philadelphia-positive chronic myeloid leukemia treated with interferon-alpha. Leukemia 1996;10(7):1134–8.

387. Waysbort A, Giroux M, Mansat V, Teixeira M, Dumas JC, Puel J. Experimental study of transplacental passage of alpha interferon by two assay techniques. Antimicrob Agents Chemother 1993;37(6):1232–7.

388. Haggstrom J, Adriansson M, Hybbinette T, Harnby E, Thorbert G. Two cases of CML treated with alpha-interferon during second and third trimester of pregnancy with analysis of the drug in the new-born immediately postpartum. Eur J Haematol 1996;57(1):101–2.

389. Delage R, Demers C, Cantin G, Roy J. Treatment of essential thrombocythemia during pregnancy with interferon-alpha. Obstet Gynecol 1996;87(5 Pt 2):814–7.

390. Hiratsuka M, Minakami H, Koshizuka S, Sato I. Administration of interferon-alpha during pregnancy: effects on fetus. J Perinat Med 2000;28(5):372–6.

391. Mubarak AA, Kakil IR, Awidi A, Al-Homsi U, Fawzi Z, Kelta M, Al-Hassan A. Normal outcome of pregnancy in chronic myeloid leukemia treated with interferon-alpha in 1st trimester: report of 3 cases and review of the literature. Am J Hematol 2002;69(2):115–8.

392. Trotter JF, Zygmunt AJ. Conception and pregnancy during interferon-alpha therapy for chronic hepatitis C. J Clin Gastroenterol 2001;32(1):76–8.

393. Jacobson KR, Murray K, Zellos A, Schwarz KB. An analysis of published trials of interferon monotherapy in children with chronic hepatitis C. J Pediatr Gastroenterol Nutr 2002;34(1):52–8.

394. Barlow CF, Priebe CJ, Mulliken JB, Barnes PD, Mac Donald D, Folkman J, Ezekowitz RA. Spastic diplegia as a complication of interferon Alfa-2a treatment of hemangiomas of infancy. J Pediatr 1998;132(3 Pt 1):527–30.

395. Dubois J, Hershon L, Carmant L, Belanger S, Leclerc JM, David M. Toxicity profile of interferon alfa-2b in children: a prospective evaluation. J Pediatr 1999;135(6):782–5.

396. Worle H, Maass E, Kohler B, Treuner J. Interferon alpha-2a therapy in haemangiomas of infancy: spastic diplegia as a severe complication. Eur J Pediatr 1999;158(4):344.

397. Enjolras O. Neurotoxicity of interferon alfa in children treated for hemangiomas. J Am Acad Dermatol 1998;39(6):1037–8.

398. Grether JK, Nelson KB, Dambrosia JM, Phillips TM. Interferons and cerebral palsy. J Pediatr 1999;134(3):324–332.

399. Rostaing L, Chatelut E, Payen JL, Izopet J, Thalamas C, Ton-That H, Pascal JP, Durand D, Canal P. Pharmacokinetics of alphaIFN-2b in chronic hepatitis C virus patients undergoing chronic hemodialysis or with normal renal function: clinical implications. J Am Soc Nephrol 1998;9(12):2344–8.

400. Uchihara M, Izumi N, Sakai Y, Yauchi T, Miyake S, Sakai T, Akiba T, Marumo F, Sato C. Interferon therapy for chronic hepatitis C in hemodialysis patients: increased serum levels of interferon. Nephron 1998;80(1):51–6.

401. Anonymous. Interferon alfa-2b and ribavirin combination therapy—indications extended: previously untreated hepatitis C patients. WHO Newsletter 1999;1/2:9.

402. Chamberlain MC. A phase II trial of intra-cerebrospinal fluid alpha interferon in the treatment of neoplastic meningitis. Cancer 2002;94(10):2675–80.

403. Zylberberg H, Fontaine H, Thepot V, Nalpas B, Brechot C, Pol S. Triggering of acute alcoholic hepatitis by alpha-interferon therapy. J Hepatol 1999;30(4):722–5.

404. Casato M, Pucillo LP, Leoni M, di Lullo L, Gabrielli A, Sansonno D, Dammacco F, Danieli G, Bonomo L. Granulocytopenia after combined therapy with interferon and angiotensin-converting enzyme inhibitors: evidence for a synergistic hematologic toxicity. Am J Med 1995;99(4):386–91.

405. Bauckner JC, Schomberg PJ, McGinnis WL, Cascino TL, Scheithauer BW, O'Fallon JR, Morton RF, Kuross SA, Mailliard JA, Hatfield AK, Cole JT, Steen PD, Bernath AM. A phase III study of radiation therapy plus carmustine with or without recombinant interferon-alpha

in the treatment of patients with newly diagnosed high-grade glioma. Cancer 2001;92(2):420–33.

406. Hassan M, Nilsson C, Olsson H, Lundin J, Osterborg A. The influence of interferon-alpha on the pharmacokinetics of cyclophosphamide and its 4-hydroxy metabolite in patients with multiple myeloma. Eur J Haematol 1999;63(3):163–70.

407. Chan TM, Wu PC, Lau JY, Lok AS, Lai CL, Cheng IK. Interferon treatment for hepatitis C virus infection in patients on haemodialysis. Nephrol Dial Transplant 1997;12(7):1414–9.

408. Desai RG. Drug interaction between alpha interferon and erythropoietin. J Clin Oncol 1991;9(5):893.

409. Nordio M, Guarda L, Lorenzi S, Lombini C, Marchini P, Mirandoli F. Interaction between alpha-interferon and erythropoietin in antiviral and antineoplastic therapy in uraemic patients on haemodialysis. Nephrol Dial Transplant 1993;8(11):1308.

410. Czejka MJ, Schuller J, Jager W, Fogl U, Weiss C. Influence of different doses of interferon-alpha-2b on the blood plasma levels of 5-fluorouracil. Eur J Drug Metab Pharmacokinet 1993;18(3):247–50.

411. Greco FA, Figlin R, York M, Einhorn L, Schilsky R, Marshall EM, Buys SS, Froimtchuk MJ, Schuller J, Schuchter L, Buyse M, Ritter L, Man A, Yap AK. Phase III randomized study to compare interferon alfa-2a in combination with fluorouracil versus fluorouracil alone in patients with advanced colorectal cancer. J Clin Oncol 1996;14(10):2674–81.

412. Ehrsson H, Eksborg S, Wallin I, Osterborg A, Mellstedt H. Oral melphalan pharmacokinetics: influence of interferon-induced fever. Clin Pharmacol Ther 1990;47(1):86–90.

413. Mannering GJ, Deloria LB. The pharmacology and toxicology of the interferons: an overview. Annu Rev Pharmacol Toxicol 1986;26:455–515.

414. Echizen H, Ohta Y, Shirataki H, Tsukamoto K, Umeda N, Oda T, Ishizaki T. Effects of subchronic treatment with natural human interferons on antipyrine clearance and liver function in patients with chronic hepatitis. J Clin Pharmacol 1990;30(6):562–7.

415. Tappero G, Ballare M, Farina M, Negro F. Severe anemia following combined alpha-interferon/ribavirin therapy of chronic hepatitis C. J Hepatol 1998;29(6):1033–4.

416. Sookoian S, Neglia V, Castano G, Frider B, Kien MC, Chohuela E. High prevalence of cutaneous reactions to interferon alfa plus ribavirin combination therapy in patients with chronic hepatitis C virus. Arch Dermatol 1999;135(8):1000–1.

417. Nathan PD, Gore ME, Eisen TG. Unexpected toxicity of combination thalidomide and interferon alpha-2a treatment in metastatic renal cell carcinoma. J Clin Oncol 2002;20(5):1429–30.

418. Israel BC, Blouin RA, McIntyre W, Shedlofsky SI. Effects of interferon-alpha monotherapy on hepatic drug metabolism in cancer patients. Br J Clin Pharmacol 1993;36(3):229–35.

419. Williams SJ, Baird-Lambert JA, Farrell GC. Inhibition of theophylline metabolism by interferon. Lancet 1987;2(8565):939–41.

420. Jonkman JH, Nicholson KG, Farrow PR, Eckert M, Grasmeijer G, Oosterhuis B, De Noord OE, Guentert TW. Effects of alpha-interferon on theophylline pharmacokinetics and metabolism. Br J Clin Pharmacol 1989;27(6):795–802.

421. Burger DM, Meenhorst PL, Koks CH, Beijnen JH. Drug interactions with zidovudine. AIDS 1993;7(4):445–60.

422. Krown SE, Gold JW, Niedzwiecki D, Bundow D, Flomenberg N, Gansbacher B, Brew BJ. Interferon-alpha with zidovudine: safety, tolerance, and clinical and virologic effects in patients with Kaposi sarcoma associated with the acquired immunodeficiency syndrome (AIDS). Ann Intern Med 1990;112(11):812–21.

423. Hoffmann RM, Ott S, Parhofer KG, Bartl R, Pape GR. Interferon-alpha-induced agranulocytosis in a patient on long-term clozapine therapy. J Hepatol 1998;29(1):170.

Interferon beta

General Information

Interferon beta is used in the form of natural fibroblast or recombinant preparations (interferon beta-1a and interferon beta-1b) and exerts antiviral and antiproliferative properties similar to those of interferon alfa. Although its efficacy has been debated (1), interferon beta has been approved for the treatment of relapsing–remitting multiple sclerosis, and more recently for secondary progressive multiple sclerosis.

The general toxicity of interferon beta is very similar to that of interferon alfa (2), with no apparent differences between the two recombinant preparations with any route of injection (SEDA-20, 332; 3–6). In multiple sclerosis, fatigue and a transient flu-like syndrome responsive to paracetamol or the combination of paracetamol plus prednisone have been observed in about 60% of patients during the first weeks of treatment, and tachyphylaxis usually developed after several doses (7). Patients with chronic progressive disease are more likely to discontinue treatment because of adverse effects (8).

Clinically relevant adverse effects associated with interferon beta and their management have been lengthily reviewed (9). Interferon beta-1a and beta-1b, the two recombinant available forms of interferon beta, have not been directly compared. From the results of a randomized, crossover study in 12 healthy volunteers, a single injection of interferon beta-1a 6 MU (Rebif) was suggested to produce less frequent and less severe fever than interferon beta-1b 8 MU (Betaseron), but identical pharmacodynamic effects (10).

A flu-like illness is the most common adverse effect of interferon beta. In an open, randomized study of the effects of paracetamol 1 g or ibuprofen 400 mg before and 6 hours after interferon beta injection on interferon beta-induced flu-like symptoms in 104 patients, the two drugs were equally effective (11).

Organs and Systems

Cardiovascular

Cardiovascular adverse effects of interferon beta include isolated reports of severe Raynaud's phenomenon (SEDA-22, 374) and acute myocarditis (SEDA-21, 374).

Fatal capillary leak syndrome has been reported (12).

- A 27-year-old woman had an 8-month history of relapsing–remitting neurological symptoms and a monoclonal gammopathy. She started to take interferon beta-1b for multiple sclerosis, but had marked somnolence 30 hours after a single injection. She rapidly became unresponsiveness, and hemodynamic tests showed low central venous and pulmonary capillary wedge pressures with generalized peripheral edema, ascites, and bilateral pleural effusions. She died within 80 hours after injection from multiple organ failure. At postmortem she was found to have C1 esterase inhibitor deficiency.

In the light of the possible effects of interferon beta on cytokine release and complement activation, a cytokine-mediated reaction was discussed as the cause of the capillary leak syndrome in this case.

Respiratory

Bronchiolitis obliterans with organizing pneumonia has been reported in a patient taking interferon beta (13).

- A 49-year-old man had a progressive unproductive cough and right hemithoracic pain after 3 months of interferon beta-1a 30 micrograms/week for multiple sclerosis. A CT scan showed a right basal pulmonary infiltrate and transbronchial biopsies showed features consistent with bronchiolitis obliterans with organizing pneumonia. The lesions resolved fully on interferon beta-1a withdrawal and prednisone treatment.

Nervous system

Although direct toxic effects of natural interferon beta on the nervous system have been regarded as a possible risk of intraventricular and/or intratumoral injection (14), interferon beta is considered to be markedly less neurotoxic than interferon alfa (15).

Although headache was not specifically identified as an adverse effect of interferon beta in pivotal trials, the frequency, duration, and intensity of headache increased during the first 6 months of treatment in 65 patients (16). There was a 35% probability of aggravated headaches in patients with pre-existing headaches.

The possible deleterious effects of interferon beta-1b on increased spasticity have been examined in 19 patients with primary progressive multiple sclerosis, 19 untreated matched patients, and 10 patients treated with interferon beta-1b for relapsing–remitting multiple sclerosis (17). Patients with primary progressive multiple sclerosis had frequent (68%) and clinically relevant increased spasticity (seven required oral baclofen), usually after about 2 months of treatment, whereas only two (11%) of the untreated patients and none of the patients with relapsing–remitting multiple sclerosis had similar disabling spasticity. Seven patients had to discontinue treatment after 6 months because of spasticity, and symptoms improved over several months after withdrawal. The authors suggested that this possible adverse effect should be taken into account in clinical trials because it could mask the positive clinical effects of interferon beta-1b.

Neurosarcoidosis has been reported in a patient with chronic hepatitis C who was treated with interferon beta.

- A 56-year-old woman developed numbness and difficulty in swallowing and in closing her left eye several weeks after starting interferon beta for chronic hepatitis C (18). She had facial paresthesia, a left facial nerve palsy, dysphagia, and signs of radiculopathy on the left side. Serum angiotensin-converting enzyme activity was raised. She had bilateral hilar lymphadenopathy without interstitial changes and increased radiogallium uptake in hilar lymph nodes and the parotid glands. Although the cerebrospinal fluid was normal, a diagnosis of neurosarcoidosis was considered, and she recovered completely after interferon beta withdrawal and glucocorticoid therapy.

Moderate exacerbation of multiple sclerosis sometimes occurs in the first 3 months of interferon beta treatment.

- A 21-year-old man had an acute and very severe clinical relapse, with multiple disseminated demyelinating lesions and axonal injury on MRI and cerebral biopsy, after the third injection of interferon beta-1a (19).

Whether this case was due to interferon beta or resulted from spontaneous exacerbation was open to question.

Sensory systems

Retinal complications of interferon alfa in chronic viral hepatitis patients are well known, but few cases have been described with interferon beta.

- Bilateral retinopathy with similar features to those observed with interferon alfa has been reported in a 40-year-old woman treated with interferon beta-1b for multiple sclerosis (20).

In 49 patients, there was reversible otological impairment with tinnitus, mild-to-moderate hearing loss, or both in respectively 8, 16, and 20% of patients after administration of interferon alfa or interferon beta (SEDA-19, 336). These disorders tended to occur more frequently in patients on high cumulative doses, but led to withdrawal of treatment in only two patients.

Psychological, psychiatric

There have been reports of depression, suicidal ideation, and attempted suicide in patients receiving interferon beta (2,8,21). The lifetime risk of depression in patients with multiple sclerosis is high, and there has been a lively debate about whether interferon beta causes or exacerbates depression in such patients. Impressions of a possibly raised incidence of depression among patients treated with interferon beta for multiple sclerosis should be interpreted in the light of the spontaneous tendency to depressive disorders and suicidal ideation, which is encountered even in patients with untreated multiple sclerosis. Moreover, no raised incidence of these complications has been recorded in some studies (4,5). A critical review of the methodological limitations in studies that assessed mood disorders in patients on disease-modifying drugs for multiple sclerosis may help explain the widely divergent results from one study to another (22). Some results have argued against a specific role of interferon beta in the risk of depressive disorders.

A multicenter comparison of 44 and 22 micrograms of interferon beta-1a and placebo in 365 patients showed no significant differences in depression scores between the groups over a 3-year period of follow-up (23). In 106 patients with relapsing–remitting multiple sclerosis, depression status was evaluated before and after 12 months of interferon beta-1a treatment (24). According to the Beck Depression Inventory II scale, most of the patients had minimum (53%) or mild (32%) depression at baseline, and depression scores were not significantly increased after 1 year of treatment. There were no cases of suicidal ideation. In another study of 42 patients treated with interferon beta-1b, major depression at baseline was found in 21% of patients and was associated with a past history of psychiatric illness in most cases (25). Major depression was not considered as an exclusion criterion for interferon beta treatment when patients were on antidepressant therapy. There was a three-fold reduction in the prevalence of depression over the 1-year course of interferon treatment, suggesting a possible beneficial effect of treatment on mood. Finally, a single subcutaneous injection of interferon beta-1b did not alter cognitive performance and mood states in eight healthy volunteers (26).

The emotional state of 90 patients with relapsing–remitting multiple sclerosis has been carefully assessed with a battery of psychological tests at baseline and after 1 and 2 years of treatment with interferon beta-1b (27). In contrast to what was expected, and despite the lack of controls, there was significant improvement in emotional state, as shown by significant reductions in scores of anxiety and depression over time. In addition, there was no effect of low-dose oral glucocorticoids in a subgroup of 46 patients.

Depression has been quantified by telephone interview in 56 patients with relapsing multiple sclerosis 2 weeks before treatment, at the start of treatment, and after 8 weeks of treatment (28). Patients with a high depressive score 2 weeks before treatment significantly improved on starting treatment and returned to baseline within 8 weeks, whereas the depression score in non-depressed patients remained essentially unchanged. The investigators therefore suggested that patients' expectations had temporarily resulted in improvement of depression, and that increased depression during treatment is more likely to reflect pretreatment depression.

The clinical features, management, and prognosis of psychiatric symptoms in patients with chronic hepatitis C have been reviewed using data from 943 patients treated with interferon alfa (85%) or interferon beta (15%) for 24 weeks (29). Interferon-induced psychiatric symptoms were identified in 40 patients (4.2%) of those referred for psychiatric examination. They were classified in three groups according to the clinical profile: 13 cases of generalized anxiety disorder (group A), 21 cases of mood disorders with depressive features (group B), and six cases of other psychiatric disorders, including psychotic disorders with delusions/hallucinations ($n = 4$), mood disorders with manic features ($n = 1$), and delirium ($n = 1$) (group C). The time to onset of the symptoms differed significantly between the three groups: 2 weeks in group A, 5 weeks in group B, and 11 weeks in group C. Women were more often affected than men. There was no difference in the incidence or nature of the disorder according to the type of interferon used. Whereas most patients who required psychotropic drugs were able to complete treatment, 10 had to discontinue interferon treatment because of severe psychiatric symptoms, five from group B and five from group C. Twelve patients still required psychiatric treatment for more than 6 months after interferon withdrawal. In addition, residual symptoms (anxiety, insomnia, and mild hypothymia) were still present at the end of the survey in seven patients. Delayed recovery was mostly observed in patients in group C and in patients treated with interferon beta.

One debatable case of visual pseudo-hallucinations occurred only, but not reproducibly, within 30–60 minutes after interferon beta-1a injection in a 37-year-old woman with disseminated encephalomyelitis (30).

Endocrine

While no evidence of thyroid dysfunction or antithyroid antibodies was found in 20 patients receiving interferon beta during 24 weeks for hematological malignancies (31), antithyroid antibodies were detected in 29% of patients with multiple sclerosis after a prospective follow-up performed at 6, 12, and 18 months of treatment (32). Biological thyroid abnormalities without antithyroid antibodies have also been found (SEDA-20, 332). Overall, thyroid disorders with antithyroid antibodies were reported in only three patients on long-term interferon beta treatment for multiple sclerosis (32,33).

Thyroid disorders before and during the first 9 months of interferon beta-1b treatment have been systematically investigated in eight patients with relapsing–remitting multiple sclerosis (34). Before treatment, one patient had positive thyroperoxidase antibodies and one was taking thyroxine for multinodular goiter. After 3 months three other patients developed sustained positive titers of thyroperoxidase antibodies, of whom one developed hypothyroidism after 9 months. These results are in accordance with a previous similar study and isolated case reports (SEDA-21, 374; SEDA-22, 405), and suggest that interferon beta, like interferon alfa, can cause thyroid autoimmunity.

As suggested in a more comprehensive long-term follow-up study, interferon beta-induced thyroid dysfunction is often transient or has limited clinical consequences (35). Of 31 patients with multiple sclerosis regularly assessed for 30–42 months for thyroid function, 13 developed thyroid disorders during treatment with interferon beta-1b. None withdrew because of thyroid disorders. Of the eight patients with no previous thyroid disorders, one had a persistent but isolated increase in antithyroglobulin titer, six developed transient signs of hypothyroidism or hyperthyroidism during the first year of therapy, and only one had overt hypothyroidism after 12 months of treatment and required thyroxine replacement. Of the five patients with baseline signs of Hashimoto's thyroiditis, one had a transiently positive antithyroglobulin titer, one developed transient hyperthyroidism, and the three patients who had previously had or who newly developed subclinical hypothyroidism remained stable throughout the study. Overall, thyroid disorders occurred only during the first 12 months of treatment and no additional cases were detected after the first year of therapy. In the authors' opinion, pre-existing or new thyroiditis is not a contraindication to continuing interferon beta-1b treatment. Two patients took thyroxine replacement and continued to receive interferon beta-1b (36).

Metabolism

Severe hypertriglyceridemia, a well-known adverse effect of interferon beta, has been reported and fully investigated in a 39-year-old man receiving interferon beta for chronic hepatitis C (37).

Hematologic

Moderate reductions in white blood cell count (that is lymphopenia, leukopenia, and granulocytopenia) have been observed with recombinant interferon beta, and marked eosinophilia recorded in an atopic patient (SEDA-21, 374).

- A 42-year-old woman developed aplastic anemia after using interferon beta-1a for 1 year (38). There was hematological improvement after withdrawal and immunosuppressive therapy.

Reversible autoimmune hemolytic anemia (SEDA-20, 332) has also been reported.

Liver

Adverse hepatic effects of interferon beta were usually limited to a dose-dependent increase in transaminases, but transient autoimmune hepatitis has been described in one patient (39).

It has been suspected that interferon beta can accelerate hepatocellular carcinoma (40).

- A 62-year-old man with severe chronic hepatitis and positive serum anti-HCV, HBs, and HBc antibodies underwent unsuccessful treatment with interferon alfa for 3 months and then received interferon beta for 6 months with a partial response. During treatment, his alfa-fetoprotein (normal before treatment) progressively increased to seven-fold the upper limit of the reference range. There was also a slight increase in interleukin-6 serum concentration. A hepatocellular carcinoma was diagnosed 9 months later.

Liver carcinoma is an unexpected consequence of interferon beta in patients with chronic hepatitis C. However, the authors cited other published Japanese reports of hepatocellular carcinoma during or after interferon treatment. It is worth noting that interferon beta, but not interferon alfa, significantly increased serum interleukin-

6 concentrations in patients with chronic hepatitis C (41), and that interleukin-6 has been suggested to promote the growth of hepatocellular carcinoma.

Fulminant liver failure has been attributed to interferon beta-1a (42), but it was subsequently confirmed that this case was confounded by concomitant exposure to nefazodone, which is hepatotoxic (43).

Urinary tract

Reversible hemolytic–uremic syndrome has been reported (SEDA-22, 405).

- Two women aged 24 and 44 years, whose primary diagnosis was relapsing multiple sclerosis, developed renal impairment and a thrombotic thrombocytopenic purpura-like syndrome within 2–4 weeks after starting interferon beta-1a (44). Thrombocytopenia and renal function normalized in the first patient, whereas the second patient had thrombotic angiopathy on renal biopsy and required dialysis while awaiting renal transplantation.

As interferon alfa has also been suggested to produce hemolytic–uremic syndrome with thrombotic thrombocytopenic purpura, it is tempting to speculate that either interferons or other cytokines may play a role in this syndrome.

Proteinuria, nephrotic syndrome, and various forms of renal lesions can be caused or exacerbated by interferon alfa (SED-14, 1252).

- Proteinuria with minimal–change nephrotic syndrome on renal biopsy has been attributed to interferon beta in a 64-year-old man with malignant melanoma (45). Although the proteinuria abated after withdrawal, the potential role of previous chemotherapy cannot be excluded.
- Nephrotic syndrome with segmental glomerulosclerosis has been reported in a 32-year-old woman with multiple sclerosis receiving interferon beta (46).

The clinicopathological features of proteinuria have been investigated in 23 patients with chronic hepatitis C who had new or worsened proteinuria during interferon treatment (interferon alfa 6–10 MU/day in three patients and interferon beta 6 MU/day in 20 patients (47). Renal function and urinary findings were normal before treatment in 21 subjects. Proteinuria appeared after a mean of 12 (range 5–30) days after the start of treatment, and the mean value was 2.1 g/day. There was low selective proteinuria in 78% of the patients. Renal histopathology in 11 patients showed IgA glomerulonephritis in five, mesangial proliferative glomerulonephritis in four, membranoproliferative glomerulonephritis in one, and nephrosclerosis in one. There was only trace deposition of hepatitis C virus core antigen in three of nine patients, suggesting that hepatitis C was not the primary cause of these glomerulopathies.

Skin

Injection-site reactions are common after subcutaneous injection of interferon beta-1b, and are more frequent than with any other available interferons. In a multicenter placebo-controlled trial, 65% of patients receiving interferon beta-1b had reactions at the injection site compared with 6% in the placebo group (2). In contrast, only 5% of those who received interferon beta-1a had injection site reactions (3). The clinical features of injection site reactions to interferon beta-1b mostly consist of benign inflammatory reactions, but they can sometimes be more severe, with sclerotic dermal plaques, painful erythematous nodules, and deep cutaneous ulcers with skin necrosis (SEDA-21, 374; 48). Late severe reactions have included a case of squamous cell carcinoma at the injection site (SEDA-21, 375) and a case of panniculitis (49).

Since interferon beta-1b became available, 1443 instances of injection site reactions, 212 cases of injection site necrosis, and 10 cases of non-injection site necrosis were notified to the US Food and Drug Administration, and antibiotic therapy or surgery was required in 20–30% of patients (50). Severe necrotizing cutaneous lesions have also been attributed to subcutaneous interferon beta-1a (51).

In contrast to previous claims, even low-dose interferon beta-1b can produce severe local reactions and cutaneous necrosis, with no recurrence after interferon alfa injection and expected better tolerance to interferon beta-1a (52–55). The mechanisms of interferon beta-induced local skin reaction might involve a local vascular inflammatory process or platelet-dependent thrombosis, but positive intracutaneous tests to interferon beta have also been found (56).

There have been other isolated reports of skin lesions.

- Intravascular papillary endothelial hyperplasia with multiple lesions on both hands has been attributed to interferon beta-1b in a 50-year-old man with multiple sclerosis (57).
- Granulomatous dermatitis with disseminated pruritic papules and histological features resembling those of sarcoid granulomas has been described in a 57-year-old man who received interferon beta-1b (58). The first lesions were observed after 2 months of treatment, persisted for 2 years, and slowly improved after interferon beta withdrawal and treatment with hydroxychloroquine PUVA.
- Erythromelalgia has been attributed to interferon beta-1a in a 38-year-old woman (59). Complete recovery was obtained only after interferon withdrawal.
- In one patient, there was cutaneous mucinosis on skin biopsy, and skin lesions persisted for several months before healing spontaneously (60).

Other reports include exacerbation of quiescent psoriasis or induction of psoriatic lesions at the injection sites (SED-13, 1099; SEDA-20, 332), and the development or exacerbation of lichen planus (SEDA-21, 375).

Musculoskeletal

Rhabdomyolysis associated with interferon beta has been reported (61).

- A 39-year-old man developed acute generalized myalgia and weakness in all four limbs 3 months after

starting interferon beta-1a (22 micrograms three times a week) for relapsing–remitting multiple sclerosis. Serum creatine kinase activity peaked at about 95 times the upper limit of the reference range. Infectious and metabolic causes were ruled out and there was no argument in favor of an underlying metabolic muscle disorder. He recovered fully after interferon beta withdrawal and supportive treatment.

Although rhabdomyolysis has not been previously attributed to interferon beta, this case is in keeping with those described with interferon alfa.

- A 39-year-old man developed monoarthritis in his right elbow after receiving interferon beta for 16 days for chronic hepatitis C (62).

Although the arthritis resolved after withdrawal, this report casts doubt on the causal relation, as there was no recurrence on re-administration.

Reproductive system

Mild to moderate menstrual disorders were twice as frequent in patients receiving interferon beta compared with placebo (17 versus 8%). Severe persistent vaginal bleeding has been reported in a 19-year-old woman (SEDA-21, 375).

Immunologic

Hypersensitivity reactions
Hypersensitivity reactions to interferon beta are rare, with only two cases of immediate-type reactions (SEDA-20, 332; 63), and one case of urticaria associated with exacerbation of asthma (64).

- A 21-year-old woman had a severe anaphylactic-like reaction with laryngospasm and undetectable blood pressure within 10 minutes after interferon beta-1a injection (63). It is still uncertain that anaphylaxis was definitely attributable to interferon, because rechallenge and skin tests were not performed in this patient, who had tolerated the treatment for the 6 previous months.
- Urticaria developed after 9 months of treatment with interferon beta-1b in a 32-year-old woman with a previous history of penicillin allergy (64). She also had an exacerbation of asthma shortly after starting treatment. A positive intradermal test to interferon beta-1b, but not to interferon beta-1a or the diluents, suggested a specific IgE allergic reaction.

Another isolated case history has suggested that interferon beta-1b might have favored the development of a non-IgE-mediated anaphylactic reaction to previously well-tolerated injections of methylprednisolone (65).

Autoimmune disorders
In contrast to interferon alfa, the autoimmune consequences of interferon beta treatment have been poorly evaluated. Interferon beta does not appear to be associated with the appearance or increased titres of several auto-antibodies, and no clinical features of autoimmune

disease were observed in patients receiving a 6-month course of interferon beta-1a or interferon beta-1b (66,67).

Subcutaneous lupus erythematosus reversible on withdrawal of treatment (SEDA-22, 405) and myasthenia gravis (SEDA-21, 375) have been described, but each only in a single patient receiving interferon beta.

The possible involvement of interferon beta in the occurrence of sarcoidosis has been noted in two patients (68,69).

Interferon beta antibodies

In multiple sclerosis, neutralizing antibodies to recombinant interferon beta occurred in 12–38% of patients treated for 2–3 years (3–5,70). There were no adverse consequences in patients who developed antibodies to interferon beta-1a (4), but there was reduced therapeutic efficacy in terms of clinical relapse rate or magnetic resonance imaging in several patients who had neutralizing antibodies to interferon beta-1b (SEDA-20, 332; 5,71).

The systemic availability of interferon beta-1b, measured by a myxovirus protein A assay, was completely inhibited in patients with neutralizing antibodies (72). The presence of increased titers of serum-binding antibodies increased the likelihood of neutralizing antibodies. From an in vitro study of nine patients who developed neutralizing antibodies against the available formulations of recombinant interferon beta (three on interferon beta-1a and six on interferon beta-1b), it appears that these antibodies systematically cross-react in both binding and biological assays (73). Although the sample size was small and lacked clinical confirmation, these results suggest that clinical benefit will not be obtained by switching to an alternative formulation when the absence of response or relapse during treatment is due to neutralizing antibodies.

The clinical significance of these antibodies is uncertain (74) and it has been proposed that decisions to discontinue treatment should be based on individual clinical responses and unequivocal demonstration of neutralizing antibodies with a reliable assay (70).

One study has shown that antibodies can spontaneously disappear in patients receiving long-term treatment. Of 24 of 51 patients who initially developed neutralizing antibodies, generally during the first year of treatment, only five still had antibodies after a mean treatment duration of 102 months (75). The mean time to antibody disappearance was 20 months.

A randomized study has been conducted in 161 patients to evaluate whether a monthly intravenous pulse of methylprednisolone reduces the frequency of neutralizing antibodies to interferon beta-1b (76). The patients who received both interferon beta and methylprednisolone had a 55% relative reduction in the development of neutralizing antibody and were significantly more likely to remain negative for neutralizing antibodies after 6 months of treatment compared with those who received interferon beta alone. The overall frequency of adverse effects and the number of withdrawals were similar between the groups, but headaches, fatigue, and myalgia were less frequent in the combination therapy group. A limitation of this study was that there was no difference in clinical outcome between the two groups.

Finally, possible differences in the immunogenic potential of recombinant and natural interferon beta preparations were found in a small study (77).

Second-Generation Effects

Teratogenicity

Data on outcomes in pregnancy after treatment with interferon beta-1a in patients with multiple sclerosis have been obtained from clinical trials (78). Of 29 pregnancies that occurred during or shortly after treatment withdrawal, 13 resulted in normal outcomes, two in premature births, one in fetal death, six in induced abortions, and seven in spontaneous abortions.

- A child whose mother had received interferon beta until 2.5 months before pregnancy had a right incomplete double renal pelvis and ureter (79). Although the authors discussed the possible role of interferon therapy, the timing of exposure was obviously not suggestive of a causal relation.

Although the data are still very limited, it is advisable to reassure exposed patients and to withdraw interferon beta up to the time of delivery.

Drug Administration

Drug dosage regimens

In 188 patients with relapsing–remitting multiple sclerosis assigned to receive interferon beta-1a 30 micrograms intramuscularly once a week or interferon beta-1b 44 micrograms subcutaneously three times a week, only injection site reactions and neutralizing antibodies to interferon beta were significantly more frequent in the interferon beta-1b group (80). These differences were probably related to the subcutaneous route of administration of interferon beta-1b. In contrast, there were significant differences in favor of interferon beta-1b for clinical outcomes after 2 years of treatment.

In a comparison of two regimens of interferon beta-1a (44 micrograms Rebif subcutaneously three times a week versus 30 micrograms Avonex intramuscularly once a week) in 677 patients with relapsing–remitting multiple sclerosis, Rebif was more effective on primary clinical outcomes (patients remaining relapse-free at 24 weeks), but produced significantly more frequent injection site reactions (88 versus 28%), asymptomatic and mild liver enzyme abnormalities (18 versus 9%), mild white cell abnormalities (11 versus 5%), and neutralizing antibodies to interferon beta (25 versus 2%) (81). However, the severity of adverse events and withdrawal due to an adverse event were similar in both groups.

Drug–Drug Interactions

Theophylline

Interferon beta reduced theophylline clearance by 29% in seven patients (SED-13, 1099).

References

1. Anonymous. Euromedicines evaluation: the striptease begins. Lancet 1996;347(9000):483(see also Harvey P. Why interferon beta 1b was licensed is a mystery. BMJ 1996;313(7052):297–8 and Napier JC. Reputation of interferon beta-1b. Lancet 1996;347(9006):968).

2. The IFNB Multiple Sclerosis Study GroupThe University of British Columbia MS/MRI Analysis Group. Interferon beta-1b in the treatment of multiple sclerosis: final outcome of the randomized controlled trial. Neurology 1995;45(7):1277–85.

3. Jacobs LD, Cookfair DL, Rudick RA, Herndon RM, Richert JR, Salazar AM, Fischer JS, Goodkin DE, Granger CV, Simon JH, Alam JJ, Bartoszak DM, Bourdette DN, Braiman J, Brownscheidle CM, Coats ME, Cohan SL, Dougherty DS, Kinkel RP, Mass MK, Munschauer FE 3rd, Priore RL, Pullicino PM, Scherokman BJ, Whitham RH, et al. Intramuscular interferon beta-1a for disease progression in relapsing multiple sclerosis. The Multiple Sclerosis Collaborative Research Group (MSCRG). Ann Neurol 1996;39(3):285–94.

4. Ebers GC, Hommes O, Hughes RAC, et alPRISMS (Prevention of Relapses and Disability by Interferon beta-1a Subcutaneously in Multiple Sclerosis) Study Group. Randomised double-blind placebo-controlled study of interferon beta-1a in relapsing/remitting multiple sclerosis. Lancet 1998;352(9139):1498–504.

5. European Study Group on Interferon Beta-1b in Secondary Progressive MS. Placebo-controlled multicentre randomised trial of interferon beta-1b in treatment of secondary progressive multiple sclerosis. Lancet 1998;352(9139):1491–7.

6. Weinstock-Guttman B, Rudick RA. Prescribing recommendations for interferon-beta in multiple sclerosis. CNS Drugs 1997;8:102–12.

7. Rio J, Nos C, Marzo ME, Tintore M, Montalban X. Low-dose steroids reduce flu-like symptoms at the initiation of IFNbeta-1b in relapsing-remitting MS. Neurology 1998;50(6):1910–2.

8. Neilley LK, Goodin DS, Goodkin DE, Hauser SL. Side effect profile of interferon beta-1b in MS: results of an open label trial. Neurology 1996;46(2):552–4.

9. Bayas A, Rieckmann P. Managing the adverse effects of interferon-beta therapy in multiple sclerosis. Drug Saf 2000;22(2):149–59.

10. Buraglio M, Trinchard-Lugan I, Munafo A, Macnamee M. Recombinant human interferon-beta-1a (Rebif) vs recombinant interferon-beta-1b (Betaseron) in healthy volunteers. A pharmacodynamic and tolerability study. Clin Drug Invest 1999;18:27–34.

11. Reess J, Haas J, Gabriel K, Fuhlrott A, Fiola M, Schicklmaier P. Both paracetamol and ibuprofen are equally effective in managing flu-like symptoms in relapsing-remitting multiple sclerosis patients during interferon beta-1a (AVONEX) therapy. Mult Scler 2002;8(1):15–8.

12. Schmidt S, Hertfelder HJ, von Spiegel T, Hering R, Harzheim M, Lassmann H, Deckert-Schluter M, Schlegel U. Lethal capillary leak syndrome after a single

13. administration of interferon beta-1b. Neurology 1999;53(1):220–2.

13. Ferriby D, Stojkovic T. Clinical picture: bronchiolitis obliterans with organising pneumonia during interferon beta-1a treatment. Lancet 2001;357(9258):751.

14. Matsumura S, Takamatsu H, Sato S, Ara S. [Central nervous system toxicity of local interferon-beta therapy. Report of three cases.]Neurol Med Chir (Tokyo) 1988;28(3):265–70.

15. Liberati AM, Biagini S, Perticoni G, Ricci S, D'Alessandro P, Senatore M, Cinieri S. Electrophysiological and neuropsychological functions in patients treated with interferon-beta. J Interferon Res 1990;10(6):613–9.

16. Pollmann W, Erasmus LP, Feneberg W, Then Bergh F, Straube A. Interferon beta but not glatiramer acetate therapy aggravates headaches in MS. Neurology 2002;59(4):636–9.

17. Bramanti P, Sessa E, Rifici C, D'Aleo G, Floridia D, Di Bella P, Lublin F. Enhanced spasticity in primary progressive MS patients treated with interferon beta-1b. Neurology 1998;51(6):1720–3.

18. Miwa H, Furuya T, Tanaka S, Mizuno Y. Neurosarcoidosis associated with interferon therapy. Eur Neurol 2001;45(4):288–9.

19. Von Raison F, Abboud H, Saint Val C, Brugieres P, Cesaro P. Acute demyelinating disease after interferon beta-1a treatment for multiple sclerosis. Neurology 2000;55(9):1416–7.

20. Sommer S, Sablon JC, Zaoui M, Rozot P, Hosni A. Rétinopathie à l'interféron bêta au cours d'une sclérose en plaques. [Interferon beta-1b retinopathy during a treatment for multiple sclerosis.] J Fr Ophtalmol 2001;24(5):509–12.

21. Lublin FD, Whitaker JN, Eidelman BH, Miller AE, Arnason BG, Burks JS. Management of patients receiving interferon beta-1b for multiple sclerosis: report of a consensus conference. Neurology 1996;46(1):12–8.

22. Feinstein A. Multiple sclerosis, disease modifying treatments and depression: a critical methodological review. Mult Scler 2000;6(5):343–8.

23. Patten SB, Metz LMSPECTRIMS Study Group. Interferon beta1a and depression in secondary progressive MS: data from the SPECTRIMS Trial. Neurology 2002;59(5):744–6.

24. Zephir H, De Seze J, Stojkovic T, Delisse B, Ferriby D, Cabaret M, Vermersch P. Multiple sclerosis and depression: influence of interferon beta therapy. Mult Scler 2003;9(3):284–8.

25. Feinstein A, O'Connor P, Feinstein K. Multiple sclerosis, interferon beta-1b and depression. A prospective investigation. J Neurol 2002;249(7):815–20.

26. Exton MS, Baase J, Pithan V, Goebel MU, Limmroth V, Schedlowski M. Neuropsychological performance and mood states following acute interferon-beta-1b administration in healthy males. Neuropsychobiology 2002;45(4):199–204.

27. Borras C, Rio J, Porcel J, Barrios M, Tintore M, Montalban X. Emotional state of patients with relapsing-remitting MS treated with interferon beta-1b. Neurology 1999;52(8):1636–9.

28. Mohr DC, Likosky W, Dwyer P, Van Der Wende J, Boudewyn AC, Goodkin DE. Course of depression during the initiation of interferon beta-1a treatment for multiple sclerosis. Arch Neurol 1999;56(10):1263–5.

29. Hosoda S, Takimura H, Shibayama M, Kanamura H, Ikeda K, Kumada H. Psychiatric symptoms related to interferon therapy for chronic hepatitis C: clinical features and prognosis. Psychiatry Clin Neurosci 2000;54(5):565–72.

30. Moor CC, Berwanger C, Welter FL. Visual pseudo-hallucinations in interferon-beta 1a therapy. Akt Neurol 2002;29:355–7.

31. Pagliacci MC, Pelicci G, Schippa M, Liberati AM, Nicoletti I. Does interferon-beta therapy induce thyroid autoimmune phenomena? Horm Metab Res 1991; 23(4):196–7.

32. Martinelli V, Gironi M, Rodegher M, Martino G, Comi G. Occurrence of thyroid autoimmunity in relapsing remitting multiple sclerosis patients undergoing interferon-beta treatment. Ital J Neurol Sci 1998;19(2):65–7.

33. Schwid SR, Goodman AD, Mattson DH. Autoimmune hyperthyroidism in patients with multiple sclerosis treated with interferon beta-1b. Arch Neurol 1997;54(9):1169–90.

34. Rotondi M, Oliviero A, Profice P, Mone CM, Biondi B, Del Buono A, Mazziotti G, Sinisi AM, Bellastella A, Carella C. Occurrence of thyroid autoimmunity and dysfunction throughout a nine-month follow-up in patients undergoing interferon-beta therapy for multiple sclerosis. J Endocrinol Invest 1998;21(11):748–52.

35. Monzani F, Caraccio N, Casolaro A, Lombardo F, Moscato G, Murri L, Ferrannini E, Meucci G. Long-term interferon beta-1b therapy for MS: is routine thyroid assessment always useful? Neurology 2000;55(4):549–52.

36. McDonald ND, Pender MP. Autoimmune hypothyroidism associated with interferon beta-1b treatment in two patients with multiple sclerosis. Aust NZ J Med 2000;30(2):278–9.

37. Homma Y, Kawazoe K, Ito T, Ide H, Takahashi H, Ueno F, Matsuzaki S. Chronic hepatitis C beta-interferon-induced severe hypertriglyceridaemia with apolipoprotein E phenotype E3/2. Int J Clin Pract 2000;54(4):212–6.

38. Aslam AK, Singh T. Aplastic anemia associated with interferon beta-1a. Am J Ther 2002;9(6):522–3.

39. Durelli L, Bongioanni MR, Ferrero B, Oggero A, Marzano A, Rizzetto M. Interferon treatment for multiple sclerosis: autoimmune complications may be lethal. Neurology 1998;50(2):570–1.

40. Malaguarnera M, Restuccia S, Di Fazio I, Di Marco R, Pistone G, Trovato BA. Rapid evolution of chronic viral hepatitis into hepatocellular carcinoma after beta-interferon treatment. Panminerva Med 1999;41(1):59–61.

41. Furusyo N, Hayashi J, Ohmiya M, Sawayama Y, Kawakami Y, Ariyama I, Kinukawa N, Kashiwagi S. Differences between interferon-alpha and -beta treatment for patients with chronic hepatitis C virus infection. Dig Dis Sci 1999;44(3):608–17.

42. Yoshida EM, Rasmussen SL, Steinbrecher UP, Erb SR, Scudamore CH, Chung SW, Oger JJ, Hashimoto SA. Fulminant liver failure during interferon beta treatment of multiple sclerosis. Neurology 2001;56(10):1416.

43. Francis GS, Grumser Y, Alteri E, Micaleff A, O'Brien F, Alsop J, Stam Moraga M, Kaplowitz N. Hepatic reactions during treatment of multiple sclerosis with interferon-beta-1a: incidence and clinical significance. Drug Saf 2003;26(11):815–27.

44. Herrera WG, Balizet LB, Harberts SW, Brown ST. Occurrence of a TTP-like syndrome in two women receiving beta interferon therapy for relapsing multiple sclerosis. Neurology 1999;52:135.

45. Nakao K, Sugiyama H, Makino E, Matsuura H, Ohmoto A, Sugimoto T, Ichikawa H, Wada J, Yamasaki Y, Makino H. Minimal change nephrotic syndrome developing during postoperative interferon-beta therapy for malignant melanoma. Nephron 2002;90(4):498–500.

46. Gotsman I, Elhallel-Darnitski M, Friedlander Z, Haviv YS. Beta-interferon-induced nephrotic syndrome in a patient with multiple sclerosis. Clin Nephrol 2000;54(5):425–6.

47. Ohta S, Yokoyama H, Wada T, Sakai N, Shimizu M, Kato T, Furuichi K, Segawa C, Hisada Y, Kobayashi K. Exacerbation of glomerulonephritis in subjects with chronic hepatitis C virus infection after interferon therapy. Am J Kidney Dis 1999;33(6):1040–8.

48. Elgart GW, Sheremata W, Ahn YS. Cutaneous reactions to recombinant human interferon beta-1b: the clinical and histologic spectrum. J Am Acad Dermatol 1997;37(4):553–8.

49. Heinzerling L, Dummer R, Burg G, Schmid-Grendelmeier P. Panniculitis after subcutaneous injection of interferon beta in a multiple sclerosis patient. Eur J Dermatol 2002;12(2):194–7.

50. Gaines AR, Varricchio F. Interferon beta-1b injection site reactions and necroses. Mult Scler 1998;4(2):70–3.

51. Radziwill AJ, Courvoisier S. Severe necrotising cutaneous lesions complicating treatment with interferon beta-1a. J Neurol Neurosurg Psychiatry 1999;67(1):115.

52. Berard F, Canillot S, Balme B, Perrot H. Nécrose cutanée locale après injections d'interféron béta. [Local cutaneous necrosis after injection of interferon beta.] Ann Dermatol Venereol 1995;122(3):105–7.

53. Sheremata WA, Taylor JR, Elgart GW. Severe necrotizing cutaneous lesions complicating treatment with interferon beta-1b. N Engl J Med 1995;332(23):1584.

54. Benincasa P, Bielory L. Necrotizing cutaneous lesions as a complication of subcutaneous interferon beta-1b. J Allergy Clin Immunol 1996;97:343.

55. Webster GF, Knobler RL, Lublin FD, Kramer EM, Hochman LR. Cutaneous ulcerations and pustular psoriasis flare caused by recombinant interferon beta injections in patients with multiple sclerosis. J Am Acad Dermatol 1996;34(2 Pt 2):365–7.

56. Feldmann R, Low-Weiser H, Duschet P, Gschnait F. Necrotizing cutaneous lesions caused by interferon beta injections in a patient with multiple sclerosis. Dermatology 1997;195(1):52–3.

57. Durieu C, Bayle-Lebey P, Gadroy A, Loche F, Bazex J. Hyperplasie endothéliale papillaire intravasculaire: multiples lésions apparues au cours d'un traitement par interféron bêta. [Intravascular papillary endothelial hyperplasia: multiple lesions appearing in the course of treatment with interferon beta.] Ann Dermatol Venereol 2001;128(12):1336–8.

58. Mehta CL, Tyler RJ, Cripps DJ. Granulomatous dermatitis with focal sarcoidal features associated with recombinant interferon beta-1b injections. J Am Acad Dermatol 1998;39(6):1024–8.

59. Demirkaya S, Bulucu F, Odabasi Z, Vural O. An erythromelalgia case occurred during interferon beta treatment for multiple sclerosis. Eur J Neurol 2002;9(Suppl 2):220.

60. Benito-Leon J, Borbujo J, Cortes L. Cutaneous mucinoses complicating interferon beta-1b therapy. Eur Neurol 2002;47(2):123–4.

61. Lunemann JD, Schwarzenberger B, Kassim N, Zschenderlein R, Zipp F. Rhabdomyolysis during interferon-beta 1a treatment. J Neurol Neurosurg Psychiatry 2002;72(2):274.

62. Murata K, Shiraki K, Takase K, Nakano T, Tameda Y. Mono-arthritis following intensified interferon beta therapy for chronic hepatitis C. Hepatogastroenterology 2002;49(47):1418–9.

63. Corona T, Leon C, Ostrosky-Zeichner L. Severe anaphylaxis with recombinant interferon beta. Neurology 1999;52(2):425.

64. Brown DL, Login IS, Borish L, Powers PL. An urticarial IgE-mediated reaction to interferon beta-1b. Neurology 2001;56(10):1416–7.

65. Clear D. Anaphylactoid reaction to methyl prednisolone developing after starting treatment with interferon beta-1b. J Neurol Neurosurg Psychiatry 1999;66(5):690.

66. Colosimo C, Pozzilli C, Frontoni M, Farina D, Koudriavtseva T, Gasperini C, Salvetti M, Valesini G. No increase of serum autoantibodies during therapy with recombinant human interferon-beta1a in relapsing-remitting multiple sclerosis. Acta Neurol Scand 1997;96(6):372–374.

67. Kivisakk P, Lundahl J, von Heigl Z, Fredrikson S. No evidence for increased frequency of autoantibodies during interferon-beta1b treatment of multiple sclerosis. Acta Neurol Scand 1998;97(5):320–3.

68. Abdi EA, Nguyen GK, Ludwig RN, Dickout WJ. Pulmonary sarcoidosis following interferon therapy for advanced renal cell carcinoma. Cancer 1987;59(5):896–900.

69. Bobbio-Pallavicini E, Valsecchi C, Tacconi F, Moroni M, Porta C. Sarcoidosis following beta-interferon therapy for multiple myeloma. Sarcoidosis 1995;12(2):140–2.

70. The IFNB Multiple Sclerosis Study Group and the University of British Columbia MS/MRI Analysis Group. Neutralizing antibodies during treatment of multiple sclerosis with interferon beta-1b: experience during the first three years. Neurology 1996;47(4):889–94.

71. Rudick RA, Simonian NA, Alam JA, Campion M, Scaramucci JO, Jones W, Coats ME, Goodkin DE, Weinstock-Guttman B, Herndon RM, Mass MK, Richert JR, Salazar AM, Munschauer FE 3rd, Cookfair DL, Simon JH, Jacobs LD. Incidence and significance of neutralizing antibodies to interferon beta-1a in multiple sclerosis. Multiple Sclerosis Collaborative Research Group (MSCRG). Neurology 1998;50(5):1266–72.

72. Deisenhammer F, Reindl M, Harvey J, Gasse T, Dilitz E, Berger T. Bioavailability of interferon beta 1b in MS patients with and without neutralizing antibodies. Neurology 1999;52(6):1239–43.

73. Khan OA, Dhib-Jalbut SS. Neutralizing antibodies to interferon beta-1a and interferon beta-1b in MS patients are cross-reactive. Neurology 1998;51(6):1698–702.

74. Cross AH, Antel JP. Antibodies to beta-interferons in multiple sclerosis: can we neutralize the controversy? Neurology 1998;50(5):1206–8.

75. Rice GP, Paszner B, Oger J, Lesaux J, Paty D, Ebers G. The evolution of neutralizing antibodies in multiple sclerosis patients treated with interferon beta-1b. Neurology 1999;52(6):1277–9.

76. Pozzilli C, Antonini G, Bagnato F, Mainero C, Tomassini V, Onesti E, Fantozzi R, Galgani S, Pasqualetti P, Millefiorini E, Spadaro M, Dahlke F, Gasperini C. Monthly corticosteroids decrease neutralizing antibodies to IFNbeta1 b: a randomized trial in multiple sclerosis. J Neurol 2002;249(1):50–6.

77. Fierlbeck G, Schreiner T. Incidence and clinical significance of therapy-induced neutralizing antibodies against interferon-beta. J Interferon Res 1994;14(4):205–6.

78. Sanberg-Wollhheim M. Outcome of pregnancy during treatment with interferon-beta-1a (Rebif) in patients with multiple sclerosis. Neurology 2002;58(Suppl):A445–6.

79. Watanabe M, Kohge N, Akagi S, Uchida Y, Sato S, Kinoshita Y. Congenital anomalies in a child born from a mother with interferon-treated chronic hepatitis B. Am J Gastroenterol 2001;96(5):1668–9.

80. Durelli L, Verdun E, Barbero P, Bergui M, Versino E, Ghezzi A, Montanari E, Zaffaroni MIndependent Comparison of Interferon (INCOMIN) Trial Study Group. Every-other-day interferon beta-1b versus once-weekly interferon beta-1a for multiple sclerosis: results of a 2-year prospective randomised multicentre study (INCOMIN). Lancet 2002;359(9316):1453–60.

81. Panitch H, Goodin DS, Francis G, Chang P, Coyle PK, O'Connor P, Monaghan E, Li D, Weinshenker BEVIDENCE Study Group. EVidence of Interferon Dose-response: Europian North American Compartative Efficacy; University of British Columbia MS/MRI Research Group. Randomized, comparative study of interferon beta-1a treatment regimens in MS: The EVIDENCE Trial. Neurology 2002;59(10):1496–506.

Interferon gamma

General Information

Recombinant interferon gamma (interferon gamma-1b) is currently only approved as an adjunct to antibacterial therapy in chronic granulomatous disease (1), but its immunoregulatory potential has been investigated in other diseases. Clinical experience with interferon gamma is therefore limited and the most relevant information on long-term safety has been obtained from the ICGDSCG trial (2). In this study, adverse effects that were significantly more frequent with interferon gamma-1b (1.5 micrograms/kg or 50 micrograms/m^2) than with placebo included mild fever and flu-like symptoms, headache, and moderate injection site reactions. There were no adverse consequences on growth and development in children followed for a mean of 2.5 years (3,4). Several other adverse effects have been reported to the manufacturers, but causal evaluation is lacking (1).

Interferon gamma has been investigated in 27 patients with systemic sclerosis randomized to receive interferon gamma for 12 months. Most of them complained of symptoms consistent with a flu-like syndrome, namely headache (85%), fever (81%), and arthralgia and myalgia (70%) (5). There were adverse events (one or more per patient) leading to treatment withdrawal in four cases, including arthralgia, cardiac pain, atrioventricular block, reversible loss of hearing, and impotence; however, a causal relation with interferon gamma was not documented.

Organs and Systems

Cardiovascular

Heart rate, ventricular or supraventricular extra beats, and asymptomatic cardiac events were not significantly different during treatment compared with baseline in 20 patients receiving interferon gamma (6). Interferon gamma rarely produced cardiovascular adverse effects. Hypotension, dysrhythmias, and possible coronary spasm were sometimes observed, mostly in patients receiving high doses or with previous cardiovascular disorders (SEDA-20, 333; SEDA-22, 405; 7,8).

Exacerbation of Raynaud's syndrome occurred in five of 20 patients with systemic sclerosis treated with interferon gamma (SEDA-20, 333).

Respiratory

Of 10 patients treated with interferon gamma-1b 200 micrograms three times a week for advanced idiopathic pulmonary fibrosis, four developed irreversible acute respiratory failure (9). All four patients had increasing dyspnea, fever, and rapidly progressive hypoxemia, and had new alveolar opacities on lung imaging. The symptoms occurred shortly after interferon gamma had been started in three patients, and after 35 injections in the fourth. Three patients died from refractory hypoxemia and the fourth underwent lung transplantation, but died a few weeks later. Pathological examination in two patients showed diffuse alveolar damage with pre-existing interstitial pneumonitis. Interferon gamma was suspected, as no other cause of abrupt pulmonary deterioration was found. Although the number of patients was small, the authors noted that before interferon beta pulmonary function tended to be worse in the four patients who developed acute respiratory failure than in the other six.

Psychological, psychiatric

Neuropsychiatric disturbances have not been consistently found in patients receiving interferon gamma, despite electroencephalographic monitoring and psychometric tests (10). However, careful examination led to the impression that interferon gamma can cause neurophysiological changes similar to those of interferon alfa (11), and data from the manufacturers also point to rare cases of nervous system adverse effects in patients treated with high-dose interferon gamma (1).

Endocrine

Interferon gamma can increase serum cortisol concentrations (12).

Metabolism

Reversible dose-dependent hypertriglyceridemia has been attributed to interferon gamma (13).

Hyperglycemia, reversible on interferon gamma withdrawal and a short course of insulin, has been reported in one patient (SEDA-22, 406).

Hematologic

Interferon gamma was supposedly the cause of asymptomatic non-immune hemolytic anemia in one patient receiving both interleukin-2 and interferon gamma (14).

Only minimal effects of interferon gamma on white blood cell counts have been observed (15).

Auto-immune thrombocytopenia occurred in a patient receiving interferon gamma (SEDA-22, 406).

Gastrointestinal

A convincing case of severe aphthous stomatitis has been reported in a patient receiving interferon gamma (SEDA-20, 333).

Urinary tract

Dose-related asymptomatic proteinuria was sometimes observed, and severe proteinuria with nephrotic syndrome has been reported once after low-dose interferon gamma (SED-13, 1100). Acute renal insufficiency is extremely rare (SEDA-20, 333; 16).

Skin

Induction of psoriatic lesions at the injection site has been observed in 10 of 42 patients treated with interferon gamma for psoriatic arthritis, while the joint symptoms were improved (17).

Single or multiple lesions of erythema nodosum leprosum occurred in 60% of patients given intradermal interferon gamma for lepromatous leprosy, and severe systemic symptoms required thalidomide treatment in two patients (18).

Severe erythroderma was observed in five of 10 patients after interferon gamma was added to ciclosporin for autologous bone marrow transplantation (19).

Immunologic

An anaphylactoid reaction and severe bronchospasm have been reported once after the first injection of interferon gamma (10).

Although interferon gamma is mainly used for its immunoregulatory properties, the possibility of clinical immune adverse consequences has been addressed in a limited number of prospective studies. In two studies involving patients with chronic hepatitis B treated for 4–6 months, most developed a new autoantibody (20,21), but none developed clinical evidence of autoimmune disease. However, other reports suggested that interferon gamma can either improve or aggravate immune or inflammatory conditions. Although no change in antinuclear antibodies was reported in a trial of 54 patients with rheumatoid arthritis (22), increased or new antinuclear antibodies were observed in three of six patients with rheumatoid arthritis who received interferon gamma for 2–8 months, and two patients had clinical exacerbations of the disease (23). Isolated cases of systemic lupus erythematosus have been reported in patients receiving interferon gamma for rheumatoid arthritis (24,25). Rheumatoid or lupus-like symptoms associated with raised antinuclear antibodies titers were also noted in 17% of patients receiving interferon alfa and interferon gamma for myeloproliferative disorders, and in only 8.3% of patients treated with interferon alfa alone (26). Interferon gamma was also involved in the induction or reactivation of seronegative arthritis in patients with cutaneous psoriasis (27) and the unexpected exacerbation of multiple sclerosis in 39% of patients (28). Finally, neutralizing antibodies have exceptionally been found (SEDA-20, 333).

References

1. Todd PA, Goa KL. Interferon gamma-1b. A review of its pharmacology and therapeutic potential in chronic granulomatous disease. Drugs 1992;43(1):111–22.

2. The International Chronic Granulomatous Disease Cooperative Study Group. A controlled trial of interferon gamma to prevent infection in chronic granulomatous disease. N Engl J Med 1991;324(8):509–16.

3. Bemiller LS, Roberts DH, Starko KM, Curnutte JT. Safety and effectiveness of long-term interferon gamma therapy in patients with chronic granulomatous disease. Blood Cells Mol Dis 1995;21(3):239–47.

4. Weening RS, Leitz GJ, Seger RA. Recombinant human interferon-gamma in patients with chronic granulomatous disease—European follow up study. Eur J Pediatr 1995;154(4):295–8.

5. Grassegger A, Schuler G, Hessenberger G, Walder-Hantich B, Jabkowski J, MacHeiner W, Salmhofer W, Zahel B, Pinter G, Herold M, Klein G, Fritsch PO. Interferon-gamma in the treatment of systemic sclerosis: a randomized controlled multicentre trial. Br J Dermatol 1998;139(4):639–48.

6. Friess GG, Brown TD, Wrenn RC. Cardiovascular rhythm effects of gamma recombinant DNA interferon. Invest New Drugs 1989;7(2–3):275–80.

7. Sonnenblick M, Rosin A. Cardiotoxicity of interferon. A review of 44 cases. Chest 1991;99(3):557–61.

8. Yamamoto N, Nishigaki K, Ban Y, Kawada Y. Coronary vasospasm after interferon administration. Br J Urol 1998;81(6):916–7.

9. Honore I, Nunes H, Groussard O, Kambouchner M, Chambellan A, Aubier M, Valeyre D, Crestani B. Acute respiratory failure after interferon-gamma therapy of end-stage pulmonary fibrosis. Am J Respir Crit Care Med 2003;167(7):953–7.

10. Mattson K, Niiranen A, Pyrhonen S, Farkkila M, Cantell K. Recombinant interferon gamma treatment in non-small cell lung cancer. Antitumour effect and cardiotoxicity. Acta Oncol 1991;30(5):607–10.

11. Born J, Spath-Schwalbe E, Pietrowsky R, Porzsolt F, Fehm HL. Neurophysiological effects of recombinant interferon-gamma and -alpha in man. Clin Physiol Biochem 1989;7(3–4):119–27.

12. Krishnan R, Ellinwood EH Jr, Laszlo J, Hood L, Ritchie J. Effect of gamma interferon on the hypothalamic–pituitary–adrenal system. Biol Psychiatry 1987;22(9):1163–6.

13. Kurzrock R, Rohde MF, Quesada JR, Gianturco SH, Bradley WA, Sherwin SA, Gutterman JU. Recombinant gamma interferon induces hypertriglyceridemia and inhibits post-heparin lipase activity in cancer patients. J Exp Med 1986;164(4):1093–101.

14. Rabinowitz AP, Hu E, Watkins K, Mazumder A. Hemolytic anemia in a cancer patient treated with recombinant interferon-gamma. J Biol Response Mod 1990;9(2):256–9.

15. Aulitzky WE, Tilg H, Vogel W, Aulitzky W, Berger M, Gastl G, Herold M, Huber C. Acute hematologic effects of interferon alpha, interferon gamma, tumor necrosis factor alpha and interleukin 2. Ann Hematol 1991;62(1):25–31.

16. Ault BH, Stapleton FB, Gaber L, Martin A, Roy S 3rd, Murphy SB. Acute renal failure during therapy with recombinant human gamma interferon. N Engl J Med 1988;319(21):1397–400.

17. Fierlbeck G, Rassner G, Muller C. Psoriasis induced at the injection site of recombinant interferon gamma. Results of immunohistologic investigations. Arch Dermatol 1990;126(3):351–5.

18. Sampaio EP, Moreira AL, Sarno EN, Malta AM, Kaplan G. Prolonged treatment with recombinant interferon gamma induces erythema nodosum leprosum in lepromatous leprosy patients. J Exp Med 1992;175(6):1729–37.

19. Horn TD, Altomonte V, Vogelsang G, Kennedy MJ. Erythroderma after autologous bone marrow transplantation modified by administration of cyclosporine and interferon gamma for breast cancer. J Am Acad Dermatol 1996;34(3):413–7.

20. Weber P, Wiedmann KH, Klein R, Walter E, Blum HE, Berg PA. Induction of autoimmune phenomena in patients with chronic hepatitis B treated with gamma-interferon. J Hepatol 1994;20(3):321–8.

21. Kung AW, Jones BM, Lai CL. Effects of interferon-gamma therapy on thyroid function, T-lymphocyte subpopulations and induction of autoantibodies. J Clin Endocrinol Metab 1990;71(5):1230–4.

22. Cannon GW, Emkey RD, Denes A, Cohen SA, Saway PA, Wolfe F, Jaffer AM, Weaver AL, Manaster BJ, McCarthy KA. Prospective 5-year followup of recombinant interferon-gamma in rheumatoid arthritis. J Rheumatol 1993;20(11):1867–73.

23. Seitz M, Franke M, Kirchner H. Induction of antinuclear antibodies in patients with rheumatoid arthritis receiving treatment with human recombinant interferon gamma. Ann Rheum Dis 1988;47(8):642–4.

24. Graninger WB, Hassfeld W, Pesau BB, Machold KP, Zielinski CC, Smolen JS. Induction of systemic lupus erythematosus by interferon-gamma in a patient with rheumatoid arthritis. J Rheumatol 1991;18(10):1621–2.

25. Machold KP, Smolen JS. Interferon-gamma induced exacerbation of systemic lupus erythematosus. J Rheumatol 1990;17(6):831–2.

26. Wandl UB, Nagel-Hiemke M, May D, Kreuzfelder E, Kloke O, Kranzhoff M, Seeber S, Niederle N. Lupus-like autoimmune disease induced by interferon therapy for myeloproliferative disorders. Clin Immunol Immunopathol 1992;65(1):70–4.

27. O'Connell PG, Gerber LH, Digiovanna JJ, Peck GL. Arthritis in patients with psoriasis treated with gamma-interferon. J Rheumatol 1992;19(1):80–2.

28. Panitch HS, Hirsch RL, Schindler J, Johnson KP. Treatment of multiple sclerosis with gamma interferon: exacerbations associated with activation of the immune system. Neurology 1987;37(7):1097–102.

INTERLEUKINS

Aldesleukin

General Information

Aldesleukin (interleukin-2, celmoleukin, proleukin, teceleukin) is produced by activated T lymphocytes and has pleiotropic immunological effects, including the proliferation of T lymphocytes. Non-glycosylated recombinant aldesleukin has been approved for the treatment of metastatic renal cell carcinoma (1) and is also being investigated in other malignant neoplasms. Low-dose aldesleukin is a relatively safe treatment of HIV infection (SEDA-20, 334).

The adverse effects of aldesleukin include fever, chills, malaise, skin rash, nausea, vomiting (often resistant to antiemetics), diarrhea, fluid retention, myalgia, insomnia, disorientation, life-threatening hypotension, and the capillary leak syndrome (which can be preceded by weight gain) (SEDA-15, 491; 2).

In early trials, aldesleukin was given with lymphokine-activated killer (LAK) cells or tumor-infiltrating lymphocytes. However, later data showed that the addition of LAK cells does not improve the therapeutic response in renal cell carcinoma and can produce more pulmonary toxicity and hypotension (1). Compared with aldesleukin or interferon alfa alone, the combination of aldesleukin plus interferon alfa produces a significantly longer event-free survival without effect on the overall survival, but induces substantial toxicity with severe and resistant hypotension (3). The optimal safe and effective dose and schedule of administration of aldesleukin is not yet well defined, and a variety of regimens have been tested, with doses of 600 000 units/kg by intermittent bolus intravenous infusion or 18 106 units/m^2 by continuous subcutaneous or intravenous infusion.

Considerable efforts have been made to limit the toxic effects of aldesleukin, which are dose- and schedule-dependent (4). Low-dose aldesleukin, continuous infusion, and/or subcutaneous administration are preferred by various investigators, because of their reluctance to use conventional high-dose or bolus dose administration. Such regimens were considered as effective and safe for outpatients (5,6).

A thorough analysis of 255 patients from seven phase II trials treated with the currently recommended high dose of aldesleukin for metastatic renal cell carcinoma has been presented (7). Although severe toxicity, generally attributable to the capillary leak syndrome, was found in most patients, the problems receded promptly after withdrawal of treatment. Deaths related to aldesleukin-induced toxicity were reported in 4% of patients, and were caused by myocardial infarction, respiratory failure, gastrointestinal toxicity, or sepsis.

Use in patients with HIV infection

The use, benefits, and adverse effects of aldesleukin in HIV-infected patients have been extensively reviewed (8). Aldesleukin significantly increased the $CD4^+$ cell count without an increase in viral load. However, many questions remain unanswered. In particular, it is still not known whether immunological improvements translate into clinical benefit. Regardless of how aldesleukin is administered—intravenously, subcutaneously, or as polyethylene glycol-modified (pegylated) aldesleukin—adverse effects are generally not treatment-limiting. As the duration of adverse effects was shorter with the subcutaneous route, these patients may be treated as outpatients (9).

In two randomized, controlled studies (44 patients given subcutaneous aldesleukin, 58 given a modified-release polyethylene glycol-modified formulation, 27 given continuous intravenous aldesleukin, and 50 controls), aldesleukin was well tolerated and a minority of patients required drug withdrawal because of adverse events (10,11). The overall adverse effects profile of both routes of administration was very similar, but was substantially less severe than previously described with high-dose aldesleukin. It consisted mostly of fatigue, nasal/sinus congestion, fever above 38 °C, headache, gastrointestinal disorders, stomatitis, somnolence, and mood change. Increased bilirubin and alanine transaminase activities were more frequent than in the control group. None of the patients developed the capillary leak syndrome or significant hypertension, but cardiomyopathy, attempted suicide, ulcerative colitis, and exacerbation of hepatitis B were identified in one patient each among 85 patients treated with aldesleukin (10). Erythema and injection site reactions were observed in 66–69% of patients who received subcutaneous aldesleukin, and skin biopsies showed a perivascular infiltrate with lymphocytes and some eosinophils.

Use in patients with metastatic melanoma

In an analysis of data from 270 patients with metastatic melanoma in eight clinical trials, high-dose aldesleukin (8.4–9.8 MU/kg during each cycle) produced an overall objective response rate of 16%, with 17 complete responses and 26 partial responses (12). Although the response rate was low, there was a durable response for at least 24 months in 10 of 17 complete responders. Adverse effects were primarily the same as those previously described in patients with metastatic renal cell carcinoma, and severe hypotension (64%) was the most frequent. Six patients died from bacterial sepsis, but none was taking prophylactic antibiotics.

In a randomized trial, 102 patients with metastatic melanoma had more frequent treatment-related adverse effects, particularly hematological suppression in patients treated with tamoxifen, cisplatin, and dacarbazine

Table 1 The frequencies of severe adverse effects of aldesleukin

General symptoms	
Fever and chills	24%
Weakness	4%
Edema	2%
Sepsis	6%
Cardiovascular	
Hypotension	74%
Supraventricular dysrhythmias	3%
Myocardial damage (angina, infarction)	4%
Respiratory	
Dyspnea	17%
Adult respiratory distress syndrome	<1%
Respiratory failure	2%
Nervous system	
Coma, seizures	4%
Psychiatric	
Behavioral changes	28%
Hematologic	
Thrombocytopenia	21%
Anemia	18%
Gastrointestinal	
Nausea and vomiting	25%
Diarrhea	22%
Stomatitis	4%
Gastrointestinal bleeding	4%
Intestinal perforation	<1%
Liver	
Hyperbilirubinemia	21%
Raised transaminases	10%
Raised alkaline phosphatase	9%
Urinary tract	
Oliguria or anuria	46%
Raised blood urea nitrogen	16%
Raised serum creatinine	14%
Acidosis	6%
Skin	
Pruritus and erythema	4%
Musculoskeletal	
Arthralgia	1%
Myalgia	1%
Death	4%

Table 2 The most frequent reasons for withdrawal of high-dose intravenous aldesleukin

Constitutional symptoms	17%
Cardiovascular	
Hypotension	19%
Atrial dysrhythmias	10%
Respiratory	
Pulmonary toxicity	12%
Nervous system	
Disorientation	10%
Hematologic	
Thrombocytopenia	7%
Gastrointestinal	
Nausea or vomiting	4%
Diarrhea	6%
Liver	
Hyperbilirubinemia	5%
Urinary tract	
Oliguria	9%
Raised creatinine concentration	13%

withdrawal of high-dose intravenous aldesleukin in Table 2.

High-dose aldesleukin is associated with a wide range of adverse effects, and practical guidelines for their avoidance and management have been detailed (14). Constitutional symptoms (malaise, fever, chills and asthenia) are universal in patients treated with high-dose aldesleukin (4). Although they are usually suppressed by paracetamol (acetaminophen), indometacin, or pethidine, they are one of the major reasons for stopping treatment. Myalgia and arthralgia are sometimes associated with the flu-like symptoms.

A wide range of aldesleukin-induced adverse effects is associated with the capillary leak syndrome, which is characterized by an increase in vascular permeability with subsequent leakage of fluids and proteins into the extravascular space (4). This results in a third–space clinical syndrome, generalized or peripheral edema, weight gain, cardiovascular and pulmonary complications with hypotension, pericardial, and pleural effusions, ascites, oliguria, and prerenal azotemia. Symptoms usually resolve in a few days after aldesleukin withdrawal. Studies on the mechanism have raised a number of hypotheses, such as damage to the endothelial cells, release of secondary cytokines, and activation of the complement cascade (15).

Denileukin diftitox
Denileukin diftitox is a fusion protein formed by binding human aldesleukin to the cytotoxic A chain of diphtheria toxin. This product binds to the aldesleukin receptor and inhibits protein synthesis, resulting in cell death. It has

followed by interferon alfa and aldesleukin, than in patients treated with chemotherapy alone, but there was no increase in survival (13).

General adverse effects

The frequencies of severe adverse effects of aldesleukin (7) are listed in Table 1 and the most frequent reasons for been approved for treatment of persistent or recurrent cutaneous T cell lymphoma and is being evaluated in patients with severe psoriasis.

In 71 patients with cutaneous T cell lymphomas randomized to denileukin diftitox 9 or 18 µg/kg/day, flu-like and gastrointestinal symptoms were observed in 92% (16). About 60% had an acute hypersensitivity reaction, with dyspnea, back pain, hypotension, and chest pain or tightness within 24 hours of infusion. A vascular leak syndrome, as defined by the presence of at least two of edema, hypoalbuminemia, and hypotension, occurred in 25%.

A dose-escalation study in 35 patients with psoriasis confirmed that constitutional symptoms in response to denileukin diftitox were dose-related and less frequent at lower doses (below 5 micrograms/kg/day) (17). There was only one case of mild vascular leak syndrome. Skin reactions compatible with delayed hypersensitivity reactions were noted in three patients, including one case of exfoliative dermatitis.

The more severe adverse effects of denileukin diftitox consisted of acute hypersensitivity reactions during or within 24 hours of infusion in 69% of patients, and a vascular leak syndrome in 27% of patients, which was severe in 6%. In contrast to acute hypersensitivity reactions, the vascular leak syndrome was typically delayed and occurred within the first 2 weeks of infusion (18). Whether this was due to a direct action of denileukin diftitox or to tumor lysis syndrome is unknown.

Organs and Systems

Cardiovascular

Hemodynamic and cardiac complications are the major limitations of high-dose aldesleukin and have been described in both adults (19,20) and children (21). Significant hypotension requiring meticulous maintenance therapy with intravenous fluids or low-dose vasopressors was observed in most patients (22). The clinical findings were very similar to the hemodynamic pattern seen in early septic shock. Aldesleukin-induced increases in plasma nitrate and nitrite concentrations correlated with the severity of hypotension (23).

Among other cardiovascular complications, cardiac dysrhythmias were reported in 6–10% of patients, angina pectoris or documented myocardial infarction in 3–4%, and mortality due to myocardial infarction in 1–2% (4). Severe myocardial dysfunction, myocarditis, and cardiomyopathy have been seldom reported (SED-13, 1103; SEDA-20, 334; SEDA-22, 406).

The cardiopulmonary toxicity of high-dose intravenous bolus aldesleukin has been analysed in 199 metastatic melanoma or renal cell carcinoma patients without underlying cardiac disease (24). Cardiovascular events occurred within hours after starting infusion, persisted throughout aldesleukin therapy, and normalized within 1–3 days after treatment withdrawal. Hypotension was the most frequent adverse effect (53% of treatment courses) and resolved promptly with vasopressor treatment. Unexpectedly, the response to treatment was significantly

better in patients with melanoma who had hypotension. There were cardiac dysrhythmias in 9% of patients; they mostly consisted of easily manageable atrial fibrillation or supraventricular tachycardia. Further courses of aldesleukin in 11 of these patients produced recurrent dysrhythmias in only two, and long-term treatment of dysrhythmias was never required. High-degree atrioventricular block and repetitive episodes of ventricular tachycardia were each observed once. Although 11% of patients had raised creatine kinase activity before or during treatment, only 2.5% had a documented rise in the MB isoenzyme fraction.

At-risk patients include those with pre-existing cardiac disease, whereas age, performance status, and sex are not significantly associated with cardiopulmonary toxicity. In view of this risk, it is reasonable to monitor cardiac function and creatine kinase activity closely in all patients, or to exclude those with significant underlying coronary or cardiorespiratory disease. Pretreatment cardiac screening has greatly reduced the incidence of myocardial infarction, ischemia, and related dysrhythmias, and two-dimensional and Doppler echocardiography was suggested to be helpful to anticipate cardiovascular toxicity (25). A reduction in systemic vascular resistance, stroke work index, and left ventricular ejection fraction are usually involved in the pathophysiology of cardiac dysfunction. Clinical, electrocardiographic, and radionuclide ventriculography monitoring in 22 patients undergoing a 5-day continuous intravenous infusion of aldesleukin for various cancers showed that reversible left ventricular dysfunction accounted for most of the observed hemodynamic changes (26). Indeed, significant coronary disease was usually not observed in patients undergoing cardiac catheterization, which argues for direct myocardial damage (24). In isolated reports, clinical and histological findings of eosinophilic, lymphocytic, or mixed lymphocytic–eosinophilic myocarditis also suggested an immune-mediated drug reaction (SED-13, 1103; SEDA-22, 406).

Aldesleukin-induced cardiac eosinophilic infiltration has been reported (27).

- After 25 days of treatment with continuous aldesleukin infusion (up to 150 000 units/kg/day) for stage IV Hodgkin's disease, a 26-year-old woman had increased fatigue, tachycardia, hypotension, and hypothermia. Echocardiography showed bilateral intraventricular masses. Her maximal absolute eosinophil count was $11.4 \times 10^9/l$ and the platelet count was $17 \times 10^9/l$. Despite aldesleukin withdrawal, her condition deteriorated and she died. Postmortem examination showed biventricular thrombi and prominent eosinophilic infiltration of the endomyocardium.

Of 10 subsequent patients who received prolonged infusions of aldesleukin and were monitored by echocardiography, one developed asymptomatic changes in cardiac function, with features suggestive of early thrombus formation and a reduced ejection fraction during weeks 6–8. The maximal absolute eosinophil count was $5 \times 10^9/l$. These abnormalities resolved on aldesleukin withdrawal.

Conjugates of aldesleukin with polyethylene glycol produce less cardiovascular toxicity (SEDA-20, 333).

Respiratory

Dose-related cough has been reported as the most fre quent adverse effect of inhaled aldesleukin (28).

Among 199 patients with metastatic melanoma or renal cell carcinoma treated with high-dose intravenous bolus aldesleukin, there was severe respiratory distress in 3.2% of treatment courses, but intubation was required in only one (24). This is far less common than earlier estimates that 10–30% of patients develop respiratory distress severe enough to warrant mechanical ventilation in 5–20% of cases (4). The improvement may be related to the current strict selection criteria for the evaluation of pulmonary function, limited fluid management strategy, prophylactic antibiotics, and prompt withdrawal of treatment in patients presenting with shortness of breath, rales, or persistent hypoxemia.

Pulmonary features of the adverse effects of aldesleukin include lung opacities, diffuse pulmonary interstitial edema, pleural effusions, alveolar edema, and hypoxemia, with full and rapid recovery after treatment withdrawal (29,30).

Aldesleukin-induced increase in lung capillary permeability or direct cardiac dysfunction is thought to be a likely mechanism of this adverse effect, and a localized vascular leak syndrome, attributed to activation of eosinophils in the lung and subsequent deposition of the eosinophil major basic protein, has also been suggested, as reported in a 49-year-old woman with breast cancer (31).

There is no significant association between pre-existing clinical dysfunction and radiological interstitial edema (30). Very severe adult respiratory distress syndrome requiring double lung transplantation has been reported in one patient (32).

Nervous system

Severe pain resulting from a previously asymptomatic thoracic spine metastasis has been attributed to aldesleukin in a 64-year-old man with metastatic renal cell carcinoma (33).

Fatal acute leukoencephalopathy with brain perivascular foci demyelination (34) and delayed progressive cognitive dysfunction (35) have been reported in isolated cases.

The neurotoxicity of aldesleukin is usually dose-related and can be treatment-limiting (36).

Sensory systems

Transient episodes of amaurosis or scotomata, both of which recurred after aldesleukin rechallenge, have been described (37). Three other patients had visual phenomena, including diplopia, scotomata, and palinopsia during treatment, which resolved on withdrawal of aldesleukin (38).

Psychological, psychiatric

Aldesleukin can cause moderate impairment of cognitive function, with disorientation, confusion, hallucinations, sleep disturbances, and sometimes severe behavioral changes requiring transient neuroleptic drug administration (39–41). Some of the cognitive deficits mimicked those observed in dementias, such as Alzheimer's disease. Several studies have also shown increased latency and reduced amplitude of event-related evoked potentials in patients with cognitive impairment (41,42). Other infrequent adverse effects included paranoid delusions, hallucinations, loss of interest, sleep disturbances or drowsiness, reduced energy, fatigue, anorexia, and malaise. Coma and seizures were exceptionally noted. Symptoms occurred within 1 week of treatment and complete recovery was usually noted after aldesleukin withdrawal.

In 10 patients with advanced tumors, low-dose subcutaneous aldesleukin produced significant psychological changes; increased depression scores, psychasthenia, and conversion hysteria were the most common findings (43).

The short-term occurrence of depressive symptoms has been investigated by using the Montgomery and Asberg Depression Rating Scale (MADRS) before and after 3 and 5 days of treatment in 48 patients without a previous psychiatric history and treated for renal cell carcinoma or melanoma with aldesleukin alone ($n = 20$), aldesleukin plus interferon alfa-2b ($n = 6$), or interferon alfa-2b alone ($n = 22$) (44). On day 5, patients in the aldesleukin groups had significantly higher MADRS scores, whereas there were no significant changes in the patients who received interferon alfa-2b alone. Eight of 26 patients given aldesleukin and only three of 22 given interferon alfa-2b alone had severe depressive symptoms. Depressive symptoms occurred as early as the second day of aldesleukin treatment and were more severe in the patients who received both cytokines. Early detection of mood changes can be useful in pinpointing patients at risk of subsequent severe neuropsychiatric complications.

Neuropsychiatric symptoms are less frequent with subcutaneous aldesleukin (4). No predictive or predisposing factors have been clearly identified. Whether a direct effect of aldesleukin on neuronal tissues, an increased vascular brain permeability with a subsequent increased brain water content, or an aldesleukin-induced release of neuroendocrine hormones (beta-endorphin, ACTH, or cortisol), accounted for these effects, is unknown. A possible immune-mediated cerebral vasculitis has also been reported in one patient (SEDA-20, 334).

Endocrine

Various hormonal and metabolic effects of aldesleukin are temporally related to hypotension. Transient serum rises in ACTH, cortisol, beta-endorphin, adrenaline and noradrenaline have been found, whereas there were no significant changes in the plasma concentrations of several other hormones (4).

An acute episode of adrenal insufficiency secondary to adrenal hemorrhage occurred in one patient receiving aldesleukin (45).

Thyroid

Since the first reports of hypothyroidism, a number of studies have reported the occurrence of thyroid dysfunction in patients receiving aldesleukin alone or in combination with LAK cells, interferon alfa, interferon gamma, or tumor necrosis factor alfa (SED-13, 1104; 46). Symptoms were usually observed after 2–4 months of treatment (47–49), and mostly consisted of moderate hypothyroidism, which resolved after immunotherapy withdrawal or thyroxine treatment (49,50). Patients treated with aldesleukin plus interferon alfa more commonly developed biphasic thyroiditis with subsequent hypothyroidism or hyperthyroidism (50–53).

The possibility of a positive correlation between the development of thyroid dysfunction and the probability of a favorable tumor response has been debated (47,49,54). The incidence of thyroid dysfunction did not correlate with the dose or the underlying disease, but increased with treatment duration (46). In a large survey of 281 cancer patients receiving low-dose (72 000 IU/kg) or high-dose (720 000 IU/kg) aldesleukin, up to 41% of previously euthyroid cancer patients developed thyroid dysfunction (55). Combined immunotherapy was also associated with more frequent thyroid disorders. Aldesleukin plus interferon alfa produced thyroid dysfunction in 20–91% of patients (46), and the incidence of laboratory thyroid dysfunction reached 100% in patients given five or six cycles of both cytokines (51). Aldesleukin plus interferon alfa also tended to be a risk factor for the development of biphasic thyroiditis (49).

Female sex and the presence of antithyroid antibodies correlated significantly with the development of thyroid disease (49,56). This, together with the findings of strong expression of HLA-DR antigens on thyrocytes or the presence of mononuclear cell infiltrates on histological examination of the thyroid, makes an autoimmune phenomenon likely (49,52). However, a possible direct effect of immunotherapy on thyroid hormonal function has also been suggested in patients who had no detectable thyroid antibodies. There was a significant decrease in TSH concentration, while thyroid autoantibodies were not significantly raised (57).

Metabolism

Reversible insulin-dependent diabetes mellitus has been described in a predisposed patient (SEDA-20, 334).

Aldesleukin can cause lipid disorders. Recurrent and marked hypocholesterolemia with reduced high- and low-density lipoproteins, and slight increases in plasma triglycerides have been observed after high-dose aldesleukin (SEDA-21, 375; 4).

Nutrition

Severe, but reversible hypovitaminosis C was noted in patients receiving high-dose aldesleukin plus LAK cells (58).

Hematologic

Hematological adverse effects of aldesleukin typically included transient anemia, thrombocytopenia, eosinophilia, neutropenia, extreme lymphopenia, and rebound lymphocytosis (4,59). Transient suppression of hemopoiesis by secondary cytokines, peripheral platelet destruction, and increased endothelium margination of lymphocytes are possible mechanisms.

Hematological toxicity was analysed in 199 patients treated with a high-dose intravenous bolus aldesleukin regimen for metastatic melanoma or renal cell carcinoma (60). Anemia requiring transfusions was noted in 14% of all treatment courses and severe thrombocytopenia occurred in 2.2%, with three patients suffering from serious hemorrhages. Severe leukopenia was infrequent and not associated with infectious episodes. Early transient lymphopenia (93% reduction) was followed by rebound lymphocytosis up to 198% above baseline values. Except for severe thrombocytopenia, treatment withdrawal was not required in this study. Other investigators found that reductions in platelet count correlated with a significant increase in ex vivo platelet functional activity, but there were no episodes of bleeding or thrombosis (61).

Aldesleukin can produce sustained eosinophilia, possibly mediated by interleukin-5 or GM-CSF, but this was not associated with allergic reactions (62).

In 42 patients with advanced cancer treated with aldesleukin and lymphokine-activated killer cells from autologous lymphocytes, there were reduced numbers of circulating erythroid and granulocyte/macrophage progenitors, with recovery after withdrawal (63). Patients developed severe anemia (partly due to phlebotomy, cytopheresis, and hemodilution), thrombocytopenia, lymphopenia, and eosinophilia, with mild neutropenia and rebound lymphocytosis after treatment was stopped.

The severity of hematological disorders was not affected by previous chemotherapy for metastatic melanoma or renal cell carcinoma and there was no correlation with response to treatment (60). However, others have found that moderate to severe dose-related thrombocytopenia occurred particularly in patients previously treated with cytotoxic agents (64). Subcutaneous low-dose aldesleukin therapy reduced the frequency and intensity of hematological toxicity, and the combination of aldesleukin plus interferon alfa produced either moderate additional toxicity or no significant enhancement (65).

Most patients develop significant, but promptly reversible coagulation disorders with prolongation of the partial thromboplastin time (the most frequent effect), hypoprothrombinemia, and reduced functional concentrations of several clotting factors II, IX, X, XI, and XII (60,66,67). No clear mechanism of aldesleukin-induced coagulopathy has been identified, and the efficacy of prophylactic vitamin K has been disputed (67). Other data suggest that aldesleukin may activate the coagulation and fibrinolytic system (64,68), but the clinical relevance of these findings is not clear.

A mean splenic index increase of 64% was found on computed tomography after a mean of 66 days of aldesleukin treatment for non-hematological malignancies (69). Splenomegaly persisted after an average of 215 days after the completion of aldesleukin treatment and was not associated with tumor progression.

Mouth

Oral effects of aldesleukin include xerostomia with reversible salivary gland hypofunction, a burning sensation in the mouth, taste disorders, mucosal atrophy, mucositis, glossitis, and ulcerative lesions (70,71).

Gastrointestinal

Minor gastrointestinal adverse effects, that is anorexia, nausea, vomiting, and diarrhea, were noted in about 80% of patients (4).

Incidental case reports included symptomatic exacerbation of Crohn's disease (72) and transient painful swelling of the appendix (SEDA-21, 376).

Severe and sometimes fatal intestinal complications have been described in 1.3–7% of patients receiving aldesleukin alone or in combination with LAK cells or interferon alfa, including intestinal ischemia, bowel ulceration or perforation, and colosplenic fistula (73–75). It has been suggested that severe diarrhea may be an indicator of subsequent colonic ischemia (75).

Liver

Mild liver dysfunction, hypophosphatemia, and hypomagnesmia are the most common laboratory abnormalities caused by aldesleukin (76,77). About 20% of patients develop mild to severe intrahepatic cholestasis with reversible and dose-dependent rises in bilirubin and alkaline phosphatase while serum transaminases were only slightly increased (4,78). Recurrence of cholestasis after aldesleukin rechallenge was not always observed (79). The mechanism of aldesleukin-induced intrahepatic cholestasis is unknown, but it might be mediated by activation of Kupfer cells and the subsequent release of cytokines (SEDA-20, 335). Focal fatty infiltrates of the liver mimicking metastases were also reported in a patient receiving both aldesleukin and a short course of interferon alfa (80).

Biliary tract

Gall-bladder changes have been reported in patients given aldesleukin and should be promptly recognized to avoid unnecessary intervention in symptomatic patients (SED-13, 1105; 81). Further systematic ultrasonographic examination in 25 HIV-infected patients treated with low-dose aldesleukin (6–18 MU/day) confirmed that most patients had gall-bladder wall thickening (80%), abnormal echo texture (64%), and intramural fluid (52%) or pericholecystic fluid (20%) (82). The frequency and severity of ultrasonographic abnormalities correlated with a higher dose of aldesleukin, as did complaints of right upper quadrant pain (24%). Although these findings mimicked those observed with acute cholecystitis, clinical symptoms and ultrasonographic abnormalities rapidly reversed after aldesleukin withdrawal or between two cycles.

Aldesleukin-induced cholecystopathy has been described in patients with cancer and was fully investigated in seven of 29 HIV-infected patients (81). Right upper quadrant abdominal pain and gallbladder wall thickening at sonography developed after 4–5 days of treatment and spontaneously resolved after withdrawal or dosage reduction. Similar symptoms recurred after renewed administration of aldesleukin. Although suggestive of acalculous cholecystitis, surgery is not required because this disorder is usually benign.

Pancreas

Acute pancreatitis has been described after high-dose bolus aldesleukin therapy (83).

Urinary tract

The renal toxicity associated with aldesleukin is dose-related. It manifests as uremia, oliguria, fluid retention, and pronounced renal tubular sodium reabsorption (77). No evidence of tubular dysfunction has been found. There is reduced renal plasma flow associated with reduced renal prostaglandin synthesis and increased plasma renin activity, which may explain the mechanism (84).

Oliguria or anuria, and increased serum creatinine concentrations occurred in over 90% of patients receiving high-dose aldesleukin (4).

Proteinuria, ranging in degree from traces to a frank, but reversible nephrotic syndrome (85,86), was sometimes observed, and a possible role of contaminants has been discussed (87).

In 199 patients with metastatic melanoma or renal cell carcinoma with high-dose intravenous bolus aldesleukin, severe oliguria, hypotension, and weight gain were frequent, and raised serum creatinine concentrations (mean peak 2.7 mg/dl) were the cause of treatment withdrawal in 13% of cycles (88). There were also various changes on urinalysis. The highest creatinine concentrations were found in patients with renal carcinoma and in elderly, male, or nephrectomized patients. There was no evidence of any long-term renal defect, and renal dysfunction was therefore not considered to be a treatment-limiting factor provided that patients were carefully managed for hypotension or oliguria.

It has been suggested that low-to-intermediate doses of aldesleukin alone or associated with interferon alfa may be safer under outpatient conditions (5). Patients over 60 years of age and individuals with previously raised serum creatinine concentrations have been thought to be likely to have longer-lasting and more severe renal impairment, but neither previous nephrectomy nor the interval between nephrectomy and initiation of aldesleukin therapy were associated with a higher risk of renal insufficiency (4).

A prerenal mechanism secondary to the vascular leak syndrome is commonly involved in the pathophysiology of acute renal insufficiency. In addition it has been suggested that a direct intrinsic intrarenal effect of aldesleukin with a higher than expected reduction in glomerular filtration rate or tubular dysfunction (85,89) is involved. Several isolated cases of acute interstitial or tubulo-interstitial nephritis with predominant T lymphocyte infiltration of the kidneys (90–92) and the exacerbation of a subclinical IgA glomerulonephritis (93) suggested altered cell-mediated immunity.

Risk factors for renal dysfunction have been analysed in 72 patients with metastatic renal cell cancer treated with high-dose aldesleukin (18 $MU/m^2/day$), interferon alfa (5 $MU/m^2/day$), and lymphokine-activated killer lymphocytes (94). There was some type of renal dysfunction in 97%, of whom 69% developed renal toxicity of grade 2 (creatinine 260–525 µmol/l) or grade 3 (creatinine 525–1050 µmol/l). Although renal function commonly resolved between successive treatment courses, six patients had a persistently raised creatinine concentration (more than 20% above baseline). Among the various potential risk factors, a multivariate analysis showed that the significant risk factors for severe renal dysfunction were male sex, pre-treatment hypertension, and sepsis during treatment.

Skin

Cutaneous reactions to aldesleukin generally comprise pruritus, flushing, mild to moderate erythematous macular and desquamative eruptions, while generalized erythroderma or photosensitivity have occasionally been observed (95). The severity was not dose-dependent and did not correlate with other systemic reactions. Histological and immunopathological examination of the skin showed mild infiltrates of activated T helper lymphocytes and increased expression of HLA-DR and intercellular adhesion molecule-1 on keratinocytes and endothelial cells, and a possible role of interferon gamma has been suggested (96–98). Other adverse effects included erosions in surgical scars, multiple superficial cutaneous ulcers, and telogen effluvium (95).

Injection site reactions have been noted after subcutaneous aldesleukin (SEDA-21, 376). Localized lobular panniculitis after subcutaneous injections was further exacerbated by intravenous aldesleukin in one patient (99).

An unusually high incidence of skin erythema (70–85%) was noted in patients who received aldesleukin after autologous bone marrow transplantation. Histological examination showed features of cutaneous graft-versus-host disease or T cell epidermal infiltrates, but cutaneous toxicity was not reproduced in patients receiving low-dose aldesleukin (100,101).

The potential role of localized vertebral palliative radiotherapy before aldesleukin treatment was denied, since the area of cutaneous toxicity was broader than the irradiated field.

Aldesleukin given alone or aldesleukin plus interferon alfa produced a high incidence of vitiligo in patients with metastatic melanoma, irrespective of whether or not they had received chemotherapy (102–104). A possible correlation between aldesleukin-induced vitiligo and a favorable tumor response was found (102) but has also been disputed (103).

Some isolated reports have given rise to the suggestion that aldesleukin can exacerbate cutaneous reactions compatible with an immune-mediated phenomenon (105). Case reports included recurrence of quiescent pemphigus vulgaris, fatal dermatitis exfoliativa compatible with pemphigus vulgaris, exacerbation of localized or widespread psoriasis, acute reactivation of eczema, rapid progression of scleroderma with myositis, and leukocytoclastic vasculitis (SED-13, 1106; SEDA-20, 335; SEDA-21, 376).

Immunostimulation due to aldesleukin may have also played a role in the occurrence or unmasking of erythema nodosum, linear IgA bullous dermatosis, and life-threatening extensive bullous skin eruption or toxic epidermal necrolysis (SED-13, 1106; SEDA-21, 376; 106).

Because aldesleukin stimulates T cells, it has been suggested to have favored the development of successive episodes of multifocal fixed drug eruption in response to chemically unrelated drugs (paracetamol, ondansetron, and tropisetron) in a 43-year-old patient (107).

Musculoskeletal

Joint or muscle pains have sometimes been reported in patients receiving aldesleukin, as has shoulder arthralgia with normal radiography and scintigraphic imaging consistent with bilateral synovitis (4,108).

Rare reports have suggested that aldesleukin can reactivate or cause rheumatoid arthritis (109) or cause necrotizing myositis with positive antinuclear antibodies (SEDA-20, 335).

Interstitial edema and local fluid retention resulting from increased vascular permeability has been suggested to cause unilateral or bilateral carpal tunnel syndrome with sensorimotor median neuropathy (SEDA-20, 334; 110).

Sexual function

A reversible reduction in testosterone concentrations has been observed in men who have received aldesleukin (4).

Immunologic

Aldesleukin was thought to be the triggering factor in the occurrence of sarcoidosis in a 36-year-old patient with AIDS stabilized for a long time by highly active antiretroviral therapy (111).

There have been very few reports of angioedema in patients receiving aldesleukin (112).

Interleukin antibodies

Recombinant aldesleukin-binding antibodies were detected in the half of 205 patients with metastatic cancer but there were neutralizing antibodies in only 7% (113). No significant difference in incidence was found between subcutaneous and continuous intravenous administration. In another study, none of the patients receiving aldesleukin alone developed neutralizing antibodies, whereas 18% of patients treated with aldesleukin and interferon alfa-2b had antibodies (114). Whatsoever, the clinical relevance of recombinant aldesleukin-neutralizing antibodies has not been accurately evaluated and a loss of response was apparently documented in only one patient (115).

Autoimmune disorders

Aldesleukin sometimes causes acute exacerbation of latent autoimmune disease, as has been further exemplified by the following description, which also included the first report of aldesleukin-induced myasthenia gravis (116).

- A 64-year-old man with non-insulin-dependent diabetes was given 14 large doses of aldesleukin (600 000 IU/kg every 8 hours) for metastatic renal cell carcinoma. One week after the completion of the first cycle he had a reversible episode of hyperosmolar, non-ketotic hyperglycemia, and insulin was started. A second cycle 3 months later was associated with hypotension, mild weakness of the right shoulder, and increased activity of creatine kinase (CK)-MB fraction. After four doses of the third cycle he again had hypotension and a raised CK-MB fraction. Two weeks later, he developed typical features of myasthenia gravis and required mechanical ventilation. Acetylcholine receptor antibodies were found and there was an inflammatory primary myositis on muscle biopsy. He gradually recovered with prednisone, pyridostigmine, and daily insulin.

In this case, which was marked by three autoimmune complications (insulin-dependent diabetes mellitus, myositis, and myasthenia gravis) in a single patient, a retrospective analysis of the patient's serum before aldesleukin therapy showed the presence of antibodies against glutamic acid decarboxylase, insulin, islet cell antigen, and striated muscle, but was negative for acetylcholine receptor antibodies. Immune stimulation by aldesleukin was therefore thought to have caused broken tolerance to self-antigens and enhanced latent autoimmunity.

Infection risk

Clinically relevant infectious complications occurred with an incidence of 10–40% after intravenous aldesleukin (4). A retrospective study showed a 13% incidence of confirmed bacterial infections during 935 treatment courses of high-dose aldesleukin; opportunistic infections were not more frequent (117). The most commonly isolated pathogens were *Staphylococcus aureus*, *Staphylococcus epidermidis*, and *Escherichia coli*. Documented infections affected mostly the catheter site or the urinary tract. Infections were usually noted during the first (68%) or second (21%) course of aldesleukin therapy, that is 4–9 days and 13–18 days after the start of treatment. Bacterial sepsis was mostly related to the use of central venous catheters and fatal septic shock was rarely recorded. There was also an increased incidence of infectious complications in patients receiving subcutaneous aldesleukin plus interferon alfa (118), but these findings were not confirmed in patients who received subcutaneous aldesleukin alone (119,120). Previous colonization of the skin with *S. aureus* and skin desquamation increased the risk of nosocomial bacteremia (117). Age, underlying tumor, source, dose and duration of intravenous aldesleukin, or the concomitant use of LAK cells were not risks factors, and severe neutropenia was not associated with bacteremia. The prophylactic use of antibiotics and

systematic screening led to a significant reduction in the frequency of infections, from 22 to 7% of patients over 3 years (117).

The mechanism of these complications is not fully understood. A reduction in neutrophil chemotaxis, superoxide production, and/or neutrophil Fc receptor expression have been suggested to be involved. Impaired cell-mediated or humoral immune responses have also been shown after high-dose aldesleukin, but the clinical consequences of these findings are unknown.

Long-Term Effects

Tumorigenicity

Isolated case reports have described relapses of acute myeloid leukemia or the proliferation of leukemic blasts cells with phenotypic changes in a patient with acute myelocytic leukemia; a high percentage of blasts expressed the CD25 antigen in both reports (121,122). A reversible increase in peripheral monoclonal B cell lymphocyte count in a patient with B cell lymphocytic lymphoma and Hodgkin's disease in a woman receiving aldesleukin for metastatic melanoma were also documented in single reports.

Drug–Drug Interactions

General

The potential of aldesleukin to participate in drug interactions has been investigated in 18 patients who underwent surgical resection of hepatic metastases (123). Compared with seven control patients who did not receive aldesleukin before surgery, six patients who received 9 or 12 MU/m^2 from days 7–3 before hepatectomy had a significant fall in the activities of total cytochromes and several mono-oxygenases. No such effect was found in five patients treated with 3 or 6 MU/m^2 before hepatectomy. This suggests that high-dose aldesleukin might cause drug interactions by inhibiting hepatic drug metabolism.

Contrast media

More frequent allergic reactions to iodinated and non-ionic contrast media injection were observed when radiological examination was performed within a period ranging from 2 to 6 weeks up to 2 years after withdrawal of aldesleukin in patients who had previously tolerated contrast media well (124,125). These reactions usually appeared within 1–4 hours after contrast media injection, but delayed reactions up to 24 hours were sometimes noted. The most frequent symptoms were diarrhea, vomiting, influenza-like symptoms, skin rash, pruritus, and facial edema, and rarely included hypotension, dyspnea, and oliguria. The overall incidence was 5–15%, but as high as 28% of patients receiving aldesleukin via arterial infusion (126). This incidence is therefore about 3–4 times higher than in the general population undergoing contrast media examination. "Recall" reactions to aldesleukin have been suggested as an explanation, since these complications more closely resemble immediate adverse effects to aldesleukin than typical contrast media reactions. Putative enhancement of the immune response to iodine-containing contrast media after aldesleukin has also been suggested.

Cytotoxic drugs

An unexpected high incidence of type I allergic reactions to cisplatin and dacarbazine has been observed, several hours after administration to patients on a combination of aldesleukin and interferon alfa (127). The reactions occurred at least after the first cycle and increased in incidence thereafter, suggesting that immunotherapy can sensitize patients to several chemotherapeutic agents.

In a phase III trial in 190 patients with metastatic melanoma, sequential chemotherapy with dacarbazine, cisplatin, and vinblastine plus interferon alfa and aldesleukin modestly increased the response rates and produced considerably more frequent and severe adverse effects than chemotherapy alone (128). In particular, severe episodes of anemia and thrombocytopenia that required blood or platelet transfusions were 2–6 times more frequent in the chemotherapy group.

Morphine

Acute encephalopathy with typical signs of morphine intoxication occurred in a patient taking aldesleukin (129).

Non-steroidal anti-inflammatory agents

Non-steroidal anti-inflammatory agents used to reduce fever and other aldesleukin adverse effects can theoretically potentiate aldesleukin nephrotoxicity by inhibiting prostaglandin synthesis. However this effect was deemed unlikely by several authors (85).

References

1. Law TM, Motzer RJ, Mazumdar M, Sell KW, Walther PJ, O'Connell M, Khan A, Vlamis V, Vogelzang NJ, Bajorin DF. Phase III randomized trial of interleukin-2 with or without lymphokine-activated killer cells in the treatment of patients with advanced renal cell carcinoma. Cancer 1995;76(5):824–32.
2. Javadpour N, Lalehzarian M. A phase I-II study of high-dose recombinant human interleukin-2 in disseminated renal-cell carcinoma. Semin Surg Oncol 1988;4(3):207–9.
3. Negrier S, Escudier B, Lasset C, Douillard JY, Savary J, Chevreau C, Ravaud A, Mercatello A, Peny J, Mousseau M, Philip T, Tursz T. Recombinant human interleukin-2, recombinant human interferon alfa-2a, or both in metastatic renal-cell carcinoma. Groupe Francais d'Immunotherapie. N Engl J Med 1998;338(18):1272–8.
4. Vial T, Descotes J. Clinical toxicity of interleukin-2. Drug Saf 1992;7(6):417–33.
5. Schomburg A, Kirchner H, Atzpodien J. Renal, metabolic, and hemodynamic side-effects of interleukin-2 and/or interferon alpha: evidence of a risk/benefit advantage of subcutaneous therapy. J Cancer Res Clin Oncol 1993;119(12):745–55.
6. Stadler WM, Vogelzang NJ. Low-dose interleukin-2 in the treatment of metastatic renal-cell carcinoma. Semin Oncol 1995;22(1):67–73.
7. Fyfe G, Fisher RI, Rosenberg SA, Sznol M, Parkinson DR, Louie AC. Results of treatment of 255 patients with metastatic renal cell carcinoma who received high-dose recombinant interleukin-2 therapy. J Clin Oncol 1995;13(3):688–96.
8. Piscitelli SC, Bhat N, Pau A. A risk-benefit assessment of interleukin-2 as an adjunct to antiviral therapy in HIV infection. Drug Saf 2000;22(1):19–31.
9. Levy Y, Capitant C, Houhou S, Carriere I, Viard JP, Goujard C, Gastaut JA, Oksenhendler E, Boumsell L, Gomard E, Rabian C, Weiss L, Guillet JG, Delfraissy JF, Aboulker JP, Seligmann MANRS 048 study group. Comparison of subcutaneous and intravenous interleukin-2 in asymptomatic HIV-1 infection: a randomised controlled trial. Lancet 1999;353(9168):1923–9.
10. Carr A, Emery S, Lloyd A, Hoy J, Garsia R, French M, Stewart G, Fyfe G, Cooper DAAustralian IL-2 Study Group. Outpatient continuous intravenous interleukin-2 or subcutaneous, polyethylene glycol-modified interleukin-2 in human immunodeficiency virus-infected patients: a randomized, controlled, multicenter study. J Infect Dis 1998;178(4):992–9.
11. Hengge UR, Goos M, Esser S, Exner V, Dotterer H, Wiehler H, Borchard C, Muller K, Beckmann A, Eppner MT, Berger A, Fiedler M. Randomized, controlled phase II trial of subcutaneous interleukin-2 in combination with highly active antiretroviral therapy (HAART) in HIV patients. AIDS 1998;12(17):F225–34.
12. Atkins MB, Lotze MT, Dutcher JP, Fisher RI, Weiss G, Margolin K, Abrams J, Sznol M, Parkinson D, Hawkins M, Paradise C, Kunkel L, Rosenberg SA. High-dose recombinant interleukin 2 therapy for patients with metastatic melanoma: analysis of 270 patients treated between 1985 and 1993. J Clin Oncol 1999;17(7):2105–16.
13. Rosenberg SA, Yang JC, Schwartzentruber DJ, Hwu P, Marincola FM, Topalian SL, Seipp CA, Einhorn JH, White DE, Steinberg SM. Prospective randomized trial of the treatment of patients with metastatic melanoma using chemotherapy with cisplatin, dacarbazine, and tamoxifen alone or in combination with interleukin-2 and interferon alfa-2b. J Clin Oncol 1999;17(3):968–75.
14. Schwartzentruber DJ. Guidelines for the safe administration of high-dose interleukin-2. J Immunother 2001;24(4):287–93.
15. Baluna R, Vitetta ES. Vascular leak syndrome: a side effect of immunotherapy. Immunopharmacology 1997;37(2–3):117–32.
16. Olsen E, Duvic M, Frankel A, Kim Y, Martin A, Vonderheid E, Jegasothy B, Wood G, Gordon M, Heald P, Oseroff A, Pinter-Brown L, Bowen G, Kuzel T, Fivenson D, Foss F, Glode M, Molina A, Knobler E, Stewart S, Cooper K, Stevens S, Craig F, Reuben J, Bacha P, Nichols J. Pivotal phase III trial of two dose levels of denileukin diftitox for the treatment of cutaneous T cell lymphoma. J Clin Oncol 2001;19(2):376–88.
17. Martin A, Gutierrez E, Muglia J, McDonald CJ, Guzzo C, Gottlieb A, Pappert A, Garland WT, Bagel J, Bacha P. A multicenter dose-escalation trial with denileukin diftitox (ONTAK, DAB(389)IL-2) in patients with severe psoriasis. J Am Acad Dermatol 2001;45(6):871–81.
18. Railan D, Fivenson DP, Wittenberg G. Capillary leak syndrome in a patient treated with interleukin 2 fusion

toxin for cutaneous T cell lymphoma. J Am Acad Dermatol 2000;43(2 Pt 1):323–4.

19. Sosman JA, Kohler PC, Hank JA, Moore KH, Bechhofer R, Storer B, Sondel PM. Repetitive weekly cycles of interleukin-2. II. Clinical and immunologic effects of dose, schedule, and addition of indomethacin. J Natl Cancer Inst 1988;80(18):1451–61.

20. Richards JM, Barker E, Latta J, Ramming K, Vogelzang NJ. Phase I study of weekly 24-hour infusions of recombinant human interleukin-2. J Natl Cancer Inst 1988;80(16):1325–8.

21. Nasr S, McKolanis J, Pais R, Findley H, Hnath R, Waldrep K, Ragab AH. A phase I study of interleukin-2 in children with cancer and evaluation of clinical and immunologic status during therapy. A Pediatric Oncology Group Study. Cancer 1989;64(4):783–8.

22. Groeger JS, Bajorin D, Reichman B, Kopec I, Atiq O, Pierri MK. Haemodynamic effects of recombinant interleukin-2 administered by constant infusion. Eur J Cancer 1991;27(12):1613–6.

23. Citterio G, Pellegatta F, Lucca GD, Fragasso G, Scaglietti U, Pini D, Fortis C, Tresoldi M, Rugarli C. Plasma nitrate plus nitrite changes during continuous intravenous infusion interleukin 2. Br J Cancer 1996;74(8):1297–301.

24. White RL Jr, Schwartzentruber DJ, Guleria A, MacFarlane MP, White DE, Tucker E, Rosenberg SA. Cardiopulmonary toxicity of treatment with high dose interleukin-2 in 199 consecutive patients with metastatic melanoma or renal cell carcinoma. Cancer 1994;74(12):3212–22.

25. Citterio G, Fragasso G, Rossetti E, Di Lucca G, Bucci E, Foppoli M, Guerrieri R, Matteucci P, Polastri D, Scaglietti U, Tresoldi M, Chierchia SL, Rugarli C. Isolated left ventricular filling abnormalities may predict interleukin-2-induced cardiovascular toxicity. J Immunother Emphasis Tumor Immunol 1996;19(2):134–41.

26. Fragasso G, Tresoldi M, Benti R, Vidal M, Marcatti M, Borri A, Besana C, Gerundini PP, Rugarli C, Chierchia S. Impaired left ventricular filling rate induced by treatment with recombinant interleukin 2 for advanced cancer. Br Heart J 1994;71(2):166–9.

27. Junghans RP, Manning W, Safar M, Quist W. Biventricular cardiac thrombosis during interleukin-2 infusion. N Engl J Med 2001;344(11):859–60.

28. Huland E, Heinzer H, Huland H. Treatment of pulmonary metastatic renal-cell carcinoma in 116 patients using inhaled interleukin-2 (IL-2). Anticancer Res 1999;19(4A):2679–83.

29. Davis SD, Berkmen YM, Wang JC. Interleukin-2 therapy for advanced renal cell carcinoma: radiographic evaluation of response and complications. Radiology 1990;177(1):127–31.

30. Saxon RR, Klein JS, Bar MH, Blanc P, Gamsu G, Webb WR, Aronson FR. Pathogenesis of pulmonary edema during interleukin-2 therapy: correlation of chest radiographic and clinical findings in 54 patients. Am J Roentgenol 1991;156(2):281–5.

31. O'Hearn DJ, Leiferman KM, Askin F, Georas SN. Pulmonary infiltrates after cytokine therapy for stem cell transplantation. Massive deposition of eosinophil major basic protein detected by immunohistochemistry. Am J Respir Crit Care Med 1999;160(4):1361–5.

32. Brichon PY, Barnoud D, Pison C, Perez I, Guignier M. Double lung transplantation for adult respiratory distress syndrome after recombinant interleukin 2. Chest 1993;104(2):609–10.

33. Trufflandier N, Gille O, Palussiere J, Prie L, Pointillart V, Ravaud A. Symptomatic neurological epidural metastasis with interleukin-2 therapy in metastatic renal cell carcinoma. Tumori 2002;88(4):338–40.

34. Vecht CJ, Keohane C, Menon RS, Punt CJ, Stoter G. Acute fatal leukoencephalopathy after interleukin-2 therapy. N Engl J Med 1990;323(16):1146–7.

35. Meyers CA, Yung WK. Delayed neurotoxicity of intraventricular interleukin-2: a case report. J Neurooncol 1993;15(3):265–7.

36. Buter J, de Vries EG, Sleijfer DT, Willemse PH, Mulder NH. Neuropsychiatric symptoms during treatment with interleukin-2. Lancet 1993;341(8845):628.

37. Bernard JT, Ameriso S, Kempf RA, Rosen P, Mitchell MS, Fisher M. Transient focal neurologic deficits complicating interleukin-2 therapy. Neurology 1990;40(1):154–5.

38. Friedman DI, Hu EH, Sadun AA. Neuro-ophthalmic complications of interleukin 2 therapy. Arch Ophthalmol 1991;109(12):1679–80.

39. Denicoff KD, Rubinow DR, Papa MZ, Simpson C, Seipp CA, Lotze MT, Chang AE, Rosenstein D, Rosenberg SA. The neuropsychiatric effects of treatment with interleukin-2 and lymphokine-activated killer cells. Ann Intern Med 1987;107(3):293–300.

40. Caraceni A, Martini C, Belli F, Mascheroni L, Rivoltini L, Arienti F, Cascinelli N. Neuropsychological and neurophysiological assessment of the central effects of interleukin-2 administration. Eur J Cancer 1993;29A(9):1266–9.

41. Walker LG, Wesnes KP, Heys SD, Walker MB, Lolley J, Eremin O. The cognitive effects of recombinant interleukin-2 (rIL-2) therapy: a controlled clinical trial using computerised assessments. Eur J Cancer 1996;32A(13):2275–83.

42. Pace A, Pietrangeli A, Bove L, Rosselli M, Lopez M, Jandolo B. Neurotoxicity of antitumoral IL-2 therapy: evoked cognitive potentials and brain mapping. Ital J Neurol Sci 1994;15(7):341–6.

43. Pizzi C, Caraglia M, Cianciulli M, Fabbrocini A, Libroia A, Matano E, Contegiacomo A, Del Prete S, Abbruzzese A, Martignetti A, Tagliaferri P, Bianco AR. Low-dose recombinant IL-2 induces psychological changes: monitoring by Minnesota Multiphasic Personality Inventory (MMPI). Anticancer Res 2002;22(2A):727–32.

44. Capuron L, Ravaud A, Dantzer R. Early depressive symptoms in cancer patients receiving interleukin 2 and/or interferon alfa-2b therapy. J Clin Oncol 2000;18(10):2143–51.

45. VanderMolen LA, Smith JW 2nd, Longo DL, Steis RG, Kremers P, Sznol M. Adrenal insufficiency and interleukin-2 therapy. Ann Intern Med 1989;111(2):185.

46. Vial T, Descotes J. Immune-mediated side-effects of cytokines in humans. Toxicology 1995;105(1):31–57.

47. Kruit WH, Bolhuis RL, Goey SH, Jansen RL, Eggermont AM, Batchelor D, Schmitz PI, Stoter G. Interleukin-2-induced thyroid dysfunction is correlated with treatment duration but not with tumor response. J Clin Oncol 1993;11(5):921–4.

48. Preziati D, La Rosa L, Covini G, Marcelli R, Rescalli S, Persani L, Del Ninno E, Meroni PL, Colombo M, Beck-Peccoz P. Autoimmunity and thyroid function in patients with chronic active hepatitis treated with recombinant interferon alpha-2a. Eur J Endocrinol 1995;132(5):587–93.

49. Vialettes B, Guillerand MA, Viens P, Stoppa AM, Baume D, Sauvan R, Pasquier J, San Marco M, Olive D,

Maraninchi D. Incidence rate and risk factors for thyroid dysfunction during recombinant interleukin-2 therapy in advanced malignancies. Acta Endocrinol (Copenh) 1993;129(1):31–8.

50. Schwartzentruber DJ, White DE, Zweig MH, Weintraub BD, Rosenberg SA. Thyroid dysfunction associated with immunotherapy for patients with cancer. Cancer 1991;68(11):2384–90.

51. Jacobs EL, Clare-Salzler MJ, Chopra IJ, Figlin RA. Thyroid function abnormalities associated with the chronic outpatient administration of recombinant interleukin-2 and recombinant interferon-alpha. J Immunother 1991;10(6):448–55.

52. Pichert G, Jost LM, Zobeli L, Odermatt B, Pedia G, Stahel RA. Thyroiditis after treatment with interleukin-2 and interferon alpha-2a. Br J Cancer 1990;62(1):100–4.

53. Reid I, Sharpe I, McDevitt J, Maxwell W, Emmons R, Tanner WA, Monson JR. Thyroid dysfunction can predict response to immunotherapy with interleukin-2 and interferon-2 alpha. Br J Cancer 1991;64(5):915–8.

54. Weijl NI, Van der Harst D, Brand A, Kooy Y, Van Luxemburg S, Schroder J, Lentjes E, Van Rood JJ, Cleton FJ, Osanto S. Hypothyroidism during immunotherapy with interleukin-2 is associated with antithyroid antibodies and response to treatment. J Clin Oncol 1993;11(7):1376–83.

55. Krouse RS, Royal RE, Heywood G, Weintraub BD, White DE, Steinberg SM, Rosenberg SA, Schwartzentruber DJ. Thyroid dysfunction in 281 patients with metastatic melanoma or renal carcinoma treated with interleukin-2 alone. J Immunother Emphasis Tumor Immunol 1995;18(4):272–8.

56. Kung AW, Lai CL, Wong KL, Tam CF. Thyroid functions in patients treated with interleukin-2 and lymphokine-activated killer cells. Q J Med 1992;82(297):33–42.

57. Monig H, Hauschild A, Lange S, Folsch UR. Suppressed thyroid-stimulating hormone secretion in patients treated with interleukin-2 and interferon-alpha 2b for metastatic melanoma. Clin Investig 1994;72(12):975–8.

58. Marcus SL, Dutcher JP, Paietta E, Ciobanu N, Strauman J, Wiernik PH, Hutner SH, Frank O, Baker H. Severe hypovitaminosis C occurring as the result of adoptive immunotherapy with high-dose interleukin 2 and lymphokine-activated killer cells. Cancer Res 1987;47(15):4208–12.

59. Aulitzky WE, Tilg H, Vogel W, Aulitzky W, Berger M, Gastl G, Herold M, Huber C. Acute hematologic effects of interferon alpha, interferon gamma, tumor necrosis factor alpha and interleukin 2. Ann Hematol 1991;62(1):25–31.

60. MacFarlane MP, Yang JC, Guleria AS, White RL Jr, Seipp CA, Einhorn JH, White DE, Rosenberg SA. The hematologic toxicity of interleukin-2 in patients with metastatic melanoma and renal cell carcinoma. Cancer 1995;75(4):1030–7.

61. Oleksowicz L, Zuckerman D, Mrowiec Z, Puszkin E, Dutcher JP. Effects of interleukin-2 administration on platelet function in cancer patients. Am J Hematol 1994;45(3):224–31.

62. Macdonald D, Gordon AA, Kajitani H, Enokihara H, Barrett AJ. Interleukin-2 treatment-associated eosinophilia is mediated by interleukin-5 production. Br J Haematol 1990;76(2):168–73.

63. Ettinghausen SE, Moore JG, White DE, Platanias L, Young NS, Rosenberg SA. Hematologic effects of immunotherapy with lymphokine-activated killer cells and recombinant interleukin-2 in cancer patients. Blood 1987;69(6):1654–60.

64. Fleischmann JD, Shingleton WB, Gallagher C, Ratnoff OD, Chahine A. Fibrinolysis, thrombocytopenia, and coagulation abnormalities complicating high-dose interleukin-2 immunotherapy. J Lab Clin Med 1991;117(1):76–82.

65. Schomburg A, Kirchner H, Atzpodien J. Hematotoxicity of interleukin-2 in man: clinical effects and comparison of various treatment regimens. Acta Haematol 1993;89(3):119–31.

66. Birchfield GR, Rodgers GM, Girodias KW, Ward JH, Samlowski WE. Hypoprothrombinemia associated with interleukin-2 therapy: correction with vitamin K. J Immunother 1992;11(1):71–5.

67. Oleksowicz L, Strack M, Dutcher JP, Sussman I, Caliendo G, Sparano J, Wiernik PH. A distinct coagulopathy associated with interleukin-2 therapy. Br J Haematol 1994;88(4):892–4.

68. Baars JW, de Boer JP, Wagstaff J, Roem D, Eerenberg-Belmer AJ, Nauta J, Pinedo HM, Hack CE. Interleukin-2 induces activation of coagulation and fibrinolysis: resemblance to the changes seen during experimental endotoxaemia. Br J Haematol 1992;82(2):295–301.

69. Ratcliffe MA, Roditi G, Adamson DJ. Interleukin-2 and splenic enlargement. J Natl Cancer Inst 1992;84(10):810–1.

70. Marmary Y, Shiloni E, Katz J. Oral changes in interleukin-2 treated patients: a preliminary report. J Oral Pathol Med 1992;21(5):230–1.

71. Nagler A, Nagler R, Ackerstein A, Levi S, Marmary Y. Major salivary gland dysfunction in patients with hematological malignancies receiving interleukin-2-based immunotherapy post-autologous blood stem cell transplantation (ABSCT). Bone Marrow Transplant 1997;20(7):575–80.

72. Sparano JA, Brandt LJ, Dutcher JP, DuBois JS, Atkins MB. Symptomatic exacerbation of Crohn disease after treatment with high-dose interleukin-2. Ann Intern Med 1993;118(8):617–8.

73. Post AB, Falk GW, Bukowski RM. Acute colonic pseudo-obstruction associated with interleukin-2 therapy. Am J Gastroenterol 1991;86(10):1539–41.

74. Rahman R, Bernstein Z, Vaickus L, Penetrante R, Arbuck S, Kopec I, Vesper D, Douglass HO Jr, Foon KA. Unusual gastrointestinal complications of interleukin-2 therapy. J Immunother 1991;10(3):221–5.

75. Sparano JA, Dutcher JP, Kaleya R, Caliendo G, Fiorito J, Mitsudo S, Shechner R, Boley SJ, Gucalp R, Ciobanu N, et al. Colonic ischemia complicating immunotherapy with interleukin-2 and interferon-alpha. Cancer 1991;68(7):1538–44.

76. Sondel PM, Kohler PC, Hank JA, Moore KH, Rosenthal NS, Sosman JA, Bechhofer R, Storer B. Clinical and immunological effects of recombinant interleukin 2 given by repetitive weekly cycles to patients with cancer. Cancer Res 1988;48(9):2561–7.

77. Webb DE, Austin HA 3rd, Belldegrun A, Vaughan E, Linehan WM, Rosenberg SA. Metabolic and renal effects of interleukin-2 immunotherapy for metastatic cancer. Clin Nephrol 1988;30(3):141–5.

78. Fisher B, Keenan AM, Garra BS, Steinberg SM, White DE, DiBisceglie AM, Hoofnagle JH, Yolles P, Rosenberg SA, Lotze MT. Interleukin-2 induces profound reversible cholestasis: a detailed analysis in treated cancer patients. J Clin Oncol 1989;7(12):1852–62.

79. Punt CJ, Henzen-Logmans SC, Bolhuis RL, Stoter G. Hyperbilirubinaemia in patients treated with recombinant human interleukin-2 (rIL-2). Br J Cancer 1990;61(3):491.

80. Lilenbaum RC, Lilenbaum AM, Hryniuk WM. Interleukin 2-induced focal fatty infiltrate of the liver that mimics metastases. J Natl Cancer Inst 1995;87(8):609–10.

81. Powell FC, Spooner KM, Shawker TH, Premkumar A, Thakore KN, Vogel SE, Kovacs JA, Masur H, Feuerstein IM. Symptomatic interleukin-2-induced cholecystopathy in patients with HIV infection. Am J Roentgenol 1994;163(1):117–21.

82. Premkumar A, Walworth CM, Vogel S, Daryanani KD, Venzon DJ, Kovacs JA, Feuerstein IM. Prospective sonographic evaluation of interleukin-2-induced changes in the gallbladder. Radiology 1998;206(2):393–6.

83. Birchfield GR, Ward JH, Redman BG, Flaherty L, Samlowski WE. Acute pancreatitis associated with high-dose interleukin-2 immunotherapy for malignant melanoma. West J Med 1990;152(6):714–6.

84. Christiansen NP, Skubitz KM, Nath K, Ochoa A, Kennedy BJ. Nephrotoxicity of continuous intravenous infusion of recombinant interleukin-2. Am J Med 1988;84(6):1072–5.

85. Shalmi CL, Dutcher JP, Feinfeld DA, Chun KJ, Saleemi KR, Freeman LM, Lynn RI, Wiernik PH. Acute renal dysfunction during interleukin-2 treatment: suggestion of an intrinsic renal lesion. J Clin Oncol 1990;8(11):1839–46.

86. Hisanaga S, Kawagoe H, Yamamoto Y, Kuroki N, Fujimoto S, Tanaka K, Kurokawa M. Nephrotic syndrome associated with recombinant interleukin-2. Nephron 1990;54(3):277–8.

87. Heslan JM, Branellec AI, Lang P, Lagrue G. Recombinant interleukin-2-induced proteinuria: fact or artifact? Nephron 1991;57(3):373–4.

88. Guleria AS, Yang JC, Topalian SL, Weber JS, Parkinson DR, MacFarlane MP, White RL, Steinberg SM, White DE, Einhorn JH, et al. Renal dysfunction associated with the administration of high-dose interleukin-2 in 199 consecutive patients with metastatic melanoma or renal carcinoma. J Clin Oncol 1994;12(12):2714–22.

89. Heys SD, Eremin O, Franks CR, Broom J, Whiting PH. Lithium clearance measurements during recombinant interleukin 2 treatment: tubular dysfunction in man. Ren Fail 1993;15(2):195–201.

90. Diekman MJ, Vlasveld LT, Krediet RT, Rankin EM, Arisz L. Acute interstitial nephritis during continuous intravenous administration of low-dose interleukin-2. Nephron 1992;60(1):122–3.

91. Feinfeld DA, D'Agati V, Dutcher JP, Werfel SB, Lynn RI, Wiernik PH. Interstitial nephritis in a patient receiving adoptive immunotherapy with recombinant interleukin-2 and lymphokine-activated killer cells. Am J Nephrol 1991;11(6):489–92.

92. Vlasveld LT, van de Wiel-van Kemenade E, de Boer AJ, Sein JJ, Gallee MP, Krediet RT, Mellief CJ, Rankin EM, Hekman A, Figdor CG. Possible role for cytotoxic lymphocytes in the pathogenesis of acute interstitial nephritis after recombinant interleukin-2 treatment for renal cell cancer. Cancer Immunol Immunother 1993;36(3):210–3.

93. Chan TM, Cheng IK, Wong KL, Chan KW, Lai CL. Crescentic IgA glomerulonephritis following interleukin-2 therapy for hepatocellular carcinoma of the liver. Am J Nephrol 1991;11(6):493–6.

94. Kruit WH, Schmitz PI, Stoter G. The role of possible risk factors for acute and late renal dysfunction after high-dose interleukin-2, interferon alpha and lymphokine-activated killer cells. Cancer Immunol Immunother 1999;48(6):331–335.

95. Asnis LA, Gaspari AA. Cutaneous reactions to recombinant cytokine therapy. J Am Acad Dermatol 1995;33(3):393–410.

96. Blessing K, Park KG, Heys SD, King G, Eremin O. Immunopathological changes in the skin following recombinant interleukin-2 treatment. J Pathol 1992;167(3):313–9.

97. Dummer R, Miller K, Eilles C, Burg G. The skin: an immunoreactive target organ during interleukin-2 administration? Dermatologica 1991;183(2):95–9.

98. Wolkenstein P, Chosidow O, Wechsler J, Guillaume JC, Lescs MC, Brandely M, Avril MF, Revuz J. Cutaneous side effects associated with interleukin 2 administration for metastatic melanoma. J Am Acad Dermatol 1993;28(1):66–70.

99. Baars JW, Coenen JL, Wagstaff J, van der Valk P, Pinedo HM. Lobular panniculitis after subcutaneous administration of interleukin-2 (IL-2), and its exacerbation during intravenous therapy with IL-2. Br J Cancer 1992;66(4):698–9.

100. Costello R, Blaise D, Jacquemier J, Monges G, Stoppa AM, Viens P, Olive D, Bouabdallah M, Brandely, Gastaut JA. Induction of cutaneous "graft-versus-host like" reaction by recombinant IL-2 after autologous bone marrow transplantation. Bone Marrow Transplant 1995;16(1):199–200.

101. Massumoto C, Benyunes MC, Sale G, Beauchamp M, York A, Thompson JA, Buckner CD, Fefer A. Close simulation of acute graft-versus-host disease by interleukin-2 administered after autologous bone marrow transplantation for hematologic malignancy. Bone Marrow Transplant 1996;17(3):351–6.

102. Richards JM, Gilewski TA, Ramming K, Mitchel B, Doane LL, Vogelzang NJ. Effective chemotherapy for melanoma after treatment with interleukin-2. Cancer 1992;69(2):427–9.

103. Wolkenstein P, Revuz J, Guillaume JC, Avril MF, Chosidow O. Autoimmune disorders and interleukin-2 therapy: a step toward "unanswered questions". Arch Dermatol 1995;131(5):615–6.

104. Scheibenbogen C, Hunstein W, Keilholz U. Vitiligo-like lesions following immunotherapy with IFN alpha and IL-2 in melanoma patients. Eur J Cancer 1994;30A(8):1209–11.

105. Gustafsson LL, Eriksson LS, Dahl ML, Eleborg L, Ericzon BG, Nyberg A. Cyclophosphamide-induced acute liver failure requiring transplantation in a patient with genetically deficient debrisoquine metabolism: a causal relationship? J Intern Med 1996;240(5):311–4.

106. Segura Huerta AA, Tordera P, Cercos AC, Yuste AL, Lopez-Tendero P, Reynes G. Toxic epidermal necrolysis associated with interleukin-2. Ann Pharmacother 2002;36(7–8):1171–4.

107. Bernand S, Scheidegger EP, Dummer R, Burg G. Multifocal fixed drug eruption to paracetamol, tropisetron and ondansetron induced by interleukin 2. Dermatology 2000;201(2):148–50.

108. Baron NW, Davis LP, Flaherty LE, Muz J, Valdivieso M, Kling GA. Scintigraphic findings in patients with shoulder pain caused by interleukin-2. Am J Roentgenol 1990;154(2):327–30.

109. Massarotti EM, Liu NY, Mier J, Atkins MB. Chronic inflammatory arthritis after treatment with high-dose interleukin-2 for malignancy. Am J Med 1992;92(6):693–697.

110. Heys SD, Mills KL, Eremin O. Bilateral carpal tunnel syndrome associated with interleukin 2 therapy. Postgrad Med J 1992;68(801):587–8.

111. Blanche P, Gombert B, Rollot F, Salmon D, Sicard D. Sarcoidosis in a patient with acquired immunodeficiency syndrome treated with interleukin-2. Clin Infect Dis 2000;31(6):1493–4.

112. Baars JW, Wagstaff J, Hack CE, Wolbink GJ, Eerenberg-Belmer AJ, Pinedo HM. Angioneurotic oedema and urticaria during therapy with interleukin-2 (IL-2). Ann Oncol 1992;3(3):243–4.

113. Scharenberg JGM, Stam AGM, von Blomberg BME, et al. The development of anti-interleukin-2 (IL-2) antibodies in patient treated with recombinant IL-2 does not interfere with clinical responsiveness. Proc Am Assoc Cancer Res 1993;34:464.

114. Atzpodien J, Hanninen EL, Kirchner H, Knuver-Hopf J, Poliwoda H. Human antibodies to recombinant interleukin-2 in patients with hypernephroma. J Interfer Res 1994;14:177–8.

115. Kirchner H, Korfer A, Evers P, Szamel MM, Knuver-Hopf J, Mohr H, Franks CR, Pohl U, Resch K, Hadam M, et al. The development of neutralizing antibodies in a patient receiving subcutaneous recombinant and natural interleukin-2. Cancer 1991;67(7):1862–4.

116. Fraenkel PG, Rutkove SB, Matheson JK, Fowkes M, Cannon ME, Patti ME, Atkins MB, Gollob JA. Induction of myasthenia gravis, myositis, and insulin-dependent diabetes mellitus by high-dose interleukin-2 in a patient with renal cell cancer. J Immunother 2002;25(4):373–8.

117. Pockaj BA, Topalian SL, Steinberg SM, White DE, Rosenberg SA. Infectious complications associated with interleukin-2 administration: a retrospective review of 935 treatment courses. J Clin Oncol 1993;11(1):136–47.

118. Jones AL, Cropley I, O'Brien ME, Lorentzos A, Moore J, Jameson B, Gore ME. Infectious complications of subcutaneous interleukin-2 and interferon-alpha. Lancet 1992;339(8786):181–2.

119. Buter J, de Vries EG, Sleijfer DT, Willemse PH, Mulder NH. Infection after subcutaneous interleukin-2. Lancet 1992;339(8792):552.

120. Schomburg AG, Kirchner HH, Atzpodien J. Cytokines and infection in cancer patients. Lancet 1992;339(8800):1061.

121. Macdonald D, Jiang YZ, Swirsky D, Vulliamy T, Morilla R, Bungey J, Barrett AJ. Acute myeloid leukaemia relapsing following interleukin-2 treatment expresses the alpha chain of the interleukin-2 receptor. Br J Haematol 1991;77(1):43–9.

122. Spiekermann K, O'Brien S, Estey E. Relapse of acute myelogenous leukemia during low dose interleukin-2 (IL-2) therapy. Phenotypic evolution associated with strong expression of the IL-2 receptor alpha chain. Cancer 1995;75(7):1594–7.

123. Elkahwaji J, Robin MA, Berson A, Tinel M, Letteron P, Labbe G, Beaune P, Elias D, Rougier P, Escudier B, Duvillard P, Pessayre D. Decrease in hepatic cytochrome P450 after interleukin-2 immunotherapy. Biochem Pharmacol 1999;57(8):951–4.

124. Choyke PL, Miller DL, Lotze MT, Whiteis JM, Ebbitt B, Rosenberg SA. Delayed reactions to contrast media after interleukin-2 immunotherapy. Radiology 1992;183(1):111–4.

125. Shulman KL, Thompson JA, Benyunes MC, Winter TC, Fefer A. Adverse reactions to intravenous contrast media in patients treated with interleukin-2. J Immunother 1993;13(3):208–12.

126. Zukiwski AA, David CL, Coan J, Wallace S, Gutterman JU, Mavligit GM. Increased incidence of

hypersensitivity to iodine-containing radiographic contrast media after interleukin-2 administration. Cancer 1990;65(7):1521–4.

127. Heywood GR, Rosenberg SA, Weber JS. Hypersensitivity reactions to chemotherapy agents in patients receiving chemoimmunotherapy with high-dose interleukin-2. J Natl Cancer Inst 1995;87(12):915–22.

128. Eton O, Legha SS, Bedikian AY, Lee JJ, Buzaid AC, Hodges C, Ring SE, Papadopoulos NE, Plager C, East MJ, Zhan F, Benjamin RS. Sequential biochemotherapy versus chemotherapy for metastatic melanoma: results from a phase III randomized trial. J Clin Oncol 2002;20(8):2045–52.

129. Bortolussi R, Fabiani F, Savron F, Testa V, Lazzarini R, Sorio R, De Conno F, Caraceni A. Acute morphine intoxication during high-dose recombinant interleukin-2 treatment for metastatic renal cell cancer. Eur J Cancer 1994;30A(12):1905–7.

Anakinra

General Information

Anakinra is an interleukin-1 receptor antagonist. It has been used to treat rheumatoid arthritis (1,2). It has been tried in graft-versus-host disease, but without success (3). According to published trial data, moderate injection site reactions were the primary adverse effect and required treatment withdrawal in under 5% of patients. An erythematous rash was seldom observed. Although a few patients have developed antibodies to anakinra, these have not so far been associated with lack of efficacy or allergic skin reactions.

Drug–Drug Interactions

Etanercept

Regulatory agencies have issued an important postmarketing warning of an increased risk of serious infections and neutropenia in patients who receive concomitant anakinra and etanercept (4). This warning was based on an analysis of a randomized clinical trial in 242 patients with rheumatoid arthritis, in which 7% of patients receiving concomitant treatment had serious infections, compared with none in those treated with etanercept alone. Concurrent administration of these two drugs was therefore not recommended.

References

1. Cohen SB. The use of anakinra, an interleukin-1 receptor antagonist, in the treatment of rheumatoid arthritis. Rheum Dis Clin North Am 2004;30(2):365–80.

2. Bresnihan B. The safety and efficacy of interleukin-1 receptor antagonist in the treatment of rheumatoid arthritis. Semin Arthritis Rheum 2001;30(5 Suppl 2):17–20.

3. Antin JH, Weisdorf D, Neuberg D, Nicklow R, Clouthier S, Lee SJ, Alyea E, McGarigle C, Blazar BR, Sonis S, Soiffer RJ, Ferrara JL. Interleukin-1 blockade does not

prevent acute graft-versus-host disease: results of a randomized, double-blind, placebo-controlled trial of interleukin-1 receptor antagonist in allogeneic bone marrow transplantation. Blood 2002;100(10):3479–82.
4. EMEA/31631/02 Public Statement. Increased risk of serious infection and neutropenia in patients treated concurrently with Kineret (anakinra) and Enbrel (etanercept). http://www.emea.eu.int/pdfs/human/press/pus/3163102en.pdf.

Interleukin-1

General Information

Interleukin-1-alfa and interleukin-1-beta are produced by two distinct genes with only 25% homology, but they act through the same receptor and share similar in vitro biological properties. Interleukin-1 on its own has modest antitumor activity and limited hemopoietic effects. It also acts synergistically with other colony-stimulating factors (for example GM-CSF, G-CSF, interleukin-3, or interleukin-6) to promote colony formation and stimulate hemopoietic recovery in patients undergoing autologous bone marrow transplantation or receiving cytotoxic anticancer treatment (1).

General adverse effects

Both forms of interleukin-1 have been investigated in humans, and they produce a wide and very similar spectrum of adverse effects (SED-13, 1101; 2). Whatever the dose, fever and chills are universal but only occasionally treatment-limiting. Tachyphylaxis can develop during prolonged administration. Other frequent but moderate adverse effects include transient fatigue, myalgia, arthralgia, dose-dependent headache, nausea, vomiting, diarrhea, and abdominal pain. Injection site reactions included local phlebitis, while subcutaneous injection of interleukin-1-beta can cause local pain and erythema. Interleukin-1-alfa can cause transient and moderate increases in bilirubin, aspartate transaminase, and serum creatinine concentrations.

Organs and Systems

Cardiovascular

The most significant adverse effect of both forms of interleukin-1 is dose-limiting hypotension resulting from a capillary leak phenomenon with clinical features of septic shock (2). Although mild weight gain, dyspnea, and pulmonary infiltrates can occur, severe capillary leak syndrome is usually not observed. Shortness of breath requiring oxygen and benign supraventricular dysrhythmias were sometimes noted. The maximum tolerated dose of interleukin-1 with pressors is therefore 0.3 micrograms/kg/day. The most probable mechanism underlying these complications is an interleukin-1-induced increase in nitric oxide production by vascular smooth muscle.

Nervous system

A few patients given interleukin-1 complain of somnolence, agitation, delusional ideation, photophobia or subjective blurred vision, but at high doses some patients experienced a greater degree of central nervous system toxicity, with complaints of confusion, severe somnolence and seizures (3).

Endocrine

Various endocrinological effects have been observed, but without clinically apparent endocrinopathies (SEDA-20, 333).

Metabolism

Interleukin-1-beta has been associated with transient hypoglycemia (4).

Mouth and teeth

Interleukin-1-alfa can cause mucositis and xerostomia (3) and can increase the severity of chemotherapy-induced oral mucositis and erythema (5).

References

1. Curti BD, Smith JW 2nd. Interleukin-1 in the treatment of cancer. Pharmacol Ther 1995;65(3):291–302.
2. Vial T, Descotes J. Clinical toxicity of cytokines used as haemopoietic growth factors. Drug Saf 1995;13(6):371–406.
3. Smith JW 2nd, Urba WJ, Curti BD, Elwood LJ, Steis RG, Janik JE, Sharfman WH, Miller LL, Fenton RG, Conlon KC, et al. The toxic and hematologic effects of interleukin-1 alpha administered in a phase I trial to patients with advanced malignancies. J Clin Oncol 1992;10(7):1141–52.
4. Crown J, Jakubowski A, Kemeny N, Gordon M, Gasparetto C, Wong G, Sheridan C, Toner G, Meisenberg B, Botet J, et al. A phase I trial of recombinant human interleukin-1 beta alone and in combination with myelosuppressive doses of 5-fluorouracil in patients with gastrointestinal cancer. Blood 1991;78(6):1420–7.
5. Prussick R, Horn TD, Wilson WH, Turner MC. A characteristic eruption associated with ifosfamide, carboplatin, and etoposide chemotherapy after pretreatment with recombinant interleukin-1 alpha. J Am Acad Dermatol 1996;35(5 Pt 1):705–9.

Interleukin-2

See Aldesleukin.

Interleukin-3

General Information

Interleukin-3 is produced by activated T lymphocytes and stimulates the proliferation and differentiation of the granulocyte, macrophage, eosinophil, basophil, erythroid, megakaryocyte, and mast cell lineages (1).

Observational studies

Subcutaneous recombinant interleukin-3 has been investigated in patients with chemotherapy-induced myelotoxicity, in the setting of autologous bone marrow transplantation or peripheral stem cell harvesting, or in patients with myelodysplastic syndrome, aplastic anemia, and Diamond–Blackfan anemia (1,2). Interleukin-3 given alone has limited clinical effects, but an enhanced hemopoietic response has been obtained with a genetically engineered GM-CSF/interleukin-3 fusion protein, PIXY321 (SEDA-21, 376; 3).

The specific toxicity of subcutaneous recombinant human interleukin-3 derived from *Escherichia coli* has been addressed in a 4-day study performed in healthy volunteers (4). All had mild-to-moderate dose-independent symptoms; flu-like symptoms, including fever, chills, headache, conjunctival congestion, myalgia, and diffuse aching, were the most frequent. Minor erythematous reactions at the injection site were also consistently described, and one patient had histological features of an allergic vasculitis resembling that reported with GM-CSF (SEDA-20, 335). Mild-to-severe skin rashes or urticaria were also sometimes observed, and there were bullae with hemorrhagic necrosis of the skin in one patient (5). In preliminary clinical trials, malaise, eye pain, nasal congestion, weakness or lethargy, tachycardia, and gastrointestinal disorders occurred in under 16% of patients (6). None of these effects was clearly related to dose, and withdrawal of treatment was not required. A similar safety profile was reported in patients who subsequently developed tachyphylaxis, and the adverse effect profile of yeast or interleukin-3 derived from *E. coli* did not appear to be different (6). Overall, the rate of withdrawal of treatment because of adverse effects was 17–50% in patients receiving 10 micrograms/kg/day. Constitutional symptoms, generalized skin reactions, and facial edema were the most frequent dose-limiting adverse events. In autologous bone marrow transplantation, the maximum tolerated dose was only 2 micrograms/kg/day. Interleukin-3-associated fever is supposedly the result of a dose-dependent increase in interleukin-6 and acute phase protein production.

Adverse effects related to interleukin-3 were observed in a comparison of G-CSF alone, GM-CSF alone, and sequential interleukin-3 and GM-CSF in 48 patients with cancer (16 in each group) receiving high-dose cyclophosphamide (7). In particular, fever above 38.5 °C, skin rash, and headaches were more frequent during interleukin-3 administration. As a result, 90% of patients receiving interleukin-3 required pharmacological treatment for adverse effects.

Placebo-controlled studies

The potential hemopoietic benefits of postchemotherapy interleukin-3 are limited. In a phase III trial in 185 ovarian cancer patients treated with carboplatin and cyclophosphamide, premature withdrawal was significantly more frequent in patients randomized to received recombinant interleukin-3 (5 micrograms/kg from day 3 to day 12) than

in the placebo group (8). The most frequent adverse effects were allergic reactions (50 versus 23%), which required interleukin-3 withdrawal in 21 patients compared with one in the placebo group, and headache (46 versus 19%). In this setting, interleukin-3 stimulated hemopoiesis, but did not reduce platelet transfusions or increase adherence to the chemotherapeutic regimen.

The benefit of interleukin-3 in promoting hemopoietic reconstitution after autologous bone marrow transplantation has been investigated in 198 patients with malignant lymphoma who received either interleukin-3 (10 micrograms/kg for 4 weeks, 130 patients) or placebo (68 patients) (9). There was no significant advantage of interleukin-3 over placebo in regard to the number of platelet transfusions before engraftment, the time to platelet engraftment, or the incidence of hemorrhagic complications. This confirms that interleukin-3 alone has limited clinical effects. In contrast, significantly more patients who received interleukin-3 had to discontinue treatment because of adverse events (26 versus 7%). Adverse events that were significantly more frequent with interleukin-3 than with placebo included mucositis (69 versus 44%), headache (38 versus 13%), and rash (25 versus 12%). It is not yet known whether the initial route of administration (continuous intravenous infusion for 7 days followed by subcutaneous administration for 21 days) might account for these findings.

General adverse effects

Constitutional symptoms, generalized skin reactions, and facial edema are the most frequent. Although they are not easily attributable to interleukin-3, other significant adverse events noted during treatment have included exacerbation of arthralgia in a seronegative patient (5) and transient thrombocytopenia in patients with myelodysplastic syndrome or aplastic anemia (10). Signs of meningism with neck rigidity were sometimes found (10).

As with G-CSF and GM-CSF, the presence of interleukin-3 receptors on leukemia cells suggests a theoretical risk of disease aggravation. However, accelerated tumor growth has not been noted in patients with non-hemopoietic tumors or newly diagnosed non-Hodgkin's lymphoma (6). Overall, some types of disease progression were observed in 11 of 86 patients with myelodysplastic syndrome, but no clear relation between interleukin-3 and disease acceleration can be assessed at the moment.

PIXY321

The clinical and hematological effects of PIXY321, a genetically engineered GM-CSF/interleukin-3 fusion protein, have been evaluated in 71 women with breast cancer (11). In addition to chemotherapy (four cycles of fluorouracil, doxorubicin, and cyclophosphamide), the patients received either PIXY321 or placebo from days 3–15. Although the incidence and/or duration of chemotherapy-induced severe neutropenia was significantly reduced by PIXY321, there were more frequent systemic adverse effects (fever, chills, abdominal pain, arthralgia, and injection-site reactions) and more severe thrombocytopenia during cycles 3 and 4. Based on these results and the lack of a demonstrable advantage of PIXY321 over GM-CSF (12), the development of PIXY321 as an adjuvant treatment in cancer was halted. In one study only insomnia and rash were more common in patients treated with subcutaneous PIXY321 compared with intravenous GM-CSF alone after autologous bone marrow transplantation (13).

Organs and Systems

Cardiovascular

Hypotension, exacerbation or new onset of atrial fibrillation, and dyspnea were infrequently observed in clinical trials (6). Although weight gain and peripheral edema can develop, only one fatal case, compatible with a capillary vascular leak syndrome, has been reported (SEDA-20, 335).

Thrombophlebitis was recorded in 45% of patients treated for advanced ovarian cancer who also received intravenous interleukin-3 (14), and deep venous thromboses were reported in children treated with maintenance interleukin-3 for Diamond–Blackfan anemia (15). In addition, one smoking breast-cancer patient developed severe hypotension and cerebellar and superior mesenteric thrombosis after subcutaneous interleukin-3 administration (SEDA-19, 340). Collectively, these case reports suggest that interleukin-3 may contribute to the development of thrombosis, but a possible increased risk of thrombosis with interleukin-3 remains to be demonstrated.

Hematologic

Interleukin-3 caused a transient rise in circulating atypical B lymphocytes, with enlargement of the spleen and lymph nodes in two patients with large-cell lymphoma and the development of a clonally-related transient plasmocytosis in one patient with relapsing follicular non-Hodgkin's lymphoma (SED-13, 1109; 10,16).

There has been one case of bone marrow histiocytosis in a patient treated with interleukin-3 for refractory aplastic anemia (SED-13, 1109).

Immunologic

An anaphylactoid reaction to recombinant human interleukin-3 (rHu interleukin-3) has been described (17).

- A 66-year-old man with radiation-induced aplastic anemia and myelodysplastic features failed to respond to multiple therapeutic regimens. A trial of recombinant human interleukin-3 was begun, but he had transient shortness of breath and hypotension after the first subcutaneous injection. On the next day, 2 hours after the second dose, he had restlessness, dyspnea, spasticity, wheezing, cyanosis, hyperthermia, tachycardia, and hypotension (70/50 mmHg). Full recovery was obtained with fluids, adrenaline, promethazine, and glucocorticoids.

Histamine release from circulating basophils was the suggested mechanism.

Drug–Drug Interactions

Angiotensin-converting enzyme (ACE) inhibitors

Severe hypotension within hours after interleukin-3 injection has been observed in three of 26 patients treated with angiotensin-converting enzyme inhibitors (SEDA-19, 340). Indirect synergy between ACE and interleukin-3 on nitric oxide production was suggested to be involved.

Carboplatin

In patients with ovarian cancer, the combination of interleukin-3 with high-dose carboplatin was poorly tolerated; severe fever, malaise, protracted nausea, vomiting, severe hypotension, and nephrotoxicity required withdrawal of interleukin-3 in 60% of patients when interleukin-3 was given only 24 hours after high-dose carboplatin (18).

GM-CSF

Combined sequential administration of interleukin-3 plus GM-CSF in patients treated for myelodysplastic syndrome suggested unacceptable toxicity (19).

Interleukin-2

Prior interleukin-2 therapy can induce atypical contrast medium hypersensitivity in the form of toxic recall reactions of various types (SEDA-17, 537), and these cannot be prevented by glucocorticoid premedication (20).

References

1. Gianella-Borradori A. Present and future clinical relevance of interleukin 3. Stem Cells 1994;12(Suppl 1):241–8.
2. de Vries EG, van Gameren MM, Willemse PH. Recombinant human interleukin 3 in clinical oncology. Stem Cells 1993;11(2):72–80.
3. Vadhan-Raj S. PIXY321 (GM-CSF/IL-3 fusion protein): biological and clinical effects of a novel cytokine. Forum Trends Exp Clin Med 1995;5:110–8.
4. Huhn RD, Yurkow EJ, Kuhn JG, Clarke L, Gunn H, Resta D, Shah R, Myers LA, Seibold JR. Pharmacodynamics of daily subcutaneous recombinant human interleukin-3 in normal volunteers. Clin Pharmacol Ther 1995;57(1):32–41.
5. Nimer SD, Paquette RL, Ireland P, Resta D, Young D, Golde DW. A phase I/II study of interleukin-3 in patients with aplastic anemia and myelodysplasia. Exp Hematol 1994;22(9):875–80.
6. Vial T, Descotes J. Clinical toxicity of cytokines used as haemopoietic growth factors. Drug Saf 1995;13(6):371–406.
7. Ballestrero A, Ferrando F, Garuti A, Basta P, Gonella R, Stura P, Mela GS, Sessarego M, Gobbi M, Patrone F. Comparative effects of three cytokine regimens after high-dose cyclophosphamide: granulocyte colony-stimulating factor, granulocyte–macrophage colony-stimulating factor (GM-CSF), and sequential interleukin-3 and GM-CSF. J Clin Oncol 1999;17(4):1296.
8. Hofstra LS, Kristensen GB, Willemse PH, Vindevoghel A, Meden H, Lahousen M, Oberling F, Sorbe B, Crump M, Sklenar I, Sluiter WJ, Kiese B, Trope CG, de Vries EG. Randomized trial of recombinant human interleukin-3 versus placebo in prevention of bone marrow depression

during first-line chemotherapy for ovarian carcinoma. J Clin Oncol 1998;16(10):3335–44.

9. Brouwer RE, Vellenga E, Zwinderman KH, Bezwoda WR, Durrant ST, Herrmann RP, Kiese B, Maraninchi D, Milligan DW, Sklenar I, Tabilio A, Volonte JL, Winfield DA, Fibbe WE. Phase III efficacy study of interleukin-3 after autologous bone marrow transplantation in patients with malignant lymphoma. Br J Haematol 1999;106(3):730–6.

10. Ganser A, Seipelt G, Lindemann A, Ottmann OG, Falk S, Eder M, Herrmann F, Becher R, Hoffken K, Buchner T, et al. Effects of recombinant human interleukin-3 in patients with myelodysplastic syndromes. Blood 1990;76(3):455–62.

11. Jones SE, Khandelwal P, McIntyre K, Mennel R, Orr D, Kirby R, Agura E, Duncan L, Hyman W, Roque T, Regan D, Schuster M, Dimitrov N, Garrison L, Lange M. Randomized, double-blind, placebo-controlled trial to evaluate the hematopoietic growth factor PIXY321 after moderate-dose fluorouracil, doxorubicin, and cyclophosphamide in stage II and III breast cancer. J Clin Oncol 1999;17(10):3025–32.

12. Schuh JC, Morrissey PJ. Development of a recombinant growth factor and fusion protein: lessons from GM-CSF. Toxicol Pathol 1999;27(1):72–7.

13. Vose JM, Pandite AN, Beveridge RA, Geller RB, Schuster MW, Anderson JE, LeMaistre CF, Ahmed T, Granena A, Keating A, Fernandez Ranada JM, Stiff PJ, Tabbara I, Longo W, Copelan EA, Nichols C, Smith A, Topolsky DL, Bierman PJ, Lebsack ME, Lange M, Garrison L. Granulocyte–macrophage colony-stimulating factor/interleukin-3 fusion protein versus granulocyte–macrophage colony-stimulating factor after autologous bone marrow transplantation for non-Hodgkin's lymphoma: results of a randomized double-blind trial. J Clin Oncol 1997;15(4):1617–23.

14. Biesma B, Willemse PH, Mulder NH, Sleijfer DT, Gietema JA, Mull R, Limburg PC, Bouma J, Vellenga E, de Vries EG. Effects of interleukin-3 after chemotherapy for advanced ovarian cancer. Blood 1992;80(5):1141–8.

15. Gillio AP, Faulkner LB, Alter BP, Reilly L, Klafter R, Heller G, Young DC, Lipton JM, Moore MA, O'Reilly RJ. Treatment of Diamond–Blackfan anemia with recombinant human interleukin-3. Blood 1993;82(3):744–51.

16. Kramer MH, Kluin PM, Wijburg ER, Fibbe WE, Kluin-Nelemans HC. Differentiation of follicular lymphoma cells after autologous bone marrow transplantation and haematopoietic growth factor treatment. Lancet 1995;345(8948):488–90.

17. Mittelman M, Zeidman A, Fradin Z, Menachem Y. Anaphylactic shock due to recombinant human interleukin-3. Eur J Haematol 1999;62(3):199–200.

18. Dercksen MW, Hoekman K, ten Bokkel Huinink WW, Rankin EM, Dubbelman R, van Tinteren H, Wagstaff J, Pinedo HM. Effects of interleukin-3 on myelosuppression induced by chemotherapy for ovarian cancer and small cell undifferentiated tumours. Br J Cancer 1993;68(5):996–1003.

19. Nand S, Sosman J, Godwin JE, Fisher RI. A phase I/II study of sequential interleukin-3 and granulocyte–macrophage colony-stimulating factor in myelodysplastic syndromes. Blood 1994;83(2):357–60.

20. Shulman KL, Thompson JA, Benyunes MC, Winter TC, Fefer A. Adverse reactions to intravenous contrast media in patients treated with interleukin-2. J Immunother 1993;13(3):208–12.

Interleukin-4

General Information

Interleukin-4 is a pleiotropic cytokine, mostly produced by activated T cells, which acts on the proliferation and differentiation of B and T lymphocytes and enhances the function of natural killer cells, eosinophils, and mast cells (1). It is being investigated for potential antitumoral and hemopoietic actions.

General adverse effects

Moderate fever with flu-like symptoms, arthralgias, fatigue, anorexia, nausea, vomiting, headache, and transient hypotension were frequent at all doses and by all routes of administration, but were more severe and prolonged at high doses (2). Periorbital, facial, and peripheral edema were also noted. Frequent discomfort caused by severe and resistant nasal congestion, supposedly due to edema and vascular engorgement from histamine stimulation, was sometimes dose-limiting. Mild asymptomatic increases in liver enzymes and minimal changes in serum creatinine concentrations can occur. No significant effects on serum hormone (ACTH, cortisol, thyrotropin, thyroxine, prolactin) or lipid concentrations have been noted (SEDA-20, 336). Other adverse events, as yet not clearly related to interleukin-4, included reversible Coomb's-positive hemolytic anemia, transient partial blindness, photophobia, and visual hallucinations. At the moment, only one report has suggested that long-term interleukin-4 may have stimulated the development of multiple myeloma (SEDA-21, 376).

Of 49 patients with advanced renal cell carcinoma treated with subcutaneous interleukin-4 (4 micrograms/kg/day for 28 days followed by a 7-day rest), nine had 13 episodes of grade 4 toxicity (3). Severe unexpected toxic effects included three cases of Bell's palsy and one episode of severe hypoglycemia in a previously well-controlled patient with diabetes mellitus.

Organs and Systems

Cardiovascular

The vascular leak syndrome was observed at a dose of 15 micrograms/kg by bolus or continuous intravenous administration, but a moderate capillary leak syndrome was also noted at lower subcutaneous doses (4).

Cardiac toxicity, consistent with myocardial infarction, was observed in three of seven patients with metastatic cancer receiving intravenous bolus interleukin-4 to a daily total of 800 micrograms/m^2 (5). A unique pattern of myocarditis with predominant polymorphonuclear, eosinophil, and mast cell infiltration was the possible cause of death in one case and suggested an allergic inflammatory myocardial process.

Endocrine

Permanent hypothyroidism associated with vitiligo was reported in a woman treated with interleukin-4 for metastatic malignant melanoma (SEDA-20, 336).

Hematologic

Unexpected severe neutropenia has been found in 33% of patients with AIDS-related Kaposi's sarcoma given interleukin-4 (SEDA-21, 376).

Isolated coagulation abnormalities with minor prolongation of prothrombin time were consistently observed, in patients given interleukin-4, particularly those with pre-existing liver disease (2).

Gastrointestinal

Significant gastrointestinal toxicity was described in patients who received interleukin-4 alone or in combination with interleukin-2 for advanced malignancy (6).

Antral or prepyloric ulcers and erosive gastritis were identified after 12 of 84 courses of interleukin-4 in 72 patients, of whom three suffered from life-threatening bleeding. There were no treatment-related deaths and no clear correlation with the dose of interleukin-4. A possible protective effect of interleukin-2 on the gastrointestinal mucosa was suggested. Although all but one of these patients also took indometacin, there was no recurrence of symptoms in several patients who developed ulcers during interleukin-4 treatment and further received interleukin-2 and indometacin. The ability of interleukin-4 to affect prostaglandin E_2 synthesis strongly suggests that interleukin-4 alone can contribute to the development of digestive mucosal injury.

Skin

Rare dermatological adverse effects have been noticed and consisted of a papular eruption. One patient had a pruritic papulovesicular eruption, which recurred after interleukin-4 re-administration and was compatible with transient acantholytic dermatosis (7).

Vitiligo associated with permanent hypothyroidism was reported in a woman treated with interleukin-4 for metastatic malignant melanoma (SEDA-20, 336).

References

1. Peyron E, Banchereau J. Interleukin-4: structure, function and clinical aspects. Eur J Dermatol 1994;4:181–8.
2. Vial T, Descotes J. Clinical toxicity of cytokines used as haemopoietic growth factors. Drug Saf 1995;13(6):371–406.
3. Whitehead RP, Lew D, Flanigan RC, Weiss GR, Roy V, Glode ML, Dakhil SR, Crawford ED. Phase II trial of recombinant human interleukin-4 in patients with advanced renal cell carcinoma: a Southwest Oncology Group study. J Immunother 2002;25(4):352–8.
4. Prendiville J, Thatcher N, Lind M, McIntosh R, Ghosh A, Stern P, Crowther D. Recombinant human interleukin-4 (rhu IL-4) administered by the intravenous and subcutaneous routes in patients with advanced cancer—a phase I toxicity study and pharmacokinetic analysis. Eur J Cancer 1993;29A(12):1700–7.
5. Trehu EG, Isner JM, Mier JW, Karp DD, Atkins MB. Possible myocardial toxicity associated with interleukin-4 therapy. J Immunother 1993;14(4):348–51.
6. Rubin JT, Lotze MT. Acute gastric mucosal injury associated with the systemic administration of interleukin-4. Surgery 1992;111(3):274–80.
7. Mahler SJ, De Villez RL, Pulitzer DR. Transient acantholytic dermatosis induced by recombinant human interleukin 4. J Am Acad Dermatol 1993;29(2 Pt 1):206–9.

Interleukin-6

General Information

Interleukin-6 is produced by T cells, monocytes, fibroblasts, endothelial cells, and keratinocytes, and regulates pleiotropic biological functions. Recombinant interleukin-6 is being evaluated for thrombopoietic and antitumoral properties (1).

General adverse effects

During clinical trials, intravenous and subcutaneous interleukin-6 produced universal moderate fever and flu-like symptoms (2). Mild nausea, weight loss, and taste disorders sometimes occurred, and central nervous system symptoms (somnolence, restlessness, confusion, hallucinations) were dose-limiting in patients with advanced malignant cancer (SEDA-21, 376), but no clear dose-related effects have been demonstrated. Moderate injection site reactions usually followed subcutaneous interleukin-6 administration, and a diffuse maculopapular erythema occurred in one patient. In contrast to several other cytokines, interleukin-6 has not been associated with signs of vascular leak syndrome or hypotension. Neutralizing antibodies to interleukin-6 were rarely evidenced (SEDA-20, 336).

Whereas no major signs of toxicity appeared at doses up to 20 micrograms/kg/day in patients with malignant disease, the maximum tolerated dose of interleukin-6 was 5 micrograms/kg/day in patients with myelodysplasia or thrombocytopenia, and only 1 microgram/kg/day in autologous bone marrow transplant patients who developed hyperbilirubinemia and severe maculopapular rash with microvesicular steatosis as treatment-limiting adverse effects (2). Combination of interleukin-6 with G-CSF or GM-CSF was not associated with significant synergism or new forms of toxicity.

Biochemical effects of interleukin-6 included asymptomatic increases in liver function tests, transient proteinuria, and increased serum creatinine concentrations. Reductions in serum albumin and cholesterol concentrations, and increases in blood glucose concentrations were dose-related (SEDA-21, 376; 2).

Organs and Systems

Sensory systems

One isolated report documented reduced visual acuity and bilateral uveitis in a patient receiving a 2-week regimen of interleukin-3 and interleukin-6 for secondary myelodysplastic syndrome (SEDA-19, 341).

Endocrine

Interleukin-6 reduced serum thyrotropin and thyroid hormone concentrations and increased LH concentrations (SEDA-20, 336).

Hematologic

Dose-dependent and reversible normochromic normocytic anemia was consistently noted within several days after starting interleukin-6, and required blood transfusion at the highest dose (3). Hemodilution was considered as the primary mechanism.

Skin

Diffuse maculopapular erythema with histological features consisting of epidermal spongiosis and interstitial mixed inflammatory cell infiltrate was reported in one patient, and a causal role was suggested by the recurrence of symptoms after interleukin-6 re-administration (SEDA-19, 341).

Long-Term Effects

Tumorigenicity

The possibility of interleukin-6 might accelerate tumor growth was suggested by findings in two patients with solid tumors (SEDA-19, 341).

References

1. Veldhuis GJ, Willemse PH, Mulder NH, Limburg PC, De Vries EG. Potential use of recombinant human interleukin-6 in clinical oncology. Leuk Lymphoma 1996;20(5–6):373–9.
2. Vial T, Descotes J. Clinical toxicity of cytokines used as haemopoietic growth factors. Drug Saf 1995;13(6):371–406.
3. Nieken J, Mulder NH, Buter J, Vellenga E, Limburg PC, Piers DA, de Vries EG. Recombinant human interleukin-6 induces a rapid and reversible anemia in cancer patients. Blood 1995;86(3):900–5.

Interleukin-10

General Information

Interleukin-10 is a potent anti-inflammatory and immunosuppressive cytokine with beneficial effects expected in a wide range of diseases (1). In healthy volunteers, its adverse effect profile mostly consisted of flu-like symptoms at the highest dose (SEDA-20, 336). First-degree atrioventricular block was noted in a few patients. Due to immunomodulating properties, potential adverse immunological effects, namely an increased risk of infections, autoimmune disorders, or B cell lymphoproliferative disorders, can be anticipated.

Organs and Systems

Hematologic

The mechanisms of mild thrombocytopenia after multiple doses of interleukin-10 have been extensively explored in 12 healthy volunteers, of whom four received placebo and eight received subcutaneous interleukin-10 (8 micrograms/kg/day for 10 days) (2). Compared with placebo, there was a 40% fall in platelet count during interleukin-10 treatment and prompt normalization after interleukin-10 withdrawal. There were also moderate changes in hemoglobin concentration. Bone marrow function, platelet production, and serum thrombopoietin concentrations suggested that a reduction in bone marrow platelet production was the primary cause.

References

1. Goldman M, Velu T, Pretaloni M. Interleukin-10. Actions and therapeutic potential. Biodrugs 1997;7:6–14.
2. Sosman JA, Verma A, Moss S, Sorokin P, Blend M, Bradlow B, Chachlani N, Cutler D, Sabo R, Nelson M, Bruno E, Gustin D, Viana M, Hoffman R. Interleukin-10 induced thrombocytopenia in normal healthy adult volunteers: evidence for decreased platelet production. Br J Haematol 2000;111(1):104–11.

Interleukin-11

See Oprelvekin.

Interleukin-12

General Information

Interleukin-12, an immunomodulatory cytokine, has potential effects in several cancer and infectious diseases. Although interleukin-12 was considered to be reasonably safe in early clinical trials, severe and sometimes fatal multiple organ adverse effects have been described in subsequent studies (SEDA-20, 336). This unexpected profile of toxicity was later shown to result from schedule-dependent toxicity, which occurred only in patients with cancer who received multiple high doses without an initial single dose of interleukin-12 (1). This severe toxicity has since been avoided.

Organs and Systems

Hematologic

Single cases of agranulocytosis and Coombs' negative hemolytic anemia have been attributed to twice-weekly interleukin-12 in 28 patients with renal cell cancer or melanoma (2). The patients responded only to cyclophosphamide and/or glucocorticoids, and the causative role of interleukin-12 was therefore inconclusive.

Immunologic

Interleukin-12 has been involved in the pathogenesis of several autoimmune disorders.

- A 53-year-old woman with previously mild and stable rheumatoid disease had an exacerbation of severe rheumatoid arthritis after each course of interleukin-12 for cervical carcinoma (3).

References

1. Leonard JP, Sherman ML, Fisher GL, Buchanan LJ, Larsen G, Atkins MB, Sosman JA, Dutcher JP, Vogelzang NJ, Ryan JL. Effects of single-dose interleukin-12 exposure on interleukin-12-associated toxicity and interferon-gamma production. Blood 1997;90(7):2541–8.
2. Gollob JA, Veenstra KG, Mier JW, Atkins MB. Agranulocytosis and hemolytic anemia in patients with renal cell cancer treated with interleukin-12. J Immunother 2001;24(1):91–8.
3. Peeva E, Fishman AD, Goddard G, Wadler S, Barland P. Rheumatoid arthritis exacerbation caused by exogenous interleukin-12. Arthritis Rheum 2000;43(2):461–3.

Oprelvekin

General Information

Oprelvekin has thrombopoietic activity and has been licensed to prevent severe thrombocytopenia and reduce the need for platelet transfusion after myelosuppressive chemotherapy (1). Common adverse effects included myalgia and arthralgias, fatigue, headache, and conjunctival injection. Peripheral edema, dyspnea, pleural effusions, tachycardia, and anemia were supposedly the result of oprelvekin-induced fluid retention (SEDA-20, 336; SEDA-21, 376). Atrial flutter or fibrillation were sometimes noted.

Severe fluid retention resistant to furosemide and fluid restriction was observed in 10 patients randomized to receive subcutaneous oprelvekin 50 µg/kg/day to prevent mucositis and acute graft-versus-host disease after allogeneic stem cell transplantation (2). One patient also had a large but reversible increase in serum transaminases.

A preliminary study of the thrombopoietic effect of oprelvekin (50 µg/kg/day for 21 days) in patients with refractory immune thrombocytopenic purpura was halted, since all of the first seven patients had adverse effects without significant changes in the platelet count (3). Adverse effects consisted of conjunctival injection, diffuse aches and joint pains, marked pedal edema, petechiae, and mild anemia. In addition, one patient had a neuropathy, which resolved more than 1 month after oprelvekin withdrawal.

References

1. Dorner AJ, Goldman SJ, Keith JC. Interleukin-11. Biological activity and clinical studies. BioDrugs 1997;8:418–29.
2. Antin JH, Lee SJ, Neuberg D, Alyea E, Soiffer RJ, Sonis S, Ferrara JL. A phase I/II double-blind, placebo-controlled study of recombinant human interleukin-11 for mucositis and acute GVHD prevention in allogeneic stem cell transplantation. Bone Marrow Transplant 2002;29(5):373–7.
3. Bussel JB, Mukherjee R, Stone AJ. A pilot study of rhuIL-11 treatment of refractory ITP. Am J Hematol 2001;66(3):172–7.

MYELOID COLONY-STIMULATING FACTORS

General Information

Around 10 glycoprotein myeloid hemopoietic growth factors or colony-stimulating factors (CSFs) have so far been identified and purified; their genes have been cloned and active recombinant proteins have been produced. Recombinant factors produced by yeast or mammalian cells are glycosylated, as they are in their native state, whereas those expressed in bacterial systems are not. Glycosylation may be clinically relevant with regard to the efficacy and antigenicity of the molecule, although antibody formation has not been observed, even after prolonged therapy (1). Most clinical studies with CSFs have hitherto been performed with granulocyte-macrophage colony-stimulating factor (GM-CSF) and granulocyte colony-stimulating factor (G-CSF), although clinical trials of other colony-stimulating factors have also been initiated in a number of centers. GM-CSF leads to a dose-related sustained increase in peripheral neutrophil numbers, with a delayed increase in circulating monocytes and eosinophils. The effect of G-CSF appears to be more restricted to neutrophils. Multi-CSF (IL-3) stimulates the production of all types of leukocytes, as well as platelets and reticulocytes (2).

Both granulocyte colony-stimulating factor (G-CSF) and granulocyte-macrophage colony-stimulating factor (GM-CSF) have been extensively investigated for the treatment of chemotherapy-induced neutropenia, reducing the duration of neutropenia after bone marrow transplantation, or mobilizing peripheral blood progenitor cells after myelosuppressive chemotherapy (3). Other clinical uses are indicated in the monographs on the individual growth factors.

Two reviews have examined the available data on the effects of hemopoietic growth factors on the duration of neutropenia and mortality in drug-induced agranulocytosis, which mostly consists of isolated case reports or small series of patients (4,5). The authors reached contrasting opinions, suggesting that hemopoietic growth factors might or might not be of interest in patients with severe drug-induced agranulocytosis. Adverse effects were noted in 13 of 118 case reports (4). Although most of them were benign, pulmonary toxicity or acute respiratory distress syndrome occurred in a few patients.

Comparative studies

There were no major differences in the adverse effect profiles in 42 patients with breast cancer randomized to filgrastim (G-CSF) or molgramostim (GM-CSF) (SEDA-22, 407). There were no significant differences in the adverse effects profiles and severity of adverse effects in 181 patients with cancers randomized to receive filgrastim (G-CSF) or sargramostim (GM-CSF) for chemotherapy-induced myelosuppression (6).

The effects and the safety of a 5-day regimen of G-CSF ($n = 9$) or GM-CSF ($n = 8$) have been compared (7).

Most patients complained of flu-like symptoms in both groups (six and seven respectively), but rash at the injection site was observed only in four patients treated with GM-CSF. In the G-CSF group, there was a fall in platelet count (below $150 \times 10^9/l$) in five patients, raised serum lactic dehydrogenase activity, and raised uric acid concentrations; three patients required transient treatment with allopurinol.

The frequency and severity of adverse effects associated with the prophylactic use of filgrastim or sargramostim have been assessed in a retrospective review of the medical records of 490 cancer patients from ten centers (8). Sargramostim-treated patients had significantly more frequent non-infectious fever, fatigue, diarrhea, injection site reactions, edema, and dermatological adverse effects, whereas skeletal pain was more frequent with filgrastim. In addition, switching to the alternative treatment was more frequent in the sargramostim group (18% of patients) than in the filgrastim group (none of the patients). The authors tried to minimize selection bias, but the strength of the results was limited by the retrospective nature of the study.

Susceptibility Factors

Age

Guidelines for the appropriate use of hemopoietic growth factors in children have been proposed by a panel of European experts, who carefully summarized the potential indications and recommendations, and concluded that adult guidelines are applicable to children in most cases (9). The authors considered that growth factors should be used in children for only a limited number of circumstances: prophylaxis or treatment in low-risk patients treated with chemotherapy, routine use in aplastic anemia, and mobilization of peripheral blood progenitor cells in healthy pediatric donors.

References

1. Sieff CA. Haemopoietic growth factors: in vitro and in vivo studies. In: Hoffbrand AV, editor. Recent Advances in Haematology. London: Churchill Livingstone, 1988:1.
2. Klingemann HG, Shepherd JD, Eaves CJ, Eaves AC. The role of erythropoietin and other growth factors in transfusion medicine. Transfus Med Rev 1991;5(1):33–47.
3. Vose JM, Armitage JO. Clinical applications of hematopoietic growth factors. J Clin Oncol 1995;13(4):1023–35.
4. Beauchesne MF, Shalansky SJ. Nonchemotherapy drug-induced agranulocytosis: a review of 118 patients treated with colony-stimulating factors. Pharmacotherapy 1999;19(3):299–305.
5. Vial T, Gallant C, Choquet-Kastylevsky G, Descotes J. Treatment of drug-induced agranulocytosis with haematopoietic growth factors. A review of the clinical experience. BioDrugs 1999;11:185–200.

6. Beveridge RA, Miller JA, Kales AN, Binder RA, Robert NJ, Harvey JH, Windsor K, Gore I, Cantrell J, Thompson KA, Taylor WR, Barnes HM, Schiff SA, Shields JA, Cambareri RJ, Butler TP, Meister RJ, Feigert JM, Norgard MJ, Moraes MA, Helvie WW, Patton GA, Mundy LJ, Henry D, Sheridan MJ, et al. A comparison of efficacy of sargramostim (yeast-derived RhuGM-CSF) and filgrastim (bacteria-derived RhuG-CSF) in the therapeutic setting of chemotherapy-induced myelosuppression. Cancer Invest 1998;16(6):366–73.

7. Fischmeister G, Kurz M, Haas OA, Micksche M, Buchinger P, Printz D, Ressmann G, Stroebel T, Peters C, Fritsch G, Gadner H. G-CSF versus GM-CSF for stimulation of peripheral blood progenitor cells (PBPC) and leukocytes in healthy volunteers: comparison of efficacy and tolerability. Ann Hematol 1999;78(3):117–23.

8. Milkovich G, Moleski RJ, Reitan JF, Dunning DM, Gibson GA, Paivanas TA, Wyant S, Jacobs RJ. Comparative safety of filgrastim versus sargramostim in patients receiving myelosuppressive chemotherapy. Pharmacotherapy 2000;20(12):1432–40.

9. Schaison G, Eden OB, Henze G, Kamps WA, Locatelli F, Ninane J, Ortega J, Riikonen P, Wagner HP. Recommendations on the use of colony-stimulating factors in children: conclusions of a European panel. Eur J Pediatr 1998;157(12):955–66.

Granulocyte colony-stimulating factor (G-CSF)

General Information

Granulocyte colony-stimulating factor (G-CSF) primarily increases the production and function of neutrophils by stimulating the proliferation of committed myeloid precursors, rather than pluripotential stem cells (1).

Recombinant human forms of G-CSF that have been developed include filgrastim, lenograstim, nartograstim, and pegfilgrastim and pegnartograstim, which are pegylated derivatives of filgrastim and nartograstim.

Besides common therapeutic indications, G-CSF has also been used in severe chronic neutropenic diseases (congenital, cyclic, idiopathic), aplastic anemia, and neonatal neutropenia. G-CSF is sometimes used in healthy volunteers to mobilize blood progenitor cells or granulocytes before infusion into neutropenic patients.

Observational studies

In all clinical studies carried out to date, G-CSF has been well tolerated, whether given subcutaneously or intravenously. At the recommended doses (5–10 micrograms/ kg), generalized musculoskeletal and transient bone pains, headache, and mild rash are the commonest adverse effects (2). No additional adverse effects or delayed consequences have been so far reported in neonates treated at birth for presumed bacterial sepsis (SEDA-20, 337). An increase in the size of the spleen has been reported (3,4). Transient rises in alkaline phosphatase, lactate dehydrogenase, and uric acid are

considered to be normal physiological consequences of the rise in the neutrophil count (5). Long-term G-CSF administration in patients with severe congenital neutropenia has also been considered to be relatively safe, with discontinuation or temporary withdrawal in only seven of 44 patients (6).

Two reviews have examined the available data on the effects of hemopoietic growth factors on the duration of neutropenia and mortality in drug-induced agranulocytosis, which mostly consists of isolated case reports or small series of patients (7,8). The authors reached contrasting opinions, suggesting that hemopoietic growth factors might or might not be of interest in patients with severe drug-induced agranulocytosis. Adverse effects were noted in 13 of 118 case reports (7). Although most of them were benign, pulmonary toxicity or acute respiratory distress syndrome have been noted in a few patients.

Comparative studies

Few studies have directly compared the safety of the various available colony-stimulating factors. The frequency and severity of adverse effects associated with the prophylactic use of filgrastim (a bacterial cell-derived G-CSF) or sargramostim (a yeast cell-derived GM-CSF) have been assessed in a retrospective review of the medical records of 490 cancer patients from 10 centers (9). Sargramostim-treated patients had significantly more frequent non-infectious fever, fatigue, diarrhea, injection site reactions, edema, and dermatological adverse effects, whereas skeletal pain was more frequent with filgrastim. In addition, switching to the alternative treatment was more frequent in the sargramostim group (18% of patients) than in the filgrastim group (none of the patients). The authors tried to minimize selection bias, but the strength of the results was limited by the retrospective nature of the study.

The effects and the safety of a 5-day regimen of G-CSF ($n = 9$) or GM-CSF ($n = 8$) have been compared (10). Most patients complained of flu-like symptoms in both groups (six and seven respectively), but rash at the injection site was observed only in four patients treated with GM-CSF. In the G-CSF group, there was a fall in platelet count (below 150×10^9/l) in five patients, raised serum lactic dehydrogenase activity, and raised uric acid concentrations; three patients required transient treatment with allopurinol.

Use in healthy volunteers

The G-CSF is sometimes used in healthy volunteers to mobilize blood progenitor cells or granulocytes before infusion into neutropenic patients (11).

The safety of filgrastim in healthy donors has been evaluated in a large prospective multicenter study (12). The interim results, obtained from the first 150 enrolled donors aged 18–64 years who received either 10 or 16 micrograms/kg/day, have shown that 99 patients had at least one adverse effect graded as mild (grade I) in 35% of cases, moderate (grade II) in 62%, and severe (grade III) in 3%. Bone pain and headaches were the most common acute adverse events, and all the patients completely recovered after withdrawal of filgrastim. There were no apparent differences in the proportion, the severity, or the type of adverse effects according to the administered regimen.

That the use of G-CSF in healthy donors of peripheral blood progenitor cells is reasonably safe has been confirmed in an analysis of adverse effects in 737 evaluable patients included in three independent databases from Spain, the USA, and Japan (13–15). In one study, the overall incidence of adverse effects was 67%. The most common adverse effects were bone pain (71–90%), headache (17–54%), fatigue (6–33%), insomnia (up to 14%), nausea/vomiting (3–13%), and low-grade fever (6%). Although most adverse effects were rated as moderate, about two-thirds of the patients required analgesics for bone pain or headache. Other adverse events, such as non-cardiac chest pain, paresthesia, itching, or minor injection site reactions, were rare. Very few patients discontinued G-CSF because of clinical toxicity. Doses higher than 8.8 micrograms/kg/day, patients younger than 35 years of age, and female sex were significant risk factors for bone pain, headache, and nausea/vomiting respectively (15).

Moderate thrombocytopenia was common after apheresis; there was more severe but asymptomatic and promptly reversible thrombocytopenia (below $50 \times 10^{12}/$ l) in up to 3.9% of patients (14,15). However, the respective contributions of apheresis and G-CSF in thrombocytopenia are difficult to assess. There was also a fall in the absolute neutrophil count to less than $1 \times 10^9/$l in 3% of patients 9–16 days after G-CSF withdrawal (15). Serum alkaline phosphatase and lactate dehydrogenase activities were increased about two-fold compared with pre-treatment, a finding that was explicable by G-CSF-induced neutrophilia (14,15). Symptoms of hypercoagulability have also been found in healthy donors.

However, more severe or unexpected consequences, including spontaneous splenic rupture, anaphylactoid reactions, deep necrotizing folliculitis, a psoriasiform eruption, acute gouty arthritis, iritis or episcleritis, and unexpectedly prolonged thrombocytopenia have been mentioned (SEDA-20, 337; SEDA-21, 378; SEDA-22, 407).

Among 90 healthy donors given 10 and 16 micrograms/kg/day of filgrastim for stem cell mobilization, severe adverse effects were mostly found in patients who had been given the higher dose (16), but one obese patient (body weight 170 kg) who received 10 micrograms/kg/day had a non-traumatic spleen rupture that resolved spontaneously.

Sufficient data on the potential long-term effects of G-CSF in healthy volunteers are still lacking. In one study, 101 healthy donors who had received filgrastim for a median of 6 days were questioned after a median of 43 (range 34–74) months to assess their current health; 70 donors also had a complete blood count (17). No unusual disease was detected and the blood counts were within the reference range. In 20 donors followed for 6–12 months after peripheral blood progenitor cell collection, there were no particular symptoms or hematological abnormalities (15).

The possible carcinogenic effects of G-CSF have also been discussed. There is as yet no indication of an increased risk of cancer, and no cases of acute or chronic leukemia were detected in a telephone interview study performed after a median of 39 months after peripheral blood progenitor cell donation in 281 donors (18).

Organs and Systems

Cardiovascular

Cardiovascular events have seldom been described in patients given colony-stimulating factors. However, possible excesses of cardiovascular events and unexpected deaths have been suggested (SED-13, 1115; 19), although the actual risk was not fully evaluated. In three isolated reports, acute arterial thrombosis or angina pectoris were deemed to have resulted from hypercoagulability with extreme leukocytosis and G-CSF-induced abnormalities in platelet aggregation (SEDA-20, 337; SEDA-21, 377; 20). Increased platelet aggregation has also been found in healthy volunteers (21). Although the relevance of these findings is unclear, caution is warranted in patients predisposed to thromboembolic events.

- A 46-year-old donor denied pre-existing cardiac symptoms, but smoking and a family history of coronary artery disease were noted as possible risk factors (22). The pre-treatment electrocardiogram was normal. Six hours after the second and the third doses of G-CSF 10 micrograms/kg before peripheral blood progenitor cell collection, he developed symptoms and signs of cardiac ischemia, including palpitation, chest discomfort, trigeminy, and T wave inversion. However, troponin was unchanged. Cardiac catheterization showed severe coronary artery occlusion and he underwent percutaneous transluminal coronary angioplasty. He finally admitted mild exertional chest discomfort 2 weeks before the first dose of G-CSF.

Although not described during clinical trials, typical capillary leak syndrome has been anecdotally observed after G-CSF administration, illustrating the possible consequences of accelerated release of activated granulocytes (SEDA-22, 407; 23).

Microthrombotic necrotizing panniculitis has been reported (24).

- A 49-year-old woman received subcutaneous filgrastim 300 micrograms/day into the upper thighs for neutropenia prophylaxis after treatment of relapsing Hodgkin's disease with mitoguazone, etoposide, vinorelbine, and ifosfamide. After 3 days she suddenly developed fever, painful livedo, deeply infiltrated edema on the legs and thighs, and inflamed livedoid erythema on both soles. Deep biopsy specimens showed small vessel thrombosis with subcutaneous necrosis and hemorrhage. She recovered over the next 4 weeks after filgrastim withdrawal and prednisone treatment.

Although a causal relation was difficult to ascertain in the context of malignancy and cytotoxic chemotherapy, the short time to occurrence after G-CSF favored a causative role.

Respiratory

Pulmonary toxicity in patients receiving chemotherapy
Whether G-CSF can cause pulmonary toxicity or enhance chemotherapy-induced pulmonary toxicity is a matter of continuing debate (SED-13, 1115; SEDA-21, 377). Some studies have suggested an increased risk of pulmonary complications in patients with hematological malignancies treated with various chemotherapeutic regimens who received G-CSF. In a review of 20 cases of interstitial pneumonia (including three that were fatal) observed during or within 10 days of G-CSF treatment, the chemotherapy regimen consisted of cyclophosphamide (95%), bleomycin (55%), methotrexate (25%), and etoposide (20%); most patients had non-Hodgkin's lymphoma (25). In another report, acute febrile interstitial pneumonitis occurred in five patients with non-Hodgkin's lymphoma who were receiving prophylactic G-CSF ($n = 3$) or GM-CSF ($n = 2$) within less than 48 hours after the second to fourth cycles of chemotherapy (doxorubicin, cyclophosphamide, bleomycin, methotrexate, plus methylprednisolone) (26). Lymphocytic alveolitis was confirmed in four of these patients, and all three patients tested had an increased number of CD8+ T cells. Even though all the patients received high-dose methylprednisolone, two died as a result of diffuse and extensive interstitial pulmonary fibrosis, identified at postmortem.

Several epidemiological studies have more accurately focused on this potential problem, but the results are conflicting. Unfortunately, most of them were retrospective and involved historical controls. Interstitial pneumonia was identified in eight of 40 patients treated with antineoplastic drugs (mostly methotrexate and bleomycin) plus G-CSF, while no such cases were found before the use of G-CSF among 35 historical controls (27). Severe pulmonary toxicity was observed in four of 12 patients treated with BACOP (bleomycin, doxorubicin, cyclophosphamide, vincristine, plus prednisone) plus G-CSF compared with one of 24 historical controls who did not receive G-CSF (28). Of 52 patients treated with CHOP (cyclophosphamide, doxorubicin, vincristine, plus prednisolone), pulmonary symptoms were found in six who received G-CSF compared with none of 49 patients treated before the availability of G-CSF (29). This last study also raised the possibility that the intensified schedule of CHOP administration (every 2 weeks instead of every 3 weeks) allowed in patients undergoing G-CSF is a possible explanation for increased pulmonary toxicity. In contrast, other investigators failed to confirm that G-CSF increases the pulmonary toxicity of antineoplastic drugs, at least bleomycin (SEDA-21, 377). This was particularly exemplified by French authors who were unable to find an increased incidence of pulmonary complications in an analysis of two randomized controlled trials in 278 patients who received a bleomycin-containing regimen plus G-CSF or placebo (30).

Other predisposing factors have been suggested in five of 310 patients who developed acute adult respiratory distress syndrome (ARDS) after receiving G-CSF after allogeneic bone marrow transplantation or conventional chemotherapy (31). All had also been exposed to drugs or procedures with significant pulmonary toxicity. Respiratory symptoms developed suddenly, in conjunction with rapid recovery of the white blood cell count. Retrospective investigations showed that all five patients had the HLA-B51 or HLA-B52 antigens. In addition, plasma concentrations of tumor necrosis factor alfa and interleukin-8 were high at the onset of the ARDS. These effects did not occur in 45 patients who did not develop ARDS. The authors suggested that the risk of G-CSF-induced ARDS increases when the white blood cell count rises rapidly in patients who have the following conditions: HLA-B51 or HLA-B52 antigens, treatment with drugs with pulmonary toxicity, and a concomitant infection before recovery from granulocytopenia.

Whatever the truth of the matter, G-CSF should be regarded as a possible cause of pulmonary complications. The abrupt increase in the number of activated neutrophils after G-CSF may account for exacerbation of latent chemotherapy-induced pulmonary damage. Endothelial damage subsequent to increased neutrophil activity (that is, enhanced superoxide release and increased adhesion molecule expression and adherence) or the release of cytokines (IL-1, IL-6, TNF) has been advanced as possible mechanisms. In addition, transient slight hypoxia was found in G-CSF users, although no relation with specific cytotoxic drug treatment or previous radiotherapy was identified (32). A sudden increase in neutrophil count, a rise in LDH and C reactive protein, and the occurrence of dyspnea or fever in G-CSF-treated patients were proposed as possible early signs of the subsequent development of interstitial pneumonia.

Pulmonary toxicity in patients not receiving chemotherapy
The G-CSF can cause severe pulmonary toxicity in patients who are not receiving concomitant chemotherapy. For example, several reports have suggested that G-CSF administration for drug-induced agranulocytosis can play a role in the development or worsening of the adult respiratory distress syndrome (ARDS) (33).

- Fatal non-cardiac pulmonary edema has been reported in a 59-year-old man with renal amyloidosis who received G-CSF for 3 days for stem cell mobilization (34).

The authors extensively reviewed the available experimental and clinical data on the pulmonary toxicity of growth factors.

Another case suggested that G-CSF alone can cause severe pulmonary toxicity (35).

- A 72-year-old man with a normal chest X-ray was unnecessarily treated with G-CSF (5 micrograms/kg/day) for very moderate cytopenia. Five days later, he complained of dyspnea and fatigue, but without fever.

His chest X-ray showed diffuse bilateral alveolar opacities and he had a low oxygen saturation. Blood cultures were negative, and infectious pneumonitis (with *Mycobacterium tuberculosis*, *Pneumocystis jiroveci*, *Herpes simplex*, and cytomegalovirus) was ruled out. Despite glucocorticoid and antibiotic treatment, he required mechanical ventilation and died 12 days after the onset of symptoms.

Nervous system

There is no clear evidence of specific central nervous system adverse effects due to G-CSF. In one patient, neurological symptoms, such as blurred vision, weakness, and headache, were attributed to G-CSF-induced extreme hyperleukocytosis with subsequent hyperviscosity (SEDA-21, 377). Encephalopathy, cortical blindness and seizures have also been mentioned in single case report (SEDA-21, 377).

Sensory systems

Severe retinal hemorrhage with a slowly reversible loss of visual acuity, and massive vitreous hemorrhage recurring after further G-CSF treatment and resulting in irreversible loss of vision in the affected eye have each been reported in single patients (SEDA-21, 378; SEDA-22, 408). Concomitant hyperleukocytosis was suggested as a possible cause in the first patient, whereas G-CSF-induced reactivation of primary ocular inflammation (probably infectious in origin) was advanced as an explanation in the second case.

- A 61-year-old healthy donor developed marginal keratitis with associated mild uveitis after being given injections of filgrastim and sargramostim for 3 days (36). Topical prednisolone and withdrawal of sargramostim produced improvement within 24 hours, while filgrastim injections were continued.

Iritis and episcleritis have also been mentioned in healthy donors of blood progenitor cells.

Endocrine

Several studies have suggested that single or short-term administration of G-CSF did not produce significant changes in the serum concentrations of cortisol, growth hormone, prolactin, follicle-stimulating hormone, luteinizing hormone, or thyrotropin (SEDA-20, 337; SEDA-21, 378).

Thyroid function and thyroid antibodies were not modified in 20 breast cancer patients (37), and only one case of hypothyroidism with increased thyroid antibodies has been reported (SEDA-20, 337). G-CSF had no effect on thyroid function in 33 patients with cancer, even in patients with pre-existing antibodies (38). Subclinical and spontaneously reversible hyperthyroidism occurred in eight patients without thyroid antibodies and with normal thyroid function before treatment, but this was felt to be related to stressful procedures.

Metabolism

Reductions in serum cholesterol concentrations have been sometimes noted in patients receiving G-CSF (2).

Hematologic

Erythrocytes

In a healthy woman, G-CSF was suggested to have transiently reactivated an alloantibody to an erythrocyte antigen (anti-Jka antibody) (39). This antibody was apparently passively transferred to the transplant recipient, who developed a high-titer of anti-Jka antibody during the first month after transplantation. This report raised the possibility that transplant recipients may develop hemolytic reactions to G-CSF subsequent to erythrocyte transfusion.

Leukocytes

The transient and moderate rises in leukocyte alkaline phosphatase and uric acid serum concentrations that are often observed after G-CSF treatment are considered to arise from an increased neutrophil count (SEDA-17, 396). Similarly, serum lactate dehydrogenase and alkaline phosphatase activities are often increased, and this should be interpreted as the consequence of enzyme release after growth factor-induced leukocyte recovery (SED-13, 1115).

Eosinophilia can occur in patients receiving long-term G-CSF for congenital neutropenia (6). Patients with congenital neutropenia or Felty's syndrome may also be susceptible to anemia and/or thrombocytopenia (6,40).

Platelets and clotting factors

There have been isolated reports of arterial thrombosis in patients or donors treated with G-CSF. In one study, there was more frequent and significantly more severe thrombocytopenia in patients who received G-CSF until 2 days before chemotherapy compared with controls, who had post-chemotherapy G-CSF only (41). This suggests that administration of G-CSF before chemotherapy can increase the bone marrow toxicity of the latter, a potentially relevant finding in patients undergoing intensification of chemotherapy with shortening treatment intervals. Isolated cases of thrombocytopenia have been reported in HIV-infected patients (SEDA-20, 337), and a reduced platelet count, sometimes associated with coagulation abnormalities, was retrospectively identified in nine of 28 patients who received prolonged G-CSF with antiretroviral drugs (42). Emperipolesis of neutrophils within megakaryocytes, an unusual feature of thrombocytopenia, was also reported in one patient receiving high-dose G-CSF (43).

Although abnormalities in platelet aggregation have been described in healthy volunteers (21), coagulation disorders are not typical features in patients who receive G-CSF. Only one HIV-infected patient treated with zidovudine and increasing G-CSF doses had a disseminated intravascular coagulopathy (42).

Hemostatic changes due to G-CSF have been investigated in 22 healthy donors (44). The patients received

G-CSF 5 micrograms/kg bd for 5 days and underwent a series of laboratory tests before and 96 hours after G-CSF administration, that is, immediately before leukapheresis. The results suggested possible hypercoagulability, including significant increases in Von Willebrand factor and factor VIII and evidence of thrombin generation. The clinical relevance of these findings and of the previously reported effects of G-CSF on platelet aggregation (SED-14, 1270) is unknown.

Treatment with G-CSF in 26 healthy donors for 5–7 days produced transient changes in endothelial cell and clotting activation markers (45). Although these abnormalities may indicate a risk of thrombotic complications, their clinical relevance to healthy donors is unknown.

- A 53-year-old man with aplastic anemia had clinically asymptomatic and reversible hypercoagulability after the transfusion of granulocytes obtained from G-CSF-stimulated donors (46).

The authors stressed the recurrence of the disorder after each of the three granulocyte transfusions that the patient had received and suggested that adverse effects might occur after transfusion performed with G-CSF-mobilized granulocytes, even though the patient has not been given G-CSF.

The differential effects of G-CSF and GM-CSF on several coagulation parameters have been compared in 34 patients who received the colony-stimulating factors after bone marrow transplantation (47). The data suggested activation of the coagulation system in patients treated with GM-CSF, which resulted in a tendency to more frequent veno-occlusive disease of the liver and a significantly higher incidence of hemorrhage.

Hemopoietic tissues

Asymptomatic but significant increases in spleen volume (up to 150%) concomitant with neutrophilia have been reported in about 25% of patients treated with G-CSF for severe chronic neutropenia (6,48).

Of 13 patients with glycogen storage disease type 1b and neutropenia or neutrophil dysfunction treated with G-CSF, all developed splenomegaly, usually after 3 months of treatment (49). Hypersplenism, as defined by moderate thrombocytopenia on at least two consecutive blood counts, was found in five patients, but none required specific interventions. In one carefully documented case, splenomegaly with extramedullary hemopoiesis was deemed to result from the mobilization of early hemopoietic progenitors from the marrow to the spleen (50). Experimental data suggested that reseeding of hemopoietic cells from the bone marrow may account for this phenomenon (51).

Splenic rupture has been reported in patients with cancer and in healthy donors, and should be anticipated by regular assessment of splenic size during prolonged treatment.

- Spontaneous splenic rupture, with histological evidence of massive extramedullary myelopoiesis after splenectomy, has been reported in a 33-year-old healthy donor who received G-CSF for 6 days (52).

- Life-threatening splenic rupture occurred in a 22-year-old woman with acute myeloid leukemia (53). The rupture was diagnosed in the presence of abdominal pain and signs of hypovolemic shock, 10 days after she started G-CSF treatment to support peripheral blood stem cell transplantation. Histology after splenectomy showed only small clusters of myeloblasts and no specific cause for the rupture. In particular, she was still pancytopenic at the time of splenic rupture.

One patient also had rapid and generalized lymph node enlargement and lymphopenia with recurrence of lymphadenopathy after a further course of G-CSF (54).

Liver

Clinical trials did not suggest G-CSF-induced hepatotoxicity, and very few cases of liver abnormalities have been reported (SED-13, 1116; SEDA-19, 343). Although it may have been coincidental, the chronological features were in keeping with drug-induced hepatotoxicity in at least two patients, since increases in serum liver enzymes or acute hepatitis associated with pancreatitis recurred after renewed administration of G-CSF. One additional case of fatal fulminant hepatitis could have been due to alcohol abuse and the use of several concomitant drugs.

Urinary tract

No evidence of nephrotoxicity emerged from clinical trials, but a transient increase in serum creatinine concentration has been described (SEDA-20, 337).

- A 4-year-old girl was given filgrastim (30 micrograms/kg/day) for severe congenital neutropenia diagnosed at birth (55). Two months later she developed microscopic hematuria and recurrent episodes of macroscopic hematuria and proteinuria. Renal ultrasonography was normal and no obvious cause was found, but filgrastim was continued. Microscopic hematuria and multiple episodes of macroscopic hematuria with mild proteinuria persisted for 4 years. At this stage, she had an acute episode of macroscopic hematuria with more severe proteinuria and an increase in serum creatinine concentration (202 µmol/l). There were features of membranoproliferative glomerulonephritis type I on renal biopsy. Her renal function improved after filgrastim withdrawal and again deteriorated after reintroduction, with a persistent increase in serum creatinine concentration. Hematuria and proteinuria partially responded to glucocorticoids. Filgrastim was finally replaced by lenograstim when she was 13 years old, and this resulted in reduced proteinuria and improved renal function.

Although the girl also had hepatitis C virus infection during the course of her disease, renal dysfunction preceded this. The persistence of hematuria and proteinuria after the disappearance of hepatitis C virus RNA also argued against a role of hepatitis C infection.

Isolated and reversible hematuria was noted in several patients receiving long-term treatment for congenital neutropenia (6).

Although suggested in one report, G-CSF does not appear to increase the risk of renal allograft rejection (SEDA-20, 337).

Skin

A wide range of cutaneous reactions have been reported in patients receiving G-CSF. Most skin disorders were minor with a skin rash or itching in about 8% of patients (56).

Injection-site reactions

Localized cutaneous lesions were sometimes noted after subcutaneous injection and mimicked those described with GM-CSF. Injection-site subcutaneous nodules infiltrated by leukemic cells have been found in patients treated for acute leukemia (SEDA-19, 343), but in two other patients, inflammatory macrophages were misinterpreted as malignant cells (SEDA-20, 337).

The G-CSF can cause a lichenoid reaction at injection sites (57).

- A 40-year-old woman with metastatic breast cancer received cyclic subcutaneous G-CSF for chemotherapy-induced neutropenia. After 5 months she had a pruritic rash at injection sites. She did not change the injection sites and the lesions recurred after each injection. Biopsy showed a lichenoid reaction and the lesions healed with residual pigmentation after topical steroid application and G-CSF discontinuation. GM-CSF was well tolerated.

- Erythema exsudativum multiforme developed in a 40-year-old healthy donor 3 days after lenograstim was started for peripheral blood stem cell mobilization (58). The lesions were on the hips, apart from the site of lenograstim injection, and resolved 1 week after withdrawal.

Neutrophilic dermatitis

The possible role of G-CSF in inducing or exacerbating neutrophilic dermatitis (Sweet's syndrome) is in keeping with its stimulant effects on the production and functions of neutrophils. Although the ability of G-CSF to induce Sweet's syndrome (acute febrile neutrophilic dermatosis) is disputed, because the underlying malignant disease is a possible confounding factor, several reports of biopsy-proven Sweet's syndrome have been convincing; they have shown variously a close temporal relation between G-CSF treatment and the variations in neutrophil count or the recurrence of the lesions after G-CSF re-administration; one report concerned two patients with chronic neutropenia (SED-13, 1116; SEDA-20, 338; SEDA-21, 378). Localized Sweet's syndrome can also occur (SEDA-20, 338). The spectrum of forms of G-CSF-induced neutrophilic dermatitis is wide. In two children with painful erythematous lesions attributed to G-CSF, histology showed microscopic, sterile, neutrophilic abscesses in one and neutrophilic panniculitis in the other (59). Other forms of neutrophilic dermatitis mentioned in G-CSF-treated patients have included isolated cases of bullous pyoderma gangrenosum and neutrophilic

eccrine hidradenitis (SEDA-21, 378; SEDA-22, 408; 60. Sweet's syndrome has also been described in a case of hairy cell leukemia (61).

Other skin complications

Disseminated vesiculopustular lesions, generalized and indurated erythematous papules or plaques, severe exacerbation of acne, and lenograstim-induced erythema nodosum, with recurrence on filgrastim administration, were mentioned in isolated patients (SED-13, 1116; SEDA-20, 337). Finally, several reports convincingly involved G-CSF in exacerbations of chronic psoriasis or psoriatic arthritis, suggesting that activated neutrophils play an important role in the occurrence and propagation of skin inflammation (SEDA-21, 378; 62).

Musculoskeletal

Transient bone and musculoskeletal pain preceding myeloid recovery by 2–3 days are the commonest adverse effects of G-CSF, and occur in up to 25% of patients. Bone pain usually disappears despite continued treatment, but severe, narcotic-resistant, generalized bone pain was attributed to bone marrow necrosis in one patient (63).

The G-CSF-induced exacerbation of pseudogout occurred in two patients (SEDA-20, 337; SEDA-22, 408).

- A 69-year-old man with a non-small-cell lung cancer treated with paclitaxel and nedaplatin developed polyarthralgia and myalgia with rising fever after receiving G-CSF for 5 days (64). Similar symptoms recurred after the second cycle of chemotherapy and on retreatment with G-CSF. Synovial biopsy showed acute synovitis with a foreign body-type giant cell reaction.

Worsening of rheumatoid symptoms has been reported in patients receiving G-CSF, particularly in patients with neutropenia due to Felty's syndrome (SEDA-19, 344; SEDA-20, 338). Although concern about the short-term safety of G-CSF has been raised in these patients, other investigators feel that G-CSF can be used for a prolonged period in most patients without a flare-up of rheumatoid symptoms (SEDA-22, 408). Similar conclusions were reached in patients with underlying rheumatoid arthritis (SEDA-21, 378). The mechanisms of rheumatological flare-up are unclear. G-CSF-induced localized neutrophil activation or G-CSF-mediated increases in local neutrophil responses to TNF-alfa have both been suggested as underlying processes.

Several investigators have diagnosed bone mineral loss, with features of osteopenia/osteoporosis on radiography, quantitative computed tomography, or absorptiometry, in patients receiving long-term G-CSF for severe congenital neutropenia (6,65). In one child there was significant improvement in bone mineral density with pamidronate (66). In another child, who had osteoporotic vertebral collapse, extensive investigations showed reduced bone mineral content, reduced concentrations of osteocalcin, and features of osteoporosis on bone biopsy (SEDA-19, 344). The role of G-CSF was unclear, because bone mineral loss is a possible complication of the underlying disease. Indeed, improvement or stabilization during G-CSF treatment was noted in several patients (6). Furthermore, there was no apparent effect on height, head circumference, or weight in patients under 18 years of age (6). In another study, there was bone mineral loss with features of osteopenia/osteoporosis in 15 of 30 patients treated with G-CSF for a mean of 5.8 years for severe chronic neutropenia (65). However, six of nine patients investigated before G-CSF treatment had evidence of osteopenia/osteoporosis.

These reports and the findings of G-CSF-induced mobilization of osteoclastic progenitors in healthy volunteers (67) support a possible role of G-CSF in bone changes.

Immunologic

Leukocytoclastic vasculitis is a well-described and confirmed adverse effect of G-CSF, as documented in several reports, with recurrence after renewed administration of G-CSF (SEDA-19, 343). Most cases were confined to the skin, and renal insufficiency with hematuria and proteinuria was noted in only very few patients. Based on 18 cases reported in the literature or to the manufacturers, vasculitis was thought to have occurred in 6% of patients with chronic benign neutropenia, but in only six of about 200 000 patients with malignant disease (68). Vasculitis usually developed when the neutrophil count rose above $800 \times 10^6/l$, suggesting that an increase in neutrophil count may play a role in necrotic vasculitis. Against this background, the occurrence of vasculitis is not considered as treatment-limiting and does not preclude further G-CSF administration if the absolute neutrophil count is lower than $1000 \times 10^6/l$.

Antibodies to rG-CSF have not so far been reported, even in patients on long-term treatment.

Exacerbation of lupus-like symptoms, with seizures, psychosis, and vasculitis, has been noted during three of 12 treatment courses in neutropenic patients with severe systemic lupus erythematosus (69).

Type I reactions

Although IgE-specific antibodies have not been yet detected, filgrastim is undoubtedly associated with type I allergic reactions. This has been illustrated in well-documented reports of anaphylactic reactions, urticaria, and angioedema, with positive intradermal tests in several patients (SEDA-20, 338; 70,71). However, anaphylaxis to G-CSF is supposedly rare and the manufacturer is aware of only two cases of anaphylactoid reactions among 20 000 patients treated with filgrastim (72). One report has suggested possible cross-reactivity between filgrastim and other products derived from *Escherichia coli* (73). Although one patient who developed an anaphylactic-like reaction, with dyspnea, hypotension, and a pruritic erythematous skin rash, within minutes of G-CSF injection, later tolerated GM-CSF uneventfully (74), possible cross-reactivity between G-CSF and GM-CSF has been reported in at least one patient (75).

Long-Term Effects

Tumorigenicity

G-CSF-induced leukemia and myelodysplasia in patients with aplastic anemia or congenital neutropenia
Concerns have arisen over the prolonged use of G-CSF in patients with aplastic anemia, congenital neutropenia, or similar disorders and a possible increased or accelerated risk of myelodysplasia or acute leukemia (SED-14, 1274). Several investigators have noted reversible increases in circulating blasts during G-CSF treatment, and isolated reports have indicated a shortened delay in the occurrence of myelodysplasia and/or acute myeloid leukemia in this setting (SED-13, 1117; SEDA-20, 338; 76). An abnormal karyotype (mostly monosomy 7) was sometimes found, and in vitro proliferation of myeloblasts by G-CSF was obtained in several patients. In addition, the potential role of point mutations on the G-CSF receptor has been also discussed as regards four of 28 patients with congenital neutropenia, two of whom developed acute myeloid leukemia (77). Myelodysplastic syndrome with monosomy 7 was also associated with G-CSF in another patient, with a reduction in the number of monosomy 7 positive cells after G-CSF withdrawal and a further increase after readministration (78).

This has been analysed in a number of epidemiological studies, most of which involved historical controls. The underlying predisposition of patients with aplastic anemia to develop myeloid malignancy has usually confounded attempts to determine whether growth factors are contributing factors.

In a retrospective study of 72 adults with aplastic anemia, of whom 18 received G-CSF and 23 received ciclosporin, five developed myelodysplastic syndrome (79). Four of them had received G-CSF + ciclosporin and all four had monosomy 7. The hematological disease was diagnosed within 16–31 months after the diagnosis of aplastic anemia and 12–20 months after the start of G-CSF treatment. Two died from acute leukemia. The incidence of myelodysplastic syndrome in this subgroup of patients was therefore 8.3% after 2 years and 39% after 3 years, whereas no case was observed over a 20-year period in patients not receiving this combined treatment. Univariate analysis showed that G-CSF + ciclosporin and G-CSF alone for more than 1 year were the most significant risk factors for the short-term development of monosomy 7 myelodysplastic syndrome.

In a prospective, multicenter, cohort study of 113 patients with aplastic anemia under 18 years of age, 12 developed myelodysplastic syndrome after a median of 37 months after the diagnosis of aplastic anemia and four others developed other cytogenetic clonal changes, of which the most common abnormality was monosomy 7 (80). From a multivariate analysis, G-CSF treatment duration and non-response to immunosuppressive therapy at 6 months were statistically significant risk factors for the development of myelodysplastic syndrome. The risk increased in proportion to the duration of G-CSF treatment, and the relative risks of the myelodysplastic syndrome were respectively 4.4 and 8.7 times higher in patients who received G-CSF for more than 120 and 180 days, compared with those who received it for less.

In contrast, a number of other studies did not confirm that the G-CSF increases the risk of myelodysplasia or acute leukemia, but the authors did not rule out a possible leukemogenic effect. In a study of patients with severe aplastic anemia the frequencies of cytogenetic abnormalities and myelodysplasia or leukemia were similar in 87 patients treated with G-CSF in addition to immunosuppressive treatment compared with 57 patients who did not receive G-CSF (81). Although the authors stated that a leukemogenic effect of G-CSF was unlikely, they mentioned that the median interval of appearance of cytogenetic abnormalities was shorter in the G-CSF group.

In another study the data from an international register of patients with severe chronic neutropenia were analysed (82). Of 352 patients treated with G-CSF for congenital neutropenia and followed for a mean of 6 years (maximum 11 years), 31 developed myelodysplasia or leukemia, whereas there were no cases in 344 patients with idiopathic or cyclic neutropenia. Associated cytogenetic clonal changes consisted of partial or complete loss of chromosome seven in 18 patients and abnormalities in chromosome 21 in nine. Isolated cytogenetic abnormalities were also found in nine other patients. None of the patients had abnormal marrow cytogenetic changes before G-CSF therapy. A more complete analysis failed to identify any correlation between G-CSF dose and treatment duration in patients who developed myelodysplasia or leukemia compared with those who were not affected. Although this argues against a role of G-CSF in the conversion of congenital neutropenia to myelodysplasia or leukemia, the authors recognized that a direct leukemogenic role of G-CSF could not be completely ruled out.

After a median follow-up of 43 months in 123 children treated with G-CSF, there was no difference in the incidence of secondary myelodysplasia or acute myeloid leukemia, in patients with aplastic anemia who survived longer than 2 years compared with the expected rate calculated before the use of G-CSF (83). Similarly, there was no evidence of an increased risk of myelodysplasia or acute myeloid leukemia in 54 patients treated with G-CSF for 4–6 years for severe congenital neutropenia (6).

Finally, in a randomized study in 102 patients of the safety and efficacy of lenograstim (5 micrograms/kg/day for 14 weeks) combined with standard immunosuppressants, there were no differences between the groups in survival, hematological response, or the occurrence of secondary leukemia (one case of myelodysplastic syndrome in each group) at a median follow-up of 5 years (84).

The role of G-CSF in leukemic transformation therefore remains unproven, primarily because these patients might be otherwise predisposed or have a previous history of immunosuppressive therapy. Although the clinical benefits of G-CSF probably outweigh any hazard of leukemogenesis, the possibility of an increased risk of myelodysplastic syndrome or acute myeloid leukemia under the influence of G-CSF should be borne in mind.

Careful monitoring of morphological bone marrow changes and cytogenetic studies are therefore recommended, and large randomized trials with long-term follow-up are still awaited to clarify these findings.

Stimulation of tumors or leukemic cells in patients with cancer

Because growth factor receptors are found on several tumor cell lines, there has been great concern that G-CSF may stimulate tumor progression (SED-13, 1117; SEDA-20, 338; SEDA-21, 378), with some anecdotal evidence of a temporal relation between G-CSF administration and the development or acceleration of malignancies, such as gastric cancer or Hodgkin's diseaseodgkin's disease (SED-13, 1117; 85–87). However, early clinical data and the results of several randomized controlled trials in patients with various malignancies provided no evidence for increased relapse rates (88,89).

With the demonstration of growth factor receptors on leukemic cells, the question has also been raised of whether there could be stimulation of leukemic cell growth with promotion of malignancies, or acceleration in the progression of myelodysplastic syndromes to acute myeloid leukemias. Although there has been some reluctance to use G-CSF in acute myeloid leukemia, no clear evidence of disease acceleration or recurrence was found in several trials (SED-13, 1117; SEDA-21, 379). Based on an analysis of available in vitro data and published clinical trials, the risk of significant stimulation of leukemia or leukemic clone with an increased incidence of leukemia regrowth is currently estimated to be very low (90). Although clinical benefits are still debated in this setting, growth factors are considered to be safe in reducing the duration of neutropenia in patients with acute myeloid leukemia.

Although G-CSF is not believed to stimulate malignant lymphoid cells, G-CSF receptors have been found in patients with T cell leukemia, and this was associated with a significant increase in T cell leukemia cells in several patients (SEDA-21, 379). Other uncommon consequences of G-CSF have included blast mobilization with a phenotype change from common acute lymphoblastic leukemia to biphenotypic leukemia in one patient (87).

The risk of secondary cancer has been assessed in 412 children treated with etoposide and anthracyclines for acute lymphoblastic leukemia, 99 of whom also received G-CSF and 58 of whom received cranial irradiation (91). Overall, 20 children developed myeloid leukemia and myelodysplastic syndrome at a median of 2.3 years after treatment. The 6-year cumulative incidence of these secondary cancers was 11% among patients who received G-CSF, close to that observed in those who received cranial irradiation (12%), but significantly higher than in those who received neither irradiation nor G-CSF (2.7%).

Acceleration of myelodysplastic syndrome

A reversible increase in circulating blasts has been noted during G-CSF treatment in several patients with myelodysplastic syndrome, and other reports have documented a reversible secondary myelodysplastic syndrome or accelerated progression of a previous myelodysplastic syndrome (SEDA-21, 379; 89). In other instances, pseudoleukemia features or transient leukoerythroblastosis were evidenced on bone marrow biopsy (SEDA-19, 344; SEDA-20, 338). Although there was no increased incidence of acute myeloblastic leukemia in G-CSF-treated patients with myelodysplastic syndrome, it has been considered that patients whose bone marrow contains more than 20% of blast cells should be regarded as being at higher risk of leukemic transformation (89).

Myeloma

The safety of growth factors in patients with myeloma is also of concern, as they can stimulate the proliferation of myeloma cells through IL-6 expression. Only isolated case reports, including accounts of the mobilization of clonal myeloma cells into the peripheral circulation, rapid progression of a multiple myeloma, or the new onset of a monoclonal gammopathy, directly or indirectly support the view that caution should be exercised in patients with multiple myeloma (SED-13, 1118; 92).

Susceptibility Factors

Renal disease

A hemodialysis patient developed refractory pleural effusion with prolonged leukopenia and thrombocytopenia, and another developed sudden cyanotic dyspnea with subsequent death after G-CSF administration for drug-induced neutropenia (93). The authors suggested that hemodialysis patients receiving G-CSF may have an increased risk of adverse effects.

Drug Administration

Drug formulations

Pegfilgrastim was developed by adding a polyethylene glycol molecule to the *N*-terminus of filgrastim. In a phase III study in 301 patients with advanced breast cancer who underwent myelosuppressive chemotherapy a single injection of pegfilgrastim had similar efficacy and safety profile to repeated injections of filgrastim (94).

Drug–Drug Interactions

Theophylline

A 30% increase in theophylline clearance occurred after the administration of G-CSF or GM-CSF (SEDA-20, 338).

Vincristine

In one study there was a synergistic effect of GM-CSF or G-CSF and cumulative doses of vincristine in causing severe atypical neuropathy (SEDA-20, 339).

Interference with Diagnostic Tests

Blood glucose analysis

Artifactual hypoglycemia occurred in patients taking G-CSF when blood glucose was analysed on the Ektachem 700 analyser (SEDA-20, 339).

Hepatitis B surface antigen

A single dose of G-CSF in a healthy donor produced a false positive test for hepatitis B surface antigen using an enzyme immunoassay (95).

References

1. Lieschke GJ, Burgess AW. Granulocyte colony-stimulating factor and granulocyte-macrophage colony-stimulating factor. N Engl J Med 1992;327(2):99–106.
2. Vial T, Descotes J. Clinical toxicity of cytokines used as haemopoietic growth factors. Drug Saf 1995;13(6):371–406.
3. Kojima S, Fukuda M, Miyajima Y, Matsuyama T, Horibe K. Treatment of aplastic anemia in children with recombinant human granulocyte colony-stimulating factor. Blood 1991;77(5):937–41.
4. Sheridan WP, Morstyn G, Wolf M, Dodds A, Lusk J, Maher D, Layton JE, Green MD, Souza L, Fox RM. Granulocyte colony-stimulating factor and neutrophil recovery after high-dose chemotherapy and autologous bone marrow transplantation. Lancet 1989;2(8668):891–5.
5. Herrmann F. G-CSF: status quo and new indications. Infection 1992;20(4):183–8.
6. Bonilla MA, Dale D, Zeidler C, Last L, Reiter A, Ruggeiro M, Davis M, Koci B, Hammond W, Gillio A, et al. Long-term safety of treatment with recombinant human granulocyte colony-stimulating factor (r-metHuG-CSF) in patients with severe congenital neutropenias. Br J Haematol 1994;88(4):723–30.
7. Beauchesne MF, Shalansky SJ. Nonchemotherapy drug-induced agranulocytosis: a review of 118 patients treated with colony-stimulating factors. Pharmacotherapy 1999;19(3):299–305.
8. Vial T, Gallant C, Choquet-Kastylevsky G, Descotes J. Treatment of drug-induced agranulocytosis with haematopoietic growth factors. A review of the clinical experience. BioDrugs 1999;11:185–200.
9. Milkovich G, Moleski RJ, Reitan JF, Dunning DM, Gibson GA, Paivanas TA, Wyant S, Jacobs RJ. Comparative safety of filgrastim versus sargramostim in patients receiving myelosuppressive chemotherapy. Pharmacotherapy 2000;20(12):1432–40.
10. Fischmeister G, Kurz M, Haas OA, Micksche M, Buchinger P, Printz D, Ressmann G, Stroebel T, Peters C, Fritsch G, Gadner H. G-CSF versus GM-CSF for stimulation of peripheral blood progenitor cells (PBPC) and leukocytes in healthy volunteers: comparison of efficacy and tolerability. Ann Hematol 1999;78(3):117–23.
11. Anderlini P, Przepiorka D, Champlin R, Korbling M. Biologic and clinical effects of granulocyte colony-stimulating factor in normal individuals. Blood 1996;88(8):2819–25.
12. Beelen DW, Ottinger H, Kolbe K, Ponisch W, Sayer HG, Knauf W, Stockschlader M, Scheid C, Schaefer UW. Filgrastim mobilization and collection of allogeneic blood progenitor cells from adult family donors: first interim report of a prospective German multicenter study. Ann Hematol 2002;81(12):701–9.

13. Anderlini P, Donato M, Chan KW, Huh YO, Gee AP, Lauppe MJ, Champlin RE, Korbling M. Allogeneic blood progenitor cell collection in normal donors after mobilization with filgrastim: the M.D. Anderson Cancer Center experience Transfusion 1999;39(6):555–60.

14. de la Rubia J, Martinez C, Solano C, Brunet S, Cascon P, Arrieta R, Alegre A, Bargay J, de Arriba F, Canizo C, Lopez J, Serrano D, Verdeguer A, Torrabadella M, Diaz MA, Insunza A, de la Serna J, Espigado I, Petit J, Martinez M, Benlloch L, Sanz M. Administration of recombinant human granulocyte colony-stimulating factor to normal donors: results of the Spanish National Donor Registry. Spanish Group of Allo-PBT. Bone Marrow Transplant 1999;24(7):723–8.

15. Murata M, Harada M, Kato S, Takahashi S, Ogawa H, Okamoto S, Tsuchiya S, Sakamaki H, Akiyama Y, Kodera Y. Peripheral blood stem cell mobilization and apheresis: analysis of adverse events in 94 normal donors. Bone Marrow Transplant 1999;24(10):1065–71.

16. Kroger N, Renges H, Sonnenberg S, Kruger W, Gutensohn K, Dielschneider T, Cortes-Dericks L, Zander AR. Stem cell mobilisation with 16 microg/kg vs 10 microg/kg of G-CSF for allogeneic transplantation in healthy donors Bone Marrow Transplant 2002;29(9):727–30.

17. Cavallaro AM, Lilleby K, Majolino I, Storb R, Appelbaum FR, Rowley SD, Bensinger WI. Three to six year follow-up of normal donors who received recombinant human granulocyte colony-stimulating factor. Bone Marrow Transplant 2000;25(1):85–9.

18. Anderlini P, Chan FA, Champlin RE, Korbling M, Strom SS. Long-term follow-up of normal peripheral blood progenitor cell donors treated with filgrastim: no evidence of increased risk of leukemia development. Bone Marrow Transplant 2002;30(10):661–3.

19. Lindemann A, Rumberger B. Vascular complications in patients treated with granulocyte colony-stimulating factor (G-CSF). Eur J Cancer 1993;29A(16):2338–9.

20. Conti JA, Scher HI. Acute arterial thrombosis after escalated-dose methotrexate, vinblastine, doxorubicin, and cisplatin chemotherapy with recombinant granulocyte colony-stimulating factor. A possible new recombinant granulocyte colony-stimulating factor toxicity. Cancer 1992;70(11):2699–702.

21. Kuroiwa M, Okamura T, Kanaji T, Okamura S, Harada M, Niho Y. Effects of granulocyte colony-stimulating factor on the hemostatic system in healthy volunteers. Int J Hematol 1996;63(4):311–6.

22. Vij R, Adkins DR, Brown RA, Khoury H, DiPersio JF, Goodnough T. Unstable angina in a peripheral blood stem and progenitor cell donor given granulocyte-colony-stimulating factor. Transfusion 1999;39(5):542–3.

23. Oeda E, Shinohara K, Kamei S, Nomiyama J, Inoue H. Capillary leak syndrome likely the result of granulocyte colony-stimulating factor after high-dose chemotherapy. Intern Med 1994;33(2):115–9.

24. Dereure O, Bessis D, Lavabre-Bertrand T, Exbrayat C, Fegueux N, Biron C, Guilhou JJ. Thrombotic and necrotizing panniculitis associated with recombinant human granulocyte colony-stimulating factor treatment. Br J Dermatol 2000;142(4):834–6.

25. Niitsu N, Iki S, Muroi K, Motomura S, Murakami M, Takeyama H, Ohsaka A, Urabe A. Interstitial pneumonia in patients receiving granulocyte colony-stimulating factor during chemotherapy: survey in Japan 1991–96. Br J Cancer 1997;76(12):1661–6.

26. Couderc LJ, Stelianides S, Frachon I, Stern M, Epardeau B, Baumelou E, Caubarrere I, Hermine O. Pulmonary toxicity of chemotherapy and G/GM-CSF: a report of five cases. Respir Med 1999;93(1):65–8.

27. Iki S, Yoshinaga K, Ohbayashi Y, Urabe A. Cytotoxic drug-induced pneumonia and possible augmentation by G-CSF—clinical attention. Ann Hematol 1993;66(4):217–8.

28. Lei KI, Leung WT, Johnson PJ. Serious pulmonary complications in patients receiving recombinant granulocyte colony-stimulating factor during BACOP chemotherapy for aggressive non-Hodgkin's lymphoma. Br J Cancer 1994;70(5):1009–13.

29. Yokose N, Ogata K, Tamura H, An E, Nakamura K, Kamikubo K, Kudoh S, Dan K, Nomura T. Pulmonary toxicity after granulocyte colony-stimulating factor-combined chemotherapy for non-Hodgkin's lymphoma. Br J Cancer 1998;77(12):2286–90.

30. Bastion Y, Reyes F, Bosly A, Gisselbrecht C, Yver A, Gilles E, Maral J, Coiffier B. Possible toxicity with the association of G-CSF and bleomycin. Lancet 1994;343(8907):1221–2.

31. Takatsuka H, Takemoto Y, Mori A, Okamoto T, Kanamaru A, Kakishita E. Common features in the onset of ARDS after administration of granulocyte colony-stimulating factor. Chest 2002;121(5):1716–20.

32. White K, Cebon J. Transient hypoxaemia during neutrophil recovery in febrile patients. Lancet 1995;345(8956):1022–4.

33. Demuynck H, Zachee P, Verhoef GE, Schetz M, Van den Berghe G, Lauwers P, Boogaerts MA. Risks of rhG-CSF treatment in drug-induced agranulocytosis. Ann Hematol 1995;70(3):143–7.

34. Gertz MA, Lacy MQ, Bjornsson J, Litzow MR. Fatal pulmonary toxicity related to the administration of granulocyte colony-stimulating factor in amyloidosis: a report and review of growth factor-induced pulmonary toxicity. J Hematother Stem Cell Res 2000;9(5):635–43.

35. Ruiz-Arguelles GJ, Arizpe-Bravo D, Sanchez-Sosa S, Rojas-Ortega S, Moreno-Ford V, Ruiz-Arguelles A. Fatal G-CSF-induced pulmonary toxicity. Am J Hematol 1999;60(1):82–3.

36. Esmaeli B, Ahmadi MA, Kim S, Onan H, Korbling M, Anderlini P. Marginal keratitis associated with administration of filgrastim and sargramostim in a healthy peripheral blood progenitor cell donor. Cornea 2002;21(6):621–2.

37. Van Hoef ME, Howell A. Risk of thyroid dysfunction during treatment with G-CSF. Lancet 1992;340(8828):1169–70.

38. Duarte R, De Luis DA, Lopez-Jimenez J, Roy G, Garcia A. Thyroid function and autoimmunity during treatment with G-CSF. Clin Endocrinol (Oxf) 1999;51(1):133–4.

39. Norol F, Bonin P, Charpentier F, Bierling P, Beaujean F, Cartron JP, Bories D, Kuentz M. Apparent reactivation of a red cell alloantibody in a healthy individual after G-CSF administration. Br J Haematol 1998;103(1):256–8.

40. Wun T. The Felty syndrome and G-CSF-associated thrombocytopenia and severe anemia. Ann Intern Med 1993;118(4):318–9.

41. de Wit R, Verweij J, Bontenbal M, Kruit WH, Seynaeve C, Schmitz PI, Stoter G. Adverse effect on bone marrow protection of prechemotherapy granulocyte colony-stimulating factor support. J Natl Cancer Inst 1996;88(19):1393–8.

42. Mueller BU, Burt R, Gulick L, Jacobsen F, Pizzo PA, Horne M. Disseminated intravascular coagulation associated with granulocyte colony-stimulating factor therapy in a child with human immunodeficiency virus infection. J Pediatr 1995;126(5 Pt 1):749–52.

43. Migita M, Fukunaga Y, Watanabe A, Maruyama K, Ohta K, Kaneko K, Kaneda M, Kakinuma K, Yamatoto M. Emperipolesis of neutrophils by megakaryocytes and thrombocytopenia observed in a case of Kostmann's syndrome during intravenous administration of high-dose rhG-CSF. Br J Haematol 1992;80(3):413–5.

44. LeBlanc R, Roy J, Demers C, Vu L, Cantin G. A prospective study of G-CSF effects on hemostasis in allogeneic blood stem cell donors. Bone Marrow Transplant 1999;23(10):991–6.

45. Falanga A, Marchetti M, Evangelista V, Manarini S, Oldani E, Giovanelli S, Galbusera M, Cerletti C, Barbui T. Neutrophil activation and hemostatic changes in healthy donors receiving granulocyte colony-stimulating factor. Blood 1999;93(8):2506–14.

46. Mizuno S, Okamura T, Iwasaki H, Ohno Y, Akashi K, Inaba S, Niho Y. Hypercoagulable state following transfusions of granulocytes obtained from granulocyte colony-stimulating factor-stimulated donors. Int J Hematol 2000;72(1):115–7.

47. Bonig H, Burdach S, Gobel U, Nurnberger W. Growth factors and hemostasis: differential effects of GM-CSF and G-CSF on coagulation activation—laboratory and clinical evidence. Ann Hematol 2001;80(9):525–30.

48. Dale DC, Bonilla MA, Davis MW, Nakanishi AM, Hammond WP, Kurtzberg J, Wang W, Jakubowski A, Winton E, Lalezari P, et al. A randomized controlled phase III trial of recombinant human granulocyte colony-stimulating factor (filgrastim) for treatment of severe chronic neutropenia. Blood 1993;81(10):2496–502.

49. Calderwood S, Kilpatrick L, Douglas SD, Freedman M, Smith-Whitley K, Rolland M, Kurtzberg J. Recombinant human granulocyte colony-stimulating factor therapy for patients with neutropenia and/or neutrophil dysfunction secondary to glycogen storage disease type 1b. Blood 2001;97(2):376–82.

50. Litam PP, Friedman HD, Loughran TP Jr. Splenic extramedullary hematopoiasis in a patient receiving intermittently administered granulocyte colony-stimulating factor. Ann Intern Med 1993;118(12):954–5.

51. Nakayama T, Kudo H, Suzuki S, Sassa S, Mano Y, Sakamoto S. Splenomegaly induced by recombinant human granulocyte-colony stimulating factor in rats. Life Sci 2001;69(13):1521–9.

52. Falzetti F, Aversa F, Minelli O, Tabilio A. Spontaneous rupture of spleen during peripheral blood stem-cell mobilisation in a healthy donor. Lancet 1999;353(9152):555.

53. Kasper C, Jones L, Fujita Y, Morgenstern GR, Scarffe JH, Chang J. Splenic rupture in a patient with acute myeloid leukemia undergoing peripheral blood stem cell transplantation. Ann Hematol 1999;78(2):91–2.

54. Kawachi Y, Ozaki S, Sakamoto Y, Uchida T, Mori M, Setsu K, Tani K, Asano S. Richter's syndrome showing pronounced lymphadenopathy in response to administration of granulocyte colony-stimulating factor. Leuk Lymphoma 1994;13(5–6):509–14.

55. Magen D, Mandel H, Berant M, Ben-Izhak O, Zelikovic I. MPGN type I induced by granulocyte colony stimulating factor. Pediatr Nephrol 2002;17(5):370–2.

56. Asnis LA, Gaspari AA. Cutaneous reactions to recombinant cytokine therapy. J Am Acad Dermatol 1995;33(3):393–410.

57. Viallard AM, Lavenue A, Balme B, Pincemaille B, Raudrant D, Thomas L. Lichenoid cutaneous drug reaction at injection sites of granulocyte colony-stimulating factor (filgrastim). Dermatology 1999;198(3):301–3.

58. Mori T, Sato N, Watanabe R, Okamoto S, Ikeda Y. Erythema exsudativum multiforme induced by granulocyte colony-stimulating factor in an allogeneic peripheral blood stem cell donor. Bone Marrow Transplant 2000;26(2):239–40.

59. Prendiville J, Thiessen P, Mallory SB. Neutrophilic dermatoses in two children with idiopathic neutropenia: association with granulocyte colony-stimulating factor (G-CSF) therapy. Pediatr Dermatol 2001;18(5):417–21.

60. Johnson ML, Grimwood RE. Leukocyte colony-stimulating factors. A review of associated neutrophilic dermatoses and vasculitides. Arch Dermatol 1994;130(1):77–81.

61. Glaspy JA, Baldwin GC, Robertson PA, Souza L, Vincent M, Ambersley J, Golde DW. Therapy for neutropenia in hairy cell leukemia with recombinant human granulocyte colony-stimulating factor. Ann Intern Med 1988;109(10):789–95.

62. Couderc LJ, Philippe B, Franck N, Balloul-Delclaux E, Lessana-Leibowitch M. Necrotizing vasculitis and exacerbation of psoriasis after granulocyte colony-stimulating factor for small cell lung carcinoma. Respir Med 1995;89(3):237–8.

63. Katayama Y, Deguchi S, Shinagawa K, Teshima T, Notohara K, Taguchi K, Omoto E, Harada M. Bone marrow necrosis in a patient with acute myeloblastic leukemia during administration of G-CSF and rapid hematologic recovery after allotransplantation of peripheral blood stem cells. Am J Hematol 1998;57(3):238–40.

64. Tsukadaira A, Okubo Y, Takashi S, Kobayashi H, Kubo K. Repeated arthralgia associated with granulocyte colony stimulating factor administration. Ann Rheum Dis 2002;61(9):849–50.

65. Yakisan E, Schirg E, Zeidler C, Bishop NJ, Reiter A, Hirt A, Riehm H, Welte K. High incidence of significant bone loss in patients with severe congenital neutropenia (Kostmann's syndrome). J Pediatr 1997;131(4):592–7.

66. Sekhar RV, Culbert S, Hoots WK, Klein MJ, Zietz H, Vassilopoulou-Sellin R. Severe osteopenia in a young boy with Kostmann's congenital neutropenia treated with granulocyte colony-stimulating factor: suggested therapeutic approach. Pediatrics 2001;108(3):E54.

67. Purton LE, Lee MY, Torok-Storb B. Normal human peripheral blood mononuclear cells mobilized with granulocyte colony-stimulating factor have increased osteoclastogenic potential compared to nonmobilized blood. Blood 1996;87(5):1802–8.

68. Jain KK. Cutaneous vasculitis associated with granulocyte colony-stimulating factor. J Am Acad Dermatol 1994;31(2 Pt 1):213–5.

69. Euler HH, Harten P, Zeuner RA, Schwab UM. Recombinant human granulocyte colony stimulating factor in patients with systemic lupus erythematosus associated neutropenia and refractory infections. J Rheumatol 1997;24(11):2153–7.

70. Jaiyesimi I, Giralt SS, Wood J. Subcutaneous granulocyte colony-stimulating factor and acute anaphylaxis. N Engl J Med 1991;325(8):587.

71. Sasaki O, Yokoyama A, Uemura S, Fujino S, Inoue Y, Kohno N, Hiwada K. Drug eruption caused by recombinant human G-CSF. Intern Med 1994;33(10):641–3.

72. Brown SL, Hill E. Subcutaneous granulocyte colony-stimulating factor and acute anaphylaxis. N Engl J Med 1991;325:587.

73. Stone HD Jr, DiPiro C, Davis PC, Meyer CF, Wray BB. Hypersensitivity reactions to *Escherichia coli*-derived polyethylene glycolated-asparaginase associated with subsequent immediate skin test reactivity to *E. coli*-derived

granulocyte colony-stimulating factor. J Allergy Clin Immunol 1998;101(3):429–31.

74. Keung YK, Suwanvecho S, Cobos E. Anaphylactoid reaction to granulocyte colony-stimulating factor used in mobilization of peripheral blood stem cell. Bone Marrow Transplant 1999;23(2):200–1.

75. Shahar E, Krivoy N, Pollack S. Effective acute desensitization for immediate-type hypersensitivity to human granulocyte–monocyte colony stimulating factor. Ann Allergy Asthma Immunol 1999;83(6 Pt 1):543–6.

76. Dantal J, Hourmant M, Cantarovich D, Giral M, Blancho G, Dreno B, Soulillou JP. Effect of long-term immunosuppression in kidney-graft recipients on cancer incidence: randomised comparison of two cyclosporin regimens. Lancet 1998;351(9103):623–8.

77. Tidow N, Pilz C, Teichmann B, Muller-Brechlin A, Germeshausen M, Kasper B, Rauprich P, Sykora KW, Welte K. Clinical relevance of point mutations in the cytoplasmic domain of the granulocyte colony-stimulating factor receptor gene in patients with severe congenital neutropenia. Blood 1997;89(7):2369–75.

78. Nishimura M, Yamada T, Andoh T, Tao T, Emoto M, Ohji T, Matsuda K, Kameda N, Satoh Y, Matsutani A, Azuno Y, Oka Y. Granulocyte colony-stimulating factor (G-CSF) dependent hematopoiesis with monosomy 7 in a patient with severe aplastic anemia after ATG/CsA/G-CSF combined therapy. Int J Hematol 1998;68(2):203–11.

79. Kaito K, Kobayashi M, Katayama T, Masuoka H, Shimada T, Nishiwaki K, Sekita T, Otsubo H, Ogasawara Y, Hosoya T. Long-term administration of G-CSF for aplastic anaemia is closely related to the early evolution of monosomy 7 MDS in adults. Br J Haematol 1998;103(2):297–303.

80. Kojima S, Ohara A, Tsuchida M, Kudoh T, Hanada R, Okimoto Y, Kaneko T, Takano T, Ikuta K, Tsukimoto IJapan Childhood Aplastic Anemia Study Group. Risk factors for evolution of acquired aplastic anemia into myelodysplastic syndrome and acute myeloid leukemia after immunosuppressive therapy in children. Blood 2002;100(3):786–90.

81. Locasciulli A, Arcese W, Locatelli F, Di Bona E, Bacigalupo AItalian Aplastic Anaemia Study Group. Treatment of aplastic anaemia with granulocyte-colony stimulating factor and risk of malignancy. Italian Aplastic Anaemia Study Group. Lancet 2001;357(9249):43–4.

82. Freedman MH, Bonilla MA, Fier C, Bolyard AA, Scarlata D, Boxer LA, Brown S, Cham B, Kannourakis G, Kinsey SE, Mori PG, Cottle T, Welte K, Dale DC. Myelodysplasia syndrome and acute myeloid leukemia in patients with congenital neutropenia receiving G-CSF therapy. Blood 2000;96(2):429–36.

83. Imashuku S, Hibi S, Nakajima F, Mitsui T, Yokoyama S, Kojima S, Matsuyama T, Nakahata T, Ueda K, Tsukimoto I, et al. A review of 125 cases to determine the risk of myelodysplasia and leukemia in pediatric neutropenic patients after treatment with recombinant human granulocyte colony-stimulating factor. Blood 1994;84(7):2380–1.

84. Gluckman E, Rokicka-Milewska R, Hann I, Nikiforakis E, Tavakoli F, Cohen-Scali S, Bacigalupo A. European Group for Blood and Marrow Transplantation Working Party for Severe Aplastic Anemia. Results and follow-up of a phase III randomized study of recombinant human-granulocyte stimulating factor as support for immunosuppressive therapy in patients with severe aplastic anaemia. Br J Haematol 2002;119(4):1075–82.

85. Soutar RL. Acute myeloblastic leukemia and recombinant granulocyte colony stimulating factor. BMJ 1991;303(6794):123–4.

86. Stathopoulos GP, Moschopoulos N, Apostolopoulou E, Papakostas P, Samelis GF. Acute non-lymphocytic leukaemia complicating gastric cancer treated with epipodophyllotoxin containing chemotherapy and G-CSF. Acta Oncol 1994;33(6):713–4.

87. Matsuzaki A, Ohga S, Ueda K, Okamuras. Induction of CD33-positive blasts by granulocyte colony-stimulating factor in a child with common acute lymphoblastic leukemia. Int J Ped Hematol Oncol 1994;1:339–41.

88. Vose JM, Armitage JO. Clinical applications of hematopoietic growth factors. J Clin Oncol 1995;13(4):1023–35.

89. Schriber JR, Negrin RS. Use and toxicity of the colony-stimulating factors. Drug Saf 1993;8(6):457–68.

90. Rowe JM, Liesveld JL. Hematopoietic growth factors in acute leukemia. Leukemia 1997;11(3):328–41.

91. Relling MV, Boyett JM, Blanco JG, Raimondi S, Behm FG, Sandlund JT, Rivera GK, Kun LE, Evans WE, Pui CH. Granulocyte colony-stimulating factor and the risk of secondary myeloid malignancy after etoposide treatment. Blood 2003;101(10):3862–7.

92. Kobbe G, Germing U, Soehngen D, Aul C, Heyll A. Massive extramedullary disease progression in a patient with stable multiple myeloma during G-CSF priming for peripheral blood progenitor mobilization. Oncol Rep 1999;6(5):1151–2.

93. Nakamura M, Sakemi T, Fujisaki T, Matsuo S, Ikeda Y, Nishimoto A, Ohtsuka Y, Tomiyoshi Y. Sudden death or refractory pleural effusion following treatment with granulocyte colony-stimulating factor in two hemodialysis patients. Nephron 1999;83(2):178–9.

94. Holmes FA, O'Shaughnessy JA, Vukelja S, Jones SE, Shogan J, Savin M, Glaspy J, Moore M, Meza L, Wiznitzer I, Neumann TA, Hill LR, Liang BC. Blinded, randomized, multicenter study to evaluate single administration pegfilgrastim once per cycle versus daily filgrastim as an adjunct to chemotherapy in patients with high-risk stage II or stage III/IV breast cancer. J Clin Oncol 2002;20(3):727–31.

95. Warren K, Eastlund T. False-reactive test for hepatitis B surface antigen following administration of granulocyte-colony-stimulating factor. Vox Sang 2002;83(3):247–9.

Granulocyte–macrophage colony-stimulating factor (GM-CSF)

General Information

Granulocyte–macrophage colony-stimulating factor (GM-CSF) primarily increases the production and activity of neutrophils, and stimulates the proliferation of monocytes and eosinophils.

Recombinant human forms of GM-CSF that are in use include molgramostim and sargramostim. Based on a retrospective review and historical comparison, the safety of molgramostim has been thought to be less than that of sargramostim (1). However, there were no significant differences in the adverse effects profiles and severity of adverse effects with GM-CSF and G-CSF in 181 patients with cancers randomized to receive sargramostim (a yeast cell-derived GM-CSF) or filgrastim (a bacterial cell-derived G-CSF) for chemotherapy-induced myelosuppression (2).

Uses

The potential clinical applications of GM-CSF have been lengthily reviewed (3). It is used:

- to reduce chemotherapy-induced myelosuppression in patients with metastatic sarcoma, breast cancer, or melanoma.
- to facilitate the harvesting of peripheral blood stem cells for autologous bone marrow transplantation.
- in cyclic neutropenia.
- to aid recovery after high doses of ionizing radiation, and less successfully, for severe aplastic anemia.

GM-CSF has also been approved for the alleviation of neutropenia following myeloablative treatment with autologous bone marrow transplantation and ganciclovir-induced neutropenia in patients with AIDS (4).

General adverse effects

The adverse effects of GM-CSF are dose-related and have usually been tolerable. At the doses usually recommended, systemic adverse effects develop in 25–30% of patients, but they are rarely treatment-limiting (5). Doses over 250 micrograms/m^2 and the intravenous route are associated with more frequent adverse effects.

Bone pain and flu-like symptoms, with fever, myalgia, chills, and headache, are the most frequent adverse effects (5–7). These reactions occur in 40–60% of all treated patients (8) and are probably due to the activation of secondary cytokines (such as TNF-alfa and IL-1) (9). Other frequently reported adverse effects include erythematous eruptions at the injection site, thrombophlebitis, nausea, facial flushing, dyspnea, and gastrointestinal disorders with anorexia and weight loss. Severe fatigue and weakness are rare.

The first dose of GM-CSF can be followed within 3 hours by flushing, hypotension, tachycardia, dyspnea, musculoskeletal pain, and nausea and vomiting (6). At very high doses (generally over 16 micrograms/kg/day), erythroderma, weight gain, and edema with pleuropericardial effusions and ascites have been reported (10). Renal symptoms have also been described (11,12), as have various biochemical abnormalities, possibly due to secondary hyperaldosteronism (13–15).

Fever was observed in up to 50% of patients at doses over 3 micrograms/kg. The fact that the fever peaks at a constant time after GM-CSF injection, the lack of clinical and biological signs of infection, and a prompt response to paracetamol have been proposed as criteria to recognize GM-CSF-induced iatrogenic fever (16), but this concept is still disputed (17).

Organs and Systems

Cardiovascular

Mild local phlebitis sometimes occurs at intravenous sites of administration of GM-CSF. Central venous catheter site thrombosis, inferior vena cava thrombosis, and possible pulmonary embolism have sometimes been observed (5,18). Although chemotherapy for breast cancer is associated with a higher risk of developing vascular thrombosis, iliac artery thrombosis was attributed to GM-CSF in two patients (19).

Raynaud's phenomenon has been reported, but confounding factors including the use of high-dose antineoplastic drugs are possible (5).

A rapidly reversible first-dose syndrome (dyspnea, hypoxia, tachycardia, and hypotension) can occur within the first hour after the first continuous infusion in 15–30% of patients (5). A dose-limiting vascular leak syndrome was consistently described in patients receiving GM-CSF 30 micrograms/kg/day or more, but lower doses were also reported to induce a clinically relevant capillary leak syndrome (SEDA-22, 408) (20,21). Continuation of GM-CSF treatment at the same dose or lower and careful management was possible in some patients. Endothelial cell damage with an increase in the transcapillary escape rate of albumin and the possible role of IL-1 and TNF production by GM-CSF-activated monocytes were suggested as possible mechanisms. This was consistent with the observation of marked hypoalbuminemia in some instances associated with edema and ascites after GM-CSF in four of nine patients treated for myelodysplastic syndrome or aplastic anemia (22).

Respiratory

It has been suggested that, as in the case of G-CSF, GM-CSF can increase the pulmonary toxicity of bleomycin and facilitate the development of the adult respiratory distress syndrome (ARDS), but evidence is still very sparse (SED-13, 1112; SEDA-19, 342).

Acute febrile interstitial pneumonitis occurred within less than 48 hours after the second to fourth cycles of chemotherapy (doxorubicin, cyclophosphamide, bleomycin, methotrexate, plus methylprednisolone) in five patients with non-Hodgkin's lymphoma who were receiving prophylactic G-CSF (n = 3) or GM-CSF (n = 2) (23). Lymphocytic alveolitis was confirmed in four of these patients and all three patients tested had an increased number of CD8+ T cells. Even though all the patients received high-dose methylprednisolone, two died as a result of diffuse and extensive interstitial pulmonary fibrosis, demonstrated at postmortem. Although both G-CSF and GM-CSF can cause acute pneumonitis in patients with cancers, it is still unknown to what extent hemopoietic growth factors are involved in this complication.

In one patient, interstitial pulmonary edema with pulmonary failure was supposedly a first-dose reaction (24).

Reversible eosinophilic pneumonia has also been reported (SEDA-19, 342).

One patient had acute bronchospasm after a subcutaneous injection of GM-CSF around a lower limb ulcer (25).

Nervous system

Very few neurological adverse effects have been associated with GM-CSF.

- Mania occurred in a 41-year-old woman taking GM-CSF who had previously tolerated G-CSF (SEDA-20, 339).
- A 49-year-old woman with chronic hepatitis C received filgrastim (G-CSF) for interferon-alfa-induced leukopenia (26). Filgrastim was withdrawn after 3 months, because of leg cramps and back pain. She later received sargramostim (GM-CSF) 500 micrograms twice weekly and she noticed gait unsteadiness and headaches within 2 weeks. During the next 3 months, she developed progressive confusion, forgetfulness, and lethargy, and both interferon alfa and sargramostim were withdrawn. She rapidly deteriorated and died from central hypoventilation 6 days later. Autopsy showed atypical, perivascular, lymphoid infiltrates in the white matter, basal ganglia, hypothalamus, brain stem, cerebellum, and spinal cord. Serum hepatitis C virus DNA sequences were not detected.

This case of fulminant perivascular lymphocytic proliferation suggests that some of the effects of GM-CSF on white blood cell proliferation can sometimes produce unexpected adverse effects.

Endocrine

Three patients with positive thyroid antibodies before GM-CSF treatment developed hypothyroidism or biphasic thyroiditis (27,28), whereas no similar thyroid dysfunction has been observed in patients without pre-existing thyroid antibodies (27). Based on these reports, GM-CSF has been thought to exacerbate underlying autoimmune thyroiditis.

Metabolism

Serum cholesterol concentrations have reportedly fallen in patients given GM-CSF (29).

Electrolyte balance

Severe symptomatic hypokalemia was thought to have resulted from increased intracellular potassium uptake linked to massive leukocytosis after GM-CSF (15).

Hematologic

Acute exacerbation of autoimmune thrombocytopenia (30) or hemolytic anemia has been linked to macrophage activation (31), and it has been suggested that patients with previous autoimmune blood disorders are at increased risk of hematological toxicity from GM-CSF.

A transient, moderate, and reversible rise in leukocyte alkaline phosphatase, lactate dehydrogenase (LDH) and serum uric acid concentrations is usually observed in cancer patients receiving supportive treatment with GM-CSF or G-CSF. Serum LDH increased from 37 to 85% and there was a linear relation between increased leukocyte production and the rise in serum LDH (32). Increases in serum LDH activity should therefore not be interpreted as indicative of disease progression, unless LDH activity remains high after growth factor withdrawal.

Erythrocytes

A typical vaso-occlusive crisis with increased hemolysis was noted within minutes after intracutaneous injection of GM-CSF in a patient with stable sickle cell disease (SEDA-19, 342). Topical GM-CSF was later uneventful.

Leukocytes

Dose-related and sometimes marked eosinophilia has been noted after GM-CSF (33). Although usually not associated with symptoms, excessive eosinophilia with fatal necrotizing pneumonia and Loeffler's endocarditis has been described (34).

Clotting factors

A marked reduction in vitamin K-dependent coagulation factors, which was prevented by vitamin K administration, has been described in patients with acute myeloid leukemia who were given GM-CSF (SEDA-19, 342).

The differential effects of G-CSF and GM-CSF on several coagulation parameters have been compared in 34 patients who received the colony-stimulating factors after bone marrow transplantation (35). The data suggested activation of the coagulation system in patients treated with GM-CSF, which resulted in a tendency to more frequent veno-occlusive disease of the liver and a significantly higher incidence of hemorrhage.

Hemopoietic tissues

Although GM-CSF acts primarily on neutrophils, stimulating effects on the myeloid lineage and other cells or cytokines of the immune system can be associated with deleterious consequences, as illustrated in several case reports. Splenomegaly with histologically documented splenic extramedullary hemopoiesis of all three lineages and histiocytic bone marrow proliferation have been described (36–38). More severe outcomes have been described, such as reactive hemophagic histiocytosis resulting in fatal pancytopenia in two bone marrow transplant patients (39). Extensive and persistent bone marrow histiocytosis was considered the likely cause of delayed bone marrow engraftment and subsequent death in both patients. These effects may have been the consequences of GM-CSF-induced proliferation and activation of the monocyte/macrophage system.

Liver

A moderate increase in serum transaminase activities sometimes occurs in patients receiving GM-CSF. More severe hepatotoxicity has been briefly reported in patients who received GM-CSF after autologous bone marrow transplantation (SEDA-19, 342). Hyperbilirubinemia was also found in 8% of bone marrow transplant patients and considered as possible ground for molgramostim withdrawal (1).

Urinary tract

There was no evidence of nephrotoxicity secondary to GM-CSF during clinical trials, but the possible occurrence of transient renal insufficiency has been discussed (1).

Skin

Cutaneous reactions to GM-CSF occur in about 50% of patients and have been reviewed (40); there is concern that autoimmune skin diseases, psoriasis, and other dermatoses might be exacerbated.

GM-CSF often causes erythema and itching at subcutaneous injection sites, with a particularly high incidence of relapsing macular pruritic infiltrates at sites of injection in patients with inflammatory breast cancer (SEDA-20, 339). Based on a retrospective review, molgramostim-induced rash was the most common treatment-limiting adverse event in bone marrow transplant patients, but further administration of sargramostim may be well tolerated (1).

Cutaneous reactions in 57 cancer patients given GM-CSF have been described in detail. They included localized immediate angioedema (8%), generalized cutaneous reactions (21%), or both (16%) (41). Generalized reactions consisted mostly of maculopapular, exfoliative, and urticarial eruptions, which resolved after topical treatment, dosage reduction, or treatment withdrawal. There was usually hyperkeratosis, mild spongiosis, lymphocytic exocytosis, and perivascular infiltration by lymphocytes, neutrophils, and eosinophils. Eosinophil activation was supposedly involved in the pathogenesis of these lesions, as was also suggested in the report of atopic dermatitis-like eruptions in two patients (42) or the acute revelation of an underlying epidermolysis bullosa acquisita in a previously asymptomatic patient (43).

As with G-CSF, GM-CSF-induced activation of neutrophils can play a critical role in the occurrence of neutrophilic dermatoses and other skin disorders. Other reports have described acute exacerbation of previous pyoderma gangrenosum (44) and subcorneal pustular dermatosis around injection sites (SEDA-19, 342).

Additional isolated reports suggesting an immunological response or inappropriate cytokine secretion subsequent to GM-CSF administration include accounts of erythema multiforme (SEDA-19, 342) and acutely generalized exacerbation of pre-existing psoriasis (45). The latter report is in keeping with the finding that GM-CSF is sometimes raised in patients with psoriasis.

Musculoskeletal

Transient bone pain is common with GM-CSF. Prompt reactivation or worsening of rheumatoid symptoms has been observed in several patients with Felty's syndrome and in one seropositive rheumatoid arthritic patient (SED-13, 1113) (46,47). GM-CSF-induced acute IL-6 release and an increase in acute phase proteins were thought to be involved.

Immunologic

Hypersensitivity reactions

Although anaphylactic reactions without any documented immune-mediated mechanism have been reported in about 8% of patients with testicular cancer given GM-CSF (48), GM-CSF has only otherwise rarely been associated with allergic reactions. Of two patients who had possible immune-mediated reactions (SEDA-19, 342) one had an immediate recurrent local reaction followed by systemic hypersensitivity reaction after sargramostim, and the other had a maculopapular pruritic eruption after molgramostim. Cross-reaction between the two recombinant forms of GM-CSF was suggested by the results of skin prick tests in one patient, but both patients thereafter tolerated filgrastim uneventfully.

However, cross-sensitivity and possible desensitization have been documented.

- A 42-year-old woman with defective immunological function had generalized pruritus, flushing, shortness of breath, and general discomfort within 30 minutes of her 16th intravenous injection of molgramostim (49). Her symptoms resolved with adrenaline, hydrocortisone, and promethazine. Despite the prophylactic use of glucocorticoids and antihistamines, she developed a similar reaction after molgramostim readministration and 4 hours after the fourth injection of filgrastim. Positive skin prick tests to molgramostim and filgrastim suggested IgE-mediated hypersensitivity. An acute desensitization protocol starting with molgramostim 0.0008 micrograms increasing to 320 micrograms was successful, and molgramostim was later continued uneventfully.

Vasculitis

GM-CSF can cause or exacerbate cutaneous leukocytoclastic vasculitis with possible renal or pulmonary involvement (SED-13, 1113). This adverse effect was substantiated by the prompt recurrence of vasculitis after drug re-administration in several patients or the report of relapsing necrotizing vasculitis at all GM-CSF injection sites.

Antibodies to GM-CSF

Formation of antibodies to recombinant GM-CSF has been detected in 31% of patients treated with sargramostim and in 95% of patients treated with molgramostim derived from *Escherichia coli* (50,51). Although the clinical relevance of this is uncertain, a significant modification of exogenous GM-CSF pharmacokinetics, a reduction in the rise in leukocyte count, and a reduction in the frequency of GM-CSF-associated adverse effects have been suggested as possible consequences. Use of the subcutaneous route and repeated administration were deemed to increase the likelihood of antibody occurrence (51). However, the fact that most patients receiving growth factors are already likely to be immunocompromised as a result of intensive chemotherapy might also account for discrepancies between the widespread use of growth factors and the paucity of reports on antibodies against growth factors. In fact only one of eight potentially immunocompromised patients had anti-GM-CSF antibody titers and they were very low (51). Antibodies to GM-CSF have not been found after prolonged use in patients with AIDS (52).

Death

There were more frequent adverse effects and an increased death rate due to pulmonary complications, sepsis, or arterial thrombosis in lung cancer patients treated with chemotherapy plus radiotherapy and GM-CSF (SEDA-20, 339).

Long-Term Effects

Tumorigenicity

Previous fears that GM-CSF might give rise to progression of pre-leukemic conditions have not been substantiated (53).

The possibility that growth factors can stimulate the growth of malignant and leukemic cells, or accelerate the progression of myelodysplastic syndrome to acute myeloid leukemia has been discussed in the monograph on G-CSF section. At the moment, there is no indication from clinical trials that GM-CSF actually increases the risk of tumor growth or the relapse rate in patients with various malignancies (29,54–56). Isolated reports have referred to delayed occurrence of B cell non-Hodgkin's lymphoma after GM-CSF treatment for aplastic anemia and de novo occurrence of diffuse oligoclonal plasmocytosis after both GM-CSF and G-CSF for high-grade glioma (SEDA-19, 342).

Although reversible increases in circulating blasts during GM-CSF treatment are sometimes noted and have raised concern on the possible accelerated occurrence of acute leukemia, the progression of myelodysplastic syndromes to acute myeloid leukemia has been only anecdotally reported (SEDA-19, 342) (57). There was no evidence of significant leukemic cell proliferation in patients with acute myeloid leukemia, and no increased risk of graft failure, leukemogenesis, relapse, or death after a median follow-up of 36 months in 128 patients who underwent autologous bone marrow transplantation for lymphoid malignancies (29,58). Finally, one report has suggested that a GM-CSF-induced abrupt rise in peripheral blasts may have caused diffuse infiltration and proliferation of leukemic blast cells in the spleen, and subsequent fatal hemorrhagic spleen rupture (59).

Susceptibility Factors

Age

In a large, randomized, placebo-controlled trial in 264 very low birth weight neonates, treatment with GM-CSF for 28 days was not associated with specific toxic effects, but the incidence of nosocomial infections was not reduced (60).

Other features of the patient

Bone marrow transplantation

Because the production of cytokines (for example IL-1 or TNF-alfa) involved in the stimulation of cells responsible for graft-versus-host disease can be enhanced by hemopoietic growth factors, the use of growth factors after allogeneic transplantation is theoretically risky. However, in reviews of trials of G-CSF or GM-CSF in allogeneic bone marrow transplantation there were no increases in late engraftment failures, relapse rates, or exacerbation of graft-versus-host disease (54,61).

HIV infection

The safety and activity of subcutaneous GM-CSF (300 micrograms/day for 1 week and 150 micrograms twice weekly for 11 weeks) has been compared with no treatment in 244 leukopenic HIV-infected patients (62). Adverse effects were reported in most of the patients treated with GM-CSF and consisted of flu-like symptoms (98%), bone pain (42%), and injection site reactions (85%). There was a two-fold increase in serum transaminase and alkaline phosphatase activities in 5.7% of patients. There was a moderate, but not significant, increase in HIV p24 antigen concentration. The few relevant clinical trials have provided no convincing evidence that GM-CSF enhances HIV replication or accelerates HIV-associated diseases (for example infections or neoplasms) in patients with AIDS (63). Only one patient with AIDS and ultrasonographic confirmation of enhanced Kaposi's sarcoma lesions temporally related to GM-CSF used for interferon- and zidovudine-related severe neutropenia has been reported (SEDA-19, 343).

Drug–Drug Interactions

Theophylline

A 30% increase in theophylline clearance occurred after the administration of G-CSF or GM-CSF (SEDA-20, 338).

Vincristine

In one study there was a synergistic effect of GM-CSF or G-CSF and cumulative doses of vincristine in causing severe atypical neuropathy (SEDA-20, 339).

References

1. Ippoliti C, Przepiorka D, Smith T, Maiese S, Giralt S, Andersson BS, Deisseroth AB, Champlin RE. Adverse effects of molgramostim in marrow transplant recipients. Clin Pharm 1993;12(7):520–5.
2. Beveridge RA, Miller JA, Kales AN, Binder RA, Robert NJ, Harvey JH, Windsor K, Gore I, Cantrell J, Thompson KA, Taylor WR, Barnes HM, Schiff SA, Shields JA, Cambareri RJ, Butler TP, Meister RJ, Feigert JM, Norgard MJ, Moraes MA, Helvie WW, Patton GA, Mundy LJ, Henry D, Sheridan MJ, et al. A comparison of efficacy of sargramostim (yeast-derived RhuGM-CSF) and filgrastim (bacteria-derived RhuG-

CSF) in the therapeutic setting of chemotherapy-induced myelosuppression. Cancer Invest 1998;16(6):366–73.

3. Armitage JO. Emerging applications of recombinant human granulocyte–macrophage colony-stimulating factor. Blood 1998;92(12):4491–508.

4. Brito-Babapule F. Therapeutic applications of the myeloid haematopoietic growth factors. Transfus Sci 1991;12:25.

5. Vial T, Descotes J. Clinical toxicity of cytokines used as haemopoietic growth factors. Drug Saf 1995;13(6):371–406.

6. Neumanaitis J. Granulocyte–macrophage-colony-stimulating factor: a review from preclinical development to clinical application. Transfusion 1993;33(1):70–83.

7. Devereux S, Linch DC. Granulocyte–macrophage colony-stimulating factor. Biotherapy 1990;2(4):305–13.

8. Klingemann HG, Shepherd JD, Eaves CJ, Eaves AC. The role of erythropoietin and other growth factors in transfusion medicine. Transfus Med Rev 1991;5(1):33–47.

9. Devereux S, Bull HA, Campos-Costa D, Saib R, Linch DC. Granulocyte macrophage colony stimulating factor induced changes in cellular adhesion molecule expression and adhesion to endothelium: in-vitro and in-vivo studies in man. Br J Haematol 1989;71(3):323–30.

10. Goldstone AH, Khwaja A. The role of haemopoietic growth factors in bone marrow transplantation. Leuk Res 1990;14(8):721–9.

11. Brandt SJ, Peters WP, Atwater SK, Kurtzberg J, Borowitz MJ, Jones RB, Shpall EJ, Bast RC Jr, Gilbert CJ, Oette DH. Effect of recombinant human granulocyte–macrophage colony-stimulating factor on hematopoietic reconstitution after high-dose chemotherapy and autologous bone marrow transplantation. N Engl J Med 1988;318(14):869–76.

12. Herrmann F, Lindemann Mertelsmann R. Polypeptides controlling hemopoietic blood cell development and activation. Blut 1987;58:173.

13. Kojima S, Fukuda M, Miyajima Y, Matsuyama T, Horibe K. Treatment of aplastic anemia in children with recombinant human granulocyte colony-stimulating factor. Blood 1991;77(5):937–41.

14. Potter MN, Mott MG, Oakhill A. Granulocyte–macrophage colony-stimulating factor (GM-CSF), hypocalcemia, and hypomagnesemia. Ann Intern Med 1990;112(9):715.

15. Viens P, Thyss A, Garnier G, Ayela P, Lagrange M, Schneider M. GM-CSF treatment and hypokalemia. Ann Intern Med 1989;111(3):263.

16. Gluck S, Gagnon A. Neutropenic fever in patients after high-dose chemotherapy followed by autologous haematopoietic progenitor cell transplantation and human recombinant granulocyte–macrophage colony stimulating factor. Bone Marrow Transplant 1994;14(6):989–90.

17. Khwaja A, Choppa R, Goldstone AH, Linch DC. Acute-phase response in patients given rhIL-3 after chemotherapy. Lancet 1992;339(8809):1617.

18. Stephens LC, Haire WD, Schmit-Pokorny K, Kessinger A, Kotulak G. Granulocyte macrophage colony stimulating factor: high incidence of apheresis catheter thrombosis during peripheral stem cell collection. Bone Marrow Transplant 1993;11(1):51–4.

19. Tolcher AW, Giusti RM, O'Shaughnessy JA, Cowan KH. Arterial thrombosis associated with granulocyte–macrophage colony-stimulating factor (GM-CSF) administration in breast cancer patients treated with dose-intensive chemotherapy: a report of two cases. Cancer Invest 1995;13(2):188–92.

20. Arning M, Kliche KO, Schneider W. GM-CSF therapy and capillary-leak syndrome. Ann Hematol 1991;62(2–3):83.

21. Emminger W, Emminger-Schmidmeier W, Peters C, Susani M, Hawliczek R, Hocker P, Gadner H. Capillary leak syndrome during low dose granulocyte–macrophage colony-stimulating factor (rh GM-CSF) treatment of a patient in a continuous febrile state. Blut 1990;61(4):219–21.

22. Kaczmarski RS, Mufti GJ. Hypoalbuminaemia after prolonged treatment with recombinant granulocyte macrophage colony stimulating factor. BMJ 1990;301(6764):1312–3.

23. Couderc LJ, Stelianides S, Frachon I, Stern M, Epardeau B, Baumelou E, Caubarrere I, Hermine O. Pulmonary toxicity of chemotherapy and G/GM-CSF: a report of five cases. Respir Med 1999;93(1):65–8.

24. Miniero R, Madon E, Artesani L, Busca A, Sandri A, Aglietta M, Ramenghi U. Acute pulmonary failure after the first administration of recombinant human granulocyte–macrophage colony-stimulating factor. Leukemia 1992;6(4):352–3.

25. Dupre D, Schoenlaub P, Coloigner M, Plantin P. Réaction anaphylactique après injection locale de GM-CSF au cours d'un ulcère veineux de jambe. [Anaphylactic reaction after local injection of GM-CSF in venous leg ulcer.] Ann Dermatol Venereol 1999;126(2):161.

26. Riggs JE, Mansmann PT, Cook LL, Schochet SS Jr, Hogg JP. Fulminant CNS perivascular lymphocytic proliferation: association with sargramostim, a hematopoietic growth factor. Clin Neuropharmacol 1999;22(5):288–91.

27. Hoekman K, von Blomberg-van der Flier BM, Wagstaff J, Drexhage HA, Pinedo HM. Reversible thyroid dysfunction during treatment with GM-CSF. Lancet 1991;338(8766):541–2.

28. Hansen PB, Johnsen HE, Hippe E. Autoimmune hypothyroidism and granulocyte–macrophage colony-stimulating factor. Eur J Haematol 1993;50(3):183–4.

29. Schriber JR, Negrin RS. Use and toxicity of the colony-stimulating factors. Drug Saf 1993;8(6):457–68.

30. Lieschke GJ, Maher D, Cebon J, O'Connor M, Green M, Sheridan W, Boyd A, Rallings M, Bonnem E, Metcalf D, et al. Effects of bacterially synthesized recombinant human granulocyte–macrophage colony-stimulating factor in patients with advanced malignancy. Ann Intern Med 1989;110(5):357–64.

31. Nathan FE, Besa EC. GM-CSF and accelerated hemolysis. N Engl J Med 1992;326(6):417.

32. Sarris AH, Majlis A, Dimopoulos MA, Younes A, Swann F, Rodriguez MA, McLaughlin P, Cabanillas F. Rising serum lactate dehydrogenase often caused by granulocyte- or granulocyte–macrophage colony stimulating factor and not tumor progression in patients with lymphoma or myeloma. Leuk Lymphoma 1995;17(5–6):473–7.

33. Gonzales-Chambers R, Rosenfeld C, Winkelstein A, Dameshek L. Eosinophilia resulting from administration of recombinant granulocyte–macrophage colony-stimulating factor (rhGM-CSF) in a patient with T-gamma lymphoproliferative disease. Am J Hematol 1991;36(2):157–9.

34. Donhuijsen K, Haedicke C, Hattenberger S, Hauswaldt C, Freund M. Granulocyte–macrophage colony-stimulating factor-related eosinophilia and Loeffler's endocarditis. Blood 1992;79(10):2798.

35. Bonig H, Burdach S, Gobel U, Nurnberger W. Growth factors and hemostasis: differential effects of GM-CSF and G-CSF on coagulation activation—laboratory and clinical evidence. Ann Hematol 2001;80(9):525–30.

36. Lindemann A, Herrmann F, Mertelsmann R, Gamm H, Rumpelt HJ. Splenic hematopoiesis following GM-CSF therapy in a patient with hairy cell leukemia. Leukemia 1990;4(8):606–7.

37. Lang E, Cibull ML, Gallicchio VS, Henslee-Downey PJ, Davey DD, Messino MJ, Harder EJ. Proliferation of abnormal bone marrow histiocytes, an undesired effect of granulocyte macrophage-colony-stimulating factor therapy in a patient with Hurler's syndrome undergoing bone marrow transplantation. Am J Hematol 1992;41(4):280–4.

38. Wilson PA, Ayscue LH, Jones GR, Bentley SA. Bone marrow histiocytic proliferation in association with colony-stimulating factor therapy. Am J Clin Pathol 1993;99(3):311–3.

39. Al-Homaidhi A, Prince HM, Al-Zahrani H, Doucette D, Keating A. Granulocyte–macrophage colony-stimulating factor-associated histiocytosis and capillary-leak syndrome following autologous bone marrow transplantation: two case reports and a review of the literature. Bone Marrow Transplant 1998;21(2):209–14.

40. Wakefield PE, James WD, Samlaska CP, Meltzer MS. Colony-stimulating factors. J Am Acad Dermatol 1990;23(5 Pt 1):903–12.

41. Mehregan DR, Fransway AF, Edmonson JH, Leiferman KM. Cutaneous reactions to granulocyte-monocyte colony-stimulating factor. Arch Dermatol 1992;128(8):1055–9.

42. Yamada H, Tubaki K, Ashida T, et al. Does recombinant granulocyte–macrophage colony-stimulating factor (GM-CSF) play a crucial role in the pathogenesis of atopic dermatitis after bone marrow transplantation (BMT). Med Science Res 1991;19:395.

43. Ward JC, Gitlin JB, Garry DJ, Jatoi A, Luikart SD, Zelickson BD, Dahl MV, Skubitz KM. Epidermolysis bullosa acquisita induced by GM-CSF: a role for eosinophils in treatment-related toxicity. Br J Haematol 1992;81(1):27–32.

44. Perrot JL, Benoit F, Segault D, Jaubert J, Guyotat D, Claudy A. Pyoderma gangrenosum aggravé par administration de GM-CSF. [Pyoderma gangrenosum aggravated by GM-CSF administration.] Ann Dermatol Venereol 1992;119(11):846–8.

45. Kelly R, Marsden RA, Bevan D. Exacerbation of psoriasis with GM-CSF therapy. Br J Dermatol 1993;128(4):468–9.

46. Hazenberg BP, Van Leeuwen MA, Van Rijswijk MH, Stern AC, Vellenga E. Correction of granulocytopenia in Felty's syndrome by granulocyte–macrophage colony-stimulating factor. Simultaneous induction of interleukin-6 release and flare-up of the arthritis. Blood 1989;74(8):2769–70.

47. de Vries EG, Willemse PH, Biesma B, Stern AC, Limburg PC, Vellenga E. Flare-up of rheumatoid arthritis during GM-CSF treatment after chemotherapy. Lancet 1991;338(8765):517–8.

48. Bokemeyer C, Schmoll HJ, Harstrick A. Side-effects of GM-CSF treatment in advanced testicular cancer. Eur J Cancer 1993;29A(6):924.

49. Shahar E, Krivoy N, Pollack S. Effective acute desensitization for immediate-type hypersensitivity to human granulocyte-monocyte colony stimulating factor. Ann Allergy Asthma Immunol 1999;83(6 Pt 1):543–6.

50. Gribben JG, Devereux S, Thomas NS, Keim M, Jones HM, Goldstone AH, Linch DC. Development of antibodies to unprotected glycosylation sites on recombinant human GM-CSF. Lancet 1990;335(8687):434–7.

51. Ragnhammar P, Friesen HJ, Frodin JE, Lefvert AK, Hassan M, Osterborg A, Mellstedt H. Induction of anti-recombinant human granulocyte–macrophage colony-stimulating factor (Escherichia coli-derived) antibodies and clinical effects in nonimmunocompromised patients. Blood 1994;84(12):4078–87.

52. Scadden DT, Agosti J. No antibodies to granulocyte macrophage colony-stimulating factor with prolonged use in AIDS. AIDS 1993;7(3):438.

53. Negrin RS, Haeuber DH, Nagler A, Olds LC, Donlon T, Souza LM, Greenberg PL. Treatment of myelodysplastic syndromes with recombinant human granulocyte colony-stimulating factor. A phase I-II trial. Ann Intern Med 1989;110(12):976–84.

54. Vose JM, Armitage JO. Clinical applications of hematopoietic growth factors. J Clin Oncol 1995;13(4):1023–35.

55. Rowe JM, Liesveld JL. Hematopoietic growth factors in acute leukemia. Leukemia 1997;11(3):328–41.

56. Terpstra W, Lowenberg B. Application of myeloid growth factors in the treatment of acute myeloid leukemia. Leukemia 1997;11(3):315–27.

57. Yoshida Y, Nakahata T, Shibata A, Takahashi M, Moriyama Y, Kaku K, Masaoka T, Kaneko T, Miwa S. Effects of long-term treatment with recombinant human granulocyte–macrophage colony-stimulating factor in patients with myelodysplastic syndrome. Leuk Lymphoma 1995;18(5–6):457–63.

58. Estey EH. Use of colony-stimulating factors in the treatment of acute myeloid leukemia. Blood 1994;83(8):2015–9.

59. Zimmer BM, Berdel WE, Ludwig WD, Notter M, Reufi B, Thiel E. Fatal spleen rupture during induction chemotherapy with rh GM-CSF priming for acute monocytic leukemia. Clinical case report and in vitro studies. Leuk Res 1993;17(3):277–83.

60. Cairo MS, Agosti J, Ellis R, Laver JJ, Puppala B, deLemos R, Givner L, Nesin M, Wheeler JG, Seth T, van de Ven C, Fanaroff A. A randomized, double-blind, placebo-controlled trial of prophylactic recombinant human granulocyte–macrophage colony-stimulating factor to reduce nosocomial infections in very low birth weight neonates. J Pediatr 1999;134(1):64–70.

61. Lazarus HM, Rowe JM. Clinical use of hematopoietic growth factors in allogeneic bone marrow transplantation. Blood Rev 1994;8(3):169–78.

62. Barbaro G, Di Lorenzo G, Grisorio B, Soldini M, Barbarini G. Effect of recombinant human granulocyte-macrophage colony-stimulating factor on HIV-related leukopenia: a randomized, controlled clinical study. AIDS 1997;11(12):1453–61.

63. \Ross SD, DiGeorge A, Connelly JE, Whiting GW, McDonnell N. Safety of GM-CSF in patients with AIDS: a review of the literature. Pharmacotherapy 1998;18(6):1290–7.

Macrophage colony-stimulating factor (M-CSF)

General Information

Macrophage colony-stimulating factor (M-CSF) stimulates the growth and differentiation of the monocyte lineage, and promotes the survival, proliferation, and functions of mature monocytes/macrophages (1). It also enhances myelopoiesis through the amplified production of G-CSF and GM-CSF by monocytes, and has antitumor activity. Purified human urinary M-CSF and recombinant human M-CSF are under investigation in humans.

The safety of human M-CSF (hM-CSF) in allogeneic and syngeneic bone marrow transplantation was evaluated in a randomized, double-blind, placebo-controlled trial in 119 patients (2). There was mild transient fever in 6.7% of patients and there were no significant adverse effects on the platelet count. The incidence of graft-versus-host disease or graft rejection and the leukemic relapse rate were not affected compared with placebo. There was a similar safety profile in patients with autologous bone marrow transplants (3).

Glycosylated mammalian-derived recombinant human M-CSF (rhM-CSF) has been used in several trials. Constitutional symptoms (malaise, fatigue, insomnia, headache, nausea, fever, and chills) sometimes occurred. There was no evidence of long-term toxicity during follow-up of patients who received rhM-CSF after allogeneic bone marrow transplantation (4).

Organs and Systems

Sensory systems

Subclinical conjunctival injection occurred in 50% of patients in one series, with moderate but symptomatic episcleritis and blurred vision in one patient (SEDA-19, 345). Asymptomatic retinal or perilimbal hemorrhages were sometimes noted, but there was no clear correlation with platelet count. Subjective ophthalmological symptoms, ocular inflammation, iridocyclitis, or malaise have also occurred as dose- or treatment-limiting adverse effects in other studies (5,6).

Hematologic

The most significant adverse effect of glycosylated mammalian-derived rhM-CSF is a transient, dose- and schedule-related severe thrombocytopenia, which correlates with monocytosis and typically occurs after 7–10 days of treatment (7). Thrombocytopenia sometimes resolves despite continued administration of rhM-CSF and has usually not been sufficiently severe to cause bleeding. In other cases, a 50% reduction in the dose of rhM-CSF should be considered to allow treatment to be continued. The mechanism of rhM-CSF-induced thrombocytopenia does not involve suppression of hemopoiesis, but rather increased activity of the monocyte/macrophage system in the liver and spleen (8).

Urinary tract

Acute nephrotic syndrome has been reported in a patient with a previous history of mild proteinuria (SEDA-20, 339), but the origin of the M-CSF (recombinant or human) was not stated.

Skin

Mild local toxicity sometimes occurs after subcutaneous injection of M-CSF (SED-13, 1118; 7). In one patient,

multiple subcutaneous nodules consistent with a panniculitis occurred after each administration (SEDA-19, 345).

In one study, severe erythroderma and a dramatic proliferation of blast cells after each dose of hM-CSF were the only significant severe adverse effects, reported in one patient each (SEDA-19, 345).

References

1. Kelley TW, Graham MM, Doseff AI, Pomerantz RW, Lau SM, Ostrowski MC, Franke TF, Marsh CB. Macrophage colony-stimulating factor promotes cell survival through Akt/protein kinase B. J Biol Chem 1999;274(37):26393–8.
2. Masaoka T, Shibata H, Ohno R, Katoh S, Harada M, Motoyoshi K, Takaku F, Sakuma A. Double-blind test of human urinary macrophage colony-stimulating factor for allogeneic and syngeneic bone marrow transplantation: effectiveness of treatment and 2-year follow-up for relapse of leukaemia. Br J Haematol 1990;76(4):501–5.
3. Khwaja A, Yong K, Jones HM, Chopra R, McMillan AK, Goldstone AH, Patterson KG, Matheson C, Ruthven K, Abramson SB, et al. The effect of macrophage colony-stimulating factor on haemopoietic recovery after autologous bone marrow transplantation. Br J Haematol 1992;81(2):288–95.
4. Nemunaitis J, Shannon-Dorcy K, Appelbaum FR, Meyers J, Owens A, Day R, Ando D, O'Neill C, Buckner D, Singer J. Long-term follow-up of patients with invasive fungal disease who received adjunctive therapy with recombinant human macrophage colony-stimulating factor. Blood 1993;82(5):1422–7.
5. Sanda MG, Yang JC, Topalian SL, Groves ES, Childs A, Belfort R Jr, de Smet MD, Schwartzentruber DJ, White DE, Lotze MT, et al. Intravenous administration of recombinant human macrophage colony-stimulating factor: clinical and immunomodulatory effects. J Clin Oncol 1994;12:97–106.
6. Bukowski RM, Budd GT, Gibbons JA, Bauer RJ, Childs A, Antal J, Finke J, Tuason L, Lorenzi V, McLain D, et al. Phase I trial of subcutaneous recombinant macrophage colony-stimulating factor: clinical and immunomodulatory effects. J Clin Oncol 1994;12(1):97–106.
7. Cole DJ, Sanda MG, Yang JC, Schwartzentruber DJ, Weber J, Ettinghausen SE, Pockaj BA, Kim HI, Levin RD, Pogrebniak HW, et al. Phase I trial of recombinant human macrophage colony-stimulating factor administered by continuous intravenous infusion in patients with metastatic cancer. J Natl Cancer Inst 1994;86(1):39–45.
8. Baker GR, Levin J. Transient thrombocytopenia produced by administration of macrophage colony-stimulating factor: investigations of the mechanism. Blood 1998;91(1):89–99.

Stem cell factor

General Information

Stem cell factor amplifies the proliferation and mobilization of myeloid, erythroid, and megakaryocyte colonies when combined with a lineage-specific hemopoietic growth factor (for example G-CSF, IL-3). Stem cell factor, added to other recombinant hemopoietic cytokines, is used to increase the mobilization of peripheral blood progenitor cells.

In preliminary trials, transient allergic-type reactions, that is urticaria, respiratory symptoms, and injection-site reactions, resulting from dose-dependent mast cell degranulation, were easily prevented by classical premedication (1).

In 102 patients with multiple myeloma, stem cell factor plus G-CSF produced more frequent injection site reactions and more frequent skin reactions (25 versus 2%), namely rash, erythema, urticaria, pruritus, and abnormal pigmentation, compared with G-CSF alone (2). These reactions occurred despite systemic prophylactic antihistamines. Other adverse effects occurred with similar frequency in the two groups of patients.

Organs and Systems

Immunologic

Stem cell factor produces direct mast cell stimulation with subsequent allergic-type reactions. Despite careful premedication with diphenhydramine, ranitidine, inhaled

salbutamol, and pseudoephedrine, such reactions were still observed in 3% of patients (3).

References

1. Maslak P, Nimer SD. The efficacy of IL-3, SCF, IL-6, and IL-11 in treating thrombocytopenia. Semin Hematol 1998;35(3):253–60.
2. Facon T, Harousseau JL, Maloisel F, Attal M, Odriozola J, Alegre A, Schroyens W, Hulin C, Schots R, Marin P, Guilhot F, Granena A, De Waele M, Pigneux A, Meresse V, Clark P, Reiffers J. Stem cell factor in combination with filgrastim after chemotherapy improves peripheral blood progenitor cell yield and reduces apheresis requirements in multiple myeloma patients: a randomized, controlled trial. Blood 1999;94(4):1218–25.
3. Shpall EJ, Wheeler CA, Turner SA, Yanovich S, Brown RA, Pecora AL, Shea TC, Mangan KF, Williams SF, LeMaistre CF, Long GD, Jones R, Davis MW, Murphy-Filkins R, Parker WR, Glaspy JA. A randomized phase 3 study of peripheral blood progenitor cell mobilization with stem cell factor and filgrastim in high-risk breast cancer patients. Blood 1999;93(8):2491–501.

TUMOR NECROSIS FACTOR ALFA AND ITS ANTAGONISTS

Tumor necrosis factor alfa

General Information

Tumor necrosis factor alfa is naturally produced by activated macrophages and monocytes and has pleiotropic effects on normal and malignant cells. Unfortunately, the systemic administration of tumor necrosis factor alfa as a single agent gave disappointing results with severe adverse effects and no significant clinical antitumor effect (SED-13, 1110; 1,2). However, tumor necrosis factor alfa combined with interferon gamma, interleukin-2, or cytotoxic drugs produced positive clinical results, and these combinations reduced the maximum tolerated dose of tumor necrosis factor alfa two to four-fold.

Severe hypotension, thought to be nitrous oxide-mediated, is the main dose-limiting toxicity at all doses. Other frequent and sometimes dose-limiting adverse effects included fever, chills and rigors, myalgias, diarrhea, nausea or vomiting, and local reactions at the injection site. During combination therapy with tumor necrosis factor alfa, hyperbilirubinemia, neurotoxicity, severe febrile reactions, and hypotension were the most frequent complications (SED-13, 1110; 1–4). Transient liver dysfunction, oliguria, and raised creatinine concentrations are common.

Organs and Systems

Cardiovascular

Hypotension, perhaps nitrous oxide-mediated, is a dose-limiting adverse effect of tumor necrosis factor alfa (5).

Severe hypophosphatemia with myocardial dysfunction was noted in patients receiving tumor necrosis factor alfa by continuous hepatic arterial infusion (SEDA-17, 433).

Congestive cardiomyopathy has been attributed to tumor necrosis factor alfa in isolated patients (SED-13, 1110; 6).

Respiratory

A reversible reduction in pulmonary diffusing capacity (7) and pulmonary hemorrhage have been attributed to tumor necrosis factor alfa in isolated patients (SED-13, 1110; 8).

Nervous system

Tumor necrosis factor alfa is considered to be a major neurotoxic agent, and most patients who received large doses developed central nervous system symptoms, most commonly headache, lethargy, fatigue, confusion, disorientation, and reduced performance. Seizures, transient amnesia, aphasia, hallucinations, and diplopia sometimes occur (9).

Psychological, psychiatric

Evaluation of cognitive function in patients receiving tumor necrosis factor alfa alone or combined with interleukin-2 showed reversible attentional deficits, memory disorders, deficits in motor coordination and frontal lobe executive functions (9). There was reversible hypoperfusion in the frontal lobes.

Endocrine

Exacerbation of hypothyroidism was noted in one patient with chronic thyroiditis who received tumor necrosis factor alfa (10).

Metabolism

Metabolic effects of tumor necrosis factor alfa include a reduction in cholesterol and high-density lipoproteins, increases in triglycerides and very low-density lipoproteins, and hyperglycemia.

Hematologic

The hematological effects of tumor necrosis factor alfa mostly consist of dose-related thrombocytopenia and granulocytopenia, and decreased monocyte or lymphocyte counts (SED-13, 1111; 11,12). Septic episodes are sometimes associated with leukopenia. Coagulopathy with laboratory evidence of disseminated intravascular coagulopathy was found in 30% of patients and was sometimes associated with thromboembolic events (13). Other coagulation disorders include transient alterations in prothrombin time, and a rise in the plasma concentrations of von Willebrand factor was found in healthy volunteers (14).

Gastrointestinal

Hemorrhagic gastritis has been attributed to tumor necrosis factor alfa (15).

Immunologic

Anaphylactic-like reactions, dyspnea, or acute bronchospasm have been attributed to tumor necrosis factor alfa in patients also treated with interleukin-2 (16).

Drug Administration

Drug administration route

Local (intralesional, intra-arterial, or intraperitoneal) administration of tumor necrosis factor alfa may well prove to be a more promising and less toxic route of administration. Although mild adverse effects, namely fever, hypotension, and fatigue, were similar to those reported after intravenous administration, coagulation disorders, pulmonary, central nervous system, liver, and renal forms of toxicity were usually not observed (17).

The most interesting and encouraging experience has been obtained using hyperthermic isolated limb perfusion (HILP) of tumor necrosis factor alfa combined with cytostatic drugs (for example melphalan) in melanoma and sarcoma (18). Although systemic toxicity was moderate in this setting, there was still a risk of severe hemodynamic changes, with clinical features of septic shock and a direct nephrotoxic effect of tumor necrosis factor alfa (19,20). A mild neuropathy, marked by transient paresthesia, is also frequent (21). Other rare adverse effects included lung infiltrates, fever, neutropenia, thrombocytopenia, coagulation disorders, transient rise in transaminases and bilirubin, and an increased risk of more severe rhabdomyolysis (SED-13, 1111; 22).

References

1. Sidhu RS, Bollon AP. Tumor necrosis factor activities and cancer therapy—a perspective. Pharmacol Ther 1993;57(1):79–128.
2. Hieber U, Heim ME. Tumor necrosis factor for the treatment of malignancies. Oncology 1994;51(2):142–53.
3. Schiller JH, Witt PL, Storer B, Alberti D, Tombes MB, Arzoomanian R, Brown RR, Proctor RA, Voss SD, Spriggs DR, et al. Clinical and biologic effects of combination therapy with gamma-interferon and tumor necrosis factor. Cancer 1992;69(2):562–71.
4. Smith JW 2nd, Urba WJ, Clark JW, Longo DL, Farrell M, Creekmore SP, Conlon KC, Jaffe H, Steis RG. Phase I evaluation of recombinant tumor necrosis factor given in combination with recombinant interferon-gamma. J Immunother 1991;10(5):355–62.
5. Hanson DS, Leggette CT. Severe hypotension following inadvertent intravenous administration of interferon alfa-2a. Ann Pharmacother 1997;31(3):371–2.
6. Hegewisch S, Weh HJ, Hossfeld DK. TNF-induced cardiomyopathy. Lancet 1990;335(8684):294–5.
7. Kuei JH, Tashkin DP, Figlin RA. Pulmonary toxicity of recombinant human tumor necrosis factor. Chest 1989;96(2):334–8.
8. Schilling PJ, Murray JL, Markowitz AB. Novel tumor necrosis factor toxic effects. Pulmonary hemorrhage and severe hepatic dysfunction. Cancer 1992;69(1):256–60.
9. Meyers CA, Valentine AD, Wong FC, Leeds NE. Reversible neurotoxicity of interleukin-2 and tumor necrosis factor: correlation of SPECT with neuropsychological testing. J Neuropsychiatry Clin Neurosci 1994;6(3):285–8.
10. Miyakoshi H, Ohsawa K, Yokoyama H, Nagai Y, Ieki Y, Bando YI, Kobayashi K. Exacerbation of hypothyroidism following tumor necrosis factor-alpha infusion. Intern Med 1992;31(2):200–3.
11. Mittelman A, Puccio C, Gafney E, Coombe N, Singh B, Wood D, Nadler P, Ahmed T, Arlin Z. A phase I pharmacokinetic study of recombinant human tumor necrosis factor administered by a 5-day continuous infusion. Invest New Drugs 1992;10(3):183–90.
12. Logan TF, Kaplan SS, Bryant JL, Ernstoff MS, Krause JR, Kirkwood JM. Granulocytopenia in cancer patients treated in a phase I trial with recombinant human tumor necrosis factor. J Immunother 1991;10(2):84–95.
13. Muggia FM, Brown TD, Goodman PJ, Macdonald JS, Hersh EM, Fleming TR, Leichman L. High incidence of coagulopathy in phase II studies of recombinant tumor necrosis factor in advanced pancreatic and gastric cancers. Anticancer Drugs 1992;3(3):211–7.
14. van der Poll T, van Deventer SJ, Pasterkamp G, van Mourik JA, Buller HR, ten Cate JW. Tumor necrosis factor induces von Willebrand factor release in healthy humans. Thromb Haemost 1992;67(6):623–6.
15. Krigel RL, Padavic-Shaller KA, Rudolph AA, Young JD, Weiner LM, Konrad M, Comis RL. Hemorrhagic gastritis as a new dose-limiting toxicity of recombinant tumor necrosis factor. J Natl Cancer Inst 1991;83(2):129–31.
16. Negrier MS, Pourreau CN, Palmer PA, Ranchere JY, Mercatello A, Viens P, Blaise D, Jasmin C, Misset JL, Franks CR, et al. Phase I trial of recombinant interleukin-2 followed by recombinant tumor necrosis factor in patients with metastatic cancer. J Immunother 1992;11(2):93–102.
17. Watanabe N, Yamauchi N, Maeda M, Neda H, Tsuji Y, Okamoto T, Tsuji N, Akiyama S, Sasaki H, Niitsu Y. Recombinant human tumor necrosis factor causes regression in patients with advanced malignancies. Oncology 1994;51(4):360–5.
18. Eggermont AM, Schraffordt Koops H, Klausner JM, Kroon BB, Schlag PM, Lienard D, van Geel AN, Hoekstra HJ, Meller I, Nieweg OE, Kettelhack C, Ben-Ari G, Pector JC, Lejeune FJ. Isolated limb perfusion with tumor necrosis factor and melphalan for limb salvage in 186 patients with locally advanced soft tissue extremity sarcomas. The cumulative multicenter European experience. Ann Surg 1996;224(6):756–65.
19. Eggimann P, Chiolero R, Chassot PG, Lienard D, Gerain J, Lejeune F. Systemic and hemodynamic effects of recombinant tumor necrosis factor alpha in isolation perfusion of the limbs. Chest 1995;107(4):1074–82.
20. Zwaveling JH, Hoekstra HJ, Maring JK, v Ginkel RJ, Schraffordt Koops H, Smit AJ, Girbes AR. Renal function in cancer patients treated with hyperthermic isolated limb perfusion with recombinant tumor necrosis factor-alpha and melphalan. Nephron 1997;76(2):146–52.
21. Drory VE, Lev D, Groozman GB, Gutmann M, Klausner JM. Neurotoxicity of isolated limb perfusion with tumor necrosis factor. J Neurol Sci 1998;158(1):1–4.
22. Hohenberger P, Haier J, Schlag PM. Rhabdomyolysis and renal function impairment after isolated limb perfusion—comparison between the effects of perfusion with rhTNF alpha and a "triple-drug" regimen. Eur J Cancer 1997;33(4):596–601.

Adalimumab

See Monoclonal antibodies (p. 457).

Etanercept

General Information

Etanercept is a dimeric fusion protein consisting of two recombinant p75 tumor necrosis factor receptors fused with the Fc portion of human IgG1. It inhibits the binding of tumor necrosis factor alfa to its receptor and thereby neutralizes its biological activity. It has been used in the treatment of moderate to severe active rheumatoid arthritis, ankylosing spondylitis, psoriatic arthropathy, and juvenile rheumatoid arthritis in patients who have failed to respond to previous disease-modifying antirheumatic drugs. The clinical pharmacology and adverse effects of etanercept in patients with rheumatoid disorders have been reviewed (1).

Comparative studies

In a study of weekly oral methotrexate in two different doses (10 or 25 mg) or twice-weekly etanercept in 632 patients, etanercept produced fewer systemic adverse effects than methotrexate, but a higher incidence of injection site reactions (2). Despite theoretical concerns about the development of autoimmune reactions in patients taking etanercept, no evidence of clinical autoimmune disease emerged from this large trial.

General adverse effects

The therapeutic use and safety of etanercept have been reviewed (3). Mild-to-moderate injection site reactions were the most common adverse effects (42–49%), with a frequency 3.8 to 6 times greater than with placebo. Non-neutralizing antibodies to etanercept were rarely detected. Etanercept-treated patients more often developed new antinuclear antibodies or anti-double-stranded DNA antibodies, but no patient developed symptoms suggestive of an autoimmune disease during clinical trials.

Organs and Systems

Respiratory

The typical histological morphology of pulmonary rheumatoid nodules that developed during etanercept treatment has been reported (4,5). Pulmonary granulomas during etanercept treatment can be coincidental and difficult to distinguish from other pulmonary complications, such as relapse of tuberculosis. In two patients with rheumatoid arthritis who underwent lung biopsy for etanercept-associated pulmonary granulomas, there were non-caseating granulomas containing birefringent particulate in one (6) and caseating necrosis in the other (7). Infectious causes were ruled out. After etanercept withdrawal, the lesions resolved completely with steroid treatment in the first patient but persisted over 1 year despite antituberculosis treatment in the other.

Nervous system

Postmarketing warnings about etanercept that have been issued by regulatory agencies and the manufacturers relate to a possible increased risk of demyelinating disorders, such as multiple sclerosis, myelitis, and optic neuritis, in patients with pre-existing or a recent history of demyelinating disorders (SEDA-26, 399). This was in keeping with the results obtained in a placebo-controlled trial of lenercept, another recombinant tumor necrosis factor alfa receptor immunoglobulin fusion protein, in 168 patients with multiple sclerosis; compared with placebo, significantly more patients randomized to lenercept

had exacerbation of multiple sclerosis, and exacerbation also occurred earlier (8).

Transverse myelitis of abrupt onset has also been reported (9).

- A 45-year-old woman with resistant rheumatoid arthritis was given etanercept 25 mg twice weekly. Nine days later she developed total acute sensory loss, with flaccid paraplegia, fecal incontinence, and urinary retention. MRI imaging and cerebrospinal fluid analysis were consistent with a diagnosis of transverse myelitis. She also had positive antinuclear and anticardiolipin antibodies. After etanercept withdrawal and treatment with dexamethasone and cyclophosphamide, her motor function improved with no change in sensory function.

Neurological events suggestive of demyelinating disorders in patients treated with tumor necrosis factor alfa antagonists and reported to the FDA's Adverse Events Reporting System have been reviewed (10). These included 17 cases temporarily associated with etanercept and two with infliximab, but complete information was lacking in a number of cases. One additional case with etanercept was more extensively detailed. The first symptoms occurred after a large range of delay after first drug administration (1 week to 15 months; mean 5 months) and mostly included paresthesia, optic neuritis, and confusion. MRI scans in 19 patients showed demyelination in various brain areas in 16. Although a causal relation was not proven, it is noteworthy that most patients improved after withdrawal and one patient had recurrent neurological symptoms after etanercept readministration. The various hypothetical mechanisms by which tumor necrosis factor alfa antagonists might produce demyelinating events have been discussed elsewhere (11). Briefly, they cause increased peripheral T cell autoreactivity, and their inability to cross the blood–brain barrier may account for exacerbation of central demyelinating disorders.

Endocrine

- Transient hyperthyroidism occurred after 6 months of etanercept treatment in a 37-year-old woman with rheumatoid arthritis (12).

However, a direct causal relation with etanercept was debatable, because there was complete resolution with propranolol and despite continuation of etanercept.

Metabolism

Type 1 diabetes mellitus occurred after 5 months treatment with etanercept for juvenile rheumatoid arthritis in a 7-year-old girl (13). Antiglutamic acid decarboxylase antibodies were positive both before and during treatment, suggesting that etanercept may have prematurely triggered an underlying disease.

Hematologic

Postmarketing warnings about etanercept that have been issued by regulatory agencies and the manufacturers relate to a possible risk of aplastic anemia and pancytopenia (10 reported cases, of which 5 ended in fatal sepsis) (8).

Etanercept has reportedly caused abrupt exacerbation of the macrophage activation syndrome (14).

- A 22-year-old woman with adult-onset Still's disease developed symptoms suggestive of the macrophage activation syndrome. After initial glucocorticoid treatment, she received two doses of etanercept, and within 6 days her white blood cell count fell from $6.4 \times 10^9/l$ to $2.5 \times 10^9/l$ and the neutrophil count from $0.8 \times 10^9/l$ to $0.2 \times 10^9/l$. There was also thrombocytopenia and impaired coagulation and her liver enzymes were raised. A bone marrow aspirate showed delayed myelopoiesis. She received multiple transfusions, intravenous immunoglobulin, and granulocyte-macrophage colony-stimulating factor. The macrophage activation syndrome was diagnosed at that time and she was successfully treated with pulse methylprednisolone and ciclosporin. Epstein–Barr virus infection was subsequently confirmed.

Because soluble tumor necrosis factor alfa receptors are supposedly involved in the macrophage activation syndrome, the authors speculated that the administration of additional soluble receptors may have been the cause of a prolonged and exacerbated syndrome.

Urinary tract

Glomerulonephritis has been discussed as a possible consequence of etanercept treatment in two patients, with biopsy-proven mesangial deposits of IgA in one (15).

Skin

Injection site reactions are very common during the first month of treatment with etanercept. Histological findings in one patient showed a mild transient inflammatory response that did not suggest sensitization (16). The clinical and histological characteristics of these lesions have been analysed in a retrospective review of 103 etanercept-treated patients and in three other patients assessed prospectively (17). Of 103 patients, 21 had injection site reactions (erythema, pain, pruritus, or edema) within the first 2 months of treatment, and typically within 1–2 days after the last injection. In addition, eight patients developed recall reactions while continuing to take etanercept. Skin biopsies and immunohistological analysis of reaction sites in three patients showed an inflammatory infiltrate consistent with a T cell-mediated delayed hypersensitivity reaction.

There have been several descriptions of new cutaneous or pulmonary nodulosis in patients with rheumatoid arthritis treated with etanercept (4,18); concomitant cutaneous vasculitis was also reported in two patients (18). Although this may have been due to the natural history of rheumatoid arthritis or a lack of response to treatment, the short time to the occurrence of cutaneous nodulosis after the start of therapy in some patients implicated the etanercept.

Cutaneous vasculitis can also be the sole cutaneous manifestation of etanercept treatment (19). Purpuric lesions with histological features of leukocytoclastic vasculitis have been reported in a 58-year-old man (20) and a necrotizing vasculitis with eosinophils in a skin biopsy in a woman with rheumatoid arthritis (21). However, it is not known whether this resulted from the deposition of specific immune complexes.

- A 13-year-old girl developed a slowly reversible purpuric rash after 6 weeks of etanercept treatment, and the lesions recurred on re-administration (22). However, further administration of a gradually increasing dose of etanercept, with concomitant high-dose glucocorticoids, and antihistamines, was well tolerated, suggesting that tolerance can be obtained.

One patient who had separate episodes of vascular purpura during each of three sequences of treatment with etanercept, with leukocytoclastic vasculitis during the third episode, later developed similar cutaneous lesions after a third injection of infliximab (19).

Other types of skin reactions that have been described in isolated reports include urticaria-like eruptions with prurigo in two patients with juvenile arthritis (23) and discoid lupus erythematosus in a woman with rheumatoid arthritis (21). Erythema multiforme in three patients and a lichenoid eruption in one were attributed to infliximab; however, one patient had similar lesions after etanercept (24).

Musculoskeletal

Painless orbital myositis has been reported in a 42-year-old woman taking etanercept, but a causal relation was not established (25).

Immunologic

Although patients treated with etanercept commonly develop new antinuclear antibodies or anti-double-stranded DNA antibodies, there were no reports of cutaneous or systemic lupus erythematosus in early clinical trials. However, since then, at least eight cases have been reported, including five patients with a lupus-like syndrome, two with acute discoid lupus, and one with subacute cutaneous lupus erythematosus (26–29). All were women and they developed their first symptoms 6 weeks to 14 months after the first injection of etanercept. Antinuclear and/or anti-DNA antibodies were positive in most of them. Etanercept was withdrawn in all patients with features of systemic lupus erythematosus, and the symptoms resolved within 2–8 weeks. The skin lesions also improved with local glucocorticoids, despite continued etanercept treatment in two patients with discoid lupus or subacute cutaneous lupus erythematosus. This suggests that etanercept-induced autoantibodies are sometimes associated with clinical autoimmune disease.

Infection risk

In contrast to infliximab, etanercept is rarely associated with severe infectious complications. This has been attributed to different mechanisms of tumor necrosis factor alfa neutralization by the two drugs. Indeed, only nine cases of tuberculosis have previously been reported to the FDA from more than 100 000 patients treated worldwide (30). However, severe or uncommon infectious complications (severe viral pneumonia, fatal pneumococcal sepsis due to necrotizing fasciitis, osteoarticular tuberculosis) have been described in patients taking etanercept and long-term glucocorticoids (31–33).

Long-Term Effects

Tumorigenicity

There is great concern about the potential development of malignancy after blockade of tumor necrosis factor alfa, and it is biologically plausible. The FDA received reports of 26 cases of lymphoproliferative disorders in patients treated with etanercept ($n = 18$) or infliximab ($n = 8$) over 20 months (34). Although this reporting rate does not exceed the age-adjusted incidence of lymphomas in the USA, spontaneous reporting underestimates the true incidence. In addition, several findings were similar to those reported in patients taking immunosuppressive drugs after transplantation. For example, 81% of the reported cases were non-Hodgkin's lymphomas. Also, the median time to occurrence after the start of anti-TNF-alfa treatment was only 8 weeks. Finally, lymphoma regressed in two patients after withdrawal and without specific cytotoxic therapy. Although the actual incidence of neoplasia was low, additional long-term data that take into account concomitant or previous immunosuppressive treatment are needed before firm conclusions can be reached.

Susceptibility Factors

Age

In eight children with juvenile rheumatoid arthritis, who had failed to respond to disease-modifying anti-rheumatic drugs, high-dose etanercept was well tolerated (35). None withdrew because of etanercept-related adverse events. One child reported transient erythema at the injection site after the first injection. Three had mild transient upper respiratory tract infections. There were no laboratory abnormalities.

Interference with Diagnostic Tests

Troponin concentration

Non-neutralizing antibodies to etanercept have been identified in clinical trials. Although there was no correlation between these antibodies and the development of adverse effects (2), their presence was suggested as a likely explanation of false-positive rises in troponin concentrations in an assay that used mouse antihuman troponin (36).

References

1. Culy CR, Keating GM. Etanercept: an updated review of its use in rheumatoid arthritis, psoriatic arthritis and juvenile rheumatoid arthritis. Drugs 2002;62(17):2493–537.
2. Bathon JM, Martin RW, Fleischmann RM, Tesser JR, Schiff MH, Keystone EC, Genovese MC, Wasko MC, Moreland LW, Weaver AL, Markenson J, Finck BK. A comparison of etanercept and methotrexate in patients with early rheumatoid arthritis. N Engl J Med 2000;343(22):1586–93.
3. Jarvis B, Faulds D. Etanercept: a review of its use in rheumatoid arthritis. Drugs 1999;57(6):945–66.
4. Kekow J, Welte T, Kellner U, Pap T. Development of rheumatoid nodules during anti-tumor necrosis factor alpha therapy with etanercept. Arthritis Rheum 2002;46(3):843–4.
5. Hubscher O, Re R, Iotti R. Pulmonary rheumatoid nodules in an etanercept-treated patient. Arthritis Rheum 2003;48(7):2077–8.
6. Peno-Green L, Lluberas G, Kingsley T, Brantley S. Lung injury linked to etanercept therapy. Chest 2002;122(5):1858–60.
7. Vavricka SR, Wettstein T, Speich R, Gaspert A, Bachli EB. Pulmonary granulomas after tumour necrosis factor alpha antagonist therapy. Thorax 2003;58(3):278–9.
8. Arnason BGWThe Lenercept Multiple Sclerosis Study GroupThe University of British Columbia MS/MRI Analysis Group. TNF neutralization in MS: results of a randomized, placebo-controlled multicenter study. Neurology 1999;53(3):457–65.
9. van der Laken CJ, Lems WF, van Soesbergen RM, van der Sande JJ, Dijkmans BA. Paraplegia in a patient receiving anti-tumor necrosis factor therapy for rheumatoid arthritis: comment on the article by Mohan et al. Arthritis Rheum 2003;48(1):269–70.
10. Mohan N, Edwards ET, Cupps TR, Oliverio PJ, Sandberg G, Crayton H, Richert JR, Siegel JN. Demyelination occurring during anti-tumor necrosis factor alpha therapy for inflammatory arthritides. Arthritis Rheum 2001;44(12):2862–9.
11. Robinson WH, Genovese MC, Moreland LW. Demyelinating and neurologic events reported in association with tumor necrosis factor alpha antagonism: by what mechanisms could tumor necrosis factor alpha antagonists improve rheumatoid arthritis but exacerbate multiple sclerosis? Arthritis Rheum 2001;44(9):1977–83.
12. Allanore Y, Bremont C, Kahan A, Menkes CJ. Transient hyperthyroidism in a patient with rheumatoid arthritis treated by etanercept. Clin Exp Rheumatol 2001;19(3):356–7.
13. Bloom BJ. Development of diabetes mellitus during etanercept therapy in a child with systemic-onset juvenile rheumatoid arthritis. Arthritis Rheum 2000;43(11):2606–8.
14. Stern A, Buckley L. Worsening of macrophage activation syndrome in a patient with adult onset Still's disease after initiation of etanercept therapy. J Clin Rheumatol 2001;7:252–6.
15. Kemp E, Nielsen H, Petersen LJ, Gam AN, Dahlager J, Horn T, Larsen S, Olsen S. Newer immunomodulating drugs in rheumatoid arthritis may precipitate glomerulonephritis. Clin Nephrol 2001;55(1):87–8.
16. Murphy FT, Enzenauer RJ, Battafarano DF, David-Bajar K. Etanercept-associated injection-site reactions. Arch Dermatol 2000;136(4):556–7.
17. Zeltser R, Valle L, Tanck C, Holyst MM, Ritchlin C, Gaspari AA. Clinical, histological, and immunophenotypic

characteristics of injection site reactions associated with etanercept: a recombinant tumor necrosis factor alpha receptor: Fc fusion protein. Arch Dermatol 2001;137(7):893–9.

18. Cunnane G, Warnock M, Fye KH, Daikh DI. Accelerated nodulosis and vasculitis following etanercept therapy for rheumatoid arthritis. Arthritis Rheum 2002;47(4):445–9.

19. McCain ME, Quinet RJ, Davis WE. Etanercept and infliximab associated with cutaneous vasculitis. Rheumatology (Oxford) 2002;41(1):116–7.

20. Galaria NA, Werth VP, Schumacher HR. Leukocytoclastic vasculitis due to etanercept. J Rheumatol 2000;27(8):2041–4.

21. Brion PH, Mittal-Henkle A, Kalunian KC. Autoimmune skin rashes associated with etanercept for rheumatoid arthritis. Ann Intern Med 1999;131(8):634.

22. Livermore PA, Murray KJ. Anti-tumour necrosis factor therapy associated with cutaneous vasculitis. Rheumatology (Oxford) 2002;41(12):1450–2.

23. Skytta E, Pohjankoski H, Savolainen A. Etanercept and urticaria in patients with juvenile idiopathic arthritis. Clin Exp Rheumatol 2000;18(4):533–4.

24. Vergara G, Silvestre JF, Betlloch I, Vela P, Albares MP, Pascual JC. Cutaneous drug eruption to infliximab: report of 4 cases with an interface dermatitis pattern. Arch Dermatol 2002;138(9):1258–9.

25. Caramaschi P, Biasi D, Carletto A, Bambara LM. Orbital myositis in a rheumatoid arthritis patient during etanercept treatment. Clin Exp Rheumatol 2003;21(1):136–7.

26. Bleumink GS, ter Borg EJ, Ramselaar CG, Ch Stricker BH. Etanercept-induced subacute cutaneous lupus erythematosus. Rheumatology (Oxford) 2001;40(11):1317–9.

27. De Bandt MJ, Descamps V, Meyer O. Two cases of etanercept-induced systemic lupus erythematosus in patients with rheumatoid arthritis. Ann Rheum Dis 2001;60:175.

28. Misery L, Perrot JL, Gentil-Perret A, Pallot-Prades B, Cambazard F, Alexandre C. Dermatological complications of etanercept therapy for rheumatoid arthritis. Br J Dermatol 2002;146(2):334–5.

29. Shakoor N, Michalska M, Harris CA, Block JA. Drug-induced systemic lupus erythematosus associated with etanercept therapy. Lancet 2002;359(9306):579–80.

30. Keane J, Gershon S, Wise RP, Mirabile-Levens E, Kasznica J, Schwieterman WD, Siegel JN, Braun MM. Tuberculosis associated with infliximab, a tumor necrosis factor alpha-neutralizing agent. N Engl J Med 2001;345(15):1098–104.

31. Baghai M, Osmon DR, Wolk DM, Wold LE, Haidukewych GJ, Matteson EL. Fatal sepsis in a patient with rheumatoid arthritis treated with etanercept. Mayo Clin Proc 2001;76(6):653–6.

32. Myers A, Clark J, Foster H. Tuberculosis and treatment with infliximab. N Engl J Med 2002;346(8):623–6.

33. Smith D, Letendre S. Viral pneumonia as a serious complication of etanercept therapy. Ann Intern Med 2002;136(2):174.

34. Brown SL, Greene MH, Gershon SK, Edwards ET, Braun MM. Tumor necrosis factor antagonist therapy and lymphoma development: twenty-six cases reported to the Food and Drug Administration. Arthritis Rheum 2002;46(12):3151–8.

35. Takei S, Groh D, Bernstein B, Shaham B, Gallagher K, Reiff A. Safety and efficacy of high dose etanercept in treatment of juvenile rheumatoid arthritis. J Rheumatol 2001;28(7):1677–80.

36. Russell E, Zeihen M, Wergin S, Litton T. Patients receiving etanercept may develop antibodies that interfere with monoclonal antibody laboratory assays. Arthritis Rheum 2000;43(4):944.

Infliximab

See Monoclonal antibodies (p. 457).

MONOCLONAL ANTIBODIES

General Information

Human monoclonal antibody immunotherapy in clinical medicine has been an exciting prospect for some time, and increasing numbers of such antibodies have gradually become available (1,2).

An illustration of the potential of human monoclonal antibodies was provided by the HA-1A antibody, a human monoclonal IgM specific for the core/lipid A part of endotoxin. Among 291 patients with Gram-negative bacteremia treated with this antibody there was a significant reduction in mortality (3). Since then other patient groups have been treated, and apart from local urticaria, flushing, and mild transient hypotension, no adverse reactions were noted (4,5). No patient has developed antibodies to HA-1A. Although the initial results seem promising, more trials are needed to substantiate the therapeutic efficacy of HA-1A.

Numerous investigators have reported and reviewed the clinical application of monoclonal antibodies in various areas, including organ transplantation, neoplastic diseases, severe sepsis, and chronic inflammatory diseases. Collectively, these antibodies generally did not produce major adverse effects. The rapid development of antibodies against murine monoclonal antibodies is one of the most important clinical limitations to their therapeutic use, but the development of humanized (chimeric human/murine) monoclonal antibodies has improved their safety. Monoclonal antibodies have also been used in non-immune mediated diseases, such as cancer, septic shock, reperfusion, and as antiplatelet drugs. Treatment of neoplastic diseases with monoclonal antibodies is theoretically attractive. Unfortunately none of the monoclonal antibodies available at present has been demonstrated to be strictly tumor-specific, and binding of antibody to normal cells has been shown to be the major unknown factor for toxicity (6).

Monoclonal antibodies that are dealt with in separate monographs are abciximab, alemtuzumab, anti-CD4 antibody, basiliximab, daclizumab, edrecolomab, gemtuzumab ozogamicin, ibritumomab, muromonab-CD3, omalizumab, palivizumab, rituximab, and trastuzumab.

Nomenclature

Modern international non-proprietary drug names have two parts. The suffix, or stem, tells you what group the drug belongs to, ideally chosen to reflect its pharmacological action. For instance, -vastatin denotes HMG Co-A reductase inhibitors (-stat- often being used for enzyme inhibitors); -olol denotes beta-blockers (but beware stanozolol); and -mycins are antibiotics. The prefix is chosen at will. It might reflect the structure or source of the drug (for example diclofenac, virginiamycin), the inventor's love of opera or the cinema (for example, mimimycin, rifampicin (7)), or just whimsy.

The monoclonal antibodies have a prefix and three substems. All, with one exception (muromonab), end in -mab for monoclonal antibody. The penultimate syllable (or substem) indicates the animal source and the prepenultimate syllable indicates the target (Table 1). The prefix (one or two syllables) is chosen at random. Finally, if the antibody is conjugated to a toxin, an extra word is added; aritox, for example, denotes the A chain of ricin.

For example, trastuzumab can be parsed as follows: trastu-zu-mab. The -zu- denotes a humanized antibody and the -tu- a tumor target. If you wanted to show that it targets the breast specifically, you could call it tramazumab.

Uses

The uses of some monoclonal antibodies are listed in Table 2.

Several anti-human T cell monoclonal antibodies have undergone preliminary trials in the treatment of renal allograft rejection. Most of these monoclonal antibodies were not effective than muromonab (1). T10B9, an anti-human pan-T lymphocyte monoclonal antibody, had similar efficacy but caused less fever, severe infection, respiratory, gastrointestinal, or neurological symptoms than muromonab (SEDA-22, 409). Other monoclonal antibodies, such as chimeric anti-CD7 and murine anti-ICAM-1 (CD54; enlimomab), were devoid of adverse effects or produced only minimal and transient adverse effects (SED-13, 1134).

Anti-CD4 monoclonal antibodies, for example OKT4A, BF-5, cM-T412 (clenoliximab, keliximab), are continuously being investigated, although in small numbers of patients, after transplantation or in chronic inflammatory diseases, such as rheumatoid arthritis (SEDA-20, 340; SEDA-21, 379; 2,8,9). Significant clinical immunomodulation has sometimes been obtained, with only transient and self-limiting, first-dose effects, namely headache, fever and chills, gastrointestinal disorders, hypotension, and tachycardia (SEDA-21, 379). Whereas most other adverse effects were not specifically associated with these monoclonal antibodies, mild skin

Table 1 The components of the names of monoclonal antibodies

Prepenultimate syllable (general target)	Prepenultimate syllable (specific tumor target)	Penultimate syllable (species source)
-ba(c)- = bacterium	-co(l)- = colon	-a- = rat
-ci(r)- = cardiovascular	-go-(t)- = gonad (testis)	-e- = hamster
-le(s)- = infectious lesions	-go-(v)- = gonad (ovary)	-i- = primate
-li(m)- = immunomodulation	-ma-(r)- = mammary	-o- = mouse
-vi(r)- = virus	-me(l)- = melanoma	-u- = human
-pr(o) = prostate		-xi- = chimeric
-tu(m)- = tumor (unspecified)		-zu- = humanized

Table 2 Some monoclonal antibodies and their uses

Monoclonal antibody	Target	Uses
Abciximab (p. 462)	Platelet glycoprotein IIb/IIIa	Prevention of ischemic cardiac complications during percutaneous coronary interventions; short-term prevention of myocardial infarction
Adalimumab	Tumor necrosis factor alfa	Crohn's disease; psoriasis; rheumatoid arthritis, ankylosing spondylitis
Alemtuzumab (p. 465)	Lymphocyte CD52 receptors	Chronic lymphocytic leukemia
Apolizumab	Lymphocyte HLA-DR	Chronic lymphocytic leukemia
Basiliximab (p. 467)	CD25 antigen of interleukin receptors on T lymphocytes	Prevention of acute renal allograft rejection
Bevacizumab	Vascular endothelial growth factor	Metastatic breast and colrectal cancer; age-related macular degeneration
Clenoliximab	CD4 cell surface glycoprotein on T lymphocytes	Rheumatoid arthritis
Daclizumab (p. 468)	CD25 antigen of interleukin receptors on T lymphocytes	Prevention of acute renal allograft rejection
Edrecolomab (p. 468)	Human tumor-associated antigen Ep-CAM (17-1A)	Adjuvant therapy for cancer after colorectal surgery
Efalizumab	CD11a component of integrin (lymphocyte function-associated antigen-1)	Severe plaque psoriasis
Enlimomab	Human intercellular adhesion molecule 1 (ICAM-1)	Burns; prevention of acute rejection and delayed onset of graft function in cadaveric renal transplantation
Epratuzumab	CD22 cell surface glycoprotein on B lymphocytes	Non-Hodgkin's lymphoma
Gemtuzumab (p. 469)	CD33 receptors on myeloid cells	CD33-positive acute myelogenous leukemia
Infliximab (p. 470)	Tumor necrosis factor alfa	Crohn's disease; rheumatoid arthritis, ankylosing spondylitis
Inolimomab	Interleukin-2 (IL-2) receptors	Prevention of graft rejection
Keliximab	CD4 cell surface glycoprotein on T lymphocytes	Rheumatoid arthritis
Muromonab (p. 477)	Immunoglobuilin G2a	Prevention of acute renal allograft rejection
Natalizumab	Intercellular adhesion molecule α4-integrin	Acute relapse in multiple sclerosis; Crohn's disease
Odulimomab	Integrin (lymphocyte function-associated antigen-1)	Prevention of ischemic renal damage during kidney transplantation
Omalizumab (p. 482)	Immunoglobulin E	Prevention of allergic asthma and seasonal rhinitis
Palivizumab (p. 482)	Respiratory syncytial virus	Prevention of respiratory syncytial virus infection
Ranibizumab	Vascular endothelial growth factor	Age-related macular degeneration
Rituximab (p. 483)	CD20 receptors on tumor cells	Chemotherapy-resistant advanced follicular lymphoma; diffuse non-Hodgkin's lymphoma
Trastuzumab (p. 487)	Human epidermal growth factor receptor II (HER2)	HER2 receptor-positive breast cancer
Visilizumab	CD3 receptors on T lymphocytes	Glucocorticoid-refractory acute graft-versus-host disease

eruptions and transient increases in hepatic enzymes, with one reversible case of liver failure, have been attributed to B-F5, a murine IgG1 CD4 monoclonal antibody (10).

Various monoclonal antibodies have been developed to be used as carrier molecules or as immunoconjugates to target drugs, enzymes, isotopes, or toxins to tumor cells. Some of the available data have been summarized (11), but there is still insufficient evidence of clinical benefit.

Rodent monoclonal antibodies

Compared with the therapeutic use of human monoclonal antibodies, the use of rodent (mouse or rat) monoclonal antibodies in vivo is disadvantageous because the xenogeneic antibody can induce immune responses that will mitigate the effectiveness of the antibody and/or cause adverse reactions in the recipient. Thus, the authors of

one report concluded that antimouse immunoglobulin responses in human patients have limited the usefulness of murine monoclonal antibodies in more than half of those treated (12). The formation of human antimouse antibodies has been described both when murine monoclonal antibodies are used as a diagnostic tool in vivo and when they are used therapeutically (13–16).

Common adverse effects of treatment with murine monoclonal antibodies include fever, chills, and malaise in 21–23% of cases and urticaria and pruritus in 15–18% (17).

The murine monoclonal antibody muromonab directed against the CD3 structure on T lymphocytes has proved to be an important therapeutic agent with potent immunosuppressive actions, and its extensive use provides examples of the adverse effects of rodent monoclonal antibodies. It is used to reverse acute rejection episodes in kidney, heart, liver, or pancreas allografts and for graft-versus-host disease in bone marrow transplant recipients, when glucocorticoids have failed, or to avoid ciclosporin nephrotoxicity and the inconvenience of polyclonal antilymphocyte globulins (18). Despite its efficacy in over 90% of cases, muromonab causes a number of adverse effects, such as fluid retention and acute pulmonary edema (19), while marked early adverse effects include fever, chills, nausea, vomiting, headache, and hypotension, the last being attributed to systemic vasodilatation.

Other rodent monoclonal antibodies against cell membrane markers (CD molecules) have been described. The adverse effects of such antibodies can be ascribed to the general adverse effects of a heterologous protein, or to effects of the cell-targeting mechanisms (for example cell lysis).

General adverse effects

Although the adverse effects of most monoclonal antibodies were very few or benign, the possibility of more severe or unusual late complications should be considered, as illustrated by several case reports. In one patient, both immediate and delayed injection site reactions were noted after injections of a type I recombinant human interleukin-1 receptor (rhu IL-1RI), and positive cutaneous tests and specific IgE antibodies strongly suggested an immune-mediated allergic reaction (20).

Severe migratory polyarthritis with fever, an urticarial rash, and renal involvement have been reported after the first dose of CAMPATH-1G, a rat antihuman monoclonal antibody reactive against CDw52 antigens, used before marrow transplantation in a 25-year-old patient (21). In patients with renal transplants or rheumatoid arthritis, alemtuzumab, a humanized monoclonal antibody directed against the CDw52 antigen found on lymphocytes, produced only mild to moderate first-dose symptoms, such as fever and rigors, nausea and vomiting, bone pain, dyspnea, and headache (SED-13, 1134) (SEDA-20, 380). By contrast, there was a high incidence of severe lymphopenia associated with infectious complications during the intravenous administration for low-grade lymphoma (22). Finally, several patients with rheumatoid arthritis treated with infliximab (a chimeric monoclonal anti-TNF-alfa antibody) or CDP-571 (a human anti-TNF-alfa antibody) developed various autoantibodies (23). Although there were no clinical consequences in these patients, the possible delayed development of overt autoimmune diseases should still be considered.

The mechanisms of adverse effects of monoclonal antibodies include sensitization due to the xenogeneic nature of the product, specific suppression of physiological functions, and secondary activation of inflammatory cells or mediators, which might be characterized by the cytokine release syndrome, as observed with muromonab-CD3 or rituximab (24). Although sensitization may be frequent, its clinical relevance is still limited, with only rare cases of allergic reactions. Although this has been strongly debated with muromonab-CD3 (orthoclone) (SED-14, 1309), the available information on the risk of infections or cancers with other monoclonal antibodies is still limited, but does not suggest an increased risk.

References

1. Cosimi AB. Future of monoclonal antibodies in solid organ transplantation. Dig Dis Sci 1995;40(1):65–72.
2. Delmonico FL, Cosimi AB. Anti-CD4 monoclonal antibody therapy. Clin Transplant 1996;10(5):397–403.
3. Ziegler EJ, Fisher CJ Jr, Sprung CL, Straube RC, Sadoff JC, Foulke GE, Wortel CH, Fink MP, Dellinger RP, Teng NN, et alThe HA-1A Sepsis Study Group. Treatment of gram-negative bacteremia and septic shock with HA-1A human monoclonal antibody against endotoxin. A randomized, double-blind, placebo-controlled trial. N Engl J Med 1991;324(7):429–36.
4. Fisher CJ Jr, Zimmerman J, Khazaeli MB, Albertson TE, Dellinger RP, Panacek EA, Foulke GE, Dating C, Smith CR, LoBuglio AF. Initial evaluation of human monoclonal anti-lipid A antibody (HA-1A) in patients with sepsis syndrome. Crit Care Med 1990;18(12):1311–5.
5. Kappos L, Polman C, Pozzilli C, et alEuropean Study Group on interferon beta-1b in secondary progressive MS. Placebo-controlled multicentre randomised trial of interferon beta-1b in treatment of secondary progressive multiple sclerosis. Lancet 1998;352(9139):1491–7.
6. Lightner DJ, Vessella RL, Chiou RK, Palme DF, Lange PH. Immunotherapy for renal cell carcinoma: recent results. World J Urol 1986;4:222.
7. Aronson J. That's show business. BMJ 1999;319(7215):972.
8. Delmonico FL, Cosimi AB, Covlin R, et al. Murine OKT4A immunosuppression in cadaver donor renal allograft recipients: a Cooperative Clinical Trials in Transplantation pilot study. Transplantation 1997;63(8):1087–95.
9. Perosa F, Scudeletti M, Imro MA, Dammacco F, Luccarelli G, Indiveri F. Anti-CD4 monoclonal antibody (mAb) and anti-idiotypic mAb to anti-CD4 in the therapy of autoimmune diseases. Clin Exp Rheumatol 1997;15(2):201–10.
10. Dantal J, Ninin E, Hourmant M, Boeffard F, Cantarovich D, Giral M, Wijdenes J, Soulillou JP, Le Mauff B. Anti-CD4 MoAb therapy in kidney transplantation—a pilot study in early prophylaxis of rejection. Transplantation 1996;62(10):1502–6.
11. Panousis C, Pietersz GA. Monoclonal antibody-directed cytotoxic therapy: potential in malignant diseases of aging. Drugs Aging 1999;15(1):1–13.
12. Larrick JW, Bourla JM. Prospects for the therapeutic use of human monoclonal antibodies. J Biol Response Mod 1986;5(5):379–93.
13. Courtenay-Luck NS, Epenetos AA, Moore R, Larche M, Pectasides D, Dhokia B, Ritter MA. Development of primary and secondary immune responses to mouse monoclonal antibodies used in the diagnosis and therapy of malignant neoplasms. Cancer Res 1986;46(12 Pt 1):6489–93.
14. Reynolds JC, Vecchio SD, Sakara H, et al. Antimurine antibody response to mouse monoclonal antibodies: clinical findings and implications. Nucl Med Biol 1989;16:121.
15. Schroff RW, Foon KA, Beatty SM, Oldham RK, Morgan AC Jr. Human anti-murine immunoglobulin responses in patients receiving monoclonal antibody therapy. Cancer Res 1985;45(2):879–85.
16. Shawler DL, Bartholomew RM, Smith LM, Dillman RO. Human immune response to multiple injections of murine monoclonal IgG. J Immunol 1985;135(2):1530–5.

17. Dillman RO, Beauregard JC, Halpern SE, Clutter M. Toxicities and side effects associated with intravenous infusions of murine monoclonal antibodies. J Biol Response Mod 1986;5(1):73–84.

18. Burke GW 3rd, Vercellotti GM, Simmons RL, Howe RB, Canafax DM, Najarian JS. Reversible pancytopenia following OKT3. Use in the context of multidrug immunosuppression for kidney allografting. Transplantation 1989;48(3):403–8.

19. Lee CW, Logan JL, Zukoski CF. Cardiovascular collapse following orthoclone OKT3 administration: a case report. Am J Kidney Dis 1991;17(1):73–5.

20. Grammer LC, Roberts M. Cutaneous allergy to recombinant human type I IL-1 receptor (rhu IL-1RI). J Allergy Clin Immunol 1997;99(5):714–5.

21. Varadi G, Or R, Rund D, Orbach H, Slavin S, Nagler A. Severe migratory polyarthritis following in vivo CAMPATH-1G. Bone Marrow Transplant 1995;16(6):843–5.

22. Tang SC, Hewitt K, Reis MD, Berinstein NL. Immunosuppressive toxicity of CAMPATH1H monoclonal antibody in the treatment of patients with recurrent low grade lymphoma. Leuk Lymphoma 1996;24(1–2):93–101.

23. Rankin ECC, Isenberg DA. Monoclonal antibody therapy in rheumatoid arthritis. An update on recent progress. Clin Immunother 1996;6:143–53.

24. Breedveld FC. Therapeutic monoclonal antibodies. Lancet 2000;355(9205):735–40.

Abciximab

General Information

Abciximab is a Fab fragment of the chimeric human-murine monoclonal antibody 7E3, which binds to the platelet glycoprotein IIb/IIIa receptor and inhibits platelet aggregation (1).

Abciximab is used for prevention of cardiac ischemic events in patients undergoing percutaneous coronary intervention and to prevent myocardial infarction in patients with unstable angina who do not respond to conventional treatment. It has also been used for thrombolysis in patients with peripheral arterial occlusive disease and arterial thrombosis (2).

Besides bleeding, other adverse reactions that have been associated with abciximab include back pain, hypotension, nausea, and chest pain (but with an incidence not significantly different from that observed with placebo).

Organs and Systems

Respiratory

Lung hemorrhage is a rare but potentially lethal complication of antithrombotic and antiplatelet therapy. The incidence of spontaneous pulmonary hemorrhage after the use of platelet glycoprotein IIb/IIIa inhibitors has been analysed from the medical records of 1020 consecutive patients who underwent coronary interventions (3). Diffuse pulmonary hemorrhage developed in seven patients, two of whom died and five of whom had activated clotting times greater than 250 seconds during the

procedure. Activated partial thromboplastin time measured at the time of lung hemorrhage was raised in all cases (mean 85, range 69–95 seconds). All had a history of congestive heart failure, and had raised pulmonary capillary wedge pressures and/or left ventricular end-diastolic pressures at the time of the procedure. Six patients also had evidence of baseline radiographic abnormalities.

Nervous system

Seven patients undergoing neurointerventional procedures who received abciximab developed fatal intracerebral hemorrhages (4). The procedures included angioplasty and stent placement in the cervical internal carotid artery ($n = 4$), angioplasty of the intracranial carotid artery ($n = 1$), and angioplasty of the middle cerebral artery ($n = 2$). Aggressive antithrombotic treatment is used as adjuvant to angioplasty and/or stent placement to reduce the rate of ischemic and thrombotic complications associated with these procedures. Intravenous abciximab has a short life (10 minutes), but its inhibitory effect on platelets lasts for 48 hours. The exact cause of abciximab-associated intracerebral hemorrhage is unclear.

Hematologic

Bleeding

The primary risk associated with abciximab is bleeding. In the EPIC trial in high-risk angioplasty, 14% of patients who received a bolus of abciximab followed by an infusion had a major bleeding complication rate, versus 7% in the placebo group (5). The most marked excess of major bleeding episodes occurred at the site of vascular puncture, but there were also a substantial number of gastrointestinal haemorrhages. However, the therapeutic regimen used was not adjusted for body weight, and the risk of major bleeding was also related to the heparin dose per kg and not only to the use of abciximab (6).

In 7800 patients with chest pain and either ST segment depression or a positive troponin test, the addition of abciximab to unfractionated heparin or low molecular weight heparin in the treatment of acute coronary syndrome was not associated with any significant reduction in cardiac events, but a doubled risk of bleeding (7).

An analysis of data from the EPIC trial identified a series of factors that predicted vascular access site bleeding or the need for vascular access site surgery in abciximab-treated patients (8). They comprised larger vascular access sheath size, the presence of acute myocardial infarction at enrolment, female sex, higher baseline hematocrits, lower body weight, and a longer time spent in the catheterization laboratory.

It must be emphasized that patients in the EPIC trial received high-dose heparin and that vascular access site sheaths were left in place for 12–16 hours. In subsequent studies, the risk of vascular site bleeding was probably reduced by using lower doses of heparin and removing sheaths sooner. This was the case in the EPILOG trial in which heparin was withdrawn immediately after the coronary procedure and vascular sheaths were removed as soon as possible (9). The incidence of major bleeding in this study was not significantly higher with abciximab than with placebo. Nevertheless, the incidence of minor bleeding complications was significantly higher in the abciximab plus standard dose heparin group (but not in the abciximab plus low dose heparin group) compared with placebo. In the EPISTENT trial, all patients received low dose, body weight-adjusted heparin: Here the incidence of both major and minor bleeding complications was low and not significantly different between treatment groups (10).

It would therefore seem possible to reduce the incidence of bleeding complications when using abciximab during prophylactic coronary revascularization procedures. This is unfortunately not the case so far in the setting of primary angioplasty for myocardial infarction after intense anticoagulation (17% of major hemorrhagic complications versus 9.5 in placebo recipients) (11). The risk of serious bleeding complications is also increased in rescue situations when high doses of heparin have been used (12), but here it can be reduced by giving protamine to reverse heparin anticoagulation before abciximab therapy (13). There is also a high incidence of major bleeding in patients who receive abciximab during percutaneous coronary revascularization after unsuccessful thrombolytic therapy. It has been suggested that abciximab should not be administered within 18 hours after thrombolytic therapy (14).

It must be emphasized that very few episodes of abciximab-related bleeding are life-threatening and that in none of the trials with abciximab as well as with other glycoprotein IIb/IIIa antagonists has there been an excess of intracranial hemorrhage (15).

However, the bleeding risk in patients enrolled in trials may not be representative of the population actually being given abciximab. To clarify this, a review of adverse events in patients receiving glycoprotein IIb/IIIa inhibitors reported to the FDA has been undertaken (16,17). The FDA received 450 reports of deaths related to treatment with glycoprotein IIb/IIIa inhibitors between November 1, 1997 and December 31, 2000; these were reviewed and a standard rating system for assessing causation was applied to each event. Of the 450 deaths, 44% were considered to be definitely or probably attributable to glycoprotein IIb/IIIa inhibitors. The mean age of patients who died was 69 years and 47% of the deaths were in women. All of the deaths that were deemed to be definitely or probably associated with glycoprotein IIb/IIIa inhibitors were associated with excessive bleeding, most often in the nervous system.

Thrombocytopenia

The other significant risk associated with abciximab is thrombocytopenia. Data pooled from three major trials showed that thrombocytopenia (under $100 \times 10^9/l$) was significantly more frequent in those who received a bolus dose of abciximab followed by an infusion than in placebo recipients (3.7 versus 2%). Severe thrombocytopenia (under $50 \times 10^9/l$) was also more frequent with abciximab (1.1 versus 0.5%) (18). Very acute and profound thrombocytopenia (under $20 \times 10^9/l$) within 24 hours after administration has been observed in 0.3–0.7% of patients treated with abciximab for the first time (15,18–20).

During postmarketing surveillance of the first 4000 patients treated with abciximab in France, 25 cases of thrombocytopenia (0.6%) were reported, with five severe cases (0.15%) and three acute profound forms (0.08%). In all cases reported, the role of heparin must be taken into account. The thrombocytopenia associated with abciximab differs with that associated with heparin by its rapid onset (within 24 hours), its reversal after platelet transfusion, and its possible association with hemorrhage but not with thrombosis.

Positive human anti-chimeric antibodies have been detected in 6% of patients (generally in low titers) but were not associated with hypersensitivity or allergic reactions. Preliminary data indicate that abciximab can be safety readministered, although a greater incidence of thrombocytopenia after administration has been reported with a lesser efficacy of platelet transfusion (12).

Thrombocytopenia due to abciximab usually occurs within 12–96 hours, but there has been a report of acute profound thrombocytopenia after 7 days (21).

- A 65-year-old woman with type 2 diabetes mellitus and coronary artery disease received a 0.25 mg/kg bolus of abciximab at the time of intervention followed by an infusion of 10 micrograms/minute for 12 hours. Her baseline platelet counts were $286 \times 10^9/l$ before use, $385 \times 10^9/l$ at 2 hours, and $296 \times 10^9/l$ at 18 hours. On day 7 she developed petechiae over her legs and her platelet count was $1 \times 10^9/l$. Coagulation tests were normal and there was no evidence of heparin-induced thrombocytopenia. She received 10 units of single-donor platelets and recovered slowly over the next 4 days. The platelet count was $114 \times 10^9/l$ on day 12.

In another case of profound thrombocytopenia after abciximab there was a delayed onset (6 days after therapy) (22). The authors speculated that preceding treatment with methylprednisolone may have delayed the onset of thrombocytopenia. The mechanism of severe thrombocytopenia associated with abciximab is unclear. Further administration should be avoided, but other glycoprotein IIb/IIIa inhibitors (eptifibatide and tirofiban) have been successfully used in patients with history of abciximab-induced thrombocytopenia.

Thrombocytopenia after a second exposure to abciximab in nine patients showed that each had a strong immunoglobulin IgG antibody that recognized platelets sensitized with abciximab (23). Five patients also had IgM antibodies. Thrombocytopenia occurred four times as often as after the first exposure. The mechanism is not understood, but these findings suggest that it may be antibody-mediated. These antibodies were also found in 77 of 104 healthy patients, but in the patients the antibodies were specific for murine sequences in abciximab, causing the life-threatening thrombocytopenia.

Nine patients who developed profound thrombocytopenia after a second exposure to abciximab had an IgG antibody that recognized platelets sensitized with abciximab. In contrast, in 104 healthy subjects, in whom IgG antibodies reactive with abciximab-coated platelets were found in 77, the antibodies were specific for murine sequences in abciximab and were capable of causing life-threatening thrombocytopenia (23).

Ethylenediaminetetra-acetate can cause pseudothrombocytopenia by activating platelet agglutination, resulting in a spuriously low platelet count (SEDA-21, 250). Of 66 patients who received abciximab after coronary revascularization, 17 developed thrombocytopenia and 9 developed severe thrombocytopenia (24). However, of these 26 patients, 18 had pseudothrombocytopenia. True thrombocytopenia occurred at 4 hours after infusion whereas pseudothrombocytopenia occurred within the first 24 hours. The mechanism of pseudothrombocytopenia may be the effect of EDTA on the calcium-dependant glycoprotein IIb/IIIa complex, which frees the antigenic binding site on glycoprotein IIb available to IgM antibody. This increased antibody binding may cause platelet clumping and lead to false thrombocytopenia. True thrombocytopenia did not lead to hemorrhagic complications, but the patients required platelet transfusion.

Immunologic

Human antichimeric antibodies, specific to the murine epitope of Fab antibody fragments, have been observed in patients treated with abciximab. These antibodies are IgG antibodies and have so far not correlated with any adverse effects (12).

Because of its antigenic potential, there are theoretical concerns about the readministration of abciximab, and this has been studied in 1342 patients, who underwent percutaneous coronary interventions and received abciximab at least twice (25). There were no cases of anaphylaxis, and there were only five minor allergic reactions, none of which required termination of the infusion. There was clinically significant bleeding in 31 patients, including one with intracranial hemorrhage. There was thrombocytopenia (platelet count below 100×10^9/l) in 5% and profound thrombocytopenia (platelet count below 20×10^9/l) in 2%. In patients who received abciximab within 1 month of a previous treatment (n = 115), the risks of thrombocytopenia and profound thrombocytopenia were 17 and 12% respectively. Human chimeric antibody titers before readministration did not correlate with adverse outcomes or bleeding, but were associated with thrombocytopenia and profound thrombocytopenia.

An anaphylactic reaction to abciximab has been reported (26).

- An obese 46-year-old woman with prolonged angina pectoris underwent coronary angiography. She had no known drug allergies, but on administration of an iodinated contrast media she developed anaphylactic shock. After successful resuscitation angiography was completed and she was given aspirin, ticlopidine for a month, and metoprolol. Five months later she developed chest pain again, and angiography was repeated after pretreatment with prednisone and diphenhydramine and she was given abciximab. Within 5 minutes she had an anaphylactic reaction, requiring resuscitation.

This case shows that anaphylactic reactions to abciximab can occur even after pretreatment with prednisone and diphenhydramine for a known allergy to iodine.

Susceptibility Factors

Renal disease

The available data do not suggest an increased risk of bleeding with abciximab among patients with mild to moderate renal insufficiency (19), even though there is reduced platelet aggregation in renal insufficiency.

References

1. Ibbotson T, McGavin JK, Goa KL. Abciximab: an updated review of its therapeutic use in patients with ischaemic heart disease undergoing percutaneous coronary revascularisation. Drugs 2003;63(11):1121–63.
2. Schweizer J, Kirch W, Koch R, Muller A, Hellner G, Forkmann L. Use of abciximab and tirofiban in patients with peripheral arterial occlusive disease and arterial thrombosis. Angiology 2003;54(2):155–61.
3. Ali A, Hashem M, Rosman HS, Kazmouz G, Gardin JM, Schrieber TL. Use of platelet glycoprotein IIb/IIIa inhibitors and spontaneous pulmonary hemorrhage. J Invasive Cardiol 2003;15(4):186–8.
4. Qureshi AI, Saad M, Zaidat OO, Suarez JI, Alexander MJ, Fareed M, Suri K, Ali Z, Hopkins LN. Intracerebral hemorrhages associated with neurointerventional procedures using a combination of antithrombotic agents including abciximab. Stroke 2002;33(7):1916–9.
5. The EPIC Investigation. Use of a monoclonal antibody directed against the platelet glycoprotein IIb/IIIa receptor in high-risk coronary angioplasty. N Engl J Med 1994;330(14):956–61.
6. Aguirre FV, Topol EJ, Ferguson JJ, Anderson K, Blankenship JC, Heuser RR, Sigmon K, Taylor M, Gottlieb R, Hanovich G, et al. Bleeding complications with the chimeric antibody to platelet glycoprotein IIb/IIIa integrin in patients undergoing percutaneous coronary intervention. EPIC Investigators. Circulation 1995;91(12):2882–90.
7. James S, Armstrong P, Califf R, Husted S, Kontny F, Niemminen M, Pfisterer M, Simoons ML, Wallentin L. Safety and efficacy of abciximab combined with dalteparin in treatment of acute coronary syndromes. Eur Heart J 2002;23(19):1538–45.
8. Blankenship JC, Hellkamp AS, Aguirre FV, Demko SL, Topol EJ, Califf RM. Vascular access site complications after percutaneous coronary intervention with abciximab in the Evaluation of c7E3 for the Prevention of Ischemic Complications (EPIC) trial. Am J Cardiol 1998;81(1):36–40.
9. The EPILOG Investigators. Platelet glycoprotein IIb/IIIa receptor blockade and low-dose heparin during percutaneous coronary revascularization. N Engl J Med 1997;336(24):1689–96.
10. The EPISTENT Investigators. Evaluation of Platelet IIb/IIIa Inhibitor for Stenting. Randomised placebo-controlled and balloon-angioplasty-controlled trial to assess safety of coronary stenting with use of platelet glycoprotein-IIb/IIIa blockade. Lancet 1998;352(9122):87–92.
11. Brener SJ, Barr LA, Burchenal JE, Katz S, George BS, Jones AA, Cohen ED, Gainey PC, White HJ, Cheek HB,

Moses JW, Moliterno DJ, Effron MB, Topol EJ. Randomized, placebo-controlled trial of platelet glycoprotein IIb/IIIa blockade with primary angioplasty for acute myocardial infarction. ReoPro and Primary PTCA Organization and Randomized Trial (RAPPORT) Investigators. Circulation 1998;98(8):734–41.

12. Ferguson JJ, Kereiakes DJ, Adgey AA, Fox KA, Hillegass WB Jr, Pfisterer M, Vassanelli C. Safe use of platelet GP IIb/IIIa inhibitors. Am Heart J 1998;135(4):S77–89.

13. Kereiakes DJ, Broderick TM, Whang DD, Anderson L, Fye D. Partial reversal of heparin anticoagulation by intravenous protamine in abciximab-treated patients undergoing percutaneous intervention. Am J Cardiol 1997;80(5):633–4.

14. Kleiman NS. A risk-benefit assessment of abciximab in angioplasty. Drug Saf 1999;20(1):43–57.

15. Pinton P. Thrombopénies sous abciximab dans le traitement des syndromes coronariens aigus par angioplastie. [Abciximab-induced thrombopenia during treatment of acute coronary syndromes by angioplasty.] Ann Cardiol Angeiol (Paris) 1998;47(5):351–8.

16. Brown DL. Deaths associated with platelet glycoprotein IIb/IIIa inhibitor treatment. Heart 2003;89(5):535–7.

17. McLenachan JM. Who would I not give IIb/IIIa inhibitors to during percutaneous coronary intervention? Heart 2003;89(5):477–8.

18. Berkowitz SD, Harrington RA, Rund MM, Tcheng JE. Acute profound thrombocytopenia after C7E3 Fab (abciximab) therapy. Circulation 1997;95(4):809–13.

19. Foster RH, Wiseman LR. Abciximab. An updated review of its use in ischaemic heart disease. Drugs 1998;56(4):629–65.

20. Joseph T, Marco J, Gregorini L. Acute profound thrombocytopenia after abciximab therapy during coronary angioplasty. Clin Cardiol 1998;21(11):851–2.

21. Sharma S, Bhambi B, Nyitray W, Sharma G, Shambaugh S, Antonescu A, Shukla P, Denny E. Delayed profound thrombocytopenia presenting 7 days after use of abciximab (ReoPro). J Cardiovasc Pharmacol Ther 2002;7(1):21–4.

22. Schwarz S, Schwab S, Steiner HH, Hacke W. Secondary hemorrhage after intraventricular fibrinolysis: a cautionary note: a report of two cases. Neurosurgery 1998;42(3):659–63.

23. Curtis BR, Swyers J, Divgi A, McFarland JG, Aster RH. Thrombocytopenia after second exposure to abciximab is caused by antibodies that recognize abciximab-coated platelets. Blood 2002;99(6):2054–9.

24. Schell DA, Ganti AK, Levitt R, Potti A. Thrombocytopenia associated with c7E3 Fab (abciximab). Ann Hematol 2002;81(2):76–9.

25. Dery JP, Braden GA, Lincoff AM, Kereiakes DJ, Browne K, Little T, George BS, Sane DC, Cines DB, Effron MB, Mascelli MA, Langrall MA, Damaraju L, Barnathan ES, Tcheng JEReoPro Readministration Registry Investigators. Final results of the ReoPro readministration registry. Am J Cardiol 2004;93(8):979–84.

26. Pharand C, Palisaitis DA, Hamel D. Potential anaphylactic shock with abciximab readministration. Pharmacotherapy 2002;22(3):380–3.

Alemtuzumab

General Information

Alemtuzumab (campath-1H) is a humanized monoclonal antibody specific for the CDw52 antigen, present on cell membranes of lymphocytes and monocytes. It has been used for treatment of patients with rheumatoid arthritis and vasculitis, is being investigated for the treatment of chronic lymphocytic leukemia, and has been used to deplete circulating lymphocytes in patients with multiple sclerosis (1). In 2001, alemtuzumab was approved in Europe for the treatment of chronic B cell lymphocytic leukemia that had been treated previously with alkylating agents and was refractory to fludarabine (2). It has also been used for induction of immunosuppression/tolerance in liver transplant recipients (3,4) and kidney/pancreas transplant recipients (5).

The major adverse effects (fever, nausea, skin rash, and hypotension) may well be related to the release of cytokines as a consequence of lysis of the target lymphocytes (6). Of four patients treated with alemtuzumab, three developed antibodies against it, but without affecting the plasma concentrations and without obvious clinical consequences. Other adverse effects have included mild renal impairment and transient thrombocytopenia.

Organs and Systems

Respiratory

Of 22 patients, median age 61 years, who had received a median of three previous types of therapy for mycosis fungoides or Sézary syndrome and were given alemtuzumab in increasing doses (from 3 to 30 mg three times a week for 12 weeks), 11 had no infectious complications, one had fatal pulmonary aspergillosis 2.5 months after the end of treatment, and another contracted fatal *Mycobacterium* pneumonia 10 months after the end of treatment (7).

Endocrine

Nine of 27 patients with multiple sclerosis developed antibodies against the thyrotropin receptor and carbimazole-responsive autoimmune hyperthyroidism after a 5-day pulse of alemtuzumab, a finding that was not reported in patients treated for other disorders (1).

Hematologic

In 50 patients with advanced, low-grade, non-Hodgkin's lymphoma alemtuzumab produced marked lymphopenia and neutropenia, which were the probable cause of frequent severe infections (8). Seven patients developed opportunistic infections and nine had bacterial septicemia; three patients died from infectious complications. Severe resistant autoimmune thrombocytopenia has also been noted in one patient, but the evidence that alemtuzumab was involved was limited (9).

Immunologic

Reactivation of cytomegalovirus is a frequent complication during treatment with alemtuzumab in patients with chronic lymphocytic leukemia (10), and other organisms are occasionally described.

- A 52-year-old man with B cell chronic lymphocytic leukemia had weight loss and a steadily rising blood lymphocyte count (11). He received alemtuzumab as first-line treatment as part of a clinical trial. After 12 weeks the leukemia completely remitted. Three years later he received chlorambucil for progressive disease and had a partial remission. After another 2 years his chemotherapy regimen was change to fludarabine and cyclophosphamide. After a further year his disease became rapidly progressive, with anemia, splenomegaly, and lymphadenopathy. Alemtuzumab was reintroduced and standard prophylaxis treatment was started with co-trimoxazole, valaciclovir, and fluconazole. After 8 weeks he developed fever up to 39 °C. There was no evidence of bacterial or viral infection. His general condition worsened rapidly and he showed signs of acute hepatitis, renal insufficiency, disseminated intravascular coagulation, and finally respiratory failure. He died 14 days after the start of the fever. Adenovirus 5 was recovered from the lung, spleen, liver, and blood.

Among 18 patients with chronic lymphocytic leukemia, one with a long-lasting lymphocytopenia died 3 months after treatment, owing to progressive multifocal leukoencephalopathy; papovavirus was isolated from the cerebrospinal fluid (12).

References

1. Coles AJ, Wing M, Smith S, Coraddu F, Greer S, Taylor C, Weetman A, Hale G, Chatterjee VK, Waldmann H, Compston A. Pulsed monoclonal antibody treatment and autoimmune thyroid disease in multiple sclerosis. Lancet 1999;354(9191):1691–5.
2. Robak T. Alemtuzumab in the treatment of chronic lymphocytic leukemia. BioDrugs 2005;19(1):9–22.
3. Calne RY. Prope tolerance with alemtuzumab. Liver Transpl 2005;11(3):361–3.
4. Marcos A, Eghtesad B, Fung JJ, Fontes P, Patel K, Devera M, Marsh W, Gayowski T, Demetris AJ, Gray EA, Flynn B, Zeevi A, Murase N, Starzl TE. Use of alemtuzumab and tacrolimus monotherapy for cadaveric liver transplantation: with particular reference to hepatitis C virus. Transplantation 2004;78(7):966–71.
5. Keven K, Basu A, Tan HP, Thai N, Khan A, Marcos A, Starzl TE, Shapiro R. Cytomegalovirus prophylaxis using oral ganciclovir or valganciclovir in kidney and pancreas-kidney transplantation under antibody preconditioning. Transplant Proc 2004;36(10):3107–12.
6. Watts RA, Isaacs JD, Hale G, Hazleman BL, Waldmann H. CAMPATH-1H in inflammatory arthritis. Clin Exp Rheumatol 1993;11(Suppl 8):S165–7.
7. Lundin J, Hagberg H, Repp R, Cavallin-Stahl E, Freden S, Juliusson G, Rosenblad E, Tjonnfjord G, Wiklund T, Osterborg A. Phase 2 study of alemtuzumab (anti-CD52 monoclonal antibody) in patients with advanced mycosis fungoides/Sezary syndrome. Blood 2003;101(11):4267–72.
8. Lundin J, Osterborg A, Brittinger G, Crowther D, Dombret H, Engert A, Epenetos A, Gisselbrecht C, Huhn D, Jaeger U, Thomas J, Marcus R, Nissen N, Poynton C, Rankin E, Stahel R, Uppenkamp M, Willemze R, Mellstedt H. CAMPATH-1H monoclonal antibody in therapy for previously treated low-grade non-Hodgkin's lymphomas: a phase II multicenter study. European Study Group of CAMPATH-1H Treatment in Low-Grade Non-Hodgkin's Lymphoma. J Clin Oncol 1998;16(10):3257–63.
9. Otton SH, Turner DL, Frewin R, Davies SV, Johnson SA. Autoimmune thrombocytopenia after treatment with Campath 1H in a patient with chronic lymphocytic leukaemia. Br J Haematol 1999;106(1):261–2.
10. Laurenti L, Piccioni P, Cattani P, Cingolani A, Efremov D, Chiusolo P, Tarnani M, Fadda G, Sica S, Leone G. Cytomegalovirus reactivation during alemtuzumab therapy for chronic lymphocytic leukemia: incidence and treatment with oral ganciclovir. Haematologica 2004;89(10):1248–52.
11. Cavalli-Bjorkman N, Osby E, Lundin J, Kalin M, Osterborg A, Gruber A. Fatal adenovirus infection during alemtuzumab (anti-CD52 monoclonal antibody) treatment of a patient with fludarabine-refractory B cell chronic lymphocytic leukemia. Med Oncol 2002;19(4):277–80.
12. Uppenkamp M, Engert A, Diehl V, Bunjes D, Huhn D, Brittinger G. Monoclonal antibody therapy with CAMPATH-1H in patients with relapsed high- and low-grade non-Hodgkin's lymphomas: a multicenter phase I/II study. Ann Hematol 2002;81(1):26–32.

Anti-CD4 monoclonal antibodies

General Information

Anti-CD4 monoclonal antibodies are used to treat various autoimmune diseases, such as rheumatoid arthritis, asthma, and psoriasis (1–3). Keliximab (IDEC CE9.1) is a human-cynomolgus monkey chimeric (primatized) antibody with specificity for human and chimpanzee CD4. Clenoliximab is an immunoglobulin G4 derivative of keliximab. These antibodies induce a more than 80% down-regulation of CD4 molecules on the surface of T lymphocytes.

Observational studies

In an open, dose-escalating study, 24 patients were allocated to five consecutive daily doses of a humanized IgG1 anti-CD4 monoclonal antibody (4162W94) (4). There was at least one predefined infusion-related adverse effect (for example fever, chills/rigors, headache, nausea, vomiting, diarrhea, dyspnea, or hypotension) in 17 patients. Most of these events were mild or moderate in intensity, occurred on the first day of dosing, and resolved within 8 hours. In some patients the adverse events were associated with the appearance of TNF alfa in the plasma during the 3 hours after the start of antibody infusion, suggesting that they resulted from cytokine release. There was systolic hypotension, defined as a systolic pressure below 90 mmHg and a fall of at least 20 mmHg, in one patient who was given 10 mg. There were non-specific skin rashes in one patient in each of the groups who were given 10, 30, and 100 mg and in three of those given 300 mg. There were three serious adverse events: fatal rupture of an aortic aneurysm, thought to be unrelated to the drug, an episode of severe reversible airways obstruction in a patient with asthma, and an episode of unexplained collapse, presumed to be vasovagal, followed by full recovery several hours after the end of the first infusion. No opportunistic or other infections were reported.

Placebo-controlled studies

In a placebo-controlled study in 48 patients with active rheumatoid arthritis, CD4 blockade produced clinical benefit (5). Adverse events were reported in 97% of the patients, compared with 73% of those given placebo. In both groups most of the events were mild to moderate. Serious adverse events were reported in five patients who received anti-CD4; syncope/vasovagal attacks ($n = 3$), back pain ($n = 1$), abdominal pain/rectal bleeding ($n = 1$). Skin rashes occurred in 62% of the patients who received the antibody. In five cases a skin biopsy was performed, and showed a cellular infiltration centered on the blood vessels, suggesting a drug-induced vasculitis.

In a randomized, dose-ranging, placebo-controlled study of keliximab in chronic severe asthma, there were no serious adverse effects related to treatment (1).

References

1. Kon OM, Sihra BS, Loh LC, Barkans J, Compton CH, Barnes NC, Larche M, Kay AB. The effects of an anti-CD4 monoclonal antibody, keliximab, on peripheral blood CD4+ T cells in asthma. Eur Respir J 2001;18(1):45–52.
2. Hepburn TW, Totoritis MC, Davis CB. Antibody-mediated stripping of CD4 from lymphocyte cell surface in patients with rheumatoid arthritis. Rheumatology (Oxford) 2003;42(1):54–61.
3. Skov L, Kragballe K, Zachariae C, Obitz ER, Holm EA, Jemec GB, Solvsten H, Ibsen HH, Knudsen L, Jensen P, Petersen JH, Menne T, Baadsgaard O. HuMax-CD4: a fully human monoclonal anti-CD4 antibody for the treatment of psoriasis vulgaris. Arch Dermatol 2003;139(11):1433–9.
4. Choy EH, Connolly DJ, Rapson N, Jeal S, Brown JC, Kingsley GH, Panayi GS, Johnston JM. Pharmacokinetic, pharmacodynamic and clinical effects of a humanized IgG1 anti-CD4 monoclonal antibody in the peripheral blood and synovial fluid of rheumatoid arthritis patients. Rheumatology (Oxford) 2000;39(10):1139–46.
5. Choy EH, Panayi GS, Emery P, Madden S, Breedveld FC, Kraan MC, Kalden JR, Rascu A, Brown JC, Rapson N, Johnston JM. Repeat-cycle study of high-dose intravenous 4162W94 anti-CD4 humanized monoclonal antibody in rheumatoid arthritis. A randomized placebo-controlled trial. Rheumatology (Oxford) 2002;41(10):1142–8.

Basiliximab

General Information

Basiliximab is a chimeric (human/mouse) anti-interleukin-2 receptor monoclonal antibody used in the prophylaxis of acute renal transplant rejection. It acts by binding the alpha chain of interleukin-2 receptors on activated T lymphocytes. Initially positive results in phase III trials have not been generally confirmed (1,2).

Compared with placebo, basiliximab was not associated with any specific adverse effects in early studies (3). However, severe hypersensitivity reactions can occur and can be associated with the cytokine release syndrome.

Organs and Systems

Respiratory

There have been reports of non-cardiogenic pulmonary edema in three adolescent renal transplant recipients, one of whom died (4).

Immunologic

Basiliximab is composed of murine sequences (30%), which can cause IgE-mediated hypersensitivity reactions. Important warnings have been released by the manufacturers regarding the possible risk of severe hypersensitivity reactions within 24 hours of initial exposure or after re-exposure after several months, based on 17 reports that included cardiac and/or respiratory failure, bronchospasm, urticaria, cytokine release syndrome, and capillary leak syndrome.

- A 42-year-old Hispanic woman, with end-stage renal disease, anemia, hypertension, and a history of an anaphylactic reaction to basiliximab, was scheduled to receive a living donor transplant and received basiliximab uneventfully (5). However, owing to donor infection the procedure was cancelled and rescheduled for 2 weeks later. Within 10 minutes after basiliximab reinduction she developed an anaphylactic reaction. In an attempt to find another induction therapy for this patient, skin testing was performed for daclizumab without response. She therefore received full-dose induction with daclizumab before her organ transplant without adverse effect.
- A child had anaphylactic shock when he received a second course of basiliximab at the time of a second renal transplantation (6). There were antibasiliximab IgE antibodies in the serum, but no IgE reactivity toward a control murine IgG_{2a} monoclonal antibody, suggesting that the IgE response was directed exclusively against basiliximab idiotypes. There was no IgE reactivity against the humanized anti-interleukin-2 receptor monoclonal antibody daclizumab. The patient's basophils harvested months after the anaphylactic shock produced leukotrienes in vitro on exposure to basiliximab.

Daclizumab, a humanized monoclonal antibody, is composed of only 10% murine antibody sequences and therefore is less immunogenic. These findings suggest that despite the similar compositions of human and mouse antibody protein sequences the IgE responsiveness is significantly different.

Drug–Drug Interactions

Ciclosporin

Basiliximab can inhibit ciclosporin metabolism transiently in children with renal transplants (7). Despite the use of lower daily doses, ciclosporin trough concentrations were significantly higher during the first 10 days after transplantation in 24 children who received basiliximab at days 0 and 4 after transplantation compared with 15 children who did not receive basiliximab. Ciclosporin dosage requirements again increased by 20% to achieve the target blood concentration at days 28–50 after transplantation. It is noteworthy that all seven acute episodes of rejection in the basiliximab group occurred during this period of time. However, these results have been debated, and there were no changes in ciclosporin dosage requirements in 54 children with liver transplants (8).

References

1. Crompton JA, Somerville T, Smith L, Corbett J, Nelson E, Holman J, Shihab FS. Lack of economic benefit with basiliximab induction in living related donor adult renal transplant recipients. Pharmacotherapy 2003;23(4):443–50.
2. Webster AC, Playford EG, Higgins G, Chapman JR, Craig J. Interleukin 2 receptor antagonists for kidney transplant recipients. Cochrane Database Syst Rev 2004;(1):CD003897.
3. Nashan B, Moore R, Amlot P, Schmidt AG, Abeywickrama K, Soulillou JPCHIB 201 International Study Group. Randomised trial of basiliximab versus placebo for control of acute cellular rejection in renal allograft recipients. Lancet 1997;350(9086):1193–8.
4. Bamgbola FO, Del Rio M, Kaskel FJ, Flynn JT. Non-cardiogenic pulmonary edema during basiliximab induction in three adolescent renal transplant patients. Pediatr Transplant 2003;7(4):315–20.
5. Leonard PA, Woodside KJ, Gugliuzza KK, Sur S, Daller JA. Safe administration of a humanized murine antibody after anaphylaxis to a chimeric murine antibody. Transplantation 2002;74(12):1697–700.
6. Baudouin V, Crusiaux A, Haddad E, Schandene L, Goldman M, Loirat C, Abramowicz D. Anaphylactic shock caused by immunoglobulin E sensitization after retreatment with the chimeric anti-interleukin-2 receptor monoclonal antibody basiliximab. Transplantation 2003;76(3):459–63.
7. Strehlau J, Pape L, Offner G, Nashan B, Ehrich JH. Interleukin-2 receptor antibody-induced alterations of ciclosporin dose requirements in paediatric transplant recipients. Lancet 2000;356(9238):1327–8.
8. Ganschow R, Grabhorn E, Burdelski M. Basiliximab in paediatric liver-transplant recipients. Lancet 2001;357(9253):388.

Daclizumab

General Information

Daclizumab, a humanized antibody directed against the alfa chain of the interleukin-2 receptor, has been used for initial immunosuppression in transplant patients. In a phase III trial in 275 patients who received ciclosporin, glucocorticoids, and daclizumab or placebo, there were no specific adverse effects associated with daclizumab (1). In particular, the cytokine-release syndrome did not occur, and there was no difference in the incidence of fungal or cytomegalovirus infections between the two groups.

Organs and Systems

Immunologic

The efficacy of daclizumab in acute and chronic glucocorticoid-refractory graft-versus-host disease has been studied in 16 patients, of whom nine responded (2). However 14 developed infectious complications during treatment, with a high incidence of cytomegalovirus reactivation; there were three infection-related deaths.

References

1. Charpentier B, Thervet E. Placebo-controlled study of a humanized anti-TAC monoclonal antibody in dual therapy for prevention of acute rejection after renal transplantation. Transplant Proc 1998;30(4):1331–2.
2. Willenbacher W, Basara N, Blau IW, Fauser AA, Kiehl MG. Treatment of steroid refractory acute and chronic graft-versus-host disease with daclizumab. Br J Haematol 2001;112(3):820–3.

Edrecolomab

General Information

Edrecolomab (17-1A antibody), a mouse monoclonal antibody, has been used in the adjuvant treatment of colorectal cancer.

Organs and Systems

Immunologic

Severe exacerbation of Wegener's granulomatosis with multiorgan involvement has been reported after the first infusion of edrecolomab (500 mg over 2 hours) in a 64-year-old man (1).

Hypersensitivity and anaphylactic reactions have been noted, and urticaria prolonged over a 4-month period was reported in one patient (2).

References

1. Franz A, Bewersdorf H, Hartung G, Dencausse Y, Queisser W. Exacerbation of Wegener's granulomatosis following single administration of monoclonal antibody 17-1A (Panorex®) during adjuvant immunotherapy of colon cancer. Onkologie 2000;23(5):472–4.
2. Sizmann N, Korting HC. Prolonged urticaria with 17-1A antibody. BMJ 1998;317(7173):1631.

Gemtuzumab ozogamicin

General Information

Gemtuzumab ozogamicin (Mylotarg) consists of a humanized anti-CD33 monoclonal antibody conjugated to the cytotoxic enediyne antibiotic calicheamicin. It has been used to treat a subset of patients with acute myeloid leukemia in association with topotecan + cytarabine. Its most common adverse effects are myelosuppression, increased hepatic enzyme activity, infections, fever and chills, bleeding, nausea and vomiting, and dyspnea.

Infusion-related adverse effects of gemtuzumab ozogamicin can be treated with a brief course of an intravenous glucocorticoid. Of 143 patients with refractory myeloid leukemia treated with gemtuzumab ozogamicin, 110 received paracetamol 650 mg orally with diphenhydramine 50 mg intravenously and 33 received the same premeditations plus methylprednisolone sodium succinate 50 mg intravenously before the infusion and repeated 1 hour later (1). There were grade 2 or worse infusion-related adverse events in 32 (29%) of the former, but in only one of the latter (3%).

Organs and Systems

Liver

Hepatotoxicity, with raised bilirubin and liver enzymes, is common with gemtuzumab (30–50%) and is mostly reversible. A more severe complication, hepatic veno-occlusive disease, a syndrome consisting of hyperbilirubinemia, painful hepatomegaly, and fluid retention or ascites, is less common and is mostly seen in patients previously undergoing bone marrow transplantation (4–5%). It occurs most commonly after high-dose chemotherapy and hemopoietic stem cell transplantation. Patients with severe veno-occlusive disease die from progressive multi-organ failure. Close monitoring of patients receiving gemtuzumab is necessary, even if they have not had previous bone marrow transplantation (2).

In 119 patients (92 with acute myeloid leukemia, 25 with advanced myelodysplastic syndrome, and two with chronic myeloid leukemia), who did not receive concomitant stem cell transplantation, 14 developed veno-occlusive disease (3). Five of these 14 patients had not received prior antileukemic therapy, and in two cases gemtuzumab ozogamicin was used as single-agent chemotherapy.

Of eight patients who were given an infusion of gemtuzumab 9 months after hemopoietic stem cell transplantation, seven had normal serum bilirubin concentrations, and all eight had transaminase and alkaline phosphatase activities that were less than 1.5 times the upper limit of the reference range (4). Six had no evidence of hepatotoxicity. One developed abdominal pain, ascites, and mildly raised transaminases. A CT scan showed no evidence of hepatic disease. This patient did not meet the criteria of veno-occlusive disease. Patient 8 did meet the criteria of veno-occlusive disease 3 days after infusion

with gemtuzumab. She developed multi-organ failure and died.

Of 17 patients who were given gemtuzumab, three developed grade 3 hyperbilirubinemia, and five developed grade 3–4 hepatic transaminitis after a median of 13 days, including one who developed veno-occlusive disease (4). This patient had abrupt onset of weight gain, associated with ascites, abdominal distension, acute hepatic failure, and right upper quadrant pain, and died. As a possible mechanism gemtuzumab may selectively target CD33-expressing cells in hepatic sinusoids, activate stellated cells, damage sinusoidal endothelial cells, and cause sinusoidal vasoconstriction or ischemic hepatocyte necrosis. Liver histology showed sinusoidal injury with extensive sinusoidal fibrosis, centrilobular congestion, and hepatocyte necrosis (5).

Immunologic

There has been one report of an anaphylactic reaction in a patient receiving gemtuzumab (6).

References

1. Giles FJ, Cortes JE, Halliburton TA, Mallard SJ, Estey EH, Waddelow TA, Lim JT. Intravenous corticosteroids to reduce gemtuzumab ozogamicin infusion reactions. Ann Pharmacother 2003;37(9):1182–5.
2. Voutsadakis IA. Gemtuzumab Ozogamicin (CMA-676, Mylotarg) for the treatment of CD33+ acute myeloid leukemia. Anticancer Drugs 2002;13(7):685–92.
3. Giles FJ, Kantarjian HM, Kornblau SM, Thomas DA, Garcia-Manero G, Waddelow TA, David CL, Phan AT, Colburn DE, Rashid A, Estey EH. Mylotarg (gemtuzumab ozogamicin) therapy is associated with hepatic venoocclusive disease in patients who have not received stem cell transplantation. Cancer 2001;92(2):406–13.
4. Cohen AD, Luger SM, Sickles C, Mangan PA, Porter DL, Schuster SJ, Tsai DE, Nasta S, Gewirtz AM, Stadtmauer EA. Gemtuzumab ozogamicin (Mylotarg) monotherapy for relapsed AML after hematopoietic stem cell transplant: efficacy and incidence of hepatic veno-occlusive disease. Bone Marrow Transplant 2002;30(1):23–8.
5. Rajvanshi P, Shulman HM, Sievers EL, McDonald GB. Hepatic sinusoidal obstruction after gemtuzumab ozogamicin (Mylotarg) therapy. Blood 2002;99(7):2310–4.
6. Reinhardt D, Diekamp S, Fleischhack G, Corbacioglu C, Jurgens H, Dworzak M, Kaspers G, Creutzig U, Zwaan CM. Gemtuzumab ozogamicin (Mylotarg) in children with refractory or relapsed acute myeloid leukemia. Onkologie 2004;27(3):269–72.

Ibritumomab

General Information

Ibritumomab is a murine IgG$_1$ anti-CD20 antibody, the parent of the engineered chimeric antibody rituximab, a monoclonal antibody with mouse variable and human constant regions. It induces apoptosis and has antiproliferative effects. Ibritumomab tiuxetan (Zevalin) is composed of the monoclonal antibody ibritumomab, the linking chelator tiuxetan, and the radioisotope ^{90}yttrium (1).

General adverse effects

A wide range of adverse effects of ibritumomab has been reported. Most were hematological, thrombocytopenia being the most common, followed by a low hemoglobin and leukopenia. The most common non-hematological events were related to infusion and were similar to those reported with rituximab; they included weakness (54%), nausea (35%), chills (15%), and fever (21%) (2,3). Infectious complications during treatment with ibritumomab are rare, pneumonia being the most common. There is no obvious hepatotoxicity.

Organs and Systems

Immunologic

There has been one report of an anti-antibody response to ibritumomab (2).

Long-Term Effects

Tumorigenicity

Acute myelogenous leukemia has been attributed to ibritumomab (4).

- An 80-year-old woman with a small B cell extranodal lymphoma was initially given chlorambucil for 10 months, with complete remission for 2 years. When she developed recurrent lymph node swelling she was given ibritumomab tiuxetan, with near-complete remission. When she developed progressive disease 14 months later, she received cyclophosphamide, vincristine, and prednisone for one cycle. She had persistent pancytopenia, and a bone marrow biopsy showed extensive infiltration by acute myelogenous leukemia.

This seems to be the first case of drug-related acute myelogenous leukemia. Fluorescent in-situ hybridization studies on the bone marrow showed a signal consistent with rearrangement of the mixed myeloid leukemia (MLL) gene on chromosome 11. This abnormality was not present before treatment.

References

1. Krasner C, Joyce RM. Zevalin: ^{90}Yttrium labeled anti-CD20 (ibritumomab tiuxetan), a new treatment for non-Hodgkin's lymphoma. Curr Pharm Biotechnol 2001;2(4):341–9.
2. Witzig TE, White CA, Wiseman GA, Gordon LI, Emmanouilides C, Raubitschek A, Janakiraman N, Gutheil J, Schilder RJ, Spies S, Silverman DH, Parker E, Grillo-Lopez AJ. Phase I/II trial of IDEC-Y2B8 radioimmunotherapy for treatment of relapsed or refractory CD20(+) B cell non-Hodgkin's lymphoma. J Clin Oncol 1999;17(12):3793–803.
3. Witzig TE, Flinn IW, Gordon LI, Emmanouilides C, Czuczman MS, Saleh MN, Cripe L, Wiseman G, Olejnik T, Multani PS, White CA. Treatment with ibritumomab tiuxetan radioimmunotherapy in patients with rituximab-refractory follicular non-Hodgkin's lymphoma. J Clin Oncol 2002;20(15):3262–9.
4. Nabhan C, Peterson LA, Kent SA, Tallman MS, Dewald G, Multani P, Gordon LI. Secondary acute myelogenous leukemia with MLL gene rearrangement following radioimmunotherapy (RAIT) for non-Hodgkin's lymphoma. Leuk Lymphoma 2002;43(11):2145–9.

Infliximab

General Information

Infliximab, a monoclonal chimeric human/murine antibody directed against tumor necrosis alfa, has been used in the treatment of severe active Crohn's disease (1,2), rheumatoid arthritis (3), and ankylosing spondylitis (4). From the available data submitted for Crohn's disease to the US and European regulatory agencies, the most significant acute adverse reactions were infusion reactions, defined as symptoms within 2 hours after intravenous infusion. The symptoms consisted of fever, chills, urticaria, dyspnea, chest pain, or hypotension, and occurred in 16% of infliximab-treated patients versus 6–7% of placebo-treated patients. Several adverse effects, such as upper respiratory tract infections, headaches, rash, or cough, were more common than with placebo, but severe adverse effects were only slightly more frequent (3.6 versus 2.6%). Clinical trials also showed an increase in the prevalence of antinuclear antibodies or the development of double-stranded DNA antibodies (9% of patients). Although there were clinical features suggestive of the lupus-like syndrome in only very few patients, this issue needs to be further investigated. Also of great concern is the report in several patients of lymphoma (5) or severe opportunistic infections (6). Patients taking concomitant immunosuppressive drugs should be carefully observed for such complications.

Organs and Systems

Cardiovascular

The preliminary results of a phase II trial in patients with moderate to severe congestive heart failure showed a higher incidence of worsening congestive heart failure and death in patients treated with infliximab compared with placebo (7). This led to warnings from regulatory agencies and to the limited use of infliximab in patients with congestive heart failure.

Death due to worsening of cardiac insufficiency in patients with congestive heart failure has been reported (SEDA-26, 401).

Respiratory

Allergic granulomatosis of the lung has been described after a second infusion of infliximab in one of 35 patients with active ankylosing spondylitis (8). The clinical and radiological symptoms resolved 8 weeks after withdrawal, but no other details were given.

- A 32-year-old man with Crohn's disease developed an eosinophilic pleural effusion soon after a second infusion of infliximab (9). He recovered within 8 weeks, but the effusion recurred after infliximab re-treatment 1 year later.

Nervous system

Features of aseptic meningitis have been reported after multiple infliximab injections (10).

- A 53-year-old man with severe rheumatoid arthritis and mixed type III cryoglobulinemia received his first four injections of infliximab uneventfully, but 4 hours after the fifth injection had severe muscle pain in the lower limbs, which required morphine and abated within 3 days. Similar symptoms were observed after the sixth injection. There were no signs of meningitis, the cerebrospinal fluid contained lymphocytes and increased concentrations of protein and IgG. Cultures were negative and MRI scans of the brain and the spine were normal. The CSF was normal 1 month later.

The authors speculated that the most likely explanation for these observations was linked to the lack of transfer of high-molecular weight soluble receptors and IgG across the blood–brain barrier, implying that control of brain tumor necrosis factor alfa cannot be obtained with monoclonal antibodies. They thought that neurological complications in diseases other than multiple sclerosis might be related to control of tumor necrosis factor alfa in the periphery, resulting in an enhanced contribution of brain-derived tumor necrosis factor alfa or other cytokines, such as interleukin-1.

Neurological events suggestive of demyelinating disorders in patients treated with tumor necrosis factor alfa antagonists and reported to the FDA's Adverse Events Reporting System have been reviewed (11). These included 17 cases temporarily associated with etanercept and two with infliximab, but complete information was lacking in a number of cases. The various hypothetical mechanisms by which tumor necrosis factor alfa antagonists might produce demyelinating events have been discussed (12). Briefly, they cause an increase in peripheral T cell autoreactivity, and their inability to cross the blood–brain barrier may account for exacerbation of central demyelinating disorders.

Sensory systems

Optic neuropathy has been described in patients with rheumatoid arthritis taking infliximab. In three patients aged 54–62 years, blurred vision or visual field loss in one or both eyes occurred after the third dose (13). Ophthalmic examination showed anterior optic neuropathy in all three patients and MRI scanning ruled out demyelinating optic neuritis. In one patient an additional infusion of infliximab produced similar symptoms in the previously unaffected eye; vision failed to improve despite infliximab withdrawal and steroid treatment.

- Retrobulbar optic neuritis was diagnosed after the ninth dose of infliximab in a 55-year-old woman (14). MRI scanning showed demyelination of the left optic nerve and the visual field defect improved after treatment with prednisone.

Hematologic

The possible role of infliximab in the development of hypercoagulability disorders has been discussed in the context of a case of arterial thrombosis (15).

- A 72-year-old woman with refractory sarcoidosis developed venous thrombosis at a catheter site and extensive multiple thromboses in small arteries in her legs after receiving a third dose of infliximab for severe enteropathy. Anticardiolipin antibodies were detected, but antinuclear and anti-double-stranded DNA antibodies were negative.

Although infliximab has been associated with autoantibody production, it is not known whether it contributed to hypercoagulability in this patient.

Liver

Acute hepatitis with infliximab has been described (16).

- A 44-year-old woman, who had used oral contraceptives for many years and had taken mesalazine, mercaptopurine, and prednisone for Crohn's disease for 7 years, developed clinical and biological signs of acute mixed hepatitis 19 days after a single dose of infliximab 5 mg/kg. There were no symptoms suggestive of hypersensitivity and liver histology showed cholestasis without inflammation or eosinophilia. Other causes, such as a recent viral infection (hepatitis A, B, C, cytomegalovirus, *Herpes simplex*) or gallstones, were ruled out. Among various autoantibodies, only antinuclear antibody titers were slightly raised. Complete normalization was observed 2 months later.

Although the patient took other potentially hepatotoxic drugs, the time-course suggested that infliximab was the cause.

Skin

Skin reactions, including erythema multiforme in three patients and a lichenoid eruption in one, were attributed to infliximab (17). One patient had similar lesions after etanercept. Patch tests with infliximab in three patients were negative, but produced a flare-up of lesions in one patient and recurrence of malaise and nausea in another patient, suggesting that infliximab is well absorbed percutaneously.

- A 72-year-old man developed bullous skin lesions the day after receiving his fourth dose of infliximab for rheumatoid arthritis (18). Human antichimeric antibodies were positive, as were antinuclear antibodies, and he completely recovered after treatment with prednisone.

In three patients with severe Crohn's disease who required digestive surgery, infliximab before or immediately after surgery was discussed as an additional possible cause of postoperative poor wound healing with serious complications (19).

Patients with congestive heart failure has been reported (SEDA-26, 401).

Immunologic

Antibodies to infliximab

Treatment with infliximab can be associated with the formation of human antichimeric antibodies. Such antibodies were rarely detected in patients with rheumatoid arthritis who were also taking methotrexate, and low titers were detected in about 13% of patients with Crohn's disease. Their clinical relevance is unclear, although their presence has sometimes been associated with an increased risk of infusion reactions, the occurrence of serum sickness-like reactions after delayed retreatment, and a shorter duration of response.

In a randomized, placebo-controlled trial in 573 patients with Crohn's disease, who responded to an initial infusion of infliximab and were then given repeated infusions, antibodies to infliximab were found in 14%; there was a trend toward a lower incidence of antibodies in patients taking concurrent glucocorticoids and immunosuppressive drugs (20). The incidence of infusion reactions was also higher in patients positive for antibodies to infliximab compared with patients without antibodies (16 versus 8%) and lower in patients who were taking both glucocorticoids and immunosuppressants compared with patients who were receiving neither (8 versus 32%).

The clinical significance of antibodies to infliximab has also been explored in 125 patients with Crohn's disease who were given infliximab, of whom 61% had antibodies after the fifth infusion; however, there was no further increase in incidence after subsequent treatment (21). The presence of antibodies was associated with a 2.4-fold increase in the risk of infusion reactions, lower serum infliximab concentrations, and a shorter duration of clinical response, compared with patients with no infliximab antibodies. Patients who received concomitant immunosuppressive therapy had a lower incidence of infliximab antibodies, higher infliximab serum concentrations, and a longer duration of clinical response. Pretreatment with glucocorticoids may reduce the risk of antibody formation, but it is not known whether a pretreatment test for human antichimeric antibodies has a predictive value for adverse reactions (22). However, there were technical issues relating to the antibody assay and definition of clinically relevant antibody titers in this study.

Autoantibodies and autoimmunity

Infliximab may increase the risk of autoimmunity, but the presence of antibodies did not predict the risk of lupus-like syndrome. In trials, the incidence of infliximab-induced anti-double-stranded DNA antibodies ranged from 5 to 34% of patients, depending on the assay method used and the duration of exposure (20–24). However, these abnormalities were rarely associated with clinical manifestations. In two large randomized trials in more than 900 infliximab-treated patients, only three developed a lupus-like syndrome, with no evidence of systemic organ involvement (20–24). However, since then, several reports have detailed infliximab-induced, lupus-like syndrome in patients with Crohn's colitis or rheumatoid arthritis, with improvement on withdrawal of infliximab (25,26).

Of 40 patients who had received multiple doses of an investigational liquid formulation of infliximab 2–4 years before, 10 had a severe delayed hypersensitivity reaction within 3–12 days after the first or the second re-infusion (27). This reaction mostly included myalgia, rash, fever, polyarthralgia, and pruritus. Although the six patients tested were negative for antibodies to infliximab before re-infusion, these antibodies were consistently raised after the reaction.

Infliximab binds to tumor necrosis factor alfa on cell surfaces and produces apoptotic cell death, releasing the nucleosomal autoantigens that induce autoantibody formation (28).

- A 69-year-old woman with a 5-year history of rheumatoid arthritis developed drug-induced lupus after receiving infliximab for 23 weeks. She had initially been given methotrexate and prednisone for 4 years. Then, because of lack of efficacy, infliximab was introduced. After three infusions of infliximab and only partial remission the dose was increased to 5 mg/kg, with success. However, before the sixth infusion she developed fever, polyarthralgia, myalgia, and general malaise. Serology excluded viral infection. Autoantibody assessment was positive, confirming the diagnosis of drug-induced lupus.

Hypersensitivity reactions

Both acute and delayed hypersensitivity reactions to infliximab have been reported in clinical trials (SEDA-24, 439).

Immediate infusion reactions to infliximab are usually defined by any significant adverse effect that occurs during or within 1–2 hours after the infusion. The symptoms mostly consist of flushing, rash, shortness of breath, wheeze, hotness, chest pain, vomiting, and abdominal pain.

Delayed reactions are defined by the occurrence of arthralgia and joint stiffness (that is a serum sickness-like reaction) in the days after infliximab administration; they have mostly been observed in patients with Crohn's disease who have received episodic treatment. In one patient the complication was associated with acute respiratory distress syndrome, which only became evident 10 days after re-treatment (22).

Incidence

Immediate hypersensitivity reactions to infliximab occur in 6–19% of adults.

In a retrospective evaluation of 165 patients (479 infliximab infusions) with Crohn's disease, the overall incidence of infusion reactions was 6.1% (29 episodes) (29).

Acute infusion reactions within 24 hours of infusion were the most frequent (26 episodes) and delayed infusion reactions from 1 to 14 days after treatment were noted in three instances only. Prophylaxis with diphenhydramine and paracetamol and the use of a test dose of infliximab allowed additional infusions without consequences in patients with mild or moderate previous acute infusion reactions. Three of the four patients who had acute severe reactions received the same prophylaxis plus corticosteroids before re-treatment: one had a similar severe acute reaction, while the other two had no recurrences. This study also suggested that acute infusion reactions are probably not IgE-mediated, as tryptase and IgE serum concentrations were not raised.

Of 86 patients with Crohn's disease receiving infliximab 14% of patients experienced severe systemic reactions, with a significant difference between adults (21%) and children (3%), the reason for which was unclear (30).

There were severe infusion reactions, defined by any significant change in vital signs or the development of chest pain, wheeze, dyspnea, vomiting, abdominal pain, or rash, in 16 of 100 patients with refractory Crohn's disease (31). Half of them occurred during the first infusion, and the rate of infusion reactions was similar in patients taking concurrent immunosuppressants or glucocorticoids compared with those who were not. One patient had anaphylactic shock, five had significant hypotension, six had acute pulmonary symptoms, two had pruritus, flushing, or rash, and one had vomiting. The final patient, who had a previous history of chronic pancreatitis, had acute pancreatitis within 1 hour of treatment.

Immediate hypersensitivity reactions

Acute hypersensitivity reactions can mimic an anaphylactic reaction, but specific IgE antibodies have not so far been identified. A dose-escalation protocol has been proposed to desensitize patients who have had acute systemic reactions (32), but this has not always been successful (33). Although most reported anaphylactic reactions to infliximab have been mild, severe reactions can occur.

- A 36-year-old man with Crohn's disease became refractory to standard anti-inflammatory treatment (glucocorticoids, mercaptopurine, methotrexate, ciclosporin, tacrolimus) (33). Remission over 8 months was achieved with a single infusion of infliximab. With the onset of relapse he was given another infusion of infliximab and had an anaphylactic-like reaction within 1 minute.
- A 35-year-old woman with known hypersensitivity to mesalazine had severe symptoms, namely chest pain, dyspnea, productive cough, skin rash, and hypotension, during a third infusion of infliximab, and died 6 hours later from refractory hypotension and respiratory failure (34). Specific IgE or human antichimeric antibodies were not checked.
- A 33-year-old man with a 3-year history of Crohn's disease had previously received a well-tolerated single infusion of infliximab. When, 14 months later, he received a second infusion for exacerbation of the

disease he had no immediate adverse effects, but complained of myalgia, arthralgia, nausea, and vomiting 7 days later and received diphenhydramine. After 3 days he had dyspnea, fever, and chills. An open lung biopsy showed features of eosinophilic pneumonia and no infections or other obvious causes were found. He subsequently worsened and required intubation and mechanical ventilation for 13 days. He was given glucocorticoids and quadruple antituberculosis drug therapy and recovered completely within 2 months. Human antichimeric antibodies were raised (13 times normal).
- A 73-year-old woman had three separate episodes of vascular purpura (with leukocytoclastic vasculitis during the third episode) during each sequence of treatment with etanercept; she later developed similar cutaneous lesions after a third injection of infliximab (35).

Delayed hypersensitivity reactions

Delayed hypersensitivity reactions were mostly observed in patients with Crohn's disease who received episodic treatment. In one patient, this complication was associated with acute respiratory distress syndrome, which became evident only 10 days after retreatment (22).

Susceptibility factors

Susceptibility factors for the development of severe systemic reactions after infliximab retreatment have been analysed in 52 adults and 34 children with Crohn's disease (30). Acute severe systemic reactions were defined by symptoms of anaphylactic reactions that required pharmacological treatment, and delayed severe systemic reactions were defined by the occurrence of arthralgia and joint stiffness (that is serum sickness-like symptoms) requiring glucocorticoids in the days after infliximab retreatment. According to these definitions, severe systemic reactions developed in 14% of patients (four acute and eight delayed) during retreatment. They were significantly more frequent in adults than in children (21 versus 3%), and delayed systemic reactions were observed exclusively in adults. These reactions mostly occurred during the second infusion of infliximab, and particularly when retreatment was distant from the first infusion, that is beyond a 20-week interval. This suggested a higher potential for delayed hypersensitivity reactions when repeated doses are given within a longer time interval, and led the authors to recommend multiple early infusions if future infliximab retreatment is anticipated.

In a retrospective review of 361 infliximab infusions in 57 children with inflammatory bowel disease there were 35 episodes of infusion reactions (36). Female sex, previous episodes of infusion reactions, and the use of immunosuppressive therapy for less than 4 months were significant predictors of subsequent infusion reactions.

Infection risk

Infliximab can increase the susceptibility of patients to severe infections, and in particular opportunistic infections (SEDA-26, 402). In patients who received repeated infusions of infliximab, infections requiring antimicrobial treatment occurred in about 30% of patients and severe infections in 4% (20).

Bacterial infections

Blockade of tumor necrosis factor alfa impairs resistance to infections with intracellular pathogens such as mycobacteria, *Pneumocystis jiroveci*, *Listeria monocytogenes*, and *Legionella pneumophila* (37,38). Severe streptococcal and staphylococcal infections have also been observed. Case reports with very severe or fatal outcomes have usually been reported in patients taking concomitant immunosuppressants and have included:

- necrotizing fasciitis due to streptococcal infection (39)
- septicemia due to *Staphylococcus aureus* (40)
- *Listeria monocytogenes* infection (41)
- disseminated tuberculosis (42)
- listeriosis (37).

The safety and efficacy of infliximab have been assessed in 40 patients with severe active spondylarthropathy in a double-blind, randomized, placebo-controlled trial (43). One 65-year-old patient improved but 3 weeks after the third infusion developed a systemic illness. He had enlarged mediastinal lymph nodes and nodular lesion of the liver and spleen. Biopsy of the mediastinal lymph nodes showed tuberculosis, which was confirmed by culture. He was treated and recovered slowly.

Reactivation of latent tuberculosis is a major concern with infliximab (SEDA-26, 402), and accounts for about one-third of infections in these patients. According to data from the manufacturers, 130 cases of active tuberculosis were notified up to October 2001. Many of the cases were disseminated or extrapulmonary tuberculosis, and several patients died. Several case reports have provided detailed information in at least seven other patients, including three who developed miliary tuberculosis and one who developed *Mycobacterium tuberculosis* enteritis (44–48). A detailed analysis of 70 cases of tuberculosis reported to the FDA has been published (49). Two-thirds of the cases were noted after three or fewer infusions and 57% of the patients had extrapulmonary disease. There were 64 cases from countries with a low incidence of tuberculosis. From these reports and the number of patients treated with infliximab, the estimated rate of tuberculosis in patients with rheumatoid arthritis treated with infliximab was four times higher than the background rate. Patients with evidence of active infection should not receive infliximab until the infection is under control; all should be screened for tuberculosis before starting infliximab (50). From these and other data it has been estimated that the risk of tuberculosis in the first year of infliximab treatment is 0.035 in US citizens and 0.2% in non-US citizens. Further investigations, such as a chest X-ray and a Mantoux test, and prophylactic treatment with isoniazid, will show whether the incidence can be reduced in patients taking anti-TNF treatment (51).

In a multicenter trial in 70 patients with ankylosing spondylitis given infliximab, treatment had to be withdrawn in three patients because of systemic tuberculosis, allergic granulomatosis of the lung, or mild leukopenia;

after withdrawal all three recovered (8). However, the allergic granulomatosis of the lung was probably due to a hypersensitivity reaction.

- An 11-year-old boy with Crohn's disease received infliximab and 3 days later developed fever, signs of cardiac failure, and *S. aureus* sepsis (52). At surgery an intramyocardial para-aortic abscess with destruction of the aortic valve was found, suggesting chronic infection, possibly activated by the use of infliximab.

Crohn's disease can lead to vasculitic changes of the aorta, which may have favored the development of the intramyocardial abscess in this case. The size of the abscess suggested persistence for several weeks.

Severe necrotizing fasciitis has been reported in a patient who was given infliximab (39).

- A 54-year-old man with rheumatoid arthritis for 12 years was given infliximab, with remission. He then developed a painful, confluent, erythematous, pustular rash over his trunk and limbs. Skin biopsy showed an acute pustular dermatitis. Five hours later he collapsed with a tachycardia (140/minute) and a blood pressure of 120/70 mmHg. He was apyrexial. His left leg was very tense, painful, and swollen, and he had a disseminated intravascular coagulopathy. There was marked necrosis of his adductor compartment and fascia of his left thigh and necrotic muscles were debrided. Blood cultures and skin swabs grew group A hemolytic streptococci. He then became unstable and died, despite efforts at resuscitation.

Viral infections

Infliximab can compromise antiviral defence mechanisms. There have been detailed reports of cytomegalovirus retinitis (53) and life-threatening disseminated cytomegalovirus infection (54). Most of these patients were taking concomitant immunosuppressants at the time of diagnosis.

- A 67-year-old woman with a 5-year history of rheumatoid arthritis, who had taken prednisone and methotrexate, was given infliximab (55). Her rheumatoid arthritis improved, but she developed multiple bilateral lesions of molluscum contagiosum on the upper and lower eyelids, despite normal CD4 and CD8 counts. She had had similar lesions during a previous course of infliximab. Excision biopsy confirmed the diagnosis.

Protozoal infections

There has been a detailed report of *P. jiroveci* pneumonia (56).

Fungal infections

In a review of 10 cases of histoplasmosis in patients treated with infliximab ($n = 9$) or etanercept ($n = 1$) the infection occurred within 1 week to 6 months after the first dose (57). Of these 10 patients, nine required treatment in an intensive care unit and one died. All lived in regions in which histoplasmosis was endemic. It was not possible to determine which patients had new infections or reactivation of previous infections.

In 41 patients with rheumatic disease who received a total of 300 infusions of infliximab over 9 months there were severe adverse effects in 15%, one of which was a case of histoplasmosis (58).

- A 28-year-old woman with unresponsive rheumatic disease developed histoplasmosis after a second infusion of infliximab. She had pet birds, and the authors thought that she had had reactivation of an infection rather than a new infection.

There have been other reports of histoplasmosis (59), invasive pulmonary aspergillosis (60), and extensive pulmonary coccidioidomycosis (61).

Death

- A 64-year-old man without heart failure was found dead 18 hours after a single infusion of infliximab for rheumatoid arthritis (62). No obvious cause was found at autopsy, except that the patient was known to have had frequent intervention by a pacemaker that had been implanted for several years.

Long-Term Effects

Tumorigenicity

There is great concern about the potential development of malignancy after blockade of tumor necrosis factor alfa, and it is biologically plausible. However, it is unclear whether this is a drug-related or a disease-related phenomenon.

There have been several cases of lymphoproliferative disease (B cell non-Hodgkin's lymphoma and nodular sclerosing Hodgkin's disease) in the 9 months after infliximab infusion in patients with Crohn's disease (63). The FDA received reports of 26 cases of lymphoproliferative disorders in patients treated with etanercept ($n = 18$) or infliximab ($n = 8$) over 20 months (64). Although this reporting rate does not exceed the age-adjusted incidence of lymphomas in the USA, spontaneous reporting underestimates the true incidence. In addition, several findings were similar to those reported in patients taking immunosuppressive drugs after transplantation. For example, 81% of the reported cases were non-Hodgkin's lymphomas. Also, the median time to occurrence after the start of anti-TNF-alfa treatment was only 8 weeks. Finally, lymphoma regressed in two patients after withdrawal and without specific cytotoxic therapy. Although the actual incidence of neoplasia was low, additional long-term data that take into account concomitant or previous immunosuppressive treatment are needed before firm conclusions can be reached.

References

1. Bell S, Kamm MA. Antibodies to tumour necrosis factor alpha as treatment for Crohn's disease. Lancet 2000;355(9207):858–60.
2. Wall GC, Heyneman C, Pfanner TP. Medical options for treating Crohn's disease in adults: focus on antitumor necrosis factor-alpha chimeric monoclonal antibody. Pharmacotherapy 1999;19(10):1138–52.
3. Maini R, St Clair EW, Breedveld F, Furst D, Kalden J, Weisman M, Smolen J, Emery P, Harriman G, Feldmann M, Lipsky PATTRACT Study Group. Infliximab (chimeric anti-tumour necrosis factor alpha monoclonal antibody) versus placebo in rheumatoid arthritis patients receiving concomitant methotrexate: a randomised phase III trial. Lancet 1999;354(9194):1932–9.
4. Keeling S, Oswald A, Russell AS, Maksymowych WP. Prospective observational analysis of the efficacy and safety of low-dose (3 mg/kg) infliximab in ankylosing spondylitis: 4-year follow up J Rheumatol 2006;33(3):558–61.
5. Bickston SJ, Lichtenstein GR, Arseneau KO, Cohen RB, Cominelli F. The relationship between infliximab treatment and lymphoma in Crohn's disease. Gastroenterology 1999;117(6):1433–7.
6. Morelli J, Wilson FA. Does administration of infliximab increase susceptibility to listeriosis? Am J Gastroenterol 2000;95(3):841–2.
7. Weisman MH. What are the risks of biologic therapy in rheumatoid arthritis? An update on safety. J Rheumatol Suppl 2002;65:33–8.
8. Braun J, Brandt J, Listing J, Zink A, Alten R, Golder W, Gromnica-Ihle E, Kellner H, Krause A, Schneider M, Sorensen H, Zeidler H, Thriene W, Sieper J. Treatment of active ankylosing spondylitis with infliximab: a randomised controlled multicentre trial. Lancet 2002;359(9313):1187–93.
9. Baig I, Storch I, Katz S. Infliximab induced eosinophilic pleural effusion in inflammatory bowel disease. Am J Gastroenterol 2002;97(Suppl):177.
10. Marotte H, Charrin JE, Miossec P. Infliximab-induced aseptic meningitis. Lancet 2001;358(9295):1784.
11. Mohan N, Edwards ET, Cupps TR, Oliverio PJ, Sandberg G, Crayton H, Richert JR, Siegel JN. Demyelination occurring during anti-tumor necrosis factor alpha therapy for inflammatory arthritides. Arthritis Rheum 2001;44(12):2862–9.
12. Robinson WH, Genovese MC, Moreland LW. Demyelinating and neurologic events reported in association with tumor necrosis factor alpha antagonism: by what mechanisms could tumor necrosis factor alpha antagonists improve rheumatoid arthritis but exacerbate multiple sclerosis? Arthritis Rheum 2001;44(9):1977–83.
13. ten Tusscher MP, Jacobs PJ, Busch MJ, de Graaf L, Diemont WL. Bilateral anterior toxic optic neuropathy and the use of infliximab. BMJ 2003;326(7389):579.
14. Foroozan R, Buono LM, Sergott RC, Savino PJ. Retrobulbar optic neuritis associated with infliximab. Arch Ophthalmol 2002;120(7):985–7.
15. Yee AM, Pochapin MB. Treatment of complicated sarcoidosis with infliximab anti-tumor necrosis factor-alpha therapy. Ann Intern Med 2001;135(1):27–31.
16. Menghini VV, Arora AS. Infliximab-associated reversible cholestatic liver disease. Mayo Clin Proc 2001;76(1):84–6.

17. Vergara G, Silvestre JF, Betlloch I, Vela P, Albares MP, Pascual JC. Cutaneous drug eruption to infliximab: report of 4 cases with an interface dermatitis pattern. Arch Dermatol 2002;138(9):1258–9.

18. Kent PD, Davis JM 3rd, Davis MD, Matteson EL. Bullous skin lesions following infliximab infusion in a patient with rheumatoid arthritis. Arthritis Rheum 2002;46(8):2257–8.

19. Griffin SP, Selby WS. Poor wound healing following surgery in three patients who received infliximab for Crohn's disease. J Gastroenterol Hepatol 2000;15(Suppl):78.

20. Hanauer SB, Feagan BG, Lichtenstein GR, Mayer LF, Schreiber S, Colombel JF, Rachmilewitz D, Wolf DC, Olson A, Bao W, Rutgeerts PACCENT I Study Group. Maintenance infliximab for Crohn's disease: the ACCENT I randomised trial. Lancet 2002;359(9317):1541–9.

21. Baert F, Noman M, Vermeire S, Van Assche G, D' Haens G, Carbonez A, Rutgeerts P. Influence of immunogenicity on the long-term efficacy of infliximab in Crohn's disease. N Engl J Med 2003;348(7):601–8.

22. Riegert-Johnson DL, Godfrey JA, Myers JL, Hubmayr RD, Sandborn WJ, Loftus EV Jr. Delayed hypersensitivity reaction and acute respiratory distress syndrome following infliximab infusion. Inflamm Bowel Dis 2002;8(3):186–91.

23. Charles PJ, Smeenk RJ, De Jong J, Feldmann M, Maini RN. Assessment of antibodies to double-stranded DNA induced in rheumatoid arthritis patients following treatment with infliximab, a monoclonal antibody to tumor necrosis factor alpha: findings in open-label and randomized placebo-controlled trials. Arthritis Rheum 2000;43(11):2383–90.

24. Mikuls TR, Moreland LW. Benefit-risk assessment of infliximab in the treatment of rheumatoid arthritis. Drug Saf 2003;26(1):23–32.

25. Ali Y, Shah S. Infliximab-induced systemic lupus erythematosus. Ann Intern Med 2002;137(7):625–6.

26. Klapman JB, Ene-Stroescu D, Becker MA, Hanauer SB. A lupus-like syndrome associated with infliximab therapy. Inflamm Bowel Dis 2003;9(3):176–8.

27. Hanauer SB, Rutgeerts PJ, D'Haens G, Targan SR, Kam L, Present DH, Wagner C, LaSorda J, Sands B, Livingstone RA. Delayed hypersensitivity to infliximab (Remicade) re-infusion after a 2-4 year interval without treatment. Gastroenterology 1999;116:A731.

28. Favalli EG, Sinigaglia L, Varenna M, Arnoldi C. Drug-induced lupus following treatment with infliximab in rheumatoid arthritis. Lupus 2002;11(11):753–5.

29. Cheifetz A, Smedley M, Martin S, Reiter M, Leone G, Mayer L, Plevy S. The incidence and management of infusion reactions to infliximab: a large center experience. Am J Gastroenterol 2003;98(6):1315–24.

30. Kugathasan S, Levy MB, Saeian K, Vasilopoulos S, Kim JP, Prajapati D, Emmons J, Martinez A, Kelly KJ, Binion DG. Infliximab retreatment in adults and children with Crohn's disease: risk factors for the development of delayed severe systemic reaction. Am J Gastroenterol 2002;97(6):1408–14.

31. Farrell RJ, Shah SA, Lodhavia PJ, Alsahli M, Falchuk KR, Michetti P, Peppercorn MA. Clinical experience with infliximab therapy in 100 patients with Crohn's disease. Am J Gastroenterol 2000;95(12):3490–7.

32. Puchner TC, Kugathasan S, Kelly KJ, Binion DG. Successful desensitization and therapeutic use of infliximab in adult and pediatric Crohn's disease patients with prior anaphylactic reaction. Inflamm Bowel Dis 2001;7(1):34–7.

33. O'Connor M, Buchman A, Marshall G. Anaphylaxis-like reaction to infliximab in a patient with Crohn's disease. Dig Dis Sci 2002;47(6):1323–5.

34. Lankarani KB. Mortality associated with infliximab. J Clin Gastroenterol 2001;33(3):255–6.

35. McCain ME, Quinet RJ, Davis WE. Etanercept and infliximab associated with cutaneous vasculitis. Rheumatology (Oxford) 2002;41(1):116–7.

36. Crandall WV, Mackner LM. Infusion reactions to infliximab in children and adolescents: frequency, outcome and a predictive model. Aliment Pharmacol Ther 2003;17(1):75–84.

37. Kamath BM, Mamula P, Baldassano RN, Markowitz JE. *Listeria* meningitis after treatment with infliximab. J Pediatr Gastroenterol Nutr 2002;34(4):410–2.

38. Shanahan JC, St Clair W. Tumor necrosis factor-alpha blockade: a novel therapy for rheumatic disease. Clin Immunol 2002;103(3 Pt 1):231–42.

39. Chan AT, Cleeve V, Daymond TJ. Necrotising fasciitis in a patient receiving infliximab for rheumatoid arthritis. Postgrad Med J 2002;78(915):47–8.

40. Matzkies FG, Manger B, Schmitt-Haendle M, Nagel T, Kraetsch HG, Kalden JR, Schulze-Koops H. Severe septicaemia in a patient with polychondritis and Sweet's syndrome after initiation of treatment with infliximab. Ann Rheum Dis 2003;62(1):81–2.

41. Gluck T, Linde HJ, Scholmerich J, Muller-Ladner U, Fiehn C, Bohland P. Anti-tumor necrosis factor therapy and *Listeria monocytogenes* infection: report of two cases. Arthritis Rheum 2002;46(8):2255–7.

42. Liberopoulos EN, Drosos AA, Elisaf MS. Exacerbation of tuberculosis enteritis after treatment with infliximab. Am J Med 2002;113(7):615.

43. Van Den Bosch F, Kruithof E, Baeten D, Herssens A, de Keyser F, Mielants H, Veys EM. Randomized double-blind comparison of chimeric monoclonal antibody to tumor necrosis factor alpha (infliximab) versus placebo in active spondylarthropathy. Arthritis Rheum 2002;46(3):755–65.

44. Mayordomo L, Marenco JL, Gomez-Mateos J, Rejon E. Pulmonary miliary tuberculosis in a patient with anti-TNF-alpha treatment. Scand J Rheumatol 2002;31(1):44–5.

45. Nunez Martinez O, Ripoll Noiseux C, Carneros Martin JA, Gonzalez Lara V, Gregorio Maranon HG. Reactivation tuberculosis in a patient with anti-TNF-alpha treatment. Am J Gastroenterol 2001;96(5):1665–6.

46. Roth S, Delmont E, Heudier P, Kaphan R, Cua E, Castela J, Verdier JM, Chichmanian RM, Fuzibet JG. Anticorps anti-TNF alpha (infliximab) et tuberculose: à propos de 3 cas. Rev Med Interne 2002;23(3):312–6.

47. Rovere Querini P, Vecchio M, Sabbadini MG, Ciboddo G. Miliary tuberculosis after biological therapy for rheumatoid arthritis. Rheumatology 2002;41(2):231.

48. Wagner TE, Huseby ES, Huseby JS. Exacerbation of *Mycobacterium tuberculosis* enteritis masquerading as Crohn's disease after treatment with a tumor necrosis factor-alpha inhibitor. Am J Med 2002;112(1):67–9.

49. Keane J, Gershon S, Wise RP, Mirabile-Levens E, Kasznica J, Schwieterman WD, Siegel JN, Braun MM. Tuberculosis associated with infliximab, a tumor necrosis factor alpha-neutralizing agent. N Engl J Med 2001;345(15):1098–104.

50. Sandborn WJ, Hanauer SB. Infliximab in the treatment of Crohn's disease: a user's guide for clinicians. Am J Gastroenterol 2002;97(12):2962–72.

51. Antoni C, Braun J. Side effects of anti-TNF therapy: current knowledge. Clin Exp Rheumatol 2002;20(6 Suppl 28):S152–7.

52. Reichardt P, Dahnert I, Tiller G, Hausler HJ. Possible activation of an intramyocardial inflammatory process

(*Staphylococcus aureus*) after treatment with infliximab in a boy with Crohn disease. Eur J Pediatr 2002;161(5):281–3.

53. Haerter G, Manfras B, Schmitt M, Wendland T, Moch B. Severe CMV retinitis in a patient with HLA-B27 associated spondylarthropathy following immunosuppressive therapy with anti-TNF alpha (infliximab). Infection 2003;31(Suppl 1):150.

54. Helbling D, Breitbach TH, Krause M. Disseminated cytomegalovirus infection in Crohn's disease following anti-tumour necrosis factor therapy. Eur J Gastroenterol Hepatol 2002;14(12):1393–5.

55. Cursiefen C, Grunke M, Dechant C, Antoni C, Junemann A, Holbach LM. Multiple bilateral eyelid molluscum contagiosum lesions associated with TNFalpha-antibody and methotrexate therapy. Am J Ophthalmol 2002;134(2):270–1.

56. Tai TL, O'Rourke KP, McWeeney M, Burke CM, Sheehan K, Barry M. *Pneumocystis carinii* pneumonia following a second infusion of infliximab. Rheumatology (Oxford) 2002;41(8):951–2.

57. Lee JH, Slifman NR, Gershon SK, Edwards ET, Schwieterman WD, Siegel JN, Wise RP, Brown SL, Udall JN Jr, Braun MM. Life-threatening histoplasmosis complicating immunotherapy with tumor necrosis factor alpha antagonists infliximab and etanercept. Arthritis Rheum 2002;46(10):2565–70.

58. Fitzcharles MA, Clayton D, Menard HA. The use of infliximab in academic rheumatology practice: an audit of early clinical experience. J Rheumatol 2002;29(12):2525–30.

59. Nakelchik M, Mangino JE. Reactivation of histoplasmosis after treatment with infliximab. Am J Med 2002;112(1):78.

60. Warris A, Bjorneklett A, Gaustad P. Invasive pulmonary aspergillosis associated with infliximab therapy. N Engl J Med 2001;344(14):1099–100.

61. Ramzan NN, Shapiro MS, Robinson E, Smilack JD. Use of infliximab leading to extensive pulmonary coccidioidomycosis. Am J Gastroenterol 2002;97(Suppl):157.

62. de' Clari F, Salani I, Safwan E, Giannacco A. Sudden death in a patient without heart failure after a single infusion of 200 mg infliximab: does TNF-alpha have protective effects on the failing heart, or does infliximab have direct harmful cardiovascular effects? Circulation 2002;105(21):E183.

63. Drewe E, Powell RJ. Clinically useful monoclonal antibodies in treatment. J Clin Pathol 2002;55(2):81–5.

64. Brown SL, Greene MH, Gershon SK, Edwards ET, Braun MM. Tumor necrosis factor antagonist therapy and lymphoma development: twenty-six cases reported to the Food and Drug Administration. Arthritis Rheum 2002;46(12):3151–8.

Muromonab

General Information

Muromonab (orthoclone, OKT3) is a murine monoclonal antibody targeted against the human CD3-receptor–T cell complex. This powerful immunosuppressive agent is used in the treatment of acute transplant rejection. Its use during initial rejection prophylaxis is subject to debate because excessive immunosuppression can increase the risk of infections and secondary malignancies (1). Renal transplant patients with a high risk of rejection have been suggested as possible candidates for muromonab prophylaxis (2). Excessive immunosuppression and unexpected over-activation of the immune system are the main adverse effects.

Cytokine release syndrome

A complex of acute systemic symptoms referred to as the "cytokine-release syndrome" is the most typical adverse effect of muromonab (3). A flu-like reaction is the key component of this complex syndrome, including fever, chills, headache, myalgia, tachycardia, and gastrointestinal symptoms. Other systemic and severe manifestations of the syndrome include acute pulmonary edema and neurological, renal, and hematological disorders. Symptoms occur within 1 hour after the initial doses of muromonab and last for several hours. A lower incidence and less severity were observed after subsequent doses (4). The cytokine-release syndrome was also less frequent after low doses or a 2-hour infusion of muromonab (instead of conventional doses or single bolus infusion) and it was thought to be more severe and of longer duration in patients with moderate-to-severe graft rejections (5–9).

Considerable efforts have been made to prevent or control the cytokine-release syndrome and its consequences (10). High-dose methylprednisolone (8 mg/kg) given before muromonab remains the basis of prophylaxis, and two separate doses are more effective than a single bolus (11). In a retrospective comparison of 345 renal transplant patients, other investigators found that the use of diltiazem allowed a reduction in the dosage of methylprednisolone, reduced nephrotoxicity, and reduced both delayed graft function and postoperative intragraft thrombosis (12). Indometacin, even at low doses, has also been successfully used without impairing rejection reversal or renal function (13). In contrast, prophylaxis with pentoxifylline was not supported in one carefully controlled study (14).

Although the release of a wide range of cytokines was increased after muromonab administration, tumor necrosis factor alfa and interleukin-6 were suggested to play a pivotal role, and monoclonal anti-TNF-alfa antibody administration reduced the acute clinical symptoms (15). A role for the activation of complement and neutrophils was also suggested.

Several humanized CD3 antibodies have been produced and tested, with the aim of reducing the adverse effects associated with the murine orthoclone antibody. The first results in renal transplant patients were encouraging, with promising clinical results, no evidence of anti-globulin response, and no or very few and minimal adverse effects attributable to various humanized monoclonal CD3 antibodies (16,17). In particular, careful patient monitoring failed to identify any significant cytokine release syndrome.

Organs and Systems

Cardiovascular

Cardiovascular manifestations are usually observed during the cytokine-release syndrome. They mostly included tachycardia and transient hypertension or hypotension (4). Fluid overload or volume depletion can also play a role. Chest pain or severe dysrhythmias are infrequent (18).

Muromonab has been thought to exert procoagulant activity and activate fibrinolysis, probably as a result of TNF-alfa release of other cytokines and cellular adhesion to the vascular endothelium (19,20). Accordingly, retrospective studies have pointed to an increased risk of intragraft thromboses with thromboses in the renal artery, renal vein, or glomerular capillaries, or thrombotic microangiopathy, leading to a higher incidence of rejection episodes in patients receiving high or conventional doses of muromonab (19,21). Among 231 kidney transplant recipients who received muromonab prophylaxis, intragraft thromboses were found in 13 (5.6%), and the use of very high-dose methylprednisolone (30 mg/kg) was suggested to be a major risk factor (22). In contrast, and despite the evidence of procoagulant activity, some investigators have failed to identify evidence that muromonab increases the risk of thromboembolic complications (20,23).

Respiratory

Dyspnea and pulmonary edema sometimes develop during the cytokine-release syndrome. Pulmonary toxicity was mostly observed in patients who had fluid retention and weight gain before receiving muromonab. The incidence has been markedly reduced by the formulation of guidelines for management (3). Cytokine release and complement activation with further neutrophil activation and pulmonary vascular endothelium damage were suggested to be involved (24).

Nervous system

Self-limiting and benign central nervous system manifestations mimicking those of aseptic meningitis, that is fever, headache, nuchal rigidity, cognitive disorders, and photophobia, were observed in 3–10% of patients who received muromonab (3). The symptoms were usually delayed for 2–3 days and resolved spontaneously despite continuation of treatment. More severe neurological disorders requiring withdrawal have been observed in up to 7% of patients (25). The various reported symptoms consisted of slowly reversible diffuse encephalopathy with mental changes, neurosensory hallucinations, tinnitus with reversible hearing loss, transient hemiparesis, cerebral infarction, generalized or focal seizures, cortical blindness, psychotic symptoms, obtundation, and coma (SED-13, 1132; SEDA-21, 380; 25). Diabetes and severely impaired renal function were possibly significant risk factors (SEDA-19, 353; SEDA-21, 380). Neurotoxic symptoms were supposedly mediated by cytokine release and potentiated by uremic toxins. Raised concentrations of

tumor necrosis factor alfa in the cerebrospinal fluid were suggested to play a major role in muromonab-induced aseptic meningitis and encephalopathy (26).

Muromonab-induced aseptic meningitis is relatively common and is usually benign, with prompt recovery despite continuation of treatment.

- In a 28-year-old man the clinical features of aseptic meningitis were prolonged over 1 month after the administration of muromonab, and persistent severe headaches resolved only after several aspirations of cerebrospinal fluid (27).

This case was described as a syndrome of headache with neurological deficits and CSF lymphocytosis (HaNDL syndrome).

Sensory systems

Eyes

Spontaneously reversible mild conjunctivitis and episcleritis have been noted in 75 and 10% of patients respectively.

Diffuse anterior scleritis responding to an increased dosage of prednisone was mentioned in one patient (28).

Isolated visual loss (persistent in one patient) shortly after muromonab administration is rare (SEDA-20, 340; 29).

Ears

Ototoxicity from muromonab has been described, but the incidence is unknown (SEDA-21, 380). Audiograms performed before and 48–72 hours after administration of muromonab showed sensorineural hearing loss of at least 15 db in five of seven renal transplant patients (30). A third audiogram 2 weeks after muromonab treatment showed amelioration or complete recovery in all four of the patients who were tested.

Hematologic

Acute thrombocytopenia has been reported in one patient (SEDA-21, 380).

Liver

Hepatitis has been attributed to cytokine release from muromonab (31).

- A 31-year-old man underwent renal transplantation for end-stage renal disease secondary to hypertension. He was given basiliximab for induction immunosuppression. At 13 months after transplantation he had evidence of transplant rejection. His creatinine concentration rose acutely from 83 to 165 µmol/l over 1 week. This was his first rejection episode (Banff IIa). There was no evidence of viral infection. He received muromonab with conventional prophylaxis (antihistamines, paracetamol, and corticosteroids) to reduce the severity of cytokine release. This was his first exposure to muromonab. Initially he complained of fever and nausea, and the following day he was somnolent and had right upper quadrant tenderness. Liver function tests, which had been normal on the day of admission, were abnormal. Hepatitis serology showed positive hepatitis B core antibody (IgM and IgG), positive hepatitis A antibody, negative hepatitis surface antigen, and negative hepatitis C antibody. The hepatitis B core antibody (IgM and IgG) had been positive before transplantation 16 months before. Muromonab was withdrawn and he showed signs of clinical and chemical improvement. Rejection was successfully treated with glucocorticoids and antithymocyte globulin.

Urinary tract

Spontaneously reversible increases in serum creatinine concentrations occurred in 8–18% of muromonab-treated patients, and were thought to have resulted from inhibition of renal prostaglandin synthesis and release of cytokines (32,33). There were no adverse consequences on short-term graft survival or graft function (32).

Isolated cases of hemolytic-uremic syndrome have been reported (SED-13, 1133; SEDA-21, 380).

Immunologic

An antibody response to muromonab has been detected in 40% of patients undergoing a 14-day induction regimen of muromonab 5 mg/day (10). It has been suggested that the incidence of antimuromonab antibodies depended on the immunosuppressive regimen, but this was based on a retrospective study in a limited number of patients (SEDA-22, 409). Furthermore, sensitization was not relevant in most patients. Only raised IgG anti-idiotypic antibodies in high enough titers (over 1:1000) significantly neutralize the binding of muromonab to the CD3 receptor and reduce clinical efficacy, thus precluding further muromonab administration.

Antimuromonab IgE antibodies have been identified after 10–25 days of treatment in six of 181 patients, and only in those with high titers of antimuromonab IgG antibodies (34). Immediate IgE-mediated anaphylactic reactions, namely anaphylactic shock, bronchospasm, urticaria, have been rarely reported and have sometimes been difficult to differentiate from the cytokine-release syndrome (35,36). Late-onset reactions after the first week of treatment, including cutaneous erythema, a fall in blood pressure, or serum sickness-like reactions, are infrequent (37).

Rare anaphylactic reactions with antimuromonab IgE antibodies have been reported (SED-14, 1309). Anaphylactoid reactions to muromonab can also occur (38).

- A 15-year-old girl underwent uneventful renal transplantation. On the third postoperative day she received her first dose of muromonab for a presumptive diagnosis of graft rejection. Despite premedication with diphenhydramine, paracetamol, and high-dose methylprednisolone, within 20 seconds after intravenous muromonab, she developed shortness of breath, digital paresthesia, facial edema, laryngeal stridor, reduced oxygen saturation, and a fall in blood pressure. She

recovered after intubation and appropriate vasopressor administration, but required transplant nephrectomy for hemorrhagic and coagulative necrosis of the transplanted kidney.

This acute reaction was supposedly mediated by non-immunologic mast cell degranulation, as screening for IgE antimuromonab antibodies was negative.

As with other potent immunosuppressive drugs, muromonab has been suspected to increase the risk of infections. Multiple possible biases in studies of the incidence of muromonab-associated infections have been discussed (3); there were no differences among patients who received muromonab compared with those who received other immunosuppressive regimens. Since then, several other investigators have reported their findings, indicating that this debate continues.

In patients with renal transplants, the overall incidence of infections during the first three posttransplantation months was significantly higher in one trial of patients treated with prophylactic muromonab or ciclosporin (39), but there was no significant difference in the severity of infections in another similar trial (40). Both studies failed to identify any adverse impact of infectious episodes on patient survival. In a comparison of prophylactic ATG-Fresenius with muromonab there were more common minor infections (for example, cutaneous mycosis, *Herpes simplex* virus infections) in the muromonab arm, but a similar incidence of life-threatening or severe infections (41). In contrast to these findings, a large retrospective study showed a significantly higher incidence of infection-related deaths among patients who received muromonab for induction therapy compared with those who did not receive muromonab (42). However, renal graft survival was significantly improved in patients treated with muromonab, and there were no subsequent viral deaths after the routine use of appropriate anti-infectious prophylaxis.

In patient with liver transplants (43,44) or heart transplants (45), retrospective studies have shown that muromonab treatment is an additional or independent risk factor for symptomatic cytomegalovirus infections in cytomegalovirus-seropositive patients or in recipients of cytomegalovirus-seropositive donors, suggesting that cytomegalovirus prophylaxis should be implemented in these patients. It has also been suggested that early muromonab administration in the posttransplant period increases the likelihood of invasive cytomegalovirus disease after liver transplantation (46). In contrast, other investigators failed to show an increased incidence of cytomegalovirus infections after muromonab versus triple drug therapy in heart transplant patients (47). Based on a retrospective study of 154 liver transplant patients, muromonab was suggested as a risk factor for *Pneumocystis jiroveci* pneumonia (48).

These results suggest that the incidence and severity of infections is more likely to be related to the degree of immunosuppression than to the effect of an individual drug.

Long-Term Effects

Tumorigenicity

As expected from its pronounced immunosuppressive activity, muromonab is a significant risk factor for secondary neoplasia, especially when high doses, increased treatment duration, sequential courses, or early retreatment are used (49). Whether the increased risk of neoplasia after muromonab-based immunosuppression is due to the drug itself or reflects the overall degree of immunosuppression is a matter of debate, and conflicting results have emerged. Several retrospective or controlled studies did not show more frequent malignancies after muromonab compared with other immunosuppressive regimens (50–52). On the other hand, the rate of non-Hodgkin's lymphomas was higher in kidney and heart transplant recipients who received muromonab prophylaxis rather than antithymocyte/antilymphocyte globulin (53). Using data from the manufacturers and the literature, the rate of malignancies after muromonab was estimated to be 0.57% (54), but potential under-reporting strongly limited the validity of this estimation. Although the roles of high cumulative doses or repeated courses as risk factors are not definitely proven, it is usually recommended not to exceed 14 days of treatment with cumulative doses of 70 mg (3).

An analysis of the Australia and New Zealand Dialysis and Transplant Registry (7953 patients with 9460 renal transplants) has confirmed that immunosuppression with polyclonal and monoclonal muromonab antibodies independently increases the risk of virus-mediated cancer (55). The increased risk was about 60% for non-Hodgkin's lymphoma and 75% for non-Hodgkin's lymphoma plus, in women, carcinoma of the cervix, vagina, and vulva.

References

1. Wilde MI, Goa KL. Muromonab CD3: a reappraisal of its pharmacology and use as prophylaxis of solid organ transplant rejection. Drugs 1996;51(5):865–94.
2. Abramowicz D, Norman DJ, Goldman M, De Pauw L, Kinnaert P, Kahana L, Thistlethwaite JR, Shield CF, Monaco AP, Vanherweghem JL, et al. OKT3 prophylaxis improves long-term renal graft survival in high-risk patients as compared to cyclosporine: combined results from the prospective, randomized Belgian and US studies. Transplant Proc 1995;27(1):852–3.
3. Kreis H. Adverse events associated with OKT3 immunosuppression in the prevention or treatment of allograft rejection. Clin Transplant 1993;7:431–46.
4. Jeyarajah DR, Thistlethwaite JR Jr. General aspects of cytokine-release syndrome: timing and incidence of symptoms. Transplant Proc 1993;25(2 Suppl 1):16–20.
5. Brown M, Korb S, Light JA, Light T, Jonsson J, Aquino A. Low-dose OKT3 induction therapy following renal transplantation leads to improved graft function and decreased adverse effects. Transplant Proc 1993;25(1 Pt 1):553–5.
6. Norman DJ, Kimball JA, Bennett WM, Shihab F, Batiuk TD, Meyer MM, Barry JM. A prospective, double-blind, randomized study of high-versus low-dose OKT3 induction immunosuppression in cadaveric renal transplantation. Transpl Int 1994;7(5):356–61.
7. Parlevliet KJ, Bemelman FJ, Yong SL, Hack CE, Surachno J, Wilmink JM, ten Berge IJ, Schellekens PT. Toxicity of OKT3 increases with dosage: a controlled study in renal transplant recipients. Transpl Int 1995;8(2):141–6.
8. Vasquez EM, Fabrega AJ, Pollak R. OKT3-induced cytokine-release syndrome: occurrence beyond the second dose and association with rejection severity. Transplant Proc 1995;27(1):873–4.
9. Buysmann S, Hack CE, van Diepen FN, Surachno J, ten Berge IJ. Administration of OKT3 as a two-hour infusion attenuates first-dose side effects. Transplantation 1997;64(11):1620–3.
10. Norman DJ, Chatenoud L, Cohen D, Goldman M, Shield CF 3rd. Consensus statement regarding OKT3-induced cytokine-release syndrome and human antimouse antibodies. Transplant Proc 1993;25(2 Suppl 1):89–92.
11. Bemelman FJ, Buysmann S, Wilmink JM, Surachno S, Hack CE, Schellekens PT, ten Berge RJ. Effects of divided doses of steroids on side effects, cytokines, and activation of complement and granulocytes, coagulation and fibrinolysis after OKT3. Transplant Proc 1994;26(6):3096–7.
12. Abramowicz D, De Pauw L, Le Moine A, Sermon F, Surquin M, Doutrelepont JM, Ickx B, Depierreux M, Vanherweghem JL, Kinnaert P, Goldman M, Vereerstraeten P. Prevention of OKT3 nephrotoxicity after kidney transplantation. Kidney Int Suppl 1996;53:S39–43.
13. Gaughan WJ, Francos BB, Dunn SR, Francos GC, Burke JF. A retrospective analysis of the effect of indomethacin on adverse reactions to orthoclone OKT3 in the therapy of acute renal allograft rejection. Am J Kidney Dis 1994;24(3):486–90.
14. Vincenti F, Danovitch GM, Neylan JF, Steiner RW, Everson MP, Gaston RS. Pentoxifylline does not prevent the cytokine-induced first dose reaction following OKT3—a randomized, double-blind placebo-controlled study. Transplantation 1996;61(4):573–7.
15. Chatenoud L. OKT3-induced cytokine-release syndrome: prevention effect of anti-tumor necrosis factor monoclonal antibody. Transplant Proc 1993;25(2 Suppl 1):47–51.
16. Friend PJ, Hale G, Chatenoud L, Rebello P, Bradley J, Thiru S, Phillips JM, Waldmann H. Phase I study of an engineered aglycosylated humanized CD3 antibody in renal transplant rejection. Transplantation 1999;68(11):1632–7.
17. Woodle ES, Xu D, Zivin RA, Auger J, Charette J, O'Laughlin R, Peace D, Jollife LK, Haverty T, Bluestone JA, Thistlethwaite JR Jr. Phase I trial of a humanized, Fc receptor nonbinding OKT3 antibody, huOKT3gamma1(Ala-Ala) in the treatment of acute renal allograft rejection. Transplantation 1999;68(5):608–16.
18. Hall KA, Dole EJ, Hunter GC, Zukoski CF, Putnam CW. Hyperpyrexia-related ventricular tachycardia during OKT3 induction therapy. Transplantation 1992;54(6):1112–3.
19. Abramowicz D, Pradier O, Marchant A, Florquin S, De Pauw L, Vereerstraeten P, Kinnaert P, Vanherwehem JL, Goldman M. Induction of thromboses within renal grafts by high-dose prophylactic OKT3. Lancet 1992;339(8796):777–8.
20. Raasveld MH, Hack CE, ten Berge IJ. Activation of coagulation and fibrinolysis following OKT3 administration to renal transplant recipients: association with distinct mediators. Thromb Haemost 1992;68(3):264–7.
21. Gomez E, Aguado S, Gago E, Escalada P, Alvarez-Grande J. Main graft vessels thromboses due to conventional-dose OKT3 in renal transplantation. Lancet 1992;339(8809):1612–3.

22. Abramowicz D, Pradier O, De Pauw L, Kinnaert P, Mat O, Surquin M, Doutrelepont JM, Vanherweghem JL, Capel P, Vereerstraeten P, et al. High-dose glucocorticosteroids increase the procoagulant effects of OKT3. Kidney Int 1994;46(6):1596–602.

23. Hollenbeck M, Westhoff A, Bach D, Grabensee B, Kolvenbach R, Kniemeyer HW. Doppler sonography and renal graft vessel thromboses after OKT3 treatment. Lancet 1992;340(8819):619–20.

24. Raasveld MH, Bemelman FJ, Schellekens PT, van Diepen FN, van Dongen A, van Royen EA, Hack CE, ten Berge IJ. Complement activation during OKT3 treatment: a possible explanation for respiratory side effects. Kidney Int 1993;43(5):1140–9.

25. Shihab F, Barry JM, Bennett WM, Meyer MM, Norman DJ. Cytokine-related encephalopathy induced by OKT3: incidence and predisposing factors. Transplant Proc 1993;25(1 Pt 1):564–5.

26. Reiss R, Makoff D, Rodriguez H, Graham S, Mittleman J, Jordan S. Encephalopathy and cerebral infarction in OKT3-treated patients with concomitant elevation of cerebrospinal fluid tumour necrosis factor alpha. Nephrol Dial Transplant 1993;8(5):464–8.

27. Thomas MC, Walker R, Wright A. HaNDL syndrome after "benign" OKT3-induced meningitis. Transplantation 1999;67(10):1384–5.

28. McCarthy JM, Sullivan K, Keown PA, Rollins DT. Diffuse anterior scleritis during OKT3 monoclonal antibody therapy for renal transplant rejection. Can J Ophthalmol 1992;27(1):22–4.

29. Dukar O, Barr CC. Visual loss complicating OKT3 monoclonal antibody therapy. Am J Ophthalmol 1993;115(6):781–5.

30. Hartnick CJ, Smith RV, Tellis V, Greenstein S, Ruben RJ. Reversible sensorineural hearing loss following administration of muromonab-CD3 (OKT3) for cadaveric renal transplant immunosuppression. Ann Otol Rhinol Laryngol 2000;109(1):45–7.

31. Go MR, Bumgardner GL. OKT3 (muromonab-CD3) associated hepatitis in a kidney transplant recipient. Transplantation 2002;73(12):1957–9.

32. Batiuk TD, Bennett WM, Norman DJ. Cytokine nephropathy during antilymphocyte therapy. Transplant Proc 1993;25(2 Suppl 1):27–30.

33. First MR, Schroeder TJ, Hariharan S. OKT3-induced cytokine-release syndrome: renal effects (cytokine nephropathy). Transplant Proc 1993;25(2 Suppl 1):25–6.

34. Abramowicz D, Crusiaux A, Niaudet P, Kreis H, Chatenoud L, Goldman M. The IgE humoral response in OKT3-treated patients. Incidence and fine specificity. Transplantation 1996;61(4):577–81.

35. Abramowicz D, Crusiaux A, Goldman M. Anaphylactic shock after retreatment with OKT3 monoclonal antibody. N Engl J Med 1992;327(10):736.

36. Georgitis JW, Browning MC, Steiner D, Lorentz WB. Anaphylaxis and desensitization to the murine monoclonal antibody used for renal graft rejection. Ann Allergy 1991;66(4):343–7.

37. Turner M, Holman J. Late reactions during initial OKT3-treatment. Clin Transplant 1993;7:1–3.

38. Berkowitz RJ, Possidente CJ, McPherson BR, Guillot A, Braun SV, Reese JC. Anaphylactoid reaction to muromonab-CD3 in a pediatric renal transplant recipient. Pharmacotherapy 2000;20(1):100–4.

39. Abramowicz D, Goldman M, De Pauw L, Vanherweghem JL, Kinnaert P, Vereerstraeten P. The long-term effects of prophylactic OKT3 monoclonal antibody in cadaver kidney transplantation—a single-center, prospective, randomized study. Transplantation 1992;54(3):433–7.

40. Norman DJ, Kahana L, Stuart FP Jr, Thistlethwaite JR Jr, Shield CF 3rd, Monaco A, Dehlinger J, Wu SC, Van Horn A, Haverty TP. A randomized clinical trial of induction therapy with OKT3 in kidney transplantation. Transplantation 1993;55(1):44–50.

41. Bock HA, Gallati H, Zurcher RM, Bachofen M, Mihatsch MJ, Landmann J, Thiel G. A randomized prospective trial of prophylactic immunosuppression with ATG-fresenius versus OKT3 after renal transplantation. Transplantation 1995;59(6):830–40.

42. Petrie JJ, Rigby RJ, Hawley CM, Suranyi MG, Whitby M, Wall D, Hardie IR. Effect of OKT3 in steroid-resistant renal transplant rejection. Transplantation 1995;59(3):347–52.

43. Hadley S, Samore MH, Lewis WD, Jenkins RL, Karchmer AW, Hammer SM. Major infectious complications after orthotopic liver transplantation and comparison of outcomes in patients receiving cyclosporine or FK506 as primary immunosuppression. Transplantation 1995;59(6):851–9.

44. Portela D, Patel R, Larson-Keller JJ, Ilstrup DM, Wiesner RH, Steers JL, Krom RA, Paya CV. OKT3 treatment for allograft rejection is a risk factor for cytomegalovirus disease in liver transplantation. J Infect Dis 1995;171(4):1014–8.

45. Wechsler ME, Giardina EG, Sciacca RR, Rose EA, Barr ML. Increased early mortality in women undergoing cardiac transplantation. Circulation 1995;91(4):1029–35.

46. Hooks MA, Perlino CA, Henderson JM, Millikan WJ Jr, Kutner MH. Prevalence of invasive cytomegalovirus disease with administration of muromonab CD-3 in patients undergoing orthotopic liver transplantation. Ann Pharmacother 1992;26(5):617–20.

47. Lake K, Anderson D, Milfred S, Love K, Pritzker M, Emery R. The incidence of cytomegalovirus disease is not increased after OKT3 induction therapy. J Heart Lung Transplant 1993;12(3):537–8.

48. Hayes MJ, Torzillo PJ, Sheil AG, McCaughan GW. Pneumocystis carinii pneumonia after liver transplantation in adults. Clin Transplant 1994;8(6):499–503.

49. Swinnen LJ, Costanzo-Nordin MR, Fisher SG, O'Sullivan EJ, Johnson MR, Heroux AL, Dizikes GJ, Pifarre R, Fisher RI. Increased incidence of lymphoproliferative disorder after immunosuppression with the monoclonal antibody OKT3 in cardiac-transplant recipients. N Engl J Med 1990;323(25):1723–8.

50. Anderson P, Schroeder T, Hariharan S, First M. Incidence of posttransplant lymphoproliferative disease in OKT-3 treated renal transplant recipients. Clin Transplant 1993;7:582–5.

51. Batiuk TD, Barry JM, Bennett WM, Meyer MM, Tolzman D, Norman DJ. Incidence and type of cancer following the use of OKT3: a single center experience with 557 organ transplants. Transplant Proc 1993;25(1 Pt 2):1391.

52. McAlister V, Grant D, Roy A, Yilmaz Z, Ghent C, Wall W. Posttransplant lymphoproliferative disorders in liver recipients treated with OKT3 or ALG induction immunosuppression. Transplant Proc 1993;25(1 Pt 2):1400–1.

53. Opelz G, Henderson R. Incidence of non-Hodgkin lymphoma in kidney and heart transplant recipients. Lancet 1993;342(8886–8887):1514–6.
54. Bertin D, Haverty T, Sanders M, et al. Posttransplant development of lymphoproliferative disroders and other malignancies following orthoclone OKT3 therapy. In: Lieberman R, Mukherjee A, editors. Principles of Drug Development in Transplantation and Autoimmunity 1996:633–41.
55. Hibberd AD, Trevillian PR, Wlodarzcyk JH, Gillies AH, Stein AM, Sheil AG, Disney AP. Cancer risk associated with ATG/OKT3 in renal transplantation. Transplant Proc 1999;31(1–2):1271–2.

Omalizumab

General Information

Omalizumab (formerly rhuMab-E25) is a humanized monoclonal antibody against IgE, which blocks the interaction of IgE with mast cells. Several phase I and phase II trials have demonstrated its efficacy in patients with allergic asthma (1–4).

In a placebo-controlled study of subcutaneous omalizumab (50, 150, and 300 mg before the ragweed season and every 3 or 4 weeks during the pollen season) in 536 patients with seasonal allergic rhinitis, injection site reactions were mild and infrequent, there were no clinically significant alterations in laboratory values, and anti-idiotypic antibodies to omalizumab were not detected; there was no evidence of immune complex-related adverse events (5–7).

In another placebo-controlled trial in 525 patients with severe asthma, the adverse effects profiles were similar in the treatment and placebo groups (8).

In an extension study in 225 children there were no anaphylactic reactions or adverse events suggestive of serum sickness or immune complex formation; anti-omalizumab antibodies were not detected (9). In cases of retreatment there were no severe adverse events related to omalizumab (10).

Organs and Systems

Skin

The safety of subcutaneous omalizumab has been assessed in 334 boys and premenarchic girls aged 6–12 years with moderate to severe allergic asthma requiring inhaled glucocorticoids in a randomized, placebo-controlled, double-blind trial (11). There were no serious treatment-related adverse events, and the frequencies of most adverse events were similar with omalizumab and placebo. However, urticaria was more frequent with omalizumab (4 versus 0.9%). It usually resolved spontaneously or with antihistamine therapy and did not recur with subsequent treatment. Urticaria was also reported in a small number of adults (0.5%) given omalizumab for allergic rhinitis (12).

References

1. Busse W, Corren J, Lanier BQ, McAlary M, Fowler-Taylor A, Cioppa GD, van As A, Gupta N. Omalizumab, anti-IgE recombinant humanized monoclonal antibody, for the treatment of severe allergic asthma. J Allergy Clin Immunol 2001;108(2):184–90.
2. Asnis LA, Gaspari AA. Cutaneous reactions to recombinant cytokine therapy. J Am Acad Dermatol 1995;33(3):393–410.
3. Tosti A, Misciali C, Bardazzi F, Fanti PA, Varotti C. Telogen effluvium due to recombinant interferon alpha-2b. Dermatology 1992;184(2):124–5.
4. Andry P, Weber-Buisset MJ, Fraitag S, Brechot C, De Prost Y. Toxidermie bulleuse à l'Introna. [Bullous drug eruption caused by Introna.] Ann Dermatol Venereol 1993;120(11):843–5.
5. Casale TB, Condemi J, LaForce C, Nayak A, Rowe M, Watrous M, McAlary M, Fowler-Taylor A, Racine A, Gupta N, Fick R, Della Cioppa G. Omalizumab Seasonal Allergic Rhinitis Trail Group. Effect of omalizumab on symptoms of seasonal allergic rhinitis: a randomized controlled trial. JAMA 2001;286(23):2956–67.
6. Bang LM, Plosker GL. Omalizumab: a review of its use in the management of allergic asthma. Treat Respir Med 2004;3(3):183–99.
7. Bang LM, Plosker GL. Spotlight on omalizumab in allergic asthma. BioDrugs 2004;18(6):415–8.
8. Boushey HA Jr. Experiences with monoclonal antibody therapy for allergic asthma. J Allergy Clin Immunol 2001;108(Suppl 2):S77–83.
9. Berger W, Gupta N, McAlary M, Fowler-Taylor A. Evaluation of long-term safety of the anti-IgE antibody, omalizumab, in children with allergic asthma. Ann Allergy Asthma Immunol 2003;91(2):182–8.
10. Nayak A, Casale T, Miller SD, Condemi J, McAlary M, Fowler-Taylor A, Della Cioppa G, Gupta N. Tolerability of retreatment with omalizumab, a recombinant humanized monoclonal anti-IgE antibody, during a second ragweed pollen season in patients with seasonal allergic rhinitis. Allergy Asthma Proc 2003;24(5):323–9.
11. Milgrom H, Berger W, Nayak A, Gupta N, Pollard S, McAlary M, Taylor AF, Rohane P. Treatment of childhood asthma with anti-immunoglobulin E antibody (omalizumab). Pediatrics 2001;108(2):E36.
12. Casale TB. Experience with monoclonal antibodies in allergic mediated disease: seasonal allergic rhinitis. J Allergy Clin Immunol 2001;108(Suppl 2):S84–8.

Palivizumab

General Information

Palivizumab is a humanized monoclonal antibody that inhibits an epitope at the A antigenic site of the F protein of respiratory syncytial virus subtypes A and B (1).

Palivizumab is generally well tolerated (2). Its most common adverse effects (over 5%) are rhinitis, cough, fever, pharyngitis, bronchiolitis, and diarrhea (3).

In 565 patients with respiratory syncytial virus infections palivizumab caused injection site reactions (2.3%), fever (1.5%), and nervousness/irritability (under 1%); no other adverse effects were reported (4).

Organs and Systems

Immunologic

The estimated risk of anaphylactic reactions to palivizumab is under one per 100 000 infants (5). No second-season subjects had a significant antipalivizumab antibody response (titer over 1:80) (6).

References

1. Scott LJ, Lamb HM. Palivizumab. Drugs 1999;58(2):305–11.
2. Mejias A, Chavez-Bueno S, Rios AM, Fonseca-Aten M, Gomez AM, Jafri HS, Ramilo O. Asma y virus respiratorio sincitial. Nuevas oportunidades de intervencion terapeutica. [Asthma and respiratory syncytial virus. New opportunities for therapeutic intervention.] An Pediatr (Barc) 2004;61(3):252–60.
3. Groothuis JR. Safety of palivizumab in preterm infants 29 to 32 weeks' gestational age without chronic lung disease to prevent serious respiratory syncytial virus infection. Eur. J Clin Microbiol Infect Dis 2003;22(7):414–7.
4. Groothuis JR, Simpson SJNorthern Hemisphere Expanded Access Study Group. Safety and tolerance of palivizumab administration in a large Northern Hemisphere trial. Pediatr Infect Dis J 2001;20(6):628–30.
5. Anonymous. Palivizumab: new indication. Moderate reduction in hospitalisation rate. Prescrire Int 2004;13(74):213–6.
6. Lacaze-Masmonteil T, Seidenberg J, Mitchell I, Cossey V, Cihar M, Csader M, Baarsma R, Valido M, Pollack PF, Groothuis JRSecond Season Safety Study Group. Evaluation of the safety of palivizumab in the second season of exposure in young children at risk for severe respiratory syncytial virus infection. Drug Saf 2003;26(4):283–91.

Rituximab

General Information

Rituximab, a chimeric monoclonal antibody directed against the CD20 antigen of normal and malignant B lymphocytes, produces prolonged depletion of B lymphocytes. It has been used to treat refractory or relapsing follicular non-Hodgkin's lymphoma and has been tried in other B cell malignancies, including low-grade non-Hodgkin's lymphoma and diffuse large B cell lymphoma. There has also been interest in its use to treat autoimmune diseases (1–3) and in reducing anti-HLA antibodies in patients awaiting renal transplantation (4).

A wide range of adverse events has been reported in most patients (5). A transient flu-like syndrome is very common (50–90%), particularly after the first infusion of rituximab, and is often associated with various hypersensitivity-like symptoms (5–20%). In the most severe cases, patients had life-threatening cytokine release syndrome with dyspnea, bronchospasm, hypoxia, hypotension, urticaria, and angioedema. Deaths have been reported in eight of 12 000–14 000 patients after drug launch.

Severe reactions to rituximab are rare, but are seen in patients with bulky tumors or with leukemic involvement with high numbers of CD20 positive cells (6,7) and were ascribed to a rapid tumor lysis syndrome (6,8,9). In 11 patients with malignant B cell leukemia, first-dose reactions were significantly more severe in patients whose baseline lymphocyte count was higher than $50 \times 10^6/l$ and were also associated with raised peak serum concentrations of tumor necrosis factor alfa and interleukin-6 (10).

Organs and Systems

Cardiovascular

Cardiac dysrhythmias have been reported in 8% of patients treated with rituximab in patients with lymphomas (11).

Respiratory

Desquamative alveolitis has been reported in a 55-yearold woman with mantle-cell lymphoma given rituximab (12).

Sensory systems

A variety of ocular adverse effects, including conjunctivitis, transient ocular edema, and visual changes, occurred in 7% of patients receiving rituximab (11).

Hematologic

The factors associated with toxicity in patients with B cell lymphoma receiving rituximab have been studied in Japan (13). By univariate analysis overall non-hematological toxic effects (grade 2 or greater) were more frequent in patients with extranodal disease and especially in those with bone marrow involvement. Fever was more frequent in patients with raised LDH activity, whereas chills/rigors and vomiting were more frequent in patients with extranodal disease. Patients with raised LDH activity or extranodal disease may therefore require closer monitoring. Hematological toxic effects of grade 3 or worse were more common in women.

- A 26-year-old woman with a diffuse large B cell lymphoma received CHOP (cyclophosphamide, hydroxydaunomycin, Oncovin, and prednisone), rituximab, and radiotherapy (14). She developed a transfusion-dependent anemia. Bone marrow biopsy confirmed pure red cell aplasia and parvovirus infection. She had no antibodies to parvovirus, suggesting that she never had a previous exposure. Intravenous immunoglobulin resulted in a reticulocytosis and recovery of her hemoglobin.

The authors suggested that rituximab had depleted her primary B cells, resulting in an inability to mount a primary immune response to parvovirus infection. Parvovirus is pathogenic to red cell precursors, causing their destruction before release from the bone marrow.

Depletion of B lymphocytes by rituximab was suggested as a likely explanation for the occurrence of chronic parvovirus B19 infection complicated by pure red cell aplasia in a 45-year-old patient (15).

Thrombocytopenia leading to gastrointestinal bleeding has been attributed to rituximab (16).

Skin

Stevens–Johnson syndrome has been attributed to rituximab (17).

- A 33-year-old man with a follicular non-Hodgkin lymphoma entered a phase II trial of rituximab. The first two cycles were given without infusion-related toxicity, but during the second cycle mucositis was noticed. Before the third cycle he developed a pruritic rash on the trunk, grade 2 mucositis, and weight loss. He was given oral fluconazole, aciclovir, and antihistamines, which led to improvement. One week after the third infusion of rituximab he had grade 3 orogenital mucositis and the maculopapular rash on the trunk worsened, with areas of ulceration. Rituximab was withdrawn. Stevens–Johnson syndrome was confirmed by biopsy.

Immunologic

Infusion reactions with rituximab are generally well tolerated, as with most monoclonal antibodies. Most reactions are limited to the first infusion, including nausea, chills, and fever. They occur in over 90% of patients. More serious is the cytokine-release syndrome, which occurs within 60–90 minutes and is characterized by fever, chills, rigors, bronchospasm, hypoxia, hypotension, urticaria, and angioedema. Infusion must be discontinued, and the patient carefully monitored with chest radiography and fluid and electrolyte assessment and treated with oxygen and bronchodilators.

A rapid tumor clearance syndrome can occur within 30–60 minutes, with similar symptoms. Lymphocytes rapidly disappear from the peripheral blood and uric acid and lactate dehydrogenase increase markedly. Treatment includes interruption of the infusion, hydration, allopurinol, oxygen, and bronchodilators. It mainly occurs in patients with high white blood cell counts, such as those with chronic lymphatic leukemia.

Severe viral infections/reactivation that have been reported in patients given rituximab have included fulminant hepatitis B (18), parvovirus-induced red cell aplasia (15), and fatal *Varicella zoster* infection (19). There was a high incidence of reactivation of cytomegalovirus and *V. zoster* virus when rituximab was combined with high-dose chemotherapy in high-risk patients with non-Hodgkin's lymphoma (20).

Long-Term Effects

Tumorigenicity

A second cancer is possible when treating a tumor by mutagenicity or immunosuppression. There may be a link between the therapy given and the development of Merkel cell carcinoma (21).

- A 54-year-old man with stage I follicular lymphocytic lymphoma with cervical lymph nodes underwent splenectomy followed by chemotherapy with chlorambucil and had a partial response. Five months later, when he developed generalized lymphadenopathy and bone marrow involvement, he received fludarabine, cyclophosphamide, and rituximab, with complete remission. Ten months later he developed a Merkel cell carcinoma involving the liver and lymph nodes. The disseminated tumor was chemoresistant and he died. His lymphoma remained in complete clinical remission throughout this time.

Two patients developed a peripheral T cell non-Hodgkin's lymphoma after rituximab therapy, one after 15 months and the other after 18 months (22).

Rituximab was suggested as a possible cause of aggressive peripheral T cell lymphoma in two patients 15 and 18 months after the use of rituximab for low-grade B cell non-Hodgkin's lymphoma (23,24).

Second-Generation Effects

Pregnancy

There are few data on the use of rituximab in pregnancy, but one case has been reported.

- A pregnant woman with relapsed follicular non-Hodgkin's lymphoma took rituximab unintentionally during the first trimester (25). The disease stabilized and following an uncomplicated pregnancy a healthy child was born at full term. Careful hematological and immunological monitoring showed no adverse effects from exposure to rituximab.

References

1. Levine TD. Rituximab in the treatment of dermatomyositis: an open-label pilot study. Arthritis Rheum 2005;52(2):601–7.
2. Keogh KA, Wylam ME, Stone JH, Specks U. Induction of remission by B lymphocyte depletion in eleven patients with refractory antineutrophil cytoplasmic antibody-associated vasculitis. Arthritis Rheum 2005;52(1):262–8.
3. Gottenberg JE, Guillevin L, Lambotte O, Combe B, Allanore Y, Cantagrel A, Larroche C, Soubrier M, Bouillet L, Dougados M, Fain O, Farge D, Kyndt X, Lortholary O, Masson C, Moura B, Remy P, Thomas T, Wendling D, Anaya JM, Sibilia J, Mariette X. Club Rheumatismes et Inflammation (CRI). Tolerance and short term efficacy of rituximab in 43 patients with systemic autoimmune diseases. Ann Rheum Dis 2005;64(6):913–20.
4. Vieira CA, Agarwal A, Book BK, Sidner RA, Bearden CM, Gebel HM, Roggero AL, Fineberg NS, Taber T, Kraus MA, Pescovitz MD. Rituximab for reduction of anti-HLA antibodies in patients awaiting renal transplantation: 1. Safety, pharmacodynamics, and pharmacokinetics. Transplantation 2004;77(4):542–8.
5. Onrust SV, Lamb HM, Balfour JA. Rituximab. Drugs 1999;58(1):79–88.

6. Byrd JC, Waselenko JK, Maneatis TJ, Murphy T, Ward FT, Monahan BP, Sipe MA, Donegan S, White CA. Rituximab therapy in hematologic malignancy patients with circulating blood tumor cells: association with increased infusion-related side effects and rapid blood tumor clearance. J Clin Oncol 1999;17(3):791–5.

7. Davis TA, White CA, Grillo-Lopez AJ, Velasquez WS, Link B, Maloney DG, Dillman RO, Williams ME, Mohrbacher A, Weaver R, Dowden S, Levy R. Single-agent monoclonal antibody efficacy in bulky non-Hodgkin's lymphoma: results of a phase II trial of rituximab. J Clin Oncol 1999;17(6):1851–7.

8. Yang H, Rosove MH, Figlin RA. Tumor lysis syndrome occurring after the administration of rituximab in lymphoproliferative disorders: high-grade non-Hodgkin's lymphoma and chronic lymphocytic leukemia. Am J Hematol 1999;62(4):247–50.

9. van der Kolk LE, Grillo-Lopez AJ, Baars JW, Hack CE, van Oers MH. Complement activation plays a key role in the side-effects of rituximab treatment. Br J Haematol 2001;115(4):807–11.

10. Winkler U, Jensen M, Manzke O, Schulz H, Diehl V, Engert A. Cytokine-release syndrome in patients with B-cell chronic lymphocytic leukemia and high lymphocyte counts after treatment with an anti-CD20 monoclonal antibody (rituximab, IDEC-C2B8). Blood 1999;94(7):2217–24.

11. Foran JM, Rohatiner AZ, Cunningham D, Popescu RA, Solal-Celigny P, Ghielmini M, Coiffier B, Johnson PW, Gisselbrecht C, Reyes F, Radford JA, Bessell EM, Souleau B, Benzohra A, Lister TA. European phase II study of rituximab (chimeric anti-CD20 monoclonal antibody) for patients with newly diagnosed mantle-cell lymphoma and previously treated mantle-cell lymphoma, immunocytoma, and small B cell lymphocytic lymphoma. J Clin Oncol 2000;18(2):317–24.

12. Zerga M, Cerchetti L, Cicco J, Constantini P, De Riz M. Desquamative alveolitis: an unusual complication of treatment with Mabthera. Blood 1999;94(Suppl 1):271.

13. Igarashi T, Kobayashi Y, Ogura M, Kinoshita T, Ohtsu T, Sasaki Y, Morishima Y, Murate T, Kasai M, Uike N, Taniwaki M, Kano Y, Ohnishi K, Matsuno Y, Nakamura S, Mori S, Ohashi Y, Tobinai KIDEC-C2B8 Study Group in Japan. Factors affecting toxicity, response and progression-free survival in relapsed patients with indolent B-cell lymphoma and mantle cell lymphoma treated with rituximab: a Japanese phase II study. Ann Oncol 2002;13(6):928–43.

14. Song KW, Mollee P, Patterson B, Brien W, Crump M. Pure red cell aplasia due to parvovirus following treatment with CHOP and rituximab for B-cell lymphoma. Br J Haematol 2002;119(1):125–7.

15. Sharma VR, Fleming DR, Slone SP. Pure red cell aplasia due to parvovirus B19 in a patient treated with rituximab. Blood 2000;96(3):1184–6.

16. Hagberg H, Lundholm L. Rituximab, a chimaeric anti-CD20 monoclonal antibody, in the treatment of hairy cell leukaemia. Br J Haematol 2001;115(3):609–11.

17. Lowndes S, Darby A, Mead G, Lister A. Stevens–Johnson syndrome after treatment with rituximab. Ann Oncol 2002;13(12):1948–50.

18. Dervite I, Hober D, Morel P. Acute hepatitis B in a patient with antibodies to hepatitis B surface antigen who was receiving rituximab. N Engl J Med 2001;344(1):68–9.

19. Bermudez A, Marco F, Conde E, Mazo E, Recio M, Zubizarreta A. Fatal visceral varicella-zoster infection following rituximab and chemotherapy treatment in a patient with follicular lymphoma. Haematologica 2000;85(8):894–5.

20. Ladetto M, Zallio F, Vallet S, Ricca I, Cuttica A, Caracciolo D, Corradini P, Astolfi M, Sametti S, Volpato F, Bondesan P, Vitolo U, Boccadoro M, Pileri A, Gianni AM, Tarella C. Concurrent administration of high-dose chemotherapy and rituximab is a feasible and effective chemo/immunotherapy for patients with high-risk non-Hodgkin's lymphoma. Leukemia 2001;15(12):1941–9.

21. Cohen Y, Amir G, Polliack A. Development and rapid dissemination of Merkel-cell carcinomatosis following therapy with fludarabine and rituximab for relapsing follicular lymphoma. Eur J Haematol 2002;68(2):117–9.

22. Cheson BD. Rituximab: clinical development and future directions. Expert Opin Biol Ther 2002;2(1):97–110.

23. Micallef IN, Kirk A, Norton A, Foran JM, Rohatiner AZ, Lister TA. Peripheral T-cell lymphoma following rituximab therapy for B-cell lymphoma. Blood 1999;93(7):2427–8.

24. Tetreault S, Abler SL, Robbins B, Saven A. Peripheral T-cell lymphoma after anti-CD20 antibody therapy. J Clin Oncol 1998;16(4):1635–7.

25. Kimby E, Sverrisdottir A, Elinder G. Safety of rituximab therapy during the first trimester of pregnancy: a case history. Eur J Haematol 2004;72(4):292–5.

TGN1412

General Information

TGN1412 is an agonistic anti-CD28 monoclonal antibody. CD28 is a co-stimulatory receptor on CD4 T lymphocytes and on many CD8 T lymphocytes. TGN1412 was genetically engineered by a company called Te Genera, by transfer of the complementarity determining regions (CDRs) from heavy and light chain variable region sequences of a monoclonal mouse anti-human CD28 antibody into human heavy and light chain variable region frameworks. Humanized variable regions were subsequently recombined with two human genes, one coding for the IgG4 γ chain and one coding for a κ chain. The intention was that TGN1412 would activate and expand regulatory T lymphocytes and induce anti-inflammatory cytokines. The proposed indicatins were B-cell chronic lymphocytic leukemia and rheumatoid arthritis.

Organs and Systems

Autacoids

At a research unit in Northwick Park Hospital in North London on 13 March2006 six healthy volunteers received TGN1412 and two received placebo in a first-in-man study run by a contract research company called Parexel. Within hours all six who had been given TGN1412 were in intensive care with severe inflammatory reactions that progressed to multiorgan failure (1). Their symptoms were as follows: headache within 50–90 minutes; lumbar myalgia, rigors within 1–2 hours, and a fever over 38 °C within 2.5–6.5 hours. They subsequently developed hypotension and tachycardia, dyspnea, tachypnea, and respiratory failure, radiological pulmonary infiltrates, and evidence of disseminated intravascular coagulation; two had peripheral limb ischemia and one developed dry gangrene of the fingers and toes. All developed lymphopenia, with significant falls in CD3, CD4 + , and CD8 + counts All recovered, but had prolonged memory problems, headaches, and inability to concentrate.

This syndrome was due to a massive cytokine storm. Serum concentrations of TNFα rose markedly within 1 hour, and TNFγ, IL-2, IL-4, IL-6, and IL-10 all increased over days 1 and 2; there were very large increases in interferon gamma at 4 hours and on day 2.

T lymphocytes normally require both antigen receptor stimulation and co-stimulation of CD28 receptors to become fully activated. However, TGN1412 was a super-agonist, and it stimulated T (and B) lymphocyte activity without the need for concurrent antigen receptor stimulation. In vitro experiments had not predicted this effect.

Following an enquiry by an independent expert scientific group, chaired by Sir Gordon Duff, Chairman of the Commission on Human Medicines (CHM, which was formed in February 2005 by conjoining the former Medicines Commission and the Committee on Safety of Medicines, CSM), the following 22 recommendations were made (2):

1. The strategy for preclinical development of a new medicine and the experimental approaches used to assemble information relevant to the safety of phase one trials must be regarded as science-based decisions, made and justified case-by-case by investigators with appropriate training.
2. Developers of medicines, research funding bodies, and regulatory authorities should expedite the collection of information on unpublished preclinical studies and phase one trials, and explore the feasibility of open access to this database.
3. Regulatory authorities should consider ways to expedite the sharing between regulators worldwide of information on Suspected Unexpected Serious Adverse Reactions (SUSARs) in phase one trials, and explore the feasibility of open access to this data.
4. A broader approach to dose calculation, beyond reliance on 'No Effect Level' or 'No Adverse Effect Level' in animal studies, should be taken. The calculation of starting dose should utilise all relevant information. Factors to be taken into account include the novelty of the agent and its mechanism of action, the degree of species-specificity of the agent, the dose-response curves of biological effects in human and animal cells, dose-response data from in vivo animal studies where relevance to human has been validated, the calculation of receptor occupancy versus concentration and the calculated exposure of targets or target cells in humans in vivo. The 'MABEL' approach is a good option for achieving this.
5. If different methods give different estimates of a safe dose in humans, the lowest value should be taken as the starting point in first-in-man trials and a margin of safety introduced.
6. When it is likely that preclinical information, for any reason, may be a poor guide to human responses in vivo, the starting dose in first-in-man trials should be calculated to err on the side of caution.
7. Careful consideration should be given to the route and the rate of administration of the first dose in first-in-man trials, with careful monitoring for an exaggerated response.
8. Decisions on starting dose and dose escalation should be made on a case-by-case basis, and should be scientifically justifiable, taking account of all relevant information.
9. The decision whether to conduct a first-in-man trial in healthy volunteers or in volunteer patients should be carefully considered and fully justified, taking into account all factors relevant to the safety of the subjects and the value of the scientific information that is likely to be obtained.
10. Principal Investigators in first-in-man trials should always be appropriately qualified and satisfy themselves that they know enough about the agent, its target and mechanism of action to be in a position to make informed clinical judgements.
11. In first-in-man studies where there is a predictable risk of certain types of severe adverse reaction, a treatment strategy should be considered beforehand. This should include the availability of specific antidotes where they exist and a clear plan of supportive treatment, including the pre-arranged contingency availability of ITU facilities.
12. First-in-man studies of higher risk medicines should always be conducted in an appropriate clinical environment supervised by staff with appropriate levels of training and expertise with immediate access to facilities for the treatment and stabilisation of individuals in an acute emergency and with pre-arranged contingency availability of ITU facilities.
13. New agents in first-in-man trials should be administered sequentially to subjects with an appropriate period of observation between dosing.
14. The interval of observation between sequential dosing of the subjects should be related to the kind of adverse reactions that might be anticipated based on the nature of the agent, its target and the recipient.
15. A similar period of monitoring should occur between sequential dosing of subjects during dose escalation.
16. More communication should be encouraged between developers and the regulator at an earlier stage before an application is filed, especially for higher risk agents, to ensure that there is time for an appropriate consideration of any safety concerns without introducing undue delay to product development. Ways to increase communication between the regulator and research ethics committees should also be considered.
17. For appraisal of applications for trials of higher risk agents, as defined by the nature of the agent, its degree of novelty, its intended pharmacological target, and its intended recipient, the regulator should have access to additional opinion from independent, specialist experts with research knowledge of their fields.
18. An Expert Advisory Group (EAG) of the Commission on Human Medicines, or a similar

body, might undertake this role with a core membership of appropriate experts and the ability to co-opt additional experts as the need dictates.

19. Consideration should be given to introducing some flexibility in the time-scale of clinical trial appraisal in exceptional cases of unusual complexity.

20. The availability of "hands-on" experience in the planning and conduct of clinical trials should be widened, for example by secondment periods to commercial organisations within postgraduate training programmes, or the development of specialist centres within the NHS and Universities (see next recommendation).

21. The feasibility of developing specialist centres for phase one clinical trials of higher risk agents and advanced medicinal products should be explored.

22. The regulatory process for first-in-man trials of higher risk agents and advanced medicinal products based on innovative technologies should be subject to frequent review.

References

1. Medicines and Healthcare products Regulatory Agency. Investigations into adverse incidents during clinical trials of TGN1412. 25 May 2006. http://www.mhra.gov.uk/NewsCentre/Pressreleases/CON2023822.

2. Department of Health. Expert Group on Phase One Clinical Trials. Final report. http://www.dh.gov.uk/en/Publicationsandstatistics/Publications/PublicationsPolicyAndGuidance/DH_063117.

Trastuzumab

General Information

Trastuzumab is a recombinant humanized monoclonal antibody that binds to the proto-oncogene, HER-2/neu gene product, which is expressed in 25–30% of primary breast cancers. It has been used to treat selected patients with metastatic breast cancer whose tumors overexpress the HER2 protein, which is amplified in 25–30% of breast cancers and is associated with an aggressive form of disease (1). Adverse effects mostly consisted of infusion-related constitutional symptoms, digestive disorders (diarrhea, vomiting), pain, cough, headache, dyspnea, mild infections, and insomnia. Compared with chemotherapy alone, the addition of trastuzumab more often produced moderately severe adverse hematological effects (leukopenia and anemia) and diarrhea. Severe congestive cardiac failure is a major adverse effect of trastuzumab. According to the product labelling, severe cardiac failure was observed in 5–19% of patients (trastuzumab alone versus trastuzumab plus anthracycline and cyclophosphamide). Other serious adverse events, including death, have occurred in 0.25% of patients treated with trastuzumab. They fall into three categories: infusion reactions; hypersensitivity reactions, including fatal anaphylaxis; and pulmonary events, including adult respiratory distress syndrome.

Organs and Systems

Cardiovascular

Cardiotoxicity is a major concern with trastuzumab, particularly as it is often used in patients who are receiving or who have previously received anthracycline antibiotics (2). It occurs in 5% of patients given trastuzumab alone, in 13% of patients given trastuzumab with paclitaxel, and in 27% of patients given trastuzumab in combination with anthracyclines and cyclophosphamide (3).

The efficacy and safety of trastuzumab have been evaluated in 235 women with metastatic breast cancer receiving standard chemotherapy (4). The most important adverse event was cardiac failure, which occurred in 27% of those who were given anthracycline, cyclophosphamide, and trastuzumab, 8% of those who were given anthracycline and cyclophosphamide alone, 13% of those who were given paclitaxel and trastuzumab, and 1% of those who were given paclitaxel alone. The incidence of cardiac failure of New York Heart Association class III or class IV was highest among patients who had received an anthracycline, cyclophosphamide, and trastuzumab. The mechanism is unknown. In a retrospective analysis of all patients with cardiac failure by an independent review and evaluation committee, the only significant risk factor was older age. Although the cardiotoxicity was severe, and in some cases life-threatening, the symptoms improved with standard medical management.

Seven phase II and III clinical trials of trastuzumab in patients with metastatic breast cancer have been reviewed (5). The physiopathology of trastuzumab-associated cardiac disease is poorly understood, and baseline MUGA scanning is recommended to identify cardiac disease. The rates of cardiac disease were highest when trastuzumab was given in combination with anthracyclines or when there had been previous exposure to anthracyclines. Given the 25% improvement in overall survival in these patients with metastatic disease, the use of trastuzumab is justified.

- A 60-year-old woman with coronary heart disease and hypertension developed breast cancer and a core biopsy showed ER+/PR+/HER2-3+ (3). She enrolled in an institutional study with neoadjuvant trastuzumab with docetaxel. A pretreatment blood pool radionuclide angiography (MUGA) scan revealed a left ventricular ejection fraction of 56%. She had a good clinical response to treatment at 3 months. Before surgery a repeat MUGA showed a dilated left ventricle and a reduced ejection fraction (35%). She underwent surgery and 2 months later her ejection fraction was 44%.
- An overweight 59-year-old woman with hypertension and asthma developed breast cancer (ER+/PR+/HER2-2+) (3). Her MUGA scan showed a left ventricular ejection fraction of 57%. She was given trastuzumab with docetaxel and had a good response after 4

months. Before surgery she became dyspneic, and a MUGA scan showed an ejection fraction of 24%; even 7 months after surgery her MUGA scan showed no improvement.

The efficacy and tolerability of trastuzumab in clinical trials has been reviewed (6). Of the first 48 patients treated in Sweden with or without chemotherapy, two had serious cardiac events and both had previously been treated with an anthracycline. As not all patients who received trastuzumab had echocardiography, the number of cardiac events was probably underestimated. It has been postulated that HER2 pathways may be involved in myocyte repair, and that concomitant administration of trastuzumab may interfere with the repair of anthracycline-damaged myocytes (7). Evidence from 20 patients has shown that cardiotoxicity is related to trastuzumab uptake in the myocardium, suggesting that the extent of HER2 receptor expression, or a related cross-reactive antigen in the myocardium, may be the underlying mechanism.

Respiratory

The toxicity of five escalating doses of trastuzumab (1–8 mg/kg) when combined with a fixed dose of interleukin-2 has been determined in 45 patients with non-hematological malignancies that overexpressed HER2 (8). There was no evidence of increasing toxicity related to the dose of trastuzumab. Five patients had pulmonary toxicity of grade 3 or higher; these were primarily attributed to interleukin-2, as the patients improved on reduction of the dose of interleukin-2.

Drug–Drug Interactions

Doxorubicin

An interaction of doxorubicin with the anti-HER$_2$ receptor humanized monoclonal antibody, trastuzumab (Herceptin), has been reported. Most patients who received trastuzumab in early trials had been pretreated with anthracyclines. Despite this, preliminary information suggested that reduced systolic cardiac function was an adverse effect of trastuzumab (10). More recently, this problem has been further highlighted in a study of women with metastatic breast cancer (11). Patients who had not received prior anthracycline-containing adjuvant chemotherapy were at greater risk of cardiotoxicity when they received trastuzumab in combination with doxorubicin or cyclophosphamide (27 and 75% respectively), compared with only 11% of patients who received trastuzumab in combination with paclitaxel (11,12). The risk of cardiac events in patients treated with doxorubicin, cyclophosphamide, and trastuzumab increased markedly after a cumulative doxorubicin dose of 360 mg/m^2. This suggests synergistic cardiotoxicity with trastuzumab and doxorubicin. Trastuzumab is therefore currently licensed only for use in conjunction with paclitaxel or docetaxel and not with conventional doxorubicin.

The mechanism of trastuzumab-induced cardiotoxicity and its synergy with doxorubicin is as yet unknown. However, the cardiac failure responds to standard medical management (13).

Since trastuzumab is active as a single agent and in combination with chemotherapy in patients whose tumors overexpress HER$_2$, the interaction with doxorubicin is clearly of concern. Although it is possible to avoid this problem by not combining trastuzumab with doxorubicin, there are compelling reasons for further exploring its use with anthracyclines. For example, follow-up results from the CALGB 8541 study have shown that patients who received high and moderate (standard) doses of cyclophosphamide plus doxorubicin plus fluorouracil survived longer than those who received low doses (14). Moreover, examination of patients' HER$_2$ status in this trial showed that those whose tumors expressed large amounts of the HER$_2$ protein had a significantly worse survival if treated with moderate or low doses of cyclophosphamide plus doxorubicin plus fluorouracil, compared with high doses (15). These results suggest that patients whose tumors express large amounts of the HER$_2$ receptor protein may require high-dose anthracyclines, presenting the problem of how then to treat them with trastuzumab without causing cardiotoxicity.

In an attempt to avoid cardiotoxicity after the administration of trastuzumab with doxorubicin, alternative adjuvant regimens have been suggested. Trastuzumab could be combined with other anthracyclines (epirubicin or liposomal formulations), which are inherently less cardiotoxic, or given sequentially rather than concomitantly with the anthracycline. Alternatively, non-anthracycline combinations, such as cyclophosphamide plus doxorubicin plus fluorouracil or based around taxanes, cisplatin, and vinorelbine are being investigated (16).

Caution should of course be exercised when giving other cytotoxic drugs, especially myelotoxic agents or agents that cause significant mucositis/stomatitis, in combination with anthracyclines.

Paclitaxel

In primates, trastuzumab clearance was reduced when it was administered with paclitaxel (9).

References

1. Goldenberg MM. Trastuzumab, a recombinant DNA-derived humanized monoclonal antibody, a novel agent for the treatment of metastatic breast cancer. Clin Ther 1999;21(2):309–18.
2. Seidman AD, Fornier MN, Esteva FJ, Tan L, Kaptain S, Bach A, Panageas KS, Arroyo C, Valero V, Currie V, Gilewski T, Theodoulou M, Moynahan ME, Moasser M, Sklarin N, Dickler M, D'Andrea G, Cristofanilli M, Rivera E, Hortobagyi GN, Norton L, Hudis CA. Weekly trastuzumab and paclitaxel therapy for metastatic breast cancer with analysis of efficacy by HER2 immunophenotype and gene amplification. J Clin Oncol 2001;19(10):2587–95.
3. Tham YL, Verani MS, Chang J. Reversible and irreversible cardiac dysfunction associated with trastuzumab in breast cancer. Breast Cancer Res Treat 2002;74(2):131–4.

4. Slamon DJ, Leyland-Jones B, Shak S, Fuchs H, Paton V, Bajamonde A, Fleming T, Eiermann W, Wolter J, Pegram M, Baselga J, Norton L. Use of chemotherapy plus a monoclonal antibody against HER2 for metastatic breast cancer that overexpresses HER2. N Engl J Med 2001;344(11):783–92.

5. Seidman A, Hudis C, Pierri MK, Shak S, Paton V, Ashby M, Murphy M, Stewart SJ, Keefe D. Cardiac dysfunction in the trastuzumab clinical trials experience. J Clin Oncol 2002;20(5):1215–21.

6. Andersson J, Linderholm B, Greim G, Lindh B, Lindman H, Tennvall J, Tennvall-Nittby L, Pettersson-Skold D, Sverrisdottir A, Soderberg M, Klaar S, Bergh J. A population-based study on the first forty-eight breast cancer patients receiving trastuzumab (Herceptin) on a named patient basis in Sweden. Acta Oncol 2002;41(3):276–81.

7. Leonard DS, Hill AD, Kelly L, Dijkstra B, McDermott E, O'Higgins NJ. Anti-human epidermal growth factor receptor 2 monoclonal antibody therapy for breast cancer. Br J Surg 2002;89(3):262–71.

8. Fleming GF, Meropol NJ, Rosner GL, Hollis DR, Carson WE 3rd, Caligiuri M, Mortimer J, Tkaczuk K, Parihar R, Schilsky RL, Ratain MJ. A phase I trial of escalating doses of trastuzumab combined with daily subcutaneous interleukin 2: report of cancer and leukemia group B 9661. Clin Cancer Res 2002;8(12):3718–27.

9. McKeage K, Perry CM. Trastuzumab: a review of its use in the treatment of metastatic breast cancer overexpressing HER2. Drugs 2002;62(1):209–43.

10. Cobleigh MA, Vogel CL, Tripathy D, Robert NJ, Scholl S, Fehrenbacher L, Wolter JM, Paton V, Shak S, Lieberman G, Slamon DJ. Multinational study of the efficacy and safety of humanized anti-HER2 monoclonal antibody in women who have HER2-overexpressing metastatic breast cancer that has progressed after chemotherapy for metastatic disease. J Clin Oncol 1999;17(9):2639–48.

11. Slamon DJ, Leyland-Jones B, Shak S, Fuchs H, Paton V, Bajamonde A, Fleming T, Eiermann W, Wolter J, Pegram M, Baselga J, Norton L. Use of chemotherapy plus a monoclonal antibody against HER2 for metastatic breast cancer that overexpresses HER2. N Engl J Med 2001;344(11):783–92.

12. Slamon D, Leyland-Jones B, Shak S, Paton V, Bajamonde A, Flemiong T, Eirmann W, Wolter J, Baselga J, Norton L. Addition of Herceptin (humanized anti-HER2 antibody) to first line chemotherapy for HER2 overexpressing metastatic breast cancer (HER2+/MBC) markedly increases anticancer activity: a randomised, multinational, controlled phase III trial (Abstract 377). Proc Am Soc Clin Oncol 1998;17:98a.

13. Gianni L. Tolerability in patients receiving trastuzumab with or without chemotherapy. Ann Oncol 2001;12(Suppl 1):S63–8.

14. Budman DR, Berry DA, Cirrincione CT, Henderson IC, Wood WC, Weiss RB, Ferree CR, Muss HB, Green MR, Norton L, Frei E 3rd. Dose and dose intensity as determinants of outcome in the adjuvant treatment of breast cancer. The Cancer and Leukemia Group B. J Natl Cancer Inst 1998;90(16):1205–11.

15. Thor AD, Berry DA, Budman DR, Muss HB, Kute T, Henderson IC, Barcos M, Cirrincione C, Edgerton S, Allred C, Norton L, Liu ET. erbB-2, p53, and efficacy of adjuvant therapy in lymph node-positive breast cancer. J Natl Cancer Inst 1998;90(18):1346–60.

16. Smith I. Future directions in the adjuvant treatment of breast cancer: the role of trastuzumab. Ann Oncol 2001;12(Suppl 1):S75–9.

IMMUNE MODULATORS

IMMUNOSUPPRESSANTS

Azathioprine and mercaptopurine

General Information

Azathioprine, a prodrug converted to 6-mercaptopurine, is widely used as a post-transplant immunosuppressant and in various autoimmune or chronic inflammatory disorders, such as rheumatoid arthritis, dermatomyositis, systemic lupus erythematosus, skin diseases, and inflammatory bowel diseases.

Adverse effects usually occur during the first two months of treatment, do not correlate with the daily dose, and result in treatment withdrawal in 14–18% of patients, mainly because of bone marrow suppression, gastrointestinal symptoms, hypersensitivity reactions, and infections (1–3). Immediate or long-term adverse effects are of particular concern outside the field of immunosuppression where other treatment options are frequently available, but in any field of use the adverse effects of these drugs weigh heavily.

Observational studies

In a follow-up study of 157 patients receiving azathioprine or mercaptopurine for Crohn's disease, the long-term risks (mainly hematological toxicity and malignancies) over 4 years of treatment were deemed to outweigh the therapeutic benefit (4). In contrast to these findings, both drugs were considered efficacious and reasonably safe in patients with inflammatory bowel disease, provided that patients are carefully selected and regularly investigated for bone marrow toxicity (5). Similar opinions were expressed regarding renal transplant patients. Conversion from ciclosporin to azathioprine in selected and carefully monitored patients had beneficial effects, by improving renal function, reducing cardiovascular risk factors, and reducing financial costs, without increasing the incidence of chronic rejection and graft loss (6).

Experience in children with juvenile chronic arthritis or chronic inflammatory bowel disease has also accumulated, and the toxicity profile of azathioprine or mercaptopurine appears to be very similar to that previously found in the adult population (SEDA-21, 381; SEDA-22, 410).

The "azathioprine hypersensitivity syndrome"

The complex of azathioprine-associated multisystemic adverse effects is referred to by the misnomer "azathioprine hypersensitivity syndrome." This well-characterized reaction has been described in numerous case reports and includes various symptoms which can occur separately or concomitantly; they comprise fever and rigors, arthralgia, myalgia, leukocytosis, cutaneous reactions, gastrointestinal disturbances, hypotension, liver injury, pancreatitis, interstitial nephritis, pneumonitis, and pulmonary hemorrhage (SED-13, 1121; SEDA-20, 341; SEDA-21, 381; SEDA-22, 410; 7). Isolated fever and rigors are sometimes observed, and severe renal and cardiac toxicity or leukocytoclastic cutaneous vasculitis are infrequent. Symptoms usually occur within the first 6 weeks of treatment and can mimic sepsis. The initial febrile reaction is often misdiagnosed as infectious, and could be associated with acute exacerbation of the underlying disease, for example myasthenia gravis (SEDA-21, 381; SEDA-22, 410). Hypersensitivity associated with reversible interstitial nephritis can also be mistaken for an acute rejection episode (8). This syndrome should therefore be promptly recognized to avoid unnecessary and costly investigations, and further recurrence on azathioprine rechallenge.

Organs and Systems

Respiratory

Although azathioprine-associated pulmonary toxicity mostly occurs as part of the azathioprine hypersensitivity reaction, isolated interstitial pneumonitis has been reported in a 13-year-old girl with autoimmune chronic active hepatitis (9).

Acute upper airway edema has been observed after a single dose of azathioprine (10).

- A 57-year-old woman with a history of several drug allergies underwent renal transplantation for end-stage polycystic kidney disease and 1 hour later was given intravenous azathioprine 400 mg. She developed profound hypotension and bradycardia within 30 minutes, reversed by sympathomimetics. Shortly after extubation, she had severe breathing difficulties with loss of consciousness. Laryngoscopy showed massive swelling of the tongue and upper airways. Later, while still taking glucocorticoids, she was rechallenged with azathioprine and had milder hypotension and edema of the airways.

Even if no clear mechanism can account for this adverse effect, positive rechallenge strongly suggested that azathioprine was the culprit.

Hematologic

Hematological toxicity is the most commonly reported severe adverse effect of azathioprine, and is marked by predominant leukopenia, thrombocytopenia, and pancytopenia (SED-13, 1120). In a 27-year survey of 739 patients treated with azathioprine 2 mg/kg for inflammatory bowel disease, dosage reduction or withdrawal of the drug because of bone marrow toxicity was necessary in 37 patients (5%) (11). There was moderate or severe leukopenia in 3.8% of patients; in three patients pancytopenia resulted in severe sepsis or death.

Leukopenia is the most serious adverse effect of azathioprine in patients with inflammatory bowel disease (12). It is variable and unpredictable and occurs 2 weeks to 11 years after the start of treatment (median 9 months); most cases recover 1 month after withdrawal.

Dual therapy with ciclosporin and prednisone has been compared with triple therapy with ciclosporin, prednisone, and azathioprine in a randomized trial in 250 renal transplant patients (13). Patients in the triple therapy group had less frequent severe episodes of acute rejection and more frequent episodes of leukopenia than the double therapy group (28% versus 4%). There were no other differences in the adverse effects profiles, in particular the incidence of infectious complications.

Macrocytic anemia and isolated thrombocytopenia without severe clinical consequences have sometimes been observed. Pure red cell aplasia can occur, but the few relevant reports concern only isolated instances involving renal transplant patients (14,15). The facts in one patient suggested that parvovirus B19 infection resulting from the immunosuppressive effects of azathioprine should also be considered as a possible indirect cause (16). Although blood cell disorders usually occur in the first 4 weeks of treatment, strict and regular surveillance of blood cell counts continuing for as long as treatment is maintained is usually recommended, since delayed hematological toxicity remains possible.

- Immune hemolytic anemia has been reported in a 67-year-old man taking mercaptopurine for chronic myelomonocytic leukemia (17). Serology showed a positive direct antiglobulin test and confirmed the presence of mercaptopurine drug-dependent antibodies. He improved and the direct antiglobulin test was no longer positive 20 days after mercaptopurine withdrawal.

Aplastic anemia due to azathioprine therapy after corneal transplantation has reportedly caused bilateral macular hemorrhage (18).

- A 38-year-old man underwent therapeutic penetrating keratoplasty for non-healing fungal keratitis in his left eye. Although the infection was controlled, he underwent a second corneal transplantation after 2 years. Since there was corneal vascularization in three quadrants, he was given oral azathioprine postoperatively. Four months later he developed gastrointestinal bleeding and a sudden reduction in vision in both eyes. His platelet count was less than $30 \times 10^9/l$, his hemoglobin 4.1 g/dl, and a bone marrow aspirate was hypocellular. There were macular hemorrhages in both eyes. The hemorrhages resolved within 2 months.

Gastrointestinal

Gastrointestinal disturbances with nausea, vomiting, and diarrhea are frequent in patients taking azathioprine or mercaptopurine. Diarrhea may be isolated or part of the azathioprine hypersensitivity syndrome. In two patients with azathioprine-induced diarrhea proven by positive rechallenge, the period of sensitization ranged from 1 week to 1 year (19).

In two cases, azathioprine caused severe gastrointestinal symptoms that could have been easily confused with an acute exacerbation of the underlying inflammatory bowel disease (20).

- A 32-year-old man with ulcerative colitis improved with prednisolone, mesalazine, and antibiotics. The dose of prednisolone was reduced and the disease flared up again. He was therefore given azathioprine and an increased dose of prednisolone, with rapid clinical improvement. After 3 weeks, he reported increasing abdominal pain, worse diarrhea, and weight loss of 3 kg. He stopped taking azathioprine and the pain improved. Because of progressive disease and active pancolitis at colonoscopy, he was given high-dose prednisolone, mesalazine, and ciprofloxacin, without improvement. He was therefore given intravenous azathioprine, but developed devastating diarrhea and weight loss of more than 6 kg in 24 hours, his CRP rose from 5 to 305 µg/ml, and he developed hypovolemic shock. He recovered after treatment with parenteral nutrition for 7 days.
- A 50-year-old woman with Crohn's disease and active disease throughout the colon was given prednisolone, mesalazine, and azathioprine 50 mg/day. After 3 weeks, the dose of azathioprine was increased to 100 mg/day, but she developed nausea, severe diarrhea, and abdominal tenderness. The symptoms subsided after azathioprine was withdrawn. She was then given mercaptopurine, without significant adverse effects.

Liver

Although rarely severe, any increase in liver enzyme activity justifies careful and regular monitoring of liver function and the results may be a reason for withdrawing treatment (SED-8, 1118; 21). In a retrospective study, hepatitis was found in 21 (2%) of 1035 renal transplant patients, and it was suggested that hepatitis B or C infection increases the risk of azathioprine hepatotoxicity (22). In 29 cardiac transplant recipients who had had probable azathioprine-induced liver dysfunction, cyclophosphamide was given, with improvement of liver enzyme activities and no increase in the rate of graft rejection or significant changes in the doses of other immunosuppressive drugs (23).

Azathioprine can cause reversible cholestasis (24), perhaps due to bile duct injury (25).

Direct hepatocellular injury with acute cytolytic hepatitis has been reported rarely (SEDA-21, 381).

In one patient, azathioprine-induced lymphoma with massive liver infiltration was the probable cause of fulminant hepatic failure (SEDA-21, 381).

Other histological features that have been described include lesions of the hepatic venous system (peliosis hepatis, sinusoidal dilatation, perivenous fibrosis, and nodular regenerative hyperplasia) and these can be associated with portal hypertension (SEDA-16, 520; SED-13, 1120; 21). Particularly severe and potentially fatal veno-occlusive liver disease has been reported in patients with renal and allogeneic bone marrow transplants taking chronic treatment (SEDA-12, 386; 26), but complete histological reversal can be observed (SEDA-20, 341).

- In a 33-year-old man azathioprine-induced veno-occlusive disease was treated with a transjugular intrahepatic portosystemic shunt over 26 months, with progressive worsening 15 months after renal transplantation (27).

Four patients with renal transplants developed hepatic veno-occlusive disease after immunosuppression with azathioprine. The diagnosis was based on typical histopathological findings: perivenular fibrosis, trilobular sinusoidal dilatation and congestion, and perisinusoidal fibrosis. The patients presented with severe progressive portal hypertension followed by fulminant liver failure and death. The disease was associated with cytomegalovirus infection, and it was not related to the dose of azathioprine (26). Veno-occlusive liver disease has also been described shortly after liver transplantation (28,29). A history of acute liver rejection affecting the hepatic veins was supposedly a contributing factor in these patients, and the presence of non-inflammatory small hepatic vein lesions was a possible early indicator of hepatotoxicity. Liver biopsy should therefore be considered in liver recipients who have biological features of hepatitis, so that treatment can be withdrawn rapidly if necessary.

Azathioprine allergy can be associated with biochemical hepatitis and a normal liver biopsy, apart form marked lipofuscin deposition (30). These findings, combined with patchy isotope uptake on technetium scintigraphy, are suggestive of focal hepatocellular necrosis.

It has been suggested that there is an increased risk of azathioprine-induced liver damage in renal transplant patients with chronic viral hepatitis (SEDA-20, 341; SEDA-23, 402).

- Fatal fibrosing cholestatic hepatitis has been reported in a 63-year-old cardiac transplant patient with acquired post-transplant hepatitis C virus infection whose immunosuppressive regimen included azathioprine (31). Histology showed several features of azathioprine hepatotoxicity, namely veno-subocclusive lesions and nodular regenerative diffuse hyperplasia, suggesting a pathogenic role of azathioprine.

In 79 renal transplant patients with chronic viral hepatitis, azathioprine maintenance treatment ($n = 34$) was associated with a poorer outcome than in 45 patients who discontinued azathioprine (32). Cirrhosis was more frequent in the first group (six versus one), and more patients died with a functioning graft (14 versus two), mostly because of liver dysfunction ($n = 5$) or infection ($n = 6$). These results suggest that azathioprine further accelerates the course of the liver disease in these patients.

- A 50-year-old woman with nodular sclerosis developed azathioprine-induced hepatotoxicity within the first weeks of treatment (33), the usual time-course. Positive rechallenge confirmed the role of azathioprine.

However, delayed occurrence of hepatitis is also possible.

- Canalicular cholestasis with portal fibrosis and ductal proliferation has been reported after 24 years of azathioprine in a 57-year-old woman with myasthenia gravis (34).

An unusual diffuse liver disease with sinusoidal dilatation (SEDA-11, 392) has been described.

Pancreas

Pancreatitis due to azathioprine or mercaptopurine has usually been reported as part of the hypersensitivity syndrome (SEDA-16, 520; SEDA-20, 341). It has mostly been observed in patients with inflammatory bowel disease, and required withdrawal of treatment in 1.3% of patients with Crohn's disease (3). Pancreatitis was not dose-related within the therapeutic range of doses and often recurred in patients who were rechallenged with either drug (SEDA-20, 341; 35). Fatal hemorrhagic pancreatitis occurred in one patient, but a role of concomitant drugs was also possible (SEDA-20, 341). Pancreatitis or hyperamylasemia were not significantly different in renal transplant patients randomly assigned to receive azathioprine or ciclosporin, and other causative factors were found in most patients with pancreatitis (36).

In a review of definite or probable drug-associated pancreatitis spontaneously reported to the Dutch adverse drug reactions system during 1977–98, azathioprine was the suspected drug in four of 34 patients, two of whom had positive rechallenge (37). Although most of the carefully described reports of azathioprine-induced pancreatitis were found in patients with inflammatory bowel disease, transplant recipients can also suffer this complication.

- Over a year after renal transplantation, a 48-year-old man, who took azathioprine, ciclosporin, and prednisolone, developed acute necrotizing pancreatitis (38). Improvement was obtained after azathioprine withdrawal, but he again took azathioprine and had similar symptoms within 30 hours after a single dose.
- Pancreatitis has been reported after a progressive increase in dose of 6-thioguanine in a 10-year-old infant (39). She had had two previous episodes of pancreatitis after mercaptopurine.

The chemical structure of 6-thioguanine, which results from the metabolism of azathioprine/mercaptopurine, is very similar to that of mercaptopurine. Therefore, a history of previous adverse effects with mercaptopurine should be anticipated in patients considered for 6-thioguanine treatment.

Skin

Rashes or other allergic-type cutaneous reactions are usually noted during the azathioprine hypersensitivity syndrome. Isolated but convincing reports point to the occurrence of vasculitis with microscopic polyarteritis (SEDA-21, 381) and Sweet's syndrome, which recurred after subsequent azathioprine exposure (SEDA-22, 410).

Pellagra with a photosensitivity-like rash and skin peeling syndrome has also been noted (SEDA-21, 381).

Musculoskeletal

Severe myalgia and symmetrical polyarthritis are sometimes reported in patients taking azathioprine. Eight cases of azathioprine-associated arthritis were identified in the WHO Drug Monitoring Database, including six cases with a typical hypersensitivity syndrome and two cases in whom joint involvement was the only reported symptom (40). Rhabdomyolysis has also been reported as a possible feature of the azathioprine hypersensitivity syndrome (SEDA-20, 341).

In two patients with Crohn's disease, azathioprine was suspected to have caused severe gait disorders with an inability to walk (41). Within 1 month of treatment, both had joint pains or diffuse arthralgias that were the presumed cause of pseudoparalysis of the legs. In one patient other causes were carefully ruled out and similar symptoms recurred shortly after azathioprine was re-introduced.

Immunologic

The distinction between relapse of the treated disease, systemic sepsis, and acute azathioprine allergy can be difficult, as has been shown in three patients with vasculitic disorders (42).

Allergic reactions to azathioprine were recorded in 2% of patients with Crohn's disease taking azathioprine (3), and there was no evidence to suggest that the incidence depended on the underlying disease. The more rapid recurrence and/or the severity of symptoms following rechallenge were in keeping with a putative immune-mediated reaction, but no immunological mechanism has been conclusively demonstrated (SED-13, 1121; 43,44). In one patient, progressively rising doses of azathioprine were successfully administered, despite positive skin prick tests (SEDA-21, 382). Anaphylactic shock has been occasionally reported (45). Delayed contact hypersensitivity with a positive patch test was described in a pharmaceutical handler of azathioprine (46).

Allergic reactions to mercaptopurine or azathioprine are well described, but a true immunoallergic reaction has never been convincingly demonstrated. Desensitization has been successfully performed in isolated patients (47), and this has been more extensively addressed in a retrospective analysis of the charts of patients treated for inflammatory bowel disease (48). Of 591 patients observed over a 28-year period, 16 (2.7%) developed allergic reactions, which mostly consisted of fever ($n = 14$), joint pains ($n = 6$), or severe back pain ($n = 5$). Symptoms commonly appeared within 1 month and lasted 5 days on average. All nine patients rechallenged with mercaptopurine had similar but less severe symptoms. Further rechallenge with azathioprine in six of these patients caused symptoms in five of them. Careful desensitization with mercaptopurine or azathioprine was attempted in five patients, and resulted in tolerance and therapeutic success in four. The last patient, who had a previous history of mercaptopurine-induced sepsis-like syndrome with renal insufficiency, had a similar reaction only after one-quarter of the dose of azathioprine. This study suggests that a direct switch from mercaptopurine to the parent drug azathioprine cannot be recommended in patients who developed allergic reactions to mercaptopurine, and that desensitization should not be attempted in patients with previous life-threatening hypersensitivity reactions.

A genetic predisposition is suspected, with a possible association between the hypersensitivity syndrome and the Bw4 and Bw6 phenotypes (SED-13, 1121). Mercaptopurine has sometimes been re-administered safely after a severe hypersensitivity reaction to azathioprine (49), suggesting a major role for the imidazole moiety of azathioprine. However, typical allergic reactions to mercaptopurine can also occur (SEDA-21, 381).

Infection risk

Infections, in particular bacterial and viral (cytomegalovirus, *Herpes simplex* virus, Epstein–Barr virus), and also protozoal and fungal infections, are major causes of morbidity and mortality in the post-transplantation period, whatever the immunosuppressive regimen used (50–52). Based on an analysis of medical and autopsy records, infections were found to be the cause of death in 70% of transplant patients, with bacteria (50%) or fungi (29%) the most common pathogens (53).

The frequency, course, and severity of *Herpes zoster* infection have been retrospectively evaluated in a sample of 550 patients treated with 6-mercaptopurine for inflammatory bowel disease (54). Twelve patients aged 14–73 years developed shingles after an average of 921 days, an incidence that was about two-fold higher than in the general population. Only three patients were still taking glucocorticoids at the time of onset of the shingles, and leukopenia was not associated with the occurrence of the infection. In nine patients, the course of the infection was 7–71 days and was uncomplicated. Two patients had more severe symptoms and suffered from postherpetic neuralgia. The last patient, a 14-year-old boy, had a brief episode of *H. zoster* during initial treatment and had *H. zoster* encephalitis at the age of 23 years, 16 months after 6-mercaptopurine had been restarted. From this report, it appears that 6-mercaptopurine can be restarted after brief discontinuation in patients who are expected to benefit from it.

- Fatal Epstein–Barr virus-associated hemophagocytic syndrome was reported in a young man taking azathioprine and prednisone for Crohn's disease (55).

Donor-specific blood transfusion in the preparation for transplantation was complicated by a higher incidence of cytomegalovirus infection in patients receiving azathioprine (56).

Long-Term Effects

Tumorigenicity

Because of the varied indications for azathioprine and mercaptopurine, it is difficult to determine whether there is an increased incidence of cancer specifically related to prolonged drug exposure. Data from the Cincinnati Transplant Tumor Registry, published in 1993, helped to define comprehensively the characteristics of neoplasms observed in organ transplant recipients (57). Skin and lip cancers were the most common, and non-Hodgkin's lymphomas represent the majority of lymphoproliferative disorders, with an incidence some 30- to 50-fold higher than in controls. An excess of Kaposi's sarcomas, carcinomas of the vulva and perineum, hepatobiliary tumors, and various sarcomas has also been reported. In contrast, the incidence of common neoplasms encountered in the general population is not increased. In renal transplant patients, the actuarial cumulative risk of cancer was 14–18% at 10 years and 40–50% at 20 years (58,59). Skin cancers accounted for about half of the cases. Very similar figures were found in later studies (SEDA-20, 341).

While there is no doubt that the incidence of malignancies is increased in the transplant population, there have been controversies as to which factors (duration of treatment, total dosage, the degree of immunosuppression, or the type of immunosuppressive regimens) are the most relevant in determining risk. Partial or complete regression of lymphoproliferative disorders and Kaposi's sarcomas after reduction of immunosuppressive therapy argues strongly for the role of the degree of immunosuppression (57). The incidence of cancer was also significantly higher in renal transplant patients taking triple therapy regimens compared with dual therapy (60). Similarly, aggressive immunosuppressive therapy may account for the higher incidence of lymphomas in patients with cardiac versus renal allografts.

In a large multicenter study in more than 52 000 kidney or heart transplant patients between 1983 and 1991, the rate of non-Hodgkin's lymphomas in the first post-transplantation year was 0.2% in kidney and 1.2% in heart recipients, and fell substantially thereafter (61). Initial immunosuppression with azathioprine and ciclosporin and prophylactic treatment with antilymphocyte antibodies or muromonab were associated with a significantly increased incidence of non-Hodgkin's lymphomas compared with other immunosuppressive regimens, which confirmed the major role of the level of immunosuppression. Later studies confirmed that immunosuppression per se rather than a single agent is responsible for the increased risk of cancer (SEDA-20, 340). Finally, the most striking difference between conventional and modern immunosuppressive regimens, including ciclosporin, was the average time to the appearance of tumors, in particular skin cancers and lymphomas, which was shorter in ciclosporin-treated patients (62,63). There was an increased incidence of non-Hodgkin's lymphomas in patients receiving long-term azathioprine and prednisolone for rheumatoid disease, although the latent period was longer than in other patients, perhaps reflecting a different pathogenesis (64).

Multiple factors with complex interactions are involved in the observed pattern and increased incidence of neoplasms. They include severely depressed immunity with an impaired immune surveillance against various carcinogens, the activation of several oncogenic viruses, and a possible mutagenic effect of the drugs. Viruses, such as papillomavirus, cytomegalovirus, and Epstein–Barr virus, are believed to play an important role in the development of several post-transplant cancers. From a theoretical point of view, the use of antiviral drugs active against herpes viruses, which are commonly implicated as co-factors, can be expected to produce a reduction in the incidence of post-transplant lymphoproliferative disorders.

Long-term treatment with azathioprine has been associated with transitional carcinoma of the bladder and non-Hodgkin's lymphoma in a single case (65).

- A 59-year-old man who had had a testicular non-Hodgkin's lymphoma for 9 years, developed diplopia and ptosis due to myasthenia gravis with antibodies to the acetylcholine receptor. He was given pyridostigmine and prednisolone. After 6 months he developed pernicious anemia, and he was given vitamin B_{12} injections. An attempt to reduce the dose of prednisolone failed, and he was therefore given azathioprine and the dose of prednisone was progressively reduced. Two years later he developed a transitional carcinoma of the bladder (pTa g1), which was removed by transurethral resection. Seven years later he developed a swollen tender right testis due to a B cell lymphoma. He tolerated chemotherapy (CHOP) poorly and died 2 months later.

In renal transplant recipients, premalignant dysplastic keratotic lesions increased in frequency by 6.8% per year after the first 3.5 years after transplantation, and were ultimately observed in all 167 patients within 16 years of transplantation (66). No relation with sun exposure or skin type was found. The great majority of these patients were taking prednisolone and azathioprine, but azathioprine was considered as the main causative factor, possibly due to a carcinogenic effect rather than to immunosuppression itself.

Several isolated reports and epidemiological studies have addressed the risk of cancer in non-transplant patients treated with azathioprine. Promptly reversible Epstein–Barr virus-associated lymphomas have been reported as single cases, as have reports of acute myeloid leukemia with 7q deletion, rapidly aggressive squamous cell carcinomas, soft tissue carcinomas, or fatal Merkel cell carcinomas in patients taking long-term azathioprine maintenance (SED-13, 1122; SEDA-20, 342; SEDA-21, 382; SEDA-22, 410). Although epidemiological studies allow a more accurate estimate, conflicting results have emerged and there is as yet no definite evidence that azathioprine actually increases the risk of cancer.

An increased risk of non-Hodgkin's lymphomas, possibly related to treatment duration, has been found in patients with rheumatoid arthritis (67). There was no evidence that azathioprine increased the overall incidence of any cancer in 259 patients with rheumatoid arthritis on immunosuppressive treatment (azathioprine in 223) and matched for age and sex (but not for disease duration and severity) with unexposed patients (68). However, death more often resulted from malignancies in those taking azathioprine.

In cases of inflammatory bowel disease, no overall increased incidence of cancer was noted after a median of 9 years follow-up in 755 patients who had taken less than 2 mg/kg/day of azathioprine over a median period of 12.5 years (69). Only colorectal cancers (mostly adenocarcinoma) were more frequent, but their incidence was also increased in chronic inflammatory bowel diseases. More specifically, there was no excess of non-Hodgkin's lymphoma, but the power of the study to detect an increased risk of this disorder was low.

Another group of investigators has estimated that the potential long-term risk of malignancies outweighs the therapeutic benefit, but this conclusion was based on the follow-up of only 157 patients treated for Crohn's disease (4).

In 626 patients with inflammatory bowel disease who had taken azathioprine for a mean duration of 27 months (mean follow-up 6.9 years), there was no increased risk of cancer (colorectal or other) (70).

In a case-control study using a database of 1191 patients with multiple sclerosis, 23 cancers (17 solid tumors, two skin tumors, and four hemopoietic cancers) were found. The relative risk of cancer was 1.3 in patients treated for less than 5 years, 2.0 in those treated for 5–10 years, and 4.4 in those treated for more than 10 years; however, none of these later changes was significant (71). Nevertheless, there was a significant association for cumulative dosages in excess of 600 g. Taken together, these results suggest a low risk of cancer in non-transplant patients, but they cannot exclude a possible dose-related increase in risk during long-term treatment.

Skin carcinoma (predominantly squamous-cell carcinoma), cancer of the lip, Kaposi's sarcoma, and carcinoma of the cervix and anus are reported to be more common following azathioprine than in the general population (72).

Mercaptopurine is not considered to be leukemogenic, but this assumption has been disputed in a study of 439 children who received mercaptopurine as part of their maintenance therapy for acute lymphoblastic leukemia (73). Five patients developed secondary myelodysplasia or acute myeloid leukemia 23–53 months after diagnosis, a consequence that was attributed to mercaptopurine. These five patients had significantly lower TPMT activity, and two were classified as heterozygous for TPMT deficiency on genotype analysis. Although the number of evaluable patients was small, the suggestion was that a subset of patients with low TMPT activity might have an increased leukemogenic risk when exposed to mercaptopurine with other cytotoxic agents. Whether these findings can be extrapolated to patients without cancers is not known.

Of 550 patients with inflammatory bowel disease treated for a mean of 8 years, 25 (4.5%) developed a malignancy, with an overall incidence of 2.7 neoplasms per 1000 years of follow-up (74). The numbers of the most commonly observed cancers, such as bowel cancers ($n = 8$), breast cancers ($n = 3$), or single cases of other cancers, did not seem to be higher than expected in the general population or in the inflammatory bowel disease population. Although mercaptopurine was suspected in two cases of testicular carcinoma, two cases of lymphoma, and one case of leukemia, the authors emphasized the small risk of malignancies compared with the beneficial results of mercaptopurine in inflammatory bowel disease.

Second-Generation Effects

Pregnancy

Even though azathioprine is teratogenic in animals, human experience allows no firm conclusions, being limited to single case reports of birth defects after first trimester exposure to azathioprine. More convincingly, there was no evidence of increased risk or of a specific pattern of congenital anomalies among hundreds of infants born to azathioprine-treated transplant patients (75–77), but large series with adequate long-term follow-up are still lacking. The absence of inosinate pyrophosphorylase, an enzyme that converts azathioprine to its active metabolites, in the fetus was suggested to account for these reassuring data. Other potential risks, that is miscarriages or stillbirths, were also within the normal range, and intrauterine growth retardation did not appear to be specifically related to azathioprine use. Potential neonatal consequences of maternal azathioprine maintenance during the whole pregnancy should be borne in mind, in view of isolated reports of immunohematological immunosuppression, pancytopenia, cytomegalovirus infection, and chromosome aberrations. Unfortunately, the extent of this risk has not been carefully evaluated.

Teratogenicity

Maternal azathioprine treatment during pregnancy is clearly teratogenic in animals, but the mechanisms are not known. A large number of reports have described the outcome of pregnancies following the use of immunosuppressant drugs, in particular in renal transplant patients, and hundreds of pregnancies have been analysed (75). The largest experience is that derived from the National Transplantation Pregnancy Registry which has been built up in the USA since 1991 (76). This registry has accumulated data on more than 900 pregnancies, of which 83% followed kidney transplantation. Overall, the immunosuppressant drug regimens commonly used in transplant patients (azathioprine or ciclosporin) do not appear to increase the overall risk of congenital malformations or produce a specific pattern of malformation. Risk factors associated with adverse pregnancy outcomes included a short time interval between transplantation and pregnancy (that is less than 1–2 years), graft dysfunction before or during pregnancy, and hypertension (78).

Possible long-term effects of in utero exposure to immunosuppressants are still seldom investigated. There have been no reports that physical and mental development or renal function are altered. In one study, there were changes in T lymphocyte development in seven children born to mothers who had taken azathioprine or ciclosporin, but immune function assays were normal, suggesting that development of the fetal immune system was not affected (79).

In 27 clinical series, the frequency of congenital anomalies among infants of patients who took azathioprine after renal transplantation ranged from 0 to 11% (80).

The consequences of paternal mercaptopurine exposure on the outcome of pregnancies have been retrospectively studied in 57 men with inflammatory bowel disease: 23 men had fathered 50 pregnancies and had taken mercaptopurine before conception; of these, 13 pregnancies were conceived within 3 months of paternal mercaptopurine use (group 1A) and 37 pregnancies were conceived at least 3 months after paternal mercaptopurine withdrawal (group 1B); the other 34 men, who fathered 90 pregnancies, had not been exposed to mercaptopurine before conception (group II) (81). Of the 140 conceptions, two resulted in congenital anomalies in group 1A, whereas there were no congenital anomalies in the other groups. One child had a missing thumb, and the other had acrania with multiple digital and limb abnormalities. The overall number of complications (spontaneous abortion and congenital anomalies) was significantly higher in group 1A (4/13) compared with both group IB (1/37) and group II (2/90). Although the retrospective nature of this study and the limited number of evaluable patients precluded any definitive conclusion, the observed congenital anomalies were similar to those found in the offspring of female rabbits treated with mercaptopurine during pregnancy, and suggested that paternal mercaptopurine treatment should ideally be discontinued at least 3 months before planned conception.

Whereas neutropenia and immune deficiencies can affect neonates born to transplant patients, the exact role of azathioprine is difficult to establish. A report has suggested that such effects should also be expected in neonates born to patients taking azathioprine for other conditions (82).

- A 27-year-old woman, who took azathioprine (125 mg/day) and mesalazine (3 g/day) during her whole pregnancy, delivered a normal boy who had febrile respiratory distress after 36 hours. Chest X-ray showed interstitial pneumonitis and thymus hypoplasia. There was severe neutropenia (20×10^6/l), lymphopenia (24×10^6/l), and hypogammaglobulinemia. His clinical condition improved over the next 26 days with immunoglobulin treatment and antibiotics, but B lymphocytes and IgM were still undetectable.

Lactation

Very few data on breastfed infants from azathioprine-treated mothers are available. Breastfeeding is not recommended owing to the potential risk of immunosuppression, growth retardation, and carcinogenesis.

Susceptibility Factors

Genetic factors

The complex metabolism of azathioprine and mercaptopurine is subject to a pharmacogenetic polymorphism that is relevant to the degree of efficacy and toxicity attained in a given individual. Thiopurine methyltransferase (TPMT) is one of the key enzymes regulating the catabolism of thiopurine drugs to inactive products. Owing to an inherited autosomal codominant trait, a significant number of patients have intermediate (11%) to low or undetectable (0.3%) TPMT activity (83). These patients produce larger amounts of the active 6-thioguanine nucleotides and may therefore be unusually sensitive to commonly used dosages and an increased risk of myelotoxicity (SED-13, 1120; SEDA-21, 381).

Monitoring azathioprine therapy by measuring erythrocyte 6-thioguanine concentrations and TPMT activity is thought to ensure optimal immunosuppressive effects and to reduce the likelihood of hematological toxicity (84,85). Low or completely absent erythrocyte TPMT activity and high concentrations of erythrocyte 6-thioguanine metabolites have been found in patients with severe azathioprine-induced bone marrow toxicity, as compared to those without bone marrow toxicity (86,87). However, intracellular concentrations of thiopurine nucleotides alone did not always correlate with hematological toxicity (88). In patients in whom TPMT deficiency was not clearly demonstrated, low lymphocyte 5'-nucleotidase activity and xanthine oxidase deficiency or other factors have been postulated as possible causes of hemotoxicity, suggesting that bone marrow toxicity is probably multifactorial (87,89,90). Although not all investigators recommend systematic pretreatment screening for purine enzyme activities, evidence of deficiency of purine enzymes could well be sought when early bone marrow toxicity occurs.

In a retrospective analysis of 106 patients with inflammatory bowel disease, to evaluate the importance of thiopurine methyl transferase (TPMT) activity in the management of azathioprine therapy in inflammatory bowel disease, the relation between inherited variations in TPMT enzyme activity and azathioprine toxicity was confirmed (91).

In 3291 patients receiving azathioprine, 10% had a low TPMT activity and 15 (1 in 220 or 0.46%) had no detectable enzymatic activity at all (92), slightly more common than has been reported in other studies (1 in 300). This makes the economics of screening, to avoid myelosuppression in patients receiving azathioprine, attractive.

Of 78 patients treated with azathioprine for systemic lupus erythematosus, 10 developed azathioprine-associated reversible neutropenia (93). Only one of these patients was homozygous for TPMT deficiency, but he had the most severe episode (aplastic anemia).

In one study, 14 of 33 patients with rheumatoid arthritis had severe adverse effects (mostly gastrointestinal toxicity, flu-like reactions or fever, pancytopenia, and hepatotoxicity) within 1–8 weeks after azathioprine was started (94). The adverse effects subsided after withdrawal in all patients, but all eight patients who were rechallenged developed the same adverse effect. A baseline reduction in TPMT activity was significantly associated with the occurrence of these adverse effects in seven of eight patients, with a relative risk of 3.1 (95% CI = 1.6–6.2) compared with patients with high TPMT activity (seven of 25 patients). Another prospective evaluation in 67 patients with rheumatic disorders showed that

TPMT genotype analysis is useful in identifying patients at risk of azathioprine toxicity (95). Treatment duration was significantly longer in patients with the wild-type TPMP alleles than in those with mutant alleles, and that was due to the early occurrence of leukopenia in the latter.

In 22 children with renal transplants, high erythrocyte TPMT activity, measured 1 month after transplantation, correlated positively with rejection episodes during the first 3 months, and this was probably due to more rapid azathioprine catabolism (96). As suggested in a study of 180 patients with acute lymphoblastic leukemia, determination of genetic polymorphisms in TMPT can be useful in predicting potential toxicity and in optimizing the determination of an appropriate dose in patients who are homozygous or heterozygous for TMPT deficiency (97).

In 30 heart transplant patients taking azathioprine, the myelosuppressive effects of azathioprine/mercaptopurine were predicted by systematic genotypic screening of thiopurine methyltransferase deficiency (98). However, myelosuppression can also be observed in patients without the thiopurine methyltransferase mutation. Of 41 patients with leukopenia or thrombocytopenia taking azathioprine/mercaptopurine for Crohn's disease, four were classified as low methylators, seven as intermediate methylators, and 30 as high methylators by genotypic analysis (99). Thus, only 27% of the patients had the typical mutations associated with enzyme deficiency and a risk of myelosuppression. The delay in bone marrow toxicity was shorter in the four homozygous patients (median 1 month) than in the others (median 3–4 months). Many other causes, including viral infections, associated drugs, or another azathioprine/mercaptopurine metabolic pathway, were suggested to account for most of the cases of late hemotoxicity. This confirmed that continuous hematological monitoring is required, even in patients with no thiopurine methyltransferase mutations.

Drug–Drug Interactions

Allopurinol

Allopurinol inhibits xanthine oxidase, which is involved in the inactivation of azathioprine and mercaptopurine, and bone marrow suppression is a well-known complication of the concomitant use of allopurinol and azathioprine (SEDA-16, 114; SEDA-20, 342). A reduction in the dosage of azathioprine or mercaptopurine by at least two-thirds and careful hematological monitoring during the first weeks of the combination has been proposed if combined use with allopurinol is required. However, compliance with these above guidelines was observed in only 58% of 24 patients with heart or lung transplants (100). In addition, although adequate azathioprine dosage reduction reduces the incidence of cytopenias, the risk persists even after the first month of the combination.

Because of the possible risks of reduced immunosuppression if the dose of azathioprine is reduced when allopurinol is given, cyclic urate oxidase can be given instead, as has been shown in six hyperuricemic transplant patients treated with azathioprine (101).

Aminosalicylates

In vitro studies have suggested that sulfasalazine and other aminosalicylates can inhibit TPMT activity, predisposing to an increased risk of bone marrow suppression in patients taking azathioprine or mercaptopurine. This was not clinically substantiated until an extensively investigated case was reported of leukopenia and anemia in a patient treated with both olsalazine and mercaptopurine (SEDA-21, 382). A further inhibiting effect of olsalazine was suggested in this patient, who had a relatively low baseline TPMT activity.

In 16 patients with Crohn's disease taking a stable dose of azathioprine, plus sulfasalazine or mesalazine, mean 6-thioguanine nucleotide concentrations fell significantly over 3 months; withdrawal of the aminosalicylates had no effect on the clinical and biological evolution of Crohn's disease in these patients (102).

In a prospective, parallel-group study in 34 patients with Crohn's disease taking azathioprine or mercaptopurine, co-administration of mesalazine 4 g/day, sulfasalazine 4 g/day, or balsalazide 6.75 g/day for 8 weeks resulted in an increase in whole blood 6-thioguanine nucleotide concen-trations and a high frequency of leukopenia (107).

Coumarin anticoagulants

Azathioprine or mercaptopurine have been sometimes involved in reduced warfarin and acenocoumarol activity, and increased warfarin dosages may be necessary (103). Similar findings were found in a patient taking maintenance phenprocoumon (SEDA-21, 382).

- Two patients required an approximate three-fold increase in the weekly anticoagulant dosage while taking azathioprine or mercaptopurine (104,105).

A pharmacokinetic interaction is the most likely cause, but the mechanism (impaired absorption or enhanced anticoagulant metabolism) is unknown.

Isotretinoin

The combination of isotretinoin and azathioprine was reported to have a synergistic effect on the occurrence of curly hair in three transplant patients with ciclosporin-induced acne (SEDA-20, 342).

Methotrexate

In 43 patients with rheumatoid arthritis, methotrexate was thought to have increased the risk of the azathioprine-induced hypersensitivity syndrome (106).

References

1. Savolainen HA, Kautiainen H, Isomaki H, Aho K, Verronen P. Azathioprine in patients with juvenile chronic arthritis: a longterm followup study. J Rheumatol 1997;24(12):2444–50.
2. Kirschner BS. Safety of azathioprine and 6-mercaptopurine in pediatric patients with inflammatory bowel disease. Gastroenterology 1998;115(4):813–21.

3. Pearson DC, May GR, Fick GH, Sutherland LR. Azathioprine and 6-mercaptopurine in Crohn disease. A meta-analysis. Ann Intern Med 1995;123(2):132–42.

4. Bouhnik Y, Lemann M, Mary JY, Scemama G, Tai R, Matuchansky C, Modigliani R, Rambaud JC. Long-term follow-up of patients with Crohn's disease treated with azathioprine or 6-mercaptopurine. Lancet 1996;347(8996):215–9.

5. Sandborn WJ. A review of immune modifier therapy for inflammatory bowel disease: azathioprine, 6-mercaptopurine, cyclosporine, and methotrexate. Am J Gastroenterol 1996;91(3):423–33.

6. Hollander AAMJ, Van der Woude FJ. Efficacy and tolerability of conversion from cyclosporin to azathioprine after kidney transplantation. A review of the evidence. BioDrugs 1998;9:197–210.

7. Saway PA, Heck LW, Bonner JR, Kirklin JK. Azathioprine hypersensitivity. Case report and review of the literature. Am J Med 1988;84(5):960–4.

8. Parnham AP, Dittmer I, Mathieson PW, McIver A, Dudley C. Acute allergic reactions associated with azathioprine. Lancet 1996;348(9026):542–3.

9. Perreaux F, Zenaty D, Capron F, Trioche P, Odievre M, Labrune P. Azathioprine-induced lung toxicity and efficacy of cyclosporin A in a young girl with type 2 autoimmune hepatitis. J Pediatr Gastroenterol Nutr 2000;31(2):190–2.

10. Jungling AS, Shangraw RE. Massive airway edema after azathioprine. Anesthesiology 2000;92(3):888–90.

11. Connell WR, Kamm MA, Ritchie JK, Lennard-Jones JE. Bone marrow toxicity caused by azathioprine in inflammatory bowel disease: 27 years of experience. Gut 1993;34(8):1081–5.

12. Cunliffe RN, Scott BB. Review article: monitoring for drug side-effects in inflammatory bowel disease. Aliment Pharmacol Ther 2002;16(4):647–62.

13. Amenabar JJ, Gomez-Ullate P, Garcia-Lopez FJ, Aurrecoechea B, Garcia-Erauzkin G, Lampreabe I. A randomized trial comparing cyclosporine and steroids with cyclosporine, azathioprine, and steroids in cadaveric renal transplantation. Transplantation 1998;65(5):653–61.

14. Creemers GJ, van Boven WP, Lowenberg B, van der Heul C. Azathioprine-associated pure red cell aplasia. J Intern Med 1993;233(1):85–7.

15. Pruijt JF, Haanen JB, Hollander AA, den Ottolander GJ. Azathioprine-induced pure red-cell aplasia. Nephrol Dial Transplant 1996;11(7):1371–3.

16. Higashida K, Kobayashi K, Sugita K, Karakida N, Nakagomi Y, Sawanobori E, Sata Y, Aihara M, Amemiya S, Nakazawa S. Pure red blood cell aplasia during azathioprine therapy associated with parvovirus B19 infection. Pediatr Infect Dis J 1997;16(11):1093–5.

17. Pujol M, Fernandez F, Sancho JM, Ribera JM, Milla F, Feliu E. Immune hemolytic anemia induced by 6-mercaptopurine. Transfusion 2000;40(1):75–6.

18. Sudhir RR, Rao SK, Shanmugam MP, Padmanabhan P. Bilateral macular hemorrhage caused by azathioprine-induced aplastic anemia in a corneal graft recipient. Cornea 2002;21(7):712–4.

19. Santiago M. Diarrhoea secondary to azathioprine in two patients with SLE. Lupus 1999;8(7):565.

20. Marbet U, Schmid I. Severe life-threatening diarrhea caused by azathioprine but not by 6-mercaptopurine. Digestion 2001;63(2):139–42.

21. Kowdley KV, Keeffe EB. Hepatotoxicity of transplant immunosuppressive agents. Gastroenterol Clin North Am 1995;24(4):991–1001.

22. Pol S, Cavalcanti R, Carnot F, Legendre C, Driss F, Chaix ML, Thervet E, Chkoff N, Brechot C, Berthelot P, Kreis H. Azathioprine hepatitis in kidney transplant recipients. A predisposing role of chronic viral hepatitis. Transplantation 1996;61(12):1774–6.

23. Wagoner LE, Olsen SL, Bristow MR, O'Connell JB, Taylor DO, Lappe DL, Renlund DG. Cyclophosphamide as an alternative to azathioprine in cardiac transplant recipients with suspected azathioprine-induced hepatotoxicity. Transplantation 1993;56(6):1415–8.

24. Ramalho HJ, Terra EG, Cartapatti E, Barberato JB, Alves VA, Gayotto LC, Abbud-Filho M. Hepatotoxicity of azathioprine in renal transplant recipients. Transplant Proc 1989;21(1 Pt 2):1716–7.

25. Horsmans Y, Rahier J, Geubel AP. Reversible cholestasis with bile duct injury following azathioprine therapy. A case report. Liver 1991;11(2):89–93.

26. Read AE, Wiesner RH, LaBrecque DR, Tifft JG, Mullen KD, Sheer RL, Petrelli M, Ricanati ES, McCullough AJ. Hepatic veno-occlusive disease associated with renal transplantation and azathioprine therapy. Ann Intern Med 1986;104(5):651–5.

27. Azoulay D, Castaing D, Lemoine A, Samuel D, Majno P, Reynes M, Charpentier B, Bismuth H. Successful treatment of severe azathioprine-induced hepatic veno-occlusive disease in a kidney-transplanted patient with transjugular intrahepatic portosystemic shunt. Clin Nephrol 1998;50(2):118–22.

28. Mion F, Cloix P, Boillot O, Gille D, Bouvier R, Paliard P, Berger F. Maladie veino-occlusive après transplantation hépatique. Association d'un rejet aiguë cellulaire et de la toxicité de l'azathioprine. [Veno-occlusive disease after liver transplantation. Association of acute cellular rejection and toxicity of azathioprine.] Gastroenterol Clin Biol 1993;17(11):863–7.

29. Sterneck M, Wiesner R, Ascher N, Roberts J, Ferrell L, Ludwig J, Lake J. Azathioprine hepatotoxicity after liver transplantation. Hepatology 1991;14(5):806–10.

30. Cooper C, Cotton DW, Minihane N, Cawley MI. Azathioprine hypersensitivity manifesting as acute focal hepatocellular necrosis. J R Soc Med 1986;79(3):171–3.

31. Delgado J, Munoz de Bustillo E, Ibarrola C, Colina F, Morales JM, Rodriguez E, Aguado JM, Fuertes A, Gomez MA. Hepatitis C virus-related fibrosing cholestatic hepatitis after cardiac transplantation: is azathioprine a contributory factor? J Heart Lung Transplant 1999;18(6):607–10.

32. David-Neto E, da Fonseca JA, de Paula FJ, Nahas WC, Sabbaga E, Ianhez LE. Is azathioprine harmful to chronic viral hepatitis in renal transplantation? A long-term study on azathioprine withdrawal. Transplant Proc 1999;31(1–2):1149–50.

33. Eaton VS, Casanova JM, Kupa A. Azathioprine hepatotoxicity confirmed by rechallenge. Aust J Hosp Pharm 2000;30:58–9.

34. Muszkat M, Pappo O, Caraco Y, Haviv YS. Hepatocanalicular cholestasis after 24 years of azathioprine administration for myasthenia gravis. Clin Drug Invest 2000;19:75–8.

35. Present DH, Meltzer SJ, Krumholz MP, Wolke A, Korelitz BI. 6-Mercaptopurine in the management of inflammatory bowel disease: short- and long-term toxicity. Ann Intern Med 1989;111(8):641–9.

36. Frick TW, Fryd DS, Goodale RL, Simmons RL, Sutherland DE, Najarian JS. Lack of association between

azathioprine and acute pancreatitis in renal transplantation patients. Lancet 1991;337(8735):251–2.

37. Eland IA, van Puijenbroek EP, Sturkenboom MJ, Wilson JH, Stricker BH. Drug-associated acute pancreatitis: twenty-one years of spontaneous reporting in The Netherlands. Am J Gastroenterol 1999;94(9):2417–22.

38. Siwach V, Bansal V, Kumar A, Rao Ch U, Sharma A, Minz M. Post-renal transplant azathioprine-induced pancreatitis. Nephrol Dial Transplant 1999;14(10):2495–8.

39. Bisschop D, Germain ML, Munzer M, Trenque T. Thioguanine, pancréatotoxicité?. [Thioguanine, pancreatotoxicity?.] Therapie 2001;56(1):67–9.

40. Pillans PI, Tooke AF, Bateman ED, Ainslie GM. Acute polyarthritis associated with azathioprine for interstitial lung disease. Respir Med 1995;89(1):63–4.

41. Bellaiche G, Cosnes J, Nouts A, Ley G, Slama JL. Troubles de la marche secondaires à la prise d'azathioprine chez 2 malades ayant une maladie de Crohn. [Gait disorders secondary to azathioprine treatment in 2 patients with Crohn's disease.] Gastroenterol Clin Biol 1999;23(4):533–4.

42. Stratton JD, Farrington K. Relapse of vasculitis, sepsis, or azathioprine allergy? Nephrol Dial Transplant 1998;13(11):2927–8.

43. Jeurissen ME, Boerbooms AM, van de Putte LB, Kruijsen MW. Azathioprine induced fever, chills, rash, and hepatotoxicity in rheumatoid arthritis. Ann Rheum Dis 1990;49(1):25–7.

44. Meys E, Devogelaer JP, Geubel A, Rahier J, Nagant de Deuxchaisnes C. Fever, hepatitis and acute interstitial nephritis in a patient with rheumatoid arthritis. Concurrent manifestations of azathioprine hypersensitivity. J Rheumatol 1992;19(5):807–9.

45. Jones JJ, Ashworth J. Azathioprine-induced shock in dermatology patients. J Am Acad Dermatol 1993;29(5 Pt 1):795–6.

46. Burden AD, Beck MH. Contact hypersensitivity to azathioprine. Contact Dermatitis 1992;27(5):329–30.

47. Dominguez Ortega J, Robledo T, Martinez-Cocera C, Alonso A, Cimarra M, Chamorro M, Plaza A. Desensitization to azathioprine. J Investig Allergol Clin Immunol 1999;9(5):337–8.

48. Korelitz BI, Zlatanic J, Goel F, Fuller S. Allergic reactions to 6-mercaptopurine during treatment of inflammatory bowel disease. J Clin Gastroenterol 1999;28(4):341–4.

49. Godeau B, Paul M, Autegarden JE, Leynadier F, Astier A, Schaeffer A. Hypersensitivity to azathioprine mimicking gastroenteritis. Absence of recurrence with 6-mercaptopurine. Gastroenterol Clin Biol 1995;19(1):117–9.

50. Garcia VD, Keitel E, Almeida P, Santos AF, Becker M, Goldani JC. Morbidity after renal transplantation: role of bacterial infection. Transplant Proc 1995;27(2):1825–6.

51. Wade JJ, Rolando N, Hayllar K, Philpott-Howard J, Casewell MW, Williams R. Bacterial and fungal infections after liver transplantation: an analysis of 284 patients. Hepatology 1995;21(5):1328–36.

52. Singh N, Yu VL. Infections in organ transplant recipients. Curr Opin Infect Dis 1996;9:223–9.

53. Reis MA, Costa RS, Ferraz AS. Causes of death in renal transplant recipients: a study of 102 autopsies from 1968 to 1991. J R Soc Med 1995;88(1):24–7.

54. Korelitz BI, Fuller SR, Warman JI, Goldberg MD. Shingles during the course of treatment with 6-mercaptopurine for inflammatory bowel disease. Am J Gastroenterol 1999;94(2):424–6.

55. Posthuma EF, Westendorp RG, van der Sluys Veer A, Kluin-Nelemans JC, Kluin PM, Lamers CB. Fatal infectious mononucleosis: a severe complication in the treatment of Crohn's disease with azathioprine. Gut 1995;36(2):311–3.

56. Suassuna JH, Machado RD, Sampaio JC, Leite LL, Villela LH, Ruzany F, Souza ER, Moraes JR. Active cytomegalovirus infection in hemodialysis patients receiving donor-specific blood transfusions under azathioprine coverage. Transplantation 1993;56(6):1552–4.

57. Penn I. Tumors after renal and cardiac transplantation. Hematol Oncol Clin North Am 1993;7(2):431–45.

58. Gaya SB, Rees AJ, Lechler RI, Williams G, Mason PD. Malignant disease in patients with long-term renal transplants. Transplantation 1995;59(12):1705–9.

59. London NJ, Farmery SM, Will EJ, Davison AM, Lodge JP. Risk of neoplasia in renal transplant patients. Lancet 1995;346(8972):403–6.

60. Kehinde EO, Petermann A, Morgan JD, Butt ZA, Donnelly PK, Veitch PS, Bell PR. Triple therapy and incidence of de novo cancer in renal transplant recipients. Br J Surg 1994;81(7):985–6.

61. Opelz G, Henderson R. Incidence of non-Hodgkin lymphoma in kidney and heart transplant recipients. Lancet 1993;342(8886–8887):1514–6.

62. Gruber SA, Gillingham K, Sothern RB, Stephanian E, Matas AJ, Dunn DL. De novo cancer in cyclosporine-treated and non-cyclosporine-treated adult primary renal allograft recipients. Clin Transplant 1994;8(4):388–95.

63. Hiesse C, Kriaa F, Rieu P, Larue JR, Benoit G, Bellamy J, Blanchet P, Charpentier B. Incidence and type of malignancies occurring after renal transplantation in conventionally and cyclosporine-treated recipients: analysis of a 20-year period in 1600 patients. Transplant Proc 1995;27(1):972–4.

64. Pitt PI, Sultan AH, Malone M, Andrews V, Hamilton EB. Association between azathioprine therapy and lymphoma in rheumatoid disease. J R Soc Med 1987;80(7):428–9.

65. Barthelmes L, Thomas KJ, Seale JR. Prostatic involvement of a testicular lymphoma in a patient with myasthenia gravis on long-term azathioprine. Leuk Lymphoma 2002;43(12):2425–6.

66. Taylor AE, Shuster S. Skin cancer after renal transplantation: the causal role of azathioprine. Acta Dermatol Venereol 1992;72(2):115–9.

67. Silman AJ, Petrie J, Hazleman B, Evans SJ. Lymphoproliferative cancer and other malignancy in patients with rheumatoid arthritis treated with azathioprine: a 20 year follow up study. Ann Rheum Dis 1988;47(12):988–92.

68. Jones M, Symmons D, Finn J, Wolfe F. Does exposure to immunosuppressive therapy increase the 10 year malignancy and mortality risks in rheumatoid arthritis? A matched cohort study. Br J Rheumatol 1996;35(8):738–45.

69. Connell WR, Kamm MA, Dickson M, Balkwill AM, Ritchie JK, Lennard-Jones JE. Long-term neoplasia risk after azathioprine treatment in inflammatory bowel disease. Lancet 1994;343(8908):1249–52.

70. Fraser AG, Orchard TR, Robinson EM, Jewell DP. Long-term risk of malignancy after treatment of inflammatory bowel disease with azathioprine. Aliment Pharmacol Ther 2002;16(7):1225–32.

71. Confavreux C, Saddier P, Grimaud J, Moreau T, Adeleine P, Aimard G. Risk of cancer from azathioprine therapy in multiple sclerosis: a case-control study. Neurology 1996;46(6):1607–12.

72. Penn I. Cancers in cyclosporine-treated vs azathioprine-treated patients. Transplant Proc 1996;28(2):876–8.

73. Bo J, Schroder H, Kristinsson J, Madsen B, Szumlanski C, Weinshilboum R, Andersen JB, Schmiegelow K. Possible carcinogenic effect of 6-mercaptopurine on bone marrow stem cells: relation to thiopurine metabolism. Cancer 1999;86(6):1080–6.

74. Korelitz BI, Mirsky FJ, Fleisher MR, Warman JI, Wisch N, Gleim GW. Malignant neoplasms subsequent to treatment of inflammatory bowel disease with 6-mercaptopurine. Am J Gastroenterol 1999;94(11):3248–53.

75. Ramsey-Goldman R, Schilling E. Immunosuppressive drug use during pregnancy. Rheum Dis Clin North Am 1997;23(1):149–67.

76. Armenti VT, Moritz MJ, Davison JM. Drug safety issues in pregnancy following transplantation and immunosuppression: effects and outcomes. Drug Saf 1998;19(3):219–32.

77. Cararach V, Carmona F, Monleon FJ, Andreu J. Pregnancy after renal transplantation: 25 years experience in Spain. Br J Obstet Gynaecol 1993;100(2):122–5.

78. Armenti VT, Ahlswede BA, Moritz MJ, Jarrell BE. National Transplantation Pregnancy Registry: analysis of pregnancy outcomes of female kidney recipients with relation to time interval from transplant to conception. Transplant Proc 1993;25(1 Pt 2):1036–7.

79. Pilarski LM, Yacyshyn BR, Lazarovits AI. Analysis of peripheral blood lymphocyte populations and immune function from children exposed to cyclosporine or to azathioprine in utero. Transplantation 1994;57(1):133–44.

80. Polifka JE, Friedman JM. Teratogen update: azathioprine and 6-mercaptopurine. Teratology 2002;65(5):240–61.

81. Rajapakse RO, Korelitz BI, Zlatanic J, Baiocco PJ, Gleim GW. Outcome of pregnancies when fathers are treated with 6-mercaptopurine for inflammatory bowel disease. Am J Gastroenterol 2000;95(3):684–8.

82. Cissoko H, Jonville-Bera AP, Lenain H, Riviere MF, Saugier J, Casanova JL, Autret-Leca E. Agranulocytose et déficit immunitaire transitoires après expostition ftale à l'azathioprine et mésalazine. [Agranulocytosis and transitory immune deficiency after fetal exposure to azathioprine and mesalazine.] Arch Pediatr 1999;6(10):1136–7.

83. Cuffari C, Hunt S, Bayless T. Utilisation of erythrocyte 6-thioguanine metabolite levels to optimise azathioprine therapy in patients with inflammatory bowel disease. Gut 2001;48(5):642–6.

84. Bergan S. Optimisation of azathioprine immunosuppression after organ transplantation by pharmacological measurements. BioDrugs 1997;8:446–56.

85. Meggitt SJ, Reynolds NJ. Azathioprine for atopic dermatitis. Clin Exp Dermatol 2001;26(5):369–75.

86. Schutz E, Gummert J, Mohr FW, Armstrong VW, Oellerich M. Azathioprine myelotoxicity related to elevated 6-thioguanine nucleotides in heart transplantation. Transplant Proc 1995;27(1):1298–300.

87. Kerstens PJ, Stolk JN, De Abreu RA, Lambooy LH, van de Putte LB, Boerbooms AA. Azathioprine-related bone marrow toxicity and low activities of purine enzymes in patients with rheumatoid arthritis. Arthritis Rheum 1995;38(1):142–5.

88. Boulieu R, Lenoir A, Bertocchi M, Mornex JF. Intracellular thiopurine nucleotides and azathioprine myelotoxicity in organ transplant patients. Br J Clin Pharmacol 1997;43(1):116–8.

89. Soria-Royer C, Legendre C, Mircheva J, Premel S, Beaune P, Kreis H. Thiopurine-methyl-transferase activity to assess azathioprine myelotoxicity in renal transplant recipients. Lancet 1993;341(8860):1593–4.

90. Serre-Debeauvais F, Bayle F, Amirou M, Bechtel Y, Boujet C, Vialtel P, Bessard G. Hématotoxicité de l'azathioprine à déterminisme génétique aggravé par un déficit en xanthine oxyase chez une transplantée rénale. [Hematotoxicity caused by azathioprine genetically determined and aggravated by xanthine oxidase deficiency in a patient following renal transplantation.] Presse Méd 1995;24(21):987–8.

91. Ansari A, Hassan C, Duley J, Marinaki A, Shobowale-Bakre EM, Seed P, Meenan J, Yim A, Sanderson J. Thiopurine methyltransferase activity and the use of azathioprine in inflammatory bowel disease. Aliment Pharmacol Ther 2002;16(10):1743–50.

92. Holme SA, Duley JA, Sanderson J, Routledge PA, Anstey AV. Erythrocyte thiopurine methyl transferase assessment prior to azathioprine use in the UK. QJM 2002;95(7):439–44.

93. Naughton MA, Battaglia E, O'Brien S, Walport MJ, Botto M. Identification of thiopurine methyltransferase (TPMT) polymorphisms cannot predict myelosuppression in systemic lupus erythematosus patients taking azathioprine. Rheumatology (Oxford) 1999;38(7):640–4.

94. Stolk JN, Boerbooms AM, de Abreu RA, de Koning DG, van Beusekom HJ, Muller WH, van de Putte LB. Reduced thiopurine methyltransferase activity and development of side effects of azathioprine treatment in patients with rheumatoid arthritis. Arthritis Rheum 1998;41(10):1858–66.

95. Black AJ, McLeod HL, Capell HA, Powrie RH, Matowe LK, Pritchard SC, Collie-Duguid ES, Reid DM. Thiopurine methyltransferase genotype predicts therapy-limiting severe toxicity from azathioprine. Ann Intern Med 1998;129(9):716–8.

96. Dervieux T, Medard Y, Baudouin V, Maisin A, Zhang D, Broly F, Loirat C, Jacqz-Aigrain E. Thiopurine methyltransferase activity and its relationship to the occurrence of rejection episodes in paediatric renal transplant recipients treated with azathioprine. Br J Clin Pharmacol 1999;48(6):793–800.

97. Relling MV, Hancock ML, Rivera GK, Sandlund JT, Ribeiro RC, Krynetski EY, Pui CH, Evans WE. Mercaptopurine therapy intolerance and heterozygosity at the thiopurine S-methyltransferase gene locus. J Natl Cancer Inst 1999;91(23):2001–8.

98. Sebbag L, Boucher P, Davelu P, Boissonnat P, Champsaur G, Ninet J, Dureau G, Obadia JF, Vallon JJ, Delaye J. Thiopurine S-methyltransferase gene polymorphism is predictive of azathioprine-induced myelosuppression in heart transplant recipients. Transplantation 2000;69(7):1524–7.

99. Colombel JF, Ferrari N, Debuysere H, Marteau P, Gendre JP, Bonaz B, Soule JC, Modigliani R, Touze Y, Catala P, Libersa C, Broly F. Genotypic analysis of thiopurine S-methyltransferase in patients with Crohn's disease and severe myelosuppression during azathioprine therapy. Gastroenterology 2000;118(6):1025–30.

100. Cummins D, Sekar M, Halil O, Banner N. Myelosuppression associated with azathioprine–allopurinol interaction after heart and lung transplantation. Transplantation 1996;61(11):1661–2.

101. Ippoliti G, Negri M, Campana C, Vigano M. Urate oxidase in hyperuricemic heart transplant recipients treated with azathioprine. Transplantation 1997;63(9):1370–1.

102. Dewit O, Vanheuverzwyn R, Desager JP, Horsmans Y. Interaction between azathioprine and aminosalicylates: an in vivo study in patients with Crohn's disease. Aliment Pharmacol Ther 2002;16(1):79–85.
103. Singleton JD, Conyers L. Warfarin and azathioprine: an important drug interaction. Am J Med 1992;92(2):217.
104. Fernandez MA, Regadera A, Aznar J. Acenocoumarol and 6-mercaptopurine: an important drug interaction. Haematologica 1999;84(7):664–5.
105. Rotenberg M, Levy Y, Shoenfeld Y, Almog S, Ezra D. Effect of azathioprine on the anticoagulant activity of warfarin. Ann Pharmacother 2000;34(1):120–2.
106. Blanco R, Martinez-Taboada VM, Gonzalez-Gay MA, Armona J, Fernandez-Sueiro JL, Gonzalez-Vela MC, Rodriguez-Valverde V. Acute febrile toxic reaction in patients with refractory rheumatoid arthritis who are receiving combined therapy with methotrexate and azathioprine. Arthritis Rheum 1996;39(6):1016–20.
107. Lowry PW, Franklin CL, Weaver AL, Szumlanski CL, Mays DC, Loftus EV, Tremaine WJ, Lipsky JJ, Weinshilboum RM, Sandborn WJ. Leucopenia resulting from a drug interaction between azathioprine or 6-mercaptopurine and mesalamine, sulphasalazine, or balsalazide. Gut 2001;49(5):656–64.

Brequinar

General Information

Brequinar (DUP 785, NSC 368390) is a quinoline carboxylic acid derivative that inhibits pyrimidine synthesis by inhibiting dihydro-orotate dehydrogenase. It was originally developed as an anticancer drug, but has also been investigated for its immunosuppressant activity after transplantation. Some data suggest that that the immunosuppressant activity of brequinar may be partly due to inhibition of tyrosine phosphorylation in lymphocytes (1).

Significant adverse effects of brequinar include thrombocytopenia, maculopapular dermatitis, mucositis, and gastrointestinal disorders (2).

Susceptibility Factors

In patients with renal, hepatic, and cardiac transplants the clearance of a single oral dose of brequinar was lower than expected from previous studies (3), perhaps due to an interaction with ciclosporin, as has been shown in rats (4). Overall safety results suggest that brequinar is well tolerated in stable transplant recipients (3).

Drug–Drug Interactions

Cisplatin

Brequinar was synergistic with cisplatin in preclinical models. However, co-administration of brequinar with cisplatin does not affect the pharmacokinetics of either drug (5).

References

1. Xu X, Williams JW, Shen J, Gong H, Yin DP, Blinder L, Elder RT, Sankary H, Finnegan A, Chong AS. In vitro and in vivo mechanisms of action of the antiproliferative and immunosuppressive agent, brequinar sodium. J Immunol 1998;160(2):846–53.
2. Philip AT, Gerson B. Toxicology and adverse effects of drugs used for immunosuppression in organ transplantation. Clin Lab Med 1998;18(4):755–65.
3. Joshi AS, King SY, Zajac BA, Makowka L, Sher LS, Kahan BD, Menkis AH, Stiller CR, Schaefle B, Kornhauser DM. Phase I safety and pharmacokinetic studies of brequinar sodium after single ascending oral doses in stable renal, hepatic, and cardiac allograft recipients. J Clin Pharmacol 1997;37(12):1121–8.
4. Pally C, Smith D, Jaffee B, Magolda R, Zehender H, Dorobek B, Donatsch P, Papageorgiou C, Schuurman HJ. Side effects of brequinar and brequinar analogues, in combination with cyclosporine, in the rat. Toxicology 1998;127(1–3):207–22.
5. Burris HA 3rd, Raymond E, Awada A, Kuhn JG, O'Rourke TJ, Brentzel J, Lynch W, King SY, Brown TD, Von Hoff DD. Pharmacokinetic and phase I studies of brequinar (DUP 785; NSC 368390) in combination with cisplatin in patients with advanced malignancies. Invest New Drugs 1998;16(1):19–27.

Ciclosporin

General Information

Ciclosporin is an immunosuppressant drug that primarily inhibits T cell activation, therefore down-regulating the T cell responses that mediate graft rejection. Myelotoxic effects are therefore not expected. Ciclosporin has also been used in a wide range of chronic inflammatory or autoimmune diseases.

Considerable efforts have been devoted to defining the optimal dose to ensure minimal toxicity while retaining efficacy. In transplant patients, the daily maintenance dose is 2–6 mg/kg/day. In non-transplant patients, daily doses of 2.5 mg/kg up to a maximum of 4 mg/kg are usually recommended.

In renal transplantation, ciclosporin maintenance monotherapy can be effectively achieved in a subset of patients with the aim of reducing adverse effects associated with glucocorticoids or azathioprine, but this should be carefully balanced against the risks of acute or chronic allograft rejection. This approach was again emphasized, based on data from 100 adults and a review of the most recent literature (1). According to the authors, clinical predictors of successful ciclosporin maintenance therapy included compliant patients over 25 years old with a donor age younger than 40 years, patients with later azathioprine withdrawal, patients with serum creatinine concentrations of 125 μmol/l or less, patients without a history of rejection (or one rejection episode responding favorably to glucocorticoids), and patients who have successfully discontinued glucocorticoids 6 months before.

Comparative studies

Although the pattern of long-term toxicity of ciclosporin and tacrolimus is remarkably similar for most serious adverse effects (particularly nephrotoxicity), a higher incidence of several minor adverse effects with ciclosporin, namely hirsutism, gingivitis or gum hyperplasia, has been thought to underlie a moderate but significant decrease in the quality of life with ciclosporin compared with tacrolimus (2).

General adverse effects

As regards long-term toxicity, particularly nephrotoxicity, and frequent drug interactions, the benefit-to-harm balance of ciclosporin is still debatable. Whereas the adverse effects have generally been deemed acceptable, although occasionally treatment-limiting in patients with rheumatoid arthritis given low-dose ciclosporin rather than conventional antirheumatic drugs, conflicting opinions have been expressed on the acceptability of the risks in patients with psoriasis (SEDA-20, 343).

Of 20 patients with chronic idiopathic thrombocytopenic purpura refractory to glucocorticoids or splenectomy treated with ciclosporin, six withdrew owing to toxicity (3). The target blood concentration range was identical to that aimed at in the first 3 months after kidney transplantation. The most common adverse effects were hypertension, headache, and severe myalgia.

The antileukemic effect of ciclosporin has been harnessed in the treatment of cytopenias associated with chronic lymphatic leukemia. In 31 patients the most common adverse effect was a raised serum creatinine concentration of grade 2 or worse in six patients (19%); three patients developed opportunistic infections (4).

Drug interactions with ciclosporin have been comprehensively reviewed (5).

Organs and Systems

Cardiovascular

Compared with azathioprine, hypertension has been considered one of the main long-term risks in patients taking ciclosporin, with major concerns about the post-transplantion increase in cardiovascular morbidity and mortality. However, there are many susceptibility factors for cardiovascular disease in transplant patients (6), and it is difficult to take into account their complex interplay. Ciclosporin-associated hypertension appears to be dose-related, and higher whole-blood ciclosporin concentrations were found during the preceding months in patients who had thromboembolic complications compared with patients who did not (7).

De novo or aggravated hypertension is very common in patients taking ciclosporin, with the highest incidence in cases of heart transplant (71–100%) and the lowest incidence in bone marrow transplant recipients (33–60%) (8). In addition, 30–45% of patients with psoriasis, rheumatoid arthritis, or uveitis had hypertension, suggesting that ciclosporin is a significant cause of hypertension in organ

transplantation. Ciclosporin-associated hypertension can cause acute vascular injury, with microangiopathic hemolysis, encephalopathy, seizures, and intracranial hemorrhage.

The incidence, clinical features, consequences, and management of ciclosporin-induced hypertension have been reviewed (9). The prevalence was 29–54% in non-transplant patients and 65–100% in heart and liver transplant patients also taking glucocorticoids. Disturbed circadian rhythm with a loss of nocturnal blood pressure fall was the main characteristic, and patients therefore had higher risks of left ventricular hypertrophy, cerebrovascular damage, microalbuminuria, and other target organ damage.

The pathophysiology of ciclosporin-induced hypertension is complex and not yet fully elucidated. Increased systemic vascular resistance subsequent to altered vascular endothelium function, renal vasoconstriction with reduced glomerular filtration and sodium-water retention, and/or increased activity of the sympathetic nervous system were suggested, while only a minor role or none was attributed to the renin–angiotensin system (10). However, hypertension often occurs before changes in renal function or sodium balance can be demonstrated, and ciclosporin nephrotoxicity alone does not explain ciclosporin-associated hypertension (8,11).

The effects of antihypertensive agents have been evaluated in patients taking ciclosporin. Collectively, dihydropyridine calcium channel blockers that do not affect ciclosporin blood concentrations substantially or at all (felodipine, isradipine, and nifedipine) are usually considered to be the drugs of choice. However, the risk of gingival hyperplasia with nifedipine, which ciclosporin also causes, should be borne in mind. Combination therapy with angiotensin-converting enzyme inhibitors or beta-blockers, or the use of other calcium channel blockers (verapamil or diltiazem) should also be considered, but careful monitoring of ciclosporin blood concentrations is recommended with the latter because they inhibit ciclosporin metabolism.

A possible role of ciclosporin in the exacerbation or development of Raynaud's disease has been suggested on one occasion; such an effect could be linked to endothelial damage or changes in platelet function (12).

A capillary leak syndrome with subsequent pulmonary edema has also been reported after intravenous ciclosporin (SEDA-21, 383).

Infusion phlebitis has been attributed to intravenous ciclosporin (13).

Respiratory

Adult respiratory distress syndrome has been described after intravenous ciclosporin. It was thought that a high concentration of the drug in the pulmonary vasculature due to administration through a central vein was responsible for capillary leakage, but in one patient the pulmonary capillary leak resolved rapidly when the intravenous ciclosporin was changed to oral (14). This suggested that Cremophor (polyoxyethylated castor oil), the solvent for parenteral ciclosporin, was responsible. However, there has been a report of an adult who developed respiratory distress syndrome in association with oral ciclosporin given after renal transplantation (15).

Hypersensitivity pneumonitis has been attributed to ciclosporin (16).

- A 35-year-old woman taking glibenclamide and mesalazine for Crohn's colitis was given ciclosporin for severe disease exacerbation. Within 6 weeks, she developed arthralgia and moderate thrombocytopenia, and ciclosporin was discontinued. Acute fever (41°C) and dyspnea were noted several days later, and a chest X-ray showed diffuse bilateral infiltrates. Bronchoalveolar lavage showed neutrophil preponderance and plasma cells, and a lung biopsy strongly suggested an acute hypersensitivity pneumonitis. All her symptoms subsided after a short course of prednisolone and oxygen.

Both the absence of an infectious cause and the rapid improvement without withdrawal of other drugs suggested that ciclosporin was the likely cause.

Nervous system

Neurological adverse effects of ciclosporin have been reported in up to 39% of all transplant patients. Most are mild. The most frequent is a fine tremor, the mechanism of which is not known. From many case reports or studies in transplant patients, the pattern of ciclosporin neurotoxicity ranges from common and mild to moderate symptoms, such as headaches, tremors, paresthesia, restlessness, mood changes, sleep disturbances, confusion, agitation, and visual hallucinations, to rare but severe or life-threatening disorders, including acute psychotic episodes, cerebellar disorders, cortical blindness (permanent in one report), spasticity or paralysis of the limbs, catatonia, speech disorders or mutism, chorea, seizures, leukoencephalopathy, and coma (SED-13, 1124; SEDA-16, 516; SEDA-17, 520; SEDA-20, 343; SEDA-21, 383; 17–19).

A 19% incidence of central nervous system toxicity with ciclosporin has been reported in pediatric renal transplantation patients; the symptoms included seizures, drowsiness, confusion, hallucinations, visual disturbances, and mental changes (20).

Neurological symptoms were observed in 12–25% of liver-transplant patients and in 29% of bone marrow transplant patients, but severe neurotoxicity occurred only in about 1% (18,19,21). They usually appeared within the first month of treatment, but were sometimes delayed (19). Particular attention should be paid to prompt recognition of severe neurotoxicity, because abnormalities of the white matter can occur. Patients usually improved rapidly after temporary ciclosporin withdrawal or dosage reduction, and tacrolimus has sometimes been used successfully instead (SEDA-21, 383; 18). However, recurrence of seizures and persistent electroencephalographic abnormalities were found in 46 and 70% of pediatric transplant patients respectively who had had ciclosporin acute encephalopathy and seizure syndrome and who were followed-up for 49 months (22).

Although the role of many other factors should be considered when neurological symptoms occur in transplant recipients, isolated reports of neurotoxicity in non-transplanted patients are in keeping with a causal role of ciclosporin. There are many susceptibility factors in ciclosporin neurotoxicity. Blood ciclosporin concentrations are sometimes raised, but severe neurological symptoms have been observed in some patients with concentrations in the usual target range (18). Other possible susceptibility factors for ciclosporin neurotoxicity include hypocholesterolemia, hypomagnesemia, aluminium overload, concomitant high-dose glucocorticoid therapy, hypertension, and concomitant microangiopathic hemolytic anemia (SED-13, 1124; SEDA-21, 383). Acute graft-versus-host disease or HLA-mismatched and unrelated donor transplants were also potential susceptibility factors in recipients of bone marrow transplants (SEDA-22, 383; 19).

Ciclosporin-induced vasculopathy, with endothelial injury and derangement of the blood–brain barrier, is the postulated mechanism of neurological damage. Transient cerebral perfusion abnormalities, demonstrable in SPECT scans of the brain, have been suggested as a reliable indicator of ciclosporin neurotoxicity (SEDA-20, 344). Clinical symptoms as well as CT and/or MRI scans were very similar to those observed in hypertensive encephalopathy, with predominant and reversible white-matter occipital lesions (23). There was complete neurological recovery in most patients after blood pressure was normalized, and deaths due to intracranial hemorrhage are reported only exceptionally.

A retrospective study identified a significantly higher incidence of central nervous system symptoms in patients with Behçet's disease (24). Headache, fever, paralysis, ataxia, dysarthria, or disturbed consciousness occurred in 12 of 47 ciclosporin-treated patients compared with nine of 270 patients not treated or taking other drugs. CT and/or MRI scans were abnormal in all 12. As the clinical findings were very similar to the neurological effects of Behçet's disease, it was suggested that ciclosporin can promote the development of neurological complications in this population.

Ciclosporin neurotoxicity is particularly frequent in liver and bone marrow transplant patients, who usually recover after temporary dosage reduction or withdrawal. However, a fatal outcome has been reported (25).

- A 54-year-old man was given ciclosporin and methotrexate after allogeneic bone marrow transplantation. He noted blurred vision during several days and became confused 11 weeks after transplantation. Generalized tonic-clonic seizures occurred the day after and he was given phenytoin and antibiotics. His neurological condition deteriorated during the next 5 days, despite ciclosporin withdrawal, and he died from respiratory failure. Postmortem examination showed white matter edema and astrocyte injury without demyelination.

Most studies have focused on the central nervous system adverse effects of ciclosporin, and there have been few reports of peripheral neuropathy.

- In two patients, ciclosporin was suggested as a possible cause of an entrapment neuropathy, and surgery was required in both (26).

However, the report did not provide sufficient evidence to assess the causal relation fully.

- Another patient developed a symmetric polyneuropathy with flaccid paraplegia while her ciclosporin serum concentrations were about twice normal (27). Electromyography showed features of axonal degeneration in the peripheral nerves and neurological symptoms improved on ciclosporin dosage reduction.

Migraine associated with ciclosporin is sometimes resistant to classical treatment and the consequences can be even more severe.

- Three young adult renal transplant patients, including two with a previous history of moderate migraine, had severe attacks of unilateral throbbing migraine associated with vomiting during ciclosporin treatment (28). In two patients, vomiting was severe enough to reduce compliance with the immunosuppressive regimen, and both subsequently lost their grafts. The same sequence of events was again observed after retransplantation.

Substitution by tacrolimus may be beneficial in such cases.

Severe ciclosporin neurotoxicity has mostly been reported in transplant patients, but should also be considered in non-transplanted patients.

- An 87-year-old patient with resistant nodular prurigo was successfully treated with ciclosporin (3 mg/kg/day) and prednisone (10 mg/day) (29). Bilateral numbness and distal limb weakness developed after 18 months. Clinical examination, electromyography, and nerve conduction studies confirmed a diffuse axonal neuropathy which rapidly progressed over the next 2 months. Ciclosporin alone was withdrawn and complete remission was observed within 3 months.

Unfortunately, ciclosporin blood concentrations and renal function at the time of diagnosis were not reported.

Very severe or fatal neurotoxicity has been reported in isolated patients only.

- Based on postmortem findings in a 32-year-old woman who died with an acute encephalopathy (30) and another report of two patients investigated with transcranial Doppler ultrasound and MRI for symptoms of ciclosporin neurotoxicity (31), vascular changes with vasospasm and dissection of the vascular intima strongly suggest that vasculopathy is a possible mechanism of ciclosporin-induced encephalopathy.

Prolonged confusion is a recognized complication of ciclosporin, and can be due to non-convulsive status epilepticus (32). Three patients who developed neurotoxicity following treatment with ciclosporin manifested with generalized tonic-clonic seizures and dysarthria. The plasma ciclosporin concentration in these patients increased as the neurological signs appeared, and the signs resolved quickly after dosage reduction (33). Tonic-clonic seizures have been reported in a child taking ciclosporin (34).

- A 13-year-old boy with severe Crohn's disease developed hematochezia and required blood transfusion. He was given ciclosporin on day 22 because of persistent rectal bleeding and diarrhea, despite high-dose intravenous glucocorticoids. After 6 days he developed multiple episodes of generalized tonic-clonic seizures, with MRI findings typical but not pathognomonic of ciclosporin: prominent meningeal enhancement, bifrontal, bitemporal, biparietal, and bioccipital cortical and subcortical white matter high-signal changes, and swelling of the gyri, which obliterated the sulci.

This case illustrates that severe ciclosporin neurotoxicity can develop in patients with predisposing factors, such as hypomagnesemia, hypocholesterolemia, hypertension, and glucocorticoid therapy.

There is still debate about whether ciclosporin crosses the blood–brain barrier and enters the cerebrospinal fluid. Ciclosporin could not be identified in cerebrospinal fluid from 14 patients with liver transplants who had various neurological complications (35). Ciclosporin metabolites were measurable in the cerebrospinal fluid in only four patients, who had evidence of acute renal insufficiency, cholestasis, and raised blood concentrations of ciclosporin metabolites but identical ciclosporin parent drug blood concentrations compared with 10 patients with undetectable concentrations of ciclosporin metabolites in the cerebrospinal fluid. Ciclosporin metabolites enter the cerebrospinal fluid, and direct neurotoxicity is therefore possible in at least some patients with renal or hepatic dysfunction.

Endogenous ligands for ciclosporin and tacrolimus, known as immunophilins, are found in very high concentrations in the basal ganglia, and ciclosporin can alter dopamine phosphorylation in the medium-sized neurons in the striatum. Changes in basal ganglia glucose metabolism have been studied in a patient with severe ciclosporin-related tremor (36).

- A 37-year-old man received ciclosporin after bone marrow transplantation for chronic myelogenous leukemia. Soon afterwards he developed a severe tremor, which persisted despite dosage reduction. A brain MRI scan was normal. After 22 months he developed a personality change. A high resolution PET scan showed symmetrical increases in ^{18}F-deoxyglucose uptake in both caudate and putamen.

These results confirm that ciclosporin can modulate dopaminergic transmission in the striatum, presumably by inhibition of calcineurin.

- A 16-year-old girl with end-stage renal insufficiency underwent successful renal transplantation and was given ciclosporin on day 1 (37). On day 10 she complained of tinnitus and tremor and had a right facial nerve palsy. An MRI scan showed areas of increased signal in the white matter of the periventricular region. The dose of ciclosporin was reduced, since no other cause could be determined. Her tremor and tinnitus resolved, but the facial nerve palsy persisted. She was given tacrolimus, but the tremor and tinnitus recurred. She was then given mycophenolate mofetil and prednisone, and the tremor and tinnitus disappeared, although the facial nerve palsy persisted. The MRI scan 3 months later was normal.

The serum magnesium concentration was below the reference range in this case, which may have favored the development of neurotoxicity.

Sensory systems

Controversial reports of ocular symptoms have been published in patients taking oral ciclosporin, with ptosis and diplopia attributed to unilateral or bilateral sixth nerve palsies in four patients (who had also taken ganciclovir), and nystagmus in one patient (SEDA-21, 383). Peripheral optic neuropathy, with visual loss, nystagmus, and ophthalmoplegia, has also been reported (38). Acute cerebral cortical blindness complicating ciclosporin therapy in a 5-year-old girl (39) and transient cortical blindness and occipital seizures with visual impairment (40,41) have also been reported in association with ciclosporin.

Bilateral optic disc edema is sometimes associated with ciclosporin given for bone marrow transplantation, but unilateral papilledema with otherwise asymptomatic raised intracranial pressure can occur (42). Eight cases of optic disc edema have been reported in bone marrow transplant patients taking ciclosporin. In two of the patients there were other possible explanations, but in all cases withdrawal of ciclosporin resulted in resolution of the papilledema (43).

Ciclosporin eye-drops have been used after keratoplasty, in high-risk cases, to prevent graft rejection and to treat severe vernal conjunctivitis, keratoconjunctivitis sicca, and various immune-related corneal disorders. Despite its severe adverse effects after systemic use, topical ciclosporin can generally be used without serious adverse reactions (44,45).

Ciclosporin oil-in-water emulsion has been used in the local treatment of moderate to severe dry eye disease. Chronic dry eye disease results from inflammation mediated by cytokines and receptors for autoimmune antibodies in the lacrimal glands. It affects the lacrimal gland acini and ducts, leading to abnormalities in the tear film, and ultimately disrupting the homeostasis of the ocular surface. Topical ciclosporin reduces the cell-mediated inflammatory response associated with inflammatory ocular surface diseases.

In two large, randomized controlled trials in 977 patients, the adverse effects associated with ciclosporin ophthalmic emulsion for the treatment of dry eye disease were minimal and consisted mostly of mild ocular burning and stinging (46). However, topical application of ciclosporin eye-drops was the suspected cause of severe visual loss with bilateral white corneal deposits in a 45-year-old patient with dry eye syndrome caused by graft-versus-host disease (47). Infrared spectroscopy and X-ray analysis suggested that the deposits contained ciclosporin. A reduction in tear clearance and compromised epithelial barrier function caused by the concomitant use of oxybuprocaine may have precipitated this adverse effect.

The efficacy, safety, tolerability, and optimal dose of ciclosporin eye-drops have been studied in a randomized, double-masked, vehicle-controlled multicenter trial in 162 patients with keratoconjunctivitis sicca with or without Sjögren's disease and refractory to conventional treatment (48). Ciclosporin ophthalmic emulsion 0.05, 0.1, 0.2, or 0.4%, or the vehicle alone was instilled twice daily into both eyes for 12 weeks, followed by a 4-week observation period. There was no clear dose–response relation; ciclosporin 0.1% emulsion produced the most consistent improvement in objective and subjective endpoints and ciclosporin 0.05% gave the most consistent improvement in symptoms. The vehicle also performed well, perhaps because of its long residence time on the ocular surface. There were no significant adverse effects, no microbial overgrowth, and no residence time of the vehicle emulsion on the ocular surface. All treatments were well tolerated and the highest ciclosporin blood concentration detected was 0.16 ng/ml.

To study the efficacy and safety of ciclosporin 0.05 and 0.1% ophthalmic emulsions and their vehicle in patients with moderate to severe dry eye disease, two identical multicenter, randomized, double-masked, vehicle-controlled trials have been performed in 877 patients for 6 months (46). More than 76% completed the course. Ciclosporin 0.05 or 0.1% eye-drops gave significantly greater improvement than the vehicle in two objective signs of dry eye disease (corneal staining and Schirmer values). Ciclosporin 0.05% also gave significantly greater improvement in three subjective measures (blurred vision, need for concomitant artificial tears, and the physician's evaluation of global response to treatment). There was no dose–response effect and there were no topical or systemic adverse findings.

Corneal deposition of ciclosporin can occur (47).

- A 45-year-old woman with dry eye syndrome caused by graft-versus-host disease after bone marrow transplantation for acute leukemia was given systemic ciclosporin and topical 0.1% sodium hyaluronate, 0.3% ofloxacin, 0.1% fluorometholone, and isotonic saline. She was also given 0.4% oxybuprocaine for the relief of severe ocular pain. The bilateral corneal epithelial defects persisted even after the application of punctal plugs, and 2% ciclosporin in olive oil was added as eye-drops three times a day bilaterally. Five days later she complained of severe visual loss in association with bilateral corneal opacities, which covered the pupil and the punctal plugs bilaterally. As she did not agree to keratectomy, infrared spectroscopy and X-ray analysis were conducted on the deposits on the plugs. The spectroscopic pattern and X-ray analysis showed that the deposits had the properties of ciclosporin.

As the corneal deposits did not abate after withdrawal of the ciclosporin eye-drops, the systemic ciclosporin as well as its topical use may have contributed to the deposits. One should be aware that precipitation of ciclosporin on a compromised cornea can lead to severe visual impairment.

Metabolism

Diabetes mellitus

Diabetes mellitus after transplantation is recognized as an important adverse effect of immunosuppressants, and has been extensively reviewed (49). However, the use of ciclosporin in immunosuppressive regimens is not associated with diabetes mellitus after transplantation (10–20%) (50).

Hyperlipidemia

Ciclosporin is potentially more toxic in patients with altered LDL concentrations or a low total serum cholesterol (51). Ciclosporin therapy itself significantly raises plasma lipoprotein concentrations by increasing the total serum cholesterol; this is due to an increase in LDL cholesterol, demonstrated in a prospective, double-blind, randomized, placebo-controlled trial in 36 men with amyotrophic lateral sclerosis (52). In 22 patients there were significant increases in mean serum triglycerides and cholesterol 2 weeks after they started to take low-dose ciclosporin (53). Hypertriglyceridemia developed in seven patients taking ciclosporin 2.0–7.5 mg/kg/day for psoriasis during the first month of therapy; the values were greater than the upper limit in age- and sex-matched controls (54).

The pathology of hyperlipidemia after transplantation is multifactorial, but it is clearly dose-dependently related to immunosuppressive therapy (55). This results in cardiovascular disease, which is one of the most common causes of morbidity and mortality in long-term survivors of organ transplantation (56). Hyperlipidemia can also cause renal atheroma, resulting in graft rejection. The possible impact of ciclosporin on lipids includes an increase in total cholesterol, LDL cholesterol, and apolipoprotein B concentrations, and a reduction in HDL cholesterol (SED-13, 1124). The influence of ciclosporin on lipoprotein(a) concentrations has been debated (SEDA-21, 383; 57). Post-transplant hyperlipidemia is multifactorial and can be affected by impaired renal function, diuretics and beta-blockers, increased age, and female sex. A combination of lipid-lowering drugs and optimization of immunosuppressive regimens compatible with long-term allograft survival is probably required to reduce post-transplantation hyperlipidemia.

Whereas azathioprine is considered to play no role, glucocorticoid use correlates positively with increased serum cholesterol concentrations. It is uncertain whether these lipid changes reflect primarily an effect of ciclosporin alone or an additive/synergistic effect of the drug plus glucocorticoids. Ciclosporin has been considered as a possible independent susceptibility factor by several investigators, but others were unable to find an association between hyperlipidemia and ciclosporin (SEDA-20, 344). There was indirect evidence for a causal role of ciclosporin in several studies; hyperlipidemia developed in non-transplant patients taking ciclosporin alone; there was a transient reduction in hyperlipidemia after ciclosporin withdrawal; there was a significant correlation between ciclosporin blood concentrations and lipid abnormalities; and there was a higher incidence of lipid abnormalities in patients taking ciclosporin alone compared with patients taking azathioprine and prednisolone (SED-8, 1131; SEDA-17, 524; SEDA-21, 383; 55,58). Other studies have provided striking evidence that

hyperlipidemia is more frequent in patients taking ciclosporin than in those taking tacrolimus, with more patients classified as having high cholesterol concentrations in the ciclosporin group or a significant fall in total cholesterol or LDL cholesterol in patients switched from ciclosporin to tacrolimus (59,60). Although the glucocorticoid-sparing effect of tacrolimus may account for these differences, the concept that the glucocorticoid dose is a confounding factor has been disputed (SEDA-22, 412). Whether these differences translate to a higher risk of cardiovascular complications in patients taking ciclosporin has not been carefully assessed. The treatment of hyperlipidemia in transplant patients may represent a major dilemma, because of several drug interactions, with an increased risk of myopathy and rhabdomyolysis after the combined use of ciclosporin and several lipid-lowering drugs.

Hyperuricemia

Significant hyperuricemia has been observed in as many as 80% of patients taking ciclosporin (61). In one series, hyperuricemia occurred in 72% of male and 82% of female patients taking ciclosporin after cardiac transplantation; there was also an increased incidence of gouty arthritis in these patients (62). Episodes of gout developed mostly in men taking diuretics, but the incidence was lower than in the hyperuricemic population. In renal transplant patients, the incidence of gout was 5–24% and tophi sometimes developed rapidly after the onset of gout (63). The potential mechanisms of hyperuricemia include reduced renal function and impaired tubular secretion of acid uric, with hypertension and diuretics as confounding factors (SEDA-21, 383).

Nutrition

Higher plasma homocysteine concentrations, which may contribute to atherosclerosis, have been found in patients taking ciclosporin, compared with both transplant patients not taking ciclosporin and non-transplant patients with renal insufficiency (SEDA-20, 344).

Electrolyte balance

Mild and uncomplicated hyperkalemia is commonly observed in patients taking ciclosporin and is generally prevented by a low potassium diet. A reduction in distal nephron potassium secretion and tubular flow rate, with insensitivity to exogenous mineralocorticoids, and leakage of cellular potassium into the extracellular fluid are possible mechanisms (SED-13, 1124; 64).

Mineral balance

Hypomagnesemia and hypercalcemia occur infrequently during ciclosporin treatment (SED-13, 1124).

• In a 43-year-old renal transplant patient, hypomagnesemia was associated with muscle weakness and a near four-fold increase in serum creatine kinase activity (65). Both disorders resolved after magnesium supplementation, and ciclosporin was continued.

Renal magnesium wasting occurred in 24% of a series of renal transplant patients taking ciclosporin; other indicators of renal function were normal (66,67).

Hypomagnesemia in the early post-transplant period has been cited as a possible risk factor for acute ciclosporin neurotoxicity. Ciclosporin-induced sustained magnesium depletion has been investigated in 109 ciclosporin-treated patients with renal transplants who had been stable for more than 6 months (68). Total and ionized plasma magnesium concentrations were significantly lower than in 21 healthy volunteers and in 15 patients with renal transplants who were not taking ciclosporin. Ciclosporin-treated patients who were also taking hypoglycemic drugs had lower plasma magnesium concentrations, but patients taking diuretics did not.

Hematologic

A very few cases of ciclosporin-induced immune hemolytic anemia have been reported (SED-13, 1125; 69,70), but a direct causal relation with ciclosporin is difficult to establish. Ciclosporin-induced hypercoagulability was suggested in patients with aplastic anemia (SEDA-20, 344). Higher whole-blood ciclosporin concentrations were found during the preceding months in patients who experienced thromboembolic complications compared with patients who had not.

Ciclosporin-associated thrombotic microangiopathy occurs in 3–14% of patients with a renal transplant and can cause allograft loss. Renal impairment, reflected by an increase in serum creatinine concentration, is often the only change found, and hemolysis is not always present. Plasmapheresis has been used to treat this complication (71).

- A 47-year-old multiparous Hispanic woman received a living-unrelated kidney transplant for end-stage renal disease secondary to polycystic kidney disease. On the day of transplantation she received intravenous daclizumab 1 mg/kg plus methylprednisolone 300 mg and mycophenolate mofetil 3 g/day, and on day 3 ciclosporin emulsion 4 mg/kg/day. On day 8 she developed thrombotic microangiopathy without evidence of rejection. Ciclosporin was withdrawn. Plasmapheresis with fresh frozen plasma was started. Daclizumab on day 14 was postponed for 24 hours and plasmapheresis was stopped to avoid clearance of daclizumab. Thereafter she was given tacrolimus, without recurrence of hemolysis.

Mouth and teeth

Ciclosporin-induced gingival hyperplasia was noted in the early 1980s, and subsequent studies investigated the prevalence and pathophysiology of this adverse effect (SED-13, 1127). The reported incidence was 7–70%, and clinically significant gingival overgrowth, that is to say requiring treatment or surgical excision, affected about 30% of patients within the first 6 months of treatment (72). Clinical and histological features are similar to those associated with phenytoin or nifedipine. Compared with control specimens, ultrastructural gingival examinations in patients taking ciclosporin showed many fibroblasts, abundant amorphous substance, and marked plasma cell infiltration (73). Although an imbalance between the production and removal of collagen is supposed to account for gingival hyperplasia, the mechanism of ciclosporin-induced gingival overgrowth has not yet been clearly established. Possible local lymphocyte resistance to ciclosporin resulting in an increasing number of several inflammatory cells in the gingival lamina propria and ciclosporin-induced inhibition of prostaglandin I_2 synthesis have also been suggested (74,75).

There are many susceptibility factors for ciclosporin-induced gingival hyperplasia. The duration of treatment and the cumulative dose during the first 6 months play a major role. Accordingly, reduction of the ciclosporin dose can lessen the risk, and the use of lower doses is thought to reduce the overall incidence (76,77). There is also a positive correlation between the degree of gingival hyperplasia and changes in renal function (78). There are conflicting findings regarding the effects of blood concentrations on the incidence of gingival hyperplasia, and no clear relation between saliva and blood ciclosporin concentrations has been found. Lower age correlated significantly with the presence of gingival hyperplasia and children under 6 years of age are more susceptible to the complication in severe form (76,79). Male sex is a predisposing factor, a finding supported by the report of an increased androgen metabolism in gingival hyperplasia induced by ciclosporin (80). There has been also speculation concerning genetic differences in the susceptibility to develop these changes (SEDA-21, 384; 72). Finally, the combination of ciclosporin and nifedipine is additive with an increased prevalence and/or severity of gingival hyperplasia (SED-13, 1127; 76,77,80–82). As several other calcium channel blockers can produce gingival overgrowth, more frequent gingival hyperplasia should be expected, at least theoretically, when these drugs are combined with ciclosporin.

It is not yet clearly established whether bacterial plaque, gingival bleeding index, or inflammation are the cause or result of gingival hyperplasia. Certainly, poor oral health with subsequent local inflammation appears to be a contributing factor. Consequently, careful dental hygiene with plaque control is often sufficient to improve or resolve hyperplasia, but surgical treatment is sometimes necessary. Preliminary case reports have suggested that azithromycin or metronidazole can improve ciclosporin-induced gingival hyperplasia (SEDA-19, 350). This has been confirmed for azithromycin, with no indication that ciclosporin blood concentrations are modified during a short course of azithromycin (SEDA-22, 414).

Gastrointestinal

Gastrointestinal symptoms due to ciclosporin are usually mild and transient. In rheumatoid arthritis, gastrointestinal intolerance has been reported in 50% of patients, being the main cause for withdrawal of ciclosporin in 8% (83). Whereas worsening colitis did not occur in patients with inflammatory bowel disease, ciclosporin was involved in the development of acute colitis in isolated reports (SED-13, 1125).

Liver

There was at least one episode of hepatotoxicity in 228 of 466 patients (49%) with renal transplants who took ciclosporin; 110 (48%) had hyperalbuminemia, 108 (47%) a raised aspartate transaminase, and 167 (59%) a raised alkaline phosphatase (84). Ciclosporin dosage reduction resulted in resolution of hepatotoxicity in 185 patients (81%), while 32 (14%) had recurrent or persistent liver function abnormalities. Eleven (2.4%) developed biliary calculous disease. The serum ciclosporin concentration was high among the patients with hepatotoxicity. Pharmacokinetic studies showed an increased AUC in the patients with hepatotoxicity, probably due to reduced drug clearance.

A causal association has been shown between the hepatotoxicity of ciclosporin and cold ischemic liver damage that can occur during preservation before liver transplantation (85). This presents a problem when ciclosporin is used after liver transplantation. In more than 1000 patients there was an incidence of mild reversible hepatotoxicity of 40% in patients taking 5-fluorouracil and levamisole as adjuvants for more than 1 year; the incidence of mild hepatotoxicity in those taking levamisole alone and amongst those receiving no treatment at all was the same, a little over 16% (86).

Experiments with isolated human hepatocytes have shown that ciclosporin competitively inhibits the uptake of cholate and glycocholate bile acids; the biological features of ciclosporin-associated hepatotoxicity are therefore mostly those of cholestasis, with reduced bile excretion (87). The presence of underlying chronic viral hepatitis can increase the severity of ciclosporin-induced cholestasis (88).

Ciclosporin can cause cholestasis and cellular necrosis by an inhibitory effect on hepatocyte membrane transport proteins at both sinusoidal and canalicular levels. It induces oxidative stress by accumulation of various free radicals. Ademetionine (S-adenosylmethionine) is a naturally occurring substance that is involved in liver detoxification processes. The efficacy of ademetionine in the treatment and prevention of ciclosporin-induced cholestasis has been studied in 72 men with psoriasis (89). The patients who were given ciclosporin plus ademetionine had low plasma and erythrocyte concentrations of oxidants and high concentrations of antioxidants. The authors concluded that ademetionine may protect the liver against hepatotoxic substances such as ciclosporin.

A possible consequence of bile acid abnormalities and cholestasis associated with ciclosporin is the development of cholelithiasis in liver transplant patients when the donor has pre-existing susceptibility for cholesterol gallstone formation or abnormalities of bile composition.

- A young patient who received a liver from a 78-year-old donor subsequently developed cholesterol gallstones (SEDA-21, 383).

In a retrospective study in 50 consecutive patients who received both parenteral nutrition and glucocorticoids, with or without the addition of ciclosporin, at some stage in their management, there was no evidence that ciclosporin caused more liver dysfunction than that associated with parenteral nutrition (90).

Urinary tract

The renal toxicity of ciclosporin has been described as being an adverse effect of the drug on the compensatory mechanisms of the kidney, without effects on proximal tubular function (urea and sodium reabsorption) (91). A rise in serum creatinine concentration may be adequate to identify acute-onset ciclosporin nephrotoxicity, but it is not suitable for identification of chronic, late-onset ciclosporin nephrotoxicity (92).

Presentation
Acute renal impairment
Acute ciclosporin-induced nephrotoxicity, causing reduced renal function, develops within the first month, and includes a dose-related rise in serum creatinine concentrations and hyperkalemia. Fatal acute tubular necrosis has also been noted after very high intravenous doses (SEDA-19, 345). Although it is clinically often difficult to differentiate from acute allograft rejection in renal transplant patients, the alteration in renal function promptly resolves on ciclosporin withdrawal or dosage reduction, and initial acute renal insufficiency is not clearly associated with the development of subsequent chronic renal dysfunction (93). Several conditions, such as pre-existing hypovolemia, concomitant diuretic treatment, or renal artery stenosis, are susceptibility factors. Hypothyroidism was thought to be involved in one patient (94), and the transplanted kidney itself rather than interindividual differences between recipients was thought to play a role (SEDA-21, 384).

Hemolytic–uremic syndrome and thrombotic microangiopathy
Hemolytic–uremic syndrome, with histological findings of thrombotic microangiopathy and possible evolution to graft loss or death, is another instance of very severe acute nephrotoxicity (SED-13, 1125). It usually occurs at between the second and fourth weeks after transplant, with associated fever, thrombocytopenia, erythrocyte fragmentation, neurotoxicity, and renal impairment. Uncommon clinical features have been reported.

- In two women, hemolytic–uremic syndrome was apparently revealed by an episode of severe acute depression (95).
- In another patient, a single injection of ciclosporin may have induced the development of fibrin thrombi seen in the perioperative graft biopsy (96). Later on, she was confirmed to have clinical and biological features of hemolytic–uremic syndrome, which reversed after ciclosporin withdrawal.

Hemolyti–uremic syndrome has also been reported during ciclosporin treatment for Behçet's disease (SEDA-21, 384). Both early and delayed hemolytic–uremic syndrome can occur after transplantation, and its actual incidence may have been underestimated. Thrombotic microangiopathy with clinical features of hemolytic–uremic syndrome was found in 3.5–5% of renal transplant patients (97,98). Graft loss was mostly found in patients who developed hemolytic–uremic syndrome early after transplantation, and the clinical distinction from acute rejection can be very difficult. Hemolytic–uremic syndrome does not recur after initial withdrawal and further ciclosporin reintroduction, once renal function has normalized, or even despite ciclosporin maintenance with dosage reduction (SED-13, 1125; SEDA-20, 345). In some cases, the patient was successfully switched to tacrolimus, and only one case of hemolytic–uremic syndrome with recurrence on ciclosporin rechallenge has been reported (SEDA-21, 384). In contrast, both ciclosporin and tacrolimus were significant susceptibility factors for recurrence of hemolytic–uremic syndrome in patients who had undergone renal transplantation for end-stage renal disease (99).

The factors that contribute to the development of thrombotic microangiopathy have been retrospectively investigated in 50 of 188 patients with kidney or kidney + pancreas allografts who underwent graft biopsies and in 19 control patients who had never had renal graft dysfunction or a biopsy (100). There were definite histological features of thrombotic microangiopathy 4 days to 6 years after transplantation in 26 patients, of whom 24 were taking ciclosporin and two were taking tacrolimus, showing that this complication can occur at any time after transplantation. Eight patients had graft loss, but only two had associated systemic evidence of microangiopathy, that is thrombocytopenia and intravascular hemolysis, suggesting that thrombotic microangiopathy should be considered in any patients with renal graft dysfunction, even if there are no suggestive systemic symptoms. Although the more frequent use of the microemulsion form of ciclosporin (Neoral) in patients with confirmed thrombotic microangiopathy than in controls suggested a possible role of this formulation, this issue remains to be further investigated, because the number of evaluable patients was small. None of the other investigated variables (age, sex, race, living-related or cadaveric donor status, the degree of HLA mismatch, the type of allograft, or the incidence of urinary tract infections after transplantation) was significantly associated with the occurrence of thrombotic microangiopathy compared with patients without thrombotic microangiopathy. Finally, the most successful strategy was a switch from ciclosporin to tacrolimus, which resulted in normalization of graft function in 81% of these patients.

Chronic renal insufficiency

Chronic renal impairment, as first reported in cardiac transplant patients (101), is of major concern, because of possible irreversible renal dysfunction. A considerable amount of work has subsequently accumulated on the development of progressive renal dysfunction in patients receiving long-term ciclosporin for organ transplantation or chronic inflammatory disease (SED-13, 1125; SEDA-20, 345; SEDA-21, 384; SEDA-22, 413), and there have been several comprehensive reviews (102–105). About one-third of all patients have increased serum creatinine concentrations and reduced glomerular filtration rate during ciclosporin maintenance therapy. The histopathological features of chronic nephropathy consist mostly of non-specific tubular atrophy and interstitial fibrosis (106); arteriolar lesions are considered very suggestive of ciclosporin nephrotoxicity. The prevalence of renal damage due to ciclosporin has fallen considerably since the use of lower doses. Arteriolopathy sometimes improves after reducing or withdrawing ciclosporin. Morphological features in patients with autoimmune diseases are non-specific, and include a wide range of lesions, mostly characterized by tubulointerstitial changes and arteriolopathy. There is no significant correlation between histological findings and ciclosporin dose. Severe histological lesions can be identified in some patients with normal renal function (107); the severity of tubulointerstitial lesions has been deemed to be a better index than the glomerular filtration rate for predicting the occurrence of chronic nephropathy, but in one study there was no correlation between histological renal findings and various measures of renal function (108).

Because the possibility of irreversible renal dysfunction is a major problem in ciclosporin maintenance in both transplant and non-transplant patients, this issue continues to receive attention. Even though many studies have been performed, the long-term prognosis is a source of conflicting opinions, and the initial assumption that long-term use of ciclosporin will sooner or later cause irreversible chronic nephropathy is hotly debated. It is still unclear to what extent long-term ciclosporin contributes to progressive renal insufficiency and whether chronic ciclosporin nephropathy is irreversible or improves after dosage reduction. A retrospective analysis of more than 12 000 renal transplant patients showed that long-term maintenance with a glucocorticoid-free ciclosporin regimen (ciclosporin alone or with azathioprine) significantly increased renal graft and patient survival, compared with patients taking other immunosuppressive regimens (109). This allowed the use of higher doses of ciclosporin without increasing the frequency of nephrotoxicity. In contrast, several investigators have considered a change to a ciclosporin-free regimen in 40% of patients, because of progressive renal deterioration with histological signs of nephrotoxicity (110). The incidence of end-stage renal insufficiency requiring dialysis or renal transplantation ranges from 1% in renal transplant patients to 3–6% in heart-transplant patients (111–114). Nevertheless, several investigators have shown that despite an initial reduction in renal function, serum creatinine concentrations stabilized with no strong evidence of progressive nephropathy after several years of surveillance in various organ transplant patients (93,112,115–117).

The potential long-term consequences of ciclosporin nephrotoxicity constitute a major disadvantage in non-transplant patients. Renal function was assessed 7 years after the end of a 1-year ciclosporin treatment period in 36 young patients from a randomized, placebo-controlled trial of ciclosporin in diabetes mellitus, 19 taking ciclosporin, and 17 taking placebo (118). Blood pressure did not differ between the groups. Compared with baseline values, urinary albumin excretion rate was significantly higher and estimated glomerular filtration rate significantly lower with ciclosporin. The results in the placebo group showed no change or increases. In addition, there was progression to micro- or macro-albuminuria in four patients taking ciclosporin, and two of five patients who underwent renal biopsy had arteriolar hyalinosis. It is not known whether these changes will translate to an increased risk of nephropathy, but they suggest that ciclosporin might enhance it. Of 91 consecutive patients with renal transplants with a minimum graft survival of 1 year who were followed for 7–8 years, 65% had stable renal function despite ciclosporin serum concentrations of 200–250 ng/ml (119). In addition, none of the 26 patients with worsening renal function had features of ciclosporin nephrotoxicity on renal biopsy.

Frequency
In a meta-analysis of 18 trials involving ciclosporin doses below 10 mg/kg/day for at least 2 months in autoimmune diseases, the weighted percentage increase in serum creatinine concentrations was 17% in ciclosporin-treated patients and 1.7% in controls (120). The corrected risk difference for an increase of more than 50% of pretreatment serum creatinine concentrations between the two groups was 21% (95% CI = 12, 30) (120). This meta-analysis did not fully consider the long-term outcome, but clinical and histological evidence of sustained or progressive ciclosporin nephropathy in this population continues to accumulate. Unfortunately, some of the findings are discordant (107,121–130).

In a retrospective study of 106 patients following renal transplantation who had been treated with ciclosporin, 85% were hypertensive compared with 54% of patients taking azathioprine (131). Renal function was significantly better in hypertensive patients treated with nifedipine than with other antihypertensive medication (beta-blockers and vasodilators), and it was similar to that of normotensive patients treated with ciclosporin.

Pathophysiology
The pathogenesis of chronic ciclosporin nephrotoxicity is not fully understood (105). Intrarenal afferent arteriolar vasoconstriction may play an important part, particularly in acute nephrotoxicity (132), in which a marked reduction in renal blood flow associated with an increase in renal vascular resistance, probably due to postglomerular vasoconstriction, has been demonstrated (133,134). The supposed mechanism is primarily an imbalance between several regulatory mechanisms of renal vasodilatation and vasoconstriction, leading to increased renal vasoconstriction, and the explanations that have been proposed include activation of the renin–angiotensin system, prostaglandin inhibition, and sympathetic nervous system activation

(135). However, it is unclear whether a continuous increase in renal vascular resistance can account for chronic renal dysfunction in patients taking long-term ciclosporin. There are many possible mediators of renal vasoconstriction, for example nitric oxide, the renin–angiotensin and kallikrein–kinin systems, endothelin-1 release, and stimulation of sympathetic nervous system activity. A major effect of ciclosporin is to promote calcium accumulation in the mitochondrial matrix, which in turn reduces ATP synthesis (136). The main morphological abnormality that has been demonstrated in the kidneys of patients taking long-term ciclosporin is interstitial fibrosis. Vascular lesions, predominantly arteriolar, with arterial intimal fibrosis have been noted in renal biopsies from patients with chronic ciclosporin nephrotoxicity (137).

Renal morphology has been studied in 17 patients who received ciclosporin for sight-threatening uveitis. Most had not received other potentially nephrotoxic drugs. Variable interstitial fibrosis, frequently associated with tubular atrophy, was noted in all 17. The extent of the pathological changes did not correlate with the age, treatment duration, or average cumulative dose (138). Ciclosporin nephrotoxicity mimics the histological features of acute allograft rejection and tubular necrosis. It is important to be able to distinguish clinically between ciclosporin toxicity on the one hand (necessitating a reduction in dose) and rejection (requiring an increase in dose) on the other.

The long-term effects of ciclosporin on renal function in 11 liver transplant recipients were evaluated over a follow-up period of 6–26 months (135). Immediately postoperatively, glomerular filtration rate (GFR) and effective renal plasma flow (ERPF) fell by 60%, subsequently settling at 45–60% of normal. There were additional toxic effects on renal tubular function. Histopathological findings were mild to moderate; notably, arterial and arteriolar nephrosclerosis. Renal function improved as the dose of ciclosporin was reduced, despite continued administration of the drug. This suggests a persistent, potentially reversible, functional component to chronic ciclosporin nephrotoxicity.

The respective roles of organ preservation and ciclosporin in the pathogenesis of post-transplant renal damage have been studied in an in vitro model that simulates the hypothermic kidney preserved before surgery in Collins' solution and exposed after transplantation to ciclosporin (139). The results showed that preservation sensitizes the kidney to ciclosporin injury, which is consistent with clinical experience (140). If the preserved kidney cells were given a period of repair before administration of ciclosporin, further injury did not happen. In animal experiments, prolonged cold preservation causes progressive deterioration in the renal cortical microcirculation; concentration of ciclosporin in the renal cortex of hypoperfused kidneys markedly potentiates the vascular damage caused by cold preservation (131).

Large-scale studies with long periods of follow-up have emphasized the major role of graft arteriopathy (chronic graft rejection) rather than chronic ciclosporin nephrotoxicity as the primary cause of graft failure (111,116,141).

Severe ciclosporin nephropathy was the cause of renal transplant failure in less than 1% of patients.

Susceptibility factors and prediction

Many factors have been postulated as being relevant to ciclosporin nephrotoxicity. Whereas in several studies initial high doses of ciclosporin increased the risk of chronic nephrotoxicity (115,121), others suggested that patients maintained on relatively high ciclosporin concentrations had no more chance than others of developing toxic nephropathy (116). Neither the daily dose nor the duration of ciclosporin treatment reasonably predicts the risk of chronic renal insufficiency. Chronic renal dysfunction can be observed, despite the maintenance of ciclosporin blood concentrations below 400 ng/ml. However, age, sustained hypertension, hypertriglyceridemia, low HDL cholesterol concentrations, and recurrent episodes of severe acute nephrotoxicity increase susceptibility to chronic ciclosporin nephrotoxicity (122,142).

From a prospective study in 36 heart transplant patients with stable renal function for at least 6 months after transplantation, it was suggested that high urinary retinol-binding protein concentrations may indicate tubulointerstitial damage and therefore detect patients who are at risk of ciclosporin nephrotoxicity (143). At the start of the study, 13 patients had high urinary retinol-binding protein concentrations and 23 had normal concentrations. After 5 years of follow-up, five of the 13 patients developed end-stage renal insufficiency requiring dialysis, whereas none of the 23 other patients had terminal renal insufficiency. Although these data await confirmation, the authors suggested that ciclosporin dosage reduction should be considered in patients with high urinary retinol-binding protein concentrations, in order to limit renal damage.

Ciclosporin can cause tubulointerstitial lesions, the pathogenesis of which is unclear. In 37 patients, the duration of ciclosporin treatment and of heavy proteinuria were independent risk factors for ciclosporin-induced tubulointerstitial disease (144).

Management

The possible risk of precipitating end-stage renal insufficiency should not be regarded as a major limitation to ciclosporin treatment in organ-transplant patients, and no matter how defective our knowledge of the susceptibility factors is, attempts must be made to prevent or manage ciclosporin nephrotoxicity. Delaying the introduction of ciclosporin until post-transplant renal function has returned to normal and reducing the dose of ciclosporin when increases in serum creatinine concentrations are more than 30% above baseline values are measures that may well reduce the risk of acute nephrotoxicity. In the long term, switching patients from ciclosporin to azathioprine, reducing ciclosporin doses, or even electively withdrawing ciclosporin have been suggested as helpful measures, but they should be regarded cautiously and set against the risk of rejection (145–149). Once-daily dosing of ciclosporin in the morning improves glomerular filtration rate and renal blood flow compared with half the dose taken twice daily (150). Despite evidence for a very similar profile of nephrotoxicity, conversion from ciclosporin to tacrolimus has been used successfully (SEDA-20, 342).

Finally, several drugs have been investigated in experimental and clinical studies to prevent ciclosporin nephrotoxicity. Calcium channel blockers, such as nifedipine, diltiazem, or verapamil, have repeatedly been proposed as reliable adjunctive drugs to minimize the long-term nephrotoxic effects of ciclosporin in renal transplant patients. Among anti-ischemic drugs, trimetazidine might be a good choice, because it prevents the loss of ATP synthesis caused by ciclosporin in rat kidney cells. S-15176 and S-16950 are trimetazidine derivatives that antagonize the mitochondrial toxicity of ciclosporin without changing its immunosuppressive effects.

Viewing the evidence as a whole, it appears that the use of lower doses of ciclosporin is probably the most important factor accounting for the fact that the majority of patients on long-term ciclosporin do not today have evidence of progressive nephrotoxicity.

Skin

Mild flushing often occurs during ciclosporin treatment, but more severe extensive erythema is uncommon.

- Recurrent episodes of diffuse flushing of the arms, the face, and the trunk reportedly occurred about 2 hours after each dose of ciclosporin in a 24-year-old man who had received a renal transplant 6 years before (151). These episodes were noted from the beginning of treatment, but worsened after he changed to Neoral, the microemulsion form of ciclosporin, and completely resolved after ciclosporin was replaced by tacrolimus.

Ciclosporin sometimes causes chronic inflammatory dermatitis, and there have been two reports of four male transplant recipients who developed clinical and histopathological features of keloid acne of the posterior scalp or neck (152,153). *Staphylococcus aureus* infection was identified in three. Ciclosporin-induced hypertrichosis was suggested as a possible cause, with local bacterial infection and immunosuppression as trigger factors.

- Multiple, large epidermoid cysts have been described in a 23-year-old man taking ciclosporin (154).

Acute generalized pustular psoriasis occurred 1 week after ciclosporin withdrawal in a 32-year-old woman who had taken ciclosporin for 12 weeks for chronic plaque psoriasis (155). This is in keeping with a similar phenomenon sometimes observed after glucocorticoid withdrawal.

Coarsening of facial features and a possibly more frequent occurrence of acne vulgaris and keratosis pilaris have been described in children taking ciclosporin (SED-8, 1125; 156). In 19 children who took ciclosporin and prednisone after renal transplantion, there was coarsening of facial features with thickening of the nares, lips, and ears, puffiness of the cheeks, prominence of the supraorbital ridges, and mandibular prognathism; this was found in all the children who had been treated for 6 months (157). Although the concurrent use of glucocorticoids may play a role in the development of acne, resolution of severe acne was in one reported case attained only after ciclosporin withdrawal (SEDA-20, 345). Convincing but anecdotal evidence of the worsening of subcutaneous sarcoidosis has been reported (SEDA-22, 384).

Sebaceous glands

Juxtaclavicular beaded lines are unique malformation of sebaceous glands or a variant of sebaceous hyperplasia.

- A 63-year-old man developed small, asymptomatic, linear papules over the neck and clavicles. He had taken prednisone and ciclosporin for 30 months after kidney transplantation (158). A skin biopsy showed sebaceous hyperplasia.

The pathogenesis of juxtaclavicular beaded lines is unclear. Some authors have reported a prevalence of 16% in heart transplant patients, but only in men. Because ciclosporin is highly lipophilic, it has many adverse effects associated with alterations of pilosebaceous follicles, such as hypertrichosis and acne. In this case the authors postulated that the combined effect of prednisone and ciclosporin may have induced sebaceous gland hyperplasia.

Hair

Widespread hypertrichosis is one of the most common complications of ciclosporin, and distichiasis (accessory eyelashes) has been reported in one patient (SEDA-20, 345). Ciclosporin-associated soft tissue proliferation with an abnormal hyperplastic reaction has been suggested to account for the development of hyperplastic pseudofolliculitis barbae (159).

Alopecia areata or alopecia totalis has been noted in isolated cases (SEDA-21, 384).

A white-headed man noted progressive darkening of the hair while taking ciclosporin (160).

Nails

Several nail changes (excess granulation tissue or ingrowing toenails) have been attributed to ciclosporin (SED-13, 1127).

- Marked pitting with Mees' lines (homogeneous transverse white lines in the nail plates) in the fingernails, a disorder that has not been previously reported, was attributed to ciclosporin-associated kidney dysfunction in a 41-year-old man who inadvertently took ciclosporin 300 mg/day for psoriasis (161).

Musculoskeletal

Muscle disorders attributed to ciclosporin have been mostly described in anecdotal case reports (SED-14, 1291). In an analysis of published or spontaneous case reports, the manufacturers found 29 cases of muscle disorders in patients taking ciclosporin; the complications fell into two categories (162). Myopathic symptoms, that is myalgia and muscle weakness without rhabdomyolysis,

were reported in 0.17% of patients and abated after dose reduction or treatment withdrawal. Rhabdomyolysis occurred in under 0.05% of patients and was mostly observed in patients taking other drugs, such as lovastatin or colchicine.

This topic has been re-analysed in a systematic review of published papers, in which relevant information from a total of 34 patients was identified (163). All but two patients were also taking concomitant drugs known to affect the muscles, among which glucocorticoids, simvastatin, lovastatin, colchicine, and pyrazinamide were the most frequently cited. Ciclosporin is therefore difficult to implicate in most patients, but at least one case with positive ciclosporin re-administration supported a causative role. The clinical picture was non-specific, with myalgia, cramps, and muscle weakness, sometimes associated with raised serum creatine kinase activity, and heterogeneous histopathology. Finally, skeletal muscle abnormalities have rarely been described in patients without muscle symptoms.

Ciclosporin is increasingly cited as a possible cause of severe bone and joint pain (164). Acute bilateral deep bone pain, mostly involving the legs, has been retrospectively identified in 19% of patients taking ciclosporin, with the highest prevalence in renal transplant recipients (165). In addition, about half of the patients with osteonecrosis had a history of episodic bone pains. Another study showed features of acute bone marrow edema on MRI in six patients who had bone pain, including one patient who further developed avascular necrosis (SEDA-21, 385). Calcium channel blockers dramatically improved bone pain in prospectively evaluated transplant patients, suggesting a possible vascular etiology (165).

Osteopenia is another potential adverse effect after renal transplantation, but the possible contribution of ciclosporin to bone loss and subsequent osteoporosis is controversial (SEDA-19, 350; SEDA-20, 345). Moreover, ciclosporin did not appear to have a negative influence on post-transplantation growth in prepubertal children (166).

Both ciclosporin and tacrolimus cause increased bone turnover and significant reductions in bone mass, more marked with tacrolimus (FK506). As most transplantation regimens include glucocorticoids, the individual effects of ciclosporin and tacrolimus are uncertain. As tacrolimus is the more potent immunosuppressant, theoretically, its use after transplantation should allow reduction in glucocorticoid doses, which would be associated with higher bone mineral density. Preliminary data suggest that there is a lower rate of vertebral fractures in patients taking tacrolimus compared with those taking ciclosporin. In 18 men who underwent liver transplantation and took ciclosporin and seven patients who took tacrolimus, bone mineral density in the lumbar spine and proximal femur was prospectively measured before and at 6, 12, and 24 months after transplantation (167). Serum concentrations of parathyroid hormone and 25-hydroxycolecalciferol were determined at the same time. Although the two groups had the same pattern of rapid early bone loss, tacrolimus was associated with lower doses of glucocorticoids and a trend to faster lumbar bone mass recovery. This may have a favorable effect on long-term bone mass evolution, especially in the femoral neck.

Reproductive system

Benign mammary hyperplasia occurs in 0.7% of women taking ciclosporin (168). The mechanism is poorly understood, but it may be related to trophic effects in the breast through ciclosporin receptors on fibroblasts (169), to an effect of ciclosporin on the hypothalamic-pituitary axis (170), or to antagonism at prolactin receptor sites on B and T (171,172).

Immunologic

Anaphylactoid reactions can occur with intravenous ciclosporin, sometimes after the first dose. Reported symptoms included pruritic rash, respiratory symptoms, chest pain, and, rarely, cardiopulmonary arrest. The presence of Cremophor EL, polyoxyethylated castor oil used as a solvent, is likely to account for this life-threatening reaction. The mechanism is still unclear, and results of skin tests were available in only three of 22 previously published patients.

In a report of an anaphylactic reaction, positive intradermal tests suggested a possible IgE-mediated reaction, most probably directed against Cremophor EL, as the patient subsequently tolerated the corn-oil-based soft gelatin formulation (173).

During a Phase I/II trial of high-dose intravenous ciclosporin, there was a high incidence of anaphylactoid reactions associated with improper mixing during preparation of the infusions, perhaps due to large initial bolus infusions of the vehicle, Cremophor EL (174).

Infection risk

Infections, in particular bacterial and viral (cytomegalovirus, *Herpes simplex* virus, Epstein–Barr virus), and also protozoal and fungal infections, are major causes of morbidity and mortality after transplantation, whatever the immunosuppressive regimen used (175–177). Based on an analysis of medical and autopsy records, infections were found to be the cause of death in 70% of transplant patients, with bacteria (50%) or fungi (29%) the most common pathogens (178).

Body temperature

Recurrent episodes of fever, which disappeared after ciclosporin withdrawal, have only been reported in one patient (SEDA-22, 414).

Long-Term Effects

Mutagenicity

An increase in chromosomal abnormalities correlated with serum ciclosporin concentrations in one study (179).

Tumorigenicity

Because of the varied indications for azathioprine and mercaptopurine, it is difficult to determine whether there is an increased incidence of cancer specifically related to prolonged drug exposure. Data from the Cincinnati Transplant Tumor Registry, published in 1993, helped to define comprehensively the characteristics of neoplasms observed in organ transplant recipients (180). Skin and lip cancers were the most common, and non-Hodgkin's lymphomas represent the majority of lymphoproliferative disorders, with an incidence some 30- to 50-fold higher than in controls. There is also an excess of Kaposi's sarcomas (181), carcinomas of the vulva and perineum, hepatobiliary tumors, various sarcomas, and renal cell carcinomas (182–184). In one case, complete regression of Kaposi's sarcoma followed withdrawal of ciclosporin (185). In contrast, the incidence of common neoplasms encountered in the general population is not increased. In renal transplant patients, the actuarial cumulative risk of cancer was 14–18% at 10 years and 40–50% at 20 years (186,187). Skin cancers accounted for about half of the cases. Very similar figures were found in later studies (SEDA-20, 341).

In patients with transplanted organs ciclosporin is associated with a small but significant risk of Epstein–Barr virus-associated lymphoproliferative disorders.

- A 39-year-old man with atopic eczema was given ciclosporin for an exacerbation, which responded well (188). After 2 years he developed a large ulcerated erythematous nodule, a CD30+ lymphoma of the skin. Ciclosporin was withdrawn and the lesion resolved within 2 months.

Of all transplant-related lymphomas 15% are of T cell origin and are unrelated to Epstein–Barr virus infection. Cutaneous T cell lymphomas are rare and carry a good prognosis, with a 90%, 4-year survival rate. Regression is often observed when immunosuppression is withdrawn or reduced.

While there is no doubt that the incidence of malignancies is increased in the transplant population, there has been controversy as to which factors (namely duration of treatment, total dosage, the degree of immunosuppression, or the type of immunosuppressive regimens) are the most relevant in determining risk. Partial or complete regression of lymphoproliferative disorders and Kaposi's sarcomas after reduction of immunosuppressive therapy argues strongly for the role of the degree of immunosuppression (180). The incidence of cancer was also significantly higher in renal transplant patients taking triple therapy regimens compared with dual therapy (189). Similarly, aggressive immunosuppressive therapy may account for the higher incidence of lymphomas in patients with cardiac versus renal allografts.

In a large, multicenter study in more than 52 000 kidney or heart transplant patients between 1983 and 1991, the rate of non-Hodgkin's lymphomas in the first post-transplantation year was 0.2% in kidney and 1.2% in heart recipients, and fell substantially thereafter (190). Initial immunosuppression with azathioprine and ciclosporin, and prophylactic treatment with antilympho- cyte antibodies or muromonab was associated with a sig- nificantly increased incidence of non-Hodgkin's lymphomas compared with other immunosuppressive regimens, which confirmed the major role of the level of immunosuppression. Later studies confirmed that immu- nosuppression per se rather than a single agent is respon- sible for the increased risk of cancer (SEDA-20, 340). Finally, the most striking difference between conven- tional and modern immunosuppressive regimens, includ- ing ciclosporin, was the average time to the appearance of tumors, in particular skin cancers and lymphomas, which was shorter in ciclosporin-treated patients (191,192).

Multiple factors with complex interactions are involved in the observed pattern and increased incidence of neo- plasms. They include severely depressed immunity with an impaired immune surveillance against various carcino- gens, the activation of several oncogenic viruses, and a possible mutagenic effect of the drugs. Viruses, such as papillomavirus, cytomegalovirus, and Epstein–Barr virus, are believed to play an important role in the development of several post-transplant cancers. From a theoretical point of view, the use of antiviral drugs active against herpes viruses which are commonly implicated as co-fac- tors can be expected to produce a reduction in the inci- dence of post-transplant lymphoproliferative disorders.

In an in vitro and in vivo experiment, ciclosporin pro- moted tumor growth by a direct cellular effect (193). This was suggested to be due to increased synthesis of trans- forming growth factor beta (TGF beta); anti-TGF beta antibodies blocked the increased spread of cancer cells. The clinical relevance of these data awaits further careful clinical confirmation. Continuing analysis of clinical experience has not provided clear evidence for a ciclo- sporin-specific effect and has instead supported an immu- nosuppressive effect (194).

Fibroadenomata are the most common solid breast masses in young women. Between 1997 and 2000, five women who had had transplant surgery and who were taking ciclosporin developed new breast masses, which were histologically confirmed to be fibroadenomata (195).

Ciclosporin-associated soft tissue proliferation with an abnormal hyperplastic reaction has been suggested to account for the development of eruptive angiomatosis (196).

Second-Generation Effects

Pregnancy

Pregnancies in women who took ciclosporin resulted in live neonates in 68%; half were premature while the other half were of low birth weights (197). Reduced renal graft function during pregnancy was associated with greater risks of neonates of lower birth weights and graft loss. In another study, a ciclosporin-based regimen was associated with more frequent miscarriage, preterm birth and intrau- terine growth retardation, compared with previous experience (198).

It has been suggested that ciclosporin is more likely to induce maternal renal dysfunction or pre-eclampsia than tacrolimus, but this view was based on a comparison involving only a small number of patients (SEDA-22, 414).

Teratogenicity

Maternal azathioprine treatment during pregnancy is clearly teratogenic in animals, but the mechanisms are not known. A large number of reports have described the outcome of pregnancies following the use of immuno- suppressant drugs, in particular in renal transplant patients, and hundreds of pregnancies have been analysed (199). The largest experience is that derived from the National Transplantation Pregnancy Registry which has been built up in the USA since 1991 (200). This registry has accumulated data on more than 900 pregnancies, of which 83% followed kidney transplantation and in this and other studies there was no difference in the rate of malformations when comparing ciclosporin with other immunosuppressive regimens (197,198,201). Ectopic pregnancies and miscarriages seemed to occur at a similar rate as in the general population. The most common complications were frequent prematurity and more frequent intrauterine growth retardation with low birth- weight. Risk factors associated with adverse pregnancy outcomes included a short time interval between trans- plantation and pregnancy (that is less than 1–2 years), graft dysfunction before or during pregnancy, and hyper- tension (202).

There have been no reports that physical and mental development or renal function are altered. In one study, there were changes in T lymphocyte development in seven children born to mothers who had taken azathiopr- ine or ciclosporin, but immune function assays were nor- mal (203). Thus, development of the fetal immune system is not affected by ciclosporin (204).

Renal function in 14 children born to women with transplants treated throughout pregnancy with a ciclo- sporin-based regimen has been extensively investigated at a mean of 2.6 years after delivery (205). No renal function abnormalities were found. In particular, glomerular filtra- tion rate was within the reference range. Renal function was found to be normal in 22 children evaluated after a mean of 39 months after birth (206), and no adverse effects on the immune function were identified in the few infants examined in this respect (203).

In a meta-analysis of the effects of exposure to ciclo- sporin during pregnancy, 15 studies (total 410 patients; 6 studies with control groups who were not given ciclo- sporin) met inclusion criteria for malformations, 10 for preterm delivery, and five for low birth weight (207). Ciclosporin did not appear to be a major human tera- togen, but was associated with increased rates of prematurity.

Lactation

Ciclosporin is excreted into human breast milk and because of potential immunosuppression, breastfeeding is usually regarded as contraindicated. Reassuring reports are now however available (SEDA-21, 385). After follow-up for 12–36 months in seven breast-fed infants (duration 4–12 months) whose mothers were treated with ciclosporin, none of them experienced renal or other long-term adverse consequences (208). Although ciclosporin concentrations measured in breast milk from six mothers were close to those measured in blood samples, it was calculated that the infants ingested less than 300 µg/day, and ciclosporin was not detectable in random blood samples.

Drug Administration

Drug formulations

In an attempt to overcome the poor and unpredictable absorption of the standard oral formulation, a microemulsion-based formulation (Neoral) has been developed. The benefit-to-harm balance of conversion from the standard to the microemulsion formulation have been discussed at length and guidelines for conversion have been proposed (209).

From the results of a retrospective study of 227 liver transplant patients who took Neoral as the primary immunosuppressant, it was suggested that this formulation may reduce the risk of severe neurotoxicity (210). Mild-to-moderate symptoms, that is headache ($n = 24$), mild hand tremor ($n = 13$), and paresthesia ($n = 5$), were the most frequent, whereas generalized seizures were reported in only two patients.

In one large study in 1097 patients, there was a significantly higher incidence of neurological complications, gastrointestinal disturbances, and increased serum creatinine concentrations during the first month of treatment with Neoral, compared with conventional ciclosporin (211). However, a meta-analysis showed that the adverse events profile was similar with the two formulations, while primary immunosuppression with Neoral produced significant benefit in terms of a lower incidence of rejection (212). In particular, in liver transplant patients treated with Neoral from the start, the incidence of adverse events was halved. All the same, because dosage adjustments were often required and often hazardous, owing to the risk of adverse effects and transplant rejection, other investigators concluded that switching to Neoral may be of little benefit, at least in previously stable liver transplant patients (213).

As the data from this meta-analysis were subject to many potential biases, the same authors reanalysed their results, taking into account only randomized, prospective studies (214). The incidence of adverse effects was higher with Sandimmune in open-label studies (840 patients) and higher with Neoral in blinded studies (3006 patients). In accordance with other investigators, these authors concluded that de novo immunosuppression with Neoral is beneficial, without significant differences in the incidence of adverse effects, whereas conversion from Sandimmune to Neoral in previously stable patients is associated with significantly more adverse effects with Neoral.

Drug dosage regimens

Several authors were unable to find convincing evidence that ciclosporin specifically increases the risk of tumors in transplant patients compared with previously used immunosuppressive regimens, and some even suggested a possibly lower incidence in ciclosporin-treated patients (191,192,215). However, in analyses from Japan and France (3454 patients), the average time that elapsed until the occurrence of cancer was significantly shorter in patients treated with ciclosporin compared with those taking conventional immunosuppressive treatment, that is 43–452 months versus 92–96 months (216,217). In addition, French authors found a higher cumulative risk of cancer after 10 years in ciclosporin-treated patients (14 versus 8.4%), and this was mostly due to an increased incidence of skin carcinomas (216). Other significant risk factors included age, a shorter duration of pretransplant dialysis and the combination with azathioprine treatment. The occurrence of cancer in ciclosporin-treated patients is thought to be dose-related, and one study found a significantly higher frequency of cancer in the normal than in the low-dose group (218). These positive findings were limited by the more frequent occurrence of acute rejection in the low-dose group.

Long-term ciclosporin also carries the risk of malignancies in non-transplant patients, and the overall incidence of lymphoma was estimated to be 0.14% among 3700 patients treated for autoimmune disease (219). However, the available studies are again conflicting. They are mostly based on a limited number of patients or a short duration of follow-up. Patients with rheumatoid arthritis receiving ciclosporin had an increased relative risk of malignancies compared with those given glucocorticoids, but it was similar to the risk in patients treated with disease-modifying antirheumatic drugs (220). Another study showed no increased risk of malignancies in ciclosporin-treated patients compared with controls who had never received ciclosporin (221). The spontaneous occurrence of cancers unrelated to the treatment cannot be excluded, and an increased risk of lymphomas has been repeatedly found in patients with rheumatoid arthritis. In patients with psoriasis and as compared to the expected incidence rate of cancer in this population, the relative risk of malignancies was 5.6 (95% CI = 3.9, 8.0) in a cohort of 1223 ciclosporin-treated patients (222). This was comparable to the increased risk of cancer in patients treated with other immunosuppressants.

Drug overdose

Experience with ciclosporin overdose has been reviewed by the manufacturers using published data or cases spontaneously reported (223). Accidental overdose was the most common, with doses of 20–400 mg/kg. In adults, no serious clinical consequences were observed with doses up to 100 mg/kg, and there were only minor clinical or biological effects (transient hypertension, tachycardia, headache, gastrointestinal symptoms, or slight increases in serum creatinine concentrations). However, life-threatening reactions occurred in three neonates, of whom one died after severe metabolic acidosis and renal insufficiency. Subchronic ciclosporin overdose over 8 days did not appear to cause any additional risk (224).

Taken together, the available data suggest that the acute toxicity of ciclosporin is low in adults, but that more severe intoxication could be expected in neonates. However, two reports, including one fatal case, have shown that accidental intoxication sometimes produces severe complications in adults (225,226).

- A 29-year-old man received a double lung transplantation for end-stage cystic fibrosis. After uneventful surgery, he was accidentally given ten times the intended dose of ciclosporin (30 instead of 3 mg/kg) and 18 hours later became anuric. His blood ciclosporin concentration was 4100 ng/ml. Hemodialysis was required for 6 weeks. A renal biopsy 7 weeks later showed typical features of acute tubular necrosis and lesions that resembled chronic nephrotoxicity. Renal function was still abnormal when he died from another cause 14 weeks after the accidental overdose.
- A 51-year-old man underwent double lung transplantation for pulmonary fibrosis, accidentally received an infusion of ciclosporin 30 mg/hour instead of 3 mg/hour, and 3 hours later had bilateral reactive mydriasis and absence of tendon reflexes. A CT brain scan showed diffuse cerebral edema, and massive intracranial hypertension rapidly developed. He died 5 hours later from brainstem compression, and pathological examination showed diffuse cerebral edema with neuronal necrosis.

The first of these cases suggested that acute renal dysfunction secondary to acute overdose can lead to renal sequelae. In the second patient, an isolated neurotoxic effect of ciclosporin was suggested because no predisposing factor except overdose was identified.

Drug–Drug Interactions

Ciclosporin is absorbed to a variable extent from the gastrointestinal tract and almost completely metabolized in both the liver and small intestine by CYP3A, which metabolizes a large number of drugs. Inducers, inhibitors, or substrates of CYP3A therefore have the potential to interact with ciclosporin. In addition, ciclosporin has wide pharmacokinetic variability and a narrow therapeutic index. Conversely, ciclosporin can inhibit the hepatic metabolism of other drugs that share the same CYP3A metabolic pathway.

Drugs that increase the systemic availability of ciclosporin do not always have negative effects, and several ciclosporin-sparing agents have indeed been used for the purpose of improving efficacy while reducing the cost of treatment. However, use of such combinations should be balanced against their potential risks (273).

Table 1 lists drugs that have proven or possible clinically relevant drug interactions with ciclosporin.

Acetazolamide

The interaction of ciclosporin with acetazolamide was previously supported by a single case report only. In three further patients, the addition of acetazolamide produced a near seven-fold increase in ciclosporin blood concentrations within 3 days (227).

Aciclovir

In an analysis of changes in ciclosporin clearance and systemic availability obtained from the medical records of 100 transplant patients, aciclovir altered ciclosporin pharmacokinetics (228).

The coadministration of ciclosporin with drugs with nephrotoxic effects carries a risk of increased renal dysfunction. Although a possible enhancement of nephrotoxicity has been suggested in patients also taking aciclovir (229), there were no such findings in a retrospective analysis of a double-blind study (230).

Adenosine and adenosine triphosphate (ATP)

Endogenous plasma adenosine concentrations were measured in 14 kidney transplant recipients taking ciclosporin and compared with five transplant recipients not taking ciclosporin, two taking sirolimus (FK506), six patients with chronic renal insufficiency, and ten controls (306). Plasma adenosine concentrations were significantly higher in those taking ciclosporin and sirolimus and in the patients taking ciclosporin the plasma adenosine concentrations correlated with serum ciclosporin concentrations. An in vitro study showed that ciclosporin inhibited the uptake of adenosine by erythrocytes. The authors concluded that since adenosine is immunosuppressant, the raised concentrations of adenosine in patients taking ciclosporin might contribute to the immunosuppressive action of ciclosporin. A further mechanism of the increase in adenosine concentration was possibly increased tissue release secondary to ciclosporin-induced vasoconstriction. The relevance of these results to the use of therapeutic intravenous adenosine in patients already taking ciclosporin is not clear.

Allopurinol

Two well-documented reports have described a marked increase in ciclosporin serum concentrations when allopurinol was co-administered (SEDA-18, 108).

Aminoglycoside antibiotics

Severe nephrotoxicity has been reported in three renal transplant patients who received ciclosporin and gentamicin, and in others receiving both drugs before surgical procedures, even though toxic serum concentrations of either drug were not reached (231).

Amiodarone

Amiodarone can increase the blood concentrations of ciclosporin and thus impair renal function.

Table 1 A summary of major interactions with ciclosporin

Pharmacokinetic	Pharmacodynamic
Anticonvulsants	**Increased risk of nephrotoxicity**
Carbamazepine*	ACE inhibitors
Phenobarbital*	Aciclovir (see text)
Phenytoin*	Aminoglycosides
Primidone*	Amphotericin
Antidepressants	Co-trimoxazole
Fluoxetine (unproven; see text)	Diuretics
Fluvoxamine	Foscarnet
Nefazodone	Melphalan
St. John's wort	Nafcillin
Antimicrobial drugs	NSAIDs (unproven)
Antifungal drugs	**Increased risk of muscle toxicity**
Ketoconazole, fluconazole, itraconazole, metronidazole	Colchicine
Chloramphenicol (unproven)	Fibric acid derivatives
Clindamycin*	HMG CoA reductase inhibitors (statins)
Fluoroquinolones	Pyrazinamide (SEDA-20, 346)
Griseofulvin*	**Increased risk of gingival hyperplasia**
Macrolides or related drugs	Nifedipine
Clarithromycin, erythromycin, josamycin, midecamycin, miocamycin, pristinamycin	**Increased risk of neurotoxicity**
Protease inhibitors	Imipenem/cilastatin
Ritonavir, saquinavir	**Increased risk of hepatotoxicity**
Pyrazinamide*	Androgens
Quinupristin/dalfopristin(SEDA-21, 386)	Norethandrolone, oxymetholone
Rifamycins*	Parenteral nutrition (see text)
Sulfadiazine*	**Increased risk of hyperkalemia**
Terbinafine* (SEDA-21, 386)	Potassium salts
Cardiovascular drugs	Potassium-sparing diuretics
Amiodarone	
Calcium channel blockers	
Amlodipine, diltiazem, nicardipine, nifedipine verapamil	
Carvedilol (SEDA-22, 415)	
Clonidine	
Propafenone	
Hypoglycemic drugs	
Glibenclamide	
Glipizide	
Troglitazone*	
Miscellaneous drugs	
Acetazolamide	
Allopurinol	
Bezafibrate	
Bile acid resin*	
Chloroquine	
Danazol	
Glucocorticoids	
Grapefruit juice	
Modafinil*	
Muromonab (SEDA-21, 386)	
Octreotide*	
Oral contraceptives (unproven)	
Orlistat*	
Probucol*	
Sulfasalazine*	
Sulfinpyrazone*	
Tacrolimus	
Ticlopidine*	
Vitamin E (water-soluble) (SEDA-20, 346)	

*These drugs reportedly reduce ciclosporin blood concentrations; the rest increase them

- A 66-year-old developed a ventricular tachycardia after kidney transplantation and was given amiodarone. Maintenance immunosuppression included prednisone, azathioprine, and ciclosporin. Ciclosporin concentrations before amiodarone initiation were stable (range 100–150 ng/ml). During amiodarone therapy, the ciclosporin concentration increased more than two-fold.

The authors proposed that changes in protein binding or metabolism might have explained this interaction.

Angiotensin receptor blockers

In an analysis of changes in ciclosporin clearance and systemic availability obtained from the medical records of 100 transplant patients, losartan and valsartan altered ciclosporin pharmacokinetics (228).

Antifungal azoles

Numerous case reports or studies have shown that ketoconazole, fluconazole, and itraconazole can inhibit ciclosporin metabolism and increase blood ciclosporin concentrations (264). Ketoconazole, which is undoubtedly the most potent inhibitor, has been used to reduce the dose, and therefore the cost or adverse effects, of ciclosporin (265–267). There was also a beneficial effect on the rate of rejection or infection. In contrast, interactions with metronidazole and miconazole have only been described in isolated case histories (SEDA-19, 351) (5).

Fluconazole

Fluconazole can increase concentrations of ciclosporin by inhibiting CYP3A4. In some studies, minimal or no effects were recorded, but in others ciclosporin concentrations were increased by fluconazole. Differences in the dosage and duration of fluconazole treatment could have explained these discrepancies (SED-12, 682) (21,84–337). For example, there was no interaction at a fluconazole dosage of 100 mg/day, but high dosages of fluconazole (400 mg/day or more) increase blood ciclosporin and tacrolimus concentrations (343,344).

The interaction of ciclosporin with fluconazole has been retrospectively evaluated in 19 kidney and pancreas/kidney transplant recipients (345). Both intravenous and oral fluconazole altered the blood concentration of ciclosporin. Five subjects did not have a significant interaction and 15 did. No patient had nephrotoxicity or transplant rejection related to antifungal therapy.

The effects of higher dosages of fluconazole on ciclosporin immunosuppression have been investigated in six renal transplant patients in a prospective, unblinded, crossover study (346). Baseline renal function, ciclosporin AUC, C_{max}, C_{min}, t_{max}, and clearance were compared with those 2, 4, and 7 days after starting fluconazole orally in a dosage of 200 mg/day. From day 8 onwards the ciclosporin dose was reduced by 50% and the above parameters were repeated on day 14. The results are shown in Table 2. On repeated-measures ANOVA only the AUC and C_{max} on day 4 of fluconazole were significantly higher than on day 0. There were no significant changes in ciclosporin clearance and t_{max}. The authors concluded

Table 2 Changes in ciclosporin kinetics during co-administration of fluconazole

Parameter	Day 0	Day 4	Day 7	Day 14
AUC (hours.ng/ml)	2887	4750	4052	2330
C_{max} (ng/ml)	701	941	768	498
C_{min} (ng/ml)	207	274	293	174
Clearance (ml/minute/kg)	17	13	12	30
t_{max} (hours)	3.0	2.0	2.5	3.0

that changes in C_{min} may not be sensitive enough to detect the described interaction and suggested monitoring the AUC near day 4 of treatment to guide ciclosporin dosage adjustments in all patients taking concomitant fluconazole.

Itraconazole

The combination of itraconazole with ciclosporin leads to a marked increase in blood ciclosporin concentrations, and this can result in a rise in serum creatinine, clearly pointing to renal damage as a result of the high ciclosporin concentrations (SED-12, 681) (69,349–351). However, an interaction has not been demonstrated in all cases (352).

Two cases of rhabdomyolysis caused by itraconazole in heart transplant recipients taking long-term ciclosporin and simvastatin have been reported (353,354). To avoid severe myopathy, ciclosporin concentrations should be monitored frequently and statins should be withdrawn or the dosage should be reduced, as long as azoles need to be prescribed in transplant recipients. Patients need to be educated about signs and symptoms that require immediate physician intervention.

Ketoconazole

The fact that ketoconazole inhibits cytochrome P450 accounts for some of its interactions. Ketoconazole increases ciclosporin concentrations, enhancing the risk of renal impairment, as shown by a fall in creatinine clearance (SED-12, 678) (6,13,25,356).

The effect of ketoconazole in ciclosporin-treated kidney transplant recipients has been the subject of a prospective randomized study (357). In 51 ketoconazole-treated patients and 49 controls there was a similar frequency of acute rejection episodes. However, in the control group, rejection episodes were more recurrent, with a poorer response to treatment. Acute ciclosporin nephrotoxicity was more common in the ketoconazole group, but this was encountered more at induction and rapidly reversed on further reduction of the dose of ciclosporin. Chronic graft dysfunction was significantly less in the ketoconazole group during the first year, but by the end of the study the difference was not statistically significant. Hepatotoxicity was similar in the two groups. Serum concentrations of cholesterol, low-density lipoprotein, and triglycerides were lower in the ketoconazole group. The authors concluded that long-term low-dose ketoconazole in ciclosporin-treated kidney transplant recipients is safe and cost-saving.

Voriconazole

The interaction of voriconazole with ciclosporin has been investigated in a randomized, double-blind, placebo-controlled, crossover study in kidney transplant recipients with stable renal function (268). During the first study period (7.5 days), subjects taking ciclosporin 150 mg/day received either concomitant voriconazole (200 mg every 12 hours) or a matching placebo. After a washout period of at least 4 days, they were switched to the other treatment. In the seven subjects who completed both regimens, concomitant administration with voriconazole resulted in a 1.7-fold increase (90% CI = 1.47, 1.96) in mean ciclosporin AUC during a dosage interval. Ciclosporin C_{max} and t_{max} were not significantly affected, but C_{min} was increased by voriconazole by a mean of 2.48 (range 1.88–3.03) times. Seven subjects withdrew during voriconazole administration, six for reasons that were considered to be drug-related; most were attributable to increased ciclosporin concentrations. Although not serious, all causality-related adverse events were more frequent during voriconazole administration than during placebo administration. Thus, when voriconazole is initiated or withdrawn in patients who are already taking ciclosporin, blood ciclosporin concentrations should be carefully monitored and the dose of ciclosporin adjusted as necessary.

Basiliximab

Basiliximab can inhibit ciclosporin metabolism transiently in children with renal transplants (332). Despite the use of lower daily doses, ciclosporin trough concentrations were significantly higher during the first 10 days after transplantation in 24 children who received basiliximab at days 0 and 4 after transplantation compared with 15 children who did not receive basiliximab. Ciclosporin dosage requirements again increased by 20% to achieve the target blood concentration at days 28–50 after transplantation. It is noteworthy that all seven acute episodes of rejection in the basiliximab group occurred during this period of time. However, these results have been debated, and there were no changes in ciclosporin dosage requirements in 54 children with liver transplants (333).

Bisphosphonates

In an analysis of changes in ciclosporin clearance and systemic availability obtained from the medical records of 100 transplant patients, alendronic acid altered ciclosporin pharmacokinetics (228).

Calcium channel blockers

A large amount of data has accumulated on the effects of various calcium channel blockers on ciclosporin metabolism or a possible renal protective effect. Diltiazem, nicardipine, and verapamil inhibit ciclosporin metabolism, and this has been investigated as a potential beneficial combination for ciclosporin-sparing effects, particularly for

diltiazem or verapamil (232,233). Any change in the formulation of calcium channel blockers in patients previously stabilized should be undertaken cautiously because unpredictable changes in ciclosporin concentrations can occur (234). In contrast, nifedipine, isradipine, or felodipine do not significantly affect ciclosporin pharmacokinetics (SED-13, 1129). Results obtained with amlodipine are conflicting; some studies have shown no effect, while others indicate an increase of up to 40% in ciclosporin blood concentrations (SEDA-19, 351) (SEDA-20, 345). Co-administration of calcium channel blockers is also regarded as a valuable option in the treatment of ciclosporin-induced hypertension, or to prevent ciclosporin nephrotoxicity.

There are conflicting results from studies on the protective role of calcium channel blockers in patients taking ciclosporin in regard to blood pressure and preservation of renal graft function. In a multicenter, randomized, placebo-controlled study in 131 de novo recipients of cadaveric renal allografts, lacidipine improved graft function from 1 year onwards, but had no effect on acute rejection rate, trough blood ciclosporin concentrations, blood pressure, number of antihypertensive drugs, hospitalization rate, or rate of adverse events (235).

However, some calcium channel blockers have pharmacokinetic interactions: diltiazem, verapamil, nicardipine, and amlodipine increase ciclosporin concentrations, whereas nifedipine, felodipine, and isradipine do not (SED-14, 604; SEDA-21, 210; SEDA-21, 212; SEDA-22, 216). Two confirmations of these observations have been published. In a retrospective study of 103 transplant patients verapamil and diltiazem, but not nifedipine or isradipine, caused a significant increase in plasma ciclosporin concentrations (305). The effect of verapamil and diltiazem on ciclosporin concentrations was independent of dosage. In a crossover comparison between verapamil, felodipine, and isradipine in 22 renal transplant recipients, verapamil interacted pharmacokinetically with ciclosporin but felodipine and isradipine did not (306).

Nine kidney transplant recipients had an increase in trough whole blood ciclosporin concentrations of 24–341% after introduction of nicardipine (307). A similar interaction has been reported with diltiazem (308) and verapamil (309).

Diltiazem

Many studies have shown an interaction of ciclosporin with diltiazem: concomitant administration allows reduction of the daily dose of ciclosporin. However, according to a study in eight renal transplant recipients, the low systemic availability and high degree of variation in diltiazem metabolism within and between patients can give unpredictable results (322).

Diltiazem abolishes the acute renal hypoperfusion and vasoconstriction induced by ciclosporin in renal transplant patients. Plasma endothelin-1 may be a mediator of ciclosporin-induced renal hypoperfusion, but is not affected by diltiazem (323). This interaction has been confirmed with a new microemulsion formulation of ciclosporin in nine patients with renal transplants who took diltiazem

90–120 mg bd for 4 weeks (324). Diltiazem caused a 51% increase in the AUC of ciclosporin and a 34% increase in peak concentration, without altering the time to peak concentration. However, the ciclosporin microemulsion did not significantly affect the pharmacokinetics of diltiazem.

- Ciclosporin-induced encephalopathy was precipitated by diltiazem in a 76-year-old white woman with corticosteroid-resistant aplastic anemia and thrombocytopenia, type 2 diabetes, and coronary artery disease, who was taking diltiazem for hypertension (325). She became comatose after 13 days of therapy with ciclosporin, and clinical examination and electroencephalography showed diffuse encephalopathy of moderate severity. Ciclosporin was withdrawn and she regained consciousness after 36 hours.

Concomitant diltiazem without proper dosage adjustment of ciclosporin can cause adverse neurological events.

Nifedipine
Ciclosporin significantly inhibits the metabolism of nifedipine, leading to increased effects (326).

The combination of ciclosporin with nifedipine produces an additive on gingival hyperplasia, with an increased prevalence and/or severity (SED-13, 1127) in both children (77,81) and adults (76,80,82). In contrast, verapamil had no significant additional effects on the prevalence or severity of ciclosporin-induced gingival overgrowth (SEDA-21, 385).

Nifedipine has been used to treat ciclosporin-induced hypertension, although amlodipine may be just as effective (304).

Nitrendipine
Nitrendipine had a small but significant nephroprotective effect independent of its antihypertensive action in patients treated for 2 years with ciclosporin and no adverse effect on renal allografts (327). Nitrendipine did not affect blood concentrations of ciclosporin. Thus, nitrendipine, in contrast to most other calcium channel blockers, does not affect ciclosporin blood concentrations and can be safely added in transplant recipients.

Verapamil
Calcium channel blockers are given to transplant patients for their protective effect against ciclosporin-induced nephrotoxicity. Verapamil has been particularly preferred, as it causes a significant increase in plasma ciclosporin concentrations and also seems to have a direct immunosuppressive action. However, in a study in 152 kidney transplant recipients, verapamil increased the incidence of postoperative infections (334). The patients, all of whom were taking ciclosporin, were assigned either to verapamil 240 mg/day or to no verapamil; during a postoperative period of 2–14 months, the incidence of infections was 22% (17/77) of those given verapamil compared with 5% (4/75) of the others. However, since the study was not randomized, it is not possible to draw reliable conclusions.

Carbapenems
The addition of imipenem + cilastatin to long-term ciclosporin provoked seizures in patients without a corresponding history (310). In general, nervous system toxicity occurred shortly after the start of the antibiotic therapy and drug concentrations were stable, suggesting a synergistic effect.

However, there was no significant increase in the frequency of seizures among 77 patients with bone marrow transplants who were taking ciclosporin alone (three seizures), 45 patients taking ciclosporin plus imipenem/cilastatin (two seizures), and 44 patients taking imipenem/cilastatin alone (no seizures) (269).

Ciclosporin-induced acute nephrotoxicity was reduced by cilastatin, an inhibitor of active tubular resorption (311). Reduced renal parenchymal accumulation of the drug may account for this effect. Serum ciclosporin concentrations were unchanged or insignificantly reduced. A similar protective effect against tacrolimus is possible, but unproven (312).

Cephalosporins
Ceftriaxone reportedly increases ciclosporin blood concentrations (313).

Chloramphenicol
Chloramphenicol was suspected of causing a dramatic increase in ciclosporin blood concentrations in a single patient.

- A morbidly obese 17-year-old Hispanic girl, who had a cadaveric renal transplantation 5 years before, took ciclosporin and prednisone for stabilization. She was treated with chloramphenicol 875 mg qds and ceftazidime 2 g tds for vancomycin-resistant enterococcal sinusitis (334). There was a substantial and sustained increase in ciclosporin concentrations after chloramphenicol was added. Normalization was achieved after withdrawal of chloramphenicol.

However, multiple concomitant confounding factors made this interaction purely speculative.

Chloroquine and hydroxychloroquine
Chloroquine can increase ciclosporin blood concentrations (335).

Clusiaceae

Hypericum perforatum (St. John's wort)
St. John's wort is a hepatic enzyme inducer (311) and can lower the plasma concentrations of various prescribed drugs, including oral anticoagulants and ciclosporin.

Hypericum perforatum caused a rapid dramatic fall in ciclosporin blood concentrations, resulting in acute heart transplant rejection in two patients aged 61 and 63 years (262). It produces an average 50% reduction in ciclosporin blood concentrations (263).

In 30 patients a fall in ciclosporin concentrations by 33–62% after self-medication with St. John's wort necessitated a gradual increase in the dose of ciclosporin of

187% (range 84–292%) (312). No patient suffered any permanent consequences as a result.

There have also been anecdotal reports of interactions of ciclosporin with St. John's wort.

- A 29-year-old woman, who had received a cadaveric kidney and pancreas transplant, had stable organ function with ciclosporin when she decided to take St. John's wort (315). Subsequently her ciclosporin concentrations became subtherapeutic and she developed signs of organ rejection. St. John's wort was withdrawn and her ciclosporin concentrations returned to the target range. However, she developed chronic kidney rejection and had to return to dialysis.
- A 63-year-old patient with a liver allograft developed severe acute rejection 14 months after transplantation (317). Two weeks before he had taken St. John's wort, which significantly reduced his ciclosporin concentration. The dose of ciclosporin was doubled, at the expense of adverse effects. He recovered fully after St. John's wort was withdrawn.
- A 55-year-old woman, who had received a kidney transplant and had stable organ function with ciclosporin, took St. John's wort and 4 weeks later her ciclosporin concentration fell sharply (318). The concentration rose again on withdrawal of St. John's wort and fell on rechallenge. As the problem was identified early enough, the patient incurred no serious consequences.
- Two patients who took ciclosporin after kidney transplantation self-medicated with St. John's wort, and their ciclosporin concentrations became subtherapeutic (319). One subsequently had an acute transplant rejection. Withdrawal of St. John's wort resulted in normalization of ciclosporin concentrations.
- After a kidney transplant for end-stage renal insufficiency a 58-year-old man was given ciclosporin, azathioprine, and prednisolone (320). Four years later he started to take St. John's wort (300 mg bd) for depression, and 2 weeks later his previously stable ciclosporin concentrations had halved. Withdrawal of the St. John's wort resulted in normalization of his ciclosporin concentrations.

In a systematic review of all reports of interactions of St. John's wort with ciclosporin, 11 case reports and two case series were found (321). In most cases there was little doubt about causality.

Colchicine

The combination of colchicine with ciclosporin increased the risk of myopathy. In a retrospective study of 221 renal transplant patients, five of 10 patients who took both drugs developed acute or chronic proximal myopathy, whereas none of the 30 controls matched for age, sex, transplant duration, ciclosporin use, and cumulative dose of glucocorticoids had similar symptoms (238).

Acute reversible ciclosporin toxicity occurred in a renal transplant patient a few days after colchicine was administered for an acute attack of gout (SEDA-16, 115). Other potential adverse effects of combining colchicine with ciclosporin include diarrhea, increases in serum liver

enzymes, bilirubin, and creatinine, and less often severe myalgia (SEDA-19, 101). Acute myopathy, associated with neuropathy in one case, has been observed in two young renal transplant recipients (SEDA-22, 119).

Corticosteroids—glucocorticoids

Glucocorticoids cause additive immunosuppression when they are given with other immunosuppressants, such as ciclosporin (SEDA-22, 451) (337).

Cytotoxic drugs

See also individual names

High-dose chemotherapy with cyclophosphamide, vincristine, prednisolone, and intrathecal methotrexate given for post-transplant lymphoproliferative disease was suggested to have favored the occurrence of acute ciclosporin neurotoxicity (headache, fever, seizures, and visual agnosia) in a 9-year-old cardiac transplant patient (239). Ciclosporin serum concentrations were normal and a further similar episode occurred on ciclosporin readministration.

Several studies have shown that ciclosporin reduces the clearance or increases the AUC of dactinomycin, etoposide, mitoxantrone, and vincristine (5,243).

Digoxin

In an analysis of changes in ciclosporin clearance and systemic availability obtained from the medical records of 100 transplant patients, digoxin increased ciclosporin systemic availability (228).

Doxorubicin

High-dose ciclosporin increased the AUC of doxorubicin and doxorubicinol and produced greater doxorubicin-related myelotoxicity (244).

Echinocandins

Ciclosporin increased the AUC of caspofungin by about 35%, but caspofungin did not increase the plasma concentrations of ciclosporin. Because of transient rises in hepatic transaminases not exceeding 2–3 times the upper limit of the reference range in single-dose interaction studies, concomitant use of caspofungin with ciclosporin should be undertaken with care (339), although limited experience in patients studied by the manufacturers suggests that it may be safe.

Efavirenz

Efavirenz causes increased requirements of ciclosporin by inducing CYP3A4.

- A 39-year-old man took ciclosporin 200 mg bd after a kidney transplant (340). The blood ciclosporin concentration was 307 ng/ml. The co-administration of prednisone caused the blood ciclosporin concentration to rise to 372 ng/ml, but it fell to 203 ng/ml when the dose was reduced to 175 mg bd. Efavirenz 600 mg/day, zidovudine 300 mg bd, and lamivudine 150 mg bd were added, and 7 days later the blood ciclosporin concentration fell to 80 ng/ml and later to 50 ng/ml.

Everolimus

Both everolimus and ciclosporin are extensively biotransformed by CYP3A and are substrates for P-glycoprotein. However, in a multicenter randomized double-blind study in 101 patients, 1 year after kidney transplantation, who were randomly assigned to receive everolimus 0.5, 1, and 2 mg bd plus ciclosporin and prednisone, the pharmacokinetics of ciclosporin were similar to published values in patients not taking everolimus (341).

Fibrates

A possible synergistic risk of muscle disorders should be considered in patients taking ciclosporin with fibric acid derivatives (SEDA-19, 351).

Fluoroquinolones

Although ciprofloxacin was initially thought to increase ciclosporin blood concentrations and enhance ciclosporin nephrotoxicity, no definite evidence to support this interaction has been found (245).

In 42 patients who had received a kidney transplant, cases were treated with ciprofloxacin in the first 1–6 months after transplantation, and matched controls (two per case) were not. The proportion of cases with at least one episode of biopsy-proven rejection 1–3 months after transplantation (45%) was significantly higher than in the controls (19%). The authors speculated that ciprofloxacin increases rejection rates in renal transplant recipients by antagonizing ciclosporin-dependent inhibition of interleukin-2 production (336).

A norfloxacin-induced increase in ciclosporin blood concentrations has been reported in children (5,246), while ofloxacin did not appear to alter ciclosporin metabolism (247).

Foscarnet

Foscarnet (248), but not ganciclovir (249), has also been involved in reversible renal insufficiency after concomitant use with ciclosporin.

Griseofulvin

Ciclosporin blood concentrations halved in a patient who took griseofulvin 500 mg/day, despite an increase in ciclosporin dose by 70% (347). When griseofulvin was withdrawn, the ciclosporin concentration rose. This interaction is attributable to induction of cytochrome P450 by griseofulvin.

Heparins

Measured ciclosporin concentrations differ according to the use of heparin or EDTA as anticoagulant (348).

Histamine H$_2$ receptor antagonists

The available data on a possible interaction between histamine H$_2$ receptor antagonists and ciclosporin are inconclusive. Whereas neither cimetidine nor ranitidine significantly altered ciclosporin pharmacokinetics, there was an increase in serum creatinine concentration in patients taking both ciclosporin and cimetidine, but not ranitidine. The clinical significance of this interaction is probably limited, and it has been attributed to competition of cimetidine with creatinine for tubular secretion (251).

HMG-CoA reductase inhibitors (statins)

Dosages of statins should be reduced in patients taking ciclosporin, because of pharmacodynamic and pharmacokinetic interactions.

Pharmacodynamic interactions
Patients taking ciclosporin with conventional dosages of lovastatin or simvastatin can develop acute muscle toxicity (SED-14, 1296; SEDA-19, 351). Among 110 ciclosporin-treated patients with heart transplants, four of 18 patients taking simvastatin 20 mg/day developed rhabdomyolysis, whereas none of the patients taking simvastatin 10 mg/day (26 patients) or pravastatin 20 mg/day (66 patients) had similar symptoms (252). Inhibition of CYP3A by ciclosporin was the most likely mechanism. In another study, there was a five-fold higher AUC of lovastatin (10 mg/day for 10 days) in 16 patients taking ciclosporin compared with 13 patients not taking ciclosporin (253).

- The addition of atorvastatin (10 mg/day) to a multidrug regimen including ciclosporin in a 40-year-old patient with a renal transplant resulted in rhabdomyolysis within 2 months (254).

In a patient with glucocorticoid-resistant nephrotic syndrome taking simvastatin and ciclosporin, there was an increase in lactic dehydrogenase activity, suggesting tissue injury, in the absence of an increase in creatine kinase (329).

Similar interactions are expected with other HMG-CoA reductase inhibitors such as cerivastatin and rosuvastatin.

Pharmacokinetic interactions
Plasma concentrations of lovastatin- or simvastatin-active metabolites were increased in several patients and in a pharmacokinetic study, suggesting that ciclosporin can inhibit their metabolism (255–257). Lower doses of lovastatin and simvastatin can be safely administered (258). Fluvastatin or pravastatin may offer some advantages, as no significant drug interactions have been documented with ciclosporin, at least for pravastatin (259).

From an analysis of changes in ciclosporin clearance and systemic availability obtained from the medical records of 100 transplant patients, atorvastatin, fluvastatin, pravastatin, and simvastatin were found to affect ciclosporin pharmacokinetics (228).

In a study of the safety and efficacy of simvastatin in hyperlipidemia after renal transplantation in 15 patients, the C_{max} and AUC of simvastatin were increased seven-fold by ciclosporin (260). In contrast, in 17 patients, tacrolimus had no effect. Although there were no complications, such as myopathy or rhabdomyolysis, creatine kinase activity must be monitored during co-administration of simvastatin and ciclosporin.

Ciclosporin produced a three- to five-fold increase in the plasma concentrations of cerivastatin and its metabolites in 12 patients with renal transplants who took cerivastatin 0.2 mg/day for 7 days compared with a single dose in 12 healthy controls (261).

Hypericum perforatum

See Clusiaceae

Idarubicin

In 27 patients, ciclosporin caused a marked increase in the AUC of idarubicin and its main metabolite idarubicinol, perhaps due to inhibition of the multidrug transporter P-glycoprotein (240).

Lincosamides

In two lung-transplant patients aged 39 and 48 years, blood ciclosporin concentrations fell after the addition of oral clindamycin (1.8 g/day), and both patients required temporary increases in daily ciclosporin dose until clindamycin withdrawal (237).

Lithium

In rats, lithium chloride alone had no significant renal toxicity, but when it was combined with ciclosporin, the renal toxicity of the latter was worsened (358). There was also a strong ciclosporin dose-dependent increase in serum lithium concentrations (tenfold at the highest dose).

Macrolide antibiotics

The pharmacokinetics of ciclosporin can be altered by macrolides. Commonly observed changes include increases in ciclosporin AUC and peak plasma concentration and reductions in the time to peak and clearance (102,104,354,356). Ciclosporin concentrations should therefore be monitored, to minimize the risk of toxicity in patients taking certain macrolides. When azithromycin is used concomitantly with ciclosporin, blood ciclosporin concentrations need to be monitored (331). Dirithromycin has a small effect on ciclosporin concentrations but to a clinically insignificant extent (338).

Erythromycin increases ciclosporin blood concentrations, and increased serum creatinine concentrations have been consistently demonstrated; isolated reports have also suggested possible interactions with clarithromycin, josamycin, midecamycin, or pristinamycin (SEDA-21, 385) (271). Midecamycin 1600 mg/day increased the steady-state concentration of ciclosporin two-fold (366). A two-fold increase in ciclosporin concentrations has been reported in patients receiving miocamycin. In contrast, spiramycin or roxithromycin did not significantly affect ciclosporin concentrations, and a single report involving azithromycin (SEDA-19, 351) was not substantiated by several prospective studies.

Methylphenidate

Potential drug–drug interactions of ciclosporin with methylphenidate and amfebutamone (bupropion) have been described (362).

- A 10-year-old boy with a heart transplant had a potentially life-threatening reduction in ciclosporin blood concentrations with amfebutamone. He subsequently had an increase in ciclosporin concentrations while taking methylphenidate.

These interactions merit further systematic investigation.

Metoclopramide

It has been suggested that metoclopramide increases the systemic availability of ciclosporin (SED-11, 783) (363).

Metronidazole

An interaction with metronidazole and ciclosporin, in which ciclosporin blood concentrations rise, has been suggested, though only in isolated case histories (SEDA-19, 351) (364).

It has been confirmed that metronidazole can produce a two-fold increase in blood concentrations of ciclosporin and tacrolimus, with a subsequent increase in serum creatinine in both cases (365).

The interaction of metronidazole with ciclosporin significantly increased blood ciclosporin and tacrolimus concentrations in two patients (365). Since both of these immunosuppressive drugs are toxic in overdosage, and since patients taking them are prone to infections, this is potentially a serious interaction.

Mycophenolate mofetil

The interaction of ciclosporin with mycophenolate mofetil was investigated in 52 renal transplant patients taking triple therapy (ciclosporin, mycophenolate mofetil, and prednisone), who continued taking the same treatment (*n* = 19) or underwent elective ciclosporin withdrawal (*n* = 19) or prednisolone withdrawal (*n* = 14) 6 months after transplantation (272). Median mycophenolate mofetil trough concentrations 3 months later were about two-fold higher in patients who had discontinued ciclosporin compared with patients who continued to take triple therapy and patients who had discontinued prednisone. No clear mechanism readily explains these changes.

Nefazodone

Nefazodone can alter blood ciclosporin concentrations (273,274). In one case there was nearly a 10-fold increase in whole-blood ciclosporin concentrations in a cardiac transplant patient shortly after the addition of nefazodone (275).

Oxycodone

In an analysis of changes in ciclosporin clearance and systemic availability obtained from the medical records of 100 transplant patients, oxycodone reduced ciclosporin systemic availability (228).

Pancuronium bromide

Ciclosporin can cause considerable prolongation of the neuromuscular paralysis induced by pancuronium (363) in one patient (and also in another given vecuronium). Reversal required both neostigmine and edrophonium. Subsequently, recurarization occurred (SEDA-14, 116). Contributing factors could have been the solvent Cremophor EL in the ciclosporin formulation (Sandimmun) and minor renal dysfunction.

Penicillins

In a study in lung transplant recipients, ciclosporin nephrotoxicity was potentiated by nafcillin (328).

Protease inhibitors

Interactions of ciclosporin with protease inhibitors should be expected, particularly with ritonavir, a potent inhibitor of CYP3A.

- Despite a prophylactic reduction in the dose of ciclosporin (100 mg/day) before antiretroviral treatment, a 40-year-old woman had an acute increase in ciclosporin trough concentrations (over 1000 ng/ml) and serum creatinine concentration (from 84 to 228 µmol/l) after taking zidovudine (600 mg/day), saquinavir (800 mg/day), and ritonavir (800 mg/day) for 11 days (286). Despite ciclosporin withdrawal, ciclosporin and creatinine blood concentrations remained high for over 10 days until triple drug therapy was withdrawn. Ritonavir was the most likely suspect.

In an HIV-1-positive kidney transplant recipient, saquinavir increased the trough concentration of ciclosporin three-fold, resulting in fatigue, headache, and gastrointestinal discomfort. Ciclosporin, like saquinavir, is metabolized by CYP3A. Saquinavir plasma concentrations were likewise increased by ciclosporin. All the symptoms disappeared after downward adjustment of the doses of both ciclosporin and saquinavir (377).

Proton pump inhibitors

Conflicting data have emerged on the interaction of omeprazole with ciclosporin, with isolated case reports suggesting that omeprazole can increase or reduce ciclosporin concentrations, whereas no effect of omeprazole was demonstrated in a controlled trial (287–289).

Rifamycins

Rifampicin 600 mg/day had no effect on the pharmacokinetics of clonidine 0.4 mg/day in six healthy subjects (369,370).

St John's wort

See Clusiaceae

NSAIDs

Based on the theoretical possibility of additive nephrotoxic effects, the combined use of NSAIDs with ciclosporin is expected to reduce renal function and therefore to increase ciclosporin-induced nephrotoxicity.

- In an 8-year-old girl with rheumatoid arthritis, the combination of ciclosporin with NSAIDs (indometacin and diclofenac) was suggested to have caused biopsy-proven, non-specific colitis, because her symptoms occurred only when the combination was used (276).

From several studies performed in healthy volunteers, repeated doses of diclofenac, aspirin, indometacin, or piroxicam did not significantly alter ciclosporin single-dose pharmacokinetics, but the AUC of diclofenac was increased by ciclosporin (277). In a further study of 20 patients with rheumatoid arthritis who took ciclosporin for 4 weeks, there was a two-fold increase in diclofenac AUC, and a small but significant increase in serum creatinine concentrations (278). Changes in renal function were easily managed by dosage titration of both drugs. In another study of 32 patients who received a 4-week course of paracetamol, indometacin, ketoprofen, or sulindac, changes in the calculated creatinine clearance were minimal (279). There were no striking differences among different NSAIDs. Taken together, the results of these studies and previous findings suggested that the clinical relevance of this interaction is limited.

Orlistat

Orlistat reduces plasma ciclosporin concentrations.

- A 29-year-old woman with increased body weight after renal transplantation was unable to adhere to a low-fat diet and took orlistat, which gave her severe diarrhea (280). Her plasma ciclosporin concentrations fell to subtherapeutic, even though she took the orlistat 2 hours before the ciclosporin and even though the daily dose of orlistat was reduced to 240 mg/day.
- There was a two-fold reduction in blood ciclosporin concentrations 2 weeks after orlistat was given to a 61-year-old patient with a heart transplant (281).

The FDA has received six reports of subtherapeutic blood ciclosporin concentrations soon after transplant recipients started to take orlistat (282). Reduced absorption of ciclosporin is the most likely mechanism (283,284) by reduction in fat absorption rather than by a direct drug–drug interaction.

Oxcarbazepine

A possible interaction of oxcarbazepine with ciclosporin has been reported after renal transplantation in a 32-yearold man (367). The ciclosporin trough serum concentration and serum sodium concentration fell after oxcarbazepine was added.

Selective serotonin reuptake inhibitors

Fluvoxamine and fluoxetine have been involved in isolated cases of increased blood ciclosporin concentrations, but fluoxetine was not confirmed to affect ciclosporin concentrations significantly in 13 patients (SEDA-20, 345) (SEDA-22, 385–386). In an analysis of changes in ciclosporin clearance and systemic availability obtained from the medical records of 100 transplant patients, sertraline altered ciclosporin pharmacokinetics (228).

Sirolimus

Combination of sirolimus with ciclosporin virtually eliminates acute rejection. However, the adverse effects of both drugs are potentiated, increasing the nephrotoxicity of ciclosporin (371).

In a single-dose, open, crossover study in 15 men and six women, the systemic availability of sirolimus 10 mg was markedly increased by concomitant ciclosporin 300 mg, Cmax, tmax, and AUC being increased by 116, 92, and 230% respectively (372,373). However, when sirolimus was given 4 hours after ciclosporin, the increases were only 37, 58, and 80%. Ciclosporin did not affect the half-life or mean residence time of sirolimus. Sirolimus did not significantly affect the systemic availability of ciclosporin.

Somatropin

Growth hormone increases the activity and regulates the gene expression of hepatic CYP3A4 (374). Mean blood concentrations of ciclosporin were lower during somatropin therapy in an open study in 16 prepubertal kidney transplant recipients, despite stable weight-related doses, suggesting that the metabolism of ciclosporin was increased by somatropin. Two patients had acute episodes of rejection during somatropin therapy; one of these may have been related to the fall in ciclosporin concentration (375).

Statins

See HMG Co-A reductase inhibitors.

Sulfasalazine

In a 51-year-old woman with a renal transplant who had been stable for the past 13.5 months with ciclosporin (9.6 mg/kg) and sulfasalazine (1.5 g/day) for ulcerative colitis, sulfasalazine withdrawal resulted in an almost two-fold increase in ciclosporin blood concentrations over the next 10 days (291).

Sulfinpyrazone

In 120 heart transplant patients, sulfinpyrazone (200 mg/day) for ciclosporin-associated hyperuricemia was associated with lowered blood ciclosporin concentrations despite an increase in the daily dose (292). The authors cited evidence (293) that sulfinpyrazone induces ciclosporin metabolism.

Sulfonylureas

Both glipizide and glibenclamide increase ciclosporin concentrations significantly (294).

Taxanes

There was a dramatic increase in the systemic availability of paclitaxel when ciclosporin was administered concomitantly (241) and in a phase I study of the pharmacokinetics of twice-daily oral paclitaxel 60–160 mg/m^2 in 15 patients in combination with ciclosporin (15 mg/kg) there was a seven-fold increase in the systemic exposure to paclitaxel; the plasma concentration increased from negligible to therapeutic concentrations (242). The inhibitory effect of ciclosporin on the gastrointestinal multidrug transporter P-glycoprotein was suggested to account for these interactions.

Thiazide diuretics

Patients taking diuretics and ciclosporin may be at higher risk of hyperuricemia and gouty complications, perhaps because of tissue breakdown caused by ciclosporin (376).

Ticlopidine

Although there was no interaction between ciclosporin and ticlopidine in a pharmacokinetic study, a 64-year-old patient with a renal transplant had a reduction in the concentration:dose ratio of ciclosporin after each of two successive courses of ticlopidine (295).

Topoisomerase inhibitors

The coadministration of etoposide and high-dose ciclosporin resulted in increased etoposide serum concentrations (330). Lower doses of etoposide were therefore recommended when combined with high-dose ciclosporin.

Troglitazone

Case reports and a retrospective evaluation of seven renal transplant patients showed that troglitazone can increase ciclosporin metabolism with a subsequent reduction of 15–45% in ciclosporin trough concentrations (296). The interaction of ciclosporin with troglitazone has been confirmed in four heart transplant patients with a 30–60% fall in ciclosporin concentrations within days of taking troglitazone 200 mg/day (297).

Vecuronium bromide

Ciclosporin can cause considerable prolongation of the neuromuscular paralysis induced by vecuronium (378), causing difficulties with reversal (SEDA-14, 116) (379). Potentiation of vecuronium in cats has also been described (SEDA-12, 188) (379).

Food-Drug Interactions

Grapefruit juice

Following the observation that grapefruit juice ingestion can increase the systemic bioavailability of ciclosporin, there was considerable interest in its possible use to reduce ciclosporin doses (SEDA-19, 351). However, this has been strongly criticized and considered hazardous because of large interindividual variability and the commercial availability of different formulations of grapefruit juice with potentially different effects on ciclosporin pharmacokinetics (250).

Parenteral nutrition

Cholestasis from other causes can increase the accumulation of ciclosporin or its metabolites, which in turn worsens hepatic cholestasis. This mechanism has been suggested in patients with bowel diseases who experienced an aggravation of hyperbilirubinemia or an increased incidence of hepatotoxicity from the combination of total parenteral nutrition and ciclosporin (SEDA-19, 348) (285).

Monitoring Therapy

Ciclosporin pharmacokinetics vary considerably between patients, and even in an individual patient from time to time, with changes in the clinical condition and treatment, particularly with administration of other drugs (298). Inadequate exposure to ciclosporin is a key factor in acute rejection and contributes to the development of chronic rejection and graft failure. Monitoring of ciclosporin concentrations is widely adopted as an accurate and practical measure of drug exposure (299).

In an open, randomized, parallel-group study in 307 patients, ciclosporin blood concentrations measured 2 hours after a dose were compared with conventional trough ciclosporin blood concentrations (300). The traditional predose blood concentration did not correlate well with drug exposure, and the 2-hour concentration was superior in preventing acute rejection. This is important, because data derived from the database of the United Network for Organ Sharing Scientific Liver Transplant Registry has shown that moderate and more severe grades of rejection are associated with poor graft function and outcome in liver transplant recipients.

Of 53 bone marrow transplant recipients in whom ciclosporin was used to suppress graft-versus-host disease, 63% developed acute nephrotoxicity (301). These patients had significantly higher plasma ciclosporin concentrations during the first month after transplantation than those who did not develop acute nephrotoxicity,

even though they received the same cumulative dose. Children received a higher cumulative dose, but their plasma concentrations did not differ significantly from the adults, and they suffered less nephrotoxicity.

Although a correlation between early post-transplantation whole-blood concentrations of ciclosporin and the occurrence of ciclosporin-induced toxicity has been suggested, blood concentrations in most patients are in the target range, and the identification of patients susceptible to adverse effects has yet to be achieved (302).

References

1. Touchard G, Verove C, Bridoux F, Bauwen F. Cyclosporin maintenance monotherapy after renal transplantation. What factors predict success? BioDrugs 1999;12:91–113.
2. Shield CF III, McGrath MM, Goss TFFK506 Kidney Transplant Study Group. Assessment of health-related quality of life in kidney transplant patients receiving tacrolimus (FK506)-based versus cyclosporine-based immunosuppression. Transplantation 1997;64(12):1738–43.
3. Kappers-Klunne MC, van't Veer MB. Cyclosporin A for the treatment of patients with chronic idiopathic thrombocytopenic purpura refractory to corticosteroids or splenectomy. Br J Haematol 2001;114(1):121–5.
4. Cortes J, O'Brien S, Loscertales J, Kantarjian H, Giles F, Thomas D, Koller C, Keating M. Cyclosporin A for the treatment of cytopenia associated with chronic lymphocytic leukemia. Cancer 2001;92(8):2016–22.
5. Campana C, Regazzi MB, Buggia I, Molinaro M. Clinically significant drug interactions with cyclosporin. An update. Clin Pharmacokinet 1996;30(2):141–79.
6. Kasiske BL, Guijarro C, Massy ZA, Wiederkehr MR, Ma JZ. Cardiovascular disease after renal transplantation. J Am Soc Nephrol 1996;7(1):158–65.
7. Kronenberg F, Lhotta K, Konigsrainer A, Konig P. Renal artery thromboembolism and immunosuppressive therapy. Nephron 1996;72(1):101.
8. Textor SC, Canzanello VJ, Taler SJ, Wilson DJ, Schwartz LL, Augustine JE, Raymer JM, Romero JC, Wiesner RH, Krom RA, et al. Cyclosporine-induced hypertension after transplantation. Mayo Clin Proc 1994;69(12):1182–93.
9. Taler SJ, Textor SC, Canzanello VJ, Schwartz L. Cyclosporin-induced hypertension: incidence, pathogenesis and management. Drug Saf 1999;20(5):437–49.
10. Ventura HO, Mehra MR, Stapleton DD, Smart FW. Cyclosporine-induced hypertension in cardiac transplantation. Med Clin North Am 1997;81(6):1347–57.
11. Sturrock ND, Lang CC, Struthers AD. Cyclosporin-induced hypertension precedes renal dysfunction and sodium retention in man. J Hypertens 1993;11(11):1209–16.
12. Davenport A. The effect of renal transplantation and treatment with cyclosporin A on the prevalence of Raynaud's phenomenon. Clin Transplant 1993;7:4–8.
13. Rottenberg Y, Fridlender ZG. Recurrent infusion phlebitis induced by cyclosporine. Ann Pharmacother 2004;38(12):2071–3.
14. Blaauw AA, Leunissen KM, Cheriex EC, Wolters J, Kootstra G, Van Hooff JP. Disappearance of pulmonary capillary leak syndrome when intravenous cyclosporine is replaced by oral cyclosporine. Transplantation 1987;43(5):758–9.

15. Carbone L, Appel GB, Benvenisty AI, Cohen DJ, Kunis CL, Hardy MA. Adult respiratory distress syndrome associated with oral cyclosporine. Transplantation 1987;43(5):767–8.

16. Roelofs PM, Klinkhamer PJ, Gooszen HC. Hypersensitivity pneumonitis probably caused by cyclosporine. A case report. Respir Med 1998;92(12):1368–70.

17. Hauben M. Cyclosporine neurotoxicity. Pharmacotherapy 1996;16(4):576–83.

18. Wijdicks EF, Wiesner RH, Krom RA. Neurotoxicity in liver transplant recipients with cyclosporine immunosuppression. Neurology 1995;45(11):1962–4.

19. Erer B, Polchi P, Lucarelli G, Angelucci E, Baronciani D, Galimberti M, Giardini C, Gaziev D, Maiello A. CsA-associated neurotoxicity and ineffective prophylaxis with clonazepam in patients transplanted for thalassemia major: analysis of risk factors. Bone Marrow Transplant 1996;18(1):157–62.

20. Bohlin AB, Berg U, Englund M, Malm G, Persson A, Tibell A, Tyden G. Central nervous system complications in children treated with ciclosporin after renal transplantation. Child Nephrol Urol 1990;10(4):225–30.

21. de Groen PC, Aksamit AJ, Rakela J, Forbes GS, Krom RA. Central nervous system toxicity after liver transplantation. The role of cyclosporine and cholesterol. N Engl J Med 1987;317(14):861–6.

22. Gleeson JG, duPlessis AJ, Barnes PD, Riviello JJ Jr. Cyclosporin A acute encephalopathy and seizure syndrome in childhood: clinical features and risk of seizure recurrence. J Child Neurol 1998;13(7):336–44.

23. Schwartz RB, Bravo SM, Klufas RA, Hsu L, Barnes PD, Robson CD, Antin JH. Cyclosporine neurotoxicity and its relationship to hypertensive encephalopathy: CT and MR findings in 16 cases. Am J Roentgenol 1995;165(3):627–31.

24. Kotake S, Higashi K, Yoshikawa K, Sasamoto Y, Okamoto T, Matsuda H. Central nervous system symptoms in patients with Behçet disease receiving cyclosporine therapy. Ophthalmology 1999;106(3):586–9.

25. Gopal AK, Thorning DR, Back AL. Fatal outcome due to cyclosporine neurotoxicity with associated pathological findings. Bone Marrow Transplant 1999;23(2):191–3.

26. Kaito K, Kobayashi M, Otsubo H, Ogasawara Y, Sekita T, Shimada T, Hosoya T. Cyclosporine and entrapment neuropathy. Report of two cases. Acta Haematol 1998;100(3):159.

27. Terrovitis IV, Nanas SN, Rombos AK, Tolis G, Nanas JN. Reversible symmetric polyneuropathy with paraplegia after heart transplantation. Transplantation 1998;65(10):1394–5.

28. Maghrabi K, Bohlega S. Cyclosporine-induced migraine with severe vomiting causing loss of renal graft. Clin Neurol Neurosurg 1998;100(3):224–7.

29. Braun R, Arechalde A, French LE. Reversible ascending motor neuropathy as a side effect of systemic treatment with ciclosporine for nodular prurigo. Dermatology 1999;199(4):372–3.

30. Koide T, Yamada M, Takahashi T, Igarashi S, Masuko M, Furukawa T, Kuroha T, Koike T, Sato M, Tanaka R, Tsuji S, Takahashi H. Cyclosporine A-associated fatal central nervous system angiopathy in a bone marrow transplant recipient: an autopsy case. Acta Neuropathol (Berl) 2000;99(6):680–4.

31. Shbarou RM, Chao NJ, Morgenlander JC. Cyclosporin A-related cerebral vasculopathy. Bone Marrow Transplant 2000;26(7):801–4.

32. Delpont E, Thomas P, Gugenheim J, Chichmanian RM, Mahagne MH, Suisse G, Dolisi C. Syndrome confusionnel prolongé au cours d'un traitement par ciclosporine: etat de mal à expression confusionnelle?. [Prolonged confusion syndrome in the course of cyclosporine treatment: a state of confusion?.] Neurophysiol Clin 1990;20(3):207–15.

33. Labar B, Bogdanic V, Plavsic F, Francetic I, Dobric I, Kastelan A, Grgicevic D, Vrtar M, Grgic-Markulin L, Balabanic-Kamauf B, et al. Cyclosporin neurotoxicity in patients treated with allogeneic bone marrow transplantation. Biomed Pharmacother 1986;40(4):148–50.

34. Rosencrantz R, Moon A, Raynes H, Spivak W. Cyclosporine-Induced neurotoxicity during treatment of Crohn's disease: lack of correlation with previously reported risk factors. Am J Gastroenterol 2001;96(9):2778–82.

35. Bronster DJ, Chodoff L, Yonover P, Sheiner PA. Cyclosporine levels in cerebrospinal fluid after liver transplantation. Transplantation 1999;68(9):1410–3.

36. Meyer MA. Elevated basal ganglia glucose metabolism in cyclosporine neurotoxicity: a positron emission tomography imaging study. J Neuroimaging 2002;12(1):92–3.

37. Ozkaya O, Kalman S, Bakkaloglu S, Buyan N, Soylemezoglu O. Cyclosporine-associated facial paralysis in a child with renal transplant. Pediatr Nephrol 2002;17(7):544–6.

38. Porges Y, Blumen S, Fireman Z, Sternberg A, Zamir D. Cyclosporine-induced optic neuropathy, ophthalmoplegia, and nystagmus in a patient with Crohn disease. Am J Ophthalmol 1998;126(4):607–9.

39. Rubin AM, Kang H. Cerebral blindness and encephalopathy with cyclosporin A toxicity. Neurology 1987;37(6):1072–6.

40. Rubin AM. Transient cortical blindness and occipital seizures with cyclosporine toxicity. Transplantation 1989;47(3):572–3.

41. Wilson SE, de Groen PC, Aksamit AJ, Wiesner RH, Garrity JA, Krom RA. Cyclosporin A-induced reversible cortical blindness. J Clin Neuroophthalmol 1988;8(4):215–20.

42. Saito J, Kami M, Taniguchi F, Kanda Y, Takeda N, Mitani K, Hirai H, Araie M, Fujino Y. Unilateral papilledema after bone marrow transplantation. Bone Marrow Transplant 1999;23(9):963–5.

43. Avery R, Jabs DA, Wingard JR, Vogelsang G, Saral R, Santos G. Optic disc edema after bone marrow transplantation. Possible role of cyclosporine toxicity. Ophthalmology 1991;98(8):1294–301.

44. BenEzra D, Pe'er J, Brodsky M, Cohen E. Cyclosporine eyedrops for the treatment of severe vernal keratoconjunctivitis. Am J Ophthalmol 1986;101(3):278–82.

45. Zierhut M, Thiel HJ, Weidle EG, Waetjen R, Pleyer U. Topical treatment of severe corneal ulcers with cyclosporin A. Graefes Arch Clin Exp Ophthalmol 1989;227(1):30–5.

46. Sall K, Stevenson OD, Mundorf TK, Reis BLCsA Phase 3 Study Group. Two multicenter, randomized studies of the efficacy and safety of cyclosporine ophthalmic emulsion in moderate to severe dry eye disease. Ophthalmology 2000;107(4):631–9.

47. Kachi S, Hirano K, Takesue Y, Miura M. Unusual corneal deposit after the topical use of cyclosporine as eyedrops. Am J Ophthalmol 2000;130(5):667–9.

48. Stevenson D, Tauber J, Reis BL. Efficacy and safety of cyclosporin A ophthalmic emulsion in the treatment of moderate-to-severe dry eye disease: a dose-ranging, randomized trial. The Cyclosporin A Phase 2 Study Group. Ophthalmology 2000;107(5):967–74.

49. Jindal RM, Sidner RA, Milgrom ML. Post-transplant diabetes mellitus. The role of immunosuppression. Drug Saf 1997;16(4):242–57.

50. Copstein LA, Zelmanovitz T, Goncalves LF, Manfro RC. Posttransplant patients: diabetes mellitus in cyclosporine-treated renal allograft a case-control study. Transplant Proc 2004;36(4):882–3.

51. Raine AE, Carter R, Mann JI, Morris PJ. Adverse effect of cyclosporin on plasma cholesterol in renal transplant recipients. Nephrol Dial Transplant 1988;3(4):458–63.

52. Ballantyne CM, Podet EJ, Patsch WP, Harati Y, Appel V, Gotto AM Jr, Young JB. Effects of cyclosporine therapy on plasma lipoprotein levels. JAMA 1989;262(1):53–6.

53. Stiller MJ, Pak GH, Kenny C, Jondreau L, Davis I, Wachsman S, Shupack JL. Elevation of fasting serum lipids in patients treated with low-dose cyclosporine for severe plaque-type psoriasis. An assessment of clinical significance when viewed as a risk factor for cardiovascular disease. J Am Acad Dermatol 1992;27(3):434–8.

54. Grossman RM, Delaney RJ, Brinton EA, Carter DM, Gottlieb AB. Hypertriglyceridemia in patients with psoriasis treated with cyclosporine. J Am Acad Dermatol 1991;25(4):648–51.

55. Hricik DE. Posttransplant hyperlipidemia: the treatment dilemma. Am J Kidney Dis 1994;23(5):766–71.

56. Massy ZA. Hyperlipidemia and cardiovascular disease after organ transplantation. Transplantation 2001;72(Suppl 6):S13–5.

57. Webb AT, Reaveley DA, O'Donnell M, O'Connor B, Seed M, Brown EA. Does cyclosporin increase lipoprotein(a) concentrations in renal transplant recipients? Lancet 1993;341(8840):268–70.

58. Kuster GM, Drexel H, Bleisch JA, Rentsch K, Pei P, Binswanger U, Amann FW. Relation of cyclosporine blood levels to adverse effects on lipoproteins. Transplantation 1994;57(10):1479–83.

59. Claesson K, Mayer AD, Squifflet JP, Grabensee B, Eigler FW, Behrend M, Vanrenterghem Y, van Hooff J, Morales JM, Johnson RW, Buchholz B, Land W, Forsythe JL, Neumayer HH, Ericzon BG, Muhlbacher F. Lipoprotein patterns in renal transplant patients: a comparison between FK 506 and cyclosporine A patients. Transplant Proc 1998;30(4):1292–4.

60. McCune TR, Thacker LR II, Peters TG, Mulloy L, Rohr MS, Adams PA, Yium J, Light JA, Pruett T, Gaber AO, Selman SH, Jonsson J, Hayes JM, Wright FH Jr, Armata T, Blanton J, Burdick JF. Effects of tacrolimus on hyperlipidemia after successful renal transplantation: a Southeastern Organ Procurement Foundation multicenter clinical study. Transplantation 1998;65(1):87–92.

61. Lin HY, Rocher LL, McQuillan MA, Schmaltz S, Palella TD, Fox IH. Cyclosporine-induced hyperuricemia and gout. N Engl J Med 1989;321(5):287–92.

62. Burack DA, Griffith BP, Thompson ME, Kahl LE. Hyperuricemia and gout among heart transplant recipients receiving cyclosporine. Am J Med 1992;92(2):141–6.

63. Ben Hmida M, Hachicha J, Bahloul Z, Kaddour N, Kharrat M, Jarraya F, Jarraya A. Cyclosporine-induced hyperuricemia and gout in renal transplants. Transplant Proc 1995;27(5):2722–4.

64. Laine J, Holmberg C. Renal and adrenal mechanisms in cyclosporine-induced hyperkalaemia after renal transplantation. Eur J Clin Invest 1995;25(9):670–6.

65. Cavdar C, Sifil A, Sanli E, Gulay H, Camsari T. Hypomagnesemia and mild rhabdomyolysis in living

66. Scoble JE, Freestone A, Varghese Z, Fernando ON, Sweny P, Moorhead JF. Cyclosporin-induced renal magnesium leak in renal transplant patients. Nephrol Dial Transplant 1990;5(9):812–5.

67. Nozue T, Kobayashi A, Kodama T, Uemasu F, Endoh H, Sako A, Takagi Y. Pathogenesis of cyclosporine-induced hypomagnesemia. J Pediatr 1992;120(4 Pt 1):638–40.

68. Vannini SD, Mazzola BL, Rodoni L, Truttmann AC, Wermuth B, Bianchetti MG, Ferrari P. Permanently reduced plasma ionized magnesium among renal transplant recipients on cyclosporine. Transpl Int 1999;12(4):244–9.

69. Faure JL, Causse X, Bergeret A, Meyer F, Neidecker J, Paliard P. Cyclosporine induced hemolytic anemia in a liver transplant patient. Transplant Proc 1989;21(1 Pt 2):2242–3.

70. Rougier JP, Viron B, Ronco P, Khayat R, Michel C, Mignon F. Autoimmune haemolytic anaemia after ABO-match, ABDR full match kidney transplantation. Nephrol Dial Transplant 1994;9(6):693–7.

71. Trimarchi H, Freixas E, Rabinovich O, Schropp J, Pereyra H, Bullorsky E. Cyclosporine-associated thrombotic microangiopathy during daclizumab induction: a suggested therapeutic approach. Nephron 2001;87(4):361–4.

72. Seymour RA. Drug-induced gingival overgrowth. Adverse Drug React Toxicol Rev 1993;12(4):215–32.

73. Mariani G, Calastrini C, Carinci F, Marzola R, Calura G. Ultrastructural features of cyclosporine A-induced gingival hyperplasia. J Periodontol 1993;64(11):1092–7.

74. O'Valle F, Mesa FL, Gomez-Morales M, Aguilar D, Caracuel MD, Medina-Cano MT, Andujar M, Lopez-Hidalgo J, Garcia del Moral R. Immunohistochemical study of 30 cases of cyclosporin A-induced gingival overgrowth. J Periodontol 1994;65(7):724–30.

75. Nell A, Matejka M, Solar P, Ulm C, Sinzinger H. Evidence that cyclosporine inhibits periodontal prostaglandin I2 synthesis. J Periodontal Res 1996;31(2):131–4.

76. Thomason JM, Seymour RA, Ellis JS, Kelly PJ, Parry G, Dark J, Idle JR. Iatrogenic gingival overgrowth in cardiac transplantation. J Periodontol 1995;66(8):742–6.

77. Wondimu B, Dahllof G, Berg U, Modeer T. Cyclosporin-A-induced gingival overgrowth in renal transplant children. Scand J Dent Res 1993;101(5):282–6.

78. Wondimu B, Berg U, Modeer T. Renal function in cyclosporine-treated pediatric renal transplant recipients in relation to gingival overgrowth. Transplantation 1997;64(1):92–6.

79. Kilpatrick NM, Weintraub RG, Lucas JO, Shipp A, Byrt T, Wilkinson JL. Gingival overgrowth in pediatric heart and heart-lung transplant recipients. J Heart Lung Transplant 1997;16(12):1231–7.

80. Sooriyamoorthy M, Gower DB, Eley BM. Androgen metabolism in gingival hyperplasia induced by nifedipine and cyclosporin. J Periodontal Res 1990;25(1):25–30.

81. Bokenkamp A, Bohnhorst B, Beier C, Albers N, Offner G, Brodehl J. Nifedipine aggravates cyclosporine A-induced gingival hyperplasia. Pediatr Nephrol 1994;8(2):181–5.

82. Thomason JM, Seymour RA, Rice N. The prevalence and severity of cyclosporin and nifedipine-induced gingival overgrowth. J Clin Periodontol 1993;20(1):37–40.

83. Landewe RB, Goei The HS, van Rijthoven AW, Rietveld JR, Breedveld FC, Dijkmans BA. Cyclosporine

in common clinical practice: an estimation of the benefit/ risk ratio in patients with rheumatoid arthritis. J Rheumatol 1994;21(9):1631–6.

84. Lorber MI, Van Buren CT, Flechner SM, Williams C, Kahan BD. Hepatobiliary and pancreatic complications of cyclosporine therapy in 466 renal transplant recipients. Transplantation 1987;43(1):35–40.

85. Harihara Y, Sanjo K, Idezuki Y. Cyclosporine hepatotoxicity and cold ischemia liver damage. Transplant Proc 1992;24(5):1984.

86. Moertel CG, Fleming TR, Macdonald JS, Haller DG, Laurie JA. Hepatic toxicity associated with fluorouracil plus levamisole adjuvant therapy. J Clin Oncol 1993;11(12):2386–90.

87. Kowdley KV, Keeffe EB. Hepatotoxicity of transplant immunosuppressive agents. Gastroenterol Clin North Am 1995;24(4):991–1001.

88. Myara A, Cadranel JF, Dorent R, Lunel F, Bouvier E, Gerhardt M, Bernard B, Ghoussoub JJ, Cabrol A, Gandjbakhch I, Opolon P, Trivin F. Cyclosporin A-mediated cholestasis in patients with chronic hepatitis after heart transplantation. Eur J Gastroenterol Hepatol 1996;8(3):267–71.

89. Neri S, Signorelli SS, Ierna D, Mauceri B, Abate G, Bordonaro F, Cilio D, Malaguarnera M. Role of admethionine (S-adenosylmethionine) in cyclosporin-induced cholestasis. Clin Drug Invest 2002;22:191–5.

90. Chicharro M, Guarner L, Vilaseca J, Planas M, Malagelada J. Does cyclosporin A worsen liver function in patients with inflammatory bowel disease and total parenteral nutrition? Rev Esp Enferm Dig 2000;92(2):68–77.

91. Laskow DA, Curtis JJ, Luke RG, Julian BA, Jones P, Deierhoi MH, Barber WH, Diethelm AG. Cyclosporine-induced changes in glomerular filtration rate and urea excretion. Am J Med 1990;88(5):497–502.

92. Mobb GE, Veitch PS, Bell PR. Are serum creatinine levels adequate to identify the onset of chronic cyclosporine A nephrotoxicity? Transplant Proc 1990;22(4):1708–10.

93. Greenberg A, Thompson ME, Griffith BJ, Hardesty RL, Kormos RL, el-Shahawy MA, Janosky JE, Puschett JB. Cyclosporine nephrotoxicity in cardiac allograft patients—a seven-year follow-up. Transplantation 1990;50(4):589–93.

94. Leong SO, Lye WC, Tan CC, Lee EJ. Acute cyclosporine A nephrotoxicity in a renal allograft recipient with hypothyroidism. Am J Kidney Dis 1995;25(3):503–5.

95. van der Molen LR, van Son WJ, Tegzess AM, Stegeman CA. Severe vital depression as the presenting feature of cyclosporin-A-associated thrombotic microangiopathy. Nephrol Dial Transplant 1999;14(4):998–1000.

96. Kohli HS, Sud K, Jha V, Gupta KL, Minz M, Joshi K, Sakhuja V. Cyclosporin-induced haemolytic–uraemic syndrome presenting as primary graft dysfunction. Nephrol Dial Transplant 1998;13(11):2940–2.

97. Wiener Y, Nakhleh RE, Lee MW, Escobar FS, Venkat KK, Kupin WL, Mozes MF. Prognostic factors and early resumption of cyclosporin A in renal allograft recipients with thrombotic microangiopathy and hemolytic uremic syndrome. Clin Transplant 1997;11(3):157–62.

98. Bren AF, Kandus A, Buturovic J, Koselj M, Kaplan Pavlovcic S, Ponikvar R, Kovac D, Lindic J, Vizjak A, Ferluga D. Cyclosporine-related hemolytic–uremic syndrome in kidney graft recipients: clinical and histomorphologic evaluation. Transplant Proc 1998;30(4):1201–3.

99. Ducloux D, Rebibou JM, Semhoun-Ducloux S, Jamali M, Fournier V, Bresson-Vautrin C, Chalopin JM. Recurrence of hemolytic–uremic syndrome in renal transplant recipients: a meta-analysis. Transplantation 1998;65(10):1405–7.

100. Zarifian A, Meleg-Smith S, O'donovan R, Tesi RJ, Batuman V. Cyclosporine-associated thrombotic microangiopathy in renal allografts. Kidney Int 1999;55(6):2457–66.

101. Myers BD, Ross J, Newton L, Luetscher J, Perlroth M. Cyclosporine-associated chronic nephropathy. N Engl J Med 1984;311(11):699–705.

102. Bennett WM, DeMattos A, Meyer MM, Andoh T, Barry JM. Chronic cyclosporine nephropathy: the Achilles' heel of immunosuppressive therapy. Kidney Int 1996;50(4):1089–100.

103. Mihatsch MJ, Ryffel B, Gudat F. The differential diagnosis between rejection and cyclosporine toxicity. Kidney Int Suppl 1995;52:S63–9.

104. Shihab FS. Cyclosporine nephropathy: pathophysiology and clinical impact. Semin Nephrol 1996;16(6):536–47.

105. Ader JL, Rostaing L. Cyclosporin nephrotoxicity: pathophysiology and comparison with FK-506. Curr Opin Nephrol Hypertens 1998;7(5):539–45.

106. Mihatsch MJ, Antonovych T, Bohman SO, Habib R, Helmchen U, Noel LH, Olsen S, Sibley RK, Kemeny E, Feutren G. Cyclosporin A nephropathy: standardization of the evaluation of kidney biopsies. Clin Nephrol 1994;41(1):23–32.

107. Habib R, Niaudet P. Comparison between pre- and post-treatment renal biopsies in children receiving ciclosporine for idiopathic nephrosis. Clin Nephrol 1994;42(3):141–6.

108. Jacobson SH, Jaremko G, Duraj FF, Wilczek HE. Renal fibrosis in cyclosporin A-treated renal allograft recipients: morphological findings in relation to renal hemodynamics. Transpl Int 1996;9(5):492–8.

109. Opelz G. Effect of the maintenance immunosuppressive drug regimen on kidney transplant outcome. Transplantation 1994;58(4):443–6.

110. Thiel G, Bock A, Spondlin M, Brunner FP, Mihatsch M, Rufli T, Landmann J. Long-term benefits and risks of cyclosporin A (Sandimmun)—an analysis at 10 years. Transplant Proc 1994;26(5):2493–8.

111. Mihatsch MJ, Morozumi K, Strom EH, Ryffel B, Gudat F, Thiel G. Renal transplant morphology after long-term therapy with cyclosporine. Transplant Proc 1995;27(1):39–42.

112. Gonwa TA, Klintmalm GB, Levy M, Jennings LS, Goldstein RM, Husberg BS. Impact of pretransplant renal function on survival after liver transplantation. Transplantation 1995;59(3):361–5.

113. Kuo PC, Luikart H, Busse-Henry S, Hunt SA, Valantine HA, Stinson EB, Oyer PE, Scandling JD, Alfrey EJ, Dafoe DC. Clinical outcome of interval cadaveric renal transplantation in cardiac allograft recipients. Clin Transplant 1995;9(2):92–7.

114. Goldstein DJ, Zuech N, Sehgal V, Weinberg AD, Drusin R, Cohen D. Cyclosporine-associated end-stage nephropathy after cardiac transplantation: incidence and progression. Transplantation 1997;63(5):664–8.

115. Almond PS, Gillingham KJ, Sibley R, Moss A, Melin M, Leventhal A, Manivel C, Kyriakides P, Payne WD, Dunn DL, et al. Renal transplant function after ten years of cyclosporine. Transplantation 1992;53(2):316–23.

116. Burke JF Jr, Pirsch JD, Ramos EL, Salomon DR, Stablein DM, Van Buren DH, West JC. Long-term efficacy and safety of cyclosporine in renal-transplant recipients. N Engl J Med 1994;331(6):358–63.

117. Ruggenenti P, Perico N, Amuchastegui CS, Ferrazzi P, Mamprin F, Remuzzi G. Following an initial decline, glomerular filtration rate stabilizes in heart transplant patients on chronic cyclosporine. Am J Kidney Dis 1994;24(4):549–53.

118. Parving HH, Tarnow L, Nielsen FS, Rossing P, Mandrup-Poulsen T, Osterby R, Nerup J. Cyclosporine nephrotoxicity in type 1 diabetic patients. A 7-year follow-up study. Diabetes Care 1999;22(3):478–83.

119. Lipkowitz GS, Madden RL, Mulhern J, Braden G, O'Shea M, O'Shaughnessy J, Nash S, Kurbanov A, Freeman J, Rennke H, Germain M. Long-term maintenance of therapeutic cyclosporine levels leads to optimal graft survival without evidence of chronic nephrotoxicity. Transpl Int 1999;12(3):202–7.

120. Vercauteren SB, Bosmans JL, Elseviers MM, Verpooten GA, De Broe ME. A meta-analysis and morphological review of cyclosporine-induced nephrotoxicity in auto-immune diseases. Kidney Int 1998;54(2):536–45.

121. Feutren G, Mihatsch MJ. Risk factors for cyclosporine-induced nephropathy in patients with autoimmune diseases. International Kidney Biopsy Registry of Cyclosporine in Autoimmune Diseases. N Engl J Med 1992;326(25):1654–60.

122. Pei Y, Scholey JW, Katz A, Schachter R, Murphy GF, Cattran D. Chronic nephrotoxicity in psoriatic patients treated with low-dose cyclosporine. Am J Kidney Dis 1994;23(4):528–36.

123. Korstanje MJ, Bilo HJ, Stoof TJ. Sustained renal function loss in psoriasis patients after withdrawal of low-dose cyclosporin therapy. Br J Dermatol 1992;127(5):501–4.

124. Young EW, Ellis CN, Messana JM, Johnson KJ, Leichtman AB, Mihatsch MJ, Hamilton TA, Groisser DS, Fradin MS, Voorhees JJ. A prospective study of renal structure and function in psoriasis patients treated with cyclosporin. Kidney Int 1994;46(4):1216–22.

125. Shupack J, Abel E, Bauer E, Brown M, Drake L, Freinkel R, Guzzo C, Koo J, Levine N, Lowe N, McDonald C, Margolis D, Stiller M, Wintroub B, Bainbridge C, Evans S, Hilss S, Mietlowski W, Winslow C, Birnbaum JE. Cyclosporine as maintenance therapy in patients with severe psoriasis. J Am Acad Dermatol 1997;36(3 Pt 1):423–32.

126. van den Borne BE, Landewe RB, The HS, Breedveld FC, Dijkmans BA. Low dose cyclosporine in early rheumatoid arthritis: effective and safe after two years of therapy when compared with chloroquine. Scand J Rheumatol 1996;25(5):307–16.

127. Zachariae H, Kragballe K, Hansen HE, Marcussen N, Olsen S. Renal biopsy findings in long-term cyclosporin treatment of psoriasis. Br J Dermatol 1997;136(4):531–5.

128. Lowe NJ, Wieder JM, Rosenbach A, Johnson K, Kunkel R, Bainbridge C, Bourget T, Dimov I, Simpson K, Glass E, Grabie MT. Long-term low-dose cyclosporine therapy for severe psoriasis: effects on renal function and structure. J Am Acad Dermatol 1996;35(5 Pt 1):710–9.

129. Rodriguez F, Krayenbuhl JC, Harrison WB, Forre O, Dijkmans BA, Tugwell P, Miescher PA, Mihatsch MJ. Renal biopsy findings and followup of renal function in rheumatoid arthritis patients treated with cyclosporin A. An update from the International Kidney Biopsy Registry. Arthritis Rheum 1996;39(9):1491–8.

130. Landeweld RB, Dijkmans BA, van der Woude FJ, Breedveld FC, Mihatsch MJ, Bruijn JA. Longterm low dose cyclosporine in patients with rheumatoid arthritis: renal function loss without structural nephropathy. J Rheumatol 1996;23(1):61–4.

131. Feehally J, Walls J, Mistry N, Horsburgh T, Taylor J, Veitch PS, Bell PR. Does nifedipine ameliorate cyclosporin A nephrotoxicity? BMJ (Clin Res Ed) 1987;295(6593):310.

132. Tindall RS, Rollins JA, Phillips JT, Greenlee RG, Wells L, Belendiuk G. Preliminary results of a double-blind, randomized, placebo-controlled trial of cyclosporine in myasthenia gravis. N Engl J Med 1987;316(12):719–24.

133. Hadj-Aissa A, Labeeuw M, Lareal MC, et al. Effets de la cyclosporine (CyA) sur le rein isole: comparaison avec l'excipient (Exc). Nephrologie 1987;8:73.

134. Hoyer PF, Krohn HP, Offner G, Byrd DJ, Brodehl J, Wonigeit K, Pichlmayr R. Renal function after kidney transplantation in children. A comparison of conventional immunosuppression with cyclosporine. Transplantation 1987;43(4):489–93.

135. Wheatley HC, Datzman M, Williams JW, Miles DE, Hatch FE. Long-term effects of cyclosporine on renal function in liver transplant recipients. Transplantation 1987;43(5):641–7.

136. Albengres E, Le Louet H, d'Athis P, Tillement JP. S15176 and S16950 interaction with cyclosporin A antiproliferative effect on cultured human lymphocytes. Fundam Clin Pharmacol 2001;15(1):41–6.

137. Mihatsch MJ, Thiel G, Ryffel B. Brief review of the morphology of cyclosporin A nephropathy. Nephrologie 1987;8(3):143–5.

138. Palestine AG, Austin HA 3rd, Balow JE, Antonovych TT, Sabnis SG, Preuss HG, Nussenblatt RB. Renal histopathologic alterations in patients treated with cyclosporine for uveitis. N Engl J Med 1986;314(20):1293–8.

139. Raphael L, Fish JC. An in vitro model for analyzing the nephrotoxicity of cyclosporine and preservation injury. Transplantation 1987;43(5):703–8.

140. Anaise D, Waltzer WC, Arnold AN, Rapaport FT. Adverse effects of cyclosporine A on the microcirculation of the cold preserved kidney. NY State J Med 1987;87(3):141–2.

141. Lewis RM. Long-term use of cyclosporine A does not adversely impact on clinical outcomes following renal transplantation. Kidney Int Suppl 1995;52:S75–8.

142. Sehgal V, Radhakrishnan J, Appel GB, Valeri A, Cohen DJ. Progressive renal insufficiency following cardiac transplantation: cyclosporine, lipids, and hypertension. Am J Kidney Dis 1995;26(1):193–201.

143. Camara NO, Matos AC, Rodrigues DA, Pereira AB, Pacheco-Silva A. Early detection of heart transplant patients with increased risk of ciclosporin nephrotoxicity. Lancet 2001;357(9259):856–7.

144. Iijima K, Hamahira K, Tanaka R, Kobayashi A, Nozu K, Nakamura H, Yoshikawa N. Risk factors for cyclosporine-induced tubulointerstitial lesions in children with minimal change nephrotic syndrome. Kidney Int 2002;61(5):1801–5.

145. Hollander AAMJ, Van der Woude FJ. Efficacy and tolerability of conversion from cyclosporin to azathioprine after kidney transplantation. A review of the evidence. BioDrugs 1998;9:197–210.

146. Kasiske BL, Heim-Duthoy K, Ma JZ. Elective cyclosporine withdrawal after renal transplantation. A meta-analysis. JAMA 1993;269(3):395–400.

147. Heim-Duthoy KL, Chitwood KK, Tortorice KL, Massy ZA, Kasiske BL. Elective cyclosporine withdrawal 1 year after renal transplantation. Am J Kidney Dis 1994;24(5):846–53.

148. Smith SR, Minda SA, Samsa GP, Harrell FE Jr, Gunnells JC, Coffman TM, Butterly DW. Late withdrawal

of cyclosporine in stable renal transplant recipients. Am J Kidney Dis 1995;26(3):487–94.

149. Mourad G, Vela C, Ribstein J, Mimran A. Long-term improvement in renal function after cyclosporine reduction in renal transplant recipients with histologically proven chronic cyclosporine nephropathy. Transplantation 1998;65(5):661–7.

150. Bunke M, Sloan R, Brier M, Ganzel B. An improved glomerular filtration rate in cardiac transplant recipients with once-a-day cyclosporine dosing. Transplantation 1995;59(4):537–40.

151. Ramsay HM, Harden PN. Cyclosporin-induced flushing in a renal transplant recipient resolving after substitution with tacrolimus. Br J Dermatol 2000;142(4):832–3.

152. Azurdia RM, Graham RM, Weismann K, Guerin DM, Parslew R. Acne keloidalis in caucasian patients on cyclosporin following organ transplantation. Br J Dermatol 2000;143(2):465–7.

153. Carnero L, Silvestre JF, Guijarro J, Albares MP, Botella R. Nuchal acne keloidalis associated with cyclosporin. Br J Dermatol 2001;144(2):429–30.

154. Gupta S, Radotra BD, Kumar B, Pandhi R, Rai R. Multiple, large, polypoid infundibular (epidermoid) cysts in a cyclosporin-treated renal transplant recipient. Dermatology 2000;201(1):78.

155. Mahendran R, Grech C. Generalized pustular psoriasis following a short course of cyclosporin (Neoral). Br J Dermatol 1998;139(5):934.

156. Halpert E, Tunnessen WW Jr, Fivush B, Case B. Cutaneous lesions associated with cyclosporine therapy in pediatric renal transplant recipients. J Pediatr 1991;119(3):489–91.

157. Reznik VM, Jones KL, Durham BL, Mendoza SA. Changes in facial appearance during cyclosporin treatment. Lancet 1987;1(8547):1405–7.

158. Lee MO, Park SK, Choi JH, Sung KJ, Moon KC, Koh JK. Juxta-clavicular beaded lines in a kidney transplant patient receiving immunosuppressants. J Dermatol 2002;29(4):235–7.

159. Lear J, Bourke JF, Burns DA. Hyperplastic pseudofolliculitis barbae associated with cyclosporin. Br J Dermatol 1997;136(1):132–3.

160. Rebora A, Delmonte S, Parodi A. Cyclosporin A-induced hair darkening. Int J Dermatol 1999;38(3):229–30.

161. Siragusa M, Alberti A, Schepis C. Mees' lines due to cyclosporin. Br J Dermatol 1999;140(6):1198–9.

162. Arellano F, Krupp P. Muscular disorders associated with cyclosporin. Lancet 1991;337(8746):915.

163. Breil M, Chariot P. Muscle disorders associated with cyclosporine treatment. Muscle Nerve 1999;22(12):1631–6.

164. Stevens JM, Hilson AJ, Sweny P. Post-renal transplant distal limb bone pain. An under-recognized complication of transplantation distinct from avascular necrosis of bone? Transplantation 1995;60(3):305–7.

165. Barbosa LM, Gauthier VJ, Davis CL. Bone pain that responds to calcium channel blockers. A retrospective and prospective study of transplant recipients. Transplantation 1995;59(4):541–4.

166. Hokken-Koelega AC, Van Zaal MA, de Ridder MA, Wolff ED, De Jong MC, Donckerwolcke RA, De Muinck Keizer-Schrama SM, Drop SL. Growth after renal transplantation in prepubertal children: impact of various treatment modalities. Pediatr Res 1994;35(3):367–71.

167. Monegal A, Navasa M, Guanabens N, Peris P, Pons F, Martinez de Osaba MJ, Rimola A, Rodes J, Munoz-Gomez J. Bone mass and mineral metabolism in liver transplant patients treated with FK506 or cyclosporine A. Calcif Tissue Int 2001;68(2):83–6.

168. Baildam AD, Higgins RM, Hurley E, Furlong A, Walls J, Venning MC, Ackrill P, Mansel RE. Cyclosporin A and multiple fibroadenomas of the breast. Br J Surg 1996;83(12):1755–7.

169. Foxwell BM, Woerly G, Husi H, Mackie A, Quesniaux VF, Hiestand PC, Wenger RM, Ryffel B. Identification of several cyclosporine binding proteins in lymphoid and non-lymphoid cells in vivo. Biochim Biophys Acta 1992;1138(2):115–21.

170. Lopez-Calderon A, Soto L, Villanua MA, Vidarte L, Martin AI. The effect of cyclosporine administration on growth hormone release and serum concentrations of insulin-like growth factor-I in male rats. Life Sci 1999;64(17):1473–83.

171. Russell DH, Kibler R, Matrisian L, Larson DF, Poulos B, Magun BE. Prolactin receptors on human T and B lymphocytes: antagonism of prolactin binding by cyclosporine. J Immunol 1985;134(5):3027–31.

172. Larson DF. Cyclosporin. Mechanism of action: antagonism of the prolactin receptor. Prog Allergy 1986;38:222–38.

173. Volcheck GW, Van Dellen RG. Anaphylaxis to intravenous cyclosporine and tolerance to oral cyclosporine: case report and review. Ann Allergy Asthma Immunol 1998;80(2):159–63.

174. Liau-Chu M, Theis JG, Koren G. Mechanism of anaphylactoid reactions: improper preparation of high-dose intravenous cyclosporine leads to bolus infusion of Cremophor EL and cyclosporine. Ann Pharmacother 1997;31(11):1287–91.

175. Garcia VD, Keitel E, Almeida P, Santos AF, Becker M, Goldani JC. Morbidity after renal transplantation: role of bacterial infection. Transplant Proc 1995;27(2):1825–6.

176. Wade JJ, Rolando N, Hayllar K, Philpott-Howard J, Casewell MW, Williams R. Bacterial and fungal infections after liver transplantation: an analysis of 284 patients. Hepatology 1995;21(5):1328–36.

177. Singh N, Yu VL. Infections in organ transplant recipients. Curr Opin Infect Dis 1996;9:223–9.

178. Reis MA, Costa RS, Ferraz AS. Causes of death in renal transplant recipients: a study of 102 autopsies from 1968 to 1991. J R Soc Med 1995;88(1):24–7.

179. Fukuda M, Ohmori Y, Aikawa I, Yoshimura N, Oka T. Mutagenicity of cyclosporine in vivo. Transplant Proc 1988;20(3 Suppl 3):929–30.

180. Penn I. Tumors after renal and cardiac transplantation. Hematol Oncol Clin North Am 1993;7(2):431–45.

181. Qunibi WY, Akhtar M, Ginn E, Smith P. Kaposi's sarcoma in cyclosporine-induced gingival hyperplasia. Am J Kidney Dis 1988;11(4):349–52.

182. Penn I. Cancers after cyclosporine therapy. Transplant Proc 1988;20(1 Suppl 1):276–9.

183. Penn I. Posttransplant malignancies. World J Urol 1988;6:125.

184. Penn I, Brunson ME. Cancers after cyclosporine therapy. Transplant Proc 1988;20(3 Suppl 3):885–92.

185. Pilgrim M. Spontane Manifestation und Regression eines Kaposi-Sarkoms unter Cyclosporin A. [Spontaneous manifestation and regression of a Kaposi's sarcoma under cyclosporin A therapy.] Hautarzt 1988;39(6):368–70.

186. Gaya SB, Rees AJ, Lechler RI, Williams G, Mason PD. Malignant disease in patients with long-term renal transplants. Transplantation 1995;59(12):1705–9.

187. London NJ, Farmery SM, Will EJ, Davison AM, Lodge JP. Risk of neoplasia in renal transplant patients. Lancet 1995;346(8972):403–6.

188. Kirby B, Owen CM, Blewitt RW, Yates VM. Cutaneous T cell lymphoma developing in a patient on cyclosporin therapy. J Am Acad Dermatol 2002;47(Suppl 2):S165–7.

189. Kehinde EO, Petermann A, Morgan JD, Butt ZA, Donnelly PK, Veitch PS, Bell PR. Triple therapy and incidence of de novo cancer in renal transplant recipients. Br J Surg 1994;81(7):985–6.

190. Opelz G, Henderson R. Incidence of non-Hodgkin lymphoma in kidney and heart transplant recipients. Lancet 1993;342(8886–8887):1514–6.

191. Gruber SA, Gillingham K, Sothern RB, Stephanian E, Matas AJ, Dunn DL. De novo cancer in cyclosporine-treated and non-cyclosporine-treated adult primary renal allograft recipients. Clin Transplant 1994;8(4):388–95.

192. Hiesse C, Kriaa F, Rieu P, Larue JR, Benoit G, Bellamy J, Blanchet P, Charpentier B. Incidence and type of malignancies occurring after renal transplantation in conventionally and cyclosporine-treated recipients: analysis of a 20-year period in 1600 patients. Transplant Proc 1995;27(1):972–4.

193. Hojo M, Morimoto T, Maluccio M, Asano T, Morimoto K, Lagman M, Shimbo T, Suthanthiran M. Cyclosporine induces cancer progression by a cell-autonomous mechanism. Nature 1999;397(6719):530–4.

194. Jensen P, Hansen S, Moller B, Leivestad T, Pfeffer P, Geiran O, Fauchald P, Simonsen S. Skin cancer in kidney and heart transplant recipients and different long-term immunosuppressive therapy regimens. J Am Acad Dermatol 1999;40(2 Pt 1):177–86.

195. Weinstein SP, Orel SG, Collazzo L, Conant EF, Lawton TJ, Czerniecki B. Cyclosporin A-induced fibroadenomas of the breast: report of five cases. Radiology 2001;220(2):465–8.

196. De Felipe I, Redondo P. Eruptive angiomas after treatment with cyclosporine in a patient with psoriasis. Arch Dermatol 1998;134(11):1487–8.

197. Armenti VT, Ahlswede KM, Ahlswede BA, Cater JR, Jarrell BE, Mortiz MJ, Burke JF Jr. Variables affecting birthweight and graft survival in 197 pregnancies in cyclosporine-treated female kidney transplant recipients. Transplantation 1995;59(4):476–9.

198. Cararach V, Carmona F, Monleon FJ, Andreu J. Pregnancy after renal transplantation: 25 years experience in Spain. Br J Obstet Gynaecol 1993;100(2):122–5.

199. Ramsey-Goldman R, Schilling E. Immunosuppressive drug use during pregnancy. Rheum Dis Clin North Am 1997;23(1):149–67.

200. Armenti VT, Moritz MJ, Davison JM. Drug safety issues in pregnancy following transplantation and immunosuppression: effects and outcomes. Drug Saf 1998;19(3):219–32.

201. Armenti VT, Ahlswede KM, Ahlswede BA, Jarrell BE, Moritz MJ, Burke JF. National Transplantation Pregnancy Registry—outcomes of 154 pregnancies in cyclosporine-treated female kidney transplant recipients. Transplantation 1994;57(4):502–6.

202. Armenti VT, Ahlswede BA, Moritz MJ, Jarrell BE. National Transplantation Pregnancy Registry: analysis of pregnancy outcomes of female kidney recipients with relation to time interval from transplant to conception. Transplant Proc 1993;25(1 Pt 2):1036–7.

203. Pilarski LM, Yacyshyn BR, Lazarovits AI. Analysis of peripheral blood lymphocyte populations and immune function from children exposed to cyclosporine or to azathioprine in utero. Transplantation 1994;57(1):133–44.

204. Baarsma R, Kamps WA. Immunological responses in an infant after cyclosporine A exposure during pregnancy. Eur J Pediatr 1993;152(6):476–7.

205. Giudice PL, Dubourg L, Hadj-Aissa A, Said MH, Claris O, Audra P, Martin X, Cochat P. Renal function of children exposed to cyclosporin in utero. Nephrol Dial Transplant 2000;15(10):1575–9.

206. Shaheen FA, al-Sulaiman MH, al-Khader AA. Long-term nephrotoxicity after exposure to cyclosporine in utero. Transplantation 1993;56(1):224–5.

207. Bar Oz B, Hackman R, Einarson T, Koren G. Pregnancy outcome after cyclosporine therapy during pregnancy: a meta-analysis. Transplantation 2001;71(8):1051–5.

208. Nyberg G, Haljamae U, Frisenette-Fich C, Wennergren M, Kjellmer I. Breast-feeding during treatment with cyclosporine. Transplantation 1998;65(2):253–5.

209. Olyaei AJ, deMattos AM, Bennett WM. Switching between cyclosporin formulations. What are the risks? Drug Saf 1997;16(6):366–73.

210. Wijdicks EF, Dahlke LJ, Wiesner RH. Oral cyclosporine decreases severity of neurotoxicity in liver transplant recipients. Neurology 1999;52(8):1708–10.

211. Keown P, Landsberg D, Halloran P, Shoker A, Rush D, Jeffery J, Russell D, Stiller C, Muirhead N, Cole E, Paul L, Zaltzman J, Loertscher R, Daloze P, Dandavino R, Boucher A, Handa P, Lawen J, Belitsky P, Parfrey P. A randomized, prospective multicenter pharmacoepidemiologic study of cyclosporine microemulsion in stable renal graft recipients. Report of the Canadian Neoral Renal Transplantation Study Group. Transplantation 1996;62(12):1744–52.

212. Shah MB, Martin JE, Schroeder TJ, First MR. Evaluation of the safety and tolerability of Neoral and Sandimmune: a meta-analysis. Transplant Proc 1998;30(5):1697–700.

213. Freise CE, Galbraith CA, Nikolai BJ, Ascher NL, Lake JR, Stock PG, Roberts JP. Risks associated with conversion of stable patients after liver transplantation to the microemulsion formulation of cyclosporine. Transplantation 1998;65(7):995–7.

214. Shah MB, Martin JE, Schroeder TJ, First MR. Validity of open labeled versus blinded trials: a meta-analysis comparing Neoral and Sandimmune. Transplant Proc 1999;31(1–2):217–9.

215. Sheil AG, Disney AP, Mathew TH, Amiss N, Excell L. Cancer development in cadaveric donor renal allograft recipients treated with azathioprine (AZA) or cyclosporine (CyA) or AZA/CyA. Transplant Proc 1991;23(1 Pt 2):1111–2.

216. Hiesse C, Rieu P, Kriaa F, Larue JR, Goupy C, Neyrat N, Charpentier B. Malignancy after renal transplantation: analysis of incidence and risk factors in 1700 patients followed during a 25-year period. Transplant Proc 1997;29(1–2):831–3.

217. Hoshida Y, Tsukuma H, Yasunaga Y, Xu N, Fujita MQ, Satoh T, Ichikawa Y, Kurihara K, Imanishi M, Matsuno T, Aozasa K. Cancer risk after renal transplantation in Japan. Int J Cancer 1997;71(4):517–20.

218. Dantal J, Hourmant M, Cantarovich D, Giral M, Blancho G, Dreno B, Soulillou JP. Effect of long-term immunosuppression in kidney-graft recipients on cancer incidence: randomised comparison of two cyclosporin regimens. Lancet 1998;351(9103):623–8.

219. Feutren G. The optimal use of cyclosporin A in autoimmune diseases. J Autoimmun 1992;5(Suppl A):183–95.

220. Arellano F, Krupp P. Malignancies in rheumatoid arthritis patients treated with cyclosporin A. Br J Rheumatol 1993;32(Suppl 1):72–5.

221. van den Borne BE, Landewe RB, Houkes I, Schild F, van der Heyden PC, Hazes JM, Vandenbroucke JP, Zwinderman AH, Goei The HS, Breedveld FC, Bernelot Moens HJ, Kluin PM, Dijkmans BA. No increased risk of malignancies and mortality in cyclosporin A-treated patients with rheumatoid arthritis. Arthritis Rheum 1998;41(11):1930–7.

222. Arellano F. Risk of cancer with cyclosporine in psoriasis. Int J Dermatol 1997;36(Suppl 1):15–7.

223. Arellano F, Monka C, Krupp PF. Acute cyclosporin overdose. A review of present clinical experience. Drug Saf 1991;6(4):266–76.

224. Sketris IS, Onorato L, Yatscoff RW, Givner M, Nicol D, Abraham I. Eight days of cyclosporine overdose: a case report. Pharmacotherapy 1993;13(6):658–60.

225. Dussol B, Reynaud-Gaubert M, Saingra Y, Daniel L, Berland Y. Acute tubular necrosis induced by high level of cyclosporine A in a lung transplant. Transplantation 2000;70(8):1234–6.

226. de Perrot M, Spiliopoulos A, Cottini S, Nicod L, Ricou B. Massive cerebral edema after I.V. cyclosporin overdose Transplantation 2000;70(8):1259–60.

227. Tabbara KF, Al-Faisal Z, Al-Rashed W. Interaction between acetazolamide and cyclosporine. Arch Ophthalmol 1998;116(6):832–3.

228. Lill J, Bauer LA, Horn JR, Hansten PD. Cyclosporine-drug interactions and the influence of patient age. Am J Health Syst Pharm 2000;57(17):1579–84.

229. Ahmed T, Fenton T, McGraw M. Reversible renal failure in renal transplant patients receiving acyclovir. Pediatr Nephrol 1993;7:C58.

230. Dugandzic RM, Sketris IS, Belitsky P, Schlech WF 3rd, Givner ML. Effect of coadministration of acyclovir and cyclosporine on kidney function and cyclosporine concentrations in renal transplant patients. DICP 1991;25(3):316–7.

231. Termeer A, Hoitsma AJ, Koene RA. Severe nephrotoxicity caused by the combined use of gentamicin and cyclosporine in renal allograft recipients. Transplantation 1986;42(2):220–1.

232. Sketris IS, Methot ME, Nicol D, Belitsky P, Knox MG. Effect of calcium-channel blockers on cyclosporine clearance and use in renal transplant patients. Ann Pharmacother 1994;28(11):1227–31.

233. Smith CL, Hampton EM, Pederson JA, Pennington LR, Bourne DW. Clinical and medicoeconomic impact of the cyclosporine–diltiazem interaction in renal transplant recipients. Pharmacotherapy 1994;14(4):471–81.

234. Jones TE, Morris RG, Mathew TH. Formulation of diltiazem affects cyclosporin-sparing activity. Eur J Clin Pharmacol 1997;52(1):55–8.

235. Kuypers DR, Neumayer HH, Fritsche L, Budde K, Rodicio JL, Vanrenterghem YLacidipine Study Group. Calcium channel blockade and preservation of renal graft function in cyclosporine-treated recipients: a prospective randomized placebo-controlled 2-year study. Transplantation 2004;78(8):1204–11.

236. Bui L, Huang DD. Possible interaction between cyclosporine and chloramphenicol. Ann Pharmacother 1999;33(2):252–3.

237. Thurnheer R, Laube I, Speich R. Possible interaction between clindamycin and cyclosporin. BMJ 1999;319(7203):163.

238. Ducloux D, Schuller V, Bresson-Vautrin C, Chalopin JM. Colchicine myopathy in renal transplant recipients on cyclosporin. Nephrol Dial Transplant 1997;12(11):2389–92.

239. Tweddle DA, Windebank KP, Hewson QC, Yule SM. Cyclosporin neurotoxicity after chemotherapy. BMJ 1999;318(7191):1113.

240. Pea F, Damiani D, Michieli M, Ermacora A, Baraldo M, Russo D, Fanin R, Baccarani M, Furlanut M. Multidrug resistance modulation in vivo: the effect of cyclosporin A alone or with dexverapamil on idarubicin pharmacokinetics in acute leukemia. Eur J Clin Pharmacol 1999;55(5):361–8.

241. Meerum Terwogt JM, Beijnen JH, ten Bokkel Huinink WW, Rosing H, Schellens JH. Co-administration of cyclosporin enables oral therapy with paclitaxel. Lancet 1998;352(9124):285.

242. Malingre MM, Beijnen JH, Rosing H, Koopman FJ, van Tellingen O, Duchin K, Ten Bokkel Huinink WW, Swart M, Lieverst J, Schellens JH. A phase I and pharmacokinetic study of bi-daily dosing of oral paclitaxel in combination with cyclosporin A. Cancer Chemother Pharmacol 2001;47(4):347–54.

243. Bisogno G, Cowie F, Boddy A, Thomas HD, Dick G, Pinkerton CR. High-dose cyclosporin with etoposide—toxicity and pharmacokinetic interaction in children with solid tumours. Br J Cancer 1998;77(12):2304–9.

244. Rushing DA, Raber SR, Rodvold KA, Piscitelli SC, Plank GS, Tewksbury DA. The effects of cyclosporine on the pharmacokinetics of doxorubicin in patients with small cell lung cancer. Cancer 1994;74(3):834–41.

245. Hoey LL, Lake KD. Does ciprofloxacin interact with cyclosporine? Ann Pharmacother 1994;28(1):93–6.

246. McLellan RA, Drobitch RK, McLellan H, Acott PD, Crocker JF, Renton KW. Norfloxacin interferes with cyclosporine disposition in pediatric patients undergoing renal transplantation. Clin Pharmacol Ther 1995;58(3):322–7.

247. Wynckel A, Toupance O, Melin JP, David C, Lavaud S, Wong T, Lamiable D, Chanard J. Traitement des légionelloses par ofloxacine chez le transplanté rénal. Absence d'interférence avec la ciclosporine A. [Treatment of legionellosis with ofloxacin in kidney transplanted patients. Lack of interaction with cyclosporin A.] Presse Méd 1991;20(7):291–3.

248. Morales JM, Munoz MA, Fernandez Zatarain G, Garcia Canton C, Garcia Rubiales MA, Andres A, Aguado JM, Gonzalez Pinto I. Reversible acute renal failure caused by the combined use of foscarnet and cyclosporin in organ transplanted patients. Nephrol Dial Transplant 1995;10(6):882–3.

249. Cantarovich M, Latter D. Effect of prophylactic ganciclovir on renal function and cyclosporine levels after heart transplantation. Transplant Proc 1994;26(5):2747–8.

250. Johnston A, Holt DW. Effect of grapefruit juice on blood cyclosporin concentration. Lancet 1995;346(8967):122–3.

251. Lewis SM, McCloskey WW. Potentiation of nephrotoxicity by H2-antagonists in patients receiving cyclosporine. Ann Pharmacother 1997;31(3):363–5.

252. Rodriguez JA, Crespo-Leiro MG, Paniagua MJ, Cuenca JJ, Hermida LF, Juffe A, Castro-Beiras A. Rhabdomyolysis in heart transplant patients on HMG-

CoA reductase inhibitors and cyclosporine. Transplant Proc 1999;31(6):2522–3.

253. Gullestad L, Nordal KP, Berg KJ, Cheng H, Schwartz MS, Simonsen S. Interaction between lovastatin and cyclosporine A after heart and kidney transplantation. Transplant Proc 1999;31(5):2163–5.

254. Maltz HC, Balog DL, Cheigh JS. Rhabdomyolysis associated with concomitant use of atorvastatin and cyclosporine. Ann Pharmacother 1999;33(11):1176–9.

255. East C, Alivizatos PA, Grundy SM, Jones PH, Farmer JA. Rhabdomyolysis in patients receiving lovastatin after cardiac transplantation. N Engl J Med 1988;318(1):47–8.

256. Campana C, Iacona I, Regazzi MB, Gavazzi A, Perani G, Raddato V, Montemartini C, Vigano M. Efficacy and pharmacokinetics of simvastatin in heart transplant recipients. Ann Pharmacother 1995;29(3):235–9.

257. Cheung AK, DeVault GA Jr, Gregory MC. A prospective study on treatment of hypercholesterolemia with lovastatin in renal transplant patients receiving cyclosporine. J Am Soc Nephrol 1993;3(12):1884–91.

258. Wanner C, Kramer-Guth A, Galle J. Use of HMG-CoA reductase inhibitors after kidney and heart transplantation. BioDrugs 1997;8:387–93.

259. Olbricht C, Wanner C, Eisenhauer T, Kliem V, Doll R, Boddaert M, O'Grady P, Krekler M, Mangold B, Christians U. Accumulation of lovastatin, but not pravastatin, in the blood of cyclosporine-treated kidney graft patients after multiple doses. Clin Pharmacol Ther 1997;62(3):311–21.

260. Ichimaru N, Takahara S, Kokado Y, Wang JD, Hatori M, Kameoka H, Inoue T, Okuyama A. Changes in lipid metabolism and effect of simvastatin in renal transplant recipients induced by cyclosporine or tacrolimus. Atherosclerosis 2001;158(2):417–23.

261. Muck W, Mai I, Fritsche L, Ochmann K, Rohde G, Unger S, Johne A, Bauer S, Budde K, Roots I, Neumayer HH, Kuhlmann J. Increase in cerivastatin systemic exposure after single and multiple dosing in cyclosporine-treated kidney transplant recipients. Clin Pharmacol Ther 1999;65(3):251–61.

262. Ruschitzka F, Meier PJ, Turina M, Luscher TF, Noll G. Acute heart transplant rejection due to Saint John's wort. Lancet 2000;355(9203):548–9.

263. Breidenbach T, Hoffmann MW, Becker T, Schlitt H, Klempnauer J. Drug interaction of St. John's wort with cyclosporin. Lancet 2000;355(9218):1912.

264. Schroeder TJ, Melvin DB, Clardy CW, Wadhwa NK, Myre SA, Reising JM, Wolf RK, Collins JA, Pesce AJ, First MR. Use of cyclosporine and ketoconazole without nephrotoxicity in two heart transplant recipients. J Heart Transplant 1987;6(2):84–9.

265. First MR, Schroeder TJ, Michael A, Hariharan S, Weiskittel P, Alexander JW. Cyclosporine–ketoconazole interaction. Long-term follow-up and preliminary results of a randomized trial. Transplantation 1993;55(5):1000–4.

266. Keogh A, Spratt P, McCosker C, Macdonald P, Mundy J, Kaan A. Ketoconazole to reduce the need for cyclosporine after cardiac transplantation. N Engl J Med 1995;333(10):628–33.

267. Sobh M, el-Agroudy A, Moustafa F, Harras F, el-Bedewy M, Ghoneim M. Coadministration of ketoconazole to cyclosporin-treated kidney transplant recipients: a prospective randomized study. Am J Nephrol 1995;15(6):493–9.

268. Romero AJ, Pogamp PL, Nilsson LG, Wood N. Effect of voriconazole on the pharmacokinetics of cyclosporine in renal transplant patients. Clin Pharmacol Ther 2002;71(4):226–34.

269. Turhal NS. Cyclosporin A and imipenem associated seizure activity in allogeneic bone marrow transplantation patients. J Chemother 1999;11(5):410–3.

270. Jones TE. The use of other drugs to allow a lower dosage of cyclosporin to be used. Therapeutic and pharmacoeconomic considerations. Clin Pharmacokinet 1997;32(5):357–67.

271. Amsden GW. Macrolides versus azalides: a drug interaction update. Ann Pharmacother 1995;29(9):906–17.

272. Gregoor PJ, de Sevaux RG, Hene RJ, Hesse CJ, Hilbrands LB, Vos P, van Gelder T, Hoitsma AJ, Weimar W. Effect of cyclosporine on mycophenolic acid trough levels in kidney transplant recipients. Transplantation 1999;68(10):1603–6.

273. Helms-Smith KM, Curtis SL, Hatton RC. Apparent interaction between nefazodone and cyclosporine. Ann Intern Med 1996;125(5):424.

274. Garton T. Nefazodone and CYP450 3A4 interactions with cyclosporine and tacrolimus1. Transplantation 2002;74(5):745.

275. Wright DH, Lake KD, Bruhn PS, Emery RW Jr. Nefazodone and cyclosporine drug–drug interaction. J Heart Lung Transplant 1999;18(9):913–5.

276. Constantopoulos A. Colitis induced by interaction of cyclosporine A and non-steroidal anti-inflammatory drugs. Pediatr Int 1999;41(2):184–6.

277. Kovarik JM, Mueller EA, Gerbeau C, Tarral A, Francheteau P, Guerret M. Cyclosporine and nonsteroidal antiinflammatory drugs: exploring potential drug interactions and their implications for the treatment of rheumatoid arthritis. J Clin Pharmacol 1997;37(4):336–43.

278. Kovarik JM, Kurki P, Mueller E, Guerret M, Markert E, Alten R, Zeidler H, Genth-Stolzenburg S. Diclofenac combined with cyclosporine in treatment refractory rheumatoid arthritis: longitudinal safety assessment and evidence of a pharmacokinetic/dynamic interaction. J Rheumatol 1996;23(12):2033–8.

279. Tugwell P, Ludwin D, Gent M, Roberts R, Bensen W, Grace E, Baker P. Interaction between cyclosporin A and nonsteroidal antiinflammatory drugs. J Rheumatol 1997;24(6):1122–5.

280. Barbaro D, Orsini P, Pallini S, Piazza F, Pasquini C. Obesity in transplant patients: case report showing interference of orlistat with absorption of cyclosporine and review of literature. Endocr Pract 2002;8(2):124–6.

281. Nagele H, Petersen B, Bonacker U, Rodiger W. Effect of orlistat on blood cyclosporin concentration in an obese heart transplant patient. Eur J Clin Pharmacol 1999;55(9):667–9.

282. Colman E, Fossler M. Reduction in blood cyclosporine concentrations by orlistat. N Engl J Med 2000;342(15):1141–2.

283. Le Beller C, Bezie Y, Chabatte C, Guillemain R, Amrein C, Billaud EM. Co-administration of orlistat and cyclosporine in a heart transplant recipient. Transplantation 2000;70(10):1541–2.

284. Schnetzler B, Kondo-Oestreicher M, Vala D, Khatchatourian G, Faidutti B. Orlistat decreases the plasma level of cyclosporine and may be responsible for the development of acute rejection episodes. Transplantation 2000;70(10):1540–1.

285. Actis GC, Debernardi-Venon W, Lagget M, Marzano A, Ottobrelli A, Ponzetto A, Rocca G, Boggio-Bertinet D, Balzola F, Bonino F, et al. Hepatotoxicity of intravenous cyclosporin A in patients with acute ulcerative colitis on total parenteral nutrition. Liver 1995;15(6):320–3.

286. Gregoor PJ, van Gelder T, van der Ende ME, Ijzermans JN, Weimar W. Cyclosporine and triple-drug treatment with human immunodeficiency virus protease inhibitors. Transplantation 1999;68(8):1210.

287. Schouler L, Dumas F, Couzigou P, Janvier G, Winnock S, Saric J. Omeprazole–cyclosporin interaction. Am J Gastroenterol 1991;86(8):1097.

288. Arranz R, Yanez E, Franceschi JL, Fernandez-Ranada JM. More about omeprazole–cyclosporine interaction. Am J Gastroenterol 1993;88(1):154–5.

289. Blohme I, Idstrom JP, Andersson T. A study of the interaction between omeprazole and cyclosporine in renal transplant patients. Br J Clin Pharmacol 1993;35(2):156–60.

290. Brinkman K, Huysmans F, Burger DM. Pharmacokinetic interaction between saquinavir and cyclosporine. Ann Intern Med 1998;129(11):914–5.

291. Du Cheyron D, Debruyne D, Lobbedez T, Richer C, Ryckelynck JP, Hurault de Ligny B. Effect of sulfasalazine on cyclosporin blood concentration. Eur J Clin Pharmacol 1999;55(3):227–8.

292. Caforio AL, Gambino A, Tona F, Feltrin G, Marchini F, Pompei E, Testolin L, Angelini A, Dalla Volta S, Casarotto D. Sulfinpyrazone reduces cyclosporine levels: a new drug interaction in heart transplant recipients. J Heart Lung Transplant 2000;19(12):1205–8.

293. Pichard L, Fabre I, Fabre G, Domergue J, Saint Aubert B, Mourad G, Maurel P. Cyclosporin A drug interactions. Screening for inducers and inhibitors of cytochrome P-450 (cyclosporin A oxidase) in primary cultures of human hepatocytes and in liver microsomes. Drug Metab Dispos 1990;18(5):595–606.

294. Islam SI, Masuda QN, Bolaji OO, Shaheen FM, Sheikh IA. Possible interaction between cyclosporine and glibenclamide in posttransplant diabetic patients. Ther Drug Monit 1996;18(5):624–6.

295. Verdejo A, de Cos MA, Zubimendi JA, Lopez-Lazaro L. Drug points. Probable interaction between cyclosporin A and low dose ticlopidine. BMJ 2000;320(7241):1037.

296. Kaplan B, Friedman G, Jacobs M, Viscuso R, Lyman N, DeFranco P, Bonomini L, Mulgaonkar SP. Potential interaction of troglitazone and cyclosporine. Transplantation 1998;65(10):1399–400.

297. Park MH, Pelegrin D, Haug MT 3rd, Young JB. Troglitazone, a new antidiabetic agent, decreases cyclosporine level. J Heart Lung Transplant 1998;17(11):1139–40.

298. Le Bigot JF, Lavene D, Kiechel JR. Pharmacocinétique et métabolisme di la cyclosporine: interaction médicamenteuse. [Pharmacokinetics and metabolism of cyclosporin; drug interactions.] Nephrologie 1987;8(3):135–41.

299. Keown PA. New concepts in cyclosporine monitoring. Curr Opin Nephrol Hypertens 2002;11(6):619–26.

300. Levy G, Burra P, Cavallari A, Duvoux C, Lake J, Mayer AD, Mies S, Pollard SG, Varo E, Villamil F, Johnston A. Improved clinical outcomes for liver transplant recipients using cyclosporine monitoring based on 2-hr post-dose levels (C2). Transplantation 2002;73(6):953–9.

301. Lindholm A, Ringden O, Lonnqvist B. The role of cyclosporine dosage and plasma levels in efficacy and toxicity in bone marrow transplant recipients. Transplantation 1987;43(5):680–4.

302. Azoulay D, Lemoine A, Dennison A, Gries JM, Dolizy I, Castaing D, Beaune P, Bismuth H. Incidence of adverse reactions to cyclosporine after liver transplantation is predicted by the first blood level. Hepatology 1993;17(6):1123–6.

303. Joos AA, Frank UG, Kaschka WP. Pharmacokinetic interaction of clozapine and rifampicin in a forensic patient with an atypical mycobacterial infection. J Clin Psychopharmacol 1998;18(1):83–85.

304. Venkat-Raman G, Feehally J, Elliott HL, Griffin P, Moore RJ, Olubodun JO, Wilkinson R. Renal and haemodynamic effects of amlodipine and nifedipine in hypertensive renal transplant recipients. Nephrol Dial Transplant 1998;13(10):2612–2616.

305. Jacob LP, Malhotra D, Chan L, Shapiro JI. Absence of a dose-response of cyclosporine levels to clinically used doses of diltiazem and verapamil. Am J Kidney Dis 1999;33(2):301–303.

306. Yildiz A, Sever MS, Turkmen A, Ecder T, Turk S, Akkaya V, Ark E. Interaction between cyclosporine A and verapamil, felodipine, and isradipine. Nephron 1999;81(1):117–118.

307. Bourbigot B, Guiserix J, Airiau J, Bressollette L, Morin JF, Cledes J. Nicardipine increases cyclosporin blood levels. Lancet 1986;1(8495):1447.

308. Pochet JM, Pirson Y. Cyclosporin–diltiazem interaction. Lancet 1986;1(8487):979.

309. Citterio F, Serino F, Pozzetto U, Fioravanti P, Caizzi P, Castagneto M. Verapamil improves Sandimmune immunosuppression, reducing acute rejection episodes. Transplant Proc 1996;28(4):2174–2176.

310. Bosmuller C, Steurer W, Konigsrainer A, Willeit J, Margreiter R. Increased risk of central nervous system toxicity in patients treated with ciclosporin and imipenem/cilastatin. Nephron 1991;58(3):362–364.

311. Carmellini M, Frosini F, Filipponi F, Boggi U, Mosca F. Effect of cilastatin on cyclosporine-induced acute nephrotoxicity in kidney transplant recipients. Transplantation 1997;64(1):164–166.

312. Paterson DL, Singh N. Interactions between tacrolimus and antimicrobial agents. Clin Infect Dis 1997;25(6):1430–1440.

313. Soto Alvarez J, Sacristan Del Castillo JA, Alsar Ortiz MJ. Interaction between ciclosporin and ceftriaxone. Nephron 1991;59(4):681–682.

314. Ernst E. Second thoughts about safety of St. John's wort. Lancet 1999;354(9195):2014–2016.

315. Breidenbach T, Kliem V, Burg M, Radermacher J, Hoffmann MW, Klempnauer J. Profound drop of cyclosporin A whole blood trough levels caused by St. John's wort (*Hypericum perforatum*). Transplantation 2000;69(10):2229–2230.

316. Barone GW, Gurley BJ, Ketel BL, Lightfoot ML, AbulEzz SR. Drug interaction between St. John's wort and cyclosporine. Ann Pharmacother 2000;34(9):1013–1016.

317. Karliova M, Treichel U, Malago M, Frilling A, Gerken G, Broelsch CE. Interaction of *Hypericum perforatum* (St. John's wort) with cyclosporin A metabolism in a patient after liver transplantation. J Hepatol 2000;33(5):853–855.

318. Mai I, Kruger H, Budde K, Johne A, Brockmoller J, Neumayer HH, Roots I. Hazardous pharmacokinetic interaction of Saint John's wort (*Hypericum perforatum*) with the immunosuppressant cyclosporin. Int J Clin Pharmacol Ther 2000;38(10):500–502.

319. Turton-Weeks SM, Barone GW, Gurley BJ, Ketel BL, Lightfoot ML, Abul-Ezz SR. St. John's wort: a hidden risk for transplant patients. Prog Transplant 2001;11(2):116–120.

320. Moschella C, Jaber BL. Interaction between cyclosporine and *Hypericum perforatum* (St. John's wort) after organ transplantation. Am J Kidney Dis 2001;38(5):1105–1107.

321. Ernst E. St. John's wort supplements endanger the success of organ transplantation. Arch Surg 2002;137(3):316–319.

322. Morris RG, Jones TE. Diltiazem disposition and metabolism in recipients of renal transplants. Ther Drug Monit 1998;20(4):365–370.

323. Asberg A, Christensen H, Hartmann A, Berg KJ. Diltiazem modulates cyclosporin A induced renal hemodynamic effects but not its effect on plasma endothelin-1. Clin Transplant 1998;12(5):363–370.

324. Asberg A, Christensen H, Hartmann A, Carlson E, Molden E, Berg KJ. Pharmacokinetic interactions between microemulsion formulated cyclosporine A and diltiazem in renal transplant recipients. Eur J Clin Pharmacol 1999;55(5):383–387.

325. Jiang TT, Huang W, Patel D. Cyclosporine-induced encephalopathy predisposed by diltiazem in a patient with aplastic anemia. Ann Pharmacother 1999;33(6):750–751.

326. McFadden JP, Pantin JE, Parkes AV, et al. Cyclosporin decreases nifedipine metabolism. BMJ 1989;299:1224.

327. Rahn KH, Barenbrock M, Fritschka E, Heinecke A, Lippert J, Schroeder K, Hauser I, Wagner K, Neumayer HH. Effect of nitrendipine on renal function in renal-transplant patients treated with cyclosporin: a randomised trial. Lancet 1999;354(9188):1415–1420.

328. Jahansouz F, Kriett JM, Smith CM, Jamieson SW. Potentiation of cyclosporine nephrotoxicity by nafcillin in lung transplant recipients. Transplantation 1993;55(5):1045–1048.

329. Ogawa D, Maruyama K, Miyatake N, Kashihara N, Makino H. Concomitant use of simvastatin and cyclosporin A increases LDH in nephrotic syndrome. Nephron 1998;80(3):351–352.

330. Lum BL, Kaubisch S, Yahanda AM, Adler KM, Jew L, Ehsan MN, Brophy NA, Halsey J, Gosland MP, Sikic BI. Alteration of etoposide pharmacokinetics and pharmacodynamics by cyclosporine in a phase I trial to modulate multidrug resistance. J Clin Oncol 1992;10(10):1635–1642.

331. Guieu R, Dussol B, Devaux C, Sampol J, Brunet P, Rochat H, Bechis G, Berland YF. Interactions between cyclosporine A and adenosine in kidney transplant recipients. Kidney Int 1998;53(1):200–204.

332. Strehlau J, Pape L, Offner G, Nashan B, Ehrich JH. Interleukin-2 receptor antibody-induced alterations of ciclosporin dose requirements in paediatric transplant recipients. Lancet 2000;356(9238):1327–1328.

333. Ganschow R, Grabhorn E, Burdelski M. Basiliximab in paediatric liver-transplant recipients. Lancet 2001;357(9253):388.

334. Nanni G, Panocchia N, Tacchino R, Foco M, Piccioni E, Castagneto M. Increased incidence of infection in verapamil-treated kidney transplant recipients. Transplant proc 2000;32(3):551–3.

335. Ljutic D, Rumboldt Z. Possible interaction between azithromycin and cyclosporin: a case report. Nephron 1995;70(1):130.

336. Wrishko RE, Levine M, Primmett DR, Kim S, Partovi N, Lewis S, Landsberg D, Keown PA. Investigation of a possible interaction between ciprofloxacin and cyclosporine in renal transplant patients. Transplantation 1997;64(7):996–9.

337. Quan VA, Saunders BP, Hicks BH, Sladen GE. Cyclosporin treatment for ulcerative colitis complicated by fatal Pneumocystis carinii pneumonia. BMJ 1997;314(7077):363–364.

338. Bachmann K, Sullivan TJ, Reese JH, Jauregui L, Miller K, Scott M, Sides GD, Shapiro R. The influence of dirithromycin on the pharmacokinetics of cyclosporine in healthy subjects and in renal transplant patients. Am J Ther 1995;2(7):490–498.

339. Groll AH, Walsh TJ. Caspofungin: pharmacology, safety and therapeutic potential in superficial and invasive fungal infections. Expert Opin Investig Drugs 2001;10(8):1545–1558.

340. Tseng A, Nguyen ME, Cardella C, Humar A, Conly J. Probable interaction between efavirenz and cyclosporine. AIDS 2002;16(3):505–506.

341. Kovarik JM, Kahan BD, Kaplan B, Lorber M, Winkler M, Rouilly M, Gerbeau C, Cambon N, Boger R, Rordorf CEverolimus Phase 2 Study Group. Longitudinal assessment of everolimus in de novo renal transplant recipients over the first post-transplant year: pharmacokinetics, exposure-response relationships, and influence on cyclosporine. Clin Pharmacol Ther 2001;69(1):48–56.

342. Lyman CA, Walsh TJ. Systemically administered antifungal agents. A review of their clinical pharmacology and therapeutic applications. Drugs 1992;44(1):9–35.

343. Osowski CL, Dix SP, Lin LS, Mullins RE, Geller RB, Wingard JR. Evaluation of the drug interaction between intravenous high-dose fluconazole and cyclosporine or tacrolimus in bone marrow transplant patients. Transplantation 1996;61(8):1268–1272.

344. Lopez-Gil JA. Fluconazole–cyclosporine interaction: a dose-dependent effect? Ann Pharmacother 1993;27(4):427–430.

345. Mathis AS, DiRenzo T, Friedman GS, Kaplan B, Adamson R. Sex and ethnicity may chiefly influence the interaction of fluconazole with calcineurin inhibitors. Transplantation 2001;71(8):1069–1075.

346. Sud K, Singh B, Krishna VS, Thennarasu K, Kohli HS, Jha V, Gupta KL, Sakhuja V. Unpredictable cyclosporin–fluconazole interaction in renal transplant recipients. Nephrol Dial Transplant 1999;14(7):1698–1703.

347. Abu-Romeh SH, Rashed A. Cyclosporin A and griseofulvin: another drug interaction. Nephron 1991;58(2):237.

348. Prasad R, Maddux MS, Mozes MF, Biskup NS, Maturen A. A significant difference in cyclosporine blood and plasma concentrations with heparin or EDTA anticoagulant. Transplantation 1985;39(6):667–669.

349. Kramer MR, Marshall SE, Denning DW, Keogh AM, Tucker RM, Galgiani JN, Lewiston NJ, Stevens DA, Theodore J. Cyclosporine and itraconazole interaction in heart and lung transplant recipients. Ann Intern Med 1990;113(4):327–329.

350. Kwan JT, Foxall PJ, Davidson DG, Bending MR, Eisinger AJ. Interaction of cyclosporin and itraconazole. Lancet 1987;2(8553):282.

351. Trenk D, Brett W, Jahnchen E, Bixnbaum D. Time course of cyclosporin/itraconazole interaction. Lancet 1987;2(8571):1335–1336.

352. Navakova I, Donnelly P, de Witte T, de Pauw B, Boezeman J, Veltman G. Itraconazole and cyclosporin nephrotoxicity. Lancet 1987;2(8564):920–921.

353. Vlahakos DV, Manginas A, Chilidou D, Zamanika C, Alivizatos PA. Itraconazole-induced rhabdomyolysis and acute renal failure in a heart transplant recipient treated with simvastatin and cyclosporine. Transplantation 2002;73(12):1962–1964.

354. Maxa JL, Melton LB, Ogu CC, Sills MN, Limanni A. Rhabdomyolysis after concomitant use of cyclosporine, simvastatin, gemfibrozil, and itraconazole. Ann Pharmacother 2002;36(5):820–823.

355. Sugar AM, Stern JJ, Dupont B. Overview: treatment of cryptococcal meningitis. Rev Infect Dis 1990;12(Suppl 3):S338–S348.

356. McLellan RA, Drobitch RK, McLellan H, Acott PD, Crocker JF, Renton KW. Norfloxacin interferes with cyclosporine disposition in pediatric patients undergoing renal transplantation. Clin Pharmacol Ther 1995;58(3):322–327.

357. Sobh MA, Hamdy AF, El Agroudy AE, El Sayed K, ElDiasty T, Bakr MA, Ghoneim MA. Coadministration of ketoconazole and cyclosporine for kidney transplant recipients: long-term follow-up and study of metabolic consequences. Am J Kidney Dis 2001;37(3):510–517.

358. Tariq M, Morais C, Sobki S, Al Sulaiman M, Al Khader A. Effect of lithium on cyclosporin induced nephrotoxicity in rats. Ren Fail 2000;22(5):545–560.

359. Azanza J, Catalan M, Alvarez P, Honorato J, Herreros J, Llorens R. Possible interaction between cyclosporine and josamycin. J Heart Transplant 1990;9(3 Pt 1):265–266.

360. Wadhwa NK, Schroeder TJ, O'Flaherty E, Pesce AJ, Myre SA, Munda R, First MR. Interaction between erythromycin and cyclosporine in a kidney and pancreas allograft recipient. Ther Drug Monit 1987;9(1):123–125.

361. Ljutic D, Rumboldt Z. Possible interaction between azithromycin and cyclosporin: a case report. Nephron 1995;70(1):130.

362. Lewis BR, Aoun SL, Bernstein GA, Crow SJ. Pharmacokinetic interactions between cyclosporine and bupropion or methylphenidate. J Child Adolesc Psychopharmacol 2001;11(2):193–198.

363. Wadhwa NK, Schroeder TJ, O'Flaherty E, Pesce AJ, Myre SA, First MR. The effect of oral metoclopramide on the absorption of cyclosporine. Transplantation 1987;43(2):211–213.

364. Campana C, Regazzi MB, Buggia I, Molinaro M. Clinically significant drug interactions with cyclosporin. An update. Clin Pharmacokinet 1996;30(2):141–179.

365. Herzig K, Johnson DW. Marked elevation of blood cyclosporin and tacrolimus levels due to concurrent metronidazole therapy. Nephrol Dial Transplant 1999;14(2):521–523.

366. Couet W, Istin B, Seniuta P, Morel D, Potaux L, Fourtillan JB. Effect of ponsinomycin on cyclosporin pharmacokinetics. Eur J Clin Pharmacol 1990;39(2):165–167.

367. Rosche J, Froscher W, Abendroth D, Liebel J. Possible oxcarbazepine interaction with cyclosporine serum levels: a single case study. Clin Neuropharmacol 2001;24(2):113–116.

368. Crosby E, Robblee JA. Cyclosporine–pancuronium interaction in a patient with a renal allograft. Can J Anaesth 1988;35(3 Pt 1):300–302.

369. Baciewicz AM, Self TH. Rifampin drug interactions. Arch Intern Med 1984;144(8):1667–1671.

370. Affrime MB, Lowenthal DT, Rufo M. Failure of rifampin to induce the metabolism of clonidine in normal volunteers. Drug Intell Clin Pharm 1981;15(12):964–966.

371. Johnson RW. Sirolimus (Rapamune) in renal transplantation. Curr Opin Nephrol Hypertens 2002;11(6):603–607.

372. Zimmerman JJ, Harper D, Getsy J, Jusko WJ. Pharmacokinetic interactions between sirolimus and microemulsion cyclosporine when orally administered jointly and 4 hours apart in healthy volunteers. J Clin Pharmacol 2003;43(10):1168–1176.

373. Bottiger Y, Sawe J, Brattstrom C, Tollemar J, Burke JT, Hass G, Zimmerman JJ. Pharmacokinetic interaction between single oral doses of diltiazem and sirolimus in healthy volunteers. Clin Pharmacol Ther 2001;69(1):32–40.

374. Liddle C, Goodwin BJ, George J, Tapner M, Farrell GC. Separate and interactive regulation of cytochrome P450 3A4 by triiodothyronine, dexamethasone, and growth hormone in cultured hepatocytes. J Clin Endocrinol Metab 1998;83(7):2411–2416.

375. Sanchez CP, Salem M, Ettenger RB. Changes in cyclosporine A levels in pediatric renal allograft recipients receiving recombinant human growth hormone therapy. Transplant Proc 2000;32(8):2807–2810.

376. Tiller DJ, Hall BM, Horvarth JS, Duggin GG, Thompson JF, Sheil AG. Gout and hyperuricaemia in patients on cyclosporin and diuretics. Lancet 1985;1(8426):453.

377. Crosby E, Robblee JA. Cyclosporine–pancuronium interaction in a patient with a renal allograft. Can J Anaesth 1988;35(3 Pt 1):300–302.

378. Wood GG. Cyclosporine-vecuronium interaction. Can J Anaesth 1989;36(3 Pt 1):358.

379. Gramstad L, Gjerlow JA, Hysing ES, Rugstad HE. Interaction of cyclosporin and its solvent, Cremophor, with atracurium and vecuronium. Studies in the cat. Br J Anaesth 1986;58(10):1149–1155.

Everolimus

General Information

Everolimus is an immunosuppressive macrolide that also has synergistic actions with ciclosporin and interrupts the proliferative responses of vascular and bronchial smooth muscle cells. In a phase I trial, its safety profile and pharmacokinetics were assessed during a 4-week course of once-daily sequential ascending doses (0.75, 2.5, or 7.5 mg/day) in renal transplant recipients on a stable regimen of ciclosporin and prednisone (1). Pharmacokinetic data showed dose proportionality, a good correlation between trough and AUC concentrations, and moderate accumulation (2.5-fold). Absorption was within 2 hours, and the half-life was 16–19 hours. There was no evidence of a pharmacokinetic interaction of ciclosporin with everolimus. Virtually every patient in this study had at least one adverse event and 43% of patients treated with everolimus 7.5 mg/day had serious adverse events. In all everolimus groups there was an increased incidence of infectious episodes (*Herpes simplex*, upper respiratory infections, pharyngitis, pneumonia, and sinusitis). Similarly, adverse events involving the gastrointestinal system (diarrhea, nausea, and vomiting) were more common. Serum concentrations of triglycerides and total cholesterol increased significantly over time. Individuals treated with everolimus 7.5 mg/day had significant falls in white cell count (−2.6%) and platelet count (−51%); the nadir occurred on day 19 and the cell counts recovered spontaneously without withdrawal of the drug. Serum creatinine concentrations and blood pressure did not change.

Drug–Drug Interactions

Ciclosporin

Both everolimus and ciclosporin are extensively biotransformed by CYP3A and are substrates for P-glycoprotein. However, in a multicenter randomized double-blind study in 101 patients, 1 year after kidney transplantation, who were randomly assigned to receive everolimus 0.5, 1, and 2 mg bd plus ciclosporin and prednisone, the pharmacokinetics of ciclosporin were similar to published values in patients not taking everolimus (2).

References

1. Kahan BD, Wong RL, Carter C, Katz SH, Von Fellenberg J, Van Buren CT, Appel-Dingemanse S. A phase I study of a 4-week course of SDZ-RAD (RAD) quiescent cyclosporine–prednisone-treated renal transplant recipients. Transplantation 1999;68(8):1100–6.
2. Kovarik JM, Kahan BD, Kaplan B, Lorber M, Winkler M, Rouilly M, Gerbeau C, Cambon N, Boger R, Rordorf CEverolimus Phase 2 Study Group. Longitudinal assessment of everolimus in de novo renal transplant recipients over the first post-transplant year: pharmacokinetics, exposure-response relationships, and influence on cyclosporine. Clin Pharmacol Ther 2001;69(1):48–56.

Gusperimus

General Information

Gusperimus is a guanidine derivative with antitumor and immunosuppressive properties. Its mechanism of action is not well understood and may involve blockade of the maturation of B and T lymphocytes and monocytes, with inhibition of both cell-mediated and antibody-mediated immunity. In preliminary clinical trials in transplant patients, adverse effects at low doses included mild-to-moderate leukopenia, facial and perioral numbness, anorexia, gastrointestinal disturbances, facial flushing, and weakness (1–3). Bone marrow suppression has been observed at high doses.

References

1. Philip AT, Gerson B. Toxicology and adverse effects of drugs used for immunosuppression in organ transplantation. Clin Lab Med 1998;18(4):755–65.
2. First MR. An update on new immunosuppressive drugs undergoing preclinical and clinical trials: potential applications in organ transplantation. Am J Kidney Dis 1997;29(2):303–17.
3. Birck R, Warnatz K, Lorenz HM, Choi M, Haubitz M, Grunke M, Peter HH, Kalden JR, Gobel U, Drexler JM, Hotta O, Nowack R, Van Der Woude FJ. 15-Deoxyspergualin in patients with refractory ANCA-associated systemic vasculitis: a six-month open-label trial to evaluate safety and efficacy. J Am Soc Nephrol 2003;14(2):440–7.

Leflunomide

General Information

The prodrug leflunomide (*N*-(4′-trifluoromethylphenyl)-5-methylisoxazole-4-carboxamide) is an isoxazole derivative. Its main metabolite is the active compound, A77 1726 (1).

Mechanism of action

A77 1726 inhibits dihydro-rate dehydrogenase, the rate-limiting enzyme in pyrimidine synthesis. It inhibits the proliferation of T and B cells, and probably acts via the production and action of interleukin-2. Besides its immunomodulatory action, A77 1726 also has an anti-inflammatory action by inhibition of nuclear factor kappa B (NFκB), tumor necrosis factor alfa (TNF-α), and interleukin 1 beta (IL-1β), and increased production of transforming growth factor beta-1 (TGF-β1) (2–5).

Pharmacokinetics

After oral administration, leflunomide undergoes rapid metabolism in the gut wall, plasma, and liver to A77 1726 (M1), peak plasma concentrations of which are reached after 6–12 hours. A77 1726 is highly (99%) bound to plasma proteins. Its pharmacokinetics are not affected by food, and dosage requirements are not influenced by age or sex. Enterohepatic recirculation and biliary recycling contribute to the long half-life of 2 weeks. About 90% of a single dose of leflunomide is eliminated, 43% in the urine, primarily as leflunomide glucuronides and an oxalinic acid derivative of A77 1726, and 48% in the feces, primarily as A77 1726. Impaired renal function can result in increased plasma concentrations of A77 1726. Elimination of A77 1726 can be dramatically increased by using colestyramine or activated charcoal (6,7).

Indications and clinical efficacy

Leflunomide has anti-inflammatory, immunosuppressive, and virustatic effects. Its efficacy has been demonstrated in patients with rheumatoid arthritis and psoriatic arthritis and other conditions in randomized, double-blind, placebo-controlled trials and other studies (8–32), and it was approved for treatment of adult rheumatoid arthritis in August 1998 (Table 1) (33). In three large phase III trials (US301, *n* = 482; MN301, *n* = 358; MN302, *n* = 999), leflunomide was as effective and well tolerated as methotrexate and sulfasalazine and superior to placebo (34). These data were confirmed by a meta-analysis (35,36). Leflunomide is therefore indicated for patients with rheumatoid arthritis who have failed first-line disease modifying anti-rheumatic drug therapy on the basis of efficacy, safety, and costs (36). It is effective as monotherapy and in combination with methotrexate or infliximab (6).

Clinical experience with leflunomide in patients with other autoimmune diseases is limited. Extended indications for the use of leflunomide include treatment of Crohn's disease in patients who are intolerant of standard

Table 1 Summary of the efficacy of leflunomide in controlled trials

Disease	Type of study; duration	Intervention	Outcome	References
Rheumatoid arthritis	Double-blind, randomized, controlled trial; 24 weeks	Leflunomide 50–100 mg/day for 1 day, then 5–25 mg/day (n = 300) versus placebo (n = 102)	Leflunomide 10 and 25 mg/day was significantly more effective than placebo	[8]
Rheumatoid arthritis	Double-blind, randomized, controlled trial; 12 months	Leflunomide 100 mg/day for 3 days, thereafter 20 mg/day (n = 182) versus methotrexate 7.5–15 mg/week (n = 180) versus placebo (n = 118)	American College of Rheumatology response and success rates were: leflunomide 52% and 41%, methotrexate 46% and 35%, and placebo 26% and 19%	[9]
Rheumatoid arthritis	Double-blind, randomized, controlled trial; 24 weeks	Leflunomide 100 mg/day for 3 days, then 20 mg/day (n = 133) versus sulfasalazine 2 g/day (n = 133) versus placebo (n = 92)	American College of Rheumatology 20 response rates were: leflunomide 55%, sulfasalazine 56%, and placebo 29%	[10,11]
Rheumatoid arthritis	Double-blind, randomized, controlled trial; 52 weeks	Leflunomide 100 mg/day for 3 days, then 20 mg/day (n = 501) versus methotrexate 7.5–15 mg/day (n = 498)	Both drugs effective, although methotrexate resulted in significantly greater improvement in tender and swollen joint counts compared with leflunomide	[12]
Rheumatoid arthritis	Double-blind, randomized, controlled trial; 6 months	Leflunomide 100 mg/day for 3 days, then 20 mg/day (n = 133) versus sulfasalazine 0.5–2 g/day (n = 133), versus placebo (n = 92)	Leflunomide slowed disease progression as early as 6 months, and there was continued retardation of radiographic progression at 2 years	[13]
Rheumatoid arthritis	Follow-up study; 2 years	Leflunomide (n = 98) versus methotrexate (n = 101)	American College of Rheumatology 20, 50, and 70 response rates for leflunomide versus methotrexate were 79 versus 67%, 56 versus 43%, and 26 versus 20%	[14]
Rheumatoid arthritis	Follow-up study; 2 years	Leflunomide 20 mg/day versus sulfasalazine 2 g/day	American College of Rheumatology 20 response rates were 82% leflunomide versus 60% sulfasalazine after 24 months	[15]
Rheumatoid arthritis	Follow-up study; 5 years	Leflunomide 10–20 mg/day (phase III) continued (n = 214)	American College of Rheumatology 20, 50, and 70 response rates after 1 year were maintained for up to 5 years	[16]
Rheumatoid arthritis	Single-center experience; 32 weeks	Leflunomide 100 mg/day for 3 days, then 20 mg/day plus infliximab 3 mg/kg at 2, 4, 8, 16, and 24 weeks (n = 20)	11/20 withdrawn (four infliximab infusion reactions, one Stevens–Johnson syndrome); the other patients achieved American College of Rheumatology 20 and 70 response rates in >80% and 46%	[17]

Disease	Study design	Treatment	Results	Ref.
Rheumatoid arthritis	Double-blind randomized controlled trial; 24 weeks	Leflunomide 100 mg/day for 2 days, then 10 mg/day (n = 130) versus placebo (n = 133), both with methotrexate 10–25 mg/day	American College of Rheumatology 20 rates at 24 weeks: leflunomide + methotrexate 46% versus placebo + methotrexate 20%; similar drug withdrawal and adverse events rates	(18)
Rheumatoid arthritis	Multicenter experience; 24 weeks	Leflunomide 100 mg/day for 3 days, then 20 mg/day (n = 969)	191 withdrawn (107 adverse events, 26 lack of efficacy, 58 other reasons); 24% good and 45% moderate responses on the disease activity score, and 61%, 34%, and 9.6% achieved American College of Rheumatology 20, 50, and 70 response rates	(19)
Rheumatoid arthritis	Single-center experience; 3 months	Leflunomide 100 mg/day for 3 days, then 20 mg/day plus infliximab 3 mg/kg at 0, 6, and every 8 weeks (n = 17)	20 adverse effects in 13 patients; 8 discontinued	(20)
Rheumatoid arthritis	Single-center experience; 24 weeks,	Leflunomide 100 mg/day for 3 days, then 100 mg/week (n = 50)	American College of Rheumatology 20, 50, and 70 response rates at 24 weeks were 74%, 64%, and 28% (five withdrawn, six lost to follow-up)	(21)
Rheumatoid arthritis	Single-center experience; 6 months	Leflunomide 100 mg/day for 3 days, then 20 mg/day (n = 378)	American College of Rheumatology 20, 50, and 70 response rates at 6 months were 48%, 25%, and 12%	(22)
Rheumatoid arthritis	Extension of double-blind, randomized, controlled trial; 48 weeks	Leflunomide + methotrexate continued (n = 96) and placebo + methotrexate switched to leflunomide 10 mg/day + methotrexate (n = 96)	American College of Rheumatology 20 response rate was 59% at 24 weeks and 55% at 48 weeks in patients maintained on leflunomide + methotrexate, and patients switched from placebo to leflunomide + methotrexate increased their American College of Rheumatology 20 response rates from 25% at 24 weeks to 57% at 48 weeks	(23)
Rheumatoid arthritis	Double-blind, randomized, controlled trial; 24 weeks	Leflunomide 10 mg/day and 100 mg on day 3 (n = 202) versus 20 mg/day and 100 mg on days 1–3 (n = 200)	American College of Rheumatology (20 response rates: leflunomide 10 mg 50% and 20 mg 57%; adverse events: leflunomide 10 mg 15% and 20 mg 12%	(24)
Rheumatoid arthritis	Multicenter experience; 11–911 days	Leflunomide 100 mg/day for 3 days, then 20 mg/day (n = 136)	76% clinical response after 12 months, but 76/136 (56%) leflunomide withdrawn (29% adverse drug reactions and 13% lack of efficacy)	(25)

(Continued)

Table 1 (Continued)

Disease	Type of study; duration	Intervention	Outcome	References
Psoriatic arthropathy, psoriasis	Double-blind, randomized, controlled trial; 24 weeks	Leflunomide 100 mg/day for 3 days, then 20 mg/day (n = 95) versus placebo (n = 91)	Leflunomide 59% and placebo 30% were responders at 24 weeks according to the psoriatic arthritis response criteria	(26)
Psoriasis	Phase II study; 12 weeks	Leflunomide 20 mg/day (n = 8)	6/8 clinical effectiveness (psoriasis area and severity index score 20 at baseline versus 13 at 12 weeks)	(27)
Liver and kidney transplant recipients	Single-center experience	Leflunomide dosage adjusted to a trough concentration of 100 µg/ml (n = 53)	Immunosuppressive potency in liver and kidney transplant recipients, allowing dosage reduction of calcineurin inhibitors and glucocorticoids, but anemia might be dose-limiting after kidney transplantation	(28)
Systemic lupus erythematosus	Single-center experience, double-blind, randomized, controlled trial; 24 weeks	Leflunomide 100 mg/day for 3 days, then 100 mg/day (n = 6) versus placebo (n = 6)	Disease activity fell significantly in both groups after 6 months, and the reduction in SLE disease activity index from baseline to 24 weeks was significantly greater with leflunomide than with placebo	(29)
Wegener's granulomatosis	Phase II study; 52 weeks	Leflunomide 20–40 mg/day (n = 20)	Maintenance of complete or partial remission after cyclophosphamide + glucocorticoid therapy resulted in one major and eight minor relapses	(30)
Crohn's disease	Single-center experience; 3 years	Leflunomide 20 mg/day (n = 12)	8/12 clinical responses; seven continued maintenance therapy and one relapsed after follow-up of 6–78 weeks	(31)
Chronic sarcoidosis	Single-center experience; 1 year	Leflunomide 100 mg/day for 3 days, then 10–20 mg/day (n = 32; 17 leflunomide and 15 leflunomide + methotrexate)	Complete or partial responses in 13/17 leflunomide and in 12/15 21leflunomide + methotrexate	(32)

immunomodulator therapy (31), chronic sarcoidosis (32), maintenance therapy of complete or partial remission in Wegener's granulomatosis (30), and mild to moderate systemic lupus erythematosus (29) (Table 1).

Leflunomide has been used as an immunosuppressive agent in kidney and liver transplant recipients to spare calcineurin inhibitors and glucocorticoids and to slow progression of chronic kidney graft dysfunction (28,37) (Table 1).

In animals, leflunomide had excellent antiviral activity against cytomegalovirus (CMV). It is currently indicated as second-line therapy for CMV disease after solid organ transplantation and in recipients intolerant of ganciclovir (38). Leflunomide also reduces HIV replication by about 75% at concentrations that can be obtained with conventional dosing (39).

General adverse drug reactions

The safety profile of leflunomide has been said to be excellent, with no myelosuppressive or nephrotoxic adverse effects (40,41). Its major adverse effects are gastrointestinal symptoms (diarrhea and nausea), abnormal liver function tests, skin rashes and pruritus, allergic reactions, alopecia, infections, weight loss, and hypertension (35,42–45). Minor adverse effects are musculoskeletal disorders. Rare adverse effects include sepsis, pancytopenia, interstitial lung disease, hypertriglyceridemia, vasculitis, aseptic meningitis, reversible neuropathy, and serious skin reactions (35,46–49).

In 3325 patients who took leflunomide, the rate of drug withdrawal was 42% within 33 months after approval by the US Food and Drugs Administration, and was more likely in patients who received a loading dose. The most common causes of discontinuation were inefficacy (30%), gastrointestinal symptoms (29%), non-adherence to therapy or loss to follow-up (14%), and raised liver enzymes (5%) (50).

However, the rate of adverse effects associated with leflunomide was significantly lower than with methotrexate and other disease-modifying antirheumatic drugs (DMARDs) in an analysis of 40 594 patients with rheumatoid arthritis (8,51). The incidences of adverse events per 1000 patient-years were as follows:

- no DMARDs: 383
- methotrexate: 145
- leflunomide monotherapy: 94
- methotrexate + other DMARDs: 70
- leflunomide + other DMARDs: 59
- leflunomide + methotrexate: 43
- other DMARDs: 143.

Leflunomide monotherapy also had the lowest rate of hepatic events in the DMARD monotherapy groups.

Further developments

Synthetic malononitrilamides (MNA) have been derived from A77 1726. FK778 is the most promising derivative, because of its much shorter half-life. It also blocks replication of herpesvirus in vitro and in vivo. It has therefore been used as part of an immunosuppressive regimen and as an antiviral agent after solid organ transplantation (52).

FK778 is under investigation in a phase II trial after kidney transplantation (53).

Organs and Systems

Cardiovascular

The incidence of hypertension in patients with rheumatoid arthritis taking leflunomide 25 mg/day was 11% in a phase II trial (54). During phase III trials, there was new-onset hypertension in 2.1–3.7% (9,10). Increased sympathetic drive has been implicated in its pathogenesis, because leflunomide-induced hypertension is accompanied by an increased heart rate (55). However, this hypothesis remains to be tested.

Pulmonary hypertension has been described in association with leflunomide (56).

Respiratory

Respiratory symptoms in the MN301, US301, and MN302 trials in patients with rheumatoid arthritis included respiratory infections (21–27%), bronchitis (5–8%), increased cough (4–5%), rhinitis (2–5%), pharyngitis (2–3%), pneumonia (2–3%), and sinusitis (1–5%) (9,10,12).

In Japan, acute interstitial pneumonia due to leflunomide has been mentioned as a serious and severe adverse effect, with an incidence of 1.1% and a fatal outcome in 0.36% (57–59).

- A 49-year-old man with rheumatoid arthritis taking methotrexate developed a skin eruption and a severe non-productive cough after taking leflunomide for 17 days (58). He died of respiratory failure 128 days after the diagnosis of acute interstitial pneumonia.
- A 54-year-old woman with rheumatoid arthritis developed an interstitial pneumonia 2 weeks after the end of a 6-week course of treatment with leflunomide (60). The onset of the pneumonia was preceded by raised serum liver enzymes and hypertension. The acute respiratory failure improved with prednisolone and colestyramine.

However, clinical trials and subsequent observational studies outside Japan have not suggested that leflunomide causes an excess of pulmonary adverse effects (61).

Nervous system

Leflunomide can cause a peripheral reversible neuropathy (49,62–65). This neuropathy is usually axonal in nature, affecting multiple sensory or motor nerves of distal extremities. The mean time of onset of peripheral neuropathy was 6 months after the start of leflunomide therapy, with a range of 3 days to 3 years. Neurological improvement was more likely after drug withdrawal within 30 days after the onset of the symptoms of neuropathy compared with continuous administration (63).

Peripheral neuropathy attributed to leflunomide was observed in two patients (49).

- A 76-year-old man, with an 18-month history of sero-positive rheumatoid arthritis, chronic emphysema, and pulmonary fibrosis, developed polymyalgia and was treated with glucocorticoids and azathioprine. Azathioprine was withdrawn after a rise in aspartate transaminase. He was then given leflunomide 100 mg over 3 days followed by 10 mg/day as a maintenance dosage. After 2 weeks, he developed a sensory neuropathy with a stocking distribution up to the malleoli and leflunomide was withdrawn 4 weeks later. During this time he had also been taking prednisolone, tramadol, disodium etidronate, indoramin, and celecoxib, none of which is known to cause neuropathy. Glucose, vitamin B12, serum folate, thyroid function, serum proteins, Bence–Jones protein electrophoresis, cryoglobulins, anti-neutrophil cytoplasmic antibodies, antinuclear antibodies, the Venereal Disease Research Laboratory test, and hepatitis B and C serology were all normal or negative. Nerve conduction was consistent with motor sensory axonal peripheral neuropathy of the lower limbs. On review 3 months after withdrawal of leflunomide, there was clear subjective and objective improvement of the neuropathy, confirmed by repeat nerve conduction studies.
- A 69-year-old woman with a 10-year history of seropositive erosive rheumatoid arthritis, previously treated with gold salts followed by methotrexate, started to take leflunomide and 3 months later reported numbness in the fingertips and feet bilaterally, with a glove-and-stocking sensory neuropathy involving all fingertips and extending to the mid-shins. Leflunomide was withdrawn. Other medications included prednisolone, lansoprazole, simvastatin, losartan, and amiodarone, which she had been taking for a long time without adverse effects. Screening tests for neuropathy, as in the previous case, were normal or negative. There was no cord or nerve root compression on magnetic resonance imaging of the cervical spine. Nerve conduction studies confirmed a sensory motor peripheral neuropathy. She reported marked improvement in her symptoms 3 months after withdrawal of treatment, and this was confirmed on clinical examination and repeat nerve conduction studies.

One case of leflunomide-induced aseptic meningitis has been reported (48).

Metabolism

Life-threatening hypertriglyceridemia has been described during treatment with leflunomide (46).

Hematologic

Pancytopenia, thrombocytopenia, and anemia can occur during leflunomide treatment (21,66–68). The risk of pancytopenia is increased when it is used in combination with methotrexate and in elderly patients. Its course can be fatal and the time of onset ranges from 11 days to 4 years (66). Anemia has been reported in renal transplant recipients (28).

Leflunomide-associated thrombocytosis and leukocytosis resolved after colestyramine washout and withdrawal of leflunomide (69).

Mouth and teeth

In the MN301, US301, and MN302 trials, mouth ulceration occurred in 3–5% (9,10,12).

Gastrointestinal

In the MN301, US301, and MN302 trials, gastrointestinal symptoms consisted of diarrhea (22–27%), nausea (13%), dyspepsia (6–10%), abdominal pain (6–8%), mouth ulceration (3–5%), vomiting (3–5%), anorexia (3%), and gastroenteritis (1–3%) (9,10,12). Diarrhea and nausea are more common in patients who receive a loading dose, but the onset of action can be delayed without the loading dose (36). Gastrointestinal symptoms occur mainly during the first 6 months after initiation of leflunomide. The severity of symptoms was mild. If there is severe diarrhea and/or weight loss, withdrawal of leflunomide and endoscopic examination is advised, since ulcerative and microscopic colitis have been detected under such circumstances (70). The pathophysiology of leflunomide-associated diarrhea and weight loss is unclear. Weight loss of 9–24 kg was observed in five of 70 patients who took leflunomide, despite normal concentrations of thyroid-stimulating hormone and no other gastrointestinal complaints (44).

Liver

Leflunomide can cause abnormal liver function tests, but the risk of serious and non-serious hepatic adverse events is not higher than with methotrexate (71). In the MN301, US301, and MN302 trials, there were abnormal liver enzymes in 6–10% (9,10,12). The co-administration of methotrexate is a risk factor (18,72–74). According to the National Cancer Institute Common Toxicity Criteria, 8.9% of patients developed grade 2 or 3 hepatotoxicity within the first year, mainly within 6 months and in combination with methotrexate, after the start of leflunomide therapy based on liver enzyme determinations (72). The use of folate was also associated with less frequent changes in liver function tests (9,10,12). Nevertheless, leflunomide can cause severe liver injury (75–78), estimated at a rate of one in 200 users (79). Leflunomide is therefore not recommended in patients with significant liver impairment or evidence of infection with hepatitis B or C virus (80).

A CYP2C9 polymorphism has been implicated in the pathogenesis of leflunomide hepatotoxicity (77).

- A 67-year-old woman with rheumatoid arthritis developed diarrhea and raised liver enzymes after taking leflunomide for 15 days. Histologically, the liver showed acute hepatitis. She was homozygous for the CYP2C9*3 allele. The liver damage subsided within a few weeks.

Urinary tract

Interstitial nephritis occurred in one case of chronic overdose of leflunomide (81).

Skin

Adverse effects of leflunomide on the skin in patients with rheumatoid arthritis include alopecia (9–17%), rash (11–12%), pruritus (5–6%), dry skin (3%), and eczema (1–3%) (9,10,12). Single cases of an erythema multiforme-like drug eruption (82), exfoliative dermatitis (83), a lichenoid drug reaction (84), and skin ulceration (85) have been reported.

Immunologic

In the treatment of rheumatoid arthritis leflunomide can cause a vasculitis, and acute necrotizing vasculitis is rare but serious (47,86).

Long-Term Effects

Mutagenicity

A minor metabolite of leflunomide, 4-Trifluoromethyl-aniline, was mutagenic in vitro (87).

Tumorigenicity

Male mice had an increased incidence of lymphoma at an oral leflunomide dose of 15 mg/kg, and female mice had a dose-related increased incidence of bronchoalveolar adenomas and carcinomas beginning at 1.5 mg/kg (87).

Second-Generation Effects

Fertility

Leflunomide did not affect fertility in rats (87).

Teratogenicity

In oral embryocytotoxicity and teratogenicity studies in rats and rabbits, leflunomide was embryocytotoxic (growth retardation, embryolethality) and teratogenic (malformations of the head, rump, vertebral column, ribs, and limbs) (87). Not only is leflunomide teratogenic and fetotoxic in animals, but its active metabolite is detectable in plasma up to 2 years after withdrawal. Therefore, the fetus could have in utero exposure to leflunomide up to 2 years after the end of treatment. Leflunomide has been classified as pregnancy category X by the Food and Drug Administration (87,88). However, experience in a very small group of pregnant women who took leflunomide and continued their pregnancy to term gave no indication of an increase in teratogenesis (89). Nevertheless, the majority of 30 pregnant women were elected to interrupt their pregnancies, except three patients (87). At present, withdrawal of leflunomide is mandatory before pregnancy, and colestyramine treatment is advised to wash out leflunomide (80,87,90,91). Both men and women who want to have a

child should discontinue leflunomide and take colestyramine to wash it out. Leflunomide has not been studied in children, possibly because of its cytotoxic nature. In particular, its teratogenic potential may be a concern when treating adolescent girls (92).

Lactation

Breastfeeding by nursing mothers is not recommended, because it is unknown if leflunomide is excreted in human milk (80,87).

Drug Administration

Drug dosage regimens

Leflunomide is taken orally. In most regimens it is begun with a loading dose of 100 mg/day over 3 days followed by a maintenance dosage of 10–20 mg/day. Leflunomide 100 mg/week had similar effectiveness and less toxicity in open trials compared with daily dosing (21,93).

Drug–Drug Interactions

Infliximab

The administration of infliximab after or simultaneously with leflunomide seems to be safe and effective in patients with rheumatoid arthritis (20,94,95).

Rifampicin

Multiple doses of rifampicin increase leflunomide concentrations (96).

Warfarin

A case of probable interaction of leflunomide with warfarin has been reported (97).

- A 49-year-old man with resistant rheumatoid arthritis took leflunomide 100 mg/day for 3 days. His international normalized ratio (INR) had been stable for 1 year while he was taking warfarin, and 2 days before starting treatment with leflunomide it was 3.4. After he took the second dose of leflunomide, he developed gross hematuria. His INR had risen to 11, and warfarin was withdrawn. The hematuria resolved spontaneously several hours later, but his INR remained raised for the next 2 days, even though he had stopped taking warfarin. He was given intravenous vitamin K 1 mg on the third day, and 12 hours later the INR fell to 1.9. Subsequently he began taking warfarin again, but at a lower dose of 1 mg/day, which was sufficient to maintain his INR within the target range.

A77 1726 inhibits CYP2C9 and might increase the systemic availability of CYP2C9 substrates, such as warfarin and phenytoin (97,98).

Management of Adverse Drug Reactions

Usually, overdosage and adverse events can be managed by dosage reduction, the addition of colestyramine, and symptomatic therapy (36). However, in one study in patients with rheumatoid arthritis, leflunomide 10 mg/day compared with 20 mg/day was associated with less efficacy and more adverse events leading to treatment withdrawal (24). Colestyramine 3×8 g/day for 11 days is recommended to wash out leflunomide, if A77 1726 plasma concentrations do not fall to 0.02 mg/l or less, additional colestyramine is advised. Without this washout procedure, it can take up to 2 years to reach A77 1726 plasma concentrations of 0.02 mg/l. Oral activated charcoal 50 g every 6 hours for 24 hours also reduced plasma A77 1726 concentrations (80).

Plasma A77 1726 concentrations can be measured by high-performance liquid chromatography (99,100). Monitoring of platelets, white blood cells, hemoglobin, and alanine transaminase activity is advised at baseline, monthly for 6 months, and every 6–8 weeks thereafter. Leflunomide should be withdrawn if pulmonary symptoms such as cough and dyspnea start or worsen (80).

References

1. Bartlett RR, Schleyerbach R. Immunopharmacological profile of a novel isoxazol derivative, HWA 486, with potential antirheumatic activity—I. Disease modifying action on adjuvant arthritis of the rat. Int J Immunopharmacol 1985;7(1):7–18.

2. Imose M, Nagaki M, Kimura K, Takai S, Imao M, Naiki T, Osawa Y, Asano T, Hayashi H, Moriwaki H. Leflunomide protects from T-cell-mediated liver injury in mice through inhibition of nuclear factor kappaB. Hepatology 2004;40(5):1160–9.

3. Manna SK, Mukhopadhyay A, Aggarwal BB. Leflunomide suppresses TNF-induced cellular responses: effects on NF-kappa B, activator protein-1, c-Jun N-terminal protein kinase, and apoptosis. J Immunol 2000;165(10):5962–9.

4. Breedveld FC, Dayer JM. Leflunomide: mode of action in the treatment of rheumatoid arthritis. Ann Rheum Dis 2000;59(11):841–9.

5. Manna SK, Aggarwal BB. Immunosuppressive leflunomide metabolite (A77 1726) blocks TNF-dependent nuclear factor-kappa B activation and gene expression. J Immunol 1999;162(4):2095–102.

6. Kremer JM. What I would like to know about leflunomide. J Rheumatol 2004;31(6):1029–31.

7. Rozman B. Clinical pharmacokinetics of leflunomide. Clin Pharmacokinet 2002;41(6):421–30.

8. Mladenovic V, Domljan Z, Rozman B, Jajic I, Mihajlovic D, Dordevic J, Popovic M, Dimitrijevic M, Zivkovic M, Campion G, et al. Safety and effectiveness of leflunomide in the treatment of patients with active rheumatoid arthritis. Results of a randomized, placebo-controlled, phase II study. Arthritis Rheum 1995;38(11):1595–603.

9. Strand V, Cohen S, Schiff M, Weaver A, Fleischmann R, Cannon G, Fox R, Moreland L, Olsen N, Furst D, Caldwell J, Kaine J, Sharp J, Hurley F, Loew-Friedrich I. Treatment of active rheumatoid arthritis with leflunomide compared with placebo and methotrexate. Leflunomide Rheumatoid Arthritis Investigators Group. Arch Intern Med 1999;159(21):2542–50.

10. Smolen JS, Kalden JR, Scott DL, Rozman B, Kvien TK, Larsen A, Loew-Friedrich I, Oed C, Rosenburg REuropean Leflunomide Study Group. Efficacy and safety of leflunomide compared with placebo and sulphasalazine in active rheumatoid arthritis: a double-blind, randomised, multicentre trial. Lancet 1999;353(9149):259–66.

11. Smolen JS. Efficacy and safety of the new DMARD leflunomide: comparison to placebo and sulfasalazine in active rheumatoid arthritis. Scand J Rheumatol Suppl 1999;112:15–21.

12. Emery P, Breedveld FC, Lemmel EM, Kaltwasser JP, Dawes PT, Gomor B, Van Den Bosch F, Nordstrom D, Bjorneboe O, Dahl R, Horslev-Petersen K, Rodriguez De La Serna A, Molloy M, Tikly M, Oed C, Rosenburg R, Loew-Friedrich I. A comparison of the efficacy and safety of leflunomide and methotrexate for the treatment of rheumatoid arthritis. Rheumatology (Oxford) 2000;39(6):655–65.

13. Larsen A, Kvien TK, Schattenkirchner M, Rau R, Scott DL, Smolen JS, Rozman B, Westhovens R, Tikly M, Oed C, Rosenburg REuropean Leflunomide Study Group. Slowing of disease progression in rheumatoid arthritis patients during long-term treatment with leflunomide or sulfasalazine. Scand J Rheumatol 2001;30(3):135–42.

14. Cohen S, Cannon GW, Schiff M, Weaver A, Fox R, Olsen N, Furst D, Sharp J, Moreland L, Caldwell J, Kaine J, Strand V. Two-year, blinded, randomized, controlled trial of treatment of active rheumatoid arthritis with leflunomide compared with methotrexate. Utilization of Leflunomide in the Treatment of Rheumatoid Arthritis Trial Investigator Group. Arthritis Rheum 2001;44(9):1984–92.

15. Scott DL, Smolen JS, Kalden JR, van de Putte LB, Larsen A, Kvien TK, Schattenkirchner M, Nash P, Oed C, Loew-Friedrich IEuropean Leflunomide Study Group. Treatment of active rheumatoid arthritis with leflunomide: two year follow up of a double blind, placebo controlled trial versus sulfasalazine. Ann Rheum Dis 2001;60(10):913–23.

16. Kalden JR, Schattenkirchner M, Sorensen H, Emery P, Deighton C, Rozman B, Breedveld F. The efficacy and safety of leflunomide in patients with active rheumatoid arthritis: a five-year followup study. Arthritis Rheum 2003;48(6):1513–20.

17. Kiely PD, Johnson DM. Infliximab and leflunomide combination therapy in rheumatoid arthritis: an open-label study. Rheumatology (Oxford) 2002;41(6):631–7.

18. Kremer JM, Genovese MC, Cannon GW, Caldwell JR, Cush JJ, Furst DE, Luggen ME, Keystone E, Weisman MH, Bensen WM, Kaine JL, Ruderman EM, Coleman P, Curtis DL, Kopp EJ, Kantor SM, Waltuck J, Lindsley HB, Markenson JA, Strand V, Crawford B, Fernando I, Simpson K, Bathon JM. Concomitant leflunomide therapy in patients with active rheumatoid arthritis despite stable doses of methotrexate. A randomized, double-blind, placebo-controlled trial. Ann Intern Med 2002;137(9):726–33.

19. Dougados M, Emery P, Lemmel EM, de la Serna R, Zerbini CA, Brin S, van Riel P. Efficacy and safety of leflunomide and predisposing factors for treatment response in patients with active rheumatoid arthritis: RELIEF 6-month data. J Rheumatol 2003;30(12):2572–9.

20. Godinho F, Godfrin B, El Mahou S, Navaux F, Zabraniecki L, Cantagrel A. Safety of leflunomide plus infliximab combination therapy in rheumatoid arthritis. Clin Exp Rheumatol 2004;22(3):328–30.

21. Jaimes-Hernandez J, Robles-San Roman M, Suarez-Otero R, Davalos-Zugasti ME, Arroyo-Borrego S. Rheumatoid arthritis treatment with weekly leflunomide: an open-label study. J Rheumatol 2004;31(2):235–7.

22. Nyugen M, Kabir M, Ravaud P. Short-term efficacy and safety of leflunomide in the treatment of active rheumatoid arthritis in everyday clinical use. Clin Drug Invest 2004;24(2):103–12.

23. Kremer J, Genovese M, Cannon GW, Caldwell J, Cush J, Furst DE, Luggen M, Keystone E, Bathon J, Kavanaugh A, Ruderman E, Coleman P, Curtis D, Kopp E, Kantor S, Weisman M, Waltuck J, Lindsley HB, Markenson J, Crawford B, Fernando I, Simpson K, Strand V. Combination leflunomide and methotrexate (MTX) therapy for patients with active rheumatoid arthritis failing MTX monotherapy: open-label extension of a randomized, double-blind, placebo controlled trial. J Rheumatol 2004;31(8):1521–31.

24. Poor G, Strand V; Leflunomide Multinational Study Group. Efficacy and safety of leflunomide 10 mg versus 20 mg once daily in patients with active rheumatoid arthritis: multinational double-blind, randomized trial Rheumatology (Oxford) 2004;43(6):744–9.

25. Van Roon EN, Jansen TL, Mourad L, Houtman PM, Bruyn GA, Griep EN, Wilffert B, Tobi H, Brouwers JR. Leflunomide in active rheumatoid arthritis: a prospective study in daily practice. Br J Clin Pharmacol 2004;58(2):201–8.

26. Kaltwasser JP, Nash P, Gladman D, Rosen CF, Behrens F, Jones P, Wollenhaupt J, Falk FG, Mease PTreatment of Psoriatic Arthritis Study Group. Efficacy and safety of leflunomide in the treatment of psoriatic arthritis and psoriasis: a multinational, double-blind, randomized, placebo-controlled clinical trial. Arthritis Rheum 2004;50(6):1939–50.

27. Tlacuilo-Parra JA, Guevara-Gutierrez E, Rodriguez-Castellanos MA, Ornelas-Aguirre JM, Barba-Gomez JF, Salazar-Paramo M. Leflunomide in the treatment of psoriasis: results of a phase II open trial. Br J Dermatol 2004;150(5):970–6.

28. Williams JW, Mital D, Chong A, Kottayil A, Millis M, Longstreth J, Huang W, Brady L, Jensik S. Experiences with leflunomide in solid organ transplantation. Transplantation 2002;73(3):358–66.

29. Tam LS, Li EK, Wong CK, Lam CW, Szeto CC. Double-blind, randomized, placebo-controlled pilot study of leflunomide in systemic lupus erythematosus. Lupus 2004;13(8):601–4.

30. Metzler C, Fink C, Lamprecht P, Gross WL, Reinhold-Keller E. Maintenance of remission with leflunomide in Wegener's granulomatosis. Rheumatology (Oxford) 2004;43(3):315–20.

31. Prajapati DN, Knox JF, Emmons J, Saeian K, Csuka ME, Binion DG. Leflunomide treatment of Crohn's disease patients intolerant to standard immunomodulator therapy. J Clin Gastroenterol 2003;37(2):125–8.

32. Baughman RP, Lower EE. Leflunomide for chronic sarcoidosis. Sarcoidosis Vasc Diffuse Lung Dis 2004;21(1):43–8.

33. Kaltwasser JP, Behrens F. Leflunomide: long-term clinical experience and new uses. Expert Opin Pharmacother 2005;6(5):787–801.

34. Li EK, Tam LS, Tomlinson B. Leflunomide in the treatment of rheumatoid arthritis. Clin Ther 2004;26(4):447–59.

35. Osiri M, Shea B, Robinson V, Suarez-Almazor M, Strand V, Tugwell P, Wells G. Leflunomide for the treatment of rheumatoid arthritis: a systematic review and metaanalysis. J Rheumatol 2003;30(6):1182–90.

36. Maddison P, Kiely P, Kirkham B, Lawson T, Moots R, Proudfoot D, Reece R, Scott D, Sword R, Taggart A, Thwaites C, Williams E. Leflunomide in rheumatoid arthritis: recommendations through a process of consensus. Rheumatology (Oxford) 2005;44(3):280–6.

37. Hardinger KL, Wang CD, Schnitzler MA, Miller BW, Jendrisak MD, Shenoy S, Lowell JA, Brennan DC. Prospective, pilot, open-label, short-term study of conversion to leflunomide reverses chronic renal allograft dysfunction. Am J Transplant 2002;2(9):867–71.

38. John GT, Manivannan J, Chandy S, Peter S, Jacob CK. Leflunomide therapy for cytomegalovirus disease in renal allograft recipients. Transplantation 2004;77(9):1460–1.

39. Schlapfer E, Fischer M, Ott P, Speck RF. Anti-HIV-1 activity of leflunomide: a comparison with mycophenolic acid and hydroxyurea. AIDS 2003;17(11):1613–20.

40. First MR. An update on new immunosuppressive drugs undergoing preclinical and clinical trials: potential applications in organ transplantation. Am J Kidney Dis 1997;29(2):303–17.

41. Shoker AS. Immunopharmacologic therapy in renal transplantation. Pharmacotherapy 1996;16(4):562–75.

42. van Riel PL, Smolen JS, Emery P, Kalden JR, Dougados M, Strand CV, Breedveld FC. Leflunomide: a manageable safety profile. J Rheumatol Suppl 2004;71:21–4.

43. Hoi A, Littlejohn GO. Aminotransferase levels during treatment of rheumatoid arthritis with leflunomide in clinical practice. Ann Rheum Dis 2003;62(4):379.

44. Coblyn JS, Shadick N, Helfgott S. Leflunomide-associated weight loss in rheumatoid arthritis. Arthritis Rheum 2001;44(5):1048–51.

45. Hewitson PJ, Debroe S, McBride A, Milne R. Leflunomide and rheumatoid arthritis: a systematic review of effectiveness, safety and cost implications. J Clin Pharm Ther 2000;25(4):295–302.

46. Laborde F, Loeuille D, Chary-Valckenaere I. Life-threatening hypertriglyceridemia during leflunomide therapy in a patient with rheumatoid arthritis. Arthritis Rheum 2004;50(10):3398.

47. Macdonald J, Zhong T, Lazarescu A, Gan BS, Harth M. Vasculitis associated with the use of leflunomide. J Rheumatol 2004;31(10):2076–8.

48. Cohen JD, Jorgensen C, Sany J. Leflunomide-induced aseptic meningitis. Joint Bone Spine 2004;71(3):243–5.

49. Carulli MT, Davies UM. Peripheral neuropathy: an unwanted effect of leflunomide? Rheumatology (Oxford) 2002;41(8):952–3.

50. Siva C, Eisen SA, Shepherd R, Cunningham F, Fang MA, Finch W, Salisbury D, Singh JA, Stern R, Zarabadi SA. Leflunomide use during the first 33 months after food and drug administration approval: experience with a national cohort of 3,325 patients. Arthritis Rheum 2003;49(6):745–51.

51. Cannon GW, Holden WL, Juhaeri J, Dai W, Scarazzini L, Stang P. Adverse events with disease modifying antirheumatic drugs (DMARD): a cohort study of leflunomide compared with other DMARD. J Rheumatol 2004;31(10):1906–11.

52. Fitzsimmons WE, First MR. FK778, a synthetic malononitrilamide. Yonsei Med J 2004;45(6):1132–5.

53. Vanrenterghem Y, van Hooff JP, Klinger M, Wlodarczyk Z, Squifflet JP, Mourad G, Neuhaus P, Jurewicz A, Rostaing L, Charpentier B, Paczek L, Kreis H, Chang R, Paul LC, Grinyo JM, Short C. The effects of FK778 in combination with tacrolimus and

steroids: a phase II multicenter study in renal transplant patients. Transplantation 2004;78(1):9–14.

54. Rozman B. Clinical experience with leflunomide in rheumatoid arthritis. Leflunomide Investigators' Group. J Rheumatol Suppl 1998;53:27–32.

55. Rozman B, Praprotnik S, Logar D, Tomsic M, Hojnik M, Kos-Golja M, Accetto R, Dolenc P. Leflunomide and hypertension. Ann Rheum Dis 2002;61(6):567–9.

56. Martinez-Taboada VM, Rodriguez-Valverde V, Gonzalez-Vilchez F, Armijo JA. Pulmonary hypertension in a patient with rheumatoid arthritis treated with leflunomide. Rheumatology (Oxford) 2004;43(11):1451–3.

57. McCurry J. Japan deaths spark concerns over arthritis drug. Lancet 2004;363(9407):461.

58. Kamata Y, Nara H, Kamimura T, Haneda K, Iwamoto M, Masuyama J, Okazaki H, Minota S. Rheumatoid arthritis complicated with acute interstitial pneumonia induced by leflunomide as an adverse reaction. Intern Med 2004;43(12):1201–4.

59. Ito S, Sumida T. Interstitial lung disease associated with leflunomide. Intern Med 2004;43(12):1103–4.

60. Takeishi M, Akiyama Y, Akiba H, Adachi D, Hirano M, Mimura T. Leflunomide induced acute interstitial pneumonia. J Rheumatol 2005;32(6):1160–3.

61. Scott DL. Interstitial lung disease and disease modifying anti-rheumatic drugs. Lancet 2004;363(9416):1239–40.

62. Bharadwaj A, Haroon N. Peripheral neuropathy in patients on leflunomide. Rheumatology (Oxford) 2004;43(7):934.

63. Bonnel RA, Graham DJ. Peripheral neuropathy in patients treated with leflunomide. Clin Pharmacol Ther 2004;75(6):580–5.

64. Kopp HG, Moerike K, Kanz L, Hartmann JT. Leflunomide and peripheral neuropathy: a potential interaction between uracil/tegafur and leflunomide. Clin Pharmacol Ther 2005;78(1):89–90.

65. Martin K, Bentaberry F, Dumoulin C, Longy-Boursier M, Lifermann F, Haramburu F, Dehais J, Schaeverbeke T, Begaud B, Moore N. Neuropathy associated with leflunomide: a case series. Ann Rheum Dis 2005;64(4):649–50.

66. Chan J, Sanders DC, Du L, Pillans PI. Leflunomide-associated pancytopenia with or without methotrexate. Ann Pharmacother 2004;38(7–8):1206–11.

67. Hill RL, Topliss DJ, Purcell PM. Pancytopenia associated with leflunomide and methotrexate. Ann Pharmacother 2003;37(1):149.

68. Auer J, Hinterreiter M, Allinger S, Kirchgatterer A, Knoflach P. Severe pancytopenia after leflunomide in rheumatoid arthritis. Acta Med Austriaca 2000;27(4):131–2.

69. Koenig AS, Abruzzo JL. Leflunomide induced fevers, thrombocytosis, and leukocytosis in a patient with relapsing polychondritis. J Rheumatol 2002;29(1):192–4.

70. Verschueren P, Vandooren AK, Westhovens R. Debilitating diarrhoea and weight loss due to colitis in two RA patients treated with leflunomide. Clin Rheumatol 2005;24(1):87–90.

71. Suissa S, Ernst P, Hudson M, Bitton A, Kezouh A. Newer disease-modifying antirheumatic drugs and the risk of serious hepatic adverse events in patients with rheumatoid arthritis. Am J Med 2004;117(2):87–92.

72. van Roon EN, Jansen TL, Houtman NM, Spoelstra P, Brouwers JR. Leflunomide for the treatment of rheumatoid arthritis in clinical practice: incidence and severity of hepatotoxicity. Drug Saf 2004;27(5):345–52.

73. Cannon GW, Kremer JM. Leflunomide. Rheum Dis Clin North Am 2004;30(2):295–309.

74. Gao JS, Wu H, Tian J. [Treatment of patients with juvenile rheumatoid arthritis with combination of leflunomide and methotrexate.]Zhonghua Er Ke Za Zhi 2003;41(6):435–8.

75. Schiemann U, Kellner H. Gastrointestinale Nebenwirkungen der Therapie rheumatischer Erkrankungen. [Gastrointestinal side effects in the therapy of rheumatologic diseases.] Z Gastroenterol 2002;40(11):937–43.

76. Anonymous. Severe liver damage with leflunomide. Prescrire Int 2001;10(55):149.

77. Sevilla-Mantilla C, Ortega L, Agundez JA, Fernandez-Gutierrez B, Ladero JM, Diaz-Rubio M. Leflunomide-induced acute hepatitis. Dig Liver Dis 2004;36(1):82–4.

78. Thomasset SC, Ong SL, Large SR. Post-coronary artery bypass graft liver failure: a possible association with leflunomide. Ann Thorac Surg 2005;79(2):698–9.

79. Moynihan R. FDA officials argue over safety of new arthritis drug. BMJ 2003;326(7389):565.

80. Aventis Pharmaceuticals Inc. Arava Tablets (leflunomide) 10 mg, 20 mg, 100 mg Product information. 2005.

81. Haydar AA, Hujairi N, Kirkham B, Hangartner R, Goldsmith DJ. Chronic overdose of leflunomide inducing interstitial nephritis. Nephrol Dial Transplant 2004;19(5):1334–5.

82. Fischer TW, Bauer HI, Graefe T, Barta U, Elsner P. Erythema multiforme-like drug eruption with oral involvement after intake of leflunomide. Dermatology 2003;207(4):386–9.

83. Bandyopadhyay D. Exfoliative dermatitis induced by leflunomide therapy. J Dermatol 2003;30(11):845–6.

84. Canonne-Courivaud D, Carpentier O, Dejobert Y, Hachulla E, Delaporte E. Toxidermie lichenoïde au léflunomide (Arava). [Lichenoid drug reaction to leflunomide.] Ann Dermatol Venereol 2003;130(4):435–7.

85. McCoy CM. Leflunomide-associated skin ulceration. Ann Pharmacother 2002;36(6):1009–11.

86. Holm EA, Balslev E, Jemec GB. Vasculitis occurring during leflunomide therapy. Dermatology 2001;203(3):258–9.

87. Brent RL. Teratogen update: reproductive risks of leflunomide (Arava); a pyrimidine synthesis inhibitor: counseling women taking leflunomide before or during pregnancy and men taking leflunomide who are contemplating fathering a child. Teratology 2001;63(2):106–12.

88. De Santis M, Straface G, Cavaliere A, Carducci B, Caruso A. Paternal and maternal exposure to leflunomide: pregnancy and neonatal outcome. Ann Rheum Dis 2005;64(7):1096–7.

89. Brent RL. Utilization of animal studies to determine the effects and human risks of environmental toxicants (drugs, chemicals, and physical agents). Pediatrics 2004;113(Suppl 4):984–95.

90. Kaplan MJ. Leflunomide Aventis Pharma. Curr Opin Investig Drugs 2001;2(2):222–30.

91. Ostensen M. Disease specific problems related to drug therapy in pregnancy. Lupus 2004;13(9):746–50.

92. Ilowite NT. Current treatment of juvenile rheumatoid arthritis. Pediatrics 2002;109(1):109–15.

93. Jakez-Ocampo J, Richaud-Patin Y, Granados J, Sanchez-Guerrero J, Llorente L. Weekly leflunomide as monotherapy for recent-onset rheumatoid arthritis. Arthritis Rheum 2004;51(1):147–8.

94. Flendrie M, Creemers MC, Welsing PM, van Riel PL. The influence of previous and concomitant leflunomide on the efficacy and safety of infliximab therapy in patients with rheumatoid arthritis; a longitudinal observational study. Rheumatology (Oxford) 2005;44(4):472–8.

95. Hansen KE, Cush J, Singhal A, Cooley DA, Cohen S, Patel SR, Genovese M, Sundaramurthy S, Schiff M. The safety and efficacy of leflunomide in combination with infliximab in rheumatoid arthritis. Arthritis Rheum 2004;51(2):228–32.

96. Kale VP, Bichile LS. Leflunomide: a novel disease modifying anti-rheumatic drug. J Postgrad Med 2004;50(2):154–7.

97. Lim V, Pande I. Leflunomide can potentiate the anticoagulant effect of warfarin. BMJ 2002;325(7376):1333.

98. Rettie AE, Jones JP. Clinical and toxicological relevance of CYP2C9: drug-drug interactions and pharmacogenetics. Annu Rev Pharmacol Toxicol 2005;45:477–94.

99. Chan V, Charles BG, Tett SE. Rapid determination of the active leflunomide metabolite A77 1726 in human plasma by high-performance liquid chromatography. J Chromatogr B Analyt Technol Biomed Life Sci 2004;803(2):331–5.

100. Schmidt A, Schwind B, Gillich M, Brune K, Hinz B. Simultaneous determination of leflunomide and its active metabolite, A77 1726, in human plasma by high-performance liquid chromatography. Biomed Chromatogr 2003;17(4):276–81.

Mizoribine

General Information

Mizoribine is an immunosuppressive agent that inhibits de novo purine biosynthesis and affects both humoral and cell-mediated immunity. It has been used as an alternative to azathioprine in transplant patients, with a reduced incidence of leukopenia and hepatotoxicity.

Mizoribine is mostly well tolerated when it is used to treat different renal diseases, such as vasculitis, lupus nephritis, or nephritic syndrome (1–3). However, hemorrhagic enteritis and erosive changes in the intestinal mucosa have been found in dogs, and similar adverse effects have been reported in humans (4).

Organs and Systems

Endocrine

There has been a single case report of inappropriate secretion of antidiuretic hormone (SIADH) attributed to mizoribine (5).

A 74-year-old man with rheumatoid arthritis developed nausea and headache 1.5 months after starting to take mizoribine. His serum sodium concentration fell to 118 mmol/l, but his urinary sodium excretion was normal and there was no hypotension or hemoconcentration. His serum antidiuretic hormone concentration was raised at 0.59 pg/ml in spite of a reduced serum osmolality to 254 mosm/kg. He had no organic disease likely to cause SIADH. Despite infusion of hypertonic saline, his serum sodium concentration did not return to normal. Shortly after mizoribine withdrawal, his serum sodium increased from 128 to 139 mmol/l and his plasma osmolality from 265 to 287 mosm/kg.

Additional predisposing factors in this case were the patient's age and difficulty in micturition because of benign prostatic hyperplasia.

Metabolism

In a double-blind, placebo-controlled, multicenter study of mizoribine in 197 children aged 2–19 years with frequently relapsing nephrotic syndrome, transient hyperuricemia was the most common adverse event, occurring in 16% (6).

References

1. Hirayama K, Kobayashi M, Hashimoto Y, Usui J, Shimizu Y, Hirayama A, Yoh K, Yamagata K, Nagase S, Nagata M, Koyama A. Treatment with the purine synthesis inhibitor mizoribine for ANCA-associated renal vasculitis. Am J Kidney Dis 2004;44(1):57–63.

2. Tanaka H, Tsugawa K, Tsuruga K, Suzuki K, Nakahata T, Ito E, Waga S. Mizoribine for the treatment of lupus nephritis in children and adolescents. Clin Nephrol 2004;62(6):412–7.

3. Shibasaki T, Koyama A, Hishida A, Muso E, Osawa G, Yamabe H, Shiiki H, Makino H, Sato H, Ishikawa I, Maeda K, Tomita K, Arakawa M, Ishida M, Sato M, Nagase M, Kashihara N, Yorioka N, Koike T, Saito T, Harada T, Mitarai T, Sugisaki T, Nagasawa T, Tomino Y, Nojima Y, Kobayashi Y, Sakai O. A randomized open-label comparative study of conventional therapy versus mizoribine onlay therapy in patients with steroid-resistant nephrotic syndrome (postmarketing survey). Clin Exp Nephrol 2004;8(2):117–26.

4. First MR. An update on new immunosuppressive drugs undergoing preclinical and clinical trials: potential applications in organ transplantation. Am J Kidney Dis 1997;29(2):303–17.

5. Fujino Y, Inaba M, Imanishi Y, Nagata M, Goto H, Kumeda Y, Nakatani T, Ishimura E, Nishizawa Y. A case of SIADH induced by mizoribin administration. Nephron 2002;92(4):938–40.

6. Yoshioka K, Ohashi Y, Sakai T, Ito H, Yoshikawa N, Nakamura H, Tanizawa T, Wada H, Maki S. A multicenter trial of mizoribine compared with placebo in children with frequently relapsing nephrotic syndrome. Kidney Int 2000;58(1):317–24.

Mycophenolate mofetil

General Information

Mycophenolate mofetil, the morpholinoethyl ester of mycophenolic acid, is an antimetabolite that interferes with the synthesis of nucleic acids and selectively inhibits the proliferation of T and B lymphocytes. It has been used to treat psoriasis and to prevent acute renal allograft rejection in combination with ciclosporin and glucocorticoids.

Uses

In 16 renal transplant patients with suspected ciclosporin nephrotoxicity, the addition of mycophenolate allowed safe reduction in the dosage of ciclosporin, with subsequent improvement in renal function and arterial blood pressure over 6 months (1). It might allow the rapid withdrawal of glucocorticoids in patients taking ciclosporin or tacrolimus, and therefore reduce the incidence of glucocorticoid-induced post-transplant diabetes, hypercholesterolemia, and hypertension (2). There have been several reports of patients with ciclosporin-associated thrombotic microangiopathy/hemolytic-uremic syndrome in whom mycophenolate was successfully substituted (3,4).

When mycophenolate replaced ciclosporin in 17 renal transplant patients with ciclosporin nephropathy, serum creatinine concentrations fell by a mean of 26% (5). There were no cases of acute allograft rejection. Adverse effects of mycophenolate were not mentioned.

There were beneficial effects on blood pressure, lipid profile, and glomerular hemodynamics by switching from ciclosporin to mycophenolate in an open study in 17 renal transplant patients with stable renal function who took ciclosporin and prednisone in two steps (6). In step I mycophenolate was added and the dose of ciclosporin was progressively reduced to produce one-third of the original trough concentration; this took about 20 weeks. In step II, ciclosporin was gradually withdrawn over 6 weeks. During step I, two patients dropped out, one with severe diarrhea which reversed after mycophenolate withdrawal and one with biopsy-proven acute rejection, with recovery after mycophenolate withdrawal and an increase in the dose of ciclosporin. During step II there was no acute rejection. At 1 year after the end of the study, two patients had stopped taking mycophenolate, one because of recurrent upper airway infections (probably not related to mycophenolate) and one because of Kaposi's sarcoma of the leg. In the last case a possible role of mycophenolate could not be ruled out (SEDA-24, 429).

Mycophenolate has also been studied in various chronic inflammatory disorders, such as rheumatoid arthritis, pemphigus vulgaris, and psoriasis. In 70 patients with chronic active Crohn's disease, mycophenolate plus glucocorticoids produced benefit on disease activity comparable to azathioprine plus glucocorticoids (7). Two of the 35 patients randomized to mycophenolate had significant adverse effects that required drug withdrawal, namely rashes and vomiting.

General adverse effects

In three pivotal clinical trials of mycophenolate mofetil in kidney transplant recipients, adverse effects were in accordance with the known antiproliferative effect of mycophenolate, namely gastrointestinal disorders, leukopenia, and opportunistic infections, in particular cytomegalovirus tissue invasive disease (SED-13, 1130; SEDA-20, 346). Nephrotoxicity was not observed in clinical trials, and renal function significantly improved in six patients converted to mycophenolate for ciclosporin nephrotoxicity (8).

In one patient, mycophenolate mofetil was putatively involved in a constellation of symptoms that included fever, exudative pharyngitis, adynamic ileus, electrolytic abnormalities, and myocardial dysfunction, which resolved on withdrawal (SEDA-20, 346).

Organs and Systems

Respiratory

Interstitial pneumonitis with severe respiratory failure has been reported in two patients (SEDA-21, 389; SEDA-22, 418). One patient improved after mycophenolate mofetil was withdrawn, but interstitial fibrosis was found on serial lung biopsies. The other patient died from respiratory failure 3 months later. Although other drugs may have been involved in these two patients, one other reported case with recurrence of respiratory failure on each rechallenge of mycophenolate is particularly convincing.

There was a dry cough in five of 45 patients taking mycophenolate, associated with dyspnea and hypoxia in one patient and asthma exacerbation in another (9). As the symptoms reversed only after mycophenolate mofetil withdrawal, the authors suggested that dry cough and dyspnea should be considered as early symptoms of pulmonary toxicity.

Hematologic

There was a dose-related increase in the incidence of leukopenia in the three pivotal trials.

Abnormalities of neutrophil morphology have been reported with mycophenolate.

- In two transplant patients, changes in circulating neutrophils (nuclear hypolobulation and abnormal clumping of nuclear chromatin) were identified after 4–5 months of treatment with mycophenolate (10). A bone marrow aspirate in one patient showed hypocellularity, abnormal clumping of chromatin beyond the promyelocyte stage, and almost no segmented neutrophils. These morphological abnormalities preceded the appearance of peripheral neutropenia in both patients and normalized after mycophenolate withdrawal.

The authors suggested that neutrophil dysplasia had resulted from inhibition of guanosine nucleoside synthesis.

Gastrointestinal

Mycophenolate mofetil often causes gastrointestinal disorders, most commonly a dose-related diarrhea and more rarely esophagitis, gastritis, duodenal or colonic ulceration, and gastrointestinal hemorrhage (SEDA-22, 418). Diarrhea can be extremely severe for various reasons, such as inappropriate dosage in low-weight patients, renal insufficiency, drug interactions (for example with sulfinpyrazone) interfering with the renal tubular excretion of mycophenolate metabolites. That was the case in two patients who had frequent diarrhea with significant weight loss and electrolyte disturbances requiring parenteral nutrition (SEDA-21, 389).

Pooled data from the tricontinental and the US studies in kidney transplant patients showed incidences of diarrhea of 31 and 36% in patients taking 2 and 3 g/day respectively (11). In a retrospective study, 29% of 109 mycophenolate-treated patients had diarrhea that required hospitalization and 12% developed upper intestinal symptoms (gastritis, esophagitis) (12). Frequent dosage reduction was necessary and only 28% of patients were still taking full doses after 1 year.

Gastrointestinal toxicity was confirmed to be the most frequent adverse effect (53%) in 120 pancreas transplant patients who received a triple immunosuppressive regimen consisting of mycophenolate, tacrolimus, and prednisone (13). As a result, conversion from mycophenolate to azathioprine at 1 year was mostly due to gastrointestinal toxicity, which was significantly more frequent in recipients of pancreas transplantation alone (49%) compared with recipients of pancreas transplantation after previous kidney transplantation (26%) or recipients of simultaneous pancreas and kidney transplants (14%). In another study in 120 kidney transplant patients randomized to receive tacrolimus and prednisone with or without mycophenolate, there was a high rate of mycophenolate withdrawal (43%) during the first 6 months, mostly because of gastrointestinal toxicity (14). In both of these studies, the withdrawal rate was higher than in the pivotal trials in kidney transplant patients (4–10% after 6 months) (11). As both studies used a combination of tacrolimus plus mycophenolate rather than mycophenolate plus ciclosporin, a synergistic effect on the gastrointestinal tract, or more probably higher serum concentrations of mycophenolic acid due to an interaction with tacrolimus, could have contributed (SEDA-21, 390; SEDA-22, 421).

The mechanism of gastrointestinal toxicity is not well understood.

• A 42-year-old woman with a renal transplant taking triple immunosuppression (azathioprine, ciclosporin, and glucocorticoids) was converted after 7 years from azathioprine plus ciclosporin to mycophenolate (2 g/day) because of ciclosporin nephrotoxicity (15). Within 2 months she had developed severe persistent watery diarrhea (5–10 stools/day) and lost 7 kg over 2 months. Investigations ruled out an infectious cause and there were features of duodenal villous atrophy on histological examination. Diarrhea disappeared after mycophenolate withdrawal and two subsequent duodenal biopsies showed improvement 2 months later and further complete recovery 6 months later.

This report suggests that loss of normal villous structure is one of the possible mechanisms of mycophenolate-induced severe diarrhea.

Diarrhea is the most commonly reported adverse effect in patients with transplants taking mycophenolate. In 26 renal transplant recipients with persistent afebrile diarrhea (daily fecal output over 200 g), prospectively investigated for infections and morphological and functional integrity of the gastrointestinal tract, all but one had an erosive enterocolitis; 70% had malabsorption of nutrients, which contributed to the diarrhea (16). In about 60% an infectious origin was demonstrated and successfully treated with antimicrobial drugs without changing the immunosuppressive regimen. In about 40% there was no infection but a Crohn's disease-like pattern of inflamma-

tion. These patients also had less pronounced malabsorption of bile acids but a significantly faster colonic transit time, which correlated with trough concentrations of mycophenolic acid. Withdrawal of mycophenolate was associated with allograft rejection in one-third of these patients.

Ischemic colitis has also been attributed to mycophenolate (17).

• A 49-year-old woman taking ciclosporin, prednisolone, and mycophenolate developed acute refractory rejection 4 days after renal transplantation. After an unsuccessful glucocorticoid pulse, her immunosuppressive regimen was successively changed to muromonab and tacrolimus with mycophenolate maintenance. Twelve days after transplantation she had abdominal pain and watery/bloody diarrhea. Colonoscopy showed multiple ulcers with mucosal injection and colon edema. A biopsy suggested ischemic colitis and cytomegalovirus infection was ruled out. Her symptoms persisted until mycophenolate was withdrawn and further colonoscopy showed complete resolution.

Patients with inflammatory bowel disease unresponsive to azathioprine or intolerant of it may benefit from mycophenolate mofetil. Of 12 patients so treated, three had minor adverse effects (headache, nausea, arthralgia). Three with ulcerative colitis developed rectal bleeding while taking mycophenolate mofetil. Histological features of the mucosa were highly suggestive of drug-induced bleeding. Enterohepatic recycling results in high colonic concentrations of mycophenolic acids, which may have a direct toxic effect on the epithelium (18).

Liver

In two renal transplant patients, serum bilirubin concentrations increased to 46 and 63 µmol/l within 3–7 days of mycophenolate treatment, and further increased to 98 µmol/l in one patient after the dose was increased (19). The bilirubin concentration returned to normal or pretreatment values after withdrawal or dosage reduction. Although both patients also received ciclosporin, which has been associated with hyperbilirubinemia, the temporal relation and a possible dose-dependent effect favored a causative role of mycophenolate.

Skin

Mycophenolate-induced eczema has been reported (20).

• A 45-year-old woman with a liver transplant began to take mycophenolate mofetil (2 g/day) before planned ciclosporin withdrawal. After 3 days she developed pruritus and a bullous eruption on her hands and feet. The lesions improved after mycophenolate was withdrawn, but soon reappeared after readministration of a lower dose (500 mg/day). A skin biopsy showed dyshidrotic eczema and a skin test with mycophenolate mofetil produced recurrence.

Hair

Alopecia has been noted in two patients converted from ciclosporin to mycophenolate (SEDA-22, 418).

- Onycholysis with blisters and loose toenails has been observed in a 45-year-old man who took tacrolimus, prednisone, and mycophenolate for 3 weeks after renal transplantation (21). The lesions improved after withdrawal and recurred after two subsequent re-exposures.

Immunologic

Transplant rejection

In a randomized study, 14 patients with liver transplants were given calcineurin inhibitors and 14 were given mycophenolate mofetil monotherapy (22). Those who were given mycophenolate had reversible episodes of acute graft rejection and there were no such episodes in those who were given calcineurin inhibitors.

In 11 patients with orthotopic liver transplants who had adverse effects from ciclosporin or tacrolimus, mycophenolate mofetil monotherapy for 1 year was successful. This was followed by a randomized, controlled trial in 18 patients, of whom nine were given mycophenolate mofetil (23). Five patients completed the 3 month trial. Of these, two had an episode of acute rejection, one after 2 months and one after 3 months, which did not respond to the reintroduction of tacrolimus and intravenous glucocorticoids. One had a glucocorticoid-responsive episode of severe acute rejection after 3 weeks. The other two patients had normal liver function tests after 2 weeks and 2 months respectively, when the trial was stopped. Mycophenolate mofetil allows a reduction of the dose of calcineurin inhibitor, with a low risk of rejection and improvement in renal function. However, it is associated with an unacceptable risk of acute rejection.

Infection risk

The role of mycophenolate in the occurrence of opportunistic infections is debated. In a retrospective comparison of 358 simultaneous pancreas plus kidney transplant patients who received a ciclosporin-based immunosuppressive regimen, the rate of opportunistic infections was similar in patients treated with mycophenolate ($n = 109$) and azathioprine ($n = 249$) (12). However, very few patients taking mycophenolate were available for long-term comparison. In contrast, another retrospective comparison of 135 renal transplant patients (69 for prophylactic treatment and 66 for rescue therapy) showed that the combination of mycophenolate, tacrolimus, and prednisone ($n = 49$) produced fewer rejection episodes, but a significantly higher incidence of infectious episodes than the combination of mycophenolate, ciclosporin, and prednisone (24). In another randomized trial of 120 renal transplant patients, there was a significantly higher rate of asymptomatic or symptomatic cytomegalovirus infection in patients who took mycophenolate, tacrolimus, and prednisone than in patients who took tacrolimus plus prednisone (20 versus 5%) (14). Overall, both of these studies suggest that mycophenolate plus tacrolimus has a

more potent immunosuppressive effect, with an increased risk of infections (and theoretically lymphoproliferative disorders), as the counterpart of a possible greater effect on acute rejection prophylaxis.

Bacterial infections

- Staphylococcal septicemia complicated by endocarditis has been reported in a 50-year-old woman after 5 months of treatment with mycophenolate for atopic dermatitis (25).

As the skin of most patients with atopic dermatitis can be colonized with *Staphylococcus aureus*, the authors suggested caution in using mycophenolate, which can also cause leukopenia. This patient had previously taken ciclosporin and azathioprine, which were ineffective, but without apparent infectious complications. A specific role of mycophenolate is therefore debatable and the occurrence of bacterial septicemia may have been purely coincidental.

Mycobacterium hemophilum is a pathogen that is found in immunosuppressed patients, such as those with malignancy, AIDS, and organ transplants. Systemic lupus erythematosus can make patients more susceptible to infection.

- A 25-year-old Chinese woman with systemic lupus erythematosus had a disease course characterized by multiple flares involving the kidneys, central nervous system, and gastrointestinal tract (26). She was given mycophenolate mofetil and multiple courses of antibiotics, with a poor response. After about 9 months she developed a recurrent right leg cellulitis. Two initial skin biopsies yielded negative bacterial and mycobacterial cultures, but histopathology of the muscle of her right thigh showed acid-fast bacilli and culture subsequently grew *M. hemophilum*.

The authors concluded that this complication had been due to late diagnosis, multiple antibiotics, and immunocompromise. These points must be taken into consideration when treating a patient with mycophenolate mofetil.

Virus infections

Cytomegalovirus

The role of mycophenolate in the rate and severity of cytomegalovirus infection in transplant patients has been debated (SEDA-23, 407) and is difficult to evaluate in otherwise immunosuppressed patients. Whereas there was a dose-related increase in the incidence of cytomegalovirus disease in the three pivotal trials, a later analysis did not confirm that mycophenolate mofetil is specifically associated with an increased risk of cytomegalovirus infection, and suggested that over-immunosuppression rather than mycophenolate mofetil per se was the main contributing factor (SEDA-22, 418) (27–29).

- Severe cytomegalovirus pancolitis has been reported in a 59-year-old man taking only mycophenolate and prednisone for Wegener's granulomatosis (30).

In a retrospective study of 84 cytomegalovirus-seronegative renal transplant patients who received a kidney from a cytomegalovirus-seropositive donor without cytomegalovirus prophylaxis, the incidence of primary cytomegalovirus infection was similar in the 24 patients who took mycophenolate plus ciclosporin and prednisone, compared with the 60 patients who took ciclosporin and prednisone alone (31). However, the incidence of cytomegalovirus disease was nearly twice as high in the mycophenolate group (67 versus 30%), but with no difference in the severity of the disease. The authors speculated that the more frequent incidence of symptomatic cytomegalovirus disease might have been due to some specific effects of mycophenolate on the primary immune response to cytomegalovirus.

Mycophenolate mofetil has been compared with azathioprine in combination with ciclosporin and glucocorticoids in 65 children after kidney transplantation (32). The main adverse effects of this treatment were infections of the urinary tract and the upper respiratory tract, abdominal pain, and diarrhea. Opportunistic infections with cytomegalovirus or cytomegalovirus syndrome occurred in 20% within the first 6 months and tissue-invasive cytomegalovirus disease in 3.1%. These results were similar to those in adults.

Varicella

A retrospective study in 19 children with renal transplants identified three who developed disseminated varicella, despite a prior history of chickenpox in two and pretransplant varicella vaccination in one (33). The clinical disease was mild and responded promptly to oral aciclovir. Although this was based on very few patients, the incidence of 16% was thought to be unexpectedly higher than that reported in historic controls (0.7–1.9%), and might have resulted from the higher degree of immunosuppression achieved with mycophenolate mofetil.

Herpes simplex

To evaluate whether mycophenolate mofetil is effective in treating moderate to severe atopic dermatitis, an open pilot study was conducted in 10 patients (34). There were no serious adverse effects, but one patient had to discontinue treatment because he developed *Herpes simplex* retinitis, which resolved after treatment with aciclovir. Although there is no direct evidence that mycophenolate mofetil is a major cause of *Herpes* retinitis, in this patient it seems likely that it was due to immunosuppression. In contrast, in vivo and in vitro mycophenolate mofetil strongly potentiates the antiherpetic effects of aciclovir, ganciclovir, and penciclovir (35). It is probably therefore enough to give antiviral therapy only when clinical signs of *Herpes* infection occur.

Fungal infections

There have been two cases of intestinal microsporidiosis (36) and one case of *Nocardia asteroides* brain abscess (37) in adults taking mycophenolate mofetil.

Body temperature

- Isolated and intermittent drug fever with a spiking pattern has been attributed to mycophenolate in a 41-year-

old man with a renal transplant (38). The relation to treatment was confirmed by the exclusion of numerous infectious causes, the persistence of fever despite ciclosporin withdrawal, subsidence of fever after mycophenolate withdrawal, and the absence of further episodes of fever during follow-up.

Long-Term Effects

Tumorigenicity

- Kaposi's sarcoma recurred 4 months after starting mycophenolate in a 58-year-old renal transplant patient who 7 years before had had similar lesions that reversed on withdrawal of ciclosporin (39).
- Kaposi's sarcoma has been reported after a mean of 7 months of treatment in three renal transplant patients whose immunosuppressive regimen included mycophenolate mofetil (40).

The investigators of the second case found that the incidence of Kaposi's sarcoma in patients taking regimens containing mycophenolate mofetil was 0.8% (3/371 patients) compared with 0.1% in patients not taking it (2/1464). It was suggested that mycophenolate mofetil might increase the susceptibility to Kaposi's sarcoma.

Second-Generation Effects

Pregnancy

- A 33-year-old woman was given a living related donor kidney transplantation during the first trimester, followed by mycophenolate mofetil, tacrolimus, and prednisone (41). The mother did well, except for mild pre-eclampsia and mild renal insufficiency. The child was born prematurely during the 36th week. The only teratogenic effects detected were hypoplastic nails and a short fifth finger.

Susceptibility Factors

Age

The adverse effects of mycophenolate mofetil in children have been reviewed retrospectively in 24 renal transplant patients (mean age 14 years) switched from azathioprine to mycophenolate mofetil a mean of 4.8 years after transplantation (42). The mean dose of mycophenolate mofetil was 560 mg/m^2. After a mean of 9.6 months, 13 had to discontinue treatment because of adverse effects, namely severe and partially reversible anemia (10 patients, of whom three required transfusions), neutropenia ($n = 1$), and diarrhea ($n = 2$). The anemia was normocytic and normochromic in nine patients, and such a high incidence of severe anemia was unexpected from the available adult data. Although patients who discontinued treatment had a lower pretreatment-calculated creatinine clearance, this was not significant and probably not the major cause of anemia. The author speculated that the anemia resulted from a disproportionately high unbound plasma concentration of mycophenolate mofetil, due to reduced protein binding and impaired renal clearance.

Drug–Drug Interactions

Ciclosporin

In 52 patients taking mycophenolate mofetil 1 g bd, prednisone, and ciclosporin to a target blood concentration of 125–175 ng/ml for 6 months after transplantation, withdrawal of ciclosporin resulted in almost a doubling of mycophenolic acid trough concentrations (43). No clear mechanism readily explains these chains these chanhes.

Tacrolimus

Patients taking tacrolimus have higher mycophenolate mofetil plasma trough concentrations than patients taking ciclosporin (44). Compared with the combination of ciclosporin plus mycophenolate mofetil, tacrolimus plus similar doses of mycophenolate produced significantly higher serum concentrations of mycophenolic acid, resulting in a greater degree of in vitro immunosuppression (SEDA-21, 390).

References

1. Hueso M, Bover J, Seron D, Gil-Vernet S, Sabate I, Fulladosa X, Ramos R, Coll O, Alsina J, Grinyo JM. Low-dose cyclosporine and mycophenolate mofetil in renal allograft recipients with suboptimal renal function. Transplantation 1998;66(12):1727–31.
2. Stegall MD, Wachs ME, Everson G, Steinberg T, Bilir B, Shrestha R, Karrer F, Kam I. Prednisone withdrawal 14 days after liver transplantation with mycophenolate: a prospective trial of cyclosporine and tacrolimus. Transplantation 1997;64(12):1755–60.
3. Lecornu-Heuze L, Ducloux D, Rebibou JM, Martin L, Billerey C, Chalopin JM. Mycophenolate mofetil in cyclosporin-associated thrombotic microangiopathy. Nephrol Dial Transplant 1998;13(12):3212–3.
4. McGregor DO, Robson RA, Lynn KL. Haemolytic–uraemic syndrome in a renal transplant recipient treated by conversion to mycophenolate mofetil. Nephron 1998;80(3):365–6.
5. Houde I, Isenring P, Boucher D, Noel R, Lachanche JG. Mycophenolate mofetil, an alternative to cyclosporine A for long-term immunosuppression in kidney transplantation? Transplantation 2000;70(8):1251–3.
6. Schrama YC, Joles JA, van Tol A, Boer P, Koomans HA, Hene RJ. Conversion to mycophenolate mofetil in conjunction with stepwise withdrawal of cyclosporine in stable renal transplant recipients. Transplantation 2000;69(3):376–83.
7. Neurath MF, Wanitschke R, Peters M, Krummenauer F, Meyer zum Buschenfelde KH, Schlaak JF. Randomised trial of mycophenolate mofetil versus azathioprine for treatment of chronic active Crohn's disease. Gut 1999;44(5):625–8.
8. Ducloux D, Fournier V, Bresson-Vautrin C, Rebibou JM, Billerey C, Saint-Hillier Y, Chalopin JM. Mycophenolate mofetil in renal transplant recipients with cyclosporine-associated nephrotoxicity: a preliminary report. Transplantation 1998;65(11):1504–6.
9. Elli A, Aroldi A, Montagnino G, Tarantino A, Ponticelli C. Mycophenolate mofetil and cough. Transplantation 1998;66(3):409.
10. Banerjee R, Halil O, Bain BJ, Cummins D, Banner NR. Neutrophil dysplasia caused by mycophenolate mofetil. Transplantation 2000;70(11):1608–10.
11. Simmons WD, Rayhill SC, Sollinger HW. Preliminary risk-benefit assessment of mycophenolate mofetil in transplant rejection. Drug Saf 1997;17(2):75–92.
12. Odorico JS, Pirsch JD, Knechtle SJ, D'Alessandro AM, Sollinger HW. A study comparing mycophenolate mofetil to azathioprine in simultaneous pancreas–kidney transplantation. Transplantation 1998;66(12):1751–9.
13. Gruessner RW, Sutherland DE, Drangstveit MB, Wrenshall L, Humar A, Gruessner AC. Mycophenolate mofetil in pancreas transplantation. Transplantation 1998;66(3):318–23.
14. Shapiro R, Jordan ML, Scantlebury VP, Vivas C, Gritsch HA, Casavilla FA, McCauley J, Johnston JR, Randhawa P, Irish W, Hakala TR, Fung JJ, Starzl TE. A prospective, randomized trial to compare tacrolimus and prednisone with and without mycophenolate mofetil in patients undergoing renal transplantation: first report. J Urol 1998;160(6 Pt 1):1982–6.
15. Ducloux D, Ottignon Y, Semhoun-Ducloux S, Labbe S, Saint-Hillier Y, Miguet JP, Carayon P, Chalopin JM. Mycophenolate mofetil-induced villous atrophy. Transplantation 1998;66(8):1115–6.
16. Maes BD, Dalle I, Geboes K, Oellerich M, Armstrong VW, Evenepoel P, Geypens B, Kuypers D, Shipkova M, Geboes K, Vanrenterghem YF. Erosive enterocolitis in mycophenolate mofetil-treated renal-transplant recipients with persistent afebrile diarrhea. Transplantation 2003;75(5):665–72.
17. Kim HC, Park SB. Mycophenolate mofetil-induced ischemic colitis. Transplant Proc 2000;32(7):1896–7.
18. Skelly MM, Logan RF, Jenkins D, Mahida YR, Hawkey CJ. Toxicity of mycophenolate mofetil in patients with inflammatory bowel disease. Inflamm Bowel Dis 2002;8(2):93–7.
19. Chueh SC, Huang CY, Lai MK. Mycophenolate mofetil-induced hyperbilirubinemia in renal transplant recipients. Transplant Proc 2000;32(7):1901–2.
20. Semhoun-Ducloux S, Ducloux D, Miguet JP. Mycophenolate mofetil-induced dyshidrotic eczema. Ann Intern Med 2000;132(5):417.
21. Rault R. Mycophenolate-associated onycholysis. Ann Intern Med 2000;133(11):921–2.
22. Schlitt HJ, Barkmann A, Boker KH, Schmidt HH, Emmanouilidis N, Rosenau J, Bahr MJ, Tusch G, Manns MP, Nashan B, Klempnauer J. Replacement of calcineurin inhibitors with mycophenolate mofetil in liver-transplant patients with renal dysfunction: a randomised controlled study. Lancet 2001;357(9256):587–91.
23. Stewart SF, Hudson M, Talbot D, Manas D, Day CP. Mycophenolate mofetil monotherapy in liver transplantation. Lancet 2001;357(9256):609–10.
24. Daoud AJ, Schroeder TJ, Shah M, Hariharan S, Peddi VR, Weiskittel P, First MR. A comparison of the safety and efficacy of mycophenolate mofetil, prednisone and cyclosporine and mycophenolate mofetil, and prednisone and tacrolimus. Transplant Proc 1998;30(8):4079–81.
25. Satchell AC, Barnetson RS. Staphylococcal septicaemia complicating treatment of atopic dermatitis with mycophenolate. Br J Dermatol 2000;143(1):202–3.
26. Teh CL, Kong KO, Chong AP, Badsha H. *Mycobacterium haemophilum* infection in an SLE patient on mycophenolate mofetil. Lupus 2002;11(4):249–52.
27. Moreso F, Seron D, Morales JM, Cruzado JM, Gil-Vernet S, Perez JL, Fulladosa X, Andres A, Grinyo JM. Incidence of leukopenia and cytomegalovirus disease in

kidney transplants treated with mycophenolate mofetil combined with low cyclosporine and steroid doses. Clin Transplant 1998;12(3):198–205.

28. Sarmiento JM, Munn SR, Paya CV, Velosa JA, Nguyen JH. Is cytomegalovirus infection related to mycophenolate mofetil after kidney transplantation? A case-control study. Clin Transplant 1998;12(5):371–4.

29. Paterson DL, Singh N, Panebianco A, Wannstedt CF, Wagener MM, Gayowski T, Marino IR. Infectious complications occurring in liver transplant recipients receiving mycophenolate mofetil. Transplantation 1998;66(5):593–8.

30. Woywodt A, Choi M, Schneider W, Kettritz R, Gobel U. Cytomegalovirus colitis during mycophenolate mofetil therapy for Wegener's granulomatosis. Am J Nephrol 2000;20(6):468–72.

31. ter Meulen CG, Wetzels JF, Hilbrands LB. The influence of mycophenolate mofetil on the incidence and severity of primary cytomegalovirus infections and disease after renal transplantation. Nephrol Dial Transplant 2000;15(5):711–4.

32. Staskewitz A, Kirste G, Tonshoff B, Weber LT, Boswald M, Burghard R, Helmchen U, Brandis M, Zimmerhackl LB; German Pediatric Renal Transplantation Study Group. Mycophenolate mofetil in pediatric renal transplantation without induction therapy: results after 12 months of treatment. Transplantation 2001;71(5):638–44.

33. Rothwell WS, Gloor JM, Morgenstern BZ, Milliner DS. Disseminated varicella infection in pediatric renal transplant recipients treated with mycophenolate mofetil. Transplantation 1999;68(1):158–61.

34. Grundmann-Kollmann M, Podda M, Ochsendorf F, Boehncke WH, Kaufmann R, Zollner TM. Mycophenolate mofetil is effective in the treatment of atopic dermatitis. Arch Dermatol 2001;137(7):870–3.

35. Neyts J, Andrei G, De Clercq E. The novel immunosuppressive agent mycophenolate mofetil markedly potentiates the antiherpesvirus activities of acyclovir, ganciclovir, and penciclovir in vitro and in vivo. Antimicrob Agents Chemother 1998;42(2):216–22.

36. Guerard A, Rabodonirina M, Cotte L, Liguory O, Piens MA, Daoud S, Picot S, Touraine JL. Intestinal microsporidiosis occurring in two renal transplant recipients treated with mycophenolate mofetil. Transplantation 1999;68(5):699–707.

37. Magee CC, Halligan RD, Milford EL, Sayegh MH. Nocardial infection in a renal transplant recipient on tacrolimus and mycophenolate mofetil. Clin Nephrol 1999;52(1):44–6.

38. Chueh SC, Hong JC, Huang CY, Lai MK. Drug fever caused by mycophenolate mofetil in a renal transplant recipient—a case report. Transplant Proc 2000;32(7):1925–6.

39. Gomez E, Aguado S, Rodriguez M, Alvarez-Grande J. Kaposi's sarcoma after renal transplantation—disappearance after reduction of immunosuppression and reappearance 7 years later after start of mycophenolate mofetil treatment. Nephrol Dial Transplant 1998;13(12):3279–80.

40. Eberhard OK, Kliem V, Brunkhorst R. Five cases of Kaposi's sarcoma in kidney graft recipients: possible influence of the immunosuppressive therapy. Transplantation 1999;67(1):180–4.

41. Pergola PE, Kancharla A, Riley DJ. Kidney transplantation during the first trimester of pregnancy: immunosuppression with mycophenolate mofetil, tacrolimus, and prednisone. Transplantation 2001;71(7):994–7.

42. Butani L, Palmer J, Baluarte HJ, Polinsky MS. Adverse effects of mycophenolate mofetil in pediatric renal

transplant recipients with presumed chronic rejection. Transplantation 1999;68(1):83–6.

43. Gregoor PJ, de Sevaux RG, Hene RJ, Hesse CJ, Hilbrands LB, Vos P, van Gelder T, Hoitsma AJ, Weimar W. Effect of cyclosporine on mycophenolic acid trough levels in kidney transplant recipients. Transplantation 1999;68(10):1603–6.

44. Hubner GI, Eismann R, Sziegoleit W. Drug interaction between mycophenolate mofetil and tacrolimus detectable within therapeutic mycophenolic acid monitoring in renal transplant patients. Ther Drug Monit 1999;21(5):536–9.

Pimecrolimus

General Information

Pimecrolimus is a non-steroidal ascomycin derivative with topical anti-inflammatory activity. In a 1% cream it is effective and safe in atopic dermatitis in infants, children, and adults (1–3), although its efficacy has been questioned (4).

Organs and Systems

Skin

The main adverse effect of pimecrolimus is local skin irritation, with a stinging or burning sensation, which occurs in 30% of patients. Typically, children have less skin irritation than adults. Adverse effects such as local immunosuppression and an increased risk of local bacterial and viral infections (notably eczema herpeticum) are less common than with topical glucocorticoids (5). In addition, there is a lack of skin atrophy (6,7). However, topical corticosteroids have the advantage of better skin penetration than pimecrolimus and will therefore continue to be used for more heavily keratinized skin such as in psoriasis (8).

Tinea incognito has been attributed to pimecrolimus (9).

- A 6-year-old boy developed a small, erythematous, slightly scaly, pruritic plaque near his right eye, which was treated with twice-daily pimecrolimus cream. After 2–3 days, the itching and erythema completely resolved, but a rough scaly plaque persisted. After 1–2 weeks, the itching gradually returned and the lesion began to increase in size. Multiple similar lesions appeared several centimeters from the initially affected area. Pimecrolimus was withdrawn and topical nystatin + triamcinolone ointment was prescribed. The eruption continued to spread, with multiple annular scaly papules and plaques with central clearing. There was excoriation and mild inflammation around all affected areas. A potassium hydroxide examination of the lesions showed numerous hyphae. The nystatin + triamcinolone was withdrawn and oral griseofulvin was prescribed. The eruption improved dramatically after 3 weeks and eventually cleared completely after 5 weeks of treatment. Topical 2% ketoconazole cream was applied twice a day during the final 2 weeks of treatment.

References

1. Van Leent EJ, Graber M, Thurston M, Wagenaar A, Spuls PI, Bos JD. Effectiveness of the ascomycin macrolactam SDZ ASM 981 in the topical treatment of atopic dermatitis. Arch Dermatol 1998;134(7):805–9.
2. Eichenfield LF, Lucky AW, Boguniewicz M, Langley RG, Cherill R, Marshall K, Bush C, Graeber M. Safety and efficacy of pimecrolimus (ASM 981) cream 1% in the treatment of mild and moderate atopic dermatitis in children and adolescents. J Am Acad Dermatol 2002;46(4):495–504.
3. Weinberg JM. Formulary review of therapeutic alternatives for atopic dermatitis: focus on pimecrolimus. J Manag Care Pharm 2005;11(1):56–64.
4. Anonymous. Pimecrolimus: new preparation. Me-too: too many risks, not beneficial enough in atopic dermatitis. Prescrire Int 2004;13(74):209–12.
5. Lubbe J, Pournaras CC, Saurat JH. Eczema herpeticum during treatment of atopic dermatitis with 0.1% tacrolimus ointment Dermatology 2000;201(3):249–51.
6. Soter NA, Fleischer AB Jr, Webster GF, Monroe E, Lawrence I. Tacrolimus ointment for the treatment of atopic dermatitis in adult patients: part II, safety. J Am Acad Dermatol 2001;44(Suppl 1):S39–46.
7. Reitamo S, Wollenberg A, Schopf E, Perrot JL, Marks R, Ruzicka T, Christophers E, Kapp A, Lahfa M, Rubins A, Jablonska S, Rustin MThe European Tacrolimus Ointment Study Group. Safety and efficacy of 1 year of tacrolimus ointment monotherapy in adults with atopic dermatitis. Arch Dermatol 2000;136(8):999–1006.
8. Nghiem P. "Topical immunomodulators?" Introducing old friends and a new ally, tacrolimus J Am Acad Dermatol 2001;44(1):111–3.
9. Crawford KM, Bostrom P, Russ B, Boyd J. Pimecrolimus-induced tinea incognito. Skinmed 2004;3(6):352–3.

Sirolimus

General Information

Sirolimus is a macrocyclic lactone immunosuppressant that has anti-rejection activity through inhibition of T cell activation. In contrast to tacrolimus and ciclosporin, sirolimus has no effect on calcineurin activity.

Sirolimus is being investigated for the prophylaxis of renal rejection in combination with ciclosporin and glucocorticoids (1).

Comparative studies

In a 12-month study in 719 patients with renal transplants, the combination of sirolimus, ciclosporin, and prednisone in 558 patients (284 taking sirolimus 2 mg/day and 274 taking 5 mg/day) produced significantly more acne, diarrhea, dyslipidemia, headache, hirsutism, hyperkalemia, hypertension, lymphocele formation, and thrombocytopenia compared with 161 patients who took azathioprine, ciclosporin, and prednisone (2). Serum creatinine

concentrations were significantly higher at 6 and 12 months in those who took sirolimus. Most of these adverse effects were thought to represent exacerbations of ciclosporin adverse effects, except for diarrhea (8–32%), dyslipidemia (30–42%), lymphocele formation (12–15%), and thrombocytopenia (9–18%), which were more probably related to sirolimus.

That the adverse events profile of sirolimus is different from that of ciclosporin has been further suggested in 83 patients taking primary immunosuppressant regimens containing sirolimus (41 patients) or ciclosporin (42 patients) (3). Arthralgia (20%), hypercholesterolemia (44%), hypertriglyceridemia (51%), leukopenia (39%), thrombocytopenia (37%), and pneumonia (17%) were significantly more frequent in patients taking sirolimus, particularly during the first 2 months of treatment, that is until sirolimus trough concentrations were carefully monitored. Serum creatinine concentrations were lower in the sirolimus group, confirming that sirolimus probably has no direct nephrotoxic effect.

Organs and Systems

Respiratory

Progressive diffuse interstitial pneumonitis has been reported as a possible adverse effect of sirolimus (4), and by 2000 the FDA was aware of at least 34 cases (5). Although the reports were insufficient to conclude that sirolimus was responsible in most cases, eight patients recovered after sirolimus withdrawal.

Bronchiolitis obliterans with organizing pneumonia has been attributed to sirolimus in two renal transplant patients (6). Both improved rapidly after sirolimus withdrawal or dosage reduction.

Metabolism

The most striking consequence of treatment with sirolimus is dose-dependent hyperlipidemia with significant increases in both cholesterol and triglyceride serum concentrations, which resolve after dosage reduction or sirolimus withdrawal (7).

In a 1-year follow-up of 40 renal transplant patients treated with various dosages of sirolimus ($0.5–7$ mg/m^2/day) in addition to a ciclosporin-based regimen, there were significant increases in serum cholesterol and triglycerides, and significant falls in white blood cell and platelet counts, compared with historical controls (1). These effects correlated with sirolimus trough concentrations but not dosages. One patient had to discontinue sirolimus because of hyperlipidemia refractory to treatment.

In six patients with renal transplants treated with sirolimus, mean total plasma cholesterol, triglyceride, and apolipoprotein concentrations increased (8). The authors suggested that sirolimus increases lipase activity in adipose tissue and reduces lipoprotein lipase activity, resulting in increased hepatic synthesis of triglycerides, increased secretion of VLDL, and increased hypertriglyceridemia.

Hematologic

Thrombocytopenia, probably related to sirolimus, as well as significant reversible reductions in platelet and white blood cell counts have been found (SEDA-20, 346).

In 119 patients taking sirolimus, thrombocytopenia (defined as a platelet count below $150 \times 10^9/l$) and leukopenia (white blood cell count below $5.0 \times 10^9/l$) occurred in 78 and 63% respectively (9). The incidence, but not the severity, of these effects correlated with sirolimus whole-blood trough concentrations. Most cases occurred within the first 4 weeks of treatment and the severity was usually limited. There was spontaneous resolution in 89% of the patients and sirolimus dosage reduction or temporary withdrawal was necessary in only 7% and 4% of the patients respectively. None of the patients required permanent withdrawal.

Immunologic

Two reports have recently suggested that sirolimus can produce features of the capillary leak syndrome in patients with psoriasis (10).

- A 53-year-old woman with severe psoriasis for 3 years, who had previously taken ciclosporin, sulfasalazine, and topical glucocorticoids, was given sirolimus 8 mg/m²/day, and 3 days later had fever, leg edema, dyspnea, weight gain, anemia, and hypotension. A chest X-ray showed pulmonary congestion and cardiomegaly. Empirical antibiotics were unsuccessful, and all symptoms progressively disappeared after sirolimus withdrawal.
- A 58-year-old man took sirolimus 8 mg/m²/day for severe psoriasis with arthritis. He also took ibuprofen, co-trimoxazole, and paracetamol. Within 1 month he developed nocturnal fever, dizziness, orthostatic hypotension, leg edema, and anemia. All his symptoms subsided after sirolimus withdrawal, furosemide treatment, and erythrocyte transfusion.

No other causes were found, and the authors noted that of 34 psoriatic patients given sirolimus, three had leg edema and a reduced hematocrit. Based on limited in vitro findings, they suggested that sirolimus might enhance apoptosis of activated lymphocytes and thereby cytokine release.

Drug–Drug Interactions

Adenosine and adenosine triphosphate (ATP)

In two kidney transplant recipients taking sirolimus (FK506), plasma adenosine concentrations were significantly increased (14). The relevance of these results to the use of therapeutic intravenous adenosine in patients already taking sirolimus is not clear.

Ciclosporin

Combination of sirolimus with ciclosporin virtually eliminates acute rejection. However, the adverse effects of both drugs are potentiated, increasing the nephrotoxicity of ciclosporin (11).

In a single-dose, open, crossover study in 15 men and six women, the systemic availability of sirolimus 10 mg was markedly increased by concomitant ciclosporin 300 mg, C_{max}, t_{max}, and AUC being increased by 116, 92, and 230% respectively (12,13). However, when sirolimus was given 4 hours after ciclosporin, the increases were only 37, 58, and 80%. Ciclosporin did not affect the half-life or mean residence time of sirolimus. Sirolimus did not significantly affect the systemic availability of ciclosporin.

Diltiazem

In 18 healthy subjects, in a randomized, crossover study of the pharmacokinetics of a single oral dose of sirolimus 10 mg, a single dose of diltiazem 120 mg, and the combination, diltiazem increased exposure to sirolimus, presumably by inhibiting its first-pass metabolism (13).

The pharmacokinetic interaction of a single oral dose of diltiazem 120 mg with a single oral dose of sirolimus 10 mg has been studied in 18 healthy subjects, 12 men and 6 women, 20-43 years old, in an open, three-period, randomized, crossover study (15). The whole-blood sirolimus AUC increased by 60% and the Cmax by 43% with diltiazem co-administration; the apparent oral clearance and volume of distribution of sirolimus fell by 38 and 45% respectively, consistent with the change in half-life from 79 to 67 hours. Sirolimus had no effect on the pharmacokinetics of diltiazem or on the effects of diltiazem on either diastolic or systolic blood pressures or the electrocardiogram. Single-dose diltiazem co-administration leads to higher sirolimus exposure, presumably by the inhibition of first-pass metabolism. Because of pronounced intersubject variability in this interaction, whole-blood sirolimus concentrations should be monitored closely in patients taking the two drugs.

Tacrolimus

Combination of sirolimus with tacrolimus virtually eliminates acute rejection. However, the adverse effects of both drugs are potentiated, increasing the nephrotoxicity of tacrolimus (11).

References

1. Kahan BD, Podbielski J, Napoli KL, Katz SM, Meier-Kriesche HU, Van Buren CT. Immunosuppressive effects and safety of a sirolimus/cyclosporine combination regimen for renal transplantation. Transplantation 1998;66(8):1040–6.
2. Kahan BD The Rapamune US Study Group. Efficacy of sirolimus compared with azathioprine for reduction of acute renal allograft rejection: a randomised multicentre study. Lancet 2000;356(9225):194–202.
3. Groth CG, Backman L, Morales JM, Calne R, Kreis H, Lang P, Touraine JL, Claesson K, Campistol JM, Durand D, Wramner L, Brattstrom C, Charpentier B Sirolimus European Renal Transplant Study Group. Sirolimus (rapamycin)-based therapy in human renal transplantation: similar efficacy and different toxicity compared with cyclosporine. Transplantation 1999;67(7):1036–42.
4. Morelon E, Stern M, Kreis H. Interstitial pneumonitis associated with sirolimus therapy in renal-transplant recipients. N Engl J Med 2000;343(3):225–6.
5. Singer SJ, Tiernan R, Sullivan EJ. Interstitial pneumonitis associated with sirolimus therapy in renal-transplant recipients. N Engl J Med 2000;343(24):1815–6.

6. Mahalati K, Murphy DM, West ML. Bronchiolitis obliterans and organizing pneumonia in renal transplant recipients. Transplantation 2000;69:1531–2.
7. Brattstrom C, Wilczek H, Tyden G, Bottiger Y, Sawe J, Groth CG. Hyperlipidemia in renal transplant recipients treated with sirolimus (rapamycin). Transplantation 1998;65(9):1272–4.
8. Morrisett JD, Abdel-Fattah G, Hoogeveen R, Mitchell E, Ballantyne CM, Pownall HJ, Opekun AR, Jaffe JS, Oppermann S, Kahan BD. Effects of sirolimus on plasma lipids, lipoprotein levels, and fatty acid metabolism in renal transplant patients. J Lipid Res 2002;43(8):1170–80.
9. Hong JC, Kahan BD. Sirolimus-induced thrombocytopenia and leukopenia in renal transplant recipients: risk factors, incidence, progression, and management. Transplantation 2000;69(10):2085–90.
10. Kaplan MJ, Ellis CN, Bata-Csorgo Z, Kaplan RS, Endres JL, Fox DA. Systemic toxicity following administration of sirolimus (formerly rapamycin) for psoriasis: association of capillary leak syndrome with apoptosis of lesional lymphocytes. Arch Dermatol 1999;135(5):553–7.
11. Johnson RW. Sirolimus (Rapamune) in renal transplantation. Curr Opin Nephrol Hypertens 2002;11(6):603–7.
12. Zimmerman JJ, Harper D, Getsy J, Jusko WJ. Pharmacokinetic interactions between sirolimus and microemulsion cyclosporine when orally administered jointly and 4 hours apart in healthy volunteers. J Clin Pharmacol 2003;43(10):1168–76.
13. Bottiger Y, Sawe J, Brattstrom C, Tollemar J, Burke JT, Hass G, Zimmerman JJ. Pharmacokinetic interaction between single oral doses of diltiazem and sirolimus in healthy volunteers. Clin Pharmacol Ther 2001;69(1):32–40.
14. Guieu R, Dussol B, Devaux C, Sampol J, Brunet P, Rochat H, Bechis G, Berland YF. Interactions between cyclosporine A and adenosine in kidney transplant recipients. Kidney Int 1998;53(1):200–2004.
15. Bottiger Y, Sawe J, Brattstrom C, Tollemar J, Burke JT, Hass G, Zimmerman JJ. Pharmacokinetic interaction between single oral doses of diltiazem and sirolimus in healthy volunteers. Clin Pharmacol Ther 2001;69(1):32–40.

Tacrolimus

General Information

Tacrolimus, a macrolide derivative, has similar immunosuppressive properties to ciclosporin and has effects on T lymphocytes by inhibiting interleukin-2 production. On a weight basis, tacrolimus is about 100 times more potent than ciclosporin. In view of the outcome of several multicenter trials, it has been used as an alternative to ciclosporin as a baseline regimen for the prophylaxis of renal and liver transplant rejection and in the treatment of acute rejection (SED-13, 1130; SEDA-21, 390; 1). The clinical pharmacology, clinical use, and adverse effects profile of tacrolimus in organ transplantation have been extensively reviewed (2).

General adverse effects

The incidence of adverse effects (for example neurotoxicity, nephrotoxicity, and hyperglycemia), particularly those requiring drug withdrawal, was initially found to be higher in tacrolimus-treated liver transplant patients, but subsequently fell after the initial tacrolimus dose was reduced. This was in accordance with the results of very early trials, which showed that the initially proposed dose of tacrolimus was too high (3). In subsequent studies, tacrolimus and ciclosporin had a similar spectrum of adverse effects for nephrotoxicity, infectious complications, and lymphoproliferative disorders, and long-term adverse effects occurred at comparable rates, that is less than 2% (SED-13, 1130; SEDA-21, 390).

Even though the glucocorticoid-sparing effect of tacrolimus is greater than that of ciclosporin, the initial hope that tacrolimus might prove less toxic than ciclosporin has not been realized. In trials in renal transplant patients, increased serum creatinine concentrations, tremor, paresthesia, gastrointestinal disorders, hyperglycemia, diabetes mellitus, pruritus, and angina pectoris occurred more often with tacrolimus, whereas there was a higher incidence of dysrhythmias, hyperkalemia, gingival hyperplasia, acne, alopecia, and hirsutism with ciclosporin (SEDA-21, 390). In the European Tacrolimus Multicenter Liver Trial, there was some evidence of possible advantages for tacrolimus over ciclosporin in terms of hypertension, cytomegalovirus infection, hirsutism, and gum hyperplasia (SEDA-21, 390). The safety profile of tacrolimus is very similar in children to that in adults, but in sharp contrast to ciclosporin, gingival hyperplasia, hirsutism, and coarsening of facial features have not been observed (4,5).

As the adverse effects of tacrolimus and ciclosporin are not strictly comparable, switching a patient from one to the other can sometimes be beneficial. Severe or persistent tacrolimus-related adverse effects, for example neurotoxicity, gastrointestinal disorders, or diabetes mellitus, can abate after replacement by ciclosporin (SEDA-20, 347) (6). Conversely, the change from ciclosporin to tacrolimus has been safely and successfully undertaken in patients with adverse effects from ciclosporin, such as nephrotoxicity, hemolytic–uremic syndrome, hypertension, neurological disorders, gingival hyperplasia, hypertrichosis, and dyslipidemia (SED-13, 1130; SEDA-20, 347; 7,8). Replacing one drug by another is not always advantageous; in two patients switched to tacrolimus for ciclosporin-induced cortical blindness, visual abnormalities promptly resolved, but both patients rapidly developed thrombotic thrombocytopenic purpura and severe graft-versus-host disease, and finally died 33 days after bone marrow transplantation (9).

Long-term follow-up (mean of 93 months) of tacrolimus-based immunosuppression has been reported in 121 adult patients with liver transplants (10). Infections were the most common causes of deaths (17 patients out of 42), and half of them occurred during the first year after transplantation. Cardiovascular events (seven patients) or de novo malignancies (three patients) were also important causes of death. End-stage renal disease related to tacrolimus nephrotoxicity was noted in two patients who required renal transplantation. At 7 years, other important adverse effects included hyperkalemia (30%) or hypertension (31%) requiring treatment, and insulin-dependent diabetes mellitus (13%). Seven patients developed de novo malignancies and six had post-transplant lymphoproliferative disorders. The risks of tacrolimus in renal transplantation have been discussed (11).

Organs and Systems

Cardiovascular

The incidence of hypertension and the prevalence of antihypertensive drug use are lower with tacrolimus than with ciclosporin (5,12).

Severe recurrent, but usually reversible hypertrophic cardiomyopathy has been infrequently reported, both in adults and children (SEDA-19, 352; SEDA-20, 346). Based on experimental data and one additional case report, the interaction of tacrolimus with calcium channel blockers in the cardiac muscle has been suggested as a possible mechanism (SEDA-21, 390). However, the role of tacrolimus in the development of cardiomyopathy is still hypothetical. Echocardiographic abnormalities were relatively common before and after liver transplantation in 12 adult patients, and there was no clear evidence that oral tacrolimus specifically alters cardiac function (13). Other investigators did not show differences in heart weight, ventricular thickness, or valve circumferences between 67 liver transplant recipients treated with tacrolimus and 72 non-transplanted patients who died from end-stage liver disease (14). In addition, more than 80% of patients in both groups had left ventricular hypertrophy.

Other isolated reports and preliminary studies have suggested a possible risk of life-threatening dysrhythmias, including sinus bradycardia or sinus arrest, asymptomatic but significant mean QT/QT$_c$ interval prolongation in 33 patients (over 500 msec in seven patients), and recurrent episodes of ventricular tachycardia or torsade de pointes in two patients (SEDA-21, 391; SEDA-22, 390; 15,16).

Several reports have previously focused on the possible occurrence of cardiomyopathy in tacrolimus-treated transplant patients, particularly children. In two further liver transplant children aged 2.5 and 14 years who died from multiorgan system failure due to sepsis and end-stage liver failure, pathological examination showed prominent concentric left ventricular hypertrophy (17). Although tacrolimus was regarded as a possible cause of asymptomatic hypertrophic cardiomyopathy in these patients, a direct causal relation was difficult to establish. The cause is probably multifactorial, and potential confounding factors (for example hypertension, glucocorticoids) are numerous in this population. In a retrospective review of 89 pediatric heart transplant patients who had survived for at least 6 months, repeated echocardiography showed signs of cardiac hypertrophy, particularly early after transplantation and in very young infants (18). However, there was no evidence of progressive hypertrophy on follow-up examinations, and no significant differences in the degree of cardiac hypertrophy between patients aged over 1 year at the time of transplantation who received ciclosporin ($n = 26$) or tacrolimus ($n = 41$).

In a retrospective study, the prevalence of hypertension 2 years after adult liver transplantation was significantly lower in patients treated with tacrolimus (64% of 28 patients) than in patients treated with ciclosporin (82% of 131 patients) (19). In addition, hypertension occurred later with tacrolimus. A similar benefit of tacrolimus over ciclosporin was found in a randomized, comparative trial in 85 heart transplant patients, and 41% of 39 tacrolimus-treated patients developed new-onset hypertension requiring treatment, compared with 71% of 46 ciclosporin-treated patients (20).

In 37 patients with liver transplants there was no difference between the pre- and post-transplant QT interval in the 25 taking oral ciclosporin and the 12 taking oral tacrolimus (21).

Cardiac symptoms manifesting as myocardial ischemia are uncommon, but can occur through tacrolimus toxicity (22).

- A 20-year-old woman with chest pain, dyspnea, and protracted electrocardiographic ST depression had very high blood tacrolimus concentrations (45 ng/ml). Subsequent coronary angiography ruled out any significant organic lesions, but showed vasospastic coronary arteries. She had no other cardiac symptoms when tacrolimus was restarted with careful surveillance of serum concentrations.

Nervous system

Tacrolimus mostly produces mild to moderate neurotoxic effects that are usually not treatment-limiting and rarely clinically relevant, at least in children (23). The occurrence of neurological symptoms, sometimes severe, is a well-known complication in the early post-transplant period, particularly in liver transplant recipients. It is therefore in most cases difficult to attribute these disorders to a particular immunosuppressive regimen.

When neurological symptoms occur in patients taking tacrolimus they are very similar to those seen in patients taking ciclosporin, with more frequent insomnia, tremor, and headaches, but a similar rate of severe neurological adverse effects, such as acute psychosis, peripheral neuropathy, seizures, encephalopathy, coma, and paralysis. Persistent speech disorders (dysarthria, apraxia, expressive aphasia, akinetic mutism), and visual blurring can also occur (SEDA-21, 391; SEDA-22, 420; 24).

The higher incidence of moderate or severe late neurotoxicity from tacrolimus compared with ciclosporin was strongly associated with severe postoperative infections, multiple organ failure, and an increased bilirubin, creatinine, and transaminases (25).

It has been suggested that anxiety rather than akathisia can account for several symptoms caused by tacrolimus, such as restlessness (SEDA-21, 391).

Posterior leukoencephalopathy, with clinical, radiological, and neuropathological features resembling those previously described with ciclosporin has been reported in several patients (SEDA-22, 420; 26). Cortical blindness, generalized tonic-clonic seizures ($n = 2$), and diffuse MRI abnormalities were found in three of 50 patients taking tacrolimus after bone marrow transplantation (SEDA-20, 347); these findings have also been observed in patients taking ciclosporin. Acute neurotoxicity was fatal in one patient despite changing from tacrolimus to ciclosporin, and autopsy showed multiple cerebral hemispheric infarcts due to cerebral vasculitis (SEDA-22, 420).

Six patients taking tacrolimus (including five children) developed signs of encephalopathy with generalized or focal seizures, reduced visual acuity or cortical blindness, altered mental status, and white matter lesions on MRI scan, particularly in the parieto-occipital regions (27–29). Three patients had tacrolimus blood concentrations above the target range before the neurological adverse event. Although there was complete resolution after tacrolimus withdrawal or reduction in dosage in four patients, two children still had persistent brain imaging abnormalities and recurrent episodes of seizures.

- A chronic inflammatory demyelinating polyneuropathy was considered to have been caused by tacrolimus in a 62-year-old patient (30).
- The presence of significant tacrolimus concentrations (5.2 and 1.3 ng/ml at 8 and 72 hours after the last dose) in the cerebrospinal fluid of a 64-year-old woman with a renal transplant, who developed an extremely severe form of encephalopathy after 21 months of treatment, suggested that tacrolimus can cross the blood–brain barrier (31).

Complete resolution of tacrolimus-induced neurotoxicity does not occur after tacrolimus withdrawal or dosage reduction (32).

- A 48-year-old man developed acute loss of speech and swallowing apraxia shortly after liver transplantation. Tacrolimus serum concentrations were very high. Although there was progressive improvement after tacrolimus withdrawal, residual speech deficits were still present 3 weeks later. A PET scan showed a marked reduction in metabolic rate in the temporal lobes and the adjacent parieto-occipital region bilaterally.

Other cases of severe neurotoxicity have been seen during tacrolimus treatment for graft-versus-host disease after allogeneic bone marrow transplantation.

- A 16-year-old girl had hypertension and generalized convulsions, which recurred after tacrolimus readministration; she subsequently died from cerebral hemorrhage and respiratory failure (33).

Based on this report and a review of previously published cases, concomitant hypertension and the use of high-dose methylprednisolone were discussed as precipitating factors of tacrolimus neurotoxicity. In two other patients aged 4 and 15 years who had prolonged leukoencephalopathy, the underlying chronic graft-versus-host disease was thought to be a risk factor (34).

In children one advantage of tacrolimus is that it can reduce the dose of glucocorticoids required for immunosuppression. This in turn improves growth. When in one center the immunosuppression protocol was changed to tacrolimus plus mycophenolate mofetil and prednisone, two patients developed transient encephalopathy associated with tacrolimus (35). In both cases, the encephalopathy was managed by treating the associated hypertension and fluid overload; tacrolimus was not withdrawn.

Both tacrolimus and ciclosporin are hydrophobic and can alter the properties of the cell membrane. They bind to an intracellular peptidylprolyl isomerase that regulates T cell activation and can interfere with cytoskeletal components that prevent interleukin-2 synthesis and release. Cytotoxic edema caused by acute cerebral ischemia is associated with reduced diffusion, reflecting the failure of membrane sodium pumps. Altered electrolyte or fluid balance can precede the onset of encephalopathy. This can be shown by fluid-attenuated inversion recovery and diffusion-weighted MRI images (36).

A polymorphism of the ABCB1 gene may be associated with a risk of tacrolimus-induced neurotoxicity after liver transplantation. In six patients with neurotoxicity and 11 without neurotoxicity, high tacrolimus concentration, liver dysfunction, and a mutation in position 2677 in exon 21 were positive predictive factors for tacrolimus-induced neurotoxicity (37).

Sensory systems

Eyes

- Optic neuropathy has been reported in a 58-year-old liver transplant patient who had taken tacrolimus for 2 months (38). Further deterioration of vision occurred despite withdrawal.

Ears

Sudden hearing loss has been attributed to tacrolimus (39).

- A 38-year-old woman was switched from ciclosporin to tacrolimus 44 days after kidney and pancreas transplantation and 17 days later had sudden hearing loss with tinnitus. Her tacrolimus blood concentration 3 days later was 28 ng/ml and peaked at 35 ng/ml 8 days later. Audiograms showed bilateral hearing loss—80% for speech perception and mild to moderate sensorineural hearing loss. Her hearing improved on tacrolimus dosage reduction and after the tacrolimus blood concentration reached 15 ng/ml.

Although she was taking many other drugs, including muromonab, which was withdrawn 1 month before the hearing loss occurred, the role of tacrolimus was supported by its chemical similarity to erythromycin, which is ototoxic when given intravenously.

Endocrine

The risk of post-transplant diabetes mellitus is greater with tacrolimus than with ciclosporin, but this was mostly true in black patients and during the initial months after transplantation (40). In one study, insulin sensitivity, alpha and beta cell function, and beta cell reserve were studied in 14 hepatitis C-positive patients with liver transplants, who took tacrolimus or ciclosporin maintenance for 1 year (41). The patients were matched for low prednisolone dosage (1.1 mg/day versus 1.3 mg/day), body mass index, lean body mass, and sex, and compared with eight controls. Insulin sensitivity and insulin secretory reserve were significantly different from controls, but there was no significant difference between ciclosporin and tacrolimus.

The incidence, mechanism, and risk factors of tacrolimus-associated diabetes mellitus are still debated. In 58 patients investigated 1–3 years after liver transplantation there was a significantly higher incidence of diabetes mellitus with tacrolimus ($n = 32$) compared with ciclosporin ($n = 26$) (42). Newly-diagnosed diabetes occurred in nine of 28 tacrolimus-treated patients, of whom six required insulin, and in none of 25 ciclosporin-treated patients. Five patients taking tacrolimus also had islet cell-specific autoantibodies that correlated significantly with HLA risk haplotypes.

- A 32-year-old woman with previous autoimmune disorders and a susceptible HLA haplotype developed diabetes with newly positive glutamic acid decarboxylase antibody after taking tacrolimus for 5 months (43).

Together, these reports suggest that tacrolimus does not suppress the production of autoantibodies in patients genetically prone to develop autoimmune diabetes, with induction of an autoimmune phenomenon. This also suggests that tacrolimus treatment should be undertaken cautiously in predisposed patients.

Metabolism

Of 834 primary adult liver transplant recipients, of whom 499 were alive and taking tacrolimus, 70% were glucocorticoid-free after 1 year; this did not change over the next 5 years (44). However, glucocorticoid-associated adverse effects, such as hypertension, diabetes, and hyperlipidemia, were not statistically significantly less common in patients not taking glucocorticoids. This may have been because of the diabetogenic effect of tacrolimus.

Diabetes mellitus

Altered glucose metabolism and subsequent hyperglycemia or even insulin-dependent diabetes mellitus is an important issue in transplant patients, particularly in adults or patients taking high doses. In animals, high-dose tacrolimus causes glucose intolerance and reduced insulin release (45). This resolves after withdrawal. Diabetes mellitus after transplantation is a relatively common complication in pediatric thoracic organ recipients taking tacrolimus (46). Specific risk factors have not been identified. A switch from tacrolimus to ciclosporin for other reasons in two patients did not resolve the problem.

The incidence of hyperglycemia or diabetes mellitus requiring insulin at some point during treatment was 10–20% in adults (2% in children), an incidence about 2–3 times higher than with ciclosporin (SEDA-20, 347). However, more recent studies and case reports have

shown that children could be also very sensitive to the diabetogenic effects of tacrolimus, with an incidence possibly higher than previously thought (47,48). While the diabetes mellitus tends to improve or abate after the dose of tacrolimus or glucocorticoid has been reduced, glucose intolerance was more frequent in the tacrolimus group after a median of 23 months (49). However, post-transplant diabetes mellitus requiring permanent insulin treatment was as frequent in patients with liver grafts taking ciclosporin or tacrolimus after 1 year (50). Finally, there was a possible correlation between impaired glucose tolerance or a diabetic pattern detected by a pretransplant 75 g oral glucose tolerance test and the later development of post-transplant diabetes mellitus (51).

In a pooled analysis of four randomized trials of tacrolimus versus ciclosporin after renal transplantation, the prevalence of post-transplant diabetes mellitus at 1 year (two studies, 532 patients) was five times higher with tacrolimus than with ciclosporin (OR = 5.0; 95% CI = 2.0, 12.4) (52). In the opinion of the US FDA, diabetes mellitus after transplantation was a significant hazard in tacrolimus-treated patients, even though about half of the patients were no longer taking insulin at 2 years after transplantation (53).

The exact mechanisms of tacrolimus-induced diabetes are unknown. In one renal transplant patient with genetic susceptibility, tacrolimus was associated with insulin-dependent diabetes mellitus and the simultaneous occurrence of anti-glutamic acid decarboxylase antibody (54). Within 2 months after conversion from tacrolimus to ciclosporin, the antibody was no longer detected and the patient's insulin requirements fell dramatically. Tacrolimus-induced direct beta cell toxicity, with subsequent development of beta cell autoimmunity, was therefore suggested as a possible mechanism in patients with genetic susceptibility for type I diabetes.

Hepatitis C virus infection has been associated with diabetes and is a significant risk in patients with renal transplants. In 427 patients with renal transplants and no previous diabetes mellitus, diabetes after transplantation occurred more often in hepatitis C virus-positive than hepatitis C virus-negative patients (39 versus 9.8%) (55). Diabetes mellitus after transplantation occurred more often in hepatitis C virus-positive patients taking tacrolimus than in those taking ciclosporin (58 versus 7.7%). In hepatitis C virus-negative patients, the rates of diabetes mellitus were similar. The authors concluded that hepatitis C is strongly associated with diabetes mellitus after renal transplantation because of the greater diabetogenicity of tacrolimus.

In 17 patients, in whom fasting blood samples were taken immediately before transplantation and at 1 and 3 months after transplantation for measurement of HbA, insulin, C-peptide, free fatty aids, lipids, urea, and creatinine, the incidence of diabetes mellitus was high (47%) (56). Diabetes was more common in black patients, but owing to the small number of patients the difference was not statistically significant. Insulin resistance seems to be the main pathogenic mechanism involved.

Lipid metabolism

In contrast to its effects on glucose metabolism, tacrolimus offers potential advantages over ciclosporin for lipid disorders (57). Compared with ciclosporin-based immunosuppressive regimens, total cholesterol and LDL cholesterol serum concentrations were lower in patients taking tacrolimus for 1 year (58). Both findings were considered to result from a significant glucocorticoid-sparing effect of tacrolimus.

Hematologic

Acute hemolysis occurred in eight of 1400 patients (59). Although multiple other causal factors could have been relevant, further hematological investigations suggested that tacrolimus can cause or promote hemolysis, particularly in patients with acquired anti-erythrocyte antibodies.

Pure red cell aplasia is an occasional complication of treatment (SED-13, 1131; SEDA-20, 347; 60). In one case, tacrolimus was thought to have caused reversible pancytopenia with severely reduced granulopoiesis and megakaryocytopoiesis on bone marrow examination (SEDA-21, 391).

- The prothrombin time was prolonged to 36 seconds, with isolated factor V deficiency (5%), 2 weeks after a 46-year-old patient with a liver transplant was given tacrolimus and oxacillin (61). Factor V antigen was lower than 5%. In vitro investigations of the patient's plasma showed dose-dependent factor V inhibitory activity in the presence of tacrolimus. Factor V activity and the coagulation profile returned to normal after withdrawal.

The development of this transiently acquired inhibitor of coagulation factor V may have been due to either tacrolimus or oxacillin.

Microangiopathy and the resulting thrombotic thrombocytopenic purpura-like syndrome has been reported in three transplant patients taking tacrolimus, including one with a severe form (62). Microangiopathy was associated with high trough tacrolimus concentrations (over 24 ng/ml) and raised concentrations of endothelin and various cytokines, namely interleukin-8, interleukin-10, interleukin-12, tumor necrosis factor alfa, and interferon gamma.

Mouth and teeth

A brief case report has suggested that tacrolimus can cause gingival hyperplasia (63).

Gastrointestinal

Severe gastrointestinal toxicity with anorexia and weight loss is sometimes observed in patients taking tacrolilmus (SEDA-19, 352).

Tacrolimus-associated *Clostridium difficile* diarrhea has been reported (64).

- A 29-year-old man was given mycophenolate and tacrolimus for an episode of renal transplant rejection that occurred 6.5 years after transplantation. Four weeks after tacrolimus was begun, he had diarrhea, nausea, and malaise. There was *C. difficile* toxin in the stools,

and his symptoms abated with metronidazole. About 1 month later, he developed diarrhea, fever, and severe dehydration. *Clostridium difficile* toxin was again detected in the stools, and his symptoms completely resolved with oral vancomycin and withdrawal of tacrolimus.

Similar cases have been reported to the manufacturers. A possible relation between the macrolide molecular structure of tacrolimus and the development of *C. difficile* colitis remains to be established.

Liver

In children 0.1% tacrolimus ointment has been used daily without major adverse effects.

- In a 3-year-old African-American boy with moderate atopic dermatitis, tacrolimus caused raised transaminase and lactate dehydrogenase activities. Tacrolimus was withdrawn on day 29, but no further information was given about their liver function tests (65).

The finding of mild to moderate liver function test abnormalities that normalized on dosage reduction or withdrawal of tacrolimus has suggested possible dose-related hepatotoxicity (66). In liver transplant patients, liver biopsy showed a centrilobular hepatocellular dropout with sinusoidal dilatation and congestion, and no features of cellular rejection or acute hepatitis.

Pancreas

Acute pancreatitis has rarely been reported in clinical trials, but no detailed cases were available before the following report (67).

- A 28-year-old woman was switched from ciclosporin to tacrolimus for prophylaxis of graft-versus-host disease after allogeneic stem cell transplantation for chronic myelogenous leukemia. She also took methylprednisolone and inhaled pentamidine. After 2 weeks she developed acute abdominal pain, tachypnea, hypoxia, and oliguria. Amylase and lipase peaked at about four and five times the upper limits of the reference ranges, and urinary analysis was consistent with acute tubular necrosis. An abdominal CT scan showed an enlarged edematous pancreas with a peripancreatic inflammatory exudate. There was no biliary obstruction or dyslipidemia. Shortly after tacrolimus withdrawal, she became anuric and had an episode of acute respiratory distress, but then improved over the next few days.

Although treatment with methylprednisolone, pentamidine, and total parenteral nutrition could have contributed in this patient, they were either continued or readministered without ill effect.

Urinary tract

Tacrolimus nephrotoxicity has been reviewed (68) and is considered to be very similar to that described with ciclosporin. The clinical and histological characteristics of acute tacrolimus nephrotoxicity have been described from a retrospective analysis of 67 patients with renal transplants, of whom 27 developed acute nephrotoxicity, in seven of whom underlying moderate-to-severe renal arteriosclerosis might have predisposed to tacrolimus nephrotoxicity (69).

Tacrolimus-induced chronic nephrotoxicity has clinical and histopathological features very similar to those induced by ciclosporin, that is tubular lesions, hyaline arteriolopathy, and hemolytic–uremic syndrome-like changes in glomeruli and vessels (70). Isolated glomerular microthrombosis has also been described (71). Although tacrolimus was successfully used in several patients suffering from ciclosporin-induced hemolytic–uremic syndrome, thrombocytopenic purpura and hemolytic–uremic syndrome, including one fatal case, have also been reported in patients taking tacrolimus (SED-13, 1131; SEDA-20, 347). In addition, ciclosporin and tacrolimus were significant risk factors for recurrence of hemolytic–uremic syndrome in patients who had undergone renal transplantation for end-stage renal disease (72). Late nephrotoxicity evaluated by the mean serum creatinine concentration and/or glomerular filtration rate at 1 year was similar in patients taking ciclosporin or tacrolimus (73,74). However, compared with ciclosporin, tacrolimus appears to be associated with more frequent and severe proximal or distal tubular acidosis 6 months after renal transplantation, although this conclusion is based on work with only a few patients in each group (SEDA-19, 352; 75). Overall, the reported incidence of tacrolimus-associated nephrotoxicity varies from 18 to 42% in liver transplant patients; among 128 patients who had early and late episodes of renal allograft dysfunction (1–156 weeks after transplantation) requiring biopsy, tacrolimus nephrotoxicity was estimated to account for only 17% of cases (76). There were higher than expected serum tacrolimus concentrations in most patients, and the highest concentrations were detected 1.6 days before the peak serum creatinine. However, renal histological lesions were independent of tacrolimus dosage or blood concentrations (77).

The nephrotoxic adverse effects of tacrolimus and ciclosporin are clinically indistinguishable. The pathological features of renal biopsies at 2 years of treatment in patients enrolled in a large multicenter comparison of tacrolimus and ciclosporin in renal transplantation have been reported (78). Of 412 patients initially randomized, renal biopsies were available from 79 taking tacrolimus and 65 taking ciclosporin. There were features of tacrolimus or ciclosporin nephrotoxicity (hyaline arteriolar change, tubular vacuolization) in 19 and 11 patients respectively. There were no differences in the rates of biopsy-proven acute rejection (8.9 versus 9.2%) or chronic allograft nephropathy (62 and 72%). In addition, the histological features of chronic allograft nephropathy were very similar. An older age of the donor, acute rejection, cytomegalovirus infection, and ciclosporin- and tacrolimus-associated nephrotoxicity during the first year of transplantation were the most significant factors associated with the occurrence of chronic nephropathy.

As with ciclosporin, tacrolimus used as a primary immunosuppressant has sometimes been associated with de novo thrombotic microangiopathy/hemolytic–uremic syndrome. Its role has been clearly confirmed in a 52-year-old heart transplant patient in whom hemolytic–uremic syndrome recurred 6 days after tacrolimus readministration (79). From a report of two additional cases and a review of 19 other reported cases, the incidence of tacrolimus-associated thrombotic microangiopathy has been suggested to be 1.0–4.7%; 15 cases were reported in renal transplant patients (80). The mean time to diagnosis was 9 months (4 days to 31 months), and the tacrolimus trough concentrations were usually within the target range. Most patients had the clinical features of hemolytic–uremic syndrome. Final outcomes were known in 18 patients: 10 had tacrolimus dosage reduction only (six recovered, three had an acute cellular rejection, one lost his renal graft); one stopped taking tacrolimus and recovered; seven had tacrolimus dosage reduction or withdrawal and underwent plasmapheresis, fresh-frozen plasma exchange, high-dose glucocorticoids, or anticoagulation (three died of sepsis and multiorgan failure, one lost her renal graft, and three recovered). Furthermore, and in contrast to previous reports (SEDA-19, 353), a change from ciclosporin to tacrolimus in patients with ciclosporin-associated hemolytic–uremic syndrome is not always successful.

- Two renal transplant patients developed resistant late acute rejection while taking ciclosporin (81). After a switch to tacrolimus, they had clinical and histological features of hemolytic–uremic syndrome, with biopsy-proven thrombotic microangiopathy within 2 and 12 days after conversion. Both finally required explantation of their renal allografts.

Skin

The long-term safety of topical tacrolimus ointment 0.1% for 6–12 months has been assessed in 316 patients with atopic dermatitis (82). The most common adverse effects clearly attributed to tacrolimus were a local burning sensation (47%), pruritus (24%), and erythema (12%); the incidences fell with time. The observed incidence of infections did not exceed the expected incidence in patients with atopic dermatitis, and there were no effects on circulating cell-mediated immunity.

In 631 adult patients with moderate to severe atopic dermatitis enrolled in a randomized, double-blind, multicenter comparison of tacrolimus (0.03% or 0.1%) with a vehicle applied twice-daily for 12 weeks, the most common adverse events were skin burning, erythema, and pruritus (83). Others were flu-like symptoms and headache. Withdrawal was required in 50 patients because of adverse events, twice as many as in the vehicle group. There was pruritus in 30 patients, skin burning in 19, skin erythema in 12, and skin infections in two. Skin burning and pruritus have consistently been observed with tacrolimus ointment, typically during the first days of treatment, reducing in incidence within the first week; they tend to be mild or moderate.

In 255 children with atopic dermatitis, tacrolimus 0.1% ointment caused transient skin burning and itching as the most common adverse events (65). Two patients required hospital admittance to control skin infections. A flu-like syndrome was the major non-topical adverse event.

- A diffuse, follicular, erythematous eruption has been reported in a 45-year-old patient with a previous history of allergies to multiple medications, including clarithromycin (84). It resolved after tacrolimus withdrawal.

The authors speculated on possible cross-sensitivity between tacrolimus and clarithromycin, which are both macrolides, but confirmatory skin-testing was not performed. In addition, the patient had taken many other drugs that might have been responsible.

Hair

In several studies, alopecia has been found more often with tacrolimus than ciclosporin, and severe alopecia has sometimes followed replacement of ciclosporin by tacrolimus. However, in the light of one detailed case report, and bearing in mind the minimal effect of tacrolimus on hair growth, it is not unlikely that alopecia has sometimes been mistakenly attributed to tacrolimus rather than to concomitant glucocorticoid-induced hair loss in the absence of the counteracting effects of ciclosporin (SEDA-21, 391).

Musculoskeletal

Severe acute rhabomyolysis with subsequent fatal acute renal insufficiency has been reported in an 18-month-old girl (SEDA-19, 353).

Like ciclosporin, tacrolimus has been thought to reduce bone mineral density, but this conclusion was based on a series of seven patients, all of whom had also taken azathioprine and glucocorticoids (85).

- Severe bone pain, previously reported in ciclosporin-treated patients (SED-14, 1291), also occurred as a possible consequence of tacrolimus treatment in a 50-year-old woman (86). Bilateral knee pain occurred within 2 months after renal transplantation and bone scintigraphy showed increased uptake in both knees. Calcitonin was ineffective, and she improved only after the dose of tacrolimus was reduced.

Sexual function

Priapism has been described in a patient with a liver transplant (87).

- One month after transplantation, a 19-year-old man who was taking tacrolimus, azathioprine, and prednisone, developed nausea and vomiting. He reported a 2-week history of painful spontaneous penile erections lasting 2–3 minutes and had had no previous episodes of priapism. An episode of spontaneous erection was confirmed during a medical examination that found no physical abnormalities. The tacrolimus blood concentration was 28 ng/ml. The digestive symptoms and priapism resolved after the tacrolimus concentration had fallen. Sickle cell disease was ruled out.

The authors discussed several mechanisms, including tacrolimus-induced vasodilatation, platelet aggregation, an increase in serotonin, or a fall in endothelin concentrations, based on in vitro data only.

Immunologic

Tacrolimus reduces IgE antibody synthesis, with a subsequent dramatic increase in IgE serum concentrations. This phenomenon has been reported in one asymptomatic patient but has also been advanced as an explanation for a case in which an infant girl treated with tacrolimus had milk hypersensitivity (SEDA-21, 391).

Fish allergy with increased IgE total concentrations and specific IgE antibodies against various fish products have been reported in two children with liver transplants (88). Even though both patients had a personal or familial history of allery, this again suggested a possible relation between tacrolimus and food allergy.

An increasing blood eosinophil count was associated with *Pneumocystis jiroveci* pneumonia in patients taking tacrolimus (89). The mean absolute eosinophil count was significantly higher and absolute eosinophilia (over 350×10^6/l) was more frequent in six patients who developed *P. jiroveci* pneumonia while taking tacrolimus compared with six patients with *P. jiroveci* pneumonia who were taking ciclosporin and eight patients without *P. jiroveci* pneumonia who were taking tacrolimus. A retrospective analysis also showed that the increase in eosinophil count preceded the diagnosis of *P. jiroveci* pneumonia.

Infection risk

Tacrolimus-based immunosuppression may be associated with a lower incidence of major infectious complications, namely CMV and pneumonia compared with other drugs (90). However, this hypothesis is based on a single paper, and other studies have been unable to find significant differences in the incidence of major infections between tacrolimus and ciclosporin (5,91). In addition, and as a direct consequence of excessive immunosuppression, a further retrospective study found an increased incidence of symptomatic Epstein–Barr virus infections and related lymphoproliferative disorders in children under 5 years of age who had taken tacrolimus rather than ciclosporin (92).

An unexplained change in the pattern of microbial causes of pneumonia has been noted in liver transplant patients taking tacrolimus, with an unexpectedly high incidence of *Legionella* and fungal pneumonia, the latter being involved in all deaths directly due to pneumonia (93).

In a randomized, double-blind, placebo-controlled study at 23 centers in the USA, children with moderate to severe atopic dermatitis applied the vehicle, tacrolimus ointment 0.03%, or tacrolimus ointment 0.1% for 12 weeks (94). Burning and pruritus were the main adverse effects. *Varicella* infection and vesiculobullous rashes on non-application areas occurred, but with a low incidence (below 5%). Since they occurred in those who used tacrolimus 0.03%, it is likely that they were random events rather than drug-related. Regardless of dose, there were some age-related differences in the incidence of individual adverse events. For example, otitis media was more common in younger children (2–6 years). Tacrolimus ointment had no age-selective effect that was not also observed with the vehicle. Each of the adverse events resolved without sequelae.

Long-Term Effects

Tumorigenicity

It has generally been considered that the incidence and pathological features of tacrolimus-induced cancers after transplantation are similar to those observed with other immunosuppressive agents, in particular ciclosporin (95). However, in a retrospective study in 392 children, who survived for more than 6 months after liver transplantation and were followed for a mean of 4.3 years, there was a five-fold higher rate of lymphoproliferative disease after transplantation in children who took tacrolimus ($n = 141$) than in those who took ciclosporin ($n = 251$) (96). As a result, the incidence density rate of lymphoproliferative disease was 4.8 per 100 person-years in tacrolimus-treated patients, with no difference among age groups. In addition, the mean time to lymphoproliferative disease (12.6 months) was five-fold shorter with tacrolimus than with ciclosporin. Most of the patients with lymphoproliferative disease had a primary Epstein–Barr virus infection after transplantation. The authors suggested that the 10-fold higher in vivo immunosuppressive effect of tacrolimus might have accounted for these findings.

Tacrolimus-induced post-transplant lymphoproliferative diseases are similar to those of the conditions induced by other immunosuppressants, particularly ciclosporin (SED-13, 1131). However, additional data from prolonged follow-up are still awaited. In children who are frequently Epstein–Barr virus-negative, the incidence of post-transplant lymphoproliferative disease varies from 6–11% to 22% after liver transplantation (97). In 89 children, the incidence of post-transplant lymphoproliferative disease at 1 year was 20% (possibly related to Epstein–Barr virus in 89% of patients) (98). Excessive immunosuppression, for example as a result of prior muromonab or antithymocyte globulin administration and high tacrolimus blood concentrations during the period preceding Epstein–Barr virus infection are regarded as significant risk factors, emphasizing the need to secure low trough tacrolimus concentrations after the first post-transplant month. An increase in total gammaglobulin and the development of oligoclonal or polyclonal immunoglobulins were thought to be preliminary signs of this syndrome.

Second-Generation Effects

Pregnancy

Among 25 infants born after 27 pregnancies in tacrolimus-treated liver transplant patients there was an unexpectedly low incidence of hypertension, pre-eclampsia, and allograft function abnormalities, whereas preterm delivery, low birth weight, and transient mild renal impairment with hyperkalemia in neonates occurred at a similar rate (99).

It has been suggested that tacrolimus may be less likely than ciclosporin to cause maternal renal dysfunction or pre-eclampsia, but this hypothesis is based only on retrospective work in a small number of patients (100).

- Congestive heart failure with dilated cardiomyopathy occurred in twin boys born to a woman with a renal transplant who had taken tacrolimus throughout her pregnancy (101). One twin died from irreversible cardiac failure, and autopsy findings showed thrombogenic cardiomyopathy and degeneration of cardiac muscle. The other twin was more actively treated and had only mild tricuspid insufficiency on follow-up.

This report is in keeping with the possible and debated role of tacrolimus in the development of cardiomyopathy in children.

Teratogenicity

In the National Transplantation Pregnancy Registry, there was no evidence of an increased incidence of congenital malformations among 25 infants born after 27 pregnancies in tacrolimus-treated liver transplant patients (99).

Fetotoxicity

Among 25 infants born after 27 pregnancies in tacrolimus-treated liver transplant patients, there were two neonatal deaths whose conception had been close to the time of transplantation, and very high tacrolimus cord levels were found in one child who presented with neonatal anuria (99).

Drug Administration

Drug overdose

Acute tacrolimus overdosage usually produces only moderate toxicity or none at all. From the data available in 16 children or adults, overdosage up to 30 times the intended dose produced no symptoms in seven patients and reversible moderate increases in serum creatinine concentrations, or transaminase activities, nausea, and mild tremors in eight patients who underwent gastric decontamination and conservative measures only (102,103). An additional patient on maintenance treatment developed renal insufficiency, histoplasmosis, and sepsis within two days of overdosage. Continuous hemofiltration dramatically increased the rate of elimination of tacrolimus in two other patients who experienced acute renal and liver failure with high plasma tacrolimus blood concentrations (104).

Even large accidental overdosage of tacrolimus does not result in marked acute toxicity (105).

- The inadvertent administration of 25 times the intended dose in a 22-month-old infant produced minimal consequences, with only a five-fold reversible increase in serum amylase activity.

Drug–Drug Interactions

Amphotericin

Tacrolimus (FK 506), a macrolide immunosuppressant, has adverse effects similar to those of ciclosporin, including nephrotoxicity. Increased nephrotoxicity can be expected when it is given with amphotericin (126).

Antimicrobial agents

The hepatic metabolism of tacrolimus is primarily mediated by CYP3A, and experimental evidence suggests a theoretical potential for numerous interactions with drugs that induce or inhibit CYP3A. However, very few formal drug interaction studies have been carried out, and most of our current knowledge is based on case reports and small series of patients, or is derived from experience accumulated with ciclosporin. Among antimicrobial agents, erythromycin, chloramphenicol, clarithromycin, clotrimazole, danazol, oral (but not intravenous) fluconazole, itraconazole, and ketoconazole increase tacrolimus serum concentrations and can cause subsequent nephrotoxicity, whereas rifampicin reduces tacrolimus concentrations (SED-13, 1131; SEDA-20, 348; SEDA-22, 419; 106–109).

- A potential interaction with pristinamycin has been described in a 41-year-old renal transplant patient who had an approximate five-fold increase in tacrolimus trough concentrations within 4 days of pristinamycin treatment (110).
- A 10-fold increase in tacrolimus dosage was required in a 61-year-old patient with a renal transplant who took concomitant rifampicin (111).

The interaction of tacrolimus with rifampicin has been convincingly confirmed in six healthy volunteers who took a single oral or intravenous dose of tacrolimus (112). Rifampicin 600 mg/day for 18 days produced a significant 47% increase in tacrolimus clearance after intravenous administration and a 51% reduction in its oral systemic availability, consistent with induction by rifampicin of both hepatic and intestinal metabolism of tacrolimus.

Calcium channel blockers

A 3-day course of diltiazem 90 mg/day produced a four-fold increase in tacrolimus trough concentrations in a 68-year-old patient with a liver transplant (113).

In a non-randomized, pharmacokinetic study, four patients taking tacrolimus after kidney and liver transplantation were given diltiazem in seven incremental dosages of 0–180 mg at 2-week intervals (114). The mean tacrolimus-sparing effect was similar to the ciclosporin-sparing effect previously reported. This effect occurred at a lower dose of diltiazem in renal transplant patients than in liver transplant patients. Tacrolimus is metabolized by CYP3A4 and is also a substrate for P

glycoprotein, and this interaction could have occurred by inhibition of these mechanisms.

A retrospective study has shown a significant improvement in kidney function and a 38% reduction in tacrolimus dosage requirements in patients taking both nifedipine and tacrolimus compared to patients not taking nifedipine (115).

Chloramphenicol

Inhibition of tacrolimus clearance has been observed in an adolescent renal transplant recipient who was treated with standard doses of chloramphenicol for vancomycin-resistant enterococci. Toxic concentrations of tacrolimus were observed on the second day of chloramphenicol treatment, requiring an 83% reduction in the dose of tacrolimus (127).

A significant interaction has also been reported in an adult (128).

- A 47-year-old white man with a cadaveric liver transplant took chloramphenicol for a urinary tract infection due to a vancomycin-resistant *Enterococcus* and inadvertently received 1850 mg qds (roughly twice the maximum recommended dose). On day 4 he had a 12-hour trough tacrolimus concentration of over 60 ng/ml, and complained of fatigue, lethargy, headache, and tremor, symptoms consistent with tacrolimus toxicity.It was suggested that the underlying mechanism might be inhibition of CYP3A4 by chloramphenicol.

Clarithromycin

Clarithromycin can increase the steady-state concentrations of drugs that depend primarily on CYP3A metabolism.

- Steady-state tacrolimus concentrations rose in a 32-year-old African-American man who took clarithromycin 500 mg bd for 4 days (129).
- In two women aged 37 and 69, acute and reversible tacrolimus nephrotoxicity developed after the addition of clarithromycin for an upper respiratory tract infection (130).

Echinocandins

While tacrolimus had no effect on the plasma pharmacokinetics of caspofungin, chronic caspofungin reduced the AUC of tacrolimus by about 20% (131).

Fluconazole

Since tacrolimus (FK506) is meta-bolized by intestinal and hepatic CYP3A4, drugs that inhibit CYP3A4 can reduce the metabolism of tacrolimus and increase tacrolimus blood concentrations (132). The effect of fluconazole on the blood concentrations of tacrolimus have been investigated in eight liver transplant patients in whom prophylactic fluconazole (200 mg/day) was withdrawn because of rises in hepatic transaminases ($n = 6$), renal dysfunction, or eosinophilia ($n = 1$ each) (133). Calculated tacrolimus concentrations fell by 13–81%

(median 41%) between the fourth and ninth days after withdrawal of fluconazole. Tacrolimus blood concentrations should be carefully monitored and dosages increased as necessary after withdrawal of fluconazole.

The interaction of tacrolimus with fluconazole has been retrospectively evaluated in 19 kidney and pancreas/kidney transplant recipients (90). Both intravenous and oral fluconazole altered the blood concentration of tacrolimus. Five subjects did not have a significant interaction and 15 did. No patient had nephrotoxicity or transplant rejection related to antifungal therapy.

- A 17-year-old man with cystic fibrosis who took itraconazole after a lung-liver transplant had high trough concentrations of tacrolimus, despite the relatively low dosage (0.1–0.3 mg/kg/day) (134).
- A patient taking tacrolimus 0.085 mg/kg bd with itraconazole 200–400 mg/day developed ketoacidosis, neutropenia, and thrombocytopenia, requiring the withdrawal of both drugs (135).
- A 34-year-old renal transplant recipient taking a stable regimen of tacrolimus and methylprednisolone was given itraconazole 100 mg bd for a yeast infection of the urinary tract (136). Concomitant therapy with itraconazole led to a marked increase in tacrolimus trough concentrations on the second day of therapy (from 13 to 21 ng/ml) and an increase in serum creatinine concentrations, necessitating dosage reduction of tacrolimus by 50%.

When itraconazole was withdrawn the effect of itraconazole on the kinetics of tacrolimus took 12 days to reverse.

The inhibitory effect of itraconazole occurred quickly, while the time of disappearance was much longer, which is important for clinical management. Thus, during coadministration of itraconazole with tacrolimus, close monitoring of tacrolimus blood concentrations and careful dosage adjustments are essential to avoid toxicity.

Ibuprofen

Acute renal insufficiency in association with the use of ibuprofen and tacrolimus has been reported in two liver transplant recipients (116), and the relevance of this interaction is probably similar to that reported with ciclosporin.

Itraconazole

Tacrolimus concentrations and toxicity are affected by itraconazole (137).

- In a 17-year-old man with cystic fibrosis who received a hepato-pulmonary transplant, there was an interaction of itraconazole 600 mg bd with tacrolimus (138). High trough concentrations of tacrolimus were noted, despite the relatively low dosage (0.1–0.3 mg/kg/day).
- Another patient experienced an interaction of tacrolimus 0.085 mg /kg bd with itraconazole 200–400 mg per day, with resulting ketoacidosis, neutropenia, and thrombocytopenia, requiring the withdrawal of both drugs (139).
- A 30-year-old man with a renal transplant had a more than two-fold increase in blood tacrolimus concentrations after starting to take itraconazole 200 mg/day,

accompanied by a reduced glomerular filtration rate and biopsy-proven tacrolimus-associated tubulopathy (140).

Because of the narrow therapeutic index of tacrolimus, blood concentrations should be monitored particularly carefully when itraconazole is co-dministered, and the dosage of tacrolimus may have to be altered (141).

The interaction of itraconazole (100 mg bd) with tacrolimus has been studied in 28 heart or lung transplant recipients (142). Tacrolimus blood concentrations were monitored on alternate days for up to 21 days after the start of itraconazole therapy ($n = 18$) or withdrawal ($n = 10$). The dose of tacrolimus was adjusted with the aim of keeping the 12-hour trough blood concentration at 7–12 micrograms/ml. The mean dose of tacrolimus during itraconazole therapy fell significantly from 8.4 to 2.9 mg/day. There was no significant change in serum creatinine or liver function tests. In patients in whom itraconazole was withdrawn, the mean dose of tacrolimus required increased significantly from 4.7 to 8.8 mg/day. Thus, substantial changes in the dose of tacrolimus were required both when itraconazole was begun and when it was withdrawn, and it was difficult to maintain tacrolimus blood concentrations within the target range during the first 2 weeks. However, major toxicity or rejection did not occur. Co-administration of itraconazole may reduce the cost of post-transplant immunosuppression. This interaction is probably due to inhibition of CYP3A4 by itraconazole.

Metronidazole

Metronidazole can produce a two-fold increase in blood concentrations of ciclosporin and tacrolimus, with a subsequent increase in serum creatinine in both cases (117).

Mibefradil

Mibefradil, a potent inhibitor of CYP3A, increased tacrolimus blood concentrations dramatically (118).

Nefazodone

Nefazodone may inhibit the metabolism of tacrolimus (119).

- A 16-year-old boy had a five-fold increase in tacrolimus blood concentrations and a two-fold increase in creatinine concentrations within 4 weeks of nefazodone treatment. Complete normalization occurred after replacement with paroxetine and a transient reduction in tacrolimus dosage.

Protease inhibitors

Various protease inhibitors are metabolic inhibitors and are predicted to have deleterious effects on tacrolimus metabolism.

- In a 52-year-old liver transplant patient with HIV infection, successive treatment with various antiretroviral combinations containing nelfinavir, ritonavir, or saquinavir increased tacrolimus blood concentrations and caused severe prolonged neurological symptoms suggestive of tacrolimus toxicity (120). The patient was finally stabilized with a regimen containing nelfinavir, stavudine, and lamivudine, and a more than 95% reduction in the dosage of tacrolimus.

- An acute drug interaction with nelfinavir has been described in a 49-year-old liver transplant man with HIV and hepatitis C infections (121). The patient had three consecutive episodes of increased blood tacrolimus concentrations during nelfinavir administration. Both drugs were finally continued, but the dose of tacrolimus was only one-seventieth of the usual dose.

Sildenafil

The effects of sildenafil can be potentiated by drugs that are metabolized by CYP3A4. Tacrolimus is an example. When sildenafil was given to patients with kidney transplants taking regular tacrolimus, peak concentrations were much higher and the half-life much longer than expected from data in healthy volunteers (143). However, an effect of the underlying disease and other concomitant drugs obviously could not be excluded.

Theophylline

An increase in tacrolimus trough blood concentrations has been attributed to concomitant theophylline therapy

- A 33-year-old man with end-stage renal disease due to diabetic nephropathy received a cadaveric kidney graft. Immunosuppressive therapy after transplantation included tacrolimus (7 mg/day), azathioprine (75 mg/day), and prednisone (7.5 mg/day). He developed erythrocytosis 3 months later and was given drugs that reduce erythropoietin production, first enalapril, without success, and then theophylline (600 mg/day). After 1 month, his serum creatinine and tacrolimus concentrations were raised. The dosage of theophylline was therefore reduced to 300 mg/day four times a week. One month later, his serum creatinine and tacrolimus trough blood concentrations increased further. On withdrawal of theophylline, both renal function and tacrolimus trough blood concentration rapidly normalized. Theophylline was then reintroduced in a lower dose and increased the AUC of tacrolimus.

CYP3A4 is primarily responsible for tacrolimus biotransformation in the liver, but it has only a minor role in theophylline metabolism. It is therefore surprising that this tacrolimus-theophylline interaction occurred. The authors suggested that as long as renal function remains stable, low-dose theophylline can be used in transplant patients with erythrocytosis, provided that tacrolimus concentrations are closely monitored.

Voriconazole

In a patient who took tacrolimus after liver transplant, co-administration of voriconazole resulted in raised trough tacrolimus concentrations (nearly 10-fold); there were no changes in another patient, who took a placebo (123).

Voriconazole inhibits the metabolism of tacrolimus in liver microsomes by 50% in vitro.

Monitoring Therapy

In 14 patients with renal transplants, there was a closed relation between individual tacrolimus whole blood trough concentrations and the occurrence of adverse effects (124). The incidence of tacrolimus adverse effects was 76% with tacrolimus concentrations above 30 ng/ml and only 5.3% with concentrations below 10 ng/ml. This relation was found in all separate groups of adverse effects analysed, that is nephrotoxicity, neurotoxicity, infections, and others. In contrast, there was no relation between tacrolimus concentrations and rejection episodes. Accordingly, the authors stressed that tacrolimus whole blood trough concentrations should be strictly kept under 20 ng/ml.

There is no relation between tacrolimus blood concentrations and the occurrence of major neurotoxicity (125).

References

1. Spencer CM, Goa KL, Gillis JC. Tacrolimus. An update of its pharmacology and clinical efficacy in the management of organ transplantation. Drugs 1997;54(6):925–75.
2. Plosker GL, Foster RH. Tacrolimus: a further update of its pharmacology and therapeutic use in the management of organ transplantation. Drugs 2000;59(2):323–89.
3. Alessiani M, Cillo U, Fung JJ, Irish W, Abu-Elmagd K, Jain A, Takaya S, Van Thiel D, Starzl TE. Adverse effects of FK 506 overdosage after liver transplantation. Transplant Proc 1993;25(1 Pt 1):628–34.
4. Asante-Korang A, Boyle GJ, Webber SA, Miller SA, Fricker FJ. Experience of FK506 immune suppression in pediatric heart transplantation: a study of long-term adverse effects. J Heart Lung Transplant 1996;15(4):415–22.
5. Pham SM, Kormos RL, Hattler BG, Kawai A, Tsamandas AC, Demetris AJ, Murali S, Fricker FJ, Chang HC, Jain AB, Starzl TE, Hardesty RL, Griffith BP. A prospective trial of tacrolimus (FK 506) in clinical heart transplantation: intermediate-term results. J Thorac Cardiovasc Surg 1996;111(4):764–72.
6. Mor E, Sheiner PA, Schwartz ME, Emre S, Guy S, Miller CM. Reversal of severe FK506 side effects by conversion to cyclosporine-based immunosuppression. Transplantation 1994;58(3):380–2.
7. Pratschke J, Neuhaus R, Tullius SG, Haller GW, Jonas S, Steinmueller T, Bechstein WO, Neuhaus P. Treatment of cyclosporine-related adverse effects by conversion to tacrolimus after liver transplantation. Transplantation 1997;64(6):938–40.
8. Busque S, Demers P, St-Louis G, Boily JG, Tousignant J, Lemieux F, Smeesters C, Corman J, Daloze P. Conversion from Neoral (cyclosporine) to tacrolimus of kidney transplant recipients for gingival hyperplasia or hypertrichosis. Transplant Proc 1998;30(4):1247–8.
9. Tezcan H, Zimmer W, Fenstermaker R, Herzig GP, Schriber J. Severe cerebellar swelling and thrombotic thrombocytopenic purpura associated with FK506. Bone Marrow Transplant 1998;21(1):105–9.
10. Jain AB, Kashyap R, Rakela J, Starzl TE, Fung JJ. Primary adult liver transplantation under tacrolimus:

more than 90 months actual follow-up survival and adverse events. Liver Transpl Surg 1999;5(2):144–50.

11. Kliem V, Brunkhorst R. Tacrolimus in kidney transplantation. A clinical review. Nephron 1998;79(1):8–20.

12. Hohage H, Bruckner D, Arlt M, Buchholz B, Zidek W, Spieker C. Influence of cyclosporine A and FK506 on 24 h blood pressure monitoring in kidney transplant recipients Clin Nephrol 1996;45(5):342–4.

13. Dollinger MM, Plevris JN, Chauhan A, MacGilchrist AJ, Finlayson ND, Hayes PC. Tacrolimus and cardiotoxicity in adult liver transplant recipients. Lancet 1995;346(8973):507.

14. Jain AB, Fung JJ. Cyclosporin and tacrolimus in clinical transplantation. A comparative review. Clin Immunother 1996;5:351–73.

15. Johnson MC, So S, Marsh JW, Murphy AM. QT prolongation and torsades de pointes after administration of FK506. Transplantation 1992;53(4):929–30.

16. Sanoski CA, Vasquez EM, Bauman JL. QT interval prolongation associated with the use of tacrolimus in transplant recipients. Pharmacotherapy 1998;18:427.

17. Chang RK, Alzona M, Alejos J, Jue K, McDiarmid SV. Marked left ventricular hypertrophy in children on tacrolimus (FK506) after orthotopic liver transplantation. Am J Cardiol 1998;81(10):1277–80.

18. Scott JS, Boyle GJ, Daubeney PE, Miller SA, Law Y, Pigula F, Griffith BP, Webber SA. Tacrolimus: a cause of hypertrophic cardiomyopathy in pediatric heart transplant recipients? Transplant Proc 1999;31(1–2):82–3.

19. Canzanello VJ, Textor SC, Taler SJ, Schwartz LL, Porayko MK, Wiesner RH, Krom RA. Late hypertension after liver transplantation: a comparison of cyclosporine and tacrolimus (FK 506). Liver Transpl Surg 1998;4(4):328–34.

20. Taylor DO, Barr ML, Radovancevic B, Renlund DG, Mentzer RM Jr, Smart FW, Tolman DE, Frazier OH, Young JB, VanVeldhuisen P. A randomized, multicenter comparison of tacrolimus and cyclosporine immunosuppressive regimens in cardiac transplantation: decreased hyperlipidemia and hypertension with tacrolimus. J Heart Lung Transplant 1999;18(4):336–45.

21. Gonzalez MG, Hernandez-Madrid A, Sanroman AL, Monge G, De Vicente E, Barcena R. Comparison of post-liver transplantation electrocardiographic alterations between cyclosporine- and tacrolimus-treated patients. Transplant Proc 1999;31(6):2423–4.

22. Uchida N, Taniguchi S, Harada N, Shibuya T. Myocardial ischemia following allogeneic bone marrow transplantation: possible implication of tacrolimus overdose. Blood 2000;96(1):370–2.

23. Neu AM, Furth SL, Case BW, Wise B, Colombani PM, Fivush BA. Evaluation of neurotoxicity in pediatric renal transplant recipients treated with tacrolimus (FK506). Clin Transplant 1997;11(5 Pt 1):412–4.

24. Wijdicks EF, Wiesner RH, Dahlke LJ, Krom RA. FK506-induced neurotoxicity in liver transplantation. Ann Neurol 1994;35(4):498–501.

25. Mueller AR, Platz KP, Bechstein WO, Schattenfroh N, Stoltenburg-Didinger G, Blumhardt G, Christe W, Neuhaus P. Neurotoxicity after orthotopic liver transplantation. A comparison between cyclosporine and FK506. Transplantation 1994;58(2):155–70.

26. Small SL, Fukui MB, Bramblett GT, Eidelman BH. Immunosuppression-induced leukoencephalopathy from tacrolimus (FK506). Ann Neurol 1996;40(4):575–80.

27. Steg RE, Kessinger A, Wszolek ZK. Cortical blindness and seizures in a patient receiving FK506 after bone marrow transplantation. Bone Marrow Transplant 1999;23(9):959–62.

28. Tomura N, Kurosawa R, Kato K, Takahashi S, Watarai J, Takeda O, Watanabe A, Takada G. Transient neurotoxicity associated with FK506: MR findings. J Comput Assist Tomogr 1998;22(3):505–7.

29. Torocsik HV, Curless RG, Post J, Tzakis AG, Pearse L. FK506-induced leukoencephalopathy in children with organ transplants. Neurology 1999;52(7):1497–500.

30. Haviv YS, Friedlaender M, Dranitzki-Elhallel M. Chronic inflammatory demyelinating polyneuropathy possibly associated with tacrolimus. Clin Drug Invest 1999;18:169–72.

31. Grimbert P, Azema C, Pastural M, Dhamane D, Remy P, Salomon L, Schortgen F, Baron C, Lang P. Tacrolimus (FK506)-induced severe and late encephalopathy in a renal transplant recipient. Nephrol Dial Transplant 1999;14(10):2489–91.

32. Bronster DJ, Gurkan A, Buchsbaum MS, Emre S. Tacrolimus-associated mutism after orthotopic liver transplantation. Transplantation 2000;70(6):979–82.

33. Mori A, Tanaka J, Kobayashi S, Hashino S, Yamamoto Y, Ota S, Asaka M, Imamura M. Fatal cerebral hemorrhage associated with cyclosporin-A/FK506-related encephalopathy after allogeneic bone marrow transplantation. Ann Hematol 2000;79(10):588–92.

34. Misawa A, Takeuchi Y, Hibi S, Todo S, Imashuku S, Sawada T. FK506-induced intractable leukoencephalopathy following allogeneic bone marrow transplantation. Bone Marrow Transplant 2000;25(3):331–4.

35. Parvex P, Pinsk M, Bell LE, O'Gorman AM, Patenaude YG, Gupta IR. Reversible encephalopathy associated with tacrolimus in pediatric renal transplants. Pediatr Nephrol 2001;16(7):537–42.

36. Furukawa M, Terae S, Chu BC, Kaneko K, Kamada H, Miyasaka K. MRI in seven cases of tacrolimus (FK-506) encephalopathy: utility of FLAIR and diffusion-weighted imaging. Neuroradiology 2001;43(8):615–21.

37. Yamauchi A, Ieiri I, Kataoka Y, Tanabe M, Nishizaki T, Oishi R, Higuchi S, Otsubo K, Sugimachi K. Neurotoxicity induced by tacrolimus after liver transplantation: relation to genetic polymorphisms of the ABCB1 (MDR1) gene. Transplantation 2002;74(4):571–2.

38. Brazis PW, Spivey JR, Bolling JP, Steers JL. A case of bilateral optic neuropathy in a patient on tacrolimus (FK506) therapy after liver transplantation. Am J Ophthalmol 2000;129(4):536–8.

39. Min DI, Ku YM, Rayhill S, Corwin C, Wu YM, Hunsicker LG. Sudden hearing loss associated with tacrolimus in a kidney–pancreas allograft recipient. Pharmacotherapy 1999;19(7):891–3.

40. Weir MR, Fink JC. Risk for posttransplant diabetes mellitus with current immunosuppressive medications. Am J Kidney Dis 1999;34(1):1–13.

41. Fernandez LA, Lehmann R, Luzi L, Battezzati A, Angelico MC, Ricordi C, Tzakis A, Alejandro R. The effects of maintenance doses of FK506 versus cyclosporin A on glucose and lipid metabolism after orthotopic liver transplantation. Transplantation 1999;68(10):1532–41.

42. Lohmann T, List C, Lamesch P, Kohlhaw K, Wenzke M, Schwarz C, Richter O, Hauss J, Seissler J. Diabetes mellitus and islet cell specific autoimmunity as adverse effects of immunosuppressive therapy by FK506/tacrolimus. Exp Clin Endocrinol Diabetes 2000;108(5):347–52.

43. Kawai T, Shimada A, Kasuga A. FK506-induced autoimmune diabetes. Ann Intern Med 2000;132(6):511.

44. Jain A, Kashyap R, Marsh W, Rohal S, Khanna A, Fung JJ. Reasons for long-term use of steroid in primary

adult liver transplantation under tacrolimus. Transplantation 2001;71(8):1102–6.

45. Tze WJ, Tai J, Murase N, Tzakis A, Starzl TE. Effect of FK 506 on glucose metabolism and insulin secretion in normal rats. Transplant Proc 1991;23(6):3158–60.

46. Paolillo JA, Boyle GJ, Law YM, Miller SA, Lawrence K, Wagner K, Pigula FA, Griffith BP, Webber SA. Posttransplant diabetes mellitus in pediatric thoracic organ recipients receiving tacrolimus-based immunosuppression. Transplantation 2001;71(2):252–6.

47. Furth S, Neu A, Colombani P, Plotnick L, Turner ME, Fivush B. Diabetes as a complication of tacrolimus (FK506) in pediatric renal transplant patients. Pediatr Nephrol 1996;10(1):64–6.

48. Moxey-Mims MM, Kay C, Light JA, Kher KK. Increased incidence of insulin-dependent diabetes mellitus in pediatric renal transplant patients receiving tacrolimus (FK506). Transplantation 1998;65(5):617–9.

49. Krentz AJ, Dmitrewski J, Mayer D, McMaster P, Buckels J, Dousset B, Cramb R, Smith JM, Nattrass M. Postoperative glucose metabolism in liver transplant recipients. A two-year prospective randomized study of cyclosporine versus FK506. Transplantation 1994;57(11):1666–9.

50. Jindal RM, Popescu I, Schwartz ME, Emre S, Boccagni P, Miller CM. Diabetogenicity of FK506 versus cyclosporine in liver transplant recipients. Transplantation 1994;58(3):370–2.

51. Tanabe K, Koga S, Takahashi K, Sonda K, Tokumoto T, Babazono T, Yagisawa T, Toma H, Kawai T, Fuchinoue S, Teraoka S, Ota K. Diabetes mellitus after renal transplantation under FK 506 (tacrolimus) as primary immunosuppression. Transplant Proc 1996;28(3):1304–5.

52. Knoll GA, Bell RC. Tacrolimus versus cyclosporin for immunosuppression in renal transplantation: meta-analysis of randomised trials. BMJ 1999;318(7191):1104–7.

53. Cavaille-Coll MW, Elashoff MR. Commentary on a comparison of tacrolimus and cyclosporine for immunosuppression after cadaveric renal transplantation. Transplantation 1998;65(1):142–5.

54. Yoshioka K, Sato T, Okada N, Ishii T, Imanishi M, Tanaka S, Kim T, Sugimoto T, Fujii S. Post-transplant diabetes with anti-glutamic acid decarboxylase antibody during tacrolimus therapy. Diabetes Res Clin Pract 1998;42(2):85–9.

55. Bloom RD, Rao V, Weng F, Grossman RA, Cohen D, Mange KC. Association of hepatitis C with posttransplant diabetes in renal transplant patients on tacrolimus. J Am Soc Nephrol 2002;13(5):1374–80.

56. Panz VR, Bonegio R, Raal FJ, Maher H, Hsu HC, Joffe BI. Diabetogenic effect of tacrolimus in South African patients undergoing kidney transplantation. Transplantation 2002;73(4):587–90.

57. Gomez E, Aguado S, Rodriguez M, Alvarez-Grande J. Kaposi's sarcoma after renal transplantation—disappearance after reduction of immunosuppression and reappearance 7 years later after start of mycophenolate mofetil treatment. Nephrol Dial Transplant 1998;13(12):3279–80.

58. Aboujoud MS, Levy MF, Klintmalm GB; US Multicenter Study Group. Hyperlipidemia after liver transplantation: long-term results of the FK506/cyclosporine A US Multicenter Trial. Transplant Proc 1995;27(1):1121–3.

59. Abu-Elmagd KM, Bronsther O, Kobayashi M, Yagihashi A, Iwaki Y, Fung J, Alessiani M, Bontempo F, Starzl T. Acute hemolytic anemia in liver and bone marrow transplant patients under FK 506 therapy. Transplant Proc 1991;23(6):3190–2.

60. Misra S, Moore TB, Ament ME, Busuttil RW, McDiarmid SV. Red cell aplasia in children on tacrolimus after liver transplantation. Transplantation 1998;65(4):575–7.

61. Leroy-Matheron C, Mallat A, Duvoux C, Metreau JM, Cherqui D, Dhumeaux D, Gouault-Heilmann M. Inhibitor against coagulation factor V after liver transplantation. Transplantation 1999;68(7):1054–6.

62. Burke GW, Ciancio G, Cirocco R, Markou M, Olson L, Contreras N, Roth D, Esquenazi V, Tzakis A, Miller J. Microangiopathy in kidney and simultaneous pancreas/kidney recipients treated with tacrolimus: evidence of endothelin and cytokine involvement. Transplantation 1999;68(9):1336–42.

63. Basile C, Marangi AL, Montanaro A, Giordano R, De Padova F, Ligorio VA, Santese D, Di Marco L, Semeraro A, Vernaglione L. Tacrolimus and gingival hyperplasia. Nephrol Dial Transplant 1998;13(11):2980–1.

64. Sharma AK, Holder FE. Clostridium difficile diarrhea after use of tacrolimus following renal transplantation. Clin Infect Dis 1998;27(6):1540–1.

65. Kang S, Lucky AW, Pariser D, Lawrence I, Hanifin JM. Long-term safety and efficacy of tacrolimus ointment for the treatment of atopic dermatitis in children. J Am Acad Dermatol 2001;44(Suppl 1):S58–64.

66. Fisher A, Mor E, Hytiroglou P, Emre S, Boccagni P, Chodoff L, Sheiner P, Schwartz M, Thung SN, Miller C. FK506 hepatotoxicity in liver allograft recipients. Transplantation 1995;59(11):1631–2.

67. Nieto Y, Russ P, Everson G, Bearman SI, Cagnoni PJ, Jones RB, Shpall EJ. Acute pancreatitis during immunosuppression with tacrolimus following an allogeneic umbilical cord blood transplantation. Bone Marrow Transplant 2000;26(1):109–11.

68. Finn WF. FK506 nephrotoxicity. Ren Fail 1999;21(3–4):319–29.

69. Shimizu T, Tanabe K, Tokumoto T, Ishikawa N, Shinmura H, Oshima T, Toma H, Yamaguchi Y. Clinical and histological analysis of acute tacrolimus (TAC) nephrotoxicity in renal allografts. Clin Transplant 1999;13(Suppl 1):48–53.

70. Ader JL, Rostaing L. Cyclosporin nephrotoxicity: pathophysiology and comparison with FK-506. Curr Opin Nephrol Hypertens 1998;7(5):539–45.

71. Antoine C, Thakur S, Daugas E, Fraoui R, Boudjeltia S, Julia P, Nochy D, Glotz D. Vascular microthrombosis in renal transplant recipients treated with tacrolimus. Transplant Proc 1998;30(6):2813–4.

72. Ducloux D, Rebibou JM, Semhoun-Ducloux S, Jamali M, Fournier V, Bresson-Vautrin C, Chalopin JM. Recurrence of hemolytic–uremic syndrome in renal transplant recipients: a meta-analysis. Transplantation 1998;65(10):1405–7.

73. Platz KP, Mueller AR, Blumhardt G, Bachmann S, Bechstein WO, Kahl A, Neuhaus P. Nephrotoxicity following orthotopic liver transplantation. A comparison between cyclosporine and FK506. Transplantation 1994;58(2):170–8.

74. Porayko MK, Gonwa TA, Klintmalm GB, Wiesner RH U.S. Multicenter Liver Study Group. Comparing nephrotoxicity of FK 506 and cyclosporine regimens after liver transplantation: preliminary results

from US Multicenter trial. Transplant Proc 1995;27(1):1114–6.

75. Heering P, Ivens K, Aker S, Grabensee B. Distal tubular acidosis induced by FK506. Clin Transplant 1998;12(5):465–71.

76. Katari SR, Magnone M, Shapiro R, Jordan M, Scantlebury V, Vivas C, Gritsch A, McCauley J, Starzl T, Demetris AJ, Randhawa PS. Clinical features of acute reversible tacrolimus (FK 506) nephrotoxicity in kidney transplant recipients. Clin Transplant 1997;11(3):237–42.

77. Gaber LW, Moore LW, Reed L, Russell W, Alloway R, Hathaway D, Shokouh-Amiri MH, Gaber AO. Renal histology with varying FK506 blood levels. Transplant Proc 1997;29(1–2):186.

78. Solez K, Vincenti F, Filo RS. Histopathologic findings from 2-year protocol biopsies from a U.S. multicenter kidney transplant trial comparing tarolimus versus cyclosporine: a report of the FK506 Kidney Transplant Study Group Transplantation 1998;66(12):1736–40.

79. Walder B, Ricou B, Suter PM. Tacrolimus (FK 506)-induced hemolytic uremic syndrome after heart transplantation. J Heart Lung Transplant 1998;17(10):1004–6.

80. Trimarchi HM, Truong LD, Brennan S, Gonzalez JM, Suki WN. FK506-associated thrombotic microangiopathy: report of two cases and review of the literature. Transplantation 1999;67(4):539–44.

81. Schmidt RH, Lenz T, Grone HJ, Geiger H, Scheuermann EH. Haemolytic–uraemic syndrome after tacrolimus rescue therapy for cortisone-resistant rejection. Nephrol Dial Transplant 1999;14(4):979–83.

82. Reitamo S, Wollenberg A, Schopf E, Perrot JL, Marks R, Ruzicka T, Christophers E, Kapp A, Lahfa M, Rubins A, Jablonska S, Rustin MThe European Tacrolimus Ointment Study Group. Safety and efficacy of 1 year of tacrolimus ointment monotherapy in adults with atopic dermatitis. Arch Dermatol 2000;136(8):999–1006.

83. Soter NA, Fleischer AB Jr, Webster GF, Monroe E, Lawrence I. Tacrolimus ointment for the treatment of atopic dermatitis in adult patients: part II, safety. J Am Acad Dermatol 2001;44(Suppl 1):S39–46.

84. Riley L, Mudd L, Baize T, Herzig R. Cross-sensitivity reaction between tacrolimus and macrolide antibiotics. Bone Marrow Transplant 2000;25(8):907–8.

85. Stempfle HU, Werner C, Echtler S, Assum T, Meiser B, Angermann CE, Theisen K, Gartner R. Rapid trabecular bone loss after cardiac transplantation using FK506 (tacrolimus)-based immunosuppression. Transplant Proc 1998;30(4):1132–3.

86. Villaverde V, Cantalejo M, Balsa A, Mola EM, Sanz A. Leg bone pain syndrome in a kidney transplant patient treated with tacrolimus (FK506). Ann Rheum Dis 1999;58(10):653–4.

87. Harmon JD, Ginsberg PC, Nachmann MM, Manzarbeita C, Harkaway RC. Stuttering priapism in a liver transplant patient with toxic levels of FK506. Urology 1999;54(2):366.

88. Inui A, Komatsu H, Fujisawa T, Matsumoto H, Miyagawa Y. Food allergy and tacrolimus. J Pediatr Gastroenterol Nutr 1999;28(3):355–6.

89. Dickenmann MJ, Tamm M, Tsinalis D, Binet I, Thiel G, Steiger J. Blood eosinophilia in tacrolimus-treated patients: an indicator of Pneumocystis carinii pneumonia. Transplantation 1999;68(10):1606–8.

90. Hadley S, Samore MH, Lewis WD, Jenkins RL, Karchmer AW, Hammer SM. Major infectious complications after orthotopic liver transplantation and comparison

91. of outcomes in patients receiving cyclosporine or FK506 as primary immunosuppression. Transplantation 1995;59(6):851–9.

91. Vincenti F, Laskow DA, Neylan JF, Mendez R, Matas AJ. One-year follow-up of an open-label trial of FK506 for primary kidney transplantation. A report of the U.S. Multicenter FK506 Kidney Transplant Group Transplantation 1996;61(11):1576–81.

92. Cox KL, Lawrence-Miyasaki LS, Garcia-Kennedy R, Lennette ET, Martinez OM, Krams SM, Berquist WE, So SK, Esquivel CO. An increased incidence of Epstein–Barr virus infection and lymphoproliferative disorder in young children on FK506 after liver transplantation. Transplantation 1995;59(4):524–9.

93. Singh N, Gayowski T, Wagener M, Marino IR, Yu VL. Pulmonary infections in liver transplant recipients receiving tacrolimus. Changing pattern of microbial etiologies. Transplantation 1996;61(3):396–401.

94. Paller A, Eichenfield LF, Leung DY, Stewart D, Appell M. A 12-week study of tacrolimus ointment for the treatment of atopic dermatitis in pediatric patients. J Am Acad Dermatol 2001;44(Suppl 1):S47–57.

95. Penn I. Post-transplant malignancy: the role of immunosuppression. Drug Saf 2000;23(2):101–13.

96. Younes BS, McDiarmid SV, Martin MG, Vargas JH, Goss JA, Busuttil RW, Ament ME. The effect of immunosuppression on posttransplant lymphoproliferative disease in pediatric liver transplant patients. Transplantation 2000;70(1):94–9.

97. McDiarmid SV. The use of tacrolimus in pediatric liver transplantation. J Pediatr Gastroenterol Nutr 1998;26(1):90–102.

98. Sokal EM, Antunes H, Beguin C, Bodeus M, Wallemacq P, de Ville de Goyet J, Reding R, Janssen M, Buts JP, Otte JB. Early signs and risk factors for the increased incidence of Epstein–Barr virus-related post-transplant lymphoproliferative diseases in pediatric liver transplant recipients treated with tacrolimus. Transplantation 1997;64(10):1438–42.

99. Jain A, Venkataramanan R, Fung JJ, Gartner JC, Lever J, Balan V, Warty V, Starzl TE. Pregnancy after liver transplantation under tacrolimus. Transplantation 1997;64(4):559–65.

100. Casele HL, Laifer SA. Association of pregnancy complications and choice of immunosuppressant in liver transplant patients. Transplantation 1998;65(4):581–3.

101. Vyas S, Kumar A, Piecuch S, Hidalgo G, Singh A, Anderson V, Markell MS, Baqi N. Outcome of twin pregnancy in a renal transplant recipient treated with tacrolimus. Transplantation 1999;67(3):490–2.

102. Curran CF, Blahunka PC, Lawrence ID. Acute overdoses of tacrolimus. Transplantation 1996;62(9):1376–7.

103. Mrvos R, Hodgman M, Krenzelok EP. Tacrolimus (FK 506) overdose: a report of five cases. J Toxicol Clin Toxicol 1997;35(4):395–9.

104. Hopp L, Lombardozzi S, Gilboa N, et al. Removal of FK 506 by continuous hemofiltration: report of two allograft recipients with renal and liver failures. Clin Transplant 1993;7:546–51.

105. Odoul F, Talbotec C, Boussa N, Le Guellec C, Furet Y, Maurage C, Breteau M. Massive ingestion of tacrolimus in a young liver transplant patient. Transplant Proc 1998;30(8):4327–9.

106. Mignat C. Clinically significant drug interactions with new immunosuppressive agents. Drug Saf 1997;16(4):267–78.

107. Capone D, Gentile A, Imperatore P, Palmiero G, Basile V. Effects of itraconazole on tacrolimus blood concentrations in a renal transplant recipient. Ann Pharmacother 1999;33(10):1124–5.

108. Gomez G, Alvarez ML, Errasti P, Lavilla FJ, Garcia N, Ballester B, Garcia I, Purroy A. Acute tacrolimus nephrotoxicity in renal transplant patients treated with clarithromycin. Transplant Proc 1999;31(6):2250–1.

109. Moreno M, Latorre A, Manzanares C, Morales E, Herrero JC, Dominguez-Gil B, Carreno A, Cubas A, Delgado M, Andres A, Morales JM. Clinical management of tacrolimus drug interactions in renal transplant patients. Transplant Proc 1999;31(6):2252–3.

110. Billaud EM, Chebassier C, Antoine C, Glotz D. Tacrolimus–pristinamycin drug interaction in renal transplant patient. Fundam Clin Pharmacol 1999;13:354.

111. Chenhsu RY, Loong CC, Chou MH, Lin MF, Yang WC. Renal allograft dysfunction associated with rifampin–tacrolimus interaction. Ann Pharmacother 2000;34(1):27–31.

112. Hebert MF, Fisher RM, Marsh CL, Dressler D, Bekersky I. Effects of rifampin on tacrolimus pharmacokinetics in healthy volunteers. J Clin Pharmacol 1999;39(1):91–6.

113. Hebert MF, Lam AY. Diltiazem increases tacrolimus concentrations. Ann Pharmacother 1999;33(6):680–2.

114. Jones TE, Morris RG. Pharmacokinetic interaction between tacrolimus and diltiazem: dose-response relationship in kidney and liver transplant recipients. Clin Pharmacokinet 2002;41(5):381–8.

115. Seifeldin RA, Marcos-Alvarez A, Gordon FD, Lewis WD, Jenkins RL. Nifedipine interaction with tacrolimus in liver transplant recipients. Ann Pharmacother 1997;31(5):571–5.

116. Sheiner PA, Mor E, Chodoff L, Glabman S, Emre S, Schwartz ME, Miller CM. Acute renal failure associated with the use of ibuprofen in two liver transplant recipients on FK506. Transplantation 1994;57(7):1132–3.

117. Herzig K, Johnson DW. Marked elevation of blood cyclosporin and tacrolimus levels due to concurrent metronidazole therapy. Nephrol Dial Transplant 1999;14(2):521–3.

118. Krahenbuhl S, Menafoglio A, Giostra E, Gallino A. Serious interaction between mibefradil and tacrolimus. Transplantation 1998;66(8):1113–5.

119. Campo JV, Smith C, Perel JM. Tacrolimus toxic reaction associated with the use of nefazodone: paroxetine as an alternative agent. Arch Gen Psychiatry 1998;55(11):1050–2.

120. Sheikh AM, Wolf DC, Lebovics E, Goldberg R, Horowitz HW. Concomitant human immunodeficiency virus protease inhibitor therapy markedly reduces tacrolimus metabolism and increases blood levels. Transplantation 1999;68(2):307–9.

121. Schvarcz R, Rudbeck G, Soderdahl G, Stahle L. Interaction between nelfinavir and tacrolimus after orthoptic liver transplantation in a patient coinfected with HIV and hepatitis C virus (HCV). Transplantation 2000;69(10):2194–5.

122. Boubenider S, Vincent I, Lambotte O, Roy S, Hiesse C, Taburet AM, Charpentier B. Interaction between theophylline and tacrolimus in a renal transplant patient. Nephrol Dial Transplant 2000;15(7):1066–8.

123. Venkataramanan R, Zang S, Gayowski T, Singh N. Voriconazole inhibition of the metabolism of tacrolimus in a liver transplant recipient and in human liver microsomes. Antimicrob Agents Chemother 2002;46(9):3091–3.

124. Bottiger Y, Brattstrom C, Tyden G, Sawe J, Groth CG. Tacrolimus whole blood concentrations correlate closely to side-effects in renal transplant recipients. Br J Clin Pharmacol 1999;48(3):445–8.

125. Burkhalter EL, Starzl TE, Van Thiel DH. Severe neurological complications following orthotopic liver transplantation in patients receiving FK 506 and prednisone. J Hepatol 1994;21(4):572–7.

126. Peters DH, Fitton A, Plosker GL, Faulds D. Tacrolimus. A review of its pharmacology, and therapeutic potential in hepatic and renal transplantation. Drugs 1993;46(4):746–94.

127. Schulman SL, Shaw LM, Jabs K, Leonard MB, Brayman KL. Interaction between tacrolimus and chloramphenicol in a renal transplant recipient. Transplantation 1998;65(10):1397–8.

128. Taber DJ, Dupuis RE, Hollar KD, Strzalka AL, Johnson MW. Drug-drug interaction between chloramphenicol and tacrolimus in a liver transplant recipient. Transplant Proc 2000;32(3):660–2.

129. Ibrahim RB, Abella EM, Chandrasekar PH. Tacrolimusclarithromycin interaction in a patient receiving bone marrow transplantation. Ann Pharmacother 2002;36(12):1971–2.

130. Gomez G, Alvarez ML, Errasti P, Lavilla FJ, Garcia N, Ballester B, Garcia I, Purroy A. Acute tacrolimus nephrotoxicity in renal transplant patients treated with clarithromycin. Transplant Proc 1999;31(6):2250–1.

131. Groll AH, Walsh TJ. Caspofungin: pharmacology, safety and therapeutic potential in superficial and invasive fungal infections. Expert Opin Investig Drugs 2001;10(8):1545–58.

132. Moreno M, Latorre A, Manzanares C, Morales E, Herrero JC, Dominguez-Gil B, Carreno A, Cubas A, Delgado M, Andres A, Morales JM. Clinical management of tacrolimus drug interactions in renal transplant patients. Transplant Proc 1999;31(6):2252–3.

133. Hairhara Y, Makuuchi M, Kawarasaki H, Takayama T, Kubota K, Ito M, Tanaka H, Yoshino H, Hirata M, Kita Y, Kusaka K, Sano K, Saiura A, Ijichi M, Matsukura A, Watanabe M, Hashizume K, Nakatsuka T. Effect of fluconazole on blood levels of tacrolimus. Transplant Proc 1999;31(7):2767.

134. Billaud EM, Guillemain R, Tacco F, Chevalier P. Evidence for a pharmacokinetic interaction between itraconazole and tacrolimus in organ transplant patients. Br J Clin Pharmacol 1998;46(3):271–2.

135. Furlan V, Parquin F, Penaud JF, Cerrina J, Ladurie FL, Dartevelle P, Taburet AM. Interaction between tacrolimus and itraconazole in a heart-lung transplant recipient. Transplant Proc 1998;30(1):187–8.

136. Capone D, Gentile A, Imperatore P, Palmiero G, Basile V. Effects of itraconazole on tacrolimus blood concentrations in a renal transplant recipient. Ann Pharmacother 1999;33(10):1124–.

137. Katari SR, Magnone M, Shapiro R, Jordan M, Scantlebury V, Vivas C, Gritsch A, McCauley J, Starzl T, Demetris AJ, Randhawa PS. Clinical features of acute reversible tacrolimus (FK 506) nephrotoxicity in kidney transplant recipients. Clin Transplant 1997;11(3):237–42.

138. Billaud EM, Guillemain R, Tacco F, Chevalier P. Evidence for a pharmacokinetic interaction between itraconazole and tacrolimus in organ transplant patients. Br J Clin Pharmacol 1998;46(3):271–2.

139. Furlan V, Parquin F, Penaud JF, Cerrina J, Ladurie FL, Dartevelle P, Taburet AM. Interaction between tacrolimus and itraconazole in a heart-lung transplant recipient. Transplant Proc 1998;30(1):187–8.

140. Ideura T, Muramatsu T, Higuchi M, Tachibana N, Hora K, Kiyosawa K. Tacrolimus/itraconazole interactions: a case

report of ABO-incompatible living-related renal transplantation. Nephrol Dial Transplant 2000;15(10):1721–3.

141. Outeda Macias M, Salvador P, Hurtado JL, Martin I. Tacrolimus–itraconazole interaction in a kidney transplant patient. Ann Pharmacother 2000;34(4):536.
142. Banerjee R, Leaver N, Lyster H, Banner NR. Coadministration of itraconazole and tacrolimus after thoracic organ transplantation. Transplant Proc 2001;33(1–2):1600–2.
143. Christ B, Brockmeier D, Hauck EW, Friemann S. Interactions of sildenafil and tacrolimus in men with erectile dysfunction after kidney transplantation. Urology 2001;58:589–93.

IMMUNOSTIMULANTS AND OTHER IMMUNE MODULATORS

Abetimus

General Information

Abetimus is a selective immunomodulator for the treatment of systemic lupus erythematosus. It induces tolerance in B lymphocytes directed against double-stranded DNA by cross-linking surface antibodies. It also reduces serum double-stranded DNA antibodies and splenic double-stranded DNA antibody-producing cells in BXSB mice, giving improved renal function and histopathology, as well as prolonged survival (1).

In a phase-2, partly randomized, double-blind, placebo-controlled study of three different doses of abetimus in 58 patients, seven did not receive all doses because of adverse events (2). Five withdrew because of adverse events related to their lupus erythematosus: non-renal exacerbations ($n = 2$), hematuria and hypertension ($n = 1$), worsening rash ($n = 1$), and nephritis ($n = 1$). One patient withdrew because of cellulitis and another because of a localized *Herpes zoster* infection. None of the reported adverse events was considered to be definitely related to the drug.

Subsequently, La Jolla Pharmaceuticals terminated two previously established licensing agreements for abetimus (3). One of the agreements was with Leo Pharmaceutical Products of Denmark, which was licensed to market abetimus in Europe and the Middle East, and the other was with Abbott Laboratories. Abbott returned all rights to abetimus to La Jolla Pharmaceuticals in September 1999, based on the results of an analysis of a phase-2/phase-3 trial of abetimus in patients with systemic lupus erythematosus and a history of renal disease, which had been stopped in May 1999 because the primary end-point (the time to worsening of renal function) was much shorter than expected. A further analysis then showed that the number of exacerbations in responders treated with abetimus was less than half the number in the patients treated with placebo. Responders also had a significant reduction in the use of high-dose glucocorticoids and cyclophosphamide.

Another phase-3 placebo-controlled trial called PEARL (Program Enabling Antibody Reduction in Lupus) was conducted in the USA in 317 patients with lupus nephritis, who were treated with abetimus 100 mg/week. The trial was completed in December 2002 and preliminary results were reported in February 2003. However, in April 2003, La Jolla Pharmaceuticals ended the trial, in order to conserve resources for the continued development of the drug.

In September 2000, the US FDA granted orphan drug status to abetimus for the treatment of lupus nephritis; the EU did likewise in November 2001.

References

1. Coutts SM, Plunkett ML, Iverson GM, Barstad PA, Berner CM. Pharmacological intervention in antibody mediated disease. Lupus 1996;5(2):158–9.
2. Furie RA, Cash JM, Cronin ME, Katz RS, Weisman MH, Aranow C, Liebling MR, Hudson NP, Berner CM, Coutts S, de Haan HA. Treatment of systemic lupus erythematosus with LJP 394. J Rheumatol 2001;28(2):257–65.
3. Anonymous. Abetimus: Abetimus sodium, LJP 394. BioDrugs 2003;17(3):212–5.

Bropirimine

General Information

Oral bropirimine is an immunostimulant that has been used in the management of transitional cell carcinoma of the bladder and upper urinary tract. It is supposedly an interferon inducer. In clinical trials, bropirimine produced mild adverse effects in about 30% of patients. Nausea or vomiting were the most common (21% of patients), and headache, transient liver enzyme rises, skin rash, and arthralgia were observed in 5–14% (1). Tachycardia or chest pain occurred in 5%. Adverse effects required drug withdrawal in 15% of patients (2).

Oral bropirimine (3 g/day thrice weekly for 1 year) has been compared with weekly intravesical Bacillus Calmette-Guérin (2 cycles of 6 weeks) in 55 patients with newly diagnosed bladder carcinoma (3). Whereas the response to treatment was not significantly different between the two groups, adverse effects resulted in more withdrawals with BCG than bropirimine (14 versus 4%). Bropirimine produced more frequent systemic reactions (in particular diarrhea, fever, flu-like syndrome, headache, nausea/vomiting) but less frequent and less severe local complications.

References

1. Sarosdy MF, Lowe BA, Schellhammer PF, Lamm DL, Graham SD Jr, Grossman HB, See WA, Peabody JO, Moon TD, Flanigan RC, Crawford ED, Morganroth J. Oral bropirimine immunotherapy of carcinoma in situ of the bladder: results of a phase II trial. Urology 1996;48(1):21–7.
2. Sarosdy MF, Manyak MJ, Sagalowsky AI, Belldegrun A, Benson MC, Bihrle W, Carroll PR, Ellis WJ, Hudson MA, Sharkey FE. Oral bropirimine immunotherapy of bladder carcinoma in situ after prior intravesical bacille Calmette-Guérin. Urology 1998;51(2):226–31.
3. Witjes WP, Konig M, Boeminghaus FP, Hall RR, Schulman CC, Zurlo M, Fittipaldo A, Riggi M, Debruyne FMEuropean Bropirimine Study Group. Results of a European comparative randomized study comparing oral bropirimine versus intravesical BCG treatment in BCG-naive patients with carcinoma in situ of the urinary bladder. Eur Urol 1999;36(6):576–81.

Bryostatins

General Information

Bryostatins are naturally occurring antineoplastic macrocyclic lactones derived from the marine invertebrate *Bugula neritina*, different varieties being isolated from different populations of the same species. More than 13 structurally related compounds have been isolated (1,2), and there is a variety of synthetic analogues (3). The bryostatins modulate the activity of protein kinase C.

Bryostatin 1 binds to the regulatory domain of protein kinase C; short-term exposure promotes activation of protein kinase C, whereas prolonged exposure promotes significant down-regulation (4). In preclinical and phase I clinical studies it had promising antitumor and immunomodulating effects. It amplifies expansion of myeloid and erythroid progenitor cells stimulated by the cytokines GM-CSF, M-CSF, and IL-3. Similarly, it induces the production of peripheral blood mononuclear cells with enhanced lymphokine-activated killer cell activity and proliferation in the presence of IL-2 (5).

In a phase II study, 17 patients with progressive indolent non-Hodgkin's lymphoma, previously treated with chemotherapy, received bryostatin 1 (5). Phlebitis was initially due to the 60% ethanol formulation used for administration, and the subsequent use of another formulation (60% polyethylene glycol, 30% ethanol, 10% Tween 80) reduced the incidence. In one patient, bryostatin 1 was withdrawn because of grade 2 thrombocytopenia. The dose-limiting adverse effect was myalgia, which occurred in eight patients.

Other adverse effects include fatigue, nausea, headache, vomiting, dyspnea, ataxia, anorexia, anemia, and lymphopenia (6–8).

In a phase-II study, 14 patients with metastatic cervical cancer or recurrent disease not eligible for surgery or radiation received bryostatin 1 50–65 $\mu g/m^2$ + cisplatin 50 mg/m^2. The most common adverse effects were myalgia, anemia, and nausea or vomiting; one patient had a hypersensitivity reaction and one developed grade 3 nephrotoxicity (9).

Organs and Systems

Skin

Adverse effects of bryostatin 1 on the skin reported during phase I and II studies were alopecia, mucositis, nonspecific rashes, bronzing, and hyperpigmentation in sunexposed areas; a morbilliform eruption has also been reported (10).

Musculoskeletal

In a phase-I trial of bryostatin 1 as a 24-hour continuous infusion followed by bolus vincristine in 24 patients with refractory B cell malignancies other than acute leukemias, the dose-limiting adverse effect was myalgia (11).

References

1. Davidson SK, Haygood MG. Identification of sibling species of the bryozoan *Bugula neritina* that produce different anticancer bryostatins and harbor distinct strains of the bacterial symbiont "*Candidatus endobugula sertula*". Biol Bull 1999;196(3):273–80.
2. Mutter R, Wills M. Chemistry and clinical biology of the bryostatins. Bioorg Med Chem 2000;8(8):1841–60.
3. Wender PA, Hinkle KW, Koehler MF, Lippa B. The rational design of potential chemotherapeutic agents: synthesis of bryostatin analogues. Med Res Rev 1999;19(5):388–407.
4. Kortmansky J, Schwartz GK. Bryostatin-1: a novel PKC inhibitor in clinical development. Cancer Invest 2003;21(6):924–36.
5. Blackhall FH, Ranson M, Radford JA, Hancock BW, Soukop M, McGown AT, Robbins A, Halbert G, Jayson GCCancer Research Campaign Phase I/II Committee. A phase II trial of bryostatin 1 in patients with non-Hodgkin's lymphoma. Br J Cancer 2001;84(4):465–9.
6. Madhusudan S, Protheroe A, Propper D, Han C, Corrie P, Earl H, Hancock B, Vasey P, Turner A, Balkwill F, Hoare S, Harris AL. A multicentre phase II trial of bryostatin-1 in patients with advanced renal cancer. Br J Cancer 2003;89(8):1418–22.
7. Armstrong DK, Blessing JA, Rader J, Sorosky JI; Gynecologic Oncology Group Study. A randomized phase II evaluation of bryostatin-1 (NSC #339555) in persistent or recurrent squamous cell carcinoma of the cervix: a Gynecologic Oncology Group Study. Invest New Drugs 2003;21(4):453–7.
8. Haas NB, Smith M, Lewis N, Littman L, Yeslow G, Joshi ID, Murgo A, Bradley J, Gordon R, Wang H, Rogatko A, Hudes GR. Weekly bryostatin-1 in metastatic renal cell carcinoma: a phase II study. Clin Cancer Res 2003;9(1):109–14.
9. Nezhat F, Wadler S, Muggia F, Mandeli J, Goldberg G, Rahaman J, Runowicz C, Murgo AJ, Gardner GJ. Phase II trial of the combination of bryostatin-1 and cisplatin in advanced or recurrent carcinoma of the cervix: a New York Gynecologic Oncology Group study. Gynecol Oncol 2004;93(1):144–8.
10. Krejci-Manwaring JM, Bogle MA, Diwan HA, Duvic MA. Morbilliform drug reaction with histologic features of pustular dermatosis associated with bryostatin-1. J Drugs Dermatol 2003;2(5):557–61.
11. Dowlati A, Lazarus HM, Hartman P, Jacobberger JW, Whitacre C, Gerson SL, Ksenich P, Cooper BW, Frisa PS, Gottlieb M, Murgo AJ, Remick SC. Phase I and correlative study of combination bryostatin 1 and vincristine in relapsed B cell malignancies. Clin Cancer Res 2003;9(16 Pt 1):5929–35.

Corynebacterium parvum

General Information

Inactivated *Corynebacterium parvum* has been tried as an adjuvant in patients with cancer and in the treatment of malignant pleural effusions. Fever and chills were frequent, with sustained fever and chest or abdominal pain in several patients (1,2).

References

1. Ludwig Lung Cancer Study Group. Adverse effect of intra-pleural *Corynebacterium parvum* as adjuvant therapy in resected stage I and II non-small cell carcinoma of the lung. J Thorac Cardiovasc Surg 1985;89(6):842–7.
2. Foresti V. Intrapleural *Corynebacterium parvum* for recurrent malignant pleural effusions. Respiration 1995;62(1):21–6.

Imiquimod

General Information

Imiquimod is an immune response enhancer that induces production of interferon and several other cytokines. It is used, in formulations containing 5%, to treat external genital and perianal warts/condylomata acuminata in adults (1). As imiquimod-treated warts regress, serum concentrations of interferon-alfa, interferon-beta, interferon-gamma, and tumor necrosis factor rise (2). Trials of imiquimod have failed to identify any particular systemic or laboratory abnormalities.

In one study, there was no deleterious effect on disease progression in HIV-infected patients, and the incidence of local adverse events with imiquimod (5% three times a week) for the treatment of anogenital warts was lower than has previously been reported in healthy individuals (3). In an uncontrolled trial of topical imiquimod 5% for the treatment of common warts and molluscum contagiosum in otherwise healthy patients, fever, healing with scarring, and healing with hyperpigmentation were each reported by one participant (4).

Organs and Systems

Skin

In randomized, double-blind studies, the most common adverse effects were inflammatory reactions at the injection site (mostly erythema and itching), which usually occurred after 2–5 weeks of treatment (5–7). These local reactions included erythema, erosions, excoriation, flaking, edema, scabbing, and induration, and were rarely severe enough to warrant withdrawal. Mild to moderate irritation has to be expected in up to 70% of patients if a 5% imiquimod cream is applied three times per week (6).

References

1. Czelusta AJ, Evans T, Arany I, Tyring SK. A guide to immunotherapy of genital warts. Focus on interferon and imiquimod. BioDrugs 1999;11:319–32.
2. Tyring SK, Arany I, Stanley MA, Tomai MA, Miller RL, Smith MH, McDermott DJ, Slade HB. A randomized, controlled, molecular study of condylomata acuminata clearance during treatment with imiquimod. J Infect Dis 1998;178(2):551–5.
3. Gilson RJ, Shupack JL, Friedman-Kien AE, Conant MA, Weber JN, Nayagam AT, Swann RV, Pietig DC, Smith MH, Owens MLImiquimod Study Group. A randomized, controlled, safety study using imiquimod for the

topical treatment of anogenital warts in HIV-infected patients. AIDS 1999;13(17):2397–404.

4. Hengge UR, Esser S, Schultewolter T, Behrendt C, Meyer T, Stockfleth E, Goos M. Self-administered topical 5% imiquimod for the treatment of common warts and molluscum contagiosum. Br J Dermatol 2000;143(5):1026–31.
5. Beutner KR, Tyring SK, Trofatter KF Jr, Douglas JM Jr, Spruance S, Owens ML, Fox TL, Hougham AJ, Schmitt KA. Imiquimod, a patient-applied immune-response modifier for treatment of external genital warts. Antimicrob Agents Chemother 1998;42(4):789–94.
6. Ferenczy A. Immune response modifiers: imiquimod. J Obstet Gynaecol 1998;18(Suppl 2):76–8.
7. Syed TA, Ahmadpour OA, Ahmad SA, Ahmad SH. Management of female genital warts with an analogue of imiquimod 2% in cream: a randomized, double-blind, placebo-controlled study. J Dermatol 1998;25(7):429–33.

Inosine pranobex

General Information

Inosine pranobex is a synthetic product, also known as isoprinosine or inosine dimepranol acedobene, with antiviral properties that are assumed to be related to its effect on T cell-mediated immunity rather than to direct antiviral activity. It has been tried in a wide range of viral diseases and also in rheumatoid arthritis (1), multiple sclerosis (2), and alopecia (3). However, clinical trials have mostly shown only modest therapeutic benefit or none at all (1,4), and no specific adverse effects, except for an increase in serum uric acid concentrations (5), reflecting the metabolic pathways of purines (6).

Organs and Systems

Immunologic

Anecdotal reports have attributed aggravation of polymyositis (7) and generalized *Herpes zoster* virus infection to inosine pranobex (8).

Drug–Drug Interactions

Zidovudine

Inosine pranobex increased zidovudine plasma concentrations and half-life (9).

References

1. Brzeski M, Madhok R, Hunter JA, Capell HA. Randomised, double blind, placebo controlled trial of inosine pranobex in rheumatoid arthritis. Ann Rheum Dis 1990;49(5):293–5.
2. Milligan NM, Miller DH, Compston DA. A placebo-controlled trial of isoprinosine in patients with multiple sclerosis. J Neurol Neurosurg Psychiatry 1994;57(2):164–8.
3. Galbraith GM, Thiers BH, Jensen J, Hoehler F. A randomized double-blind study of inosiplex (isoprinosine) therapy

in patients with alopecia totalis. J Am Acad Dermatol 1987;16(5 Pt 1):977–83.
4. Kinghorn GR, Woolley PD, Thin RN, De Maubeuge J, Foidart JM, Engst R. Acyclovir vs isoprinosine (Immunovir) for suppression of recurrent genital Herpes simplex infection. Genitourin Med 1992;68(5):312–6.
5. Sarciron ME, Delabre I, Walbaum S, Raynaud G, Petavy AF. Effects of multiple doses of isoprinosine on Echinococcus multilocularis metacestodes. Antimicrob Agents Chemother 1992;36(1):191–4.
6. Thorsen S, Pedersen C, Sandstrom E, Petersen CS, Norkrans G, Gerstoft J, Karlsson A, Christensen KC, Hakansson C, Pehrson PO, et alScandinavian Isoprinosine Study Group. One-year follow-up on the safety and efficacy of isoprinosine for human immunodeficiency virus infection. J Intern Med 1992;231(6):607–15.
7. Chuck AJ, Lloyd Jones JK, Dunn NA. Is inosine pranobex contraindicated in autoimmune disease? BMJ (Clin Res Ed) 1988;296(6622):646.
8. Revuz J, Guillaume JC, Roujeau JC, Perroud AM. Généralisation d'un zona chez un sujet non immunodéprime recevant de l'isoprinosine et de la rifamycine S. V. [Generalization of zona in a nonimmunosuppressed patient receiving isoprinosine and rifamycin SV.] Ann Dermatol Venereol 1983;110(6–7):563.
9. De Simone C, Famularo G, Tzantzoglou S, Moretti S, Jirillo E. Inosine pranobex in the treatment of HIV infection: a review. Int J Immunopharmacol 1991;13(Suppl 1):19–27.

Lentinan

General Information

Lentinan is an immunomodulating glucan that is extracted from the mushroom *Lentinus edodes*. It has been used in small numbers of patients with gastric cancers (1–3) and malignant effusions (4). It has also been used in HIV-positive patients (5) and to ameliorate impairment of natural killer cell activity after cardiopulmonary bypass (6).

General adverse effects

The incidence of adverse effects due to lentinan, particularly those requiring withdrawal, is low (5). Of 98 patients with HIV infection, treatment had to be withdrawn in four because of adverse effects; other adverse effects included one case each of an anaphylactoid reaction, back pain, leg pain, depression, rigors, fever, chills, granulocytopenia, and raised liver enzymes (5).

Organs and Systems

Hematologic

Leukopenia occurred in one of 19 patients with unresectable or recurrent gastric cancers when they were given lentinan 2 mg/kg intravenously together with TS-1 (tegafur + gimestat + otastat potassium in a molar ratio of 10:4:10) 80 mg/m^2/day (7).

Skin

Skin rashes have been noted in 4% of patients treated with lentinan (8).

References

1. Taguchi T. Clinical efficacy of lentinan on patients with stomach cancer: end point results of a four-year follow-up survey. Cancer Detect Prev Suppl 1987;1:333–49.
2. Qing ZJ, Ming QX, Zhong TF. Clinical evaluation of antitumor effects of lentinan combined with chemotherapy in the treatment of various malignancies. Gan To Kagaku Ryoho 1997;24(Suppl 1):1–8.
3. Nakano H, Namatame K, Nemoto H, Motohashi H, Nishiyama K, Kumada K. A multi-institutional prospective study of lentinan in advanced gastric cancer patients with unresectable and recurrent diseases: effect on prolongation of survival and improvement of quality of life. Kanagawa Lentinan Research Group. Hepatogastroenterology 1999;46(28):2662–8.
4. Kawaoka T, Yoshino S, Hazama S, Tangoku A, Oka M. [Clinical evaluation of intrapleural or peritoneal administration of lentinan and OK-432 for malignant effusion.] Gan To Kagaku Ryoho 2003;30(11):1562–5.
5. Gordon M, Guralnik M, Kaneko Y, Mimura T, Goodgame J, DeMarzo C, Pierce D, Baker M, Lang W. A phase II controlled study of a combination of the immune modulator, lentinan, with didanosine (ddI) in HIV patients with CD4 cells of 200–500/mm^3. J Med 1995;26(5–6):193–207.
6. Hamano K, Gohra H, Katoh T, Fujimura Y, Zempo N, Esato K. The preoperative administration of lentinan ameliorated the impairment of natural killer activity after cardiopulmonary bypass. Int J Immunopharmacol 1999;21(8):531–40.
7. Nimura H, Mitsumori N, Tsukagoshi S, Nakajima M, Atomi Y, Suzuki S, Kusano M, Yoshiyuki T, Tokunaga A. [Pilot study of TS-1 combined with lentinan in patients with unresectable or recurrent advanced gastric cancer.] Gan To Kagaku Ryoho 2003;30(9):1289–96.
8. Chihara G, Tagushi T. Lentinan: biological activities and possible clinical use. EOS Riv Immunol Immunofarmacol 1982;2:93.

Muramyl tripeptide

General Information

The antitumor properties of muramyl tripeptide are thought to be related to its immunoenhancing effects, in particular on the monocyte/macrophage system. Its most common adverse effect is a flu-like syndrome, usually during the first administration. In one trial in nine patients, four had mild to moderate respiratory distress, two of whom had pre-existing asthma and symptoms suggestive of asthma exacerbation (1).

Reference

1. Kleinerman ES, Meyers PA, Raymond AK, Gano JB, Jia SF, Jaffe N. Combination therapy with ifosfamide and liposome-encapsulated muramyl tripeptide: tolerability, toxicity, and immune stimulation. J Immunother Emphasis Tumor Immunol 1995;17(3):181–93.

Picibanil

General Information

Picibanil (OK 432) is derived from *Streptococcus pyogenes* and has been used in the treatment of cancers, lymphangiomas, and viral infections. Low-grade fever, nausea and vomiting, and an inflammatory reaction at the injection site were commonly reported, whereas joint pain and mild liver dysfunction were seldom described.

Organs and Systems

Fluid balance

Hyponatremia due to the syndrome of inappropriate secretion of antidiuretic hormone (SIADH) has been attributed to picibanil (1).

- A 59-year-old woman with a previous history of squamous cell carcinoma of the esophagus developed a metastatic lung tumor 4 years later. A right lower lobectomy was performed, and intrapleural picibanil was instilled on postoperative days 4, 5, and 9 for pulmonary fistula with prolonged air leakage. On day 13 she had fatigue, nausea, and drowsiness. Her serum sodium concentration was 106 mmol/l and there was a 2.5-fold increase in serum antidiuretic hormone concentration. She recovered completely after fluid restriction and sodium supplementation.

The author thought that SIADH had resulted from severe pleurisy secondary to intrapleural administration of picibanil rather than to direct stimulation of antidiuretic hormone release.

Hematologic

Hemolytic anemia, presumably of immune origin, has been reported in a patient taking picibanil (2).

References

1. Hanagiri T, Muranaka H, Hashimoto M, Nagashima A. A syndrome of inappropriate secretion of antidiuretic hormone associated with pleuritis caused by OK-432. Respiration 1998;65(4):310–2.
2. Nomura S, Kanoh T. Immune hemolytic anemia associated with streptococcal preparation OK-432. Cancer 1987;59(8):1409–11.

Ribonucleic acid

General Information

Ribonucleic acid has been used to enhance immune function in patients with cancer. Of 83 patients who received subcutaneous injections of ribonucleic acid (10 mg every other day) for various skin diseases, three developed an erythematous edematous reaction around the injection sites after the 7th to 15th injections (1). Although patch tests were negative in all three patients, lesions were reproduced after intradermal injection in one patient.

Reference

1. Li LF. Erythematous skin reaction to subcutaneous injection of ribonucleic acid. Contact Dermatitis 1999;41(4):239.

Thalidomide

General Information

Thalidomide was synthesized in 1953 by Wilhelm Kunz and Herbert Keller, working for Chemie Grünenthal. Kunz was preparing a series of peptides for antibiotic synthesis and in doing so isolated a non-peptide by-product, which Keller recognized as an analogue of the hypnotic glutethimide. They prepared a series of further analogues, one of which was thalidomide. It was introduced as a hypnotic in the late 1950s, as a supposedly safe sedative for children and pregnant women. Besides West Germany, Great Britain was the only country in which formulations containing thalidomide were sold on a large scale during the period 1959–60 inclusive. Following the discovery of its major teratogenic effects, thalidomide was withdrawn from the market in the early 1960s.

Modern uses

Since its withdrawal, thalidomide has been found to be effective in the treatment of erythema nodosum leprosum, and in 1997 it was marketed in the USA for this indication. The mechanism of action of thalidomide is still unclear (1,2), but it has many anti-inflammatory and immunomodulatory actions in vitro and in vivo (3,4).

In dermatological practice, thalidomide has also been used to treat patients with various diseases that are unresponsive to conventional therapy. Among these are aphthous stomatitis, Behçet's disease, discoid and systemic lupus erythematosus, uremic pruritus, actinic prurigo, prurigo nodularis, sarcoidosis, adult Langerhans cell histiocytosis, erosive lichen planus, and pyoderma gangrenosum (5). There has also been research on a possible antineoplastic action of thalidomide (6), which may be produced via antiangiogenic effects or direct effects on tumor cells, such as induction of apoptosis or G1 arrest of the cell cycle, inhibition of growth factor production, regulation of interactions between tumor and stromal cells, modulation of tumor immunity, modulation of adhesion molecules, and inhibition of cyclooxygenase type 2 (7,8). The malignancies in which thalidomide has been used include multiple myeloma, glioblastoma multiforme, renal cell carcinoma, and malignant melanoma.

The use of thalidomide in dermatology is based on its immunomodulatory properties. In vitro it inhibits leukocyte chemotaxis and reduces phagocytosis by monocytes and polymorphonuclear leukocytes, without signs of cytotoxicity (9,10). The production of TNF-alpha in human monocytes is selectively inhibited by enhanced degradation of TNF-alpha messenger RNA (11). In phytohemagglutinin-activated cultures of peripheral blood mononuclear cells the production of interleukin-4 and interleukin-5 (cytokines for type 2 T helper cells) is enhanced, while interferon-gamma production is inhibited by thalidomide (12). Its antiangiogenic activity is probably the cause of its teratogenic effects (13). There is evidence that angiogenesis is increased in multiple myeloma and that thalidomide is active in refractory myeloma (14). In organ bath experiments thalidomide antagonizes the actions of histamine, 5-hydroxytryptamine, acetylcholine, and prostaglandins; neither the mechanisms nor the clinical relevance of these effects is known (15).

Stereopharmacology of thalidomide

Thalidomide is given in a racemic mixture of its two enantiomers, R-thalidomide and S-thalidomide; the former is responsible for its hypnotic effects and the latter for its immunomodulatory and teratogenic effects (16).

Formulations

The full chemical name of thalidomide is α-(N-phthalimido)glutarimide or N-(2,6-dioxopiperid-3-yl)phthalimide. It has been marketed under a wide variety of brand names, including Contergan, Distaval, Glutanon, Hippuzon, Isomin, Kedavon, Kevadon, Neurosedine, Neurosedyn, Proban M, Sedalis, Softenon, Telagan, and Telargon. It has also been used in combination with various other drugs, for example in the proprietary combinations Tensival, Valgraine (with ergotamine tartrate), and Asmaval (with ephedrine).

The development of an intravenous formulation of rac-thalidomide is problematic, because of its poor solubility and rapid degradation in aqueous media (17). However, a chemically stable solution of the separate enantiomers of thalidomide for intravenous infusion has been described.

Pharmacokinetics

Thalidomide is slowly absorbed after oral administration; after an oral dose of 100 mg the t_{max} is 2–4 hours and the C_{max} is around 1 µg/ml (16). At larger doses its poor solubility in intestinal fluids reduces its rate of absorption even further. Co-administration with a high-fat meal causes small (<10%) changes in the AUC and C_{max} but prolongs the t_{max} markedly, to about 6 hours (18).

Thalidomide is slowly and variably absorbed after rectal administration (19). The mean availability of several formulations relative to oral administration was less than 40%.

The two enantiomers of thalidomide, R and S, undergo fast chiral interconversion at physiological pH (16). The apparent clearance rates in adults are 10 l/hour for R-thalidomide and 21 l/hour for S-thalidomide; however, each has a half-life of about 5 hours, implying different volumes of distribution (70 liters for the R-enantiomer and 150 liters for the S-enantiomer). Because of rapid

interconversion, administration of R-thalidomide alone as a hypnotic would not avoid the teratogenic affects of S-thalidomide. Thalidomide does not induce its own metabolism. Its plasma protein binding is low.

The clearance of thalidomide is not altered in hepatic disease or in renal insufficiency, but hemodialysis increases it two-fold (20). Very small amounts of hydroxylated metabolites are detected in the blood and urine.

General adverse effects

Aside from teratogenicity, the main adverse effects of thalidomide include somnolence, dizziness, fatigue, tremor, rash, constipation, and edema. Although these adverse effects are generally mild and reversible, more severe adverse effects, such as peripheral neuropathy, deep vein thrombosis, and neutropenia, have occasionally been reported.

Organs and Systems

Cardiovascular

Bradycardia, hypotension, orthostatic hypotension, and dizziness have been reported with thalidomide; these effects may have been due to its central sedative effects or to vasovagal activation (21).

Of 96 patients taking thalidomide 52 had a heart rate below 60/minute at some time during follow-up and 10 developed symptomatic bradycardia; the symptoms abated with reduction of the dose in most cases (22).

Diabetic microvascular disease has been attributed to thalidomide (23).

- A 57-year-old man with type I diabetes mellitus started taking thalidomide after failed stem cell transplantation for multiple myeloma and after 10 months developed a sensory neuropathy with loss of pain sensation and ischemic changes in the legs.

The authors suggested that the antiangiogenic properties of thalidomide were implicated in the pathogenesis of diabetic foot disease in this patient.

Thromboembolic disease

> DoTS classification (BMJ 2003;327:1222–5)
> Adverse effect: Deep venous thrombosis with thalidomide
> Dose-relation: collateral effect
> Time-course: intermediate
> Susceptibility factors: genetic; diseases (multiple myeloma, lupus erythematosus); drugs (chemotherapy, especially doxorubicin; darbepoetin)

Deep venous thrombosis is a common complication of thalidomide, especially when it is used in combination with chemotherapy and in patients with multiple myeloma (24–26).

Arterial thrombosis has also been reported. Of 23 patients with myeloma who took thalidomide 150 mg/day for 142 patient-months there were seven cases of thrombosis, five venous and two arterial; in a historical control group of 18 similar patients who did not take thalidomide there was only one case over 289 months (26,27).

Incidence

Of 50 patients with multiple myeloma, 14 developed a deep venous thrombosis after taking thalidomide 400 mg/day, compared with two of 50 patients who did not take it (24) All the episodes occurred during the first 3 cycles of therapy. One patient taking thalidomide had a pulmonary embolus. Most of the patients continued to take thalidomide with the addition of low molecular weight heparin followed by warfarin and there was no progression of deep venous thrombosis.

Of 23 men with advanced androgen-dependent prostatic cancer who received docetaxel alone, none developed a venous thrombosis, compared with nine of 47 men who received docetaxel + thalidomide (28).

Susceptibility factors

The risk of thrombosis from thalidomide may be increased in certain conditions, such as malignancies, cicatricial pemphigoid (29), and systemic lupus erythematosus. Four episodes of thrombosis (two arterial, two venous) occurred in three patients with systemic lupus erythematosus and one with severe atopic dermatitis within 10 weeks of starting treatment with thalidomide 50–100 mg/day (30). All four had at least one risk factor for thrombosis, but none had thrombosis before or after treatment with thalidomide.

The incidence of deep venous thrombosis is increased by the co-administration of doxorubicin, as suggested by a study in 232 patients with multiple myeloma who received a combination of thalidomide and chemotherapy in two protocols that differed only by the inclusion of doxorubicin in one: DT-PACE (dexamethasone + thalidomide + cisplatin + doxorubicin + cyclophosphamide + etoposide) and DCEP-T (dexamethasone + cyclophosphamide + etoposide + cisplatin + thalidomide) (25). There was an increased risk of deep venous thrombosis in those who received DT-PACE but not in those who received DCEP-T. Multivariate analysis confirmed that those who received thalidomide + doxorubicin had an increased risk of deep venous thrombosis. In two separate trials in patients taking thalidomide for multiple myeloma, deep venous thrombosis occurred in four of 15 patients who received concomitant treatment with doxorubicin + dexamethasone compared with three of 45 who received dexamethasone only (26).

Of 535 patients who received thalidomide with or without cytostatic chemotherapy, 82 developed a deep venous thrombosis (31). Multivariate analysis showed that the combination of thalidomide with chemotherapy that contained doxorubicin was associated with the highest odds ratio (OR = 4.3). Newly diagnosed disease (OR = 2.5) and chromosome 11 abnormalities (OR = 1.8) were also independent predictors. After a median period of 2.9 years, survival was worse in those with chromosome 13

abnormalities, aged over 60 years, with a raised lactate dehydrogenase activity, and a raised serum creatinine concentration.

Three episodes of thrombosis occurred in patients who had taken thalidomide (25–100 mg/day) for up to 2 years (32). However, all had other risk factors (heterozygous protein C resistance in one and surgical intervention or trauma in the others), so a causal role of thalidomide was debatable.

In a trial of thalidomide in Behçet's disease there was superficial thrombophlebitis in 10 of 32 patients taking thalidomide 100 mg/day, two of 31 patients taking thalidomide 300 mg/day, and three of 32 patients taking placebo (33). The fact that this apparent increase in the incidence of thrombophlebitis in those taking 100 mg/day was not reproduced at the higher dosage suggests that the effect occurred by chance.

Management

Of 256 patients with myeloma randomized to thalidomide or not, 221 received no prophylactic anticoagulation and 35 received low-dose warfarin 1 mg/day (31). The incidence of deep venous thrombosis was higher in those who took thalidomide (hazard ratio 4.5). Warfarin did not reduce the risk, and prophylactic subcutaneous enoxaparin 40 mg/day was therefore introduced in 68 patients of a subsequent group of 130 patients who received thalidomide. This intervention eliminated the difference in the incidence of deep venous thrombosis between those who took thalidomide and those who did not.

Pulmonary hypertension

Pulmonary hypertension has been reported in one patient taking thalidomide (34).

- A 51-year-old man with multiple myeloma and a history of cardiovascular disease took thalidomide 100 mg/day and developed reversible pulmonary hypertension (pulmonary artery pressure 70 mmHg) with normal mitral valve and left ventricular function. After withdrawal of thalidomide for 2 months the pulmonary artery pressure fell to 47 mmHg. Rechallenge with a lower dose of thalidomide was again associated with a rise in pulmonary artery pressure.

Respiratory

In some early cases an increased incidence of asthmatic attacks was reported by asthmatic patients (35).

- A 65-year-old man with IgG multiple myeloma was given thalidomide and after 37 days developed acute cough, sweating, general malaise, and dyspnea at rest (36). There was an interstitial and alveolar pattern on the right side of a chest X-ray and arterial blood gases showed partial respiratory insufficiency (pH 7.40, $PaCO_2$ 40 mmHg, PaO_2 47 mmHg). Microbiology was negative (sputum and blood cultures and urinary antigen detection for *Streptococcus pneumoniae* and *Legionella pneumophila*). He recovered when thalidomide was withdrawn and oxygen and intravenous glucocorticoids were given. A chest X-ray and arterial blood gases were normal 4 days later.

Nervous system

Somnolence is very common in patients taking thalidomide, and headache, dizziness, paresthesia, and peripheral neuropathy are common. Stupor, coma, and seizures have also been reported (21). The sedative effect possibly occurs through activation of the sleep center in the brainstem. However, even when it is taken in large doses, thalidomide is not associated with lack of coordination or respiratory depression (3).

In patients with leprosy, HIV infection, and multiple myeloma, the incidences of somnolence, fatigue, and weakness were 36–43%, 48%, and 6–22% respectively (21). Administration of thalidomide at bedtime minimizes appreciation of the drowsiness that it produces, and daytime drowsiness usually abates over several weeks.

Stupor has been reported in six patients with advanced refractory malignancies, complicated by severe weakness, anemia, nausea, vomiting, and dehydration, or tumor lysis syndrome with renal insufficiency; three developed fever, neutropenia, sepsis, and/or pneumonia, but the contribution of thalidomide was uncertain (21).

Seizures, including generalized tonic-clonic seizures, have been reported in patients taking thalidomide, 18 during the first 18 months of its availability in the USA; there was a past history of seizures or pre-existing nervous system disease in 11 (21).

Polyneuropathy

DoTS classification (BMJ 2003;327:1222–5)
Adverse effect: Polyneuropathy with thalidomide
Dose-relation: Collateral reaction
Time-course: Long-term
Susceptibility factors: sex (women more susceptible); age (elderly people more susceptible)

A chronic polyneuropathy was described soon after thalidomide was introduced. It is predominantly sensory, affecting distal nerves. Anatomically the lesion is a degeneration of the axis cylinder (37).

Mechanism

In six patients with multiple myeloma who developed a thalidomide-induced sensory polyneuropathy, spinal cord MRI showed high-signal intensity in the posterior columns in only one patient, with abnormal central conduction time at somatosensory-evoked potentials (38). These results suggest that thalidomide can induce either an axonal length-dependent neuropathy or, less often, a ganglionopathy.

Clinical features

The common symptoms are tingling of the hands, gradually increasing sensory disturbances, and finally motor disturbances, usually of the hands, although only after

thalidomide has been taken over a lengthy period. A positive Babinsky reflex and disturbed vibration sense have also been reported (39). Unless the drug is discontinued promptly at the start of symptoms the polyneuropathy can be irreversible (40,41).

In 35 patients with polyneuropathy, mostly of the sensory type, which occurred after about 9 months of ingestion of thalidomide 100–200 mg/day, the principal symptoms were paresthesia and distal sensory disturbances in the feet. Withdrawal of the drug led to partial improvement, but complete resolution was not observed (42–45).

In 114 patients with thalidomide polyneuropathy other features included toxic psychosis, amnesic and aphasic symptoms, cerebellar syndromes, and autonomic dysfunction. An attempt was made to relate thalidomide toxicity to daily or total dose and duration of therapy but no association was found. The severity of the polyneuropathy was related to the age of the patient (46).

In 22 patients with thalidomide polyneuropathy, who were followed for 4–6 years after withdrawal, the symptoms and signs remained unchanged in 50% and improved in 25%; the rest recovered. Improvement was usually slow, and in some patients did not begin for 3 years (47).

- A 68-year-old woman took 20 tablets of thalidomide per month for 6 months and developed a severe peripheral neuropathy, which persisted for 3 years. Electromyography showed irreversible damage to several nerve trunks (48).

The distinguishing features of thalidomide polyneuropathy and of leprous polyneuropathy have been described. In thalidomide polyneuropathy the longest nerve fibers are affected first and the condition progressively involves fibers of decreasing length. Thus, the upper border of sensory loss in the limbs is roughly the same distance from the dorsal root ganglion cells; this can be estimated using a tape measure. Loss of tendon reflexes is also characteristic. In leprous polyneuropathy, the cells first affected are those in the coolest tissues, as *Mycobacterium leprae* is temperature-sensitive. This leads to the early involvement of the lobes of the ears, the nose, and the digits. Typically, deep reflexes are preserved (49).

Restlessness, agitation, queer sensations, difficulty in memorizing (40), and vertigo and convulsions (50) have also been reported. In nearly all cases there was a concomitant polyneuropathy. Muscle weakness or cramps, mild ataxia, carpal tunnel syndrome, and signs of pyramidal tract involvement have also been described (51).

Deterioration of the sensory nerve action potentials more than 40% from baseline may predict the development of neuropathy (51).

After withdrawal of thalidomide, symptoms are usually slow to recover, if they eventually do (3). The first symptoms of peripheral neuropathy can develop even after the withdrawal of thalidomide (33).

Incidence and susceptibility factors

The incidence of peripheral neuropathy, with symmetrical painful paresthesia of the hands and feet often accompanied by sensory loss in the legs, seems to vary with the condition that is being treated, and ranges from under 1% in patients with leprosy to over 70% in patients with prurigo nodularis (41,52). The symptoms do not correlate with either the duration of treatment or the dose. Women and elderly people seem to have an increased risk of neuropathy (53).

Incidences of 21–100% have been reported after treatment for up to 5 years (38,54–57).

Some have found no correlation between the occurrence of neuropathy and the cumulative dose (56); while others have found correlations with total dose (41,57) or daily dose. In 135 patients treated with thalidomide for various skin diseases, there were no cases in those who took daily doses of 25 mg/day or less, but the relative risk of neuropathy was 8.2 at a daily dose of 50–75 mg/day, and 20 at a daily dose of over 75 mg/day (54). It has been suggested that the risk increases at total doses over 20 g (58). Below this dose the risk of neuropathy is about 10% (57).

The incidence and susceptibility factors for thalidomide neuropathy have been studied in a prospective cohort study in 135 patients (54). Structured questionnaires were administered, standardized neurological and electrophysiological examinations were performed, and neuropathic signs and symptoms were classified by investigators who did not know the dose of thalidomide or the treatment duration. Definite thalidomide neuropathy occurred in 25% of patients, and another 30% developed atypical neuropathy, discordant clinical and electrophysiological features, or typical clinical signs without electrophysiological investigation. The only significant susceptibility factor was the daily dose: neuropathy did not develop at dosages below 25 mg/day.

Diagnosis and monitoring

Changes in nerve conductivity are frequent and predictable in thalidomide-induced neuropathy. Nerve conduction studies are required before and during therapy, irrespective of dose (55).

In 135 patients treated with thalidomide for various skin diseases who were prospectively monitored for 2 years there was clinical and electrophysiological evidence of a thalidomide-induced neuropathy in 25%; however, the neuropathy was subclinical in nearly a quarter of patients and when all potential cases were included, the rate was 56% (54). The incidence was maximal during the first year of treatment (20%).

Peripheral nerve function should be monitored by reviewing symptoms, regular neurological examination, and periodic screening of sensory nerve electrophysiology (58). If there is evidence of neuropathy, withdrawal of thalidomide should be considered; the decision should be made on an individual basis and should take into account the seriousness and severity of the underlying condition and the severity of the neuropathy.

Psychological, psychiatric

Mood changes are common with thalidomide (3). Three cases of paranoid reactions have been reported in patients with multiple myeloma taking thalidomide; however, causality was not proved (21).

- Reversible dementia occurred in a patient with multiple myeloma taking thalidomide 200 mg/day plus dexamethasone (59). Memory deficit and mania occurred about 2 months after the start of therapy and did not resolve on withdrawal of dexamethasone and administration of risperidone. The memory loss worsened and proceeded to disorientation, apraxia, and tremor 4 months after the start of therapy. The dementia resolved completely within 48 hours after withdrawal of thalidomide.

Endocrine

Hypothyroidism has occasionally been reported in patients taking thalidomide (60,61).

- A 44-year-old man with an initial TSH concentration within the reference range took thalidomide 400 mg/day for multiple myeloma and within 4 weeks developed cold intolerance, fatigue, depression, dizziness, and bradycardia, and had a markedly raised TSH (62). He was given levothyroxine and the dose of thalidomide was reduced to 200 mg/day, after which he became euthyroid.

This case prompted further investigation of thyroid function in patients with multiple myeloma. TSH concentrations were measured in 174 patients who had been randomly assigned to chemotherapy plus thalidomide 400 mg/day ($n = 92$) or chemotherapy alone ($n = 82$). After 3–4 months 18 of the patients taking thalidomide had a serum TSH concentration over 5 IU/ml, including six with a concentration over 10 IU/ml (range 12–114 IU/ml), while seven receiving chemotherapy alone had a serum TSH concentration over 5 IU/ml and none had a concentration over 10 IU/ml. In 169 patients with relapsing multiple myeloma who took thalidomide 200–800 mg/day, of those with a serum TSH concentration in the reference range to begin with, 61 had increases after 2–6 months.

Metabolism

In a placebo-controlled study in six patients with type 2 diabetes mellitus thalidomide 150 mg/day for 3 weeks reduced insulin-stimulated glucose uptake by 31% and glycogen synthesis by 48% (63). However, it had no effect on rates of glycolysis, carbohydrate oxidation, non-oxidative glycolysis, lipolysis, free fatty acid oxidation, or re-esterification. The authors concluded that thalidomide increases insulin resistance in obese patients with type 2 diabetes.

This effect can have clinical consequences. For example, in patients with prostate cancer, reducing the dose of thalidomide improved hyperglycemia, suggesting that thalidomide may have exacerbated it in the first place (64).

- A 70-year-old man with no family history of diabetes or known diabetes took thalidomide 400 mg/day for refractory multiple myeloma. He developed hyperglycemia, which had to be treated with insulin and later with glipizide GITS 5 mg/day and which responded despite continuation of thalidomide (65).

Weight gain and edema have been reported in patients taking thalidomide (3). In 13 patients with minimally symptomatic HIV disease thalidomide for 14 days caused an increase in weight of 3.6% (66).

Electrolyte balance

Severe hyperkalemia occurred in six of eight patients with multiple myeloma and moderate to severe renal insufficiency who took thalidomide 100–200 mg/day for up to 12 days; three died and one recovered after withdrawal of thalidomide (67). Hyperkalemia occurred despite the fact that most of the patients also took dexamethasone.

Fluid balance

Thalidomide can cause painful edema of the legs, which is transitory and disappears as treatment continues (68). Peripheral edema was reported in 4.2% of patients with erythema nodosum leprosum, in patients with HIV infection (3.1% of those taking 100 mg/day and 8.3% of those taking 200 mg/day), and in up to 22% of patients with refractory multiple myeloma (21).

Hematologic

Thalidomide can cause leukopenia. In controlled trials in patients with HIV infection the incidences of neutropenia were 9%, 17%, and 25% in those who took placebo, thalidomide 100 mg/day, and thalidomide 200 mg/day respectively (21).

Neutropenia occurred in 14 of 80 patients treated with thalidomide for refractory chronic graft-versus-host disease (69). The median thalidomide dose at which neutropenia developed was 200 mg qds. Erythrocyte and platelet counts were not affected. After withdrawal of thalidomide the neutropenia resolved within a month (except in three patients, who died with refractory graft-versus-host disease). Six patients were rechallenged with thalidomide and again became neutropenic.

Of 44 patients who took thalidomide for refractory multiple myeloma, 10 developed grade 3 or 4 neutropenia, usually in the first or second week of treatment (70). There was concomitant progression of thrombocytopenia in five cases and bone marrow hypoplasia without a significant increase in myeloma cell numbers in five. Neutropenia was more common in patients with low neutrophil and platelet counts, anemia, or a high percentage of plasma cells in the bone marrow before thalidomide treatment.

Of 50 Taiwanese patients with relapsed and/or refractory multiple myeloma who took thalidomide on a dose-escalation schedule, 100–800 mg/day, 18 of 22 responders had reduced leukocyte counts before there was significant reduction in M proteins, compared with only four of the 28 non-responders (71). The median time from the start of thalidomide treatment to the minimum leukocyte count was 28 (range 7–150) days, with a mean cell count of 2.19 (range 0.96–3.35) $\times 10^9$/l. The leukopenia was generally

transient, with rapid recovery despite continuation of thalidomide.

Myeloproliferative reactions have been reported in three patients with myelofibrosis taking thalidomide 200 mg/day (72). Thalidomide-associated leukemic transformation has also been reported in five patients with multiple myeloma (73).

Mouth

Xerostomia is common in patients taking thalidomide (2,3).

- An oral lichenoid eruption occurred in a 33-year-old woman after she had taken thalidomide 200 mg/day for a few days for graft-versus-host disease after bone marrow transplantation for chronic myeloid leukemia (74).

Gastrointestinal

Constipation is common in patients taking thalidomide (2,3).

Liver

Severe hepatotoxicity has been attributed to thalidomide in multiple myeloma (75) and hepatic failure can occur (21,76,77).

Four post-marketing reports of hepatic failure have been reported; one patient with multiple myeloma developed severe jaundice, hepatic failure, and coma, and died 1 month after the start of thalidomide therapy; three other patients had pre-existing liver disease, and hepatic failure and death were probably not drug-related (21).

- A 50-year-old man with history of chronic hepatitis B had transient rises in serum transaminases after two successive episodes of autologous stem cell transplantation, with spontaneous resolution; at that time PCR for hepatitis B virus was negative (76). Later he was given thalidomide and after 5 months suddenly experienced dizziness and jaundice. The concentration of hepatitis B virus DNA was 1641 pg/ml and serological tests for other viruses were negative. Despite conventional supportive care, he died of septicemic shock caused by *Klebsiella* pneumonia. Other hepatotoxic agents were excluded.
- A 58-year-old woman, with a history of chronic stable hepatitis C infection, was given thalidomide 200 mg/day for end-stage plasma cell leukemia (77). Within 1 week she developed jaundice, light-coloured stools, and marked rises in serum transaminases, which had been stable before the introduction of thalidomide. The jaundice resolved promptly on withdrawal of all drugs; other drugs besides thalidomide that might have been implicated were reintroduced without ill effects.

Skin

Rash due to thalidomide is commonly described as erythematous, macular, and pruritic; it occurs over the back, trunk, and limbs and most commonly occurs 10–14 days after the start of treatment (21). In trials of thalidomide in patients with erythema nodosum leprosum the incidence of rash was 25%, in patients with HIV infection it was 42%, and in patients with myeloma it was up to 26%.

Other skin reactions to thalidomide include pustuloderma, exfoliative reactions, and hypersensitivity reactions, including toxic epidermal necrolysis (3). The frequency of erythema nodosum was increased compared with placebo during the first 8 weeks of thalidomide therapy for Behçet's syndrome, but not thereafter (33).

Redness of the palms was observed in four of 13 patients treated with thalidomide (43). Erythroderma and peripheral eosinophilia occurred in two patients with chronic renal insufficiency who were taking thalidomide for prurigo nodularis (78).

Three of forty patients taking thalidomide for leprosy developed dermatitis herpetiformis, which was thought to have been caused by the treatment (79).

In 87 patients with multiple myeloma in an open trial given thalidomide alone ($n = 50$) or thalidomide + dexamethasone ($n = 37$), there were minor to moderate skin eruptions in 23 patients taking thalidomide alone and in 16 of those taking thalidomide + dexamethasone (80). These included morbilliform, seborrheic, maculopapular, and non-specific dermatitis. Three patients taking thalidomide + dexamethasone had severe skin reactions (exfoliative erythroderma, erythema multiforme, and toxic epidermal necrolysis) that required hospitalization and withdrawal of thalidomide.

Worsening of psoriasis has been reported in a 46-year-old woman taking thalidomide for Behçet's disease (81).

Nails

Brittle nails occurred in three patients who took thalidomide (43), and in another case brittleness was accompanied by marked ridging of the nails (82). This last patient also had amenorrhea. She was taking 50–100 mg nightly at the time.

Sexual function

Erectile dysfunction and loss of libido have occasionally been attributed to thalidomide (83).

Reproductive system

Amenorrhea

In women taking thalidomide there have been occasional reports of amenorrhea (84–89).

Four of 13 women with cutaneous lupus erythematosus (either discoid or associated with systemic disease) treated with thalidomide 100–300 mg/day had amenorrhea during the first 4–5 months of treatment (85). They had high serum concentrations of pituitary gonadotrophins, normal prolactin concentrations, and low estradiol concentrations; antiovary antibodies were not detected. In one woman an ovarian biopsy showed severe ovarian atrophy and absence of ova or follicles. In all four women menstruation resumed 2–3 months after withdrawal of thalidomide. In two women thalidomide was reintroduced: one developed oligomenorrhea again after 5 months, with high concentrations of pituitary gonadotrophins; withdrawal of thalidomide resulted in remission.

Other cases of ovarian failure in women taking thalidomide for aphthous ulcers have been described (87).

Among 21 women who took thalidomide, secondary amenorrhea occurred in four who took it for refractory cutaneous lupus erythematosus and in one who took it for aphthous ulcers (84). Menstruation resumed 2–3 months after withdrawal of thalidomide, and in one case amenorrhea recurred after reintroduction, in association with raised serum concentrations of pituitary gonadotrophins.

Four of thirteen women who took thalidomide for cutaneous lupus erythematosus developed amenorrhea (85). In one case a biopsy showed severe ovarian atrophy and absence of ova or follicles. In another case rechallenge with thalidomide 50 mg/day resulted in amenorrhea, which resolved on withdrawal.

Two young women with discoid lupus erythematosus developed amenorrhea after taking thalidomide 100–150 mg/day (86). In one patient the menstrual cycle returned to normal within 5 months after withdrawal of thalidomide; in another the dosage was reduced to 50 mg on alternate days but menstruation had not returned 6 months later.

Of seven women who took thalidomide for aphthous ulcers three developed amenorrhea (87).

- A 28-year-old woman took thalidomide 100 mg/day for Behçet's disease and after 3 months developed amenorrhea (89). She took an oral contraceptive for 8 months, but then had a deep vein thrombosis in association with a factor V Leiden mutation; the oral contraceptive was withdrawn and she was given warfarin. She remained amenorrheic. She had a raised serum concentration of follicle-stimulating hormone but all other laboratory tests were normal. Ultrasonography showed a normal uterus and an endometrial lining of 4 mm. The amenorrhea was attributed to thalidomide, which she decided to continue taking; she remained amenorrheic.

Thalidomide may destroy follicular cells by an action at follicle stimulating hormone receptors, either by directly inhibiting the binding of follicle stimulating hormone or by a post-receptor mechanism (87).

Gynecomastia

In men taking thalidomide there have been occasional reports of gynecomastia.

- A 69-year-old man developedsided gynecomastia after taking thalidomide 200 mg/day for 2 years (90). Mammography showed diffuse dense glandular right breast tissue in the retroareolar area with no discrete masses or microcalcification. He had taken no other drugs and had serum concentrations of prolactin, estradiol, and testosterone in the reference ranges. Thalidomide was withdrawn but the gynecomastia did not change during the following 3 months.
- A 55-year-old man developed unilateral gynecomastia after taking thalidomide 200 mg/day for 2 weeks (91). Mammography and ultrasonography showed an enlarged but otherwise normal mammary gland. He continued to take thalidomide for 4 months and the gynecomastia persisted.

Immunologic

Leukocytoclastic vasculitis has been reported in one of 260 patients (92).

Of 54 patients randomized to either placebo ($n = 26$) or thalidomide 200 mg/day ($n = 28$) starting 80 days after allogeneic bone marrow transplantation chronic graft-versus-host disease was significantly more common in those who took thalidomide; there was also a significant overall survival advantage in those who took placebo (93). These results suggest that while thalidomide is effective in treating chronic graft-versus-host disease, its use to prevent chronic graft-versus-host disease results in a paradoxical outcome.

Tumor lysis syndrome has been attributed to thalidomide in a 59-year-old woman with myeloma (94).

Infection risk

Disseminated infection with *Herpes simplex* virus and *Varicella zoster* virus occurred in a patient taking thalidomide for relapsed multiple myeloma (95).

Body temperature

Febrile reactions are common in patients taking thalidomide. In one study of 56 patients with HIV infection who took thalidomide for 14–21 days, 24 discontinued therapy owing to adverse reactions. Cutaneous and/or febrile reactions, which occurred in 20 patients, were the most frequent adverse effects (96).

Death

A randomized, placebo-controlled study of thalidomide in toxic epidermal necrolysis, undertaken because of the potent in vitro TNF-alpha-inhibitory properties of thalidomide, was stopped because of excess mortality in the thalidomide group (10 of 12 patients died compared with three of 10 in the placebo group) (97). There was an insignificant increase in plasma TNF-alpha in the thalidomide-treated patients on day 2.

Second-Generation Effects

Teratogenicity

Thalidomide should not be used during pregnancy because of its teratogenic effects (61,98–109). In 46 examined cases of malformations, 41 of the mothers had taken thalidomide, while in the other five cases the possibility could not be ruled out, while among 300 normal controls none of the mothers had taken thalidomide (110).

History

In the late 1950s and early 1960s thalidomide was used as a sedative in pregnant women in several countries in Europe and also distributed for trials in the USA, but was then identified as a cause of severe congenital limb malformations in many of the babies whose mothers had taken it while pregnant. The thalidomide disaster produced deep distrust in the way the public control of the effects of drugs was carried out. Suddenly, the edifices for the public control of drugs were in many countries perceived as gravely deficient and barely adapted to their purposes. People realized that drugs that were not safe could be produced by respected pharmaceutical companies, prescribed by trusted doctors, and sold by authorized pharmacies. It also became widely known that many marketed drugs were not providing their purported benefits and that claims of efficacy were barely checked by the drug regulatory authorities.

The outrage over thalidomide stimulated considerable reinforcement of the public control of drugs. In the USA, an amendment of the Food, Drug, and Cosmetic Act was approved by Congress in 1962 (111). Not only the safety but also the efficacy of drugs would henceforth be part of the criteria that the FDA used as benchmarks in decisions over whether drugs should be allowed on to the market. Since then pharmaceutical companies have had to show premarketing proof of both the safety and the efficacy of any new drug they want to introduce. Moreover, manufacturers of drugs in the USA have since 1962 had a duty to report to the FDA any information on adverse effects of their products.

At that time, existing drugs on the US market also came under scrutiny, and a review of their efficacy conducted by the US National Academy of Sciences (112) led to the voluntary withdrawal by pharmaceutical manufacturers of about two-thirds of the approximately 7100 products that the FDA had previously approved (113).

Similar legislative changes were called for in other countries, with a strong emphasis on applying the principle of premarket testing of drugs, rather than relying on random, more or less voluntary, postmarket surveillance and monitoring.

In Britain the thalidomide tragedy led to calls for a revision of the existing drug safety regulations. However, the government's position was ambiguous. It expressed a belief in the value of premarket testing of all new drugs, but did not want to move against the interests of the pharmaceutical industry. The "goose which has laid so many golden therapeutic eggs" (114) was important for the economy. Instead of creating new legislation with far-reaching requirements on the testing of new drugs, a Committee on Safety of Drugs (CSD) was appointed in 1964, expecting voluntary cooperation from the pharmaceutical industry, and its chairman asserted that it was not going to impose unnecessary restraints on the industry. Moreover, a flexible approach was to be taken regarding the efficacy of medicines. The CSD would invite reports on the toxicological testing of drugs, consider whether clinical trials should be undertaken, and assess the results in terms of safety and efficacy. It pledged that information submitted to it by the manufacturers of new drugs would be kept confidential. In its first year the CSD received 600 submissions for new drugs from pharmaceutical manufacturers. Its reviews were rapid and it rejected only a small proportion of the submissions (115).

In 1967 the Association of the British Pharmaceutical Industry (ABPI) was facing radical political proposals to abolish brand names of drugs and introduce mandatory labeling with therapeutic classifications on all medicines. To avoid legislation with mandatory rules, the ABPI revised its Code of Practice to cover the inclusion in promotional material of information on adverse effects, precautions, and contraindications (116). When the Medicines Commission was established in 1969, under the 1968 Medicines Act, to regulate the quality, safety, efficacy, and promotion of drugs, the rules of confidentiality regarding data on the effects of drugs remained in place. The Medicines Commission saw its task as integrating consideration of the pharmaceutical industry's interests with the interest of public safety (115).

In Sweden, public outrage eased the acceptance of proposals for new legislation on drug control that were pending in the Riksdag (the Swedish Parliament). A new law in 1962 (115), and subsequent regulations issued in 1963 (117), stressed the importance of controlling drug safety and efficacy. Mandatory premarket testing, with results examined by the Swedish national drug control agency, was to be the main instrument in controlling the drug market.

The thalidomide disaster led to other initiatives in many countries to create mechanisms by which doctors could easily alert colleagues to illnesses that they suspected were due to drug exposure. Such national schemes eventually led to the establishment in 1968 of the WHO Collaborating Center for International Drug Monitoring, which receives national data on adverse drug reactions and uses them to issue warnings about hazards to the medical community.

Features

Birth defects associated with the use of thalidomide during the first trimester include phocomelia, duodenal stenosis, esophageal fistula, neural tube defects, microphthalmia, deformities of the pinnae of the ears, and mid-line hemangiomas (118). A simple nevus extending from the forehead over the nose down to the upper lip is a characteristic feature. Before the introduction of thalidomide, phocomelia was a rare malformation (119).

A summary of the types of malformations that can occur is given in Table 1, based on 14 necropsies at the Pathological Institute, University of Hamburg (120).

The commonest abnormalities are agenesis or malformations of the upper and lower limbs; the eyes, ears, and internal organs can also be involved (108). Of 285 cases, 251 had upper-limb defects and 146 upper-limb defects alone. In 92 cases both the upper and lower limbs were affected and in five cases only the lower limbs were involved. Syndactyly and polydactyly were common. In some cases the hands and feet were attached directly to the trunk. Occasionally all four limbs are virtually absent. In 21 cases the ears were imperfectly developed without impaired hearing. In another series, in 50% of cases only the arms were involved; in 25% both arms and legs; in 16% the external ear was absent (121). In 303 cases, 37 other defects were observed, the biggest single group being cardiac abnormalities; congenital anomalies of the gut were also noted (119,122).

Of 96 children with congenital limb deformities who were born in 1962–63, 68 had a history of thalidomide administration during the first trimester (123). The results are summarized in Table 2. In addition, electroencephalographic examination of 71 of the children showed abnormalities in 32 of 48 cases with a history of thalidomide administration, and 12 of 23 in those who had not been exposed to the drug.

In another series of 22 cases there were anomalies of the heart ($n = 5$), anomalies of the external ear ($n = 4$), duodenal atresia ($n = 6$), anomalies of the urinary tract ($n = 5$), and microphthalmia, imperforate anus, and internal hydrocephalus ($n = 1$ each) (102,104).

Three cases of congenital limb deformity after the administration of thalidomide-containing formulations during the first trimester were the first of this kind to be reported from the UAR and Kuwait(124).

Children exposed to thalidomide appear to be shorter than normal children, but growth rates are relatively normal (125).

Duodenal stenosis and left-sided hydronephrosis and hydroureter due to an abnormal opening of the left ureter into the bladder have been reported associated with phocomelia in a 5-month-old male infant. The mother had taken thalidomide in early pregnancy (126).

The differential diagnosis between the Stilling–Türk–Duanesches syndrome and thalidomide embryopathy has been detailed, following a review of the case history of a boy with multiple congenital abnormalities (127).

Cardiovascular

- A 29-year-old primipara was delivered of a female infant who died 30 hours later after increasingly severe attacks of cyanosis. Postmortem a cor triloculare was found. The mother had taken thalidomide 25 mg on the day of conception and afterwards on average 3 tablets a week for 5 weeks, the last tablet on the 35th day of pregnancy (128).

Ear, nose, and throat

Ear defects occurred in a child whose mother took a thalidomide-containing formulation in the early months of pregnancy. The abnormalities included absence of both auricles, hypoplasia of the middle ear, deafness, ophthalmoplegia of the right eye, and retarded mental development (129).

Nervous system

In some cases the central nervous system may have been affected (109,130,131), and cranial nerve palsies have been reported (132). In a survey of ear deformities attributed to thalidomide (133) there were also 19 cases of seventh cranial nerve lesions and 18 cases of sixth nerve lesions (134).

Sensory systems

Ocular malformations, including aplasia of the macula, choroidal colobomata, microphthalmos, and extraocular muscle paresis have been attributed to thalidomide taken in early pregnancy (135). Ocular defects have been

Table 1 A summary of the malformations caused by thalidomide

Abnormality		Number
Cardiovascular	Anomalies of the heart and arteries	10
	Fallot's tetralogy	5
	Ventricular septal defect	4
Respiratory	Bilobed right lung	5
Ear, nose, and throat	Anomalies of the external ear	7
Sensory systems	Microphthalmia	2
Gastrointestinal	Duodenal atresia	4
	Agenesis of appendix and cecum	5
	Malrotation	7
	Imperforate anus	1
Liver	Abnormal lobulation of the right lobe of the liver	5
Biliary tract	Absent gallbladder	8
	Atresia of the common bile duct	3
Urinary tract	Anomalies of the urinary tract	10
Skin	Facial nevus	1
Musculoskeletal	Hypogenesis or agenesis of long bones	5
	Phocomelia	4
	Defects of metacarpal and phalanges only	3
	Amelia	2
Reproductive function	Bicornuate uterus	5 (of 8 female children)
	Atresia or absence of the vagina	3

Table 2 Abnormalities in children with congenital limb deformities

	Thalidomide taken in first trimester	No history of thalidomide exposure
Number of cases	68	28
Limb abnormality alone	13	17
Congenital heart disease	14	1
Abnormality of urogenital system	43	3
Abnormality of alimentary system	18	5
Hydrocephalus and meningocele	4	2

reported in four of 21 thalidomide children examined in Canada; there was strabismus in two cases, congenital blepharoptosis in one, and ocular muscle palsies associated with other central nervous system damage in one (136).

Hematologic
Panmyelophthisis, with additional features resembling the Fanconi syndrome, has been reported after the administration of thalidomide in the first months of pregnancy (137).

Mouth, teeth
Dental examination of 40 children in Stockholm with thalidomide embryopathy showed hypodontia and disturbances of mineralization. In addition, children with very shortened forelimbs are more susceptible to tooth injury when they fall (138,139).

Cleft deformities of the face are more common in thalidomide children than in other children. Two cases of cleft lip and palate have been attributed to thalidomide taken in early pregnancy (140). There was a cleft lip and/or palate in three of 161 cases in Hamburg and in six of 918 cases seen in other centers. These deformities are usually associated with ear deformities, an association that was observed before the introduction of thalidomide (141).

Gastrointestinal
Agenesis of the appendix due to thalidomide can cause acute abdominal pain and tenderness (142,143). In two cases of anal stenosis the malformation was isolated and of the type due to incomplete rupture of the anal membrane; there were no malformations of the extremities (144).

Excessive sweating has been seen in thalidomide-deformed children (143,145). In some patients, small doses of ascorbic acid (50 mg daily) are helpful in this condition (143).

Musculoskeletal
Two cases of Perthe's disease have been reported in children with congenital abnormalities after thalidomide ingestion by the mother during the first trimester (146).

Thalidomide can cause growth disturbance at the upper end of the femur.

Frequency

The numbers of babies with phocomelia seen in university clinics in Germany and a few clinics in England are listed in Table 3 (119).

However, it is difficult to calculate how often dysmelic malformations occur in relation to the number of pregnant women who have taken thalidomide (101,103). In Hamburg 0.17% of all neonates had such malformations. Other reports state that about 20% of expectant mothers who had taken thalidomide in the early months gave birth to an abnormal infant (104,147).

The total number of afflicted children in the Rhineland and Westphalia alone before thalidomide was withdrawn was estimated at 1500–2000 (104,119,147). In England and Wales the number of cases was calculated to be at least 800 (148).

The frequency in Bonn in 1962 was 3.56 per 1000 of all newborn children (200 times the frequency in 1960–61). In Liverpool, the frequency during 1960 and 1961 was lower (0.778 per 1000), but nevertheless considerably higher than in other countries. Cases have been reported from Australia, Scotland, and Sweden(149). The USA was relatively free from this adverse effect, since thalidomide (as Kevadon) failed to pass the Food and Drug Administration because of another adverse effect, namely polyneuropathy(119).

It was estimated that 10 000 deformed children were born in West Germany before thalidomide was withdrawn; of these, 4000 are believed to have survived. In Japan there were believed to be 1000 thalidomide children; in England 400; in the Scandinavian countries 280; in Canada 200; in Belgium 60; and 25 in the Netherlands. From 1958 to 1961, 223 kg of thalidomide were marketed in Austria; during this period 19 children were born showing abnormalities compatible with the dysmelia syndrome.

Dose relation

The actual dose of thalidomide taken is not as important as the fact of its ingestion (103,104,147). Neither the duration of administration of thalidomide nor the total dose was related to the teratogenic risk (77,119). Some cases have been observed after the ingestion of only 1, 2, or 3 tablets (150).

A baby with micromelia of all four limbs was born to a woman who had taken only a single dose of thalidomide 200 mg in the first weeks of pregnancy (151). In two other cases the total dose was less than 125 mg (152).

In one case the question arose as to whether ingestion of thalidomide by the father previous to or at the time of conception could have played a role (153).

- A baby was born with bilateral absence of radii and thumbs. The mother denied having taken thalidomide or any other drug. The father had been receiving thalidomide for some six months before the conception of the child.

However, the taking of a single sleeping tablet by the mother could easily have been forgotten in this case. Nevertheless, in one study in rabbits the effect on the offspring of the administration of thalidomide to the male parent was studied (154). It was concluded that in rabbits of a cross-bred colony of high fertility there was a deleterious effect on the progeny ascribable to paternal treatment with thalidomide.

Time course

During a 1-year period, 10 babies with major limb defects were born in Stirlingshire maternity units. At least eight of the mothers had had thalidomide prescribed in the early weeks of pregnancy (59,98–101).

The critical phase for teratogenic effects of thalidomide is from the 27th to the 40th day after conception or from the 37th to the 54th day after the first day of the last menstrual period (155). In 12 of 86 cases the date of conception was fairly well known and the narrowest interval of time that spanned the taking of thalidomide was from the 27th to the 44th day after conception (150). In 205 cases, the mothers that were able to give precise accounts of the timing of administration of thalidomide had taken it from the 31st to 39th day from the first day of

Table 3　Numbers of babies with phocomelia in Germany and Britain

Place	1949–59	1959	1960	1961	Total (1959–61)
Bonn	—	2	19	50	71
Bremen	—	—	4	20	24
Frankfurt	—	1	4	11	16
Göttingen	—	3	1	10	14
Hamburg (Lens)	—	1	16	57	74
Hamburg (clinics)	—	1	30	154	185
Heidelberg	—	2	5	9	16
Kiel	—	2	4	26	32
Munich	3	2	14	44	60
Munster	4	3	27	96	126
Birmingham	—	—	4	13	17
Liverpool	—	—	8	25	33
Stirling	—	—	—	—	—

their last menstrual period, and in two cases they had taken only two tablets at 36–39 days (156).

In contrast, one woman gave birth to a baby with typical abnormalities after having taken thalidomide for 2 months before conception but only during the first 3 weeks of pregnancy (157).

Experimental data

Experimental work on thalidomide is complicated by the fact that different species respond in different ways to the drug (158). For example, oral thalidomide 25–200 mg/kg/day in rabbits produced a large number of fetal abnormalities, whereas very few occurred in rats. In contrast, after intravenous injection of thalidomide dissolved in propylene glycol or dimethylsulfoxide, abnormalities were produced in both species with doses as low as 2.5–10 mg/kg/day in rabbits, and 10 mg/kg/day in rats (159).

In vitro experiments

In leukocyte cultures, thalidomide is a potential antimitotic agent (160). There was a reduction in the percentage of lymphocytes transformed into the "blast" and "intermediate" types. The cells showed morphological abnormalities: pyknotic changes, chromatin clumping, and perinuclear pink halo of cytoplasm.

Mesanephric tissue from human embryos is normally capable of producing cartilage in vitro. However, when chondrogenic tissues from human embryos aged 5–8.5 weeks were exposed to thalidomide, it interfered with this process and the authors suggested that it may have a specific effect on similar tissues in vivo, accounting for the types of malformation of the fetus that have been observed (161).

Chickens

When chick eggs were injected with thalidomide, gross malformations were found only in the thalidomide-treated group after breeding; they affected 20% of the chickens and included encephalocele, anencephaly, microphthalmia, beak malformations, deformities of the jaw and legs (128).

In chick embryos, malformations were induced by introducing thalidomide into the amniotic cavity. However, other types of traumatic procedures similarly resulted in abnormalities (162).

Changes in the mitochondria of the endothelial cells of the axial limb bud artery occurred in chick embryos after treatment with thalidomide (163). However, there were no macroscopic abnormalities in chicks after thalidomide administration.

Thalidomide caused profound alterations in the morphogenesis of the encephalon in the developing chick embryo in vitro. Platyneuria occurred in 82% compared with 23% in the control group. Thalidomide has an inhibitory effect on growth, as measured by failure of closure of the neural plate, which can be reversed by the addition of ATP to the cultures (164).

The action of thalidomide on the production of limb abnormalities in the chick are similar to those produced by nitrogen mustard(165). Only mesodermal tissues are affected; differentiation is arrested and the mesodermal cells regroup beneath the ectodermal cap. The latter no longer induces development of the proximal portion of the limb, but only of its terminal part, which explains the occurrence of phocomelia.

Dogs

Of nine dogs treated with thalidomide 100 mg/kg/day in the first 3 weeks of pregnancy, three had no litters at all. Of a total of 30 pups, 19 appeared normal, two were stillborn and four died within 48 hours (of these six, two had malformations), and five survived for some days but had an abnormal tail bone (166).

Mice

In mice treated with thalidomide there was a marked reduction in litter size (167). The young had congenital anomalies, such as cleft lip, microphthalmia and malformation of the tail, in a frequency of 5–10%.

There was a high incidence (17.5%) of abnormal embryos in mice treated during the sixth to eighth days of pregnancy, whilst thalidomide-treated animals had a higher incidence of fetal resorption (168). Others, however, failed to find any malformations or other adverse effects when using doses ranging from 2 mg/kg up to 400 mg/kg (169).

In random-bred Charles River strain albino mice, thalidomide 1000 mg/kg/day given from the first day of mating failed to produce gross malformations of the offspring (170).

Monkeys

In seven pregnancies in monkeys, one normal fetus was obtained, four had deformities, and two had teratomas (171).

Rabbits

In rabbits treated with thalidomide there was a marked reduction in litter size (167). The frequency of malformations (encephalocele, anencephaly) was 30%. Experiments with thalidomide on pregnant rabbits showed that the young invariably showed deformities similar to those seen in humans (172).

In rabbits, malformations were found with doses of 5 mg/kg/day, 150 mg/kg/day, and 500 mg/day, given between the seventh and eleventh days of pregnancy. There were abnormalities of the extremities, skull, nose, and palate, as well as malformations of the kidneys. There seemed to be an increase in frequency with higher doses (173).

When 10 pregnant New Zealand white rabbits were fed thalidomide from the eighth to the eleventh days of pregnancy in doses of 150 mg/kg, 59 fetuses were produced, of which 56 were malformed. The 11 control rabbits gave birth to 94 normal fetuses (174).

In six male rabbits of proven fertility treated with 0.75–2.5 g of thalidomide for 10–21 days before mating, three of forty experimental matings did not result in pregnancies; six litters had five or fewer offspring; there was gross abnormality of one male offspring in each of two different litters fathered by the same male; eight litters showed total loss of young and in another eight litters there was marked loss of young by day 14 of the postnatal period (154).

Rabbits have been found to be very sensitive to the action of thalidomide, but the types of abnormality produced vary with the strain of rabbit. In hybrid rabbits, in which the pregnant doe received thalidomide in a dose of 150 mg/kg on days 7–13, 13% of the young were deformed (175). Apart from the femur, only preaxial structures of both forelimbs and hind limbs were affected. Abnormalities were of both the supernumerary and reduction types. In contrast, only abnormalities of the forelimbs occurred in the New Zealand white strain of rabbits under the same dosage schedule (176). The pattern of these limb defects bore no resemblance to spontaneously occurring deformities, and it is suggested it is a characteristic pattern for the drug.

In Chinchilla and New Zealand white rabbits, thalidomide 150 mg/kg on days 6–15 of pregnancy caused increased incidences of conceptions undergoing resorption and of fetal malformations, and reductions in litter size and body weight of the 28-day fetuses; 22% of fetuses were deformed, with abnormalities affecting the locomotor, nervous, cutaneous, ocular, respiratory, and renal systems (177).

In liver-damaged rabbits, thalidomide 150 mg/kg on days 7–12 of pregnancy produced an 80% rate of fetal abnormalities. The teratogenic activity correlated with high blood and tissue concentrations of thalidomide (178). There was no correlation between the dose of thalidomide and blood thalidomide concentration in healthy rabbits (179).

Experimental work in six strains of rabbit showed that defective evolution of the spiral septum underlay many of the cardiac abnormalities. Incomplete evidence in the literature suggests the same effect may be present in human cardiac deformities (180).

A synthetic analogue of thalidomide, methyl-4-phthalimido-DL-glutamate, was teratogenic in rabbits (181).

Rats

In rats treated with thalidomide, congenital malformations were not seen, but the number of young per litter was reduced by 33% (167).

In rats thalidomide produced abnormalities of the ossification centers of the sternum and cervical vertebrae (182). These changes in ossification centers were more easily found after small doses than with large doses, since in the latter many of the young do not survive until birth.

In Wistar rats that received thalidomide 0.5–1% in the diet for periods from 9 days before mating up to the 20th day of pregnancy, 1% thalidomide produced the greatest number of fetal resorptions and extensive defects of ossification of thoracic centers, sternebrae, and pelvic girdles. Of 170 observed malformations, 150 (82%) occurred in rats treated with thalidomide before mating. The authors

suggested that thalidomide may have a gonadal effect (183).

A histochemical study of the development of the sternum in thalidomide-treated rats showed increased storage of glycogen and reduced or absent alkaline phosphatase activity. These changes resulted in a delay in calcification of cartilage (184).

There were no macroscopic abnormalities in rats after thalidomide administration, although the number of resorption sites in the latter after 18 days gestation was increased (171).

Mechanisms

The mechanism by which thalidomide causes fetal abnormalities is not known. There is a high incidence of fetal resorption, but the cause of this is not known; it could be secondary to an abnormality of the fetus.

The more marked effect of thalidomide on some systems, for example the nervous system, the fetus, and erythrocytes, may be due to differing membrane permeabilities of different tissues to the drug (185). From a study of five head autopsies, and electroencephalographic and neurological findings in 17 individuals with the thalidomide embryopathy, it has been suggested that the action of thalidomide is not confined to mesoblastic tissue (186). This is especially true in children with an aural embryopathy. Cytogenic examination of mitotic cells in five children with ear deformities showed that the proportion of non-modal chromosomes was not greater than 10% and there were no structural changes in single chromosomes (187).

The abnormality of the ossification centers found in the rat could be connected with abnormal development of long bones. Radiographs of the limbs of 92 children with deformities due to thalidomide showed joint changes similar to those in neuropathic (Charcot's) joints in adults. The authors suggested that thalidomide causes joint changes by causing an embryonic sensory neuropathy. This hypothesis can be extended to explain other visceral and congenital malformations (188).

Thalidomide prolongs the survival time of skin homografts in the mouse, and the mechanism involved is thought to be immunosuppressive, because of the inhibition of the appearance of immunoblasts in the regional lymph nodes (189). The fetus is immunogenetically a homograft, and an early spontaneous abortion is homograft rejection. Thalidomide may therefore act by preventing spontaneous abortions, allowing damaged fetuses to reach term. If this were so, the abortion rate of those women who took thalidomide should be reduced (190). However, thalidomide has a direct toxic action on the pre-implantation blastocyst, especially the embryonic disc, and the immunological theory also cannot be reconciled with the fact that thalidomide produced teratogenic effects when given to the male rabbit before mating (191).

It has been suggested that thalidomide acts by a toxic action on the initial nerve impulses in the organogenetic phase of development due to accumulation of the drug in the nervous system of the embryo (192).

It has been suggested that in some way, thalidomide interferes with the action of certain of the B vitamins, that as a result of this antagonism fetal damage can occur, and that in the adult there may be a link between this effect and the polyneuropathy that thalidomide can cause (193). Thalidomide and its two isoglutamine derivatives caused an increase in sensitivity of intracellular hemoglobin to oxidation by nitrite ions in rats; simultaneous administration of pyridoxine and riboflavin prevented or corrected this change (185).

Prevention

Women of child-bearing age should take steps not to become pregnant while taking thalidomide, for example by using reliable contraception. If a woman taking thalidomide misses a menstrual period, thalidomide should be withdrawn for at least 9 weeks (120). Counseling about therapeutic abortion will be necessary.

Susceptibility Factors

The incidences of polyneuropathy and hypersensitivity reactions seem to be higher in HIV-infected patients (2,93).

Drug–Drug Interactions

Darbepoetin

In a study of the combination of thalidomide 100 mg/day with darbepoetin alfa 2.25 mg/kg/day in patients with myelodysplastic syndromes, there was an unexpectedly high incidence of thromboembolic events (194). Of the first seven patients enrolled, two developed deep vein thromboses and one died of a massive pulmonary embolus. The authors concluded that thalidomide may increase the thromboembolic risk associated with erythropoietic proteins in patients with myelodysplastic syndromes.

Dexamethasone

An interaction of thalidomide with dexamethasone has been postulated (195).

- A 64-year-old man with myeloma took dexamethasone and thalidomide 200 mg/day for 14 days and had no adverse effects. The dosage was increased to 400 mg/day and 10 days later a rash occurred; thalidomide was withdrawn. Within 3 days he developed toxic epidermal necrolysis.

Two other patients of eight who received thalidomide plus dexamethasone for multiple myeloma had unexpected severe skin rashes, including one who became seriously ill with erythroderma. Both recovered fully after thalidomide was withdrawn.

Docetaxel

The increased risk of venous thromboembolism in patients taking thalidomide and docetaxel is discussed in the cardiovascular section.

Sedative drugs

Thalidomide enhances the sedative actions of alcohol, barbiturates, chlorpromazine, and reserpine (118), perhaps by additive effects on their several pharmacodynamic actions (196), although other mechanisms have been described (197).

Sex steroids

Thalidomide does not interact with ethinylestradiol or norethindrone (198).

References

1. Calabrese L, Fleischer AB. Thalidomide: current and potential clinical applications. Am J Med 2000;108(6):487–95.
2. Gunzler V. Thalidomide in human immunodeficiency virus (HIV) patients. A review of safety considerations. Drug Saf 1992;7(2):116–34.
3. Tseng S, Pak G, Washenik K, Pomeranz MK, Shupack JL. Rediscovering thalidomide: a review of its mechanism of action, side effects, and potential uses. J Am Acad Dermatol 1996;35(6):969–79.
4. Koch HP. Thalidomide and congeners as anti-inflammatory agents. Prog Med Chem 1985;22:165–242.
5. Stirling DI. Thalidomide and its impact in dermatology. Semin Cutan Med Surg 1998;17(4):231–42.
6. Woodyatt B. Thalidomide. Lancet 1962;1:750.
7. Hattori Y, Iguchi T. Thalidomide for the treatment of multiple myeloma. Congenit Anom (Kyoto) 2004;44(3):125–36.
8. Fanelli M, Sarmiento R, Gattuso D, Carillio G, Capaccetti B, Vacca A, Roccaro AM, Gasparini G. Thalidomide: a new anticancer drug? Expert Opin Investig Drugs 2003;12(7):1211–25.
9. Faure M, Thivolet J, Gaucherand M. Inhibition of PMN leukocytes chemotaxis by thalidomide. Arch Dermatol Res 1980;269(3):275–80.
10. Barnhill RL, Doll NJ, Millikan LE, Hastings RC. Studies on the anti-inflammatory properties of thalidomide: effects on polymorphonuclear leukocytes and monocytes. J Am Acad Dermatol 1984;11(5 Pt 1):814–9.
11. Moreira AL, Sampaio EP, Zmuidzinas A, Frindt P, Smith KA, Kaplan G. Thalidomide exerts its inhibitory action on tumor necrosis factor alpha by enhancing mRNA degradation. J Exp Med 1993;177(6):1675–80.
12. McHugh SM, Rifkin IR, Deighton J, Wilson AB, Lachmann PJ, Lockwood CM, Ewan PW. The immunosuppressive drug thalidomide induces T helper cell type 2 (Th2) and concomitantly inhibits Th1 cytokine production in mitogen- and antigen-stimulated human peripheral blood mononuclear cell cultures. Clin Exp Immunol 1995;99(2):160–7.
13. D'Amato RJ, Loughnan MS, Flynn E, Folkman J. Thalidomide is an inhibitor of angiogenesis. Proc Natl Acad Sci USA 1994;91(9):4082–5.
14. Rajkumar SV, Witzig TE. A review of angiogenesis and antiangiogenic therapy with thalidomide in multiple myeloma. Cancer Treat Rev 2000;26(5):351–62.
15. Hastings RC, Morales MJ, Shannon EJ. Studies on the mechanism of action of thalidomide in leprosy. Pharmacologist 1976;18:218.
16. Eriksson T, Bjorkman S, Hoglund P. Clinical pharmacology of thalidomide. Eur J Clin Pharmacol 2001;57(5):365–76.
17. Eriksson T, Bjorkman S, Roth B, Hoglund P. Intravenous formulations of the enantiomers of thalidomide:

pharmacokinetic and initial pharmacodynamic characterization in man. J Pharm Pharmacol 2000;52(7):807–17.

18. Teo SK, Scheffler MR, Kook KA, Tracewell WG, Colburn WA, Stirling DI, Thomas SD. Thalidomide dose proportionality assessment following single doses to healthy subjects. J Clin Pharmacol 2001;41(6):662–7.

19. Eriksson T, Wallin R, Hoglund P, Roth B, Qi Z, Ostraat O, Bjorkman S. Low bioavailability of rectally administered thalidomide. Am J Health Syst Pharm 2000;57(17):1607–10.

20. Eriksson T, Hoglund P, Turesson I, Waage A, Don BR, Vu J, Scheffler M, Kaysen GA. Pharmacokinetics of thalidomide in patients with impaired renal function and while on and off dialysis. J Pharm Pharmacol 2003;55(12):1701–6.

21. Clark TE, Edom N, Larson J, Lindsey LJ. Thalomid (thalidomide) capsules: a review of the first 18 months of spontaneous postmarketing adverse event surveillance, including off-label prescribing. Drug Saf 2001;24(2):87–117.

22. Fahdi IE, Gaddam V, Saucedo JF, Kishan CV, Vyas K, Deneke MG, Razek H, Thorn B, Bissett JK, Anaissie EJ, Barlogie B, Mehta JL. Bradycardia during therapy for multiple myeloma with thalidomide. Am J Cardiol 2004;93(8):1052–5.

23. Pitini V, Arrigo C, Aloi G, Azzarello D, La Gattuta G. Diabetic foot disease in a patient with multiple myeloma receiving thalidomide. Haematologica 2002;87(2):ELT07.

24. Zangari M, Anaissie E, Barlogie B, Badros A, Desikan R, Gopal AV, Morris C, Toor A, Siegel E, Fink L, Tricot G. Increased risk of deep-vein thrombosis in patients with multiple myeloma receiving thalidomide and chemotherapy. Blood 2001;98(5):1614–5.

25. Zangari M, Siegel E, Barlogie B, Anaissie E, Saghafifar F, Fassas A, Morris C, Fink L, Tricot G. Thrombogenic activity of doxorubicin in myeloma patients receiving thalidomide: implications for therapy. Blood 2002;100(4):1168–71.

26. Osman K, Comenzo R, Rajkumar SV. Deep venous thrombosis and thalidomide therapy for multiple myeloma. N Engl J Med 2001;344(25):1951–2.

27. Bowcock SJ, Rassam SM, Ward SM, Turner JT, Laffan M. Thromboembolism in patients on thalidomide for myeloma. Hematology 2002;7(1):51–3.

28. Horne MK 3rd, Figg WD, Arlen P, Gulley J, Parker C, Lakhani N, Parnes H, Dahut WL. Increased frequency of venous thromboembolism with the combination of docetaxel and thalidomide in patients with metastatic androgen-independent prostate cancer. Pharmacotherapy 2003;23(3):315–8.

29. Howell E, Johnson SM. Venous thrombosis occurring after initiation of thalidomide for the treatment of cicatricial pemphigoid. J Drugs Dermatol 2004;3(1):83–5.

30. Flageul B, Wallach D, Cavelier-Balloy B, Bachelez H, Carsuzaa F, Dubertret L. Thalidomide et thromboses. [Thalidomide and thrombosis.] Ann Dermatol Venereol 2000;127(2):171–4.

31. Zangari M, Barlogie B, Thertulien R, Jacobson J, Eddleman P, Fink L, Fassas A, Van Rhee F, Talamo G, Lee CK, Tricot G. Thalidomide and deep vein thrombosis in multiple myeloma: risk factors and effect on survival. Clin Lymphoma 2003;4(1):32–5.

32. Pouaha J, Martin S, Trechot P, Truchetet F, Barbaud A, Schmutz JL. Thalidomide et thromboses: trois observations. [Thalidomide and thrombosis: three observations.] Presse Méd 2001;30(20):1008–9.

33. Hamuryudan V, Mat C, Saip S, Ozyazgan Y, Siva A, Yurdakul S, Zwingenberger K, Yazici H. Thalidomide in the treatment of the mucocutaneous lesions of the Behçet

syndrome. A randomized, double-blind, placebo-controlled trial. Ann Intern Med 1998;128(6):443–50.

34. Younis TH, Alam A, Paplham P, Spangenthal E, McCarthy P. Reversible pulmonary hypertension and thalidomide therapy for multiple myeloma. Br J Haematol 2003;121(1):191–2.

35. Mellin GW, Katzenstein M. The saga of thalidomide. Neuropathy to embryopathy, with case reports of congenital anomalies. N Engl J Med 1962;267:1184–92.

36. Carrion Valero F, Bertomeu Gonzalez V. Toxicidad pulmonar por talidomida. [Lung toxicity due to thalidomide.] Arch Bronconeumol 2002;38(10):492–4.

37. Seitelberger F. Thalidomid-poly-neuropathie. [Thalidomide polyneuropathy. Clinical biopsy studies.] Wien Klin Wochenschr 1968;80(3):41–3.

38. Isoardo G, Bergui M, Durelli L, Barbero P, Boccadoro M, Bertola A, Ciaramitaro P, Palumbo A, Bergamasco B, Cocito D. Thalidomide neuropathy: clinical, electrophysiological and neuroradiological features. Acta Neurol Scand 2004;109(3):188–93.

39. Broser F. [Polyneuritis and funicular myelosis after Contergan use.]Med Klin 1962;57:53–7.

40. Frenkel H. [Contergan—side effects. Central nervous system manifestations and polyneuritic symptoms in long-term medication with N-phthalyl glutamic acid imide.]Med Welt 1961;18:970–5.

41. Wulff CH, Hoyer H, Asboe-Hansen G, Brodthagen H. Development of polyneuropathy during thalidomide therapy. Br J Dermatol 1985;112(4):475–80.

42. Voss R. Nil nocere! Contergan–Polyneuritis. [Nil nocere. Contergan polyneuritis.] Münch Med Wochenschr 1961;103:1431–2.

43. Fullerton PM, Kremer M. Neuropathy after intake of thalidomide (Distaval). BMJ 1961;5256:855–8.

44. Hultsch EG, Hartmann J. Nil nocere! Die Thalidomid (Contergan) Polyneuritis. [Nil nocere. Thalidomide (Contergan) polyneuritis.] Münch Med Wochenschr 1961 Nov 3;103:2141–4.

45. Becker J. [Polyneuritis due to contergan.] Nervenarzt 1961;32:321–3.

46. Gibbels E. Toxische Schäden bei der Thalidomid-Medikation. [Toxic injuries in thalidomide medication.] Fortschr Neurol Psychiatr Grenzgeb 1967;35(8):393–411.

47. Fullerton PM, O'Sullivan DJ. Thalidomide neuropathy: a clinical electrophysiological, and histological follow-up study. J Neurol Neurosurg Psychiatry 1968;31(6):543–51.

48. Broser F, Hopf HC, Hohl J. Frage der Dauerschädigung bei der Contergan–Polyneuropathie und bei anderen Polyneuropathien bzw. Polyneuritiden. [Problems of permanent damage in Contergan polyneuropathy and other polyneuropathies or polyneuritides. Results of clinical and electromyographic follow ups.] Nervenarzt 1969;40(1):33–5.

49. Sabin TD. Thalidomine neuropathy and leprous neuritis. Lancet 1974;1(7849):165–6.

50. Schiefer I. [On clinical experiences with Contergan in tuberculous children.]Med Welt 1960;52–53:2765–8.

51. Gardner-Medwin JM, Smith NJ, Powell RJ. Clinical experience with thalidomide in the management of severe oral and genital ulceration in conditions such as Behçet's disease: use of neurophysiological studies to detect thalidomide neuropathy. Ann Rheum Dis 1994;53(12):828–32.

52. Clemmensen OJ, Olsen PZ, Andersen KE. Thalidomide neurotoxicity. Arch Dermatol 1984;120(3):338–41.

53. Ochonisky S, Verroust J, Bastuji-Garin S, Gherardi R, Revuz J. Thalidomide neuropathy: incidence and clinico-

electrophysiologic findings in 42 patients. Arch Dermatol 1994;130(1):66–9.

54. Bastuji-Garin S, Ochonisky S, Bouche P, Gherardi RK, Duguet C, Djerradine Z, Poli F, Revuz JThalidomide Neuropathy Study Group. Incidence and risk factors for thalidomide neuropathy: a prospective study of 135 dermatologic patients. J Invest Dermatol 2002;119(5):1020–6.

55. Harland CC, Steventon GB, Marsden JR. Thalidomide-induced neuropathy and genetic differences in drug metabolism. Eur J Clin Pharmacol 1995;49(1–2):1–6.

56. Briani C, Zara G, Rondinone R, Della Libera S, Ermani M, Ruggero S, Ghirardello A, Zampieri S, Doria A. Thalidomide neurotoxicity: prospective study in patients with lupus erythematosus. Neurology 2004;62(12):2288–90.

57. Cavaletti G, Beronio A, Reni L, Ghiglione E, Schenone A, Briani C, Zara G, Cocito D, Isoardo G, Ciaramitaro P, Plasmati R, Pastorelli F, Frigo M, Piatti M, Carpo M. Thalidomide sensory neurotoxicity: a clinical and neurophysiologic study. Neurology 2004;62(12):2291–3.

58. Apfel SC, Zochodne DW. Thalidomide neuropathy: too much or too long? Neurology 2004;62(12):2158–9.

59. Morgan AE, Smith WK, Levenson JL. Reversible dementia due to thalidomide therapy for multiple myeloma. N Engl J Med 2003;348(18):1821–2.

60. Simpson JA. Myxoedema after thalidomide. BMJ 1962;1:55.

61. Lillicrap DA. Myxoedema after thalidomide (Distaval). BMJ 1962;1:477.

62. Badros AZ, Siegel E, Bodenner D, Zangari M, Zeldis J, Barlogie B, Tricot G. Hypothyroidism in patients with multiple myeloma following treatment with thalidomide. Am J Med 2002;112(5):412–3.

63. Iqbal N, Zayed M, Boden G. Thalidomide impairs insulin action on glucose uptake and glycogen synthesis in patients with type 2 diabetes. Diabetes Care 2000;23(8):1172–6.

64. Figg WD, Arlen P, Gulley J, Fernandez P, Noone M, Fedenko K, Hamilton M, Parker C, Kruger EA, Pluda J, Dahut WL. A randomized phase II trial of docetaxel (Taxotere) plus thalidomide in androgen-independent prostate cancer. Semin Oncol 2001;28(4 Suppl 15):62–6.

65. Pathak RD, Jayaraj K, Blonde L. Thalidomide-associated hyperglycemia and diabetes: case report and review of literature. Diabetes Care 2003;26(4):1322–3.

66. Haslett P, Hempstead M, Seidman C, Diakun J, Vasquez D, Freedman VH, Kaplan G. The metabolic and immunologic effects of short-term thalidomide treatment of patients infected with the human immunodeficiency virus. AIDS Res Hum Retroviruses 1997;13(12):1047–54.

67. Harris E, Behrens J, Samson D, Rahemtulla A, Russell NH, Byrne JL. Use of thalidomide in patients with myeloma and renal failure may be associated with unexplained hyperkalaemia. Br J Haematol 2003;122(1):160–1.

68. Jonquieres ED, Mosto SJ, Brusco CM. Talidomida y reacción leprosa lepromatosa. [Thalidomide and lepromatous leprosy reaction.] Arch Argent Dermatol 1967;17(3):279–86.

69. Parker PM, Chao N, Nademanee A, O'Donnell MR, Schmidt GM, Snyder DS, Stein AS, Smith EP, Molina A, Stepan DE, Kashyap A, Planas I, Spielberger R, Somlo G, Margolin K, Zwingenberger K, Wilsman K, Negrin RS, Long GD, Niland JC, Blume KG, Forman SJ. Thalidomide as salvage therapy for chronic graft-versus-host disease. Blood 1995;86(9):3604–9.

70. Hattori Y, Kakimoto T, Okamoto S, Sato N, Ikeda Y. Thalidomide-induced severe neutropenia during treatment of multiple myeloma. Int J Hematol 2004;79(3):283–8.

71. Huang SY, Tang JL, Yao M, Ko BS, Hong RL, Tsai W, Wang CH, Tien HF, Shen MC, Chen YC. Reduction of leukocyte count is associated with thalidomide response in treatment of multiple myeloma. Ann Hematol 2003;82(9):558–64.

72. Tefferi A, Elliot MA. Serious myeloproliferative reactions associated with the use of thalidomide in myelofibrosis with myeloid metaplasia. Blood 2000;96(12):4007.

73. Badros A, Morris C, Zangari M, Barlogie B, Tricot G. Thalidomide paradoxical effect on concomitant multiple myeloma and myelodysplasia. Leuk Lymphoma 2002;43(6):1267–71.

74. Bez C, Lodi G, Sardella A, Della Volpe A, Carrassi A. Oral lichenoid lesions after thalidomide treatment. Dermatology 1999;199(2):195.

75. Trojan A, Chasse E, Gay B, Pichert G, Taverna C. Severe hepatic toxicity due to thalidomide in relapsed multiple myeloma. Ann Oncol 2003;14(3):501–2.

76. Bang SM, Kim SS, Park SH, Ahn JY, Cho EK, Shin DB, Lee JH. Acute exacerbation of chronic hepatitis B during thalidomide therapy for multiple myeloma: a case report. Korean J Intern Med 2004;19(3):196–8.

77. Fowler R, Imrie K. Thalidomide-associated hepatitis: a case report. Am J Hematol 2001;66(4):300–2.

78. Bielsa I, Teixido J, Ribera M, Ferrandiz C. Erythroderma due to thalidomide: report of two cases. Dermatology 1994;189(2):179–81.

79. Sheskin J, Sagher F. Erupción tipo dermatitis herpetiforme en enfermos del mal de Hansen tratados con talidomida. [Dermatitis herpetiformis-like eruption in patients with Hansen disease treated with thalidomide.] Fontilles (Alicante) 1968;7:229.

80. Hall VC, El-Azhary RA, Bouwhuis S, Rajkumar SV. Dermatologic side effects of thalidomide in patients with multiple myeloma. J Am Acad Dermatol 2003;48(4):548–52.

81. Dobson CM, Parslew RA. Exacerbation of psoriasis by thalidomide in Behçet's syndrome. Br J Dermatol 2003;149(2):432–3.

82. Heathfield KW. Neuropathy after thalidomide ("Distaval"). BMJ 1961;2:1084.

83. Grosshans E, Illy G. Thalidomide therapy for inflammatory dermatoses. Int J Dermatol 1984;23(9):598–602.

84. Frances C, El Khoury S, Gompel A, Becherel PA, Chosidow O, Piette JC. Transient secondary amenorrhea in women treated by thalidomide. Eur J Dermatol 2002;12(1):63–5.

85. Ordi J, Cortes F, Martinez N, Mauri M, De Torres I, Vilardell M. Thalidomide induces amenorrhea in patients with lupus disease. Arthritis Rheum 1998;41(12):2273–5.

86. Passeron T, Lacour JP, Murr D, Ortonne JP. Thalidomide-induced amenorrhoea: two cases. Br J Dermatol 2001;144(6):1292–3.

87. Gompel A, Frances C, Piette JC, Blanc AS, Cordoliani F, Piette AM. Ovarian failure with thalidomide treatment in complex aphthosis: comment on the concise communication by Ordi, et al. Arthritis Rheum 1999;42(10):2259–60.

88. Gutierrez-Rodriguez O, Starusta-Bacal P, Gutierrez-Montes O. Treatment of refractory rheumatoid arthritis—the thalidomide experience. J Rheumatol 1989;16(2):158–63.

89. Dharia SP, Steinkampf MP, Cater C. Thalidomide-induced amenorrhea: case report and literature review. Fertil Steril 2004;82(2):460–2.

90. Mourad YA, Shamseddine A, Taher A. Thalidomide-associated gynecomasty in a patient with multiple myeloma. Hematol J 2003;4(5):372.

91. Pulik M, Genet P, Lionnet F, Touahri T. Thalidomide-associated gynecomasty in a patient with multiple myeloma. Am J Hematol 2002;70(3):265.

92. Witzens M, Moehler T, Neben K, Fruehauf S, Hartschuh W, Ho AD, Goldschmidt H. Development of leukocytoclastic vasculitis in a patient with multiple myeloma during treatment with thalidomide. Ann Hematol 2004;83(7):467–70.

93. Chao NJ, Parker PM, Niland JC, Wong RM, Dagis A, Long GD, Nademanee AP, Negrin RS, Snyder DS, Hu WW, Gould KA, Tierney DK, Zwingenberger K, Forman SJ, Blume KG. Paradoxical effect of thalidomide prophylaxis on chronic graft-vs.-host disease Biol Blood Marrow Transplant 1996;2(2):86–92.

94. Cany L, Fitoussi O, Boiron JM, Marit G. Tumor lysis syndrome at the beginning of thalidomide therapy for multiple myeloma. J Clin Oncol 2002;20(8):2212.

95. Curley MJ, Hussein SA, Hassoun PM. Disseminated herpes simplex virus and varicella zoster virus coinfection in a patient taking thalidomide for relapsed multiple myeloma. J Clin Microbiol 2002;40(6):2302–4.

96. Haslett P, Tramontana J, Burroughs M, Hempstead M, Kaplan G. Adverse reactions to thalidomide in patients infected with human immunodeficiency virus. Clin Infect Dis 1997;24(6):1223–7.

97. Wolkenstein P, Latarjet J, Roujeau JC, Duguet C, Boudeau S, Vaillant L, Maignan M, Schuhmacher MH, Milpied B, Pilorget A, Bocquet H, Brun-Buisson C, Revuz J. Randomised comparison of thalidomide versus placebo in toxic epidermal necrolysis. Lancet 1998;352(9140):1586–9.

98. Kohler G, Fisher AM, Dunn PM. Thalidomide and congenital abnormalities. Lancet 1962;1:326.

99. Morgan BC. Thalidomide ("Distaval") and foetal abnormalities. BMJ 1962;1:792.

100. Ferguson AW, Rogerson G. Thalidomide and congenital abnormalities. Lancet 1962;1:691.

101. Speirs AL. Thalidomide and congenital abnormalities. Lancet 1962;1:303–5.

102. Pfeiffer RA, Kosenow W. Zur Frage einer exogenen Verursachung von schweren Extremitätenmißbildungen. [On the problem of exogenous causes of severe malformations of the extremities.] Munch Med Wochenschr 1962;104:68–74.

103. Burley DM, Lenz W. Thalidomide and congenital abnormalities. Lancet 1962;1:271.

104. Lenz W, Pfeiffer RA, Kosenow W, Hayman DJ. Thalidomide and congenital abnormalities. Lancet 1962;1:45–6.

105. Wiedemann HR. [Indications of a current increase of hypoplastic and aplastic deformities of the extremities.] Med Welt 1961;37:1863–6.

106. Yang TS, Shen Cheng CC, Wang CM. A survey of thalidomide embryopathy in Taiwan. Taiwan Yi Xue Hui Za Zhi 1977;76(7):546–62.

107. Edwards DH, Nichols PJ. The spinal abnormalities in thalidomide embryopathy. Acta Orthop Scand 1977;48(3):273–6.

108. Newman CG. Clinical observations on the thalidomide syndrome. Proc R Soc Med 1977;70(4):225–7.

109. McBride WG. Thalidomide embryopathy. Teratology 1977;16(1):79–82.

110. Lenz W. Kindliche Mißbildungen nach Medikament-Einnahme während der Gravidität?. [Congenital abnormalities after drug use during pregnancy?] Dtsch Med Wochenschr 1961;86:2555–6.

111. USA, 76 Statute. 780, 87th Congress, 2nd session, October 10, 1962.

112. US National Academy of Sciences. Drug Efficacy Study. A Report to the Commissioner of Food and DrugsWashington DC: National Academy of Sciences;. 1969.

113. Bryan PA. "DESI Who?". FDA Consumer. DHEW Publication No 73-3031, 1972.

114. PSGB. Industry, Safety, Sainsbury and the Bill. Pharm J 1968;200:274–5.

115. Abraham J. In: Science, Politics and the Pharmaceutical Industry: Controversy and Bias in the Drug Regulation. New York: St Martin's Press, 1995:66–80.

116. PSGB. New ABPI code of practice. Pharm J 1967;198:692–3.

117. Riksdagen, Sweden. Kungl Maj:ts läkemedelsförordning. Svensk Författningssamling 1962;701.

118. Beckman DA, Brent RL. Mechanisms of teratogenesis. Annu Rev Pharmacol Toxicol 1984;24:483–500.

119. Taussig HB. A study of the German outbreak of phocomelia. The thalidomide syndrome. JAMA 1962;180:1106–14.

120. Pliess G. Thalidomide and congenital abnormalities. Lancet 1962;1:1128.

121. Lenz W, Knapp K. Die Thalidomid–Embryopathie. [Thalidomide embryopathy.] Dtsch Med Wochenschr 1962;87:1232–42.

122. Franklin AW. Thalidomide babies. Memorandum from the British Paediatric Association. BMJ 1962;5303:522–4.

123. Ciciliani J, Tolks H. Ergebnisse systematischer Untersuchungen bei 96 Dysmeliekindern. [Results of systematic studies of 96 dysmelia children.] Med Welt 1966;43:2301–7.

124. Sakr R, el-Zawahry K, Khalifa AS, Aboul Hassan A, Khalil M. Hazards to the newlyborn infant from thalidomide-containing drugs administered to pregnant mothers. (Report on three cases). J Egypt Med Assoc 1966;49(1):78–87.

125. Brook CG, Jarvis SN, Newman CG. Linear growth of children with limb deformities following exposure to thalidomide in utero. Acta Paediatr Scand 1977;66(6):673–5.

126. Lecutier MA. Phocomelia and internal defects due to thalidomide. BMJ 1962;5317:1447–8.

127. Petersen CE. Thalidomidembryopathie mit seltener Symptomatik. Pädiatr Prax 1967;6:625.

128. Kemper F. Thalidomide and congenital abnormalities. Lancet 1962;2:836.

129. Rasore-Quartino A, Rovei S. Un caso di anotia talidomidica. [A case of thalidomide anotia.] Minerva Pediatr 1967;19(46):2056–60.

130. Archer J. Thalidomide and neurological damage revisited. JAMA 1978;239(16):1608–9.

131. Murphy R, Mohr P. Two congenital neurological abnormalities caused by thalidomide. BMJ 1977;2(6096):1191.

132. D Avignon M, Barr B. Ear abnormalities and cranial nerve palsies in thalidomide children. Arch Otolaryngol 1964;80:136–40.

133. Phelps PD. Congenital lesions of the inner ear, demonstrated by tomography. Arch Otolaryngol 1974;100(1):11–8.

134. Phelps PD, Roland PE. Thalidomide and cranial nerve abnormalities. BMJ 1977;2(6103):1672.

135. Zetterstrom B. Ocular malformations caused by thalidomide. Acta Ophthalmol (Copenh) 1966;44(3):391–5.

136. Rafuse EV, Arstikaitis M, Brent HP. Ocular findings in thalidomide children. Can J Ophthalmol 1967;2(3):222–5.

137. Canani MB, Raganati M, Tropodi V. Su di un caso di panmieloftsi con malformazioni multiple e probabile genesi talidomidica. [On a case of pan-myelophthisis with multiple malformations probably caused by thalidomide.] Pediatrica (Napoli) 1966;74(6):1009.

138. Axrup K, et al. Children with thalidomide embryopathy: odontologic observations and aspects. Dent Dig 1966;72(9):403.

139. Axrup K, D'Avignon M, Hellgren K, Henrikson C-O, Juhlin I-M, Larsson KS, Persson GE, Welander E. Children with thalidomide embryopathy: odontological observations and aspects. Acta Odontol Scand 1966;24(1):3–21.

140. Fogh-Andersen P. Thalidomide and congenital cleft deformities. Acta Chir Scand 1966;131(3):197–200.

141. Immeyer F. Lippen- Kiefer- Gaumen-spalten bei Thalidomid-geschädigten Kindern. [Cleft lip and palate in thalidomide-induced embryopathies.] Acta Genet Med Gemellol (Roma) 1967;16(3):244–74.

142. Bremner DN, Mooney G. Agenesis of appendix: a further thalidomide anomaly. Lancet 1978;1(8068):826.

143. Smithells RW. Thalidomide, absent appendix, and sweating. Lancet 1978;1(8072):1042.

144. Ives EJ. Thalidomide and anal abnormalities. Can Med Assoc J 1962;87:670–2.

145. McBride WG. Excessive sweating and reduction deformities. Lancet 1978;1(8068):826.

146. Stainsby GD, Quibell EP. Perthes-like changes in the hips of children with thalidomide deformities. Lancet 1967;2:242.

147. McBride WG. Thalidomide and congenital abnormalities. Lancet 1961;2:1358.

148. Smithells RW. Thalidomide and malformations in Liverpool. Lancet 1962;1:1270–3.

149. Weicker H, Hungerland H. Thalidomid–Embryopathie. [Thalidomide embryopathy. I. Incidence inside and outside Germany.] Dtsch Med Wochenschr 1962;87:992–8passim.

150. Anonymous. Properties of thalidomide. BMJ 1962;2:785–6.

151. Tomsa DA, Hunter TAA, Ashley DJB, Woollam DHM, Applebey M. Thalidomide and congenital abnormalities. Lancet 1962;2:400.

152. Saunders H, Wright R, Hodgkin K. Thalidomide and congenital deformities. BMJ 1962;5307:796.

153. Jacobs J. Drugs and foetal abnormalities. BMJ 1962;2(5301):407.

154. Lutwak-Mann C. Observations on progeny of thalidomide-treated male rabbits. BMJ 1964;5390:1090–1.

155. Lenz W, Knapp K. Die Thalidomid–Embryopathie. [Thalidomide embryopathy.] Dtsch Med Wochenschr 1962;87:992.

156. Weicker H, Bachmann KD, Pfeiffer RA, Gleiss J. [Thalidomide embryopathy. II. Results of individual anamnestic findings in the areas of inquiry of the universities of Bonn, Cologne, Muenster and Duesseldorf pediatric clinics.]Dtsch Med Wochenschr 1962;87:1597–607.

157. Ward SP. Thalidomide and congenital abnormalities. BMJ 1962;5305:646–7.

158. Helm F. Tierexperimentelle Untersuchungen und Dysmeliesyndrom. [Studies in experiment animals and dysmelia syndrome.] Arzneimittelforschung 1966;16(9):1232–44.

159. Schumacher H, Blake DA, Gurian JM, Gillette JR. A comparison of the teratogenic activity of thalidomide in rabbits and rats. J Pharmacol Exp Ther 1968;160(1):189–200.

160. Roath S, Wales MB, Elves MW, Israels MCG. Effect of thalidomide on leucocyte cultures. Lancet 1962;2:812.

161. Lash JW, Saxen L. Human teratogenesis: invitro studies on thalidomide-inhibited chondrogenesis. Dev Biol 1972;28(1):61–70.

162. Williamson AP, Blattner RJ, Lutz HR. Abnormalities in chick embryos following thalidomide and other insoluble compounds in the amniotic cavity. Proc Soc Exp Biol Med 1963;112:1022–5.

163. Jurand A. Early changes in limb buds of chick embryos after thalidomide treatment. J Embryol Exp Morphol 1966;16(2):289–300.

164. Ruano Gil D. The influence of thalidomide on the development of chick embryos cultivated in vitro. Acta Anat (Basel) 1967;66(2):226–37.

165. Wolff E. La production des monstruosités par des substances chimiques et leur explication. [The induction of monstrosities by chemical substances and their explanation.] Ann Pharm Fr 1968;26(6):473–92.

166. Weidman WH, Young HH, Zollman PE. The effect of thalidomide on the unborn puppy. Mayo Clin Proc 1963;38:518–22.

167. Giroud A, Tuchmann-Duplessis H, Mercier-Parot L. Influence de la thalidomide sur le développement foetal. [Influence of thalidomide on fetal development.] Bull Acad Natl Med 1962;146:343–5.

168. DiPaolo JA, Buffalo PD. Congenital malformation in strain A mice. Its experimental production by thalidomide. JAMA 1963;183:139–41.

169. Mauss HJ, Stumpe K. Tierexperimentelle Untersuchungen zur Frage der Thalidomid–Embryopathie. [Animal experiments on the question of thalidomide embryopathy.] Klin Wschr 1963;41(1):21–5.

170. Szabo KT, Steelman RL. Effects of maternal thalidomide treatment on pregnancy, fetal development, and mortality of the offspring in random-bred mice. Am J Vet Res 1967;28(127):1823–8.

171. Delahunt CS, Lassen LJ, Rieser N. Some comparative teratogenic studies with thalidomide. Proc Eur Soc Study Drug Tox 1966;7:229.

172. Somers GF. Thalidomide and congenital abnormalities. Lancet 1962;1:912–3.

173. Ingalis TH, Curley FJ, Zappasodi P. Thalidomide embryopathy in hybrid rabbits. N Engl J Med 1964;271:441–4.

174. Dekker A, Mehrizi A. Use of thalidomide as a teratogenic agent in rabbits. Bull Johns Hopkins Hosp 1964;115(3):223–30.

175. Vickers TH. The thalidomide embryopathy in hybrid rabbits. Br J Exp Pathol 1967;48(1):107–17.

176. Pearn JH, Vickers TH. The rabbit thalidomide embryopathy. Br J Exp Pathol 1966;47(2):186–92.

177. Fabro S, Smith RL. The teratogenic activity of thalidomide in the rabbit. J Pathol Bacteriol 1966;91(2):511–9.

178. Heine W. Thalidomidembryopathie im Tierversuch. III. Teratologische Testung von Thalidomidabbauprodukten. [Thalidomide embryopathy in animal experiments. 3. Teratologic tests of thalidomide catabolic products.] Z Kinderheilkd 1966;96(2):141–6.

179. Heine W, Stuwe W. Thalidomidembryopathie im Tierversuch. II. Thalidomidblutspiegelwerte bei lebergesunden und lebergeschädigten Versuchstieren. [Thalidomide embryopathy in animal experiments. II. Thalidomide blood level in experimental animals with normal and damaged liver.] Z Kinderheilkd 1966;96(1):14–8.

180. Vickers TH. The cardiovascular malformations in the rabbit thalidomide embryopathy. Br J Exp Pathol 1968;49(2):179–96.

181. Wuest HM, Fox RR, Crary DD. Relationship between teratogeny and structure in the thalidomide field. Experientia 1968;24(10):993–4.

182. Klein Obbink HJ, Dalderup LM. Effects of thalidomide on the skeleton of the rat foetus. Experientia (Basel) 1964;20(5):283–4.

183. Cook MJ, Moore DF. The effect of thalidomide on the developing rat foetus. Br J Exp Pathol 1967;48(2):150–8.

184. Globus M, Gibson MA. A histological and histochemical study of the development of the sternum in thalidomide-treated rats. Teratology 1968;1(3):235–55.

185. Metcalf WK. The relation of vitamin-B complex to the effect of thalidomide on the sensitivity of intracellular haemoglobin to oxidation. Dev Med Child Neurol 1967;9(1):87–97.

186. Horstmann W. Hinweise auf zentral nervöse Schäden im Rahmen der Thalidomid–Embryopathie. [Reference to central nervous system damage within the context of thalidomide embryopathy. Pathological–anatomic, electroencephalographic and neurologic findings.] Z Kinderheilkd 1966;96(4):291–307.

187. Ahrens K. Cytogenische und klinische Untersuchungen bei thalidomidgeschädigten Kindern mit Ohrmissbildungen. [Cytogenetic and clinical studies in thalidomide damaged children with ear malformations.] Arch Klin Exp Ohren Nasen Kehlkopfheilkd 1966;186(3):264–78.

188. McCredie J. Thalidomide and congenital Charcot's joints. Lancet 1973;2(7837):1058–61.

189. Turk JL, Hellmann K, Duke DI. Effect of thalidomide on the immunological response in local lymph nodes after a skin homograft. Lancet 1966;1(7447):1134–6.

190. Hellmann K. Immunosuppression by thalidomide: implications for teratology. Lancet 1966;1(7447):1136–7.

191. Chard T. Immunosuppression by thalidomide. Lancet 1966;1:1373.

192. Gordon G. The mechanism of thalidomide deformities correlated with the pathogenic effects of prolonged dosage in adults. Dev Med Child Neurol 1966;8(6):761–7.

193. Evered DF, Randall HG. Thalidomide and B vitamins. BMJ 1963;1(5330):610.

194. Steurer M, Sudmeier I, Stauder R, Gastl G. Thromboembolic events in patients with myelodysplastic syndrome receiving thalidomide in combination with darbepoietin-alpha. Br J Haematol 2003;121(1):101–3.

195. Rajkumar SV, Gertz MA, Witzig TE. Life-threatening toxic epidermal necrolysis with thalidomide therapy for myeloma. N Engl J Med 2000;343(13):972–3.

196. Frederickson RC, Slater IH, Dusenberry WE, Hewes CR, Jones GT, Moore RA. A comparison of thalidomide and pentobarbital—new methods for identifying novel hypnotic drugs. J Pharmacol Exp Ther 1977;203(1):240–51.

197. Somers GF. Pharmacological properties of thalidomide (alpha-phthalimido glutarimide), a new sedative hypnotic drug. Br J Pharmacol Chemother 1960;15:111–6.

198. Trapnell CB, Donahue SR, Collins JM, Flockhart DA, Thacker D, Abernethy DR. Thalidomide does not alter the pharmacokinetics of ethinyl estradiol and norethindrone. Clin Pharmacol Ther 1998;64(6):597–602.

199. Nathan PD, Gore ME, Eisen TG. Unexpected toxicity of combination thalidomide and interferon alpha-2a treatment in metastatic renal cell carcinoma. J Clin Oncol 2002;20(5):1429–30.

Mutagenic effects of drugs other than anticancer drugs and drugs used in immunology

Benznidazole

Like metronidazole, benznidazole is mutagenic. In tests for chromosomal aberrations and induction of micronuclei in cultures of peripheral lymphocytes from children with Chagas' disease, there were increases in micronucleated interphase lymphocytes and of chromosomal aberrations after treatment with benznidazole (1).

Benzodiazepines

In 18 patients taking benzodiazepines and/or neuroleptic drugs, there were increased chromosomal aberrations and increased sister chromatid exchange, but there were no significant differences between this group and another group of 18 patients taking lithium in addition to benzodiazepines and/or antipsychotic drugs (2).

Bromocriptine

No chromosomal changes were found in 19 children born after bromocriptine-induced ovulation (3).

Ciclosporin

An increase in chromosomal abnormalities correlated with serum ciclosporin concentrations in one study (4).

Estrogens

A finding that needs further study is that when estrogens are used for the treatment of osteoporosis they may have some genotoxic potential, as evidenced by their ability to cause an increased frequency of sister chromatid exchange (5).

Ethylene Oxide

There is overwhelming evidence that ethylene oxide produces genetic damage in a wide range of organisms and cells, including somatic cells of exposed humans (6,7). Ethylene oxide is a germ-cell mutagen in rodents. In male mice it induces chromosome breakage, leading to dominant lethal mutations and heritable translocations. Sensitive stages appear to be restricted to late spermatocytes and early spermatozoa.

The International Agency for Research on Cancer (IARC) Working Group reviewed the published studies of workers exposed to ethylene oxide in hospital and factory sterilization units and in ethylene manufacturing and processing plants (8). The studies consistently showed chromosomal damage in peripheral blood lymphocytes, including chromosomal aberrations in 11 of 14 studies, sister chromatid exchange in 20 of 23 studies, micronuclei

in three of eight studies, and gene mutation in one study. In general, the degree of damage is correlated with the degree and duration of exposure. The induction of sister chromatid exchange appears to be more sensitive to exposure to ethylene oxide than is induction of either chromosomal aberrations or micronuclei. In one study, chromosomal aberrations were observed in the peripheral lymphocytes of workers 2 years after cessation of exposure to ethylene oxide, and sister chromatid exchanges 6 months after cessation of exposure. However, in one study, incidental exposure to high concentrations of ethylene oxide did not cause any measurable permanent mutational/cytogenetic damage in lymphocytes of exposed persons (9).

The effects of glutathione-S-transferase T1 and M1 genotypes on hemoglobin adducts in erythrocytes and sister chromatid exchange in lymphocytes have been examined in 58 hospital operators of sterilizers that used ethylene oxide and non-exposed workers (10). The results suggested that the glutathione-S-transferase T1 null genotype was associated with increased formation of ethylene oxide-hemoglobin adducts in relation to occupational exposure. This suggests that individuals with the glutathione-S-transferase T1 null genotype may be more susceptible to the genotoxic effects of ethylene oxide.

In females, ethylene oxide also induces presumed, dominant, lethal mutations. When females are exposed shortly after mating or during the early pronuclear stage of the zygote, high frequencies of fetal anomalies are induced.

Ethylene oxide was ineffective in inducing morphological-specific locus mutations in spermatogonial stem cells; however, it produced dominant visible and electrophoresis-specific locus mutants in male mice, assumed to be derived from poststem cells.

The effectiveness of ethylene oxide in inducing chromosome breakage in germ cells of male mice is strongly influenced by varying degrees or rates of exposure. Since there was a dose-rate effect for ethylene oxide-induced, dominant, lethal mutations at high concentrations and over long exposure periods, considering the short burst exposure and low TWA exposure in humans, the question of whether significant dose-rate effects also exist at low exposures is unanswered.

Formaldehyde

Formaldehyde is mutagenic in many laboratory test systems, for example fruit flies (Drosophila), grasshoppers, flowering plants, fungi, bacteria, and cultured human bronchial fibroblasts.

Marked chromosomal abnormalities and chromosomal breaks were found in metaphases in direct bone marrow preparations from 40 patients undergoing maintenance hemodialysis (SEDA-11, 477; 11). During the period of these cytogenetic studies, the dialysers were reused after sterilization with formaldehyde, and each patient may have received residual amounts of as much as 127 (sd 51) mg of formaldehyde during each dialysis.

Formaldehyde may be genotoxic by a dual mechanism: direct damage to DNA and inhibition of repair of mutagenic and carcinogenic DNA lesions by other chemical and physical carcinogens.

Hycanthone

Experimentally, hycanthone has been reported to be mutagenic in *Salmonella typhimurium* and *Escherichia coli*, but no human data are available (12,13).

Isoflurane

Genetic damage was demonstrated in 10 non-smoking veterinary surgeons exposed to isoflurane and nitrous oxide compared with 10 non-smoking, non-exposed veterinary physicians acting as controls (14). The surgeons were monitored for 1 week in a working environment comparable to that of pediatric anesthesia, with the use of uncuffed endotracheal tubes and open-circuit breathing systems during operations on small animals. The overall calculated 8-hour time-weighted average exposure of cases was 5.3 ppm for isoflurane and 13 ppm for nitrous oxide. The European exposure limits are 10 ppm and 100 ppm respectively, and the corresponding values recommended by USA-NIOSH are 2 ppm and 25 ppm respectively. These values therefore violated the USA-NIOSH limit for isoflurane. The mean frequency of sister chromatid exchanges in peripheral blood lymphocytes was significantly higher in exposed workers than in controls (10 versus 7.4) and the proportion of micronuclei was also significantly higher in exposed workers (8.7 versus 6.8 per 500 binucleated cells). These measures reflect the mutagenicity of isoflurane and nitrous oxide. The findings are comparable to smoking 11–20 cigarettes a day. However, this study did not distinguish between the potential genotoxic effects of isoflurane and nitrous oxide; nor did it show a dose-dependency of genotoxicity, owing to the small sample size.

Isoniazid

Isoniazid is not mutagenic (SEDA-6, 276), but patients taking combined isoniazid and rifampicin therapy for 3–10 months developed an increased rate of chromosomal aberrations in peripheral blood lymphocytes (SEDA-9, 276). However, this effect is not known to have clinical consequences.

Isotretinoin

The reported occurrence of sarcomas in some patients treated with isotretinoin may be a chance finding (SEDA-21, 164); retinoids may prevent or even cure certain malignancies (14a).

Leflunomide

A minor metabolite of leflunomide, 4-Trifluoromethylaniline, was mutagenic in vitro (15).

Lomefloxacin

In vitro lomefloxacin photochemically produced oxidative DNA damage, an effect known to be of mutagenic potential (6). This may be the basis of the photochemical mutagenicity and photochemical carcinogenicity of quinolones.

Metronidazole

Mutagenicity of metronidazole has been demonstrated in some bacterial systems (SEDA-13, 832). Studies on breakages in single-stranded DNA in the lymphocytes of patients treated with metronidazole for *Trichomonas vaginitis* have suggested that such breakages were repaired after withdrawal. Another study reported chromosomal aberrations in the lymphocytes of ten volunteers taking metronidazole (SEDA-21, 301). A mutagenic effect would theoretically be possible in patients with a DNA repair defect (SEDA-16, 310).

The genotoxic effects of metronidazole (250 mg bd for 10 days) and nalidixic acid (400 mg bd for 10 days) have been assessed in women with *Trichomonas vaginalis* infections (16). The genotoxic potential of these drugs was evaluated using a sister chromatid exchange test in peripheral blood lymphocytes. Metronidazole had no effect but nalidixic acid caused an increase in sister chromatid exchange frequency. This result confirms that there is little evidence of genotoxicity with metronidazole.

Nalidixic acid

The genotoxic effects of nalidixic acid (400 mg bd for 10 days) and metronidazole (250 mg tds for 10 days) have been investigated in a prospective randomized study in 20 patients with *Trichomonas vaginalis* infections (17). Evaluation was by the sister-chromatid exchange test, in which an increased number of exchanges in lymphocytes reflects mutagenic action. Metronidazole had no effect but there was a significant increase with nalidixic acid.

Neuroleptic drugs

There was an increase in markers of genotoxicity in patients receiving long-term neuroleptic drugs in combination with other psychotropic drugs (n = 36) compared with controls (n = 36) (18). In another study there was an association between the frequency of chromosomal aberrations in lymphocytes and the probability of tumor induction (19).

Nifurtimox

Chromosomal aberrations were significantly increased in cultures of peripheral lymphocytes from a small group of children with Chagas' disease treated with nifurtimox. G-binding analysis of chromosomal aberration sites showed that treated patients presented coincidence in the chromosome regions affected (SEDA-15, 298).

Niridazole

Niridazole should not be used in pregnancy; mutagenic effects have been seen in bacteria (20).

Nitrofurantoin

In vitro, nitrofurantoin acts as a mutagen by inhibiting DNA synthetase. In human fibroblast cultures it damages DNA (21). Treatment with nitrofurantoin for 12 months caused a significant increase in chromosome aberrations and sister chromatid exchanges in the lymphocytes of 69 children (22).

Noscapine

In vitro experiments have shown that noscapine can produce spindle inhibition and polyploidy, suggesting that it may be genotoxic or carcinogenic (SEDA-17, 210) The degree of risk to humans when noscapine is used in a cough mixture remains to be established. Nevertheless, as there are alternative drugs, noscapine should not be given to given to women of childbearing potential.

Paracetamol

Animal studies have indicated a carcinogenic effect when paracetamol has been administered for prolonged periods in relatively high dosages. However, no clinical data are so far available to corroborate this. The matter cannot be dismissed entirely for the time being, in view of a report (23) of the development of chromosomal aberrations after prolonged use.

Penicillamine

In one experimental study it has been suggested that penicillamine may be mutagenic (24).

Phenylbutazone

Phenylbutazone infusion for 10 days induced chromosomal abnormalities in patients with rheumatoid arthritis (39), although the significance of this finding is not clear.

Radio contrast use

An increased frequency of chromosomal aberrations and sister chromatid exchanges has been found in lymphocytes up to 1 week after intravenous urography; diatrizoate produced more changes than ioxaglate (SEDA-19, 430) (25). Earlier it was reported that the incidence of chromosomal aberrations in the lymphocytes of seven infants who underwent angiocardiography was higher than expected. Whether this means that contrast media produce significant cytogenetic damage is not at all clear.

Radio-iodine

Mutagenic effects on the sexual organs are difficult to determine in practice. However, while the radiation dose to the ovary and testes is rather small after ^{131}I treatment for hyperthyroidism (maximum 5 roentgens) it can be substantial after the higher amounts of ^{131}I that are used for thyroid cancer. In any case, children born to mothers previously treated with ^{131}I did not have an increased incidence of congenital malformations. The number of such observations is too small, however, to allow definite conclusions about its safety (26). In patients treated for thyroid carcinoma there was no differences in fertility rate, birth weight, prematurity, or congenital malformations compared with healthy subjects, providing reassurance about the use of radioiodine to treat hyperthyroidism in women of child-bearing age (SEDA-20, 394).

Sparfloxacin

DNA damage produced by sparfloxacin and UVA in retinal pigment epithelial cells in vitro was remedied by antioxidants, suggesting a possible in vivo strategy for preventing or minimizing retinal damage in humans (27).

Theophylline

Genetic effects of theophylline are not well known. Theophylline suppresses phosphodiesterase and cyclic AMP activity, and increases calcium transport in animals (SEDA-4, 25), suggesting a potential for teratogenicity. An increased rate of sister chromatid exchange rate, an indication of mutagenicity, has also been reported (SEDA-17, 1).

Trimethoprim

Genotoxic effects of trimethoprim on cultured human lymphocytes have been described (28). Chromosome studies performed in cultures of peripheral blood lymphocytes did not show significant differences before and after treatment. Cytogenetic studies on bone marrow cells from 12 patients with urinary tract infections treated with cotrimoxazole did not show structural chromosomal aberrations; however, there was an increased number of micronuclei in these patients compared with controls (29).

Vidarabine

Vidarabine is oncogenic and mutagenic in animals (30).

References

1. Villar JC, Marin-Neto JA, Ebrahim S, Yusuf S. Trypanocidal drugs for chronic asymptomatic *Trypanosoma cruzi* infection. Cochrane Database Syst Rev 2002;(1):CD003463.

2. Bigatti MP, Corona D, Munizza C. Increased sister chromatid exchange and chromosomal aberration frequencies in psychiatric patients receiving psychopharmacological therapy. Mutat Res 1998;413(2):169–75.

3. Schellekens LA, Snuiverink H, Van den Berghe H. Chromosomal patterns of children born after induction of ovulation with bromocriptine. Arzneimittelforschung 1977;27(11):2151–3.

4. Fukuda M, Ohmori Y, Aikawa I, Yoshimura N, Oka T. Mutagenicity of cyclosporine in vivo. Transplant Proc 1988;20(3 Suppl 3):929–30.

5. Sahin FI, Sahin I, Ergun MA, Saracoglu OF. Effects of estrogen and alendronate on sister chromatid exchange (SCE) frequencies in postmenopausal osteoporosis patients. Int J Gynaecol Obstet 2000;71(1):49–52.

6. WHO International Agency for Research of Cancer. Ethylene oxide. IARC Monogr Eval Carcinog Risks Hum 1994;60:73–159.

7. Dellarco VL, Generoso WM, Sega GA, Fowle JR 3rd, Jacobson-Kram D. Review of the mutagenicity of ethylene oxide. Environ Mol Mutagen 1990;16(2):85–103.

8. Schroder JM, Hoheneck M, Weis J, Deist H. Ethylene oxide polyneuropathy: clinical follow-up study with morphometric and electron microscopic findings in a sural nerve biopsy. J Neurol 1985;232(2):83–90.

9. Tates AD, Boogaard PJ, Darroudi F, Natarajan AT, Caubo ME, van Sittert NJ. Biological effect monitoring in industrial workers following incidental exposure to high concentrations of ethylene oxide. Mutat Res 1995;329(1):63–77.

10. Yong LC, Schulte PA, Wiencke JK, Boeniger MF, Connally LB, Walker JT, Whelan EA, Ward EM. Hemoglobin adducts and sister chromatid exchanges in hospital workers exposed to ethylene oxide: effects of glutathione S-transferase T1 and M1 genotypes. Cancer Epidemiol Biomarkers Prev 2001;10(5):539–50.

11. IARC Monographs updating of Vol. 1 to 42, Supplement, 1987:211–16.

12. Hartman PE. Early years of the *Salmonella* mutagen tester strains: lessons from hycanthone. Environ Mol Mutagen 1989;14(Suppl 16):39–45.

13. Cook TM, Goldman CK. Hycanthone and its congeners as bacterial mutagens. J Bacteriol 1975;122(2):549–56.

14. Hoerauf K, Lierz M, Wiesner G, Schroegendorfer K, Lierz P, Spacek A, Brunnberg L, Nusse M. Genetic damage in operating room personnel exposed to isoflurane and nitrous oxide. Occup Environ Med 1999;56(7):433–7.

14a. Peck GL. Therapy and prevention of skin cancer. In: Saurat JH, editor. Retinoids. Basel S. Karger 1985;345.

15. Brent RL. Teratogen update: reproductive risks of leflunomide (Arava); a pyrimidine synthesis inhibitor: counseling women taking leflunomide before or during pregnancy and men taking leflunomide who are contemplating fathering a child. Teratology 2001;63(2):106–12.

16. Akyol D, Mungan T, Baltaci V. A comparative study of genotoxic effects in the treatment of *Trichomonas vaginalis* infection: metronidazole or nalidixic acid. Arch Gynecol Obstet 2000;264(1):20–3.

17. Akyol D, Mungan T, Baltaci V. A comparative study of genotoxic effects in the treatment of *Trichomonas vaginalis* infection: metronidazole or nalidixic acid. Arch Gynecol Obstet 2000;264(1):20–3.

18. Bigatti MP, Corona D, Munizza C. Increased sister chromatid exchange and chromosomal aberration frequencies in psychiatric patients receiving psychopharmacological therapy. Mutat Res 1998;413(2):169–75.

19. Bonassi S, Abbondandolo A, Camurri L, Dal Pra L, De Ferrari M, Degrassi F, Forni A, Lamberti L, Lando C, Padovani P, Sbrana I, Vecchio D, Puntoni R. Are chromosome aberrations in circulating lymphocytes predictive of future cancer onset in humans? Preliminary results of an Italian cohort study. Cancer Genet Cytogenet 1995;79(2):133–5.

20. McCalla DR, Voutsinos D, Olive PL. Mutagen screening with bacteria: niridazole and nitrofurans. Mutat Res 1975;31(1):31–7.

21. Hirsch-Kauffmann M, Herrlich P, Schweiger M. Nitrofurantoin damages DNA of human cells. Klin Wochenschr 1978;56(8):405–7.

22. Slapsyte G, Jankauskiene A, Mierauskiene J, Lazutka JR. Cytogenetic analysis of peripheral blood lymphocytes of children treated with nitrofurantoin for recurrent urinary tract infection. Mutagenesis 2002;17(1):31–5.

23. Fyfe AI, Wright JM. Chronic acetaminophen ingestion associated with (1;7) (p11) translocation and immune deficiency syndrome. Am J Med 1990;88(4):443–4.

24. Speit G, Haupter S. Cytogenetic effects of penicillamine. Mutat Res 1987;190(3):197–203.

25. Nunez ME, Sinues B. Cytogenic effects of diatrizoate and ioxaglate on patients undergoing excretory urography. Invest Radiol 1990;25(6):692–7.

26. Maxon HR, Thomas SR, Chen IW. The role of nuclear medicine in the treatment of hyperthyroidism and well-differentiated thyroid adenocarcinoma. Clin Nucl Med 1981;6(10S):P87–98.

27. Verna LK, Holman SA, Lee VC, Hoh J. UVA-induced oxidative damage in retinal pigment epithelial cells after H_2O_2 or sparfloxacin exposure. Cell Biol Toxicol 2000;16(5):303–12.

28. Abou-Eisha A, Creus A, Marcos R. Genotoxic evaluation of the antimicrobial drug, trimethoprim, in cultured human lymphocytes. Mutat Res 1999;440(2):157–62.

29. Sorensen PJ, Jensen MK. Cytogenetic studies in patients treated with trimethoprim–sulfamethoxazole. Mutat Res 1981;89(1):91–4.

30. Chang TW, Snydman DR. Antiviral agents: action and clinical use. Drugs 1979;18(5):354–76.

Tumorigenic effects of drugs other than anticancer drugs and drugs used in immunology

Acesulfame

The studies on the basis of which acesulfame gained approval showed no evidence in animals of mutagenicity, teratogenicity, or adverse reproductive effects; a 2-year toxicology study in beagles showed no untoward adverse effects. The incidence of lymphocytic leukemia was slightly increased in high-dosed female mice, but not beyond the spontaneous variation with this strain. No other evidence of potential carcinogenicity was obtained, and it has been concluded that at the estimated level of exposure, acesulfame and its metabolites are not a health hazard (1).

Aminophenazone

Aminophenazone and its derivatives may be metabolized to carcinogenic nitrosamines. The clinical importance of this is not clear (SEDA-2, 389) (2).

Androgens and anabolic steroids

There is no essential difference between androgens and so-called anabolic steroids. High doses of either, such as can be used in refractory anemias, have been associated with the induction of benign liver tumors and primary hepatocellular carcinoma. The fact that primary hepatoma, liver adenoma, and peliosis are uncommon conditions and that there is a considerable overlap between the patients concerned and the tiny fraction of the population taking high-dose androgens strongly suggests that the association of both events is more than coincidental (3). Some animal studies and in vitro studies have also pointed to a hepatic carcinogenic effect of anabolic steroids. No cases seem to have been described in sportsmen who have used high-dose androgens or in girls suffering from precocious puberty, but the former at least often use these drugs for relatively short periods; furthermore, such use is likely to be surreptitious and thus poorly documented. Most of the widely used compounds in this class, including methyltestosterone, have been reported to induce liver tumors. The apparent exceptions are the nortestosterone derivatives without 17-alpha substitution. Whether these drugs are indeed safer or whether they have merely been used less often in high doses is not known.

The incidence of liver tumors following the use of androgens and anabolic steroids still cannot be calculated. What is clear is that if these products are used in high doses or over long periods of time (and there is now much doubt about whether they are more than marginally effective in such conditions as osteoporosis and aplastic anemia), techniques such as CT scanning and ultrasonography should be used routinely to ensure early detection of liver lesions.

In a prospective study of 1200 infertile women in Israel, including a subgroup of women who developed breast cancer, there was no statistical association with the use of fertility-inducing drugs (4).

A subfertile man treated with human menopausal gonadotropin + human chorionic gonadotropin (hMG + hCG) developed a malignant teratoma of the testis; however, in view of his history a cause-and-effect relation was dubious (5).

Anthranoids

Several anthranoid derivatives (notably the aglycones aloe-emodin, chrysophanol, emodin, and physicon) are genotoxic in bacterial and/or mammalian test systems (SEDA-12, 409), and two anthranoid compounds (the synthetic laxative dantron and the naturally occurring l-hydroxyanthraquinone) have carcinogenic activity in rodents. In an epidemiological study, chronic abusers of anthranoid laxatives (identified by the presence of pseudomelanosis coli) had an increased relative risk of 3.04 (95% CI = 1.18, 4.90) for colorectal cancer (6). The German health authorities therefore restricted the indication of herbal anthranoid laxatives to constipation which has not responded to bulk-forming therapy (which rules out their inclusion in slimming aids). In addition, they imposed restrictions on the laxative use of anthranoid-containing herbs (for example not to be used for more than 1–2 weeks without medical advice, not to be used in children under 12 years of age, and not to be used during pregnancy and lactation) (6,7).

- A 73-year-old man with a 5-year history of centrocytic non-Hodgkin's lymphoma presented with subcutaneous nodules in the abdominal wall at the sites where he had previously received subcutaneous injections of mistletoe (8). The nodules turned out to be infiltrations by the centrocytic lymphoma. The patient died 6 weeks later of bilateral pneumonia. The authors hypothesized that mistletoe has a growth-promoting action on lymphoma cells, mediated by high local concentrations of interleukin-6 liberated from the skin by mistletoe lectins.

Antiretroviral drugs

- Eruptive angiolipomata occurred in a 49-year-old woman after she had taken stavudine 30 mg bd, lamivudine 150 mg bd, and saquinavir 600 mg 8-hourly for 3 months (9). This has also been reported with other protease inhibitors (10,11) and the mechanism is not known. In one case lipomata regressed after the introduction of indinavir (12).

Aristolochia

Aristolochic acid I and aristolochic acid II are mutagenic in several test systems. A mixture of these two compounds was so highly carcinogenic in rats that even homeopathic *Aristolochia* dilutions have been banned from the German market. The closely related aristolactam I and aristolactam II have not been submitted to carcinogenicity testing, but these compounds similarly show mutagenic activity in bacteria.

When 19 kidneys and urethras removed from 10 patients with Chinese herb nephropathy who required kidney transplantation were examined histologically, there were conclusive signs of neoplasms in 40% (13).

One patient who had a urothelial malignancy 6 years after the onset of Chinese herb nephropathy later developed a breast carcinoma that metastasised to the liver (14). The urothelial malignancy contained aristolochic acid-DNA adducts and mutations in the p53 gene, and the same mis-sense mutation in codon 245 of exon 7 of p53 was found in DNA from the breast and liver tumors. However, DNA extracted from the urothelial tumor also showed a mutation in codon 139 of exon 5, which was not present in the breast and liver.

BCG Vaccine

The effects of immunization with BCG have been studied extensively (15–18) (SEDA-7, 323) (470,471). On the whole the results are inconclusive, with little good evidence of either preventive or tumor-inducing effects.

Bromocriptine

In rats (but not in mice) high doses of bromocriptine induced malignant uterine tumors within 2 years (SEDA-3, 122). Tumor induction has not been seen in man, but enlargement of a non-invasive pituitary tumor has been observed on more than one occasion.

Calcium channel blockers

A retrospective cohort study in 5052 elderly subjects, of whom 451 were taking verapamil, diltiazem, or nifedipine, showed that these drugs were associated with a cancer risk of 1.72 (95% CI = 1.27, 2.34), and there was a significant dose–response relation (339). A small risk of cancer (RR = 1.27; 95% CI = 0.98, 1.63) with calcium channel blockers was reported in a nested case-control retrospective study involving 446 cases of cancers in hypertensive patients (340). However, the authors concluded that this finding may have been spurious, as there was no relation between the cancer risk and the duration of drug use. Another study did not show any excess cancer risk with short-acting nifedipine after myocardial infarction in patients followed up for 10 years, although there were only 22 cancer deaths in 2607 patients (19). Neither did the much larger Bezafibrate Infarction Prevention (BIP) Study, which reported cancer incidence data in 11 575 patients followed for a mean period of 5.2 years, with

246 incident cancer cases, 129 among users (2.3%) and 117 (2.1%) among non-users of calcium channel blockers (20). Others also failed to find a positive link between calcium channel blockers and cancer (21,22). However, elderly women taking estrogens and short-acting calcium channel blockers had a significantly increased risk of breast carcinoma (hazard ratio = 8.48; 95% CI = 2.99, 24) (23). This controversy can perhaps only be resolved by prospective studies with longer follow-up periods (24), although ideal studies are unlikely ever to be conducted.

Cannabinoids

THC does not appear to be carcinogenic, but there is plenty of evidence that the tar derived from cannabis smoke is. Bacteria exposed to cannabis tar develop mutations in the standard Ames test for carcinogenicity (25), and hamster lung cells in tissue culture develop accelerated malignant transformations within 3–6 months of exposure to tobacco or cannabis smoke (26).

Carbamazepine

Carbamazepine and phenytoin have previously been associated with lymphoproliferative disorders, including dermatopathic lymphadenitis, atypical lymphoid proliferation, and cutaneous pseudolymphoma. In most reported cases, regression follows withdrawal of treatment with the causative drug. However, rarely true lymphoma can develop.

- A 13-year-old girl who had taken carbamazepine for about 8 months developed multiple painless reddish skin nodules, which grew and quickly ulcerated (27). The nodules were on the neck, trunk, and arms and varied in size. Neither lymphadenopathy nor splenomegaly was detected. Histology showed a CD30, primary, cutaneous, anaplastic, large-cell lymphoma. Carbamazepine was withdrawn, she received radiotherapy, and the lesions regressed. At 3 years after diagnosis she was still in complete remission.

The development of liver tumors in mice and an increased incidence of mammary fibroadenomata in female rats at one time caused concern in the USA, although animal studies elsewhere and clinical studies have shown no evidence of tumor-forming potential.

Pseudolymphomatous reactions, pseudomalignant histiocytosis, a reaction resembling mycosis fungoides, and malignant lymphoma have been noted in individual cases (SED-13, 144) (28,29).

Chromium

Hexavalent chromium compounds have no medical uses and are known as mutagens and carcinogens (30). In an in vitro study the coordination of chromium by picolinate ligands made chromium picolinate more toxic to cultured cells, leading to enhanced apoptosis (31). These observations support the hypothesis that chromium pico-linate is a human carcinogen.

A mortality study among workers engaged in producing chromium compounds from chromite, performed using retrospective data (32), showed a significantly increased risk of lung cancer, despite cessation of exposure. The risk of nasal cavity/sinus cancer was also significantly increased.

Clomiphene

Concern that the drug treatment of female infertility might predispose the user to malignant melanoma was first engendered by a US study published in 1995 (33). Among women who had used clomiphene citrate for infertility, the incidence of melanoma was higher (RR = 1.8; 95% CI = 0.8, 3.5) than among American women in general. However, in a case-cohort study of nearly 4000 infertile women there was a similar increase in the incidence of melanoma among those who had been treated with human chorionic gonadotropin compared with the rest; there was no association with the use of clomiphene.

Quite apart from the inherent discrepancy in these findings, several pieces of evidence have confused the debate. In the first place, the cohort of melanoma cases was small—barely a handful. In the second place, some earlier papers had suggested that infertility in women might of itself have an association with melanoma. The same impression came from various studies, in which the incidences of cancers in infertile women were examined (34–36). If that were true, it could affect the initial find-ings in either direction: a high spontaneous incidence might mask a real drug effect, or it might provide a pre-disposition to melanoma, which the drugs might then more readily trigger.

In the meantime, data from Australia have shown no greater incidence of melanoma among women who had used fertility drugs and undergone in vitro fertilization than in the country's general female population (37). Since then there has been one more significant paper, again from Australia, using data from a specialized ferti-lity clinic in Queensland, relating to all women who attended the center over a decade (38). Whenever possi-ble, the women were traced and their subsequent history noted. Originally intended as a retrospective case-cohort study using a subcohort, the approach had to be amended because no cases of melanoma were found in the subco-hort. The work therefore proceeded as a matched case-control study; all the data were taken and set against publicly available figures on melanoma in Queensland. After some necessary exclusions, 3186 women were included; care was taken to minimize recall bias. Fourteen women developed melanoma after fertility treatment, eight cases being invasive. The expected inci-dence in the general population would have been 15.8 cases in the same period. The incidence actually observed was therefore only 0.89 of that anticipated (95%

CI = 0.54, 1.48). The numbers of women who had used clomiphene or human menopausal gonadotropin were too small to make more differentiated calculations, but the incidence of melanoma seemed to correspond to that in the general population.

On current evidence there seems no reason to discou-rage fertility-promoting drug treatments because of any risk of melanoma; they may even reduce it to some extent. However, this does not alter the fact that the data are deficient in various ways. Quite apart from the small numbers of melanoma cases that have been recorded, all the work to date has been performed in relatively sunny parts of the world; it is not known what would happen in other climates. Within countries there are sharp differ-ences in melanoma figures; in the USA, where about 32 000 new cases of skin melanoma were projected for 1994 (39), the highest melanoma rates occur among light-skinned populations in areas of intense sunlight, for exam-ple Arizona; the same applies to Queensland, Australia. In the USA as a whole there is a melanoma incidence among whites of 12.4 per 100 000 (40), while mortality rates vary inversely with latitude (41). Furthermore, in whites, there has been a recent increase in the incidence of melanoma, during the precise period that this type of treatment has become popular, but probably for entirely different reasons, which may be associated with lifestyles and holiday habits; the reported incidence in whites rose by no less than 102% from 1973 to 1991 (41). Finally, as the Australian authors themselves stressed, the fact that the Queensland clinic was a private institution specializing in IVF/GIFT therapy means that women with endocrine-associated or ovulation-associated infertility may not have been referred to it so readily.

All this makes it very difficult to find a baseline inci-dence for melanoma with which cases treated for inferti-lity can be compared. It is to be hoped that data of this type will continue to arrive from other centers, so that a definitive judgement will become possible.

Mammary cancer in the mother has been suspected as a risk of clomiphene, but specific investigations into the mat-ter have not supported this suspicion (SED-12, 1034; 42).

A case of testicular seminoma in a man receiving both clomiphene and mesterolone for 15 months for oligosper-mia has been described (43), but it is unlikely that the drug was responsible.

Cocaine

Chronic cocaine use, which is associated with immuno-suppression, may be carcinogenic. The possible associa-tion between chronic cocaine exposure and pancreatic adenocarcinoma has been investigated (44,45). A study of hospital records in Brazil for the years 1986–1998 showed that of 198 patients with pancreatic adenocarci-noma, 13 (6.5%) were younger than 40 years; of these, five had a history of chronic cocaine inhalation and one had abused marijuana.

Danazol

Danazol is a weak androgen and also has a series of other hormonal and anti-hormonal properties. It inhibits pituitary gonadotropin and has been used in the treatment of endometriosis, fibrocystic disease of the breast, idiopathic thrombocytopenic purpura, and hereditary angioedema. Its hepatotoxic effects include reversible rises in serum transaminases and cholestatic hepatitis; a few cases of hepatocellular tumors have been reported.

- A 34-year-old woman who had taken danazol 400 mg/day for 13 years for hereditary angioedema developed a mass in the right hypochondrium. Her alcohol intake was under 20 g/day. She had a large heterogeneous hepatic tumor, a well-differentiated hepatocellullar carcinoma in a non-cirrhotic liver.

The hypothesis that hepatocellular carcinoma had been caused by danazol was accepted in the absence of other causes (46).

Deferoxamine

Deferoxamine is used experimentally in a variety of diseases, including Kaposi's sarcoma, and in vitro tests have suggested that it inhibits the growth of sarcoma-derived cells (47). Unfortunately, the intralesional injection of deferoxamine led to paradoxical exacerbation of Kaposi's sarcoma of the skin and the development of numerous sarcomatous papules in the area of injection, whereas there were no changes in untreated lesions (48).

Diuretics

See also Spironolactone

There is an association between diuretic use and renal cell carcinoma (49). Some of the studies that support this association can be dismissed, since the epidemiological data on which they were based were not suitably adjusted for confounding variables, including obesity, hypertension, age, and cigarette smoking. However, other case-control studies have shown a small risk of renal cell carcinoma in patients taking long-term diuretics after adjustment of the data for potentially confounding variables.

The carcinogenic mechanism of diuretics is not known, but could be related to a carcinogenic action of N-nitroso metabolic derivatives of thiazide and loop diuretics or structural changes in the transporting tubular epithelia, which provoke different stages of apoptosis. Rats and mice treated with diuretics have been reported to develop nephropathies and renal adenomas. Renal cell carcinoma arises in renal tubular cells, which are the principal site of action of diuretics. Contact over years or decades may have a low-grade carcinogenic effect. However, most prospective randomized trials provide too short a period of observation to assess the potential for carcinogenicity unequivocally. Furthermore, the findings may have been confounded by other risk factors

for renal cell carcinoma. Adjustment for confounders greatly attenuated the risk (to non-significance) in one study, and in another the association with diuretic use disappeared completely. Therefore, the findings from these observational studies may have resulted from uncontrolled confounding by known or unrecognized risk factors.

The relation between diuretic therapy and the risk of malignancies has been examined in a review of pertinent publications between 1966 and 1998 (50). In nine case control studies (4185 cases), the odds ratio for renal cell carcinoma in patients treated with diuretics was 1.55 (95% CI = 1.42, 1.71) compared with non-users of diuretics. In three cohort studies of 1 226 229 patients (802 cases), patients taking diuretics had a more than two-fold risk of renal cell carcinoma compared with patients not taking diuretics. Women had an odds ratio of 2.01 (CI = 1.56, 1.67) compared with 1.96 (CI = 1.34, 2.13) in men. Thus, the cumulative evidence suggests that long-term use of diuretics may be associated with renal cell carcinoma.

The findings linking diuretic therapy with renal cell carcinoma need careful scrutiny. The strength of evidence provided by observational studies is limited, and such studies have yielded contradictory and controversial results in the past. An accompanying editorial (51) pointed out that some of the studies reviewed appear to have been designed to evaluate predictors of renal cell carcinoma without an a priori hypothesis that diuretics might be implicated. Statistical significance (set at $P < 0.05$) may have emerged merely by chance if 20 risk factors were examined.

Another commentary (52) emphasized the potential bias of observational studies and also publication bias in meta-analysis. The contemporary relevance of the findings is further reduced, since many of the studies included patients taking very high doses of thiazides. It is difficult to disentangle a drug-related effect from the association between hypertension and renal cell carcinoma.

Since renal cell carcinoma is rare, the practical importance of these observations is small: one extra case of renal cell carcinoma in 1500 patients treated for 20 years. If the hypothesis is correct, antihypertensive therapy with diuretics will prevent 20–40 strokes, 3–28 heart attacks, 3–10 cardiovascular deaths, and 4–14 deaths overall for every extra case of renal cell carcinoma. Even middle-aged women would be spared six strokes for each potential case of renal cell carcinoma. If a low grade carcinogen is involved, most patients will not live long enough for its effect to be expressed. The available information does not support a change in current prescription practices for diuretics in the treatment of hypertension and cardiac failure. Physicians should be more concerned about controlling blood pressure rather than concerning themselves with what at best might be a small risk of renal cell carcinoma.

Other cancer types have been evaluated for their association with diuretic therapy. The development of colon cancer has been studied in 14 166 patients aged 45–74 years with a previous myocardial infarction and/or stable angina, screened for participation in the Bezafibrate

Infarction Prevention Study (53). Of these, 2153 used diuretics and 12 013 did not. Multivariate analysis identified diuretics as an independent predictor of an increased incidence of colon cancer (hazard ratio 2.0) and colon cancer mortality (hazard ratio 3.7). However, the association between diuretic therapy and a higher incidence of colon cancer was observed only among non-users of aspirin. There was a relatively lower incidence of colon cancer in furosemide users and a higher incidence in the small combined subgroup of those who took amiloride and/or hydrochlorothiazide. Further studies to test the association between diuretics and colon cancer, as well as the potential protective effects of aspirin, are needed. Until these data become available, physicians should be aware of the potential effects of diuretics, especially when choosing long-term treatment for young patients with mild hypertension.

Estrogens

The complexity of the relation between hormonal replacement therapy and breast cancer has been stressed (SED-14, 1454) (SEDA-22, 465), and much depends on the type of replacement therapy given and the class of tumor studied. This latter point has been underscored by a US study that provided evidence that the use of combined hormonal replacement therapy increases the risk of lobular, but not ductal, breast carcinoma in middle-aged women (54).

An American cohort study designed to determine whether increases in risk associated with an estrogen + progestogen regimen are greater than those associated with estrogen alone has been carried out based on follow-up data for 1980–1995 from the National Breast Cancer Detection Demonstration Project (55). From 46 355 postmenopausal women, mean age at the start of follow-up was 58 years, 2082 cases of breast cancer were identified. Increases in risk with estrogen only and estrogen + progestogen were restricted to use within the previous 4 years, the relative risks being 1.2 and 1.4 respectively. The relative risk increased by 0.01 with each year of estrogen use and by 0.08 with each year of estrogen + progestogen use. Among women with a BMI of 24.4 kg/m^2 or less, the mean increases in relative risk were 0.03 and 0.12 with each year of estrogen use and estrogen + progestogen use respectively. These associations were evident for the majority of invasive tumors with ductal histology and regardless of the extent of invasive disease. The risk in heavier women did not increase with the use of estrogen only or estrogen + progestogen. These data suggest that estrogen + progestogen increases the risk of breast cancer beyond that associated with estrogen alone.

Exposure to diethylstilbestrol during pregnancy in 4836 women has been reported to carry a relative risk of 1.27 of breast cancer later in life. However, the authors found no evidence to support the link between diethylstilbestrol exposure and ovarian, endometrial, or other cancers.

In a 25-year follow-up study there were very slightly more breast tumors in women using diethylstilbestrol in pregnancy and significantly more cancer deaths (56).

In one study there was a six-fold risk of endometrial cancer among estrogen users compared with non-users; long-term users (over 5 years) had a 15-fold risk; there were excess risks for both diethylstilbestrol and conjugated estrogens (57).

Diethylstilbestrol can cause hepatic adenomas and carcinomas in experimental animals (58), and hepatocellular carcinoma has been reported in a man who took a total of 668 g over 12 years for suspected carcinoma of the prostate (59).

For the sake of simplicity the carcinogenic effects of estrogens in all formulations, including the combined oral contraceptives, are included here.

Knowledge of tumor induction by sex steroids is largely based on interpretation of epidemiological data, with careful exclusion of possible confounding elements. Hepatic tumors have given rise to most concerns, but some evidence also indicates an increased incidence of various other malignancies, including carcinomas of the breast, endometrium, and prostate (60).

The overall incidence of reproductive cancers attributable to oral contraceptive use has been estimated in a modeling analysis (61). The authors assumed a 50% reduction in ovarian and endometrial cancers associated with 5 years or more of tablet use, and used two alternative scenarios for breast and cervical cancer effects. If oral contraceptive use produces a 20% increase in breast cancer before age 50 and the same increase in cervical cancer, then for every 100 000 tablet users there would be 44 fewer reproductive cancers and these users would gain one more day free of cancer. If instead the increase in risk of early breast cancer and of cervical cancer is 50%, oral contraceptive users would have 11 fewer cancer-free days.

In dealing with liver tumors, it is essential to consider all the various types of sex steroids in a single review since they seem to resemble one another closely in their long-term effects on this organ. The nomenclature used in the literature is unfortunately confusing: most reports differentiate between "hepatic adenoma" and "focal nodular hyperplasia," but the latter term is also sometimes used to cover the whole range. Other terms that have been used are "focal cirrhosis," "regenerative hyperplasia," "hamartoma," "mixed adenoma," and "benign hepatoma," while "peliosis" may constitute a precancerous state.

Ethylene oxide

Ethylene oxide is carcinogenic, assigned to Group 1 of the IARC (62). There is limited evidence of carcinogenicity in humans, but much evidence in experimental animals, and the IARC has classified ethylene oxide in category 1 ("carcinogenic in humans"), based primarily on evidence in animals and genotoxic considerations. The overall evaluation of the Working group of the IARC, updated in 1995, is based on the following supporting evidence.

Ethylene oxide is a directly acting alkylating agent that:

- induces a sensitive, persistent, dose-related increase in the frequency of chromosomal aberrations and sister chromatid exchange in peripheral lymphocytes and micronuclei in bone marrow cells of exposed workers;
- has been associated with malignancies of the lymphatic and hemopoietic systems in both humans and experimental animals;
- induces a dose-related increase in the frequency of hemoglobin adducts in exposed humans and a dose-related increase in the numbers of adducts in both DNA and hemoglobin in exposed rodents;
- induces gene mutations and heritable translocations in germ cells of exposed rodents;
- is a powerful mutagen and clastogen at all phylogenetic levels.

In 1979, three cases of hemopoietic cancer that had occurred between 1972 and 1977 were reported in workers at a Swedish factory where 50% ethylene oxide and 50% methyl formate had been used since 1968 to sterilize hospital equipment (63).

In epidemiological studies of exposure to ethylene oxide, the most frequently reported association has been with lymphatic and hemopoietic cancer. Two populations were studied: people using ethylene oxide as a sterilizing agent and chemical workers manufacturing or using ethylene oxide. Of studies of sterilization personnel, the largest and most informative is that conducted in the USA (64,65). Overall, mortality from lymphatic and hemopoietic cancers was only marginally raised, but there was a significant trend, especially for lymphatic leukemia and non-Hodgkin's lymphoma, in relation to estimated cumulative exposure. For exposure to 1 ppm (1.8 mg/m^3) over a working lifetime of 45 years, a ratio of 1.2 was estimated for lymphatic and hemopoietic cancers. The other studies of workers involved in sterilization in Sweden (66–68) and in the UK (69) each showed non-significant excesses of lymphatic and hemopoietic cancers. An assessment based on epidemiological data showed no increase in leukemia in those who had been exposed to ethylene oxide (70).

Because of the possibility of confounding occupational exposure in the studies of chemical workers exposed to ethylene oxide (71,66,67,69,72–80), less weight can be given to the positive findings. Nevertheless, they are compatible with a small but consistent excess of lymphatic and hemopoietic cancers found in studies of sterilization personnel. Some of the epidemiological studies have shown an additional risk of cancer of the stomach, which was significant only in one study from Sweden (66,67,72).

Fluoroquinolones

Results of carcinogenicity studies have suggested that the risk of neoplastic disease is minimal, even during long-term use (81). However, the risk may be increased by exposure to UVA light. Skin tumors, only a minority of them malignant, developed in mice after treatment with various quinolones for up to 78 weeks and exposure to

UV light. It therefore appears that fluoroquinolones have the potential to enhance the UVA-induced phototumorigenic effect (82).

Folic acid

In a large US cohort study folic acid was associated with an increased risk of cancer in general and of cancers of the oropharynx and hypopharynx (83). However, the authors pointed to the possibility that the observed association could have depended on confounding by alcohol and smoking.

Formaldehyde

There is evidence of possible carcinogenicity of formaldehyde from two inhalation studies on rats and mice (SEDA-10, 423; SEDA-11, 477; SEDA-12, 571) (84).

In man, a number of epidemiological studies using different designs have been conducted (85) on the health risks of non-medical exposure to formaldehyde and also in health-care professionals (86–91), with contradictory results. Cancers in excess in more than one study were: Hodgkin's disease (92,93), leukemia (86,87,90,91,94), cancers of the buccal cavity and pharynx (particular the nasopharynx) (86,87,93,95,96), lung (86,92,95,97–99), nose (100–104), prostate (87,92,94), bladder (87,91,94), brain (105), colon (86–88,93,95), skin (86,93), and kidney (95).

There was no association between formaldehyde exposure and lung cancer in a case-referral study among Danish physicians working in departments of pathology, forensic medicine, and anatomy (89).

Mortality from prostatic cancer was increased among embalmers (87) and industrial workers (92,94), but the excess was statistically significant only among embalmers (87). A slight excess of mortality from bladder cancer (87,90,94), a significant excess of colon cancers (86,87,95), and a significant excess mortality from skin cancer (86,93) were noted among British pathologists (90), embalmers (86,87), and industrial workers (93–95).

Excess mortality from leukemia and cancer of the brain was generally not seen among industrial workers, which suggests that the increased rates of these cancers among professionals (anatomists (105), pathologists (90), embalmers (86,87), and undertakers (91)) is due to factors other than just formaldehyde.

It is of course possible that the studies that have provided positive evidence of a link between formaldehyde and cancer related to more intensive exposure; for example, reports on the risk associated with chronic exposure to low concentrations of formaldehyde suggest that formaldehyde cannot be a potent carcinogen; if it were, the high degree of environmental exposure would result in much clearer evidence of risk. However, any compound that produces cancer in experimental animals or mutagenicity in several test systems should be considered as a potential cancer risk to human subjects, even though humans and animals may differ in their susceptibility to formaldehyde. The contradictory evidence from human studies should therefore be taken seriously and efforts should be made to reduce exposure.

The need to re-evaluate the rationale underlying the use of formaldehyde, formocresol, and paraformaldehyde in dentistry has been stressed, since the clinical use and delivery of these products are considered to be arbitrary and unscientific (106).

Glucocorticoids

Direct tumor-inducing effects of the glucocorticoids are not known, but the particular risk that malignancies in patients undergoing immunosuppression with these or other drugs will spread more rapidly is a well-recognized problem.

- Progressive endometrial carcinoma associated with azathioprine and prednisone therapy has been reported (107).
- Rapid progression of Kaposi's sarcoma 10 weeks after combined treatment with glucocorticoids and cyclophosphamide has been described; marked improvement of the skin lesions was noted after discontinuation of prednisone therapy (108).

Patients (mean age 39 years, $n = 1862$) who underwent 1924 renal transplantations from March 1995 to May 1997 were followed for 3–150 months. They received one of the following regimens: prednisolone plus azathioprine (group 1; $n = 100$); prednisolone plus azathioprine plus ciclosporin (group 2; $n = 1464$); and the same therapy as group 2 plus either muromonab-CD3 or antithymocyte globulin as induction or antirejection therapy (group 3; $n = 298$). The mean time to appearance of neoplasia after renal transplantation was 48 months. Malignancies developed earlier in group 3 patients (mean time to appearance 31 months) than in group 2 (39 months) and in group 1 (90 months). Seven of the patients who developed malignancies had also received pulse methylprednisolone for acute rejection. The authors concluded that the treatment of acute rejection with pulsed methylprednisolone and the use of muromonab-CD3 and antithymocyte globulin may lead to an increased incidence of malignancies after renal transplantation. They recommended that strategies be implemented for the early detection of malignancy (109).

In seven patients, accelerated growth of Kaposi's sarcoma lesions during glucocorticoid therapy suggested that glucocorticoids can alter the biological behavior of this malignant disease (110). Hydrocortisone accelerates the growth of cell lines derived from Kaposi's sarcoma cells cultured in vitro and this may partially explain these findings. Reports continue to point to the reversibility of the condition when glucocorticoids are withdrawn (111).

Kaposi's sarcoma has been associated with prednisolone therapy in two elderly women (112).

- An 84-year-old woman with polymyalgia rheumatica and a 79-year-old woman with undifferentiated connective tissue disease and leukocytoclastic vasculitis were given prednisolone 20 mg/day with subsequent dosage reductions. The first patient developed a raised

purpuric rash and lymphedema of the left leg within 5 months and the second developed large purple nodules on the soles of her feet and the backs of her hands accompanied by periorbital and peripheral edema. Skin biopsies showed Kaposi's sarcoma, and both patients had raised IgG antibody titers to human herpesvirus-8.

Prior infection with herpesvirus-8 is a requisite for the development of Kaposi's sarcoma. The question arises as to how glucocorticoid treatment alone can lead to the emergence of this malignancy. In vitro evidence supports the hypothesis that glucocorticoids have a direct role in stimulating tumor development and the activation of herpesvirus-8.

A possible relation between systemic glucocorticoid use and a risk of esophageal cancer has been described in a population-based study in Denmark, in which the prescriptions database and the Danish cancer registry were linked (113). There was an increase in the number of cases observed ($n = 36$) compared with the number expected ($n = 19$), with a standardized incidence ratio of 1.92 (95% CI = 1.34, 2.65).

Gonadorelin

Tumor flare occurs in up to 30% of treated patients after the first 4–7 days of gonadorelin therapy, due to an initial surge in gonadotropin concentrations (114). For this reason antiandrogen treatment is often given before gonadorelin in men with prostate cancer. However, despite tumor flare there was no difference in survival in a prospective, multicenter comparison of gonadorelin and surgical oophorectomy in 136 patients (115).

Granulocyte colony-stimulating factor

Concerns have arisen over the prolonged use of G-CSF in patients with aplastic anemia, congenital neutropenia, or similar disorders and a possible increased or accelerated risk of myelodysplasia or acute leukemia (SED-14, 1274). Several investigators have noted reversible increases in circulating blasts during G-CSF treatment, and isolated reports have indicated a shortened delay in the occurrence of myelodysplasia and/or acute myeloid leukemia in this setting (SED-13, 1117; SEDA-20, 338) (116). An abnormal karyotype (mostly monosomy 7) was sometimes found, and in vitro proliferation of myeloblasts by G-CSF was obtained in several patients. In addition, the potential role of point mutations on the G-CSF receptor has been also discussed as regards four of 28 patients with congenital neutropenia, two of whom developed acute myeloid leukemia (117). Myelodysplastic syndrome with monosomy 7 was also associated with G-CSF in another patient, with a reduction in the number of monosomy 7 positive cells after G-CSF withdrawal and a further increase after readministration (118).

This has been analysed in a number of epidemiological studies, most of which involved historical controls. The underlying predisposition of patients with aplastic anemia to develop myeloid malignancy has usually confounded attempts to determine whether growth factors are contributing factors.

In a retrospective study of 72 adults with aplastic anemia, of whom 18 received G-CSF and 23 received ciclosporin, five developed myelodysplastic syndrome (119). Four of them had received G-CSF + ciclosporin and all four had monosomy 7. The hematological disease was diagnosed within 16–31 months after the diagnosis of aplastic anemia and 12–20 months after the start of G-CSF treatment. Two died from acute leukemia. The incidence of myelodysplastic syndrome in this subgroup of patients was therefore 8.3% after 2 years and 39% after 3 years, whereas no case was observed over a 20-year period in patients not receiving this combined treatment. Univariate analysis showed that G-CSF + ciclosporin and G-CSF alone for more than 1 year were the most significant risk factors for the short-term development of monosomy 7 myelodysplastic syndrome.

In a prospective, multicenter, cohort study of 113 patients with aplastic anemia under 18 years of age, 12 developed myelodysplastic syndrome after a median of 37 months after the diagnosis of aplastic anemia and four others developed other cytogenetic clonal changes, of which the most common abnormality was monosomy 7 (120). From a multivariate analysis, G-CSF treatment duration and non-response to immunosuppressive therapy at 6 months were statistically significant risk factors for the development of myelodysplastic syndrome. The risk increased in proportion to the duration of G-CSF treatment, and the relative risks of the myelodysplastic syndrome were respectively 4.4 and 8.7 times higher in patients who received G-CSF for more than 120 and 180 days, compared with those who received it for less.

In contrast, a number of other studies did not confirm that the G-CSF increases the risk of myelodysplasia or acute leukemia, but the authors did not rule out a possible leukemogenic effect. In a study of patients with severe aplastic anemia the frequencies of cytogenetic abnormalities and myelodysplasia or leukemia were similar in 87 patients treated with G-CSF in addition to immunosuppressive treatment compared with 57 patients who did not receive G-CSF (121). Although the authors stated that a leukemogenic effect of G-CSF was unlikely, they mentioned that the median interval of appearance of cytogenetic abnormalities was shorter in the G-CSF group.

In another study the data from an international register of patients with severe chronic neutropenia were analysed (122). Of 352 patients treated with G-CSF for congenital neutropenia and followed for a mean of 6 years (maximum 11 years), 31 developed myelodysplasia or leukemia, whereas there were no cases in 344 patients with idiopathic or cyclic neutropenia. Associated cytogenetic clonal changes consisted of partial or complete loss of chromosome seven in 18 patients and abnormalities in chromosome 21 in nine. Isolated cytogenetic abnormalities were also found in nine other patients. None of the patients had abnormal marrow cytogenetic changes before G-CSF therapy. A more complete analysis failed to identify any correlation between G-CSF dose and treatment duration in patients who developed myelodysplasia or leukemia compared with those who were not affected. Although this argues against a role of G-CSF in the conversion of congenital neutropenia to myelodysplasia or leukemia, the authors recognized that a direct leukemogenic role of G-CSF could not be completely ruled out.

After a median follow-up of 43 months in 123 children treated with G-CSF, there was no difference in the incidence of secondary myelodysplasia or acute myeloid leukemia, in patients with aplastic anemia who survived longer than 2 years compared with the expected rate calculated before the use of G-CSF (123). Similarly, there was no evidence of an increased risk of myelodysplasia or acute myeloid leukemia in 54 patients treated with G-CSF for 4–6 years for severe congenital neutropenia (124).

Finally, in a randomized study in 102 patients of the safety and efficacy of lenograstim (5 micrograms/kg/day for 14 weeks) combined with standard immunosuppressants, there were no differences between the groups in survival, hematological response, or the occurrence of secondary leukemia (one case of myelodysplastic syndrome in each group) at a median follow-up of 5 years (125).

The role of G-CSF in leukemic transformation therefore remains unproven, primarily because these patients might be otherwise predisposed or have a previous history of immunosuppressive therapy. Although the clinical benefits of G-CSF probably outweigh any hazard of leukemogenesis, the possibility of an increased risk of myelodysplastic syndrome or acute myeloid leukemia under the influence of G-CSF should be borne in mind. Careful monitoring of morphological bone marrow changes and cytogenetic studies are therefore recommended, and large randomized trials with long-term follow-up are still awaited to clarify these findings.

Carcinogenetic effects of nickel, recognized from occupational medicine, can involve the upper or lower respiratory tract.

Previous fears that GM-CSF might give rise to progression of pre-leukemic conditions have not been substantiated (126).

The possibility that growth factors can stimulate the growth of malignant and leukemic cells, or accelerate the progression of myelodysplastic syndrome to acute myeloid leukemia has been discussed in the monograph on G-CSF section. At the moment, there is no indication from clinical trials that GM-CSF actually increases the risk of tumor growth or the relapse rate in patients with various malignancies (127,128–130). Isolated reports have referred to delayed occurrence of B cell non-Hodgkin's lymphoma after GM-CSF treatment for aplastic anemia and de novo occurrence of diffuse oligoclonal plasmocytosis after both GM-CSF and G-CSF for high-grade glioma (SEDA-19, 342).

Although reversible increases in circulating blasts during GM-CSF treatment are sometimes noted and have raised concern on the possible accelerated occurrence of acute leukemia, the progression of myelodysplastic syndromes to acute myeloid leukemia has been only anecdotally reported (SEDA-19, 342) (131). There was no evidence of significant leukemic cell proliferation in patients with acute myeloid leukemia, and no increased risk of graft failure, leukemogenesis, relapse, or death after a median follow-up of 36 months in 128 patients who underwent autologous bone marrow transplantation for lymphoid malignancies (127,132). Finally, one report has suggested that a GM-CSF-induced abrupt rise in peripheral blasts may have caused diffuse infiltration and proliferation of leukemic blast cells in the spleen, and subsequent fatal hemorrhagic spleen rupture (133).

Growth hormone

The incidence of malignancy is increased in acromegaly, in which growth hormone is present in excess. Patients treated with growth hormone have therefore been carefully monitored. The first report of leukemia in Japanese children treated with growth hormone (341) prompted a worldwide survey. There have been reports of 44 new cases of leukemia in growth hormone recipients, of which only 20 were acute lymphoblastic leukemia. This is much less than the expected 80–85% of new childhood leukemia (134).

A review of Japanese patients found that of the 15 patients who had developed hematological malignancies since 1975, 6 had other risk factors for leukemia, such as Fanconi's syndrome or prior chemotherapy or radiotherapy. The incidence of leukemia in this study was 3 per 100 000, similar to that in the general population of the same age (135). The National Cooperative Growth Study (NCGS—a postmarketing database that includes 19 846 patient-years since the time of growth hormone exposure) similarly reported no increase in the incidence of new leukemia when patients with other risk factors were excluded from the analysis (136).

The recurrence rate of intracranial tumors has been addressed in a number of large observational studies. Reports from the NCGS database (which includes 1262 children with brain tumors) and from England have shown no increase in intracranial tumor recurrence in patients treated with growth hormone (137,138). For patients with craniopharyngioma, postoperative irradiation reduced the recurrence rate, but growth hormone therapy did not increase the risk (139).

In the NCGS study extracranial non-leukemia malignancy rates were similarly not increased in patients treated with growth hormone compared with those who were not (140).

Despite theoretical concerns, there is no evidence that either intracranial or extracranial malignancy, new or recurrent, is increased in subjects treated with growth hormone (137,139,140). Despite this, certain precautions are still recommended for children who have previously been treated for cancer. The diagnosis of growth hormone deficiency should be clearly established (134) and it is recommended that treatment be delayed for at least 1 year after tumor therapy has been completed (141).

In a cohort study in 1848 British patients who received human pituitary-derived growth hormone from 1959 to 1985 (30 000 patient-years), there were two cases of colorectal cancer (0.25 expected) and two cases of Hodgkin's disease (0.85 expected); the standardized mortality ratios were 10.8 and 11.4 respectively (142). However, the number of cancers was small and the doses used were higher than typically today, and these results should be interpreted with caution.

Hair dyes

In a review of cohort and case-control studies of occupational exposure to hair dyes among hairdressers, barbers, and beauticians, the relative risk of bladder cancer was 1.4 from cohort studies, and somewhat over 1.0 from case-control studies; however, there were confounding factors, particularly since allowance for smoking was lacking or inadequate in most studies (143). In five case-control studies of personal use of hair dyes, there was no evidence of an increased risk of bladder cancer. In nine cohort studies the relative risk of lymphoid neoplasms overall was 1.2 (1.5 for non-Hodgkin's lymphomas and 1.1 for multiple myeloma). Of five case-control studies, three reported some association with lymphoid neoplasms, but the estimates of relative risk were only moderately above 1.0 and there was insufficient allowance for potential confounding factors, including social class and greying hair, which could correlate with both hair dye use and lymphoid neoplasms. No other neoplasms, including those of breast, skin, and lung were related to the use of hair dyes. In another study there was an increased risk of Hodgkin's disease among women who reported the use of hair coloring products before 1980 (OR = 1.3; CI = 1, 1.8) (144).

Histamine (H₂) receptor antagonists

Tumor-inducing effects have been much discussed ever since the introduction of the H_2 receptor antagonists but their existence has not been clearly established. The discussion was seeded by:

- findings of intestinal metaplasia of the gastric epithelium in rats used for chronic toxicity studies, though only at extraordinarily high doses, followed by the appearance of intramucosal carcinomas in the pyloric region after 11 months of study;
- reports of patients taking cimetidine in whom gastric carcinoma was diagnosed; however, the drug has been widely (and sometimes without careful prior diagnosis) used in patients with a range of gastric disorders, and some of these are believed to have had early carcinomas at the time when cimetidine was started (145);
- the fact that cimetidine can undergo nitrosylation to form a mutagen;
- the structural resemblance of cimetidine to tiotidine, which can cause gastric carcinoma in animals.

In a retrospective case-control assessment of medical records of 56 patients who died of cardio-esophageal adenocarcinoma and 56 age- and sex-matched controls who died of myocardial infarction, subjects who died of cardio-esophageal adenocarcinoma were more likely to have consumed H_2 receptor antagonists (RR = 7.5; 95% CI = 1.3,42) (146).

However, there is still no valid reason for considering the H_2 receptor antagonists to be tumorigenic, and when studies have detected some excess incidence of gastric cancer in long-term users of H_2 receptor antagonists this was attributable to selection bias (147). The fact that drugs of this type have now been released for self-medication in many countries seems very likely to lead to an increase in the incidence of cases in which an H_2 receptor antagonist is used without prior exclusion of premalignant or malignant change, thus confusing the situation further.

- A gastric carcinoid tumor was found in a man of 62 taking ranitidine (148). The dosage had been unusually high and there was pre-existing chronic renal insufficiency as well as diabetes, but the tumor was similar in type to that seen in animals; it was successfully removed by partial gastrectomy and did not recur.

HMG Co–enzyme A reductase inhibitors

It has been suspected that low concentrations of serum cholesterol might be associated with an increased risk of cancer or overall mortality. All fibrates and statins cause cancer in rodents, but the relevance of this finding to man has been questioned (149). In an epidemiological study these risks were almost non-existent after adjusting for confounding factors. However, in the CARE study, breast cancer occurred in one patient in the control group and 12 in the pravastatin group (150). The incidence of cancers, both during clinical studies and up to 9 years after, has been reassuring (151).

Hycanthone

Experimentally, hycanthone has been reported to be carcinogenic in mice (152,153), but no human data are available.

Hydroxytoluene

Although it has been suggested that butylated hydroxytoluene induces tumors in rats, others have suggested that it may protect tissues against the carcinogenic effects of many different substances.

Insulin–like growth factor

A non-Hodgkin's lymphoma developed in the right femur of a 58-year-old man who had used IGF-I 40 micrograms bd (154) in a study of the effect of adding IGF to insulin therapy (SEDA-23, 457).

Iron

The risk of colorectal cancer due to iron has been specifically examined in a prospective investigation in more than 14 000 patients (155). Iron appears to confer an increased risk of colorectal cancer, and the localization of risk may be attributable to the mode of epithelial exposure. It seems that luminal exposure to oral iron increases the risk proximally, whereas an increased serum iron concentration increases the risk distally.

Genetic hemochromatosis constitutes a high risk factor for the development of hepatocellular carcinoma. It is widely accepted that venesection prevents the evolution of cirrhosis in hemochromatosis and indirectly protects against the development of hepatocellular carcinoma. However, three cases did not conform to the "siderosis-cirrhosis-carcinoma" sequence, and prompt and adequate iron depletion did not protect against the development of cancer (156).

- A 39-year-old army officer had bouts of palpitation and dizziness. There were no risk factors for chronic liver disease apart from a family history of hemochromatosis. His cardiovascular and nervous systems were normal but there was 5 cm hepatomegaly. Percutaneous liver biopsy showed grade 4 siderosis in parenchymal and non-parenchymal liver cells and a mild inflammatory infiltrate with minimal portal fibrosis. He had 45 liters of blood venesected over the next 18 months and a repeat biopsy 3 years later showed a non-cirrhotic liver with no stainable iron. He developed a non-resectable primary hepatocellular clear cell carcinoma 17 years after the initial diagnosis.
- The other two cases were male siblings. One presented with atypical chest pain and had 3 cm hepatomegaly. Liver biopsy showed parenchymal grade 4 siderosis with normal architecture. He had 170 liters of blood venesected over the next 27 years, but then his iron indices indicated reaccumulation. Ultrasound showed a hyperechoic lesion in the liver due to a moderately differentiated hepatocellular carcinoma. His elder sibling, who had grade 4 siderosis and normal hepatic architecture, also developed a well-differentiated hepatocellular carcinoma.

Lithium

There is no evidence that lithium causes of promotes the growth of tumors. Since tumors are not rare events over a lifetime, and since lithium is taken for long periods of time, any apparent association is likely to be coincidental.

Medroxyprogesterone

The effects of depot medroxyprogesterone acetate on reproductive cancers appear to be similar to those of combined oral contraceptives. Most notably, despite initial concerns about breast cancer in beagle dogs that were given large doses of medroxyprogesterone, a pooled analysis of epidemiological studies concluded that women using medroxyprogesterone are not at increased risk of breast cancer (157). Furthermore, the risk did not increase with increasing duration of use. However, women who had begun use within the past 5 years had significantly increased risk, perhaps because of accelerated growth of pre-existing tumors or increased surveillance.

Another review, dating from 1994, concluded that depot medroxyprogesterone acetate has a protective effect against endometrial cancer that is at least as strong as for combined oral contraceptives, but that, based on the limited available evidence, there is no association with ovarian cancer (158). Regarding cervical neoplasia, studies of depot medroxyprogesterone acetate do not show a strong adverse effect, but as with combined oral contraceptives it is uncertain whether there is no association or a slightly increased risk (159).

Mepacrine

The possibility of a relation of mepacrine to the incidence of squamous cell carcinoma was suspected in Australian ex-servicemen, but causality is not clear (SEDA-13, 818; SEDA-14, 241). Extensive sun exposure could have been a factor, and that would explain the difference in findings around the world.

Methapyrilene

Tumor-inducing effects have been reported in animal studies on methapyrilene; the significance of this finding is not clear (SEDA-4, 171). An association between antihistamine exposure and accelerated tumor growth seen in experimental animal models has found no support in an epidemiological study (160).

Methylxanthines

A possible association between the use of methylxanthine consumption and the occurrence of fibrocystic breast disease has been suggested (SEDA-6, 8) (161). It was concluded that in women who are predisposed to fibrocystic disease, methylxanthines are factors in its development. The mechanism of this effect might be an inhibitory action on the activity of cyclic AMP and cyclic GMP phosphodiesterases.

Metronidazole

Prolonged high-dose exposure of mice to metronidazole leads to an increased incidence of lung tumors, and in one study there was an increase in lymphoreticular neoplasia in female animals. These results, which caused much concern when first published, are probably non-specific and not relevant to humans; these and other neoplasms have also been induced in mice merely by varying the diet. Several long-term follow-up studies in man have failed to demonstrate an excess cancer risk (SEDA-13, 831). There has been a single report of cancers in three patients with Crohn's disease who had taken metronidazole for years (SEDA-11, 595) (162), but they had also taken sulfasalazine and glucocorticoids, and this cannot be regarded as constituting reasonable evidence of a causal link.

Neuroleptic drugs

Since neuroleptic drugs raise prolactin concentrations, there is concern that this may increase the risk of breast cancer. Although studies have failed to show an association, it would be best to avoid neuroleptic drugs in a patient with a hormone-dependent breast tumor.

There is concern that neuroleptic drugs may increase the risk of breast cancer because of raised prolactin concentrations. For a long time, findings did not confirm this association (163), but a Danish cohort study of 6152 patients showed a slight increase in the risk of breast cancer among schizophrenic women (164).

Nitrofurantoin

Some studies have shown similar metabolism of nitrofurantoin and other (carcinogenic) nitrofurans. Formation of carcinogenic nitrofurantoin metabolites is therefore possible (165). However, a carcinogenic effect has not been proven for nitrofurantoin (166).

Nitric oxide

In view of the hypothesis that nitric oxide can have mutagenic or carcinogenic effects, chromosomal alterations have been sought in blood lymphocytes from patients taking chronic nitrates and after in vitro exposure to a nitric oxide donor (167). No structural alterations were found in vivo or in vitro, only an increased frequency of micronucleus formation, a nuclear morphological change that has been suggested to be associated with a risk of cancer. However, this first report of a genotoxic effect of nitrates probably has no clinical relevance.

Paraffin

There have been many reports of so-called paraffinomas, benign tumors due to granulomatous reactions, in patients using paraffin.

Paraffin used for breast enhancement can cause mammary paraffinomas, and there have been many such reports in men and women (177–197). The tumors can calcify but are benign; in one case there was no evidence of malignant transformation after 60 years (198), although in another case there was an associated malignancy (199). Lymphatic spread of paraffin has been described (200), as has sarcoid formation (201).

Paraffinomas have also been reported after the use of paraffin to enhance the male and female external genitalia (197,202–217).

When liquid paraffin is used as a laxative, paraffinomas can occur in the colon and rectum (218–221).

Paraffin used as packing after nasal surgery can cause nasal paraffinomas (222–227).

Other tissues in which paraffinomas have been reported include the orbit and eyelids (228–232), the lungs (233–240), the limbs (241–243), sometimes with subsequent calcification (244), the face (245–247), nose (248), and scalp (249), muscle (250), the bladder (251), and the ureter (252).

Although in most cases paraffinomas occur at the site of injection, remote deposition can occur, for example in the mediastinum (253–255).

- A 55-year-old woman, who had undergone intrapleural injection of paraffin for pulmonary tuberculosis 15 years before, developed a large left-sided chest wall mass and spinal paralysis (256). A paraffinoma had invaded the vertebral canal.

Paraffin deposition has also been reported in the retinal fundi, the liver, and the spleen, in addition to the lungs (257).

There is epidemiological evidence linking the use of liquid paraffin to gastrointestinal cancer (258). Malignant transformation of a paraffinoma has occasionally been suggested.

- An 82-year-old woman who had taken long-term liquid paraffin as a laxative, developed a lipoid pneumonia and a mesothelioma (259).

Parathyroid hormone

The rate of osteosarcoma in animal and human trials of parathyroid hormone has been reviewed (260). Rats treated with parathyroid hormone for 2 years had a high dose-dependent rate of osteosarcoma, up to 48% in animals given 75 micrograms/kg; human trials were therefore interrupted (261). However, the anabolic effect of parathyroid hormone is much greater and occurs much earlier in rats than in humans, possibly because of fundamental differences in bone biology: moreover, osteosarcoma has never been associated with primary, secondary, or tertiary hyperparathyroidism in humans (260). There has been no evidence of osteosarcoma in several hundred patients involved in parathyroid hormone clinical trials lasting up to 3 years, after 5 years minimum follow-up (260).

Penicillamine

There are a few case reports of lymphatic malignancies in patients using penicillamine, but epidemiological data in support of the association are lacking (SEDA-7, 259) (262–264).

Phenacetin

Studies on the tumor-inducing effects of heavy use of analgesics, especially those that contain phenacetin, have given contrasting results (SEDA-21, 100; 265,266). There

has been a case-control study of the role of habitual intake of aspirin on the occurrence of urothelial cancer and renal cell carcinoma (267). In previous studies there was a consistent association between phenacetin and renal cell carcinoma, but inconclusive results with respect to non-phenacetin analgesics. In 1024 patients with renal cell carcinoma and an equal number of matched controls, regular use of analgesics was a significant risk factor for renal cell carcinoma (OR = 1.6; CI = 1.4, 1.9). The risk was significantly increased by aspirin, NSAIDs, paracetamol, and phenacetin, and within each class of analgesic the risk increased with increasing exposure. Individuals in the highest exposure categories had about a 2.5-fold increase in risk relative to non-users or irregular users of analgesics. However, exclusive users of aspirin who took aspirin 325 mg/day or less for cardiovascular problems were not at an increased risk of renal cell carcinoma (OR = 0.9; CI = 0.6, 1.4).

Phenelzine

A single case of angiosarcoma in the liver has been reported in a patient taking phenelzine (268); similar tumors have occurred in mice treated with phenelzine.

Phenytoin

Pseudolymphoma and a condition resembling malignant lymphoma occur very rarely with phenytoin (SED-13, 142). There is no evidence of a significant increase in the incidence of other tumors. There have also been reports of pseudolymphoma with other antiepileptic drugs, including carbamazepine (269–271), lamotrigine (272), phenobarbital (273), and valproic acid (273).

Photochemotherapy

In a review of the English language literature on the risk of non-melanoma skin cancer from photochemotherapy in the treatment of psoriasis (274) the following were the conclusions:

(a) PUVA is an independent dose-related carcinogen in humans and can initiate and promote the formation of squamous cell carcinoma (275). The relation of basal cell carcinoma to PUVA alone is not well established.

(b) The carcinogenic risk of PUVA is not simply dose-related and skin type; geographic location and other well-established co-carcinogenic risk factors must be taken into account.

(c) Three factors are important co-carcinogens with PUVA: a history of arsenic exposure, ionizing radiation therapy, and skin cancer. Other factors believed to be related to increased risk include skin types I and II.

(d) Factors that appear to be associated with little or no risk of PUVA-related carcinogenesis include methotrexate (although a study from Sweden (276) has suggested otherwise), topical tar, and ultraviolet B

(UVB). Exceptions to this include simultaneous use of methotrexate and PUVA, and high exposure of the genital skin to UVB/tar. Retinoids may prove to be negatively correlated with skin cancer.

(e) The dose-related increased risk of cutaneous squamous cell carcinoma from PUVA is independent of skin type (I–IV), although the absolute risk is much higher in skin types I and II.

(f) Men treated with PUVA without genital protection are at high risk of developing dose-related invasive squamous cell carcinoma of the penis and the scrotum (SEDA-15, 141).

(g) PUVA-induced squamous cell carcinoma is not biologically aggressive. Nevertheless, metastases have been observed in some patients, emphasizing the need for continued monitoring (277).

(h) There is no definitive degree of cumulative PUVA exposure above which carcinogenicity can be predicted. However, the risk of squamous cell carcinoma is less in patients with skin types II, III, and IV, no risk factors, and a cumulative exposure below 1000 J/cm^2. Of patients treated with over 2000 J/cm^2, even those without risk factors, at least 20% will develop squamous cell carcinomas and 50% atypical squamous keratoses (275). Patients with skin type I should be monitored more rigorously than others.

The following recommendations were made

(a) Whenever possible, exclude patients with a history of ionizing radiation therapy, skin cancer, or arsenic exposure.

(b) Shield the male genital skin at all times during PUVA treatment.

(c) Use the European dosage protocol (lower doses and less frequent irradiations than the US protocol) whenever possible.

(d) Reduce PUVA dosage by combining or cycling with other treatments. Avoid maintenance therapy if possible.

(e) Use PUVA in younger patients only when necessary.

(f) Monitor patients with skin type I closely.

(g) Monitor patients prospectively and at least annually for keratoses and cutaneous carcinoma, particularly after cumulative exposure of more than 1000 J/cm^2.

Polyurethane

In a study of the mortality (1958–98) and cancer morbidity (1971–94) in a cohort of 8288 male and female employees from 11 factories in England and Wales engaged in the manufacture of flexible polyurethane foams, mortality from lung cancer in female employees was significantly increased (standardized mortality ratio 181) (278). There was no excess among male employees (standardized mortality ratio 107). There were no significantly increased cause-specific standardized mortality ratios among the subcohort ($n = 1782$) with some period of isocyanate exposure.

Proton pump inhibitors

There has been concern about the potential for proton pump inhibitors to cause enterochromaffin-like cell hyperplasia, gastric carcinoid tumors and gastric cancers, colorectal polyps and adenocarcinoma, atrophic gastritis, and intestinal metaplasia in patients with *H. pylori* infection, and bacterial overgrowth.

Carcinoid nodules were detected in the stomach of rats given large doses of omeprazole over prolonged periods. A variety of evidence, however, suggests that these findings were neither specific to omeprazole nor likely to indicate material risks to man (279), and that other arguments for a tumor-inducing effect of proton pump inhibitors are equally unconvincing. Firstly, similar carcinoid change has been detected with secretory antagonists and the fibrates, which are anti-secretory in rats. Secondly carcinoidogenesis can be inhibited by antrectomy, presumably by removing an antral gastrin drive, and it can be enhanced by partial fundectomy, when relative anacidity increases antral gastrin release. Thirdly, although omeprazole treatment can raise serum gastrin levels quite markedly in man, they do so by a level of magnitude less than in pernicious anemia, in which carcinoid tumors are recorded, albeit rarely. Fourthly, despite close searching, carcinoids have not been detected complicating ordinary ulcer treatment in man. Others have claimed on the basis of tissue work in vitro that omeprazole may itself be a mitogen or mutagen; it has been counterclaimed that the technique used in the studies concerned is inherently unreliable and that other standard techniques have failed to reveal mutagenic potential (SED-12, 943). Finally, selective and important actions on a cytochrome which would activate carcinogens have been claimed, but seem unlikely experimentally. This is one of the situations in which there is inherent difficulty in disproving a postulated relationship. Currently it seems very unlikely that an appreciable risk exists, but most experts would now recommend that any patient requiring long-term treatment with a proton pump inhibitor should take treatment to eradicate *H. pylori* infection (SEDA-20, 318).

Therapeutic doses of proton pump inhibitors usually produce somewhat higher serum gastrin concentrations than histamine receptor antagonists. However, except for small intestinal bacterial overgrowth, there is no convincing evidence yet to implicate proton pump inhibitors in the development of malignant or premalignant lesions in the human gastrointestinal tract. Nevertheless, although omeprazole has been used for more than 14 years and lansoprazole for more than 10 years, longer-term data are required to completely rule out the possibility of increased risk of gastric tumor formation.

An increasing number of gastric polyps is being reported in patients taking proton pump inhibitors. Although these may be coincidental and may only account for a minority of sporadic cases (280), it is too early to disregard the possibility that they are treatment induced (281). Long-term prospective controlled trials including investigation of the effects of stopping and restarting proton pump inhibitors on the evolution of gastric polyps will have to be done before a firm causal relation can be established.

An uncontrolled retrospective study of patients who had taken proton pump inhibitors for an average of 33 months found gastric polyps in 17 of 231 patients who underwent two or more endoscopies for complicated gastro-esophageal reflux disease (282). The polyps were generally small (under 1 cm), sessile, and multiple, and were present in the proximal or mid gastric body. Of the 15 polyps removed endoscopically, nine were fundic gland type, four were hyperplastic, and two were inflammatory. None had any dysplasia or carcinoma.

A gastric carcinoid tumor, detected during long-term anti-ulcer therapy with a histamine receptor antagonist and proton pump inhibitors, has been reported (283).

- A 31 year old Japanese man with recurrent duodenal ulcer was treated with famotidine, omeprazole, and lansoprazole at different times over 3 years. Gastroscopy showed a small carcinoid tumor in the upper cardia after 35 months. The lesion became larger while the patient was taking lansoprazole.

Radio contrast media

Some have suggested that the passage of contrast agents through malignant lymph nodes may facilitate metastases; one relevant case relates to Hodgkin's disease (284) and another to melanoma (460). There is also some animal evidence of this. However, it has generally been considered that lymphography is unlikely to be a significant factor in malignant dissemination and that its diagnostic value in planning treatment far outweighs any theoretical risk. Computed tomography and magnetic resonance imaging have now largely replaced lymphography for the demonstration of malignant lymph nodes.

Radio-iodine

The total number of case reports of thyroid cancer after ^{131}I is very small (under 30 cases) (285) in relation to the estimated number of patients treated with ^{131}I since 1941 (over 1 000 000 patients). Moreover, systematic follow-up or retrospective studies did not show an increased risk of thyroid carcinoma in patients treated with ^{131}I for hyperthyroidism. The results of two such studies are shown in more detail in Table 1 (286) and Table 2 (287).

In another follow-up study of 1005 women treated with ^{131}I there was no increase in total morbidity or in the incidence of thyroid cancer (288).

In 10 552 Swedish patients (mean age 57 years) who received ^{131}I for hyperthyroidism (mean follow-up 15 years) there were increases in overall cancer mortality and deaths due to carcinoma of the stomach, lung, and kidney. While the findings for stomach cancer may be of significance, for tumors at other sites, because of an association with time after ^{131}I treatment (58 cases at 10 years or more of follow-up against the expected 44 cases), the lack of a relation between cancer mortality and either the time from radioiodine treatment or the dose administered argues against a carcinogenic effect of radioiodine (SEDA-17, 475) (289).

The use of very high amounts of ^{131}I for thyroid cancer imposes special care and risks: the frequency of radiation thyroiditis is much higher (more than 20%) and similar symptoms of pain and swelling can also be observed in the salivary glands. Nausea and vomiting may also occur. The incidence of leukemia is increased: 15 cases being reported in 5000 patients treated with ^{131}I for thyroid cancer (290); it therefore seems wise to limit the total dose of ^{131}I in a single patient to 500 mCi unless the thyroid disease activity permits higher long-term risks. It is also important to keep such patients well hydrated to allow rapid elimination of ^{131}I not retained by thyroid tissue.

Table 1 ^{131}I treatment and thyroid cancer: a comparison with thyroidectomy and antithyroid drugs

Incidence of thyroid cancer	Thyroidectomy (n = 11 732)	^{131}I(n = 21 714)	Antithyroid drugs (n = 1238)
Within 1 year of treatment	50	9	0
After 1 year of treatment	4	19	4
Total	54 (4.6%)	28 (11.3%)	4 (3.2%)
Number of deaths from thyroidcancer	4	6	0

Table 2 ^{131}I treatment and thyroid cancer

Number of patients treated with^{131}I	3000
Mean age	57 years
Mean dose of ^{131}I	13.3 mCi
Mean observation period	13 years
Thyroid cancer	
Observed incidence	4%
Expected incidence	3.2%
Thyroid cancer more than 5 years after ^{131}I	
Observed incidence	2.1%
Expected incidence	3%

The radiation dose to the ovaries is not negligible, being approximately 200 roentgens after 500 mCi of ^{131}I, a dose sufficient to increase slightly the subsequent risk of miscarriage or congenital abnormalities. However, no apparent increase in the rate of abnormalities has been observed in the outcome of pregnancies among women previously treated for thyroid cancer.

The use of ^{131}I in children is different from its use in adults. Experience worldwide is much more limited as regards both the number of children treated and the total number of years of observation (SEDA-20, 394). The risk of eventual tumor-inducing effects in the thyroid or other tissues is real. The young thyroid is very sensitive to external radiation or to nuclear fallout: 66% of young adults developed thyroid lesions 25 years after such exposure (291). One report on a high prevalence of hypothyroidism after ^{131}I showed no cases of thyroid or other malignancies after a mean follow-up period of almost 15 years (292). However, others found an increased frequency of thyroid nodules: among case reports on thyroid cancer after ^{131}I in the world literature the younger age group is largely over-represented, owing to the frequency of ^{131}I use in this age group (285). In view of the small number of long-term results in a young population with probably higher susceptibility for thyroid tumors it seems unwise to use ^{131}I as preferred treatment for adolescents or young adults with hyperthyroidism. Much longer follow-up periods will be necessary, preferably with central registration to allow a definite conclusion about treatment (290,293). However, many experts consider the current follow-up period sufficiently long to extend the use of ^{131}I to all patients with Graves' disease above the age of 25 (SEDA-14, 368) (294). There are, however, large discrepancies in treatment strategies globally.

A possible link between breast cancer in women and thyroid hormone therapy was suggested on the basis of a retrospective study of patients with breast cancer (SEDA-3, 340). A subsequent statistical re-analysis of the original data failed, as did later studies, to confirm such a relation (SEDA-3, 340; SEDA-4, 294) (295).

Reserpine

Early retrospective studies suggested that reserpine was associated with breast cancer, but prospective studies and meta-analyses of case-control studies have shown only a weak association (296). In vitro studies have shown that rauwolfia alkaloids are not genotoxic or mutagenic (297).

Sclerosants

A number of case reports have suggested that sclerosant therapy could be carcinogenic (SEDA-15, 401).

Senna

A well-defined purified senna extract was not carcinogenic, when administered orally to rats in daily doses up to 25 mg/kg for 2 years (298).

Spironolactone

Spironolactone is antiandrogenic and increases the peripheral metabolism of testosterone to estradiol (299). It often causes gynecomastia in men and breast enlargement and soreness in women. Five cases of mammary carcinoma have been reported. Potential human metabolic products of spironolactone are carcinogenic in rodents, and the UK Committee on Safety of Medicines in 1988 restricted the approved indications for the drug, removing the indications of essential hypertension and idiopathic edema (300).

Talc

Ovarian cancer has been increasing in frequency over the past 40 years, and a role for environmental factors in its etiology has been inferred from its higher incidence in industrialized countries. Cosmetic talc, deposited in the vagina after direct application to the perineum or to undergarments, sanitary napkins, or diaphragms, or through use of a talc-dusted condom during intercourse, may play an important role. In a case-control study of the use of talc in genital hygiene the risk of ovarian cancer was significantly increased in women who applied talc directly as a body powder, on a daily basis, for more than 10 years (301). The greatest risk of ovarian cancer was in the subgroup of women estimated to have made more than 10 000 talc applications during years when they were ovulating. However, this exposure was found in only 14% of women with ovarian cancer. The authors concluded that a life-time pattern of perineal talc use may increase the risk of epithelial ovarian cancer, but that it is unlikely to be the cause of most cases of epithelial ovarian cancers.

Tamoxifen

Several authors (302,303) have described a variety of cases, seven in all, of malignancies secondary to therapeutic dosages of tamoxifen given for 6 months to 10 years.

Uterine fibroids and endometrial polyps (sometimes with bleeding) have been reported in menopausal women who had taken tamoxifen for periods of months or years (SEDA-16, 466) (304,305). In view of this, the question of whether tamoxifen increases the risk of endometrial cancer has been widely discussed. The authors of a 1993 review of the outcome of six major trials tended strongly to the conclusion that tamoxifen can cause both endometrial hyperplasia and endometrial cancer proportional to the total dose (306); the figures pointed to an overall incidence of endometrial cancer of 0.5% in tamoxifen users and 0.1% in controls. Another major review up to 1992 concluded that in the world literature there were 70 cases of uterine malignancies with tamoxifen, including

61 cases of adenocarcinoma of the endometrium and four cases of uterine sarcoma (307).

Six cases of endometrial carcinoma were subsequently reported from France (308), and 36 cases in all had been reported up to that time (309). Although the effect can be caused by tamoxifen alone in women aged over 55, in younger women it is more likely to be an additive one, attributable to use of both tamoxifen and pelvic irradiation in the same subject.

Two distinct patterns of uterine cancer have been shown using magnetic resonance imaging of the tamoxifen-exposed uterus in 35 women (310). Patients with pattern 1 had homogeneous high signal intensity of the endometrium on T2-weighted images and enhancement of the endometrial–myometrial interface and a signal void in the lumen on gadolinium-enhanced images (18 patients). Patients with pattern 2 had heterogeneous endometrial signal intensity on T2-weighted images with enhancement of the endometrial–myometrial interface and lattice-like enhancement traversing the endometrial canal on gadolinium-enhanced images (17 patients).

Although the endometrial cancers associated with tamoxifen are usually pure adenocarcinomas, other types of rare tumors have also been reported. A pure uterine rhabdomyosarcoma has been reported (311), and a mesodermal mixed tumor of the endometrium occurred 5 years after 5 years of tamoxifen therapy (312). The tumor responded only to combined treatment with doxorubicin, cyclophosphamide, 5-fluorouracil, and carboplatin. It is possible that this type of tumor arises later than adenocarcinomas and should be looked for during long-term use of tamoxifen.

- Two well-documented cases of uterine carcinosarcoma have been reported in elderly women after 6 and 7 years of tamoxifen treatment (313). At laparotomy, a heterologous malignant mixed Mullerian tumor with peritoneal spread was found in each case and rapidly proved fatal; large uterine polyps with special histological features may represent an intermediate step in the formation of such tumors (314).

Ten similar cases have been described before.

When assessing the risk of endometrial malignancy in women with breast cancer taking tamoxifen, it is worth taking into account evidence that patients with breast cancer may at the outset have some endometrial pathology. In women with breast cancer scheduled for tamoxifen there were endometrial polyps in 9.3%, endometrial cysts in 16%, and synechiae in 12% at the outset. Tamoxifen significantly increased the incidence of these benign endometrial lesions, usually after less than 1 year of treatment. There were no cases of endometrial carcinoma in 34 patients who had taken tamoxifen for 12–24 months, and only one in 78 patients who had taken it for 5–72 months (315).

The risk that tamoxifen may cause endometrial cancer has been the subject of lively correspondence in the Lancet (316), fired by the paper published in 2000 by Bergman and her colleagues, who had concluded that the endometrial cancers seen with tamoxifen are unusually aggressive (317). Concern was expressed that such a conclusion could lead to even wider hesitation to use tamoxifen in breast cancer, despite the fact that it is already used very selectively, for example in women with positive estrogen receptors. A contradiction between Bergman's results and those of the NSABP P-1 were also highlighted, and doubts expressed whether Bergman's findings justify restricting the use of tamoxifen as a preventive agent. However, a Canadian group adduced its own work to support Bergman's findings, while French workers suggested that her unfavorable results, which were not seen in their own patients, could have been due to selection bias. It was also argued that a progestogen-releasing intrauterine contraceptive device might be used to counter the undesirable effects of tamoxifen on the endometrium. Clearly the issue raised by Bergman is still subject to debate, but it is obvious that physicians who use tamoxifen in advanced breast cancer or as a preventive agent should continue to do so selectively and that ways of protecting the endometrium during tamoxifen therapy need to be found.

The effects of norethisterone on endometrial abnormalities have been studied in 463 postmenopausal women taking tamoxifen or placebo (318). As in other studies, the results showed that any increased risk of endometrial cancer caused by tamoxifen is low and that transvaginal ultrasound screening is probably not justified for asymptomatic women taking tamoxifen. The authors found that 26% of women taking tamoxifen have endometrial thickening of 8 mm or more. It is possible to identify cysts in 7% of these women, polyps in 3%, and both cysts and polyps in 8%. These changes are characteristic of tamoxifen and unlike those seen with estrogen replacement therapy.

The usefulness of transvaginal ultrasound in detecting serious uterine changes in tamoxifen users has been disputed. According to one group it is a dependable diagnostic method (319), whereas others found it disappointing, with a high proportion of false positive results, even when the assessment criteria were chosen so as to exclude mild endometrial thickening (320). Setting these two papers beside one another it seems that one can detect marked endometrial changes but that ultrasound is not a dependable means of determining whether there is malignancy.

Titanium

A rhabdomyosarcoma has been reported near the site of a pacemaker (321).

- An 85-year-old man developed a voluminous, rapidly evolving tumor beneath the right clavicle where a titanium pacemaker had been implanted 5 years before. Immunohistochemistry showed that it was a rhabdomyosarcoma.

The role of the pacemaker and especially of titanium in the development of this tumor was not clear.

Trichloroethylene

The incidence of cancer among 803 Danish workers exposed to trichloroethylene has been evaluated (322). There was no overall increase. However, the standardized incidence ratio was significantly higher in men with non-Hodgkin's lymphoma or esophageal cancer and in women with cervical cancer.

Vitamin A (carotenoids)

Negative outcomes in several supplementation trials of beta-carotene, especially the results of the Finnish Alpha-Tocopherol Beta-Carotene (ATBC) Cancer Prevention Study (323) (SEDA-20, 363), have again revived discussion about the carcinogenic potential of beta-carotene. The ATBC trial showed that there was a statistically significant increase in the incidence of lung cancer in heavy smokers who took beta-carotene.

Problems concerning the interactions of cigarette smoking, cancer, and carotenoids have been reviewed (324).

Over several decades, evidence has accumulated that a diet rich in fruit and vegetables is associated with a lower risk of cardiovascular disease and various forms of cancer, principally cancer of the lung and stomach, but also esophageal, oral, breast, and prostate cancer (325,326). It is possible that this effect is in part due to their beta-carotene content.

Beta-carotene and other micronutrients have been claimed to counteract oxidative processes that participate in various stages of carcinogenesis, and increased consumption of fruit and vegetables rich in carotenoids lowered urinary indices of oxidized lipids and DNA in healthy subjects (327). Although beta-carotene and other carotenoids are excellent in vitro quenchers of singulett oxygen and beta-carotene, and may also protect lipids from radical-initiated peroxidation under certain conditions, evidence for antioxidant properties of beta-carotene in vivo is much less compelling (328). Assessment of the antioxidant benefit of beta-carotene is especially complicated by the fact that carcinogenesis is a very complex multistage process, in which oxidative pathways play variable and incompletely understood roles. While a few early supplementation trials suggested a beneficial role of beta-carotene (326), many other studies did not show such an effect. The proposed beneficial properties of carotenoids appear to be consistent with findings that cigarette smokers generally have subnormal serum concentrations of various carotenoids and other micronutrients, such as vitamin C, supposed to be caused by the increased oxidative stress associated with smoking and its attendant activation of the inflammatory and immune systems. On the other hand, the low concentrations in smokers could also result from lower intake of these micronutrients. Lower concentrations of carotenoids and other micronutrients are also observed in passive smokers (329,330).

The constituents of cigarette smoke can degrade beta-carotene (331,332), but the conclusion that smoking causes increased carotenoid metabolism demands the demonstration of raised carotenoid oxidation products. Moreover, the consistent observation of subnormal carotenoid concentrations but unchanged alpha-tocopherol concentrations (330) suggests that factors other than oxidative stress contribute to the relative carotenoid deficiency.

The assumption that remedying the carotenoid deficit would minimize the risks of cancer and heart disease associated with passive smoking has not been supported by several large randomized supplemention trials. In two major trials there was an increased incidence of cancer with beta-carotene supplementation in both smokers and asbestos workers. Of course, both high-risk groups might already have been in the early stages of cancer development at the start of the studies (323,324).

These surprising findings have raised an interesting apparent paradox: how can supplementation with beta-carotene, a presumed antioxidant and possible chemoprotective agent, enhance cancer formation, even though this is thought to involve oxidative processes? In some experimental systems carotenoids have pro-oxidant properties at high concentrations, but these are not reached in vivo (329,330). Another mechanism is an increase or alteration in carotenoid metabolism in high-risk groups, resulting in the formation of metabolites or oxidation products that could be procarcinogenic (for instance by interfering with retinoid signaling pathways, by promoting DNA damage, or by inducing cytochrome P450 enzymes that might promote carcinogen activation) (326,333). Such induction of cytochrome P450 enzymes might also enhance the catabolism of retinoic acid, which plays an important role in lung epithelial proliferation and differentiation. Downregulation of the retinoic acid receptor, RARb, by beta-carotene supplementation has been shown in recent studies in ferrets (333). RARb may act as a tumor suppressor gene. Moreover, lung expression of the proto-oncogenes c-jun and c-fos was increased in animals exposed to cigarette smoke and also receiving beta-carotene supplements (333).

In general, the negative outcomes of several supplementation trials and the lack of proof that carotenoids form the primary beneficial component of fruit and vegetables should serve as a warning against unregulated supplementation with these individual micronutrients, especially in view of the potential carcinogenic effect of carotenoids.

The carcinogenic effect of beta-carotene has recently been found to be reduced by vitamin E (334), suggesting that, rather than individual micronutrient supplementation, combinations of various such substances might be more advantageous.

Vitamin K

The relation between neonatal vitamin K administration and childhood cancer has been investigated in three case-control studies.

In a retrospective study 685 children who developed cancer before their 15th birthday were compared with

3442 controls matched for date and hospital of birth (335). There was no association between the administration of vitamin K and the development of all childhood cancers (unadjusted odds ratio 0.89; 95% CI = 0.69, 1.15) or of all cases of acute lymphoblastic leukemia (1.20; 0.75, 1.92), but there was a raised odds ratio for acute lymphoblastic leukemia 1–6 years after birth (1.79; 1.02, 3.15).

However, no such association was seen in a separate cohort-based study not dependent on case-note retrieval, in which the rates of acute lymphoblastic leukemia in children born in hospital units in which all babies received vitamin K were compared with those born in units in which less than a third received prophylaxis. It was concluded that on the basis of currently published evidence neonatal intramuscular vitamin K administration does not increase the risk of early childhood leukemia.

In another study children aged 0–14 years with leukemia ($n = 150$), lymphomas ($n = 46$), central nervous system tumors ($n = 79$), a range of other solid tumours ($n = 142$), and a subset of acute lymphoblastic leukemia ($n = 129$) were compared with 777 children matched for age and sex (336). Odds ratios showed no significant positive association for leukemias (1.30; 0.83, 2.03), acute lymphoblastic leukemia (1.21; 0.74, 1.97), lymphomas (1.06; 0.46, 2.42), central nervous system tumors (0.74; 0.40, 1.34), and other solid tumors (0.59; 0.37, 0.96). There was no association with acute lymphoblastic leukemia in children aged 1–6 years. The authors concluded that they had not confirmed the observation of an increased risk of childhood leukemia and cancer associated with intramuscular vitamin K.

In another study 597 cases and matched controls were compared. The association between cancer generally and intramuscular vitamin K was of borderline significance (odds ratio 1.44); the association was strongest for acute lymphoblastic leukemia (1.73) (337). However, there was also an effect of abnormal delivery. The authors suggested from the lack of consistency between the various studies so far published, including their own, and the low relative risks found in most of them, that the risk, if any, attributable to the use of vitamin K cannot be large, but that the possibility that there is some risk cannot be excluded. They recommended that prophylaxis using the commonly used intramuscular dose of 1 mg should be restricted to babies at particularly high risk of vitamin K deficiency; alternatively, a lower dose might be given to a larger proportion of those at risk.

Ecological studies of the relation between hospital policies on neonatal vitamin K administration and subsequent occurrences of childhood cancer have been analysed using data from selected large maternity units in Scotland, England, and Wales (338). The study covered 94 hospitals, with a total of 2.3 million births during periods when intramuscular vitamin K was routinely used and 1.4 million births when a selective policy was in operation. An increased risk was occasionally associated with vitamin K

(highest odds ratio 1.25 for acute lymphoblastic leukemia in one hospital), but the overall results were not significant, and there was no evidence to support the previously suggested doubling of the risk of childhood cancer.

On the basis of all these results it is unlikely that there is a greatly increased risk of childhood cancer attributable to intramuscular vitamin K given to newborns, if indeed there is any risk at all.

References

1. FAO/WHO. Evaluation of certain food additives and contaminants. Twenty-sixth report of the Joint FAO/WHO Expert Committee on Food Additives. World Health Organ Tech Rep Ser 1982;683:7–51.
2. World Health Organisation. Aminophenazone a possible cancer hazard? WHO Drug Info 1977;9Jul-Sep.
3. Oda K, Oguma N, Kawano M, Kimura A, Kuramoto A, Tokumo K. Hepatocellular carcinoma associated with long-term anabolic steroid therapy in two patients with aplastic anemia. Nippon Ketsueki Gakkai Zasshi 1987;50(1):29–36.
4. Potashnik G, Lerner-Geva L, Genkin L, Chetrit A, Lunenfeld E, Porath A. Fertility drugs and the risk of breast and ovarian cancers: results of a long-term follow-up study. Fertil Steril 1999;71(5):853–9.
5. Rubin SO. Malignant teratoma of testis in a subfertile man treated with HCG and HMG. A case report. Scand J Urol Nephrol 1973;7(1):81–4.
6. Siegers CP, von Hertzberg-Lottin E, Otte M, Schneider B. Anthranoid laxative abuse—a risk for colorectal cancer? Gut 1993;34(8):1099–101.
7. Kommission E. Aufbereitungsmonographien. Dtsch Apoth Ztg 1993;133:2791–4.
8. Hagenah W, Dorges I, Gafumbegete E, Wagner T. Subkutane Manifestationen eines zentrozytischen Non-Hodgkin-Lymphoms an Injektionsstellen eines Mistelpräparats. [Subcutaneous manifestations of a centrocytic non-Hodgkin lymphoma at the injection site of a mistletoe preparation.] Dtsch Med Wochenschr 1998;123(34–35):1001–4.
9. Dauden E, Alvarez S, Garcia-Diez A. Eruptive angiolipomas associated with antiretroviral therapy. AIDS 2002;16(5):805–6.
10. Dank JP, Colven R. Protease inhibitor-associated angiolipomatosis. J Am Acad Dermatol 2000;42(1 Pt 1):129–31.
11. Bornhovd E, Sakrauski AK, Bruhl H, Walli R, Plewig G, Rocken M. Multiple circumscribed subcutaneous lipomas associated with use of human immunodeficiency virus protease inhibitors? Br J Dermatol 2000;143(5):1113–4.
12. Bates D. Valacyclovir neurotoxicity: two case reports and a review of the literature. Can J Hosp Pharm 2002;55:123–7.
13. Cosyns JP, Jadoul M, Squifflet JP, Wese FX, van Ypersele de Strihou C. Urothelial lesions in Chinese-herb nephropathy. Am J Kidney Dis 1999;33(6):1011–7.
14. Lord GM, Hollstein M, Arlt VM, Roufosse C, Pusey CD, Cook T, Schmeiser HH. DNA adducts and p53 mutations in a patient with aristolochic acid-associated nephropathy. Am J Kidney Dis 2004;43(4):e11–7.
15. Skegg DC. BCG vaccination and the incidence of lymphomas and leukaemia. Int J Cancer 1978;21(1):18–21.

16. Lilienfeld AM, Pedersen E, Dowd JE. In: Cancer Epidemiology: Methods of Study. Baltimore, MD: Johns Hopkins Press, 1967:72.

17. Snider DE, Comstock GW, Martinez I, Caras GJ. Efficacy of BCG vaccination in prevention of cancer: an update. J Natl Cancer Inst 1978;60(4):785–8.

18. Kendrick MA, Comstock GW. BCG vaccination and the subsequent development of cancer in humans. J Natl Cancer Inst 1981;66(3):431–7.

19. Jonas M, Goldbourt U, Boyko V, Mandelzweig L, Behar S, Reicher-Reiss H. Nifedipine and cancer mortality: ten-year follow-up of 2607 patients after acute myocardial infarction. Cardiovasc Drugs Ther 1998;12(2):177–81.

20. Braun S, Boyko V, Behar S, Reicher-Reiss H, Laniado S, Kaplinsky E, Goldbourt U. Calcium channel blocking agents and risk of cancer in patients with coronary heart disease. Benzafibrate Infarction Prevention (BIP) Study Research Group. J Am Coll Cardiol 1998;31(4):804–8.

21. Rosenberg L, Rao RS, Palmer JR, Strom BL, Stolley PD, Zauber AG, Warshauer ME, Shapiro S. Calcium channel blockers and the risk of cancer. JAMA 1998;279(13):1000–4.

22. Hole DJ, Gillis CR, McCallum IR, McInnes GT, MacKinnon PL, Meredith PA, Murray LS, Robertson JW, Lever AF. Cancer risk of hypertensive patients taking calcium antagonists. J Hypertens 1998;16(1):119–24.

23. Fitzpatrick AL, Daling JR, Furberg CD, Kronmal RA, Weissfeld JL. Use of calcium channel blockers and breast carcinoma risk in postmenopausal women. Cancer 1997;80(8):1438–47.

24. Howes LG, Edwards CT. Calcium antagonists and cancer. Is there really a link? Drug Saf 1998;18(1):1–7.

25. Wehner FC, van Rensburg SJ, Thiel PG. Mutagenicity of marijuana and Transkei tobacco smoke condensates in the *Salmonella*/microsome assay. Mutat Res 1980;77(2):135–42.

26. Leuchtenberger C, Leuchtenberger R. Cytological and cyto-chemical studies of the effects of fresh marihuana smoke on growth and DNA metabolism of animal and human lung cultures. In: Braude MC, Szara S, editors. The Pharmacology of Marijuana. New York: Raven Press, 1976:595–612.

27. Di Lernia V, Viglio A, Cattania M, Paulli M. Carbamazepine-induced, CD30+, primary, cutaneous, anaplastic large-cell lymphoma. Arch Dermatol 2001;137(5):675–6.

28. Gutierrez-Rave Pecero VM, Luque Marquez R, Ayerza Lerchundi MA, Fernandez Jurado A. Phenytoin-induced hemocytophagic histiocytosis indistinguishable from malignant histiocytosis. South Med J 1991;84(5):649–50.

29. Jeng YM, Tien HF, Su IJ. Phenytoin-induced pseudolymphoma: reevaluation using modern molecular biology techniques. Epilepsia 1996;37(1):104–7.

30. Bagchi D, Stohs SJ, Downs BW, Bagchi M, Preuss HG. Cytotoxicity and oxidative mechanisms of different forms of chromium. Toxicology 2002;180(1):5–22.

31. Manygoats KR, Yazzie M, Stearns DM. Ultrastructural damage in chromium picolinate-treated cells: a TEM study. Transmission electron microscopy. J Biol Inorg Chem 2002;7(7-8):791–8.

32. Rosenman KD, Stanbury M. Risk of lung cancer among former chromium smelter workers. Am J Ind Med 1996;29(5):491–500.

33. Rossing MA, Daling JR, Weiss NS, Moore DE, Self SG. Risk of cutaneous melanoma in a cohort of infertile women. Melanoma Res 1995;5(2):123–7.

34. Ron E, Lunenfeld B, Menczer J, Blumstein T, Katz L, Oelsner G, Serr D. Cancer incidence in a cohort of infertile women. Am J Epidemiol 1987;125(5):780–90.

35. Brinton LA, Melton LJ 3rd, Malkasian GD Jr, Bond A, Hoover R. Cancer risk after evaluation for infertility. Am J Epidemiol 1989;129(4):712–22.

36. Modan B, Ron E, Lerner-Geva L, Blumstein T, Menczer J, Rabinovici J, Oelsner G, Freedman L, Mashiach S, Lunenfeld B. Cancer incidence in a cohort of infertile women. Am J Epidemiol 1998;147(11):1038–42.

37. Venn A, Watson L, Lumley J, Giles G, King C, Healy D. Breast and ovarian cancer incidence after infertility and in vitro fertilisation. Lancet 1995;346(8981):995–1000.

38. Young P, Purdie D, Jackman L, Molloy D, Green A. A study of infertility treatment and melanoma. Melanoma Res 2001;11(5):535–41.

39. Boring CC, Squires TS, Tong T, Montgomery S. Cancer statistics, 1994. CA Cancer J Clin 1994;44(1):7–26.

40. In: Rees LAG, Eisner MP, Kosary CL, Hankey BF, Miller BA, Clegg L, Edwards BK, editors. SEER Cancer Statistics Review, 1973–1999. Bethesda MD: National Cancer Institute, 2002:72 http://seer.cancer.gov/csr/1973-1999/.

41. Glass AG, Hoover RN. The emerging epidemic of mela-noma and squamous cell skin cancer. JAMA 1989;262(15):2097–100.

42. Kimbel HK. Inquiry of the 'Arzneimittelkommission der Deutschen Arzteschaft'. Personal communication. 1978.

43. Neoptolemos JP, Locke TJ, Fossard DP. Testicular tumour associated with hormonal treatment for oligospermia. Lancet 1981;2(8249):754.

44. Duarte JG, do Nascimento AF, Pantoja JG, Chaves CP. Chronic inhaled cocaine abuse may predispose to the development of pancreatic adenocarcinoma. Am J Surg 1999;178(5):426–7.

45. Nahrwold DL. Editorial comment. Am J Surg 1999;178:427.

46. Crampon D, Barnoud R, Durand M, Ponard D, Jacquot C, Sotto JJ, Letoublon C, Zarski JP. Danazol therapy: an unusual aetiology of hepatocellular carcinoma. J Hepatol 1998;29(6):1035–6.

47. Simonart T, Degraef C, Andrei G, Mosselmans R, Hermans P, Van Vooren JP, Noel JC, Boelaert JR, Snoeck R, Heenen M. Iron chelators inhibit the growth and induce the apoptosis of Kaposi's sarcoma cells and of their putative endothelial precursors. J Invest Dermatol 2000;115(5):893–900.

48. Simonart T, Boelaert JR, Van Vooren JP. Enhancement of classic Kaposi's sarcoma growth after intralesional injec-tions of desferrioxamine. Dermatology 2002;204(4):290–2.

49. Young JB, Brownjohn AM, Lee MR. Diuretics and idio-pathic oedema. Nephron 1986;43(4):311–2.

50. Marty H. Pseudo-Bartter Syndrom bei Diuretika-Abusus. [Pseudo-Bartter syndrome in diuretics abuse.] Schweiz Med Wochenschr 1985;115(7):250–2.

51. Lopez Jimenez M, Barbado FJ, Mateos F, Pena JM, Gil A, Arnalich F, Tovar I, Alonso FG, Vazquez Rodriguez JJ. Sindrome de Bartter factitio inducido por la ingestion subrepticia de diureticos. [Factitious Bartter's syndrome induced by the surreptitious ingestion of diuretics.] Med Clin (Barc) 1985;84(1):23–6.

52. Schmieder RE, Delles C, Messerli FH. Diuretic therapy and the risk for renal cell carcinoma. J Nephrol 2000;13(5):343–6.

53. Grossman E, Messerli FH, Goldbourt U. Does diuretic therapy increase the risk of renal cell carcinoma? Am J Cardiol 1999;83(7):1090–3.

54. Li CI, Weiss NS, Stanford JL, Daling JR. Hormone replacement therapy in relation to risk of lobular and ductal breast carcinoma in middle-aged women. Cancer 2000;88(11):2570–7.

55. Schairer C, Lubin J, Troisi R, Sturgeon S, Brinton L, Hoover R. Menopausal estrogen and estrogen-progestin replacement therapy and breast cancer risk. JAMA 2000;283(4):485–91.

56. In: Herbst AL, editor. Intrauterine exposure to diethylstilbestrol in the human. Proceedings, "Symposium on DES". Chicago: American College of Obstetricians and Gynecologists, 1977:265–70.

57. Antunes CM, Strolley PD, Rosenshein NB, Davies JL, Tonascia JA, Brown C, Burnett L, Rutledge A, Pokempner M, Garcia R. Endometrial cancer and estrogen use. Report of a large case-control study. N Engl J Med 1979;300(1):9–13.

58. Williams GM, Iatropoulos M, Cheung R, Radi L, Wang CX. Diethylstilbestrol liver carcinogenicity and modification of DNA in rats. Cancer Lett 1993;68(2–3):193–8.

59. Rosinus V, Maurer R. [Diättylstilböstrol-induziertes Leberzellkarzinom? Diethylstilbestrol-induced liver cancer?.]Schweiz Med Wochenschr 1981;111(30):1139–42.

60. Ford LG, Brawley OW, Perlman JA, Nayfield SG, Johnson KA, Kramer BS. The potential for hormonal prevention trials. Cancer 1994;74(Suppl 9):2726–33.

61. Coker AL, Harlap S, Fortney JA. Oral contraceptives and reproductive cancers: weighing the risks and benefits. Fam Plann Perspect 1993;25(1):17–2136.

62. WHO International Agency for Research of Cancer. Ethylene oxide. IARC Monogr Eval Carcinog Risks Hum 1994;60:73–159.

63. Hogstedt C, Malmqvist N, Wadman B. Leukemia in workers exposed to ethylene oxide. JAMA 1979;241(11):1132–3.

64. Stayner L, Steenland K, Greife A, Hornung R, Hayes RB, Nowlin S, Morawetz J, Ringenburg V, Elliot L, Halperin W. Exposure-response analysis of cancer mortality in a cohort of workers exposed to ethylene oxide. Am J Epidemiol 1993;138(10):787–98.

65. Steenland K, Stayner L, Greife A, Halperin W, Hayes R, Hornung R, Nowlin S. Mortality among workers exposed to ethylene oxide. N Engl J Med 1991;324(20):1402–7.

66. Hogstedt C, Aringer L, Gustavsson A. Epidemiologic support for ethylene oxide as a cancer-causing agent. JAMA 1986;255(12):1575–8.

67. Hogstedt C. Epidemiological studies on ethylene oxide and cancer: an updating. In: Bartsch H, Hemminki K, O'Neill, editors. Methods for Detecting DNA Damaging Agents in Humans: Applications in Cancer Epidemiology and Prevention 89. Lyon: IARC, 1988:265–70.

68. Hagmar L, Welinder H, Linden K, Attewell R, Osterman-Golkar S, Tornqvist M. An epidemiological study of cancer risk among workers exposed to ethylene oxide using hemoglobin adducts to validate environmental exposure assessments. Int Arch Occup Environ Health 1991;63(4):271–7.

69. Gardner MJ, Coggon D, Pannett B, Harris EC. Workers exposed to ethylene oxide: a follow up study. Br J Ind Med 1989;46(12):860–5.

70. Baca D, Drexler C, Cullen E. Obstructive laryngotracheitis secondary to gentian violet exposure. Clin Pediatr (Phila) 2001;40(4):233–5.

71. Tates AD, Boogaard PJ, Darroudi F, Natarajan AT, Caubo ME, van Sittert NJ. Biological effect monitoring in industrial workers following incidental exposure to high concentrations of ethylene oxide. Mutat Res 1995;329(1):63–77.

72. Hogstedt C, Rohlen O, Berndtsson BS, Axelson O, Ehrenberg L. A cohort study of mortality and cancer incidence in ethylene oxide production workers. Br J Ind Med 1979;36(4):276–80.

73. Morgan RW, Claxton KW, Divine BJ, Kaplan SD, Harris VB. Mortality among ethylene oxide workers. J Occup Med 1981;23(11):767–70.

74. Shore RE, Gardner MJ, Pannett B. Ethylene oxide: an assessment of the epidemiological evidence on carcinogenicity. Br J Ind Med 1993;50(11):971–97.

75. Kiesselbach N, Ulm K, Lange HJ, Korallus U. A multicentre mortality study of workers exposed to ethylene oxide. Br J Ind Med 1990;47(3):182–8.

76. Benson LO, Teta MJ. Mortality due to pancreatic and lymphopoietic cancers in chlorohydrin production workers. Br J Ind Med 1993;50(8):710–6.

77. Teta MJ, Benson LO, Vitale JN. Mortality study of ethylene oxide workers in chemical manufacturing: a 10 year update. Br J Ind Med 1993;50(8):704–9.

78. Bisanti L, Maggini M, Raschetti R, Alegiani SS, Ippolito FM, Caffari B, Segnan N, Ponti A. Cancer mortality in ethylene oxide workers. Br J Ind Med 1993;50(4):317–24.

79. Thiess AM, Schwegler H, Fleig I, Stocker WG. Mutagenicity study of workers exposed to alkylene oxides (ethylene oxide/propylene oxide) and derivatives. J Occup Med 1981;23(5):343–7.

80. Greenberg HL, Ott MG, Shore RE. Men assigned to ethylene oxide production or other ethylene oxide related chemical manufacturing: a mortality study. Br J Ind Med 1990;47(4):221–30.

81. Fort FL. Mutagenicity of quinolone antibacterials. Drug Saf 1992;7(3):214–22.

82. Klecak G, Urbach F, Urwyler H. Fluoroquinolone antibacterials enhance UVA-induced skin tumors. J Photochem Photobiol B 1997;37(3):174–81.

83. Selby JV, Friedman GD, Fireman BH. Screening prescription drugs for possible carcinogenicity: eleven to fifteen years of follow-up. Cancer Res 1989;49(20):5736–47.

84. Shelley WB. Immediate sunburn-like reaction in a patient with formaldehyde photosensitivity. Arch Dermatol 1982;118(2):117–8.

85. IARC Monographs updating of Vol. 1 to 42, Supplement, 1987:211–16.

86. Walrath J, Fraumeni JF Jr. Mortality patterns among embalmers. Int J Cancer 1983;31(4):407–11.

87. Walrath J, Fraumeni JF Jr. Cancer and other causes of death among embalmers. Cancer Res 1984;44(10):4638–41.

88. Stroup NE, Blair A, Erikson GE. Brain cancer and other causes of death in anatomists. J Natl Cancer Inst 1986;77(6):1217–24.

89. Jensen OM, Andersen SK. Lung cancer risk from formaldehyde. Lancet 1982;1(8277):913.

90. Harrington JM, Oakes D. Mortality study of British pathologists 1974–80. Br J Ind Med 1984;41(2):188–91.

91. Levine RJ, Andjelkovich DA, Shaw LK. The mortality of Ontario undertakers and a review of formaldehyde-related mortality studies. J Occup Med 1984;26(10):740–6.

92. Blair A, Stewart P, O'Berg M, Gaffey W, Walrath J, Ward J, Bales R, Kaplan S, Cubit D. Mortality among industrial workers exposed to formaldehyde. J Natl Cancer Inst 1986;76(6):1071–84.

93. Stayner L, Smith AB, Reeve G, Blade L, Elliott L, Keenlyside R, Halperin W. Proportionate mortality study of workers in the garment industry exposed to formaldehyde. Am J Ind Med 1985;7(3):229–40.

94. Fayerweather WE, Pell S, Bender JB. Case-control study of cancer deaths in DuPont workers with potential exposure to formaldehyde. In: Clary JJ, Gibson JE, Waritz RS, editors. Formaldehyde: Toxicology, Epidemiology, Mechanisms. New York: Marcel Dekker, 1983:47–125.

95. Liebling T, Rosenman KD, Pastides H, Griffith RG, Lemeshow S. Cancer mortality among workers exposed to formaldehyde. Am J Ind Med 1984;5(6):423–8.

96. Vaughan TL, Strader C, Davis S, Daling JR. Formaldehyde and cancers of the pharynx, sinus and nasal cavity: I. Occupational exposures. Int J Cancer 1986;38(5):677–83.

97. Partanen T, Kauppinen T, Nurminen M, Nickels J, Hernberg S, Hakulinen T, Pukkala E, Savonen E. Formaldehyde exposure and respiratory and related cancers. A case-referent study among Finnish woodworkers. Scand J Work Environ Health 1985;11(6):409–15.

98. Coggon D, Pannett B, Acheson ED. Use of job-exposure matrix in an occupational analysis of lung and bladder cancers on the basis of death certificates. J Natl Cancer Inst 1984;72(1):61–5.

99. Bertazzi PA, Pesatori AC, Radice L, Zocchetti C, Vai T. Exposure to formaldehyde and cancer mortality in a cohort of workers producing resins. Scand J Work Environ Health 1986;12(5):461–8.

100. Hayes RB, Raatgever JW, de Bruyn A, Gerin M. Cancer of the nasal cavity and paranasal sinuses, and formaldehyde exposure. Int J Cancer 1986;37(4):487–92.

101. Olsen JH, Jensen SP, Hink M, Faurbo K, Breum NO, Jensen OM. Occupational formaldehyde exposure and increased nasal cancer risk in man. Int J Cancer 1984;34(5):639–44.

102. Olsen JH, Asnaes S. Formaldehyde and the risk of squamous cell carcinoma of the sinonasal cavities. Br J Ind Med 1986;43(11):769–74.

103. Acheson ED, Barnes HR, Gardner MJ, Osmond C, Pannett B, Taylor CP. Formaldehyde in the British chemical industry. An occupational cohort study. Lancet 1984;1(8377):611–6.

104. Vaughan TL, Strader C, Davis S, Daling JR. Formaldehyde and cancers of the pharynx, sinus and nasal cavity: II. Residential exposures. Int J Cancer 1986;38(5):685–8.

105. Lewis BB, Chestner SB. Formaldehyde in dentistry: a review of mutagenic and carcinogenic potential. J Am Dent Assoc 1981;103(3):429–34.

106. Lewis BB, Chestner SB. Formaldehyde in dentistry: a review of mutagenic and carcinogenic potential. J Am Dent Assoc 1981;103(3):429–34.

107. Hodgkinson DJ, Williams TJ. Endometrial carcinoma associated with azathioprine and cortisone therapy. A case report. Gynecol Oncol 1977;5(3):308–12.

108. Erban SB, Sokas RK. Kaposi's sarcoma in an elderly man with Wegener's granulomatosis treated with cyclophosphamide and corticosteroids. Arch Intern Med 1988;148(5):1201–3.

109. Thiagarajan CM, Divakar D, Thomas SJ. Malignancies in renal transplant recipients. Transplant Proc 1998;30(7):3154–5.

110. Gill PS, Loureiro C, Bernstein-Singer M, Rarick MU, Sattler F, Levine AM. Clinical effect of glucocorticoids on Kaposi sarcoma related to the acquired immunodeficiency syndrome (AIDS). Ann Intern Med 1989;110(11):937–40.

111. Tebbe B, Mayer-da-Silva A, Garbe C, von Keyserlingk HJ, Orfanos CE. Genetically determined coincidence of Kaposi sarcoma and psoriasis in an HIV-negative patient after prednisolone treatment. Spontaneous regression 8 months after discontinuing therapy. Int J Dermatol 1991;30(2):114–20.

112. Vincent T, Moss K, Colaco B, Venables PJ. Kaposi's sarcoma in two patients following low-dose corticosteroid treatment for rheumatological disease. Rheumatology (Oxford) 2000;39(11):1294–6.

113. Sorensen HT, Mellemkjaer L, Friis S, Olsen JH. Use of systemic corticosteroids and risk of esophageal cancer. Epidemiology 2002;13(2):240–1.

114. Mahler C. Is disease flare a problem? Cancer 1993;72(Suppl 12):3799–802.

115. Taylor CW, Green S, Dalton WS, Martino S, Rector D, Ingle JN, Robert NJ, Budd GT, Paradelo JC, Natale RB, Bearden JD, Mailliard JA, Osborne CK. Multicenter randomized clinical trial of goserelin versus surgical ovariectomy in premenopausal patients with receptor-positive metastatic breast cancer: an intergroup study. J Clin Oncol 1998;16(3):994–9.

116. Dantal J, Hourmant M, Cantarovich D, Giral M, Blancho G, Dreno B, Soulillou JP. Effect of long-term immunosuppression in kidney-graft recipients on cancer incidence: randomised comparison of two cyclosporin regimens. Lancet 1998;351(9103):623–8.

117. Tidow N, Pilz C, Teichmann B, Muller-Brechlin A, Germeshausen M, Kasper B, Rauprich P, Sykora KW, Welte K. Clinical relevance of point mutations in the cytoplasmic domain of the granulocyte colony-stimulating factor receptor gene in patients with severe congenital neutropenia. Blood 1997;89(7):2369–75.

118. Nishimura M, Yamada T, Andoh T, Tao T, Emoto M, Ohji T, Matsuda K, Kameda N, Satoh Y, Matsutani A, Azuno Y, Oka Y. Granulocyte colony-stimulating factor (G-CSF) dependent hematopoiesis with monosomy 7 in a patient with severe aplastic anemia after ATG/CsA/G-CSF combined therapy. Int J Hematol 1998;68(2):203–11.

119. Kaito K, Kobayashi M, Katayama T, Masuoka H, Shimada T, Nishiwaki K, Sekita T, Otsubo H, Ogasawara Y, Hosoya T. Long-term administration of G-CSF for aplastic anaemia is closely related to the early evolution of monosomy 7 MDS in adults. Br J Haematol 1998;103(2):297–303.

120. Kojima S, Ohara A, Tsuchida M, Kudoh T, Hanada R, Okimoto Y, Kaneko T, Takano T, Ikuta K, Tsukimoto I. Japan Childhood Aplastic Anemia Study Group. Risk factors for evolution of acquired aplastic anemia into myelodysplastic syndrome and acute myeloid leukemia after immunosuppressive therapy in children. Blood 2002;100(3):786–90.

121. Locasciulli A, Arcese W, Locatelli F, Di Bona E, Bacigalupo A. Italian Aplastic Anaemia Study Group. Treatment of aplastic anaemia with granulocyte-colony stimulating factor and risk of malignancy. Italian Aplastic Anaemia Study Group. Lancet 2001;357(9249):43–4.

122. Freedman MH, Bonilla MA, Fier C, Bolyard AA, Scarlata D, Boxer LA, Brown S, Cham B, Kannourakis G, Kinsey SE, Mori PG, Cottle T, Welte K, Dale DC. Myelodysplasia syndrome and acute myeloid leukemia in patients with congenital neutropenia receiving G-CSF therapy. Blood 2000;96(2):429–36.

123. Imashuku S, Hibi S, Nakajima F, Mitsui T, Yokoyama S, Kojima S, Matsuyama T, Nakahata T, Ueda K, Tsukimoto I, et al. A review of 125 cases to determine the risk of myelodysplasia and leukemia in pediatric neutropenic patients after treatment with recombinant human granulocyte colony-stimulating factor. Blood 1994;84(7):2380–1.

124. Aguirre FV, Topol EJ, Ferguson JJ, Anderson K, Blankenship JC, Heuser RR, Sigmon K, Taylor M, Gottlieb R, Hanovich G, et al. Bleeding complications with the chimeric antibody to platelet glycoprotein IIb/IIIa integrin in patients undergoing percutaneous coronary intervention. EPIC Investigators. Circulation 1995;91(12):2882–90.

125. Gluckman E, Rokicka-Milewska R, Hann I, Nikiforakis E, Tavakoli F, Cohen-Scali S, Bacigalupo A. European Group for Blood and Marrow Transplantation Working Party for Severe Aplastic Anaemia. Results and follow-up of a phase III randomized study of recombinant human-granulocyte stimulating factor as support for immunosuppressive therapy in patients with severe aplastic anaemia. Br J Haematol 2002;119(4):1075–82.

126. Negrin RS, Haeuber DH, Nagler A, Olds LC, Donlon T, Souza LM, Greenberg PL. Treatment of myelodysplastic syndromes with recombinant human granulocyte colony-stimulating factor. A phase I-II trial. Ann Intern Med 1989;110(12):976–84.

127. Schriber JR, Negrin RS. Use and toxicity of the colony-stimulating factors. Drug Saf 1993;8(6):457–68.

128. Vose JM, Armitage JO. Clinical applications of hematopoietic growth factors. J Clin Oncol 1995;13(4):1023–35.

129. Rowe JM, Liesveld JL. Hematopoietic growth factors in acute leukemia. Leukemia 1997;11(3):328–41.

130. Terpstra W, Lowenberg B. Application of myeloid growth factors in the treatment of acute myeloid leukemia. Leukemia 1997;11(3):315–27.

131. Yoshida Y, Nakahata T, Shibata A, Takahashi M, Moriyama Y, Kaku K, Masaoka T, Kaneko T, Miwa S. Effects of long-term treatment with recombinant human granulocyte–macrophage colony-stimulating factor in patients with myelodysplastic syndrome. Leuk Lymphoma 1995;18(5–6):457–63.

132. Estey EH. Use of colony-stimulating factors in the treatment of acute myeloid leukemia. Blood 1994;83(8):2015–9.

133. Zimmer BM, Berdel WE, Ludwig WD, Notter M, Reufi B, Thiel E. Fatal spleen rupture during induction chemotherapy with rh GM-CSF priming for acute monocytic leukemia. Clinical case report and in vitro studies. Leuk Res 1993;17(3):277–83.

134. Moshang T Jr. Use of growth hormone in children surviving cancer. Med Pediatr Oncol 1998;31(3):170–2.

135. Nishi Y, Tanaka T, Takano K, Fujieda K, Igarashi Y, Hanew K, Hirano T, Yokoya S, Tachibana K, Saito T, Watanabe S. Recent status in the occurrence of leukemia in growth hormone-treated patients in Japan. GH Treatment Study Committee of the Foundation for Growth Science, Japan. J Clin Endocrinol Metab 1999;84(6):1961–5.

136. Allen DB, Rundle AC, Graves DA, Blethen SL. Risk of leukemia in children treated with human growth hormone: review and reanalysis. J Pediatr 1997;131(1 Pt 2):S32–6.

137. Moshang T Jr, Rundle AC, Graves DA, Nickas J, Johanson A, Meadows A. Brain tumor recurrence in children treated with growth hormone: the National Cooperative Growth Study experience. J Pediatr 1996;128(5 Pt 2):S4–7.

138. Ogilvy-Stuart AL, Ryder WD, Gattamaneni HR, Clayton PE, Shalet SM. Growth hormone and tumour recurrence. BMJ 1992;304(6842):1601–5.

139. Price DA, Wilton P, Jonsson P, Albertsson-Wikland K, Chatelain P, Cutfield W, Ranke MB. Efficacy and safety of growth hormone treatment in children with prior craniopharyngioma: an analysis of the Pharmacia and Upjohn International Growth Database (KIGS) from 1988 to 1996. Horm Res 1998;49(2):91–7.

140. Tuffli GA, Johanson A, Rundle AC, Allen DB. Lack of increased risk for extracranial, nonleukemic neoplasms in recipients of recombinant deoxyribonucleic acid growth hormone. J Clin Endocrinol Metab 1995;80(4):1416–22.

141. Frisch H. Pharmacovigilance: the use of KIGS (Pharmacia and Upjohn International Growth Database) to monitor the safety of growth hormone treatment in children. Endocrinol Metabol 1997;4(Suppl B):83–6.

142. Swerdlow AJ, Higgins CD, Adlard P, Preece MA. Risk of cancer in patients treated with human pituitary growth hormone in the UK, 1959–85: a cohort study. Lancet 2002;360(9329):273–7.

143. La Vecchia C, Tavani A. Epidemiological evidence on hair dyes and the risk of cancer in humans. Eur J Cancer Prev 1995;4(1):31–43.

144. Zhang Y, Holford TR, Leaderer B, Boyle P, Zahm SH, Flynn S, Tallini G, Owens PH, Zheng T. Hair-coloring product use and risk of non-Hodgkin's lymphoma: a population-based case-control study in Connecticut. Am J Epidemiol 2004;159(2):148–54.

145. Colin-Jones DG, Langman MJ, Lawson DH, Vessey MP. Cimetidine and gastric cancer: preliminary report from post-marketing surveillance study. BMJ (Clin Res Ed) 1982;285(6351):1311–3.

146. Suleiman UL, Harrison M, Britton A, McPherson K, Bates T. H2-receptor antagonists may increase the risk of cardio-oesophageal adenocarcinoma: a case-control study. Eur J Cancer Prev 2000;9(3):185–91.

147. Moller H, Nissen A, Mosbech J. Use of cimetidine and other peptic ulcer drugs in Denmark 1977–1990 with analysis of the risk of gastric cancer among cimetidine users. Gut 1992;33(9):1166–9.

148. Rao SS, Nayak KS, Swarnalata G, Goyal DN, Rao KP, Mitros FA. Gastric carcinoid associated with ranitidine in a patient with renal failure. Am J Gastroenterol 1993;88(8):1273–4.

149. Cattley RC. Carcinogenicity of lipid-lowering drugs. JAMA 1996;275(19):1479.

150. Sacks FM, Pfeffer MA, Moye LA, Rouleau JL, Rutherford JD, Cole TG, Brown L, Warnica JW, Arnold JM, Wun CC, Davis BR, Braunwald E. The effect of pravastatin on coronary events after myocardial infarction in patients with average cholesterol levels. Cholesterol and Recurrent Events Trial investigators. N Engl J Med 1996;335(14):1001–9.

151. Dalen JE, Dalton WS. Does lowering cholesterol cause cancer? JAMA 1996;275(1):67–9.

152. Botros SS. Effect of praziquantel versus hycanthone on deoxyribonucleic acid content of hepatocytes in murine schistosomiasis mansoni. Pharmacol Res 1990;22(2):219–29.

153. Bulay O, Urman H, Patil K, Clayson DB, Shubik P. Carcinogenic potential of hycanthone in mice and hamsters. Int J Cancer 1979;23(1):97–104.

154. Mayer-Davis EJ. Cancer in a patient receiving IGF-I therapy. Diabetes Care 2000;23:433–4.

155. Wurzelmann JI, Silver A, Schreinemachers DM, Sandler RS, Everson RB. Iron intake and the risk of colorectal cancer. Cancer Epidemiol Biomarkers Prev 1996;5(7):503–7.

156. Goh J, Callagy G, McEntee G, O'Keane JC, Bomford A, Crowe J. Hepatocellular carcinoma arising in the absence of cirrhosis in genetic haemochromatosis: three case reports and review of literature. Eur J Gastroenterol Hepatol 1999;11(8):915–9.

157. Skegg DC, Noonan EA, Paul C, Spears GF, Meirik O, Thomas DB. Depot medroxyprogesterone acetate and breast cancer. A pooled analysis of the World Health Organization and New Zealand studies. JAMA 1995;273(10):799–804.

158. Lumbiganon P. Depot-medroxyprogesterone acetate (DMPA) and cancer of the endometrium and ovary. Contraception 1994;49(3):203–9.

159. La Vecchia C. Depot-medroxyprogesterone acetate, other injectable contraceptives, and cervical neoplasia. Contraception 1994;49(3):223–30.

160. Meltzer EO, Storms WW, Pierson WE, Cummins LH, Orgel HA, Perhach JL, Hemsworth GR. Efficacy of azelastine in perennial allergic rhinitis: clinical and rhinomanometric evaluation. J Allergy Clin Immunol 1988;82(3 Pt 1):447–55.

161. Boyle CA, Berkowitz GS, LiVolsi VA, Ort S, Merino MJ, White C, Kelsey JL. Caffeine consumption and fibrocystic breast disease: a case-control epidemiologic study. J Natl Cancer Inst 1984;72(5):1015–9.

162. Krause JR, Ayuyang HQ, Ellis LD. Occurrence of three cases of carcinoma in individuals with Crohn's disease treated with metronidazole. Am J Gastroenterol 1985;80(12):978–82.

163. Schyve PM, Smithline F, Meltzer HY. Neuroleptic-induced prolactin level elevation and breast cancer: an emerging clinical issue. Arch Gen Psychiatry 1978;35(11):1291–301.

164. Mortensen PB. The incidence of cancer in schizophrenic patients. J Epidemiol Community Health 1989;43(1):43–7.

165. Boyd MR, Stiko AW, Sasame HA. Metabolic activation of nitrofurantoin—possible implications for carcinogenesis. Biochem Pharmacol 1979;28(5):601–6.

166. Hasegawa R, Murasaki G, St John MK, Zenser TV, Cohen SM. Evaluation of nitrofurantoin on the two stages of urinary bladder carcinogenesis in the rat. Toxicology 1990;62(3):333–47.

167. Andreassi MG, Picano E, Del Ry S, Botto N, Colombo MG, Giannessi D, Lubrano V, Vassalle C, Biagini A. Chronic long-term nitrate therapy: possible cytogenetic effect in humans? Mutagenesis 2001;16(6):517–21.

177. Gumrich H. Die röntgenologische Darstellung eines Mammaparaffinoms. [Roentgenologic representation of mammary paraffinomas.] Medizinische 1955;14:500.

178. Tinckler LF, Stock FE. Paraffinoma of the breast. Aust NZ J Surg 1955;25(2):142–4.

179. Clarkson P. Local mastectomy and augmentation mammaplasty for bilateral paraffinoma of breasts. Nurs Mirror Midwives J 1965;121(152):13–6.

180. Munchow H. Paraffinolschaden im Gewebe am Beispiel verkalkter Paraffinome in den Mammae. [Paraffin-oil damage to tissue as in the example of calcified paraffinomas in mammae.] Radiol Diagn (Berl) 1966;7(6):743–7.

181. Bonvallet JM. Paraffinome des deux seins chez un homme. [Paraffinoma of both breasts in a man.] Chirurgie 1971;97(3):190–2.

182. Brombart JC. Un paraffinome du sein. Aspects radiologiques. [Breast paraffinoma. Radiological aspects.] J Belge Radiol 1972;55(5):585–7.

183. Alagaratnam TT, Ong GB. Paraffinomas of the breast. J R Coll Surg Edinb 1983;28(4):260–3.

184. Raven RW. Paraffinoma of the breast. Clin Oncol 1981;7(2):157–61.

185. Kay SP, Saad MN. Paraffinoma of the male breast: a case report. Br J Plast Surg 1983;36(4):522–3.

186. Tepavicharova P, Popmikhailova Kh, Videnov L. [Paraffinoma of the breasts.] Khirurgiia (Sofiia) 1988;41(4):90–3.

187. Czeti I, Siko PP. Removal of both breasts for paraffinoma and subsequent replacement. Acta Chir Plast 1988;30(2):122–4.

188. Yang WT, Suen M, Ho WS, Metreweli C. Paraffinomas of the breast: mammographic, ultrasonographic and radiographic appearances with clinical and histopathological correlation. Clin Radiol 1996;51(2):130–3.

189. Zekri A, Ho WS, King WW. Paraffinomes déstructifs des seins et de la paroi thoracique dus a l'injection de paraffine pour augmentation mammaire. A propos de trois cas et revue de la littérature. [Destructive paraffinoma of the breast and thoracic wall caused by paraffin injection for mammary increase. Apropos of 3 cases with review of the literature.] Ann Chir Plast Esthet 1996;41(1):90–3.

190. Alagaratnam TT, Ng WF. Paraffinomas of the breast: an oriental curiosity. Aust NZ J Surg 1996;66(3):138–40.

191. Sinclair DS, Freedy L, Spigos DG. Case 3. Altered breast: paraffin injection with development of paraffinomas. AJR Am J Roentgenol 2000;175(3):861864–5.

192. Khong PL, Ho LW, Chan JH, Leong LL. MR imaging of breast paraffinomas. AJR Am J Roentgenol 1999;173(4):929–32.

193. Ho WS, Chan AC, Law BK. Management of paraffinoma of the breast: 10 years' experience. Br J Plast Surg 2001 Apr;54(3):232–4.

194. Wang J, Shih TT, Li YW, Chang KJ, Huang HY. Magnetic resonance imaging characteristics of paraffinomas and siliconomas after mammoplasty. J Formos Med Assoc 2002;101(2):117–23.

195. Peng NJ, Chang HT, Tsay DG, Liu RS. Technetium-99m-sestamibi scintimammography to detect breast cancer in patients with paraffinomas or siliconomas after breast augmentation. Cancer Biother Radiopharm 2003;18(4):573–80.

196. Chen JS, Liu WC, Yang KC, Chen LW, Huang JS, Chang HT. Reconstruction with bilateral pedicled TRAM flap for paraffinoma breast. Plast Reconstr Surg 2005;115(1):96–104.

197. Rintala A. Ulcerating paraffinoma. Ann Chir Gynaecol 1976;65(5):356–60.

198. Thiels C, Dumke K. Mammaverkalkung nach Paraffininjektion. [Breast calcinosis following paraffin injection.] Rofo 1977;126(2):173–4.

199. Pennisi VR. Obscure carcinoma encountered in subcutaneous mastectomy in silicone- and paraffin-injected breasts: two patients. Plast Reconstr Surg 1984;74(4): 535–8.

200. Ooi GC, Peh WC, Ip M. Migration and lymphatic spread of calcified paraffinomas after breast augmentation. Australas Radiol 1996;40(4):404–7.

201. Montagnac R, Collet E, Schillinger F, Chapelon C. Sarcoidose secondaire a un paraffinome mammaire bilateral. [Sarcoidosis secondary to bilateral breast paraffinoma.] Presse Méd 1993;22(33):1707.

202. Bradley RH Jr, Ehrgott WA. Paraffinoma of the penis: case report. J Urol 1951;65(3):453-9.

203. May JA, Pickering PP. Paraffinoma of the penis. Calif Med 1956;85(1):42-4.

204. Masse R. Paraffinome peno-scrotal. [Paraffinoma of the penis and scrotum.] Ann Med Leg Criminol Police Sci Toxicol 1967;47(6):704-6.

205. Foucar E, Downing DT, Gerber WL. Sclerosing lipogranuloma of the male genitalia containing vitamin E: a comparison with classical "paraffinoma". J Am Acad Dermatol 1983;9(1):103-10.

206. Akkus E, Iscimen A, Tasli L, Hattat H. Paraffinoma and ulcer of the external genitalia after self-injection of Vaseline. J Sex Med 2006;3(1):170-2.

207. Podluzhnyi GA, Tigov AD, Braganets AM, Iakimenko VA. [The clinical picture, classification and surgical treatment of paraffinomas of the external genitalia.] Urol Nefrol (Mosk) 1991;(4):69-73.

208. Lee T, Choi HR, Lee YT, Lee YH. Paraffinoma of the penis. Yonsei Med J 1994;35(3):344-8.

209. Gfesser M, Worret WI. Paraffinome de pénis. [Paraffinoma of the penis.] Hautarzt 1996;47(9):705-7.

210. Jeong JH, Shin HJ, Woo SH, Seul JH. A new repair technique for penile paraffinoma: bilateral scrotal flaps. Ann Plast Surg 1996;37(4):386-93.

211. Muraro GB, Dami A, Farina U. Paraffinoma of the penis: one-stage repair. Arch Esp Urol 1996;49(6):648-50.

212. Steffens J, Kosharskyy B, Hiebl R, Schonberger B, Rottger P, Loening S. Paraffinoma of the external genitalia after autoinjection of Vaseline. Eur Urol 2000;38(6):778-781.

213. Cohen JL, Keoleian CM, Krull EA. Penile paraffinoma: self-injection with mineral oil. J Am Acad Dermatol 2001;45(6 Suppl):S222-4.

214. Cohen JL, Keoleian CM, Krull EA. Penile paraffinoma: self-injection with mineral oil. J Am Acad Dermatol 2002;47(5 Suppl):S251-3.

215. Moon du G, Yoo JW, Bae JH, Han CS, Kim YK, Kim JJ. Sexual function and psychological characteristics of penile paraffinoma. Asian J Androl 2003;5(3):191-4.

216. Santos P, Chaveiro A, Nunes G, Fonseca J, Cardoso J. Penile paraffinoma. J Eur Acad Dermatol Venereol 2003;17(5):583-4.

217. Eo SR, Kim KS, Kim DY, Lee SY, Cho BH. Paraffinoma of the labia. Plast Reconstr Surg 2004;113(6):1885-7.

218. Nairn RC, Woodruff MF. Paraffinoma of the rectum. Ann Surg 1955;141(4):536-40.

219. Bennett DH, Wade JS. Rectal paraffinoma. Proc R Soc Med 1969;62(8):818.

220. Nishio T, Sasai Y. [Paraffinoma.]Ryoikibetsu Shokogun Shirizu 1994;(4):268-70.

221. Yanagi H, Furukawa Y, Kusunoki M, Utsunomiya J. [Colorectal paraffinoma.] Ryoikibetsu Shokogun Shirizu 1994;(6):549-50.

222. Broadbent TR. Nasal paraffinoma following rhinoplasty. Northwest Med 1957;56(7):814-5.

223. Becker H. Paraffinoma as a complication of nasal packing. Plast Reconstr Surg 1983;72(5):735-6.

224. Montgomery PQ, Khan JI, Feakins R, Nield DV. Paraffinoma revisited: a post-operative condition following rhinoplasty nasal packing. J Laryngol Otol 1996;110(8):785-6.

225. Bachor E, Dost P, Unger A, Ruwe M. Paraffinome—eine seltene Komplikation nach endonasaler Chirurgie. [Paraffinoma—a rare complication following endonasal surgery.] Laryngorhinootologie 1999;78(6):307-12.

226. Mehendale FV, Sommerlad BC. Paraffinoma—a complication of Jelonet packs following rhinoplasty. Br J Plast Surg 2001;54(2):179-80.

227. Gryskiewicz JM. Paraffinoma or postrhinoplasty mucous cyst of the nose: which is it? Plast Reconstr Surg 2001;108(7):2160-1.

228. Mouly R, Dufourmentel C, Grupper C, Arouete J, Pailheret JP, Crehange JR. Huilome palpebral après injection intralacrymale. [Palpebral paraffinoma following intralacrim injection.] Ann Chir Plast 1972;17(1):61-6.

229. Lieb W. Paraffingranulom des Unterlides. [Paraffin granuloma of the lower lid.] Klin Monatsbl Augenheilkd 1987;190(2):125-6.

230. Feldmann R, Harms M, Chavaz P, Salomon D, Saurat JH. Orbital and palpebral paraffinoma. J Am Acad Dermatol 1992;26(5 Pt 2):833-5.

231. Hintschich CR, Beyer-Machule CK, Stefani FH. Paraffinoma of the periorbit—a challenge for the oculoplastic surgeon. Ophthal Plast Reconstr Surg 1995;11(1):39-43.

232. Keefe MA, Bloom DC, Keefe KS, Killian PJ. Orbital paraffinoma as a complication of endoscopic sinus surgery. Otolaryngol Head Neck Surg 2002;127(6):575-7.

233. Berg R Jr, Burford TH. Pulmonary paraffinoma (lipoid pneumonia); a critical study. J Thorac Surg 1950;20(3):418-28.

234. McLetchie NG, De Profio FR, O'Rafferty FM. [Paraffinoma of the lung.] Treat Serv Bull 1952;7(9):410-8.

235. Wood Ga, Mitchell SP. Pulmonary paraffinoma verified at thoracotomy; report of two cases. Calif Med 1953;79(6):452-4.

236. Nelson LM. Lipiodol swallow and paraffinoma of the lung. Br J Tuberc Dis Chest 1954;48(1):60-2.

237. Bordet F, Daumet P, Garnier C, Paillas J. [Pulmonary paraffinoma complicated by suppuration.] J Fr Med Chir Thorac 1959;13:547-54.

238. Vaidya MP. Oil granuloma (paraffinoma) of the lung. Postgrad Med J 1962;38:355-8.

239. Mouly R, Dufourmentel C. Les paraffinomes des membres. [Limb paraffinomas.] Ann Chir Plast 1964;16:210-8.

240. Borrie J, Gwynne JF. Paraffinoma of lung: lipoid pneumonia. Report of two cases. Thorax 1973;28(2):214-21.

241. Fasal P. Paraffinoma of the arms with granulomatous lesions over the elbows. AMA Arch Derm Syphilol 1950;62(6):928-9.

242. Rivas Diez B. Parafinomas ulcerados de ambas piernas; veinticinco anos de evolucion. [Ulcerating paraffinoma of both legs; 25 years of evolution.] Bol Tr Soc Argent Cir 1952;36(22):64015.

243. Thiers H, Croisille M. Paraffinome des parties molles de la jambe (à propos d'un cas). [Paraffinoma of the soft parts of the leg (apropos of a case).] J Radiol Electrol Med Nucl 1969;50(1):83-4.

244. Galland MC, Cohen M, Aquaron R, Maurin R, Duick JP, Bouteiller JC, Sauget Y, Manez R, Pizzi-Anselme M, Pelissier JL, et al. Lipogranulome calcifie après injection d'huile gomenolée: un "paraffinome" 60 ans après. [Calcified lipogranuloma after gomenoleo oil injection: "paraffinoma" 60 years later.] Therapie 1990;45(1):27-32.

245. Duperrat B, Recht P, Lenoir JC. [Paraffinoma of the face caused by work accident.] Presse Méd 1960;68:691-2.

246. van der Waal I. Paraffinoma of the face: a diagnostic and therapeutic problem. Oral Surg Oral Med Oral Pathol 1974;38(5):675–80.

247. Vazquez-Martinez OT, Ocampo-Candiani J, Mendez-Olvera N, Sanchez Negron FA. Paraffinomas of the facial area: treatment with systemic and intralesional steroids. J Drugs Dermatol 2006;5(2):186–9.

248. Sinrachtanant C, Tantinikorn W, Warnnissorn M, Assanasen P. Sclerosing lipogranuloma of the nose: a new treatment using adipose tissue transplantation. Facial Plast Surg 2003;19(4):363–7.

249. Klein JA, Cole G, Barr RJ, Bartlow G, Fulwider C. Paraffinomas of the scalp. Arch Dermatol 1985;121(3):382–5.

250. Dumont-Fruytier M, Tennstedt D, Lachapelle JM. Paraffinomes multiples thoraco-abdominaux. [Multiple thoraco-abdominal paraffinomas.] Dermatologica 1980;160(3):208–14.

251. Moon WK, Kim SH, Lee SJ, Han MC. Paraffinoma in the urinary bladder: CT findings. J Comput Assist Tomogr 1992;16(2):308–10.

252. Kelleher J, Wilson S, Witherow RO. Paraffinoma of the ureter. Br J Urol 1987;59(1):92–3.

253. Kergin FG. Esophageal obstruction due to paraffinoma of mediastinum; reconstruction by intrathoracic colon graft. Ann Surg 1953;137(1):91–7.

254. Deck KA, Ruiz-Ayuso F, Steinbruck HG. Paraffinom im vorderen Mediastinum. [Paraffinoma in the anterior mediastinum.] Med Klin 1969;64(4):160–4.

255. Franks RE, Cleland WP. Mediastinal fibrosis from paraffin wax. Proc Thorac Cardiovasc Soc 1978;240:1515.

256. Shiiku C, Harada H, Yamamoto N, Ito T, Koizumi J, Matsui T, Abe T. [A case of paraffinoma after plombage with spinal paralysis.] Kyobu Geka 2002;55(2):178–80.

257. Lewis PD, Dayan AD. "Paraffinosis" secondary to bilateral oleothorax. Thorax 1965;20(5):436–40.

258. Boyd JT, Doll R. Gastro-intestinal cancer and the use of liquid paraffin. Br J Cancer 1954;8(2):231–7.

259. Meyniard O, Boissonnas A, Laisne MJ, Laroche C, Abelanet R. Pneumopathie chronique a l'huile de paraffine et modifications pleurales: hyperplasie mesotheliale et mesotheliome. [Chronic pneumonia caused by paraffin oil and pleural modifications: mesothelial hyperplasia and mesothelioma.] Rev Fr Mal Respir 1980;8(3):259–63.

260. Tashjian AH Jr, Chabner BA. Commentary on clinical safety of recombinant human parathyroid hormone 1–34 in the treatment of osteoporosis in men and postmenopausal women. J Bone Miner Res 2002;17(7):1151–61.

261. Vahle JL, Sato M, Long GG, Young JK, Francis PC, Engelhardt JA, Westmore MS, Linda Y, Nold JB. Skeletal changes in rats given daily subcutaneous injections of recombinant human parathyroid hormone (1–34) for 2 years and relevance to human safety. Toxicol Pathol 2002;30(3):312–21.

262. Gilman PA, Holtzman NA. Acute lymphoblastic leukemia in a patient receiving penicillamine for Wilson's disease. JAMA 1982;248(4):467–8.

263. Sheldon P, Wood JK. Remission of arthritis and radiological improvement after combination therapy for non-Hodgkin's lymphoma in a patient with rheumatoid arthritis undergoing treatment with D-penicillamine. Ann Rheum Dis 1985;44(8):556–8.

264. Anonymous. Neoplasms in rheumatoid arthritis: update on clinical and epidemiologic data. Am J Med 1985;78(1A):1–83.

265. Dubach UC, Rosner B, Pfister E. Epidemiologic study of abuse of analgesics containing phenacetin. Renal morbidity and mortality (1968-1979). N Engl J Med 1983;308(7):357–62.

266. Dubach UC, Rosner B, Sturmer T. An epidemiologic study of abuse of analgesic drugs. Effects of phenacetin and salicylate on mortality and cardiovascular morbidity (1968 to 1987). N Engl J Med 1991;324(3):155–60.

267. Gago-Dominguez M, Yuan JM, Castelao JE, Ross RK, Yu MC. Regular use of analgesics is a risk factor for renal cell carcinoma. Br J Cancer 1999;81(3):542–8.

268. Daneshmend TK, Scott GL, Bradfield JW. Angiosarcoma of liver associated with phenelzine. BMJ 1979;1(6179):1679.

269. Cogrel O, Beylot-Barry M, Vergier B, Dubus P, Doutre MS, Merlio JP, Beylot C. Sodium valproate-induced cutaneous pseudolymphoma followed by recurrence with carbamazepine. Br J Dermatol 2001;144(6):1235–8.

270. Saeki H, Etoh T, Toda K, Mihm MC Jr. Pseudolymphoma syndrome due to carbamazepine. J Dermatol 1999;26(5):329–31.

271. Sinnige HA, Boender CA, Kuypers EW, Ruitenberg HM. Carbamazepine-induced pseudolymphoma and immune dysregulation. J Intern Med 1990;227(5):355–8.

272. Pathak P, McLachlan RS. Drug-induced pseudolymphoma secondary to lamotrigine. Neurology 1998;50(5):1509–10.

273. Knowles SR, Shapiro LE, Shear NH. Anticonvulsant hypersensitivity syndrome: incidence, prevention and management. Drug Saf 1999;21(6):489–501.

274. Studniberg HM, Weller P. PUVA, UVB, psoriasis, and nonmelanoma skin cancer. J Am Acad Dermatol 1993;29(6):1013–22.

275. Lever LR, Farr PM. Skin cancers or premalignant lesions occur in half of high-dose PUVA patients. Br J Dermatol 1994;131(2):215–9.

276. Lindelof B, Sigurgeirsson B. PUVA and cancer: a case-control study. Br J Dermatol 1993;129(1):39–41.

277. Stern R. Metastatic squamous cell cancer after psoralen photochemotherapy. Lancet 1994;344(8937):1644–5.

278. Sorahan T, Nichols L. Mortality and cancer morbidity of production workers in the UK flexible polyurethane foam industry: updated findings, 1958–98. Occup Environ Med 2002;59(11):751–8.

279. Langman MJ. Omeprazole. BMJ 1991;303(6801):481–2.

280. Declich P, Ferrara A, Galati F, Caruso S, Baldacci MP, Ambrosiani L. Do fundic gland polyps develop under long-term omeprazole therapy? Am J Gastroenterol 1998;93(8):1393.

281. Naegels S, Urbain D. Omeprazole and fundic gland polyps. Am J Gastroenterol 1998;93(5):855.

282. Choudhry U, Boyce HW Jr, Coppola D. Proton pump inhibitor-associated gastric polyps: a retrospective analysis of their frequency, and endoscopic, histologic, and ultrastructural characteristics. Am J Clin Pathol 1998;110(5):615–21.

283. Haga Y, Nakatsura T, Shibata Y, Sameshima H, Nakamura Y, Tanimura M, Ogawa M. Human gastric carcinoid detected during long-term antiulcer therapy of H2 receptor antagonist and proton pump inhibitor. Dig Dis Sci 1998;43(2):253–7.

284. Engeset A. In: Ruttmann E, editor. Dissemination f tumor cells by lymphangiography Proceedings, International Symposium on Lymphology, Zurich, 1966. Stuttgart: Georg Thieme Verlag, 1967:308.

285. McDougall IR, Nelsen TS, Kempson RL. Papillary carcinoma of the thyroid seven years after I-131 therapy for Graves' disease. Clin Nucl Med 1981;6(8):368–71.

286. Wolff J. Risks for stable and radioactive iodine in radiation protection of the thyroid. In: Hall R, Kobberling J, editors. Thyroid Disorders Associated with Iodine Deficiency and Excess. Serono Symposia Publications 22. New York: Raven Press, 1985:111.

287. Holm LE, Dahlqvist I, Israelsson A, Lundell G. Malignant thyroid tumors after iodine-131 therapy: a retrospective cohort study. N Engl J Med 1980;303(4):188–91.

288. Hoffman DA, McConahey WM, Diamond EL, Kurland LT. Mortality in women treated for hyperthyroidism. Am J Epidemiol 1982;115(2):243–54.

289. Holm LE, Hall P, Wiklund K, Lundell G, Berg G, Bjelkengren G, Cederquist E, Ericsson UB, Hallquist A, Larsson LG, et al. Cancer risk after iodine-131 therapy for hyperthyroidism. J Natl Cancer Inst 1991;83(15):1072–7.

290. Blahd WH. Treatment of malignant thyroid disease. Semin Nucl Med 1979;9(2):95–9.

291. Larsen PR, Conard RA, Knudsen K. Thyroid hypofunction appearing as a delayed manifestation of accidental exposure to radioactive fallout in a Marshallese population. In: Biological Effects of Ionizing Radiation 1. Vienna: International Atomic Energy Agency, 1978:101.

292. Freitas JE, Swanson DP, Gross MD, Sisson JC. Iodine-131: optimal therapy for hyperthyroidism in children and adolescents? J Nucl Med 1979;20(8):847–50.

293. Maxon HR, Thomas SR, Chen IW. The role of nuclear medicine in the treatment of hyperthyroidism and well-differentiated thyroid adenocarcinoma. Clin Nucl Med 1981;6(10S):P87–98.

294. Graham GD, Burman KD. Radioiodine treatment of Graves' disease. An assessment of its potential risks. Ann Intern Med 1986;105(6):900–5.

295. Gorman CA, Becker DV, Greenspan FS, Levy RP, Oppenheimer JH, Rivlin RS, Robbins J, Vanderlaan WP. Breast cancer and thyroid therapy. Statement by the American Thyroid Association. JAMA 1977;237(14):1459–60.

296. Grossman E, Messerli FH, Goldbourt U. Carcinogenicity of antihypertensive therapy. Curr Hypertens Rep 2002;4(3):195–201.

297. von Poser G, Andrade HH, da Silva KV, Henriques AT, Henriques JA. Genotoxic, mutagenic and recombinogenic effects of rauwolfia alkaloids. Mutat Res 1990;232(1):37–43.

298. Lyden-Sokolowski A, Nilsson A, Sjoberg P. Two-year carcinogenicity study with sennosides in the rat: emphasis on gastro-intestinal alterations. Pharmacology 1993;47(Suppl 1):209–15.

299. Rose LI, Underwood RH, Newmark SR, Kisch ES, Williams GH. Pathophysiology of spironolactone-induced gynecomastia. Ann Intern Med 1977;87(4):398–403.

300. Committee on Safety of Medicines. Spironolactone. Curr Probl 1988;21.

301. Harlow BL, Cramer DW, Bell DA, Welch WR. Perineal exposure to talc and ovarian cancer risk. Obstet Gynecol 1992;80(1):19–26.

302. Clement PB, Oliva E, Young RH. Mullerian adenosarcoma of the uterine corpus associated with tamoxifen therapy: a report of six cases and a review of tamoxifen-associated endometrial lesions. Int J Gynecol Pathol 1996;15(3):222–9.

303. Orbo A, Lindal S, Mortensen E. Tamoxifen og endometriecancer. En kasuistikk. [Tamoxifen and endometrial cancer. A case report.] Tidsskr Nor Laegeforen 1996;116(16):1877–8.

304. Boudouris O, Ferrand S, Guillet JL, Madelenat P. Efféts paradoxaux du tamoxifène sur l'utérus de la femme. [Paradoxical effects of tamoxifen on the woman's uterus.

Apropos of 7 cases of myoma that appeared while under anti-estrogen treatment.] J Gynecol Obstet Biol Reprod (Paris) 1989;18(3):372–8.

305. Nuovo MA, Nuovo GJ, McCaffrey RM, Levine RU, Barron B, Winkler B. Endometrial polyps in postmenopausal patients receiving tamoxifen. Int J Gynecol Pathol 1989;8(2):125–31.

306. Rutqvist LE, Mattsson A. Cardiac and thromboembolic morbidity among postmenopausal women with early-stage breast cancer in a randomized trial of adjuvant tamoxifen. The Stockholm Breast Cancer Study Group. J Natl Cancer Inst 1993;85(17):1398–406.

307. Seoud MA, Johnson J, Weed JC Jr. Gynecologic tumors in tamoxifen-treated women with breast cancer. Obstet Gynecol 1993;82(2):165–9.

308. Treilleux T, Mignotte H, Clement-Chassagne C, Guastalla P, Bailly C. Tamoxifen and malignant epithelial-nonepithelial tumours of the endometrium: report of six cases and review of the literature. Eur J Surg Oncol 1999;25(5):477–82.

309. Ramondetta LM, Sherwood JB, Dunton CJ, Palazzo JP. Endometrial cancer in polyps associated with tamoxifen use. Am J Obstet Gynecol 1999;180(2 Pt 1):340–1.

310. Ascher SM, Johnson JC, Barnes WA, Bae CJ, Patt RH, Zeman RK. MR imaging appearance of the uterus in postmenopausal women receiving tamoxifen therapy for breast cancer: histopathologic correlation. Radiology 1996;200(1):105–10.

311. Okada DH, Rowland JB, Petrovic LM. Uterine pleomorphic rhabdomyosarcoma in a patient receiving tamoxifen therapy. Gynecol Oncol 1999;75(3):509–13.

312. Dumortier J, Freyer G, Sasco AJ, Frappart L, Zenone T, Romestaing P, Trillet-Lenoir V. Endometrial mesodermal mixed tumor occurring after tamoxifen treatment: report on a new case and review of the literature. Ann Oncol 2000;11(3):355–8.

313. Jessop FA, Roberts PF. Mullerian adenosarcoma of the uterus in association with tamoxifen therapy. Histopathology 2000;36(1):91–2.

314. Fotiou S, Hatjieleftheriou G, Kyrousis G, Kokka F, Apostolikas N. Long-term tamoxifen treatment: a possible aetiological factor in the development of uterine carcinosarcoma: two case-reports and review of the literature. Anticancer Res 2000;20(3B):2015–20.

315. Andia D, Lafuente P, Matorras R, Usandizaga JM. Uterine side effects of treatment with tamoxifen. Eur J Obstet Gynecol Reprod Biol 2000;92(2):235–40.

316. Tempfer C, Kubista E, Atkins CD, Narod SA, Pal T, Graham T, Mitchell M, Fyles A, Lasset C, Bonadona V, Mignotte H, Bremond A, Van Leeuwen FE, Bergman L, Beelen MLR, Gallee MPW, Hollema H, Dickson MJ, Pandiarajan T, Kairies P, Marsh F, Mayfield M. Tamoxifen and risk of endometrial cancer. Lancet 2001;357(9249):65–8.

317. Bergman L, Beelen ML, Gallee MP, Hollema H, Benraadt J, van Leeuwen FE. Risk and prognosis of endometrial cancer after tamoxifen for breast cancer. Comprehensive Cancer Centres' ALERT Group. Assessment of Liver and Endometrial cancer Risk following Tamoxifen. Lancet 2000;356(9233):881–7.

318. Powles TJ, Bourne T, Athanasiou S, Chang J, Grubock K, Ashley S, Oakes L, Tidy A, Davey J, Viggers J, Humphries S, Collins W. The effects of norethisterone on endometrial abnormalities identified by transvaginal ultrasound screening of healthy post-menopausal

women on tamoxifen or placebo. Br J Cancer 1998;78(2):272–5.

319. Strauss HG, Wolters M, Methfessel G, Buchmann J, Koelbl H. Significance of endovaginal ultrasonography in assessing tamoxifen-associated changes of the endometrium. A prospective study. Acta Obstet Gynecol Scand 2000;79(8):697–701.

320. Gerber B, Krause A, Muller H, Reimer T, Kulz T, Makovitzky J, Kundt G, Friese K. Effects of adjuvant tamoxifen on the endometrium in postmenopausal women with breast cancer: a prospective long-term study using transvaginal ultrasound. J Clin Oncol 2000;18(20):3464–70.

321. Carpentier O, Dubost-Brama A, Martin De Lassalle E, Piette F, Delaporte E. Rhabdomyosarcome sur site d'implantation d'un stimulateur cardiaque. [Rhabdomyosarcoma at site of pacemaker implantation.] Ann Dermatol Venereol 2000;127(10):837–40.

322. Hansen J, Raaschou-Nielsen O, Christensen JM, Johansen I, McLaughlin JK, Lipworth L, Blot WJ, Olsen JH. Cancer incidence among Danish workers exposed to trichloroethylene. J Occup Environ Med 2001;43(2):133–9.

323. The Alpha-Tocopherol, Beta Carotene Cancer Prevention Study Group. The effect of vitamin E and beta carotene on the incidence of lung cancer and other cancers in male smokers. N Engl J Med 1994;330(15):1029–35.

324. van der Vliet A. Cigarettes, cancer, and carotenoids: a continuing, unresolved antioxidant paradox. Am J Clin Nutr 2000;72(6):1421–3.

325. Block G, Patterson B, Subar A. Fruit, vegetables, and cancer prevention: a review of the epidemiological evidence. Nutr Cancer 1992;18(1):1–29.

326. Pryor WA, Stahl W, Rock CL. Beta carotene: from biochemistry to clinical trials. Nutr Rev 2000;58(2 Pt 1):39–53.

327. Thompson HJ, Heimendinger J, Haegele A, Sedlacek SM, Gillette C, O'Neill C, Wolfe P, Conry C. Effect of increased vegetable and fruit consumption on markers of oxidative cellular damage. Carcinogenesis 1999;20(12):2261–6.

328. Krinsky NI. The antioxidant and biological properties of the carotenoids. Ann NY Acad Sci 1998;854:443–7.

329. Cross CE, Traber M, Eiserich J, van der Vliet A. Micronutrient antioxidants and smoking. Br Med Bull 1999;55(3):691–704.

330. Alberg AJ, Chen JC, Zhao H, Hoffman SC, Comstock GW, Helzlsouer KJ. Household exposure to passive cigarette smoking and serum micronutrient concentrations. Am J Clin Nutr 2000;72(6):1576–82.

331. Handelman GJ, Packer L, Cross CE. Destruction of tocopherols, carotenoids, and retinol in human plasma by cigarette smoke. Am J Clin Nutr 1996;63(4):559–65.

332. Baker DL, Krol ES, Jacobsen N, Liebler DC. Reactions of beta-carotene with cigarette smoke oxidants. Identification of carotenoid oxidation products and evaluation of the prooxidant/antioxidant effect. Chem Res Toxicol 1999;12(6):535–43.

333. Wang XD, Russell RM. Procarcinogenic and anticarcinogenic effects of beta-carotene. Nutr Rev 1999;57(9 Pt 1):263–72.

334. Perocco P, Mazzullo M, Broccoli M, Rocchi P, Ferreri AM, Paolini M. Inhibitory activity of vitamin E and alpha-naphthoflavone on beta-carotene-enhanced transformation of BALB/c 3T3 cells by benzo(a)pyrene and cigarette-smoke condensate. Mutat Res 2000;465(1–2):151–8.

335. Parker L, Cole M, Craft AW, Hey EN. Neonatal vitamin K administration and childhood cancer in the north of England: retrospective case-control study. BMJ 1998;316(7126):189–93.

336. McKinney PA, Juszczak E, Findlay E, Smith K. Case-control study of childhood leukaemia and cancer in Scotland: findings for neonatal intramuscular vitamin K. BMJ 1998;316(7126):173–7.

337. Passmore SJ, Draper G, Brownbill P, Kroll M. Case-control studies of relation between childhood cancer and neonatal vitamin K administration. BMJ 1998;316(7126):178–84.

338. Passmore SJ, Draper G, Brownbill P, Kroll M. Ecological studies of relation between hospital policies on neonatal vitamin K administration and subsequent occurrence of childhood cancer. BMJ 1998;316(7126):184–9.

339. Pahor M, Guralnik JM, Ferrucci L, Corti MC, Salive ME, Cerhan JR, Wallace RB, Havlik RJ. Calcium-channel blockade and incidence of cancer in aged populations. Lancet 1996;348(9026):493–7.

340. Jick H, Jick S, Derby LE, Vasilakis C, Myers MW, Meier CR. Calcium-channel blockers and risk of cancer. Lancet 1997;349(9051):525–8.

341. Anonymous. Leukaemia in patients treated with growth hormone. Lancet 1988;1(8595):1159–60.

Adverse immunological effects of drugs other than anticancer drugs and drugs used in immunology

Abacavir

The risk of allergic reactions to abacavir may be as high as 10% (1). However, the incidence is more usually reported to be 3–5% (2,3). Allergic reactions usually occur within the first 28 days of therapy and rarely thereafter. They are characterized by non-specific complaints suggestive of an upper respiratory tract infection, fever, rash, nausea, and vomiting. Resolution of the symptoms occurs within days of withdrawal. Severe and even fatal reactions to readministration have been observed, and it has been suggested that rechallenge is contraindicated in any patients who have had an allergic reaction (4). However, it is safe to rechallenge patients who have stopped treatment because of other types of adverse reaction. Of 1201 patients treated in clinical trials, 219 interrupted abacavir therapy for reasons other than allergy; on reintroduction there were no cases of allergy or anaphylaxis (5).

The susceptibility factors associated with allergic reactions have been sought in an analysis of all protocols conducted by GlaxoSmithKline that involved abacavir exposure for at least 24 weeks with a quality-assured or validated clinical database by 30 June 2000 ($n = 5332$) (6). There were 197 allergic reactions (3.7%). The risks of allergic reactions were lower in black people (OR = 0.59; 95% CI = 0.38, 0.91) than in other ethnic groups, and in patients who had received previous therapy for HIV-1 infection with other antiretroviral agents (OR = 0.58; 95% CI = 0.44, 0.78) compared with those receiving therapy for the first time.

Genetic factors affecting the immune response to abacavir have been sought in patients who had taken abacavir for more than 6 weeks, 18 with hypersensitivity reactions and 167 without (7). HLA-B*5701 was present in 14 of the 18 patients with abacavir hypersensitivity, and in four of the 167 others (OR = 117; 95% CI = 29, 481). The combination of HLA-DR7 and HLA-DQ3 was found in 13 of the 18 and five of the 167 (OR = 73; CI = 20, 268). HLA-B*5701, HLA-DR7, and HLA-DQ3 were present in combination in 13 of the 18 and none of the 167 (OR = 822; CI = 43, 15 675). Other MHC markers also present on the 57.1 ancestral haplotype to which these three markers belong confirmed the presence of haplotype-specific linkage disequilibrium, and mapped potential susceptibility loci to a region bounded by C4A6 and HLA-C. HLA-B*5701, HLA-DR7, and HLA-DQ3 had a positive predictive value for hypersensitivity of 100%, and a negative predictive value of 97%. The authors concluded that susceptibility to abacavir hypersensitivity is carried on the 57.1 ancestral haplotype and that withholding abacavir from those with HLA-B*5701, HLA-DR7, and HLA-DQ3 should reduce the prevalence of hypersensitivity

from 9% to 2.5% without inappropriately denying abacavir to any patient.

In a retrospective case-control study of patients with allergic reactions, HLA-B57 was present in 39 of 84 patients compared with 4 of 113 controls (8). However, there were few women and other ethnic groups in the study, and so these findings relate largely to white men.

In a multicenter trial, 128 children were randomly assigned to zidovudine + lamivudine ($n = 36$), to zidovudine + abacavir ($n = 45$), or to lamivudine + abacavir ($n = 47$) (9). One child had an allergic reaction to abacavir and stopped taking it, as did three with possible reactions.

Abciximab

Human antichimeric antibodies, specific to the murine epitope of Fab antibody fragments, have been observed in patients treated with abciximab. These antibodies are IgG antibodies and have so far not correlated with any adverse effects (10).

Because of its antigenic potential, there are theoretical concerns about the readministration of abciximab, and this has been studied in 1342 patients, who underwent percutaneous coronary interventions and received abciximab at least twice (11). There were no cases of anaphylaxis, and there were only five minor allergic reactions, none of which required termination of the infusion. There was clinically significant bleeding in 31 patients, including one with intracranial hemorrhage. There was thrombocytopenia (platelet count below 100×10^9/l) in 5% and profound thrombocytopenia (platelet count below 20×10^9/l) in 2%. In patients who received abciximab within 1 month of a previous treatment (n = 115), the risks of thrombocytopenia and profound thrombocytopenia were 17 and 12% respectively. Human chimeric antibody titers before readministration did not correlate with adverse outcomes or bleeding, but were associated with thrombocytopenia and profound thrombocytopenia.

An anaphylactic reaction to abciximab has been reported (12).

- An obese 46-year-old woman with prolonged angina pectoris underwent coronary angiography. She had no known drug allergies, but on administration of an iodinated contrast media she developed anaphylactic shock. After successful resuscitation angiography was completed and she was given aspirin, ticlopidine for a month, and metoprolol. Five months later she developed chest pain again, and angiography was repeated after pretreatment with prednisone and diphenhydramine and she was given abciximab. Within 5 minutes she had an anaphylactic reaction, requiring resuscitation.

This case shows that anaphylactic reactions to abciximab can occur even after pretreatment with prednisone and diphenhydramine for a known allergy to iodine.

Acebutolol

Patients taking acebutolol relatively commonly develop antinuclear antibodies (13,14).

Acecainide

The main advantage of acecainide over procainamide is the lower incidence of the lupus-like syndrome. Many fewer patients develop antinuclear antibodies during long-term treatment with acecainide than during long-term treatment with procainamide (15).

There are also reports of remission of lupus-like syndrome without recurrence in patients in whom acecainide has been used as a replacement for procainamide (16,1479,1480). Furthermore, patients in whom procainamide has previously caused a lupus-like syndrome have been reported not to suffer from the syndrome on subsequent long-term treatment with acecainide (16). However, one patient suffered mild arthralgia while taking acecainide, having had a more severe arthropathy while taking procainamide (16).

Aceclofenac

A hypersensitivity reaction characterized by multiple purpuric lesions and reduced renal function has been described in an elderly patient (SEDA-18, 103), and there have been reports of hypersensitivity vasculitis (SEDA-20, 91; SEDA-21, 103).

Acetylcholinesterase inhibitors

Severe urticaria and anaphylaxis associated with pyridostigmine (an unspecified dose) occurred in a 54-year-old woman with myasthenia gravis (17). Urticaria started almost immediately after introduction of the drug but was partially controlled by the antihistamine cetirizine. However, pyridostigmine was stopped after 2 months and the urticaria resolved completely. Rechallenge with oral pyridostigmine led to an anaphylactic reaction that was treated with subcutaneous adrenaline. There were no sequelae.

Acetylcysteine

Hypersensitivity reactions have been reported when acetylcysteine is given intravenously in paracetamol overdose. A generalized erythematous rash can develop, and itching, nausea, vomiting, dizziness, and severe breathlessness with bronchospasm and tachycardia have been reported (SEDA-5, 170). Angioedema with hypotension and bronchospasm have also been described (1478). Wheal responses to high concentrations of acetylcysteine

(20 mg/ml) were significantly greater in those who reacted to the drug. In two patients with a positive reaction the response could be inhibited by prior therapy with an antihistamine. As hypersensitivity reactions have been reported in up to 3% of patients receiving intravenous acetylcysteine for paracetamol overdose, physicians need to be prepared for these reactions (18). A pseudo-allergic reaction on the basis of histamine liberation, rather than an immunological etiology, is suggested as the mechanism (19,20).

Management guidelines for the treatment of anaphylactoid reactions to intravenous acetylcysteine have been developed. Patients who develop only flushing of the skin require no treatment. Urticaria should be treated with diphenhydramine and acetylcysteine infusion can be continued. If angioedema or respiratory distress occur, diphenhydramine should be given and the acetylcysteine infusion stopped; it can be restarted 1 hour after the administration of diphenhydramine if no symptoms are present (SEDA-22, 195).

Acetylsalicylic acid

Aspirin hypersensitivity

Of adult asthmatics 2–20% have aspirin hypersensitivity (1307). The mechanism is related to a deficiency in bronchodilator prostaglandins; prostaglandin inhibition may make arachidonic acid produce more leukotrienes with bronchoconstrictor activity. Oral challenge in asthmatic patients is an effective but potentially dangerous method for establishing the presence of aspirin hypersensitivity (21).

The term "aspirin allergy" is better avoided, in the absence of identification of a definite antigen–antibody reaction. This topic has been reviewed (SEDA-17, 94) (SEDA-18, 90).

Aciclovir

Although allergy to aciclovir is unusual, it can occur; in one case it resulted in a skin rash (22).

- A 38-year-old woman of African descent, with a history of atopy and mild asthma, developed a periumbilical, erythematous, maculopapular rash and generalized pruritus after starting aciclovir. The reaction resolved within a few days after withdrawal, recurred when famciclovir was used, and again resolved when famciclovir was withdrawn. She was successfully stabilized on suppressive therapy after a graded challenge with aciclovir four times a day for 5 days.

Cross-reactivity between aciclovir and famciclovir is unusual. Aciclovir desensitization may be a novel method of treating patients with aciclovir allergy.

Contact sensitization to aciclovir is rare, but frequent application to inflamed skin in relapsing *Herpes simplex* may increase the risk of allergy. Severe contact dermatitis in a teenager has been reported.

- A 16-year-old girl with an 11-year history of frequent cold sores developed an erythematous rash and severe contact dermatitis during oral and topical aciclovir therapy (23). Patch tests showed contact sensitization to aciclovir and to the related compound ganciclovir.
- In a 44-year-old woman who used topical aciclovir for genital herpes, aciclovir contact allergy was associated with a systemic contact allergic reaction with an erythematous vesiculobullous eruption in the labial and perioral skin and a rash on the upper trunk and extremities (24). Patch tests were positive to aciclovir, valaciclovir, and ganciclovir, but not to famciclovir.

Pre-existing vesicular edematous cheilitis (probably due to contact allergy to the protecting lip salve) was aggravated after application of Zovirax cream (25). Patch tests to the lip salve were positive, but in addition there were positive photopatch tests to Zovirax cream, but not to its separate constituents.

Acrylic bone cement

Methylmethacrylate is essentially an immunologically inert implant material, but it induces an inflammatory mononuclear cell migration (26,27). Both cemented and cementless prostheses cause a foreign-body-type host response. A new connective tissue capsule is formed around the artificial joint, which is coarser than normal. The reaction is partly granulomatous, with a tendency to necrosis and loosening of the prosthesis. After an initial necrotic phase of 2–3 weeks repair follows, leading to stabilization within 2 years.

Sensitization can occur in patients, surgeons, and dentists and is occasionally reported (28). As most surgical gloves do not provide a reliable barrier, additional gloves are recommended. Contact dermatitis, dizziness, and nausea and vomiting occur. Ethylene oxide present in acrylic bone cement can cause acute allergic reactions in sensitized patients (29).

Adenosine and adenosine triphosphate (ATP)

- An anaphylactic reaction has been reported in a 75-year-old woman who was given adenosine 12 mg for a supraventricular tachycardia. She developed bronchospasm and profound inspiratory stridor, her arterial blood pressure fell to 50/30 mmHg from an arterial systolic pressure of 70 mmHg, and she recovered with appropriate treatment (30).

Ajmaline and its derivatives

Hypersensitivity to ajmaline is rare, but there has been a report of an immune interstitial nephritis in association with fever (31).

Albumin

Immunological reactions to human serum albumin tend to be non-IgE-mediated anaphylactic reactions (0.011% of cases treated), about a third of which are life-threatening (32). A case in which the mechanism seemed to be IgE-mediated anaphylaxis against native albumin has been reported (33).

A meta-analysis of 193 albumin-treated women versus 185 controls showed a significant reduction of severe OHSS after administration of human albumin; two cases of urticaria and one case of an anaphylactic reaction were reported (34).

Alcuronium

Histamine release and anaphylactoid reactions occur with alcuronium (35–37). The precise incidence is not clear. Erythema is said to occur much less frequently than after D-tubocurarine (38). A retrospective study in Australia (39) showed that 37% of serious anaphylactoid reactions reported there were associated with alcuronium; alcuronium, however, at that time accounted for almost 50% of the total muscle relaxant consumption in Australia, and if this is taken into account the likelihood of a serious reaction is less than with D-tubocurarine, as others have also concluded (40). Clinical features reported range from erythema to severe hypotension and tachycardia (41) and bronchospasm (42,43). In a large prospective surveillance study (SEDA-15, 125; SED-12, 473) involving over 1400 patients given alcuronium (initial dose 0.25 + 0.09 mg/kg), there were adverse reactions in almost 18% of the patients, with moderate hypotension (20–50% fall) in 13%, severe hypotension in 0.8%, and bronchospasm in 0.1%.

Alfentanil

A possible hypersensitivity reaction to alfentanil was reported in an atopic 13-year-old girl who developed life-threatening bronchospasm and confluent urticarial wheals (44).

Alfuzosin

Dermatomyositis has been attributed to alfuzosin.

- A 75-year-old man, who had taken alfuzosin for 1 year, developed muscle pain and weakness over 4 days, accompanied by tenderness and swelling of the deltoid muscles (45). There was erythema, with rash, periungual purpura, and erythematous plaques over the finger joints. Serum CK, LDH, and transaminase activities were raised and ANA was positive. An MRI scan showed findings consistent with inflammation of muscle and a biopsy confirmed the diagnosis of dermatomyositis. Three days after drug withdrawal there was no improvement, so prednisone was started and he recovered within a few days. The temporal relation in this case was weak.

- Dermatomyositis, with typical clinical effects, biochemical tests, electromyography, and muscle biopsy, occurred in a 75-year-old man who had taken alfuzosin for 1 year (46). There was no malignancy and he recovered fully after alfuzosin withdrawal (timing not given).

Allopurinol

Hypersensitivity reactions to allopurinol occur in about 10–15% of patients. Desensitization with both oral and intravenous allopurinol has been successful (SEDA-17, 114). In the allopurinol hypersensitivity syndrome, the skin is most prominently involved (47). Symptoms develop after 2–5 weeks of treatment. Hepatic involvement is present in 40% and renal involvement in 45%; 25% of patients have combined renal and hepatic lesions. The hypersensitivity syndrome has been estimated to occur in 1 in 1000 hospitalized patients. A major complication is an extensive cutaneous staphylococcal infection with septicemia and endocarditis. Gastrointestinal hemorrhage, disseminated intravascular coagulation, adult respiratory distress syndrome, cerebral vasculitis, and peripheral axonal neuropathy have also been described (SEDA-21, 109). Death occurs in 20–30% of patients with severe hypersensitivity syndrome.

One report has presented evidence of a possible association between severe drug-induced erythema multiforme and reactivation of infection with human herpesvirus 6. The reactivation is thought to have contributed in some way to the development of allopurinol hypersensitivity reactions (48).

Allopurinol has been associated, albeit rarely, with pANCA (antineutrophil cytoplasmic antibodies with a peripheral pattern) positivity. A generalized cutaneous vasculitis has been associated with the presence in the serum of pANCA and antimyeloperoxidase antibodies (49). A skin biopsy of a lesion showed leukocytoclastic vasculitis with eosinophilic infiltration. Allopurinol was withdrawn and the symptoms resolved completely. The possible drug causes of ANCA-positive vasculitis with high titers of antimyeloperoxidase antibodies in 30 new patients have been reviewed (50). The findings illustrate that this type of vasculitis is a predominantly drug-induced disorder. Only 12 of the 30 cases were not related to a drug. Allopurinol was implicated in two of the other 18 cases.

Treatment of the allopurinol hypersensitivity syndrome includes drug withdrawal and the administration of systemic corticosteroids (prednisone 40–200 mg/day) for several months. Desensitization strategies allow some patients to resume allopurinol therapy later without any further problem (51–53). The standard desensitization protocol consists of an initial allopurinol dosage of 50 µg/day, increasing every 3 days to a target of 50–100 mg/day. The interval between dosage increases can be extended to 5 days or more in elderly patients with multiple co-morbidity. Using this protocol, desensitization was successful in 25 out of 32 patients (78%); 28 patients completed the desensitization protocol and 21 did so without requiring deviation from the standard dosage schedule and without adverse effects. During the follow-up for 902 patient-months, seven of the 28 patients had recurrent skin eruptions after completing the desensitization protocol and after rechallenge with allopurinol. Desensitization to allopurinol is not recommended for all patients, but it can be useful in selected patients who have had a pruritic maculopapular eruption during treatment with allopurinol and who cannot be treated with other drugs.

Alpha$_1$-antitrypsin

An acute allergic reaction to alpha$_1$-protease inhibitor has been reported (54).

Aluminium

Aluminium has a non-specific immunosuppressive action, which results in a lower incidence of transplant rejection in patients with high aluminium concentrations in the tissues; in the first instance one might consider this a reason for seeking to maintain a particularly high aluminium concentration in transplant patients. However, there are good reasons not to do so. Firstly, should infection occur, this immunosuppressive effect can lead to increased risk and higher mortality; work in dialysis patients has confirmed that an increased aluminium load raises the risk of infections (55). Secondly, after transplantations there already is a high aluminium concentration because of mobilization of aluminium from the storage pool. Aluminium loading before transplantation should therefore be avoided and excessive concentrations countered (56).

Aluminium salts are currently the only widely used adjuvants in human vaccines (57). Developments in the understanding of the structure, composition, and preparation of immunostimulating complexes (ISCOMs) have been reviewed and compared.

Amfebutamone (bupropion)

Two cases of serum sickness-like reactions have been reported in association with amfebutamone when used as an aid to smoking cessation (58,59). Both patients developed localized swellings of the fingers and hands, urticaria, and arthralgia. In both cases treatment with antihistamines and corticosteroids produced rapid relief of symptoms.

In three other patients (two women, one man) a serum sickness-like reaction developed 6–21 days after the start of amfebutamone treatment (60). The symptoms, arthralgia, pruritus, and tongue swelling, abated within 2 weeks of treatment with oral corticosteroids. Serum sickness reactions to drugs are rare, and it will be important to find out whether amfebutamone carries an increased risk of this unusual reaction.

Amiloride

Sweden's National Adverse Reaction Monitoring System called the attention of physicians to a case in which a 73-year-old woman developed anaphylactic shock after taking only a single tablet of Moduretic (hydrochlorothiazi + amiloride) (61). The National System had received three other reports on anaphylactic reactions to this combination, and by 1988 the WHO center in Uppsala had received eight others from other countries. Except for mild skin reactions, hypersensitivity reactions to hydrochlorothiazide alone are highly unusual and not of this type.

Aminoglycoside antibiotics

In a prospective study of the results of skin patch testing in 149 patients who were scheduled for ear surgery, 14% of the patients had a positive skin reaction to one of the aminoglycosides (13% for gentamicin, 13% for neomycin) (62). In 16% of the patients with chronic otitis media and 6.7% of the patients with otosclerosis there was allergy to one of the aminoglycosides commonly found in antibiotic ear-drops. Patients who had previously received more than five courses of antibiotic ear-drops had a greater tendency to develop allergy to the aminoglycosides (35%).

Cross-reactivity between aminoglycoside antibiotics has long been known. Aminoglycoside antibiotics can be categorized in two groups, depending on the aminocyclotol nucleus: streptidine (streptomycin) and deoxystreptamine (neomycin, kanamycin, gentamicin, paromomycin, spectinomycin, and tobramycin). Another antigenic determinant is neosamine, a diamino sugar present in neomycin and, with minor changes, also in paromomycin, kanamycin, tobramycin, amikacin, and isepamicin. Streptomycin shares no common antigenic structures with the other aminoglycoside antibiotics, and cross-sensitivity with streptomycin has not been reported. Acute contact dermatitis was described in a 30-year-old man after rechallenge with gentamicin 80 mg; a patch test was positive for gentamicin, neomycin, and amikacin (63).

Occasional cases of anaphylactic shock have been reported, most of which have been due to streptomycin; other aminoglycosides have rarely been implicated, such as gentamicin (64,65) and neomycin (66).

Aminophenazone

A range of allergic skin reactions, acute anaphylactic shock, acute bronchospasm (in predisposed patients), and cross-sensitivity to aspirin have been attributed to aminophenazone (67).

Aminosalicylates

The causes of ANCA-positive vasculitis with high titers of antimyeloperoxidase antibodies in 30 new patients have been reviewed (68). The findings illustrate that this type of vasculitis is predominantly drug-induced. Only 12 of the 30 cases were not related to a drug. The most frequently implicated drug was hydralazine ($n = 10$); the others were propylthiouracil ($n = 3$), penicillamine ($n = 2$), allopurinol ($n = 2$), and sulfasalazine ($n = 1$).

Treatment with sulfasalazine was associated with lupus-like symptoms and systemic lupus erythematosus-related autoantibody production in 10% of patients with early rheumatoid arthritis; risk factors included a systemic lupus erythematosus-related HLA haplotype, increased serum interleukin-10 concentrations, and a speckled pattern of antinuclear antibodies (69).

Sulfasalazine-induced angioimmunoblastic lymphadenopathy has been reported in a patient with juvenile chronic arthritis (70).

A Kawasaki-like syndrome has been reported in a patient taking sulfasalazine, who later reacted in the same way to mesalazine (SEDA-16, 427).

The possibility of allergic reactions to mesalazine has been suggested, but they may be rather less of a problem than with sulfasalazine.

- Angioedema has been reported in a 23-year-old man with inflammatory bowel disease 48 hours after he was given mesalazine 4 g/day (71).

A lupus-like syndrome has been described on several occasions (SEDA-15, 400) (72).

Amiodarone

Lupus-like syndrome has rarely been attributed to amiodarone.

- A 71-year-old woman, who had been taking amiodarone 200 mg bd for 2 years, developed malaise, intermittent fever, arthralgia, and weight loss (73). She had a malar rash and hypoventilation at both lung bases. Her erythrocyte sedimentation rate was markedly raised (90 mm/hour), there was a mild normochromic normocytic anemia (10 g/dl), a slight lymphopenia, and otherwise normal routine tests. Her rheumatoid factor was raised in a titer of 1:320, and circulating complexes of IgG-C1q were positive. Antinuclear antibody was positive (1:640), but all other antibodies were negative. There was progressive improvement on withdrawal of amiodarone and all the biochemical tests returned to normal.
- A 59-year-old man, who had taken amiodarone 200 mg/day for 2 years, developed fever, pleuritic chest pain, dyspnea at rest, a non-productive cough, malaise, and joint pains (74). He had a verrucous endocarditis and a pleuropericardial effusion. He had raised titers of antinuclear antibodies (1:320) with anti-Ro specificity. Serum complement was normal and there were no circulating immune complexes, no cryoglobulins, and no anti-dsDNA, anti-La, anti-U1 ribonucleoprotein, anti-Sm, anti-Sc1, 70, anti-Jo 1, antihistone, antiphospholipid, anticentromere, anticardiolipin, or anticytoplasmic antibodies. Within 7 days of withdrawal of amiodarone the signs and symptoms started to resolve,

and he recovered fully with the addition of predniso-lone.

Angioedema has been reported in a 70-year-old woman who had taken amiodarone 200 mg/day for 8 years (75). The amiodarone was withdrawn and the symptoms disappeared. Rechallenge produced facial flush and facial angioedema within 20 minutes of a 200 mg dose.

Amphetamines

An anaphylactic reaction after the injection of crushed tablets equivalent to 45 mg of amfetamine occurred in a young woman; in others injected with the same solution and at the same time there were no adverse effects (SED-9, 8). The reaction may have involved amfetamine or excipients. Scleroderma is a potential consequence of various stimulants used for appetite control (76).

Amphotericin

A literature review found no support for the routine use of a test dose of amphotericin before the first therapeutic dose of amphotericin deoxycholate, as is still recommended by the manufacturers (77). The mechanism of common infusion-related adverse effects does not appear to be allergic in nature, and true allergic reactions are rare. Moreover, the absence of a reaction to a test dose does not necessarily indicate that patients will not have a severe infusion-related reaction later in the course of therapy, and the procedure of administering a test dose can lead to a detrimental delay in adequate antifungal therapy. The authors recommended starting therapy with amphotericin deoxycholate at the full therapeutic target dose, with careful bedside monitoring for infusion-related adverse events throughout therapy.

Anaphylaxis is rare with amphotericin (78). It is important to note that a patient may tolerate one formulation and respond with anaphylaxis to another.

- Anaphylaxis after ABCD occurred in a patient who had previously been treated with both amphotericin deoxycholate and ABLC without infusion-related adverse effects (79). During the first infusion of ABCD he developed spontaneously reversible severe back pain and then swelling of his lips, respiratory distress, and left-sided hemiparesis, which resolved after 24 hours. An MRI scan suggested an ischemic event in the right putamen, lending support to the hypothesis that he had had an anaphylactic reaction to ABCD, hypoperfusion, and a subsequent stroke.
- In another patient, serious adverse events (fever, severe rigors, a fall in blood pressure, worsening mental status, increasing creatinine concentration, and leukocytosis) occurred after unrecognized substitution of one amphotericin formulation (ABLC) by another (ABCD) (80).

After discovery of the switch, ABLC therapy was reinstituted and tolerated without incident.

These cases underscore the need to monitor patients closely when infusing the first dose of a different formulation of amphotericin.

Angiotensin-converting enzyme inhibitors

Angioedema

Angioedema is a potentially fatal complication that has been associated with several different ACE inhibitors, with a reported incidence of 0.1–0.5%.

Angioedema due to ACE inhibitors can manifest as recurrent episodes of facial swelling, which resolves on withdrawal, or as acute oropharyngeal edema and airways obstruction, which requires emergency treatment with an antihistamine and corticosteroids. It may be life-threatening (81) and may need tracheostomy (82). It is occasionally fatal (83). An unusual presentation with subglottic stenosis has also been reported (84). A variant form is angioedema of the intestine, which tends to occur within the first 24–48 hours of treatment (85,86).

- Two patients presented with isolated visceral angioedema with episodes of recurrent abdominal symptoms (87). Each had undergone surgical procedures for symptoms that persisted after surgery and were ultimately relieved by withdrawal of their ACE inhibitors.
- Another similar case was diagnosed as angioedema of the small bowel after an abdominal CT scan (88). Angioedema occurred in a 58-year-old woman 3 hours after biopsy of a hypopharyngeal mass under general anesthesia and was accompanied by transient electrocardiographic features of anterior myocardial infarction with severe hypokinesis of the anterior wall regions on echocardiography but no significant change in creatinine kinase activity (89). Only T wave inversion persisted on follow-up. Repeat echocardiography showed significant spontaneous improvement and coronary angiography showed normal coronary arteries. Hypotension and hypoxemia did not seem to occur, and the authors could not therefore speculate on the mechanism of the concomitant cardiac changes.
- Recurrent episodes of tongue swelling have been reported with cilazapril (90) and perindopril (91).
- A 74-year-old man with a permanent latex condom catheter developed penile swelling that was non-pitting and involved the subcutaneous tissue of a normal scrotum, after taking lisinopril 5 mg/day for 6 days (92). Removal of the catheter had no effect. After other possible causes were ruled out, ACE inhibitor-induced angioedema was suspected and lisinopril was withdrawn. Within a few days, the swelling, which had not spread, resolved.

Captopril

Lupus–like syndrome has been reported with captopril (93). The authors believed their patient to be the fifth such published case.

- A 54-year-old Caucasian man presented with a 4-week history of chills, fever, malaise, and generalized arthralgia. Following an aortic valve replacement, he had taken aspirin, coumadin, and captopril 25 mg tds for 1 year. He was febrile (temperature 39.4 °C), normotensive, with diffuse livedo reticularis, and the physical signs of aortic valve disease. Infective endocarditis was ruled out by appropriate investigations. He had a raised erythrocyte sedimentation rate (142 mm/hour) and a positive antinuclear antibody test (FANA 1:2560) with a negative antinative DNA test. Captopril was withdrawn and he was given prednisone for 5 days. His symptoms resolved rapidly and the livedo reticularis cleared within 2 days. The FANA and ESR returned to normal and remained so at follow-up 6 months later.

During early drug development, the occurrence of antinuclear antibodies in 10 of 37 patients taking high doses of captopril was described (94).

Enalapril

Eosinophilic gastroenteritis after enalapril has been described (97). The authors briefly reviewed this rare condition, which is diagnosed on the basis of the presence of gastrointestinal symptoms, eosinophilic infiltration of the gastrointestinal tract, and the absence of parasitic or extra-intestinal disease. It has also been reported after clofazimine and naproxen.

- A 63-year-old hypertensive woman, who had a carcinoma of the distal esophagus resected 19 months earlier, developed chronic diarrhea. *Clostridium difficile* toxin was identified in her stools and the diarrhea resolved after treatment with metronidazole. Enalapril was added to her antihypertensive treatment, and 3 months later the diarrhea recurred. Stool examination was negative and there was no *Clostridium difficile* toxin. Her condition worsened and she lost 5 kg in weight. She had marked eosinophilia (2.4×10^9/l), and a small bowel biopsy showed mild chronic inflammation and edema, partial villous atrophy, and large clusters of eosinophils in the lamina propria with some focal infiltration of the epithelium. She stopped taking enalapril and her diarrhea promptly abated and the eosinophil count fell to 0.5×10^9/l at 3 weeks and 0.1×10^9/l at 2 months.

Angiotensin II receptor antagonists

Because ACE inhibitor-induced anaphylaxis is thought to be related to accumulation of bradykinin, it was assumed that angiotensin II receptor antagonists would not cause this reaction. However, angioedema has been described within 30 minutes of a first dose of losartan 50 mg in a 52-year-old man (95). The author also referred to a single case of losartan-induced angioedema mentioned in the manufacturers' package insert from among 4058 patients

treated with losartan. In an international safety update report based on 200 000 patients there were 13 cases of angioedema (96). Two had also taken an ACE inhibitor and three others had previously developed angioedema when taking ACE inhibitors.

Losartan

Angioedema has been reported with angiotensin II receptor antagonists (98,99).

- An African-American developed swelling of the lips and shortness of breath within 24 hours of starting losartan. However, similar reactions had been noted before, while the patient was taking captopril. It was therefore unclear whether the reaction was related to losartan or was a carry-over reaction to captopril.
- A 45-year-old white man, who had taken losartan, hydrochlorothiazide, allopurinol, and colchicine for 9 months, developed facial urticaria, eyelid swelling, shortness of breath, and upper chest tightness, which resolved quickly with famotidine, methylprednisolone, and adrenaline. He had a recurrence 7 hours later, not having taken another dose of losartan. The patient had no history of allergy and was well after losartan withdrawal.

The late onset and recurrence of symptoms after initial resolution are the unique original features of this case report. Patients with such reactions should be kept under observation after the resolution of initial symptoms.

Anticholinergic drugs

See also individual names
Allergic reactions to local application in the eye can occur, usually in the form of contact dermatitis and conjunctival redness and are more common with hyoscine than with atropine, although contact dermatitis is less likely (100).

Anticoagulant proteins

In two of 370 patients treated with drotrecogin alfa during a phase III trial, antibodies to activated protein C were found, but these were not inhibitory; no cases of neutralizing antibodies have been found (101).

Because activated drotrecogin alfa reduces inflammation, it is theoretically possible that there is an increased risk of infection. However, a phase III trial did not show an increased rate of infection in the drotrecogin alfa-treated patients compared with placebo (102).

Antiepileptic drugs

See also individual names
The anticonvulsant hypersensitivity syndrome is a potentially fatal reaction to arene oxide-producing anticonvulsants, such as phenytoin, carbamazepine, and phenobarbital (103,104). It occurs in 1 : 1000 to 1 : 10 000 exposures and its main manifestations include fever, rash,

and lymphadenopathy, accompanied by multisystem abnormalities. Cross-reactivity among drugs is as high as 70–80%. The reaction may be genetically determined, and siblings of affected patients may be at increased risk. Management includes rapid withdrawal of the offending agent and care of conjunctival and skin lesions; the use of steroids is controversial, as is the value of cyclophosphamide and intravenous immunoglobulin (105). Early identification is essential for proper management, and it has been suggested that Bayesian analysis, especially when coupled with a lymphocyte toxicity assay, can improve the differential diagnosis (SEDA-19, 62).

- Within 5 days of being switched to valproate after developing a rash ascribed to carbamazepine, a 55-year-old man developed anticonvulsant hypersensitivity syndrome (maculopapular rash, fever, hepatitis, and eosinophilia) and ocular manifestations consistent with bilateral anterior uveitis (106).

Although mild conjunctivitis is common in the anticonvulsant hypersensitivity syndrome, uveitis has not been reported before in this context.

Antimony and antimonials

As an industrial and environmental toxin, antimony trioxide can cause disturbances of immune homeostasis. Workers in antimony trioxide manufacture had reduced serum concentrations of cytokines (interleukin 2, gamma interferon) and immunoglobulin (IgG1, IgE) (107).

Antituberculosis drugs

See also individual names
In allergic reactions, the drug most probably responsible can be difficult to identify, since the same kind of reaction can occur independently of the chemical nature of the drug. For evaluation of allergic drug reactions, the analysis of time relations (duration of exposure, reaction time, drug-free interval before re-exposure) is extremely important. Particularly in allergic reactions to rifampicin, intermittent treatment or re-exposure after a drug free-interval favors sensitization and occurrence. Depending on the severity of the adverse effects, one, two, or all drugs must be stopped until the adverse reaction has completely disappeared. The use of second-line antituberculosis drugs may sometimes be necessary. In patients with drug fever or common rashes, specific desensitization may be attempted, at least with isoniazid (108). In more severe reactions, with anaphylactic shock, agranulocytosis, thrombocytopenia, toxic epidermal necrolysis, or Stevens–Johnson syndrome, specific desensitization should not be considered and the drug should be discarded from the combination.

Aprotinin

As might be expected with a bovine protein, allergic reactions can occur, and repeated exposure can even result in anaphylactic reactions. In view of this, some have advocated a strategy of using aprotinin only if excessive bleeding is a problem after surgery (109).

- An aphylactic reaction has been described after the use of fibrin glue as a sealant after mastectomy, probably due to the presence of bovine aprotinin (110).

In one study of 248 patients undergoing cardiac surgery, seven had allergic reactions, ranging from skin flushing to severe circulatory depression (111). Most of the reactions occurred when aprotinin was given a second time within 6 months after the first exposure. However, anaphylaxis has been documented after primary exposure (112). The reported incidence of anaphylactic reactions in other studies has ranged from 0.3 to 0.6% after a single exposure, rising to almost 5% with prior aprotinin exposure (113).

Up to 1980, 32 cases of non-fatal shock attributed to aprotinin had been reported to the Japanese Ministry of Health and Welfare, most concerning patients treated for pancreatitis (114). Although these patients survived, fatal anaphylaxis has been reported (115). Other apparently allergic reactions reported include erythema, urticaria, bronchospasm, nausea and vomiting, diarrhea, muscle pains, and blood pressure changes (116). A case of allergic pancreatitis attributed to aprotinin has also been reported (117).

There is evidence that severe allergic reactions to aprotinin are mediated by IgE, and preoperative screening for the presence of aprotinin-specific IgE antibodies can be of value in identifying patients at risk (118,119).

The sera of 150 patients who had undergone cardiac surgery and were receiving aprotinin for the first time have been studied before and after the operation. At 3.5 months after surgery, the prevalence of aprotinin-specific IgG antibodies was 33% (15/45) after local, 28% (13/46) after intravenous, and 69% (41/59) after combined exposure (120). The authors concluded that local administration of aprotinin induces a specific immune response and reinforces that of intravenous exposure; they therefore recommended that any exposure in a patient should be documented.

Allergic reactions, including anaphylaxis, can occur on re-exposure to aprotinin. The incidence rates of aprotinin-related reactions are 2.7% in re-exposed adults (5/183) and 1.2% in children (3/354), with an overall incidence of 1.8% (8/437). The following advice has been given to reduce the risk and severity of these reactions (113,121):

- give a test dose of aprotinin
- delay the first bolus injection until the surgeon starts the procedure
- give an antihistamine before re-exposure
- avoid re-exposure within the first 6 months after the last exposure.

Infection risk

Inevitably, concern has recently been expressed about the possibility of transmission of the prion believed to be responsible for bovine spongiform encephalopathy (BSE) and new variant Creutzfeldt-Jakob disease. However, the manufacturers of aprotinin have stated that the bovine lungs used as the source of aprotinin are collected in countries in South America (principally

Uruguay) in which no cases of transmissible spongiform encephalopathy have been recorded. There is no evidence that any patient with new variant Creutzfeldt-Jakob disease has received aprotinin. Furthermore, in vitro experiments involving spiking of material with mouse-associated scrapie agent have demonstrated an 18-log reduction of the added prions during the manufacturing process (122).

Apiaceae

An anaphylactic reaction has been described in a patient who was sensitized to coriander (123).

Artificial sweeteners

The role of aspartame in hypersensitivity reactions is controversial, although there have been case reports (124). In a multicenter, randomized, double-blind, placebo-controlled, crossover study, aspartame was more likely than placebo to cause urticaria or angioedema (125).

Aspartame can cause granulomatous septal panniculitis (126).

Lobular panniculitis has been described in a 57-year-old diabetic man who ingested large amounts of aspartame as a sweetener, in soft drinks and other products. He stopped taking aspartame and the tender subcutaneous nodules disappeared (127).

Ascorbic acid (vitamin C)

Ascorbic acid can sometimes cause immune reactions. Ascorbic acid and citric acid are used as food additives, ascorbic acid (E300) as an acidifier, an antioxidant, and an additive in wheat, and citric acid as an acidifying complex-binding agent. Because additives are widely used in foods, beverages, and drugs, people with allergies or intolerance have to be carefully instructed. Caution must also be taken when scratch tests are performed with these substances (128).

- A 62-year-old man had frequent angioedema, and a scratch test was performed with several food additives. Scratching with 1% ascorbic acid and 1% citric acid in vaseline resulted in a +3 reaction, and 20 minutes later he developed angioedema with swelling of the glottis, reddening of the face and hands, itching, vertigo, tachycardia, and hypotension. He was given a glucocorticoid and an antihistamine and recovered within half an hour.

Asteraceae

Intravenous administration of Echinacea has been associated with severe allergic reactions. Oral ingestion can cause allergic skin and respiratory responses (129).

Five cases of adverse drug reactions have been attributed to oral Echinacea extracts (130). Two of the patients

had anaphylaxis and one had an acute attack of asthma. The authors also tested 100 atopic subjects and found that 20 of them, who had never before taken Echinacea, had positive reactions to skin prick tests.

An anaphylactic reaction to Echinacea angustifolia has been reported (131).

- A 37-year-old woman who took various food supplements on an irregular basis self-medicated with 5 ml of an extract of E. angustifolia. She had immediate burning of the mouth and throat followed by tightness of the chest, generalized urticaria, and diarrhea. She made a full recovery within 2 hours.

The basis for this anaphylactic reaction was hypersensitivity to Echinacea, confirmed by skin prick and RAST testing. However, others have challenged the notion of a causal relation in this case (132). Nevertheless, the author affirmed his belief that Echinacea was the causal agent and reported that at that time Echinacea accounted for 22 of 266 suspected adverse reactions to complementary medicines reported to the Australian Adverse Drug Reaction Advisory Committee (133).

Sjögren's syndrome has been attributed to Echinacea (134).

Anaphylactic shock has been reported after the use of a herbal tea containing an extract of the fruit of the milk thistle (135).

Atorvastatin

See HMG coenzyme–A reductase inhibitors

Atracurium dibesilate

There have been reports of angioedema (136) and bronchospasm (137,138), attributed to histamine release. A large prospective surveillance study involving more than 1800 patients given atracurium showed a 10% incidence of adverse reactions, with bronchospasm in 0.2% of patients (139).

Extreme sensitivity to an intradermal skin test (0.003 mg), some 24 hours after a severe skin reaction to the intravenous administration of atracurium, has been described (140).

Severe systemic reactions after atracurium administration may be due to antibody-mediated anaphylaxis (1470) rather than non-specific histamine liberation. It has been suggested that systemic effects from non-specific histamine release are dose-dependent.

Atropine

Hypersensitivity to atropine is most usually seen in the form of contact dermatitis and conjunctivitis. One case of anaphylactic shock after intravenous injection of atropine has been reported (SEDA-14, 122).

Azapropazone

Patients with aspirin intolerance often also react to many other NSAIDs. Azapropazone seems to be a safe alternative in these patients, according a study that showed good tolerance of the drug in patients with aspirin intolerance (141).

Azithromycin

Occupational allergic contact dermatitis has been attributed to azithromycin (142).

- A 32-year-old pharmaceutical worker had been loading reactors at three different stages of azithromycin synthesis for the past 3 years and had been exposed to airborne powders. He wore overalls and latex gloves. His symptoms had persisted for 1 year in the form of pruritus, erythema, vesicles, and scaling of the face and forearms. A positive patch test and a positive workplace challenge were considered reliable in the diagnosis of occupational allergic contact dermatitis induced by azithromycin. After transfer to another work station that excluded exposure to azithromycin, he had no further work-related symptoms.

Hypersensitivity to azithromycin has been reported (143).

- A 79-year-old man developed fever, mental changes, a rash, acute renal insufficiency, and hepatitis after he had completed a 5-day course of oral azithromycin (500 mg initially then 250 mg/day). With intravenous hydration only, his fever abated and his urinary output and renal and hepatic function returned to normal over the next 4 days. His mental status improved significantly. The skin rash was followed by extensive desquamation.

Azithromycin has been associated with Churg–Strauss syndrome in a patient with atopy (144).

Bacille Calmette–Guérin (BCG) vaccine

The incidence of adverse effects after BCG immunization has been extensively investigated by the Committee on Prophylaxis of the International Union Against Tuberculosis and Lung Disease (IUATLD). Retrospective studies including 51 countries worldwide and collecting data from 1948–74, according to organ and system category, have been published (SED-12, 795) (145,146). The IUATLD carried out a second (prospective) 6-country study (1979–83) (147), using the classification system already used in the retrospective study. The mean risk of local complications and suppurative lymphadenitis was low: 0.387 per 1000 vaccinees or 0.093 per 1000 with positive bacteriological/histological findings, respectively. There were 21 cases of disseminated BCG infections and allergic manifestations recorded in four countries. The estimated risks of serious disseminated BCG infection were higher than calculated previously (except for bone and joint lesions), but very low when comparing the benefit and risks of BCG immunization, especially in infants (147).

Anaphylactic reactions

Allergy to BCG exceptionally occurs when intravesical BCG is used as an immunoenhancing agent. An anaphylactic reaction has been reported (148).

Three cases of anaphylactic reactions to BCG have been described in young children, one (in a 3-month-old girl) being fatal (149).

An acute shock-like syndrome developed 30 minutes after BCG immunization of a newborn girl.

Non-IgE-mediated anaphylactic (anaphylactoid) reactions suspected to be caused by dextran as used in BCG vaccines have been described (SEDA-16, 375).

Bacitracin

Bacitracin is one of the most important clinical allergens (150). Anaphylaxis rarely occurs after topical administration of bacitracin ointment (151,152).

- A 45-year-old man developed a near-fatal anaphylactic reaction after he applied bacitracin ointment to an excoriated area on his foot. He had had a similar, but less severe, episode 4 years earlier. IgE antibodies to bacitracin were positive.
- A 24-year-old man injured in a motorcycle accident was treated with viscous lidocaine and bacitracin zinc ointment for extensive abrasions on the extremities. Five minutes later, he developed symptoms of severe anaphylaxis and required adrenaline, antihistamines, intravenous fluids, and glucocorticoids. Two weeks later, only the prick test to bacitracin zinc ointment was positive.

Anaphylaxis has also been reported after bacitracin nasal packing (153).

- A 48-year-old man underwent uneventful septorhinoplasty, after which his right nostril was packed with 6 ft of vaseline gauze placed in the finger of a latex glove coated with bacitracin ointment. Within seconds, his oxygen saturation fell from 97 to 94% (and increased to 97% with 100% oxygen), but blood pressure and heart rate were unchanged. After the left nostril had been packed, his oxygen saturation fell to 89%, no pulse wave was registered and an electrocardiogram showed a heart rate of 39/minute with first-degree atrioventricular block, and the blood pressure was not obtainable by non-invasive measurement. Cardiopulmonary resuscitation was successful, but the patient remained intubated for 2 days because of concerns about facial and upper airway edema. Later he gave a history of an episode of irritation and swelling after nasal application of polymyxin B and bacitracin ointment 2–3 weeks before surgery. Skin prick testing was positive for bacitracin but negative for latex, polymyxin, cefazolin, and saline.

Cases of anaphylaxis have also been reported after bacitracin irrigation (154,155).

- A 65-year-old man undergoing elective sternal debridement and rewiring was given a prophylactic infusion of vancomycin 1 g preoperatively. Anesthesia was induced with thiopental, suxamethonium, and fentanyl, and maintained with fentanyl, vecuronium, and isoflurane. A few minutes after wound irrigation with bacitracin (about 25 U/ml), his blood pressure fell precipitously, necessitating intravenous fluids and adrenaline. His face and arms were flushed. Afterwards, he reported having had a rash several years before after the use of an over-the-counter ointment composed of polymyxin B, bacitracin, and neomycin.
- A 9-year-old child with a repaired myelomeningocele and congenital hydrocephalus who had undergone four previous shunt revisions in the past had two episodes of anaphylaxis during insertion of the ventriculoperitoneal shunt. The shunt tubing had been soaked in a solution of bacitracin 2500 U/ml. A skin prick test was positive for bacitracin.

Thiomersal, a mercury derivative of thiosalicylic acid, is a preservative used in several types of consumer products, including cosmetics, ophthalmic and otolaryngological medications, and vaccines. In a retrospective study in 574 patients, people who were allergic to thiomersal were more likely to be allergic to bacitracin (156).

Barium sulfate

Hypersensitivity reactions to products used during barium meal examinations are extremely rare. Barium sulfate is generally regarded as an inert and insoluble compound that is neither absorbed nor metabolized and is eliminated unchanged from the body. However, some studies have shown that very small amounts of barium sulfate can be absorbed from the gastrointestinal tract. Plasma and urine barium concentrations can be increased after oral barium sulfate. In addition, there are many additives in commercially prepared barium products, some of which can cause immune responses. A patient with a history of a severe reaction to barium agents should not receive barium products again (SEDA-22, 503).

Reactions to other constituents of barium sulfate enemas have been recognized (SEDA-18, 441) and could be as common as one in 1000. They vary from urticarial rashes to severe anaphylactic reactions, and can be particularly severe in patients with asthma (157). Hypersensitivity to the latex balloon catheter used in double contrast barium enemas appears to be a common mechanism (158), but hypersensitivity to glucagon, to the preservative methylparabens, or to other additives seems to be responsible in some cases. Insofar as the latex balloon is concerned, thorough washing will remove the allergen responsible for the reaction (159).

Infection risk

Transient bacteremia was recorded in 11.4% of a series of 175 patients who had undergone barium enema examination; it appeared almost at once and lasted up to 15 minutes (160). Although a second study elsewhere failed to confirm these findings, a subsequent fatal case of staphylococcal septicemia in an elderly patient with an immune deficiency suggests that the risks are not merely theoretical (161).

Benzalkonium chloride

Life-threatening anaphylactic reactions that rarely occur during general anesthesia are mostly due to neuromuscular blockers. They may be due to cross-allergy mediated by drug-specific IgE antibodies to the quaternary ammonium moiety of the neuromuscular blocker molecule, perhaps with a contribution from IgE-independent mechanisms. Quaternary ammonium compounds, such as benzalkonium, in cosmetics and toiletries may play a role in sensitization (162).

Allergic reactions can occur after topical use, but are fairly rare. Allergic contact dermatitis has been reported in some cases. Allergic rhinitis on contact has also been reported.

In a study of the efficacy and acceptability of benzalkonium chloride-containing contraceptives (vaginal sponges, pessaries, and creams) in 56 women, one developed an allergic reaction with edema of the vulva (163). Non-allergic local irritation, itching, and a burning sensation were reported in nine women and nine husbands.

Benzocaine

Benzocaine can cause sensitization, and being a para-aminobenzoic acid derivative it can cross-react with para-phenylenediamine, sulfonamides, aniline dyes, and related local anesthetics. However, in a recent retrospective study of 5464 patients it was concluded that benzocaine allergy is not common in the UK, confirming earlier reports that benzocaine should not be used as a single screening agent for local anesthetic allergy (164).

Allergic contact dermatitis has been attributed to local benzocaine (165).

- A 72-year-old woman was treated for thoracic *Herpes zoster* with oral aciclovir and topical benzocaine 20% ointment. She subsequently developed painful pruritic erythematous dermatitis in the area of the lesions, spreading to her arm. The dermatitis was initially misdiagnosed as aciclovir resistance, but on patch testing she had a positive reaction to benzocaine.

The authors highlighted the problem in diagnosing allergic contact dermatitis in patients who have other skin lesions in that area. They emphasized the importance of patch testing to identify the causative agent.

Benzoxonium chloride

Contact allergic reactions have been rarely reported with benzoxonium, with potential cross-reactivity with benzalkonium chloride and domiphen bromide (166,167).

- A 37-year-old woman developed intense burning and pruritic eczema where she had applied a cream containing benzoxonium for seborrheic dermatitis for 5 months (168). The reaction disappeared on withdrawal of the cream. Patch tests were positive to benzoxonium chloride 0.1% aqueous on days 2 and 4. Patch tests with benzalkonium chloride and benzoxonium chloride in 20 controls were negative.

Benzyl alcohol

Various allergic reactions have been attributed to benzyl alcohol.

- A 55-year-old man developed fatigue, nausea, and diffuse angioedema shortly after an intramuscular injection of vitamin B12 containing benzyl alcohol (169).
- In another male patient, fever developed, and a maculopapular rash occurred on his chest and arms after an injection of cytarabine, vincristine, and heparin in a dilution solution containing benzyl alcohol (170).

Beta$_2$-adrenoceptor agonists

The possibility of a causal relation between the administration of beta$_2$-adrenoceptor agonists and reduced serum immunoglobulin concentrations has been raised in various studies. In one study, adults with asthma taking steroids were compared with patients taking beta$_2$-adrenoceptor agonists (171). The patients who were using beta$_2$-adrenoceptor agonists had significantly lower serum IgG concentrations, irrespective of any history of steroid use. However, in patients using both treatments this depressive effect was even more pronounced; its mechanism is unclear.

Beta$_2$-adrenoceptor agonists and the response to allergens

Following inhalation of an allergen by a sensitized asthmatic, an immediate or type I response is seen. This occurs rapidly and is characterized by dyspnea, wheeze, and a fall in the FEV$_1$ or peak expiratory flow. The response can be prevented or reversed by inhalation of a beta$_2$-agonist. Several hours later, however, a proportion of asthmatics develop a delayed or type III response. This response is prolonged and associated with inflammatory changes in the airways. For some time after it resolves there is an increase in non-specific reactivity of the airways. This can be quantified by measuring the PC$_{20}$ of histamine or methacholine. This is the provocative concentration necessary to cause a 20% fall in the FEV$_1$ or peak expiratory flow. The delayed response is not prevented by prior inhalation of a beta$_2$-agonist. It can be prevented by prior treatment with cromoglicate or a corticosteroid.

Treatment with a beta$_2$-agonist aerosol, before allergen inhalation, allows inhalation of significantly greater amounts of allergen before the type I response occurs. In asthmatics who only have a type I response before treatment with a beta$_2$-agonist, a late response to the increased allergen dose results. In asthmatics who already have a type III response, this response is increased (172). Treatment with an oral beta$_2$-agonist for 2 weeks increases sensitivity to inhaled allergen. In addition, reversal of allergen-induced bronchoconstriction by an inhaled beta$_2$-agonist is significantly impaired (173). Treatment for 1 week with an inhaled beta$_2$-agonist increases the late (type III) asthmatic response to the same dose of inhaled allergen. The increase in airway reactivity to methacholine following the late response is also increased (174). Sufficient inhaled beta$_2$-agonist needs to be taken to produce this effect. The effect is seen with salbutamol 0.8 mg/day, but not with 0.2 or 0.4 mg/day (175). Pretreatment with an inhaled beta$_2$-agonist not only increases the response to allergen but also attenuates the protective effect of a beta$_2$-agonist against both allergen and methacholine, that is both specific and non-specific airway reactivity is increased (176).

Clearly, the combined use of a regular inhaled beta$_2$-agonist and allergen exposure can cause more airway inflammation than allergen exposure alone. It has been suggested that regular use of beta$_2$-agonists may induce dysfunction of beta-receptors on the mast cells making the mast cells more prone to release mediator (177). Regular treatment with beta$_2$-agonists alone will result in greater airway inflammation and persistent asthma. This emphasizes the importance of regular prophylactic medication with cromoglicate or inhaled corticosteroids.

Beta-adrenoceptor antagonists

Leukocytoclastic vasculitis has been reported with sotalol (178).

- A progressive cutaneous vasculitis occurred in a 66-year-old man taking sotalol for prevention of a symptomatic atrial fibrillation. After 7 days he noted a petechial eruption on his wrists and ankles. This progressed during the next days to palpable purpura on the hands, wrists, ankles, and feet. A biopsy specimen showed changes consistent with leukocytoclastic vasculitis. After withdrawal of sotalol the skin rash cleared completely without any other intervention.

Other beta-blockers associated with leukocytoclastic vasculitis include acebutolol, alprenolol, practolol, and propranolol.

Antinuclear antibodies in high titers were detected in a number of patients with the practolol oculomucocutaneous syndrome. Tests in patients taking acebutolol (179,180) and celiprolol (181) have also shown a high frequency of antinuclear antibodies. Positive lupus erythematosus cell preparations have been observed in patients taking acebutolol (180).

The lupus-like syndrome was part of the practolol syndrome and has also been attributed to acebutolol

(182,183), atenolol (SEDA-16, 194), labetalol (184), pindolol (185), and propranolol (186). However, apart from practolol, it seems to be very rare during treatment with beta-adrenoceptor antagonists.

Anaphylactic reactions have been attributed to beta-adrenoceptor antagonists only very infrequently (187). However, it appears that anaphylactic reactions precipitated by other agents can be particularly severe in patients taking beta-blockers, especially non-selective drugs, and may require higher-than-usual doses of adrenaline for treatment (188–191,191). The view that allergy skin testing or immunotherapy is inadvisable in patients taking beta-blockers (192) has been disputed, bearing in mind the low incidence of this adverse effect (193).

Labetalol

Antinuclear and antimitochondrial antibodies develop not uncommonly during long-term administration of labetalol (194).

Propranolol

Propranolol has been implicated in hypersensitivity pneumonitis (195,196), although other beta-blockers have also been associated with this complication.

Beta-lactam antibiotics

See also Cephalosporins, Penicillins

The adverse effects of early penicillin use consisted almost exclusively of anaphylaxis. This stimulated extensive research into the immune responses associated with penicillin and made penicillin the most prominent model for immune reactions to drugs.

The pathogenesis of many presumably immunologically mediated reactions to beta-lactam antibiotics is still unknown. Reliable and standardized tests to predict hypersensitivity only exist for a minority of allergic reactions, that is, IgE-mediated reactions. The matter is further complicated by the fact that beta-lactams can readily induce immune responses that by themselves do not necessarily result in disease. This is the case, for example, when anti-erythrocyte antibodies directed against beta-lactam bound to the erythrocyte surface are formed. This biological property (immunogenicity) has to be distinguished from allergenicity, that is, immune responses causing disease.

Cross-reactivity, that is, hypersensitivity reactions initially induced by one compound but triggered by another, is an important and as yet unresolved problem, complicated by the fact that beta-lactams undergo structural modifications after administration, and that different parts of the molecule (such as the nucleus or side chains) can be involved. Data from cross-exposed patients (skin tests or drug challenge) suggest a high degree of cross-reactivity between compounds belonging to the same class and between the penicillins and carbapenems, but a low degree of cross-reactivity between penicillins and cephalosporins and between monobactams and the other beta-lactams.

Mechanisms

Drug allergy or hypersensitivity represents an acquired capacity of the organism to mount an immunologically mediated reaction to a compound. This ultimately involves covalent or exceptionally non-covalent binding to and modification of host molecules (presumably proteins) by the drug, to which the host becomes sensitized (induction phase). Re-exposure to the sensitizing drug can trigger a series of immunological effector mechanisms (effector phase). These can be defined as pathways of inflammation or tissue injury, but they also represent mechanisms of immune protection from infectious agents.

Traditionally, the classification scheme defined by Gell and Coombs (197) distinguishes four types of reactions:

- type I reactions, which are IgE-mediated immediate hypersensitivity reactions.
- type II reactions, which are mediated by cytotoxic IgM and/or IgG.
- type III reactions, which are mediated by immune complexes.
- type IV reactions, which are cell-mediated hypersensitivity responses.

However, this classification fails to account for the complex and sequential involvement of several cell types and mediators in the immune response, as recognized today (198).

IgE-antibody-mediated adverse reactions

IgE-antibody-mediated hypersensitivity can serve as a paradigm to demonstrate some important features of beta-lactam hypersensitivity. Beta-lactams are small molecules that have to combine with a host macromolecule to be recognized by the immune system. In the case of penicillin, this reaction involves coupling of reactive degradation products to a protein-containing carrier (199). There are several degradation pathways, which result in the formation of reactive compounds, most importantly penicilloyl (200), also called the major determinant. Other less abundant degradation products include penilloate, benzylpenicilloate, and benzylpenilloate, the so-called minor determinants.

The complex contains haptens, often multiple, coupled to a protein-containing carrier molecule, and can induce T cell-dependent B cell activation, leading to the formation of antihapten antibodies. The mechanisms that govern the selection of the different immunoglobulin isotypes are reviewed elsewhere (198).

The time required for sensitization is called "latency" and is variable, depending on factors such as route of exposure, hapten dose, and chemical reactivity of the drug, as well as on genetic and acquired host factors. The period between the last exposure to the drug and the first appearance of symptoms has been termed the "reaction time." It is part of the clinical description of an adverse event and may help to attribute it to a specific drug (SED-12, 594).

Once sensitivity has been established, that is, once hapten-specific IgE-producing B cells have been formed, exposure to even small amounts of hapten can induce a cascade of events that lead to immediate reactions, such as anaphylaxis (201). Briefly, preformed IgE antibodies to drug determinants recognize the hapten-carrier complex and fix to the surface of mast cells or basophils, triggering the release of a series of mediators, such as histamine, neutral proteases, biologically active arachidonic acid products, and cytokines. This ultimately leads to a clinical spectrum that ranges from a mild local reaction to anaphylactic shock.

For more details see Meyler's Side Effects of Antimicrobial Drugs.

Beta-lactamase inhibitors

Clavulanic acid has a very low immunogenic and allergenic potential in animals. The possible impact of its co-administration with other beta-lactam antibiotics is unknown (202). Two patients with IgE-mediated hypersensitivity to oral co-amoxiclav and positive skin tests for clavulanic acid, but not for penicillins, both tolerated oral amoxicillin. One patient was also challenged with clavulanic acid and developed urticaria, conjunctivitis, and bronchial obstruction (203). Since co-amoxiclav has been widely used since its introduction in 1981, the frequency of hypersensitivity reactions is low. The clinical data available on sulbactam and tazobactam are still limited and do not allow an assessment of the frequency and pattern of associated hypersensitivity reactions (204).

Biguanides

Leukocytoclastic vasculitis and pneumonitis have been attributed to metformin (205,206).

Bismuth

Sensitization to bismuth derivatives has been reported but is rare.

- A 33-year-old woman with atopic hand eczema and allergic rhinitis was given Noviform, an eye ointment containing bibrocathol (bismuth oxide and tetrabromocathechol), for periorbital dermatitis and noticed an exacerbation of her dermatitis (207). A patch test was positive for bismuth oxide. Anaphylaxis to bismuth subsalicylate (Pepto-Bismol) has been observed (208).
- A 25-year-old man with symptoms of acute gastroenteritis took Pepto-Bismol, a total of eight caplets over 6 hours. About 30 minutes after the last dose, he developed generalized acute urticaria. He had previously tolerated Pepto-Bismol well, but had presumably become sensitized. He was successfully treated with intravenous fluids and histamine H_1 receptor antagonists.

Blood cell transfusion and bone marrow transplantation

Sensitization to HLA antigens

Sensitization to HLA antigens (209) is undesirable in patients awaiting organ transplantation and in patients who need long-term platelet transfusion. The success of protocols based on the use of leukocyte-depleted and frozen erythrocytes may be limited, since HLA antigens may be expressed on erythrocytes. In one study the erythrocytes of 50% of blood donors contained HLA-A, HLA-B, and HLA-C antibodies (but not antibodies to class II antigens or to leukocyte-specific antigens) (686). Neither storage at 4 °C for 21 days nor cryopreservation affected the expression of these antigens. The immunogenicity of HLA antigens on red cells is unknown.

Blood donation

Although no important adverse effects are associated specifically with multiple blood donations, depressed cell-mediated immunity and reduced lymphocyte proliferation responses have been reported in the past (210). This fear has been allayed, for example, by a 1992 study in 27 donors who had regularly given whole blood for at least 4 years; there were no abnormalities in lymphocyte subsets, neutrophil and monocyte receptors, or molecules important for host defences (211). In 25 volunteer donors undergoing regular platelet apheresis by a discontinuous process a large number of T4 and T8 lymphocytes, a moderate number of B lymphocytes, and a smaller number of monocytes were removed (212).

Frequent donations involving apheresis procedures have been reported to cause allergic reactions (urticaria, flushing, wheezing, chest pain, and in a few cases hypotension), probably due to exposure to ethylene oxide (213). Ethylene oxide is often used for sterilizing the polyvinyl chloride tubing, and similar allergic reactions in patients undergoing chronic hemodialysis have been attributed to sensitization to the ethylene oxide used for sterilizing the dialyser. One study has shown significant concentrations of IgE antibodies to ethylene dioxide in the sera of 78% of donors with allergic reactions but in only 12% of control sera.

Bromocriptine

- An allergic reaction was attributed to bromocriptine in a 26-year-old woman with a prolactin-secreting microadenoma (214).

Buflomedil

An anaphylactic reaction to buflomedil has been reported (215).

- A 53-year-old woman with Raynaud's phenomenon developed an urticarial rash, pruritus, and hypotension 10 minutes after the parenteral administration of buflomedil. She received corticosteroids and recovered within 6 hours. When she later underwent skin tests with buflomedil, there was an immediate positive reaction, suggesting a type I hypersensitivity mechanism.

Bupivacaine

A non-IgE-mediated allergic reaction to bupivacaine has been reported (SEDA-21, 136).

- A 69-year-old woman with a history of bronchospasm after NSAID administration had heavy feelings in her arms and itchy eyes, without any change in hemodynamics, 30 minutes after an intradermal injection of bupivacaine. The same symptoms occurred during subsequent retesting 1 month later, with the addition of coughing and sneezing.

Buprenorphine

There have been reports of anaphylactic reactions with buprenorphine (216).

Bupropion

See Amfebutamone

C1 esterase inhibitor concentrate

Allergic reactions to C1 esterase inhibitor concentrate have been observed, including possible exacerbation of angioedema (217).

Infection risk

The use of C1 esterase inhibitor concentrate has been associated with transmission of hepatitis C, but this can be prevented by heat treatment (218).

Calcipotriol

Contact allergic reactions to calcipotriol are rare. In one case patch tests with Psorcutan Salbe and calcipotriol (its active ingredient) were both positive (219).

Calcitonin

Calcitonin allergy is very rare.

- A 60-year-old woman tolerated daily intranasal calcitonin for 6 months of the year for 4 years (220). She developed nasal watering, nasal and ocular pruritus, and sweating immediately after the administration of nasal calcitonin when she restarted after a 6-month break. These symptoms recurred 2 years later, with abdominal pain and hypotension, after 10 months of intramuscular calcitonin, and were again reproduced by a lower dose intramuscularly.
- A 65-year-old woman, who had previously tolerated calcitonin nasal spray, developed eye and nose congestion, an itchy nose, and sneezing minutes after using

intranasal salmon calcitonin (221). She was later given intramuscular salmon calcitonin and developed generalized urticaria and nasal itching within minutes. Skin testing was positive with eel and salmon calcitonins but not human calcitonin, and she was treated with human calcitonin without adverse effects.

Calcium channel blockers

Verapamil, nifedipine, and diltiazem have all been associated with allergic reactions, including skin eruptions and effects on liver and kidney function. Nifedipine has also been reported to cause a febrile reaction (222), and diltiazem was associated with fever, lymphadenopathy, hepatosplenomegaly, an erythematous maculopapular rash, and eosinophilia in a 50-year-old man (223).

Nifedipine

Anaphylaxis has been attributed to sublingual nifedipine (224).

- A 71-year-old man with prostatic adenocarcinoma and a pathological vertebral fracture received sublingual nifedipine for hypertension and 15 minutes later became stuporose and complained of pruritus, generalized erythema, dizziness, and nausea. His blood pressure had fallen to 60/40 mmHg, his pulse rate was 120/minute, and his respiratory rate was 30/minute. He had cyanosis and severe bronchospasm with no focal neurological abnormalities. After treatment with subcutaneous adrenaline, intravenous fluids, hydrocortisone, and aminophylline, his blood pressure increased to 125/70 mmHg. During the following days his neurological and pulmonary status rapidly improved.

Cannabinoids

Tetrahydrocannabinol depresses lymphocyte and macrophage activity in cell cultures, while in rats in vivo it directly suppresses natural killer cell activity and impairs T lymphocyte transformation by phytohemagglutinin in concentrations of cannabinoids achievable with the usual doses (225). Variable results have been obtained in man in tests of circulating T cells and hormonal immunity (226).

In animals and man, chronic use often suppresses the immune system's response to inhaled bacterial or fungal material. In this connection it is relevant to note that a contaminant mould (*Aspergillus*) found in cannabis can predispose immunocompromised cannabis smokers to infection. It has been suggested that baking the cannabis (at 300 °F for 15 minutes) before smoking will kill the fungus and reduce the potential risk (227).

The effects of marijuana on immune function have been reviewed (228). The studies suggest that marijuana affects immune cell function of T and B lymphocytes, natural killer cells, and macrophages. In addition, cannabis appears to modulate host resistance, especially the secondary immune response to various infectious agents, both viral and bacterial. Lastly, marijuana may also affect the cytokine network, influencing the production and function of acute-phase and immune cytokines and modulating network cells, such as macrophages and T helper cells. Under some conditions, marijuana may be immunomodulatory and promote disease.

A severe allergic reaction after intravenous marijuana has been reported (229).

- A 25-year-old man with intermittent metamfetamine use developed facial edema, pruritus, and dyspnea 45 minutes after injecting a mixture of crushed marijuana leaves and heated water. He was anxious, and had tachypnea, respiratory stridor, wheezing, edema of the face and oral mucosa, and truncal urticaria. There was mild pre-renal uremia and urine toxicology was positive for metamfetamine and marijuana. Skin testing was not done. With appropriate medical intervention there was resolution of symptoms within a day.

The authors noted that marijuana may have contaminants, including *Aspergillus*, *Salmonella*, herbicides, and mercury, which can trigger allergic reactions.

Captopril

See Angiotensin converting enzyme inhibitors

Carbamazepine

Hypersensitivity reactions are relatively common with carbamazepine. Most affect the skin, but systemic reactions with fever, lymphadenopathy, and/or involvement of the bone-marrow, the liver, the heart, the gastrointestinal system, the lungs, and other organs have been described. Severe serum sickness associated with immunoblastic lymphadenopathy has been reported in one case (SED-13, 148; 230). Occasional cases of systemic lupus erythematosus have occurred within the first few months, although an unusual case with onset after 8 years has been described (SEDA-22, 83).

- A 44-year-old woman, who was allergic to phenytoin, developed fever, lymphadenopathy, pneumonitis, hepatitis, and a morbilliform eruption after taking carbamazepine for 1 month (231). A skin biopsy of the dermis showed atypical lymphocytes that were CD3+, CD30+, and L26−. She improved quickly after carbamazepine was withdrawn.

This seems to have been the first report of carbamazepine-induced histological features of cutaneous pseudolymphoma, including CD30+ cells.

Cervical lymphadenopathy, fever, and a maculopapular skin rash developed in a 17-year-old boy after he had taken carbamazepine for 3 weeks (up to 600 mg/day) (232). Lymph node biopsies showed features typical of Kikuchi disease, a rare and self-limited immune-mediated lymphadenopathy that affects mostly the cervical region. The condition cleared rapidly after withdrawal.

- A 40-year-old man who had taken carbamazepine since childhood suffered for over 10 years from a lupus-like

illness with hypocomplementemia, pancytopenia, and splenomegaly (233). He later developed cryoglobulinemia with membranoproliferative glomerulonephritis and raised ANA and pANCA titers. A causative role of carbamazepine in the latter syndrome was suggested by the observation that after withdrawal the antibodies fell and cryoglobulinemia resolved.

The carbamazepine hypersensitivity syndrome has been reviewed (234). Some of the following cases are examples of the different manifestations of this syndrome.

- A 12-year-old boy developed a maculopapular rash on two occasions after taking carbamazepine (235). A patch test was positive, but an in vitro lymphocyte transformation test was negative. However, T cells incubated with carbamazepine produced an excess of interferon-gamma.

The author proposed that this had been a delayed hypersensitivity response, perhaps mediated by a reactive metabolite.

- A 45-year-old man developed acute cardiac tamponade due to systemic lupus erythematosus associated with carbamazepine, which he had taken for 8 months (236).
- An 11-year-old girl developed a skin rash, fever, lymphadenopathy, and arthralgia after taking carbamazepine (plasma concentration 21 µmol/l) for 3 weeks (237). She had a lymphocytosis, mild thrombocytopenia, marked eosinophilia, and high transaminases. She was given betamethasone, and carbamazepine was gradually withdrawn. The fever and rash gradually abated and all the laboratory tests normalized by 2 weeks after the disappearance of the skin rash.

Carbapenems

There was a high degree of cross-reactivity between imipenem determinants, analogous to the penicillin determinants in penicillin-allergic patients. Nine of twenty patients with positive penicillin skin tests had positive skin reactions to analogous imipenem determinants (238). In view of this appreciable cross-reactivity, imipenem should not be given to patients with penicillin allergy.

Immediate hypersensitivity related to imipenem has been reported in a patient allergic to penicillin and aztreonam (239).

Carbonic anhydrase inhibitors

Fatal anaphylactic shock with massive pulmonary edema has been reported in a 66-year-old woman who was taking acetazolamide for glaucoma (240). She had a history of sulfonamide allergy, and acetazolamide is a sulfonamide derivative. Sulfonamide allergy should be regarded as a contraindication to acetazolamide.

- Non-fatal anaphylactic shock with acute pulmonary edema has been reported in a 79-year-old woman after a first dose of acetazolamide (241). There was no history of sulfonamide allergy and she had been taking hydrochlorothiazide for some time.

Anaphylactic shock with acetazolamide should be recognized to occur as a first-dose phenomenon with no prior demonstrable sulfonamide allergy.

Celastraceae

The immunosuppressive properties of Lei gong teng can promote the development of infectious diseases (242).

Cephalosporins

Type I reactions

Immediate hypersensitivity reactions, mediated through IgE antibodies to cephalosporin determinants, are a major factor limiting their use. Early cases of anaphylaxis to cephalosporins were probably due to contamination with trace amounts of penicillin (243). These studies may therefore have over-reported cross-sensitivity.

In a retrospective study the frequency of systemic anaphylaxis to cefaloridine, cefalotin, or cefalexin was two out of 9388 patients (0.02%) without a history of penicillin allergy, and two out of 450 patients (0.4%) with a history of penicillin allergy (244). In the first group, two of the 1983 patients treated with cefalotin accounted for the adverse event.

Two of 178 prospective patients, of whom 151 had a history of penicillin allergy but were negative on penicillin skin testing, had reactions to a cephalosporin (245). There were 27 who had a positive penicillin skin test but did not react to a cephalosporin. Similar results were found by others (246).

However, a history of penicillin allergy is often vague, and many studies have suggested that it is an unreliable indicator, which has been confirmed (247). In 62 penicillin skin-test-positive patients, cephalosporins produced only one reaction of mild urticaria and bronchospasm (248).

Primary cephalosporin allergy in patients not allergic to penicillin has been reported, but the exact frequency is not known (249,250). The true incidence of allergic reactions may differ among the cephalosporins. Several reports implicating particular compounds have been published (251–253,254,255).

An accurate molecular definition of cephalosporin allergy is not currently available. Relevant determinants of cephalosporin-induced anaphylaxis may not reside in the bicyclic core, but rather in the side chain (256,257).

Neither in vitro tests nor skin tests reliably predict cephalosporin allergy (258). The true frequency of allergic reactions in penicillin-allergic patients exposed to cephalosporins has been estimated to be 1 or 2% (259). Nevertheless, when there is a history of penicillin anaphylaxis or other severe IgE-mediated reactions, it is wise to avoid cephalosporins.

An acute, life-threatening, anaphylactic reaction has been described in a child who received his first intravenous injection of ceftriaxone (260).

- A 3-year-old boy developed a high fever and a petechial rash. In the past he had been treated four times with amoxicillin for upper respiratory tract infections without allergic reactions. At presentation he had multiple petechiae over the trunk and limbs. There were no signs of meningeal irritation. He was given intravenous ceftriaxone 100 mg/kg and after 1 minute developed excitation and a generalized papular urticarial rash. His heart rate increased to 160/minute and the blood pressure was not measurable. He was given subcutaneous adrenaline 0.15 mg plus intravenous clemastine fumarate 2 mg, dexamethasone 3 mg, and fluids. Within 15 minutes his circulation was restored and the urticarial rash abated. Instead of ceftriaxone, he was given chloramphenicol for 7 days, and no further allergic reaction was observed. *Neisseria meningitidis*, sensitive to chloramphenicol and ceftriaxone, was cultured from his blood and spinal fluid. He was discharged well 12 days after admission. One month later, skin tests for ceftriaxone and benzylpenicillin were negative, as was a test for ceftriaxone-specific IgE. Because hypersensitivity could not be demonstrated, a controlled intravenous challenge with ceftriaxone 100 mg/kg was performed, and 20 seconds later there was again excitation and a generalized papular urticarial rash. He was treated as before and recovered within 15 minutes.

According to the authors, anaphylaxis after a single injection of ceftriaxone without previous exposure to the drug is very rare, and they referred to only one previous report (261). However, despite the fact that hypersensitivity could not be demonstrated by skin testing or the presence of ceftriaxone-specific IgE, the outcome of the challenge to ceftriaxone very clearly pointed to an anaphylactic reaction.

An anaphylactic reaction to a subconjunctival injection of cefazolin has been described.

- A 70-year-old white woman with a history of penicillin allergy underwent an uncomplicated eye operation, at the end of which she received a subconjunctival injection of cefazolin 50 mg (262). About 90 minutes postoperatively she developed acute respiratory distress and an erythematous macular rash over the face, neck, chest, forearms, and lateral thighs. The rash became urticarial without pruritus. She was given bronchodilators and intravenous glucocorticoids, with little improvement, but repeated subcutaneous injections of adrenaline gave some improvement in breathing. However, she had to be intubated, and was weaned from the ventilator only after some hours.

The main lesson from this case is that a small amount of a beta-lactam antibiotic anywhere in the body can cause life-threatening anaphylaxis.

For more details see Meyler's Side Effects of Antimicrobial Drugs.

Chloral hydrate

Several reports have highlighted the importance of gelatin allergy in young children, with some deaths due to anaphylaxis.

- A 2-year-old boy and a 4-year-old boy developed anaphylactic symptoms after being given a chloral hydrate suppository, which contained gelatin, for sedation before electroencephalography (263).

Chloral hydrate suppositories are often used to sedate children during various examinations and the authors suggested using gelatin-free formulations.

Chloramphenicol

Systemic reactions with collapse, bronchospasm, angioedema, and urticaria occur rarely (264,265).

Infection risk

The number and types of microorganisms that constitute the normal microflora of the alimentary, respiratory, and genital tracts change during therapy with chloramphenicol. Superinfections can then develop with *Staphylococcus aureus*, *Pseudomonas*, *Proteus*, and fungi. The changes in intestinal flora may be partly responsible for a reduction in the synthesis of vitamin K-dependent clotting factors, especially in patients with severe illnesses and malnutrition or during the administration of oral anticoagulants.

Chlorhexidine

Allergic reactions, including anaphylaxis, from chlorhexidine are reported with all types of use and are well documented (1474). However, chlorhexidine may still not be suspected as a possible cause of anaphylaxis when several agents are used in the anesthetized surgical patient, and hypersensitivity to chlorhexidine may not be tested for (266). If a reaction occurs during anesthesia, there is often doubt about the exact agent responsible; patch-testing will help if there is doubt about causality.

Mechanism

The molecular basis of the recognition of chlorhexidine in a sensitive patient has been examined (267).

- A 75-year-old man had three anaphylactic events after the use of chlorhexidine. The first occurred in September 1995 during general anesthesia for coronary artery bypass grafts. Ten minutes after induction he developed a marked fall in blood pressure, bronchospasm, tachycardia, and increased pulmonary artery pressure. In July 1996, a transurethral resection of the prostate was performed under spinal anesthetic. At cystoscopy he developed a headache, a rash, and bronchospasm, which settled after treatment. He had a further cystoscopy in February 1998, during which he became flushed, wheezy, and hypotensive, and had a cardiac arrest. He was successfully resuscitated. He had raised serum tryptase activities (60.4 and 26.6 µg/l at 3.5 and 9.5 hours after the event), suggesting a true anaphylactic reaction. Since the only pharmacological

agent common to all three procedures was urethral jelly containing lidocaine 2% and chlorhexidine 0.05%, he subsequently had skin prick tests, intradermal tests, and sequential subcutaneous challenges to lidocaine without any positive or adverse effects. Because he had developed profound anaphylaxis with cardiac arrest after the topical administration of chlorhexidine, skin tests were deemed unethical, and an in vitro method for detecting sensitivity to chlorhexidine was pursued. Detailed quantitative hapten inhibition studies were carried out with chlorhexidine-reactive IgE antibodies identified in the serum of the patient.

The authors concluded that unlike most drug allergic determinants the whole chlorhexidine molecule is complementary to the IgE antibody combining sites and that the 4-chlorophenol, biguanide, and hexamethylene structures together comprise the allergenic component.

Chloroquine and hydroxychloroquine

- Allergic contact dermatitis, which progressed to generalized dermatitis and conjunctivitis, followed later by severe asthma, occurred in a 60-year-old worker in the pharmaceutical industry after exposure to hydroxychloroquine (268). Patch-testing showed delayed sensitivity to hydroxychloroquine. Equivalent tests in five healthy volunteers were negative. The patch test reactions were pustular, and a biopsy was interpreted as multiform contact dermatitis. Bronchial exposure to hydroxychloroquine dust produced delayed bronchial obstruction over the next 20 hours, progressing to fever and generalized erythema (hematogenous contact dermatitis).

Chloroxylenol

Allergic contact dermatitis can occur after sensitization to chloroxylenol, for example in medicated Vaseline or in electrocardiographic paste (269).

In a retrospective analysis of patch tests in 951 patients 1.8% had positive reactions to chloroxylenol (270). Most of the patients had been sensitized by popular proprietary formulations containing chloroxylenol (SEDA-11, 221).

Chlorprothixene

Rare disorders of connective tissue resembling systemic lupus erythematosus have been reported with chlorpromazine, perphenazine, and chlorprothixene (271).

Ciclosporin

Anaphylactoid reactions can occur with intravenous ciclosporin, sometimes after the first dose. Reported symptoms included pruritic rash, respiratory symptoms, chest pain, and, rarely, cardiopulmonary arrest. The presence of Cremophor EL, polyoxyethylated castor oil used as a solvent, is likely to account for this life-threatening reaction. The mechanism is still unclear, and results of skin tests were available in only three of 22 previously published patients.

In a report of an anaphylactic reaction, positive intradermal tests suggested a possible IgE-mediated reaction, most probably directed against Cremophor EL, as the patient subsequently tolerated the corn-oil-based soft gelatin formulation (272).

During a Phase I/II trial of high-dose intravenous ciclosporin, there was a high incidence of anaphylactoid reactions associated with improper mixing during preparation of the infusions, perhaps due to large initial bolus infusions of the vehicle, Cremophor EL (273).

Infection risk

Infections, in particular bacterial and viral (cytomegalovirus, *Herpes simplex* virus, Epstein–Barr virus), and also protozoal and fungal infections, are major causes of morbidity and mortality after transplantation, whatever the immunosuppressive regimen used (274,275,276). Based on an analysis of medical and autopsy records, infections were found to be the cause of death in 70% of transplant patients, with bacteria (50%) or fungi (29%) the most common pathogens (277).

Cinchocaine

An anaphylactic reaction to cinchocaine has been described.

- A 71-year-old man received intrathecal anesthesia using 0.3% cinchocaine 2 ml for a transurethral prostatectomy (278). He had a history of allergic rhinitis, and 2 months before had had an uneventful prostate biopsy and cystoscopy, also under spinal anesthesia with isobaric bupivacaine. Within 45 minutes of the spinal injection he complained of periorbital itching, started to shake, and developed muscle rigidity. He rapidly became unconscious, with a systolic blood pressure of 40 mmHg and widespread erythema. He was treated with hydrocortisone and antihistamines and required an infusion of adrenaline. Intradermal testing after full recovery was positive with cinchocaine.

Cinnarizine and flunarizine

Subacute cutaneous lupus erythematosus has been attributed to cinnarizine.

- A 32-year-old woman developed an erythematous, papulosquamous, annular, polycyclic skin eruption on her neck, trunk, and lateral parts of the limbs after sunbathing while taking cinnarizine and thiethylperazine (a phenothiazine) for vertigo. She had positive antinuclear antibodies (nucleolar pattern, anti-Ro/SSA). The lesions cleared without residual scars within a few weeks after stopping both drugs and starting steroids and chloroquine.

Phenothiazines can induce photosensitivity, but cinnarizine does not. The authors' arguments that cinnarizine was to blame in this case were its structural resemblance to piperazine and a similar episode of skin eruption in the same patient after sunbathing many years before while she was taking cinnarizine only but for which she did not seek medical advice (279).

Ciprofloxacin

Anaphylactoid reactions occurred in 3 of about 3200 students who took ciprofloxacin 500 mg for chemoprophylaxis of meningococcal meningitis; two had no history of atopic illness (280). Additional adverse reactions were mild skin rashes in three students and nausea and vomiting in two.

Angioimmunoblastic lymphadenopathy is a rare disorder characterized by generalized lymphadenopathy, fever, hepatosplenomegaly, immune hemolytic anemia, and polyclonal hypergammaglobulinemia. Biopsy-proven angioimmunoblastic lymphadenopathy has been reported in a 79-year-old man who had received ciprofloxacin (281).

A Jarisch–Herxheimer reaction to ciprofloxacin has been reported (282).

- A 14-year-old girl developed tachycardia, hypotension, and disseminated intravascular coagulation after her first dose of oral ciprofloxacin 500 mg for presumed pyelonephritis. A peripheral blood smear showed spirochetes consistent with *Borrelia* species.

Cisatracurium besilate

Anaphylactic reactions have been reported (283–285).

Clonidine and apraclonidine

During long-term treatment of glaucoma with apraclonidine allergic reactions can occur. In a retrospective analysis of 64 patients who used apraclonidine 1% for more than 2 weeks, 31 (48%) developed an allergic reaction that led to withdrawal of treatment, with a mean latency of 4.7 months (286). Those who had allergic reactions tended to be older and female.

- A 46-year-old woman, who took clonidine 25 mg bd for menopausal flushing, developed depigmentation and swelling of her forearms (287). A skin biopsy showed a pattern consistent with immune complex disease, with IgG, IgM, C1q, C2c, and C4 complement between muscle fibers and at the dermo-epidermal junctions. All of these abnormalities disappeared after withdrawal.

Clopidogrel

A severe allergic reaction has been associated with clopidogrel (288).

- A 57-year-old man took clopidogrel after a myocardial infarction and after 5 days developed a fever, rash, pruritus, and abdominal pain. Three days later he developed shock. He had thrombocytopenia, lymphopenia, aseptic leukocyturia, and raised serum activities of transaminases, amylase, and gamma-glutamyl transpeptidase. Blood cultures were negative. Clopidogrel was withdrawn and within 1 week he had completely recovered and all blood tests had returned to normal. One month later, he took clopidogrel again; 4 hours later the same symptoms reappeared, with aseptic leukocyturia and raised transaminases and gamma-glutamyl transpeptidase. Drug allergy was suspected and clopidogrel was withdrawn. All the symptoms disappeared within a few days and did not recur during the following year. It is highly probable that this reaction was provoked by clopidogrel because of the positive rechallenge and because the patient did not take any other drug.

Clozapine

Allergic reactions associated with clozapine are uncommon; however, a case of rash (SEDA-21, 55) and a case of pleural effusion (SEDA-22, 60) have previously been reported. Both rash and pleural effusion have been reported in a 37-year-old woman about 1 week after starting clozapine (289).

Coagulation proteins

Patients with bleeding disorders are at risk of developing antibodies against the protein that is absent, present in reduced amounts, or present in an inactive form in their blood. Such coagulation inhibitors make treatment very difficult. Inhibitors of factor VIII are the most common and develop in 5–20% of patients with hemophilia A. Inhibitors of factor IX develop in 1–4% of patients with hemophilia B (693,694). Patients with factor VIII inhibitors present clinically either as "high responders" who show a strong anamnestic response and a sharp rise in inhibitor concentrations after exposure to factor VIII, or "low responders," who show little or no anamnestic response (290).

Because of the difference in prevalence of inhibitors in hemophilia B and hemophilia A, it has been postulated that there is a correlation between mutation type and inhibitor risk (291). Of the patients with gross deletion, nonsense, or frameshift mutations, 11% developed inhibitors compared with 0% and 0.36% of patients with hemophilia B with mis-sense or other mutations.

Recombinant and high-purity coagulation factor products appear to have a greater tendency to induce inhibitors than human-derived concentrates of intermediate or low purity (292). These intermediate-purity or low-purity human-derived concentrates are probably more suitable for inducing immune tolerance in patients with hemophilia with inhibitors. It has been suggested that for immune tolerance a high content of Von Willebrand factor in factor VIII concentrates is required, although direct comparisons of different products have not been made (293).

Risk factors for developing an inhibitor are the severity of the hemophilia, age (under 30 years), genetic predisposition, antigenicity of factor replacement therapy, and race (increased prevalence among black people) (294). In addition, it has been suggested that changing from one product to another can also stimulate the development of inhibitors (295).

Inhibitor formation has been observed in only a few patients with factor XI deficiency. Like patients with hemophilia A and B, these patients may be treated with prothrombin complex concentrates or recombinant factor VIIa (296).

Cocaine

The prevalence of infection with the human immunodeficiency virus (HIV) among drug abusers, including cocaine users, is increasing (297). Two separate reports have suggested that cocaine may compromise immunological function. In one study, human mononuclear cells were stimulated in vitro with mitogens in the presence and absence of cocaine; cocaine inhibited the proliferation of the mononuclear cells (298). In a second study, cocaine amplified HIV-1 replication in co-cultures containing cytomegalovirus-activated peripheral blood mononuclear cells (299).

Two cases of connective tissue disease have been reported (300).

A case of urticarial vasculitis, a type III hypersensitivity reaction, has been reported after cocaine use (301).

- A 24-year-old man with acute malaise and fever had a pruritic rash with multiple erythematous circumscribed weals on the trunk, arms, legs, neck, and scalp. He admitted to using intranasal cocaine 6 months, 4 days, and 1 day before the onset of the symptoms. His temperature was 39 °C. His erythrocyte sedimentation rate was 80 mm in the first hour, C-reactive protein was 283 mg/l (reference range below 10), and the white blood cell count was $12.4 \times 10^9/l$ with 89% neutrophils. A biopsy of an urticarial lesion showed a perivascular inflammatory infiltrate in the upper and middle dermis. Bed rest, oral prednisone, oral hydroxyzine, and topical polidocanol led to improvement within 24 hours.

Two cases of cocaine-induced type I hypersensitivity reactions, have been reported (302).

- A 23-year-old woman developed tongue swelling and difficulty in breathing immediately after having sniffed cocaine. The anterior half of her tongue was edematous with bleeding lesions caused by her fingernails. There were cocaine metabolites in the urine. The diagnosis was angioedema of the tongue induced by cocaine or its contaminants, and it resolved with subcutaneous adrenaline, H_1 receptor antihistamines, and intravenous glucocorticoids.
- A 19-year-old man developed generalized urticaria, intense pruritus, and mild bronchospasm 30 minutes after injecting cocaine for the third time. He had weals on the face, neck, arms, and chest, and scattered wheezing

in the lungs. Urine toxicology screen was positive for cocaine metabolites. His symptoms resolved several hours after the administration of H_1 receptor antihistamines and intravenous glucocorticoids.

Cocamidopropyl betaine

Contact allergic reactions are infrequent and have been attributed to sensitizing intermediates rather than cocamidopropyl betaine itself. Of 30 patients who were allergic to cocamidopropyl betaine, all reacted to 3-dimethylaminopropylamine (303). Two studies have shown that cocamidopropylamine is the more relevant impurity (304,305).

Codeine

True allergy to opioids is extremely rare. However, a near anaphylactic reaction in a patient taking codeine has been reported; the management of true codeine allergy was discussed and agents with different structures, such as phenylpiperidines or methadone-like compounds, are recommended (SEDA-17, 80).

Collagen and gelatin

Bovine collagen is contraindicated in patients with immunological disorders and reports of delayed allergic reactions underline the need for adequate follow-up when collagen implants are used. Patients should be tested with bovine collagen and reassessed at 4 weeks. About 3% of the patients tested in this way developed hypersensitivity reactions to collagen, whereas 1% of treated patients have symptoms of hypersensitivity at treatment sites (306). In this series, erythema was the sole symptom in 24%, and erythema and induration occurred in an additional 42%. Of the patients with complications, 45% reported an onset of symptoms within 10 days while in 22% the onset was more than 30 days following treatment with collagen. Abscesses as a manifestation of hypersensitivity to bovine collagen occur rarely (four in 10 000 cases), but the possibility of contamination should always be considered. Local tissue necrosis occurs rarely after implantation (nine reported in 10 000 cases) and this is thought to be the result of local vascular interruption rather than a hypersensitivity reaction. The incidence varies widely according to the site of implantation, but more than one-half of the cases involve the glabellar region, probably because of its special vascular distribution (307).

Anaphylactic reactions to collagen have been described (308). Despite pretreatment collagen testing, anaphylactic shock has been reported in one patient, necessitating adrenergic agents and glucocorticoids.

An allergic rash has been described after collagen injection (309).

Delayed hypersensitivity reactions after bovine collagen injection for stress urinary incontinence have been reported.

- A 50-year-old woman had a negative collagen skin test for 4 weeks (310). After an injection of transurethral collagen, she developed a flare-up at the skin test site and subsequently had recurrent flares at 21–26 day intervals for six cycles, which corresponded to her menses and were thought to be hormone-related.
- A 64-year-old woman with recurrent urinary leakage elected to undergo conservative therapy with collagen injection, had no reaction to a collagen skin test, and had an uneventful transurethral injection of collagen 30 days later (311). Her postoperative course was complicated by urethritis, trigonitis, severe urge, bilateral leg arthralgias, leg pain relieved by massage, and leg edema at 6 weeks. She had a total voided volume of 300 ml and a postvoid residual of 180 ml, and was started on intermittent self-catheterization for urinary retention. Induration at the skin injection test site was noticeable 9 weeks after the injection. Her severe urge, leg edema, and pain gradually resolved after 13 months, but her stress incontinence continued without relief.
- A 50-year-old woman with stress urinary incontinence chose a trial of transurethral injection of collagen (312). A skin test showed no evidence of allergy at 1 month and collagen 2.5 ml was injected transurethrally without problems but with little improvement. A second injection of 2.5 ml 5 weeks later was again uneventful, but 2 weeks later she began to have difficulty in emptying her bladder, with a poor stream and a sense of incomplete emptying. At the same time she noticed redness and firmness at the initial skin test site on her arm, which had previously been benign.

Several reports have highlighted the importance of gelatin allergy in young children, with some deaths due to anaphylaxis. Elsewhere, anaphylactoid reactions have been reported to gelatin-containing injectables (SEDA-20, 310).

- A 2-year-old and a 4-year-old boy developed anaphylactic symptoms after being given a chloral hydrate suppository, which contained gelatin, for sedation before electroencephalography (313).

The authors suggested using gelatin-free formulations in children.

Corticotrophins (corticotropin and tetracosactide)

Although the incidence of severe allergic reactions to natural corticotropin of animal origin fell as progressively purer products were introduced, the problem remained for a small minority of patients. Exact figures are difficult to cite, but hypersensitivity reactions have sometimes even been described in patients with no history of corticotropin treatment, presumably sensitized by other animal material. Hypersensitivity to corticotropin generally causes only dizziness, nausea and vomiting, or cutaneous hypersensitivity reactions, but in several instances shock with circulatory failure has been observed (314). In a number of patients who were allergic to porcine corticotropin, no such problems were observed when tetracosactide was given. This suggests that the absence of most of the antigenic part of the original molecule reduces the risk of hypersensitivity reactions. However, the smaller synthetic molecule can still stimulate the formation of antibodies in some individuals (SEDA-12, 979) (315).

However, allergic reactions and anaphylactic shock have been observed during treatment with tetracosactide and have even proved fatal. Local reactions have even been seen after the administration of small doses for intracutaneous testing. In the early years of tetracosactide use, the frequency of local and general reactions to a long-acting acetylated tetracosactide was estimated at as little as one in 30 000 (SED-12, 979), but it is doubtful whether this figure can be supported today, unless one interprets it as referring only to major calamities. Indeed, subclinical immune reactions to both natural and tetracosactide appear to be fairly common during long-term treatment of patients with asthma, with an incidence of intradermal reactions of about 50%, a prevalence of IgE antibodies that is significantly higher than in controls, and a high incidence of low-titer agglutinating antibodies to corticotropin. The antibodies can result in a gradual loss of effect.

Infection risk

Pneumonia due to *Pneumocystis jiroveci* (formerly *Pneumocystis carinii*) has been attributed to high-dose corticotropin (316).

- An infant girl was given corticotropin 80 U/day for infantile spasms. After 5 weeks she became increasingly lethargic, with reduced oral intake, cough, an increased respiratory rate (50 breaths/minute), and a fever of 38.6 °C. Investigations were consistent with pneumonia and she was given intravenous ceftriaxone. She initially improved, but 36 hours later her respiratory distress worsened and she required intubation and mechanical ventilation. The diagnosis of *P. jiroveci* pneumonia was confirmed and she was given intravenous co-trimoxazole and glucocorticoids. Her respiratory distress resolved and she was extubated 10 days later. Immunological testing after the withdrawal of corticotropin did not show any abnormalities that could have predisposed her to *P. jiroveci* pneumonia.

The authors commented that a transient immunodeficiency related to corticotrophin may have predisposed to the development of *P. jiroveci* pneumonia.

Corticosteroids—glucocorticoids

Since the glucocorticoids have immunosuppressive and anti-inflammatory properties, one would not expect allergic reactions to be a problem, except when excipients act as allergens. Nevertheless, allergic reactions to glucocorticoids themselves have been reported (SEDA-21, 419)

(317). Urticaria after glucocorticoid treatment has been explained as a reaction of the mesenchyme. Also, an increase in eosinophilic leukocytes (which normally are diminished by glucocorticoids) has been reported as a first reaction to treatment with glucocorticoids.

Class I immune reactions

Anaphylactic shock has been described after intranasal hydrocortisone acetate, intramuscular methylprednisolone (SEDA-21, 419) (318), intravenous methylprednisolone (SEDA-22, 448) (319), intramuscular dexamethasone (SEDA-22, 448) (320), and intra-articular methylprednisolone (SEDA-22, 449) (321). A life-threatening anaphylactic-like reaction to intravenous hydrocortisone has been described in patients with asthma (322). Acute laryngeal obstruction has been described for the first time after the intravenous administration of hydrocortisone (SEDA-22, 449) (323). There is some reason to believe that sodium succinate esters are more likely to cause hypersensitivity reactions (SEDA-17, 449), but unconjugated glucocorticoids can definitely produce allergy in some cases (SEDA-16, 452).

- A 64-year-old woman with a history of bronchial asthma developed increasing shortness of breath after an upper respiratory tract infection (324). Her medication included inhaled salbutamol as necessary, theophylline 300 mg bd, and aspirin 325 mg/day. She was given nebulized salbutamol and ipratropium and hydrocortisone 200 mg intravenously. Within 30 minutes, she developed a generalized rash, fever (38.3°C), and respiratory distress. She was promptly intubated and mechanical ventilation was started. No further doses of glucocorticoid were given. Skin testing with various parenteral formulations of glucocorticoids produced a 5 mm wheal at the site of hydrocortisone and methylprednisolone injections. She was subsequently given a challenge dose of triamcinolone using a metered-dose inhaler with no reaction, and was therefore continued on this medication.

- An anaphylactoid reaction (angioedema, generalized urticaria, worsening bronchospasm, and marked hypotension) occurred in a 35-year-old man with multiple sclerosis who became allergic to methylprednisolone (dose not stated) after starting treatment with interferon beta-1b (325). He had previously been treated with different courses of methylprednisolone. Clinicians should be aware that the complexity of the effects of interferon beta-1b on the immune system can lead to unexpected outcomes. It is uncertain whether the sequence of events here was due to an effect of interferon beta-1b or to coincidence.

- A 17-year-old boy, with an 11-year history of asthma, had anaphylaxis with respiratory distress shortly after he received intravenous methylprednisolone for an exacerbation of asthma while taking a tapering course of oral prednisone 15 mg/day (326). He had been glucocorticoid-dependent for at least 1 year. He reported having received intravenous glucocorticoids previously. He was treated with inhaled salbutamol and then intravenous methylprednisolone 125 mg over 15–30 seconds, and 3–4 minutes later became flushed and dyspneic, and developed diffuse urticarial lesions on his trunk and face and an undetectable blood pressure. He was treated with adrenaline, but required intubation. Sinus bradycardia developed and then asystole. He was successfully resuscitated and a 10–15 seconds period of generalized tonic-clonic activity was treated with diazepam. He remained unresponsive to stimulation for 30 minutes. However, he awoke 1 hour after his respiratory arrest and was extubated and discharged the following day taking a tapering dosage of prednisone.

- An anaphylactoid reaction occurred in a 68-year-old woman after treatment with intravenous methylprednisolone for asthma. She had developed urticaria with methylprednisolone 1 year earlier, but the reaction had been thought to be related to the solvent in the formulation (327).

- Forty minutes after a first dose of prednisone 25 mg, a 17-year-old girl with a history of aspirin intolerance had generalized flushing, hives, hypogastric pain, and abdominal cramps, followed by vomiting and diarrhea (328). She lost consciousness and developed arterial hypotension. She responded to intravenous diphenhydramine and hydrocortisone. Intradermal skin tests were positive for prednisone and negative for methylprednisolone and hydrocortisone. An oral challenge test with prednisone led to flushing, nausea, dizziness, tachycardia, and hypotension and responded to intravenous diphenhydramine and hydrocortisone. Challenge tests with intravenous methylprednisolone and hydrocortisone were negative.

- A 30-year-old man with recurrent atopic eczema of the head and neck, generalized xerosis, keratosis pilaris of the arms, and a history of dyshidrosis was initially treated with prednisolone-21-acetate ointment (329). His skin eruption became worse. He was given oral prednisolone 25 mg, and 5 hours after the first dose developed intense generalized pruritus with erythema and swelling of the face. After 24 hours there was generalized erythema with disseminated partly follicular papules. There was an eosinophilia (1.1×10^9/l). Total IgE was not raised. Patch tests showed delayed reactions to hydrocortisone 1%, prednisolone 1%, prednisolone-21-acetate ointment, and prednisolone 2.5%. Prick and intradermal tests with methylprednisolone succinate, hydrocortisone succinate, betamethasone, and triamcinolone acetonide in concentrations up to 1 : 10 were negative at 15 minutes. However, 4 hours after intradermal testing, generalized pruritus developed and 24 hours later there was a disseminated partly follicular eczematous reaction with involvement of the flexural areas. Biopsy of the eruptions caused by prednisolone and of the positive skin reaction to methylprednisolone succinate showed superficial dermatitis with a perivascular infiltration consisting predominantly of CD4+ cells and some eosinophils. Immunofluorescence showed increased expression of HLA-DR molecules on the CD4+ and CD8+ cells. During the exanthema caused by prednisolone,

interleukin-5 (14 pg/ml), interleukin-6 (38 pg/ml), and interleukin-10 (26 pg/ml) were detected in the blood; 2 months after recovery these cytokines were not detectable.

The authors of the last report commented that generalized delayed type hypersensitivity to systemic administration of a glucocorticoid is rare. Despite the potent immunosuppressive effect of glucocorticoids on immunocompetent cells, the clinical features, the skin biopsy specimen, and the positive delayed skin test reactions strongly suggested an immunological mechanism: T cells were clearly involved and the high concentrations of interleukins 5, 6, and 10 were consistent with a T helper type 2 reaction. The raised concentrations of interleukin-5 were probably responsible for the blood and tissue eosinophilia.

Budesonide has been marketed in oral form for intestinal inflammatory disease. An non-IgE-mediated anaphylactic reaction has been associated with oral budesonide (330).

- A 32-year-old woman with Crohn's disease, who had taken prednisone 20 mg/day and azathioprine 150 mg/day, switched to budesonide 9 mg/day because of weight gain, and 5 minutes after the first capsule her tongue and throat swelled, accompanied by wheeziness and diarrhea. She was given clemastine and recovered after 4 ays. Intracutaneous tests with diluted budesonide suggested a non-IgE-mediated reaction. She had a previous history of a similar reaction to mesalazine. One year later her tongue and throat swelled after intravenous dexamethasone.

Urticaria with angioedema has been described in a patient taking deflazacort (331).

- A 64-year-old woman with allergic alveolitis caused by parakeet feathers improved with intravenous methylprednisolone, and was given oral deflazacort 60 mg/day, to be reduced progressively. After 30 days she developed generalized itchy blotches and lip edema. At that time she was mistakenly taking deflazacort in a dose of 120 mg/day. She was given an antihistamine, without any improvement. Deflazacort was then replaced by prednisolone and her symptoms disappeared immediately. Skin tests (a prick test and an epicutaneous test) were positive with deflazacort. Oral provocation with deflazacort 30 mg was positive, with the immediate appearance of the same symptoms as in the initial episode.

In an NIH workshop summary report on the relation between asthma therapy and Churg–Strauss syndrome, the authors concluded that no one compound or class of antiasthmatic agents was solely implicated. An association was found for pranlukast, montelukast, zafirlukast, the 5-lipoxygenase inhibitor zileuton, inhaled corticosteroids, and salmeterol. As corticosteroids constitute the principal therapy of Churg–Strauss syndrome, tapering of these agents may allow incipient Churg–Strauss syndrome to become manifest. In patients who develop

Churg–Strauss syndrome and do not receive corticosteroids (332–334), these various antiasthmatic medications might be used to treat asthmatic symptoms but not the underlying Churg–Strauss syndrome (335).

Corticosteroids—glucocorticoids, inhaled

Hypersensitivity to inhaled glucocorticoids is rare.

- An asthmatic patient using inhaled budesonide and salbutamol developed an acute asthma attack. Despite emergency treatment the patient deteriorated, requiring endotracheal intubation and assisted ventilation, and there was no improvement until the glucocorticoid was withdrawn, after which there was steady improvement. Skin prick tests with prednisolone, sodium hemisuccinate, and 6-methylprednisolone-sodium hemisuccinate were positive. Thirty minutes after intradermal 6-methylprednisolone-sodium hemisuccinate 4 mg, the patient developed a dry cough, dyspnea, and wheezing and a 17% fall in FEV_1.
- A 37-year-old woman who was pregnant developed Churg–Strauss syndrome after withdrawal of her usual high-dose inhaled glucocorticoid therapy (drug not stated) that she had used for 3 years for bronchial asthma (336).

The authors of the second report commented that activated eosinophils and their cytotoxic products, such as eosinophil catatonic protein, may play a part in the pathogenesis of Churg–Strauss syndrome. Measuring serum concentrations of eosinophil catatonic protein may be useful in monitoring disease activity, since concentrations were increased before treatment and normalized afterwards.

Co-trimoxazole

See Trimethoprim

Coumarin anticoagulants

Skin-test reactivity, that is induration and tissue factor generation by monocytes, is reduced by therapeutic doses of oral anticoagulants, but lymphocyte transformation activity is not. This constitutes the rationale for the use of oral anticoagulants in the treatment of immune diseases characterized by fibrin deposition, such as allograft rejection and lupus nephritis (337).

COX-2 inhibitors

There is considerable difficulty and controversy in identifying and classifying allergic reactions to NSAIDs, for many reasons (338). First, the difficulty in making a definite diagnosis in patients who have these reactions without provocative challenge with the suspected drug and other NSAIDs. Secondly, reactions are characterized by a large spectrum of target organ responses to NSAIDs,

and the same drug can cause different types of reactions in different organs in the same or different individuals. Thirdly, a patient can have a similar reaction to a structurally different NSAID. Finally, reports of these reactions include different, often imprecise, terms, making interpretation difficult. It is worth evaluating the safety of new coxibs in patients who cannot tolerate non-selective NSAIDs.

Anaphylaxis due to celecoxib has been described (SEDA 26, 121). Life-threatening anaphylaxis, with urticaria, angioedema, and bronchospasm, has also been described 30 minutes after a dose of celecoxib for arthritis of the hip (339).

Allergic vasculitis has been reported in association with various NSAIDs, and has been attributed to celecoxib (340,341), including one case with a fatal outcome (342).

Whether allergic reactions to celecoxib occur more often in patients who report a previous reaction to sulfonamides, and should therefore be contraindicated in such patients, is still unknown (343).

Angioedema has been attributed to rofecoxib (SEDA-26, 121).

- A 60-year-old man developed angioedema after taking two doses of rofecoxib 12.5 mg 18 and 12 hours before (344). Despite intensive treatment he developed pulmonary hemorrhagic edema and died a day later. He had fibrotic lung disease, which may have predisposed him to the lethal event.

The tolerability of rofecoxib in patients with cutaneous allergic and pseudoallergic adverse reactions to non-selective NSAIDs has been confirmed in a study in 139 patients with NSAID-induced adverse reactions: 60 with urticaria alone (43%), 34 with angioedema (25%), 34 with angioedema plus urticaria (2.9%), and 2 with Stevens–Johnson syndrome (1.4%) (345). They all underwent a single-blind, placebo-controlled oral challenge with increasing doses of rofecoxib, and 138 of them tolerated it without adverse reactions. Only one had mild urticaria on the arms. Rofecoxib may be a useful alternative in patients with NSAID hypersensitivity.

Anaphylaxis

Among the anaphylactic reactions to NSAIDs that result in different types of reaction (urticaria, angioedema, asthma, or hypotension), there have been very few reports of anaphylactic shock. However, anaphylaxis has been described in patients taking celecoxib (346,347) or rofecoxib (348). Rofecoxib caused anaphylaxis in a patient who had had a similar reaction to diclofenac, suggesting that COX-2 inhibitors may be not safe in all individuals who have adverse reactions to non-selective COX inhibitors. It also suggests that different mechanisms may be involved in patients with asthma and in those with anaphylactoid reactions to NSAIDs.

Cromoglicate sodium

Immunological reactions to cromoglicate can involve the pericardium, the lung, the eye, the nasal mucosa, the skin, the joints, and the liver. Rarely, a hypersensitivity reaction can cause fever (349). A survey of the world literature up to 1982 found 13 cases of facial rash, urticaria, and/or generalized dermatitis, and one of nasal congestion. In 19 patients there was bronchospasm and/or pulmonary edema, eventually culminating in shock. Four cases of eosinophilic or granulomatous pulmonary infiltration, one of liver disease and vasculitis, one of pericarditis, and three of polymyositis were reported.

IgE and/or specifically reactive lymphocytes do not mediate many of the adverse reactions to cromoglicate, which mimic allergic processes of the immediate or delayed type. These reactions fulfilled the criteria that characterize pseudo-allergic reactions (350,351). There is a much higher incidence of such adverse reactions when cromoglicate is used orally in the treatment of food allergy, as high as 29% of cases treated (350,351).

The US Food and Drug Administration has issued a report (SEDA-7, 1) on a suspected case of cromoglicate-induced lupus-like syndrome. Treatment with cromoglicate for 6 months resulted in arthritis, positive LE cells, and a positive antinuclear factor. After withdrawal of cromoglicate, the signs and symptoms regressed. Although this does not prove cause and effect, the report suggests a similarity between lupus-like syndrome and some of the adverse reactions that were listed earlier in the US data sheet (SEDA-3, 48).

Cuprammonium cellulose

Anaphylaxis as an adverse effect of hemodialysis has been analysed from records of about 260 000 courses of dialysis treatment, at three centers. There were 21 severe reactions over the 10.5-year period of the survey, all highly suggestive of anaphylaxis (352). Reactions occurred within minutes of initiating dialysis and were characterized by cardiopulmonary, mucocutaneous, and/or gastrointestinal tract symptoms. Four respiratory arrests occurred and there was one death. When the individual histories and treatments were analysed, there was strong evidence that hollow-fiber dialysers made of cuprammonium cellulose were responsible. No obvious factors could be found to identify predisposed patients; suboptimal rinsing of the cuprammonium cellulose hollow-fiber dialysers before use may have been responsible for some of the reactions. Repeated dialysis anaphylaxis in one patient has been reported (353).

Cyanoacrylates

Infection can develop in the frontal area and at the lateral base of the skull after the use of cyanoacrylates, even after a symptom-free interval of several years; the lesions can be characterized by infected granular nodules, chronic sinusitis, or otogenic meningitis (354).

Danaparoid sodium

Delayed hypersensitivity reactions have been reported in patients given danaparoid (355).

Dapsone and analogues

The sulfones occasionally exacerbate lepromatous leprosy, the so-called sulfone syndrome or dapsone syndrome, which resembles acute infectious mononucleosis (SEDA-16, 347; 356), and can develop 3–6 weeks after the start of treatment in malnourished patients. It appears to be an allergic reaction. It includes fever, malaise, pruritus, exfoliative dermatitis, photosensitivity, polyarthritis (357), jaundice and even hepatic necrosis, hepatosplenomegaly, lymphadenopathy, methemoglobinemia, and anemia. The syndrome is accompanied by the formation of atypical T lymphocytes with markedly increased spontaneous thymidine uptake (SEDA-8, 289). The full syndrome is probably rare, but it is important to recognize its partial expression (358–360). It has been suggested that it has become more common since the introduction of multidrug therapy (361), especially with rifampicin plus dapsone. The syndrome usually resolves rapidly after withdrawal of dapsone and with glucocorticoid treatment (for example prednisolone 30–60 mg/day). However, it can also end in a fatal allergic reaction (SEDA-12, 259).

Anaphylactic shock and tachycardia are among the most severe allergic reactions to dapsone (361).

Deferiprone

A few observations have suggested that deferiprone can cause a lupus-like syndrome, with antinuclear and antihistone antibodies (362,363), but this suspicion is still unproven (364,365).

Infection risk

- An 82-year-old woman with a myelodysplastic syndrome died of *Escherichia coli* septicemia after 5 months of treatment with deferiprone (366). There was no granulocytopenia.

Deferoxamine

Generalized hypersensitivity reactions and anaphylactic shock can occur but are infrequent. Hypersensitivity reactions to deferoxamine may require permanent withdrawal, worsening the prognosis in thalassemia. However, successful desensitization has been achieved in three patients with previous deferoxamine hypersensitivity, enabling continued administration of deferoxamine (367–369).

Infection risk

In many species, from mammals to microbes, iron is essential, and the extremely low free iron content of the blood is an important antimicrobial factor. Many microorganisms do not produce siderophores and are entirely dependent on the iron content of their direct environment; usually their inability to produce siderophores is associated with low infectivity. In the case of increased availability of iron, for example in iron storage diseases, patients may have increased susceptibility to infectious diseases (370–372). Furthermore, iron impairs granulocyte function (373,374) and monocytic function (375). An abundance of publications has shown that the use of deferoxamine in iron storage disease, dialysis patients, or acute iron poisoning (376) can promote the development of infections, notably with microorganisms that are iron-dependent and are known to be otherwise only slightly infective (SED-12, 553; 375–380). Besides providing iron to these microorganisms by acting as a siderophore, deferoxamine can deplete the pool of iron available to the macrophage cytotoxic system (381)

Yersinia enterocolitica or *Yersinia pseudotuberculosis*, *Pneumocystis jiroveci* (382), *Staphylococcus aureus* (384), *Cunninghamella bertholletiae* (381), and *Rhizopus* spp. have been involved. The diagnosis of these spontaneously rare infections may be even more difficult, because the deferoxamine-associated form can have an unusual and atypical course.

Many reports of fatal cases of mucormycosis have underlined the danger of acquiring disseminated fungal infection in patients receiving deferoxamine (375,384–394). Boelaert and co-workers of the International Registry of Mucormycosis in Dialysis Patients (Algemeen Ziekenhuis Sint Jan, B-8000 Brugge, Belgium) collected data on a total of 62 cases of mucormycosis, of which 59 were studied in detail (395); 78% of these patients were receiving deferoxamine. The infection presented as disseminated mucormycosis in 44%, rhinocerebral in 31%, and other forms in 25%, and ran a fatal course in 52 patients (86%). The fungus (cultured in only 36%) was always *Rhizopus* (in spite of the fact that human mucormycosis can be caused by various other fungal genera (for example *Mucor*, *Absida*, and *Cunninghamella*). The finding that the species was *R. microsporus* in all identified cases is at variance with the usual predominance of *R. oryzae* in patients with diabetes mellitus. Patients using deferoxamine who present with fever, sinusitis, dry cough, hemoptysis (396), acute loss of vision (397), or neurological symptoms should undergo evaluation for mucormycosis.

Occasionally, such conditions can start with skin lesions imitating vasculitis (387) or cutaneous infarction (375), or present with cavernous sinus or carotid arterial thrombosis (390). Although mucormycosis often has a fatal course, it can have a favorable prognosis if diagnosed early and treated aggressively with surgery and antifungal drugs (396). Many patients have several risk factors for mucormycosis in addition to deferoxamine (for example hemochromatosis, diabetes mellitus, splenectomy, immune suppression) and the contribution of deferoxamine can be difficult to prove or quantify in individual cases.

In many species, from mammals to microbes, iron is essential, and the extremely low free iron content of the blood is an important antimicrobial factor. Many microorganisms do not produce siderophores and are entirely dependent on the iron content of their direct environment; usually their inability to produce siderophores is associated with low infectivity. In the case of increased availability of iron, for example in iron storage diseases,

patients may have increased susceptibility to infectious diseases (370–372). Furthermore, iron impairs granulocyte function (373,374) and monocytic function (375). An abundance of publications has shown that the use of deferoxamine in iron storage disease, dialysis patients, or acute iron poisoning (376) can promote the development of infections, notably with microorganisms that are iron-dependent and are known to be otherwise only slightly infective (SED-12, 553) (375–380). Besides providing iron to these microorganisms by acting as a siderophore, deferoxamine can deplete the pool of iron available to the macrophage cytotoxic system (381), and adversely influence the immune system (382,383).

Delavirdine

Severe hypersensitivity reaction to delavirdine, including anaphylaxis, can occur and may necessitate drug withdrawal (398).

Dextrans

Anaphylactic reactions to dextrans have been reported, for example within 10 minutes after exposure to dextran in hysteroscopy (399). It can be fatal (400).

- A 54-year-old man developed generalized pruritus, dyspnea, and sudden hemodynamic shock, with cardiac and respiratory arrest 8 hours after the resection of a hepatic hydatid cyst, while being given dextran 40. He had no prior history of atopy or adverse drug reactions. Despite intensive resuscitation he remained unconscious and hemodynamically unstable. During the succeeding days he became septic with progressive renal function impairment and died on day 5. A range of serum tests for antibodies detected dextran-reactive antibodies. In addition, there was evidence of complement protein consumption within 6–24 hours of the clinical reaction.

The authors suggested that dextran-reactive antibodies had formed immune complexes with dextran, leading to complement activation and release of mediators of anaphylaxis. There was also evidence of mast cell degranulation. They therefore recommended that titration of dextran-reactive antibodies before administration of dextrans could provide a method of identifying those who are at risk of dextran-induced anaphylactic reactions.

- A 24-year-old healthy volunteer was given 10 ml of 6% dextran 60 during a preliminary examination (401). After about 5 minutes the first clinical symptoms of anaphylactic shock were evident, with a reduction in systolic blood pressure to 90 mmHg and an increased heart rate to over 90/minute. These returned to normal after therapy in the head-down position with clemastine 2 ml (2 mg), hydrocortisone 200 mg, and etherified starch 500 ml over about 8 minutes. During this period, responsiveness was unsatisfactory although he complained of warming of the skin, paresthesia, and nausea.

The authors suggested that this reaction had been due to a dextran-induced anaphylactic reaction, but were uncertain as to the cause of these observations, as they were not accompanied by immediate symptoms of shock. It is unclear if this case was caused by an antibody reaction.

Frequency and susceptibility factors

A large-scale prospective study was carried out in 49 public and private hospitals throughout France between June 1991 and October 1992, aimed at discovering the frequency and severity of anaphylactoid reactions to colloid plasma substitutes, looking for possible risk factors, and determining the mechanisms involved (402). In all, 19 593 patients were evaluated; 48% were given gelatins, 27% starches, 16% albumin, and 9% dextrans. There were 43 anaphylactoid reactions, an overall frequency of 0.22%, or one reaction per 456 patients. The frequency differed according to the plasma substitute used: 0.35% for gelatins, 0.27% for dextrans, 0.10% for albumin, and 0.06% for starches. The reactions were serious (grades III and IV) in 20% of cases.

Multivariate analysis showed four independent susceptibility factors: the administration of gelatins (OR = 4.81), the administration of dextrans (OR = 3.83), a history of drug allergy (OR = 3.16), and being male (OR = 1.98). The relative risks of anaphylactoid reactions due to one type of plasma substitute with respect to another were estimated to be six times less with starches than with gelatins and 4.7 times less than with dextrans. The relative risk of albumin was 3.4 times less than that of gelatins, and almost identical to that of the starches. An immunological assessment was carried out in 15 patients who had been given a gelatin (Plasmion); in seven cases an IgE-dependent reaction was proved. It was concluded that gelatins and dextrans should be avoided in patients with a known history of drug allergy; when a reaction does occur, an immunological assessment should be carried out, as the reaction may be due to specific antibodies, in which case that particular plasma substitute would be contraindicated for the rest of the patient's life.

Dextromethorphan

Dextromethorphan-induced anaphylactic symptoms have been reported (403).

- A 40-year-old woman suffered repeated hives, lip swelling, and shortness of breath on taking cough suppressants containing dextromethorphan. None was sufficient to require emergency medical intervention. On challenge with dextromethorphan 1 mg, mild transient pruritus occurred. After dextromethorphan 30 mg, hives and nasal and conjunctival congestion occurred. Vital signs and peak flow remained stable. There was no bronchospasm or angioedema. No reaction occurred to hydrocodone or codeine.

The authors noted that many opioids are potent histamine releasers and most reactions to opioids are anaphylactoid

rather than IgE-mediated. It was of particular interest that the patient was able to tolerate the opioids hydrocodone and codeine.

Diazepam

Hypersensitivity reactions after diazepam are very rare and usually mild. However, some severe reactions have been reported.

- A 50-year-old woman with chronic depression or dysthymic disorder and alcohol dependence was given oral thioridazine 100 mg/day and diazepam 10 mg qds (404). She had no history of drug allergy. Two days later she noticed an erythematous eruption on her ankles. Thioridazine was withdrawn, but the eruption became more widespread over a few hours. She was given methylprednisolone 80 mg/day, but the following day the eruption progressively became bullous and her condition worsened. She developed a fever of 39.4 ° C, felt ill, and had a neutrophilia, but blood cultures were sterile and her renal function was normal. A skin biopsy showed bullous vasculitis with numerous eosinophils in the dermis. Diazepam was then withdrawn, which led to resolution of pyrexia and gradual healing of the skin lesions over the next 2 months. The lymphocyte blast transformation test was positive for diazepam.
- A 28-year-old nurse had generalized urticaria and collapsed while she was undergoing a gastroscopy for suspected *Helicobacter pylori* infection (405). Before the start of the procedure she was given lidocaine oral spray and intravenous diazepam 10 mg, and at the end intravenous flumazenil 1 mg. Skin prick tests and intradermal tests with diazepam 5 mg/ml produced a weal-and-flare reaction; flumazenil 0.1 mg/ml and lidocaine 2% had no effect.

Although in the second case, for safety reasons, a challenge test was not performed, it was suggested that the reaction had been IgE-mediated.

Dibromopropamidine

Contact allergy is infrequently reported with dibromopropamidine.

- A 40-year-old man with genital herpes and an acute edematous vesicobullous dermatitis on his penile shaft had a positive patch test with dibromopropamidine and not the other ingredients of the cream (406).

Diclofenac

See NSAIDs

Diethylcarbamazine

Brugia malayi is more susceptible to diethylcarbamazine than *W. bancrofti*. A study of the former, undertaken to explain the very severe effects often associated with diethylcarbamazine treatment of lymphatic filariasis, provided evidence of the involvement of the cytokine interleukin-6 (IL-6), concentrations of which were raised during treatment (407).

The involvement of inflammatory mediators in the development of adverse events has recently been studied in 29 patients with *B. malayi* microfilaremia treated with diethylcarbamazine (408). Before and at serial time points after the start of treatment, plasma concentrations of the inflammatory mediators interleukin-6, interleukin-8, interleukin-10, tumor necrosis factor-alfa, and lipopolysaccharide-binding protein were measured in relation to diethylcarbamazine concentrations and adverse events. The adverse effects of diethylcarbamazine correlated well with pretreatment microfilariae counts, consistent with previous experience with diethylcarbamazine in lymphatic filariasis and onchocerciasis. Concurrent measurements of diethylcarbamazine concentrations failed to establish a clear relation between diethylcarbamazine concentrations and adverse events. Detailed kinetic studies showed the strongest association of the severity of symptoms with interleukin-6 and lipopolysaccharide-binding protein. Concentrations of interleukin-6 started to rise as early as 2–4 hours and reached a maximum after about 8 hours. Fever also occurred at 4–8 hours, consistent with the pyrogenic activity of interleukin-6. In addition, interleukin-6 plays a central role in the induction of the acute phase proteins involved in inflammatory reactions. Indeed, concentrations of the acute phase protein, lipopolysaccharide-binding protein, started to rise at 8 hours (that is after interleukin-6), and also peaked later than interleukin-6, at 24–48 hours after diethylcarbamazine. These observations suggest that the adverse effects of diethylcarbamazine result from an exaggerated host inflammatory response stimulated by a high load of antigen released from killed or degenerating microfilariae.

Diethyl sebacate

There were positive patch tests to diethyl sebacate (10 and 30% in ether and 1 and 10% in petrolatum) in a 48-year-old woman who had been using a topical antimycotic ointment (409).

Diethylstilbestrol

See also Estrogens

Diethylstilbestrol

In 13 women exposed to diethylstilbestrol in utero compared with similar control subjects with respect to the in vitro T cell response to the mitogens phytohemagglutinin, concanavalin A, and interleukin-2, incorporation of tritiated thymidine into T cells from diethylstilbestrol-exposed women was increased three-fold over a range of concentrations in response to concanavalin A, increased by 50% over a range of concentrations in response to phytohemagglutinin, and increased two-fold in response

to the endogenous mitogen interleukin-2 (439). This in vitro evidence of a change in T cell-mediated immunity clearly raises questions about the clinical consequences.

Difetarsone

Generalized angioedema occurred in a patient taking difetarsone 500 mg tds for *Entamoeba histolytica* infection (SEDA-11, 597) (410).

Dihydrocodeine

See Opioid analgesics

Diphencyprone

- Pressure-induced urticaria and widespread severe dermographism developed after the first application to the scalp of a 0.003% solution of diphencyprone in a 19-year-old Japanese man (411). Diphencyprone was withdrawn, but the symptoms persisted for almost 3 months.

An IgE-mediated hypersensitivity reaction was suggested by the authors, but skin tests were not performed and neither was specific IgE measured. A similar case has been described and the adverse events of diphencyprone reviewed (412).

Diphtheria vaccine

See Vaccines

Dipyridamole

Infusion of dipyridamole caused an acute allergic reaction during myocardial scintigraphy (413).

- A 56-year old man with a history of allergy to aspirin, tetracycline, and penicillin, including angioedema and dyspnea, was given a dipyridamole stress test. About 1 minute after the infusion was started he reported periorbital pruritus. The infusion was completed uneventfully with the administration of [99m]technetium sestamibi at 7 minutes. Twenty minutes later he had tightness in the neck, dyspnea, and generalized facial swelling. He was given oxygen and intravenous promethazine hydrochloride and hydrocortisone. He improved over the next 2 hours, with residual periorbital edema but complete recovery from the respiratory symptoms. The cardiac study was completed without further events. The result was normal.

Direct thrombin inhibitors

The effects on activated partial thromboplastin time and the incidence and clinical relevance of antihirudin antibodies in patients treated with lepirudin have been studied using data from two prospective multicenter studies, in which patients with heparin-induced thrombocytopenia received one of four intravenous lepirudin dosage regimens (414). Of 196 evaluable patients, 87 (44%) had IgG antihirudin antibodies. The development of antihirudin antibodies depended on the duration of treatment (antibody-positive patients 18.6 days versus antibody-negative patients 11.6 days). Antihirudin antibodies were not associated with increases in clinical endpoints (limb amputation, new thromboembolic complications, or major bleeding). In 23 of 51 evaluable patients in whom antihirudin antibodies developed during treatment with lepirudin, the antibodies enhanced the anticoagulatory effect of lepirudin. During prolonged treatment with lepirudin, anticoagulatory activity should be monitored daily.

Desirudin has a very low immunogenic potential. During repeated administration to 263 healthy volunteers, there were no signs or symptoms directly attributable to desirudin and only three volunteers exposed to a second course had allergic reactions with pruritic erythema attributable to desirudin in one case (415). In this study, specific antibodies directed against desirudin were detected in only one subject.

Disopyramide

Angioedema has been attributed to disopyramide (416).

Disulfiram

Allergic reactions to disulfiram tend to be limited (417). However, the possibility of hypersensitivity should be borne in mind in patients who have had allergic reactions in the past, regardless of the allergen concerned.

Doxycycline

Renal small-vessel vasculitis related to doxycycline has been reported (418).

Ecstasy

See Methylenedioxymetamphetamine

Edetic acid and its salts

Derivatives of edetic acid are allergenic and can cause allergic reactions, with rashes, fever, edema, and arthralgia. There can be cross-allergy to ethylenediamine, which is a constituent of various drug formulations (for example aminophylline, some ointments) (SED-8, 538). In addition, disodium edetate is found in small amounts in certain drugs, as a result of the removal of trace quantities of heavy metals. However, ethylenediaminetetraacetate was administered for lead poisoning without ill effects to a child with a proven allergy to ethylenediamine hydrochloride (419).

Efavirenz

The incidence of allergic reactions to efavirenz is 10–34%. They usually cause an erythematous maculopapular rash,

with or without fever, 1–3 weeks after the start of therapy. Desensitization has been reported (420).

- A 37-year-old HIV-positive white man was given efavirenz, amprenavir, stavudine, lamivudine, and didanosine after failure of a previous regimen. After 8 days he developed a generalized pruritic rash and all the drugs were withdrawn. Two weeks later he was given efavirenz, stavudine, didanosine, lamivudine, and lopinavir, but developed red itchy skin within a day. All the drugs were withdrawn. He was then successfully restarted on stavudine, didanosine, lamivudine, lopinavir, and amprenavir. Desensitization to efavirenz was undertaken, but on day 12 he again developed a rash on the trunk and limbs, which was treated with a topical steroid and diphenhydramine 45 minutes before each dose of efavirenz. The desensitization protocol was continued for another 4 days, and 16 months later he was taking full-dose efavirenz in combination with the other antiretroviral drugs.

Efavirenz can cause an allergic syndrome called the DRESS syndrome (Drug Rash with Eosinophilia and Systemic Symptoms). It is a life-threatening reaction that typically includes a rash, fever, lymphadenopathy, hepatitis, interstitial nephritis, pneumonia, myocarditis, and hematological abnormalities, particularly eosinophilia and a mononucleosis-like atypical lymphocytosis. The DRESS syndrome has been described in an HIV-infected woman taking efavirenz (421).

- A 44-year-old HIV-1 infected woman from the Ivory Coast, who was taking stavudine, lamivudine, efavirenz, and pyrimethamine plus sulfadiazine for *Toxoplasma* encephalitis, developed a maculopapular rash on both arms. The sulfadiazine was withdrawn and clindamycin was added. Ten days later her condition had worsened. Her temperature was 40 °C, pulse rate 137/minute, and respiratory rate 26/minute. She had a generalized maculopapular rash without mucosal involvement, moderate abdominal tenderness, hepatomegaly, jaundice, and bilateral crackles. Her white cell count was $16 \times 10^9/l$ with 9% eosinophils and 51% lymphocytes. A chest X-ray showed moderate bilateral interstitial pneumonitis. All drugs were withdrawn and she was given intravenous methylprednisolone. The skin rash and all systemic manifestations resolved within 1 week and HIV treatment was restarted uneventfully with lamivudine, stavudine, and nelfinavir.

Although this syndrome has been described with sulfonamides (which the patient had taken), the fact that her condition worsened after withdrawal of sulfadiazine, and the characteristic timing of the syndrome (2–6 weeks after starting a drug), suggested efavirenz as the cause.

- In a 39-year-old man efavirenz caused a confluent maculopapular rash, and pulmonary interstitial infiltrates without lymphadenopathy (422). The symptoms resolved when efavirenz was withdrawn while other antiretroviral drugs were continued. The patient was rechallenged, and the rash and fever reappeared; however, recurrence of the pulmonary infiltrates was not addressed.

A leukocytoclastic vasculitis has been attributed to efavirenz (423).

- A 44-year-old man, having taken various antiretroviral drugs, started to take efavirenz; 5 days later he developed palpable purpura on both legs, with pruritus. His white cell count was $14.4 \times 10^9/l$ and a skin biopsy showed a leukocytoclastic vasculitis. Efavirenz was withdrawn and he was given prednisolone for 3 days; the lesions disappeared, leaving only minimal hyperpigmentation.

Enalapril

See Angiotensin converting enzyme inhibitors

Ephedra, ephedrine, and pseudoephedrine

Pseudoephedrine can cause hypersensitivity, as in three cases reported by allergy specialists from Spain (424).

- A 33-year-old man developed anaphylaxis on a second exposure to pseudoephedrine, having developed urticaria after a first exposure.
- A 24-year-old woman developed severe urticaria and fever, but no other systemic reaction, after a single dose of pseudoephedrine.
- A 67-year-old woman developed urticaria and angioedema of the eyelids after a single dose of pseudoephedrine.

In all three cases skin testing was performed; it was positive in the first two instances but not the third. The authors noted that such cases are reportedly uncommon and that cross-sensitivity is to be expected between pseudoephedrine and ephedrine.

Erythropoietin, epoetin alfa, epoetin beta, epoetin gamma, and darbepoetin

Occasionally low-titer antibodies have been reported in patients treated with epoetin (425,426). Neutralizing anti-erythropoietin antibodies have been found in patients with chronic renal insufficiency who develop pure red cell aplasia after subcutaneous administration of epoetin alfa (especially Eprex). This adverse effect was probably restricted to patients with renal insufficiency because they had used subcutaneous erythropoietin for many years. The incidence was calculated as one in 10 000 patients after 1 year of use of erythropoietin (427–429).

There is no evidence of antibody formation to darbepoetin alfa, probably in part owing to the fact that carbohydrate chains are rarely immunogenic (430–432). No antibodies to darbepoetin alfa were detected in over 1534 patients treated for 2 years (433).

An allergic reaction led to early termination of epoetin treatment in one of 26 pregnant women treated with epoetin for iron deficiency anemia (434).

Anaphylaxis has been observed after the administration of epoetin that contained bovine gelatine as a stabilizer (435). Antibovine gelatine IgE antibodies were found. No anaphylactic reaction was observed after the administration of epoetin that contained human serum albumin as a stabilizer in the same patient.

Estrogens

See also Hormonal contraceptive, Hormone replacement therapy

Estrogens can have adverse immunological effects, which could predispose to infections (436).

The immunological effects of two contraceptive combinations, namely Valette (dienogest 2.0 mg + ethinylestradiol 0.03 mg) and Lovelle (desogestrel 0.15 mg + ethinylestradiol 0.02 mg), have been examined during one treatment cycle (437). Lovelle significantly increased the numbers of lymphocytes, monocytes, and granulocytes. Valette reduced the CD4 lymphocyte count after 10 days and Lovelle did the opposite. Lovelle increased CD19 and CD23 cell counts after 21 days. Phagocytic activity was unaffected by either formulation. After 10 days both contraceptives reduced serum IgA, IgG, and IgM concentrations, which remained low at day 21 with Lovelle but returned to baseline with Valette. Secretory IgA was unaffected by either contraceptive. Neither treatment affected concentrations of interleukins, except for a significant difference between the treatment groups in interleukin-6 after 10 days, which resolved after 21 days. Concentrations of non-immunoglobulin serum components fluctuated; macroglobulin was increased by Valette. However, total protein and albumin concentrations were reduced more by Lovelle than Valette. Complement factors also fluctuated. There was no evidence of sustained immunosuppression with either Valette or Lovelle.

A severe anaphylactic reaction occurred in one patient who was given an intravenous formulation of conjugated estrogens (SED-12, 1033) (438). Some formulations of conjugated estrogens contain foreign (equine) material.

Etacrynic acid

Two patients developed a Henoch-Schönlein type of necrotic hemorrhagic rash of the legs and lower part of the body accompanied by histological evidence of vasculitis (440). In both cases the lesions appeared about 2–3 weeks after the start of treatment; in another case a hemorrhagic rash was accompanied by acute gastric and duodenal ulceration (441).

Etherified starches

Starch derivatives are relatively safer in terms of adverse reactions than other colloid plasma substitutes, but there is an incidence of anaphylactic reactions of 4–6 per million.

- An anaphylactic reaction has been attributed to etherified starches during re-infusion of autologous bone marrow in a man treated for malignant lymphoma (442). The re-infused material had been processed using etherified starches. The patient reported pruritus and carpal spasm. Edema and erythema of the hands were present, together with hypotension and tachycardia. A very small amount of etherified starches was present in the processed bone autograft.

However, in this case other causes such as dimethylsulfoxide (DMSO) or plasma used while processing the autologous bone marrow for freezing could not be excluded.

- A 43-year-old male non-smoker, with a history of asthma, hypertension, and angina pectoris, was admitted to an intensive care unit for mechanical ventilation for acute severe asthma (443). He was given an inhaled bronchodilator, aminophylline, and prednisolone. His condition improved slowly but he became hypovolemic. Within 60 seconds of a fluid challenge with pentastarch 200 ml he had a severe anaphylactoid reaction.

Patients with allergy and atopy have an exaggerated response to chemical mediators released during adverse reactions. The incidence of allergy, atopy, and asthma in patients who have anaphylactic reactions is substantially greater than in non-reacting controls, which may have explained this incident. This sudden unanticipated severe reaction demanded immediate intervention, and its occurrence in a patient with pre-existing bronchospasm posed problems in maintaining ventilation and oxygenation.

Volume therapy with etherified starches in trauma patients results in a reduction in circulating adhesion molecules, an effect that is not observed with albumin infusion (444). Continuous infusion of pentoxifylline did not have a beneficial modulating action on circulating adhesion molecules. Adhesion molecules appear to play an important role in tissue damage secondary to the inflammatory process. Besides neutrophil- and endothelium-bound adhesion molecules, soluble forms have been detected in the circulating blood in trauma patients. They seem to be markers of endothelial damage, but they may also have other biological functions.

Of 1004 patients assessed at least 14 days after starch administration, using a highly sensitive enzyme-linked immunoadsorbent assay technique, one had a low titer (1:10) of etherified starch-reactive antibodies of the immunoglobulin M (IgM) class. Despite repeated infusions, no clinical reaction could be detected in this patient. The authors concluded that antibodies to etherified starches are extremely rare and that they do not necessarily cause anaphylaxis. This low antigenicity of etherified starches might explain their excellent tolerance, compared with other plasma expanders (445).

The reason for the considerable tolerability of etherified starch may be the raw material: etherified starch is synthesized from amylopectin by attaching hydroxyethyl groups. Amylopectin is very similar to glycogen, but whereas glycogen occurs in the cells of warm-blooded organisms, amylopectin is the lower-branched analogue in cells of plant

origin. The human immune system is replete with this molecular structure. This may explain why the etherified starch-induced antibody was directed against the hydroxyethyl group and not against the starch molecule itself.

Ethosuximide

Patients who develop antinuclear antibodies should be watched for the subsequent development of systemic lupus erythematosus (SEDA-19, 67; SEDA-22, 83).

Ethylenediamine

Systemic contact dermatitis is a delayed hypersensitivity skin reaction that results from systemic exposure. Exanthematous systemic contact dermatitis from ethylenediamine has been reported with aminophylline. Disodium edetate (ethylenediamine tetra-acetic acid) has caused contact dermatitis after local application (SEDA-23, 242), and ethylenediamine cross-reacted in a patch test in a patient who had had contact dermatitis with hydroxyzine, an ethylenediamine derivative (SEDA-22, 178). Prior sensitization can occur to ethylenediamine in creams and ointments (SED-14, 485).

Originally described in 1984, baboon syndrome is a form of systemic contact dermatitis involving the buttocks and adjacent skin in a distribution reminiscent of the erythematous buttocks seen in baboons (446). Areas under the underwear, the inner thighs, and the axillae can also be affected. Most cases are caused by oral agents, suggesting that excretion of the antigen may be a factor. In one case systemic administration caused a reaction at a site that may have been previously exposed to topical ethylenediamine (447).

- A 64-year-old man developed a pruritic erythematous eruption in the perineal area a few hours after a stress test, during which he received dipyridamole and intravenous aminophylline. He had a morbilliform erythema of the perineal area under his underclothing anteriorly, with still more prominent erythema posteriorly. The measles-like rash lacked epidermal changes of exudation or scaling. A series of 20 standard patch tests were negative, except for a +++ response to ethylenediamine. On being questioned, he remembered using a topical medicament prescribed for his wife on this area in the distant past. He improved uneventfully with time and avoidance.

The authors proposed that the topical medicament had contained ethylenediamine.

- A 30-year-old woman developed a generalized urticarial reaction immediately after the intravenous administration of aminophylline (448). Skin intradermal testing was positive to ethylenediamine. Rechallenge was positive with intravenous aminophylline but negative with diprophylline, which does not contain ethylenediamine.

Most reports of aminophylline hypersensitivity reactions in the English language literature were delayed reactions. However, most of the Japanese cases were immediate reactions. Acetylation is the main metabolic pathway of ethylenediamine. Most Japanese are rapid or intermediate acetylators, while 50% of Caucasians are slow acetylators. This difference suggests an explanation for the different incidences of immediate and delayed reactions to ethylenediamine in Japanese and Caucasians.

Ethylene oxide

Dialyser hypersensitivity syndrome (SEDA-11, 219; SEDA-11, 479) presents as an acute anaphylactic reaction, the symptoms of which range from mild to life-threatening. The cause of the syndrome is unknown, but affected patients appear to have a high incidence of positive radioabsorbent tests to a conjugate of human serum albumin and ethylene oxide used to sterilize artificial kidneys. This conjugate may be the allergen responsible.

Immediate hypersensitivity reactions occurred in six of 600 donors who underwent automated platelet pheresis; skin-prick testing in four of them (but in none of 40 controls) was positive when an ethylene oxide human serum albumin reagent was used (449). Radioallergosorbent testing showed that serum from four of the six donors, but only one of 145 controls, contained IgE antibodies to ethylene oxide-albumin.

Etomidate

Transient erythema has been described, but histamine release does not occur (450).

Etomidate is the induction agent of choice in atopic patients, in whom etomidate, fentanyl, and vecuronium comprise the safest combination of drugs for general anesthesia. However, non-allergic anaphylactic (anaphylactoid) reactions have been observed, even with this combination (1475,1476), and it can even be life-threatening; one patient also had a myocardial infarction (564).

Euphorbiaceae

Anaphylaxis has been attributed to consumption of whole castor beans (451).

- A 44-year-old woman chewed a castor bean seed and within minutes developed urticaria, drowsiness, Quincke's edema, and extreme hypotension. Her anaphylactic shock was treated with adrenaline, intravenous glucocorticoids, antihistamines, and intravenous fluids. She quickly recovered and a subsequent blood test demonstrated CAP-RAST to castor beans.

Fabaceae

Prolonged ingestion of alfalfa seeds or alfalfa tablets has been associated with the induction or exacerbation of a lupus-like syndrome in humans, perhaps because of the canavanine alfalfa contains (452,453).

Factor VII

The development of antibodies against recombinant factor VIIa or hypersensitivity reactions to normal doses of recombinant factor VIIa have not so far been reported (454). No antibodies against recombinant factor VIIa were observed in a group of 222 hemophilia A and 16 hemophilia B patients with inhibitors treated with high doses of factor VIIa (455). However, antibodies to factor VII have been observed in a patient with factor VII deficiency who received 40 times the recommended dose of recombinant activated factor VIIa (456). Another case of low-titer and transient factor VII antibody formation has been reported in a patient with factor VII deficiency (457).

Factor VIII

There has been some concern about the possible effects of factor VIII formulations on the immune system. In vitro experiments with coagulation factor concentrates have shown immunosuppressive effects (458,459), such as the impairment of Fc receptor-mediated phagocytosis and intracellular bacterial killing (460). Inhibition of IL-2 production, an impaired MLR, and impairment of PHA transformation have been demonstrated (461). A fall in the number of T4 lymphocytes has also been found. Whether these findings reflect functional impairment of the immune system is still unclear.

If the modulation of certain immune functions is in fact due to contaminating components in the preparations, one would expect the new generation of factor VIII preparations of very high purity to behave differently. Highly purified factor VIII with a specific activity of 100–150 U/mg protein is now available, as is factor VIII purified by immunoaffinity chromatography using mouse monoclonal antibodies.

In 58 previously treated patients with hemophilia treated with a recombinant factor VIII product for more than 5 years, there were neither allergic reactions to murine or hamster proteins nor any de novo formation of inhibitors of factor VIII (462).

Antibodies to factor VIII (factor VIII inhibitors)

Patients with bleeding disorders are at risk of developing antibodies against the coagulation protein that is absent, present in reduced amounts, or present in an inactive form in their blood. Such coagulation inhibitors make treatment very difficult. Gene deletions, truncations, and inversions of the factor VIII gene give rise to abnormal forms of the factor VIII protein, resulting in failure to induce tolerance against the normal form of factor VIII (463). Starting with factor VIII treatment at an early age is associated with an increased risk of developing inhibitors (464).

Frequency

Inhibitors of factor VIII are the most common and develop in 5–36% of patients with hemophilia A (465,466). Inhibitors of factor IX develop in 1–8% of patients with hemophilia B (466–468). Frequency varies with age (466). Patients with factor VIII inhibitors present clinically either as "high responders" who show a strong anamnestic response and a sharp rise in inhibitor concentrations after exposure to factor VIII, or "low responders", who show little or no anamnestic response (469).

Following the introduction of recombinant factor products, the incidence of antibody formation seemed to be higher than in patients using plasma products (470). However, after considering factors such as the number of exposure days, the severity of the disease, and the frequency of prospective monitoring, the prevalence and the incidence of antibody formation for both products were similar.

In two studies of previously untreated patients with severe hemophilia, who were given two different recombinant factor VIII products, the incidence of development of an inhibitor was comparable (about 30%) (471).

In 31 previously untreated and minimally treated children with severe hemophilia A, who received full-length recombinant factor VIII (formulated with sucrose) for home therapy and surgery, there was no difference in the incidence of inhibitor formation compared with other recombinant products or plasma-derived products (472).

Factor IX

Allergic and anaphylactic reactions due to factor IX inhibitor have been described (SEDA-21, 343) (473). Anaphylactic reactions occur particularly in patients with undetectable concentrations of factor IX, because of major disruptions in the factor IX gene (474). In patients with factor IX inhibitor, IgG1 subclass antibodies have been found, which may activate complement, resulting in allergic reactions (SEDA-21, 343) (474). However, it has also been suggested that allergic reactions to factor IX products are IgE-mediated.

- In two patients with severe factor IX deficiency and high concentrations of factor IX inhibitors who developed anaphylaxis to factor IX, RAST and skin test reactions to factor IX were positive (474). After desensitization, the circulating IgE antibodies to factor IX fell.

Treatment with high dosages of clotting factors to induce immune tolerance brings a risk of allergic reactions, as has been observed in a 4-year-old child with hemophilia B (475).

Antibodies to factor IX (factor IX inhibitors)

Patients with bleeding disorders are at risk of developing antibodies against the coagulation protein that is absent, present in reduced amounts, or present in an inactive form in their blood. Such coagulation inhibitors make treatment very difficult.

Inhibitors of factor VIII are the most common and develop in 5–15% of patients with hemophilia A. Inhibitors of factor IX develop in 1–4% of patients with hemophilia B (476,477). Patients with hemophilia B with complete gene deletions or derangement of the factor IX gene are particularly at risk of developing antibodies after the administration of factor IX concentrate (478). In patients with hemophilia B with antibodies, treatment with factor IX concentrate can result in an anaphylactic response.

Anaphylaxis in conjunction with inhibitor development has been described. Patients with hemophilia B with complete gene deletions have the greatest risk of anaphylaxis, with a minimum risk of 26%, whereas the risk in patients with null mutations was 2.4% and nearly zero for missense mutations (479). Predisposing factors for the development of anaphylaxis, besides mutation type, are genetic predisposition and environmental experience, such as the type and frequency of factor IX product (479).

Famotidine

See Histamine (H_2) receptor antagonists

Fazadinium

Histamine release from fazadinium is very uncommon, but hypotension associated with an urticarial rash and two cases of severe bronchospasm and cardiac arrest (in patients who had also received thiopental) have been reported (480) as probably being due to fazadinium.

Immunological investigations combined with positive intradermal tests have been used to confirm fazadinium as the causative agent in a severe reaction (481).

Fenfluramines

Shortly after starting dexfenfluramine 30 mg/day, an 18-year-old woman died of sclerodermal renal crisis (482). Although there have been reports linking long-term fenfluramine use and the development of scleroderma (483,484), this is perhaps the first report implicating dexfenfluramine.

Fibrates

Vasculitis, Raynaud's phenomenon, and polyarthritis have been reported with gemfibrozil (485).

Allergic reactions have been reported with some fibrates.

- A 61-year-old woman with penicillin allergy suffered generalized urticaria, chest tightness, wheezing, nausea, vomiting, hypotension, and loss of consciousness (486). Two hours earlier, she had taken Eulitop Retard after lunch. She had intense positive responses to intradermal Eulitop Retard and its active component, bezafibrate; skin tests in control subjects were negative. Specific IgE tests (RAST) to Eulitop Retard were negative. The positive skin tests suggested that an IgE mechanism was responsible for this adverse reaction.

- A 69-year-old woman developed a major allergic reaction after taking fenofibrate 300 mg/day for 10 days (487). The clinical features included weakness, hyperthermia, and slight muscular pain. Biological abnormalities were mildly raised muscle enzymes and pancytopenia, which developed rapidly.

Fibrin glue

An anaphylactic reaction occurred after the use of bovine fibrin glue as a sealant after mastectomy, probably due to the presence of bovine aprotinin (488).

The use of preparations of fibrin glue containing bovine thrombin resulted in the development of antibovine thrombin antibodies. In a prospective study, 13 of 34 patients developed a thrombin inhibitor and reduced factor V activity (489,490). In another study a factor V inhibitor developed after cardiac surgery (491).

Severe hypotension has been reported after the use of bovine fibrin glue for hemostasis in hepatic injury (743). In one there was cardiac arrest and death. These effects may have been the result of an anaphylactic reaction to one or more components of the glue. Of the three ingredients used to prepare fibrin glue, cryoprecipitate and bovine thrombin are antigenic and potentially the most likely causes of anaphylaxis.

Floctafenine

Floctafenine has frequently been associated with anaphylactic reactions (492).

Flucytosine

Anaphylaxis has been reported in a patient with AIDS (493).

Fluoxetine

See Selective serotonin reuptake inhibitors.

Fluoroquinolones

Fluoroquinolones have immunomodulatory effects, at least partly at the gene transcription level, demonstrated by inhibition of cytokine (IL-1α, TNF-α, IL-6, and IL-8) mRNA and cytokine (IL-1α and IL-1β) concentrations by grepafloxacin (1–30 mg/l) in vitro (494).

Anaphylactic shock associated with cinoxacin was reported in three patients by the Netherlands Center for Monitoring of Adverse Reactions to Drugs (495). Another 17 cases were reported to the WHO Collaborating Center for International Drug Monitoring. In some cases the reaction was observed immediately after the first dose of a repeat cycle of treatment. Anaphylactoid reactions to ciprofloxacin have been reported in patients with cystic fibrosis (496–498).

Organ-specific reactions attributed to hypersensitivity involve the liver and kidneys. In one instance centrilobular hepatic necrosis developed during treatment of a urinary tract infection with ciprofloxacin (499). Among 14 cases of drug-induced allergic nephritis, two were associated with quinolones (500). Isolated case reports of allergic nephropathy associated with norfloxacin and ciprofloxacin therapy suggest that this type of reaction is probably very rare (501), since the authors were able to find only 28 other reported cases. If hypersensitivity reactions occur, switching from one quinolone compound to another is probably not advisable, since oral provocation using different agents reproduced the initially observed hypersensitivity reaction (502). This clinical observation is supported by the results of in vitro lymphocyte transformation tests, which were positive with ofloxacin in two patients with allergy to ciprofloxacin (503).

Moxifloxacin

In vitro, moxifloxacin has immunomodulatory activity through its capacity to alter the secretion of IL1-α and TNF-α by human monocytes (504).

Moxifloxacin can cause anaphylactic reactions (505).

A case of simultaneous drug allergies has been reported (506).

- A 32-year-old woman had a generalized urticaria 15 minutes after taking co-amoxiclav and 1 year later developed a non-pruritic micropapular rash some hours after taking moxifloxacin 400 mg.

Pefloxacin

Pefloxacin in suprabactericidal concentrations (2.0 mg/ml and 0.4 mg/ml) markedly suppressed T lymphocyte proliferation in blast transformation; 0.08 mg/ml did not (507). Pefloxacin in a maximal effective dose (200 mg/kg) suppressed delayed hypersensitivity skin reactions in mice.

Flurbiproten

See NSAIDs

Fluvastatin

See HMG coenzyme A reductase inhibitors

Folic acid, folinic acid, and calcium folinate

There have been some reports of hypersensitivity after oral, parenteral, and intradermal administration of folic acid, and a case has recently been reported with folinic acid (508).

- An 80-year-old woman had a colonic resection for Duke's C stage adenocarcinoma and was then given fluorouracil 400 mg/m^2/day and folinic acid 200 mg/m^2/day for 5 days every 4 weeks. She later developed metastases and a second course of chemotherapy included irinotecan (180 mg/m^2), fluorouracil 400 mg/m^2, followed by a continuous infusion of 2400 mg/m^2 over 2 days, folinic acid 200 mg/m^2, ondansetron, and atropine. During the first course of chemotherapy she developed urticaria following the administration of ondansetron and folinic acid. The ondansetron was withdrawn and replaced by metoclopramide and prednisone. During the next course, just after the administration of folinic acid, metoclopramide, and prednisone, she had more urticaria and profound hypotension and required intravenous adrenaline. Folinic acid was withdrawn and subsequent courses were uneventful.

Using a published method (509) the reaction in this case was considered to be very probably due to folinic acid.

IgE-antibodies to folic acid have been demonstrated in a woman with anaphylactic reactions to two multivitamin formulations containing folic acid (510).

Formaldehyde

See also Glutaral

Aldehydes are irritating and sensitizing and cause contact dermatitis in health-care workers (SEDA-21, 254). The incidence of allergy to aldehydes has been examined in 280 health-care workers with skin lesions (511). Allergy was diagnosed in 64 (23%). Most (86%) were sensitive to only one aldehyde. Formaldehyde caused allergy slightly more often (14%) than glutaraldehyde (12%). Only five (1.9%) were sensitive to glyoxal. This hierarchy of sensitivity was also confirmed in animal testing.

Immediate-type allergy to formaldehyde mediated by ice occurred during the use of a formaldehyde reconditioned dialyser in a 20-year-old woman without a personal or familiar history of atopy.

A specific cold agglutinin cross-reacting with anti-N was detected in the sera of 68 (21%) of 325 hemodialysis patients; each had used a dialyser that had been sterilized with formaldehyde. The results of transfusion experiments suggested in vivo hemolytic activity of this antibody. The authors postulated that such in vivo exposure to formaldehyde might make the MN-receptor on erythrocytes immunogenic, thus inducing the formation of the anti-N-like antibody.

The commonly used Clinitest reaction for residual formaldehyde in reused dialysers fails to detect concentrations below 50 ppm (512). The use of Schiff reagent in ratios of 1:1 to 3:1, which can detect formaldehyde at concentrations of 3.6–5.0 ppm, has therefore been recommended (SEDA-12, 571; 513). It can also be used in combination with a glucose-containing dialysate.

Fosfomycin

The immunomodulatory effect of fosfomycin may in part be explained by an effect on cytokine production, as shown in mice in vivo (514).

Fragrances

Contact sensitivity to fragrance mix is not infrequent and reflects the ubiquitous presence of these substances (515). The frequency of positive patch tests to the fragrance mix has increased over recent years. However, the mix has been estimated to miss 15% of relevant contact allergies (516). In a study of 1855 consecutive patients, patch tests with additional fragrance allergens has shown that lyral (2.7% positive reactions), citral (1.1%), and farnesol P (0.5%) are valuable additions when patch-testing to detect a fragrance allergy. Several other compounds that were tested at the same time were positive less often (517). A similar study in 1606 consecutively tested patients showed that ylang-ylang oil I (2.6% positive patch tests), ylang-ylang oil II (2.5%), lemongrass oil (1.6%), narcissus absolute (1.3%), jasmine absolute (1.2%), and sandalwood oil (0.9%) are the most important ingredients (518). In this series, limonene was positive in 0.6% of cases, but in another series of 2273 consecutive patients it was positive in 2.8%, of whom 57% did not react to the fragrance mix (519).

These and other compounds were patch-tested in another series of fragrance-sensitive patients (520). Of the 218 subjects tested, 76% were positive to the fragrance mix. Ten fragrances were not detected by the fragrance mix: benzenepropanol; beta, beta, 3-methylhexylsalicylate; dl-citronellol; synthetic ylang-ylang oil; benzyl mixture (containing benzyl alcohol, benzyl salicylate, and benzyl acetate); cyclohexylacetate; eugenyl methyl ether; isoeugenyl methyl ether; 3-phenyl-1-propanol; and 3,7-dimethyl-7-methoxyoctan-2-ol. In earlier studies by this group, significant additional reactions were found to sandela, geranium oil bourbon, spearmint oil, galaxolide (1,3,4,6,7,8-hexahydro-4,6,6,7,8,8-hexamethyl-cyclopenta-gamma-2-benzopyran), omega-6-hexadecenlactone, and tripal (dimethyltetrahydrobenzaldehyde) (521,522).

Patients with chronic venous insufficiency and venous leg ulcers are at risk of sensitization to topical medications. The frequency of sensitization in these patients is up to 67% (523). In a study using an expanded European standard series and 20 different wound dressings for patch-testing in 36 patients with chronic venous insufficiency, sensitization to fragrance mix was found in three cases (524).

Furaltadone

Furaltadone can provoke contact allergic reactions (525). A case of contact allergy to the antibiotic in eardrops, with positive patch tests, has been reported (526).

Furosemide

It has long been thought that loop and thiazide diuretics pose a theoretical risk of cross-sensitivity in patients with sulfonamide allergy because of their common structures. However, the available literature does not provide sufficient numbers of well-documented cases to support this impression (529). It seems that careful administration of

diuretics is permissible in patients with documented sulfonamide allergy, but as always such a drug challenge
should not be attempted without careful follow-up. A
furosemide rechallenge protocol, based on a method
that has been used to rechallenge with a sulfa-containing
antimicrobial agent, safely allowed the long-term reinstitution of loop diuretic therapy with furosemide (530).

Fusidic acid

Fusidic acid may have an immunomodulatory effect that
seems to be partly mediated by suppression of cytokine
production. The effect on several diseases has been investigated, but it remains to be characterized more in detail
whether there is any therapeutic usefulness (527).

Positive patch tests occurred in three of 1119 patients
who had used topical fusidic acid (528). In the second part
of this study, all cases of positive patch tests to fusidic acid
over the previous 20 years were reviewed; the average
frequency was 1.62 patch-tested patients per year (1.45%)
of those who were patch-tested.

Gabapentin

- A hypersensitivity syndrome secondary to gabapentin
  has been described in a 72-year-old patient after 9 days
  (531). The symptoms (altered mental status, fever, diffuse macular rash, and an enlarged spleen) resolved
  after withdrawal.

However, the concomitant use of levofloxacin made the
association of gabapentin with the hypersensitivity syndrome unclear.

Gallamine triethiodide

Histamine release may be associated with the use of
gallamine more often than was previously believed,
according to several studies involving large numbers of
patients (532–534,535). There have been several reports
of reactions involving skin flushing, bronchospasm, or
cardiovascular collapse possibly due to gallamine, including anaphylactoid reactions to small precurarizing doses
(536,537).

Gallium

- A 40-year-old woman had multiple bone injuries,
  severe sepsis, and coma after a car accident; a retroperitoneal hematoma caused by lumbar fractures was
  drained, but she continued to be pyrexial (538). She had
  prominent accumulation of ^{67}Ga, which had been used
  for bone scanning, in her multiple recent fractures and
  an area of accumulation in the soft tissue related to a
  fractured vertebra. Post-traumatic paravertebral calcifications had accumulated ^{67}Ga and simulated the presence of an infected hematoma.

Gemcitabine

Two patients developed necrotizing enterocolitis after a
first cycle of chemotherapy for epithelial ovarian/perito-
neal cancer; both were due to vasculitis (539).

- In a 56-year-old man with a transitional cell carcinoma
  of the bladder gemcitabine plus cisplatin caused extensive necrotizing vasculitis with muscle damage after the
  second course of therapy (540). Chemotherapy was
  withdrawn immediately but the symptoms of severe
  myalgia and swelling persisted, and he needed additional treatment, consisting of cyclophosphamide and
  prednisolone.

Other cases of vasculitis have been reported (541).

- A 70-year-old woman with a bladder cancer was given
  gemcitabine 1700 mg on days 1 and 8 and 3–4 days later
  developed paresthesia of the fingers, Raynaud's phenomenon, an intermittent fever, digital necrosis, and
  fingertip gangrene (542). Angiography showed occlusion of the digital arteries of the second, third, and
  fourth fingers. Skin biopsy showed hyperkeratosis,
  acanthosis, and papillomatosis, with endothelioangiitis
  and non-specific arterial inflammation.

Radiation recall consists of inflammatory reactions triggered by cytotoxic drugs in previously irradiated areas;
most are skin reactions. Gemcitabine has been implicated
in several cases. The authors of a literature review discovered 12 cases of radiation recall caused by gemcitabine
and reported a case of myositis in the rectus abdominis
muscle of a patient with pancreatic adenocarcinoma as an
effect of radiation recall (543). Most of the cases had
inflammation of internal organs or tissues and 30% had
dermatitis or mucositis. This is different from the effect of
other agents that commonly cause radiation recall
(anthracyclines and taxanes), with which 63% are skin
reactions. Compared with anthracyclines and taxanes,
the interval from the completion of radiation therapy to
the start of chemotherapy is less with gemcitabine (median time 56 days, compared with 218 days for the taxanes
and 646 days for doxorubicin).

General anesthetics

The issue of hypersensitivity reactions during general
anesthesia is a matter of concern. However, despite considerable work on the subject, there is divergence in interpretation (544). In patients with no pre-anesthetic
immunological anomaly, general anesthesia is unlikely
to affect immune status significantly (545).

Widespread erythema and edema, the most dangerous
form of which affects the glottis, occur in some cases of
hypersensitivity. Hypotension is also seen, together with
compensatory tachycardia. Bronchospasm is a common
respiratory finding (546).

There were significant immunological changes in the
peripheral blood film of personnel working in

unscavenged operating theaters in Croatia (547). Some of the effects persisted beyond a 4-week period away from that environment.

In a review of 23 444 anesthetics given during 12 months, one patient in 630 had generalized erythema and edema and one in 1230 had erythema and hypotension (548). One patient died of shock. Female patients aged 15–25 with a history of allergy, subjects with excessive anxiety, and those who had previously undergone general anesthesia had a statistically significant higher risk of developing non-allergic anaphylactic reactions. The incidence of allergic anaphylactic reactions (with IgE antibodies) is said to be one in 4500–20 000 general anesthetics per year (549). However, the diagnosis is often missed (550).

The patient's history is hardly helpful; neither the presence nor the absence of a previous reaction gives guidance as to the likelihood of its occurring on future exposure. The mechanisms underlying such reactions may or may not involve histamine release, but the distinction between allergic anaphylactic and non-allergic anaphylactic (anaphylactoid) reactions is often unclear, for lack of definitive and easily available investigations. Furthermore, because anesthetic drugs are often given rapidly and in combination, it can be impossible to decide which was responsible for the reaction. Intradermal injection of a test dose is of limited predictive value (551); false-positive and false-negative results are often obtained, particularly with opiates, tubocurarine, and atracurium. What is more, the test is dose-dependent and can itself precipitate a hypersensitivity reaction (552). It has been suggested that leukocyte histamine release on exposure to drugs can be used in combination with paper radioallergosorbent testing for IgE antibodies, to detect the precise cause of any anaphylactic reaction: these techniques point to neuromuscular blocking drugs as being most commonly implicated in anaphylaxis (551).

In a French study, 1585 patients underwent diagnostic investigations after anaphylactic shock during anesthesia; 813 of them had a reaction of immunological origin. The drugs involved were muscle relaxants (70%), latex (13%), anesthetic drugs (5.6%), opioids (1.7%), colloids (4.7%), and antibiotics (2.6%) (575). Among the 45 patients in whom anesthetics were involved, the agents implicated were thiopental ($n = 18$), propofol ($n = 10$), ketamine ($n = 1$), midazolam ($n = 7$), diazepam ($n = 5$), and flunitrazepam ($n = 4$). These data did not differ from those reported in a UK study (575). In both studies there was a high proportion of cases in which muscular relaxants were used alongside anesthetics, resulting in a two-fold risk of hypersensitivity.

Gentamicin

Allergic contact dermatitis due to gentamicin is rare in patients with eyelid dermatitis, but it can occur.

- A 55-year-old housewife developed pruritic, erythematous, scaly plaques on the eyelids, spreading in a few days periorbitally after treatment with gentamicin eye-

drops (Colircusi Gentamicina) (553). A positive patch test reaction to kanamycin, to which the patient had not been previously exposed, suggested cross-reactivity.

Glafenine

Although rash has sometimes occurred (554), hypersensitivity reactions have been much more serious. Many acute anaphylactic reactions have been observed (SEDA-4, 69; SEDA-6, 98; 555,556), with shock in more than 50% of cases; it was recorded in 24 of 1517 reports on the drug collected by the Pharmacovigilance Unit in Lyons, France (554). Occasional isolated fever, confirmed by rechallenge (557), is probably also of hypersensitive origin. Interstitial nephritis, hepatitis, and pulmonary hypersensitivity have been reported.

Glues

Two patients developed severe type I allergic reactions to a hair bond.

- A 37-year-old atopic patient had generalized pruritus, diffuse urticaria, angioedema, rhinoconjunctivitis, and tachycardia within minutes of having glued a hair bond to her scalp. Skin tests with the glue (diluted 1:10 000 in saline) were positive, as was an IgE RAST on latex proteins (558).
- A 40-year-old woman noted palmar irritation, followed by generalized pruritus, a feeling of faintness, facial edema, and difficulty in breathing. A latex skin prick test was positive (559).

Glutaral

See also Formaldehyde

Aldehydes are irritating and sensitizing and cause contact dermatitis in health-care workers (SEDA-21, 254). The incidence of allergy to aldehydes has been examined in 280 health-care workers with skin lesions (560). Allergy was diagnosed in 64 (23%). Most (86%) were sensitive to only one aldehyde. Formaldehyde caused allergy slightly more often (14%) than glutaral (12%). Only 5 (1.9%) were sensitive to glyoxal. This hierarchy of sensitivity was also confirmed in animal testing.

Anaphylaxis occurred in a woman after the fourth intramuscular injection of a glutaral-containing pollen formulation (SEDA-11, 478; 561).

Glycols

Polyethylene glycol has reportedly caused anaphylaxis (SEDA-20, 440).

Propylene glycol can be used in allergic individuals, although propylene glycol itself can cause allergic skin reactions. The incidence of propylene glycol allergy among patients with eczema is thought to be greater than 2% (562). Used in dermatological formulations, propylene glycol can occasionally perpetuate eczema in hypersensitive patients (563).

Gold and gold salts

Several patients with selective IgA deficiency and even a panhypogammaglobulinemia during intramuscular gold treatment have been described (SEDA-14, 190; SEDA-15, 230; SEDA-21, 237).

Polyarteritis (564) and systemic lupus erythematosus (565) have been reported after the administration of gold compounds.

- After taking sodium aurothiomalate for 10 months (cumulative dose 550 mg) a 12-year-old girl with severe exudative polyarthritis developed pericarditis, high titers of antinuclear antibodies, and antibodies to native double-stranded DNA (565). After withdrawal her symptoms rapidly disappeared and did not recur after a follow-up period of 5 years. The titers of autoantibodies fell to normal within 1 year.

In one series of some 5500 patients with juvenile rheumatoid arthritis, 105 were found to have developed secondary amyloidosis; 37 of the latter had been receiving sodium aurothiomalate. In 12 of these children the time between withdrawal of gold (because of adverse effects) and the finding of amyloid A was less than six months (SEDA-21, 237).

- A 63-year-old woman with rheumatoid arthritis was given intramuscular gold sodium thiomalate and began to have nausea, vomiting, anorexia, and watery diarrhea (566). A year later the watery diarrhea became more frequent (more than 10 times within a day) and she developed proteinuria. Biopsies from the stomach, duodenum, and kidney showed systemic amyloidosis. This was a rare case of secondary systemic amyloidosis associated with rheumatoid arthritis. It is not clear from the report what the role of gold was in this case.

Gonadorelin

Altered immune function has been reported in several cases associated with gonadorelin agonist therapy. This is possibly related to the initial surge in sex steroids that occurs with these agents, but there is no evidence that this is the mechanism. Cardiac allograft rejection occurred in three men within months of starting gonadorelin therapy for prostate cancer. One died of heart failure, but the other two recovered cardiac function after the gonadorelin agonist was withdrawn (567).

Systemic lupus erythematosus can be exacerbated in the initial gonadotropin-stimulating phase of gonadorelin therapy: in one case this was fatal (568).

Gonadotropins

Gonadotropins of natural origin contain various allergens, which can give rise to hypersensitivity reactions.

This was a serious problem with the "PMS" gonadotropin formulations formerly made from the serum of pregnant mares but now apparently obsolete; it was also described in the past with an FSH formulation of porcine origin. However hypersensitivity reactions can also occur to extracts of human material.

- A generalized allergic reaction to human menopausal gonadotropin (Pergonal) has been described during controlled ovarian hyperstimulation (569). In this case a desensitization protocol allowed the patient to complete her treatment cycle without further problems. Subsequently recombinant follicle stimulating hormone was used successfully and uneventfully.

On occasion, there have even been such reactions to highly purified human products, notably FSH; they can be managed by changing the treatment to intramuscular recombinant follicle stimulating hormone (570).

Granulocyte colony-stimulating factor (G-CSF)

Leukocytoclastic vasculitis is a well-described and confirmed adverse effect of G-CSF, as documented in several reports, with recurrence after renewed administration of G-CSF (SEDA-19, 343). Most cases were confined to the skin, and renal insufficiency with hematuria and proteinuria was noted in only very few patients. Based on 18 cases reported in the literature or to the manufacturers, vasculitis was thought to have occurred in 6% of patients with chronic benign neutropenia, but in only six of about 200 000 patients with malignant disease (571). Vasculitis usually developed when the neutrophil count rose above $800 \times 10^6/l$, suggesting that an increase in neutrophil count may play a role in necrotic vasculitis. Against this background, the occurrence of vasculitis is not considered as treatment-limiting and does not preclude further G-CSF administration if the absolute neutrophil count is lower than $1000 \times 10^6/l$.

Antibodies to rG-CSF have not so far been reported, even in patients on long-term treatment.

Exacerbation of lupus-like symptoms, with seizures, psychosis, and vasculitis, has been noted during three of 12 treatment courses in neutropenic patients with severe systemic lupus erythematosus (572).

Type I reactions

Although IgE-specific antibodies have not been yet detected, filgrastim is undoubtedly associated with type I allergic reactions. This has been illustrated in well-documented reports of anaphylactic reactions, urticaria, and angioedema, with positive intradermal tests in several patients (SEDA-20, 338; 573,574). However, anaphylaxis to G-CSF is supposedly rare and the manufacturer is aware of only two cases of anaphylactoid reactions among 20 000 patients treated with filgrastim (575). One report has suggested possible cross-reactivity between filgrastim and other products derived from *Escherichia coli* (576). Although one patient who developed an anaphylactic-like reaction, with dyspnea, hypotension, and a pruritic erythematous skin rash, within minutes of G-CSF injection, later tolerated GM-CSF uneventfully (577), possible cross-reactivity between G-CSF and GM-CSF has been reported in at least one patient (578).

Granulocyte–macrophage colony-stimulating factor (GM-CSF)

Hypersensitivity reactions

Although anaphylactic reactions without any documented immune-mediated mechanism have been reported in about 8% of patients with testicular cancer given GM-CSF (579), GM-CSF has only otherwise rarely been associated with allergic reactions. Of two patients who had possible immune-mediated reactions (SEDA-19, 342) one had an immediate recurrent local reaction followed by systemic hypersensitivity reaction after sargramostim, and the other had a maculopapular pruritic eruption after molgramostim. Cross-reaction between the two recombinant forms of GM-CSF was suggested by the results of skin prick tests in one patient, but both patients thereafter tolerated filgrastim uneventfully.

However, cross-sensitivity and possible desensitization have been documented.

- A 42-year-old woman with defective immunological function had generalized pruritus, flushing, shortness of breath, and general discomfort within 30 minutes of her 16th intravenous injection of molgramostim (580). Her symptoms resolved with adrenaline, hydrocortisone, and promethazine. Despite the prophylactic use of glucocorticoids and antihistamines, she developed a similar reaction after molgramostim readministration and 4 hours after the fourth injection of filgrastim. Positive skin prick tests to molgramostim and filgrastim suggested IgE-mediated hypersensitivity. An acute desensitization protocol starting with molgramostim 0.0008 micrograms increasing to 320 micrograms was successful, and molgramostim was later continued uneventfully.

Griseofulvin

The triggering of a lupus-like syndrome by griseofulvin, by way of an allergic reaction, has been described, but is rare (581).

Guar gum

Guar gum can cause occupational rhinitis (582) and asthma (583). Of 162 employees at a carpet-manufacturing plant where guar gum was used to adhere dye to the fiber, 37 (23%) had a history suggestive of occupational asthma and 59 (36%) occupational rhinitis (584). Eight (5%) had immediate skin reactivity to guar gum and 11 (8.3%) had serum IgE antibodies to guar gum.

An employee of a pet food plant developed a severe cough, rhinitis, and conjunctivitis, and skin tests confirmed guar allergy. The symptoms resulted in obstructive sleep apnea which resolved after absence from work and recurred after rechallenge with guar gum dust (585).

Gum resins

In a retrospective study, 1270 patients with leg ulcers were tested for contact allergy with colophonium and the modified ester gum: 31 patients were positive to colophonium alone, 41 to the ester gum alone, and 33 to both colophonium and the ester gum (586). The authors recommended that the patch test tray for patients with leg ulcers should include both colophonium and the ester gum resin.

Two other patients with cheilitis due to contact allergy to a lipstick reacted positively to glyceryl hydrogenated rosinate, an ester gum, and the main component of the rosinate, glyceryl abietate (both patchtested at 20% in petrolatum) (587).

Hair dyes

Allergic reactions to constituents of hair dyes are not uncommon and are generally due to delayed hypersensitivity. Immediate hypersensitivity reactions have been described, but they are rare and seldom life-threatening.

Contact allergy to the paraphenylene group of hair dyes is well established (588). To test for cross-reactivity between these oxidative dyes and the new generation of hair dyes, 40 hairdressers allergic to paraphenylenediamine were selected; none reacted to any of the four acid dyes, two FD&C dyes, or four D&C dyes, suggesting that these newer hair dyes are safe alternatives to the paraphenylene-based hair dyes (589).

There is a risk of sensitization from paraphenylenediamine when it is applied to the skin in combination with henna (590–592). This can result in contact allergic reactions as well as persistent contact leukoderma, as illustrated in five patients with paint-on henna tattoos (593). All were positive on patch-testing with paraphenylenediamine. One developed erythema multiforme 4 weeks after the last application and the authors found no other causes of erythema multiforme.

The use of the combination of henna and paraphenylenediamine in 20 cases over 2 years in Khartoum (Sudan) resulted in severe toxicity (SEDA-9, 142). The initial symptoms were those of angioedema, with massive edema of the face, lips, glottis, pharynx, neck, and bronchi. These occurred within hours of the application of the dye-mix to the skin. In some the symptoms progressed on the second day to anuria and acute renal insufficiency, with death on the third day. Dialysis helped some patients, but others died from renal tubular necrosis.

The oxidation product of paratoluenediamine has been identified as a rare cause of a life-threatening immediate hypersensitivity reaction (594).

- A 45-year-old woman developed extensive urticarial lesions 30 minutes after the application of a hair dye, starting on the scalp and face, followed by abdominal cramps, watery diarrhea, vomiting, dysphonia, and loss of consciousness. A prick test with a 1/128 dilution of the hair dye showed a positive reaction, but individual dye constituents did not. Prick testing with the oxidation products of the individual dye constituents showed a strongly positive reaction to oxidized paratoluenediamine, which was weaker after addition of an antioxidant to the mixture.

Ten healthy controls had negative prick tests with the oxidized paratoluenediamine.

Halofantrine

Anaphylactic shock has been attributed to halofantrine (595).

Halothane

Halothane can suppress host defence mechanisms; the clinical consequences are unclear (SED-11, 210; SEDA-3, 101; SEDA-4, 77; SEDA-5, 121; SEDA-11, 109).

Heparins

A wide range of allergic reactions have been described in patients receiving heparin, including urticaria, conjunctivitis, rhinitis, asthma, cyanosis, tachypnea, a feeling of oppression, fever, chills, angioedema, and anaphylactic shock.

• A patient with end-stage renal disease developed recurrent anaphylaxis after receiving heparin during hemodialysis (596). There were raised concentrations of total and mature tryptase at 1 hour, but although the latter returned to normal by 24 hours the former did not. Prick tests were negative with heparin, enoxaparin, and danaparoid, but intradermal skin tests were positive with heparin and enoxaparin. Danaparoid was used as an anticoagulant during dialysis for the next 3 years without any adverse effects.

In some cases of allergy to a heparin formulation, the precipitating agent will prove to be a preservative, such as chlorocresol (597) or chlorbutol (598), rather than heparin itself.

Hepatitis vaccines

Hepatitis A

Vasculitis suspected to be caused by the first dose of hepatitis A vaccine has been reported (SEDA-21, 331).

Hexanetriol

• A 35-year-old woman had a 3-week history of pruritic erythema, edema, and linear vesiculation of the upper arms where she had applied fluocinonide cream (599).

Patch tests with the cream were positive, but the active ingredient fluocinonide (0.05% in petrolatum) was negative, while 1,2,6-hexanetriol 5% showed strong positive reactions on days 3 and 7.

Histamine (H₂) receptor antagonists

Early studies suggested an increased risk of nosocomial pneumonia associated with H_2 receptor antagonists in critically ill patients. To investigate this further, two randomized studies have been performed. One compared ranitidine (0.25 mg/kg/hour intravenously) with sucralfate (1 g every 6 hours via nasogastric tube) for prophylaxis against stress-induced gastritis in 96 severely injured patients (600). Ranitidine was associated with a 1.5 times increased risk of developing any infection compared with sucralfate. Furthermore, of the 49 patients who received ranitidine, 14 developed 26 separate episodes of pneumonia, while of the 47 patients who received sucralfate, 10 developed 14 episodes of pneumonia. The other study, placebo-controlled, compared intravenous ranitidine (50 mg tds) and pirenzepine (10 mg tds) in 158 patients who were being mechanically ventilated; the pneumonia rates were similar in the three groups (601).

In another study of stress ulcer prophylaxis, 53 critically ill patients were randomized to receive sucralfate 1 g 6-hourly, cimetidine 300 mg 8-hourly, or cimetidine 900 mg/day by continuous intravenous infusion (602). Although bacterial colonization was increasingly likely in patients with a persistent alkaline gastric environment, gastric luminal pH and the degree of bacterial colonization of the stomach were similar in the three groups.

Vasculitis occurred in a patient taking famotidine who had tolerated cimetidine well (603).

HMG coenzyme-A reductase inhibitors

Lupus-like symptoms have been reported in patients taking statins (604).

Atorvastatin

A hypersensitivity reaction to atorvastatin has been reported.

• Antinuclear and antihistone antibodies developed in a 26-year-old man who was taking atorvastatin (605). He had constitutional symptoms and slight headaches but no definite symptoms of lupus. After some months without medication he became seronegative and asymptomatic.

This case was similar to other previous reports with other statins.

Fluvastatin

• A 67-year-old woman had a fatal reaction 1 week after she started to take fluvastatin 20 mg/day. When the drug was withdrawn 10 weeks later, she had arthralgia, myalgia, an erythematous maculopapular rash, and breathlessness due to a widespread alveolitis (606).

Lovastatin

There were 25 serious hypersensitivity reactions (such as arthralgia and thrombocytopenia) among the first million patients taking lovastatin; at least some of these were considered to be due to the drug (607).

Simvastatin

Lupus-like syndrome has been associated with simvastatin, with antibodies to double-stranded DNA in the serum (608).

- Simvastatin-induced lupus erythematosus was suspected in a 79-year-old white man after 3 months (609). He had signs of pleuropericarditis that resolved within 2 weeks of withdrawal.

Hormonal contraceptives—oral

There is a sex difference in immune responsiveness, but little attention has been paid to the possible role played by sex hormones in its regulation. This lack of insight has led to the question of whether the use of oral contraceptives might affect the immune response, for better or for worse. An authoritative review of the immunological effects of estrogens and progestogens has concluded that, although understanding of any effect is incomplete, it is not likely that the low doses used in oral contraceptives would have negative effects on the immune system (610).

If that is the case, there must be another explanation for periodic reports that suggest an increased risk of systemic infections in oral contraceptive users. In a 1974 study by the British Royal College of General Practitioners oral contraceptive users had a higher than average incidence of certain infectious diseases (611).

Support for the concept that oral contraceptives might increase the risk of infection has been presented in other studies, and workers in the tropics have remarked that pregnant women appear to be unduly sensitive to malarial infestation (WHO, unpublished data).

The antibody response to tetanus toxoid in women is considerably lower in oral contraceptive users than in controls (612).

A depressed lymphocyte response to phytohemagglutinin has been observed in a series of women taking oral contraceptives (613); the reduction in phytohemagglutinin response reflects impaired T cell function, and this finding is of interest in view of the fact that a deficiency of T cell function is important in certain autoimmune diseases. Another consequence of prolonged impairment of T cell function would be an increased susceptibility to infectious diseases.

There have been several studies of the effect of sex hormones on serum immunoglobulin titers. In a study of the effect of four different oral contraceptives on the serum concentration of IgA, IgG, and IgM, the concentrations of all three immunoglobulins fell during the first course of treatment and returned to normal

during subsequent cycles (614). There was some evidence that the steroid-induced reduction in immunoglobulins was predominantly caused by the estrogenic component. Subsequently, a study was conducted in which plasma from women currently taking combined oral contraceptives, past users of such products, women who had never used them, and non-users with a history of venous thrombosis was examined for the presence of immunoglobulin G (IgG) that showed specific binding of ethinylestradiol (615). There was no increase in "specific" IgG and no evidence of ethinylestradiol binding in oral contraceptive users compared with non-users. This study therefore provided no support for the hypothesis that a significant percentage of oral contraceptive users develop a specific IgG with high binding affinity for ethinylestradiol, which might be causally linked to the development of thrombotic phenomena in oral contraceptive users.

Numerous case reports have suggested that combined oral contraceptives can cause systemic lupus erythematosus (616,617). However, systematic examination of this issue in a 1994 case-control study showed no association (618).

Aggravation of bronchial asthma, eczema, rashes, angioedema, and vasomotor rhinitis have been incidentally observed, and cold urticaria has been reported in women taking oral contraceptives (619). It is not known whether in any particular individual the hypersensitivity reaction is due to the hormones themselves or to other ingredients in the tablet. Nasal provocation tests with suspensions of contraceptive steroids in patients with allergic rhinitis or pollinosis who had been taking these products showed a positive response in one-third of cases; the same patients also reacted to topical estrogens (620). Life-threatening anaphylaxis with a positive rechallenge test occurred in a young woman using oral contraceptives, but this must be extraordinarily rare (621).

The immunological effects of two contraceptive combinations, namely Valette (ethinylestradiol 0.03 mg + dienogest 2.0 mg) and Lovelle (ethinylestradiol 0.02 mg + desogestrel 0.15 mg), have been examined during one treatment cycle (622). The latter significantly increased the numbers of lymphocytes, monocytes, and granulocytes. Valette reduced the CD4 lymphocyte count after 10 days and Lovelle did the opposite. Lovelle increased CD19 and CD23 cell counts after 21 days. Phagocytic activity was unaffected by either treatment. After 10 days, both contraceptives reduced the serum concentrations of IgA, IgG, and IgM, which remained low at day 21 with Lovelle but returned to baseline with Valette. Secretory IgA was unaffected by either contraceptive. Neither treatment affected concentrations of interleukins, except for a significant difference between the treatment groups in interleukin-6 after 10 days, which resolved after 21 days. Concentrations of non-immunoglobulin serum components fluctuated; macroglobulin was increased by Valette. However, total protein and albumin concentrations were reduced more by Lovelle than Valette. Complement factors also fluctuated. There was no evidence of sustained immunosuppression with either Valette or Lovelle.

Hormone replacement therapy—estrogens

Two healthy young women took estrogen supplements for some 3 years and then developed classic Sjögren's syndrome (623). The syndrome was most severe in the woman who had taken the higher dose. These cases seem to have confirmed earlier reports that estrogens can play a role in the pathogenesis of Sjögren's syndrome in susceptible patients.

Hyaluronic acid

Immediate and delayed hypersensitivity reactions have been reported with hyaluronic acid (624).

Hydralazine

The lupus-like syndrome (SED-9, 318) with hydralazine occurs particularly in slow acetylators (and only rarely in fast acetylators) and in patients with the HLA-DR4 antigen. Blood dyscrasias and necrotizing vasculitis are additional features.

Current knowledge about the possible mechanisms of drug-induced lupus-like syndrome has been reviewed (625). Three mechanisms seem most plausible. One involves a change, possibly caused by a reactive metabolite, in the way that antigens are processed and presented to T cells, leading to the presentation of cryptic antigens. Another possibility is that a reactive metabolite binds to the class II major histocompatibility antigen and induces an autoimmune reaction analogous to a graft-versus-host reaction. A third possibility is that hydralazine inhibits DNA methylation, leading to an increase in DNA transcription and a generalized activation of the immune system.

A variety of vasculitic diseases, including Wegener's granulomatosis, microscopic polyangiitis, Churg–Strauss syndrome, and crescentic glomerulonephritis, are associated with antineutrophil cytoplasmic antibodies (ANCA) or leukocytoclastic vasculitis. In drug-induced ANCA-positive vasculitis, antimyeloperoxidase antibodies are most often found; they produce a perinuclear pattern of staining by indirect immunofluorescence (pANCA), but antiproteinase 3 (anti-PR3) antibodies can also occur (cANCA).

The possible drug causes of ANCA-positive vasculitis with high titers of antimyeloperoxidase antibodies in 30 new patients have been reviewed (626). The findings illustrate that this type of vasculitis is a predominantly drug-induced disorder. Only 12 of the 30 cases were not related to a drug. The most frequently implicated drug was hydralazine (10 cases); the remainder involved propylthiouracil (3 cases), penicillamine (2 cases), allopurinol (2 cases), and sulfasalazine.

Hydroxycarbamide

Hydroxycarbamide has been associated with Behçet's syndrome (627).

Hydroxytoluene

It is impossible to decide from experimental findings in animals what the result will be of prolonged human exposure to low concentrations of such substances. Butylated hydroxytoluene causes various allergies; symptoms of hay fever and asthma have been reported.

Chewing gum should be considered as a possible cause of unexplained food allergy.

- Butylated hydroxytoluene in chewing gum caused disseminated urticarial eruption in a young woman (628). An adverse drug reaction was ruled out, and the only recent dietary change had been regular use of chewing-gum containing butylated hydroxytoluene. The skin lesions showed signs of vasculitis, with a perivascular cellular infiltrate, heavy extravascular deposition of fibrinogen, and intraendothelial deposits of IgM, C'9, C3, and C9. She stopped using the gum and within a week the eruption had subsided. An oral provocation test confirmed that butylated hydroxytoluene was responsible, the cutaneous signs returning within several hours of rechallenge.

Hyoscine

An isolated case of angioedema has been described during the use of hyoscine butylbromide (SEDA-8, 148).

Ibuprofen

See NSAIDs

Indometacin

See NSAIDs

Influenza vaccine

See Vaccines

Insulin

Insulin allergy is quite common (SEDA-7, 403; 629–631). Allergy has been reported to human insulin and protamine (632) and to human insulin (633,634).

- A 41-year-old woman became allergic to all types of insulin (beef, pork, human, lente, etc.). She had used insulin for the first time during pregnancy and was intermittently treated unsatisfactorily with oral agents. She used lispro insulin for more than 6 months without an allergic reaction.
- A 54-year-old woman with gestational diabetes was later found to be allergic to chromium, pollen, dust, penicillin, acarbose, and metformin (635). She was treated with diet and glibenclamide, but later required insulin. With Humulin N insulin she developed a wheal of 15 mm immediately after the injection, which resolved in a few hours. However, a painful itchy

induration appeared 2–3 hours after the injection and lasted a few days. She had an immediate reaction to isophane insulin, with induration, but insulin lispro was well-tolerated.

- A 5-year-old child with diabetes, Pierre Robin syndrome, cleft palate, allergic rhinitis, recurrent sinusitis, and obstructive sleep apnea, who had previously had skin rashes after penicillin, sulfonamides, and clindamycin, was given soluble and isophane human insulins (636). Three years later she developed local reactions, 2–5 cm areas, 30–120 minutes after injection. Skin-prick tests were negative for the diluent, isophane, and soluble insulin, but intradermal testing was positive with both insulins. Cetirizine and dexamethasone added to the insulin gave temporary relief. She was then given insulin lispro by pump. After about 8 months, she started to develop local reactions again but with cetirizine and the pump her reactions were manageable.

- A 6-year-old boy developed recurrent generalized urticaria 1 year after he started to use human Mixtard insulin (637). The rash started 10 minutes after injections in the arms, thighs, and buttocks, at sites where earlier injections had been given, and disappeared within 12 hours. When he was changed to insulin lispro he had three urticarial reactions in the first 2 weeks and then sporadically. The reactions were treated with chlorphenamine for 2 years.

Presentation

Although serious systemic reactions are rare, local reactions at the site of injection are not infrequent. They appear as reddening, swelling, heat, burning, and itching, with or without frankly painful sensations. They can set in immediately or after some hours. The lesion can extend gradually and persist for variable periods. Some immediate reactions are related to IgE (or IgE/IgG) concentrations (638), but a direct relation between allergic reactions and a specific IgG fraction cannot be established (639).

- A 45-year-old woman who had used insulin for 4 years had a biphasic hypersensitivity reaction to human insulin (or another component of the injection fluid) (640). Within 20 minutes after the injection a swelling developed and in a later phase papular lesions with lichenoid features and post-inflammatory hyperpigmentation emerged. Histologically, there was neutrophilic infiltration with erythrocyte extravasation and eosinophilic amorphous material, surrounded by neutrophilic infiltrate. Saline injection did not elicit an effect. IgE anti-insulin antibodies were not found. There was no Arthus reaction (type IV allergy).

Other reactions are of the tuberculin granulomatous type or of the local vasculitis Arthus type. The local reactions can be accompanied, preceded, or followed by a generalized reaction, such as urticaria, nausea, vomiting, diarrhea, angioedema, wheezing, or anaphylactic shock. The last of these is rare, but sometimes fatal.

Insulin can induce local, painful lumps at injection sites. Sclerosing granulomata are occasionally seen (641)

perhaps due to zinc (642). Such reactions are most commonly a consequence of an incorrect injection technique, generally the use of too short a needle or too superficial an injection. General edema (SEDA-11, 364) or abscesses (SEDA-7, 406) generated by insulin injections are extremely rare.

Lipodystrophy, lipoatrophy, or lipohypertrophy can be a consequence of chronic local insulin reactions that can be elicited by less pure as well as by highly purified preparations (643), but such reactions can also develop at sites distant to the injection.

Leukocytoclastic vasculitis has been attributed to human insulin.

- A 48-year-old woman with type 1 diabetes developed tender induration within 2–6 hours and persisting for 1–3 days after injection of both isophane and regular insulins (644). This was followed by intense itching and redness, but no wheal-and-flare reaction. Switching to semisynthetic insulin and other insulin analogues or continuous subcutaneous insulin infusion had no effect. After 3 years the condition became incapacitating. Humalog 5–6 times a day, including an injection at 0300 hours was the best tolerated regimen. Intradermal tests showed allergy to human, porcine, and bovine insulins, but no reaction to protamine or other additives. Skin biopsies showed a leukocytoclastic vasculitis. Prednisolone 10 mg/day plus azathioprine 50 mg/day, later replaced by methotrexate 7–15 mg/week, produced complete resolution within 8 weeks.

Insulin aspart

When short-acting insulins are given to patients who are allergic to regular insulin the allergic reactions can disappear. Although the short-acting insulins often have the same immunogenic epitopes, rapid dissociation of the fast-acting insulins into monomers can reduce their antigenic effects. Insulin lispro is known to be beneficial, and this has also been reported for aspart insulin (645).

- A 45-year-old man with type 2 diabetes treated with glibenclamide and metformin received combined chemotherapy for non-Hodgkin's lymphoma and was given premixed insulin. He developed local wheal-and-flare reactions immediately after the injections. Skin prick tests were positive for various types of insulin but weakly positive for lispro and negative for insulin aspart. He tolerated aspart insulin without any allergic reactions.

A few patients treated with insulin aspart developed antibodies, which cross-reacted with antibodies against human insulin and fell after 3 months (646). In lipodystrophy with lipoatrophic diabetes high insulin resistance is often found, for which leptin deficiency is one contributory factor.

Allergic reactions have been described with insulin aspart.

- A 53-year-old woman had type 2 diabetes that was not well controlled with diet and oral hypoglycemic drugs (647). She took intermediate-acting insulins, and after 2 months noticed redness and itching at injection sites. When she used insulin aspart and insulin lispro successively, the local reactions continued. She had a high serum concentration of total IgE (748 IU/ml; reference range below 400) and insulin-specific IgE (20 IU/ml; reference range below 0.34), positive insulin antibodies, and positive prick tests for insulin lispro, insulin aspart, human insulin, porcine insulin, and protamine. With intensive nutrition therapy and oral drugs her HbA$_{1c}$ fell to 5.5%.
- A 29-year-old woman with raised insulin concentrations during therapy had lipodystrophy and high insulin antibody titers with high binding capacity and high affinity (648).

Insulin antibodies are rarely found in patients with lipodystrophy.

Insulin detemir

An unspecified allergic reaction to insulin detemir has been reported (649).

Insulin glargine

Insulin glargine solved a problem in a man with type 1 diabetes after pork, beef, and human insulins had elicited allergic reactions (650). Antihistamines ameliorated the reactions but did not resolve them. Insulin glargine elicited no reactions, even when regular insulin was given. This case suggests that the A chain, which is modified in insulin glargine, is part of the allergic epitope. Tolerance to insulin glargine appeared to suppress allergy to regular insulin.

Insulin lispro

The long-term antigenicity of insulin lispro and cross-reactivity with human insulin antibodies over 4 years has been investigated in 1221 patients with both type 1 and type 2 diabetes, either insulin-naïve or with prior insulin treatment, in a multicenter combination of controlled and non-controlled open studies (651). Like recombinant human insulin, insulin lispro elicited a low immunogenic response. The reversal of amino acids in B28 and B29 is in a relatively non-immunogenic area. Moreover, antigenicity often correlates with residence of insulin in subcutaneous tissues, and insulin lispro has a short residence time. The patients did not develop increased dosage requirements. Intermittent treatment did not increase specific or cross-reactive responses. The antibody responses were slightly higher in type 1 than in type 2 diabetes. In lipodystrophy with lipoatrophic diabetes, high insulin resistance is often found, for which leptin deficiency is one contributory factor.

Insulin-like growth factor (IGF-I)

IGF-I can cause allergic reactions (652).

- A 75-year-old man with glucose intolerance, severe hyperinsulinemia, and extreme insulin resistance with anti-insulin receptor antibodies had immunosuppressive therapy and plasmapheresis to remove the antibodies, without lasting success. Treatment with hrIGF-I, 0.4 mg/kg/day, reduced HbA$_{1c}$ from 13.8% to 8.0%. After 5 months he developed a generalized skin eruption 20 minutes after the injection. When IGF-I was withdrawn the HbA$_{1c}$ rose again. After careful desensitization with hrIGF-I, 0.1 mg three times a week, IGF-I was continued, with good effect on HbA$_{1c}$.

Iodine-containing medicaments

Allergy to iodides can occur (653,654).

Of 126 participants in a study of the metabolism of radiolabelled proteins, four repeatedly developed urticaria and other symptoms after potassium iodide administration (655). Two of them were challenged with oral potassium iodide and developed urticaria, angioedema, polymyalgia, conjunctivitis, and coryza. Ten control patients were also challenged without adverse effects.

- Delayed hypersensitivity to potassium iodide occurred in a 66-year-old man who was given a cough syrup, Elixifilin, which contained potassium iodide (130 mg/15 ml), as well as theophylline and alcohol. Dyspnea, angioedema, itching, and erythema of the face and neck developed a few hours after the second dose. His symptoms disappeared 24 hours after treatment with parenteral glucocorticoids. Five hours after Elixifilin or iodide challenge, he developed edema of the face and neck, itching of the pharynx and eyes, and a sensation of heat (656).

Iodinated contrast media

French workers investigating the causes of severe reactions to iodinated contrast agents suggested that any patient who has had a severe anaphylactoid or anaphylactic reaction after the injection of a contrast agent should undergo immunological assessment (657). The diagnosis of drug anaphylaxis is usually based on the history, proof of mediator release, and the presence of drug-specific IgE antibodies or positive skin tests. In five patients with severe anaphylactoid reactions after the intravascular injection of an iodinated contrast agent, the clinical symptoms, biology, and skin tests were consistent with anaphylaxis. The authors also reported that no premedication has proved effective in preventing subsequent allergic reactions to contrast agents.

In one study iodinated contrast agents were among the top 10 drugs responsible for anaphylaxis (161 cases due to contrast media out of 1338 reports of anaphylaxis) (658). Dextran was the most common cause of anaphylaxis (418 cases). The overall death rate was significantly higher in men than in women and increased with age. The report also suggested that since the introduction of low molecular weight dextran 1 the incidence of severe anaphylaxis to dextran has fallen markedly and that radiographic contrast agents may now be the most common agents causing anaphylaxis. Most of the anaphylactic reactions and all the fatal cases were due to ionic agents.

Patients allergic to additives, such as parabens in sodium iopodate, can react to them, for example with rash (659).

Hypersensitivity reactions seem to be less common after arteriography than after urography, perhaps because the agent does not pass directly through the lungs, although the data are limited. There were mild allergic reactions in six of 167 patients who underwent arteriography with iodamide (SED-12, 1175; 660). Two severe delayed generalized cutaneous reactions with blistering occurred after lumbar aortography with iopamidol and iohexol (SED-12, 1175; 661).

Three cases of mild allergic-like reactions to oral water-soluble iodinated contrast media during CT examinations of the abdomen have been documented (662). Two patients received Gastrografin and the third received the same agents under the brand name Gastroview. The main reaction was a skin rash that resolved within 2 days. The author advised that clinicians and radiologists should be aware of the potential for adverse reactions to oral iodinated contrast agents. In another case, a severe systemic allergic reaction occurred in a patient who was given oral iohexol (663). In a patient with known allergy to iodinated contrast media it would be prudent to consider barium suspension in preference to an iodinated agent to outline the bowel.

Allergic or even anaphylactic reactions can occur after lymphography, either to the contrast agent or to the dye; in hypersensitive patients, prior use of glucocorticoids and antihistamines may fail to prevent a severe reaction (664).

Non-IgE-mediated anaphylactic (anaphylactoid) reactions

A life-threatening anaphylactoid reaction occurred in a child after intravenous administration of a non-ionic contrast medium (ioversol) (665).

- A 3-year-old girl was investigated for hypertension and a renal arteriogram was performed. Her blood pressure before the study was 125/60 mmHg. She received 30 ml of ioversol (iodine 320 mg/ml). Within 30 seconds she developed tachycardia (200/minute) and hypotension (60/20 mmHg). She developed diffuse urticaria over her entire body and there was wheezing on auscultation. Cardiopulmonary resuscitation was begun and she received a saline infusion and adrenaline 1:1000 subcutaneously, 0.01 ml/kg, intravenous diphenhydramine 1 mg/kg, and intravenous hydrocortisone 5 mg/kg. She responded rapidly. Surprisingly, the authors thought that the contrast medium had not caused this response, and the patient was subsequently given a second injection of ioversol 320 in a dose of 1 ml/kg. Within 60 seconds she again became tachycardic and hypotensive and urticaria reappeared over the whole body with wheezing. Similar treatment was offered and she responded rapidly.

The authors claimed that this was the first case report of anaphylactoid shock after the administration of ioversol in a child.

A fatal anaphylactoid reaction to an intravenous non-ionic contrast medium occurred during a CT scan (666). The authors highlighted the value of measuring serum tryptase in the diagnosis of anaphylactoid reactions.

- An 81-year-old man underwent CT scanning of the head with intravenous contrast enhancement (100 ml of the non-ionic contrast medium iopamidol). After the injection he complained of sweating and nausea and had a cardiorespiratory arrest. Immediate resuscitation and intravenous dexamethasone and adrenaline were not successful. Mast cell tryptase activity in a sample taken 4 hours after death was high. At autopsy, the coronary and pulmonary arteries were patent. The right heart chambers were moderately enlarged. The lungs were hyperemic and edematous and there was obstructive edema of the larynx.

This patient had all the features of anaphylactoid reactions, which include pulmonary and laryngeal edema and a massive rise in serum tryptase. The half-life of tryptase is about 2 hours. Moderately raised post-mortem tryptase activity in the absence of anaphylaxis has been described. Therefore, only very high serum tryptase activity, as seen in this case, should be regarded as specific for fatal anaphylactoid reactions.

Iodopropynylbutylcarbamate

Four contact allergic reactions were reported in a series of 3168 consecutively patch-tested patients (1472). In another study there were 16 positive reactions (0.3%) in 4883 consecutive patients (667).

Iron salts

Iron enhances the pathogenicity of micro-organisms, adversely affects the function of macrophages and lymphocytes, and enhances fibrogenic pathways, all of which may enhance hepatic injury due to iron itself or to iron alongside other factors.

Oral iron

Skin reactions to oral iron are extremely rare.

- A 40-year-old woman with iron deficiency anemia due to menstrual blood loss took oral iron for 3 months without any adverse effects (668). Nine months later she became anemic again and 2 hours after an oral dose of ferrous sulfate 525 g (105 mg of elemental iron) she developed generalized pruritus and an erythematous maculopapular rash. This recurred 1 week later, when she took ferrous protein succinilate 800 g (40 g of iron). Desensitization with oral iron was carried out. Skin prick tests and patch tests with iron formulations were negative. Two single-blind, placebo-controlled oral challenges were performed and she began to have similar cutaneous symptoms. A slow desensitization protocol, using increasing doses, was tolerated without adverse effects. Chronic oral iron therapy once a day for 9 months sustained the desensitized state and the anemia disappeared.

Isoflurane

Anaphylaxis has been reported in a patient who received isoflurane (669).

Isoniazid

The expansion or new development of tuberculous lesions during ultimately successful therapy has been termed a "paradoxical response." It is most often reported in relation to intracranial tuberculomata, but is probably most common in tuberculous lymphadenopathy. It is also described in tuberculous pleurisy and in parenchymal lung disease. In most cases, the problem eventually settles, but sometimes glucocorticoid therapy is used empirically.

A lupus-like syndrome or vasculitis, with arthritis, rheumatic pain, fever, pleurisy, and leukopenia, has been reported in patients taking isoniazid (670,671). Tests for antinuclear antibodies are useful to distinguish idiopathic systemic lupus erythematosus and drug-induced lupuslike syndromes. However, many patients taking isoniazid have antinuclear antibodies, usually without signs or symptoms of systemic lupus erythematosus. Isoniazid can also exacerbate pre-existing systemic lupus erythematosus (670,671). Long-term glucocorticoid treatment may be necessary if symptoms persist after withdrawal of isoniazid.

- Two Japanese patients developed pleural effusions while taking antituberculosis therapy and were believed to have isoniazid-induced lupus-like syndrome (672). This diagnosis was based on the presence of antinuclear antibody in the effusate, and in one patient, a positive lymphocyte stimulation test using isoniazid; in the other patient it was negative. Both had moderately strongly positive serum antinuclear antibodies (1:160). In the first patient, the effusion disappeared 2 weeks after withdrawal of isoniazid; in the other treatment was continued but the effusion nevertheless resolved in 10 weeks.

It is worth checking for evidence of lupus-like syndrome in patients with paradoxical responses to antituberculosis therapy but it remains to be seen how many cases would be explained by it.

Isopropamide iodide

Isopropamide iodide can cause allergic reactions in patients who are sensitive to iodine.

Isopropanolamine

- Contact dermatitis to a gel containing biphenylacetic acid, a non-steroidal anti-inflammatory agent,

carbomer, and isopropanolamine has been reported (673). Patch tests showed a positive reaction to isopropanolamine (1% aqueous) on day 4. Patch-testing of 22 patients as controls showed one case of slight irritation.

Itraconazole

Itraconazole 200 mg bd for 2 weeks caused a serum sickness-like reaction in a 53-year-old woman with Ménière's disease (674).

Japanese encephalitis vaccine

See Vaccines

Kanamycin

Sensitization (rash, drug fever) after parenteral administration of kanamycin is less frequent than with streptomycin. Anaphylaxis has only rarely been described. Cross-allergy with the other aminoglycosides is frequent (675).

Ketorolac

See NSAIDs

Labetalol

See Beta-adrenoceptor antagonists

Lamotrigine

A phenytoin-like hypersensitivity syndrome with skin rash, leukocytosis, and laboratory evidence of liver and kidney dysfunction has been attributed to lamotrigine (SEDA-22, 89).

Twenty-six lamotrigine-associated reactions consistent with the features of the anticonvulsant hypersensitivity syndrome have been reviewed, including nine previously published (676). The patients were aged 3.5–74 (mean 28) years and 14 were female. Valproate was used as co-medication in 60%. Fever was present in all patients, a skin rash in 77% (with Stevens–Johnson syndrome or toxic epidermal necrolysis in five cases), hematological abnormalities in 69% (including eosinophilia in 19%), liver abnormalities in 65%, renal involvement in 23%, disseminated intravascular coagulation in 15%, and musculoskeletal disorders in 8%. Multiorgan involvement was present in 46%. One patient died. Overall, the characteristics of the syndrome were comparable to that induced by aromatic anticonvulsants, except for a somewhat higher incidence of severe skin rashes and a lower frequency of eosinophilia and lymphadenopathy.

- A 35-year-old man with Lennox–Gastaut syndrome developed tender cervical lymphadenopathy 14 weeks after lamotrigine was introduced, when the dosage was increased to 200 mg/day (677). Frozen section examination of a biopsy specimen 10 weeks later suggested lymphoma, but further histopathological investigations documented lymphoid hyperplasia consistent with a diagnosis of pseudolymphoma, which resolved 1 month after withdrawal.

This seems to have been the first report of pseudolymphoma associated with lamotrigine.

Systemic hypersensitivity reactions to lamotrigine can be severe.

- A 27-year-old woman developed disseminated intravascular coagulation, fever, rash, and hepatic dysfunction 11 days after starting lamotrigine (678). The drug dosage was not stated.
- A 17-year-old girl with a history of bipolar disorder developed fever, lymphadenopathy, skin rash, diarrhea, and acute renal insufficiency requiring dialysis after taking lamotrigine for 4 weeks (679). Renal biopsy showed acute interstitial nephritis with focal granulomas; colonic biopsy showed colitis and ileitis with non-necrotizing epithelioid granulomas.
- Severe hypersensitivity affecting the skin, lymph nodes, and liver has been reported with lamotrigine in a 36-year-old man, who had taken high doses of sodium valproate and lamotrigine for about a month (680). Skin tests were negative with both drugs, but lymphocyte stimulation tests were twice positive with lamotrigine. Later re-exposure to sodium valproate was tolerated.

Drug-induced lupus-like syndrome has been associated with lamotrigine (681).

- A 70-year-old woman, who had taken lamotrigine 2 mg/kg/day for about 2 years developed arthralgia affecting the small joints of the hands, wrists, and knees, an erythematous skin rash, myalgia, and Raynaud's phenomenon. Serum antinuclear antibodies were positive (1:320, speckled pattern), as was anti-Ro/SSA. Rheumatoid factor and anticardiolipin antibodies were negative and serum complement was normal. Lamotrigine was withdrawn and the symptoms and abnormal tests gradually normalized.

Latex

Severe anaphylactic reactions have been reported in response to dental work (latex dental dams), barium enemas (latex enema devices), and numerous surgical procedures involving mainly latex gloves and catheters. The two major contributing factors appear to be a hereditary disposition and occupational exposure. The latter has increased rapidly owing to progress in medical technology, the associated increase in the use of medical devices, and increased awareness among health-care professionals of the need to wear protective gloves during various procedures. This increased exposure has meant that a growing number of people have become sensitized to latex proteins; in one study, 6–7% of surgical personnel and 18–40% of

patients with spina bifida were sensitive to latex (682). Particularly high-risk circumstances appear to be direct contact of a latex device or air-borne particles from a latex device (for example corn starch carrying latex proteins) with mucous membranes or with tissues exposed as a result of surgical procedures.

FDA investigations, which eventually identified natural latex/natural rubber (NLNR) allergy as an emerging public health concern, were started in response to voluntary reports submitted by physicians, nurses, and technologists (683). The first reports described deaths that occurred during barium enema procedures, before the administration of barium. Over the past decade, the FDA has received more than 1700 reports of severe allergic reactions, including 16 deaths, related to medical devices containing latex. The deaths all occurred in 1989 among children with spina bifida and were caused by a reaction to the latex cuffs used on the tip of barium enema catheters.

In Australia, regulatory changes have been proposed for the labeling and safety requirements of latex-containing devices that directly or indirectly come into contact with body tissues (684). Most latex-containing devices are in this category, and include tubes, catheters, empty containers, syringes, medical gloves, and devices such as condoms and diaphragms. The FDA is requiring all medical devices containing latex to be labeled as such and to carry a caution that latex can cause allergic reactions (685). The FDA has also urged manufacturers of latex containing medical devices to set the protein levels in their products as low as possible. The FDA also requires that "hypoallergenic" claims should not be attached to medical devices, because they incorrectly imply that the devices may be safely used by people who are sensitive to latex.

Lauromacrogols

Contact allergic reactions to lauromacrogol 400 have been reported (686). Patch-testing can yield irritant reactions. In a retrospective study of 8739 patients tested with a topical drug patch test series, 3186 patients were tested with 0.5% lauromacrogol 400 in water (687). There was slight irritation in 0.88%, weakly positive reactions in 0.97%, and strongly positive reactions in 0.25%. In 6202 patients tested with a 3% solution of lauromacrogol 400 in petrolatum, there was slight skin irritation in 0.48%, weakly positive reactions in 1.77%, and strongly positive reactions in 0.34%. Among the 649 patients tested with both formulations, concurrence was moderate.

Levofloxacin

Anaphylactic and anaphylactoid reactions are rare adverse events after the administration of fluoroquinolones (about 0.46–1.2 per 100 000 patients).

- On two occasions a 49-year-old asthmatic woman who took levofloxacin for a chest infection developed worse respiratory distress, requiring intubation (688). The second reaction was accompanied by a marked skin reaction.

An in vitro study in rat peritoneal mast cells showed that levofloxacin-mediated release of histamine may be closely linked to activation of pertussis toxin-sensitive G proteins (689).

Lidocaine

There have been 62 reports of allergic contact dermatitis to lidocaine worldwide between 1972 and 1996; 49 were in Australia and several showed cross-reactivity with other amide local anesthetics, such as bupivacaine, mepivacaine, and prilocaine (690).

Lincosamides

Although the risk of drug hypersensitivity is increased in patients with AIDS, clindamycin hypersensitivity has been considered to be relatively uncommon, despite its widespread use, with rash developing in about 9% of patients. However, in a retrospective survey of 50 patients with AIDS recruited in a European multicenter study of treatment for *Toxoplasma* encephalitis, the incidence of rash in 26 patients given pyrimethamine plus clindamycin was 58%, compared with 75% in those given pyrimethamine plus sulfadiazine, a non-significant difference (691). Treatment was initially continued throughout the duration of hypersensitivity, and was tolerated in all patients taking pyrimethamine plus clindamycin, but had to be withdrawn in half of those taking pyrimethamine plus sulfadiazine. Stevens–Johnson syndrome developed in two patients and fatal toxic epidermal necrolysis in one. Thus, the continuation of treatment despite a rash was more likely to succeed with pyrimethamine plus clindamycin but was potentially hazardous with pyrimethamine plus sulfadiazine.

In a prospective study, true-positive patch tests were seen in four of six patients with known clindamycin hypersensitivity, while 22 healthy controls were negative; there was one false positive and one false negative reaction (692).

Successful desensitization has been described in a 35-year-old woman who developed a generalized rash after taking clindamycin (600 mg 6-hourly) and pyrimethamine for 12 days for AIDS-associated cerebral toxoplasmosis; the rash resolved after withdrawal of clindamycin (693). Subsequent oral rechallenge was performed (without pre-treatment with glucocorticoids or antihistamines), starting with three doses of 20 mg on day 1, 40 mg on day 2, 80 mg on day 3, and so on, until a dose of 600 mg qds was reached on day 7. A transient rash lasting 5 hours developed after the second dose of 600 mg. She remained free from adverse reactions for the duration of follow-up (13 months).

Lindane

Henoch-Schönlein purpura, possibly caused by topical lindane, has been described (694).

Lipsticks, substances used in

The fatty acid esters have low allergenic potential but cases of contact allergy has been reported, in one case to di-isostearyl malate (patch-tested in 7.7% in petrolatum) (695), and in another case to glyceryl monoisostearate monomyristate in a 23-year-old woman, who had cheilitis from her lipstick (696).

- A 17-year-old woman developed pruritic edematous erythema on her lips after using a lipstick containing isopalmitate (697). A patch test with 10% isopalmitate in petrolatum was positive on day 3, with six negative controls.
- A 27-year-old woman developed papules, scales, and slight swelling of her lips (698). A patch test with iso-palmityl diglyceryl sebacate, 10% in petrolatum, was positive.

Lithium

Lithium is not an allergen. Allergic reactions that have been reported in patients taking lithium have been attributed to excipients in the formulation (699), as in a case of leukocytoclastic vasculitis (700).

In a brief report, evidence has been presented that short-term exposure to lithium (less than 2 months) caused alterations in the expression of histocompatibility antigens (701).

In 10 healthy volunteers, lithium caused increases in interleukin-4 and interleukin-10 concentrations and falls in interleukin-2 and interferon concentrations (702). In in vitro studies of monocytes from women with breast cancer, lithium chloride suppressed production of interleukin-8 and induced production of interleukin-15 (703,704). The clinical implications of these findings are unclear.

The immunomodulatory effects of lithium have been reviewed (705,706). Lithium

(a) stimulated the production of pro-inflammatory cytokines and negative immunoregulatory cytokines or proteins in nine healthy subjects (707);
(b) altered the expression of human leukocyte antigens (HLA) in 11 of 15 subjects (701);
(c) normalized manifestations of mild immune activation in 17 rapid cycling bipolar patients (708).

The clinical implications of these findings are unclear.

The very complex antiviral and immunomodulatory effects of lithium have been reviewed (709). In 15 inpatients, lithium produced changes in a number of histocompatibility antigens, but whether these have any clinical implications is unknown (710).

Local anesthetics

Systemic hypersensitivity reactions are not a frequent problem in local anesthesia. Systemic toxicity or allergy to additives (hyaluronidase, bisulfate, parabens) has sometimes been mistakenly classified as hypersensitivity to local anesthetics (SEDA-17, 135; 711).

Well-documented case reports are very few, relating particularly to the older aminoesters; this appears to be because these agents have the highly antigenic para-aminobenzoic acid as a metabolite (SEDA-13, 98). The incidence of true allergy is actually very low, probably less than 1% of all the adverse effects attributable to these substances (SEDA-20, 123).

Allergic reactions to aminoamide local anesthetics are unusual, but type I hypersensitivity reactions are described, and life-threatening anaphylaxis can rarely occur (SEDA-21, 136; SEDA-22, 134). Cross-reaction between amides also occurs, for example articaine, bupivacaine, lidocaine, and prilocaine (SEDA-22, 134).

Type IV delayed hypersensitivity reactions are uncommon, but allergic contact dermatitis and localized erythema and blistering have been reported (SEDA-21, 136).

- A 58-year-old man with a urological stoma used a catheter lubricated with Braum Monodose ointment (712). After almost 2 years, he developed severe pruritus and squamous erythematous plaques in the peristomal skin. Patch tests were positive with the lubricant ointment and one of its constituents, tetracaine.

Both anaphylactoid reactions and bronchospasm have occasionally been reported, although the latter may have been due to sympathetic nervous blockade leading to unopposed parasympathetic effects (SEDA-18, 143; 713).

Contact hypersensitivity also occurs. Benzocaine is a potent skin sensitizer, and several cases of contact dermatitis to lidocaine have been reported. In many cases there is no cross-reactivity between different local anesthetics.

- A 79-year-old man developed a weeping dermatitis of the perianal skin, buttocks, and proximal thighs (714). In the previous 3 weeks, he had used Proctosedyl cream which contains cinchocaine (dibucaine). Patch tests were positive with Proctosedyl cream and 5% cinchocaine in petrolatum, while benzocaine, lidocaine, and clioquinol were negative.
- A 62-year-old woman had a systemic contact dermatitis several days after topical administration of DoloPosterine ointment for hemorrhoids (715). She had erythematous vesicular lesions on her perianal area and an edematous erythematous rash on her upper thighs, elbow flexures, axillae, and face. Patch tests with the ointment and its constituents were positive with DoloPosterine and dibucaine 5% in petrolatum; patch tests with benzocaine and other local anesthetics were negative.
- A 71-year-old Japanese man developed an itchy erythematous papular eruption after using an over-the-counter medicament for skin wounds (Makiron) for 1 month (716). Patch tests with the constituents showed positive reactions to dl-chlorphenamine maleate and cinchocaine hydrochloride (both 1% in petrolatum). Patch tests with lidocaine hydrochloride and mepivacaine hydrochloride showed no cross-sensitization.

An allergic reaction has been described in a patient given mepivacaine (717).

Anaphylactic shock has been reported after spinal anesthesia with tetracaine (SED-12, 257; 718).

However, some sensitized patients do cross-react with various related local anesthetic agents or chemically similar compounds, including some muscle relaxants (SEDA-15, 117). On the other hand, cross-reactivity between aminoesters and aminoamides seems unlikely and does not appear to be on record. Although cross-reactivity between amide local anesthetics is uncommon, it has been reported.

- A 26-year-old woman, 6 months pregnant, developed local redness and itching after exposure to topical agents containing lidocaine, and a further similar reaction to bupivacaine, also with swelling, 8 hours after injection (719). She had a history of anaphylaxis to an unidentified agent, and a patch test was performed using mepivacaine, lidocaine, and ropivacaine; all resulted in strong reactions after 48 hours, while patch testing was negative with chloroprocaine. She subsequently had a cesarean section under spinal anesthesia with chloroprocaine with no adverse reaction.
- A 39-year-old man was investigated for three episodes of facial swelling following dental procedures over 2 years. The swelling always occurred on the same side as the dental procedure and about 12 hours after it, took a couple of days to resolve, did not respond to antihistamines, and was not associated with a rash, laryngeal edema, or bronchospasm. He was admitted twice and treated with intravenous antibiotics for cellulitis. He also reported a history of a rash after penicillin but no previous reactions to local anesthetics. All blood tests, including full blood count, C3 and C4 concentrations, and C1 esterase inhibitor activity and function were normal; an antinuclear antibody test was negative, IgE concentrations were not raised, and latex-specific IgE was not detected. Skin prick, intradermal, and subcutaneous tests were carried out with isotonic saline, lidocaine, prilocaine, and procaine; these did not show immediate reactions, but 2 days later a wheal appeared at the lidocaine site. There was a less intense reaction with prilocaine and none with saline or procaine.

The authors concluded that sensitization to lidocaine must have taken place during previous procedures and that cross-reactivity with another amide type local anesthetic, prilocaine, had also occurred.

Contact dermatitis was reported in three hemodialysis patients who used Emla cream repeatedly as analgesia for AV fistula cannulation (SEDA-21, 136).

Twenty patients with a prior history of generalized and/or local skin reactions after local anesthetics were examined with intradermal testing and patch testing; in 10 of them a lymphocyte transformation test was performed to investigate whether they had T cell sensitization to local anesthetics, which might have been responsible for their symptoms (720). Only two had a positive intradermal test, whereas six had a positive patch test and six had a positive lymphocyte transformation test, suggesting that allergic skin symptoms could be mediated by T cells in some patients who do not have evidence of an IgE-mediated reaction.

- A 20-year-old woman, who had had eight previous uneventful exposures to local anesthetics for dental procedures, received an injection of 1% lidocaine for treatment of an in-growing toenail; 12 hours later she developed widespread urticaria lasting a week accompanied by bronchospasm and abdominal discomfort (721). A skin prick test gave a slight positive reaction, and later a positive intradermal injection provided evidence of a true type I hypersensitivity reaction. Following negative skin and intradermal tests with prilocaine, subsequent dental treatment 12 months later was performed using prilocaine with no untoward effects.
- A 70-year-old woman received a peribulbar block using 10 ml of 2% lidocaine, 0.75% bupivacaine (50/50), and hyaluronidase 500 units for cataract extraction; 12 hours later she awoke with a painful, swollen eye (722). There was marked swelling, erythema, tenderness of the eyelids, and a tense orbit, with reduced visual acuity, marked restriction of eye movements, and conjunctival chemosis. There was no hematoma or evidence of infection, but allergy could not be ruled out. Four days later, she received tetracaine eye drops and local infiltration with lidocaine for further suturing and again developed similar symptoms and signs in that eye, with swelling extending to the cheek; follow-up showed persistent ocular dysfunction.

The second patient had had previous exposure to prilocaine, lidocaine, and bupivacaine without problems. The author proposed a diagnosis of lidocaine allergy, although hyaluronidase as the antigen could not be excluded.

- A 23-year-old woman developed an allergic contact dermatitis after applying an over-the-counter proprietary antipruritic jelly containing 0.1% cinchocaine chloride, and a "caine" mixture (5% benzocaine, 1% cinchocaine hydrochloride, 1% procaine hydrochloride) (723). She had positive patch testing to both components.

Allergic reactions attributed to local anesthetics can be due to excipients in the formulation (724).

- A 69-year-old woman developed hypesthesia of all four limbs lasting several hours after three gastroscopies using lidocaine jelly; although the symptom was not typical of an allergic reaction, intradermal tests and nasal provocation tests were performed. The intradermal tests were negative, but the nasal provocation tests were positive for carboxymethylcellulose, a suspending agent used in lidocaine jelly; this caused ipsilateral nasal congestion and dysesthesia of the tongue and the ipsilateral temporal region within 30 minutes. A drug-induced lymphocyte stimulation test was also positive for carboxymethylcellulose.

Hypersensitivity to carboxymethylcellulose may have contributed to this patient's unusual symptoms.

The use of skin testing to identify a causative drug allergen has been repeatedly advocated by several groups, but their advice has not always been followed. Intradermal testing can be helpful in distinguishing between safe and unsafe agents in patients with a history of allergy to local anesthesia.

Various types of immunodepressant effects of local anesthetics can be detected by laboratory testing, although they may have no clinical significance. Lidocaine dose-dependently inhibits EA rosetting by human lymphocytes. In vitro depression of human leukocyte random motility and phagocytosis has also been reported (SED-11, 220; 725).

When injected into the skin, local anesthetics often cause pseudo-allergic reactions, with similar symptoms to immediate type allergy (726). However, true immediate hypersensitivity to local anesthetics is extremely rare.

- A 50-year-old man had local infiltrations a few days after an injection of lidocaine and dexamethasone (727). Prick and intradermal tests were negative after 20 minutes. However, lidocaine produced a positive patch test after 2 days, with erythema and papules.

Lopinavir and ritonavir

Subcutaneous non-tuberculous granulomatous lesions developed in a 48-year-old HIV-positive man when he was given ritonavir (728).

Losartan

See Angiotensin receptor antagonists

Lovastatin

See HMG coenzyme A reductase inhibitors

Loxoprofen

See NSAIDs

Macrolide antibiotics

Immunomodulatory effects of macrolides have been repeatedly reported; for example suppression of the release of chemotactic mediators may be important for the clinical effect of roxithromycin in patients with chronic lower respiratory tract infections (729). Both clarithromycin and azithromycin altered cytokine production in human monocytes in vitro (730).

The suppressive activity of macrolide antibiotics on pro-inflammatory cytokine production has also been shown in human peripheral blood monocytes, in which roxithromycin inhibited the in vitro production of interleukin-1 beta and tumor necrosis factor alpha (731). It also suppressed cytokine production after a prolonged pretreatment period in mice. In another mouse model both roxithromycin and clarithromycin inhibited angiogenesis and enhanced the antitumor activity of some cytotoxic agents, suggesting a beneficial effect when combined with such drugs against solid tumors (732,733). Furthermore, growth suppression of human fibroblasts by roxithromycin has been demonstrated both in vitro and in vivo (734).

Azithromycin has been associated with Churg–Strauss syndrome in a patient with atopy (735).

- A 46-year-old man with asthma was treated with oral roxithromycin 300 mg/day for 5 days for purulent rhinitis and 2 weeks later developed arthritis, mononeuritis multiplex, eosinophilia (64%), eosinophilic infiltrations in the bone marrow, raised IgE concentrations, and transient pulmonary infiltrates. Churg–Strauss syndrome was diagnosed.

A similar course of disease had occurred 1 year before, after the administration of azithromycin (736).

Roxithromycin had an immunomodulatory action on peripheral blood mononuclear cells in patients with psoriasis (1473). The anti-inflammatory activity of roxithromycin is due to reduced production of proinflammatory mediators, cytokines, and co-stimulatory molecules, as has been shown in animal studies (737).

- Churg–Strauss syndrome has been reported in an 18-year-old woman taking cysteinyl leukotriene receptor antagonists and oral rokitamycin 400 mg bd for 10 days (738).

Leukocytoclastic vasculitis associated with clarithromycin has been reported in an 83-year-old woman who was treated for pneumonia. All her symptoms resolved after withdrawal and a short course of glucocorticoids (739).

- Henoch–Schönlein purpura developed in an 84-year-old Indian woman 10 days after she started to take clarithromycin (250 mg bd) for pneumonia (740). She was otherwise healthy and taking no regular medications. Histology confirmed a leukocytoclastic vasculitis of superficial vessels, with extravasation of erythrocytes, and direct immunofluorescence showed immunoglobulin A in superficial dermal vessels. Treatment with prednisone (1 mg/kg/day) was required. Most of the symptoms and signs resolved within a few days, but renal function remained impaired.The authors identified two previous case reports of clarithromycin-induced leukocytoclastic vasculitis.
- A 39-year-old man developed acute angioedema and urticaria 6 hours after taking erythromycin base 500 mg in enteric-coated pellets for acute sinusitis (741). He remembered having taken erythromycin once before without any problem. He had no known allergies and was taking no regular medications, but he had had chemotherapy for non-Hodgkin's lymphoma several years earlier.

The authors identified five previous reports of erythromycin-associated urticarial reactions. However, it was not possible to exclude a reaction to the ingredients of the coated pellets.

Malaria vaccine

See Vaccines

Measles, mumps, and rubella vaccines

See Vaccines

Medroxyprogesterone

Anaphylactic reactions to medroxyprogesterone are very rare.

- A 40-year-old woman developed anaphylactic shock after receiving depot medroxyprogesterone acetate 150 mg intramuscularly (742). She was not taking any other medications, and there was no history of allergy to food or cosmetics. She responded fully to immediate resuscitation. She had another episode when she received another dose 12 weeks later.

Mefenamic acid

See NSAIDs

Meglitinides

- A 62-year-old woman with type 2 diabetes, hypertension, and chronic hepatitis C virus infection developed palpable purpura over her legs and buttocks 3 weeks after starting to take repaglinide 500 mg qds (793). The purpura ulcerated and became infected. Repaglinide was withdrawn and the purpura resolved. A biopsy showed leukocytoclastic vasculitis.

Repaglinide, which is metabolized in the liver, is cleared more slowly in people with liver disease, and hepatitis C may have played a part in this case. Although hepatitis C can cause a leukocytoclastic vasculitis, the clinical correlation and the rapid disappearance of the purpura after the withdrawal of repaglinide makes it likely that this was an adverse effect of the drug. Caution with repaglinide in liver disease is important.

Melatonin

There has been a single report of a subject in a controlled trial of melatonin who had difficulty in swallowing and breathing within 20 minutes of taking melatonin 0.5 mg. The symptoms resolved without treatment after 45 minutes and recurred in a milder form after rechallenge (794).

Meloxicam

See NSAIDs

Menthol

Hypersensitivity reactions to menthol are well recognized and comprise urticaria and flushing. Twelve cases of contact sensitivity to the flavoring agents menthol and peppermint oil were reported in patients presenting with intra-oral symptoms in association with burning mouth syndrome, recurrent oral ulceration, or a lichenoid reaction (795). Nine patients were followed up and six of these described resolution or improvement of their symptoms as a result of avoiding menthol and peppermint.

Mercury and mercurial salts

Merthiolate was tested as a matter of routine in an extended standard series of skin tests in patients with different subtypes of eczema and varicose complex (796). Of 880 patients 53% responded positively to one or more allergens, 3.9% to merthiolate. The latest results of skin tests in adults have confirmed the persistence of contact allergy to merthiolate and justify further follow-up and systematic screening.

Attention has been given to mercury as a cause of autoimmune responses, especially in the kidney (797). Exposure to mercury can cause immune responses to various auto-antigens and autoimmune disease of the kidney and other tissues. Although epidemiological studies have shown that occupational exposure to mercury does not usually result in autoimmunity, mercury can cause the formation of antinuclear antibodies, scleroderma-like disease, lichen planus, or membranous nephropathy in some individuals. In experimental animals mercury causes autoimmune disease similar to that observed in humans, with emphasis on the importance of immunogenetic and pharmacogenetic factors.

Homeopathic medicines can cause mercury allergy (baboon syndrome).

- A 5-year-old girl developed an itchy erythematous macular rash, symmetrically distributed in the anogenital area and thighs (798). The lesions developed into a widespread maculopapular vesicular rash in 48 hours, sparing the face, palms, and soles. The eruption cleared after systemic corticosteroids and antihistamines, with scaling and post-inflammatory hypopigmentation. She had had neonatal periumbilical dermatitis associated with the application of merbromin to the cord, and 24 hours before the onset of the rash had taken a single homeopathic tablet (Mercurius Heel), which contained soluble mercury. Allergy tests to a standard series of foods and respiratory allergens were negative and total IgE was normal. Patch-testing to allergens showed positive reactions to thiomersal and metallic mercury.

Previous sensitization and the subsequent development of an allergic contact dermatitis from vaccines that contain thiomersal has received more attention than before (799). Cross-reactivity, exposure factors, and tolerance to vaccines containing thiomersal have been studied in 125 patients sensitized to mercury derivatives in a cross-sectional study (799). Childhood vaccinations, merbromin used as an antiseptic, broken thermometers, and the use of drops were the main sources of previous exposure. There was sensitization to thiomersal in 57 patients and 24 had a positive intradermal reaction. Ammoniated mercury elicited positive reactions in 78% of all patients and

merbromin in 66%. In most cases (100/125) there was cross-reactivity among different mercury derivatives. Intramuscular thiomersal caused a mild local reaction in only five patients (4% of the total, 9% of thiomersal positive reactions). Most of the patients had positive tests to both organic and inorganic mercury derivatives. Vaccination with thiomersal is relatively safe, even for individuals with delayed type hypersensitivity, since more than 90% of allergic patients tolerated intramuscular challenge tests with thiomersal. However, in such patients it would be advisable to restrict the use of mercurial antiseptics and mercury thermometers.

Methyldopa

Lupus-like syndrome has been attributed to methyldopa, causing hemolytic anemia, arthritis, photosensitivity, and high titers of antinuclear antibody (1:256) and of IgG antibodies to class I histones in a 55-year-old man who took methyldopa 250 mg bd for 13 months; the syndrome resolved spontaneously when methyldopa was withdrawn (800).

Methylene blue

See Methylthioninium chloride

Methylenedioxymetamfetamine (MDMA, ecstasy)

Four healthy male MDMA users volunteered for a randomized, double-blind, double-dummy, crossover pilot study in which they took single oral doses of MDMA 75 mg ($n = 2$) or 100 mg ($n = 2$), alcohol (0.8 mg/kg), MDMA plus alcohol, or placebo to study the effects on their immune system. The doses of MDMA were compatible with those used for recreational use (801). The baseline immunological parameters were within the reference ranges. Acute MDMA use produced time-dependent immune dysfunction, which paralleled MDMA plasma concentrations and MDMA-induced cortisol stimulation kinetics. The changes in the immune system after MDMA peaked at 1–2 hours. Although the total leukocyte count remained unchanged, there was a fall in the ratio of CD4 to CD8 T cells and in the percentage of mature T lymphocytes (CD3 cells), probably because of a fall in both the percentage and the absolute number of T helper cells. The fall in CD4 cell count and in the functional responsiveness of lymphocytes to mitogenic stimulation with phytohemagglutinin A was MDMA dose-dependent. Alcohol produced a decrease in T helper cells, B lymphocytes, and mitogen-induced lymphocyte proliferation. Combined MDMA and alcohol use produced the greatest suppressive effect on CD4 cell count and mitogen-stimulated lymphoproliferation. Immune function was partially restored at 24 hours. According to the authors, these results provided the first evidence that recreational use of MDMA alone or in combination with alcohol alters immunological status. The reaction of the immune system to MDMA appears to be an alteration of physiological homeostasis, similar to that seen in volunteers exposed to acute physiologic stress, suggesting that MDMA could be a "chemical stressor". Moreover, combined MDMA and alcohol use produced additive effects. This is an important finding, since in the general population alcohol and MDMA are commonly taken together.

Because other drugs of abuse can cause immune dysfunction in regular users, the effects of acute administration of ecstasy on the immune system have been studied in both controlled and natural settings (802). In the controlled study, 18 male ecstasy users were given two doses of ecstasy 100 mg at intervals of 4 or 24 hours. There were significant reductions in CD4 T helper cells (30%) and the lymphoproliferative response to phytohemagglutinin mitogenic stimulation (68%) 1.5 hours after the first dose, and a 103% increase in the number of natural killer cells. At 4 hours, CD4 T helper cells and lymphocyte proliferative responses were reduced by 40% and 87%, but natural killer cell numbers increased to 141%. At 24 hours, the second dose augmented the alterations in the numbers of CD4 T helper cells and natural killer cells about threefold. The authors suggested that this large effect after repeated administration of ecstasy increases the interval during which the immune response is compromised, leading to a higher risk of illness and infection in ecstasy abusers.

In the uncontrolled study, 30 recreational users of ecstasy (mean age 24 years) were observed for 2 years and had lymphocyte counts at yearly intervals. The ecstasy users tended to have lower white blood cell counts over time. Lymphocyte counts were significantly lower than in healthy controls by year 1 and significantly lower than that the following year. CD4 and CD19 cell numbers fell significantly from basal to year 1 and from year 1 to year 2. Natural killer cell numbers were always lower than in healthy controls but did not fall with time. The authors extended these results to suggest a possible role of serotonin dysregulation caused by ecstasy in compromising immune function. These findings suggest that ecstasy abusers may be at a significantly higher risk of infectious diseases.

Methylphenobarbital

Giant cell myocarditis has been reported in a patient taking phenytoin, phenobarbital, and methylphenobarbital, and in one taking primidone (803).

Giant cell myocarditis has been reported in a patient taking phenytoin, phenobarbital, and mephobarbital and in one taking primidone (804).

Methylthioninium chloride (methylene blue)

Methylthioninium chloride marking of a colonic polyp resulted in an inflammatory mass with small arteries showing both segmental and circumferential fibrinoid necrosis with thrombosis (805).

- A 68-year-old Hispanic woman had multiple polyps associated with recurrent episodes of hematochezia over several years. All but a single polyp were removed endoscopically. The region of the remaining polyp was labelled with 2 ml of methylthioninium chloride injected in divided doses to aid operative localization. Because surgery was postponed, methylthioninium chloride was again injected. At surgery the polyp and a 5 cm perirectal indurated mass were identified, and there was a blue track from the submucosal to the outer portions of muscularis propria into the adjacent fat. Microscopically, the mucosa was intact and the submucosa was edematous. There were acute inflammatory cells in the submucosa and muscularis propria. Inflammation (acute and chronic), fibroblastic proliferation, and fat necrosis were seen in areas outside the muscularis propria and extending to the connective tissue margin. A prominent finding was fibrinoid necrosis of small arteries, in some cases segmental and in others circumferential. The internal elastic lamina was destroyed and there were thromboses and vessel wall inflammation. There was no evidence of infiltrating carcinoma in the adenomatous polyp or the adjacent colon. The inflammation and vascular changes were only in the mass defined grossly by induration; sections away from this area were unremarkable. The blue track contained blue–black pigment within macrophages.

The mechanisms of the tissue damage and vascular changes in this case were unclear.

Anaphylactic shock has been attributed to methylthioninium chloride (SEDA-22, 526).

Mexiletine

Mexiletine caused an increased incidence of positive antinuclear antibody (ANA) titers in some studies (806,807), but not in others (808,809). The clinical significance of this effect is not clear. For example, there have been no reports of a lupus-like syndrome attributable to mexiletine.

Mexiletine caused increases in the serum activities of aspartate transaminase, alanine transaminase, and alkaline phosphatase in a few patients.

Minocycline

Immunoallergic reactions have been reported with minocycline and include lupus-like syndrome, autoimmune hepatitis, eosinophilic pneumonia, hypersensitivity syndrome, a serum sickness-like illness (810), and Sweet's syndrome (SEDA-21, 262J; SEDA-22, 271). Over 60 minocycline-induced cases of lupus-like syndrome and 24 cases of minocycline-induced autoimmune hepatitis were found in a review of the literature (811). In 13 patients, both disorders co-existed. These patients had symmetrical polyarthralgia/polyarthritis, raised liver enzymes, and positive antinuclear antibodies; they were also generally antihistone-negative, and only two patients had p-ANCA antibodies. Minocycline-related lupus can also occur in adolescents (812).

Lupus-like syndrome

Drug-induced lupus is a well-known phenomenon, although the mechanisms are unclear. The diagnostic features should include no prior history of systemic lupus erythematosus (SLE) before the start of treatment, at least one clinical feature of SLE, a positive antinuclear antibody during sustained drug therapy, and dramatic symptomatic improvement after drug withdrawal. Since 1970, at least 49 drugs have been reported to be associated with drug-related lupus (813), of which hydralazine and procainamide have been claimed to be the most commonly implicated. However, new reports on minocycline-induced lupus continue to appear (814–816) and it is possible that minocycline is now the most common cause.

In a retrospective nested case-control study in 27 688 young patients with acne, 711572 had used minocycline, of whom 1565 had the lupus-like syndrome (817). Minocycline was associated with an 8.5-fold risk of the lupus-like syndrome. The effect was greater in longer-term users, but the absolute risk of developing lupus-like syndrome seemed to be relatively low.

Minocycline-induced lupus usually occurs some months, or even years, after the start of therapy, and it usually resolves when the drug is withdrawn. The diagnosis can easily be overlooked, especially in patients with rheumatoid arthritis (818). It would always be wise to follow the recommendation that a patient's antinuclear antibody be checked before starting minocycline and when drug-induced lupus is suspected.

In a retrospective review of drug safety databases, minocycline was the only tetracycline derivative that caused drug-induced lupus (SEDA-22, 268; 819). The authors proposed that the propensity of minocycline to cause drug-induced lupus may be due to the presence of a functional group that is easily oxidized to a reactive metabolite. However, the chemically modified tetracycline CMT-3, which has also reportedly caused a lupus-like syndrome (820), lacks this group, so another theory is needed.

- A 16-year-old girl, who had taken minocycline for acne for more than 2 years, developed a severe cough with paroxysms (821). She had also a recent history of joint pain with swelling and stiffness, fever, general weakness, and weight loss of 9 kg. She had been treated as an outpatient for presumed pneumonia with multiple antibiotics, but developed progressive dyspnea. Pulmonary lupus was suspected, and minocycline was withdrawn. She was treated with an initial 3-day course of intravenous methylprednisolone 20 mg tds, and then prednisone for 2 weeks. She improved very rapidly, and the prednisone was gradually reduced over 7 weeks.

According to the authors, the patient fulfilled all the criteria for a diagnosis of drug-induced lupus-like syndrome, that is no history of lupus erythematosus before

minocycline therapy, the presence of antinuclear antibodies, at least one clinical feature of lupus erythematosus, and prompt recovery after withdrawal of minocycline. She also had positive antihistone antibodies, compatible with drug-induced lupus-like syndrome.

- A 54-year-old woman with a 2-week history of low-grade fever, dry cough, and dyspnea was given levofloxacin for a presumed community-acquired pneumonia (822). Five days later she developed severe respiratory failure and was mechanically ventilated and given antibiotics (imipenem and clarithromycin). Microbiological examination of tracheobronchial aspirates was negative for pathogenic organisms, as were serological tests for common agents of atypical pneumonia. She progressively improved and was taken off the ventilator after 6 days and discharged about 10 days later, but 14 days later was readmitted with rapidly progressive pulmonary failure requiring mechanical ventilation. It then transpired that 2 weeks before the first episode of respiratory failure, she had started to take oral minocycline for acne vulgaris and had started to take it again 24 hours before the second episode. The minocycline was stopped and she was given intravenous methylprednisolone. She improved rapidly, and for 12 months after minocycline withdrawal she remained free of respiratory symptoms.

It is a good rule of thumb that patients who develop minocycline-induced lupus should never be rechallenged with minocycline, as symptoms tend to recur (815,823,824). If minocycline is used to treat rheumatoid arthritis, the patient should be followed very carefully, as worsening arthritis may be erroneously attributed to the underlying disease. It should also be emphasized that in the search for a cause of joint pains, minocycline should always be considered (825).

Minoxidil

A "polymyalgia syndrome," characterized by fatigue, anorexia, weight loss, and severe pain in the shoulders and the pelvic girdle, was attributed to minoxidil in four men (826).

In 11 patients allergic to topical minoxidil lotion, patch tests showed that four were positive to minoxidil itself (827). Propylene and butylene glycol are used as solvents for minoxidil in topical formulations. Nine of the 11 patients appeared to have positive patch tests to propylene glycol and one of the 11 reacted to its alternative butylene glycol.

- A 57-year-old man developed a pigmented contact dermatitis after using topical minoxidil 5% for 2 years (828). Patch tests were negative with the European standard series and with a textile and finishes series, but positive with minoxidil 5% on days 3 and 7. However, withdrawal of the minoxidil did not lead to improvement after 10 months.
- A 24-year-old woman with androgenic alopecia became sensitized to topical minoxidil after using minoxidil 4%

with retinoic acid in a propylene glycol base (829). She subsequently also became sensitized to saw palmetto (*Serenoa repens*), a topical herbal extract commonly promoted for the treatment of hair loss.

- Allergic contact dermatitis occurred in a 54-year-old man who had used 1% minoxidil on the scalp for 8 months (830). He had positive patch tests to minoxidil in alcohol, but not to minoxidil in petrolatum, piperidine, pyrimidine, or diaminopyrimidine.

The authors of the last report suggested that the whole structure of minoxidil is required for sensitization and that propylene glycol in the formulation of minoxidil that is used therapeutically increases the penetration of minoxidil into the skin, enhancing the risk of a reaction.

Monoamine oxidase inhibitors

Rashes have been reported, but their relation to drug ingestion is poorly substantiated. The hepatocellular damage caused by hydrazine derivatives is probably mediated by an immunological mechanism.

Monobactams

Aztreonam has minor immunogenicity in animals and was associated with a 2% incidence of all presumably immunologically mediated drug reactions in early phase I and II trials (831).

When *Escherichia coli* was co-cultured with mouse peritoneal macrophages and exposed to aztreonam and ceftazidime, there was enhanced secretion of TNF-alpha; imipenem did not do this (832). Both aztreonam and ceftazidime enhanced LPS release from *E. coli* while imipenem did not, consistent with the observed differences in TNF-alpha release. All three antibiotics increased *E. coli*-induced expression of inducible nitric oxide synthase (iNOS), as assessed by both mRNA and protein.

Negligible cross-reactivity has been reported in both animal and human studies involving hapten inhibition, skin tests, and treatment of penicillin-allergic patients with therapeutic doses of aztreonam (831,833–838). Aztreonam therefore seems to be a safe alternative for patients with penicillin allergy. However, the numbers of safely treated patients reported are still small, and immediate type hypersensitivity to aztreonam has been reported in patients with penicillin allergy (839–842).

Several cephalosporins, for example ceftazidime, have the same aminothiazole side chain as aztreonam.

Sensitization with either drug involving side chain-specific antibodies may therefore predispose to allergy to the other. However, clinical data on this problem are currently not available.

Morniflumate

- A 4-year-old girl developed angioedema and urticaria 30 minutes after receiving rectal morniflumate. Her

signs and symptoms resolved in 48 hours. Skin prick and intradermal tests to morniflumate were negative, but rechallenge with rectal administration caused a recurrence (843).

Moxifloxacin

See Fluoroquinolones

Myrtaceae

Of 1017 subjects, 16 had positive skin tests to *Melaleuca quinquenervia* pollen extract (844). Six of them were subjected to double-blind nasal challenge with the pollen extract and four to single-blind bronchial challenge; 11 received 34 different *Melaleuca* odor challenges (blossoms, bark, and leaves) through a closed system for up to 30 minutes. Four inhaled an odor from cajeput oil (derived from *Melaleuca* leaves) for 1 hour. One of six nasal challenges and one of four bronchial challenges were positive. All the odor challenges with blossoms, bark, leaves, and cajeput oil were negative. A radioallergosorbent test for *Melaleuca* pollen extract correlated with the skin test results. The authors concluded that the *Melaleuca* tree is not a significant source of aeroallergens and explained the few positive results on the basis of cross-reactivity with pollen extracts from a proven aeroallergen, *Bahia* grass pollen.

Naproxen

See NSAIDs

Neuroleptic drugs

Hypogammaglobulinemia in a 22-year-old woman with brief psychotic disorder has been attributed to neuroleptic drug therapy (845). About 4 months after she had started to receive neuroleptic drugs, her serum concentrations of total protein had fallen to 58 g/l, with an IgG concentration of 3.49 g/l, an IgA concentration of 0.54 g/l, and an IgM concentration of 0.34 g/l.

Antiphospholipid syndrome is a disorder of recurrent arterial or venous thrombosis, thrombocytopenia, hemolytic anemia, or a positive Coombs' test, and in women recurrent idiopathic fetal loss, associated with raised concentrations of antiphospholipid antibodies. In systemic lupus erythematosus, the risk of this syndrome is about 40%, compared with a risk of 15% in the absence of antiphospholipid antibodies (846). However, only half of those with antiphospholipid antibodies have systemic lupus erythematosus, and the overall risk of the syndrome is about 30%. In patients who have antiphospholipid antibodies associated with chlorpromazine, there appears to be no increased risk of the syndrome. In contrast, in the primary antiphospholipid syndrome, the only clinical manifestations are the features of this syndrome.

- Symptomatic antiphospholipid syndrome has been described in a 42-year-old woman treated with chlorpromazine 260 mg/day (847). She presented with sudden-sided weakness, numbness, and headache. Examination confirmed upper motor neuron signs affecting the right arm, leg, and face, with hemiplegia and hemiparesthesia. Autoantibody screening showed positive antinuclear antibodies, with an IgG titer of 50 and an IgM titer of 1600. Anticardiolipin antibody was positive with a raised IgM titer of 24 (normal less than 9). The symptoms and the serological findings resolved after withdrawal of the phenothiazine.

Drug-induced lupus erythematosus has been reviewed (848,849). Neuroleptic drugs, particularly chlorpromazine and chlorprothixene, have often been associated with this autoimmune disorder. It is recommended that several diagnostic criteria for this condition should be met: (1) exposure to a drug suspected to cause lupus erythematosus; (2) no previous history of the condition; (3) detection of positive antinuclear antibodies; and (4) rapid improvement and a gradual fall in the antinuclear antibodies and other serological findings on drug withdrawal. Rare disorders of connective tissue resembling systemic lupus erythematosus have been reported with chlorpromazine, perphenazine, and chlorprothixene (850).

Neuromuscular blocking drugs

Hypersensitivity reactions can occur with all neuromuscular blocking agents, including the newer agents (851–853). Allergic reactions during anesthesia have been reviewed (854).

Frequency

The incidence of life-threatening anaphylactic or anaphylactoid reactions occurring during anesthesia is variably reported as being between one in 1000 and one in 10 000 anesthetics (855,856), and in one survey was one in 6500 (857). The frequency quoted depends on the criteria used. An epidemiological study (858) has suggested that the incidence is somewhat greater than one in 5000 anesthetics. The mortality from such serious reactions is reported to be in the range of 3.4–6% (856–858). Minor systemic reactions attributable to histamine release probably occur in more than 1% of anesthesia (859). Neuromuscular blocking drugs are the triggering agents in 151% or more of these reactions (860–862), and of them D-tubocurarine is the most potent histamine liberator. During the last two decades, however, several large series of patients have been investigated, and the data suggest that suxamethonium is the relaxant most likely to produce life-threatening reactions, if allowances are made for the frequency of usage of the different agents (SEDA-17, 12; 858,860,862–866). Pancuronium has repeatedly been shown to be the relaxant least often associated with anaphylactoid reactions major or minor.

The incidence of allergic reactions to several muscle relaxants has been assessed in relation to the number of vials sold in France (867). In line with a previous publication (868), the proportion of reported reactions to rocuronium was higher than its corresponding market share. Based on that, the authors suggested classifying the risk of allergic reactions to neuromuscular blocking agents as high (suxamethonium, rocuronium), intermediate (pancuronium, vecuronium, mivacurium), and low (atracurium, cisatracurium). This classification is based on the assumption that the ratio of used/sold vials is similar for each agent, which may or may not be true. The authors themselves insisted that they did not recommend one muscle relaxant over another on the basis of their allergic potential (869). As highlighted before (SEDA-26, 150), there are significant methodological and statistical problems when such rare events are compared. What we need is an international network of clinics specialized in investigating patients after suspected intraoperative allergic reactions, and the French GERAP centers are an excellent example of this.

Nickel

Nickel allergy is an adverse effect of the use of nickel-containing medical appliances, such as orthopedic metal alloys, dental materials, and implants (870), and allergic reactions are common. Nickel allergy and contact dermatitis with nickel-based appliances have been reviewed (871).

- A 13-year-old non-atopic girl with a 1-year history of recurrent itchy eyelid inflammation and conjunctivitis in both eyes had been fitted with a removable orthodontic appliance 14 months before (872). The metal wires of the orthodontic appliance were made of steel containing 10–13% nickel and 16–19% chromium. Patch-testing confirmed allergy to nickel. A low nickel diet improved the dermatitis, but it did not clear. She was advised to stop wearing the orthodontic appliance, and the ocular lesions cleared within 2 weeks.

In 700 Finnish adolescents, of whom 476 had a history of orthodontic treatment with metallic appliances and others a history of ear-piercing, the frequency of nickel sensitization was 19% (873); in other studies of adolescent girls, among whom body-piercing was popular, sensitivity has been as high as 30%. A review of the literature concerning nickel hypersensitivity in relation to orthodontic appliances has shown that the risk is very low for patients who are not nickel hypersensitive at the start of the treatment (874).

Occupational exposure explains most cases of nickel-associated asthma (875) and rhinitis (876).

Contact dermatitis as a reaction to nickel is well known but usually reflects continuing non-medical exposure, for example among hairdressers (877); nickel released from injection needles and from Dermojets can, however, also give rise to cutaneous hypersensitivity reactions.

Exceptionally, nickel contained in food has caused recurrence of an earlier contact dermatitis to the metal (878); sensitivity to nickel in food may be caused by a type

IV immunological reaction in the gut. The commonly recommended patch test procedure is not fully reliable for diagnosing nickel allergy. The lymphocyte transformation test has been suggested as a useful additional tool (879); an increased incidence of HLA-B21 was found in patients with cutaneous nickel hypersensitivity (880).

Although sensitization to nickel sulfate is common in patients with anogenital contact dermatitis and in patients with dermatitis in other body sites, the relevance to anogenital complaints of sensitization to nickel sulfate should always be doubted (881–883). However, direct transmission of nickel between the hands and the anogenital region has to be taken into account, and food can be a rare source of nickel contact in the anogenital area. In these cases relevance can be proved by oral nickel provocation and a nickel-restricted diet for a limited period may be justified (884).

The therapeutic use of intramuscular chrysotherapy has been limited by the high incidence of skin adverse effects. The pathogenic mechanisms of these are unknown, but could include allergic reactions to gold or to nickel as a contaminant. In order to investigate these mechanisms further, 15 patients who developed skin eruptions after chrysotherapy were assessed using skin biopsy and lymphocyte transformation stimulated by gold and nickel salts in vitro (885). Chrysotherapy caused two main cutaneous eruptions: lichenoid reactions and non-specific dermatitis. Peripheral blood mononuclear cells from patients with lichenoid reactions proliferated in response to gold salts in vitro, while those who developed non-specific dermatitis responded mainly to nickel. Nickel was a significant contaminant of the gold formulation (sodium aurothiomalate, Myocrisin, Rhone-Poulenc Ltd), amounting to a total dose of 650 ng over 6 months. The authors suggested that a significant percentage of skin reactions during chrysotherapy are due to nickel contamination.

- A 79-year-old woman had an abdominal aortic aneurysm repaired with a straight Vanguard R stent, mainly composed of nickel (about 55%) and titanium (about 21%) with a reinforcing thread of platinum (886). Three weeks later she developed severe erythema and eczema on the legs with continuous pruritus and excoriated papules. Patch tests were positive to nickel sulfate and cobalt chloride.The need for preoperative patch-testing for metals is controversial. Enquiry about metal allergy is recommended before endoluminal surgical procedures.

The mobile-phone culture has spread rapidly and possible effects connected with its use may still be underestimated (887).

- A 36-year-old dermatologist with a history of jewellery intolerance developed dermatitis on the right side of the chin, with red pruritic papules. The dermatitis had worsened after prolonged use of her mobile phone. Patch tests were positive to nickel sulfate. She solved the problem by covering the phone with a plastic case.

- A 32-year-old woman developed dermatitis on her left cheek and suggested that it might have been caused or worsened by her mobile phone. Patch tests showed only positive reaction to nickel sulfate. The dimethylglyoxime test for nickel on the side of her phone was positive. The skin lesion resolved rapidly after she covered the phone with a plastic case.

Nicotine replacement therapy

Leukocytoclastic vasculitis has been ascribed to nicotine patches in two patients (888). Two other patients developed vasculitis in association with the use of nicotine patches (889). The authors concluded that it was likely that the reactions in the two patients were related to the nicotine therapy. However, the possibility of a reaction to the vehicle (coconut oil and polymers) could not be excluded.

Nicotinic acid and derivatives

Anaphylactic shock can occur with nicotinic acid (890).

A pseudoallergic reaction has been reported in a patient who took several nicotinic acid-containing formulations (891).

- A previously healthy 40-year-old woman developed a generalized macular erythematous rash associated with palpitation and light-headedness, recurring every few days. The rash started behind the neck and arms, with a sensation of tingling, progressing to a general feeling of heat. She felt ill and had to lie down until the episode subsided after 45–90 minutes, with residual fatigue for several hours. Laboratory findings were all in the reference ranges. She was taking two multivitamin tablets a day, each containing nicotinic acid 20 mg, one B complex tablet containing nicotinic acid 50 mg, and 1–3 tablets of an antiemetic containing nicotinic acid 50 mg. Thus, she had unknowingly taken nicotinic acid up to 240 mg/day. Graded oral challenge with nicotinic acid 20–200 mg reproduced her symptoms.

Nifedipine

See Calcium channel blockers

Nitrofurantoin

In patients with the lupus-like syndrome at least two immunological tests (antinuclear factor, rheumatoid factor, Coombs' test, and antibodies against smooth muscle, thyroglobulin, thyroid cell cytoplasm, or glomeruli) were positive. The lymphocyte transformation test was always positive. However, the LE cell phenomenon was always negative. As in other allergic reactions to nitrofurantoin, circulating albumin IgG complexes were found by immunoelectrophoresis, with tailing of the albumin line (892). The syndrome regresses after withdrawal.

Non-steroidal anti-inflammatory drugs (NSAIDs)

There is considerable difficulty and controversy in identifying and classifying allergic reactions to NSAIDs, for many reasons (893). First, the difficulty in making a definite diagnosis in patients who have these reactions without provocative challenge with the suspected drug and other NSAIDs. Secondly, reactions are characterized by a large spectrum of target organ responses to NSAIDs, and the same drug may cause different types of reactions in different organs in the same or different individuals. Thirdly, a patient can have a similar reaction to a structurally different NSAID. Finally, reports of these reactions include different, often imprecise, terms, making interpretation difficult.

Anaphylactic or anaphylactoid reactions to NSAIDs are probably relatively rare. Even today, the only data available are from 1981, when the FDA's Division of Drug Experience was notified of 131 cases attributable to various NSAIDs (894). Tolmetin was the most frequently implicated compound. However, the figures are distorted, because some of these drugs are much more widely used than others. A retrospective cohort study using 1980–84 Medicaid billing data from three states in the USA, designed to assess the relative risk of hypersensitivity reactions from different NSAIDs, failed to confirm that tolmetin is associated with a higher risk of hypersensitivity reactions than other NSAIDs (895). However, two drugs (glafenine and zomepirac) have been withdrawn from the market because of their propensity to cause severe hypersensitivity reactions.

The clinical picture of hypersensitivity reactions varies from vasomotor rhinitis, urticaria, and angioedema to serious bronchoconstriction and in some cases anaphylactic shock.

Two pathogenic mechanisms have been proposed: an allergic immunological hypersensitivity reaction and a pseudoallergic reaction characterized by mast-cell degranulation by complement components, histamine liberation by drugs, and interference with endogenous eicosanoid biosynthesis (896). The first mechanism appears to be responsible for anaphylactic shock and/or urticaria after amidopyrine or noramidopyrine, and the second for bronchoconstriction after aspirin, noramidopyrine, or aminophenazone and other pyrazole drugs. It is important to distinguish the two mechanism, since the first type of intolerance is fairly structure-specific and can be avoided by switching from a drug to which the patient has proved sensitive to an NSAID with a distinct structure, whereas pseudoallergic aspirin-sensitive patients must avoid all drugs that inhibit fatty acid cyclo-oxygenase.

There have been reports of exaggerated responses (angioedema and malaise) to bee stings in patients taking NSAIDs (SEDA-11, 88). More recently a report of resensitization to bee stings associated with diclofenac has been received by the Centre for Adverse Reactions Monitoring in New Zealand. The patient, who had been successfully desensitized to bee venom many years before, developed life-threatening anaphylaxis after a bee sting while taking diclofenac (897).

Infection risk

NSAIDs can mask signs of infection, such as fever and pain, which can delay appropriate treatment. Furthermore they can impair the host defence mechanism against infection and can modulate the acute inflammatory response in such a way as to alter the course of infection, predisposing the patient to bacteremia, shock, and multiorgan failure (898,899). Until appropriate studies have defined the relation between NSAIDs and severe soft tissue infections, it is better to avoid using them, if possible, until the cause of the fever is known.

In 11 cases of necrotizing fasciitis (which is usually caused by *Streptococcus pyogenes*) NSAIDs were suspected to have predisposed to the infection and/or to have caused its fulminant evolution (SEDA-12, 79). Sporadic cases continue to be reported (900), but a causal link between this severe infection and NSAIDs is far from proven (901).

Diclofenac

Acute allergic reactions were reported in 48 patients, and included anaphylactic or anaphylactoid reactions and angioedema without shock. Two anaphylactic reactions, one fatal, to parenteral diclofenac have been reported (SEDA-18, 104). Hepatorenal damage (SEDA-15, 100), thrombocytopenia, and hemolytic anemia mediated by an immune mechanism have been reported (SEDA-16, 110).

Skin tests with diclofenac were not useful in diagnosing hypersensitivity in a series of 12 non-atopic patients who had severe symptoms of hypersensitivity (902). However, oral challenge in patients who had had only cutaneous symptoms was diagnostic.

Flurbiprofen

Leukocytoclastic vasculitis caused by flurbiprofen has been observed in a patient with rheumatoid arthritis (SEDA-15, 101).

Ibuprofen

Anaphylaxis after ibuprofen was reported in a patient with asthma who was also taking zafirlukast, a leukotriene receptor antagonist (SEDA-22, 116).

Indometacin

Masking of infection and abnormal immune reactions have been reported (903). It is not clear whether this has any clinical significance.

Ketorolac

Anaphylaxis and anaphylactoid reactions have been reported (SEDA-17, 112).

Loxoprofen

Three cases of a type-I hypersensitivity reaction to loxoprofen, characterized by generalized urticarial rash and dyspnea, have been reported (904,905).

Mefenamic acid

Asthma and anaphylactic shock are the most dangerous acute hypersensitivity reactions. There is cross-sensitivity with other NSAIDs (906). Rash, urticaria, and pruritus accompany more serious reactions.

Meloxicam

Meloxicam may be relatively safe when given to patients with NSAID-induced urticaria/angioedema (907,908). Of 148 NSAID-sensitive subjects with an unequivocal history of urticaria with or without angioedema, who were challenged with increasing oral doses of meloxicam (1–7 mg/day) in a single-blind placebo-controlled trial, only two had a positive test (urticaria in one and urticaria/angioedema in the other); both had chronic idiopathic urticaria (909).

Naproxen

Generalized reactions (910) include cutaneous necrotizing vasculitis (SEDA-5, 106; SEDA-17, 113), nephritis, paralytic ileus, and angiitis with cutaneous, muscular, articular, and renal involvement (911).

- A leukocytoclastic vasculitis occurred in a 62-year-old woman with skin, peripheral nerve, and renal involvement (912). Long-term corticosteroid treatment caused gradually resolution.
- Exercise-induced anaphylaxis in a girl who had been taking naproxen for 3 weeks was confirmed by rechallenge (SEDA-21, 106).

Tolmetin

From early on, the high incidence of hypersensitivity reactions with tolmetin was striking, for example in spontaneous adverse reaction reports. However, the high incidence was not confirmed in a retrospective comparative review (SEDA-6, 98; SEDA-7, 134; 913). Several factors can explain the discrepancy. For example, patients covered by the review may have persisted with treatment, since they did not experience such reactions.

Nucleoside analogue reverse transcriptase inhibitors (NRTIs)

- A man developed several erythematous plaques on his face due to borderline tuberculoid leprosy with a reversal reaction (914). He had severe CD4 T cell lymphocytopenia due to HIV infection and had been given HAART. A fall in viral load and an increase in CD4 count preceded the development of the skin lesions,

suggesting immune reconstitution as the underlying mechanism for the reversal reaction.

Paradoxical reactions are often observed in patients with pulmonary and extra-pulmonary tuberculosis being treated with HAART. Clinicians need to distinguish these from other adverse reactions related to drug therapy. Reversal reactions in leprosy are increasingly likely as more patients with HIV infection are treated with HAART in developing countries.

Nystatin

Allergic reactions to topical use are rare (SED-11, 576; 915).

Contact allergy due to topical nystatin has been reported in a woman using a combination of clobetasol and nystatin (916). The contact allergy was demonstrated with a positive patch test on day 4.

In another case, the patient developed a maculopapular rash over the trunk and limbs, associated with fever, arthralgia, malaise, and diarrhea; nystatin patch tests were positive on days 2 and 4 (917).

Oak moss resin

Oak moss resin is usually reported as a contact allergen in those who use perfumed products, but is also reported in rural and forestry workers (918). Perfumes are recognized as being potential sensitizers in soluble oils (919), but oak moss as a specific sensitizer within a coolant has not previously been reported.

- A 47-year-old atopic man gave a 3-year history of dermatitis of his hands, forearms, and face (920). He had worked for 24 years as an engineer, grinding components for printing presses. During an enforced absence from work, he noticed that his rash had resolved, but it relapsed within 2 days of his return. Further remissions were noted during his annual holidays, but the rash would always recur within 2 days of returning to work. His skin eruption continued to deteriorate until the coolant used during the grinding process was withdrawn. His rash subsequently resolved and did not recur. Patch testing with standard series, oils and coolants, the constituents of fragrance mix, and his own coolant gave strong positive reactions to fragrance mix, balsam of Peru (*Myroxylon pereirae*), sodium metabisulfite, diethanolamine, and oak moss, and a smaller reaction to his own coolant. The manufacturer of the coolant was contacted for information on the individual constituents of the oil. Further patch tests were then carried out with these components plus the individual components of the fragrance used within it. There were strong positive reactions to oak moss resin and monoethanolamine.

This case highlights the importance of patch testing with individual components of a suspected product in occupational dermatitis. This reduces the chance of false positive reactions and of missing a relevant allergen.

Ocular dyes

Most systemic reactions after intravenous fluorescein are allergic, but in the past some were due to contamination with dimethylformamide, an industrial solvent (921). It is difficult to predict adverse effects by intracutaneous testing. A delayed allergic response, developing a few hours after intravenous fluorescein dye injection, can occur (922). It is recommended that a complete allergy evaluation be performed in all patients who have adverse reactions to fluorescein, in order to differentiate true allergic reactions from other types of reactions (923).

Olanzapine

Hypersensitivity syndrome, defined as a drug-induced complex consisting of fever, rash, and internal organ involvement, has been associated with olanzapine (924).

- A 34-year-old man took clozapine for several months, but developed a cardiomyopathy. Clozapine was withdrawn and olanzapine 20 mg/day was given instead; 60 days later he developed a recurrent high fever, rash, and pruritus. There was bilateral periorbital edema and generalized erythroderma without target lesions or bullae and no mucosal involvement. He also had an eosinophilia and hepatitis.

Omeprazole

See Proton pump inhibitors

Opioid analgesics

An anaphylactic reaction to epidural fentanyl has been reported (925). Anaphylaxis has been reported with dihydrocodeine (926).

Pethidine

Pethidine causes histamine release (927). Of 16 patients given pethidine (mean dose 4.3 mg/kg), 5 had signs of the effects of histamine (hypotension, tachycardia, erythema) and raised histamine concentrations (927).

- A 42-year-old patient presented with generalized pruritus, erythema, urticaria, facial angioedema, dysphagia, dysphonia, and dizziness 95 minutes after a single intramuscular dose of pethidine 100 mg for severe renal colic (928). Prick tests and intradermal tests with pethidine and other compounds confirmed an allergic reaction to pethidine.

Orgotein

Two anaphylactic reactions have been reported, one after intra-articular injection, the other after submucosal bladder injection of orgotein. An IgE-mediated mechanism was demonstrated in the first case (SEDA-12, 94; SEDA-14, 96).

Oxamniquine

Fever occurs in about a quarter of patients taking oxamniquine (SEDA-11, 598) (929), and in some 15% of these, a Löffler-like syndrome with eosinophilia and pulmonary infiltrates was seen when it was specifically looked for.

Oxaprozin

Life-threatening respiratory distress, facial edema, and lethargy occurred in a woman with a history of severe asthma and aspirin allergy (SEDA-22, 118).

Oxitropium

Total serum IgE has been measured in 36 patients with allergic rhinitis and 11 healthy subjects given a submaximal dose of oxitropium bromide 600 micrograms by inhalation (930). FEV_1 was greater than 80% of predicted in all subjects. Baseline FEV_1 correlated negatively with serum IgE concentration. Oxitropium bromide inhalation produced an increase in FEV_1 (mean 155 ml) that was significantly greater in allergic patients with high serum IgE than in healthy subjects (64 ml) or in those with allergic rhinitis and low serum IgE (82 ml). The effect of an inhaled beta$_2$-adrenoceptor agonist (orciprenaline) was similar in all three groups. These findings may explain some of the variation in response to inhaled antimuscarinic drugs in patients with asthma. The data also suggested that IgE may itself modify airway tone by an increase in cholinergic responsiveness.

Oxygen-carrying blood substitutes

Hemoglobin solutions do not have the antigenic properties of the blood groups.

Pantothenic acid derivatives

Contact allergy to dexpanthenol is rare, but it occurs more often in some patients (for example those with eczema of the lower leg). Between 1992 and 1999, only 163 of 13 216 patients tested in the Information Network of Departments of Dermatology had a positive reaction to dexpanthenol. There have been no previous cases of occupational dexpanthenol sensitization caused by occupational exposure, but one has been reported in a junior nurse (931).

- Six weeks after starting training a 29-year-old nurse developed flushing and pruritus on the back of both hands and fingers, spreading to the forearms. Because of increased skin sensitivity she had been recommended to use skin protection measures; however, she did not use the skin protection cream that was available at the hospital but used a "Hand- und Hautsalbe" that had been designed for use especially in hairdressing salons. In addition to the lesions on her hands and arms she had periorbital shadowing, angular cheilitis, palmar hyperlinearity, and slightly generalized xerosis of the skin. She also reported seasonal rhinoconjunctivitis, intolerability of metals, and rhagades on the ears. After withdrawal of all supposed allergenic substances and local antieczematous therapy, the hand and arm lesions healed within a few days. Skin tests were positive for nickel-II-sulfate, imidazolidinyl urea, phenyl mercury acetate, and the hand cream, in which pantothenol (5% in vaseline) was identified as the allergen. She avoided the cream and the eczema did not recur.

Parabens

Parabens can cause allergic contact dermatitis that can run an insidious course, especially when the parabens are in glucocorticoid ointments. In such cases, treatment leads to a protracted dermatitis without acute exacerbation, so that neither the patient nor the physician suspects parabens as a possible cause. A sensitization index of 0.8% was found in 273 patients with chronic dermatitis (932).

In 1973, in a multicenter study of 1200 individuals carried out by the North American Contact Dermatitis Group, there was a 3% incidence of delayed hypersensitivity reactions to parabens. General allergic reactions have also been reported after the injection of parabens-containing formulations of lidocaine and hydrocortisone and after oral use of barium sulfate contrast suspension, haloperidol syrup, and an antitussive syrup, all of which contained parabens (SEDA-11, 484).

Paracetamol

Acute hypersensitivity reactions due to paracetamol are rare (SEDA-22, 114), but can be life-threatening (933).

Paraffins

Although soft paraffin has been used to treat irritant contact dermatitis (934) and to protect the skin from other sensitizers (935), hypersensitivity reactions can occur, but are rare (936–943). Yellow soft paraffin is slightly more antigenic than white soft paraffin (941). Contact sensitization to a neat cutting oil containing chlorinated paraffin occurred in 12 men (944). Contact urticaria mimicking dermatitis has also been reported (945).

Sensitization to soft paraffins can cause false-positive drug patch tests (946).

- A 31-year-old woman with a long history of presumed atopic dermatitis actually had contact dermatitis due to the soft white paraffin that was present in the several

medicaments (glucocorticoids, tacrolimus, pimecrolimus, and ciclosporin) that she had used to treat the skin (947).

Parathyroid hormone and analogues

Dose-dependent antiparathyroid hormone antibodies developed in under 10% of 1093 women in one study; however, there was no reduction in efficacy (948).

Parenteral nutrition

Parenteral nutrition can adversely affect the immune system, thereby increasing the risk of infection and sepsis, for example by impairing neutrophil function, blocking the function of the reticuloendothelial system, and altering cell-mediated immunity. However, much of the evidence has been obtained in experiments using large bolus doses; the immunological effects of more conservative doses administered as continuous infusions over 12–24 hour/day are less clear. As the chylomicron-like lipid is metabolized, increased triglyceride concentrations may alter the function of macrophages by reducing chemotaxis and phagocytic capacity, although this has not been consistently demonstrated. Excessive parenteral administration of lipid may overload the mononuclear cells of the reticuloendothelial system, resulting in an inability to clear bacteria from the bloodstream. Studies of the alterations in cellular immunity associated with intravenous infusions of lipid emulsions have produced mixed results. Increases in B lymphocyte and T lymphocyte counts, increased lymphocyte mitogenesis, and increased production of interleukin-2 have been reported in patients receiving parenteral lipids. Others have reported no change or reductions in natural killer cell counts, helper-to-suppressor cell ratios, and antibody-dependent cellular cytotoxicity compared with patients not receiving intravenous lipids. No significant changes in serum immunoglobulin or complement concentrations have been observed secondary to intravenous lipid administration.

A growing area of interest is the use of intravenous medium-chain triglycerides, which have a different metabolic fate to long-chain triglycerides and may not have similar detrimental effects on the reticuloendothelial function, leukocyte activity, and eicosanoid production. Another focus of research is the differences observed between the various lipid components and fatty acids. The polyunsaturated fatty acid content of cell membranes, an important factor in the structural and functional integrity of the cell, can be altered by the provision of increased amounts of n-3 fatty acids in place of n-6 fatty acids. In a 1987 study, the effects of different parenteral nutrition solutions on in vitro lymphocyte reactivity and measured lymphocyte responsiveness were investigated in patients during treatment (949). In vitro lymphocyte responses were significantly depressed by a fat emulsion at concentrations similar to those achieved in clinical practice, but were unaffected by dextrose or amino acid solutions. These and similar finding by others indicate that careful consideration should be given before using fat emulsions in patients whose cell-mediated immunity is already impaired.

Immune function has been studied in ten surgical infants (aged under 6 months) requiring parenteral nutrition in two consecutive phases: (a) after 31 days with no enteral feeding (parenteral nutrition) and (b) after 4.7 days from the addition to parenteral nutrition of small volumes of enteral feeding. Host bactericidal activity against coagulase-negative staphylococci, measured by an in vitro whole blood model, was lowest in the patients who received parenteral nutrition, and it increased significantly after the addition of small enteral feeds, approaching the levels measured in controls. Production of tumor necrosis factor-alfa was low during parenteral nutrition and rose significantly after the addition of small enteral feeds in patients on parenteral nutrition. The increase in killing of coagulase-negative staphylococci after the addition of small enteral feeds correlated significantly with the duration of enteral feeding. The mechanism causing impaired immune function during parenteral nutrition is not known, and it is probably multifactorial. Neither is it understood how small additional enteral feeds affect host bactericidal activity (950).

Allergic reactions

Severe allergic reactions can occur to parenterally administered lipid solutions. Such reactions may be mistaken for symptoms of the underlying disease or adverse effects of cytostatic chemotherapy (951). There is some evidence that the presence of soya bean proteins is responsible.

In 1989 the Perioperative Anaphylactic Reactions Study Group began an epidemiological survey of anaphylactoid reactions during anesthesia. Details recorded about patients who have suffered an anaphylactic reaction include demographic information and the results of allergy testing. In the most recent survey 1750 patients were reported from 27 diagnostic centers during January 1992 to June 1994 (952). Plasma substitutes accounted for 5.0% of the reactions observed. Intravenous infusions carry a comparatively small risk of anaphylaxis in the perioperative period. Other surveys come to a similar conclusion (953).

Allergic reactions have been reported infrequently in children receiving parenteral nutrition. The length of exposure before the reaction, the severity of the response, and the component responsible are variable.

- Anaphylaxis has been reported in a 4-year-old child when parenteral nutrition was resumed after a 5-day interruption in therapy after prior treatment 16 days after surgery for Wilms' tumor.

The authors considered the reaction to have been a type 1 IgE-mediated allergic response, although the causative agent was not identified. It was considered unlikely that individual amino acids had stimulated the allergic response, although the possibility of aggregated amino acids acting as a potential sensitizing agent could not be excluded. A component of the multivitamin mixture was considered the more likely explanation; the substances administered were vitamin E, vitamin K_1, the preservatives butylated hydroxyanisole (BHA) and butylated hydroxytoluene (BHT), and polysorbate emulsifiers (954).

Anaphylaxis linked to vitamin B complex in a parenteral nutrition regimen has been reported (955).

- An 8-year-old girl had a diaphragmatic hernia repaired at 7 days of age and had two episodes of adhesion ileus at 8 months. After laparotomy she was given all-in-one parenteral nutrition and after 21 days developed a reddish rash on her face and chest. The rash was pruritic and resolved quickly after intravenous diphenhydramine. She was readmitted 15 days after discharge because of malnutrition. Parenteral nutrition was restarted and she rapidly became irritable and developed an itchy rash over her face and trunk and swelling of her lips and eyelids. Parenteral nutrition was discontinued, diphenhydramine was given, and her symptoms abated rapidly. The possibility of hypersensitivity to a component of the parenteral nutrition was considered, and by a process of elimination the cause of the reaction was identified as the vitamin product MVI No 1. This was further confirmed by a skin test 1 year after the anaphylactic episode, but using a vitamin B complex solution.

Previous reports of anaphylactic reactions to parenteral nutrition have been identified as being caused by fat emulsion, vitamin K, iron dextran, and in particular multivitamins. This appears to be the first report of a reaction to vitamin B complex injection. However, neither the source of the vitamin B complex test product nor its formulation was identified by the authors, and there is doubt about the specific allergens responsible for the allergic response in this case.

Infection risk

Infection has long been recognized as a risk of parenteral nutrition and it has proved impossible to eliminate it (SEDA-22, 379). Once established, sepsis can increase the risk of fat overload syndrome. In an extensive study in Taiwan there was sepsis with positive blood cultures in 56 of 378 children receiving parenteral nutrition; the risk factors were longer duration of parenteral nutrition, age under 3 months, the use of central venous catheters, gastrointestinal disease as an indication for parenteral nutrition, low birth weight, and short gestational age in prematurity (956).

Various explanations have been offered for the occurrence of sepsis during parenteral nutrition, quite apart from the fact that the solution itself may be contaminated. Phytosterols can cause changes in neutrophil function. Cholestasis may play a role and then be further aggravated by the sepsis, creating a vicious circle. And fat emulsion may reduce hepatic phagocytosis. In vitro evidence using material from preterm infants suggests that administration of Intralipid may interfere with the binding of IL-2 to the specific receptors on their activated lymphocytes, with suppression of the immune response (957).

However, the clinical significance of these various mechanisms has been questioned. Some experimental in vitro work on human white cells suggests that the effect is markedly dose-dependent; it has been suggested that very few inhibitory effects on phagocytic cells will be found if lipid emulsion rates are kept at around 0.08 g/kg/hour (958). It is also notable that in one large series of premature very low birth weight infants in whom the use and duration of treatment with parenteral nutrition were associated with short gestational age and low birth weight, children treated with parenteral nutrition had a higher risk of sepsis usually caused by *Staphylococcus epidermidis* or *Staphylococcus aureus* (959). Thus, although the risk of sepsis in this age group appears to be significantly increased by parenteral nutrition, the causative organisms were fairly benign. It was concluded that the advantages of parenteral nutrition outweighed the risk of sepsis in this group of infants.

The incidences of bacteremia and fungemia during the first month after bone marrow transplantation for hematological malignancies have been studied in a prospective comparison in 512 patients. The patients were randomly assigned to receive 6–8% (low dose) or 25–30% (standard dose) of total energy as a 20% lipid emulsion. An adaptive randomization scheme, stratified for various treatments and transplant type, ensured that confounding treatment variables did not differ between the groups. Of 482 evaluable patients, 55 in the standard-dose group developed bacteremia or fungemia compared with 54 in the low-dose group. There was no association between the incidence of bacteremia or fungemia and intravenous lipid. Similar results were obtained when the results were analysed according to intention to treat, when bacterial or fungal infections at all sites were included, and when the observation period was extended to 60 days. These results suggest that moderate amounts of intravenous lipid rich in linoleic acid are not associated with an increased incidence of bacterial or fungal infections in patients undergoing bone marrow transplantation and receiving parenteral nutrition (960).

In infants of very low birth weight, fungal colonization and the association between fungal colonization and systemic fungal diseases was significantly linked to prolonged administration of antibiotics, parenteral nutrition, and fat emulsion (Intralipid) (961). Of 116 infants with birth weights under 1500 g, fungal colonization was detected in 25, of whom 17 developed colonization by 2 weeks of life. *Candida albicans* (61%) and *Candida parapsilosis* (29%) were the two most common organisms. The rectum (76%) was the most frequent site of colonization. Cultures were taken from the oropharynx, rectum, skin (groin and axilla), urine, and endotracheal aspirates in the first 24 hours after birth and weekly thereafter. There was an association between colonization and subsequent fungemia in one infant, representing 4% of colonized infants. It was also noted that although fungal colonization represents a risk factor for invasive candidiasis in infants of very low birth weight, candidiasis in this population is not invariably associated with prior colonization. Factors other than fungal colonization can also contribute to the occurrence of invasive candidiasis.

In a study of the independent risk factors for nosocomial coagulase-negative staphylococcal bacteremia among neonates of very low birth weight, after adjusting for the severity of the underlying illness, there was a significant association between coagulase-negative staphylococcal bacteremia and exposure during hospitalization to intravenous lipids (962). The study was conducted in 590 consecutively admitted neonates with birth weights under 1500 g, in two neonatal intensive care units, with a case-control study of 74 cases of coagulase-negative staphylococcal bacteremia and 74 pairs of matched controls. The independent risk factors for bacteremia were intravenous lipids (odds ratio 9.4), mechanical ventilation (OR = 2.0), and short peripheral venous catheters (OR = 2.6). It would appear that exposure to intravenous lipids at any time during hospitalization remains, and has possibly become an increasingly important risk factor for coagulase-negative staphylococcal bacteremia. In neonates of very low birth weight 85% of these bacteremias are now attributable to lipid therapy. In contrast, the relative importance of intravenous catheters as an independent risk factor has declined. Mechanical ventilation in the week before bacteremia has emerged as a risk factor for bacteremia.

There is evidence that lipid emulsion, which is cleared by the Kupffer cells of the reticuloendothelial system, can adversely affect reticuloendothelial function by reducing its ability to remove blood-borne bacteria. In a study of the blood clearance and organ localization of viable ^{35}S-radiolabelled *Escherichia coli* after slow intraperitoneal and more rapid intravenous administration of 20% fat emulsion in Sprague-Dawley rats, although there was rapid bacterial blood clearance in control and test animals, there was a significant change in the organ localization of bacteria as a result of the administration of lipid emulsion. There was a slight increase in lung localization of bacteria in rats that received intraperitoneal fat emulsion, and a significant increase in lung trapping of bacteria in rats that received intravenous fat emulsion. Liver localization of bacteria was reduced in all groups after fat emulsion. The data are understood to indicate that intravenous fat emulsion reduces hepatic phagocytosis and increases pulmonary localization of *E. coli*, and it is thought that this may produce greater susceptibility to infection. Patients with underlying sepsis are at greatest risk. The capacity of the lungs to kill sequestered bacteria is not known. Thus, increased bacterial lung localization may result in local inflammation and other pulmonary complications, and in the re-emergence into the blood of *E. coli*, with systemic sepsis as a result (963).

Paroxetine

See Selective serotonin reuptake inhibitors

Pefloxacin

See Fluoroquinolones

Penicillamine

Several experimental studies in humoral and cell-mediated immune systems have demonstrated numerous effects of penicillamine on the immune system; these findings are in keeping with a reduction in the overactivity of helper T lymphocyte that is found in rheumatoid arthritis (964,965). There is a fall in the numbers of immunoglobulin-secreting cells, and cultured mononuclear cells produce less IgA, IgG, and IgM. There is suppression of the autologous mixed lymphocyte reaction (966) and reduced hydroxyl radical generation from polymorphonuclear leukocytes (967). Penicillamine reduces the clearance of immune complexes and inhibits the complement cascade (968).

Penicillamine is uniquely likely among therapeutic drugs to cause autoimmune reactions (see Table 1).

Clinically and pathologically these variants of autoimmune disorders are closely similar to or indistinguishable from the spontaneous diseases. A major difference is that the patients usually recover when penicillamine is withdrawn. Differences in HLA configurations also suggest that penicillamine-induced and spontaneous autoimmune disorders occur in different populations.

During penicillamine treatment autoantibodies develop in a high proportion of patients without clinical disease (969). For example, penicillamine can be associated with the development of anticentromere antibodies (970,971). Although these are usually a marker of serious autoimmune diseases, in association with penicillamine, the phenomenon was not accompanied by clinical symptoms and disappeared after stopping the drug.

In the serum of three patients with acute hypersensitivity reactions to penicillamine, complement-binding antibodies against penicillamine were detected (972). Patients with Wilson's disease are not known to have an abnormal immune status. The striking variability of penicillamine-induced pathology, including autoimmune reactions such as SLE, is also seen in patients with Wilson's disease, but the proportion of these patients in whom withdrawal is necessary is smaller, about 2–8% (973–976).

An unusual case report showed that low back pain can be a manifestation of drug hypersensitivity (977).

Although hypersensitivity reactions are frequent, systemic anaphylaxis has only been reported rarely (978).

Penicillins

Type I reactions

Anaphylactic shock can occur, even after oral administration of penicillin and skin testing. However, anaphylactic shock is less common after oral than parenteral administration (979). In one study the incidence of anaphylactic shock was 0.04% of all patients treated with penicillin (980). It is also low in patients receiving long-term benzathine penicillin (1.2 million units every 4 weeks). Four episodes of anaphylaxis occurred in 0.012% of injections (1.2 reactions to 10 000 injections) (981). Anaphylactic shock resulting in death occurred in 0.002% of all patients treated with penicillin (1598) and in 0.003% of those treated with benzathine penicillin (981).

In nearly half of the cases, the course of anaphylactic shock, especially that induced by penicillin and other small molecular substances, is that of a cardiovascular reaction without any other effects suggestive of an allergic mechanism (982–984). There is an extensive list of articles on anaphylactic shock to penicillins (980,982,983,985–989). General anesthesia does not inhibit the development of anaphylactic shock in penicillin allergy (989).

Diagnosis

The two most important elements in the evaluation of an individual for the presence or absence of beta-lactam hypersensitivity are the drug history and skin tests. Other diagnostic tools, such as measurement of drug-specific antibodies and lymphocyte transformation tests, are investigational or restricted to specialized laboratories. Standardized and widely used protocols for skin testing only exist for the penicillins and allow assessment of IgE-mediated hypersensitivity. The most commonly used reagents are penicilloyl-polylysine (PPL, which contains multiple penicilloyl molecules coupled to a polylysine carrier) and fresh penicillin followed by minor determinant mixtures (MDM), containing penicilloate, benzylpenicilloate, and benzylpenilloate (990). A survey conducted among members of the American Academy of Allergy and Immunology reported the use of penicilloyl-polylysine and fresh penicillin by 86% and minor determinant mixtures by 40% of those responding to the questionnaire (991).

Skin tests are first applied as a prick test for safety. In the absence of a local or systemic reaction, an intradermal

Table 1 Autoimmune-like reactions reported in suspected association with penicillamine

Pemphigus (erythematosus, foliaceus, vulgaris)
Bullous pemphigoid, cicatricial pemphigoid
Graft-versus-host-like skin eruptions
Myasthenia gravis
Dermatomyositis/polymyositis
Glomerulonephritis
Lupus-like syndrome
Goodpasture's syndrome
Autoimmune hypoglycemia
Thyroiditis
Sjögren's syndrome
Aplastic anemia
Thrombocytopenia
Agranulocytosis
Thrombotic thrombocytopenic purpura (Moschcowitz's syndrome)
Evans' syndrome
Churg–Strauss syndrome
Necrotizing vasculitis
Guillain–Barré syndrome

test is performed and interpreted as described elsewhere (992,993). Experience with skin testing in penicillin allergy has been reviewed (987,994). Properly performed sequential testing is considered a safe procedure, and only an estimated 1% or less of penicillin allergic patients will have systemic symptoms while undergoing skin tests. However, at least three deaths have been reported with both epicutaneous and intradermal testing (995).

In a collaborative study in the National Institute of Allergy and Infectious Diseases (NIAID), hospitalized patients were tested with major and minor skin test reagents in order to assess the predictive value of skin testing. Among 600 history-negative patients, 568 had negative skin tests and none had a reaction to penicillin. Among 726 history-positive patients, 566 had a negative skin test and received penicillin, seven of whom (1.2%) had a possibly IgE-mediated reaction. Nine of the 167 patients with positive skin tests were exposed to penicillin, two of whom had reactions compatible with IgE-mediated reactions. These data suggest that overall, 99% of patients with negative skin tests to penicilloyl-polylysine and minor determinant mixtures can safely receive penicillin. A history of a previous reaction slightly increases the risk of an adverse reaction, to 1.2%. Most positive skin tests were detected with penicilloyl-polylysine with or without minor determinant mixtures, and a further 16% reacted to minor determinant mixtures alone (996).

In another study in an outpatient clinic for sexually transmitted diseases, 5063 consecutive patients were tested with penicilloyl-polylysine with and without minor determinant mixtures (997). The role of the history of a previous penicillin reaction was emphasized in this study: 1.7% of history-negative subjects had a positive skin test; in contrast, 7.1% of history-positive patients had a positive skin test, and a previous history of anaphylaxis or urticaria was associated with positive skin tests in 17% and 12% respectively. Penicillin was safe in more than 99% of patients with a negative history and a negative skin test. Reactions were more common (2.9%) in patients with a positive history and a negative skin test. The reactions were mild and self-limiting. Two patients with a history of severe IgE-mediated reaction had mild anaphylactic reactions.

Relatively safe doses for skin testing, provided that one begins with a prick test, are 25 nmol/ml of penicilloyl-polylysine and purified benzylpenicillin. Positive skin tests of the immediate type with penicilloyl-polylysine are usually obtained 2 weeks to 3 months after the clinical reaction (998).

The safety of such an approach has been challenged in a description of three patients who were negative in skin tests with penicilloyl-polylysine and minor determinant mixtures and who tolerated therapeutic doses of benzylpenicillin, but reacted to amoxicillin (982). In an extension of that study, 177 patients who were allergic to beta-lactams were identified using the clinical history, a skin test panel including penicilloyl-polylysine, and minor determinant mixtures, as well as ampicillin and amoxicillin and drug-specific radio-allergosorbent tests. Fifty-four

patients (31%) tolerated penicillin G but reacted to amoxicillin with anaphylaxis, urticaria, or angioedema. Skin tests with penicilloyl-polylysine and minor determinant mixtures failed to detect those patients, but tests with amoxicillin were positive in 63% (999).

Canadian data have partly confirmed these findings (1000). Benzylpenicillin derivatives and semisynthetic penicillins were applied to 112 patients with a history of an allergic reaction to penicillins. The tests were positive in 21 patients (19%), of whom 16 reacted against the semisynthetic penicillin reagents only. Reports of subjects allergic to flucloxacillin (1001), cloxacillin (1002), and cefadroxil (1003), but not penicillin, lend further support to the concept of side chain-specific allergic reactions (see the monograph on beta-lactam antibiotics).

Pentoxifylline

In an open, randomized, controlled trial in 56 children with cerebral malaria, the 26 children who received pentoxifylline 10 mg/kg/day by continuous infusion had significantly shorter periods of coma than the controls. The pentoxifylline recipients showed a trend toward a lower mortality. Pentoxifylline has an inhibitory effect on the synthesis of tumor necrosis factor alfa. The better outcome in the treated group was associated with a fall in tumor necrosis factor alfa serum concentrations on the third day of treatment in a few subjects; this was not seen in the controls (1004).

However, in a later, randomized, placebo-controlled trial pentoxifylline neither reduced tumor necrosis factor alfa serum concentrations nor affected the clinical course in 51 patients who received it as adjunctive treatment to standard antimalarial therapy in a dosage of 20 mg/kg/day over 5 days (1005).

Pertussis vaccine

See Vaccines

Pethidine

See Opioid analgesics

Phenols

Contact dermatitis in patients exposed to nonoxynols was initially considered to result from irritation, but allergic reactions have also been reported (1006). Nonoxynol contact allergy has been described in two patients who developed contact photosensitivity to nonoxynol-l0 in the antiseptic product Hexomedine transcutanée (1007). Among 32 control subjects, 13 had positive photopatch tests to Hexomedine transcutanée and four had positive photopatch tests to nonoxynol-10. Surprisingly, the authors observed that only undiluted nonoxynol was phototoxic. In another study, nonoxynol-9 was found to be rarely sensitizing and compatible with latex and silicone lubricants used in condoms (1008).

There is evidence of immunosuppressive effects due to interference by dibenzo-p-dioxin and/or dibenzofuran with the chemical properties of pentachlorphenol (SEDA-11, 485) (1009).

Phenylephrine

Phenylephrine was the drug that most often caused sensitization in patients with contact allergy after the application of mydriatic eye-drops. Since several eye-drops are often used in the same patient, it is always important to find out which drug or preservative is the allergen (1010–1013).

Phenylpropanolamine (norephedrine)

Phenylpropanolamine can give rise to severe allergic reactions with dyspnea, urticaria, and facial swelling (1014).

Phenytoin

There has been a report of hypersensitivity to phenytoin (which had been previously well tolerated) after a hypersensitivity reaction to carbamazepine (1015).

- A 19-year-old man with partial epilepsy took phenytoin 300 mg/day for over 6 months. Carbamazepine was introduced and after about 6 weeks (while taking phenytoin 300 mg/day and carbamazepine 600 mg/day) he developed fever, anorexia, a sore throat, bloody diarrhea, a diffuse, erythematous, maculopapular rash and palatal petechiae, tender cervical lymphadenopathy, and mild splenomegaly. His liver enzymes were raised and he had a leukocytosis with eosinophilia. Phenytoin and carbamazepine were withdrawn, and he was given prednisone and sodium valproate 1000 mg/day. The rash resolved, as did other manifestations of what was thought to be a hypersensitivity reaction. About a year later, phenytoin was reintroduced starting at 100 mg/day. He developed a sore throat after taking the first dose and a widespread rash after the second dose. There was no evidence of hepatic or hematological dysfunction. Phenytoin was withdrawn and the rash resolved in 1 week.

Cross-sensitivity among aromatic antiepileptic drugs occurs in about 75% of patients with a hypersensitivity reaction. It has previously been described on first exposure to each of the offending drugs (1016). However, this patient developed an allergic rash on his second exposure to phenytoin, having previously tolerated it for 6 months. This suggests that carbamazepine may have altered his response to phenytoin.

About 20 cases of a lupus-like syndrome have been described, mostly in the Scandinavian literature. The clinical picture consisted of arthralgia or, rarely, exacerbation of a pre-existing rheumatoid arthritis and generalized lymphadenopathy, mostly associated with chronic lung and/or liver reactions, such as chronic active hepatitis (1017,1018).

The phenytoin hypersensitivity syndrome ranges from a simple rash to a fulminant fatal illness with exfoliative dermatitis, vasculitis, and disseminated intravascular coagulation. Features include variable combinations of fever, eosinophilia, lymphadenopathy, hepatosplenomegaly, atypical lymphocytes, blood dyscrasias, serum sickness, hepatitis, and renal insufficiency.

IgA depression is seen in about 10% of patients (1019). There has been one report of deficiency of IgG2 and IgG4 (SEDA-17, 73) and one of panhypogammaglobulinemia (SEDA-16, 73).

- A 32-year-old man developed acute lung injury and renal insufficiency after 4 days of starting to take phenytoin (1020). The symptoms mimicked a renopulmonary syndrome, and resolved completely after withdrawal of phenytoin and the addition of steroids.

Giant cell myocarditis has been reported in a patient taking phenytoin, phenobarbital, and mephobarbital and in one taking primidone (1021).

Lupus-like syndrome has been attributed to phenytoin (1022).

- A 67-year-old white man who had taken phenytoin 300 mg/day for about 15 years developed fever, pericarditis, severe abdominal pain, malaise, and weight loss. He had a positive antinuclear antibody in a titer of 1:80 in a homogeneous pattern, a strongly positive antihistone antibody test, a raised erythrocyte sedimentation rate (115 mm/hour), and a neutrophilia (21 × 10^9/l). All these abnormalities resolved within a few weeks of withdrawal. Rechallenge was not performed.

The long delay between the start of therapy in this case and the clinical presentation makes it highly likely that phenytoin was not implicated and that recovery was spontaneous.

Photochemotherapy (PUVA)

Concerns that PUVA therapy can cause systemic lupus erythematosus (SLE) and other connective tissue diseases, such as giant cell arteritis (SEDA-6, 147), have been raised by several reports (SED-12, 336; SEDA-15, 139; SEDA-17, 183; 1023). There have been several studies of the incidence of serum antinuclear antibodies in patients who have received PUVA, with both positive and negative results. Current evidence suggests that frequent evaluation of antinuclear antibodies during treatment of patients with uncomplicated psoriasis with an initially negative antinuclear antibody test and with no symptoms of connective tissue diseases is unnecessary (1024).

Hypersensitivity reactions occur infrequently and have included drug fever, skin rashes, and bronchial asthma. Anaphylaxis to 5-methoxypsoralen has been reported (1025).

• A 36-year-old woman had been treated for a polymorphic light eruption with two annual courses of PUVA, three times weekly for 6 weeks, plus oral 5-methoxypsoralen 60 mg, without any adverse effects. However, during the fourth course, 30 minutes after taking 5-methoxypsoralen 60 mg, she developed intense pruritus of the palms, spreading to the body. This was followed by erythema of the palms and symmetrical erythematous patches and urticarial lesions on the trunk. She had dizziness and slight difficulty in breathing. Her symptoms cleared within an hour after intravenous administration of an antihistamine and cortisone. Two months later skin prick tests with 5-methoxypsoralen were negative, but placebo-controlled oral provocation with 5-methoxypsoralen 20 mg resulted in symptoms similar to those she had experienced during PUVA.

Physical contraceptives—intrauterine devices

Immunological and hypersensitivity reactions beyond the uterus are uncommon, but they can occur. Rashes, including generalized urticaria and eczematoid eruptions, have occurred as a result of allergy to the copper released from IUCDs, although they are extremely rare (SEDA-11, 204; SEDA-12, 186; SEDA-21, 234). One woman who had worn a copper-containing device for 12 months developed widespread urticaria and angioedema of the eyelids and the labia majora and minora for about 6 months (1026). She also had persistent symptoms of premenstrual and postmenstrual spotting and leukorrhea for about 6 months. A patch test was positive with 1% copper sulfate, as was an in vitro lymphocyte-stimulating test with copper. An endometrial biopsy showed vulvovaginitis, with hyperplasia of the cervical canal and T cell and eosinophilic granulocyte infiltration. Removal of the device caused complete remission.

The incidence of salpingitis and other pelvic inflammation is believed to be higher in users of IUCDs. A study of cervical smears in women using IUCD contraception compared with others using other methods of contraception showed that the incidence of cervical inflammation was higher in the former (1027).

Genital tract actinomycosis has come increasingly to the fore (1028,1029). In one study in Britain, the pelvic smears of nearly one-third of women using plastic devices were positive for *Actinomyces*-like organisms, compared with two of 165 women using copper-loaded IUCDs and none in a series of oral contraceptive users. There was a highly significant correlation between the presence of these organisms on smear and pain or other symptoms of pelvic inflammatory disease.

Current users of IUCDs suffer more often from acute rather than chronic pelvic inflammatory disease (1.51 compared with 0.54 times per 1000 woman-years). In ex-users the situation was reversed, chronic pelvic inflammatory disease being more common (0.95 compared with 0.48 times per 1000 woman-years) (1030).

Plague vaccine

See Vaccines

Plasma products

Immunological adverse effects of the administration of plasma range from mild urticaria and flushing to fatal anaphylaxis. Such reactions can occur either during the infusion or some minutes after. Mild reactions often start locally and have a tendency to spread. In more severe cases dyspnea, arthralgia, and fever occur. Stabilizers or other additives in plasma protein preparations may be of significance in provoking these reactions. In addition, protein aggregates in the preparations may participate in anaphylactoid reactions, including acute pulmonary injury. Severe reactions have occasionally been encountered.

Development of an antibody response

The development of an antibody response against a deficient or genetically different protein can cause post-transfusion complications. The main problems are antibodies against antihemophilia factors, for example directed against factor VIII or factor IX, which may be produced in hemophiliacs after repeated transfusions and inhibit the therapeutic effect. Another problem arises when antibody formation occurs in IgA-deficient subjects who receive IgA-containing products and produce anti-IgA antibodies. Inhibitors of coagulation proteins and antibodies to IgA are described in the monographs on coagulation proteins and immunoglobulins.

Frequency and susceptibility factors

A large-scale prospective study was carried out in 49 public and private hospitals throughout France between June 1991 and October 1992, aimed at discovering the frequency and severity of anaphylactoid reactions to colloid plasma substitutes, looking for possible risk factors, and determining the mechanisms involved (402). In all, 19 593 patients were evaluated; 48% were given gelatins, 27% starches, 16% albumin, and 9% dextrans. There were 43 anaphylactoid reactions, an overall frequency of 0.22%, or one reaction per 456 patients. The frequency differed according to the plasma substitute used: 0.35% for gelatins, 0.27% for dextrans, 0.10% for albumin, and 0.06% for starches. The reactions were serious (grades III and IV) in 20% of cases.

Multivariate analysis showed four independent susceptibility factors: the administration of gelatins (OR = 4.81), the administration of dextrans (OR = 3.83), a history of drug allergy (OR = 3.16), and being male (OR = 1.98). The relative risks of anaphylactoid reactions due to one type of plasma substitute with respect to another were estimated to be six times less with starches than with gelatins and 4.7 times less than with dextrans. The relative risk of albumin was 3.4 times less than that of gelatins, and almost identical to that of the starches. An immunological assessment was carried out in 15 patients who had been given a gelatin (Plasmion); in seven cases an IgE-dependent reaction was proved. It was concluded that gelatins and dextrans should be avoided in patients with a known history of drug allergy; when a reaction does occur, an immunological assessment should be carried out, as the reaction may be due to specific antibodies, in which case that particular plasma substitute would be contraindicated for the rest of the patient's life.

Pneumococcal vaccine

See Vaccines

Polyacrylonitrile

Non-IgE-mediated anaphylactic reactions to polyacrylonitrile membranes have been reported (1030,1031). The effects are enhacing in those using ACE inhibitors (1032,1033), perhaps because of an effect of bradykinin (1034), which is released by the membranes (1030,1035,1036) and whose metabolism is inhibited by ACE inhibitors. The effects also occur to a lesser extent in those taking angiotensin receptor antagonists (1037) and in those with C1 esterase inhibitor deficiency (1038). Treating the membranes with polyethyleneimine prevents bradykinin release (1039).

The FDA has issued a safety alert about life-threatening anaphylactoid reactions associated with the concurrent use of angiotensin converting enzyme (ACE) inhibitors and polyacrylonitrile dialyzers (1040). The warning was followed by increased reports in the literature and to the FDA of severe, sudden and sometimes fatal reactions. Symptoms include nausea, abdominal cramps, burning, angioedema, and shortness of breath, leading rapidly to severe hypotension. When these symptoms are recognized, dialysis should be stopped immediately and aggressive treatment for anaphylactoid reactions begun. Antihistamines do not relieve the symptoms. The mechanism of this interaction has not been established, and the incidence and scope of the problem are unknown.

Polygeline

Anaphylactic reactions associated with parenteral gelatin products are relatively common. The number of reports to the UK licensing authority now approaches 300, involving 127 patients, with 7 deaths. Most of these reactions are associated with multiconstituent gelatin-containing products, such as Gelofusine. An anaphylactic reaction due solely to the use of Gelofusine in a patient with non-hemorrhagic hypovolemia has been reported (1041).

- A 57-year-old man presented with a 3-day history of lower abdominal pain and vomiting. He was hemodynamically stable but febrile, with tenderness and guarding in the lower abdomen. He was given intravenous fluids and antibiotics and mini-laparotomy was

performed. Although 6 liters of crystalloids were given, his urine output was minimal, so 500 ml of Gelofusine was prescribed. Within 10 minutes he developed an urticarial rash, with wheals on his face and chest and difficulty in breathing. The infusion was stopped and replaced with crystalloids via a new administration set. Intravenous chlorphenamine and hydrocortisone improved his condition and the operation was completed without further complications.

Anaphylactic reactions to gelatins occur in about 0.1% of patients. Such reactions are more common in atopic patients and men and often occur within 10 minutes of starting the infusion. The authors recommended the use of allergy identification jewellery in such individuals, to reduce the possibility of life-threatening reactions.

The allergic reactions that have been described in association with polygeline are thought to be caused by direct histamine release as a result of allergenic stimulation of mast cells. These cases raise the questions of whether polygeline is appropriate for bronchoreactive patients and whether such patients should be protected by histamine receptor blockade.

- A 46-year-old man with diabetes mellitus and a history of allergy to penicillin, seafood, and soap had spinal anesthesia, and his systolic blood pressure fell to 90 mmHg (1042). He was given 500 ml of gelafundin. Within minutes, he complained of pruritus along the drip site. There was no rash or urticaria, but the infusion was stopped immediately. He became restless, had copious oral secretions, complained of dyspnea, quickly lost consciousness, and was bradycardic and hypotensive, with a systolic blood pressure of 65 mmHg. He was given Hartman's solution, Haesteril 6%, adrenaline, and atropine. He had a markedly raised IgE concentration (16 000 IU/ml). He eventually recovered.

The authors suggested that the sequence of events strongly suggested an anaphylactic reaction to gelafundin, and they concluded that while polygelines are useful volume substitutes they should be used carefully in atopic individuals or those with previous drug allergies. Etherified starch is considered a safer alternative in such patients.

- Suspected polygeline-induced anaphylaxis occurred in an 83-year-old woman within 1 minute of receiving an infusion of about 10 ml (exact dose not stated) of polygeline after induction of anesthesia for left thoracotomy (1043). Her arterial blood pressure fell to 30 mmHg and there were no palpable pulses and no detectable cardiac output, but she was successfully resuscitated. About 1 month later she showed a strongly positive reaction to polygeline on skin testing. It is believed that modification of the manufacturing process of polygeline has reduced the incidence of associated adverse reactions, although there have been no large-scale studies to estimate the current incidence.

Three cases of acute anaphylactoid reactions to polygeline have been described from Australia. The reactions were serious and the explanation for them was unclear. All three patients were either normovolemic or mildly hypovolemic at the time of the event (1044).

In a comparison of 4% human albumin solution, gelatin, and dextran 40, given as replacement fluids during plasma exchange, the gelatin solution induced two immediate allergic reactions and one delayed reaction (among 37 patients exposed). There was no cross-reactive allergy between the two colloids. Dextran 1000 injections were well tolerated. Gelatin infusions were associated with 10 times more episodes of hypovolemia (5.6 compared with 0.62%). This difference is probably explained by the faster elimination of gelatin from the vascular compartment, and it suggests that a larger volume of gelatin is required compared with dextran 40 for the same volume of plasma exchanged (1045).

An IgE-mediated anaphylactic reaction to polygeline (Haemaccel, Hoechst Marion Roussel) has been reported (1046).

- A 33-year-old woman with supraventricular tachycardia and a history of cadaveric renal transplantation for end-stage renal insufficiency, who was taking an immuno-suppressant, enalapril, and simvastatin, was given intravenous adenosine and polygeline 500 ml. After 30 minutes she developed generalized urticaria. Promethazine and hydrocortisone did not ameliorate her symptoms and an hour later she developed angioedema of the lips and tongue, but no airway obstruction, bronchospasm, or hypotension. The reaction resolved with subcutaneous adrenaline. Skin prick tests 2 weeks later showed hypersensitivity to polygeline but not to latex (a possible contaminant).

The authors suggested that the positive skin prick reaction showed that the cause was an IgE-mediated anaphylactic reaction, rather than an anaphylactoid reaction, although this was not confirmed by independent tests.

Polyhexanide

Severe anaphylaxis occurred in an 18-year-old woman and a 15-year-old man when polyhexanide was used to clean surgical wounds (1047). Immediate-type hypersensitivity to polyhexanide was suggested by positive skin prick tests. Both patients had previously been exposed to chlorhexidine, but skin tests with chlorhexidine were negative.

Polymyxins

Compared with their toxic effects, allergic reactions to the polymyxins are relatively unimportant. Nevertheless, drug fever and maculopapular eruptions and other skin lesions have been observed in few patients (1048,1049).

In 145 patients with eczema of the external ear canal, allergic contact dermatitis was diagnosed in one-third; topical therapeutic agents, especially neomycin sulfate and probably polymyxin B, were the dominating allergens (1050).

Polyvidone

Polyvidone has been reported to cause anaphylaxis (1051).

- A 32-year-old man took paracetamol (in Doregrippin) for flu-like symptoms and about 10 minutes later developed generalized urticaria, angioedema, hypotonia, and tachycardia, and became semiconscious. His symptoms were rapidly relieved by intravenous antihistamines and steroids. This was the first time he had taken Doregrippin, but he had previously taken paracetamol-containing formulations, which had been well tolerated. He was not taking any regular medications. Subsequent testing of the various constituents of the analgesic tablets identified polyvidone as the cause of the anaphylactic reaction.

This report demonstrates a rare case of a type I allergic reaction toward a commonly used ingredient of tablets and widely used disinfectants.

In principle, all forms of the well-known iodine-induced allergic reactions, such as iododerma tuberosum, dermatitis, petechiae, and sialadenitis are possible with povidone-iodine, but the incidence seems to be very low (SEDA-11, 489; SEDA-12, 586; 1052–1054).

- A severe anaphylactoid reaction occurred immediately after the instillation of a 10% solution of povidone-iodine into a hydatid cyst cavity during surgery. Severe bronchospasm developed immediately and was followed by a coagulopathy and subsequent liver and renal insufficiency (1055).

There have been only a few reports of contact allergy to povidone-iodine, despite its widespread use. In two cases there were positive patch test reactions on days 2, 3, and 7 to povidone-iodine (5% aqueous) and iodine (0.5% in petrolatum), but negative reactions to povidone itself (1056).

Pranlukast

The association of cysteinyl leukotriene receptor antagonists with eosinophilic conditions, especially Churg–Strauss syndrome, has generated widespread interest. However, evaluation of the few data is hampered by poor understanding of the underlying pathophysiology of the syndrome as well as by the limited knowledge of the effect that cysteinyl leukotriene has on the immune response and the possibility of interacting genetic polymorphisms (335).

- A 26-year-old asthmatic woman had severe acute necrotizing eosinophilic endomyocarditis while taking pranlukast, inhaled beclomethasone, and oral theophylline (1057). Oral prednisolone had been replaced by pranlukast 9 months before the event. Cardiac injury was accompanied by peripheral eosinophilia, cardiogenic shock, and pulmonary infiltrates, suggesting atypical Churg–Strauss syndrome. She recovered after intensive treatment, steroid pulse therapy, and withdrawal of pranlukast.

- A 53-year-old asthmatic woman developed p-ANCA-positive vasculitis while taking pranlukast 450 mg/day (1058). Inhaled beclomethasone dipropionate had previously been tapered from 1200 to 800 µg/day over the previous 17 months. She had a mononeuritis multiplex, eosinophilia, and sinusitis. A lymphocyte stimulation test was negative for pranlukast.

In the second case, because p-ANCA had been positive before the patient started to take pranlukast, the authors suggested that her Churg–Strauss syndrome had occurred either through unmasking of a previously unrecognized forme fruste, through tapering the inhaled corticosteroid, or had been coincidental with the natural course of a pre-existing progressive Churg–Strauss syndrome.

Praziquantel

Allergic reactions to praziquantel can be due to parasite death and include fever, urticaria, pruritic skin rashes, and eosinophilia. In one violent reaction there was marked eosinophilia, pleuritic chest pain, cardiac effusion, and ascites, pointing strongly to an exudative polyserositis (1059).

Preservatives

Preservatives are important causes of allergic contact dermatitis in cosmetics. In a 10-year analysis in 16 centers in 11 countries, 73 818 consecutive patients were patch-tested for the preservatives listed above. There were several cases of contact allergy to formaldehyde and MCI/MI. These preservatives are currently avoided in cosmetics. However, the frequency of positive reactions to MDBGN has risen, from 0.7% in 1991 to 3.5% in 2000. The authors suggested that the concentration of this preservative should be reduced in leave-on cosmetic products (1060).

DMDM hydantoin is a preservative that is used mainly in cosmetics. In 1808 consecutive patients DMDM hydantoin was patch-tested in a concentration of 2% in petroleum, and in a further 34 321 patients it was tested in a concentration of 2% in water. The proportion of positive reactions was 0.39–0.65%, with no evidence of a significant time trend. In the 180 positive cases cosmetics (30%) or topical drugs (22%) were considered causal (1061).

Hexamidine (0.15% petrolatum) (SEDA-10, 128) has rarely been reported to cause a contact allergic reaction (1062,1063). Of 1554 patients tested with polyhexamethylenebiguanide 2.5% in aqua, 6 (0.4%) had a positive reaction, indicating a very low sensitization rate (1064).

Primidone

Giant cell myocarditis has been reported in a patient taking phenytoin, phenobarbital, and mephobarbital and in one taking primidone (1065).

Procainamide

Lupus-like syndrome

DoTS classification (BMJ 2003;327:1222–5)
Dose-relation: collateral effect
Time-course: delayed
Susceptibility factors: genetic (slow acetylators)

Procainamide is one of the common causes of drug-induced lupus-like syndrome (1066), which is contrasted with idiopathic lupus erythematosus in Table 1.

Frequency

About 29–35% of patients taking procainamide for at least a year are affected and the effect is dose-related. The average age of onset is 59–68 years and 35–58% of the subjects are women. The syndrome can come on within a few weeks, but has been reported as late as 9 years after starting treatment.

Table 1   The contrast between drug-induced lupus-like syndrome and idiopathic lupus erythematosus

Feature	Idiopathic lupus erythematosus	Drug-induced lupus-like syndrome
Age and sex	Typically young women	Any (depends on use)
Acetylator status	Any	More likely in slow acetylators
Organs involved	Any	Kidneys usually spared
Antinuclear antibody	Usually present	Usually present
Complement	Can be reduced	Usually normal
Anti-DNA antibodies	Usually present (native DNA)	Only to single-stranded DNA

Propafenone

Propafenone can cause a rise in antinuclear antibody titers (1067) and has once been reported to have caused a lupus-like syndrome (1068).

Propofol

True anaphylaxis to propofol has been observed (1069).

Infection risk

Soon after the introduction of propofol in 1989, clusters of infections related to its use were reported, and there have since been several reports (1070,1071). The complications include hypotension, tachycardia, septic shock, convulsions, and death. Ethylenediaminetetra-acetic acid (EDTA) was added to the formulation to retard microbial growth. However, there have been concerns over the effects of this additive on trace element homeostasis, particularly when it is used in intensive care units for long-term sedation. Five randomized controlled trials have been reviewed, and minimal or no effects have been found on zinc, magnesium, or calcium homeostasis. However, there is no evidence to suggest that cluster infection has been or will be reduced with this formulation and there is still a need for care with sterility when using this product.

Propranolol

See Beta-adrenoceptor antagonists

Propyphenazone

Severe type I hypersensitivity reactions have been reported (SEDA-16, 108). Serious generalized urticaria with angioedema has occurred (1072). Rechallenge with oral propyphenazone caused a severe anaphylactic reaction in a patient with a negative skin test. Although the report stressed the importance of oral challenge, it also drew attention to its risks (SEDA-12, 83).

In 44 of 53 patients, all of whom developed symptoms suggestive of IgE-mediated anaphylaxis within 30 minutes of taking propyphenazone, skin tests showed typical wheal and flare reactions and significant amounts of propyphenazone-specific serum IgE was detected in 31 (1073). In seven of nine patients with negative skin tests, propyphenazone-specific IgE was detected.

Protamine

Although protamine itself was for a long time not generally considered allergenic, allergic reactions can occur in susceptible individuals. Attributed to residual fish antigens that remained after purification, they are characterized by flushing, urticaria, wheezing, angioedema, and hypotension, and they can occur even after slow intravenous administration. True anaphylaxis with bronchospasm and/or anaphylactic shock is very rare (1074).

It now seems to be widely believed that, exceptionally, protamine itself can act as an allergen. There were positive skin tests with protamine in patients who had anaphylaxis and who had all previously received protamine (1074). Cases of anaphylactic shock after slow intravenous administration of protamine sulfate to patients with diabetes mellitus suggested cross-allergy to protamine present in protamine zinc insulin (1075–1077), especially in patients with serum antiprotamine IgE or IgG antibodies (1078). Insulin-dependent patients with diabetes who use protamine insulin may be at greater risk of adverse effects when they receive protamine sulfate. A retrospective study in patients who received protamine sulfate to reverse the effects of heparin during catheterization procedures or cardiac surgery showed a relative risk of anaphylaxis four times higher in patients with diabetes who had used protamine insulin than in nondiabetic controls (1079). In these patients, the risk of anaphylaxis on administration of protamine sulfate is about 1%.

Protease inhibitors

A man developed several erythematous plaques on his face due to borderline tuberculoid leprosy with a reversal reaction (1080). He had severe CD4 T cell lymphocytopenia due to HIV infection and had been given highly active antiretroviral therapy (HAART). A fall in viral load and an increase in CD4 count preceded the development of the skin lesions, suggesting immune reconstitution as the underlying mechanism for the reversal reaction. Paradoxical reactions are often observed in patients with pulmonary and extra-pulmonary tuberculosis being treated with HAART. Clinicians need to distinguish these from other adverse reactions related to drug therapy. Reversal reactions in leprosy are increasingly likely as more patients with HIV infection are treated with HAART in developing countries.

Protein hydrolysates

Occasionally single reports of contact urticaria and of allergic contact dermatitis due to hair conditioner and skin cleanser have been published (SEDA-21, 166) (1081). Protein hydrolysates used in hair-care products have been tested in 11 hairdressers with hand dermatitis, in 2160 consecutive adults with suspected respiratory disease, and in 28 adults with chronic atopic dermatitis (1082). The hairdressers underwent both scratch tests (1% aqueous) and patch tests (5% aqueous) with 22 protein hydrolysates (collagen, keratin, elastin, milk, wheat, almond, silk). Skin prick tests with one to three hydrolysates (1% aqueous) were conducted in the other patients. All 2199 patients were tested with hydroxypropyl trimonium hydrolysed collagen (Crotein Q). There were positive scratch/prick test reactions in 12 patients to three protein hydrolysates. Remarkably, all were women with atopic dermatitis. They reacted at least to hydroxypropyl trimonium-hydrolysed collagen (Crotein Q) and 11 had positive reactions to one or more allergens in a standard prick series. In three patients, clinical relevance could be confirmed by open tests with both undiluted and diluted hair conditioner containing Crotein Q (one hairdresser with contact urticaria on the hands, two cases of contact urticaria on the head, face, and upper body from a hair conditioner containing Crotein Q). Furthermore, in seven of eight sera studied, specific IgE to Crotein Q was detected, while 11 control sera were negative. These results show that protein hydrolysates in hair-care products may be underestimated causes of contact urticaria, particularly in patients with atopy.

Prothrombin complex concentrate

In about 5% of patients with hemophilia A with antibodies to factor VIII treated with an activated prothrombin complex product (Autoplex), there was a significant increase in antibody titer (1083).

Proton pump inhibitors

Angioedema and urticaria triggered by omeprazole, but not by the enteric granules devoid of the capsule shell, has been described (SEDA-18, 373).

- Cutaneous leukocytoclastic vasculitis has been reported in a 71-year-old woman with epigastric pain who had taken omeprazole 20 mg/day for 4 weeks (1084). She made a full recovery after omeprazole was withdrawn.

Anaphylaxis has been attributed to omeprazole (1085).

- A 35-year-old alcoholic with pancreatitis developed anaphylaxis after an intravenous infusion of omeprazole. He had raised serum tryptase activity 6 hours after the onset of anaphylaxis. Total serum IgE concentrations were also raised. Intradermal tests 2 months later were positive for both omeprazole and lansoprazole, suggesting cross-reactivity.

Yersinia enterocolitica septicemia occurred in a patient taking omeprazole and heavy oral iron supplementation (1086). The authors suggested that intra-luminal iron together with a raised intestinal pH resulting from omeprazole may have contributed to the enhanced proliferation and dissemination of this organism. Since treatment with omeprazole arrests the secretion of gastric acid, it increases the risk of overgrowth with small intestinal bacteria in patients with scleroderma (SEDA-20, 318).

Pyrimethamine

Pyrimethamine + dapsone

Maloprim given for antimalarial prophylaxis was associated with immunosuppression: in military personnel in Singapore (1087). The incidence of upper respiratory tract infections was 64% higher than in the non-treated group.

Three patients developed a hypersensitivity syndrome after taking pyrimethamine 12.5 mg + dapsone 100 mg weekly as malaria prophylaxis (1088). The diagnosis was based on the presence of fever, lymphadenopathy, a maculopapular rash, and hepatitis. A mild Coombs'-positive hemolytic anemia was also observed in one of the patients. All the clinical, hematological, and biochemical abnormalities normalized within 3 months of tapering regimens of moderate-dose prednisolone.

Pyritinol

A high titer of antinuclear antibodies and anti-double-stranded native DNA antibodies occurred during treatment with pyritinol 400 mg/day in a woman with rheumatoid arthritis (1089). A clear temporal relation and a reduction in antinuclear antibody titers and disappearance of anti-DNA antibodies after drug withdrawal strongly suggested a causal relation.

Quinidine

A variety of immune syndromes have occasionally been reported with quinidine, including a lupus-like syndrome, polymyalgia rheumatica, and vasculitis (SEDA-20, 179; SEDA-23, 202).

Life-threatening vasculitis has been attributed to quinidine in a healthy volunteer taking part in a clinical trial (1090).

- A 58-year-old man took quinidine 200 mg tds for 7 days as part of an interaction study with a new alpha-blocker. He developed widespread maculopapular purpuric lesions on the limbs, trunk, and ears. His temperature rose to 38.4°C and some of the lesions on his fingers, toes, ears, and nose became necrotic. He had peripheral edema with a bluish purpuric discoloration of the hands and feet. There was mucous membrane involvement with purpuric, partially necrotic lesions on the tongue and palate. A skin biopsy showed necrotizing vasculitis with focal leukocytoclasia. Direct immunofluorescence showed microgranular deposits of IgA, IgM, and C3 around the superficial skin vessels. Quinidine was withdrawn and he was given intravenous methyl prednisolone followed by oral prednisone for one month. He recovered completely within 3 weeks.

There has been a report of a dermatomyositis-like illness in a man taking quinidine (1091).

- A previously healthy 63-year-old man, who had taken quinidine gluconate 972 mg/day for 9 months, developed diffuse edematous erythema on the extensive surfaces of the hands, arms, and face, with marked accentuation over the joints. His nail-fold capillaries were dilated and the shoulder abductors were slightly weak. His erythrocyte sedimentation rate was slightly raised (29 mm/hour) and there was a positive ANA titer (1:640) with a speckled pattern. There were no antibodies to Sm, ribonucleoprotein, SSA or SSB antigens, or histones. There was no evidence of inflammatory myopathy on electromyography, and a skin biopsy showed a mild, superficial, perivascular, lymphocytic inflammation with positive direct immunofluorescence for IgG and IgM at the dermoepidermal junction. There was no evidence of malignancy. All these abnormalities resolved rapidly after quinidine withdrawal.

Lupus-like syndrome

A lupus-like syndrome has occasionally been reported in patients taking quinidine. It usually presents with polyarthralgia, a raised erythrocyte sedimentation rate, and a raised antinuclear antibody titer. It can occasionally be associated with antihistone antibodies and a circulating coagulant. In two cases (1092) the syndrome was associated with quinidine and not with procainamide. Lupus anticoagulant has been reported with the use of quinine and quinidine, and an associated antiphospholipid syndrome has been described (1093).

Quinine

Quinine can cause a variety of immune-mediated syndromes, most commonly isolated thrombocytopenia, but rarely microangiopathic hemolytic anemia with thrombocytopenia and acute renal insufficiency (hemolytic–uremic syndrome). Two reports of immune-mediated syndromes following the use of quinine for leg cramps have helped to provide an immunopathological explanation for the diversity of such presentations (1094,1095).

- One patient presented with thrombocytopenic purpura, presumed to be idiopathic (which responded to glucocorticoids and intravenous immunoglobulin) and subsequently presented again with hemolytic–uremic syndrome, and required intensive renal replacement and immunosuppressive therapy. Analysis of serum samples from the isolated thrombocytopenic stage of the presentation showed the presence of quinine-dependent antibodies specific for platelet surface glycoprotein GPIb/IX. Quinine-dependent antibody targets widened to include glycoprotein IIb/IIIa during the hemolytic–uremic phase of the illness, with additional binding to neutrophils and lymphocytes.
- In another case of acute systemic allergy to quinine, which mimicked septic shock, with little hemolysis or renal involvement, the patient presented twice with a virtually identical clinical picture: sudden fever, rigors, and back pain, followed by hypotension, metabolic acidosis, granulocytopenia, and disseminated intravascular coagulation. On each occasion clinical and laboratory indices recovered spontaneously within 36 hours. A retrospective analysis of the patient's serum showed the presence of neutrophil-specific, quinine-dependent antibodies.

A quinine-induced lupus-like syndrome, including pericarditis and polyarthralgia, and positive antinuclear and anti-cardiolipin antibodies, and a polymyalgia rheumatica-like syndrome have been described with quinine or quinidine (SEDA-20, 261; SEDA-21, 298).

Rabies vaccine

See Vaccines

Resorcinol

Systemic allergic reactions have been reported in eight patients after topical application of a wart formulation containing resorcinol (1096). All developed a marked eczematous, sometimes bullous reaction, localized to the site of application; in four cases there were generalized urticaria and angioedema, in one pompholyx eczema, and in three generalized eczema with pompholyx. In all cases there were positive patch tests with resorcinol.

Riboflavin

Anaphylaxis has been reported in a boy who took a multivitamin tablet containing riboflavin (1097).

- A 15-year-old boy developed flushing and a generalized papular rash after taking one multivitamin tablet, followed by dizziness, dyspnea, nausea, and severe angioedema of the face 40 minutes later. He became drowsy and developed hypotension (67/48 mmHg) and tachycardia (131/minute). He was given subcutaneous adrenaline, intravenous isotonic saline, and diphenhydramine and hydrocortisone, and after 30 minutes his vital signs became stable; he recovered consciousness shortly after. He had no history of atopic diseases or adverse drug reactions, but reported that he had had dizziness many times after drinking one particular yellow-colored brand of soft drink and that he had lost consciousness twice after drinking it about 5 years before. Intradermal skin tests with the vitamins and determination of in vitro histamine release showed a strong positive response to riboflavin. He was advised to exclude riboflavin-containing products from his diet and to carry adrenaline for self-administration. During the next 13 months he had no further adverse reactions.

The multivitamin tablet that this boy took contained 100 mg of vitamins B_1, B_2, and B_6, cyanocobalamin concentrate 500 micrograms, and vitamin C 500 mg. The soft drink contained vitamin B_1 (0.6 ppm), vitamin B_2 (8.9 ppm), and vitamin C 200 micrograms/ml.

Rifamycins

There is no evidence that rifampicin causes clinically significant deleterious effects on the immune system in humans (1098), whereas it can cause immunosuppression in animals (1099). Rifampicin partially suppresses cutaneous hypersensitivity to tuberculin and T cell function (1100). In 33 patients with leprosy treated with a rifampicin drug combination, a flu-like illness or antibodies to rifampicin-conjugated proteins were not observed (1101).

A possible explanation of the association of allergic reactions with intermittent therapy is that during daily regimens the antigen–antibody complexes are continuously cleared from the plasma without reaching a critical concentration, whereas in intermittent regimens, antibody titers can increase markedly during the drug-free days. This is supported by the observation that anti-rifampicin antibodies, measured by the indirect Coombs' test, developed more commonly during intermittent than during daily therapy and that antibodies may disappear from the serum when patients change from intermittent to daily regimens.

Severe anaphylaxis has been reported in two patients with infected wounds that had been treated with topical rifamycin for several months (1102). There was urticaria, angioedema, and hypotension in one case, and urticaria, wheezing, dyspnea, and hypotensive shock in the other. In both cases, prick tests with 10% rifamycin solution were positive, while there were no positive reactions in 20 controls.

- A 36-year-old woman developed generalized urticaria during a second course of treatment with rifamycin eye-drops within a month and a 49-year-old man had systemic urticaria, bronchospasm, and hypotension shortly after his surgical wound had been washed with a solution of rifamycin (1103). Both patients had positive skin prick tests to rifamycin (1 mg/ml) when tested several weeks after the acute episode, while 10 healthy volunteers had negative tests. The woman also had a positive skin prick test to rifampicin 2 mg/ml, although she had never taken it before.

An HIV-infected patient who developed an anaphylactic reaction to rifampicin tolerated treatment with rifabutin without any adverse event.

The lupus-like syndrome has been reported in seven patients, six of them women who were taking rifampicin (*n* = 4) or rifabutin (*n* = 3) in standard dosages for mycobacterial infections (1104). None was HIV-1 positive, none was also taking isoniazid, and although they were taking other antimycobacterial drugs, their symptoms disappeared after withdrawal of the rifamycin alone. All had two or more episodes of fever, malaise, myalgia, and arthralgia, and all had positive antinuclear antibodies. All were also taking either ciprofloxacin or clarithromycin, and the authors speculated that these drugs, which are cytochrome P_{450} enzyme inhibitors, could have increased the serum concentrations of the rifamycins.

Desensitization protocols can be helpful in patients who have had anaphylactic reactions, and the detection of IgE antibodies to rifampicin may be helpful in clarifying pathogenesis. A switch to a daily regimen, when administration was previously intermittent, may allow resumption of rifampicin without further problems. In 35 HIV-positive patients with previous allergic reactions to rifampicin, oral desensitization was safe and allowed the reintroduction of rifampicin in 60% of cases (1105). However, the flu-like syndrome, hemolytic and thrombocytopenic crises, and acute renal insufficiency are not IgE-mediated, and when rifampicin is thought to be indispensable, a course of treatment may be completed under glucocorticoid cover. Four patients with reactions to rifampicin, one with rash, fever, and lymphadenopathy and one with hepatitis, completed courses of antituberculosis therapy for nervous system infections under glucocorticoid cover (1106).

Risperidone

Risperidone has been rarely associated with allergic reactions (SEDA-22, 70).

Ritodrine

A petechial rash due to vasculitis has been documented in a pregnant woman given ritodrine (SEDA-17, 165).

Ritonavir

See Lopinavir

Rocuronium bromide

Several allergic reactions to rocuronium have been reported (1107–1116). Based on data from the UK, Australia, and France, it had been suggested that the incidence of such reactions after rocuronium administration parallels its frequency of use, as assessed by its market share, implying that rocuronium does not have unusual allergenic properties (1111,1117,1118). In one hospital, the incidence of such reactions was 1 in 3000 (1111) and in another 1 in 6000 (1107). Also, the incidence of hypotension, tachycardia, or reduced oxygen saturation (which might suggest an anaphylactoid reaction) was relatively low after rocuronium administration compared with other muscle relaxants in a computerized analysis of 47 295 anesthetic records in one hospital (1119).

However, the French Group on the Study of Perianesthetic Anaphylactoid Reactions (GERAP) has reported that the proportion of anaphylactoid reactions to rocuronium was similar to suxamethonium in relation to the individual market shares of these agents (1118). There were 41 cases among 452 reported cases of anaphylaxis due to neuromuscular blocking agents that were attributed to rocuronium (1120). This would make rocuronium look unfavorable, taking into account the fact that suxamethonium is believed to trigger anaphylactoid reactions more often than any non-depolarizing neuromuscular blocker. The authors assumed that their figures might have been partly due to anesthetists' paying more attention to the effects of drugs that had become available more recently, especially in cases of mild reactions. Reporting bias has also been offered as one possible explanation of 29 reports of anaphylaxis to rocuronium among 150 000 patients in Norway, in contrast to 8 cases among 800 000 patients in the other Scandinavian countries (1121). This observation has prompted the Norwegian Medicines Agency to recommend that rocuronium be temporarily withdrawn from routine practice and that it be used for rapid-sequence induction only.

It is difficult to understand why such an increase in the number of reported cases should only be observed in France and Norway and not in other countries in which rocuronium is widely used. For the time being, it is not possible to decide whether anaphylactoid reactions are more common with rocuronium than with other non-depolarizing muscle relaxants. To get a clearer picture, a large longitudinal survey would be needed (1122), which is unlikely to be performed, owing to the large number of cases that would be required. We shall probably have to rely on national surveys, like the French one cited above. International networking and pooling of data might be the way forward. All of this will depend on clinicians chasing every case of a suspected anaphylactoid reaction by immunological testing and reporting all confirmed cases to appropriate bodies.

The Norwegian Medicines Agency has recommended that rocuronium bromide should be withdrawn from routine practice, referring to 29 reported cases of anaphylaxis or anaphylactoid reactions among 150 000 administrations over 2.5 years. In response, and with regard to the paucity of reported cases of anaphylaxis to rocuronium in other Nordic countries, the statistical problems of surveying such rare adverse drug reactions have been highlighted (1121).

One patient died after developing multiorgan failure due to a reaction to rocuronium (1123).

• A 64-year-old obese man, scheduled for a hernia repair, had had previous episodes of venous thromboembolism, for which he was still taking an oral anticoagulant. Previous general anesthesia had been uneventful. General anesthesia was induced with sufentanil 15 micrograms and propofol 400 mg. He was given rocuronium 50 mg to facilitate endotracheal intubation, and shortly after developed bronchospasm, severe hypotension, tachycardia, and generalized erythema. He was resuscitated with adrenaline, hydrocortisone, and colloid infusion. However, his further course after admission to the intensive care unit was complicated by persistent hypotension, acute respiratory distress syndrome, acute renal insufficiency, disseminated intravascular coagulation, and pancreatitis, and he died 7 days after the incident. Blood samples drawn at 30 and 60 minutes after the initial presentation showed increased concentrations of histamine and tryptase. Specific IgE antibodies against quaternary ammonium groups were detected, with a positive radioimmunoassay inhibition by rocuronium.

Death caused by an anaphylactic reaction to a muscle relaxant seems to be rare, although mortality rates from intraoperative anaphylaxis in the range of 3.4–6% have been reported (1124–1126). The incidence of cardiac arrest was 4.9% among patients with anaphylactic reactions to muscle relaxants referred to the French GERAP centers for further testing, but these patients all survived (1118).

Rokitamycin

See Macrolide antibiotics

Roxithromycin

See Macrolide antibiotics

Salbutamol

Hypersusceptibility reactions to salbutamol are extremely rare, but one well-documented allergic reaction has been described (SEDA-13, 109).

Sclerosants

Contact allergic reactions to lauromacrogol 400 have been reported (1127). Patch testing with lauromacrogol

400 may yield irritant reactions. In a retrospective study of 8739 patients tested with a topical drug patch test series, 3186 patients were tested with 0.5% lauromacrogol 400 in water (1128). There was slight irritation in 0.88%, weakly positive reactions in 0.97%, and strongly positive reactions in 0.25%. In 6202 patients tested with lauromacrogol 400 3% in petrolatum, there was slight skin irritation in 0.48%, weakly positive reactions in 1.77%, and strongly positive reactions in 0.34%. Among the 649 patients tested with both formulations, concurrence was moderate.

Selective serotonin re-uptake inhibitors (SSRIs)

Infection risk: three cases of *Herpes simplex* reactivation associated with fluoxetine have been described (SEDA-16, 10).

Fluoxetine

Vasculitis has been attributed to fluoxetine (1129,1130).

• A patient who took fluoxetine for a manic-depressive disorder developed pulmonary inflammatory nodules with non-caseating giant cell granulomas, interstitial pneumonia, and non-necrotizing vasculitis, but remained asymptomatic (1131). The diagnosis was made by open lung biopsy. The pulmonary nodules progressively resolved after withdrawal and the chest X-ray returned to normal in 9 months.

Paroxetine

A skin reaction consistent with a vasculitis has been attributed to paroxetine.

• A 20-year-old woman taking paroxetine 10 mg/day for obsessive-compulsive disorder developed multiple purple lesions on the fingers of both hands after 15 weeks (1132). The lesions disappeared after 1 week but returned in 2 days after rechallenge with paroxetine.

Selenium

Selenium can cause allergic reactions (1133–1135).

Silicone

There is a possible association between silicone breast implants and underlying connective tissue diseases (1136–1139).

In patients with symptoms of connective tissue diseases it has been assumed that rupture of the gel-filled prosthesis was the most likely cause of the symptoms. Although the prosthesis was intact in some patients, amorphous silicone-like material was identified by light microscopy in surgically removed fibrous tissue. In one study (1140), granulomatous inflammatory reactions developed when silicone elastomers were used as skin expanders. This was attributed to leakage of particles of the plastic material through the expander wall. Lymphadenitis and destructive synovitis following silicone implants (especially joint prostheses) have been described before (1141,1142), while use of silicone in dialysis tubing also led to dissemination of silicone causing splenomegaly and deposits in liver, bone marrow, skin and visceral lymph nodes. Exposure for less than 53 months did not elicit these complications (1143,1144).

Immunological abnormalities in the form of increased autoantibodies, specifically antinuclear antibodies, antithyroid antibodies, rheumatoid factor, and increased immune complexes, have been evaluated and documented (1145). In addition, abnormalities in lymphocyte subsets have been reported, with reduced lymphocytic mitogenic response, as well as abnormalities in the ratios of T-helper to T-suppressor cells (1146). Several mechanisms have been suggested, among them that silicone oozes through the intact capsule of the implants, enters the lymphatic system, and causes an immunological reaction (1147); this reaction causes further development of autoimmune disease through an adjuvant effect, with possible immune dysregulation (1148).

More evidence for the antigenicity of silicone has been provided in studies that have shown specific silicone antibodies directed against silanized albumin in the sera of two patients exposed to silastic tubing (1149). In 520 patients, aged 28–65 years, who had had silicone breast implants for 3–22 years, the most common symptoms were fatigue (96%), myalgia (86%), morning stiffness (86%), insomnia (77%), attention deficit (74%), night sweats (43%), cervical lymphadenopathy (78%), and axillary lymphadenopathy (55%).

Clinical, histopathological, and fibroblast studies have been carried out in 30 patients given subcutaneous injections of silicone (1150). The mean time between the injection and the onset of symptoms was 6 years. All the patients had sclerodermatous skin changes, subcutaneous nodules, edema, and/or hyperpigmentation at the site(s) of injection(s); five individuals also had skin changes at sites far from the injection; 13 patients had clinical features of an autoimmune disease; 11 patients gave a history of arthralgias, including four who had symmetrical nonerosive polyarthritis; 20 of 28 patients had positive antinuclear antibodies. This report confirms the association between the injection of silicon and the development of autoimmune disease (human adjuvant disease). Pneumonitis and pulmonary edema following subcutaneous injection of silicone have been reported earlier (1151–1153).

In an evaluation of the frequency and clinical characteristics of the underlying connective tissue disorders associated with silicone breast implants, 300 women with silicone breast implants were studied (1154). In addition to a history and physical examination, C reactive protein, rheumatoid factor, and autoantibodies were determined. Criteria for fibromyalgia and/or chronic fatigue syndrome were met by 54%; connective tissue diseases were detected in 11%; and undifferentiated connective tissue disease or human adjuvant disease in 10.6%. A variety of disorders, such as angioedema, frozen shoulder, and a multiple sclerosis-like syndrome, were also found. Several other miscellaneous conditions, including recurrent and unexplained low grade fever, hair loss, skin rash, symptoms of the sicca syndrome, Raynaud's phenomenon, carpal tunnel syndrome, memory loss, headaches, chest pain, and shortness of breath were also seen. Of 93 patients who underwent explantation, 70% reported improvement in their systemic symptoms.

Silver salts and derivatives

A meta-analysis of the clinical and economic effects of chlorhexidine and silver sulfadiazine antiseptic-impregnated catheters has been undertaken (1155). The costs of hypersensitivity reactions were considered as part of the analysis, and the use of catheters impregnated with antiseptics resulted in reduced costs. The analysis used the higher estimated incidence of hypersensitivity reactions occurring in Japan, where the use of chlorhexidine impregnated catheters is still banned (1156).

Snakebite antivenom

Antivenom treatment can be complicated by early reactions (anaphylaxis), pyrogenic reactions, or late reactions (serum sickness-type). The incidence and severity of early reactions is proportional to the dose of antivenom and the speed with which it enters the blood stream (1157,1158). These reactions usually develop within 10–180 minutes of starting antivenom therapy. The reported incidence of early reactions after intravenous antivenom in snakebite patients, which ranges from 43% (1159) to 81% (1160), appears to increase with the dose and decrease when refined antivenom is used and administration is by intramuscular rather than intravenous injection. Unless patients are watched carefully for 3 hours after treatment, mild reactions can be missed and deaths misattributed to the envenoming itself. In most cases symptoms are mild: urticaria, nausea, vomiting, diarrhea, headache, and fever; however, in up to 40% of cases severe systemic anaphylaxis develops, with bronchospasm, hypotension, or angioedema. However, deaths are rare (1161).

Early reactions respond well to adrenaline given by intramuscular injection of 0.5–1 ml of a 0.1% solution (1:1000, 1 mg/ml) in adults (children 0.01 ml/kg) at the first sign of trouble. Antihistamines also should be given by intravenous injection to counteract the effects of histamine released during the reaction.

Pyrogenic reactions result from contamination of antivenom by endotoxin-like compounds. High fever develops 1–2 hours after treatment and is associated with rigors, followed by vasodilatation and a fall in blood pressure. Febrile convulsions can occur in children. Patients should be cooled and given antipyretic drugs by mouth, powdered and washed down a nasogastric tube, or by suppository.

Late (serum sickness-type) reactions develop 5–24 days after treatment. Symptoms include fever, itching, urticaria, arthralgia (which can involve the temporomandibular joint), lymphadenopathy, periarticular swellings, mononeuritis multiplex, albuminuria, and rarely encephalopathy. This is an immune complex disease which responds to antihistamines or, in more severe cases, to glucocorticoids.

Early antivenom reactions are not usually Type I IgE-mediated reactions to equine serum proteins and are not predicted by hypersensitivity tests. Several methods have been used to reduce acute adverse reactions to antivenom. A small test dose of antivenom to detect patients who may develop acute adverse reactions to the antivenom has no predictive value, can itself cause anaphylaxis, and is no longer recommended (1161). Prophylactic use of hydrocortisone and antihistamines before infusion with antivenom is also practiced widely, although the theoretical basis for their use is unclear. Antihistamines counter only the effects of histamine after its release and do not prevent further release; one small randomized controlled trial showed no benefit from the routine use of antihistamines (1162). Hydrocortisone takes time to act and may be ineffective as a prophylactic against acute adverse reactions that can develop almost immediately after antivenom treatment, which is very often administered urgently to snakebite victims. One study has suggested that intravenous hydrocortisone is ineffective in preventing acute adverse reactions to antivenom, but if given together with intravenous chlorphenamine it can reduce these reactions (1163). However, this trial recruited only 52 patients and was not designed to study the efficacy of chlorphenamine alone, making it difficult to give a clear interpretation of the results and recommendations on pretreatment with glucocorticoids and antihistamines to prevent acute reactions to antivenom. In one study of 105 patients, low-dose adrenaline given subcutaneously immediately before administration of antivenom to snakebite victims significantly reduced the incidence of acute adverse reactions to the serum (1159). However, this trial did not enroll sufficient participants to establish safety adequately, a major concern regarding the use of adrenaline in a prophylactic role, particularly the risk of intra-cerebral haemorrhage. Therefore, further studies on the safety of this treatment are required before it can be recommended routinely. For the present, the only available alternative to prevention is the early detection of adverse reactions to antivenom and the ready availability of drugs such as adrenaline for their prompt treatment.

Somatostatin and analogues

Antibodies to somatostatin analogues have been reported only rarely. However, in one study octreotide antibodies were demonstrated in 63 (27%) of 231 patients treated with subcutaneous octreotide for more than 3 years, rising to 57% after 5 years and 72% after 8 years (1164). The antibodies did not reduce clinical efficacy.

- A 64-year-old woman, who had had monthly intramuscular injections of long-acting octreotide in the buttocks for 6 years, had increased uptake of ^{111}In-pentetreotide in both buttocks, thought to represent granuloma formation at the injection sites (1165). Localized granulomas have previously been described in isolated cases after intramuscular somatostatin analogues, and somatostatin receptors are expressed in high density in activated lymphocytes.

Allergic reactions to somatostatin are rare. Of 97 cirrhotic patients randomized to subcutaneous octreotide, one stopped therapy because of erythematous itchy skin, which then resolved (1166).

Somatropin

Patients treated with recombinant somatropin commonly develop antibodies against growth hormone; the incidence is 22–88% (1167). There were low titers of anti-growth hormone antibody, with no reduction in growth response, in 44% of children who used modified-release somatropin once a month and in 68% who used it twice a month (1168). Antibodies almost never have clinical significance, but the fourth case of reduced growth due to neutralizing antibodies against growth hormone has been reported in a 9-year-old boy; growth resumed after he was changed to a methionyl-free human formulation of somatropin (1166).

Systemic allergic reactions to somatropin are very rare, but can be overcome by desensitization (SEDA-13, 1308; 1169). Although early studies suggested a higher rate of renal transplant rejection in recipients of somatropin than in controls (SEDA-21, 452), this was not confirmed in a long-term prospective study (1170).

- In a 15-year-old boy with previously quiescent lupus nephritis, laboratory markers of disease activity rose during somatropin treatment and returned to baseline concentrations within 3 months after withdrawal (1171).

Spiramycin

A peculiar hypersensitivity reaction was reported in an employee of a pharmaceutical company who developed attacks of sneezing, coughing, and breathlessness while working with spiramycin; he had immediate positive skin prick tests to spiramycin and developed blood eosinophilia during asthma attacks (1172).

Henoch–Schönlein purpura occurred in a patient taking spiramycin (1173).

Statins

See HMG Coenzyme A inhibitors

Stem cell factor

Stem cell factor produces direct mast cell stimulation with subsequent allergic-type reactions. Despite careful premedication with diphenhydramine, ranitidine, inhaled salbutamol, and pseudoephedrine, such reactions were still observed in 3% of patients (1174).

Streptogramins

The combination of quinupristin + dalfopristin reduces cytokine production in stimulated monocytes from healthy volunteers, suggesting significant immunomodulatory activity (1175).

Sulfites and bisulfites

The major symptoms of an adverse reaction to a sulfite are flushing, acute bronchospasm, and hypotension (SED-11, 492; SEDA-10, 232; SEDA-11, 221; 1176). The incidence of sulfite sensitivity in an asthmatic population is estimated at about 10%. Sulfites have therefore been withdrawn from the composition of several medicines intended for asthmatic patients.

Metabisulfite-induced anaphylaxis through an IgE-mediated mechanism has been described in a patient who developed urticaria, angioedema, and nasal congestion following provocative challenge with sodium metabisulfite (1177).

The presence of sodium metabisulfite as an antioxidant in commercial lidocaine with adrenaline significantly increased discomfort during injection (1178).

Anaphylactic shock occurring during epidural anesthesia for cesarean section has been attributed to sodium metabisulfite (1179).

Reports of contact allergy to topical medicaments containing sodium metabisulfite are rare (1180). In two cases, a topical corticosteroid formulation that contained sodium metabisulfite (Trimovate cream) caused contact allergy; patch tests were positive with both sodium metabisulfite and Trimovate cream (1181).

Sulfonamides

Sulfa allergy refers to a specific hypersensitivity response to a group of chemicals containing a sulfonamide moiety covalently bound to a benzene ring; drugs structurally similar to sulfonamides may cross-react, for example sulfonylureas, thiazides, and furosemide (1182). Sulfa allergy is most consistent with an immune-mediated reaction with delayed onset, 7–14 days after the start of therapy, characterized by fever, rash, and eosinophilia. IgG antibodies may be present and directed against proteins in the endoplasmic reticulum (about 80% of patients) or against the drug covalently bound to protein (about 5% of patients). High-dose methylprednisolone sodium succinate (250 mg every 6 hours for 48 hours) may not only alleviate the signs but also markedly attenuate the antibody response, as reported in a 19-year-old man (1183).

Hypersusceptibility to sulfonamides has been proposed to be the mechanism for many adverse reactions,

including anaphylactic shock, serum sickness-like syndrome, systemic allergic vasculitis, drug fever (up to 1–2% in some series), lupus-like syndrome, myocarditis, pulmonary infiltrates, interstitial nephritis, aseptic meningitis, hepatotoxicity, blood dyscrasias (agranulocytosis, thrombocytopenia, eosinophilia, pancytopenia), and a wide variety of skin reactions (urticaria, erythema nodosum, erythema multiforme, erythroderma, toxic epidermal necrolysis, and photosensitivity).

Urticarial and maculopapular rashes are the most frequent adverse reactions to sulfonamides after gastrointestinal symptoms. Although hypersusceptibility is suspected to be the mechanism for these adverse effects, type I allergic reactions, which are induced by IgE antibodies, have been confirmed only rarely. It appears that with the older sulfonamides severe reactions were more frequent. In some patients who have immediate hypersensitivity reactions to sulfonamides, IgE has been found that can bind to an N4-sulfonamidoyl determinant (N4-SM) (1184).

It is desirable to predict hypersusceptibility reactions to sulfonamides. IgE-induced in vitro reactions to sulfonamides have mainly been studied in the last 15 years (1184–1186). A lymphocyte toxicity assay showed a positive result in about 70% of patients with a maculopapular rash, an urticarial reaction, or erythema multiforme (1187). This biochemical test determines the percent of cell death due to toxic metabolites. The same in vitro reaction using the hydroxylamine metabolite of sulfamethoxazole gave significantly different results in six patients with fever and skin rash with or without hepatitis than in control patients (1188). Unfortunately, in most adverse reactions it is not known whether the reaction is dose-related or allergic. Individual differences in metabolism predispose to idiosyncratic reactions, for example sulfonamides are metabolized by N-acetylation (mediated by a genetically determined polymorphic enzyme) and oxidation to potentially toxic metabolites (1189,1190). Fever and rash were observed significantly more often in slow than in fast acetylators. Systemic glutathione deficiency, with a consequently reduced capacity to scavenge such toxic metabolites, might contribute to these adverse reactions, particularly in patients with AIDS (1191,1192). In a child with dihydropteridine reductase deficiency, a variant of phenylketonuria, adverse drug reactions occurred to co-trimoxazole (1193). Unfortunately, there are no reliable in vitro tests to predict idiosyncratic reactions in vivo (1188–1190,1192,1194).

Sulfonylureas

Hypersensitivity vasculitis has been described with glibenclamide (1195). Glibenclamide contains a sulfa moiety and can cause allergic reactions in someone who is allergic to sulfonamides.

- A 57-year-old man with a previously undocumented sulfa allergy used atenolol 100 mg/day, hydrochlorothiazide 25 mg/day, docusate sodium 100 mg/day, and ranitidine 300 mg bd for several months (1477). He started to take celecoxib 200 mg/day, and 1 month later developed erythema multiforme and difficulty in breathing caused by swelling of the throat. He improved after withdrawal of his drugs and further treatment. He was then instructed to reintroduce his previous drugs one a day. One day later, after taking glibenclamide 5 mg, he developed new lesions and dyspnea. After 3 weeks he had another relapse when he reintroduced hydrochlorothiazide. He omitted glibenclamide, celecoxib, and hydrochlorothiazide, but continued to use insulin, metformin, ranitidine, and psyllium. The urticarial lesions disappeared.

Celecoxib and hydrochlorothiazide also have sulfa moieties and could have contributed in this case.

Sulindac

Several types of proven or suspected hypersensitivity have already been mentioned, for example in connection with the liver, but the exact mechanism of a particular adverse effect has not always been clear. One case of fever, pharyngitis, cervical lymphadenopathy, leukopenia, liver abnormalities, proteinuria, pulmonary infiltrates, and abdominal pain has been described. Another patient who previously took sulindac without problems developed pruritus, dyspnea, perioral edema, and lethargy after taking a single dose of sulindac 150 mg.

Pneumonitis is probably part of a general hypersensitivity reaction (SEDA-6, 94; 1196,1197).

An anaphylactic reaction has been described (1198). Sulindac is also thought to have been responsible for a severe multisystem reaction (possibly again anaphylactic) involving the cardiovascular, hepatic, pulmonary, and hematological systems in a patient with quiescent systemic lupus erythematosus (1199).

Sunscreens, substances used in

Photopatch-testing with sunscreens in Sweden has been reviewed (1200). Between 1990 and 1996, 355 patients with suspected photosensitivity were photopatch-tested with seven sunscreens (benzophenone-3 (Eusolex 4360), isopropyldibenzoylmethane (Eusolex 8020), butylmethoydibenzoylmethane (Parsol 1789), octylmethoxycinnamate (Parsol MCX), PABA, phenylbenzimidazole sulfonic acid (Eusolex 232), 4-methylbenzylidene camphor (Eusolex 6300); 2% petrolatum). There were 42 allergic reactions in 28 patients. The most common allergen was benzophenone-3 (Eusolex 4360), with 15 photocontact and one contact allergic reaction, followed by eight photocontact and four allergic contact reactions to isopropyl dibenzoylmethane (Eusolex 8020). In six cases, photocontact reactions were due to butylmethoxydibenzoylmethane (Parsol 1789). Phenylbenzimidazole sulfonic acid (Eusolex 232) caused two cases of photocontact allergy, and benzophenone-3 caused contact urticaria in one patient (1200). There was a similar frequency of photocontact dermatitis to Eusolex 4360, Eusolex 8020,

and Parsol 1789 in an Italian study, in which nine of 36 patients had positive reactions when photopatch-tested with sunscreens (UVA 10 J/m^2) (1201).

In 19 patients with positive photopatch tests to sunscreens among all the patients that were photopatch-tested between 1992 and 1999 (total not stated) there were 21 positive photopatch tests to sunscreen agents (1202). Nine patients reacted to oxybenzone, eight to butylmethoxydibenzoylmethane, three to methoxycinnamate, and one to benzophenone. There were no reactions to para-aminobenzoic acid (PABA), reflecting the increased use of PABA-free sunscreens. Six patients also had positive patch tests to components of the sunscreen base, such as fragrances, which can complicate the diagnosis.

Oxybenzone is the most frequently used benzophenone in sunscreens, estimated to be present in 20–30% of commercial products. Phototoxicity and allergic contact dermatitis have been described, but reports of immediate-type hypersensitivity are scarce.

- A 22-year-old woman with a history of atopy had anaphylaxis 10 minutes after widespread application of an oxybenzone-containing sunscreen (1203). Blinded patch tests with the sunscreen and its ingredients yielded wheal and flare reactions after 15 minutes to the sunscreen and to oxybenzone. Some days before skin testing the woman had had contact urticaria on the face after kissing a friend who had applied the same sunscreen.

A positive patch test to polyvinylpyrrolidone/eicosene (10% in petrolatum on days 2 and 4) was found in a patient who had used a sun block (1204).

Photo-induced contact urticaria to benzophenone-3 and benzophenone-10, possibly in combination with delayed hypersensitivity, has been described (1205). Urticaria occurred within minutes of UVA irradiation (10 J), 24 hours after the application of the benzophenones.

Octyl triazone is a UVB absorber structurally unrelated to the benzophenones. Photocontact allergy to this agent in a sunscreen has been described (1206).

Suxamethonium

From the results of intradermal injections, suxamethonium has only 1% of the histamine-releasing activity of D-tubocurarine (1207). However, through the years there have been many reports of reactions, varying from flushing and urticaria to bronchospasm (1208,1209) and severe shock (1210–1213). That suxamethonium was responsible was suggested in some cases by the fact that the patients reacted on different occasions with raised plasma histamine and catecholamine concentrations (1214–1216). The association was confirmed in other cases by repeatedly injecting the drug, thereby producing bronchospasm several times in the course of the one anesthetic (1217,1218). Skin testing has also yielded confirmation, although this can be dangerous (1211). Analysis of large series of patients (1219–1224) who have had severe anaphylactoid reactions during anesthesia, using more sophisticated laboratory and immunological investigations in addition to intradermal skin tests, suggests that suxamethonium may be much more commonly associated with such reactions than was previously believed. In 18 cases (1225) cardiovascular collapse was the predominant feature in 72% and bronchospasm in 33%; cardiac arrest occurred in five patients. In addition, two reports (1226,1227) of anaphylactic reactions involving both thiopental and suxamethonium have raised the question of "aggregate"-induced reactions (1226) occurring when drugs are given in such a way that they can interact in the injection system.

Taxaceae

Of 18 patients with seasonal allergic rhinitis, suffering mainly in April and May, five were sensitized to the pollen of *Taxus cuspidata* (1227).

Tea tree oil

Since the beginning of the 1990s, several case reports of allergic contact dermatitis to tea tree oil have been published (1228,1229). Most of these adverse effects emerged after the application of aged tea tree oil, and patients who are allergic to tea tree oil do not react to patch tests with freshly distilled tea tree oil (1230). In a review of tea tree oil focussing on the allergic compounds in detail, the authors concluded that *d*-limonen, alpha-terpenes, and the aromadendrens are important allergens, whereas 1,8-cineole was not believed to be important, as has been previously stated (1231). Tea tree oil undergoes photo-oxidation within a few days to several months, leading to degradation products, such as peroxides, epoxides, and endoperoxides, which are moderate to strong sensitizers. Experimental sensitization in guinea pigs was followed by patch tests with 15 constituents of oxidized tea tree oil in 11 patients with tea tree oil contact dermatitis (1230). All the patients reacted to alpha-terpinene, terpinolene, and ascaridol, the latter being a deterioration product of alpha-terpinene.

Many people who are allergic to tea tree oil also react to turpentine, colophony, fragrances, balsam of Peru, and plant extracts of Compositae (1232).

- A 46-year-old Chinese man developed an allergic contact dermatitis to tea tree oil, colophony, balsam of Peru, and abitol. He had used the tea tree oil under an occlusive dressing on a superficial abrasion on his left shin for 2 weeks, after which the treated area became red and itchy. During the next week, skin lesions appeared on his trunk and extremities, and were diagnosed as an erythema multiforme-like id reaction.
- A 38-year-old man developed an immediate hypersensitivity reaction, characterized by pruritus, throat constriction, and light-headedness, after topical application of tea tree oil (1233). An intradermal test with tea tree oil gave a wheal and flare reaction. Specific IgG and IgE were not detected.

Teicoplanin

Allergic reactions have been reported with teicoplanin. Erythroderma during infusion of teicoplanin with fever and hypotension was described in a single patient. Re-exposure elicited the same reaction (1234). Allergic cross-reactivity between teicoplanin and vancomycin has been reported (1235,1236). This cross-reactivity was documented by in vitro studies showing IgE release by basophils in response to stimulation by both vancomycin and teicoplanin in a further patient who had an allergic reaction to vancomycin (1237). In other studies the second drug did not elicit allergic reactions in patients known to be allergic to one of the two compounds (1238–1240). Based on these small studies and individual case reports one can conclude that allergic reactions to teicoplanin can occur in patients with known allergic reactions to vancomycin, but the frequency of occurrence of this type of cross-reaction appears to be low. Therefore, known hypersensitivity to vancomycin is not a contraindication to the use of teicoplanin.

Local reactions at the injection site, including pain, redness, or discomfort after intramuscular injection, and phlebitis after intravenous injection, occur in about 3% of patients (1241).

Terbinafine

Exacerbation of lupus erythematosus has been reported during terbinafine therapy (1242–1245). Of 21 consecutive patients with subacute cutaneous lupus erythematosus who attended an outpatient dermatology department in Germany during 1 year, 4 had terbinafine-associated disease (1246). In addition to high titers of antinuclear antibodies with a homogeneous pattern, anti-Ro(SS-A) antibodies were present; in three of the four women, anti-La(SS-B) antibodies were also found. All the patients had antihistone antibodies, as in drug-induced lupus, and showed the characteristic genetic association with the HLA-B8,DR3 haplotype; moreover, in two cases HLA-DR2 was also present. After withdrawal of terbinafine, antinuclear antibody titers fell and antihistone antibodies became undetectable within 4.5 months in three patients.

- A 66-year-old man with giant cell arteritis and hypertension developed a hypersensitivity reaction 4.5 weeks after starting to take terbinafine, with a skin eruption, fever, lymphadenopathy, and hepatic dysfunction (1247). Concomitant medications included prednisone, doxazosin, and aspirin. His symptoms and signs resolved within 6 weeks after withdrawal of terbinafine and continuation of all the other medications. The hypersensitivity syndrome reaction in this case was idiosyncratic, with no apparent predisposing factors.

Tetanus toxoid

Allergic reactions to reinforcing doses of tetanus toxoid have been described by different investigators (SEDA-8,

300; SEDA-11, 288). The association between high titers of antitoxin produced by active immunization and reactions is well established (1248,1249). Booster doses of tetanus toxoid are being given with unnecessary and indeed excessive frequency. Continuing to do this will produce a more highly toxoid-sensitive population without adding significantly to the already high protection that this immunized population has against tetanus. It is therefore recommended that routine boosters in individuals known to have had primary immunization including a reinforcing dose be given only at 10-year intervals, and that emergency boosters be given no less than 1 year apart (1250). Allergic reactions may be due to an allergy to the toxoid or the proteins of *C. tetani* that co-purify with toxoid during the precipitation process used in its conventional preparation (1251).

Tetracyclines

Based on the strategy that inhibition of angiogenesis is of importance in anticancer therapy, CMT-3 (COL-3) was used in a phase 1 study in 35 patients at the National Institutes of Health in the USA in patients with refractory metastatic cancer (1252). The patients received a test dose of CMT-3, followed by pharmacokinetic testing during daily dosing for 7 days. After a few doses, three patients developed symptoms of drug-induced lupus, and the diagnoses were verified after a few days or weeks. CMT-3 was withdrawn and there was improvement.

Thalidomide

Leukocytoclastic vasculitis has been reported in one of 260 patients (1253).

Of 54 patients randomized to either placebo (*n* = 26) or thalidomide 200 mg/day (*n* = 28) starting 80 days after allogeneic bone marrow transplantation chronic graft-versus-host disease was significantly more common in those who took thalidomide; there was also a significant overall survival advantage in those who took placebo (1254). These results suggest that while thalidomide is effective in treating chronic graft-versus-host disease, its use to prevent chronic graft-versus-host disease results in a paradoxical outcome.

Tumor lysis syndrome has been attributed to thalidomide in a 59-year-old woman with myeloma (1255).

Theophylline

Salivary IgA was significantly reduced in asthmatic children treated with theophylline compared with healthy controls or unmedicated patients with asthma (1256). This finding is in harmony with earlier statements that theophylline reduces the bactericidal capacity of leukocytes and affects suppressor T cells (SEDA-11, 6). Theophylline also interferes with basophil and eosinophil responses; these immunomodulatory effects might participate in its therapeutic efficacy (1257,1258).

Thiacetazone

Cutaneous allergic reactions to thiacetazone are very common in HIV-positive patients, in the order of 20%. Ethambutol should therefore be used instead of thiacetazone in these patients (1259).

Thiamphenicol

Thiamphenicol has immunosuppressive properties, which are ascribed to an effect on immunocompetent cells, rather than on immunoglobulin synthesis (1260). In animals, thiamphenicol prolonged the survival of skin homografts (1261).

Thiazide diuretics

It has long been thought that loop and thiazide diuretics pose a theoretical risk of cross-sensitivity in patients with sulfonamide allergy because of their common structures. However, the available literature does not provide sufficient numbers of well-documented cases to support this impression (1262). It seems that careful administration of diuretics is permissible in patients with documented sulfonamide allergy, but as always such a drug challenge should not be attempted without careful follow-up. A furosemide rechallenge protocol, based on a method that has been used to rechallenge with a sulfa-containing antimicrobial agent, safely allowed the long-term reinstitution of loop diuretic therapy with furosemide (1263).

Thiazolidinediones

- Angioedema has been reported in an obese woman after she had taken pioglitazone 30 mg/day for 7 days (1264). She developed a sore throat followed by dyspnea and swelling of the lips and tongue. There was no rash. After intravenous glucocorticoids her symptoms rapidly abated.

Thionamides

Antineutrophil cytoplasmic antibody (ANCA)-positive vasculitis is a well-described complication, particularly with propylthiouracil and to a lesser extent with carbimazole, and has been most often described in patients with Graves' disease. The possible drug-induced causes of ANCA-positive vasculitis with high titers of antimyeloperoxidase antibodies in 30 new patients have been reviewed (1265). The findings illustrated that this type of vasculitis is a predominantly drug-induced disorder. Only 12 of the 30 cases were not related to a drug. The most frequently implicated drug was hydralazine (*n* = 10); the remainder involved propylthiouracil (*n* = 3), penicillamine (*n* = 2), allopurinol (*n* = 2), and sulfasalazine (*n* = 1).

Cutaneous vasculitis is often a feature of such cases, although severe systemic manifestations often also occur. Two patients with propylthiouracil hypersensitivity presented with skin manifestations but also had renal, rheumatological, and hematological features (1266). A review of the literature showed that the symptoms and signs in patients with ANCA-associated thionamide-induced vasculitis are diverse. Acral purpuric skin lesions are typically seen; recognition of these classical clinical features may allow early diagnosis and limit associated morbidity and the requirement for other therapies, particularly immunosuppression. Several other reports have described cases of MPO-ANCA-positive cases of vasculitis presenting in a variety of ways in both adults and children treated with propylthiouracil (1267–1270).

There have been reports of propylthiouracil-induced ANCA-associated small vessel vasculitis (1271,1272), crescentic glomerulonephritis (1273), and Wegener's granulomatosis (1274). More common, however, may be a condition termed "antithyroid arthritis syndrome," which is a transient migratory polyarthritis occurring within 2 months of starting thionamides and resolving within 4 weeks of stopping therapy (1275).

ANCA-positive vasculitis in a patient with multinodular goiter has been described, together with a review of the clinical features in a further 26 cases (1276). Renal involvement, typically with crescentic or necrotizing glomerulonephritis on biopsy, and arthralgia were the most common manifestations. A few cases of diffuse proliferative lupus nephritis associated with ANCAs have been reported (SEDA-20, 394). Other cases of ANCA-associated disease in patients have been reported, including subjects presenting with neutrophilic dermatosis (1277), pyoderma gangrenosum, secondary sterile pyoarthrosis (1278), and purpura fulminans (1279). Small vessel vasculitis leading to pulmonary alveolar hemorrhage and crescentic glomerulonephritis has also been described (1279).

In 61 patients with Graves' hyperthyroidism, 32 of whom were taking propylthiouracil and 29 methimazole, there was a higher prevalence of antimyeloperoxidase ANCAs in those taking propylthiouracil than in those taking thiamazole (25 versus 3.4%) (1280). There were no significant differences in age, duration of therapy, or drug dosage in those who developed antimyeloperoxidase ANCAs compared with those who did not. Two ANCA-positive patients in this study developed rheumatoid arthritis or membranous glomerulonephritis, but none developed classical ANCA-associated vasculitis.

There have been reports of antimyeloperoxidase ANCAs associated with diffuse pulmonary alveolar hemorrhage (1281), IgA nephropathy (1282), and drug-induced neutropenia (1283) in patients who had Graves' hyperthyroidism taking propylthiouracil. Investigation using serum from the last of these patients implicated a complement-mediated mechanism. In another case ANCAs developed in two of three monozygotic triplets, both of whom had Graves' disease treated with propylthiouracil, supporting a genetic role in the development of this drug complication (1284).

Long-term outcomes in a series of seven children who developed myeloperoxidase-specific ANCA-positive necrotizing crescentic glomerulonephritis associated with propylthiouracil were studied in Japan (1285). Three had nephritis alone and four had extrarenal vasculitis. All had taken glucocorticoids, some with additional drugs, and all had achieved remission. None had progressed to end-stage renal insufficiency or death during a mean period of follow-up of 58 months. This apparently benign course, albeit with a relatively short period of follow-up, is similar to that seen in adult patients with this drug complication and implies a better prognosis than in subjects with non-drug-induced ANCA-positive vasculitic disease.

The size of this problem has been addressed using serum samples from 117 patients with Graves' disease treated either with propylthiouracil or thiamazole, and from untreated patients (1286). Myeloperoxidase ANCA and proteinase-3 antineutrophil cytoplasmic antibodies (PR3-ANCA) were tested by enzyme-linked immunosorbent assay. Myeloperoxidase ANCA was negative in all untreated patients and patients taking thiamazole, but positive in 21 of 56 patients taking propylthiouracil. In contrast, PR3-ANCA was not detected in any patient in the study. The proportion of patients who were positive for myeloperoxidase ANCA increased with the duration of propylthiouracil therapy. Of the 21 patients who were positive for myeloperoxidase ANCA, 12 had no symptoms, but nine complained of myalgia, arthralgia, or coryza-like symptoms after the appearance of the antibody; none had abnormal urinary findings. These findings suggest a specific association between propylthiouracil therapy and the development of myeloperoxidase ANCA in patients with Graves' disease.

ANCA-positive microscopic polyangiitis has been associated with propylthiouracil, with a fatal outcome despite treatment with glucocorticoids and cyclophosphamide (1287). Another patient presented atypically with acute pericarditis 10 months after starting to take propylthiouracil 100 mg tds (1288). Another patient developed ANCA-negative leukocytoclastic vasculitis of the skin (1289).

Several cases of "collagen-like" or "lupus-like" disease have been reported (joint pain, skin rash, and positive antinuclear antibodies) during treatment with either propylthiouracil or thiamazole (SEDA-8, 3; SEDA-10, 368). Some cases of general vasculitis can be fatal, although high-dose glucocorticoid therapy can be helpful (1290).

Other reports have described serious immunological complications of propylthiouracil in the absence of ANCA, including interstitial nephritis and fatal Stevens–Johnson syndrome in a 90-year-old woman treated for 5 weeks (1291) and disseminated intravascular coagulation and vasculitis 2 weeks after the introduction of propylthiouracil in a 42-year-old woman (1292). The latter was treated successfully by drug withdrawal and intravenous methylprednisolone.

Thiopental sodium

Anaphylaxis has been repeatedly reported after thiopental (SEDA-10, 190; SEDA-11, 211; 1471), but is rare, with an estimated incidence of one in 30 000.

- An extreme example reported in 1993 involved a 55-year-old obese man with no history of allergy to penicillin, who had on earlier occasions received sodium thiopental without reaction; on this occasion he stopped breathing and had severe bronchial constriction and vascular collapse requiring prolonged resuscitation and mechanical ventilation (1293).

Thiurams

Allergic contact dermatitis following exposure to thiuram compounds in rubber products, such as disposable rubber gloves, is well recognized (1294).

- A 49-year-old man developed acute pruritic dermatitis of the hand, which settled quickly with oral glucocorticoids and antibiotics (1295). Six months later he developed a similar eruption, which became more widespread, involving the trunk and limbs. He had no personal or family history of atopy, and had no known allergies or previous history of skin disease. He had a widespread dry eczematous eruption, most marked in exposed areas. The rash had developed soon after he had handled plants that had been sprayed with a fungicide. The safety data sheet for this product indicated that it contained 80% thiuram. Full blood count and serum electrolytes were normal, and autoantibodies and a porphyrin screen were negative. Biopsy of the lesion showed significantly sun-damaged skin with a superficial perivascular chronic inflammatory infiltrate, confluent surface parakeratosis, and epidermal acanthosis with moderate spongiosis, consistent with a spongiotic dermatitis. He denied any previous contact with rubber gloves in both occupational and social settings, and had not had dermatitis before. He was treated with sun protection, topical and oral glucocorticoids, and a moisturizer. He had no further contact with the fungicide and the eruption resolved completely. He was advised to avoid all thiuram products, including rubber products and fungicides, in the future. Despite this, he subsequently developed one recurrence of hand dermatitis when he again used rubber gloves for protection at work.

Three Chinese national servicemen developed an itchy postauricular rash (1296). None had a history of atopy and all three reported prior use of rubberized spectacle retainers as a curved pliable extension to the posterior ends of the earpieces of their spectacles, to stabilize them while undergoing rigorous military physical training. They were all patch-tested with the National Skin Center standard series and were positive to thiuram mix and the rubberized spectacle retainers. They were treated with topical corticosteroids and were advised to stop wearing their rubberized spectacle retainers.

Thrombolytic agents

Since streptokinase is a natural product of cultures of streptococci and therefore has similar antigenic properties, most of the population have anti-streptokinase antibodies. These antibodies may explain both the allergic reactions that can

occur and resistance to the drug, which occurs in some cases. Within 3 or 4 days of streptokinase administration, the titer of neutralizing antibodies has become sufficient to inactivate the usual doses. Persistence of these antibodies is observed in up to 80% of patients 1 year after treatment and in about 50% of patients after 2–4 years (1297,1298). If streptokinase has to be re-administered within 8 months of previous exposure, the neutralizing effects of plasma should be taken into account and the dose of streptokinase should be adjusted to overcome these effects (1299). However, the extent to which streptokinase antibodies decline after earlier exposure to streptokinase is controversial, and persistently raised titers are found in a large proportion of patients (1300). For this reason, an alternative thrombolytic agent should be recommended in patients who have already received streptokinase. In addition, it appears that allergic reactions occur more often when streptokinase is reused (1301).

Anistreplase, a compound consisting of streptokinase and anisoylated plasminogen, can also cause allergic reactions, but has a longer half-life, allowing intravenous administration in a relatively short interval of time.

Urokinase is extracted from human urine or prepared from cultures of fetal kidney cells and does not seem to cause allergic reactions.

Pro-urokinase, alteplase, reteplase, and tenecteplase, which are recombinant products, also appear to be free from allergic reactions. Pro-urokinase and alteplase have short half-lives (3–8 minutes) and require continuous infusion administration, which may in some cases be an advantage as it allows rapid surgical intervention when necessary (1302). Reteplase and tenecteplase have substantially longer half-lives, allowing bolus administration.

The incidence of acute generalized allergic reactions in patients treated with streptokinase or anistreplase was originally reported to be high, but with the introduction of more highly purified forms of streptokinase the figure has fallen to 1–5%. The most common manifestations of non-anaphylactic reactions to streptokinase or anistreplase are skin rashes and pyrexia. However, anaphylactic shock with streptokinase is also well known, although rare; it occurred in 0.1% of the patients in the GISSI trial (1303). Life-threatening angioedema has been described with streptokinase (1304,1305) and with alteplase (1306–1308). Skin rashes are seen especially with streptokinase, but rarely, if ever, with alteplase.

Several cases of low back pain associated with streptokinase or anistreplase injections for acute myocardial infarction have been described, with rapid resolution once the streptokinase was stopped (1309,1310). It is presumed that the mechanism is allergic, since no such report has been published with alteplase (1311).

Streptokinase is regularly reported to have induced an immune complex syndrome, characterized by plasmacytosis, often severe, and accompanied by fever and the development of hemolytic anemia, occurring as early as the first week after the start of treatment; in some cases, temporary alterations in renal function also occur (1312).

Vasculitis has been rarely described after streptokinase or anistreplase (1313–1316), but not after urokinase or alteplase. It is characterized by lymphocyte infiltration and deposition of immune complexes, fibrin, and complement in the skin microvasculature.

Other patients have the typical picture of serum sickness, sometimes associated with acute renal insufficiency (1317–1319) or of Henoch–Schönlein purpura (1320) with a purpuric rash, joint and abdominal pains, and sometimes hematuria (1321).

Adult respiratory distress syndromes and multisystem organ failure have been reported with streptokinase and anistreplase (1322–1325); the timing of the onset of symptoms and the antibody profile in one case suggested an immunological response (1323).

The clinical efficacy of thrombolytic drugs such as streptokinase does not appear to be compromised by the occurrence of allergic reactions, according to data from GUSTO-1 (1326).

There have been three reports of anaphylactoid reactions, mostly orolingual angioedema, after therapy of acute ischemic stroke with alteplase.

- In one patient there was marked edema of the lip about 45 minutes after a bolus dose of alteplase; it subsided within 2 hours without any intervention (1327).

Of 105 consecutive patients treated with alteplase for acute ischemic stroke, 2 developed anaphylactoid reactions (1328). The first had a rash and extensive bilateral swelling of the tongue, epiglottis, and uvula, requiring intubation. The second developed unilateral swelling of the tongue and lips without a rash or hypotension.

In 230 patients treated with alteplase for acute ischemic stroke, there were two cases of orolingual angioedema (1329). Both presented with localized symptoms only, symmetrical in one and asymmetrical in the other.

IgE-associated anaphylactic reactions can also occur.

- A 70-year-old woman was treated with intravenous alteplase for thrombolysis in acute ischemic stroke and 30 minutes later had acute sinus tachycardia and hypotension, followed by cyanosis and loss of consciousness (1330). Serum samples analysed by ELISA were positive for IgE antibodies to alteplase.

Such reactions are very rare; there have been four reported cases in over 1 million administrations.

Thyroid hormones

Fever, liver dysfunction, and eosinophilia occurred during liothyronine or levothyroxine treatment of a hypothyroid patient and disappeared after withdrawal of therapy (1331). In vitro lymphocyte testing confirmed sensitization for thyroid hormones.

Progressive re-institution of liothyronine subsequently proved possible in this patient without recurrence of hypersensitivity. Liothyronine was considered preferable because of the shorter biological half-life.

Thyrotrophin and thyrotropin

Many years ago bovine thyrotrophin was used for diagnostic purposes and to increase ^{131}I uptake. However, for diagnostic purposes it has been replaced by sensitive TSH assays, and because of antibody development and hypersensitivity reactions it is not used therapeutically. There is no evidence that thyrotropin causes allergic reactions, even after multiple injections (1332).

Rapid tumor expansion has been occasionally reported after thyrotropin, including four of 55 patients with central nervous system metastases enrolled in a compassionate use protocol (1333). Two patients with locally recurrent papillary carcinoma had tumor growth 12–48 hours after their second injection of recombinant thyrotropin (rTSH); rapid improvement in neck pain, stridor, and dysphonia after glucocorticoids suggested an inflammatory etiology (1333). There were no features to suggest an allergic reaction; only one such case has been reported and there are no reports of antibody formation even after repeated dosing (1334).

Tick-borne meningoencephalitis vaccine

See Vaccines

Ticlopidine

A lupus-like illness (fever, rash, arthritis, renal involvement, and positive antinuclear and antihistone antibodies) developed in three patients 2–8 weeks after they started to take ticlopidine (1335). After withdrawal, there was slow but complete resolution in all patients.

Tiopronin

Tiopronin can cause fever, with or without a rash (1336). In a patient with a prior hypersensitivity reaction to penicillamine, there was no cross-hypersensitivity to tiopronin (1337).

Tiopronin has occasionally been described as a cause of polymyositis (1338,1339).

- A 62-year-old woman with rheumatoid arthritis, hypothyroidism, and hypertension, treated for 6 years with tiopronin (dosage not specified), developed severe polymyositis. She had dysphagia and muscle weakness and pain in all limbs; there were no skin abnormalities. Her creatine kinase activity was 12 000 U/l (reference range 25–160) and her LDH 23 000 U/l (240–480). Her C-reactive protein was 58 µg/ml and the erythrocyte sedimentation rate 42 mm/hour (both raised). Electromyography of her proximal and distal muscles showed pseudomyotonic fibrillations. A biopsy of the deltoid muscle showed necrosis of muscle fibers and interstitial mononuclear infiltrates. There was no evidence of a paraneoplastic syndrome. Tests for toxoplasmosis, trichinosis, picornavirus, HIV, and hepatitis A, B, and C were negative, and there were no autoantibodies (anti-Jo, anti-KU, anti-PM/SCL, anti-DNA, anti-SSA, anti-SSB, anti-ECT, antithyroid, rheumatoid factor, or cryoglobulins), although ANF was positive on one occasion (1/100). Tiopronin was withdrawn, she was given glucocorticoids and methotrexate, and made a good recovery.

Titanium

Allergic reactions to titanium can occur (1340). Inflammatory reactions and contact sensitivity have been reported after insertion of titanium implants. Osseointegration of the implant tends to occur, but around the area there can be an intense inflammatory reaction and persistent irritation of soft tissues (SEDA-22, 250) (1341,1342).

Occasionally, reactions to titanium can occur at a distance from a hip implant, probably because small particles of titanium become detached and enter the system.

- Distant granulomatous reactions occurred in an elderly man, who developed symptomless lymph node histiocytosis, which was discovered incidentally.
- Another man had a visceral granulomatosis reaction (liver, spleen, and lymph node) associated with hepatic and splenic enlargement; in affected tissue specimens particles from the hip arthroplasty were detected, and titanium was found in the spleen (1343).

Despite its widespread use, titanium is only rarely linked with contact allergic reactions. A hypersensitivity reaction has been attributed to titanium in a pacemaker (1344).

- An 86-year-old Japanese man received a pacemaker for atrioventricular block, and 2 months later developed a scaly erythema over the implantation site and later widespread nummular eczema. Histologically, the lesions showed slight spongiosis, intracellular edema, moderate acanthosis in the epidermis, and perivascular infiltration with thickened capillary walls in the dermis. The pacemaker contained titanium and a variety of other metals, but patch tests were all negative. However, titanium sensitivity was demonstrated by intracutaneous and lymphocyte stimulation tests.

Titanium is so widely used that the risk of contact sensitivity to it must be very small. If a patient shows contact sensitivity to titanium, a replacement pacemaker should be completely encased in patch-tested non-allergenic material.

Tobramycin

- Hypersensitivity to inhaled tobramycin has been reported in a 9-year-old boy who developed a rash after a course of gentamicin (1345). The rash resolved after withdrawal, but returned all over his body when inhaled tobramycin was restarted. He was desensitized using escalating doses of inhaled tobramycin, tolerated the procedure well, and was still using once-a-day tobramycin 9 months after desensitization.

Tocainide

Arthralgia has been reported in two cases with positive antinuclear antibody titers, suggesting the possibility of a lupus-like syndrome (1346). In another case tocainide treatment was associated with both a lupus-like syndrome and neutropenia (1347). Cross-reactivity of tocainide with lidocaine has been reported (1348).

Tolmetin

See NSAIDs

Tolterodine

Anticholinergic drugs can rarely cause immunological reactions.

- An 81-year-old Swiss woman took immediate-release tolterodine 2 mg bd and 18 days later had fever, malaise, and nausea with vomiting (1349). Liver function tests showed a mixed hepatitic and cholestatic pattern and she also had leukocytosis and eosinophilia.

The authors suggested that this was a hypersensitivity reaction; if so it is the first of its kind to be reported with tolterodine.

Torasemide

Two possible cases of vasculitis with renal insufficiency have been reported in patients taking torasemide (1350,1351). This adverse effect is not surprising, since torasemide is structurally similar to sulfa drugs, which can cause vasculitis.

- A 70-year-old man developed heart failure secondary to ischemic heart disease and severe aortic stenosis (1350). Furosemide 20 mg/day was replaced by torasemide 5 mg/day. After the second dose he developed oliguria and an erythematous morbilliform rash with palpable violet petechial lesions on the legs. Chest X-ray showed bilateral alveolar infiltrates. Serum creatinine and potassium were raised (212 µmol/l and 6.7 mmol/l respectively). Skin biopsy showed leukocytoclastic vasculitis. After withdrawal of torasemide, his renal function improved (serum creatinine 97 µmol/l) and the skin lesions resolved (leaving residual pigmented areas) within 8 days.
- An 84-year-old man with ischemic heart disease and hypertension took torasemide 10 mg/day for persistent edema (1350). About 24 hours after the first dose of torasemide, he developed painless, non-palpable, petechial lesions on the limbs and trunk, with oliguria. His serum creatinine was 256 µmol/l and his serum potassium 6.2 mmol/l. Skin biopsy showed non-leukocytoclastic vasculitis with a mixed inflammatory infiltrate including eosinophils. He was symptom free 15 days after withdrawal of torasemide.

Neither patient had a previous history of drug hypersensitivity. Both patients had previously tolerated furosemide, another sulfonamide derivative. The temporal correlation with torasemide administration suggested a causal relation, but the mechanism was unclear.

Tosylchloramide sodium

Contact sensitization to tosylchloramide has been reported (1351).

- Urticaria, rhinitis, dyspnea, and edema of the face were reported in a female nurse after contact (SEDA-11, 492) (1352). Specific IgE antibodies to tosylchloramide were demonstrated.

Tranilast

Immune thrombocytopenia caused by tranilast has been reported in a 17-year-old man. The drug was withdrawn and oral prednisolone was started. He recovered within 1 week. Antiplatelet antibodies were not detected, but there was a platelet-associated IgG, which increased when a sample of his serum was incubated with tranilast in vitro (1353).

Triclocarban

There have been several cases of allergic contact dermatitis after the use of antiperspirants containing triclocarban and propylene glycol (1354).

Trientine

- A 44-year-old woman developed antinuclear and anti-double-stranded-DNA antibodies (without clinical signs) while taking penicillamine; the antibodies disappeared after withdrawal, but recurred when she was subsequently given trientine (1355).

Trifluridine

Trifluridine can cause allergic reactions (1356).

Trimethoprim and co-trimoxazole

The sulfonamide component of co-trimoxazole is generally believed to be more allergenic than trimethoprim. However, trimethoprim alone can cause hypersensitivity reactions more commonly than has previously been thought. Most of these reactions present as generalized skin reactions. The hydroxylamine and other metabolites of sulfamethoxazole can bind covalently to proteins because of their chemical reactivity, resulting in the induction of specific adverse immune responses. Therefore, changes in the activity of detoxification pathways are associated with a greater risk of allergic reactions to sulfonamides. Allergies to sulfonamides, particularly sulfamethoxazole, are more frequent in patients with AIDS, but the reason for this increased risk is not fully understood. No tools are available to predict which patients have a greater risk for developing allergies to sulfonamides. In a small study in HIV-positive patients with hypersensitivity syndrome reaction, the lymphocyte toxicity assay has a strong potential for use as a diagnostic tool to assess co-trimoxazole hypersensitivity (1357). Diagnosis is essential to avoid possible progression to severe reactions and readministration of the offending drug.

In patients who absolutely require further treatment, successful desensitization can be achieved (1358). Two patients with chronic granulomatous disease who had previously been intolerant of co-trimoxazole completed a 5-day desensitization protocol with a good clinical outcome (1359).

Anaphylactic shock is rare, but has been reported with co-trimoxazole (1360). However, it is possible that this reaction was due to the sulfonamide compound (1361). The case histories of 13 patients (12 women, one man, aged 22–68 years) with anaphylactic reactions to trimethoprim alone that were reported to a national drug safety unit have been analysed (1362). Nine were classified as probable anaphylaxis. The casual relation between exposure to trimethoprim and anaphylaxis was classified as definite in three reports, possible in four, and probable in six. In one patient, IgE antibodies against trimethoprim were demonstrated.

- Culture-negative arthritis, bilateral uveitis, mucocutaneous Stevens–Johnson syndrome, and eosinophilia developed in a 31-year-old woman after 3 days of therapy with oral trimethoprim 160 mg bd for a lower urinary tract infection (1363). At the start of antibiotic therapy, glucocorticoids and local anesthetics were injected into the lateral aspect of the right knee. Recovery was rapid after trimethoprim was withdrawn. Two months later she developed headache, nausea, malaise, and bilateral uveitis after taking trimethoprim again.

With sera from patients with known hypersensitivity to trimethoprim, IgE-specific recognition of three different but related metabolites has been demonstrated, including the entire molecule itself, the 3,4-dimethoxybenzyl group, and the 2,4-diamino-5-(3′,4′-dimethoxybenzyl) pyrimidine group (1364). The incidence of adverse reactions in patients with AIDS is higher than in others (1362). Most of these effects are not true allergic reactions, but are related to high doses of co-trimoxazole, and include rashes, nausea, and vomiting. They can be reduced in both frequency and severity by corticosteroids, which are often given in moderate to severe *P. jiroveci* pneumonia. The risk of hypersusceptibility reactions (Stevens–Johnson syndrome, neutropenia, hepatotoxicity, aseptic meningitis, thrombocytopenia) is also higher than in other patients. Since many rashes with co-trimoxazole are not necessarily due to allergic mechanisms, a previous rash should not prevent later re-administration. It may be prudent, however, to use a rapid test dose when co-trimoxazole is the treatment of choice (1365).

The incidence of adverse reactions to co-trimoxazole in HIV-infected patients is high. Several reports have shown that an incremental increase in drug dosage may allow a significant proportion of patients to tolerate prophylactic dosages of co-trimoxazole. Eight of 14 selected HIV-infected patients (13 men, 1 woman; patients who experienced severe reactions such as anaphylaxis or Stevens–Johnson syndrome were excluded) were successfully desensitized and after a regimen of gradual incremented exposure over 11 days as an outpatient procedure could continue to take co-trimoxazole (1366). *N*-acetyl-cysteine (3 g of a 421% liquid solution bd) did not prevent hypersensitivity reactions to co-trimoxazole in HIV-infected patients (1367). Although cross-reactivity can occur, dapsone can be used for patients with mild hypersensitivity reactions to co-trimoxazole for prophylaxis of *P. jiroveci* pneumonia (1368).

A syndrome that resembles bacterial sepsis is well recognized in patients with AIDS (1369). This reaction can occur within hours of a large dose of co-trimoxazole, but most often occurs on rechallenge.

- A sepsis-like hypersensitivity reaction occurred in 38-year-old HIV-positive Hispanic man after a 14-day course of co-trimoxazole (1370).

The mechanism of this unusual reaction is unclear.

Desensitization

Desensitization can be efficient in a large proportion of patients (88%) using a 5-day protocol, in which co-trimoxazole is administered orally in a granular formulation in increasing doses, beginning with trimethoprim 0.4 mg and sulfamethoxazole 2 mg and doubling the dose every 423 hours until the therapeutic dose is achieved (1371). Another dosage regimen (12 doses of increasing amounts of co-trimoxazole at half-hour intervals) resulted in an overall success rate of 91% at 1 month in 44 patients (1372). Such tolerance induction protocols can be adopted, even during pregnancy without risk to the mother or to the fetus (1373).

Another uncontrolled trial of a 6-day desensitization procedure in 33 cases has been reported (1374). The protocol started with a dose of 0.2 mg rising to 800 mg over 6 days and 32 of the subjects successfully completed the course. In addition,423 of 14 cases were successfully re-challenged with co-trimoxazole. However, this study lacked a clear description of follow-up or the reasons for the selection of subjects for desensitization or re-challenge, and cannot be used as a basis for recommending this desensitization technique.

Oral desensitization to co-trimoxazole was successfully achieved in patients with AIDS suffering from fever, rash, and wheezing due to the drug (1375–1378). In a randomized study of desensitization with rechallenge in HIV-positive patients with previous adverse effects of co-trimoxazole 73 patients were given a 14-day course of trimethoprim 200 mg/day (1379). Fourteen had adverse reactions to trimethoprim. The remaining 59 subjects were randomized to a 2-day desensitization technique (34 subjects) or rechallenge (25 subjects). There were seven hypersensitivity reactions in both groups. Clearly there is no advantage of this 2-day desensitization technique over rechallenge with co-trimoxazole in HIV-positive individuals.

In a randomized, double-blind study in HIV patients, gradual introduction of co-trimoxazole was associated with significantly fewer adverse drug reactions compared with standard initiation of therapy (1380).

Overall it appears that desensitization to co-trimoxazole is safe in the absence of previous serious adverse events, although it is not yet certain whether desensitization is better than re-challenge or indeed what the ideal desensitization method should be.

Tropicamide

A solution containing tropicamide 1% and benzalkonium chloride 0.01% (Mydriaticum) was introduced in 1979 to obtain mydriasis and cycloplegia for diagnostic purposes. Contact dermatitis from ophthalmic formulations is common, preservatives being the most frequent causes (1381). Allergic contact dermatitis has been reported, implicating tropicamide as a sensitizer (1382).

Vaccines

The questions of whether early childhood immunization affects the development of atopy and whether it causes allergic reactions have been reviewed (1383). The authors concluded that immunization programs do not explain the increasing incidence of allergic diseases, but that individual children may uncommonly develop an allergic reaction to a vaccine.

Non-sterile injection equipment can transmit HIV and other infectious agents, including hepatitis viruses. There is also a possibility of needle transmission from an HIV-infected person to a vaccinator. Data from the USA show that the risk of transmission of HIV through needle stick is very low, perhaps 20 times lower than in the case of hepatitis B, and in the order of one per 100 accidents. Furthermore, the types of injections given during immunization sessions do not as a rule cause bleeding. The risk of transmission is thus extremely low. No instances of immunization-related spread of HIV to other infants have been reported, and if proper sterilization of needles and syringes is performed and vaccines are administered correctly the risk of HIV transmission is zero (1384). However, the use of unsterilized or improperly sterilized needles and syringes is common, particularly in many developing countries, and contributes largely to the spread of hepatitis B and C, as well to the spread of human immunodeficiency virus and other blood-borne pathogens. These risks are recognized by the WHO as major public health problems and led the Organization to initiate a broad program of activities to ensure safe injection techniques (1385). The guidelines published by WHO and UNICEF in 1986/87 (1386,1387), which can be set out briefly as follows, are still valid. Essentially they state that:

(a) a single sterile needle and a single sterile syringe should be used with each injection;
(b) reusable needles and syringes are recommended for use in developing countries; they should be steam-sterilized between uses; boiling is an acceptable alternative procedure when steam sterilization is not available;
(c) disposable needles and syringes should only be used if an assurance can be obtained that they will be destroyed after a single use;

(d) disease transmission by use of jet injectors is theoretically possible and has been demonstrated in human beings in a single situation (SEDA-11, 296); until further studies clarify the risks of disease transmission with different types of injectors, their use should be restricted to special circumstances in which large numbers of persons need to be immunized within a short period of time.

Jet-gun-associated infections

The first outbreak of a disease in which a jet injector was implicated as the vehicle of transmission has been reported. Thirty-one attendees at a weight-reduction clinic in Southern California experienced hepatitis B after daily parenteral injections of human chorionic gonadotrophin given by jet injectors; transmission appeared to have resulted from the multiple repeated jet injections (1388). WHO and UNICEF have stated in their "Guidelines for selecting injection equipment for the Expanded Program on Immunization" that the use of jet injectors should be restricted to circumstances in which reusable or disposable equipment is not feasible because of the large number of persons to be immunized within a short period of time (1386).

A new type of needleless jet-injector (Mini-Imojet) administers liquid vaccines from a single-use, prefilled cartridge ("imule"), thereby avoiding the risk of cross-contamination. Administration of various vaccines by jet-injector has been compared with standard syringe technique. All the jet-administered vaccines were of equivalent or superior immunogenicity. The most common reactions were mild (minor bleeding, superficial papules, erythema, induration). The technical and safety advantages of the Mini-Imojet reinforce the potential use of this technique for mass immunization (1387).

Diphtheria vaccine

• A six-year-old child had anaphylaxis 30 minutes after a fifth dose of DT vaccine (1388). Skin tests, in vitro determination of specific IgE antibodies, and immunoblotting assays showed that the IgE response was directed against tetanus and diphtheria toxoids. Cross-reactivity between the two toxoids was not demonstrated, indicating the presence of co-existing but non-cross-reacting IgE and IgG antibodies.

Influenza vaccine

Changes in the lymphocyte population similar to those observed during virus infections occurred within the first 2 weeks after immunization (1389). There were no reports describing more severe courses of infectious diseases during this period.

The question of whether egg allergy is a justified contraindication to influenza immunization has been studied in 80 individuals with egg allergy and 124 control subjects, who received influenza vaccine containing ovalbumin/ovomucoid 0.02, 0.1, or 1.2 µg/ml (1390). The individuals with egg allergy received the vaccine in two doses 30 minutes apart; the first dose was one-tenth and the second dose nine-tenths of the recommended dose. The patients with egg allergy, even those with significant allergic reactions after egg ingestion, safely received influenza vaccine in this two-dose protocol with vaccine containing no more than 1.2 µg/ml of egg protein.

There have been reports of individual cases of giant cell arteritis (1391) and polymyalgia rheumatica (1392,1393) in temporal relation to influenza vaccine.

• A 70-year-old man, previously healthy, developed giant cell arteritis 5 days after influenza immunization (1394).The authors mentioned another case reported in 1976.

Japanese encephalitis vaccine

Hypersensitivity reactions (generalized urticaria or angioedema) after the use of Japanese encephalitis vaccine have been reported from some countries (see Table 1); the vaccine constituents responsible for these events have not been identified (1395). There has been a detailed report of the adverse effects, mainly allergic mucocutaneous reactions, of Biken vaccine in Danish travellers and US Marine Corps personnel (SEDA-22, 351).

Table 1 Allergic reactions after Japanese encephalitis immunization

Country	Estimated number of vaccines	Number of reactions	Estimated rate per 100 000 vaccines
Denmark	42 000	21	50
Sweden	15 000	1	7
UK	1950	1	51
Australia			
Nationwide	3400	4	118
Fairfield Hospital	601	3	499
Canada			
University of Calgary	96	1	1042
USA			
Travellers	1328	2	151
Army	526	1	190
Army and dependents (Okinawa)	35 253	220	624
Total	100 154	254	254

The Advisory Committee on Immunization Practices (ACIP) has recommended that vaccinees should be observed for 30 minutes after immunization and that medications to treat anaphylaxis should be available (1395) [http://www.cdc.gov/mmwr/PDF/rr/rr4201.pdf]. A personal history of allergic disorders should be considered when weighing the risks and benefits of the vaccine for an individual. Japanese encephalitis vaccine should not be given to persons who had a previous adverse reaction after receiving Japanese encephalitis vaccine or a previous hypersensitivity reaction to other vaccines of neural origin.

In Japan, children who had immediate-type allergic reactions to Japanese encephalitis vaccine had antigelatin IgE in their sera. However, the immunological mechanism of non-immediate-type allergic reactions that consist of cutaneous signs developing several hours or more after Japanese encephalitis immunization is not yet clear. Serum samples taken from 28 children who had non-immediate-type allergic skin reactions have been compared with serum samples taken from 10 children who had immediate-type reactions (1396). All the children who had had immediate-type reactions had antigelatin IgE and IgG. Of 28 children who had had non-immediate-type reactions, one had antigelatin IgE and nine had antigelatin IgG. These results suggest that some children who develop non-immediate-type allergic reactions have also been sensitized to gelatin.

Malaria vaccine

Immediate-type hypersensitivity reactions (acute, systemic urticaria after the third immunization) occurred in two of 39 volunteers immunized with a synthetic multi-antigen peptide vaccine (PfCS-MAP1NYU) against *P. falciparum* sporozoites, with detection of serum IgE MAP antibody (1397). Immediate pain at the injection site was associated with the adjuvant QS-21, and delayed local inflammatory reactions were associated with high titers of circulating IgG anti-MAP antibody. Skin tests using intradermal injections of diluted MAP vaccine, to identify those who were sensitized to the vaccine, were negative in seven volunteers tested 27 days after the first vaccination, but six of these developed positive wheal and flare reactions when tested 14 or 83 days after the second vaccination; IgE MAP antibody was detected in only one of them. Skin tests may help in identifying individuals who have been sensitized to malaria peptides and who are at risk of developing systemic allergic reactions after revaccination.

On the other hand, delayed-type hypersensitivity testing has been used to test T cell functional activity in 27 volunteers immunized with a synthetic multi-antigen peptide vaccine (MAP) (PfCS-MAP1NYU) against *P. falciparum* sporozoites (1398). Intradermal inoculations (0.02 ml) of several concentrations of the MAP vaccine and adjuvant control solutions were applied and induration measured 2 days after. Nine of 14 vaccinees with high serum titers of anti-MAP antibody developed positive skin tests (at least 5 mm induration), which first appeared by 29 days after immunization and persisted for at least 3–6 months after one or two more immunizations. In contrast, skin tests were negative in all of eight vaccinees with no or low antibody titers, and in all of five non-immunized volunteers. Biopsies of positive skin test sites were histologically compatible with a delayed hypersensitivity reaction. The authors concluded that the presence of T cell functional activity is reflected by a positive skin test response to the MAP antigen and may serve as another marker for vaccine immunogenicity.

Measles vaccine

It has been suggested that hydrolysed gelatin, rather than egg protein, is responsible for most episodes of anaphylaxis after measles immunization (1399). Egg allergy should no longer be a contraindication to measles immunization. However, a previous anaphylactic reaction to measles or MMR vaccine remains a contraindication.

Toxic shock syndrome was reported to have developed within 3 hours of measles immunization in four children, three of whom died. It was initially seen in women who were using tampons in the presence of vaginal colonization and/or infection with toxin-producing strains of *Staphylococcus aureus*. The hallmarks of toxic shock syndrome are high fever, diarrhea, vomiting, tachycardia, hypertension, mucocutaneous ulceration, rash, conjunctival injection, red palms and soles, and a bleeding diathesis. There was some evidence that a used vial of measles vaccine had been kept in cold water and had thereby become contaminated (1400). Similar events from various developing countries have been reported to the World Health Organization. Careful investigation pointed clearly to secondary bacterial contamination as the cause of disease and death (1401).

Pertussis vaccines

Data from the Third National Health and Nutrition Survey (1988–94) have been used to analyse the possible effects of DTP or tetanus immunization on allergies and allergy-related symptoms among 13 944 infants, children, and adolescents aged 2 months to 16 years in the USA (1402). The authors concluded that DTP or tetanus immunization increases the risk of allergies and related respiratory symptoms in children and adolescents. However, the small number of non-immunized individuals and the study design limited their ability to make firm causal inferences about the true magnitude of effect.

It has been suggested that the development of a sterile abscess represents an idiosyncratic reaction of some individuals, perhaps genetically determined, which causes a granulomatous response to antigens, irrespective of the location of the vaccine (1403). Others maintain that it is caused by a contaminated needle track or to vaccine material coating the outside of the needle, resulting from the lack of a proper injection technique.

Plague vaccine

Known allergy to any of the plague vaccine constituents (beef protein, soya, casein, phenol) contraindicates immunization. Severe local or systemic reactions following previous doses contraindicate revaccination (1404).

Pneumococcal vaccine

Arthus reactions and systemic reactions have commonly been reported after booster doses of polysaccharide vaccine and are thought to result from antigen–antibody reactions involving antibodies induced by the previous immunization (1405). Data on revaccination of children are not yet sufficient to provide a basis for recommendation.

An allergic reaction has been described to 23-valent polysaccharide pneumococcal vaccine (1406).

- A 2-year-old child developed bronchospasm and cutaneous and laryngeal edema immediately after the injection of a 23-valent polysaccharide pneumococcal vaccine. The symptoms resolved within 1 hour of treatment with antihistamines, glucocorticoids, and aerosols. Skin tests and specific IgE tests showed that the pneumococcal antigens were responsible for the anaphylaxis.

Rabies vaccine

In recipients given primary courses of third-generation rabies vaccines, only mild local and systemic reactions were reported by about 20%. Systemic allergic reactions have occurred in 11 per 10 000 vaccinees (1407). However, 2–21 days after the administration of HDC vaccine, about 5% of patients receiving booster injections for pre-exposure prophylaxis and a few receiving postexposure primary immunization develop an immune complex (serum sickness-like) reaction, including urticaria, fever, malaise, arthralgias, arthritis, nausea, and vomiting. This syndrome may prove to be less common with RVA, but direct comparisons are lacking.

Anaphylaxis has been reported rarely after HDC vaccine prophylaxis (1408).

Tick-borne meningoencephalitis vaccine

A case of facial edema and pain and swelling of the left knee following the receipt of tick-borne meningoencephalitis vaccine was suspected to be caused by thiomersal allergy (1409).

Varicella vaccine

In one case a hypersensitivity vasculitis developed 2 weeks after *Varicella* immunization (1410).

Infection risk

Spread of infection to the siblings of immunized leukemic children has been observed. Between 18 and 36 days after the receipt of *Varicella* vaccine 2–10% of exposed children developed mild *Varicella* and/or seroconversion to *Varicella* virus.

Transmission of the *Varicella* vaccine virus from a toddler (with a history of allergic diathesis) to his pregnant mother has been reported and discussed (SEDA-22, 354).

Complicated wild *Varicella* in immunized individuals has been reported (1411); among the two cases the first reported case of *Varicella* meningitis occurring in a child with documented immunization and seroconversion (1412).

Cases of zoster both in healthy and in immunosuppressed persons have been reported (1413–1415).

A 19-month-old girl was immunized against *Varicella* at 15 months of age and later developed zoster infection (1416). Viral cultures from various lesions isolated *Varicella zoster* virus. The Oka vaccine strain was revealed by polymerase chain reaction.

There have been three case reports of suspected reactivation of *Varicella zoster* through hepatitis A vaccine, influenza vaccine, and simultaneous administration of rabies and Japanese encephalitis vaccine (1417).

- A 53-year-old woman without signs of immunodeficiency developed zoster in the left T10 dermatome 14 days after influenza immunization. The rash resolved without sequelae. Five months later she received another injection of influenza vaccine and 12 days later developed zoster in the left T1 dermatome. Recovery was prolonged.
- An 80-year-old woman with carcinoma developed long-lasting left thoracic zoster 6 days after influenza immunization. Influenza vaccination before and after the event had no adverse effect.
- A 27-year-old man developed zoster in the second and third branches of the trigeminal nerve 1 day after immunization against rabies and Japanese encephalitis.

Zoster in childhood is unusual and probably even less common after *Varicella* immunization.

- A 6-year-old boy developed a zoster infection (with a vesicular rash in a left second thoracic dermatome pattern on his back extending to the back of his left arm) 15 days after the receipt of *Varicella* vaccine (Oka strain) (1418). Molecular biological analysis of the virus isolated from the vesicles showed a pattern consistent with wild-type *Varicella zoster* virus.

The authors felt that this case mandated a careful review of all cases of zoster after *Varicella* immunization. Zoster induced by *Varicella* immunization could have implications for the use of immunization to prevent zoster in the elderly, a population with almost uniform *Varicella zoster* latent virus and at higher risk of zoster.

Yellow fever vaccine

Rash, erythema multiforme, urticaria, angioedema, and asthma occur infrequently, predominantly in people with a history of allergy, especially to eggs (1419).

Severe immediate hypersensitivity reactions (type 1), sometimes accompanied by anaphylactic shock and circulatory collapse, have been described very rarely (1419). Allergic reactions of the Arthus phenomenon type, characterized by local swelling and necrosis following less than 24 hours after immunization, have occurred in rare instances. Some of these cases have been fatal.

Two episodes have been reported from the Ivory Coast (1974) and Ghana (1982) (1419). In the Ivory Coast, there were 39 cases of severe reactions with eight deaths following a mass campaign, in which 730 000 persons were immunized. The clinical features were uniform: a few hours after immunization the vaccinees developed signs of local inflammation. In severe cases, edema and inflammation were followed by cardiovascular collapse. Bacterial contamination could have been the cause: during the campaign, five-dose vaccine ampoules were pooled to prepare 50 and 100 doses for use in jet injectors. In Ghana, six vaccinees developed fulminant reactions 2–6 hours after immunization, including two deaths. The clinical features resembled those in the Ivory Coast episode. In 2001, during a mass vaccination campaign against yellow fever in Abidjan, the Ivory Coast, more than 2.6 million doses were administered and 87 adverse events were notified, of which 41 were considered to be vaccine-related. There was one case of anaphylaxis and 26 cases of urticaria, five of which were generalized (1420).

People who are known to be suffering from allergy must be tested intradermally before immunization.

Valproic acid

Hypersensitivity reactions to valproate are rare. Lupus-like syndrome has been reported occasionally with valproate (SEDA-19, 75; SEDA-20, 69) and valpromide (1430).

In vitro tests have shown that valproate can increase the viral burden in HIV-infected individuals by potentiating replication of the virus (1431). In a retrospective review of 11 HIV-positive patients with behavioral disturbances taking valproate HIV-1 viral load did not increase in six of the nine patients who had measurements between the first week and 3.5 months after the start of valproate treatment; no follow-up was available for the other three (1432). These data suggest that, contrary to in vitro data, HIV-1 viral load is not adversely affected by valproate in the presence of effective antiretroviral therapy.

Vancomycin

Allergic reactions with vancomycin, such as rashes, chills, fever, and eosinophilia, can occur in up to 5% of patients. Severe anaphylactic reactions are rare. Alpha-tryptase is only detected in the blood during systemic anaphylactic reactions, having been released by degranulation from activated mast cells. Plasma tryptase activities were unchanged, independent of increased histamine concentrations, antihistamine pretreatment, and clinical symptoms of anaphylactoid reaction in 40 patients receiving vancomycin (1 g over 10 minutes) before elective arthroplasty (1433). The authors conclude that plasma tryptase activities can be used to distinguish chemical from immunological reactions.

Vancomycin anaphylaxis is a major management problem in patients with methicillin-resistant *S. aureus* sepsis. However, desensitization in patients with previous anaphylaxis is possible (1434).

- An anaphylactic reaction occurred in a 77-year-old woman 5 minutes after the start of a vancomycin infusion, when she had received only 40 mg (1435). She became unconscious and had a severe cardiovascular collapse, from which she was resuscitated with intravenous ephedrine and adrenaline.

- A 47-year-old white woman with end-stage renal disease had had anaphylactoid shock after vancomycin 1 g intravenously infused over 1.5 hours and gentamicin 90 mg 3 years before, despite premedication with diphenhydramine (1436). She was treated with doubling doses of vancomycin every 30 minutes for methicillin-resistant *S. epidermidis*. She had no reaction.

The authors of the second report could not exclude that the previous anaphylactoid reaction had not been due to gentamicin, as no specific testing was done. Although successful vancomycin desensitization has been described, this would be the first time in a patient with a history of anaphylactoid reaction.

In some patients the clinical presentation of red man syndrome is identical to that of acute IgE-mediated anaphylaxis. Vancomycin desensitization should therefore be considered for severe red man syndrome reactions that do not respond to premedication and a slower rate of infusion, and in anaphylactic reactions to vancomycin when substitution of another antibiotic is not feasible. Rapid desensitization is preferred, as it is effective in the majority of patients and enables administration of vancomycin within 24 hours. In patients who fail rapid desensitization, a slow desensitization protocol may be tried (1437).

Vasculitic rashes have been described rarely. Two case reports have suggested that there may be cross-reactivity between vancomycin and teicoplanin with respect to biopsy-proven leukocytoclastic vasculitis (1438). In both cases, vancomycin-induced vasculitis improved after drug withdrawal. Teicoplanin was started and the rash reappeared several days later. In one case the rash faded after teicoplanin had been withdrawn. In the other, teicoplanin was continued, but the rash improved after prednisolone was given.

Varicella vaccine

See Vaccines

Viscaceae

Parenteral administration of *V. album* can cause serious allergic reactions (1439), and anaphylactic reactions have been described (1440).

Vitamin A: Carotenoids

Large doses of vitamin A in children in poor socioeconomic conditions have often for logistic reasons been combined with other health-care interventions, such as immunization. A randomized, case-control study of 336 infants receiving either 33 000 micrograms RE/day (100 000 IU) of vitamin A or placebo simultaneously with measles vaccine showed a lower seroconversion to measles in the vitamin A group (1441).

Vitamin A: Retinoids

Hypersensitivity reactions to retinoids are rare and consist of occasional drug rashes.

- Immunomodulatory effects of isotretinoin in the treatment of facial acne (40 mg/day for 4 weeks) were blamed for a recurrence of pulmonary alveolar proteinosis in a 16-year-old girl, in whom it had been in spontaneous remission for 2 years (1442).

Although the time-course of this effect was suggestive, it should be borne in mind that about 25% of patients with this disease have exacerbations without a clear cause.

Vitamin B$_6$ (thiamine)

Anaphylactic shock is a major adverse effect of thiamine, and can be life-threatening. It is IgE-mediated (1443) and usually occurs after multiple parenteral dosages (1443–1447) but occasionally also after intramuscular injection. In some cases oral challenge did not produce any reaction (1445,1448,1449).

- A 51-year-old woman with diabetes mellitus, chronic alcoholism, and anxiety disorder became acutely confused and was given 50% dextrose 25 g and thiamine hydrochloride 100 mg intravenously; 20 minutes later she became deeply cyanosed with shallow labored breathing at 28/minute, hypertensive, and tachycardic, with respiratory and metabolic acidosis and a blood alcohol concentration of 124 mg/dl (27 mmol/l) (1450). The next morning she was communicative and oriented and her vital signs and blood gases were normal. She was given thiamine hydrochloride intravenously and within moments developed shortness of breath, warmth, and tightness of the throat. She had a tachycardia, hypotension, hypoxia, and central cyanosis. She recovered within 24 hours.

In 989 consecutive patients (1070 doses) there were 12 adverse reactions (1.1% of doses), comprising local irritation in 11 cases and a major skin reaction in the 12th. The authors concluded that thiamine hydrochloride can safely be given intravenously and that intradermal test doses before administration are not warranted unless patients have had previous allergic reactions (1451).

Vitamin B$_{12}$ (cobalamins)

Allergy to vitamin B$_{12}$ injection is infrequent, but can be serious. Positive results of basophil histamine release assay and skin testing suggest an IgE-mediated mechanism (1452). Severe hypersensitivity to cyanocobalamin or hydroxocobalamin has been reported in patients who took the other cobalamin without further allergic reactions (1453).

- A 45-year-old woman with pernicious anemia was given intramuscular hydroxocobalamin and developed mild generalized pruritus (1454). Subsequent monthly injections of hydroxocobalamin 1 mg were followed by incrementally worsening pruritus and then frank urticaria. The last of nine injections was followed by urticaria, bronchospasm, and oropharyngeal angioedema, which responded to adrenaline. She underwent skin prick and intradermal testing with hydroxocobalamin and cyanocobalamin. Wheal-and-flare reactions occurred after injection of hydroxocobalamin, suggesting an IgE-mediated response. There was no reaction to cyanocobalamin. She subsequently had a reaction to subcutaneous cyanocobalamin 0.1 ml (100 micrograms) and then intramuscular cyanocobalamin 0.5 ml (500 micrograms). Her macrocytic anemia resolved with monthly cyanocobalamin. After 1 year she had an episode of delayed urticaria after a routine injection of cyanocobalamin. Skin prick and intradermal tests were again negative with cyanocobalamin, but there were wheal-and-flare reactions to hydroxocobalamin. She then tolerated monthly intramuscular cyanocobalamin for over 12 months.
- A 42-year-old woman who had received monthly intramuscular cyanocobalamin for 4 years developed Quincke's edema. She was given hydroxocobalamin instead, each injection being preceded by 4 mg of dexamethasone. After 13 years of this treatment she had not had any allergic reactions.
- A 35-year-old woman who had received monthly intramuscular hydroxocobalamin for 6 years developed anaphylactic shock immediately after a dose. Later she was given cyanocobalamin with terfenadine 120 mg/day for 2 days before each injection. After 3 years she had not had any allergic reactions.

Skin prick and intradermal tests, with increasing concentrations of hydroxocobalamin and cyanocobalamin, and histamine release tests on blood basophils with hydroxocobalamin and cyanocobalamin were negative in the second and third patients.

One way of dealing with vitamin B$_{12}$ allergy is to use the alternative compound after skin testing to exclude cross-reactivity. If cross-reactivity occurs, desensitization may be considered. Alternatively, oral B$_{12}$ can be used.

Vitamin C

See Ascorbic acid

Vitamin K analogues

Allergic reactions have been attributed to phytomenadione, menadione, and vitamin K$_4$. In mice, menadione caused marked hypodynamia and hypothermia. This effect was potentiated by riboflavin. Allergic reactions to the systemic administration of vitamin K are immunologically mediated, and generally arise in patients with coagulation or liver problems.

Intradermal tests with phytomenadione and menadione caused an allergic skin reaction 7–22 days after injection in 13 of 145 healthy subjects. The results suggested that the index of cutaneous sensitivity lies somewhere between 5.5 and 8.9%. On the other hand, the absence of adverse effects with oral phytomenadione is striking. Continuation of treatment orally can in some cases prevent dermatitis (1455). No cross-sensitivity has been seen between phytomenadione and menadione (1456). Anaphylactoid reactions, some fatal, to phytomenadione have been reported (SEDA-15, 416) mainly from intravenous use (1457).

The recommendation that prolongation of the international normalized ratio (INR) to over 6.0 should be corrected with parenteral phytomenadione (1458,1459) is not accompanied by the caveat that the intravenous route entails the risk of life-threatening, non-IgE-mediated anaphylactic reactions and even death, due to the use of polyethoxylated castor oil (Cremophor EL) as a solvent (1460). A severe reaction to intravenous phytomenadione has been reported (1461).

- A 74-year-old woman, taking warfarin, presented with an INR of 6.2. She was given a slow intravenous injection of phytomenadione (Konakion, Roche Products Ltd) 0.25 ml (500 μg) over about 60 seconds, and soon after felt profoundly unwell and complained of severe backache. She was given chlorphenamine 10 mg by rapid intravenous injection and adrenaline 1 mg in 10 ml of water over 30 minutes, with a good result.

An unusual case of allergy to vitamin K, with a relapsing and remitting eczematous reaction, has been described after an intramuscular injection of vitamin K_1 (1462).

- A 27-year-old woman with cystic fibrosis and pancreatic insufficiency was given intramuscular vitamin K_1 into her thigh. The next day transient erythema occurred over the injection site and 6 weeks later there was localized pain, erythema, and edema. She was given intravenous cefuroxime for presumed cellulitis, but over the next few days the features became more consistent with localized eczema; she was given oral prednisolone 30 mg/day, super-potent topical corticosteroids, corticosteroid injections, and corticosteroids under occlusion with Duoderm, all of which failed to result in improvement. She then also developed an eczematous reaction to the Duoderm dressing. Patch tests were positive to vitamin K_1 and cross-reacted with vitamin K_4. She was also positive to colophonium and ester gum rosin, the dressing adhesive. Recurrent angio-edema persisted for several months and 2 years later she still had symptoms at the injection sites.

In all reported cases, only the whole formulation of vitamin K_1 (in its vehicle) or vitamin K_1 alone elicited positive patch tests. When individual additives were tested the results were negative. No previous exposure to vitamin K_1 was required for the development of type IV hypersensitivity, and primary sensitization occurred within 1–2 weeks or after a longer time period, as in the patient described here.

Warfarin

See Coumarin anticoagulants

Wound dressings, substances used in

Patients with chronic venous insufficiency and venous leg ulcers are at risk of sensitization to topical medications. The frequency of sensitization in these patients is up to 67% (1463). In a study using an expanded European standard series and 20 different wound dressings for patch-testing in 36 patients with chronic venous insufficiency, sensitization to modern wound dressings was found in 8.3% (three cases) and was caused by propylene glycol as an ingredient of hydrogels (1464). However, it must be emphasized that positive patch test reactions to propylene glycol can indicate irritation rather than contact allergy. There were no cases of sensitization to hydrocolloids, alginates, or polyurethane foams. The rank order of allergens was headed by ointment bases (sensitization to wool wax alcohols in 33% of patients; amerchol 19%; cetearyl alcohol 14%; propylene glycol 8.3%), followed by plant resins/ethereal oils (balsam of Peru 22%; colophony 14%; fragrance mix 8.3%; propolis 5.6%), and topical antibiotics (neomycin sulfate 17%; chloramphenicol 14%) (1465).

Yohimbine

A lupus-like syndrome in conjunction with generalized erythroderma and progressive renal insufficiency has been attributed to yohimbine (1466,1467).

Zinc

Zinc can reportedly impair immune responses (1468).

Zomepirac

The manufacturers received 1100 reports of allergic reactions in the first 2 years after launch. Fatal anaphylactic and anaphylactoid reactions have been reported: 10% of all reports on anaphylactic reactions in the USA named zomepirac, making it second only to the much older drug tolmetin. Hypersensitivity reactions are characterized by hypotension, bronchospasm, and serious respiratory distress, with or without oropharyngeal edema. Type-III allergic reactions have also been described.

Zonisamide

Zonisamide-induced lupus erythematosus has been reported in a 5-year-old child taking zonisamide and ethosuximide (1469). He had raised titers of antinuclear antibodies and anti-DNA antibodies and presented with fever, pericarditis, pleurisy, and arthralgia. Clinical recovery and a reduction in the anti-DNA-antibody titer promptly followed withdrawal. A lymphocyte transformation test against zonisamide was positive.

References

1. Katlama C, Fenske S, Gazzard B, Lazzarin A, Clumeck N, Mallolas J, Lafeuillade A, Mamet JP, Beauvais LAZL30002 European study team. TRIZAL study: switching from successful HAART to Trizivir (abacavir–lamivudine–zidovudine combination tablet): 48 weeks efficacy, safety and adherence results. HIV Med 2003;4(2):79–86.

2. Hervey PS, Perry CM. Abacavir: a review of its clinical potential in patients with HIV infection. Drugs 2000;60(2):447–79.

3. Henry K, Wallace RJ, Bellman PC, Norris D, Fisher RL, Ross LL, Liao Q, Shaefer MSTARGET Study Team. Twice-daily triple nucleoside intensification treatment with lamivudine–zidovudine plus abacavir sustains suppression of human immunodeficiency virus type 1: results of the TARGET Study. J Infect Dis 2001;183(4):571–8.

4. Escaut L, Liotier JY, Albengres E, Cheminot N, Vittecoq D. Abacavir rechallenge has to be avoided in case of hypersensitivity reaction. AIDS 1999;13(11):1419–20.

5. Loeliger AE, Steel H, McGuirk S, Powell WS, Hetherington SV. The abacavir hypersensitivity reaction and interruptions in therapy. AIDS 2001;15(10):1325–6.

6. Symonds W, Cutrell A, Edwards M, Steel H, Spreen B, Powell G, McGuirk S, Hetherington S. Risk factor analysis of hypersensitivity reactions to abacavir. Clin Ther 2002;24(4):565–73.

7. Mallal S, Nolan D, Witt C, Masel G, Martin AM, Moore C, Sayer D, Castley A, Mamotte C, Maxwell D, James I, Christiansen FT. Association between presence of HLA-B*5701, HLA-DR7, and HLA-DQ3 and hypersensitivity to HIV-1 reverse-transcriptase inhibitor abacavir. Lancet 2002;359(9308):727–32.

8. Hetherington S, Hughes AR, Mosteller M, Shortino D, Baker KL, Spreen W, Lai E, Davies K, Handley A, Dow DJ, Fling ME, Stocum M, Bowman C, Thurmond LM, Roses AD. Genetic variations in HLA-B region and hypersensitivity reactions to abacavir. Lancet 2002;359(9312):1121–2.

9. Paediatric European Network for Treatment of AIDS (PENTA). Comparison of dual nucleoside-analogue reverse-transcriptase inhibitor regimens with and without nelfinavir in children with HIV-1 who have not previously been treated: the PENTA 5 randomised trial. Lancet 2002;359(9308):733–40.

10. Ferguson JJ, Kereiakes DJ, Adgey AA, Fox KA, Hillegass WB Jr, Pfisterer M, Vassanelli C. Safe use of platelet GP IIb/IIIa inhibitors. Am Heart J 1998;135(4):S77–89.

11. Dery JP, Braden GA, Lincoff AM, Kereiakes DJ, Browne K, Little T, George BS, Sane DC, Cines DB, Effron MB, Mascelli MA, Langrall MA, Damaraju L, Barnathan ES, Tcheng JEReoPro Readministration Registry Investigators. Final results of the ReoPro readministration registry. Am J Cardiol 2004;93(8):979–84.

12. Pharand C, Palisaitis DA, Hamel D. Potential anaphylactic shock with abciximab readministration. Pharmacotherapy 2002;22(3):380–3.

13. Booth RJ, Bullock JY, Wilson JD. Antinuclear antibodies in patients on acebutolol. Br J Clin Pharmacol 1980;9(5):515–7.

14. Cody RJ Jr, Calabrese LH, Clough JD, Tarazi RC, Bravo EL. Development of antinuclear antibodies during acebutolol therapy. Clin Pharmacol Ther 1979;25(6):800–5.

15. Lahita R, Kluger J, Drayer DE, Koffler D, Reidenberg MM. Antibodies to nuclear antigens in patients treated with procainamide or acetylprocainamide. N Engl J Med 1979;301(25):1382–5.

16. Kluger J, Leech S, Reidenberg MM, Lloyd V, Drayer DE. Long-term antiarrhythmic therapy with acetylprocainamide. Am J Cardiol 1981;48(6):1124–32.

17. Castellano A, Cabrera M, Robledo T, Martinez-Cocera C, Cimarra M, Llamazares AA, Chamorro M. Anaphylaxis by pyridostigmine. Allergy 1998;53(11):1108–9.

18. Bonfiglio MF, Traeger SM, Hulisz DT, Martin BR. Anaphylactoid reaction to intravenous acetylcysteine associated with electrocardiographic abnormalities. Ann Pharmacother 1992;26(1):22–5.

19. Bateman DN, Woodhouse KW, Rawlins MD. Adverse reactions to N-acetylcysteine. Lancet 1984;2(8396):228.

20. Tenenbein M. Hypersensitivity-like reactions to N-acetylcysteine. Vet Hum Toxicol 1984;26(Suppl 2):3–5.

21. Ward MR. Reye's syndrome: an update. Nurse Pract 1997;22(12):45–649–50, 52–3.

22. Kawsar M, Parkin JM, Forster G. Graded challenge in an aciclovir allergic patient. Sex Transm Infect 2001;77(3):204–5.

23. Wollenberg A, Baldauf C, Rueff F, Przybilla B. Allergic contact dermatitis and exanthematous drug eruption following aciclovir-cross reaction with ganciclovir. Allergo J 2000;9:96–9.

24. Lammintausta K, Makela L, Kalimo K. Rapid systemic valaciclovir reaction subsequent to aciclovir contact allergy. Contact Dermatitis 2001;45(3):181.

25. Rodriguez WJ, Bui RH, Connor JD, Kim HW, Brandt CD, Parrott RH, Burch B, Mace J. Environmental exposure of primary care personnel to ribavirin aerosol when supervising treatment of infants with respiratory syncytial virus infections. Antimicrob Agents Chemother 1987;31(7):1143–6.

26. Santavirta S, Konttinen YT, Bergroth V, Gronblad M. Lack of immune response to methyl methacrylate in lymphocyte cultures. Acta Orthop Scand 1991;62(1):29–32.

27. Santavirta S, Gristina A, Konttinen YT. Cemented versus cementless hip arthroplasty. A review of prosthetic biocompatibility. Acta Orthop Scand 1992;63(2):225–32.

28. Donaghy M, Rushworth G, Jacobs JM. Generalized peripheral neuropathy in a dental technician exposed to methyl methacrylate monomer. Neurology 1991;41(7):1112–6.

29. Rumpf KW, Rieger J, Jansen J, Scherer M, Seubert S, Seubert A, Sellin HJ. Quincke's edema in a dialysis patient after administration of acrylic bone cement: possible role of ethylene oxide allergy. Arch Orthop Trauma Surg 1986;105(4):250–2.

30. Shaw AD, Boscoe MJ. Anaphylactic reaction following intravenous adenosine. Anaesthesia 1999;54(6):608.

31. Dupond JL, Herve P, Saint-Hillier Y, Guyon B, Colas JM, Perol C, Leconte des Floris R. Anurie recidivant a 3 reprises; complication exceptionelle d'un traitement antiarythmique. J Med Besancon 1975;11:231.

32. Ring J, Messmer K. Incidence and severity of anaphylactoid reactions to colloid volume substitutes. Lancet 1977;1(8009):466–9.

33. Stafford CT, Lobel SA, Fruge BC, Moffitt JE, Hoff RG, Fadel HE. Anaphylaxis to human serum albumin. Ann Allergy 1988;61(2):85–8.

34. Aboulghar M, Evers JH, Al-Inany H. Intravenous albumin for preventing severe ovarian hyperstimulation syndrome: a Cochrane review. Hum Reprod 2002;17(12):3027–32.

35. Chan CS, Yeung ML. Anaphylactic reaction to alcuronium. Case report. Br J Anaesth 1972;44(1):103–5.

36. Rowley RW. Hypersensitivity reaction to diallyl nortoxiferine (Alloferine). Anaesth Intensive Care 1975;3:74.

37. Fisher MM, Hallowes RC, Wilson RM. Anaphylaxis to alcuronium. Anaesth Intensive Care 1978;6(2):125–8.

38. Pandit SK, Dundee JW, Stevenson HM. A clinical comparison of pancuronium with tubocurarine and alcuronium in major cardiothoracic surgery. Anesth Analg 1971;50(6):926–35.

39. Fisher MM, Munro I. Life-threatening anaphylactoid reactions to muscle relaxants. Anesth Analg 1983;62(6):559–64.

40. Galletly DC, Treuren BC. Anaphylactoid reactions during anaesthesia. Seven years' experience of intradermal testing. Anaesthesia 1985;40(4):329–33.

41. Panning B, Peest D, Kirchner E, Schedel I. Anaphylaktoider Schock nach Alloferin. [Anaphylactoid shock following Alloferin.] Anaesthesist 1985;34(4):211–2.

42. Fadel R, Herpin-Richard N, Rassemont R, Salomon J, David B, Laurent M, Henocq E. Choc anaphylactique à la diallylnortoxiferine: étude clinique et immunologique. [Anaphylactic shock from diallylnortoxiferine. Clinical and immunological studies.] Ann Fr Anesth Réanim 1982;1(5):531–4.

43. Plotz J, Schreiber W. Vergleichende Untersuchung von Atracurium und Alcuronium zur Intubation älterer Patienten in Halothannarkose. [Comparative study of atracurium and alcuronium for the intubation of older patients in halothane anesthesia.] Anaesthesist 1984;33(11):548–51.

44. Coventry DM, Stone P. Hypersensitivity reactions to alfentanil? Anaesthesia 1988;43(10):887–8.

45. Vela-Casasempere P, Borras-Blasco J, Navarro-Ruiz A. Alfuzosin-associated dermatomyositis. Br J Rheumatol 1998;37(10):1135–6.

46. Schmutz J-L, Barbaud A, Trechot PH. Alfuzosine, inducteur de dermatomyosite. [Alfuzosine-induced dermatomyositis.] Ann Dermatol Venereol 2000;127(4):449.

47. Lupton GP, Odom RB. The allopurinol hypersensitivity syndrome. J Am Acad Dermatol 1979;1(4):365–74.

48. Suzuki Y, Inagi R, Aono T, Yamanishi K, Shiohara T. Human herpesvirus 6 infection as a risk factor for the development of severe drug-induced hypersensitivity syndrome. Arch Dermatol 1998;134(9):1108–12.

49. Choi HK, Merkel PA, Niles JL. ANCA-positive vasculitis associated with allopurinol therapy. Clin Exp Rheumatol 1998;16(6):743–4.

50. Choi HK, Merkel PA, Walker AM, Niles JL. Drug-associated antineutrophil cytoplasmic antibody-positive vasculitis: prevalence among patients with high titers of antimyeloperoxidase antibodies. Arthritis Rheum 2000;43(2):405–13.

51. Tanna SB, Barnes JF, Seth SK. Desensitization to allopurinol in a patient with previous failed desensitization. Ann Pharmacother 1999;33(11):1180–3.

52. Vazquez-Mellado J, Guzman Vazquez S, Cazarin Barrientos J, Gomez Rios V, Burgos-Vargas R. Desensitisation to allopurinol after allopurinol hypersensitivity syndrome with renal involvement in gout. J Clin Rheumatol 2000;6:266–8.

53. Fam AG, Dunne SM, Iazzetta J, Paton TW. Efficacy and safety of desensitization to allopurinol following cutaneous reactions. Arthritis Rheum 2001;44(1):231–8.

54. Meyer FJ, Wencker M, Teschler H, Steveling H, Sennekamp J, Costabel U, Konietzko N. Acute allergic reaction and demonstration of specific IgE antibodies against alpha-1-protease inhibitor. Eur Respir J 1998;12(4):996–7.

55. Sulkova S, Valek A. Aluminium elimination in patients receiving regular dialysis treatment for chronic renal failure. Trace Elem Med 1991;8(Suppl 1):26–30.

56. Winterberg B, Korte R, Lison AE. Clinical impact of aluminium load in kidney transplant recipients. Trace Elem Med 1991;8(Suppl 1):46–8.

57. Sjolander A, Cox JC, Barr IG. ISCOMs: an adjuvant with multiple functions. J Leukoc Biol 1998;64(6):713–23.

58. Peloso PM, Baillie C. Serum sickness-like reaction with bupropion. JAMA 1999;282(19):1817.

59. Tripathi A, Greenberger PA. Bupropion hydrochloride induced serum sickness-like reaction. Ann Allergy Asthma Immunol 1999;83(2):165–6.

60. McCollom RA, Elbe DH, Ritchie AH. Bupropion-induced serum sickness-like reaction. Ann Pharmacother 2000;34(4):471–3.

61. Anonymous. Moduretic—anaphylactic shock. Uppsala: WHO Collaborating Centre for Adverse Drug Reaction Monitoring. Adv React Newslett 1988;(3–4).

62. Yung MW, Rajendra T. Delayed hypersensitivity reaction to topical aminoglycosides in patients undergoing middle ear surgery. Clin Otolaryngol Allied Sci 2002;27(5):365–8.

63. Paniagua MJ, Garcia-Ortega P, Tella R, Gaig P, Richart C. Systemic contact dermatitis to gentamicin. Allergy 2002;57(11):1086–7.

64. Schulze S, Wollina U. Gentamicin-induced anaphylaxis. Allergy 2003;58(1):88–9.

65. Hall FJ. Anaphylaxis after gentamycin. Lancet 1977;2(8035):455.

66. Goh CL. Anaphylaxis from topical neomycin and bacitracin. Australas J Dermatol 1986;27(3):125–6.

67. Bartoli E, Faedda in Masala R, Chiandussi L. Drug-induced asthma. Lancet 1976;1(7973):1357.

68. Choi HK, Merkel PA, Walker AM, Niles JL. Drug-associated antineutrophil cytoplasmic antibody-positive vasculitis: prevalence among patients with high titers of antimyeloperoxidase antibodies. Arthritis Rheum 2000;43(2):405–13.

69. Gunnarsson I, Nordmark B, Hassan Bakri A, Grondal G, Larsson P, Forslid J, Klareskog L, Ringertz B. Development of lupus-related side-effects in patients with early RA during sulphasalazine treatment-the role of IL-10 and HLA. Rheumatology (Oxford) 2000;39(8):886–93.

70. Pay S, Dinc A, Simsek I, Can C, Erdem H. Sulfasalazine-induced angioimmunoblastic lymphadenopathy developing in a patient with juvenile chronic arthritis. Rheumatol Int 2000;20(1):25–7.

71. Nguyen-Khac E, Le Baron F, Thevenot T, Tiry-Lescut C, Tiry F. Oedème de Quincke possiblement imputable à la mesalazine au cours de la maladie de Crohn. [Angioedema in Crohn's disease possibly due to mesalazine.] Gastroenterol Clin Biol 2002;26(5):535–6.

72. Pent MT, Ganapathy S, Holdsworth CD, Channer KC. Mesalazine induced lupus-like syndrome. BMJ 1992;305(6846):159.

73. Susano R, Caminal L, Ramos D, Diaz B. Amiodarone induced lupus. Ann Rheum Dis 1999;58(10):655–6.

74. Sheikhzadeh A, Schafer U, Schnabel A. Drug-induced lupus erythematosus by amiodarone. Arch Intern Med 2002;162(7):834–6.

75. Burches E, Garcia-Verdegay F, Ferrer M, Pelaez A. Amiodarone-induced angioedema. Allergy 2000;55(12):1199–200.

76. Aeschlimann A, de Truchis P, Kahn MF. Scleroderma after therapy with appetite suppressants. Scand J Rheumatol 1990;19(1):87–90.

77. Griswold MW, Briceland LL, Stein DS. Is amphotericin B test dosing needed? Ann Pharmacother 1998;32(4):475–7.

78. Groll AH, Piscitelli SC, Walsh TJ. Clinical pharmacology of systemic antifungal agents: a comprehensive review of agents in clinical use, current investigational compounds, and putative targets for antifungal drug development. Adv Pharmacol 1998;44:343–500.

79. Kauffman CA, Wiseman SW. Anaphylaxis upon switching lipid-containing amphotericin B formulations. Clin Infect Dis 1998;26(5):1237–8.

80. Johnson JR, Kangas PJ, West M. Serious adverse event after unrecognized substitution of one amphotericin B lipid preparation for another. Clin Infect Dis 1998;27(5):1342–3.

81. Sadeghi N, Panje WR. Life-threatening perioperative angioedema related to angiotensin-converting enzyme inhibitor therapy. J Otolaryngol 1999;28(6):354–6.

82. Maestre ML, Litvan H, Galan F, Puzo C, Villar Landeira JM. Imposibilidad de intubacion por angioedema secundario a IECA. [Impossibility of intubation due to angioedema secondary to an angiotensin-converting enzyme inhibitor.] Rev Esp Anestesiol Reanim 1999;46(2):88–91.

83. Hedner T, Samuelsson O, Lunde H, Lindholm L, Andren L, Wiholm BE. Angio-oedema in relation to treatment with angiotensin converting enzyme inhibitors. BMJ 1992;304(6832):941–6.

84. Martin DJ, Grigg RG, Tomkinson A, Coman WB. Subglottic stenosis: an unusual presentation of ACE inhibitor-induced angioedema. Aust NZ J Surg 1999;69(4):320–321.

85. Jacobs RL, Hoberman LJ, Goldstein HM. Angioedema of the small bowel caused by an angiotensin-converting enzyme inhibitor. Am J Gastroenterol 1994;89(1):127–8.

86. Dupasquier E. Une forme clinique rare d'oedème angio-neurotique sous énalapril: l'abdomen aigu. [A rare clinical form of angioneurotic edema caused by enalapril: acute abdomen.] Arch Mal Coeur Vaiss 1994;87(10):1371–4.

87. Byrne TJ, Douglas DD, Landis ME, Heppell JP. Isolated visceral angioedema: an underdiagnosed complication of ACE inhibitors? Mayo Clin Proc 2000;75(11):1201–4.

88. Chase MP, Fiarman GS, Scholz FJ, MacDermott RP. Angioedema of the small bowel due to an angiotensin-converting enzyme inhibitor. J Clin Gastroenterol 2000;31(3):254–7.

89. Blomberg PJ, Surks HK, Long A, Rebeiz E, Mochizuki Y, Pandian N. Transient myocardial dysfunction associated with angiotensin-converting enzyme inhibitor-induced angioedema: recognition by serial echocardiographic studies. J Am Soc Echocardiogr 1999;12(12):1107–9.

90. Kyrmizakis DE, Papadakis CE, Fountoulakis EJ, Liolios AD, Skoulas JG. Tongue angioedema after long-term use of ACE inhibitors. Am J Otolaryngol 1998;19(6):394–6.

91. Lapostolle F, Borron SW, Bekka R, Baud FJ. Lingual angioedema after perindopril use. Am J Cardiol 1998;81(4):523.

92. Henson EB, Bess DT, Abraham L, Bracikowski JP. Penile angioedema possibly related to lisinopril. Am J Health Syst Pharm 1999;56(17):1773–4.

93. Ratliff NB 3rd, Pieranna F, Manganelli P. Captopril induced lupus. J Rheumatol 2002;29(8):1807–8.

94. Reidenberg MM, Case DB, Drayer DE, Reis S, Lorenzo B. Development of antinuclear antibody in patients treated with high doses of captopril. Arthritis Rheum 1984;27(5):579–81.

95. Acker CG, Greenberg A. Angioedema induced by the angiotensin II blocker losartan. N Engl J Med 1995;333(23):1572.

96. Hansson L. Medical and cost-economy aspects of modern antihypertensive therapy—with special reference to 2 years of clinical experience with losartan. Blood Press Suppl 1997;1:52–5.

97. Barak N, Hart J, Sitrin MD. Enalapril-induced eosinophilic gastroenteritis. J Clin Gastroenterol 2001;33(2):157–8.

98. Cha YJ, Pearson VE. Angioedema due to losartan. Ann Pharmacother 1999;33(9):936–8.

99. Rivera JO. Losartan-induced angioedema. Ann Pharmacother 1999;33(9):933–5.

100. Havener WH. Ocular Pharmacology. 4th ed. St Louis: CV Mosby, 1978.

101. Schein RM, Kinasewitz GT. Risk-benefit analysis for drotrecogin alfa (activated). Am J Surg 2002;184(Suppl 6A):S25–38.

102. Olsen KM, Martin SJ. Pharmacokinetics and clinical use of drotrecogin alfa (activated) in patients with severe sepsis. Pharmacotherapy 2002;22(12 Pt 2):S196–205.

103. Tomson T, Kenneback G. Arrhythmia, heart rate variability, and antiepileptic drugs. Epilepsia 1997;38(Suppl 11):S48–51.

104. Schlienger RG, Shear NH. Antiepileptic drug hypersensitivity syndrome. Epilepsia 1998;39(Suppl 7):S3–7.

105. Griebel ML. Acute management of hypersensitivity reactions and seizures. Epilepsia 1998;39(Suppl 7):S17–21.

106. Ciernik IF, Thiel M, Widmer U. Anterior uveitis and the anticonvulsant hypersensitivity syndrome. Arch Intern Med 1998;158(2):192.

107. Kim HA, Heo Y, Oh SY, Lee KJ, Lawrence DA. Altered serum cytokine and immunoglobulin levels in the workers exposed to antimony. Hum Exp Toxicol 1999;18(10):607–13.

108. Hoigne R. Allergische Erkrankungen. In: Stucki P, Hess T, editors. Hadorn, Lehrbuch der Therapie. 7th ed. Berne-Stuttgart-Vienna: Verlag Hans Huber, 1983:155.

109. Cicek S, Demirkilic U, Ozal E, Kuralay E, Bingol H, Tatar H, Ozturk OY. Postoperative use of aprotinin in cardiac operations: an alternative to its prophylactic use. J Thorac Cardiovasc Surg 1996;112(6):1462–7.

110. Kon NF, Masumo H, Nakajima S, Tozawa R, Kimura M, Maeda S. [Anaphylactic reaction to aprotinin following topical use of biological tissue sealant.] Masui 1994;43(10):1606–10.

111. Dietrich W, Spath P, Ebell A, Richter JA. Prevalence of anaphylactic reactions to aprotinin: analysis of two hundred forty-eight reexposures to aprotinin in heart operations. J Thorac Cardiovasc Surg 1997;113(1):194–201.

112. Cohen DM, Norberto J, Cartabuke R, Ryu G. Severe anaphylactic reaction after primary exposure to aprotinin. Ann Thorac Surg 1999;67(3):837–8.

113. Dietrich W. Incidence of hypersensitivity reactions. Ann Thorac Surg 1998;65(Suppl 6):S60–4.

114. Japanese Ministry of Health and Welfare. Information on adverse reaction to drugs. Japan Med Gaz 1980;10April 20.

115. Proud G, Chamberlain J. Anaphylactic reaction to aprotinin. Lancet 1976;2(7975):48–9.

116. Robert S, Wagner BK, Boulanger M, Richer M. Aprotinin. Ann Pharmacother 1996;30(4):372–80.

117. Siegel M, Werner M. Allergische Pankreatitis bei einer Sensibilisierung gegen den Kallikrein-Trypsin-Inaktivator. [Allergic pancreatitis caused by sensitization to the kallikrein–trypsin inactivator.] Dtsch Med Wochenschr 1965;90(39):1712–6.

118. Wuthrich B, Schmid P, Schmid ER, Tornic M, Johansson SG. IgE-mediated anaphylactic reaction to aprotinin during anaesthesia. Lancet 1992;340(8812):173–4.

119. Scheule AM, Beierlein W, Arnold S, Eckstein FS, Albes JM, Ziemer G. The significance of preformed aprotinin-specific antibodies in cardiosurgical patients. Anesth Analg 2000;90(2):262–6.

120. Scheule AM, Beierlein W, Wendel HP, Jurmann MJ, Eckstein FS, Ziemer G. Aprotinin in fibrin tissue adhesives induces specific antibody response and increases antibody response of high-dose intravenous application. J Thorac Cardiovasc Surg 1999;118(2):348–53.

121. Faught C, Wells P, Fergusson D, Laupacis A. Adverse effects of methods for minimizing perioperative allogeneic transfusion: a critical review of the literature. Transfus Med Rev 1998;12(3):206–25.

122. Golker CF, Whiteman MD, Gugel KH, Gilles R, Stadler P, Kovatch RM, Lister D, Wisher MH, Calcagni C, Hubner GE. Reduction of the infectivity of scrapie agent as a model for BSE in the manufacturing process of Trasylol. Biologicals 1996;24(2):103–11.

123. Manzanedo L, Blanco J, Fuentes M, Caballero ML, Moneo I. Anaphylactic reaction in a patient sensitized to coriander seed. Allergy 2004;59(3):362–3.

124. Kulczycki A Jr. Aspartame-induced urticaria. Ann Intern Med 1986;104(2):207–8.

125. Geha R, Buckley CE, Greenberger P, Patterson R, Polmar S, Saxon A, Rohr A, Yang W, Drouin M. Aspartame is no more likely than placebo to cause urticaria/angioedema: results of a multicenter, randomized, double-blind, placebo-controlled, crossover study. J Allergy Clin Immunol 1993;92(4):513–20.

126. Novick NL. Aspartame-induced granulomatous panniculitis. Ann Intern Med 1985;102(2):206–7.

127. McCauliffe DP, Poitras K. Aspartame-induced lobular panniculitis. J Am Acad Dermatol 1991;24(2 Pt 1):298–300.

128. Thumm EJ, Jung EG, Bayerl C. Anaphylaktische Reaktion nach Scratchtestung mit Ascorbinsäure (E 300) und Zitronensäure (E 330). Allergologie 2000;23:354–9.

129. Anonymous. Wie verträglich sind Echinacea-haltige Präparate? Dtsch Arzteblatt 1996;93:2723.

130. Mullins RJ, Heddle R. Adverse reactions associated with echinacea: the Australian experience. Ann Allergy Asthma Immunol 2002;88(1):42–51.

131. Mullins RJ. Echinacea-associated anaphylaxis. Med J Aust 1998;168(4):170–1.

132. Myers SP, Wohlmuth H. Echinacea-associated anaphylaxis. Med J Aust 1998;168(11):583–4.

133. Logan JL, Ahmed J. Critical hypokalemic renal tubular acidosis due to Sjögren's syndrome: association with the purported immune stimulant Echinacea. Clin Rheumatol 2003;22(2):158–9.

134. Geier J, Fuchs T, Wahl R. Anaphylaktischer Schock durch einen Mariendistel-Extrakt bei Soforttyp-Allergie auf Kiwi. Allergologie 1990;13:387–8.

135. Geier J, Fuchs T, Wahl R. Anaphylaktischer Schock durch einen Mariendistel-Extrakt bei Soforttyp-Allergie auf Kiwi. Allergologie 1990;13:387–8.

136. Srivastava S. Angioneurotic oedema following atracurium. Br J Anaesth 1984;56(8):932–3.

137. Siler JN, Mager JG Jr, Wyche MQ Jr. Atracurium: hypotension, tachycardia and bronchospasm. Anesthesiology 1985;62(5):645–6.

138. Sale JP. Bronchospasm following the use of atracurium. Anaesthesia 1983;38(5):511–2.

139. Beemer GH, Dennis WL, Platt PR, Bjorksten AR, Carr AB. Adverse reactions to atracurium and alcuronium. A prospective surveillance study. Br J Anaesth 1988;61(6):680–4.

140. Aldrete JA. Allergic reaction after atracurium. Br J Anaesth 1985;57(9):929–30.

141. Gutgesell C, Fuchs T. Azapropazone in aspirin intolerance. Allergy 1999;54(8):897–8.

142. Milkovic-Kraus S, Kanceljak-Macan B. Occupational airborne allergic contact dermatitis from azithromycin. Contact Dermatitis 2001;45(3):184.

143. Cascaval RI, Lancaster DJ. Hypersensitivity syndrome associated with azithromycin. Am J Med 2001;110(4):330–1.

144. Hubner C, Dietz A, Stremmel W, Stiehl A, Andrassy H. Macrolide-induced Churg–Strauss syndrome in a patient with atopy. Lancet 1997;350(9077):563.

145. Lotte A, Wasz-Hockert O, Poisson N, Dumitrescu N, Verron M, Couvet E. BCG complications. Estimates of the risks among vaccinated subjects and statistical analysis of their main characteristics. Adv Tuberc Res 1984;21:107–93.

146. Lotte A, Wasz-Hockert O, Poisson N, Dumitrescu N, Verron M, Couvet E. A bibliography of the complications of BCG vaccination. A comprehensive list of the world literature since the introduction of BCG up to July 1982, supplemented by over 100 personal communications. Adv Tuberc Res 1984;21:194–245.

147. Lotte A, Wasz-Hockert O, Poisson N, Engbaek H, Landmann H, Quast U, Andrasofszky B, Lugosi L, Vadasz I, Mihailescu P, et al. Second IUATLD study on complications induced by intradermal BCG-vaccination. Bull Int Union Tuberc Lung Dis 1988;63(2):47–59.

148. Proctor JW, Zidar B, Pomerantz M, Yamamura Y, Eng CP, Woodside D. Anaphylactic reaction to intralesional B.C.G Lancet 1978;2(8081):162.

149. Tshabalala RT. Anaphylactic reactions to BCG in Swaziland. Lancet 1983;1(8325):653.

150. Maouad M, Fleischer AB Jr, Sherertz EF, Feldman SR. Significance–prevalence index number: a reinterpretation and enhancement of data from the North American contact dermatitis group. J Am Acad Dermatol 1999;41(4):573–6.

151. Lin FL, Woodmansee D, Patterson R. Near-fatal anaphylaxis to topical bacitracin ointment. J Allergy Clin Immunol 1998;101(1 Pt 1):136–7.

152. Saryan JA, Dammin TC, Bouras AE. Anaphylaxis to topical bacitracin zinc ointment. Am J Emerg Med 1998;16(5):512–3.

153. Gall R, Blakley B, Warrington R, Bell DD. Intraoperative anaphylactic shock from bacitracin nasal packing after septorhinoplasty. Anesthesiology 1999;91(5):1545–7.

154. Blas M, Briesacher KS, Lobato EB. Bacitracin irrigation: a cause of anaphylaxis in the operating room. Anesth Analg 2000;91(4):1027–8.

155. Carver ED, Braude BM, Atkinson AR, Gold M. Anaphylaxis during insertion of a ventriculoperitoneal shunt. Anesthesiology 2000;93(2):578–9.

156. Suneja T, Belsito DV. Thimerosal in the detection of clinically relevant allergic contact reactions. J Am Acad Dermatol 2001;45(1):23–7.

157. Stringer DA, Hassall E, Ferguson AC, Cairns R, Nadel H, Sargent M. Hypersensitivity reaction to single contrast barium meal studies in children. Pediatr Radiol 1993;23(8):587–8.

158. Ownby DR, Tomlanovich M, Sammons N, McCullough J. Anaphylaxis associated with latex allergy during barium enema examinations. Am J Roentgenol 1991;156(5):903–8.

159. Anonymous. Literature review: Allergic reactions to barium procedures and latex rubber. London: E-Z-EM Ltd.

160. Le Frock J, Ellis CA, Klainer AS, Weinstein L. Transient bacteremia associated with barium enema. Arch Intern Med 1975;135(6):835–7.

161. Hammer JL. Septicemia following barium enema. South Med J 1977;70(11):1361–3.

162. Weston A, Assem ES. Possible link between anaphylactoid reactions to anaesthetics and chemicals in cosmetics and biocides. Agents Actions 1994;41(Spec No):C138–9.

163. Meyer U, Gerhard I, Runnebaum B. Benzalkonium-chlorid zur vaginaten Kontrazeption—der Scheidenschwamm. [Benzalkonium chloride for vaginal contraception—the vaginal sponge.] Geburtshilfe Frauenheilkd 1990;50(7):542–7.

164. Sidhu SK, Shaw S, Wilkinson JD. A 10-year retrospective study on benzocaine allergy in the United Kingdom. Am J Contact Dermat 1999;10(2):57–61.

165. Roos TC, Merk HF. Allergic contact dermatitis from benzocaine ointment during treatment of *Herpes zoster*. Contact Dermatitis 2001;44(2):104.

166. de Groot AC, Conemans J, Liem DH. Contact allergy to benzoxonium chloride (Bradophen). Contact Dermatitis 1984;11(5):324–5.

167. Bruynzeel DP, de Groot AC, Weyland JW. Contact dermatitis to lauryl pyridinium chloride and benzoxonium chloride. Contact Dermatitis 1987;17(1):41–2.

168. Diaz-Ramon L, Aguirre A, Raton-Nieto JA, de Miguel M. Contact dermatitis from benzoxonium chloride. Contact Dermatitis 1999;41(1):53–4.

169. Grant JA, Bilodeau PA, Guernsey BG, Gardner FH. Unsuspected benzyl alcohol hypersensitivity. N Engl J Med 1982;306(2):108.

170. Wilson JP, Solimando DA Jr, Edwards MS. Parenteral benzyl alcohol-induced hypersensitivity reaction. Drug Intell Clin Pharm 1986;20(9):689–91.

171. Mansfield LE, Nelson HS. Effect of beta-adrenergic agents on immunoglobulin G levels of asthmatic subjects. Int Arch Allergy Appl Immunol 1982;68(1):13–6.

172. Lai CK, Twentyman OP, Holgate ST. The effect of an increase in inhaled allergen dose after rimiterol hydrobromide on the occurrence and magnitude of the late asthmatic response and the associated change in nonspecific bronchial responsiveness. Am Rev Respir Dis 1989;140(4):917–23.

173. Larsson K, Martinsson A, Hjemdahl P. Influence of beta-adrenergic receptor function during terbutaline treatment on allergen sensitivity and bronchodilator response to terbutaline in asthmatic subjects. Chest 1992;101(4):953–60.

174. Cockcroft DW, O'Byrne PM, Swystun VA, Bhagat R. Regular use of inhaled albuterol and the allergen-induced late asthmatic response. J Allergy Clin Immunol 1995;96(1):44–9.

175. Bhagat R, Swystun VA, Cockcroft DW. Salbutamol-induced increased airway responsiveness to allergen and reduced protection versus methacholine: dose response. J Allergy Clin Immunol 1996;97(1 Pt 1):47–52.

176. Cockcroft DW, McParland CP, Britto SA, Swystun VA, Rutherford BC. Regular inhaled salbutamol and airway responsiveness to allergen. Lancet 1993;342(8875):833–7.

177. Cockcroft DW. Inhaled beta2-agonists and airway responses to allergen. J Allergy Clin Immunol 1998;102(5):S96–9.

178. Rustmann WC, Carpenter MT, Harmon C, Botti CF. Leukocytoclastic vasculitis associated with sotalol therapy. J Am Acad Dermatol 1998;38(1):111–2.

179. Booth RJ, Bullock JY, Wilson JD. Antinuclear antibodies in patients on acebutolol. Br J Clin Pharmacol 1980;9(5):515–7.

180. Cody RJ Jr, Calabrese LH, Clough JD, Tarazi RC, Bravo EL. Development of antinuclear antibodies during acebutolol therapy. Clin Pharmacol Ther 1979;25(6):800–5.

181. Huggins MM, Menzies CW, Quail D, Rumfitt IW. An open multicenter study of the effect of celiprolol on serum lipids and antinuclear antibodies in patient with mild to moderate hypertension. J Drug Dev 1991;4:125–33.

182. Bigot MC, Trenque T, Moulin M, Beguin J, Loyau G. Acebutolol-induced lupus syndrome. Therapie 1984;39:571–5.

183. Hourdebaigt-Larrusse P, Grivaux M. Une nouvelle obscuration de lupus induit par un béta-bloquant. Sem Hop 1984;60:1515.

184. Griffiths ID, Richardson J. Lupus-type illness associated with labetalol. BMJ 1979;2(6188):496–7.

185. Clerens A, Guilmot-Bruneau MM, Defresne C, Bourlond A. Beta-blocking agents: side effects. Biomedicine 1979;31(8):219.

186. Harrison T, Sisca TS, Wood WH. Case report. Propranolol-induced lupus syndrome? Postgrad Med 1976;59(1):241–4.

187. Holzbach E. Ein Beta-blocker als Zusatztherapie beim Delirium tremens. [Beta-Blockers as adjuvant therapy in delirium tremens.] MMW Munch Med Wochenschr 1980;122(22):837–40.

188. Jacobs RL, Rake GW Jr, Fournier DC, Chilton RJ, Culver WG, Beckmann CH. Potentiated anaphylaxis in patients with drug-induced beta-adrenergic blockade. J Allergy Clin Immunol 1981;68(2):125–7.

189. Hannaway PJ, Hopper GD. Severe anaphylaxis and drug-induced beta-blockade. N Engl J Med 1983;308(25):1536.

190. Cornaille G, Leynadier F, Modiano, Dry J. Gravité du choc anaphylactic chez les malades traités par béta-bloqueurs. [Severity of anaphylactic shock in patients treated with beta-blockers.] Presse Med 1985;14(14):790–1.

191. Raebel MA. Potentiated anaphylaxis during chronic beta-blocker therapy. DICP Ann Pharmacother 1988;22:720.

192. Toogood JH. Beta-blocker therapy and the risk of anaphylaxis. CMAJ 1987;136(9):929–33.

193. Arkinstall WW, Toogood JH. Beta-blocker therapy and the risk of anaphylaxis. CMAJ 1987;137(5):370–1.

194. Kanto JH. Current status of labetalol, the first alpha- and beta-blocking agent. Int J Clin Pharmacol Ther Toxicol 1985;23(11):617–28.

195. Aellig WH, Clark BJ. Is the ISA of pindolol beta 2-adrenoceptor selective? Br J Clin Pharmacol 1987;24(Suppl 1):S21–8.

196. Gauthier-Rahman S, Akoun GM, Milleron BJ, Mayaud CM. Leukocyte migration inhibition in propranolol-induced pneumonitis. Evidence for an immunologic cell-mediated mechanism. Chest 1990;97(1):238–41.

197. Gell PGH, Coombs RRA. Classification of allergic reactions responsible for clinical hypersensitivity and disease. In: Gell PGH, Coombs RRA, Lachmann PJ, editors. Clinical Aspects of Immunology. Oxford: Blackwell Scientific Publications, 1975:251–4.

198. Plaut M, Zimmerman EM. Allergy and mechanisms of hypersensitivity. In: Paul WE, editor. Fundamental Immunology. 3rd ed. New York: Raven Press, 1993:1399.

199. De Weck AL. Pharmacologic and immunochemical mechanisms of drug hypersensitivity. Immunol Allergy Clin North Am 1991;11:461.

200. Lafaye P, Lapresle C. Fixation of penicilloyl groups to albumin and appearance of anti-penicilloyl antibodies in penicillin-treated patients. J Clin Invest 1988;82(1):7–12.

201. Bochner BS, Lichtenstein LM. Anaphylaxis. N Engl J Med 1991;324(25):1785–90.

202. Edwards RG, Dewdney JM, Dobrzanski RJ, Lee D. Immunogenicity and allergenicity studies on two beta-lactam structures, a clavam, clavulanic acid, and a carbapenem: structure-activity relationships. Int Arch Allergy Appl Immunol 1988;85(2):184–9.

203. Fernandez-Rivas M, Perez Carral C, Cuevas M, Marti C, Moral A, Senent CJ. Selective allergic reactions to clavulanic acid. J Allergy Clin Immunol 1995;95(3):748–50.

204. Wilson SE, Nord CE. Clinical trials of extended spectrum penicillin/beta-lactamase inhibitors in the treatment of intra-abdominal infections. European and North American experience. Am J Surg 1995;169(Suppl 5A):S21–6.

205. Klapholz L, Leitersdorf E, Weinrauch L. Leucocytoclastic vasculitis and pneumonitis induced by metformin. BMJ (Clin Res Ed) 1986;293(6545):483.

206. Dore P, Perault MC, Recart D, Dejean C, Meurice JC, Fougere MC, Vandel B, Patte F. Pneumopathie medicamenteuse a la metformine? [Pulmonary diseases induced by metformin?] Therapie 1994;49(5):472–3.

207. Wictorin A, Hansson C. Allergic contact dermatitis from a bismuth compound in an eye ointment. Contact Dermatitis 2001;45(5):318.

208. More D, Whisman B, Johns J, Hagan L. Anaphylaxis to Pepto-Bismol. Allergy 2002;57(6):558.

209. Rivera R, Scornik JC. HLA antigens on red cells. Implications for achieving low HLA antigen content in blood transfusions. Transfusion 1986;26(4):375–81.

210. Strauss RG. Apheresis donor safety—changes in humoral and cellular immunity. J Clin Apher 1984;2(1):68–80.

211. Lewis SL, Kutvirt SG, Simon TL. Investigation of the effect of long-term whole blood donation on immunologic parameters. Transfusion 1992;32(1):51–6.

212. Matsui Y, Martin-Alosco S, Doenges E, Christenson L, Shapiro HM, Yunis EJ, Page PL. Effects of frequent and sustained plateletapheresis on peripheral blood mononuclear cell populations and lymphocyte functions of normal volunteer donors. Transfusion 1986;26(5):446–52.

213. Dolovich J, Sagona M, Pearson F, Buccholz D, Hiner E, Marshall C. Sensitization of repeat plasmapheresis donors to ethylene oxide gas. Transfusion 1987;27(1):90–3.

214. Merola B, Sarnacchiaro F, Colao A, Di Sarno A, Di Somma C, Schettini G, Lombardi G. Allergy to ergot-derived dopamine agonists. Lancet 1992;339(8793):620.

215. Scala E, Guerra EC, Pirrotta L, Giani M, De Pita O, Puddu P. Anaphylactic reactions to buflomedil. Allergy 1999;54(3):288–9.

216. Peduto VA, Di Martino M, Tani R, Toscano A, Napoleone M. Reazione anafilattoide da bupreuorfina: descrizione di un caso. [Anaphylactoid reaction to buprenorphine: a case report.] Anaesthesiol Reanim 1988;38:241.

217. Nomura S, Hashimoto J, Osawa G. Can C1 esterase inhibitor concentrate be a cause of the exacerbation of hereditary angioneurotic oedema? Vox Sang 1995;69(1):85.

218. Cicardi M, Mannucci PM, Castelli R, Rumi MG, Agostoni A. Reduction in transmission of hepatitis C after the introduction of a heat-treatment step in the production of C1-inhibitor concentrate. Transfusion 1995;35(3):209–12.

219. Frosch PJ, Rustemeyer T. Contact allergy to calcipotriol does exist. Report of an unequivocal case and review of the literature. Contact Dermatitis 1999;40(2):66–71.

220. Porcel SL, Cumplido JA, de la Hoz B, Cuevas M, Losada E. Anaphylaxis to calcitonin. Allergol Immunopathol (Madr) 2000;28(4):243–5.

221. Rodriguez A, Trujillo MJ, Herrero T, Baeza ML, de Barrio M. Allergy to calcitonin. Allergy 2001;56(8):801.

222. Carraway RD. Febrile reaction following nifedipine therapy. Am Heart J 1984;108(3 Pt 1):611.

223. Scolnick B, Brinberg D. Diltiazem and generalized lymphadenopathy. Ann Intern Med 1985;102(4):558.

224. Pedro-Botet J, Minguez S, Supervia A. Sublingual nifedipine-induced anaphylaxis. Arch Intern Med 1998;158(12):1379.

225. Klein TW, Newton C, Friedman H. Inhibition of natural killer cell function by marijuana components. J Toxicol Environ Health 1987;20(4):321–32.

226. Pillai R, Nair BS, Watson RR. AIDS, drugs of abuse and the immune system: a complex immunotoxicological network. Arch Toxicol 1991;65(8):609–17.

227. Levitz SM, Diamond RD. Aspergillosis and marijuana. Ann Intern Med 1991;115(7):578–9.

228. Klein TW, Friedman H, Specter S. Marijuana, immunity and infection. J Neuroimmunol 1998;83(1–2):102–15.

229. Perez JA Jr. Allergic reaction associated with intravenous marijuana use. J Emerg Med 2000;18(2):260–1.

230. Igarashi M, Bando Y, Shimanuki K, Hosoda N, Sunaoshi W, Shirai H, Miura H. Immunosuppressive factors detected during convalescence in a patient with severe serum sickness induced by carbamazepine. Int Arch Allergy Immunol 1993;100(4):378–81.

231. Nathan DL, Belsito DV. Carbamazepine-induced pseudolymphoma with CD-30 positive cells. J Am Acad Dermatol 1998;38(5 Pt 2):806–9.

232. Ganga A, Corda D, Gallo Carrabba G, Cossu S, Massarelli G, Rosati G. A case of carbamazepine-induced lymphadenopathy resembling Kikuchi disease. Eur Neurol 1998;39(4):247–8.

233. Lhotta K, Konig P. Cryoglobulinaemia, membranoproliferative glomerulonephritis and pANCA in a patient treated with carbamazepine. Nephrol Dial Transplant 1998;13(7):1890–1.

234. Elstner S, Sperling W. Das Carbamazepin-Hypersensitivitäts-Syndrome. Differentialdiagnostische Erwagungen an einer exemplarischen Fallvorstellungo. [The carbamazepine hypersensitivity syndrome. Differential diagnosis and a representative case history.] Fortschr Neurol Psychiatr 2000;68(4):188–92.

235. Koga T, Kubota Y, Nakayama J. Interferon-gamma production in the peripheral lymphocytes of a patient with carbamazepine hypersensitivity syndrome. Acta Dermatol Venereol 2000;80(1):73.

236. Verma SP, Yunis N, Lekos A, Crausman RS. Carbamazepine-induced systemic lupus erythematosus presenting as cardiac tamponade. Chest 2000;117(2):597–8.

237. Verrotti A, Feliciani C, Morresi S, Coscione G, Morgese G, Toto P, Chiarelli F. Carbamazepine-induced hypersensitivity syndrome in a child with epilepsy. Int J Immunopathol Pharmacol 2000;13(1):49–53.

238. Saxon A, Adelman DC, Patel A, Hajdu R, Calandra GB. Imipenem cross-reactivity with penicillin in humans. J Allergy Clin Immunol 1988;82(2):213–7.

239. Hantson P, de Coninck B, Horn JL, Mahieu P. Immediate hypersensitivity to aztreonam and imipenem. BMJ 1991;302(6771):294–5.

240. Gerhards LJ, van Arnhem AC, Holman ND, Nossent GD. Fatale anafylactische reactie na inname van acetazolamide (Diamox) wegens glaucoom. [Fatal anaphylactic reaction after oral acetazolamide (Diamox) for glaucoma.] Ned Tijdschr Geneeskd 2000;144(25):1228–30.

241. Gallerani M, Manzoli N, Fellin R, Simonato M, Orzincolo C. Anaphylactic shock and acute pulmonary edema after a single oral dose of acetazolamide. Am J Emerg Med 2002;20(4):371–2.

242. Guo JL, Yuan SX, Wang XC, Xu SX, Li DD. *Tripterygium wilfordii* Hook F in rheumatoid arthritis and ankylosing spondylitis. Preliminary report. Chin Med J (Engl) 1981;94(7):405–12.

243. Pedersen-Bjergaard J. Cephalotin in the treatment of penicillin-sensitive patients. Acta Allergol 1967;22:299.

244. Petz LD. Immunologic reactions of humans to cephalosporins. Postgrad Med J 1971;47(Suppl):64–9.

245. Solley GO, Gleich GJ, Van Dellen RG. Penicillin allergy: clinical experience with a battery of skin-test reagents. J Allergy Clin Immunol 1982;69(2):238–44.

246. Van Arsdel PP Jr, Miller S. Antimicrobial treatment of patients with a penicillin allergy history. J Allergy Clin Immunol 1990;85:188.

247. Surtees SJ, Stockton MG, Gietzen TW. Allergy to penicillin: fable or fact? BMJ 1991;302(6784):1051–2.

248. Saxon A, Beall GN, Rohr AS, Adelman DC. Immediate hypersensitivity reactions to beta-lactam antibiotics. Ann Intern Med 1987;107(2):204–15.

249. Abraham GN, Petz LD, Fudenberg HH. Cephalothin hypersensitivity associated with anti-cephalothin antibodies. Int Arch Allergy Appl Immunol 1968;34(1):65–74.

250. Ong R, Sullivan T. Detection and characterization of human IgE to cephalosporin determinants. J Allergy Clin Immunol 1988;81:222.

251. Nishioka K, Katayama I, Kobayashi Y, Takijiri C. Anaphylaxis due to cefaclor hypersensitivity. J Dermatol 1986;13(3):226–7.

252. Hama R, Mori K. High incidence of anaphylactic reactions to cefaclor. Lancet 1988;1(8598):1331.

253. Levine LR. Quantitative comparison of adverse reactions to cefaclor vs. amoxicillin in a surveillance study. Pediatr Infect Dis 1985;4(4):358–61.

254. Bloomberg RJ. Cefotetan-induced anaphylaxis. Am J Obstet Gynecol 1988;159(1):125–6.

255. Hashimoto Y, Soeda A, Takarada M, Tanioka H. Anaphylaxis to moxalactam: report of a case. J Oral Maxillofac Surg 1990;48(9):1004–6.

256. Blanca M, Fernandez J, Miranda A, Terrados S, Torres MJ, Vega JM, Avila MJ, Perez E, Garcia JJ, Suau R. Cross-reactivity between penicillins and cephalosporins: clinical and immunologic studies. J Allergy Clin Immunol 1989;83(2 Pt 1):381–5.

257. Anderson JA. Cross-sensitivity to cephalosporins in patients allergic to penicillin. Pediatr Infect Dis 1986;5(5):557–61.

258. Saxon A, Beall GN, Rohr AS, et al. Immediate hypersensitivity reactions to beta-lactam antibiotics. Urology 1988;31(Suppl):14.

259. Saxon A. Antibiotic choices for the penicillin-allergic patient. Postgrad Med 1988;83(4):135–8141–2, 147–8.

260. Ernst MR, van Dijken PJ, Kabel PJ, Draaisma JM. Anaphylaxis after first exposure to ceftriaxone. Acta Paediatr 2002;91(3):355–6.

261. Romano A, Piunti E, Di Fonso M, Viola M, Venuti A, Venemalm L. Selective immediate hypersensitivity to ceftriaxone. Allergy 2000;55(4):415–6.

262. Berrocal AM, Schuman JS. Subconjunctival cephalosporin anaphylaxis. Ophthalmic Surg Lasers 2001;32(1):79–80.

263. Yamada A, Ohshima Y, Tsukahara H, Hiraoka M, Kimura I, Kawamitsu T, Kimura K, Mayumi M. Two cases of anaphylactic reaction to gelatin induced by a chloral hydrate suppository. Pediatr Int 2002;44(1):87–9.

264. Palchick BA, Funk EA, McEntire JE, Hamory BH. Anaphylaxis due to chloramphenicol. Am J Med Sci 1984;288(1):43–5.

265. Liphshitz I, Loewenstein A. Anaphylactic reaction following application of chloramphenicol eye ointment. Br J Ophthalmol 1991;75(1):64.

266. Evans P, Foxell RM. Chlorhexidine as a cause of anaphylaxis. Int J Obstet Anaesth 2002;11:145–6.

267. Pham NH, Weiner JM, Reisner GS, Baldo BA. Anaphylaxis to chlorhexidine. Case report. Implication of immunoglobulin E antibodies and identification of an allergenic determinant. Clin Exp Allergy 2000;30(7):1001–7.

268. Meier H, Elsner P, Wuthrich B. Berufsbedingtes kontaktekzem und Asthma bronchiale bei ungewohnlicher allergischer Reaktion vona Spattyp auf Hydroxychloroquin. [Occupationally-induced contact dermatitis and bronchial asthma in a unusual delayed reaction to hydroxychloroquine.] Hautarzt 1999;50(9):665–9.

269. Storrs FJ. Para-chloro-meta-xylenol allergic contact dermatitis in seven individuals. Contact Dermatitis 1975;1(4):211–213.

270. Myatt AE, Beck MH. Contact sensitivity to parachlorometaxylenol (PCMX). Clin Exp Dermatol 1985;10(5):491–4.

271. McNevin S, MacKay M. Chlorprothixene-induced systemic lupus erythematosus. J Clin Psychopharmacol 1982;2(6):411–2.

272. Volcheck GW, Van Dellen RG. Anaphylaxis to intravenous cyclosporine and tolerance to oral cyclosporine: case report and review. Ann Allergy Asthma Immunol 1998;80(2):159–63.

273. Liau-Chu M, Theis JG, Koren G. Mechanism of anaphylactoid reactions: improper preparation of high-dose intravenous cyclosporine leads to bolus infusion of Cremophor EL and cyclosporine. Ann Pharmacother 1997;31(11):1287–91.

274. Garcia VD, Keitel E, Almeida P, Santos AF, Becker M, Goldani JC. Morbidity after renal transplantation: role of bacterial infection. Transplant Proc 1995;27(2):1825–6.

275. Wade JJ, Rolando N, Hayllar K, Philpott-Howard J, Casewell MW, Williams R. Bacterial and fungal infections after liver transplantation: an analysis of 284 patients. Hepatology 1995;21(5):1328–36.

276. Singh N, Yu VL. Infections in organ transplant recipients. Curr Opin Infect Dis 1996;9:223–9.

277. Reis MA, Costa RS, Ferraz AS. Causes of death in renal transplant recipients: a study of 102 autopsies from 1968 to 1991. J R Soc Med 1995;88(1):24–7.

278. Mizuno Y, Esaki Y, Kato H. [Anaphylactoid reaction to dibucaine during spinal anesthesia.] Masui 2002;51(11):1254–6.

279. Toll A, Campo-Pisa P, Gonzalez-Castro J, Campo-Voegeli A, Azon A, Iranzo P, Lecha M, Herrero C. Subacute cutaneous lupus erythematosus associated with cinnarizine and thiethylperazine therapy. Lupus 1998;7(5):364–6.

280. Burke P, Burne SR. Allergy associated with ciprofloxacin. BMJ 2000;320(7236):679.

281. Knoops L, van den Neste E, Hamels J, Theate I, Mineur P. Angioimmunoblastic lymphadenopathy following ciprofloxacin administration. Acta Clin Belg 2002;57(2):71–3.

282. Webster G, Schiffman JD, Dosanjh AS, Amieva MR, Gans HA, Sectish TC. Jarisch–Herxheimer reaction associated with ciprofloxacin administration for tick-borne relapsing fever. Pediatr Infect Dis J 2002;21(6):571–3.

283. Clendenen SR, Harper JV, Wharen RE Jr, Guarderas JC. Anaphylactic reaction after cisatracurium. Anesthesiology 1997;87(3):690–2.

284. Toh KW, Deacock SJ, Fawcett WJ. Severe anaphylactic reaction to cisatracurium. Anesth Analg 1999;88(2):462–4.

285. Iannuzzi E, Iannuzzi M, Pedicini MS, Cirillo V, Chiefari M, Sacerdoti G. Anaphylactic reaction after cisatracurium administration. Eur J Anaesthesiol 2002;19(9):691–3.

286. Butler P, Mannschreck M, Lin S, Hwang I, Alvarado J. Clinical experience with the long-term use of 1% apraclonidine. Incidence of allergic reactions. Arch Ophthalmol 1995;113(3):293–6.

287. Petersen HH, Hansen M, Albrectsen JM. Clonidine-induced immune complex disease. Acta Dermatol Venereol 1989;69(6):519–20.

288. Sarrot-Reynauld F, Bouillet L, Bourrain JL. Severe hypersensitivity associated with clopidogrel. Ann Intern Med 2001;135(4):305–6.

289. Stanislav SW, Gonzalez-Blanco M. Papular rash and bilateral pleural effusion associated with clozapine. Ann Pharmacother 1999;33(9):1008–9.

290. Van Leeuwen EF, Mauser-Bunschoten EP, Van Dijken PJ, Kok AJ, Sjamsoedin-Visser EJ, Sixma JJ. Disappearance of factor VIII:C antibodies in patients with haemophilia A upon frequent administration of factor VIII in intermediate or low dose. Br J Haematol 1986;64(2):291–7.

291. Parquet A, Laurian Y, Rothschild C, Navarro R, Guerois C, Gay V, Durin A, Peynet J, Sultan Y. Incidence of factor IX inhibitor development in severe haemophilia B patients treated with only one brand of high purity plasma derived factor IX concentrate. Thromb Haemost 1999;82(4):1247–9.

292. Penner JA. Haemophilic patients with inhibitors to factor VIII or IX: variables affecting treatment response. Haemophilia 2001;7(1):103–8.

293. Berntorp E. Immune tolerance induction: recombinant vs. human-derived product. Haemophilia 2001;7(1):109–13.

294. Penner JA. Management of haemophilia in patients with high-titre inhibitors: focus on the evolution of activated prothrombin complex concentrate AUTOPLEX T. Haemophilia 1999;5(Suppl 3):1–9.

295. Zanon E, Zerbinati P, Girolami B, Bertomoro A, Girolami A. Frequent but low titre factor VIII inhibitors in haemophilia A patients treated with high purity concentrates. Blood Coagul Fibrinolysis 1999;10(3):117–20.

296. Bolton-Maggs PH. The management of factor XI deficiency. Haemophilia 1998;4(4):683–8.

297. Robinson AJ, Gazzard BG. Rising rates of HIV infection. BMJ 2005;330(7487):320–1.

298. Delafuente JC, DeVane CL. Immunologic effects of cocaine and related alkaloids. Immunopharmacol Immunotoxicol 1991;13(1–2):11–23.

299. Peterson PK, Gekker G, Chao CC, Schut R, Verhoef J, Edelman CK, Erice A, Balfour HH Jr. Cocaine amplifies HIV-1 replication in cytomegalovirus-stimulated peripheral blood mononuclear cell cocultures. J Immunol 1992;149(2):676–80.

300. Trozak DJ, Gould WM. Cocaine abuse and connective tissue disease. J Am Acad Dermatol 1984;10(3):525.

301. Hofbauer GF, Hafner J, Trueb RM. Urticarial vasculitis following cocaine use. Br J Dermatol 1999;141(3):600–1.

302. Castro-Villamor MA, de las Heras P, Armentia A, Duenas-Laita A. Cocaine-induced severe angioedema and urticaria. Ann Emerg Med 1999;34(2):296–7.

303. Angelini G, Foti C, Rigano L, Vena GA. 3-Dimethylaminopropylamine: a key substance in contact allergy to cocamidopropylbetaine? Contact Dermatitis 1995;32(2):96–9.

304. Fowler JF, Fowler LM, Hunter JE. Allergy to cocamidopropyl betaine may be due to amidoamine: a patch test and product use test study. Contact Dermatitis 1997;37(6):276–81.

305. McFadden JP, Ross JS, White IR, Basketter DA. Clinical allergy to cocamidopropyl betaine: reactivity to cocamidopropylamine and lack of reactivity to 3-dimethylaminopropylamine. Contact Dermatitis 2001;45(2):72–4.

306. DeLustro F, Smith ST, Sundsmo J, Salem G, Kincaid S, Ellingsworth L. Reaction to injectable collagen: results in animal models and clinical use. Plast Reconstr Surg 1987;79(4):581–94.

307. Hanke CW, Higley HR, Jolivette DM, Swanson NA, Stegman SJ. Abscess formation and local necrosis after treatment with Zyderm or Zyplast collagen implant. J Am Acad Dermatol 1991;25(2 Pt 1):319–26.

308. Mullins RJ, Richards C, Walker T. Allergic reactions to oral, surgical and topical bovine collagen. Anaphylactic risk for surgeons. Aust NZ J Ophthalmol 1996;24(3):257–60.

309. Lipsky H. Endoscopic treatment of vesicoureteral reflux with collagen. Pediatr Surg Int 1991;6:301–3.

310. Stothers L, Goldenberg SL. Delayed hypersensitivity and systemic arthralgia following transurethral collagen injection for stress urinary incontinence. J Urol 1998;159(5):1507–9.

311. Echols KT, Chesson RR, Breaux EF, Shobeiri SA. Persistence of delayed hypersensitivity following transurethral collagen injection for recurrent urinary stress incontinence. Int Urogynecol J Pelvic Floor Dysfunct 2002;13(1):52–4.

312. Ginsberg DA, Boyd SD. Permanent urinary retention after transurethral injection of collagen. J Urol 2002;167(2 Pt 1):648.

313. Yamada A, Ohshima Y, Tsukahara H, Hiraoka M, Kimura I, Kawamitsu T, Kimura K, Mayumi M. Two cases of anaphylactic reaction to gelatin induced by a chloral hydrate suppository. Pediatr Int 2002;44(1):87–9.

314. Riikonen R, Simell O, Dunkel L, Santavuori P, Perheentupa J. Hormonal background of the hypertension and fluid derangements associated with adrenocorticotrophic hormone treatment of infants. Eur J Pediatr 1989;148(8):737–41.

315. Glass D, Nuki G, Daly JR. Development of antibodies during long-term therapy with corticotrophin in rheumatoid arthritis. II. Zinc tetracosactrin (Depot Synacthen). Ann Rheum Dis 1971;30(6):593–6.

316. Dunagan DP, Rubin BK, Fasano MB. *Pneumocystis carinii* pneumonia in a child receiving ACTH for infantile spasms. Pediatr Pulmonol 1999;27(4):286–9.

317. Lopez-Serrano MC, Moreno-Ancillo A, Contreras J, Ortega N, Cabanas R, Barranco P, Munoz-Pereira M. Two cases of specific adverse reactions to systemic corticosteroids. J Invest Allergol Clin Immunol 1996;6(5):324–7.

318. Moreno-Ancillo A, Martin-Munoz F, Martin-Barroso JA, Diaz-Pena JM, Ojeda JA. Anaphylaxis to 6-alpha-methylprednisolone in an eight-year-old child. J Allergy Clin Immunol 1996;97(5):1169–71.

319. van den Berg JS, van Eikema Hommes OR, Wuis EW, Stapel S, van der Valk PG. Anaphylactoid reaction to intravenous methylprednisolone in a patient with multiple sclerosis. J Neurol Neurosurg Psychiatry 1997;63(6):813–4.

320. Figueredo E, Cuesta-Herranz JI, De Las Heras M, Lluch-Bernal M, Umpierrez A, Sastre J. Anaphylaxis to dexamethasone. Allergy 1997;52(8):877.

321. Mace S, Vadas P, Pruzanski W. Anaphylactic shock induced by intraarticular injection of methylprednisolone acetate. J Rheumatol 1997;24(6):1191–4.

322. Hayhurst M, Braude A, Benatar SR. Anaphylactic-like reaction to hydrocortisone. S Afr Med J 1978;53(7):259–60.

323. Srinivasan V, Lanham PR. Acute laryngeal obstruction – reaction to intravenous hydrocortisone? Eur J Anaesthesiol 1997;14(3):342.

324. Vaghjimal A, Rosenstreich D, Hudes G. Fever, rash and worsening of asthma in response to intravenous hydrocortisone. Int J Clin Pract 1999;53(7):567–8.

325. Clear D. Anaphylactoid reaction to methyl prednisolone developing after starting treatment with interferon beta-1b. J Neurol Neurosurg Psychiatry 1999;66(5):690.

326. Schonwald S. Methylprednisolone anaphylaxis. Am J Emerg Med 1999;17(6):583–5.

327. Vanpee D, Gillet JB. Allergic reaction to intravenous methylprednisolone in a woman with asthma. Ann Emerg Med 1998;32(6):754.

328. Polosa R, Prosperini G, Pintaldi L, Rey JP, Colombrita R. Anaphylaxis after prednisone. Allergy 1998;53(3):330–1.

329. Yawalkar N, Hari Y, Helbing A, von Greyerz S, Kappeler A, Baathen LR, Pichler WJ. Elevated serum levels of interleukins 5, 6, and 10 in a patient with drug-induced exanthem caused by systemic corticosteroids. J Am Acad Dermatol 1998;39(5 Part 1):790–3.

330. Heeringa M, Zweers P, de Man RA, de Groot H. Drug Points: Anaphylactic-like reaction associated with oral budesonide. BMJ 2000;321(7266):927.

331. Gomez CM, Higuero NC, Moral de Gregorio A, Quiles MH, Nunez Aceves AB, Lara MJ, Sanchez CS. Urticaria–angioedema by deflazacort. Allergy 2002;57(4):370–1.

332. Tuggey JM, Hosker HS. Churg–Strauss syndrome associated with montelukast therapy. Thorax 2000;55(9):805–6.

333. Reinus JF, Persky S, Burkiewicz JS, Quan D, Bass NM, Davern TJ. Severe liver injury after treatment with the leukotriene receptor antagonist zafirlukast. Ann Intern Med 2000;133(12):964–8.

334. Actis GC, Morgando A, Lagget M, David E, Rizzetto M. Zafirlukast-related hepatitis: report of a further case. J Hepatol 2001;35(4):539–41.

335. Hashimoto M, Fujishima T, Tanaka H, Kon H, Saikai T, Suzuki A, Nakatsugawa M, Abe S. Churg–Strauss syndrome after reduction of inhaled corticosteroid in a patient treated with pranlukast for asthma. Intern Med 2001;40(5):432–4.

336. Priori R, Tomassini M, Magrini L, Conti F, Valesini G. Churg–Strauss syndrome during pregnancy after steroid withdrawal. Lancet 1998;352(9140):1599–600.

337. Edwards RL, Rickles FR. Delayed hypersensitivity in man: effects of systemic anticoagulation. Science 1978;200(4341):541–3.

338. Stevenson DD, Sanchez-Borges M, Szczeklik A. Classification of allergic and pseudoallergic reactions to drugs that inhibit cyclooxygenase enzymes. Ann Allergy Asthma Immunol 2001;87(3):177–80.

339. Grob M, Pichler WJ, Wuthrich B. Anaphylaxis to celecoxib. Allergy 2002;57(3):264–5.

340. Skowron F, Berard F, Bernard N, Balme B, Perrot H. Cutaneous vasculitis related to celecoxib. Dermatology 2002;204(4):305.

341. Jordan KM, Edwards CJ, Arden NK. Allergic vasculitis associated with celecoxib. Rheumatology (Oxford) 2002;41(12):1453–5.

342. Schneider F, Meziani F, Chartier C, Alt M, Jaeger A. Fatal allergic vasculitis associated with celecoxib. Lancet 2002;359(9309):852–3.

343. Wiholm BE, Shear NH, Knowles S, Shapiro L. Should celecoxib be contraindicated in patients who are allergic to sulfonamides? Drug Saf 2002;25(4):297–9.

344. Kumar NP, Wild G, Ramasamy KA, Snape J. Fatal haemorrhagic pulmonary oedema and associated angioedema after the ingestion of rofecoxib. Postgrad Med J 2002;78(921):439–40.

345. Nettis E, Di PR, Ferrannini A, Tursi A. Tolerability of rofecoxib in patients with cutaneous adverse reactions to nonsteroidal anti-inflammatory drugs. Ann Allergy Asthma Immunol 2002;88(3):331–4.

346. Levy MB, Fink JN. Anaphylaxis to celecoxib. Ann Allergy Asthma Immunol 2001;87(1):72–3.

347. Habki R, Vermeulen C, Bachmeyer C, Charoud A, Mofredj A. Choc anaphylactique au célécoxib. [Anaphylactic shock induced by celecoxib.] Ann Med Interne (Paris) 2001;152(5):355.

348. Schellenberg RR, Isserow SH. Anaphylactoid reaction to a cyclooxygenase-2 inhibitor in a patient who had a reaction to a cyclooxygenase-1 inhibitor. N Engl J Med 2001;345(25):1856.

349. Repo UK, Nieminen P. Pulmonary infiltrates with eosinophilia and urinary symptoms during disodium cromoglycate treatment. A case report. Scand J Respir Dis 1976;57(1):1–4.

350. Kallos P, Kallos L. Pseudo-allergic reactions due to sodium cromoglycate. In: Dukor P, Kallos P, Schlumberger HD, West GB, editors. Pseudo-allergic Reactions. Involvement of Drugs and Chemicals. Basel: Karger, 1982:122–32.

351. Sheffer AL, Rocklin RE, Goetzl EJ. Immunologic components of hypersensitivity reactions to cromolyn sodium. N Engl J Med 1975;293(24):1220–4.

352. Daugirdas JT, Ing TS, Roxe DM, Ivanovich PT, Krumlovsky F, Popli S, McLaughlin MM. Severe anaphylactoid reactions to cuprammonium cellulose hemodialyzers. Arch Intern Med 1985;145(3):489–94.

353. Wenzel-Seifert K, Sharma AM, Keller F. Repeated dialysis anaphylaxia. Nephrol Dial Transplant 1990;5(9):821–4.

354. Chilla R. Histoacryl-induzierte Spatkomplikationen nach Duraplastiken an der Fronto- und Otobasis. [Late histoacryl-induced complications of dura surgery in the frontal and lateral base of the skull.] HNO 1987;35(6):250–1.

355. Koch P, Munssinger T, Rupp-John C, Uhl K. Delayed-type hypersensitivity skin reactions caused by subcutaneous unfractionated and low-molecular-weight heparins: tolerance of a new recombinant hirudin. J Am Acad Dermatol 2000;42(4):612–9.

356. Chan HL, Lee KO. Tonsillar membrane in the DDS (dapsone) syndrome. Int J Dermatol 1991;30(3):216–7.

357. Pavithran K. Dapsone syndrome with polyarthritis: a case report. Indian J Lepr 1990;62(2):230–2.

358. Kraus A, Jakez J, Palacios A. Dapsone induced sulfone syndrome and systemic lupus exacerbation. J Rheumatol 1992;19(1):178–80.

359. Johnson DA, Cattau EL Jr, Kuritsky JN, Zimmerman HJ. Liver involvement in the sulfone syndrome. Arch Intern Med 1986;146(5):875–7.

360. Mohle-Boetani J, Akula SK, Holodniy M, Katzenstein D, Garcia G. The sulfone syndrome in a patient receiving dapsone prophylaxis for *Pneumocystis carinii* pneumonia. West J Med 1992;156(3):303–6.

361. Richardus JH, Smith TC. Increased incidence in leprosy of hypersensitivity reactions to dapsone after introduction of multidrug therapy. Lepr Rev 1989;60(4):267–73.

362. Mehta J, Singhal S, Revankar R, Walvalkar A, Chablani A, Mehta BC. Fatal systemic lupus erythematosus in patient taking oral iron chelator L1. Lancet 1991;337(8736):298.

363. Mehta J, Singhal S, Mehta BC. Oral iron chelator L1 and autoimmunity. Blood 1993;81(7):1970–1.

364. Olivieri NF, Matsui D, Liu PP, Blendis L, Cameron R, McClelland RA, Templeton DM, Koren G. Oral iron chelation with 1,2-dimethyl-3-hydroxypyrid-4-one (L1) in iron loaded thalassemia patients. Bone Marrow Transplant 1993;12(Suppl 1):9–11.

365. Al-Refaie FN, Hoffbrand AV, Nortey P, Wonke B, Wickens DG. Oral iron chelator L1 and autoimmunity. Blood 1993;81(7):1971–2.

366. Kersten MJ, Lange R, Smeets ME, Vreugdenhil G, Roozendaal KJ, Lameijer W, Goudsmit R. Long-term treatment of transfusional iron overload with the oral iron chelator deferiprone (L1): a Dutch multicenter trial. Ann Hematol 1996;73(5):247–52.

367. Miller KB, Rosenwasser LJ, Bessette JA, Beer DJ, Rocklin RE. Rapid desensitisation for desferrioxamine anaphylactic reaction. Lancet 1981;1(8228):1059.

368. Cianciulli P, Sorrentino F, Maffei L, Amadori S. Continuous low-dose subcutaneous desferrioxamine (DFO) to prevent allergic manifestations in patients with iron overload. Ann Hematol 1996;73(6):279–81.

369. Bousquet J, Navarro M, Robert G, Aye P, Michel FB. Rapid desensitisation for desferrioxamine anaphylactoid reaction. Lancet 1983;2(8354):859–60.

370. Seifert A, von Herrath D, Schaefer K. Iron overload, but not treatment with desferrioxamine favours the development of septicemia in patients on maintenance hemodialysis. Q J Med 1987;65(248):1015–24.

371. Chiu HY, Flynn DM, Hoffbrand AV, Politis D. Infection with *Yersinia enterocolitica* in patients with iron overload. BMJ (Clin Res Ed) 1986;292(6513):97.

372. Mofenson HC, Caraccio TR, Sharieff N. Iron sepsis: *Yersinia enterocolitica* septicemia possibly caused by an overdose of iron. N Engl J Med 1987;316(17):1092–3.

373. Waterlot Y, Cantinieaux B, Hariga-Muller C, De Maertelaere-Laurent E, Vanherweghem JL, Fondu P. Impaired phagocytic activity of neutrophils in patients receiving haemodialysis: the critical role of iron overload. BMJ (Clin Res Ed) 1985;291(6494):501–4.

374. Emami A, Fagundus DM. Granulocyte dysfunction in patients with iron overload. Br J Haematol 1990;74(4):546–7.

375. Sane A, Manzi S, Perfect J, Herzberg AJ, Moore JO. Deferoxamine treatment as a risk factor for zygomycete infection. J Infect Dis 1989;159(1):151–2.

376. Mazzoleni G, deSa D, Gately J, Riddell RH. *Yersinia enterocolitica* infection with ileal perforation associated with iron overload and deferoxamine therapy. Dig Dis Sci 1991;36(8):1154–60.

377. Nouel O, Voisin PM, Vaucel J, Dartois-Hoguin M, Le Bris M. Association d'une septicémie à *Yersinia enterocolitica*, d'une hémochromatose idiopathique et d'un traitement par deferoxamine. [*Yersinia enterocolitica*

septicemia associated with idiopathic hemochromatosis and deferoxamine therapy. A case.] Presse Med 1991;20(31):1494–6.

378. Pierron H, Gillet R, Perrimond H, Broudeur JC, Soudry G. Yersiniose et dyshémoglobinose. Á propos de 4 observations. [*Yersinia* infection and hemoglobin disorder. Apropos of 4 cases.] Pediatrie 1990;45(6):379–82.

379. Kaneko T, Abe F, Ito M, Hotchi M, Yamada K, Okada Y. Intestinal mucormycosis in a hemodialysis patient treated with desferrioxamine. Acta Pathol Jpn 1991;41(7):561–6.

380. Abcarian PW, Demas BE. Systemic *Yersinia enterocolitica* infection associated with iron overload and deferoxamine therapy. Am J Roentgenol 1991;157(4):773–5.

381. Rex JH, Ginsberg AM, Fries LF, Pass HI, Kwon-Chung KJ. *Cunninghamella bertholletiae* infection associated with deferoxamine therapy. Rev Infect Dis 1988;10(6):1187–94.

382. Kouides PA, Slapak CA, Rosenwasser LJ, Miller KB. *Pneumocystis carinii* pneumonia as a complication of desferrioxamine therapy. Br J Haematol 1988;70(3):383–4.

383. Eijgenraam FJ, Donckerwolcke RA. Treatment of iron overload in children and adolescents on chronic haemodialysis. Eur J Pediatr 1990;149(5):359–62.

384. Hamdy NA, Andrew SM, Shortland JR, Boletis J, Raftery AT, Kanis JA, Brown CB. Fatal cardiac zygomycosis in a renal transplant patient treated with desferrioxamine. Nephrol Dial Transplant 1989;4(10):911–3.

385. Daly AL, Velazquez LA, Bradley SF, Kauffman CA. Mucormycosis: association with deferoxamine therapy. Am J Med 1989;87(4):468–71.

386. Arizono K, Fukui H, Miura H, Hayano K, Otsuka Y, Tajiri M. [A case report of rhinocerebral mucormycosis in hemodialysis patient receiving deferoxamine.] Nippon Jinzo Gakkai Shi 1989;31(1):99–103.

387. Sombolos K, Kalekou H, Barboutis K, Tzarou V. Fatal phycomycosis in a hemodialyzed patient receiving deferoxamine. Nephron 1988;49(2):169–70.

388. Goodill JJ, Abuelo JG. Mucormycosis—a new risk of deferoxamine therapy in dialysis patients with aluminum or iron overload. N Engl J Med 1987;317(1):54.

389. Boelaert JR, van Roost GF, Vergauwe PL, Verbanck JJ, de Vroey C, Segaert MF. The role of desferrioxamine in dialysis-associated mucormycosis: report of three cases and review of the literature. Clin Nephrol 1988;29(5):261–6.

390. Van Johnson E, Kline LB, Julian BA, Garcia JH. Bilateral cavernous sinus thrombosis due to mucormycosis. Arch Ophthalmol 1988;106(8):1089–92.

391. Veis JH, Contiguglia R, Klein M, Mishell J, Alfrey AC, Shapiro JI. Mucormycosis in deferoxamine-treated patients on dialysis. Ann Intern Med 1987;107(2):258.

392. Anonymous. Mucormycosis induced by deferoxamine mesylate. Information on Adverse Reactions to Drugs. Japan: Pharmaceutical Affairs Bureau, Ministry of Health and Welfare, February 1988.

393. Boelaert JR, Fenves AZ, Coburn JW. Mucormycosis among patients on dialysis. N Engl J Med 1989;321(3):190–1.

394. Nakamura M, Weil WB Jr, Kaufman DB. Fatal fungal peritonitis in an adolescent on continuous ambulatory peritoneal dialysis: association with deferoxamine. Pediatr Nephrol 1989;3(1):80–2.

395. Slade MP, McNab AA. Fatal mucormycosis therapy associated with deferoxamine. Am J Ophthalmol 1991;112(5):594–5.

396. Venkattaramanabalaji GV, Foster D, Greene JN, Muro-Cacho CA, Sandin RL, Saez R, Robinson LA. Mucormycosis associated with deferoxamine therapy

after allogeneic bone marrow transplantation. Cancer Control 1997;4(2):168–71.

397. Murray MF, Galetta SL, Raps EC, Kenyon L, Brennan PJ. Deferoxamine-associated mucormycosis in a non-dialysis patient. Infect Dis Clin Pract 1996;5:395–7.

398. Mills G, Morgan J, Hales G, Smith D. Acute hypersensitivity with delavirdine. Antivir Ther 1999;4(1):51.

399. Ahmed N, Falcone T, Tulandi T, Houle G. Anaphylactic reaction because of intrauterine 32% dextran-70 instillation. Fertil Steril 1991;55(5):1014–6.

400. Hernandez D, de Rojas F, Martinez Escribano C, Arriaga F, Cuellar J, Molins J, Barber L. Fatal dextran-induced allergic anaphylaxis. Allergy 2002;57(9):862.

401. Lehmann G, Asskali F, Forster H. Schwerer Zwischen fall nach I.V. – Applikation von 10 ml (0.6 g) 6% igem Dextran 60 bei einem gesunden Probanden. [Severe adverse event following i.v. administration of 10 ml 6% dextran 60 (0.6 g) in a healthy volunteer.] Anaesthesist 2002;51(10):820–4.

402. Laxenaire MC, Charpentier C, Feldman L. Réactions anaphylactoïdes aux substituts colloidaux du plasma: incidence, facteurs de risque, mécanismes. Enquete prospective multicentrique française. Groupe Français d'Etude de la Tolerance des Substituts Plasmatiques. [Anaphylactoid reactions to colloid plasma substitutes: incidence, risk factors, mechanisms. A French multicenter prospective study.] Ann Fr Anesth Reanim 1994;13(3):301–10.

403. Knowles SR, Weber E. Dextromethorphan anaphylaxis. J Allergy Clin Immunol 1998;102(2):316–7.

404. Olcina GM, Simonart T. Severe vasculitis after therapy with diazepam. Am J Psychiatry 1999;156(6):972–3.

405. Asero R. Hypersensitivity to diazepam. Allergy 2002;57(12):1209.

406. Selvaag E. Contact allergy to dibromopropamidine cream. Contact Dermatitis 1999;40(1):58.

407. Yazdanbakhsh M, Duym L, Aarden L, Partono F. Serum interleukin-6 levels and adverse reactions to diethylcarbamazine in lymphatic filariasis. J Infect Dis 1992;166(2):453–4.

408. Reuben R, Rajendran R, Sunish IP, Mani TR, Tewari SC, Hiriyan J, Gajanana A. Annual single-dose diethylcarbamazine plus ivermectin for control of Bancroftian filariasis: comparative efficacy with and without vector control. Ann Trop Med Parasitol 2001;95(4):361–78.

409. Kimura M, Kawada A. Contact dermatitis due to diethyl sebacate. Contact Dermatitis 1999;40(1):48–9.

410. McIntyre L, Krajden S, Keystone JS. Angioedema due to diphetarsone and a review of its toxicity. Trop Geogr Med 1983;35(1):49–51.

411. Skrebova N, Nameda Y, Takiwaki H, Arase S. Severe dermographism after topical therapy with diphenylcyclopropenone for alopecia universalis. Contact Dermatitis 2000;42(4):212–5.

412. Alam M, Gross EA, Savin RC. Severe urticarial reaction to diphenylcyclopropenone therapy for alopecia areata. J Am Acad Dermatol 1999;40(1):110–2.

413. Angelides S, Van der Wall H, Freedman SB. Acute reaction to dipyridamole during myocardial scintigraphy. N Engl J Med 1999;340(5):394.

414. Eichler P, Friesen HJ, Lubenow N, Jaeger B, Greinacher A. Antihirudin antibodies in patients with heparin-induced thrombocytopenia treated with lepirudin: incidence, effects on aPTT, and clinical relevance. Blood 2000;96(7):2373–8.

415. Close P, Bichler J, Kerry R, Ekman S, Bueller HR, Kienast J, Marbet GA, Schramm W, Verstraete M. Weak allergenicity of recombinant hirudin CGP 39393

416. (REVASC) in immunocompetent volunteers. The European Hirudin in Thrombosis Group (HIT Group). Coron Artery Dis 1994;5(11):943–9.

416. Porterfield JG, Antman EM, Lown B. Respiratory difficulty after use of disopyramide. N Engl J Med 1980;303(10):584.

417. Minet A, Frankart M, Eggers S, Lachapelle JM, Bourlond A. Réactions allergiques aux implants de disulfirame. [Allergic reactions to disulfiram implants.] Ann Dermatol Venereol 1989;116(8):543–5.

418. Goland S, Kazarsky R, Kagan A, Huszar M, Abend I, Malnick SDH. Renal vasculitis associated with doxycycline. J Pharm Technol 2001;17:220–2.

419. Fisher AA. Safety of ethylenediamine tetraacetate in the treatment of lead poisoning in persons sensitive to ethylenediamine hydrochloride. Cutis 1991;48(2):105–6.

420. Phillips EJ, Kuriakose B, Knowles SR. Efavirenz-induced skin eruption and successful desensitization. Ann Pharmacother 2002;36(3):430–2.

421. Bossi P, Colin D, Bricaire F, Caumes E. Hypersensitivity syndrome associated with efavirenz therapy. Clin Infect Dis 2000;30(1):227–8.

422. Behrens GM, Stoll M, Schmidt RE. Pulmonary hypersensitivity reaction induced by efavirenz. Lancet 2001;357(9267):1503–4.

423. Domingo P, Barcelo M. Efavirenz-induced leukocytoclastic vasculitis. Arch Intern Med 2002;162(3):355–6.

424. Venturini M, Lezaun A, Abos T, Fraj J, Monzon S, Colas C, Duce F. Immediate hypersensitivity due to pseudoephedrine. Allergy 2002;57(1):52–3.

425. Cameron JS, Barany P, Barbas J, Carrera F, Chanard J. European best practice guidelines for the management of anaemia in patients with chronic renal failure. Working Party for European Best Practice Guidelines for the Management of Anaemia in Patients with Chronic Renal Failure. Nephrol Dial Transplant 1999;14(Suppl 5):1–50.

426. Leikis MJ, Forbes IK, McMahon LP, Becker GJ. Resolution of pure red cell aplasia with continued production of low titer anti-epoetin antibodies. Clin Nephrol 2004;62(6):481–2.

427. Mercadal L, Sutton L, Casadevall N, Bagnis C, Jacobs C. Immunological reaction against erythropoietin causing red-cell aplasia. Nephrol Dial Transplant 2002;17(5):943.

428. Gershon SK, Luksenburg H, Cote TR, Braun MM. Pure red-cell aplasia and recombinant erythropoietin. N Engl J Med 2002;346(20):1584–6.

429. Casadevall N, Nataf J, Viron B, Kolta A, Kiladjian JJ, Martin-Dupont P, Michaud P, Papo T, Ugo V, Teyssandier I, Varet B, Mayeux P. Pure red-cell aplasia and antierythropoietin antibodies in patients treated with recombinant erythropoietin. N Engl J Med 2002; 346(7):469–75.

430. Locatelli F, Vecchio LD. Darbepoetin alfa. Amgen. Curr Opin Investig Drugs 2001;2(8):1097–104.

431. Smith RE Jr, Jaiyesimi IA, Meza LA, Tchekmedyian NS, Chan D, Griffith H, Brosman S, Bukowski R, Murdoch M, Rarick M, Saven A, Colowick AB, Fleishman A, Gayko U, Glaspy J. Novel erythropoiesis stimulating protein (NESP) for the treatment of anaemia of chronic disease associated with cancer. Br J Cancer 2001;84(Suppl 1):24–30.

432. Heatherington AC, Schuller J, Mercer AJ. Pharmacokinetics of novel erythropoiesis stimulating protein (NESP) in cancer patients: preliminary report. Br J Cancer 2001;84(Suppl 1):11–6.

433. Anonymous. Darbepoetin alfa: profile report. Drugs Ther Perspect 2002;18:4–5.

434. Sifakis S, Angelakis E, Vardaki E, Koumantaki Y, Matalliotakis I, Koumantakis E. Erythropoietin in the treatment of iron deficiency anemia during pregnancy. Gynecol Obstet Invest 2001;51(3):150–6.

435. Sakaguchi M, Kaneda H, Inouye S. A case of anaphylaxis to gelatin included in erythropoietin products. J Allergy Clin Immunol 1999;103(2 Pt 1):349–50.

436. Styrt B, Sugarman B. Estrogens and infection. Rev Infect Dis 1991;13(6):1139–50.

437. Klinger G, Graser T, Mellinger U, Moore C, Vogelsang H, Groh A, Latterman C, Klinger G. A comparative study of the effects of two oral contraceptives containing dienogest or desogestrel on the human immune system. Gynecol Endocrinol 2000;14(1):15–24.

438. Searcy CJ, Kushner M, Nell P, Beckmann CR. Anaphylactic reaction to intravenous conjugated estrogens. Clin Pharm 1987;6(1):74–6.

439. Burke L, Segall-Blank M, Lorenzo C, Dynesius-Trentham R, Trentham D, Mortola JF. Altered immune response in adult women exposed to diethylstilbestrol in utero. Am J Obstet Gynecol 2001;185(1):78–81.

440. Bar-On H, Eisenberg S, Eliakim M. Clinical experience with ethacrynic acid with reference to a possible complication of the Schoenlein–Henoch type. Isr J Med Sci 1967;3(1):113–8.

441. Pain AK. Acute gastric ulceration associated with drug therapy. BMJ 1967;1(540):634.

442. Putarek K, Minigo H, Planinc-Peraica A, Jaksic B. Allergic reaction during reinfusion of autologous bone marrow related to treatment of Hodgkin's lymphoma; possible role of hydroxyethyl starch—a case report. Libri Oncol 1996;25:53–5.

443. Kannan S, Milligan KR. Moderately severe anaphylactoid reaction to pentastarch (200/0.5) in a patient with acute severe asthma Intensive Care Med 1999;25(2):220–2.

444. Boldt J, Heesen M, Padberg W, Martin K, Hempelmann G. The influence of volume therapy and pentoxifylline infusion on circulating adhesion molecules in trauma patients. Anaesthesia 1996;51(6):529–35.

445. Dieterich HJ, Kraft D, Sirtl C, Laubenthal H, Schimetta W, Polz W, Gerlach E, Peter K. Hydroxyethyl starch antibodies in humans: incidence and clinical relevance. Anesth Analg 1998;86(5):1123–6.

446. Guin JD, Fields P, Thomas KL. Baboon syndrome from i.v. aminophylline in a patient allergic to ethylenediamine Contact Dermatitis 1999;40(3):170–1.

447. Andersen KE, Hjorth N, Menne T. The baboon syndrome: systemically-induced allergic contact dermatitis. Contact Dermatitis 1984;10(2):97–100.

448. Yoshizawa A, Araki Y, Kobayashi N, Kudo K. [A case of aminophylline hypersensitivity reaction due to ethylenediamine.] Arerugi 1999;48(11):1206–11.

449. Leitman SF, Boltansky H, Alter HJ, Pearson FC, Kaliner MA. Allergic reactions in healthy plateletpheresis donors caused by sensitization to ethylene oxide gas. N Engl J Med 1986;315(19):1192–6.

450. Doenicke A, Hartel U, Buttner T, Kropp W. Anaesthesien für endoskopischdiagnostische Eingriffe unter besonderer Berücksightigung von Etomidate. In: Proceedings, 8th International Anaesthesia Postgraduate Course. Vienna: H Egermann, 1977.

451. Navarro-Rouimi R, Charpin D. Anaphylactic reaction to castor bean seeds. Allergy 1999;54(10):1117.

452. Roberts JL, Hayashi JA. Exacerbation of SLE associated with alfalfa ingestion. N Engl J Med 1983;308(22):1361.

453. Alcocer-Varela J, Iglesias A, Llorente L, Alarcon-Segovia D. Effects of L-canavanine on T cells may explain the induction of systemic lupus erythematosus by alfalfa. Arthritis Rheum 1985;28(1):52–7.

454. Shapiro AD. Recombinant factor VIIa in the treatment of bleeding in hemophilic children with inhibitors. Semin Thromb Hemost 2000;26(4):413–9.

455. Hedner U. Use of high dose factor VIIa in hemophilia patients. Adv Exp Med Biol 2001;489:75–88.

456. Roberts HR. Clinical experience with activated factor VII: focus on safety aspects. Blood Coagul Fibrinolysis 1998;9(Suppl 1):S115–8.

457. Barthels M. Clinical efficacy of prothrombin complex concentrates and recombinant factor VIIa in the treatment of bleeding episodes in patients with factor VII and IX inhibitors. Thromb Res 1999;95(4 Suppl 1):S31–8.

458. Aledort LM. Blood products and immune changes: impacts without HIV infection. Semin Hematol 1988;25(2 Suppl 1):14–9.

459. Carr R, Veitch SE, Edmond E, Peutherer JF, Prescott RJ, Steel CM, Ludlam CA. Abnormalities of circulating lymphocyte subsets in haemophiliacs in an AIDS-free population. Lancet 1984;1(8392):1431–4.

460. Mannhalter JW, Ahmad R, Leibl H, Gottlicher J, Wolf HM, Eibl MM. Comparable modulation of human monocyte functions by commercial factor VIII concentrates of varying purity. Blood 1988;71(6):1662–8.

461. Thorpe R, Dilger P, Dawson NJ, Barrowcliffe TW. Inhibition of interleukin-2 secretion by factor VIII concentrates: a possible cause of immunosuppression in haemophiliacs. Br J Haematol 1989;71(3):387–91.

462. Seremetis S, Lusher JM, Abildgaard CF, Kasper CK, Allred R, Hurst D. Human recombinant DNA-derived antihaemophilic factor (factor VIII) in the treatment of haemophilia A: conclusions of a 5-year study of home therapy. The KOGENATE Study Group. Haemophilia 1999;5(1):9–16.

463. Spiegel PC Jr, Stoddard BL. Optimization of factor VIII replacement therapy: can structural studies help in evading antibody inhibitors? Br J Haematol 2002;119(2):310–22.

464. van der Bom JG, Mauser-Bunschoten EP, Fischer K, van den Berg HM. Age at first treatment and immune tolerance to factor VIII in severe hemophilia. Thromb Haemost 2003;89(3):475–9.

465. DellaCroce FJ, Kountakis S, Aguilar EF 3rd. Manifestations of factor VIII inhibitor in the head and neck. Arch Otolaryngol Head Neck Surg 1999;125(11):1258–61.

466. Darby SC, Kerling DM, Spooner RJ, Wan Kan S, Giangrande PL, Collins PW, Hill FG, Hay CR. The incidence of factor VIII and factor IX inhibitors in the hemophilia population of the UK and their effect on subsequent mortality, 1977–1999. J Thromb Haemost 2004;2(7):1047–54.

467. Hasegawa DK, Edson JR. Detection of factor VIII and IX inhibitors after first exposure to heat-treated concentrates. Lancet 1987;1(8530):449.

468. Pasi KJ, Hamon MD, Perry DJ, Hill FG. Factor VIII and IX inhibitors after exposure to heat-treated concentrates. Lancet 1987;1(8534):689.

469. Van Leeuwen EF, Mauser-Bunschoten EP, Van Dijken PJ, Kok AJ, Sjamsoedin-Visser EJ, Sixma JJ. Disappearance of factor VIII:C antibodies in patients with haemophilia A upon frequent administration of factor VIII in intermediate or low dose. Br J Haematol 1986;64(2):291–7.

470. Abshire TC, Brackmann HH, Scharrer I, Hoots K, Gazengel C, Powell JS, Gorina E, Kellermann E, Vosburgh E. Sucrose formulated recombinant human antihemophilic factor VIII is safe and efficacious for treatment of hemophilia A in home therapy—International Kogenate-FS Study Group. Thromb Haemost 2000;83(6):811–6.

471. Berntorp E. Other ongoing rFVIII PUP studies. Vox Sang 1999;77(Suppl 1):10–2.

472. Giangrande PL; KOGENATE Bayer Study Group. Safety and efficacy of KOGENATE Bayer in previously untreated patients (PUPs) and minimally treated patients (MTPs). Haemophilia 2002;8(Suppl 2):19–22.

473. Tengborn L, Hansson S, Fasth A, Lubeck PO, Berg A, Ljung R. Anaphylactoid reactions and nephrotic syndrome—a considerable risk during factor IX treatment in patients with haemophilia B and inhibitors: a report on the outcome in two brothers. Haemophilia 1998;4(6):854–9.

474. Dioun AF, Ewenstein BM, Geha RS, Schneider LC. IgE-mediated allergy and desensitization to factor IX in hemophilia B. J Allergy Clin Immunol 1998;102(1):113–7.

475. Barnes C, Brewin T, Ekert H. Induction of immune tolerance and suppression of anaphylaxis in a child with haemophilia B by simple plasmapheresis and antigen exposure: progress report. Haemophilia 2001;7(4):439–40.

476. Hasegawa DK, Edson JR. Detection of factor VIII and IX inhibitors after first exposure to heat-treated concentrates. Lancet 1987;1(8530):449.

477. Pasi KJ, Hamon MD, Perry DJ, Hill FG. Factor VIII and IX inhibitors after exposure to heat-treated concentrates. Lancet 1987;1(8534):689.

478. Shapiro AD. Recombinant factor VIIa in the treatment of bleeding in hemophilic children with inhibitors. Semin Thromb Hemost 2000;26(4):413–9.

479. Thorland EC, Drost JB, Lusher JM, Warrier I, Shapiro A, Koerper MA, Dimichele D, Westman J, Key NS, Sommer SS. Anaphylactic response to factor IX replacement therapy in haemophilia B patients: complete gene deletions confer the highest risk. Haemophilia 1999;5(2):101–5.

480. Alexander JP. Adverse reactions following fazadinium–thiopentone induction. Anaesthesia 1979;34(7):661–5.

481. Baldassare M, Mastroianni A. Su un grave caso di shock da bromuro di fazadinio. [On a severe case of shock caused by fazadinium bromide.] Acta Anaesthesiol Ital 1983;34:91.

482. Jefferson HJ, Jayne DR. Peripheral vasculopathy and nephropathy in association with phentermine. Nephrol Dial Transplant 1999;14(7):1761–3.

483. Korkmaz C, Fresko I, Yazici H. A case of systemic sclerosis that developed under dexfenfluramine use. Rheumatology (Oxford) 1999;38(4):379–80.

484. Aeschlimann A, de Truchis P, Kahn MF. Scleroderma after therapy with appetite suppressants. Report on four cases. Scand J Rheumatol 1990;19(1):87–90.

485. Smith GW, Hurst NP. Vasculitis, Raynaud's phenomenon and polyarthritis associated with gemfibrozil therapy. Br J Rheumatol 1993;32(1):84–5.

486. de Barrio M, Matheu V, Baeza ML, Tornero P, Rubio M, Zubeldia JM. Bezafibrate-induced anaphylactic shock: unusual clinical presentation. J Investig Allergol Clin Immunol 2001;11(1):53–5.

487. Rabasa-Lhoret R, Rasamisoa M, Avignon A, Monnier L. Rare side-effects of fenofibrate. Diabetes Metab 2001;27(1):66–8.

488. Kon NF, Masumo H, Nakajima S, Tozawa R, Kimura M, Maeda S. [Anaphylactic reaction to aprotinin following topical use of biological tissue sealant.] Masui 1994;43(10):1606–10.

489. Banninger H, Hardegger T, Tobler A, Barth A, Schupbach P, Reinhart W, Lammle B, Furlan M. Fibrin glue in surgery: frequent development of inhibitors of bovine thrombin and human factor V. Br J Haematol 1993;85(3):528–32.

490. Ortel TL, Charles LA, Keller FG, Marcom PK, Oldham HN Jr, Kane WH, Macik BG. Topical thrombin and acquired coagulation factor inhibitors: clinical spectrum and laboratory diagnosis. Am J Hematol 1994;45(2):128–35.

491. Muntean W, Zenz W, Finding K, Zobel G, Beitzke A. Inhibitor to factor V after exposure to fibrin sealant during cardiac surgery in a two-year-old child. Acta Paediatr 1994;83(1):84–7.

492. van der Klauw MM, Wilson JH, Stricker BH. Drug-associated anaphylaxis: 20 years of reporting in The Netherlands (1974–1994) and review of the literature. Clin Exp Allergy 1996;26(12):1355–63.

493. Kotani S, Hirose S, Niiya K, Kubonishi I, Miyoshi I. Anaphylaxis to flucytosine in a patient with AIDS. JAMA 1988;260(22):3275–6.

494. Ono Y, Ohmoto Y, Ono K, Sakata Y, Murata K. Effect of grepafloxacin on cytokine production in vitro. J Antimicrob Chemother 2000;46(1):91–4.

495. Stricker BH, Slagboom G, Demaeseneer R, Slootmaekers V, Thijs I, Olsson S. Anaphylactic reactions to cinoxacin. BMJ 1988;297(6661):1434–5.

496. Davis H, McGoodwin E, Reed TG. Anaphylactoid reactions reported after treatment with ciprofloxacin. Ann Intern Med 1989;111(12):1041–3.

497. Kennedy CA, Goetz MB, Mathisen GE. Ciprofloxacin-induced anaphylactoid reactions in patients infected with the human immunodeficiency virus. West J Med 1990;153(5):563–4.

498. Miller MS, Gaido F, Rourk MH Jr, Spock A. Anaphylactoid reactions to ciprofloxacin in cystic fibrosis patients. Pediatr Infect Dis J 1991;10(2):164–5.

499. Grassmick BK, Lehr VT, Sundareson AS. Fulminant hepatic failure possibly related to ciprofloxacin. Ann Pharmacother 1992;26(5):636–9.

500. Shibasaki T, Ishimoto F, Sakai O, Joh K, Aizawa S. Clinical characterization of drug-induced allergic nephritis. Am J Nephrol 1991;11(3):174–80.

501. Hadimeri H, Almroth G, Cederbrant K, Enestrom S, Hultman P, Lindell A. Allergic nephropathy associated with norfloxacin and ciprofloxacin therapy. Report of two cases and review of the literature. Scand J Urol Nephrol 1997;31(5):481–5.

502. Davila I, Diez ML, Quirce S, Fraj J, De La Hoz B, Lazaro M. Cross-reactivity between quinolones. Report of three cases. Allergy 1993;48(5):388–90.

503. Ronnau AC, Sachs B, von Schmiedeberg S, Hunzelmann N, Ruzicka T, Gleichmann E, Schuppe HC. Cutaneous adverse reaction to ciprofloxacin: demonstration of specific lymphocyte proliferation and cross-reactivity to ofloxacin in vitro. Acta Derm Venereol 1997;77(4):285–8.

504. Araujo FG, Slifer TL, Remington JS. Effect of moxifloxacin on secretion of cytokines by human monocytes stimulated with lipopolysaccharide. Clin Microbiol Infect 2002;8(1):26–30.

505. Aleman AM, Quirce S, Cuesta J, Novalbos A, Sastre J. Anaphylactoid reaction caused by moxifloxacin. J Investig Allergol Clin Immunol 2002;12(1):67–8.

506. Gonzalez-Mancebo E, Cuevas M, Gonzalez Gonzalez E, Lara Catedra C, Dolores Alonso M. Simultaneous drug allergies. Allergy 2002;57(10):963–4.

507. Artsimovich NG, Nastoiashchaia NN, Navashin PS. [Effect of pefloxacin on immune response.] Antibiot Khimioter 2001;46(4):11–12.

508. Benchalal M, Yahchouchy-Chouillard E, Fouere S, Fingerhut A. Anaphylactic shock secondary to intravenous administration of folinic acid: a first report. Ann Oncol 2002;13(3):480–1.

509. Moore N, Biour M, Paux G, Loupi E, Begaud B, Boismare F, Royer RJ. Adverse drug reaction monitoring: doing it the French way. Lancet 1985;2(8463):1056–8.

510. Dykewicz MS, Orfan NA, Sun W. In vitro demonstration of IgE antibody to folate–albumin in anaphylaxis from folic acid. J Allergy Clin Immunol 2000;106(2):386–9.

511. Kiec-Swierczynska M, Krecisz B, Krysiak B, Kuchowicz E, Rydzynski K. Occupational allergy to aldehydes in health care workers. Clinical observations. Experiments. Int J Occup Med Environ Health 1998;11(4):349–58.

512. Friedman EA, Lundin AP 3rd. Environmental and iatrogenic obstacles to long life on hemodialysis. N Engl J Med 1982;306(3):167–9.

513. Zasuwa G, Levin NW. Problem in hemodialysis. N Engl J. Med 1982;306(25):1550.

514. Matsumoto T, Tateda K, Miyazaki S, Furuya N, Ohno A, Ishii Y, Hirakata Y, Yamaguchi K. Fosfomycin alters lipopolysaccharide-induced inflammatory cytokine production in mice. Antimicrob Agents Chemother 1999;43(3):697–8.

515. Marren P, Wojnarowska F, Powell S. Allergic contact dermatitis and vulvar dermatoses. Br J Dermatol 1992;126(1):52–6.

516. De Groot AC, Weyland JW, Nater JP. Unwanted Effects of Cosmetics and Drugs Used in Dermatology. 3rd ed. Amsterdam: Elsevier, 1994.

517. Frosch PJ, Johansen JD, Menne T, Pirker C, Rastogi SC, Andersen KE, Bruze M, Goossens A, Lepoittevin JP, White IR. Further important sensitizers in patients sensitive to fragrances. I. Reactivity to 14 frequently used chemicals. Contact Dermatitis 2002;47(2):78–85.

518. Frosch PJ, Johansen JD, Menne T, Pirker C, Rastogi SC, Andersen KE, Bruze M, Goossens A, Lepoittevin JP, White IR. Further important sensitizers in patients sensitive to fragrances. II. Reactivity to essential oils. Contact Dermatitis 2002;47(5):279–87.

519. Matura M, Goossens A, Bordalo O, Garcia-Bravo B, Magnusson K, Wrangsjo K, Karlberg AT. Oxidized citrus oil (R-limonene): a frequent skin sensitizer in Europe. J Am Acad Dermatol 2002;47(5):709–14.

520. Larsen W, Nakayama H, Fischer T, Elsner P, Frosch P, Burrows D, Jordan W, Shaw S, Wilkinson J, Marks J, Sugawara M, Nethercott M, Nethercott J. Fragrance contact dermatitis—a worldwide multicenter investigation (Part III). Contact Dermatitis 2002;46(3):141–4.

521. Larsen W, Nakayama H, Lindberg M, Fischer T, Elsner P, Burrows D, Jordan W, Shaw S, Wilkinson J, Marks J Jr, Sugawara M, Nethercott J. Fragrance contact dermatitis: a worldwide multicenter investigation (Part I). Am J Contact Dermat 1996;7(2):77–83.

522. Larsen W, Nakayama H, Fischer T, Elsner P, Frosch P, Burrows D, Jordan W, Shaw S, Wilkinson J, Marks J Jr, Sugawara M, Nethercott M, Nethercott J. Fragrance contact dermatitis: a worldwide multicenter investigation (Part II). Contact Dermatitis 2001;44(6):344–6.

523. Wilson CL, Cameron J, Powell SM, Cherry G, Ryan TJ. High incidence of contact dermatitis in leg-ulcer patients—implications for management. Clin Exp Dermatol 1991;16(4):250–3.

524. Gallenkemper G, Rabe E, Bauer R. Contact sensitization in chronic venous insufficiency: modern wound dressings. Contact Dermatitis 1998;38(5):274–8.

525. Neldner KH. Contact dermatitis from animal feed additives. Arch Dermatol 1972;106(5):722–3.

526. Sanchez-Perez J, Cordoba S, del Rio MJ, Garcia-Dies A. Allergic contact dermatitis from furaltadone in eardrops. Contact Dermatitis 1999;40(4):222.

527. Christiansen K. Fusidic acid adverse drug reactions. Int J Antimicrob Agents 1999;12(Suppl 2):S3–9.

528. Morris SD, Rycroft RJ, White IR, Wakelin SH, McFadden JP. Comparative frequency of patch test reactions to topical antibiotics. Br J Dermatol 2002; 146(6):1047–51.

529. Phipatanakul W, Adkinson NF Jr. Cross-reactivity between sulfonamides and loop or thiazide diuretics: a theoretical or actual risk? Allergy Clin Immunol Int 2000;12:26–8.

530. Earl G, Davenport J, Narula J. Furosemide challenge in patients with heart failure and adverse reactions to sulfa-containing diuretics. Ann Intern Med 2003;138(4):358–9.

531. Ragucci MV, Cohen JM. Gabapentin-induced hypersensitivity syndrome. Clin Neuropharmacol 2001;24(2):103–5.

532. Hatton F, Tiret L, Maujol L, N'Doye P, Vourc'h G, Desmonts JM, Otteni JC, Scherpereel P. Enquête épidémiologique sur les anesthésies. [INSERM. Epidemiological survey of anesthesia. Initial results.] Ann Fr Anesth Réanim 1983;2(5):331–86.

533. Fisher MM, Munro I. Life-threatening anaphylactoid reactions to muscle relaxants. Anesth Analg 1983;62(6):559–64.

534. Laxenaire MC, Moneret-Vautrin DA, Vervloet D. The French experience of anaphylactoid reactions. Int Anesthesiol Clin 1985;23(3):145–60.

535. Galletly DC, Treuren BC. Anaphylactoid reactions during anaesthesia. Seven years' experience of intradermal testing. Anaesthesia 1985;40(4):329–33.

536. Harrison GR, Thompson ID. Adverse reaction to methohexitone and gallamine. Anaesthesia 1981;36(1):40–4.

537. Harrison JF, Bird AG. Anaphylaxis to precurarising doses of gallamine triethiodide. Anaesthesia 1986;41(6):600–4.

538. Lantsberg S, Rachinsky I, Boguslavsky L. False-positive Ga-67 uptake in a septic patient after severe automobile trauma. Clin Nucl Med 1999;24(11):890–1.

539. Geisler JP, Schraith DF, Manahan KJ, Sorosky JI. Gemcitabine associated vasculitis leading to necrotizing enterocolitis and death in women undergoing primary treatment for epithelial ovarian/peritoneal cancer. Gynecol Oncol 2004;92(2):705–7.

540. Birlik M, Akar S, Tuzel E, Onen F, Ozer E, Manisali M, Kirkali Z, Akkoc N. Gemcitabine-induced vasculitis in advanced transitional cell carcinoma of the bladder. J Cancer Res Clin Oncol 2004;130(2):122–5.

541. Voorburg AM, van Beek FT, Slee PH, Seldenrijk CA, Schramel FM. Vasculitis due to gemcitabine. Lung Cancer 2002;36(2):203–5.

542. D'Alessandro V, Errico M, Varriale A, Greco A, De Cata A, Carnevale V, Grilli M, De Luca P, Brucoli I, Susi M, Camagna A. Acronecrosi degli arti superiori da gemcitabina: segnalazione di un caso clinico. [Case report: Acro-necrosis of the upper limbs caused by gemcitabine therapy.] Clin Ter 2003;154(3):207–10.

543. Friedlander PA, Bansal R, Schwartz L, Wagman R, Posner J, Kemeny N. Gemcitabine-related radiation recall preferentially involves internal tissue and organs. Cancer 2004;100(9):1793–9.

544. Walton B. Anaesthesia, surgery and immunology. Anaesthesia 1978;33(4):322–48.

545. Ryhanen P. Effects of anaesthesia and operative surgery on the immune response of patients of different ages. Ann Clin Res 1977;19(Suppl):9.

546. Clarke RS. The clinical presentation of anaphylactoid reactions in anesthesia. Int Anesthesiol Clin 1985;23(3):1–16.

547. Peric M, Vranes Z, Marusic M. Immunological disturbances in anaesthetic personnel chronically exposed to high occupational concentrations of nitrous oxide and halothane. Anaesthesia 1991;46(7):531–7.

548. Laxenaire MC, Manel J, Borgo J, Moneret-Vautrin DA. Facteurs de risque d'histamino-libération: étude prospective dans une population anestésie. [Risk factors in histamine liberation: a prospective study in an anesthetized population.] Ann Fr Anesth Reanim 1985;4(2):158–66.

549. Watkins J. Investigation of allergic and hypersensitivity reactions to anaesthetic agents. Br J Anaesth 1987;59(1):104–11.

550. Youngman PR, Taylor KM, Wilson JD. Anaphylactoid reactions to neuromuscular blocking agents: a commonly undiagnosed condition? Lancet 1983;2(8350):597–9.

551. Assem ES. Anaphylactic anaesthetic reactions. The value of paper radioallergosorbent tests for IgE antibodies to muscle relaxants and thiopentone. Anaesthesia 1990;45(12):1032–8.

552. Assem ES, Symons IE. Anaphylaxis due to suxamethonium in a 7-year-old child: a 14-year follow-up with allergy testing. Anaesthesia 1989;44(2):121–4.

553. Sanchez-Perez J, Lopez MP, De Vega Haro JM, Garcia-Diez A. Allergic contact dermatitis from gentamicin in eyedrops, with cross-reactivity to kanamycin but not neomycin. Contact Dermatitis 2001;44(1):54.

554. Descotes J, Lery N, Vigneau C, Loupi E, Evreux JC. Bilan des effets secondaires dus a la glafénine au Centre de Pharmacovigilance de Lyon. [Overview of glafenine side-effects from the experience of Lyon Pharmacovigilance Unit.] Therapie 1980;35(3):405–8.

555. Stricker BH, de Groot RR, Wilson JH. Anaphylaxis to glafenine. Lancet 1990;336(8720):943–4.

556. Stricker BH, de Groot RR, Wilson JH. Glafenine-associated anaphylaxis as a cause of hospital admission in The Netherlands. Eur J Clin Pharmacol 1991;40(4):367–71.

557. Garre M, Youinou P, Burtin C, Rolland J, Deraedt R. Fièvre isolée: effet secondaire singulier de la glafénine. [Isolated fever: an unusual side effect of glafenine.] Therapie 1980;35(6):752–3.

558. Cogen FC, Beezhold DH. Hair glue anaphylaxis: a hidden latex allergy. Ann Allergy Asthma Immunol 2002;88(1):61–3.

559. Wakelin SH. Contact anaphylaxis from natural rubber latex used as an adhesive for hair extensions. Br J Dermatol 2002;146(2):340–1.

560. Kiec-Swierczynska M, Krecisz B, Krysiak B, Kuchowicz E, Rydzynski K. Occupational allergy to aldehydes in health care workers. Clinical observations. Experiments. Int J Occup Med Environ Health 1998;11(4):349–58.

561. Small P. Modified ragweed extract. J Allergy Clin Immunol 1982;69(6):547.

562. Catanzaro JM, Smith JG Jr. Propylene glycol dermatitis. J Am Acad Dermatol 1991;24(1):90–5.

563. Andersen KE. Hudreaktioner fremkaldt af propylenglykol. [Skin reactions caused by propylene glycol.] Ugeskr Laeger 1980;142(38):2478–80.

564. Oochi N, Kbayashi K, Nanishi F, Tsuruda H, Onoyama K, Fujishima M, Omae T. [A case of gold nephropathy associated with polyarteritis nodosa.] Nippon Jinzo Gakkai Shi 1986;28(1):87–94.

565. Korholz D, Nurnberger W, Göbel U, Wahn V. Gold-induzierter systemischer Lupus erythematodes. [Gold-induced systemic lupus erythematosus.] Monatsschr Kinderheilkd 1988;136(9):644–6.

566. Tahara K, Nishiya K, Yoshida T, Matsubara Y, Matsumori A, Ito H, Kumon Y, Hashimoto K, Moriki T, Ookubo S. [A case of secondary systemic amyloidosis associated with rheumatoid arthritis after 3-year disease duration.] Ryumachi 1999;39(1):27–32.

567. Schofield RS, Hill JA, McGinn CJ, Aranda JM. Hormone therapy in men and risk of cardiac allograft rejection. J Heart Lung Transplant 2002;21(4):493–5.

568. Casoli P, Tumiati B, La Sala G. Fatal exacerbation of systemic lupus erythematosus after induction of ovulation. J Rheumatol 1997;24(8):1639–40.

569. Harrison S, Wolf T, Abuzeid MI. Administration of recombinant follicle stimulating hormone in a woman with allergic reaction to menotropin: a case report. Gynecol Endocrinol 2000;14(3):149–52.

570. Battaglia C, Salvatori M, Regnani G, Primavera MR, Genazzani AR, Artini PG, Volpe A. Allergic reaction to a highly purified urinary follicle stimulating hormone preparation in controlled ovarian hyperstimulation for in vitro fertilization. Gynecol Endocrinol 2000;14(3):158–61.

571. Jain KK. Cutaneous vasculitis associated with granulocyte colony-stimulating factor. J Am Acad Dermatol 1994;31(2 Pt 1):213–5.

572. Euler HH, Harten P, Zeuner RA, Schwab UM. Recombinant human granulocyte colony stimulating factor in patients with systemic lupus erythematosus associated neutropenia and refractory infections. J Rheumatol 1997;24(11):2153–7.

573. Jaiyesimi I, Giralt SS, Wood J. Subcutaneous granulocyte colony-stimulating factor and acute anaphylaxis. N Engl J Med 1991;325(8):587.

574. Sasaki O, Yokoyama A, Uemura S, Fujino S, Inoue Y, Kohno N, Hiwada K. Drug eruption caused by recombinant human G-CSF. Intern Med 1994;33(10):641–3.

575. Brown SL, Hill E. Subcutaneous granulocyte colony-stimulating factor and acute anaphylaxis. N Engl J Med 1991;325:587.

576. Stone HD Jr, DiPiro C, Davis PC, Meyer CF, Wray BB. Hypersensitivity reactions to *Escherichia coli*-derived polyethylene glycolated-asparaginase associated with subsequent immediate skin test reactivity to *E. coli*-derived granulocyte colony-stimulating factor. J Allergy Clin Immunol 1998;101(3):429–31.

577. Keung YK, Suwanvecho S, Cobos E. Anaphylactoid reaction to granulocyte colony-stimulating factor used in mobilization of peripheral blood stem cell. Bone Marrow Transplant 1999;23(2):200–1.

578. Shahar E, Krivoy N, Pollack S. Effective acute desensitization for immediate-type hypersensitivity to human granulocyte–monocyte colony stimulating factor. Ann Allergy Asthma Immunol 1999;83(6 Pt 1):543–6.

579. Bokemeyer C, Schmoll HJ, Harstrick A. Side-effects of GM-CSF treatment in advanced testicular cancer. Eur J Cancer 1993;29A(6):924.

580. Shahar E, Krivoy N, Pollack S. Effective acute desensitization for immediate-type hypersensitivity to human granulocyte-monocyte colony stimulating factor. Ann Allergy Asthma Immunol 1999;83(6 Pt 1):543–6.

581. Watsky MS, Lynfield YL. Lupus erythematosus exacerbated by griseofulvin. Cutis 1976;17(2):361–3.

582. Kanerva L, Tupasela O, Jolanki R, Vaheri E, Estlander T, Keskinen H. Occupational allergic rhinitis from guar gum. Clin Allergy 1988;18(3):245–52.

583. Lagier F, Cartier A, Somer J, Dolovich J, Malo JL. Occupational asthma caused by guar gum. J Allergy Clin Immunol 1990;85(4):785–90.

584. Malo JL, Cartier A, L'Archeveque J, Ghezzo H, Soucy F, Somers J, Dolovich J. Prevalence of occupational asthma and immunologic sensitization to guar gum among employees at a carpet-manufacturing plant. J Allergy Clin Immunol 1990;86(4 Pt 1):562–9.

585. Leznoff A, Haight JS, Hoffstein V. Reversible obstructive sleep apnea caused by occupational exposure to guar gum dust. Am Rev Respir Dis 1986;133(5):935–6.

586. Salim A, Shaw S. Recommendation to include ester gum resin when patch testing patients with leg ulcers. Contact Dermatitis 2001;44(1):34.

587. Bonamonte D, Foti C, Angelini G. Contact allergy to ester gums in cosmetics. Contact Dermatitis 2001;45(2):110–1.

588. Sosted H, Agner T, Andersen KE, Menne T. 55 cases of allergic reactions to hair dye: a descriptive, consumer complaint-based study. Contact Dermatitis 2002;47(5):299–303.

589. Fautz R, Fuchs A, van der Walle H, Henny V, Smits L. Hair dye-sensitized hairdressers: the cross-reaction pattern with new generation hair dyes. Contact Dermatitis 2002;46(6):319–24.

590. Tosti A, Pazzaglia M, Corazza M, Virgili A. Allergic contact dermatitis caused by mehindi. Contact Dermatitis 2000;42(6):356.

591. Mohamed M, Nixon R. Severe allergic contact dermatitis induced by paraphenylenediamine in paint-on temporary "tattoos". Australas J Dermatol 2000;41(3):168–71.

592. Lestringant GG, Bener A, Frossard PM. Cutaneous reactions to henna and associated additives. Br J Dermatol 1999;141(3):598–600.

593. Jappe U, Hausen BM, Petzoldt D. Erythema-multiforme-like eruption and depigmentation following allergic contact dermatitis from a paint-on henna tattoo, due to paraphenylenediamine contact hypersensitivity. Contact Dermatitis 2001;45(4):249–50.

594. Pasche-Koo F, French L, Piletta-Zanin PA, Hauser C. Contact urticaria and shock to hair dye. Allergy 1998;53(9):904–5.

595. Fourcade L, Gachot B, De Pina JJ, Heno P, Laurent G, Touze JE. Choc anaphylactique associé au traitement du paludisme par halofantrine. [Anaphylactic shock related to the treatment of malaria with halofantrine.] Presse Méd 1997;26(12):559.

596. Berkun Y, Haviv YS, Schwartz LB, Shalit M. Heparin-induced recurrent anaphylaxis. Clin Exp Allergy 2004;34(12):1916–8.

597. Ainley EJ, Mackie IG, Macarthur D. Adverse reaction to chlorocresol-preserved heparin. Lancet 1977;1(8013):705.

598. Dux S, Pitlik S, Perry G, Rosenfeld JB. Hypersensitivity reaction to chlorbutol-preserved heparin. Lancet 1981;1(8212):149.

599. Miura Y, Hata M, Yuge M, Numano K, Iwakiri K. Allergic contact dermatitis from 1,2,6-hexanetriol in fluocinonide cream. Contact Dermatitis 1999;41(2):118–9.

600. O'Keefe GE, Gentilello LM, Maier RV. Incidence of infectious complications associated with the use of histamine2-receptor antagonists in critically ill trauma patients. Ann Surg 1998;227(1):120–5.

601. Hanisch EW, Encke A, Naujoks F, Windolf J. A randomized, double-blind trial for stress ulcer prophylaxis shows no evidence of increased pneumonia. Am J Surg 1998;176(5):453–7.

602. Ortiz JE, Sottile FD, Sigel P, Nasraway SA. Gastric colonization as a consequence of stress ulcer prophylaxis: a prospective, randomized trial. Pharmacotherapy 1998;18(3):486–91.

603. Andreo JA, Vivancos F, Lopez VM, Soriano J. Vasculitis leucocitoclastica y famotidina. [Leukocytoclastic vasculitis and famotidine.] Med Clin (Barc) 1990;95(6):234–5.

604. Antonov D, Kazandjieva J, Etugov D, Gospodinov D, Tsankov N. Drug-induced lupus erythematosus. Clin Dermatol 2004;22(2):157–66.

605. Jimenez-Alonso J, Jaimez L, Sabio JM, Hidalgo C, Leon L. Atorvastatin-induced reversible positive antinuclear antibodies. Am J Med 2002;112(4):329–30.

606. Sridhar MK, Abdulla A. Fatal lupus-like syndrome and ARDS induced by fluvastatin. Lancet 1998;352(9122):114.

607. Tobert JA, Shear CL, Chremos AN, Mantell GE. Clinical experience with lovastatin. Am J Cardiol 1990;65(12):F23–6.

608. Noel B, Panizzon RG. Lupus-like syndrome associated with statin therapy. Dermatology 2004;208(3):276–7.

609. Khosla R, Butman AN, Hammer DF. Simvastatin-induced lupus erythematosus. South Med J 1998;91(9):873–4.

610. Schuurs AHWM, Geurts TBP, Goorissen EM. Immunologic effects of estrogens, progestins, and estrogen–progestin combinations. In: Goldzieher JW, Fotherby K, editors. Pharmacology of the Contraceptive Steroids. New York: Raven Press, 1994:379–99.

611. Royal College of General Practitioners' Oral Contraception Study. Effect on hypertension and benign breast disease of progestagen component in combined oral contraceptives. Lancet 1977;1(8012):624.

612. Joshi UM, Rao SS, Kora SJ, Dikshit SS, Virkar KD. Effect of steroidal contraceptives on antibody formation in the human female. Contraception 1971;3:327.

613. Hagen C, Froland A. Depressed lymphocyte response to P.H.A. in women taking oral contraceptives Lancet 1972;1(7761):1185.

614. Klinger G, Schubert H, Stelzner A, Krause G, Carol W. Zum Verhalten der Serumimmunoglobulin Titer von IgA, IgG und IgM bei Kurz- und Langzeitapplikation verschiedener hormonaler Kontrazeptiva. [Serum immunoglobulin titer of IgA, IgG and IgM during short- and long-term administration of contraceptive hormones.] Dtsch Gesundheitsw 1978;33(23):1057–62.

615. Huang NH, Li C, Goldzieher JW. Absence of antibodies to ethinyl estradiol in users of oral contraceptive steroids. Fertil Steril 1984;41(4):587–92.

616. Mathur AK, Gatter RA. Chorea as the initial presentation of oral contraceptive induced systemic lupus erythematosus. J Rheumatol 1988;15(6):1042–3.

617. Kulisevsky Bojarski J, Rodriguez de la Serna A, Rovira Gols A, Roig Arnall C. Migraña acompañada como manifestaciôn del lupus eritematoso sistemicon: presentación de 2 casos. [Complicated migraine as a manifestation of systemic lupus erythematosus. Presentation of 2 cases.] Med Clin (Barc) 1986;87(3):112–4.

618. Strom BL, Reidenberg MM, West S, Snyder ES, Freundlich B, Stolley PD. Shingles, allergies, family

medical history, oral contraceptives, and other potential risk factors for systemic lupus erythematosus. Am J Epidemiol 1994;140(7):632–42.

619. Burns MR, Schoch DR, Grayzel AI. Cold urticaria and an oral contraceptive. Ann Intern Med 1983;98(6):1025–6.

620. Pelikan Z. Possible immediate hypersensitivity reaction of the nasal mucosa to oral contraceptives. Ann Allergy 1978;40(3):211–9.

621. Scinto J, Enrione M, Bernstein D, Bernstein IL. In vitro leukocyte histamine release to progesterone and pregnanediol in a patient with recurrent anaphylaxis associated with exogenous administration of progesterone. J Allergy Clin Immunol 1990;85:228.

622. Klinger G, Graser T, Mellinger U, Moore C, Vogelsang H, Groh A, Latterman C, Klinger G. A comparative study of the effects of two oral contraceptives containing dienogest or desogestrel on the human immune system. Gynecol Endocrinol 2000;14(1):15–24.

623. Nagler RM, Pollack S. Sjögren's syndrome induced by estrogen therapy. Semin Arthritis Rheum 2000;30(3):209–14.

624. Andre P. Evaluation of the safety of a non-animal stabilized hyaluronic acid (NASHA—Q-Medical, Sweden) in European countries: a retrospective study from 1997 to 2001. J Eur Acad Dermatol Venereol 2004;18(4):422–5.

625. Choi HK, Merkel PA, Walker AM, Niles JL. Drug-associated antineutrophil cytoplasmic antibody-positive vasculitis: prevalence among patients with high titers of antimyeloperoxidase antibodies. Arthritis Rheum 2000;43(2):405–13.

626. Uetrecht JP. Drug induced lupus: possible mechanisms and their implications for prediction of which new drugs may induce lupus. Exp Opin Invest Drugs 1996;5:851–60.

627. Vaiopoulos G, Terpos E, Viniou N, Nodaros K, Rombos J, Loukopoulos D. Behçet's disease in a patient with chronic myelogenous leukemia under hydroxyurea treatment: a case report and review of the literature. Am J Hematol 2001;66(1):57–8.

628. Moneret-Vautrin DA, Bene MC, Faure G. She should not have chewed. Lancet 1986;1(8481):617.

629. Kahn CR, Rosenthal AS. Immunologic reactions to insulin: insulin allergy, insulin resistance, and the autoimmune insulin syndrome. Diabetes Care 1979;2(3):283–95.

630. deShazo RD, Boehm TM, Kumar D, Galloway JA, Dvorak HF. Dermal hypersensitivity reactions to insulin: correlations of three patterns to their histopathology. J Allergy Clin Immunol 1982;69(2):229–37.

631. Ross JM. Allergy to insulin. Pediatr Clin North Am 1984;31(3):675–87.

632. Yoshino K, Takeda N, Muramatsu M, Morita H, Mune T, Ishizuka T, Yasuda K. [A case of generalized allergy to both human insulin and protamine in insulin preparation.] J Jpn Diabetes Soc 1999;42:927–30

633. Warita E, Shimuzi H, Ubukata T, Mori M. [A case of human insulin allergy.] J Jpn Diabetes Soc 1999;42:1013–5.

634. Abraham MR, al-Sharafi BA, Saavedra GA, Khardori R. Lispro in the treatment of insulin allergy. Diabetes Care 1999;22(11):1916–7.

635. Panczel P, Hosszufalusi N, Horvath MM, Horvath A. Advantage of insulin lispro in suspected insulin allergy. Allergy 2000;55(4):409–10.

636. Eapen SS, Connor EL, Gern JE. Insulin desensitization with insulin lispro and an insulin pump in a 5-year-old child. Ann Allergy Asthma Immunol 2000;85(5):395–7.

637. Sackey AH. Recurrent generalised urticaria at insulin injection sites. BMJ 2000;321(7274):1449.

638. Kumar D. Insulin allergy: differences in the binding of porcine, bovine, and human insulins with anti-insulin IgE. Diabetes Care 1981;4(1):104–7.

639. Soto-Aguilar MC, deShazo RD, Morgan JE, Mather P, Ibrahim G, Frentz JM, Lauritano AA. Total IgG and IgG subclass specific antibody responses to insulin in diabetic patients. Ann Allergy 1991;67(5):499–503.

640. Al-Sheik OA. Unusual local cutaneous reactions to insulin injections: a case report. Saudi Med J 1998;19:199–201.

641. Elte JW, van der Schroeff JG, van Leeuwen AW, Radder JK. Sclerosing granuloma after short-term administration of depot-insulin Hoechst. Case report and a review of the literature. Klin Wochenschr 1982;60(23):1461–4.

642. Jordaan HF, Sandler M. Zinc-induced granuloma—a unique complication of insulin therapy. Clin Exp Dermatol 1989;14(3):227–9.

643. Young RJ, Steel JM, Frier BM, Duncan LJ. Insulin injection sites in diabetes—a neglected area? BMJ (Clin Res Ed) 1981;283(6287):349.

644. Mandrup-Poulsen T, Molvig J, Pildal J, Rasmussen AK, Andersen L, Skov BG, Petersen J. Leukocytoclastic vasculitis induced by subcutaneous injection of human insulin in a patient with type 1 diabetes and essential thrombocytemia. Diabetes Care 2002;25(1):242–3.

645. Airaghi L, Lorini M, Tedeschi A. The insulin analogue aspart: a safe alternative in insulin allergy. Diabetes Care 2001;24(11):2000.

646. Lindholm A, Jensen LB, Home PD, Raskin P, Boehm BO, Rastam J. Immune responses to insulin aspart and biphasic insulin aspart in people with type 1 and type 2 diabetes. Diabetes Care 2002;25(5):876–82.

647. Takata H, Kumon Y, Osaki F, Kumagai C, Arii K, Ikeda Y, Suehiro T, Hashimoto K. The human insulin analogue aspart is not the almighty solution for insulin allergy. Diabetes Care 2003;26(1):253–4.

648. Usui H, Makino H, Shikata K, Sugimoto T, Wada J, Yamana J, Matsuda M, Yoneda M, Koshima I. A case of congenital generalized lipodystrophy with lipoatrophic diabetes developing anti-insulin antibodies. Diabet Med 2002;19(9):794–5.

649. Vague P, Selam JL, Skeie S, De Leeuw I, Elte JW, Haahr H, Kristensen A, Draeger E. Insulin detemir is associated with more predictable glycemic control and reduced risk of hypoglycemia than NPH insulin in patients with type 1 diabetes on a basal-bolus regimen with premeal insulin aspart. Diabetes Care 2003;26(3):590–6.

650. Moriyama H, Nagata M, Fujihira K, Yamada K, Chowdhury SA, Chakrabarty S, Jin Z, Yasuda H, Ueda H, Yokono K. Treatment with human analogue (GlyA21, ArgB31, ArgB32) insulin glargine (HOE901) resolves a generalized allergy to human insulin in type 1 diabetes. Diabetes Care 2001;24(2):411–2.

651. Fineberg SE, Huang J, Brunelle R, Gulliya KS, Anderson JH Jr. Effect of long-term exposure to insulin lispro on the induction of antibody response in patients with type 1 or type 2 diabetes. Diabetes Care 2003;26(1):89–96.

652. Yamamoto T, Sato T, Mori T, Yamakita T, Hasegawa T, Miyamoto M, Hosoi M, Ishii T, Yoshioka K, Tanaka S, Fujii S. Clinical efficacy of insulin-like growth factor-1 in a patient with autoantibodies to insulin receptors: a case report. Diabetes Res Clin Pract 2000;49(1):65–9.

653. Toman Z. Alergicka reakcepo sukcinylcholinjodidu Spofa behem celkove anestezie. [Allergic reaction after succinylcholine iodide Spofa during general anesthesia.] Rozhl Chir 1976;55(12):836–8.

654. Sicherer SH. Risk of severe allergic reactions from the use of potassium iodide for radiation emergencies. J Allergy Clin Immunol 2004;114(6):1395–7.

655. Curd JG, Milgrom H, Stevenson DD, Mathison DA, Vaughan JH. Potassium iodide sensitivity in four patients with hypocomplementemic vasculitis. Ann Intern Med 1979;91(6):853–7.

656. Munoz FJ, Bellido J, Moyano JC, Alvarez MJ, Juan JL. Adverse reaction to potassium iodide from a cough syrup. Allergy 1997;52(1):111–2.

657. Dewachter P, Mouton-Faivre C. Reactions sévères avec les produits de contraste iodes: l'anaphylaxie est-elle responsable?. [Severe reactions to iodinated contrast agents: is anaphylaxis responsible?.] J Radiol 2001;82(9 Pt 1):973–7.

658. Wang DY, Forslund C, Persson U, Wiholm BE. Drug-attributed anaphylaxis. Pharmacoepidemiol Drug Saf 1998;7(4):269–74.

659. Kuwano A, Sugai T, Mochida K. Systemic contact dermatitis induced by oral contrast media for the gallbladder. Skin Res 1993;35(Suppl 16):114–20.

660. Kaude J. Angiografi med jodamid—klinisk provning av ett trijoderat kontrastmedel. [Angiography with iodamide—clinical test of a triiodide contrast medium.] Lakartidningen 1971;68(Suppl 4):42–8.

661. Ansell G, Wilkins RA. Complications in Diagnostic Imaging. 2nd ed. Oxford: Blackwell; 1987.

662. Ridley LJ. Allergic reactions to oral iodinated contrast agents: reactions to oral contrast. Australas Radiol 1998;42(2):114–7.

663. Glover JR, Thomas BM. Case report: severe adverse reaction to oral iohexol. Clin Radiol 1991;44(2):137–8.

664. Lossef SV, Barth KH. Severe delayed hypotensive reaction after ethiodol lymphangiography despite premedication. Am J Roentgenol 1993;161(2):417–8.

665. Zuckerman GB, Riess PL, Patel L, Constantinescu AR, Rosenfeld DL. Development of a life-threatening anaphylactoid reaction following administration of ioversol in a child. Pediatr Radiol 1999;29(4):295–7.

666. Brockow K, Vieluf D, Puschel K, Grosch J, Ring J. Increased postmortem serum mast cell tryptase in a fatal anaphylactoid reaction to nonionic radiocontrast medium. J Allergy Clin Immunol 1999;104(1):237–8.

667. Schnuch A, Geier J, Brasch J, Uter W. The preservative iodopropynyl butylcarbamate: frequency of allergic reactions and diagnostic considerations. Contact Dermatitis 2002;46(3):153–6.

668. Ortega N, Castillo R, Blanco C, Alvarez M, Carrillo T. Oral iron cutaneous adverse reaction and successful desensitization. Ann Allergy Asthma Immunol 2000;84(1):43–5.

669. Slegers-Karsmakers S, Stricker BH. Anaphylactic reaction to isoflurane. Anaesthesia 1988;43(6):506–7.

670. Rothfield NF, Bierer WF, Garfield JW. Isoniazid induction of antinuclear antibodies. A prospective study. Ann Intern Med 1978;88(5):650–2.

671. Hoigne R, Biedermann HP, Naegeli HR. INH-induzierter systemischer Lupus Erythematodes: 2 Beobachtungen mit Reexposition. Schweiz Med Wochenschr 1975;105(50):1726.

672. Hiraoka K, Nagata N, Kawajiri T, Suzuki K, Kurokawa S, Kido M, Sakamoto N. Paradoxical pleural response to antituberculous chemotherapy and isoniazid-induced lupus. Review and report of two cases. Respiration 1998;65(2):152–5.

673. Cooper SM, Shaw S. Contact allergy to isopropanolamine in Traxam gel. Contact Dermatitis 1999;41(4):233–4.

674. Park H, Knowles S, Shear NH. Serum sickness-like reaction to itraconazole. Ann Pharmacother 1998;32(11):1249.

675. Chung CW, Carson TR. Cross-sensitivity of common aminoglycoside antibiotics. Arch Dermatol 1976;112(8):1101–7.

676. Schlienger RG, Knowles SR, Shear NH. Lamotrigine-associated anticonvulsant hypersensitivity syndrome. Neurology 1998;51(4):1172–5.

677. Pathak P, McLachlan RS. Drug-induced pseudolymphoma secondary to lamotrigine. Neurology 1998;50(5):1509–10.

678. Sarris BM, Wong JG. Multisystem hypersensitivity reaction to lamotrigine. Neurology 1999;53(6):1367.

679. Fervenza FC, Kanakiriya S, Kunau RT, Gibney R, Lager DJ. Acute granulomatous interstitial nephritis and colitis in anticonvulsant hypersensitivity syndrome associated with lamotrigine treatment. Am J Kidney Dis 2000;36(5):1034–40.

680. Schaub N, Bircher AJ. Severe hypersensitivity syndrome to lamotrigine confirmed by lymphocyte stimulation in vitro. Allergy 2000;55(2):191–3.

681. Sarzi-Puttini P, Panni B, Cazzola M, Muzzupappa S, Turiel M. Lamotrigine-induced lupus. Lupus 2000;9(7):555–7.

682. Anonymous. Allergic reactions to Latex-containing medical devices. FDA Med Bull 1991;91(July):2–3.

683. Dillard SF. Natural rubber latex allergy. FDA Med Bull 1997;27(2):4.

684. Anonymous. Latex in devices—regulations concerning health and safety. WHO Pharm Newslett 1995;5/6:19.

685. Anonymous. Latex containing devices—labelling required. WHO Pharm Newslett 1997;1&2:16–7.

686. Frosch PJ, Schulze-Dirks A. Kontaktallergie durch Polidocanol (Thesis). [Contact allergy caused by polidocanol (thesis).] Hautarzt 1989;40(3):146–9.

687. Uter W, Geier J, Fuchs T. IVDK Study Group. Contact allergy to polidocanol, 1992 to 1999. J Allergy Clin Immunol 2000;106(6):1203–4.

688. Smythe MA, Cappelletty DM. Anaphylactoid reaction to levofloxacin. Pharmacotherapy 2000;20(12):1520–3.

689. Mori K, Maru C, Takasuna K, Furuhama K. Mechanism of histamine release induced by levofloxacin, a fluoroquinolone antibacterial agent. Eur J Pharmacol 2000;394(1):51–5.

690. Weightman W, Turner T. Allergic contact dermatitis from lignocaine: report of 29 cases and review of the literature. Contact Dermatitis 1998;39(5):265–6.

691. Caumes E, Bocquet H, Guermonprez G, Rogeaux O, Bricaire F, Katlama C, Gentilini M. Adverse cutaneous reactions to pyrimethamine/sulfadiazine and pyrimethamine/clindamycin in patients with AIDS and toxoplasmic encephalitis. Clin Infect Dis 1995;21(3):656–8.

692. Lammintausta K, Tokola R, Kalimo K. Cutaneous adverse reactions to clindamycin: results of skin tests and oral exposure. Br J Dermatol 2002;146(4):643–8.

693. Marcos C, Sopena B, Luna I, Gonzalez R, de la Fuente J, Martinez-Vazquez C. Clindamycin desensitization in an AIDS patient. AIDS 1995;9(10):1201–2.

694. Fagan JE. Henoch-Schonlein purpura and gamma-benzene hexachloride. Pediatrics 1981;67(2):310–1.

695. Guin JD. Allergic contact cheilitis from di-isostearyl malate in lipstick. Contact Dermatitis 2001;44(6):375.

696. Asai M, Kawada A, Aragane Y, Tezuka T. Allergic contact cheilitis due to glyceryl monoisostearate monomyristate in a lipstick. Contact Dermatitis 2001;45(3):173.

697. Kimura M, Kawada A. Contact dermatitis due to 2-hexyldecanoic acid (isopalmitate) in a lipstick. Contact Dermatitis 1999;41(2):99–100.

698. Suzuki K, Matsunaga K, Suzuki M. Allergic contact dermatitis due to isopalmityl diglyceryl sebacate in a lipstick. Contact Dermatitis 1999;41(2):110.

699. Clark KJ, Jefferson JW. Lithium allergy. J Clin Psychopharmacol 1987;7(4):287–9.

700. Lowry MD, Hudson CF, Callen JP. Leukocytoclastic vasculitis caused by drug additives. J Am Acad Dermatol 1994;30(5 Part 2):854–5.

701. Kang BJ, Park SW, Chung TH. Can the expression of histocompatibility antigen be changed by lithium? Int J Neuropsychopharmacol 1999;2(Suppl 1):S55.

702. Rapaport MH, Manji HK. The effects of lithium on ex vivo cytokine production. Biol Psychiatry 2001;50(3):217–24.

703. Merendino RA, Arena A, Gangemi S, Ruello A, Losi E, Bene A, Valenti A, D'Ambrosio FP. In vitro effect of lithium chloride on interleukin-15 production by monocytes from IL-breast cancer patients. J Chemother 2000;12(3):252–7.

704. Merendino RA, Arena A, Gangemi S, Ruello A, Losi E, Bene A, D'Ambrosio FP. In vitro interleukin-8 production by monocytes treated with lithium chloride from breast cancer patients. Tumori 2000;86(2):149–52.

705. Rybakowski JK. The effect of lithium on the immune system. Hum Psychopharmacol 1999;14:345–53.

706. Harvey BH, Meyer CL, Gallicchio VS. The hemopoietic and immuno-modulating action of lithium salts: an investigation into the chemotherapy of HIV infection in South Africa. In: Lucas KC, Becker RW, Gallicchio VS, editors. Lithium-50 Years: Recent Advances in Biology and Medicine. Cheshire, Connecticut: Weidner Publishing, 1999:137–52.

707. Maes M, Song C, Lin AH, Pioli R, Kenis G, Kubera M, Bosmans E. In vitro immunoregulatory effects of lithium in healthy volunteers. Psychopharmacology (Berl) 1999; 143(4):401–7.

708. Rapaport MH, Guylai L, Whybrow P. Immune parameters in rapid cycling bipolar patients before and after lithium treatment. J Psychiatr Res 1999;33(4):335–40.

709. Rybakowski JK. Antiviral and immunomodulatory effect of lithium. Pharmacopsychiatry 2000;33(5):159–64.

710. Kang BJ, Park SW, Chung TH. Can the expression of histocompatibility antigen be changed by lithium? Bipolar Disord 2000;2(2):140–4.

711. Fisher MM, Bowey CJ. Alleged allergy to local anaesthetics. Anaesth Intensive Care 1997;25(6):611–4.

712. Fernandez-Redondo V, Leon A, Santiago T, Toribio J. Allergic contact dermatitis from local anaesthetic on peristomal skin. Contact Dermatitis 2001;45(6):358.

713. McGough EK, Cohen JA. Unexpected bronchospasm during spinal anesthesia. J Clin Anesth 1990;2(1):35–6.

714. Kearney CR, Fewings J. Allergic contact dermatitis to cinchocaine. Australas J Dermatol 2001;42(2):118–9.

715. Erdmann SM, Sachs B, Merk HF. Systemic contact dermatitis from cinchocaine. Contact Dermatitis 2001;44(4):260–1.

716. Hayashi K, Kawachi S, Saida T. Allergic contact dermatitis due to both chlorpheniramine maleate and dibucaine hydrochloride in an over-the-counter medicament. Contact Dermatitis 2001;44(1):38–9.

717. Hiyoshi K, Iwanaga Y, Kado K, Takeda K. [Allergic reactions caused by mepivacaine ECG changes after spinal anesthesia using mepivacaine.] Masui 1978;27(2):177–80.

718. Moriwaki K, Higaki A, Sasaki H, Murata K, Sumida T, Baba I. [A case report of anaphylactic shock induced by tetracaine used for spinal anesthesia.] Masui 1986;35(8):1279–84.

719. Redfern DC. Contact sensitivity to multiple local anesthetics. J Allergy Clin Immunol 1999;104(4 Pt 1):890–1.

720. Orasch CE, Helbling A, Zanni MP, Yawalkar N, Hari Y, Pichler WJ. T-cell reaction to local anaesthetics: relationship to angioedema and urticaria after subcutaneous application—patch testing and LTT in patients with adverse reaction to local anaesthetics. Clin Exp Allergy 1999;29(11):1549–54.

721. Ball IA. Allergic reactions to lignocaine. Br Dent J 1999;186(5):224–6.

722. Walters G, Georgiou T, Hayward JM. Sight-threatening acute orbital swelling from peribulbar local anesthesia. J Cataract Refract Surg 1999;25(3):444–6.

723. Nakada T, Iijima M. Allergic contact dermatitis from dibucaine hydrochloride. Contact Dermatitis 2000;42(5):283.

724. Kakuyama M, Toda H, Osawa M, Fukuda K. An adverse effect of carboxymethylcellulose in lidocaine jelly. Anesthesiology 1999;91(6):1969.

725. Hammer R, Dahlgren C, Stendahl O. Inhibition of human leukocyte metabolism and random mobility by local anaesthesia. Acta Anaesthesiol Scand 1985;29(5):520–3.

726. Gall H, Kaufmann R, Kalveram CM. Adverse reactions to local anesthetics: analysis of 197 cases. J Allergy Clin Immunol 1996;97(4):933–7.

727. Breit S, Rueff F, Przybilla B. "Deep impact" contact allergy after subcutaneous injection of local anesthetics. Contact Dermatitis 2001;45(5):296–7.

728. Kawsar M, El-Gadi S. Subcutaneous granulomatous lesions related to ritonavir therapy in a HIV infected patient. Int J STD AIDS 2002;13(4):273–4.

729. Nakamura H, Fujishima S, Inoue T, Ohkubo Y, Soejima K, Waki Y, Mori M, Urano T, Sakamaki F, Tasaka S, Ishizaka A, Kanazawa M, Yamaguchi K. Clinical and immunoregulatory effects of roxithromycin therapy for chronic respiratory tract infection. Eur Respir J 1999;13(6):1371–9.

730. Khan AA, Slifer TR, Araujo FG, Remington JS. Effect of clarithromycin and azithromycin on production of cytokines by human monocytes. Int J Antimicrob Agents 1999;11(2):121–32.

731. Suzaki H, Asano K, Ohki S, Kanai K, Mizutani T, Hisamitsu T. Suppressive activity of a macrolide antibiotic, roxithromycin, on pro-inflammatory cytokine production in vitro and in vivo. Mediators Inflamm 1999;8(4–5):199–204.

732. Yatsunami J, Fukuno Y, Nagata M, Tsuruta N, Aoki S, Tominaga M, Kawashima M, Taniguchi S, Hayashi S. Roxithromycin and clarithromycin, 14-membered ring macrolides, potentiate the antitumor activity of cytotoxic agents against mouse B16 melanoma cells. Cancer Lett 1999;147(1–2):17–24.

733. Yatsunami J, Fukuno Y, Nagata M, Tominaga M, Aoki S, Tsuruta N, Kawashima M, Taniguchi S, Hayashi S. Antiangiogenic and antitumor effects of 14-membered ring macrolides on mouse B16 melanoma cells. Clin Exp Metastasis 1999;17(4):361–7.

734. Nonaka M, Pawankar R, Tomiyama S, Yagi T. A macrolide antibiotic, roxithromycin, inhibits the growth of nasal polyp fibroblasts. Am J Rhinol 1999;13(4):267–72.

735. Hubner C, Dietz A, Stremmel W, Stiehl A, Andrassy H. Macrolide-induced Churg–Strauss syndrome in a patient with atopy. Lancet 1997;350(9077):563.

736. Dietz A, Hubner C, Andrassy K. Makrolid–Antibiotika indurierte Vaskulitis (Churg–Strauss syndrome). [Macrolide antibiotic-induced vasculitis (Churg–Strauss syndrome).] Laryngorhinootologie 1998;77(2):111–4.

737. Shimane T, Asano K, Suzuki M, Hisamitsu T, Suzaki H. Influence of a macrolide antibiotic, roxithromycin, on mast cell growth and activation in vitro. Mediators Inflamm 2001;10(6):323–32.

738. Richeldi L, Rossi G, Ruggieri MP, Corbetta L, Fabbri LM. Churg–Strauss syndrome in a case of asthma. Allergy 2002;57(7):647–8.

739. Gavura SR, Nusinowitz S. Leukocytoclastic vasculitis associated with clarithromycin. Ann Pharmacother 1998;32(5):543–5.

740. Goldberg EI, Shoji T, Sapadin AN. Henoch–Schönlein purpura induced by clarithromycin. Int J Dermatol 1999;38(9):706–8.

741. Gallardo MA, Thomas I. Hypersensitivity reaction to erythromycin. Cutis 1999;64(6):375–6.

742. Selo-Ojeme DO, Tillisi A, Welch CC. Anaphylaxis from medroxyprogesterone acetate. Obstet Gynecol 2004;103(5 Pt 2):1045–6.

793. Margolin N. Severe leucocytoclastic vasculitis induced by repaglinide in a patient with chronic hepatitis C. Clin Drug Invest 2002;22:795–6.

794. Spitzer RL, Terman M, Williams JB, Terman JS, Malt UF, Singer F, Lewy AJ. Jet lag: clinical features, validation of a new syndrome-specific scale, and lack of response to melatonin in a randomized, double-blind trial. Am J Psychiatry 1999;156(9):1392–6.

795. Morton CA, Garioch J, Todd P, Lamey PJ, Forsyth A. Contact sensitivity to menthol and peppermint in patients with intraoral symptoms. Contact Dermatitis 1995;32(5):281–4.

796. Audicana MT, Munoz D, del Pozo MD, Fernandez E, Gastaminza G, Fernandez de Corres L. Allergic contact dermatitis from mercury antiseptics and derivatives: study protocol of tolerance to intramuscular injections of thimerosal. Am J Contact Dermat 2002;13(1):3–9.

797. Pelclova D, Lukas E, Urban P, Preiss J, Rysava R, Lebenhart P, Okrouhlik B, Fenclova Z, Lebedova J, Stejskalova A, Ridzon P. Mercury intoxication from skin ointment containing mercuric ammonium chloride. Int Arch Occup Environ Health 2002;75(Suppl):S54–9.

798. Bernard S, Enayati A, Roger H, Binstock T, Redwood L. The role of mercury in the pathogenesis of autism. Mol Psychiatry 2002;7(Suppl 2):S42–3.

799. Pichichero ME, Cernichiari E, Lopreiato J, Treanor J. Mercury concentrations and metabolism in infants receiving vaccines containing thiomersal: a descriptive study. Lancet 2002;360(9347):1737–41.

800. Nordstrom DM, West SG, Rubin RL. Methyldopa-induced systemic lupus erythematosus. Arthritis Rheum 1989;32(2):205–8.

801. O'Connor A, Cluroe A, Couch R, Galler L, Lawrence J, Synek B. Death from hyponatraemia-induced cerebral oedema associated with MDMA ("Ecstasy") use. NZ Med J 1999;112(1091):255–6.

802. Hartung TK, Schofield E, Short AI, Parr MJ, Henry JA. Hyponatraemic states following 3,4-methylenedioxymethamphetamine (MDMA, "ecstasy") ingestion. Quart J Med 2002;95(7):431–7.

803. Daniels PR, Berry GJ, Tazelaar HD, Cooper LT. Giant cell myocarditis as a manifestation of drug hypersensitivity. Cardiovasc Pathol 2000;9(5):287–91.

804. Daniels PR, Berry GJ, Tazelaar HD, Cooper LT. Giant cell myocarditis as a manifestation of drug hypersensitivity. Cardiovasc Pathol 2000;9(5):287–91.

805. Borczuk AC, Petterino B, Alt E. Inflammatory mass with fibrinoid necrosis of vessels caused by methylene blue marking of a colonic polyp. Cardiovasc Pathol 1998;7:267–9.

806. Flaker GC, Beach CL, Chapman D. Adverse side effects associated with mexiletine. Clin Progr Electrophysiol Pacing 1986;4:602–7.

807. Stein J, Podrid PJ, Lampert S, Hirsowitz G, Lown B. Long-term mexiletine for ventricular arrhythmia. Am Heart J 1984;107(5 Pt 2):1091–8.

808. Johansson BW, Stavenow L. Long-term clinical effects and side effects of mexiletine in patients with ventricular arrhythmias. Clin Progr Electrophysiol Pacing 1986;4:589–94.

809. Johansson BW, Stavenow L, Hanson A. Long-term clinical experience with mexiletine. Am Heart J 1984;107(5 Pt 2):1099–102.

810. Puyana J, Urena V, Quirce S, Fernandez-Rivas M, Cuevas M, Fraj J. Serum sickness-like syndrome associated with minocycline therapy. Allergy 1990;45(4):313–5.

811. Angulo JM, Sigal LH, Espinoza LR. Coexistent minocycline-induced systemic lupus erythematosus and autoimmune hepatitis. Semin Arthritis Rheum 1998;28(3):187–92.

812. Akin E, Miller LC, Tucker LB. Minocycline-induced lupus in adolescents. Pediatrics 1998;101(5):926.

813. Hess E. Drug-related lupus. N Engl J Med 1988;318(22):1460–2.

814. Gordon MM, Porter D. Minocycline induced lupus: case series in the West of Scotland. J Rheumatol 2001;28(5):1004–6.

815. Lawson TM, Amos N, Bulgen D, Williams BD. Minocycline-induced lupus: clinical features and response to rechallenge. Rheumatology (Oxford) 2001;40(3):329–35.

816. Graham LE, Bell AL. Minocycline-associated lupus-like syndrome with ulnar neuropathy and antiphospholipid antibody. Clin Rheumatol 2001;20(1):67–9.

817. Sturkenboom MC, Meier CR, Jick H, Stricker BH. Minocycline and lupuslike syndrome in acne patients. Arch Intern Med 1999;159(5):493–7.

818. Marzo-Ortega H, Misbah S, Emery P. Minocycline induced autoimmune disease in rheumatoid arthritis: a missed diagnosis? J Rheumatol 2001;28(2):377–8.

819. Shapiro LE, Knowles SR, Shear NH. Comparative safety of tetracycline, minocycline, and doxycycline. Arch Dermatol 1997;133(10):1224–30.

820. Ghate JV, Turner ML, Rudek MA, Figg WD, Dahut W, Dyer V, Pluda JM, Reed E. Drug-induced lupus associated with COL-3: report of 3 cases. Arch Dermatol 2001;137(4):471–4.

821. Christodoulou CS, Emmanuel P, Ray RA, Good RA, Schnapf BM, Cawkwell GD. Respiratory distress due to minocycline-induced pulmonary lupus. Chest 1999;115(5):1471–3.

822. Oddo M, Liaudet L, Lepori M, Broccard AF, Schaller MD. Relapsing acute respiratory failure induced by minocycline. Chest 2003;123(6):2146–8.

823. Singer SJ, Piazza-Hepp TD, Girardi LS, Moledina NR. Lupuslike reaction associated with minocycline. JAMA 1997;277(4):295–6.

824. Masson C, Chevailler A, Pascaretti C, Legrand E, Bregeon C, Audran M. Minocycline related lupus. J Rheumatol 1996;23(12):2160–1.

825. Bonnotte B, Gresset AC, Chauffert B, Courtois JM, Martin F, Collet E, Sgro C, Lorcerie B. Symptomes évocateurs de maladie de système chez des patients prenant du chlorhydrate de minocycline. [Early signs of systemic disease in patients taking minocycline chlorhydrate.] Presse Méd 1999;28(21):1105–8.

826. Colamarino R, Dubost JJ, Brun P, Flori B, Tournilhac M, Eschalier A, Sauvezie B. Etats polyalgiques induits par le

minoxidil topique. [Polymyalgia induced by topical minoxidil.] Ann Med Interne (Paris) 1990;141(5):425–8.

827. Friedman ES, Friedman PM, Cohen DE, Washenik K. Allergic contact dermatitis to topical minoxidil solution: etiology and treatment. J Am Acad Dermatol 2002;46(2):309–12.

828. Trattner A, David M. Pigmented contact dermatitis from topical minoxidil 5%. Contact Dermatitis 2002;46(4):246.

829. Sinclair RD, Mallari RS, Tate B. Sensitization to saw palmetto and minoxidil in separate topical extemporaneous treatments for androgenetic alopecia. Australas J Dermatol 2002;43(4):311–2.

830. Suzuki K, Suzuki M, Akamatsu H, Matsungaga K. Allergic contact dermatitis from minoxidil: study of the cross-reaction to minoxidil. Am J Contact Dermat 2002;13(1):45–6.

831. Adkinson NF Jr. Immunogenicity and cross-allergenicity of aztreonam. Am J Med 1990;88(3C):S12–5; discussion S38–42.

832. Cui W, Lei MG, Silverstein R, Morrison DC. Differential modulation of the induction of inflammatory mediators by antibiotics in mouse macrophages in response to viable Gram-positive and Gram-negative bacteria. J Endotoxin Res 2003;9(4):225–36.

833. Adkinson NF Jr, Swabb EA, Sugerman AA. Immunology of the monobactam aztreonam. Antimicrob Agents Chemother 1984;25(1):93–7.

834. Saxon A, Beall GN, Rohr AS, et al. Immediate hypersensitivity reactions to beta-lactam antibiotics. Urology 1988;31(Suppl):14.

835. Saxon A, Beall GN, Rohr AS, Adelman DC. Immediate hypersensitivity reactions to beta-lactam antibiotics. Ann Intern Med 1987;107(2):204–15.

836. Adkinson NF Jr, Wheeler B Jr, Swabb EA Jr. Clinical tolerance of the monobactam aztreonam in penicillin-allergic subjects. In: Proceedings, 14th International Congress of Chemotherapy 1985:155. Abstract WS-26–4. Kyoto, Japan.

837. Loria RC, Finnerty N, Wedner HJ. Successful use of aztreonam in a patient who failed oral penicillin desensitization. J Allergy Clin Immunol 1989;83(4):735–7.

838. Jensen T, Koch C, Pedersen SS, Hoiby N. Aztreonam for cystic fibrosis patients who are hypersensitive to other beta-lactams. Lancet 1987;1(8545):1319–20.

839. Hantson P, de Coninck B, Horn JL, Mahieu P. Immediate hypersensitivity to aztreonam and imipenem. BMJ 1991;302(6771):294–5.

840. Iglesias Cadarso A, Saez Jimenez SA, Vidal Pan C, Rodriguez Mosquera M. Aztreonam-induced anaphylaxis. Lancet 1990;336(8717):746–7.

841. Soto Alvarez J, Sacristan del Castillo JA, Sampedro Garcia I, Alsar Ortiz MJ. Immediate hypersensitivity to aztreonam. Lancet 1990;335(8697):1094.

842. Moss RB, McClelland E, Williams RR, Hilman BC, Rubio T, Adkinson NF. Evaluation of the immunologic cross-reactivity of aztreonam in patients with cystic fibrosis who are allergic to penicillin and/or cephalosporin antibiotics. Rev Infect Dis 1991;13(Suppl 7):S598–607.

843. Matheu V, Sierra Z, Gracia MT, Caloto M, Alcazar MM, Martinez MI, Zapatero L. Morniflumate-induced urticaria–angioedema. Allergy 1998;53(8):812–3.

844. Stablein JJ, Bucholtz GA, Lockey RF. *Melaleuca* tree and respiratory disease. Ann Allergy Asthma Immunol 2002;89(5):523–30.

845. Abe S, Suzuki T, Hori T, Baba A, Shiraishi H. Hypogammaglobulinemia during antipsychotic therapy. Psychiatry Clin Neurosci 1998;52(1):115–7.

846. McNeil HP, Chesterman CN, Krilis SA. Immunology and clinical importance of antiphospholipid antibodies. Adv Immunol 1991;49:193–280.

847. Lillicrap MS, Wright G, Jones AC. Symptomatic antiphospholipid syndrome induced by chlorpromazine. Br J Rheumatol 1998;37(3):346–7.

848. Pramatarov KD. Drug-induced lupus erythematosus. Clin Dermatol 1998;16(3):367–77.

849. Krohn K, Bennett R. Drug-induced autoimmune disorders. Inmunol Allergy Clin North Am 1998;18:897–911.

850. McNevin S, MacKay M. Chlorprothixene-induced systemic lupus erythematosus. J Clin Psychopharmacol 1982; 2(6):411–2.

851. Krombach J, Hunzelmann N, Koster F, Bischoff A, Hoffmann-Menzel H, Buzello W. Anaphylactoid reactions after cisatracurium administration in six patients. Anesth Analg 2001;93(5):1257–9.

852. Legros CB, Orliaguet GA, Mayer MN, Labbez F, Carli PA. Severe anaphylactic reaction to cisatracurium in a child. Anesth Analg 2001;92(3):648–9.

853. Briassoulis G, Hatzis T, Mammi P, Alikatora A. Persistent anaphylactic reaction after induction with thiopentone and cisatracurium. Paediatr Anaesth 2000;10(4):429–34.

854. Mertes PM, Laxenaire MC. Allergic reactions occurring during anaesthesia. Eur J Anaesthesiol 2002;19(4):240–62.

855. Laxenaire MC, Moneret-Vautrin DA, Watkins J. Diagnosis of the causes of anaphylactoid anaesthetic reactions. A report of the recommendations of the joint Anaesthetic and Immuno-allergological Workshop, Nancy, France: 19 March 1982. Anaesthesia 1983;38(2):147–8.

856. Fisher MM, More DG. The epidemiology and clinical features of anaphylactic reactions in anaesthesia. Anaesth Intensive Care 1981;9(3):226–34.

857. Laxenaire MC. Epidémiologie des réactions anaphylactoïdes peranesthésiques. Quatrième enquête multicentrique (juillet 1994–décembre 1996). [Epidemiology of anesthetic anaphylactoid reactions. Fourth multicenter survey (July 1994–December 1996).] Ann Fr Anesth Reanim 1999;18(7):796–809.

858. Hatton F, Tiret L, Maujol L, N'Doye P, Vourc'h G, Desmonts JM, Otteni JC, Scherpereel P. INSERM. Enquête épidémiologique sur les anesthésies. Premiers résultats. [INSERM. Epidemiological survey of anesthesia. Initial results.] Ann Fr Anesth Reanim 1983;2(5):331–86.

859. Thornton JA, Lorenz W. Histamine and antihistamine in anaesthesia and surgery: report of a symposium. Anaesthesia 1983;38:373.

860. Fisher MM, Munro I. Life-threatening anaphylactoid reactions to muscle relaxants. Anesth Analg 1983;62(6):559–64.

861. Boileau S, Hummer-Sigiel M, Moeller R, Drouet N. Réévaluation des risques respectifs d'anaphylaxie et d'histaminoblitération avec les substances anesthésiologiques. [Reassessment of the respective risks of anaphylaxis and histamine liberation with anesthetic substances.] Ann Fr Anesth Reanim 1985;4(2):195–204.

862. Laxenaire MC. Substances responsables des chocs anaphylactiques peranesthésiques. Troisième enquête multicentrique française (1992–1994). [Substances responsible for peranesthetic anaphylactic shock. A third French multicenter study (1992–94).] Ann Fr Anesth Reanim 1996;15(8):1211–8.

863. Laxenaire MC, Moneret-Vautrin DA, Vervloet D, Alazia M, Francois G. Accidents anaphylactoïdes graves peranesthésiques. [Severe perianesthetic anaphylactic accidents.] Ann Fr Anesth Reanim 1985;4(1):30–46.

864. Laxenaire MC, Moneret-Vautrin DA, Vervloet D. The French experience of anaphylactoid reactions. Int Anesthesiol Clin 1985;23(3):145–60.

865. Galletly DC, Treuren BC. Anaphylactoid reactions during anaesthesia. Seven years' experience of intradermal testing. Anaesthesia 1985;40(4):329–33.

866. Pepys J, Pepys EO, Baldo BA, Whitwam JG. Anaphylactic/anaphylactoid reactions to anaesthetic and associated agents. Skin prick tests in aetiological diagnosis. Anaesthesia 1994;49(6):470–5.

867. Mertes PM, Laxenaire MC, Alla F. Groupe d'Etudes des Réactions Anaphylactoïdes Peranesthésiques. Anaphylactic and anaphylactoid reactions occurring during anesthesia in France in 1999–2000. Anesthesiology 2003;99(3):536–45.

868. Laxenaire MC, Mertes PM. Groupe d'Etudes des Réactions Anaphylactoïdes Peranesthésiques. Anaphylaxis during anaesthesïa. Results of a two-year survey in France. Br J Anaesth 2001;87(4):549–58.

869. Laxenaire M, Mertes P. Anaphylaxis during anaesthesia. Br J Anaesth 2002;88:605–6.

870. Grimaudo NJ. Biocompatibility of nickel and cobalt dental alloys. Gen Dent 2001;49(5):498–503.

871. Budinger L, Hertl M. Immunologic mechanisms in hypersensitivity reactions to metal ions: an overview. Allergy 2000;55(2):108–15.

872. Mancuso G, Berdondini RM. Eyelid dermatitis and conjunctivitis as sole manifestations of allergy to nickel in an orthodontic appliance. Contact Dermatitis 2002;46(4):245.

873. Kerosuo H, Kullaa A, Kerosuo E, Kanerva L, Hensten-Pettersen A. Nickel allergy in adolescents in relation to orthodontic treatment and piercing of ears. Am J Orthod Dentofacial Orthop 1996;109(2):148–54.

874. Lindsten R, Kurol J. Orthodontic appliances in relation to nickel hypersensitivity. A review. J Orofac Orthop 1997;58(2):100–8.

875. Block GT, Yeung M. Asthma induced by nickel. JAMA 1982;247(11):1600–2.

876. Niordson AM. Nickel sensitivity as a cause of rhinitis. Contact Dermatitis 1981;7(5):273–4.

877. Wahlberg JE. Nickel allergy in hairdressers. Contact Dermatitis 1981;7(6):358–9.

878. Di Gioacchino M, Masci S, Cavallucci E, Pavone G, Andreassi M, Gravante M, Pizzicannella G, Boscolo P. Modificazioni immuno-istopatologiche della mucosa gastro-intestinale in pazient; con allergia da contatto al nichel. [Immuno-histopathologic changes in the gastrointestinal mucosa in patients with nickel contact allergy.] G Ital Med Lav 1995;17(1–6):33–6.

879. Al-Tawil NG, Marcusson JA, Moller E. Lymphocyte transformation test in patients with nickel sensitivity: an aid to diagnosis. Acta Derm Venereol 1981;61(6):511–5.

880. Kapoor-Pillarisetti A, Mowbray JF, Brostoff J, Cronin EA. HLA dependence of sensitivity to nickel and chromium. Tissue Antigens 1981;17(3):261–4.

881. Bauer A, Geier J, Elsner P. Allergic contact dermatitis in patients with anogenital complaints. J Reprod Med 2000;45(8):649–54.

882. Marren P, Wojnarowska F, Powell S. Allergic contact dermatitis and vulvar dermatoses. Br J Dermatol 1992;126(1):52–6.

883. Lucke TW, Fleming CJ, McHenry P, Lever R. Patch testing in vulval dermatoses: how relevant is nickel? Contact Dermatitis 1998;38(2):111–2.

884. Bresser H. Orale Nickelprovokation und nickelarme Diät. Indikation und praktische Durchfuhrung. [Oral nickel provocation and a nickel-free diet. Indications and practical implementation.] Hautarzt 1992;43(10):610–5.

885. Choy EH, Gambling L, Best SL, Jenkins RE, Kondeatis E, Vaughan R, Black MM, Sadler PJ, Panayi GS. Nickel contamination of gold salts: link with gold-induced skin rash. Br J Rheumatol 1997;36(10):1054–8.

886. Gimenez-Arnau A, Riambau V, Serra-Baldrich E, Camarasa JG. Metal-induced generalized pruriginous dermatitis and endovascular surgery. Contact Dermatitis 2000;43(1):35–40.

887. Pazzaglia M, Lucente P, Vincenzi C, Tosti A. Contact dermatitis from nickel in mobile phones. Contact Dermatitis 2000;42(6):362–3.

888. Van der Klauw MM, Van Hillo B, Van den Berg WH, Bolsius EP, Sutorius FF, Stricker BH. Vasculitis attributed to the nicotine patch (Nicotinell). Br J Dermatol 1996;134(2):361–4.

889. Anonymous. Vasculitis attributed to the nicotine patch (Nicotinell). WHO Newslett 1996;7:5.

890. Britton ML, Bradberry JC, Letassy NA, Mckenney JM, Sirmans SM. ASHP Therapeutic Position Statement on the safe use of niacin in the management of dyslipidemias. American Society of Health-System Pharmacists. Am J Health Syst Pharm 1997;54(24):2815–9.

891. Grouhi M, Sussman G. Pseudoallergic toxic reaction. Ann Allergy Asthma Immunol 2000;85(4):269–71.

892. Teppo AM, Haltia K, Wager O. Immunoelectrophoretic "tailing" of albumin line due to albumin-IgG antibody complexes: a side effect of nitrofurantoin treatment? Scand J Immunol 1976;5(3):249–61.

893. Stevenson DD, Sanchez-Borges M, Szczeklik A. Classification of allergic and pseudoallergic reactions to drugs that inhibit cyclooxygenase enzymes. Ann Allergy Asthma Immunol 2001;87(3):177–80.

894. Eaton RA. A comparison of anaphylactoid reactions associated with non-steroidal anti-inflammatory drugs. ADR Highlights 1981;8116:.

895. Strom BL, Carson JL, Schinnar R, Sim E, Morse ML. The effect of indication on the risk of hypersensitivity reactions associated with tolmetin sodium vs other nonsteroidal anti-inflammatory drugs. J Rheumatol 1988;15(4):695–9.

896. Czerniawska-Mysik G, Szczeklik A. Idiosyncrasy to pyrazolone drugs. Allergy 1981;36(6):381–4.

897. Anonymous. Sensitisation to bee and wasp stings with NSAIDs/ACE inhibition. Reactions 1999;3:747.

898. Stevens DL. Could nonsteroidal antiinflammatory drugs (NSAIDs) enhance the progression of bacterial infections to toxic shock syndrome? Clin Infect Dis 1995;21(4):977–80.

899. Barnham M, Anderson AW. Non-steroidal anti-inflammatory drugs (NSAIDs). A predisposing factor for streptococcal bacteraemia? Adv Exp Med Biol 1997;418:145–7.

900. Rivey MP, Allington DR, Henry Dunham AL. Necrotising fasciitis in an elderly patient: case report. Pharm Technol 1998;14:58–62.

901. Kahn LH, Styrt BA. Necrotizing soft tissue infections reported with nonsteroidal antiinflammatory drugs. Ann Pharmacother 1997;31(9):1034–9.

902. del Pozo MD, Lobera T, Blasco A. Selective hypersensitivity to diclofenac. Allergy 2000;55(4):412–3.

903. Romanowska-Gorecka B, Oleszczak B. Maskukacy wplyw indocydu na przebieg ropnych procesow zapalnych. [Masking effect of indocin on the course of purulent inflammatory processes.] Pol Tyg Lek 1969;24(52):2019–2020.

904. Maeda K, Anan S, Akaboshi Y, Yoshida H. A case of urticarial drug eruption from loxoprofen sodium (Loxonin). Skin Res 1988;30(Suppl 4):44.

905. Nagaoka K, Ozaki S, Chinen Y, et al. Clinical effects of Loxonin in patients of rheumatoid arthritis. Jpn Arch Intern Med 1989;36:65.

906. Szczeklik A, Gryglewski RJ, Czerniawska-Mysik G. Participation of prostaglandins in pathogenesis of aspirin-sensitive asthma. Naunyn Schmiedebergs Arch Pharmacol 1977;297(Suppl 1):S99–S110.

907. Kosnik M, Music E, Matjaz F, Suskovic S. Relative safety of meloxicam in NSAID-intolerant patients. Allergy 1998;53(12):1231–3.

908. Quaratino D, Romano A, Di Fonso M, Papa G, Perrone MR, D'Ambrosio FP, Venuti A. Tolerability of meloxicam in patients with histories of adverse reactions to nonsteroidal anti-inflammatory drugs. Ann Allergy Asthma Immunol 2000;84(6):613–7.

909. Nettis E, Di Paola R, Ferrannini A, Tursi A. Meloxicam in hypersensitivity to NSAIDs. Allergy 2001;56(8):803–4.

910. Grennan DM, Jolly J, Holloway LJ, Palmer DG. Vasculitis in a patient receiving naproxen. NZ Med J 1979;89(628):48–9.

911. Plouvier B, Gosselin B, Hatron PY, Plouvier-Carrez J, Devulder B. Vasculopathie allergique systémique induite par le naproxen. [Systemic allergic vasculopathy after naproxen.] Ann Med Interne (Paris) 1979;130(3):173–6.

912. Schapira D, Balbir-Gurman A, Nahir AM. Naproxen-induced leukocytoclastic vasculitis. Clin Rheumatol 2000;19(3):242–4.

913. Strom BL, Carson JL, Schinnar R, Sim E, Morse ML. The effect of indication on the risk of hypersensitivity reactions associated with tolmetin sodium vs other nonsteroidal anti-inflammatory drugs. J Rheumatol 1988;15(4):695–9.

914. Lawn SD, Wood C, Lockwood DN. Borderline tuberculoid leprosy: an immune reconstitution phenomenon in a human immunodeficiency virus-infected person. Clin Infect Dis 2003;36(1):e5–6.

915. Pareek SS. Nystatin-induced fixed eruption. Br J Dermatol 1980;103(6):679–80.

916. Cooper SM, Shaw S. Contact allergy to nystatin: an unusual allergen. Contact Dermatitis 1999;41(2):120.

917. Cooper SM, Reed J, Shaw S. Systemic reaction to nystatin. Contact Dermatitis 1999;41(6):345–6.

918. Goncalo S, Cabral F, Goncalo M. Contact sensitivity to oak moss. Contact Dermatitis 1988;19(5):355–7.

919. Hodgson G. Eczemas associated with lubricants and metalworking fluids. Dermatol Dig 1976;11–5Oct.

920. Owen CM, August PJ, Beck MH. Contact allergy to oak moss resin in a soluble oil. Contact Dermatitis 2000;43(2):112.

921. Jacob JS, Rosen ES, Young E. Report on the presence of a toxic substance, dimethyl formamide, in sodium fluorescein used for fluorescein angiography. Br J Ophthalmol 1982;66(9):567–8.

922. Johnson RN, McDonald HR, Schatz H. Rash, fever, and chills after intravenous fluorescein angiography. Am J Ophthalmol 1998;126(6):837–8.

923. Lopez-Saez MP, Ordoqui E, Tornero P, Baeza A, Sainza T, Zubeldia JM, Baeza ML. Fluorescein-induced allergic reaction. Ann Allergy Asthma Immunol 1998;81(5 Pt 1):428–30.

924. Raz A, Bergman R, Eilam O, Yungerman T, Hayek T. A case report of olanzapine-induced hypersensitivity syndrome. Am J Med Sci 2001;321(2):156–8.

925. Zucker-Pinchoff B, Ramanathan S. Anaphylactic reaction to epidural fentanyl. Anesthesiology 1989;71(4):599–601.

926. Panos MZ, Burnett S, Gazzard BG. Use of naloxone in opioid-induced anaphylactoid reaction. Br J Anaesth 1988;61(3):371.

927. Flacke JW, Flacke WE, Bloor BC, Van Etten AP, Kripke BJ. Histamine release by four narcotics: a double-blind study in humans. Anesth Analg 1987;66(8):723–30.

928. Anibarro B, Vila C, Seoane FJ. Urticaria induced by meperidine allergy. Allergy 2000;55(3):305–6.

929. Higashi GI, Farid Z. Oxamniquine fever—drug-induced or immune-complex reaction? BMJ 1979;2(6194):830.

930. Endoh N, Ichinose M, Takahashi T, Miura M, Kageyama N, Mashito Y, Sugiura H, Ikeda K, Takasaka T, Shirato K. Relationship between cholinergic airway tone and serum immunoglobulin E in human subjects. Eur Respir J 1998;12(1):71–4.

931. Scudlik C, Schnuch A, Uter W, Schwanitz HJ. Berufsbedingtes Kontaktekzem nach Anwenung einer Dexpanthenol-haltigen Salbe und Überblick über die IVDK-Daten zu Dexpanthenol (IVDK = Informationsverbund Dermatologischer Kliniken) Aktuel Dermatol 2002;28:398–401.

932. Schorr WF. Paraben allergy. A cause of intractable dermatitis. JAMA 1968;204(10):859–62.

933. Ayonrinde OT, Saker BM. Anaphylactoid reactions to paracetamol. Postgrad Med J 2000;76(898):501–2.

934. Odio MR, O'Connor RJ, Sarbaugh F, Baldwin S. Continuous topical administration of a petrolatum formulation by a novel disposable diaper. 2. Effect on skin condition. Dermatology 2000;200(3):238–43.

935. Shulakov NA, Novikov VE, Loseva VA, Makushkina VK, Kozlov NB, Iakushev PF, Bondarev DP. [Vaseline protection of the skin from the effects of the sealant Uniherm-6.] Gig Tr Prof Zabol 1990;(12):43–4.

936. Maibach H. Chronic dermatitis and hyperpigmentation from petrolatum. Contact Dermatitis 1978;4(1):62.

937. Dooms-Goossens A, Degreef H. Sensitization to yellow petrolatum used as a vehicle for patch testing. Contact Dermatitis 1980;6(2):146–7.

938. Lawrence CM, Smith AG. Ampliative medicament allergy: concomitant sensitivity to multiple medicaments including yellow soft paraffin, white soft paraffin, gentian violet and Span 20. Contact Dermatitis 1982;8(4):240–5.

939. Dooms-Goossens A, Dooms M. Contact allergy to petrolatums. (III). Allergenicity prediction and pharmacopoeial requirements. Contact Dermatitis 1983;9(5):352–9.

940. Dooms-Goossens A, Degreef H. Contact allergy to petrolatums. (II). Attempts to identify the nature of the allergens. Contact Dermatitis 1983;9(4):247–56.

941. Dooms-Goossens A, Degreef H. Contact allergy to petrolatums. (I). Sensitizing capacity of different brands of yellow and white petrolatums. Contact Dermatitis 1983;9(3):175–85.

942. Ayadi M, Martin P. Contact allergy to petrolatum. Contact Dermatitis 1987;16(1):51.

943. Kang H, Choi J, Lee AY. Allergic contact dermatitis to white petrolatum. J Dermatol 2004;31(5):428–30.

944. Scerri L, Dalziel KL. Occupational contact sensitization to the stabilized chlorinated paraffin fraction in neat cutting oil. Am J Contact Dermat 1996;7(1):35–7.

945. Grin R, Maibach HI. Long-lasting contact urticaria from petrolatum mimicking dermatitis. Contact Dermatitis 1999;40(2):110.

946. Ulrich G, Schmutz JL, Trechot P, Commun N, Barbaud A. Sensitization to petrolatum: an unusual cause of false-positive drug patch-tests. Allergy 2004;59(9):1006–9.

947. Kundu RV, Scheman AJ, Gutmanovich A, Hernandez C. Contact dermatitis to white petrolatum. Skinmed 2004;3(5):295–6.

948. Neer RM, Arnaud CD, Zanchetta JR, Prince R, Gaich GA, Reginster JY, Hodsman AB, Eriksen EF, Ish-Shalom S, Genant HK, Wang O, Mitlak BH. Effect of parathyroid hormone (1–34) on fractures and bone mineral density in postmenopausal women with osteoporosis. N Engl J Med 2001;344(19):1434–41.

949. Francis DM, Shenton BK. Fat emulsion adversely affects lymphocyte reactivity. Aust NZ J Surg 1987;57(5):323–9.

950. Okada Y, Klein N, van Saene HK, Pierro A. Small volumes of enteral feedings normalise immune function in infants receiving parenteral nutrition. J Pediatr Surg 1998;33(1):16–9.

951. Weidmann B, Lepique C, Heider A, Schmitz A, Niederle N. Hypersensitivity reactions to parenteral lipid solutions. Support Care Cancer 1997;5(6):504–5.

952. Laxenaire MC, Cottineau C, Neidhardt M, Tunon De Lara M, Rakotoseheno JC, Bricard H, Vergnaud MC, Laroche D, Dubois F, Jacson F, Claussner-Poulignan M, Jacquot C, Zambelli P, Hautier MB, Facon A, Orsel I, Motin J, Dubost R, Courvoisier L, et al. Substances responsables des chocs anaphylactiques peranethesiques. Troisième enquête multicentrique française (1992–1994). [Substances responsible for peranesthetic anaphylactic shock. A third French multicenter study (1992–94).] Ann Fr Anesth Reanim 1996;15(8):1211–8.

953. Theissen JL, Zahn P, Theissen U, Brehler R. Allergische und pseudoallergische reaktionen in der anästhesie. Teil I: Pathogenese Risikofaktoren, substanzen. [Allergic and pseudo-allergic reactions in anesthesia. I: Pathogenesis, risk factors, substances.] Anästhesiol Intensivmed Notfallmed Schmerzther 1995;30(1):3–12.

954. Market AD, Lew DB, Schropp KP, Hak EB. Parenteral nutrition-associated anaphylaxis in a 4-year-old child. J Pediatr Gastroenterol Nutr 1998;26(2):229–31.

955. Wu SF, Chen W. Hypersensitivity to vitamin preparation in parenteral nutrition: report of one case. Acta Paediatr Taiwan 2002;43(5):285–7.

956. Yeung CY, Lee HC, Huang FY, Wang CS. Sepsis during total parenteral nutrition: exploration of risk factors and determination of the effectiveness of peripherally inserted central venous catheters. Pediatr Infect Dis J 1998;17(2):135–42.

957. Sirota L, Straussberg R, Notti I, Bessler H. Effect of lipid emulsion on IL-2 production by mononuclear cells of newborn infants and adults. Acta Paediatr 1997;86(4):410–3.

958. Waitzberg DL, Bellinati-Pires R, Salgado MM, Hypolito IP, Colleto GM, Yagi O, Yamamuro EM, Gama-Rodrigues J, Pinotti HW. Effect of total parenteral nutrition with different lipid emulsions of human monocyte and neutrophil functions. Nutrition 1997;13(2):128–32.

959. Beganovic N, Verloove-Vanhorick SP, Brand R, Ruys JH. Total parenteral nutrition and sepsis. Arch Dis Child 1988;63(1):66–7.

960. Lenssen P, Bruemmer BA, Bowden RA, Gooley T, Aker SN, Mattson D. Intravenous lipid dose and incidence of bacteremia and fungemia in patients undergoing bone marrow transplantation. Am J Clin Nutr 1998;67(5):927–33.

961. Huang YC, Li CC, Lin TY, Lien RI, Chou YH, Wu JL, Hsueh C. Association of fungal colonization and invasive disease in very low birth weight infants. Pediatr Infect Dis J 1998;17(9):819–22.

962. Avila-Figueroa C, Goldmann DA, Richardson DK, Gray JE, Ferrari A, Freeman J. Intravenous lipid emulsions are the major determinant of coagulase-negative staphylococcal bacteremia in very low birth weight newborns. Pediatr Infect Dis J 1998;17(1):10–7.

963. Katz S, Plaisier BR, Folkening WJ, Grosfeld JL. Intralipid adversely affects reticuloendothelial bacterial clearance. J Pediatr Surg 1991;26(8):921–4.

964. Joyce DA. D-penicillamine pharmacokinetics and pharmacodynamics in man. Pharmacol Ther 1989;42(3):405–27.

965. Rosada M, Fiocco U, De Silvestro G, Doria A, Cozzi L, Favaretto M, Todesco S. Effect of D-penicillamine on the T cell phenotype in scleroderma. Comparison between treated and untreated patients. Clin Exp Rheumatol 1993;11(2):143–8.

966. Panayi GS, Mills MM. Second-line drug treatment in rheumatoid arthritis associated with depressed autologous mixed lymphocyte reaction. Rheumatol Int 1986;6(1):25–9.

967. Miyachi Y, Yoshioka A, Imamura S, Niwa Y. Decreased hydroxyl radical generation from polymorphonuclear leucocytes in the presence of D-penicillamine and thiopronine. J Clin Lab Immunol 1987;22(2):81–4.

968. Sim E, Dodds AW, Goldin A. Inhibition of the covalent binding reaction of complement component C4 by penicillamine, an anti-rheumatic agent. Biochem J 1989;259(2):415–9.

969. Price EJ, Venables PJ. Drug-induced lupus. Drug Saf 1995;12(4):283–90.

970. Haberhauer G, Broll H. Drug-induced anticentromere antibody? Z Rheumatol 1989;48(2):99–100.

971. Haberhauer G. D-penicillamine (DPA)-induced anticentromere antibody (ACA). Clin Exp Rheumatol 1989;7(3):332–4.

972. Storch W. Antikörper gegen D-penicillamin bei primär biliärer Zirrhose. [Antibodies against D-penicillamine in primary biliary cirrhosis.] Immun Infekt 1990;18(1):22–3.

973. Stremmel W, Meyerrose KW, Niederau C, Hefter H, Kreuzpaintner G, Strohmeyer G. Wilson disease: clinical presentation, treatment, and survival. Ann Intern Med 1991;115(9):720–6.

974. Barbosa ER, Scaff M, Canelas HM. Degeneraçăo hepatolenticular. Avaliaçăo da evoluçăo neurologica em 76 casos tratados. [Hepatolenticular degeneration: evaluation of neurological course in 76 treated cases.] Arq Neuropsiquiatr 1991;49(4):399–404.

975. Tankanow RM. Pathophysiology and treatment of Wilson's disease. Clin Pharm 1991;10(11):839–49.

976. Yarze JC, Martin P, Munoz SJ, Friedman LS. Wilson's disease: current status. Am J Med 1992;92(6):643–54.

977. Zvulunov A, Grunwald MH, Avinoach I, Halevy S. Transient acantholytic dermatosis (Grover's disease) in a patient with progressive systemic sclerosis treated with D-penicillamine. Int J Dermatol 1997;36(6):476–7.

978. Tanphaichitr K. D-penicillamine-induced bronchial spasm. South Med J 1980;73(6):788–90.

979. Bochner BS, Lichtenstein LM. Anaphylaxis. N Engl J Med 1991;324(25):1785–90.

980. Idsoe O, Guthe T, Willcox RR, de Weck AL. Art und Ausmass der Penizillinnebenwirkungen unter besonderer Berücksichtigung von 151 Todesfällen nach anaphylaktischem Schock. [Nature and extent of penicillin side effects with special reference to 151 fatal cases after anaphylactic shock.] Schweiz Med Wochenschr 1969;99(33):1190–7contd.

981. Markowitz M, Kaplan E, Cuttica R, et al. Allergic reactions to long-term benzathine penicillin prophylaxis for rheumatic fever. International Rheumatic Fever Study Group. Lancet 1991;337(8753):1308–10.

981. Capaul R, Maibach R, Kunzi UP, et al. Atopy, bronchial asthma and previous adverse drug reactions (ADRs): risk factors for ADRs? Post Marketing Surveillance 1993;7:331.

982. Blanca M, Perez E, Garcia J, Miranda A, Fernandez J, Vega JM, Terrados S, Avila M, Martin A, Suau R. Anaphylaxis to amoxycillin but good tolerance for benzyl penicillin. In vivo and in vitro studies of specific IgE antibodies. Allergy 1988;43(7):508–10.

983. Hunziker I, Kunzi UP, Braunschweig S, Zehnder D, Hoigné R. Comprehensive hospital drug monitoring (CHDM): adverse skin reactions, a 20-year survey. Allergy 1997;52(4):388–93.

984. Hoigné R. Akute Nebenreaktionen auf Penicillinpräparate. [Acute side-reactions to penicillin preparations.] Acta Med Scand 1962;171:201–8.

985. Bertelsen K, Dalgaard JB. Penicillindodsfald. 16 secerede Danske tilfaelde. [Death due to penicillin. 16 Danish cases with autopsies.] Nord Med 1965;73:173–7.

986. Hoffman DR, Hudson P, Carlyle SJ, Massello W 3rd. Three cases of fatal anaphylaxis to antibiotics in patients with prior histories of allergy to the drug. Ann Allergy 1989;62(2):91–3.

987. Lin RY. A perspective on penicillin allergy. Arch Intern Med 1992;152(5):930–7.

988. Spark RP. Fatal anaphylaxis due to oral penicillin. Am J Clin Pathol 1971;56(3):407–11.

989. Cullen DJ. Severe anaphylactic reaction to penicillin during halothane anaesthesia. A case report. Br J Anaesth 1971;43(4):410–2.

990. Macy E, Richter PK, Falkoff R, Zeiger R. Skin testing with penicilloate and penilloate prepared by an improved method: amoxicillin oral challenge in patients with negative skin test responses to penicillin reagents. J Allergy Clin Immunol 1997;100(5):586–91.

991. Wickern GM, Nish WA, Bitner AS, Freeman TM. Allergy to beta-lactams: a survey of current practices. J Allergy Clin Immunol 1994;94(4):725–31.

992. Levine BB, Redmond AP, Fellner MJ, Voss HE, Levytska V. Penicillin allergy and the heterogenous immune responses of man to benzylpenicillin. J Clin Invest 1966;45(12):1895–906.

993. VanArsdel PP Jr, Larson EB. Diagnostic tests for patients with suspected allergic disease. Utility and limitations. Ann Intern Med 1989;110(4):304–12.

994. Barbaud A, Reichert-Penetrat S, Trechot P, Jacquin-Petit MA, Ehlinger A, Noirez V, Faure GC, Schmutz JL, Bene MC. The use of skin testing in the investigation of cutaneous adverse drug reactions. Br J Dermatol 1998;139(1):49–58.

995. Ressler C, Mendelson LM. Skin test for diagnosis of penicillin allergy—current status. Ann Allergy 1987;59(3):167–70.

996. Sogn DD, Evans R 3rd, Shepherd GM, Casale TB, Condemi J, Greenberger PA, Kohler PF, Saxon A, Summers RJ, VanArsdel PP Jr, et al. Results of the National Institute of Allergy and Infectious Diseases Collaborative Clinical Trial to test the predictive value of skin testing with major and minor penicillin derivatives in hospitalized adults. Arch Intern Med 1992;152(5):1025–32.

997. Gadde J, Spence M, Wheeler B, Adkinson NF Jr. Clinical experience with penicillin skin testing in a large inner-city STD clinic. JAMA 1993;270(20):2456–63.

998. Erffmeyer JE. Adverse reactions to penicillin. Ann Allergy 1981;47(4):288–300.

999. Vega JM, Blanca M, Garcia JJ, Carmona MJ, Miranda A, Perez-Estrada M, Fernandez S, Acebes JM, Terrados S. Immediate allergic reactions to amoxicillin. Allergy 1994;49(5):317–22.

1000. Silviu-Dan F, McPhillips S, Warrington RJ. The frequency of skin test reactions to side-chain penicillin determinants. J Allergy Clin Immunol 1993;91(3):694–701.

1001. Baldo BA, Pham NH, Weiner J. Detection and side-chain specificity of IgE antibodies to flucloxacillin in allergic subjects. J Mol Recognit 1995;8(3):171–7.

1002. Torres MJ, Blanca M, Fernandez J, Esteban A, Moreno F, Vega JM, Garcia J. Selective allergic reaction to oral cloxacillin. Clin Exp Allergy 1996;26(1):108–11.

1003. Sastre J, Quijano LD, Novalbos A, Hernandez G, Cuesta J, de las Heras M, Lluch M, Fernandez M. Clinical cross-reactivity between amoxicillin and cephadroxil in patients allergic to amoxicillin and with good tolerance of penicillin. Allergy 1996;51(6):383–6.

1004. Di Perri G, Di Perri IG, Monteiro GB, Bonora S, Hennig C, Cassatella M, Micciolo R, Vento S, Dusi S, Bassetti D, et al. Pentoxifylline as a supportive agent in the treatment of cerebral malaria in children. J Infect Dis 1995;171(5):1317–22.

1005. Hemmer CJ, Hort G, Chiwakata CB, Seitz R, Egbring R, Gaus W, Hogel J, Hassemer M, Nawroth PP, Kern P, Dietrich M. Supportive pentoxifylline in falciparum malaria: no effect on tumor necrosis factor alpha levels or clinical outcome: a prospective, randomized, placebo-controlled study. Am J Trop Med Hyg 1997;56(4):397–403.

1006. Dooms-Goossens A, Deveylder H, de Alam AG, Lachapelle JM, Tennstedt D, Degreef H. Contact sensitivity to nonoxynols as a cause of intolerance to antiseptic preparations. J Am Acad Dermatol 1989;21(4 Pt 1):723–7.

1007. Michel M, Dompmartin A, Moreau A, Leroy D. Contact photosensitivity to nonoxynol used in antiseptic preparations. Photodermatol Photoimmunol Photomed 1994;10(5):198–201.

1008. Fisher AA. Allergic contact dermatitis to nonoxynol-9 in a condom. Cutis 1994;53(3):110–1.

1009. Dickson D. PCP dioxins found to pose health risks. Nature 1980;283(5746):418.

1010. Wigger-Alberti W, Elsner P, Wuthrich B. Allergic contact dermatitis to phenylephrine. Allergy 1998;53(2):217–8.

1011. Erdmann SM, Sachs B, Merk HF. Allergic contact dermatitis from phenylephrine in eyedrops. Am J Contact Dermat 2002;13(1):37–8.

1012. Villarreal O. Reliability of diagnostic tests for contact allergy to mydriatic eyedrops. Contact Dermatitis 1998;38(3):150–4.

1013. Rafael M, Pereira F, Faria MA. Allergic contact blepharoconjunctivitis caused by phenylephrine, associated with persistent patch test reaction. Contact Dermatitis 1998;39(3):143–4.

1014. Speer F, Carrasco LC, Kimura CC. Allergy to phenylpropanolamine. Ann Allergy 1978;40(1):32–4.

1015. Klassen BD, Sadler RM. Induction of hypersensitivity to a previously tolerated antiepileptic drug by a second antiepileptic drug. Epilepsia 2001;42(3):433–5.

1016. Arroyo S, de la Morena A. Life-threatening adverse events of antiepileptic drugs. Epilepsy Res 2001;47(1–2):155–74.

1017. Rodriguez-Garcia JL, Sanchez-Corral J, Martinez J, Bellas C, Aguado M, Serrano M. Phenytoin-induced benign lymphadenopathy with solid spleen lesions mimicking a malignant lymphoma. Ann Oncol 1991;2(6):443–5.

1018. Tsund SH, Lin TI. Angioimmunoblastic lymphoadenopathy in a patient taking diphenylhydantoin. Ann Clin Lab Med 1981;11:542.

1019. Ruff ME, Pincus LG, Sampson HA. Phenytoin-induced IgA depression. Am J Dis Child 1987;141(8):858–61.

1020. Polman AJ, van der Werf TS, Tiebosch AT, Zijlstra JG. Early-onset phenytoin toxicity mimicking a renopulmonary syndrome. Eur Respir J 1998;11(2):501–3.

1021. Daniels PR, Berry GJ, Tazelaar HD, Cooper LT. Giant cell myocarditis as a manifestation of drug hypersensitivity. Cardiovasc Pathol 2000;9(5):287–91.

1022. Siragusa RJ, Ramos-Caro FA, Edwards NL, Flowers FP. Drug-induced lupus due to phenytoin. J Pharm Technol 2000;16:5–7.

1023. Bruze M, Krook G, Ljunggren B. Fatal connective tissue disease with antinuclear antibodies following PUVA therapy. Acta Dermatol Venereol 1984;64(2):157–60.

1024. Calzavara-Pinton P, Franceschini F, Rastrelli M, Manera C, Zane C, Cattaneo R, De Panfilis G. Antinuclear antibodies are not induced by PUVA treatment in patients with uncomplicated psoriasis. J Am Acad Dermatol 1994;30(6):955–8.

1025. Legat FJ, Wolf P, Kranke B. Anaphylaxis to 5-methoxypsoralen during photochemotherapy. Br J Dermatol 2001;145(5):821–2.

1026. Purello D'Ambrosio F, Ricciardi L, Isola S, Gangemi S, Cilia M, Levanti C, Marcazzo A. Systemic contact dermatitis to copper-containing IUD. Allergy 1996;51(9):658–9.

1027. Bulgaresi P, Confortini M, Galanti L, Gargano D. Inflammatory changes and cervical intraepithelial neoplasia in IUD users. Cervix Low Female Genital Tract 1989;7(3):207–12.

1028. Duguid HL, Parratt D, Traynor R. Actinomyces-like organisms in cervical smears from women using intrauterine contraceptive devices. BMJ 1980;281(6239):534–7.

1029. Leeton J. Female genital actinomycosis and the intrauterine device. Med J Aust 1980;1(11):518.

1030. Vessey MP, Yeates D, Flavel R, McPherson K. Pelvic inflammatory disease and the intrauterine device: findings in a large cohort study. BMJ (Clin Res Ed) 1981;282(6267):855–7.

1030. Creamer P, Lim K, George E, Dieppe P. Acute inflammatory polyarthritis in association with tamoxifen. Br J Rheumatol 1994;33(6):583–5.

1030. Tielemans C, Madhoun P, Lenaers M, Schandene L, Goldman M, Vanherweghem JL. Anaphylactoid reactions during hemodialysis on AN69 membranes in patients receiving ACE inhibitors. Kidney Int 1990;38:982–4.

1031. Parnes EL, Shapiro WB. Anaphylactoid reactions in hemodialysis patients treated with the AN69 dialyzer. Kidney Int 1991;40:1148–52.

1032. Brunet P, Jaber K, Berland Y, Baz M. Anaphylactoid reactions during hemodialysis and hemofiltration: role of associating AN69 membrane and angiotensin I-converting enzyme inhibitors. Am J Kidney Dis 1992;19:444–7.

1033. Rousaud BF, Garcia JM, Camps EM, Cubells TD, Comamala MR. ACE inhibitors and anaphylactoid reactions to high-flux membrane dialysis (AN69): clinical aspects. Nephron 1992;60:487.

1034. Schaefer RM, Fink E, Schaefer L, Barkhausen R, Kulzer P, Heidland A. Role of bradykinin in anaphylactoid reactions during hemodialysis with AN69 dialyzers. Am J Nephrol 1993;13:473–7.

1035. Schulman G, Hakim R, Arias R, Silverberg M, Kaplan AP, Arbeit L. Bradykinin generation by dialysis membranes: possible role in anaphylactic reaction. J Am Soc Nephrol 1993;3:1563–9.

1036. Fink E, Lemke HD, Verresen L, Shimamoto K. Kinin generation by hemodialysis membranes as a possible cause of anaphylactoid reactions. Braz J Med Biol Res 1994;27:1975–83.

1037. John B, Anijeet HK, Ahmad R. Anaphylactic reaction during haemodialysis on AN69 membrane in a patient receiving angiotensin II receptor antagonist. Nephrol Dial Transplant 2001;16:1955–6.

1038. Ebo DG, Stevens WJ, Bosmans JL. An adverse reaction to angiotensin-converting enzyme inhibitors in a patient with neglected C1 esterase inhibitor deficiency. J Allergy Clin Immunol 1997;99:425–6.

1039. Thomas M, Valette P, Mausset AL, Dejardin P. High molecular weight kininogen adsorption on hemodialysis membranes: influence of pH and relationship with contact phase activation of blood plasma. influence of pretreatment with poly(ethyleneimine). Int J Artif Organs 2000;23:20–6.

1040. Anonymous. Severe allergic reactions associated with dialysis and ACE inhibitors. FDA Med Bull 1992;22(1):4.

1041. Jenkins SC, Clifton MA. Gelofusine allergy—the need for identification jewellery. Ann R Coll Surg Engl 2002;84(3):206–7.

1042. Ong EL. A case of hypersensitivity to gelafundin. Singapore Med J 2001;42(4):176–7.

1043. Duffy BL, Harding JN, Fuller WR, Peake SL. Cardiac arrest following Haemaccel. Anaesth Intensive Care 1994;22(1):90–2.

1044. Prevedoros HP, Bradburn NT, Harrison GA. Three cases of anaphylactoid reaction to Haemaccel. Anaesth Intensive Care 1990;18(3):409–12.

1045. Bombail-Girard D, Boulechfar H, Tangre M, Landillon N, Bussel A. Etude comparative de l'efficacité et de la tolérance de deux substituts de plasma utilisés comme solution de remplissage au cours des échanges plasmatiques. [Comparative study of the efficacy and tolerability of 2 plasma substitutes used as vascular-loading solutions during plasma exchange.] Ann Med Interne (Paris) 1990;141(7):611–4.

1046. Chew GY, Phan TG, Quin JW. Anaphylactic or anaphylactoid reaction to Haemaccel? Med J Aust 1999;171(7):387–8.

1047. Olivieri J, Eigenmann PA, Hauser C. Severe anaphylaxis to a new disinfectant: polyhexanide, a chlorhexidine polymer. Schweiz Med Wochenschr 1998;128(40):1508–11.

1048. Hillen U, Geier J, Goos M. Kontaktallergien bei Patienten mit Ekzemen des ausseren Gehorgangs. Ergebnisse des Informationsverbundes Dermatologischer Kliniken und der Deutschen Kontaktallergie-Gruppe. [Contact allergies in patients with eczema of the external ear canal. Results of the Information Network of Dermatological Clinics and the German Contact Allergy Group.] Hautarzt 2000;51(4):239–43.

1049. Sasaki S, Mitsuhashi Y, Kondo S. Contact dermatitis due to sodium colistimethate. J Dermatol 1998;25(6):415–7.

1050. Zehnder D, Kunzi UP, Maibach R, Zoppi M, Halter F, Neftel KA, Muller U, Galeazzi RL, Hess T, Hoigne R. Die Häufigkeit der Antibiotika-assoziierten Kolitis bei hospitalisierten Patienten der Jahre 1974–1991 im "Comprehensive Hospital Drug Monitoring" Bern/St. Gallen. [Frequency of antibiotics-associated colitis in hospitalized patients in 1974–1991 in "Comprehensive Hospital Drug Monitoring", Bern/St. Gallen.] Schweiz Med Wochenschr 1995;125(14):676–83.

1051. Ronnau AC, Wulferink M, Gleichmann E, Unver E, Ruzicka T, Krutmann J, Grewe M. Anaphylaxis to polyvinylpyrrolidone in an analgesic preparation. Br J Dermatol 2000;143(5):1055–8.

1052. Gortz G, Haring R. Wirkung und Nebenwirkung von Polyvinylpyrrolidon-Jod (PVP-Jod). Therapiewoche 1981;31:4364.

1053. Zamora JL. Chemical and microbiologic characteristics and toxicity of povidone-iodine solutions. Am J Surg 1986;151(3):400–6.

1054. Ancona A, Suarez de la Torre R, Macotela E. Allergic contact dermatitis from povidone-iodine. Contact Dermatitis 1985;13(2):66–8.

1055. Ökten F, Oral M, Çanakiçi N, Kwtipek Ö, Öztin C, Öztames O. An anaphylactoid reaction to polyvinylpyrrolidone iodine. A case report. Turk Anesteziyol Reanim 1993;21:118–23.

1056. Erdmann S, Hertl M, Merk HF. Allergic contact dermatitis from povidone-iodine. Contact Dermatitis 1999;40(6):331–2.

1057. Katz RS, Papernik M. Zafirlukast and Churg–Strauss syndrome. JAMA 1998;279(24):1949.

1058. Green RL, Vayonis AG. Churg–Strauss syndrome after zafirlukast in two patients not receiving systemic steroid treatment. Lancet 1999;353(9154):725–6.

1059. Azher M, el-Kassimi FA, Wright SG, Mofti A. Exudative polyserositis and acute respiratory failure following praziquantel therapy. Chest 1990;98(1):241–3.

1060. Wilkinson JD, Shaw S, Andersen KE, Brandao FM, Bruynzeel DP, Bruze M, Camarasa JM, Diepgen TL, Ducombs G, Frosch PJ, Goossens A, Lachapelle JM, Lahti A, Menne T, Seidenari S, Tosti A, Wahlberg JE. Monitoring levels of preservative sensitivity in Europe. A 10-year overview (1991–2000). Contact Dermatitis 2002;46(4):207–10.

1061. Uter W, Frosch PJ. IVDK Study Group and the German Contact Dermatitis Research Group, DKG. Contact allergy from DMDM hydantoin, 1994–2000. Contact Dermatitis 2002;47(1):57–8.

1062. Revuz J, Poli F, Wechsler J, Dubertret L. Dermite de contact a l'hexamidine. [Contact dermatitis from hexamidine.] Ann Dermatol Venereol 1984;111(9):805–10.

1063. Dooms-Goossens A, Vandaele M, Bedert R, Marien K. Hexamidine isethionate: a sensitizer in topical pharmaceutical products and cosmetics. Contact Dermatitis 1989;21(4):270.

1064. Schnuch A, Geier J, Brasch J, Fuchs T, Pirker C, Schulze-Dirks A, Basketter DA. Polyhexamethylenebiguanide: a relevant contact allergen? Contact Dermatitis 2000;42(5):302–3.

1065. Daniels PR, Berry GJ, Tazelaar HD, Cooper LT. Giant cell myocarditis as a manifestation of drug hypersensitivity. Cardiovasc Pathol 2000;9(5):287–91.

1066. Yung RL, Richardson BC. Drug-induced lupus. Rheum Dis Clin North Am 1994;20(1):61–86.

1067. Gaita F, Richiardi E, Bocchiardo M, Asteggiano R, Pinnavaia A, Di Leo M, Rosettani E, Brusca A. Short- and long-term effects of propafenone in ventricular arrhythmias. Int J Cardiol 1986;13(2):163–70.

1068. Guindo J, Rodriguez de la Serna A, Borja J, Oter R, Jane F, Bayes de Luna A. Propafenone and a syndrome of the lupus erythematosus type. Ann Intern Med 1986;104(4):589.

1069. Laxenaire MC, Gueant JL, Bermejo E, Mouton C, Navez MT. Anaphylactic shock due to propofol. Lancet 1988;2(8613):739–40.

1070. Zaloga GP, Teres D. The safety and efficacy of propofol containing EDTA: a randomised clinical trial programme focusing on cation and trace metal homeostasis in critically ill patients. Intensive Care Med 2000;26(Suppl 4):S398–9.

1071. Mehta U, Gunston GD, O'Connor N. Serious consequences to misuse of propofol anaesthetic. S Afr Med J 2000;90(3):240.

1072. Kienlein-Kletschka B, Baurle G. Epicutane sofort Reaktion. Aktuelle Derm 1981;7:88.

1073. Himly M, Jahn-Schmid B, Pittertschatscher K, Bohle B, Grubmayr K, Ferreira F, Ebner H, Ebner C. IgE-mediated immediate-type hypersensitivity to the pyrazolone drug propyphenazone. J Allergy Clin Immunol 2003;111(4):882–8.

1074. Doolan L, McKenzie I, Krafchek J, Parsons B, Buxton B. Protamine sulphate hypersensitivity. Anaesth Intensive Care 1981;9(2):147–9.

1075. Gottschlich GM, Gravlee GP, Georgitis JW. Adverse reactions to protamine sulfate during cardiac surgery in diabetic and non-diabetic patients. Ann Allergy 1988;61(4):277–81.

1076. Gupta SK, Veith FJ, Ascer E, Wengerter KR, Franco C, Amar D, el-Gaweet ES, Gupta A. Anaphylactoid reactions to protamine: an often lethal complication in insulin-dependent diabetic patients undergoing vascular surgery. J Vasc Surg 1989;9(2):342–50.

1077. Stewart WJ, McSweeney SM, Kellett MA, Faxon DP, Ryan TJ. Increased risk of severe protamine reactions in NPH insulin-dependent diabetics undergoing cardiac catheterization. Circulation 1984;70(5):788–92.

1078. Weiss ME, Nyhan D, Peng ZK, Horrow JC, Lowenstein E, Hirshman C, Adkinson NF Jr. Association of protamine IgE and IgG antibodies with life-threatening reactions to intravenous protamine. N Engl J Med 1989;320(14):886–92.

1079. Vincent GM, Janowski M, Menlove R. Protamine allergy reactions during cardiac catheterization and cardiac surgery: risk in patients taking protamine–insulin preparations. Cathet Cardiovasc Diagn 1991;23(3):164–8.

1080. Florence E, Schrooten W, Verdonck K, Dreezen C, Colebunders R. Rheumatological complications associated with the use of indinavir and other protease inhibitors. Ann Rheum Dis 2002;61(1):82–4.

1081. van der Walle HB, Brunsveld VM. Dermatitis in hairdressers. (I). The experience of the past 4 years. Contact Dermatitis 1994;30(4):217–21.

1082. Niinimaki A, Niinimaki M, Makinen-Kiljunen S, Hannuksela M. Contact urticaria from protein hydrolysates in hair conditioners. Allergy 1998;53(11):1078–82.

1083. White GC 2nd. Seventeen years' experience with Autoplex/Autoplex T: evaluation of inpatients with severe haemophilia A and factor VIII inhibitors at a major haemophilia centre. Haemophilia 2000;6(5):508–12.

1084. Odeh M, Lurie M, Oliven A. Cutaneous leucocytoclastic vasculitis associated with omeprazole. Postgrad Med J 2002;78(916):114–5.

1085. Galindo PA, Borja J, Feo F, Gomez E, Garcia R, Cabrera M, Martinez C. Anaphylaxis to omeprazole. Ann Allergy Asthma Immunol 1999;82(1):52–4.

1086. Fakir M, Saison C, Wong T, Matta B, Hardin JM. Septicemia due to *Yersinia enterocolitica* in a hemodialyzed, iron-depleted patient receiving omeprazole and oral iron supplementation. Am J Kidney Dis 1992;19(3):282–4.

1087. Lee PS, Lau EY. Risk of acute non-specific upper respiratory tract infections in healthy men taking dapsone–pyrimethamine for prophylaxis against malaria. BMJ (Clin Res Ed) 1988;296(6626):893–5.

1088. Thong BY, Leong KP, Chng HH. Hypersensitivity syndrome associated with dapsone/pyrimethamine (Maloprim) antimalaria chemoprophylaxis. Ann Allergy Asthma Immunol 2002;88(5):527–9.

1089. Larbre JP, Perret P, Collet P, Llorca G. Antinuclear antibodies during pyrithioxine treatment. Br J Rheumatol 1990;29(6):496–7.

1090. Lipsker D, Walther S, Schulz R, Nave S, Cribier B. Life-threatening vasculitis related to quinidine occurring in a healthy volunteer during a clinical trial. Eur J Clin Pharmacol 1998;54(9–10):815.

1091. Gilliland WR. Quinidine-induced dermatomyositis-like illness. J Clin Rheumatol 1999;5:39.

1092. Amadio P Jr, Cummings DM, Dashow L. Procainamide, quinidine, and lupus erythematosus. Ann Intern Med 1985;102(3):419.

1093. Bird MR, O'Neill AI, Buchanan RR, Ibrahim KM, Des Parkin J. Lupus anticoagulant in the elderly may be associated with both quinine and quinidine usage. Pathology 1995;27(2):136–9.

1094. Glynne P, Salama A, Chaudhry A, Swirsky D, Lightstone L. Quinine-induced immune thrombocytopenic purpura followed by hemolytic uremic syndrome. Am J Kidney Dis 1999;33(1):133–7.

1095. Schattner A. Quinine hypersensitivity simulating sepsis. Am J Med 1998;104(5):488–90.

1096. Barbaud A, Modiano P, Cocciale M, Reichert S, Schmutz JL. The topical application of resorcinol can provoke a systemic allergic reaction. Br J Dermatol 1996;135(6):1014–5.

1097. Ou LS, Kuo ML, Huang JL. Anaphylaxis to riboflavin (vitamin B2). Ann Allergy Asthma Immunol 2001;87(5):430–3.

1098. Farr B, Mandell GL. Rifampin. Med Clin North Am 1982;66(1):157–68.

1099. Bassi L, Di Berardino L, Arioli V, Silvestri LG, Ligniere EL. Conditions for immunosuppression by rifampicin. J Infect Dis 1973;128(6):736–44.

1100. Dickinson JM, Aber VR, Mitchison DA. Bactericidal activity of streptomycin, isoniazid, rifampin, ethambutol, and pyrazinamide alone and in combination against *Mycobacterium tuberculosis*. Am Rev Respir Dis 1977;116(4):627–35.

1101. Rook GA. Absence from sera from normal individuals or from rifampin-treated leprosy patients (THELEP trials) of antibody to rifamycin-protein or rifamycin-membrane conjugates. Int J Lepr Other Mycobact Dis 1985;53(1):22–27.

1102. Baciewicz AM, Self TH, Bekemeyer WB. Update on rifampin drug interactions. Arch Intern Med 1987;147(3):565–8.

1103. Garcia F, Blanco J, Carretero P, Herrero D, Juste S, Garces M, Perez R, Fuentes M. Anaphylactic reactions to topical rifampin. Allergy 1999;54(5):527–8.

1104. Berning SE, Iseman MD. Rifamycin-induced lupus syndrome. Lancet 1997;349(9064):1521–2.

1105. Arrizabalaga J, Casas A, Camino X, Iribarren JA, Rodriguez Arrondo F, Von Wichmann MA. Utilidad de la desensibilizacion a rifampicina en el tratamiento de enfermedades producidas por micobacterias en pacientes con SIDA. [The usefulness of the desensitization to rifampin in the treatment of mycobacterial disease in patients with AIDS.] Med Clin (Barc) 1998;111(3):103–4.

1106. Morris H, Muckerjee J, Akhtar S, Abdullahi L, Harrison M, Scott G. Use of corticosteroids to suppress drug toxicity in complicated tuberculosis. J Infect 1999;39(3):237–40.

1107. Allen SJ, Gallagher A, Paxton LD. Anaphylaxis to rocuronium. Anaesthesia 2000;55(12):1223–4.

1108. Barthelet Y, Ryckwaert Y, Plasse C, Bonnet-Boyer MC, d'Athis F. Accidents anaphylactiques graves après administration de rocuronium. [Severe anaphylactic reactions after administration of rocuronium.] Ann Fr Anesth Reanim 1999;18(8):896–900.

1109. Donnelly T. Anaphylaxis to rocuronium. Br J Anaesth 2000;84(5):696.

1110. Heier T, Guttormsen AB. Anaphylactic reactions during induction of anaesthesia using rocuronium for muscle relaxation: a report including 3 cases. Acta Anaesthesiol Scand 2000;44(7):775–81.

1111. Neal SM, Manthri PR, Gadiyar V, Wildsmith JA. Histaminoid reactions associated with rocuronium. Br J Anaesth 2000;84(1):108–11.

1112. Matthey P, Wang P, Finegan BA, Donnelly M. Rocuronium anaphylaxis and multiple neuromuscular blocking drug sensitivities. Can J Anaesth 2000; 47(9):890–893.

1113. Yee R, Fernandez JA. Anaphylactic reaction to rocuronium bromide. Anaesth Intensive Care 1996;24(5):601–4.

1114. Kierzek G, Audibert J, Pourriat JL. Anaphylaxis after rocuronium. Eur J Anaesthesiol 2003;20(2):169–70.

1115. Thomas R, Wood M. Anaphylaxis to rocuronium. Anaesthesia 2003;58(2):196.

1116. Rose M, Fisher M. Rocuronium: high risk for anaphylaxis? Br J Anaesth 2001;86(5):678–82.

1117. Joseph P, Benoit Y, Gressier M, Blanc P, Lehot JJ. Accident anaphylactique après administration de rocuronium: intérêt du bilan primaire pour le diagnostic précoce. [Anaphylaxis after rocuronium: advantage of blood tests for early diagnosis.] Ann Fr Anesth Reanim 2002;21(3):221–3.

1118. Laxenaire MC, Mertes PM. Groupe d'Etudes des Réactions Anaphylactoides Peranesthésiques. Anaphylaxis during anaesthesia. Results of a two-year survey in France. Br J Anaesth 2001;87(4):549–58.

1119. Booij LH, Houweling PJ. Rocuronium: high risk for anaphylaxis? Br J Anaesth 2001;87(5):805–6.

1120. Laxenaire MC. Epidemiologie des réactions anaphylactoides peranesthesiques. Quatrieme enquete multicentrique (juillet 1994–decembre 1996). Le Groupe d'Etudes des Réactions Anaphylactoides Peranésthesiques. [Epidemiology of anesthetic anaphylactoid reactions. Fourth multicenter survey (July 1994–December 1996).] Ann Fr Anesth Reanim 1999;18(7):796–809.

1121. Laake JH, Rottingen JA. Rocuronium and anaphylaxis — a statistical challenge. Acta Anaesthesiol Scand 2001;45(10):1196–203.

1122. Fisher M, Baldo BA. Anaphylaxis during anaesthesia: current aspects of diagnosis and prevention. Eur J Anaesthesiol 1994;11(4):263–84.

1123. Baillard C, Korinek AM, Galanton V, Le Manach Y, Larmignat P, Cupa M, Samama CM. Anaphylaxis to rocuronium. Br J Anaesth 2002;88(4):600–2.

1124. Fisher MM, More DG. The epidemiology and clinical features of anaphylactic reactions in anaesthesia. Anaesth Intensive Care 1981;9(3):226–34.

1125. Hatton F, Tiret L, Maujol L, N'Doye P, Vourc'h G, Desmonts JM, Otteni JC, Scherpereel P. Enquête épidémiologique sur les anesthesies. [INSERM. Epidemiological survey of anesthesia. Initial results.] Ann Fr Anesth Reanim 1983;2(5):331–86.

1126. Mitsuhata H, Matsumoto S, Hasegawa J. [The epidemiology and clinical features of anaphylactic and anaphylactoid reactions in the perioperative period in Japan.] Masui 1992;41(10):1664–9.

1127. Frosch PJ, Schulze-Dirks A. Kontaktallergie durch Polidocanol (Thesis). [Contact allergy caused by polidocanol (thesis).] Hautarzt 1989;40(3):146–9.

1128. Uter W, Geier J, Fuchs TIVDK Study Group. Contact allergy to polidocanol, 1992 to 1999. J Allergy Clin Immunol 2000;106(6):1203–4.

1129. Roger D, Rolle F, Mausset J, Lavignac C, Bonnetblanc JM. Urticarial vasculitis induced by fluoxetine. Dermatology 1995;191(2):164.

1130. Fisher A, McLean AJ, Purcell P, Herdson PB, Dahlstrom JE, Le Couteur DG. Focal necrotising vasculitis with secondary myositis following fluoxetine administration. Aust NZ J Med 1999;29(3):375–6.

1131. de Kerviler E, Tredaniel J, Revlon G, Groussard O, Zalcman G, Ortoli JM, Espie M, Hirsch A, Frija J. Fluoxetin-induced pulmonary granulomatosis. Eur Respir J 1996;9(3):615–7.

1132. Margolese HC, Chouinard G, Beauclair L, Rubino M. Cutaneous vasculitis induced by paroxetine. Am J Psychiatry 2001;158(3):497.

1133. Mani MZ. Photosensitivity to Selsun shampoo. Indian J Dermatol Venereol Leprol 1994;60:49–50.

1134. Jirasek L, Kalensky J. Precitlivelost na platinu, rhodium, zlato, med', antimom a jine vzacne kovy a profesionalni dermatitidy zpusobene selenem. [Hypersensitivity to platinum, rhodium, gold, copper, antimony and other precious metals and occupational dermatitis caused by selenium.] Cesk Dermatol 1975;50(6):361–8.

1135. Diskin CJ, Tomasso CL, Alper JC, Glaser ML, Fliegel SE. Long-term selenium exposure. Arch Intern Med 1979;139(7):824–6.

1136. Vasey FB, Espinoza LR, Martinez-Osuna P, Seleznick MJ, Brozena SJ, Penske NA. Silicone and rheumatic disease: replace implants or not? Arch Dermatol 1991;127(6):907.

1137. Spiera H, Kerr LD. Scleroderma following silicone implantation: a cumulative experience of 11 cases. J Rheumatol 1993;20(6):958–61.

1138. Gutierrez FJ, Espinoza LR. Progressive systemic sclerosis complicated by severe hypertension: reversal after silicone implant removal. Am J Med 1990;89(3):390–2.

1139. Endo LP, Edwards NL, Longley S, Corman LC, Panush RS. Silicone and rheumatic diseases. Semin Arthritis Rheum 1987;17(2):112–8.

1140. Maturri L, Azzolini A, Campiglio GL, Tardito E. Are synthetic prostheses really inert? Preliminary results of a study on the biocompatibility of Dacron vascular prostheses and silicone skin expanders. Int Surg 1991;76(2):115–8.

1141. Atkinson RE, Smith RJ. Silicone synovitis following silicone implant arthroplasty. Hand Clin 1986;2(2):291–9.

1142. Nalbandian RM, Swanson AB, Maupin BK. Long-term silicone implant arthroplasty. Implications of animal and human autopsy findings. JAMA 1983;250(9):1195–8.

1143. Bommer J, Ritz E, Waldherr R. Silicone-induced splenomegaly: treatment of pancytopenia by splenectomy in a patient on hemodialysis. N Engl J Med 1981;305(18):1077–9.

1144. Bommer J, Waldherr R, Gastner M, Lemmes R, Ritz E. Iatrogenic multiorgan silicone inclusions in dialysis patients. Klin Wochenschr 1981;59(20):1149–57.

1145. Vojdani A, Brautbar N, Campbell AW. Antibody to silicone and native macromolecules in women with silicone breast implants. Immunopharmacol Immunotoxicol 1994;16(4):497–523.

1146. Vojdani A, Brautbar N, Campbell AW. Antibody to silicone and native macromolecules in women with silicone breast implants. Immunopharmacol Immunotoxicol 1994;16(4):497–523.

1147. McGrath MH, Burkhardt BR. The safety and efficacy of breast implants for augmentation mammaplasty. Plast Reconstr Surg 1984;74(4):550–60.

1148. Vojdani A, Campbell A, Brautbar N. Immune functional impairment in patients with clinical abnormalities and silicone breast implants. Toxicol Ind Health 1992;8(6):415–29.

1149. Goldblum RM, Pelley RP, O'Donell AA, Pyron D, Heggers JP. Antibodies to silicone elastomers and reactions to ventriculoperitoneal shunts. Lancet 1992;340(8818):510–3.

1150. Cabral AR, Alcocer-Varela J, Orozco-Topete R, Reyes E, Fernandez-Dominguez L, Alarcon-Segovia D. Clinical, histopathological, immunological and fibroblast studies in 30 patients with subcutaneous injections of modelants including silicone and mineral oils. Rev Invest Clin 1994;46(4):257–66.

1151. Chastre J, Basset F, Viau F, Dournovo P, Bouchama A, Akesbi A, Gibert C. Acute pneumonitis after subcutaneous injections of silicone in transsexual men. N Engl J Med 1983;308(13):764–7.

1152. Celli BR, Kovnat DM. Acute pneumonitis after subcutaneous injections of silicone. N Engl J Med 1983;309(14):856–7.

1153. Manresa JM, Manresa F. Silicone pneumonitis. Lancet 1983;2(8363):1373.

1154. Cuellar ML, Gluck O, Molina JF, Gutierrez S, Garcia C, Espinoza R. Silicone breast implant—associated musculoskeletal manifestations. Clin Rheumatol 1995;14(6):667–72.

1155. Veenstra DL, Saint S, Sullivan SD. Cost-effectiveness of antiseptic-impregnated central venous catheters for the prevention of catheter-related bloodstream infection. JAMA 1999;282(6):554–60.

1156. Raad I, Hanna H. Intravascular catheters impregnated with antimicrobial agents: a milestone in the prevention of bloodstream infections. Support Care Cancer 1999;7(6):386–90.

1157. Anonymous. Antivenom therapy and reactions. Lancet 1980;1(8176):1009–10.

1158. Reid HA. Antivenom reactions and efficacy. Lancet 1980;1(8176):1024–5.

1159. Premawardhena AP, de Silva CE, Fonseka MM, Gunatilake SB, de Silva HJ. Low dose subcutaneous adrenaline to prevent acute adverse reactions to antivenom serum in people bitten by snakes: randomised, placebo controlled trial. BMJ 1999;318(7190):1041–3.

1160. Ariaratnam CA, Sjostrom L, Raziek Z, Kularatne SA, Arachchi RW, Sheriff MH, Theakston RD, Warrell DA. An open, randomized comparative trial of two antivenoms for the treatment of envenoming by Sri Lankan Russell's viper *(Daboia russelii russelii)*. Trans R Soc Trop Med Hyg 2001;95(1):74–80.

1161. Malasit P, Warrell DA, Chanthavanich P, Viravan C, Mongkolsapaya J, Singhthong B, Supich C. Prediction, prevention, and mechanism of early (anaphylactic) antivenom reactions in victims of snake bites. BMJ (Clin Res Ed) 1986;292(6512):17–20.

1162. Fan HW, Marcopito LF, Cardoso JL, Franca FO, Malaque CM, Ferrari RA, Theakston RD, Warrell DA. Sequential randomised and double blind trial of promethazine prophylaxis against early anaphylactic reactions to antivenom for bothrops snake bites. BMJ 1999;318(7196):1451–2.

1163. Gawarammana IB, Kularatne SA, Dissanayake WP, Kumarasiri RP, Senanayake N, Ariyasena H. Parallel infusion of hydrocortisone +/− chlorpheniramine bolus injection to prevent acute adverse reactions to antivenom for snakebites. Med J Aust 2004;180(1):20–3.

1164. Kaal A, Orskov H, Nielsen S, Pedroncelli AM, Lancranjan I, Marbach P, Weeke J. Occurrence and effects of octreotide antibodies during nasal, subcutaneous and slow release intramuscular treatment. Eur J Endocrinol 2000;143(3):353–61.

1165. Rideout DJ, Graham MM. Buttock granulomas: a consequence of intramuscular injection of Sandostatin detected by In-111 octreoscan. Clin Nucl Med 2001;26(7):650.

1166. Erstad BL. Octreotide for acute variceal bleeding. Ann Pharmacother 2001;35(5):618–26.

1167. Pitukcheewanont P, Schwarzbach L, Kaufman FR. Resumption of growth after methionyl-free human growth hormone therapy in a patient with neutralizing antibodies to methionyl human growth hormone. J Pediatr Endocrinol Metab 2002;15(5):653–7.

1168. Reiter EO, Attie KM, Moshang T Jr, Silverman BL, Kemp SF, Neuwirth RB, Ford KM, Saenger PGenentech, Inc.-Alkermes, Inc. Collaborative Study Group. A multicenter study of the efficacy and safety of sustained release GH in the treatment of naive pediatric patients with GH deficiency. J Clin Endocrinol Metab 2001;86(10):4700–6.

1169. Walker SB, Weiss ME, Tattoni DS. Systemic reaction to human growth hormone treated with acute desensitization. Pediatrics 1992;90(1 Pt 1):108–9.

1170. Guest G, Berard E, Crosnier H, Chevallier T, Rappaport R, Broyer M. Effects of growth hormone in short children after renal transplantation. French Society of Pediatric Nephrology. Pediatr Nephrol 1998;12(6):437–46.

1171. Yap HK, Loke KY, Murugasu B, Lee BW. Subclinical activation of lupus nephritis by recombinant human growth hormone. Pediatr Nephrol 1998;12(2):133–5.

1172. Davies RJ, Pepys J. Asthma due to inhaled chemical agents—the macrolide antibiotic spiramycin. Clin Allergy 1975;5(1):99–107.

1173. Valero Prieto I, Calvo Catala J, Hortelano Martinez E, Abril L, de Medrano V, Glez-Cruz Cervellera MI, Herrera Ballester A, Orti E. Purpura de schönlein–Henoch asociada a espiramicina y con importantes manifestaciones digestiwas. [Schoenlein–Henoch purpura associated with spiramycin and with important digestive manifestations.] Rev Esp Enferm Dig 1994;85(1):47–9.

1174. Shpall EJ, Wheeler CA, Turner SA, Yanovich S, Brown RA, Pecora AL, Shea TC, Mangan KF, Williams SF, LeMaistre CF, Long GD, Jones R, Davis MW, Murphy-Filkins R, Parker WR, Glaspy JA. A randomized phase 3 study of peripheral blood progenitor cell mobilization with stem cell factor and filgrastim in high-risk breast cancer patients. Blood 1999;93(8):2491–501.

1175. Schwenger V, Mundlein E, Dagrosa EE, Fahr AM, Zeier M, Mikus G, Andrassy K. Treatment of life-threatening multiresistant staphylococcal and enterococcal infections in patients with end-stage renal failure with quinupristin/dalfopristin: preliminary report. Infection 2002;30(5):257–61.

1176. Chan TY, Critchley JA. Is chloroxylenol nephrotoxic like phenol? A study of patients with DETTOL poisoning. Vet Hum Toxicol 1994;36(3):250–1.

1177. Sokol WN, Hydick IB. Nasal congestion, urticaria, and angioedema caused by an IgE-mediated reaction to sodium metabisulfite. Ann Allergy 1990;65(3):233–8.

1178. Long CC, Motley RJ, Holt PJ. Taking the "sting" out of local anaesthetics. Br J Dermatol 1991;125(5):452–5.

1179. Soulat JM, Bouju P, Oxeda C, Amiot JF. Choc anaphylactoide aux metabisulfites au cours d'une césarienne sous anesthésie péridurale. [Anaphylactoid shock due to metabisulfites during cesarean section under peridural anesthesia.] Cah Anesthesiol 1991;39(4):257–9.

1180. Heshmati S, Maibach HI. Active sensitization to sodium metabisulfite in hydrocortisone cream. Contact Dermatitis 1999;41(3):166–7.

1181. Tucker SC, Yell JA, Beck MH. Allergic contact dermatitis from sodium metabisulfite in Trimovate cream. Contact Dermatitis 1999;40(3):164.

1182. Dwenger CS. 'Sulpha' hypersensitivity. Anaesthesia 2000;55(2):200–1.

1183. Bedard K, Smith S, Cribb A. Sequential assessment of an antidrug antibody response in a patient with a systemic delayed-onset sulphonamide hypersensitivity syndrome reaction. Br J Dermatol 2000;142(2):253–8.

1184. Carrington DM, Earl HS, Sullivan TJ. Studies of human IgE to a sulfonamide determinant. J Allergy Clin Immunol 1987;79(3):442–7.

1185. Sher MR, Suchar C, Lockey RF. Anaphylactic shock induced by oral desensitization to trimethoprim/sulfmethoxazole. J Allergy Immunol 1986;77:133.

1186. Gruchalla RS, Sullivan TJ. Detection of human IgE to sulfamethoxazole by skin testing with sulfamethoxazoylpoly-L-tyrosine. J Allergy Clin Immunol 1991;88(5):784–92.

1187. Ghajar BM, Naranjo CA, Shear NH, Lanctot KL. Improving the accuracy of the differential diagnosis of idiosyncratic adverse drug reactions (IADRs): skin eruptions and sulfonamides. Clin Pharmacol Ther 1990;47(2):127.

1188. Shear NH, Rieder MJ, Spielberg SP, et al. Hypersensitivity reactions to sulfonamide antibiotics are mediated by a hydroxylamine metabolite. Clin Res 1987;35:717.

1189. Shear NH, Spielberg SP, Grant DM, Tang BK, Kalow W. Differences in metabolism of sulfonamides predisposing to idiosyncratic toxicity. Ann Intern Med 1986;105(2):179–84.

1190. Rieder MJ, Shear NH, Kanee A, Tang BK, Spielberg SP. Prominence of slow acetylator phenotype among patients with sulfonamide hypersensitivity reactions. Clin Pharmacol Ther 1991;49(1):13–7.

1191. Delomenie C, Mathelier-Fusade P, Longuemaux S, Rozenbaum W, Leynadier F, Krishnamoorthy R, Dupret JM. Glutathione S-transferase (GSTM1) null genotype and sulphonamide intolerance in acquired immunodeficiency syndrome. Pharmacogenetics 1997;7(6):519–20.

1192. Coopman SA, Johnson RA, Platt R, Stern RS. Cutaneous disease and drug reactions in HIV infection. N Engl J Med 1993;328(23):1670–4.

1193. Woody RC, Brewster MA. Adverse effects of trimethoprim–sulfamethoxazole in a child with dihydropteridine reductase deficiency. Dev Med Child Neurol 1990;32(7):639–42.

1194. Shear NH, Spielberg SP. In vitro evaluation of a toxic metabolite of sulfadiazine. Can J Physiol Pharmacol 1985;63(11):1370–2.

1195. Clarke BF, Campbell IW, Ewing DJ, Beveridge GW, MacDonald MK. Generalized hypersensitivity reaction and visceral arteritis with fatal outcome during glibenclamide therapy. Diabetes 1974;23(9):739–42.

1196. Takimoto CH, Lynch D, Stulbarg MS. Pulmonary infiltrates associated with sulindac therapy. Chest 1990;97(1):230–2.

1197. Fein M. Sulindac and pneumonitis. Ann Intern Med 1981;95(2):245.

1198. Burrish GF, Kaatz BL. Sulindac-induced anaphylaxis. Ann Emerg Med 1981;10(3):154–5.

1199. Hyson CP, Kazakoff MA. A severe multisystem reaction to sulindac. Arch Intern Med 1991;151(2):387–8.

1200. Berne B, Ros AM. 7 years experience of photopatch testing with sunscreen allergens in Sweden. Contact Dermatitis 1998;38(2):61–4.

1201. Ricci C, Pazzaglia M, Tosti A. Photocontact dermatitis from UV filters. Contact Dermatitis 1998;38(6):343–4.

1202. Cook N, Freeman S. Report of 19 cases of photoallergic contact dermatitis to sunscreens seen at the Skin and Cancer Foundation. Australas J Dermatol 2001;42(4):257–9.

1203. Emonet S, Pasche-Koo F, Perin-Minisini MJ, Hauser C. Anaphylaxis to oxybenzone, a frequent constituent of sunscreens. J Allergy Clin Immunol 2001;107(3):556–7.

1204. Smith HR, Armstrong K, Wakelin SH, White IR. Contact allergy to PVP/eicosene copolymer. Contact Dermatitis 1999;40(5):283.

1205. Bourrain JL, Amblard P, Beani JC. Contact urticaria photoinduced by benzophenones. Contact Dermatitis 2003;48(1):45–6.

1206. Sommer S, Wilkinson SM, English JS, Ferguson J. Photoallergic contact dermatitis from the sunscreen octyl triazone. Contact Dermatitis 2002;46(5):304–5.

1207. Bourne JG, Collier HO, Somers GF. Succinylcholine (succinoylcholine), muscle-relaxant of short action. Lancet 1952;1(25):1225–9.

1208. Smith NL. Histamine release by suxamethonium. Anaesthesia 1957;12(3):293–8.

1209. Bele-Binda N, Valeri F. A case of bronchospasm induced by succinylcholine. Can Anaesth Soc J 1971;18(1):116–9.

1210. Redderson C, Perkins HM, Adler WH, Gravenstein JS. Systemic reaction to succinylcholine: a case report. Anesth Analg 1971;50(1):49–52.

1211. Sitarz L. Anaphylactic shock following injection of suxamethonium. Anaesth Resusc Intensive Ther 1974;2(1):83–6.

1212. Mandappa JM, Chandrasekhara PM, Nelvigi RG. Anaphylaxis to suxamethonium. Two case reports. Br J Anaesth 1975;47(4):523–5.

1213. James OF, Aseervatham SD, Fortunaso B, Clancy R. Anaphylactoid reaction to suxamethonium. Anaesth Intensive Care 1979;7(3):288.

1214. Kepes ER, Haimovici H. Allergic reaction to succinylcholine. JAMA 1959;171:548–9.

1215. Jerums G, Whittingham S, Wilson P. Anaphylaxis to suxamethonium. A case report. Br J Anaesth 1967;39(1):73–7.

1216. Moss J, Fahmy NR, Sunder N, Beaven MA. Hormonal and hemodynamic profile of an anaphylactic reaction in man. Circulation 1981;63(1):210–3.

1217. Fellini AA, Bernstein RL, Zauder HL. Bronchospasm due to suxamethonium; report of a case. Br J Anaesth 1963;35:657–9.

1218. Katz AM, Mulligan PG. Bronchospasm induced by suxamethonium. A case report. Br J Anaesth 1972;44(10):1097–9.

1219. Fisher MM, Munro I. Life-threatening anaphylactoid reactions to muscle relaxants. Anesth Analg 1983;62(6):559–64.

1220. Laxenaire MC, Moneret-Vautrin DA, Vervloet D, Alazia M, Francois G. Accidents anaphylactoïdes graves peranesthésiques. [Severe peranesthetic anaphylactic accident.] Ann Fr Anesth Reanim 1985;4(1):30–46.

1221. Laxenaire MC, Moneret-Vautrin DA, Vervloet D. The French experience of anaphylactoid reactions. Int Anesthesiol Clin 1985;23(3):145–60.

1222. Galletly DC, Treuren BC. Anaphylactoid reactions during anaesthesia. Seven years' experience of intradermal testing. Anaesthesia 1985;40(4):329–33.

1223. Youngman PR, Taylor KM, Wilson JD. Anaphylactoid reactions to neuromuscular blocking agents: a commonly undiagnosed condition? Lancet 1983;2(8350):597–9.

1224. Vuitton D, Neidhardt-Audion M, Girardin P, Racadot E, Geissmann C, Laurent R, Barale F. Caractéristiques épidemiologiques de 21 accidents anaphylactoïdes per-anesthésiques observés dans une population de 12,855 sujets opérés. [Epidemiologic characteristics of 21 per-anesthetic anaphylactoid accidents observed in a population of 12,855 surgically treated patients.] Ann Fr Anesth Reanim 1985;4(2):167–72.

1225. Laxenaire MC, Moneret-Vautrin DA, Boileau S. Choc anaphylactique au suxaméthonium: à propos de 18 cas. [Anaphylactic shock induced by suxamethonium.] Ann Fr Anesth Reanim 1982;1(1):29–36.

1226. Wright PJ, Shortland JR, Stevens JD, Parsons MA, Watkins J. Fatal haemopathological consequences of general anaesthesia. Br J Anaesth 1989;62(1):104–7.

1227. Maguchi S, Fukuda S. *Taxus cuspidata* (Japanese yew) pollen nasal allergy. Auris Nasus Larynx 2001;28(Suppl):S43–7.

1228. Apted JH. Contact dermatitis associated with the use of tea-tree oil. Australas J Dermatol 1991;32(3):177.

1229. Varma S, Blackford S, Statham BN, Blackwell A. Combined contact allergy to tea tree oil and lavender oil complicating chronic vulvovaginitis. Contact Dermatitis 2000;42(5):309–10.

1230. Hausen BM, Reichling J, Harkenthal M. Degradation products of monoterpenes are the sensitizing agents in tea tree oil. Am J Contact Dermat 1999;10(2):68–77.

1231. Beckmann B. Tea tree oil. Dermatosen 1998;46:120–4.

1232. de Groot AC, Weyland JW. Systemic contact dermatitis from tea tree oil. Contact Dermatitis 1992;27(4):279–80.

1233. Mozelsio NB, Harris KE, McGrath KG, Grammer LC. Immediate systemic hypersensitivity reaction associated with topical application of Australian tea tree oil. Allergy Asthma Proc 2003;24(1):73–5.

1234. Paul C, Janier M, Carlet J, Tamion F, Carlotti A, Fichelle JM, Daniel F. [Erythroderma induced by teicoplanin.] Ann Dermatol Venereol 1992;119(9):667–9.

1235. McElrath MJ, Goldberg D, Neu HC. Allergic cross-reactivity of teicoplanin and vancomycin. Lancet 1986;1(8471):47.

1236. Davenport A. Allergic cross-reactivity to teicoplanin and vancomycin. Nephron 1993;63(4):482.

1237. Knudsen JD, Pedersen M. IgE-mediated reaction to vancomycin and teicoplanin after treatment with vancomycin. Scand J Infect Dis 1992;24(3):395–6.

1238. Smith SR, Cheesbrough JS, Makris M, Davies JM. Teicoplanin administration in patients experiencing reactions to vancomycin. J Antimicrob Chemother 1989;23(5):810–2.

1239. Wood G, Whitby M. Teicoplanin in patients who are allergic to vancomycin. Med J Aust 1989;150(11):668.

1240. Schlemmer B, Falkman H, Boudjadja A, Jacob L, Le Gall JR. Teicoplanin for patients allergic to vancomycin. N Engl J Med 1988;318(17):1127–8.

1241. Campoli-Richards DM, Brogden RN, Faulds D. Teicoplanin. A review of its antibacterial activity, pharmacokinetic properties and therapeutic potential. Drugs 1990;40(3):449–86.

1242. Brooke R, Coulson IH, al-Dawoud A. Terbinafine-induced subacute cutaneous lupus erythematosus. Br J Dermatol 1998;139(6):1132–3.

1243. Murphy M, Barnes L. Terbinafine-induced lupus erythematosus. Br J Dermatol 1998;138(4):708–9.

1244. Holmes S, Kemmett D. Exacerbation of systemic lupus erythematosus induced by terbinafine. Br J Dermatol 1998;139(6):1133.

1245. Schilling MK, Eichenberger M, Maurer CA, Sigurdsson G, Buchler MW. Ketoconazole and pulmonary failure after esophagectomy: a prospective clinical trial. Dis Esophagus 2001;14(1):37–40.

1246. Bonsmann G, Schiller M, Luger TA, Stander S. Terbinafine-induced subacute cutaneous lupus erythematosus. J Am Acad Dermatol 2001;44(6):925–31.

1247. Gupta AK, Porges AJ. Hypersensitivity syndrome reaction to oral terbinafine. Australas J Dermatol 1998;39(3):171–2.

1248. Levine L, Ipsen J Jr, McComb JA. Adult immunization. Preparation and evaluation of combined fluid tetanus and diphtheria toxoids for adult use. Am J Hyg 1961;73:20–35.

1249. Relihan M. Reactions to tetanus toxoid. J Ir Med Assoc 1969;62(390):430–4.

1250. Edsall G, Elliott MW, Peebles TC, Eldred MC. Excessive use of tetanus toxoid boosters. JAMA 1967;202(1):111–3.

1251. Leen CL, Barclay GR, McClelland DB, Shepherd WM, Langford DT. Double-blind comparative trial of standard (commercial) and antibody-affinity-purified tetanus toxoid vaccines. J Infect 1987;14(2):119–24.

1252. Ghate JV, Turner ML, Rudek MA, Figg WD, Dahut W, Dyer V, Pluda JM, Reed E. Drug-induced lupus associated with COL-3: report of 3 cases. Arch Dermatol 2001;137(4):471–4.

1253. Witzens M, Moehler T, Neben K, Fruehauf S, Hartschuh W, Ho AD, Goldschmidt H. Development of leukocytoclastic vasculitis in a patient with multiple myeloma during treatment with thalidomide. Ann Hematol 2004;83(7):467–70.

1254. Chao NJ, Parker PM, Niland JC, Wong RM, Dagis A, Long GD, Nademanee AP, Negrin RS, Snyder DS, Hu WW, Gould KA, Tierney DK, Zwingenberger K, Forman SJ, Blume KG. Paradoxical effect of thalidomide prophylaxis on chronic graft-vs.-host disease Biol Blood Marrow Transplant 1996;2(2):86–92.

1255. Cany L, Fitoussi O, Boiron JM, Marit G. Tumor lysis syndrome at the beginning of thalidomide therapy for multiple myeloma. J Clin Oncol 2002;20(8):2212.

1256. Gozal D, Ben-Aryeh H, Szargel R, Colin A. Salivary composition in asthmatic children on theophylline. Isr J Med Sci 1985;21(5):460–1.

1257. Ezeamuzie CI, Al-Hage M. Effects of some anti-asthma drugs on human eosinophil superoxide anions release and degranulation. Int Arch Allergy Immunol 1998;115(2):162–8.

1258. Gibbs BF, Vollrath IB, Albrecht C, Amon U, Wolff HH. Inhibition of interleukin-4 and interleukin-13 release from immunologically activated human basophils due to the actions of anti-allergic drugs. Naunyn Schmiedebergs Arch Pharmacol 1998;357(5):573–8.

1259. Nunn P, Kibuga D, Gathua S, Brindle R, Imalingat A, Wasunna K, Lucas S, Gilks C, Omwega M, Were J, McAdam K. Cutaneous hypersensitivity reactions due to thiacetazone in HIV-1 seropositive patients treated for tuberculosis. Lancet 1991;337(8742):627–30.

1260. Vindel JA, Khoury B. Inhibition by thiamphenicol of antibody production induced by different antigens. Postgrad Med J 1974;50(Suppl 5):108–10.

1261. Ono K, Hattori T, Kusaba A, Inokuchi K. Prolongation of rat heart allograft survival by thiamphenicol. Surgery 1972;71(2):258–61.

1262. Phipatanakul W, Adkinson NF Jr. Cross-reactivity between sulfonamides and loop or thiazide diuretics: a theoretical or actual risk? Allergy Clin Immunol Int 2000;12:26–8.

1263. Earl G, Davenport J, Narula J. Furosemide challenge in patients with heart failure and adverse reactions to sulfa-containing diuretics. Ann Intern Med 2003;138(4):358–9.

1264. Shadid S, Jensen MD. Angioneurotic edema as a side effect of pioglitazone. Diabetes Care 2002;25(2):405.

1265. Choi HK, Merkel PA, Walker AM, Niles JL. Drug-associated antineutrophil cytoplasmic antibody-positive vasculitis: prevalence among patients with high titers of antimyeloperoxidase antibodies. Arthritis Rheum 2000;43(2):405–13.

1266. Chastain MA, Russo GG, Boh EE, Chastain JB, Falabella A, Millikan LE. Propylthiouracil hypersensitivity: report of two patients with vasculitis and review of the literature. J Am Acad Dermatol 1999;41(5 Pt 1):757–64.

1267. Morita S, Ueda Y, Eguchi K. Anti-thyroid drug-induced ANCA-associated vasculitis: a case report and review of the literature. Endocr J 2000;47(4):467–70.

1268. Sera N, Yokoyama N, Abe Y, Ide A, Usa T, Tominaga T, Ejima E, Kawakami A, Ashizawa K, Eguchi K. Antineutrophil cytoplasmic antibody-associated vasculitis complicating Graves' disease: report of two adult cases. Acta Med Nagasaki 2000;45:33–6.

1269. Otsuka S, Kinebuchi A, Tabata H, Yamakage A, Yamazaki S. Myeloperoxidase–antineutrophil cytoplasmic antibody-associated vasculitis following propylthiouracil therapy. Br J Dermatol 2000;142(4):828–30.

1270. Matsubara K, Nigami H, Harigaya H, Osaki M, Baba K. Myeloperoxidase antineutrophil cytoplasmic antibody positive vasculitis during propylthiouracil treatment: successful management with oral corticosteroids. Pediatr Int 2000;42(2):170–3.

1271. Harper L, Cockwell P, Savage CO. Case of propylthiouracil-induced ANCA associated small vessel vasculitis. Nephrol Dial Transplant 1998;13(2):455–8.

1272. Miller RM, Savige J, Nassis L, Cominos BI. Antineutrophil cytoplasmic antibody (ANCA)-positive cutaneous leucocytoclastic vasculitis associated with antithyroid therapy in Graves' disease. Australas J Dermatol 1998;39(2):96–9.

1273. Fujieda M, Nagata M, Akioka Y, Hattori M, Kawaguchi H, Ito K. Antineutrophil cytoplasmic antibody-positive crescentic glomerulonephritis associated with propylthiouracil therapy. Acta Paediatr Jpn 1998;40(3):286–9.

1274. Pillinger M, Staud R. Wegener's granulomatosis in a patient receiving propylthiouracil for Graves' disease. Semin Arthritis Rheum 1998;28(2):124–9.

1275. Bajaj S, Bell MJ, Shumak S, Briones-Urbina R. Antithyroid arthritis syndrome. J Rheumatol 1998;25(6):1235–9.

1276. Gunton JE, Stiel J, Caterson RJ, McElduff A. Clinical case seminar: anti-thyroid drugs and antineutrophil cytoplasmic antibody positive vasculitis. A case report and review of the literature. J Clin Endocrinol Metab 1999;84(1):13–6.

1277. Miller RM, Darben TA, Nedwich J, Savige J. Propylthiouracil-induced antineutrophil cytoplasmic antibodies in a patient with Graves' disease and a neutrophilic dermatosis. Br J Dermatol 1999;141(5):943–4.

1278. Darben T, Savige J, Prentice R, Paspaliaris B, Chick J. Pyoderma gangrenosum with secondary pyarthrosis following propylthiouracil. Australas J Dermatol 1999;40(3):144–6.

1279. Park KE, Chipps DR, Benson EM. Necrotizing vasculitis secondary to propylthiouracil presenting as purpura fulminans. Rheumatology (Oxford) 1999;38(8):790–2.

1280. Wada N, Mukai M, Kohno M, Notoya A, Ito T, Yoshioka N. Prevalence of serum anti-myeloperoxidase antineutrophil cytoplasmic antibodies (MPO-ANCA) in patients with Graves' disease treated with propylthiouracil and thiamazole. Endocr J 2002;49(3):329–34.

1281. Katayama K, Hata C, Kagawa K, Noda M, Nakamura K, Shimizu H, Fujimoto M. Diffuse alveolar hemorrhage associated with myeloperoxidase–antineutrophil cytoplasmic antibody induced by propylthiouracil therapy. Respiration 2002;69(5):473.

1282. Winters MJ, Hurley RM, Lirenman DS. ANCA-positive glomerulonephritis and IgA nephropathy in a patient on propylthiouracil. Pediatr Nephrol 2002;17(4):257–60.

1283. Akamizu T, Ozaki S, Hiratani H, Uesugi H, Sobajima J, Hataya Y, Kanamoto N, Saijo M, Hattori Y, Moriyama K, Ohmori K, Nakao K. Drug-induced neutropenia associated with anti-neutrophil cytoplasmic antibodies (ANCA): possible involvement of complement in granulocyte cytotoxicity. Clin Exp Immunol 2002;127(1):92–8.

1284. Herlin T, Birkebaek NH, Wolthers OD, Heegaard NH, Wiik A. Anti-neutrophil cytoplasmic autoantibody (ANCA) profiles in propylthiouracil-induced lupus-like manifestations in monozygotic triplets with hyperthyroidism. Scand J Rheumatol 2002;31(1):46–9.

1285. Fujieda M, Hattori M, Kurayama H, Koitabashi Y. Members and Coworkers of the Japanese Society for Pediatric Nephrology. Clinical features and outcomes in children with antineutrophil cytoplasmic autoantibody-positive glomerulonephritis associated with propylthiouracil treatment. J Am Soc Nephrol 2002;13(2):437–45.

1286. Sera N, Ashizawa K, Ando T, Abe Y, Ide A, Usa T, Tominaga T, Ejima E, Yokoyama N, Eguchi K. Treatment with propylthiouracil is associated with appearance of antineutrophil cytoplasmic antibodies in some patients with Graves' disease. Thyroid 2000;10(7):595–9.

1287. Seligman VA, Bolton PB, Sanchez HC, Fye KH. Propylthiouracil-induced microscopic polyangiitis. J Clin Rheumatol 2001;7:170–4.

1288. Colakovski H, Lorber DL. Propylthiouracil-induced perinuclear-staining antineutrophil cytoplasmic autoantibody-positive vasculitis in conjunction with pericarditis. Endocr Pract 2001;7(1):37–9.

1289. Meister LH, Guerra IR, Carvalho GD. Images in thyroidology. Vasculitis secondary to treatment with propylthiouracil. Thyroid 2001;11(2):199–200.

1290. Wing SS, Fantus IG. Adverse immunologic effects of antithyroid drugs. CMAJ 1987;136(2):121–7.

1291. Dysseleer A, Buysschaert M, Fonck C, Van Ginder Deuren K, Jadoul M, Tennstedt D, Cosyns JP, Daumerie C. Acute interstitial nephritis and fatal Stevens–Johnson syndrome after propylthiouracil therapy. Thyroid 2000;10(8):713–6.

1292. Khurshid I, Sher J. Disseminated intravascular coagulation and vasculitis during propylthiouracil therapy. Postgrad Med J 2000;76(893):185–6.

1293. Seymour DG. Anaphylactic reaction to thiopental. JAMA 1993;270:2503.

1294. von Hintzenstern J, Heese A, Koch HU, Peters KP, Hornstein OP. Frequency, spectrum and occupational relevance of type IV allergies to rubber chemicals. Contact Dermatitis 1991;24(4):244–52.

1295. Saunders H, Watkins F. Allergic contact dermatitis due to thiuram exposure from a fungicide. Australas J Dermatol 2001;42(3):217–8.

1296. Leow YH, Ng SK, Goh CL. An unusual cause of post-auricular dermatitis. Contact Dermatitis 2000;42(5):308.

1297. Elliot JM, Cross DB, Cederholm-Williams S, et al. Streptokinase titers 1 to 4 years after intravenous streptokinase. Circulation 1991;84(Suppl 2):116.

1298. Massel D, Turpie AGG, Oberhardt BJ, et al. Estimation of resistance to streptokinase: a preliminary report of a rapid bedside test. Can J Cardiol 1993;9:E134.

1299. Jalihal S, Morris GK. Antistreptokinase titres after intravenous streptokinase. Lancet 1990;335(8683):184–5.

1300. Cross DB. Should streptokinase be readministered? Insights from recent studies of antistreptokinase antibodies. Med J Aust 1994;161(2):100–1.

1301. Cross DB, White HD. Allergic reactions to streptokinase: does antibody formation prevent reuse in a second myocardial infarction? Clin Immunother 1994;2:415.

1302. Jolliet P, Magnin C, Unger PF. Pulmonary embolectomy after intravenous thrombolysis with alteplase. Lancet 1990;335(8684):290–1.

1303. Gruppo Italiano per lo Studio della Streptocochinasi nell'Infarto miocardico (GSSI). Effectiveness of intravenous thrombolytic treatment in acute myocardial infarction. Lancet 1987;1:397.

1304. Cooper JP, Quarry DP, Beale DJ, Chappell AG. Life-threatening, localized angio-oedema associated with streptokinase. Postgrad Med J 1994;70(826):592–3.

1305. Stephens MB, Pepper PV. Streptokinase therapy. Recognizing and treating allergic reactions. Postgrad Med 1998;103(3):89–90.

1306. Francis CW, Brenner B, Leddy JP, Marder VJ. Angioedema during therapy with recombinant tissue plasminogen activator. Br J Haematol 1991;77(4):562–3.

1307. Purvis JA, Booth NA, Wilson CM, Adgey AA, McCluskey DR. Anaphylactoid reaction after injection of alteplase. Lancet 1993;341(8850):966–7.

1308. Pancioli A, Brott T, Donaldson V, Miller R. Asymmetric angioneurotic edema associated with thrombolysis for acute stroke. Ann Emerg Med 1997;30(2):227–9.

1309. Dickinson RJ, Rosser A. Low back pain associated with streptokinase. BMJ 1991;302(6768):111–2.

1310. Hannaford P, Kay CR. Back pain and thrombolysis. BMJ 1992;304(6831):915.

1311. Lear J, Rajapakse R, Pohl J. Low back pain associated with streptokinase. Lancet 1992;340(8823):851.

1312. Chan NS, White H, Maslowski A, Cleland J. Plasmacytosis and renal failure after readministration of streptokinase for threatened myocardial reinfarction. BMJ 1988;297(6650):717–8.

1313. Bucknall C, Darley C, Flax J, Vincent R, Chamberlain D. Vasculitis complicating treatment with intravenous anisoylated plasminogen streptokinase activator complex in acute myocardial infarction. Br Heart J 1988;59(1):9–11.

1314. Gemmill JD, Sandler M, Hillis WS, Tillman J, Wakeel R. Vasculitis complicating treatment with intravenous anisoylated plasminogen streptokinase activator complex in acute myocardial infarction. Br Heart J 1988;60(4):361.

1315. Ong AC, Handler CE, Walker JM. Hypersensitivity vasculitis complicating intravenous streptokinase therapy in acute myocardial infarction. Int J Cardiol 1988;21(1):71–3.

1316. Sorber WA, Herbst V. Lymphocytic angiitis following streptokinase therapy. Cutis 1988;42(1):57–8.

1317. Albert F, Dubourg O, Steg G, Delorme G, Bourdarias JP. Maladie sérique après fibrinoyse par streptokinase intraveineuse au cours d'un infarctus du myocarde. [Serum sickness after fibrinolysis using intravenous streptokinase in myocardial infarction.] Arch Mal Coeur Vaiss 1988;81(8):1013–5.

1318. Davies KA, Mathieson P, Winearls CG, Rees AJ, Walport MJ. Serum sickness and acute renal failure after streptokinase therapy for myocardial infarction. Clin Exp Immunol 1990;80(1):83–8.

1319. Noel J, Rosenbaum LH, Gangadharan V, Stewart J, Galens G. Serum sickness-like illness and leukocytoclastic vasculitis following intracoronary arterial streptokinase. Am Heart J 1987;113(2 Pt 1):395–7.

1320. Verstraete M, Vermylen J, Donati MB. The effect of streptokinase infusion on chronic arterial occlusions and stenoses. Ann Intern Med 1971;74(3):377–82.

1321. Argent N, Adam PC. Proteinuria and thrombolytic agents. Lancet 1990;335(8681):106–7.

1322. Le SP, Chatterjee K, Wolfe CL. Adult respiratory distress syndrome following thrombolytic therapy with APSAC for acute myocardial infarction. Am Heart J 1992;123(5):1368–9.

1323. Tio RA, Voorbij RH, Enthoven R. Adult respiratory distress syndrome after streptokinase. Am J Cardiol 1992;70(20):1632–3.

1324. Montserrat I, Altimiras J, Dominguez M, Lamich R, Olle A, Fontcuberta J. Adverse reaction to streptokinase with multiple systemic manifestations. Pharm World Sci 1995;17(5):168–71.

1325. Montgomery HE, McIntyre CW, Almond MK, Davies K, Pumphrey CW, Bennett D. Rhabdomyolysis and multiple system organ failure with streptokinase. BMJ 1995;311(7018):1472.

1326. Tsang TS, Califf RM, Stebbins AL, Lee KL, Cho S, Ross AM, Armstrong PW. Incidence and impact on outcome of streptokinase allergy in the GUSTO-I trial. Global Utilization of Streptokinase and t-PA in Occluded Coronary Arteries. Am J Cardiol 1997;79(9):1232–5.

1327. Papamitsakis NI, Kuyl J, Lutsep HL, Clark WM. Benign angioedema after thrombolysis for acute stroke. J Stroke Cerebrovasc Dis 2000;9:79–81.

1328. Hill MD, Barber PA, Takahashi J, Demchuk AM, Feasby TE, Buchan AM. Anaphylactoid reactions and angioedema during alteplase treatment of acute ischemic stroke. CMAJ 2000;162(9):1281–4.

1329. Rudolf J, Grond M, Schmulling S, Neveling M, Heiss W. Orolingual angioneurotic edema following therapy of acute ischemic stroke with alteplase. Neurology 2000;55(4):599–600.

1330. Rudolf J, Grond M, Prince WS, Schmulling S, Heiss WD. Evidence of anaphylaxy after alteplase infusion. Stroke 1999;30(5):1142–3.

1331. Shibata H, Hayakawa H, Hirukawa M, Tadokoro K, Ogata E. Hypersensitivity caused by synthetic thyroid hormones in a hypothyroid patient with Hashimoto's thyroiditis. Arch Intern Med 1986;146(8):1624–5.

1332. Robbins RJ, Robbins AK. Clinical review 156: Recombinant human thyrotropin and thyroid cancer management. J Clin Endocrinol Metab 2003;88(5):1933–8.

1333. Braga M, Ringel MD, Cooper DS. Sudden enlargement of local recurrent thyroid tumor after recombinant human TSH administration. J Clin Endocrinol Metab 2001;86(11):5148–51.

1334. McDougall IR, Weigel RJ. Recombinant human thyrotropin in the management of thyroid cancer. Curr Opin Oncol 2001;13(1):39–43.

1335. Braun-Moscovici Y, Schapira D, Balbir-Gurman A, Sevilia R, Menachem Nahir A. Ticlopidine-induced lupus. J Clin Rheumatol 2001;7:102–5.

1336. Pak CY, Fuller C, Sakhaee K, Zerwekh JE, Adams BV. Management of cystine nephrolithiasis with alpha-mercaptopropionylglycine. J Urol 1986;136(5):1003–8.

1337. Matsukawa Y, Saito N, Nishinarita S, Horie T, Ryu J. Therapeutic effect of tiopronin following D-penicillamine toxicity in a patient with rheumatoid arthritis. Clin Rheumatol 1998;17(1):73–4.

1338. Koeger AC, Rozenberg S, Chaibi P, Camus JP, Bourgeois P. Polymyosite induite par la tiopronine, confirmée par l'histologie. [Tiopronin-induced polymyositis confirmed by histology.] Rev Rhum Ed Fr 1993;60(1):78–9.

1339. Cacoub P, Sbai A, Azizi P, Gatfosse M, Godeau P, Piette JC. Polymyosite induite par la tiopronine. [Polymyositis induced by tiopronine.] Presse Méd 1999;28(17):911–2.

1340. Farronato G, Tirafili C, Alicino C, Santoro F. Titanium appliances for allergic patients. J Clin Orthod 2002;36(12):676–9.

1341. Holgers KM, Thomsen P, Tjellstrom A. Persistent irritation of the soft tissue around an osseointegrated titanium implant. Case report. Scand J Plast Reconstr Surg Hand Surg 1994;28(3):225–30.

1342. Piattelli A, Scarano A, Piattelli M, Bertolai R, Panzoni E. Histologic aspects of the bone and soft tissues surrounding three titanium non-submerged plasma-sprayed implants retrieved at autopsy: a case report. J Periodontol 1997;68(7):694–700.

1343. Peoc'h M, Pasquier D, Ducros V, Moulin C, Bost F, Faure C, Pasquier B. Réactions granulomateuses systémiques et prothèse de hance. Deux observations anatomo-cliniques. [Systemic granulomatous reaction in hip prosthesis. Apropos of 2 anatomoclinical cases.] Rev Chir Orthop Reparatrice Appar Mot 1996;82(6):564–7.

1344. Yamauchi R, Morita A, Tsuji T. Pacemaker dermatitis from titanium. Contact Dermatitis 2000;42(1):52–3.

1345. Spigarelli MG, Hurwitz ME, Nasr SZ. Hypersensitivity to inhaled TOBI following reaction to gentamicin. Pediatr Pulmonol 2002;33(4):311–4.

1346. Mohiuddin SM, Esterbrooks D, Mooss AN, Dahl JM, Hilleman DE. Efficacy and tolerance of tocainide during long-term treatment of malignant ventricular arrhythmias. Clin Cardiol 1987;10(8):457–62.

1347. Oliphant LD, Goddard M. Tocainide-associated neutropenia and lupus-like syndrome. Chest 1988;94(2):427–8.

1348. Duff HJ, Roden DM, Marney S, Colley DG, Maffucci R, Primm RK, Oates JA, Woosley RL. Molecular basis for the antigenicity of lidocaine analogues: tocainide and mexiletine. Am Heart J 1984;107(3):585–9.

1349. Schlienger RG, Keller MJ, Krahenbuhl S. Tolterodine-associated acute mixed liver injury. Ann Pharmacother 2002;36(5):817–9.

1350. Palop-Larrea V, Sancho-Calabuig A, Gorriz-Teruel JL, Martinez-Mir I, Pallardo-Mateu LM. Vasculitis with acute kidney failure and torasemide. Lancet 1998;352(9144):1909–10.

1351. Sanfelix Genoves J, Benlloch Nieto H, Verdu Tarraga R, Costa Alcaraz AM. Erupcion purpurica compatible con vasculitis y torasemida. [Eruption of purpura compatible with vasculitis and torasemide.] Aten Primaria 1998;21(4):252–3.

1351. Metzner HH. Kontaktsensibilisierungen durch Tosylchloramidnatrium (Chloramin) und Hydroxychinolin (Sulfachin). [Contact sensitization caused by tosylchloramide sodium (chloramine) and hydroxyquinoline (Sulfachin).] Dermatol Monatsschr 1987;173(11):674–7.

1352. Dooms-Goossens A, Gevers D, Mertens A, Vanderheyden D. Allergic contact urticaria due to chloramine. Contact Dermatitis 1983;9(4):319–20.

1353. Nagae S, Hori Y. Immune thrombocytopenia due to tranilast (Rizaben): detection of drug-dependent platelet-associated IgG. J Dermatol 1998;25(11):706–9.

1354. Osmundsen PE. Concomitant contact allergy to propantheline bromide and TCC. Contact Dermatitis 1975;1(4):251–2.

1355. Demelia L, Vallebona E, Perpignano G, Pitzus F. Positivizzazione di sierologia lupica in corso di morbo di Wilson in trattamento con penicillamina. Reumatismo 1991;43:119–24.

1356. Cirkel PK, van Ketel WG. Allergic contact dermatitis to trifluorothymidine eyedrops. Contact Dermatitis 1981;7(1):49–50.

1357. Neuman MG, Malkiewicz IM, Phillips EJ, Rachlis AR, Ong D, Yeung E, Shear NH. Monitoring adverse drug reactions to sulfonamide antibiotics in human immunodeficiency virus-infected individuals. Ther Drug Monit 2002;24(6):728–36.

1358. Choquet-Kastylevsky G, Vial T, Descotes J. Allergic adverse reactions to sulfonamides. Curr Allergy Asthma Rep 2002;2(1):16–25.

1359. Hasui M, Kotera F, Tsuji S, Yamamoto A, Taniuchi S, Fujikawa Y, Nakajima M, Yoshioka A, Kobayashi Y. Successful resumption of trimethoprim–sulfamethoxazole after oral desensitisation in patients with chronic granulomatous disease. Eur J Pediatr 2002;161(6):356–7.

1360. Bijl AM, Van der Klauw MM, Van Vliet AC, Stricker BH. Anaphylactic reactions associated with trimethoprim. Clin Exp Allergy 1998;28(4):510–2.

1361. Johnson MP, Goodwin SD, Shands JW Jr. Trimethoprim–sulfamethoxazole anaphylactoid reactions in patients with AIDS: case reports and literature review. Pharmacotherapy 1990;10(6):413–6.

1362. Cribb AE, Lee BL, Trepanier LA, Spielberg SP. Adverse reactions to sulphonamide and sulphonamide–trimethoprim antimicrobials: clinical syndromes and pathogenesis. Adverse Drug React Toxicol Rev 1996;15(1):9–50.

1363. Arola O, Peltonen R, Rossi T. Arthritis, uveitis, and Stevens–Johnson syndrome induced by trimethoprim. Lancet 1998;351(9109):1102.

1364. Pham NH, Baldo BA, Manfredi M, Zerboni R. Fine structural specificity differences of trimethoprim allergenic determinants. Clin Exp Allergy 1996;26(10):1155–60.

1365. Greenberger PA, Patterson R. Management of drug allergy in patients with acquired immunodeficiency syndrome. J Allergy Clin Immunol 1987;79(3):484–8.

1366. Theodore CM, Holmes D, Rodgers M, McLean KA. Cotrimoxazole desensitization in HIV-seropositive patients. Int J STD AIDS 1998;9(3):158–61.

1367. Walmsley SL, Khorasheh S, Singer J, Djurdjev O, Schlech W, Thompson W, Duperval R, Toma E, Tsoukas C, Senay H, Wells P, Uetrecht J, Shear N, Rachlis A, Fong B, McGreer A, Smaill F, Cohen J, Ford P, Gilmour J, Mackie I, Williams K, Montaner J, Zarowny D. A randomized trial of N-acetylcysteine for prevention of trimethoprim-sulfamethoxazole hypersensitivity reactions in *Pneumocystis carinii* pneumonia prophylaxis (CTN 057). Canadian HIV Trials Network 057 Study Group. J Acquir Immune Defic Syndr Hum Retrovirol 1998;19(5):498–505.

1368. Holtzer CD, Flaherty JF Jr, Coleman RL. Cross-reactivity in HIV-infected patients switched from trimethoprim–sulfamethoxazole to dapsone. Pharmacotherapy 1998; 18(4):831–5.

1369. O'Kane EB, Schneeweiss R. Trimethoprim–sulfamethoxazole-induced sepsis-like syndrome in a patient with AIDS. J Am Board Fam Pract 1996;9(6):448–50.

1370. Moran KA, Ales NC, Hemmer PA. Newly diagnosed human immunodeficiency virus after sepsis-like reaction of trimethoprim–sulfamethoxazole. South Med J 2001;94(3):350–2.

1371. Yoshizawa S, Yasuoka A, Kikuchi Y, Honda M, Gatanaga H, Tachikawa N, Hirabayashi Y, Oka S. A 5-day course of oral desensitization to trimethoprim/sulfamethoxazole (T/S) in patients with human immunodeficiency virus type-1 infection who were previously intolerant to T/S. Ann Allergy Asthma Immunol 2000;85(3):241–4.

1372. Demoly P, Messaad D, Reynes J, Faucherre V, Bousquet J. Trimethoprim–sulfamethoxazole-graded challenge in HIV-infected patients: long-term follow-up regarding efficacy and safety. J Allergy Clin Immunol 2000;105(3):588–9.

1373. Nucera E, Schiavino D, Buonomo A, Del Ninno M, Sun JY, Patriarca G. Tolerance induction to cotrimoxazole. Allergy 2000;55(7):681–2.

1374. Lopez-Serrano MC, Moreno-Ancillo A. Drug hypersensitivity reactions in HIV-infected patients. Induction of cotrimoxazole tolerance. Allergol Immunol Clin 2000;15:347–51.

1375. Sher MR, Suchar C, Lockey RF. Anaphylactic shock induced by oral desensitization to trimethoprim/sulfmethoxazole. J Allergy Immunol 1986;77:133.

1376. Torgovnick J, Arsura E. Desensitization to sulfonamides in patients with HIV infection. Am J Med 1990;88(5):548–9.

1377. Finegold I. Oral desensitization to trimethoprim–sulfamethoxazole in a patient with acquired immunodeficiency syndrome. J Allergy Clin Immunol 1986;78(5 Pt 1):905–8.

1378. Papakonstantinou G, Fuessl H, Hehlmann R. Trimethoprim–sulfamethoxazole desensitization in AIDS. Klin Wochenschr 1988;66(8):351–3.

1379. Bonfanti P, Pusterla L, Parazzini F, Libanore M, Cagni AE, Franzetti M, Faggion I, Landonio S, Quirino T. The effectiveness of desensitization versus rechallenge treatment in HIV-positive patients with previous hypersensitivity to TMP–SMX: a randomized multicentric study. C.I.S.A.I. Group Biomed Pharmacother 2000;54(1):45–9.

1380. Leoung GS, Stanford JF, Giordano MF, Stein A, Torres RA, Giffen CA, Wesley M, Sarracco T, Cooper EC, Dratter V, Smith JJ, Frost KR. American Foundation for AIDS Research (amfAR) Community-Based Clinical Trials Network. Trimethoprim–sulfamethoxazole (TMP-SMZ) dose escalation versus direct rechallenge for *Pneumocystis carinii* pneumonia prophylaxis in human immunodeficiency virus-infected patients with previous adverse reaction to TMP–SMZ. J Infect Dis 2001;184(8):992–7.

1381. Herbst RA, Maibach HI. Allergic contact dermatitis from ophthalmics: update 1997. Contact Dermatitis 1997;37(5):252–3.

1382. Boukhman MP, Maibach HI. Allergic contact dermatitis from tropicamide ophthalmic solution. Contact Dermatitis 1999;41(1):47–8.

1383. Gruber C, Nilsson L, Bjorksten B. Do early childhood immunizations influence the development of atopy and do they cause allergic reactions? Pediatr Allergy Immunol 2001;12(6):296–311.

1384. La Force FM. Immunization of children infected with human immunodeficiency virus. WHO/EPI/GEN/86.6 Rev 1, Geneva. 1986.

1385. Kane M. Unsafe injections. Bull World Health Organ 1998;76(1):99–100.

1386. Expanded Programme on Immunization. Immunization policy. WHO/EPI/GEN/86.7 Rev 1, Geneva. 1986.

1387. Expanded Programme on Immunization. Joint WHO/UNICEF statement on immunization and AIDS. Wkly Epidemiol Rec 1987;62(9):53.

1387. Parent du Chatelet I, Lang J, Schlumberger M, Vidor E, Soula G, Genet A, Standaert SM, Saliou P, Gueye A, Julien H, Lafaix C, Lemardeley P, Monnereau A, Spiegel A, Soke M, Varichon JP. Clinical immunogenicity and tolerance studies of liquid vaccines delivered by jet-injector and a new single-use cartridge (Imule): comparison with standard syringe injection. Imule Investigators Group. Vaccine 1997;15(4):449–58.

1388. Shah RH, Mackey K, Wallace H, Yawata K, Roberto R, Meissinger J, Ascher M, Hagens S, Chin JCenters for Disease Control (CDC). Hepatitis B associated with jet gun injection—California. MMWR Morb Mortal Wkly Rep 1986;35(23):373–6.

1388. Martin-Munoz MF, Pereira MJ, Posadas S, Sanchez-Sabate E, Blanca M, Alvarez J. Anaphylactic reaction to diphtheria–tetanus vaccine in a child: specific IgE/IgG determinations and cross-reactivity studies. Vaccine 2002;20(27–28):3409–12.

1389. Gerth HG. Grippeschutzimpfung. Dtsch Med Wochenschr 1989;114:180.

1390. James JM, Zeiger RS, Lester MR, Fasano MB, Gern JE, Mansfield LE, Schwartz HJ, Sampson HA, Windom HH, Machtinger SB, Lensing S. Safe administration of influenza vaccine to patients with egg allergy. J Pediatr 1998;133(5):624–8.

1391. Perez C, Loza E, Tinture T. Giant cell arteritis after influenza vaccination. Arch Intern Med 2000;160(17):2677.

1392. Liozon E, Ittig R, Vogt N, Michel JP, Gold G. Polymyalgia rheumatica following influenza vaccination. J Am Geriatr Soc 2000;48(11):1533–4.

1393. Perez C, Maravi E. Polymyalgia rheumatica following influenza vaccination. Muscle Nerve 2000;23(5):824–5.

1394. Finsterer J, Artner C, Kladosek A, Kalchmayr R, Redtenbacher S. Cavernous sinus syndrome due to vaccination-induced giant cell arteritis. Arch Intern Med 2001;161(7):1008–9.

1395. Advisory Committee on Immunization Practices (ACIP). Inactivated Japanese encephalitis virus vaccine. MMWR Recomm Rep 1993;42(RR-1):1–15.

1396. Sakaguchi M, Miyazawa H, Inouye S. Specific IgE and IgG to gelatin in children with systemic cutaneous reactions to Japanese encephalitis vaccines. Allergy 2001;56(6):536–9.

1397. Edelman R, Wasserman SS, Kublin JG, Bodison SA, Nardin EH, Oliveira GA, Ansari S, Diggs CL, Kashala OL, Schmeckpeper BJ, Hamilton RG. Immediate-type hypersensitivity and other clinical reactions in volunteers immunized with a synthetic multi-antigen peptide vaccine (PfCS-MAP1NYU) against *Plasmodium falciparum* sporozoites. Vaccine 2002;21(3–4):269–80.

1398. Kublin JG, Lowitt MH, Hamilton RG, Oliveira GA, Nardin EH, Nussenzweig RS, Schmeckpeper BJ, Diggs CL, Bodison SA, Edelman R. Delayed-type hypersensitivity in volunteers immunized with a synthetic multi-antigen peptide vaccine (PfCS-MAP1NYU) against *Plasmodium falciparum* sporozoites. Vaccine 2002;20(13–14):1853–61.

1399. Duclos P, Ward BJ. Measles vaccines: a review of adverse events. Drug Saf 1998;19(6):435–54.

1400. Phadke MA, Joshi BN, Warerkar UV, Diwan MP, Panse GA, Sokhey J, Bhate SM. Toxic shock syndrome: an unforeseen complication following measles vaccination. Indian Pediatr 1991;28(6):663–5.

1401. Milstein J, Dittmann S. Personal communication, 1995.

1402. Hurwitz EL, Morgenstern H. Effects of diphtheria–tetanus–pertussis or tetanus vaccination on allergies and allergy-related respiratory symptoms among children and adolescents in the United States. J Manipulative Physiol Ther 2000;23(2):81–90.

1403. Vulginity V. Sterile abscesses after diphtheria–tetanus toxoids–pertussis vaccination. Pediatr Infect Dis J 1987;6:497.

1404. Committee on Immunization. In: Guide for Adult Immunization. Philadelphia: American College of Physicians, 1985:65.

1405. Centers for Disease Control (CDC). Update: pneumococcal polysaccharide vaccine usage—United States. MMWR Morb Mortal Wkly Rep 1984;33(20):273–6281.

1406. Ponvert C, Ardelean-Jaby D, Colin-Gorski AM, Soufflet B, Hamberger C, de Blic J, Scheinmann P. Anaphylaxis to the 23-valent pneumococcal vaccine in child: a case-control study based on immediate responses in skin tests and specific IgE determination. Vaccine 2001;19(32):4588–91.

1407. Committee on Immunization. Guide for Adult Immunization. Philadelphia: American College of Physicians, 1985.

1408. Anonymous. Rabies vaccine. Med Lett 1991;117–8.

1409. Ackermann R. Allergische Reaktion nach FSME-Auffrischimpfung (Anfrage und Antwort). Dtsch Med Wochenschr 1990;115:1213.

1410. Fraunfelder FW, Rosenbaum JT. Drug-induced uveitis. Incidence, prevention and treatment. Drug Saf 1997;17(3):197–207.

1411. Pillai JJ, Gaughan WJ, Watson B, Sivalingam JJ, Murphey SA. Renal involvement in association with post-vaccination *Varicella*. Clin Infect Dis 1993;17(6):1079–80.

1412. Naruse H, Miwata H, Ozaki T, Asano Y, Namazue J, Yamanishi K. *Varicella* infection complicated with meningitis after immunization. Acta Paediatr Jpn 1993;35(4):345–7.

1413. Plotkin SA, Starr SE, Connor K, Morton D. Zoster in normal children after *Varicella* vaccine. J Infect Dis 1989;159(5):1000–1.

1414. Hammerschlag MR, Gershon AA, Steinberg SP, Clarke L, Gelb LD. Herpes zoster in an adult recipient of live attenuated *Varicella* vaccine. J Infect Dis 1989;160(3):535–7.

1415. Magrath DI. Prospective vaccines for national immunization programmes. In: Proceedings, 3rd Meeting of National Programme Managers on Expanded Programme on Immunization. St Vincent, Italy 22–25 May 1990:155 ICP/EPI 023/31, 1990.

1416. Liang MG, Heidelberg KA, Jacobson RM, McEvoy MT. Herpes zoster after *Varicella* immunization. J Am Acad Dermatol 1998;38(5 Pt 1):761–3.

1417. Walter R, Hartmann K, Fleisch F, Reinhart WH, Kuhn M. Reactivation of herpesvirus infections after vaccinations? Lancet 1999;353(9155):810.

1418. Kohl S, Rapp J, La Russa P, Gershon AA, Steinberg SP. Natural *Varicella-zoster* virus reactivation shortly after varicella immunization in a child. Pediatr Infect Dis J 1999;18(12):1112–3.

1419. World Heath Organization. Prevention and Control of Yellow Fever in AfricaGeneva: WHO;. 1986.

1420. Fitzner J, Coulibaly D, Kouadio DE, Yavo JC, Loukou YG, Koudou PO, Coulombier D. Safety of the yellow fever vaccine during the September 2001 mass vaccination campaign in Abidjan, Ivory Coast. Vaccine 2004;23(2):156–62.

1430. Bonnet F, Morlat P, De Witte S, Combe C, Beylot J. Lupus-like syndrome and vasculitis induced by valpromide. J Rheumatol 2003;30(1):208–9.

1431. Jennings HR, Romanelli F. The use of valproic acid in HIV-positive patients. Ann Pharmacother 1999; 33(10):1113–6.

1432. Maggi JD, Halman MH. The effect of divalproex sodium on viral load: a retrospective review of HIV-positive patients with manic syndromes. Can J Psychiatry 2001;46(4):359–62.

1433. Renz CL, Laroche D, Thurn JD, Finn HA, Lynch JP, Thisted R, Moss J. Tryptase levels are not increased during vancomycin-induced anaphylactoid reactions. Anesthesiology 1998;89(3):620–5.

1434. Chopra N, Oppenheimer J, Derimanov GS, Fine PL. Vancomycin anaphylaxis and successful desensitization in a patient with end stage renal disease on hemodialysis by maintaining steady antibiotic levels. Ann Allergy Asthma Immunol 2000;84(6):633–5.

1435. Duffy BL. Vancomycin reaction during spinal anaesthesia. Anaesth Intensive Care 2002;30(3):364–6.

1436. Sorensen SJ, Wise SL, al-Tawfiq JA, Robb JL, Cushing HE. Successful vancomycin desensitization in a patient with end-stage renal disease and anaphylactic shock to vancomycin. Ann Pharmacother 1998;32(10):1020–3.

1437. Wazny LD, Daghigh B. Desensitization protocols for vancomycin hypersensitivity. Ann Pharmacother 2001;35(11):1458–64.

1438. Marshall C, Street A, Galbraith K. Glycopeptide-induced vasculitis—cross-reactivity between vancomycin and teicoplanin. J Infect 1998;37(1):82–3.

1439. Pichler WJ, Angeli R. Allergie auf Mistelextrakt. [An allergy to mistletoe extract.] Dtsch Med Wochenschr 1991;116(35):1333–4.

1440. Hutt N, Kopferschmitt-Kubler M, Cabalion J, Purohit A, Alt M, Pauli G. Anaphylactic reactions after therapeutic injection of mistletoe (*Viscum album* L.) Allergol Immunopathol (Madr) 2001;29(5):201–3.

1441. Semba RD, Munasir Z, Beeler J, Akib A, Muhilal, Audet S, Sommer A. Reduced seroconversion to measles in infants given vitamin A with measles vaccination. Lancet 1995;345(8961):1330–2.

1442. Khurshid I, Seymour JF, Nakata K, Downie GH. Recurrent manifestations of idiopathic pulmonary alveolar proteinosis after isotretinoin (Accutane) treatment. Chest 2001;120(Suppl):335.

1443. Fernandez M, Barcelo M, Munoz C, Torrecillas M, Blanca M. Anaphylaxis to thiamine (vitamin B1). Allergy 1997;52(9):958–60.

1444. Stephen JM, Grant R, Yeh CS. Anaphylaxis from administration of intravenous thiamine. Am J Emerg Med 1992;10(1):61–3.

1445. Leung R, Puy R, Czarny D. Thiamine anaphylaxis. Med J Aust 1993;159(5):355.

1446. Van Haecke P, Ramaekers D, Vanderwegen L, Boonen S. Thiamine-induced anaphylactic shock. Am J Emerg Med 1995;13(3):371–2.

1447. Wrenn KD, Slovis CM. Is intravenous thiamine safe? Am J Emerg Med 1992;10(2):165.

1448. Kolz R, Lonsdorf G, Burg G. Unverträglichkeitsreaktionen nach parenteraler Gabe von Vitamin B1. [Intolerance reactions following parenteral administration of vitamin B1.] Hautarzt 1980;31(12):657–9.

1449. Morinville V, Jeannet-Peter N, Hauser C. Anaphylaxis to parenteral thiamine (vitamin B1). Schweiz Med Wochenschr 1998;128(44):1743–4.

1450. Johri S, Shetty S, Soni A, Kumar S. Anaphylaxis from intravenous thiamine—long forgotten? Am J Emerg Med 2000;18(5):642–3.

1451. Wrenn KD, Murphy F, Slovis CM. A toxicity study of parenteral thiamine hydrochloride. Ann Emerg Med 1989;18(8):867–70.

1452. de Blay F, Sager MF, Hirth C, Alt M, Chamouard P, Baumann R, Pauli G. IGE-mediated reaction to hydroxocobalamin injection in patient with pernicious anaemia. Lancet 1992;339(8808):1535–6.

1453. Tordjman R, Genereau T, Guinnepain MT, Weyer A, Lortholary O, Royer I, Casassus P, Guillevin L. Reintroduction of vitamin B12 in 2 patients with prior B12-induced anaphylaxis. Eur J Haematol 1998; 60(4):269–70.

1454. Heyworth-Smith D, Hogan PG. Allergy to hydroxycobalamin, with tolerance of cyanocobalamin. Med J Aust 2002;177(3):162–3.

1455. Pigatto PD, Bigardi A, Fumagalli M, Altomare GF, Riboldi A. Allergic dermatitis from parenteral vitamin K. Contact Dermatitis 1990;22(5):307–8.

1456. Hwang SW, Kim YP, Chung BS, Kim HK. Vitamin K1 dermatitis. Korean J Dermatol 1983;21:91.

1457. ADRAC Slow down on parenteral vitamin K. Aust Adverse Drug React Bull 1991;10:3.

1458. Hirsh J, Dalen JE, Deykin D, Poller L, Bussey H. Oral anticoagulants. Mechanism of action, clinical effectiveness, and optimal therapeutic range. Chest 1995;108(Suppl 4):S231–46.

1459. Routledge PA. Practical prescribing: warfarin. Prescr J 1997;37:173–9.

1460. Martin JC. Anaphylactoid reactions and vitamin K. Med J Aust 1991;155(11–12):851.

1461. Jolobe OM, Penny E. Severe reaction to i.v. vitamin K Pharm J 1999;262:112.

1462. Sommer S, Wilkinson SM, Peckham D, Wilson C. Type IV hypersensitivity to vitamin K. Contact Dermatitis 2002;46(2):94–6.

1463. Wilson CL, Cameron J, Powell SM, Cherry G, Ryan TJ. High incidence of contact dermatitis in leg-ulcer patients—implications for management. Clin Exp Dermatol 1991;16(4):250–3.

1464. Aberer W, Fuchs T, Peters K. PJ F. Propylenglykol: Kutane Nebenwirkungen und Testmethodik. Literaturübersicht und Ergebnisse einer Multicenterstudie der Deutschen Kontaktallergiegruppe (DKG). Dermatosen 1997;36:156–8.

1465. Gallenkemper G, Rabe E, Bauer R. Contact sensitization in chronic venous insufficiency: modern wound dressings. Contact Dermatitis 1998;38(5):274–8.

1466. Sandler B, Aronson P. Yohimbine-induced cutaneous drug eruption, progressive renal failure, and lupus-like syndrome. Urology 1993;41(4):343–5.

1467. De Smet PA, Smeets OS. Potential risks of health food products containing yohimbe extracts. BMJ 1994;309(6959):958.

1468. Hunt JR. Position of the American Dietetic Association: vitamin and mineral supplementation. J Am Dietet Assoc 1996;96(1):73–7.

1469. Mutoh K, Hidaka Y, Hirose Y, Kimura M. Possible induction of systemic lupus erythematosus by zonisamide. Pediatr Neurol 2001;25(4):340–3.

1470. Kumar AA, Thys J, Van Aken HK, Stevens E, Crul JF. Severe anaphylactic shock after atracurium. Anesth Analg 1993;76(2):423–5.

1471. Moneret-Vautrin DA, Widmer S, Gueant JL, Kamel L, Laxenaire MC, Mouton C, Gerard H. Simultaneous anaphylaxis to thiopentone and a neuromuscular blocker: a study of two cases. Br J Anaesth 1990;64(6):743–5.

1472. Bryld LE, Agner T, Rastogi SC, Menne T. Iodopropynyl butylcarbamate: a new contact allergen. Contact Dermatitis 1997;36(3):156–8.

1473. Ohshima A, Takigawa M, Tokura Y. CD8+ cell changes in psoriasis associated with roxithromycin-induced clinical improvement. Eur J Dermatol 2001;11(5):410–5.

1474. Stephens R, Mythen M, Kallis P, Davies DW, Egner W, Rickards A. Two episodes of life-threatening anaphylaxis in the same patient to a chlorhexidine–sulphadiazine-coated central venous catheter. Br J Anaesth 2001;87(2):306–8.

1475. Fazackerley EJ, Martin AJ, Tolhurst-Cleaver CL, Watkins J. Anaphylactoid reaction following the use of etomidate. Anaesthesia 1988;43(11):953–4.

1476. Moorthy SS, Laurent B, Pandya P, Fry V. Anaphylactoid reaction to etomidate: report of a case. J Clin Anesth 2001;13(8):582–4.

1477. Ernst EJ, Egge JA. Celecoxib-induced erythema multiforme with glyburide cross-reactivity. Pharmacotherapy 2002;22(5):637–40.

1478. Mant TG, Tempowski JH, Volans GN, Talbot JC. Adverse reactions to acetylcysteine and effects of overdose. BMJ (Clin Res Ed) 1984;289(6439):217–9.

1479. Kluger J, Drayer DE, Reidenberg MM, Lahita R. Acetylprocainamide therapy in patients with previous procainamide-induced lupus syndrome. Ann Intern Med 1981;95(1):18–23.

1480. Stec GP, Lertora JJ, Atkinson AJ Jr, Nevin MJ, Kushner W, Jones C, Schmid FR, Askenazi J. Remission of procainamide-induced lupus erythematosus with N-acetylprocainamide therapy. Ann Intern Med 1979;90(5):799–801.

Index of drug names

A

Abacavir, **631**
Abciximab, **462–4**
  immunological effects of, **631–2**
  organs and systems
    hematologic, **462–4**
    immunologic, **464**
    nervous system, **462**
    respiratory, **462**
  susceptibility factors, **464**
Abetimus, **576**
Acebutolol, **632**
Acecainide, **632**
Aceclofenac, **632**
Acesulfame, **603**
Acetaminophen *see* paracetamol
Acetylcholinesterase inhibitors, **632**
Acetylcysteine, **632**
Acetylsalicylic acid, **632**
Aciclovir, **632–3**
Acivicin, **75**
Acrylic bone cement, **633**
Adalimumab *see* Monoclonal antibodies
Adenosine and adenosine triphosphate
  (ATP), **633**
Ajmaline and its derivatives, **633**
Albumin, **633**
Albuterol *see* Salbutamol
Alcuronium, **633**
Aldesleukin, **409–17**
  drug–drug interactions, **416–17**
  general adverse effects, **410–11**
  long-term effects, **416**
  organs and systems
    biliary tract, **414**
    cardiovascular, **411–12**
    endocrine, **412–13**
    gastrointestinal, **414**
    hematologic, **413**
    immunologic, **415–16**
    infection risk, **416**
    liver, **414**
    metabolism, **413**
    mouth, **414**
    musculoskeletal, **415**
    nervous system, **412**
    nutrition, **413**
    pancreas, **414**
    psychological, psychiatric, **412**
    respiratory, **412**
    sensory systems, **412**
    sexual function, **415**
    skin, **415**
    urinary tract, **414–15**
  use in patients with HIV infection, **409**
  use in patients with metastatic
    melanoma, **409–10**
Alemtuzumab, **465–6**
Alfentanil, **633**
Alfuzosin, **633–4**
Alkylating agents, **3, 13–35**
  alkylating agents — *N*-lost derivatives, **15**
  alkylating agents—nitrosoureas, **13–14**
  busulfan, **16–18**

cyclophosphamide, **20–7**
  dacarbazine, **30**
  ifosfamide, **30–2**
  melphalan, **32–3**
  mitomycin, **33–4**
  procarbazine, **35**
  temozolomide, **30**
Alkylating agents—nitrosoures, **13–14**
Alkylating agents—*N*-lost derivatives, **15**
Allopurinol, **634**
Alpha₁-antitrypsin, **634**
Alprostadil, **332–5**
  organs and systems
    cardiovascular, **333**
    hematologic, **333**
    immunologic, **335**
    musculoskeletal, **334**
    respiratory, **333**
    sexual function, **334–5**
    skin, **333–4**
Aluminium, **634**
Amfebutamone (bupropion), **634**
Amiloride, **635**
Aminoglycoside antibiotics, **635**
Aminophenazone
  immunological effects of, **635**
  tumorigenic effects of, **603**
Aminosalicylates, **635**
Amiodarone, **635–6**
Amphetamines, **636**
Amphotericin, **636**
Anakinra, **421**
Anaphylaxis, **694**
Anesthetics, **666–7**
Anesthetics (local), **678–80**
Angiotensin-converting enzyme
  inhibitors, **636–9**
Anthracyclines and related compounds,
  75–82
  drug administration, **80–1**
  drug–drug interactions, **81–2**
  long-term effects, **79**
  organs and systems
    cardiovascular, **75–7**
    gastrointestinal, **78–9**
    hair, **79**
    hematologic, **78**
    mouth, **78**
    nails, **79**
    sensory systems, **78**
    skin, **79**
    sweat glands, **79**
    urinary tract, **79**
  second-generation effects, **79–80**
  susceptibility factors, **80**
Anthracyclines—liposomal formulations,
  86–9
  drug administration, **89**
  drug–drug interactions, **89**
  long-term effects, **89**
  organs and systems
    cardiovascular, **86–7**
    gastrointestinal, **88**
    hair, **88**
    hematologic, **87–8**

    immunologic, **88–9**
    liver, **88**
    respiratory, **87**
    skin, **88**
  pharmacokinetics, **86**
  second-generation effects, **89**
  susceptibility factors, **89**
Anthranoids, **603**
Antiandrogens, **97–103**
  drug administration, **102–103**
  drug–drug interactions, **103**
  interference with diagnostic routines,
    103
  long-term effects, **102**
  observational studies, **97–8**
  organs and systems
    breasts, **102**
    cardiovascular, **99**
    endocrine, **99**
    gastrointestinal, **100**
    hematologic, **100**
    liver, **100**
    metabolism, **99–100**
    musculoskeletal, **101**
    pancreas, **100**
    reproductive system, **102**
    respiratory, **99**
    senses, **cataract**, **99**
    sexual function, **101–102**
    skin, **100–101**
  placebo-controlled studies, **98–9**
  susceptibility factors, **102**
  systematic reviews, **99**
Antibody response, development of, **697**
Anti-CD4 monoclonal antibodies, **466–7**
Antimetabolites, **3, 36–74**
  cytarabine, **36**
  doxifluridine, **37**
  floxuridine, **37–8**
  fludarabine, **38–9**
  fluorouracil, **40–8**
  gemcitabine, **53–4**
  methotrexate, **55–66**
  miltefosine, **71–2**
  piritrexim, **72**
  raltitrexed, **72–3**
  tioguanine, **73–4**
  trimetrexate, **74**
Antiretroviral drugs, **603**
Apiaceae, **639**
Apraclonidine, **649**
Aristolochia, **604**
Aromatase inhibitors, **108–10**
  drug-drug interactions, **110**
  long-term effects, **109**
  organs and systems, **108–109**
  susceptibility factors, **110**
Artificial sweeteners, **639**
Ascorbic acid (vitamin C), **639**
Asparaginase, **227**
Asteraceae, **639**
Atorvastatin *see* HMG coenzyme-A
  reductase inhibitors
Atracurium dibesilate, **639**
Atropine, **639**

Printed in the United States
By Bookmasters